MARVIN H. SLEISENGER, M.D.

Professor and Vice Chairman, Department of Medicine,
University of California School of Medicine, San Francisco;
Chief, Medical Services, Veterans Administration Hospital,
San Francisco

JOHN S. FORDTRAN, M.D.

Professor of Medicine, The University of
Texas Southwestern Medical School at Dallas;
Senior Attending Physician, Parkland Memorial
Hospitals, Dallas, Texas

with a foreword by

FRANZ J. INGELFINGER, M.D.

GASTROINTESTINAL DISEASE

DISEASE

Pathophysiology • Diagnosis • Management

W. B. SAUNDERS COMPANY
Philadelphia | London | Toronto

W. B. Saunders Company: West Washington Square
Philadelphia, Pa. 19105

12 Dyott Street
London, WC1A   1DB

833 Oxford Street
Toronto, Ontario M8Z 5T9, Canada

Gastrointestinal Disease: Pathophysiology, Diagnosis, Management   ISBN 0-7216-8363-0

Print No.:   9   8   7   6   5   4   3

This work is dedicated to three gastroenterologists:

THOMAS P. ALMY; MORTON I. GROSSMAN; FRANZ J. INGELFINGER

—with our deep respect and admiration.

Contributors

WILLIAM ADMIRAND, M.D. Assistant Professor of Internal Medicine, University of California School of Medicine. Chief of Gastroenterology, San Francisco General Hospital, San Francisco, California.

THOMAS P. ALMY, M.D. Nathan Smith Professor and Chairman, Department of Medicine, Dartmouth Medical School. Director of Medicine, the Dartmouth-Hitchcock Affiliated Hospitals, Hanover, New Hampshire.

JOHN AMBERG, M.D. Professor and Chairman, Department of Radiology, Vanderbilt University, Nashville, Tennessee.

JOSEPH P. BELBER, M.D. Associate Clinical Professor of Medicine, University of California School of Medicine, San Francisco. Chief, Gastroenterology Section, Medical Service, Veterans Administration Hospital, Martinez, California; Attending Endoscopist, San Francisco General Hospital, San Francisco, California.

MICHAEL D. BENDER, M.D. Instructor in Medicine, University of California School of Medicine, San Francisco, California.

JOHN A. BENSON, JR., M.D. Professor of Medicine and Head, Division of Gastroenterology, University of Oregon Medical School, Portland, Oregon.

LLOYD L. BRANDBORG, M.D. Clinical Professor of Medicine, University of California, San Francisco. Chief, Gastroenterology, Veterans Administration Hospital, San Francisco; Consultant, Gastroenterology, Letterman General Hospital and U.S. Public Health Service Hospital, San Francisco, U.S. Naval Hospital, Oakland, and David Grant U.S. Air Force Medical Center, Travis Air Force Base, California.

JAMES CHRISTENSEN, M.S., M.D. Professor of Internal Medicine, University of Iowa College of Medicine. Staff Physician, University of Iowa Hospitals; Attending Physician, Iowa City Veterans Administration Hospital, Iowa City, Iowa.

ALLAN R. COOKE, M.B., M.D.(SYD.), F.R.A.C.P. Associate Professor of Internal Medicine, University of Iowa College of Medicine. Attending Physician, University of Iowa and Veterans Administration Hospitals, Iowa City, Iowa.

KIMBERLY J. CURTIS, M.D. Assistant Professor of Medicine, University of California, San Francisco, California.

MURRAY DAVIDSON, M.D. Professer of Pediatrics, Albert Einstein College of Medicine, Yeshiva University. Director of Pediatrics, Bronx-Lebanon Hospital Center, Bronx, New York.

DAVEY RONALD DEAL, M.D. Assistant Professor of Medicine, University of California, San Francisco, California.

ROBERT M. DONALDSON, JR., M.D. Professor of Medicine, Boston University School of Medicine. Visiting Physician, University Hospital and Boston City Hospital, Boston, Massachusetts.

DAVID L. EARNEST, M.D. Assistant Professor of Medicine, University of California School of Medicine, San Francisco. Staff Gastroenterologist, University of California Service, San Francisco General Hospital, San Francisco, California.

EDWIN H. EIGENBRODT, M.D. Associate Professor of Pathology, University of Texas Southwestern Medical School. Staff, Parkland Memorial Hospital, Dallas; Consulting Staff, Presbyterian and Veterans Administration Hospitals, Dallas, and Irving Community Hospital, Irving, Texas.

JOHN S. FORDTRAN, M.D. Professor of Internal Medicine, Southwestern Medical School and Parkland Memorial Hospitals, Dallas, Texas.

HENRY I. GOLDBERG, M.D. Associate Professor of Radiology, University of California, San Francisco, California.

RICHARD J. GRAND, M.D. Assistant Professor of Pediatrics, Harvard Medical School. Associate in Medicine and Chief of Gastrointestinal Research Laboratory, Children's Hospital Medical Center, Boston, Massachusetts.

GARY M. GRAY, M.D. Associate Professor and Head, Division of Gastroenterology, Stanford University School of Medicine. Attending Physician and Gastroenterologist, Stanford University Hospital, Stanford, Veterans Administration Hospital, Palo Alto, and Santa Clara Valley Medical Center, San Jose, California.

NORTON GREENBERGER, M.D. Professor and Chairman, Department of Medicine, University of Kansas School of Medicine, Kansas City, Kansas.

DANIEL H. GREGORY, M.D. Assistant Professor of Internal Medicine, Health Sciences Division of Virginia Commonwealth University. Assistant Chief, Gastroenterology, McGuire Veterans Administration Hospital, Richmond, Virginia.

JOYCE D. GRYBOSKI, M.D. Associate Clinical Professor of Pediatrics, Yale University Medical School. Pediatrician and Attending Physician, Yale–New Haven Hospital Medical Center, New Haven; Consultant, Newington Children's Hospital, Newington, New Britain General Hospital, New Britain, and Windham Hospital, Willimantic, Connecticut.

HANS-BEAT HADORN, M.D., Ph.D. Professor of Pediatrics and Head, Gastrointestinal Unit, Department of Pediatrics, University of Berne, Switzerland.

J. R. HAMILTON, B.Sc.(MED.), M.D., F.R.C.P.(C.) Associate Professor of Pediatrics, University of Toronto. Chief, Division of Gastroenterology, Hospital for Sick Children, Toronto; Assistant Scientist, Research Institute, Hospital for Sick Children, Toronto, Ontario, Canada.

JON I. ISENBERG, M.D. Assistant Professor of Medicine, University of California at Los Angeles. Chief, Gastroenterology Section, Wadsworth Veterans Administration Hospital, Los Angeles, California.

STEVEN JACOBSOHN, M.D. Instructor in Medicine, University of California, San Francisco, California.

GRAHAM H. JEFFRIES, M.B., CH.B., D.PHIL. Professor and Chairman, Department of Medicine, Pennsylvania State University College of Medicine. Physician in Chief, Milton. S. Hershey Medical Center Hospital, Hershey, Pennsylvania.

R. SCOTT JONES, M.D. Associate Professor of Surgery, Duke University Medical Center. Attending Surgeon, Duke Hospital, and Watts Hospital, Durham; Assistant Chief, Surgical Service, Veterans Administration Hospital, Durham, North Carolina.

O. DHODANAND KOWLESSAR, M.D. Professor of Medicine and Director, Division of Gastroenterology, Jefferson Medical College and Thomas Jefferson University, Philadelphia, Pennsylvania.

CHARLES KRONE, M.D. Assistant Professor of Internal Medicine and Chief of Gastroenterology Section, University of Arizona College of Medicine. Chief of Gastroenterology Service, University Hospital, Arizona Medical Center of the University of Arizona, Tucson; Chief of Gastroenterology Service, Veterans Administration Hospital, Tucson, Arizona.

DAVID H. LAW, M.D. Professor of Medicine (Vice Chairman), University of New Mexico School of Medicine. Chief, Medical Service, Albuquerque Veterans Administration Hospital, Albuquerque, New Mexico.

PETER M. LOEB, M.D. Assistant Professor of Medicine, University of California at San Diego. Staff, University Hospital, San Diego, and Veterans Administration Hospital, La Jolla, California.

V. I. MATHAN, M.D., PH.D. Associate Professor of Medicine, Wellcome Research Unit, Christian Medical College and Hospital, Vellore, Tamilnadu, India.

ROBERT N. McCLELLAND, M.D., F.A.C.S. Professor of Surgery, University of Texas Southwestern Medical School. Senior Attending Surgeon, Parkland Memorial, Presbyterian, and Veterans Administration Hospitals, Dallas, Texas.

JAMES E. McGUIGAN, M.D. Professor of Medicine, University of Florida College of Medicine. Chief, Division of Gastroenterology, University of Florida College of Medicine, Gainesville, Florida.

CLIFFORD S. MELNYK, M.D. Associate Professor of Internal Medicine, University of Oregon Medical School, Portland, Oregon.

JAMES H. MEYER, M.D. Assistant Professor of Medicine, University of California, San Francisco, California.

WILLIAM M. MICHENER, M.D., M.S. Professor of Pediatrics, University of New Mexico School of Medicine. Assistant Chairman, Department of Pediatrics, Bernalillo County Medical Center, Albuquerque, New Mexico.

ALBERT A. MOSS, M.D. Assistant Clinical Professor, University of California, San Francisco. Staff Radiologist, Oak Knoll Naval Hospital, Oakland, California.

THOMAS F. O'BRIEN, JR., M.D. Associate Professor of Medicine, Bowman Gray School of Medicine of Wake Forest University. Attending Physician, North Carolina Baptist Hospital, Winston-Salem, North Carolina.

ROBERT K. OCKNER, M.D. Associate Professor of Medicine, University of California School of Medicine, San Francisco. Attending Physician, University of California–Moffitt, Veterans Administration, and San Francisco General Hospitals, San Francisco, California.

ROBERT L. OWEN, M.D. Instructor in Medicine, University of California Medical School, San Francisco. Staff, University of California Medical Center, San Francisco, and Cell Biology Section, Veterans Administration Hospital, San Francisco, California.

CHARLES E. POPE II, M.D. Associate Professor, Department of Medicine, University of Washington. Chief, Gastroenterology, Seattle Veterans Administration Hospital, Seattle, Washington.

STEVEN RAFFIN, M.D. Instructor in Medicine, University of California School of Medicine, San Francisco. Veterans Administration Trainee in Gastroenterology, Veterans Administration Hospital, San Francisco, California.

CHARLES T. RICHARDSON, M.D. Assistant Chief, Gastroenterology, Wilford Hall U.S. Air Force Medical Center, Lackland Air Force Base, Texas.

DAVID M. ROSEMAN, M.D. Clinical Associate Professor of Medicine, University of California, San Diego. Staff, University Hospital of San Diego County, San Diego; Acting Chief, Gastroenterology, Veterans Administration Hospital, La Jolla; Staff, Scripps Memorial Hospital, La Jolla, California.

HARRY SHWACHMAN, M.D. Professor of Pediatrics, Harvard Medical School. Senior Associate in Medicine and Chief of Clinical Nutrition Division, Children's Hospital Medical Center, Boston, Massachusetts.

MERVIN SILVERBERG, M.D. Professor of Pediatrics, Cornell University Medical College. Director, Department of Pediatrics, and Director, Pediatric Gastroenterology, North Shore Hospital, Manhasset, New York.

MARVIN H. SLEISENGER, M.D. Professor and Vice Chairman, Department of Medicine, University of California, San Francisco. Chief, Medical Service, Veterans Administration Hospital, San Francisco, California.

FREDERIC W. SMITH, M.D. Associate Professor of Medicine, University of Oregon Medical School. Section Chief, Gastroenterology, Veterans Administration Hospital, Portland, Oregon.

JOHN Q. STAUFFER, M.D. Assistant Professor of Medicine, Upstate Medical Center, Syracuse. Associate Director, Division of Gastroenterology, State University Hospital, Syracuse, New York.

M. MICHAEL THALER, M.D. Associate Professor of Pediatrics, University of California, San Francisco. Director, Pediatric Gastroenterology, University of California and Herbert C. Moffitt Hospitals, San Francisco, California.

JERRY S. TRIER, M.D. Director, Division of Gastroenterology, Peter Bent Brigham Hospital. Associate Professor of Medicine, Harvard Medical School. Consultant, Gastroenterology, West Roxbury Veterans Administration Hospital; Consultant, Gastroenterology, Boston Veterans Administration Hospital, Boston, Massachusetts.

CHARLES O. WALKER, M.D. Assistant Professor of Internal Medicine, University of Texas Southwestern Medical School at Dallas. Chief of Gastroenterology, Veterans Administration Hospital, Dallas; Attending Gastroenterologist, Parkland Memorial Hospital, Dallas, Texas.

JOHN H. WALSH, M.D. Assistant Professor of Medicine, UCLA School of Medicine. Veterans Administration Clinical Investigator, Wadsworth Veterans Administration Hospital, Los Angeles, California.

LAWRENCE W. WAY, M.D. Associate Professor of Surgery, University of California School of Medicine, San Francisco. Chief of Surgery, Ft. Miley Veterans Administration Hospital, San Francisco, California.

ELLIOT WESER, M.D. Professor of Medicine, University of Texas Medical School at San Antonio. Attending Physician, Bexar County Hospital, San Antonio, Texas.

Foreword

Textbooks serve as the foundations of medical knowledge. On the basic facts and broad overview that they provide, the student erects a framework of ideas with pieces of information culled from the pluralistic system of medical pedagogy: lectures, clinics, medical journals, audio tapes, video cassettes, and informal chit-chat. Finally, with his ever-accumulating clinical experience, he completes the conceptual structure that serves him in the exercise of his profession.

Seen in such a context, a good textbook does not depend on exhaustive detail, the nuances of diagnosis and management, or even the immediacy of its particulars, all of which are to be found in the complementary sources of information. Crucial, however, are the organization, substantiality, specificity, and accessibility of the contents. Organization must facilitate the reader's understanding, the facts marshaled should express a reasonable consensus, the penchant for convenient vaguenesses (e.g., "not infrequently," "in most cases") should be contained, and—most important, although as a rule neglected—the subject matter should be effectively indexed. In these days of sophisticated indexing and retrieval systems, a fat tome crammed with valuable data that cannot readily be found is inexcusable.

The organization of this Sleisenger-Fordtran gastroenterologic text, with a clinical section in conventional organ system arrangement preceded by a section on pathophysiology, is designed to foster understanding. Moreover, the editors appear sensitive to today's demand for relevance and practicality. Instead of beginning the volume with an analysis of molecular interaction, they have placed first a chapter written by that dean of colonology, Dr. Thomas Almy, on the effect of stress on gut function. The reader thus will not have to hunt in the back pages, where the subject is conventionally buried, to find a general discussion of the alimentary tract disorders that are by far the most common.

Another commendable feature is the editors' enterprise in putting out a basic book on gastroenterology that really deals with the gut and leaves out the liver. A number of excellent textbooks on the liver are already available, but there is a relative dearth of convenient foundation books describing the alimentary tract and its disorders. Eliminating the liver permits the editors to describe, without skimping on essentials, an organ system that, like a newly found continent, is rapidly being opened up by the new means of exploration provided by immunology, endocrinology, peroral biopsy, and fiberoptics. Pediatric gastroenterology, a long neglected field, receives its due share of page space. Broad concepts as well as the minutiae of clinical manifestations are appropriately elaborated, and adequate coverage of the basic alimentary tract phenomena—secretion, digestion, absorption, and motility—is possible.

The organization of this textbook thus augurs well: it will serve its ordained purpose of providing students with the essential foundations of gastroenterology, and the "students" served will range, as the editors hope, from the first-year matriculant in medical school to the experienced specialist.

FRANZ J. INGELFINGER

Preface

The arrangement of material and its manner of presentation in this book are based upon two principles in which the Editors believe. The first is that excellence in medical practice depends upon an understanding of medical science and that clinical advances are made for the most part along scientific routes. The second is that diseases and deranged physiological states should be critically appraised and evaluated prior to describing the disorder to any professional audience. In our view, there is no longer any justification in clinical medicine for anecdotal attitudes, and long-held views must be subjected to critical reappraisal.

Another of our guiding principles has been that all material important in the study of a clinical discipline can be written simultaneously for students at all levels—from the medical student to the accomplished and trained specialist. Hence, this work contains in a clinical context much of what is important in gastrointestinal physiology and pathophysiology and much that reflects the contributions of pathology and radiology. The more strictly clinical aspects of gastroenterology with which the practitioner, pediatrician, and surgeon are intimately concerned are critically presented. Description of clinical disease (diagnosis and management, particularly) is authoritative only insofar as the facts will permit. Statements are documented and uncertainties emphasized.

Finally, we hope to encourage a healthy skepticism and a thirst for new knowledge in the art and science of gastroenterology. Without this, students and physicians will become satisfied with the ambiguities of clinical medicine.

MARVIN H. SLEISENGER
JOHN S. FORDTRAN

Acknowledgments

First of all, we are most grateful to our friends who are also the contributors to this book for their professional expertise and for their cheerful willingness to meet our exacting deadlines. In a very real sense this book is their achievement as well as ours. Particular thanks are due to Drs. Lloyd L. Brandborg, Robert M. Donaldson, Jr., Henry I. Goldberg, James E. McGuigan, James H. Meyer, Charles E. Pope II, and Jerry S. Trier, for effective consultation and beautiful source material, and to Dr. Murray Davidson for helping us include pediatric disorders.

Another special word of gratitude goes to Nancy Stiening, our editorial assistant, whose contribution and devotion to this text from its inception have been invaluable.

Numerous of our colleagues have aided us greatly by their constant professional encouragement and support; among them, we would like especially to thank Drs. John M. Dietschy, Daniel W. Foster, Floyd C. Rector, Rudi Schmid, Donald W. Seldin, and Lloyd H. Smith, Jr.

For excellent secretarial assistance, including tasks as diverse as typing, editorial help, and packing of manuscripts, we thank Yolanda Calloway, Eva Fruit, Jean Harber, Margaret Warren, and Carolyn Wickwire.

For care and forbearance of the domestic variety, we are proud to acknowledge the aid of our wives, Lenore Sleisenger and Jewel Fordtran, and of our children, Tom Sleisenger and Bill, Bess, Joey, and Amy Fordtran.

And last but not least, we thank those devoted "pros" at the W. B. Saunders Company, John Dusseau, Ray Kersey, Dave Kilmer, and Herb Powell.

MARVIN H. SLEISENGER

JOHN S. FORDTRAN

Contents

Section 5.   The Gallbladder and Pancreas

Section 6.

Section 7.

PART II.   DIAGNOSIS AND MANAGEMENT

Section 9.   The Esophagus

Section 11. The Small Intestine

Section 12. The Biliary Tract

Section 13.   The Pancreas

Chapter 93

CHRONIC PANCREATITIS... 1185

John A. Benson, Jr.

Chapter 94

CARCINOMA OF THE PANCREAS 1198

Clifford S. Melnyk

Chapter 95

CYSTIC FIBROSIS 1206

Harry Shwachman, Richard J. Grand

Chapter 96

DISEASES OF THE PANCREAS IN CHILDHOOD................................... 1226

Hans-Béat Hadorn, M. Michael Thaler

Part I

Pathophysiology

ASPECTS OF NUTRITION AND DEFENSE

Chapter 1

The Gastrointestinal Tract in Man Under Stress

Thomas P. Almy

Most disorders of the digestive tract are first manifested by symptoms rather than physical signs. When expressed to the physician in the form of specific complaints, these symptoms constitute some of the most common problems in his practice, even though a much larger number of individuals—estimated at 50 per cent of random samples of the population—experience the same discomforts without complaint.[1] In addition to the high prevalence of such symptoms, the frequency with which the physician cannot relate them to a morphologically or biochemically recognizable disease of the gut, after the most searching clinical and laboratory examination, is impressive.

In the past this failure to find explanations for digestive complaints in objective findings on clinical examination has led to widespread confusion—to an artificial distinction between "organic" and "functional" disease,[2] and to an inadequate distinction between malingering and neurotic symptom formation. Although the scientific advances of the last 20 years still leave us ignorant of the causes of many of these symptoms, we are able, neverthe-less, to recognize with some accuracy their relationship to definable alterations in the *physiology* of the gut. In succeeding chapters the more important gastrointestinal symptoms will be individually analyzed in terms of pathophysiology. The present purpose is to offer a general concept of symptom formation in terms of altered function, adaptation to life stress, and the total behavior of the organism. This concept is justified not as an intellectual lollipop, but rather as a practical necessity in the management of this type of health problem.

EVOLUTION AND ADAPTIVE DISORDERS

Ontogeny, it is commonly said, repeats phylogeny; and both the structure and the functions of the human gastrointestinal tract reveal clear traces of the evolutionary process. One need only mention the existence of the appendix; or the fact that the anatomic adaptation of the intestines to the erect posture is, after a million years, not quite complete; or that there seems no real necessity, in the digestion of our food, for the secretion of hydrochloric acid and pepsin.

In most animals the gut must absorb all needed nutritional elements except oxygen, and its surface thus becomes an important interface with the environment. The earthworm moves through the soil, and the soil through the worm. Many lower marine forms spend most of their time filtering the water around them for suitable food, and ingest much potentially noxious matter in so doing. Self-preservation, even at this primitive level, requires the intestinal tract to serve not only as an organ of digestion but also as an organ of defense. That which cannot be digested and utilized must be either regurgitated or enveloped in mucus and passed through the gut as rapidly as possible. The likelihood of physical or chemical injury to the mucosa by ingested noxious substances makes the capacity to regenerate lining epithelial cells a prime mechanism of defense. Indeed some organisms, such as the sea cucumber, defend themselves by extruding their entire intestinal tract and growing a new one.

Higher animals have evolved increasingly complex systems for the selection of those elements in the environment which may be suitable as food; yet these defensive mechanisms of the gut are retained in various forms and are certainly useful. Riddance of ill-tasting, possibly poisonous material is accomplished by reflex vomiting or regurgitation, triggered by stimulation of the end organs for taste or smell. Flushing away of bacteria or their toxins is effected by diarrhea, the adaptive value of which is not always appreciated by the suffering—and hurrying—patient. On a less obvious plane, we are protected against many potentially noxious agents which we ingest in search of gratification or comfort, or merely in ignorance of their effects, by enzymatic mechanisms of defense resident chiefly in the liver parenchyma. Thus, alcohol dehydrogenase begins the conversion of a poison into a food, although at considerable metabolic expense; and many drugs and food additives are met with adaptive changes in the smooth endoplasmic reticulum of the liver cell, productive of detoxifying enzymes.

Whether or not one accepts a current theory that man finally evolved on the continent of Africa as a direct descendant of a killer ape,[3] it is clear that for much of the past several million years the pattern of survival of his mammalian ancestors was that of the hunter. His canine teeth, the skeletal muscle which expedites swallowing as far as his mid-esophagus, his ample glandular stomach, and the lack of a forestomach suitable for rumination would seem to testify to this. In the wild, the hunting animal must pursue, fight, kill, and eat in rapid succession. The association of increased gastric motility and secretion with sustained hostility seems plausibly related to this relatively recent phase of our evolution. Likewise, the hunter often quite suddenly becomes the hunted; and the animal eating its prey must flee a more powerful adversary attracted by the smell of carrion. It seems likely that the temporary inhibition of digestion and of the urge to defecate under conditions of stress thus acquired survival value. Although these conditions are seldom closely duplicated in the life of modern man, the author is aware of numerous clinical examples of the suspension of these functions during military combat. In one, involving total obstipation for six weeks during jungle fighting behind enemy lines, the resemblance to subhuman conditions of survival was especially striking.

In theory, then, alterations in intestinal function under stress, with relevance to symptom formation in man, are probably not uniquely human phenomena, but are as old as the evolutionary necessity of survival of the fittest. The resulting gastrointestinal disorders, in this view, are *not* "diseases of civilization," and *not* manifestations of the complexity of man's higher integrative functions, but reflections of primitive or instinctual drives deeply rooted in our animal heritage. It no longer seems reasonable to reject a "psychophysiologic" hypothesis because the disorder it attempts to explain sometimes occurs in infancy, or in the mentally defective, or in primitive tribes approximating Rousseau's setting for the "noble savage." The recent observation of what appears to be the development of ulcerative colitis in the Siamang gibbon, under social and familial conditions strangely similar to those postulated for the human disease, may be a particularly dramatic example of this principle in operation.[4]

EVIDENCE FOR ETIOLOGICAL IMPORTANCE OF REACTIONS TO STRESS

But on what empirical grounds do we base the idea that some gastrointestinal disturbances are related to life stress, and in man to emotional tension? The evidence, it must be admitted, is largely hearsay and anecdotal, the observations largely uncontrolled and subject to strong bias; yet the enormous number of reported temporal associations of these phenomena compel closer attention.

The clinician frequently hears from his patients that symptoms arising from definable changes in gastrointestinal motility, such as dysphagia, nausea, vomiting, constipation, diarrhea, and abdominal pain, have coincided in time with life situations perceived by them as stressful and giving rise to feelings of emotional conflict. A report on 60 unselected cases of "mucous colitis" established the *regularity* of these coincidences.[5] Much more rarely does the physician observe these associations directly, perhaps in part because the doctor-patient transaction is usually reassuring and separates the patient in time and space from the described threat. Almost never have efforts been made to collect similar historical data from a control group; in at least one such study, these associations were no less frequent in diseases not *believed* to be influenced by psychophysiological reactions. In another recent study based upon community-wide sampling of supposedly healthy persons and patients bearing the diagnosis of irritable colon, the patients revealed a significantly increased frequency of supposedly stressful life situations (related to family affairs, personal strivings, and work conditions) in the period of the survey.[6] Even with such systematic surveys and with maximal care to avoid observer bias, the validity of the results is limited by the accuracy of recall of symptoms by the interviewee, the variable quantitative relationship between disturbed function and gut symptoms, and the highly subjective judgment of whether

a given life situation, however readily recognized, was stressful to *that individual at that time.*

Many of the uncertainties of these clinical studies have been dispelled by direct laboratory observations of animals and man under stress. In one of the earliest investigations based upon the roentgen ray, Cannon showed that under the fluoroscope the bismuth-filled intestines of his spread-eagled laboratory cats interrupted their normal movements when the cat was threatened by a growling dog held nearby.[7] This change in motility coincided in time with erection of the hairs, arching of the back, elevation of blood pressure, and other bodily changes considered part of the "emergency reaction" in preparation of the animal for fight or flight.

Cannon's findings led him to postulate that the usual effect of stressful situations on the intestine is to inhibit its motility and other functions as part of a general mobilization of the organism mediated by the sympathetic (adrenergic) nerves. When in 1941 Wolf and Wolff made prolonged observations of the gastric function of a single human subject through a large permanent gastric fistula, they showed that in situations evoking fear or depression the motility, secretion, and vascularity of the stomach were consistently reduced,[8] which was compatible with Cannon's hypothesis. They noted, on the other hand, that in other well studied stressful circumstances to which their subject reacted with feelings of hostility and resentment the stomach's contractions became stronger, its secretion more abundant, and its vascularity increased. Thus the possibility of bidirectional changes in function, associated with stress, was first demonstrated.

The recognition of similar relationships in other segments of the gut quickly followed. C. M. Jones, conducting observations of the mucosa of the sigmoid colon of healthy subjects for other purposes, had observed in one patient a precise temporal coincidence between acute social embarrassment and marked mucosal engorgement and hyperemia (personal communication). This led Almy, Tulin, Kern, and their associates to study the effects of stressful interviews on mucosal engorgement and motility of the human sigmoid, continuously monitored by endoscopy or by kymographic recordings.[9] Both in healthy persons and in patients with irritable colon, close temporal correlations were found between induced emotional tension and colonic functional changes. Heightened sigmoid contractions were linked with feeling states of anxiety, tension, and struggling to cope with adverse circumstances, whereas depressed contractions appeared, often abruptly, with feelings of guilt, self-reproach, and despondency, at times with overt weeping. In many respects these observations and the studies of Grace et al.[10] on patients with colostomies were mutually confirmatory. In more recent years, and using more modern techniques for the recording of colonic motility, transient motor disturbances in association with emotional tension have been recorded.[11, 12] The relevance of these disturbances to the development of intestinal pain, diarrhea and constipation, and other symptoms seems highly probable.

Abbot and coworkers recorded kymographically the motility of the descending portion of the duodenum in individuals who had complained of "nervous vomiting" and observed exaggerated, unremitting contractions at times of emotional tension induced in the laboratory by stressful interview.[13] The role of this motor disturbance in the physiological mechanisms of nausea and vomiting is well established.

Wolf and Almy studied the swallowing mechanism, both in normal subjects and in patients with dysphagia, by simple observation of barium swallows.[14] In both groups they noted marked delay in the passage of barium into the stomach, apparently caused by failure of relaxation of the esophagogastric sphincter, in response to a variety of stimuli. Delay attributable to extremely cold or hot barium, or that which had been excessively seasoned with Tabasco sauce, seemed an *appropriate* defense of the body against a noxious agent. But even greater delays were observed in volunteer subjects who swallowed while enduring painful stimuli applied to the head or the hand, or who were preoccupied with problems of personal significance. These were regarded as *inappropriate* bodily reactions, as in these instances the noxious agent was not literally swallowed.

Similar questions of the biological *appropriateness* of the gastrointestinal reactions were evident in all the studies cited. The identity of the bodily reactions to appropriate and inappropriate stimuli, and the impossibility of distinguishing objectively the phenomena in previously healthy persons and in those who had complained for years of "functional" disorders of the intestine, suggested that these are fundamental or primitive *reactions to nonspecific stress*, akin to the general "emergency reaction" of Cannon. The fact that they are temporally associated with feelings of emotional tension in man simply adds another dimension to our understanding of the total experience, as the interpretation of the feeling states of other animals is, to say the least, less reliable. In this view, *emotions do not cause bodily changes*. Instead, these are concomitant manifestations of a common event, just as thunder and lightning are parallel manifestations of an electrical discharge in the skies, or as weeping and sadness are parallel reactions to bereavement. Realization of this has a practical end—we address ourselves more energetically to the relief of the social problem than to often fruitless efforts to suppress function of the end organ.

It is evident that the understanding of gastrointestinal reactions under stress is far from complete, that many gut functions in this setting remain unexplored, and that our concept of the regulatory mechanisms has been largely at the level of the autonomic nervous system. Much more insight can be expected when other elements in the end organ and other levels of integration are studied. The possible significance in these reactions of the tissue proteases, such as fibrinolysin, remains to be defined. Control mechanisms for local antibody formation may prove to be involved in stress phenomena. The demonstrations that mucin biosynthesis is inhibited by adrenocorticoids,[15] and that DNA synthesis in gastric epithelial cells is suspended during restraint stress in rodents,[16] indicate that our present conception of these intestinal reactions to stress is both an oversimplification and an understatement.

ORGAN SELECTION

The question of why in some individuals the gut is "selected" as the focal point of bodily dysfunction and symptom formation during stress has given rise to much speculation. The observation itself may be questioned in many instances, as more persistent inquiry often reveals that those whose complaints to the physician center entirely on gastric or intestinal function also suffer from headache, excessive sweating, palpitation, giddiness, and other symptoms. In the same experimental studies of stressed normal subjects which showed the reality of intestinal dysfunction under these conditions, changes in respiration, blood pressure, and skin temperature were commonly observed.[14] Yet in other patients significant extraintestinal symptoms cannot be elicited, and some are truly monosymptomatic. Such occurrences have been variously explained in accordance with prevailing psychiatric doctrine, but evidence in support of these hypotheses has been scant. For example those in the psychoanalytic school, especially Alexander and his associates, have related peptic ulcer to reaction patterns persisting from the "oral" phase of personality development, and colonic disorders to similar persistence of the "anal" phase. Regarding feces as a gift by which the child may gratify his parents, they have attributed constipation to the desire to withhold affection from supporting figures and diarrhea to the desire to appease them.[17] Members of the psychosomatic school have often referred to "organ language" as evidence of the somatization of specific emotional drives or conflicts.[18] The popular use of such expressions as "something I cannot swallow," "it burns me up," and "listen to my gripes" certainly reflects a widespread belief in the association of emotional conflict with specific gut symptoms; but it does not explain how or why. However striking the imagination and intuition upon which these concepts were based, their lack of objective support has tended to discourage proper attention to this entire field by the scientifically trained clinician.

Some clinical observers have suggested that these correlations may result from earlier experiences, perhaps in childhood, in which painful emotional crises became associated with preoccupation with gastrointestinal function, by accident or by parental design. As parent-child interaction is early focused successively on feeding patterns and on toilet training, and as these events occur too early for accurate recollection in later life, the idea of *conditioning* of visceral responses is an attractive one. Clinically, although anecdotal evidence has at times been obtained in support of this happening in specific patients, solid evidence is lacking. For example, no convincing difference has yet been shown between the childhood toilet training experiences of patients with irritable colon and those of a control group.

It has often been remarked, nevertheless, that the visceral reactions of a number of individuals to the same stressful situation are not predictable from the nature of the stress, but are strongly influenced by the attitudes of the several persons as influenced by previous experience and training. In the extreme case, severe pain is viewed by the masochist not as stress but as gratification; and anniversary flowers may produce rage or tears in a divorcée. In a unique experiment, mucosal engorgement and heightened contractility of the sigmoid were observed in a medical student who was made to believe that a carcinoma of the rectum had just been found in him, whereas these reactions were absent in an identical procedure with a subject who knew in advance it was a hoax. In this study, the knowledge and previous instruction of the students were such as to intensify their disturbance at the indirect hints at a dire diagnosis which were purposely made by the physician-investigator. The perception of the reality situation was strikingly affected by this prior experience and by the differences in their awareness of the intent of the experiments.[9]

The direct conditioning of purposeful visceral responses was first shown, of course, by Pavlov when he trained a dog to salivate at the sound of a bell. The operant conditioning of visceral responses, as a part of reward or avoidance systems, has only recently been demonstrated in man and animals by Miller and his group.[19] In their experiments, animals rewarded repetitively and promptly for spontaneous visceral reactions of the desired sort (for example, slow pulse, or increased colonic contractions) quickly "learned" to sustain these responses over long periods. This laboratory model may have its counterpart in the neurotic mechanism of "secondary gain," in which a pathophysiological state resulting in symptom formation elicits a loving, sympathetic response from a potentially supportive figure such as a parent or a physician, and the reward thus obtained becomes unconsciously fixed as a pattern of behavior. If this concept is borne out by further study, the morphological basis (or "the pathology") of these visceral disorders is to be found, as suggested earlier by Stead,[20] in the subcellular organelles of cortical neurons in which the memory trace for conditioning of experiences is stored. Whether or not the operant conditioning of visceral responses is the ultimate explanation, the concept has led already to new and fruitful procedures in therapy, to be mentioned below.

IMPLICATIONS FOR DIAGNOSIS

The demonstration that common gastrointestinal syndromes such as the irritable colon, aerophagia, nervous vomiting, and dysphagia may often be produced by biologically ingrained patterns of defense and adaptation to stress has many implications for the practical management of nearly all patients with digestive disease. For stress in some form is an inevitable fact of life, and any illness may be regarded in some degree as stressful. It follows that the clinical syndrome in a given patient may be wholly related to the general adaptive reactions, or wholly due to some intercurrent process such as an infection or a neoplasm, with the stress reaction mild enough to contribute nothing to the symptomatology. Very often, symptoms caused by an "organic" lesion of the bowel and those caused by a stress reaction are additive and intertwined. These three possibilities are illustrated by the following examples.

Case 1. Mrs. T. T., a 40-year-old mother of three children, had had a history of enuresis and nailbiting in childhood, and persistent constipation beginning at that time. Five years before admission she had begun to have epigas-

tric and right upper quadrant pain after meals. Gallstones were found on X-ray, and the gallbladder was removed. Recurrence of the same pain prompted two explorations of the common duct with negative findings. Persistent pain led to review of the history and to disclosure that the onset of pain coincided with the death of her third child from a congenital malformation, and its continuance with a series of family problems. Supportive psychotherapy brought relief.

COMMENT. Unbiased review of this patient's symptoms, unvarying in character since before the time of the first operation and related at many points to emotion-laden personal crises, compelled the conclusion that they were wholly due to irritable colon, and that the cholelithiasis had been "silent."

Case 2. R. C., a 20-year-old single woman, had been orphaned at an early age, raised in several foster homes, and spent two years (age 16 to 18) in a reformatory for delinquent behavior. Four months previously she had begun living as the mistress of a violent-tempered bartender who had several times physically abused her. For the past three months she had suffered from hypogastric pain, constipation alternating with mild diarrhea, and mucus in the stools. There were no abnormal findings on physical examination, sigmoidoscopy, and gastrointestinal X-rays. Efforts at mental health counseling yielded no symptomatic benefit, and were met with stolid insistence that her current social situation was the most secure she had had in her life. Repeated examination of the stools then revealed cysts of *Entamoeba histolytica*. Antiamebic therapy led promptly to a sustained remission of symptoms, which continued to the time of the last follow-up visit.

COMMENT. Despite a close coincidence between the onset of symptoms and what appeared to be a disturbing social situation, the latter on further study proved to be not stressful to the patient and probably of no consequence for her physical symptoms. The prompt and lasting relief from specific therapy for amebiasis afforded strong presumptive evidence for this alternative diagnosis.

Case 3. Mrs. D. L., a 47-year-old housewife, was admitted to the hospital with intractable vomiting of five days' duration. The onset had been abrupt and had followed within one hour her notification of the death of her son while leading a platoon in front-line combat. With treatment by sedation and intravenous fluids and with the continuous solicitude of her husband and family, her grief abated and her vomiting ceased in three days. Prior to her planned discharge, a gastrointestinal series was performed, and an antral carcinoma was found to narrow the gastric outlet to a diameter of about 3 mm. On repeated questioning, she acknowledged that for nearly a month before her son's death she had had an indifferent appetite and a mild sense of fullness after meals.

COMMENT. Over the time period described above, the onset and subsidence of emesis correlated precisely with the patient's bereavement and subsequent consolation. The evident organic obstruction of the pylorus, continuing both before and after that date, must be regarded as a contributory but not adequate explanation of the vomiting.

The differential diagnosis between socalled functional and organic conditions, then, is less often a matter of "either-or" than of "how much of each." The diagnosis of stress reactions cannot be based solely upon exclusion of recognizable lesions of the gut by clinical and laboratory means, both because the existence of such a lesion does not rule out a concomitant stress reaction and because the diagnostic methods themselves are far from perfect. Thus the chance of recognizing an active duodenal ulcer on a single barium meal is probably not over 50 to 70 per cent. There must be *positive support* for the diagnosis of a "functional" disorder, going beyond the mere observation that the patient is "nervous." The best available evidence begins with the recognition of *temporal coincidence* between the onset or recurrence of key symptoms and the occurrence of a stressful situation, and at times a similar correlation between amelioration of symptoms and abatement of stress and the associated feeling states. The more abrupt the onset and offset, the closer the correlations in time, and the greater the number of episodes, the more convincing is this circumstantial evidence. Such evidence is best collected, and bias avoided, by deliberately separating the taking of the symptomatic from that of the social history, recording an accurate chronology for each, and then bringing them into conjunction in a life chart (see Table 1-1). In practice it is essential to begin eliciting the social history of the patient on the first visit, or before the physical examination is completed, laboratory studies reported, or any definitive treatment offered. Unless the physician thus indicates to the patient his routine and unbiased interest in the social aspects of illness, the later emphasis he may place upon them may be regarded as a special indignity, an imputation of weakness of character, or a "brush-off." On the other hand, such confidence on the patient's part is required for full disclosure of some social situations that the life chart can rarely be completed on the first visit.

It must be emphasized that life situations prevailing at the onset of illness must be judged not for their meaning to the physician, but for their putative meaning to the patient. I have already referred to the masochist's inverted view of the experiences of pain and relief from pain; the impotence of a husband is likely to be viewed differently by an idealistic young wife and a middle-aged matron weary of callous sexual exploitation. After collection of accurate social data, then, the second requirement for diagnosis is an understanding of these life situations in terms of the patient's own attitudes and value systems. In both these phases, nondirective interviewing and the testimony of the patient's close relatives and friends provide a degree of validity unattainable by more direct approaches. The necessity for patience and persistence in history-taking for

TABLE 1-1. LIFE CHART OF L. E., A 36-YEAR-OLD NURSE ANESTHETIST

AGE	LIFE SITUATION	BOWEL FUNCTION
13–20	Home, father dead, dominating mother	Irregular constipation, given castor oil
20–23	Nursing training, living near home	Steadily constipated
23–27	Private duty nursing, away from home	Regular, without laxatives
28	Mother ill, died; patient returned home to care for her in terminal illness	Severely constipated
29–30	Returned to private duty nursing	Regular, without laxatives
31–36	Worked as nurse anesthetist	Severely constipated

Comment: This evidence prompted inquiry into the emotional significance of her work as an anesthetist. The patient then revealed that while nursing her mother in her terminal illness she had had to fight off a recurring desire to give her an overdose of morphine. Her guilt feelings about these thoughts returned painfully whenever she "put a patient to sleep" when she again held "a life in (her) hands."

these purposes can hardly be overemphasized. The writer has on occasion obtained a clear understanding of the significant dynamic factors in a patient's illness only after six to eight hours of interviewing. As many psychiatrists persist even longer in this search, and ultimately succeed, and as most physicians conclude after *less* effort that *no* socially disturbing event had any significance in their patient's illness, it must be apparent that errors of omission in this field are common. In this view, it is clearly impractical in the press of ordinary medical practice to investigate this question adequately in each patient; but negative conclusions as to the relevance of psychophysiological reactions in a given illness should be stated with a certain degree of humility.

IMPLICATIONS FOR TREATMENT AND PROGNOSIS

Finally, this all-important process of evaluation profoundly influences both the *prognosis* and the *appropriate methods of therapy.* Many years ago it was suggested that patients with "mucous colitis" be divided arbitrarily into "less neurotic" and "more neurotic" groups.[5] The distinction may be readily made by the nonpsychiatrist—the less neurotic patient with a "functional" disorder is likely to have clear-cut episodes of symptoms punctuated by remissions, and the episodes are associated in time with social problems the stressful significance of which is clear to the neutral observer. The "more neurotic" patient, on the other hand, shows less clear temporal correlations between life stress and gut disorder, and may even have continuous symptoms during periods of what appears to the physician as an agreeable condition of living. Put another way, the *threshold* of stress in the more neurotic patient is low, or the secondary gain from the symptoms is great enough that they are unlikely to be given up.

The treatment of the more neurotic patient must be undertaken with little hope of radical cure except at times through prolonged use, in carefully selected cases, of psychoanalytic techniques. The only realistic goal of the internist or primary contact physician is palliation through symptomatic and supportive management. Sympathetic reassurance, after careful study of the patient's problem, is a good beginning. It is often possible to manipulate the social situation to conform to the constricted adaptive capabilities of the patient, e.g., different living arrangements or a new job. Strong therapeutic suggestion, often efficiently reinforced by a placebo or a special diet, is the basis for the effectiveness of various quacks and cultists in dealing with such patients, and should not be rejected by the conscientious, well-trained physician. Likewise, other ritualistic practices, such as exercises, warm baths, and prescribed rest periods, are frequent reminders of the physician's protection and availability. Finally, these patients should have the special protection of periodic health examinations by the same physician or group of physicians; otherwise they may waste their own or the public's resources in unneeded repetition of expensive laboratory examinations by often-changed medical advisors, or on the other hand may fail to have proper early care for intercurrent and sometimes lethal disease.

In the less neurotic, usually well adjusted patient the goals of therapy, even in the hands of the general physician, may be set much higher, for extended remission or substantial cure is achievable. The process begins, during the history-taking, with the patient's ventilation of unexpressed feelings and his discovery of the significance of emotionally charged situations in his own illness. The possibilities of sublimation of strong feelings (for example, into aggressive sports and games) and of adopting a new attitude toward painful realities are explored. Relapses of symptoms become the occasions for new discussions with the physician and the gain of additional insight. Symptomatic therapy is accorded a distinctly secondary role, and reduction in the use of medications is set up as a goal. Reassurance is largely implied and unexpressed.

With the better understanding of the probable mechanisms of these visceral responses, new concepts of therapy are beginning to appear. Based upon the operant conditioning of reward and avoidance patterns, the possibilities of purposeful control over involuntary reactions—almost literally, of mind over matter—are beginning to be realized. The experimental animal "learns" to perpetuate desired patterns of visceral function because they lead promptly and predictably to pleasurable sensations derived from electrical stimulation of subcortical areas of the brain.[19] In well motivated human subjects, similar reward is obtained simply from the knowledge that success is being achieved and from the encouragement of the therapist. All that may be needed otherwise is the instant feedback of information on current functioning of the organ in question. Thus the patient, watching the oscilloscope monitor, may "learn" to suppress his own cardiac extrasystoles, or induce the brain-wave activity which goes with a trance-like state. Indeed, the rise of a new multitude of yoga devotees, aided by electronic feedback loops, seems a distinct possibility. What these methods may accomplish for sufferers from stress-related digestive disorders remains, of course, to be determined.

CONCLUSIONS

To sum up, the meaning of gastrointestinal symptoms is becoming increasingly well understood in terms of disturbances of physiology of the gut, its appendages, and related control mechanisms. Evidence has accumulated in the clinic and in the laboratory to show that these disturbances are part of an array of adaptive reactions to life stress. Some of these are apparently of remote biological origin, having begun in animal species much lower than man in the evolutionary scale, and are at times seemingly inappropriate to the human crises in which the physician sees them. Their relationship to emotional tension seems almost uniquely human, but only because in man such a relationship is the more readily recognizable.

The gastrointestinal disorders which seem to be wholly attributable to these adaptations to life stress are among the most common conditions with which the physician must deal. In studies of industrial absenteeism caused by illness, they rank with the common cold as one of the two most important reasons for days lost from work; thus, a single large corporation counts its losses from this cause as well in excess of one million dollars per year. Yet the problem is bigger than this; for the universality of these adaptive responses means that they may coincide with illnesses from other causes and may account in variable degree for the symptomatic picture of those illnesses. Some of these disease mechanisms have been recognized only recently, and beyond question there are others still to be discovered; the importance of each in the causation of bowel disorder in a given patient and in our total experience with functional disorders must be carefully evaluated. Thus, despite early indications that many patients previously considered as having the irritable colon actually have demonstrable intestinal lactase deficiency, the controlling influence of lactose intolerance in their illnesses is not always clear. Unitarian theories of causation should be set aside, and the psychophysiological *aspect* of illness considered along with all other pathogenetic mechanisms.

A clear understanding of these adaptive reactions of the human gastrointestinal tract is needed in the diagnosis and differential diagnosis of all patients with digestive disorders. When these reactions predominate in the etiology of the disorder in a given patient, assistance in coping with life stress should receive first priority in the therapeutic plan. The choice of treatment methods and the prognosis are usually obvious from careful study of this aspect of the illness.

REFERENCES

1. Hammond, E. C. Some preliminary findings on physical complaints from a prospective study of 1,064,004 men and women. Amer. J. Publ. Health 54:11, 1964.
2. Lipkin, M., and Mack, M. Functional or organic? A pointless question. Ann. Intern. Med. 71:1013, 1969.
3. Dart, R. The predatory transition from ape to man. Internat. Anthropol. Ling. Rev. 1:4, 1953. Cited by R. Ardrey in The Territorial Imperative. New York, Dell Publishing Company, 1966.
4. Stout, C., and Snyder, R. L. Ulcerative colitis-like lesion in Siamang gibbons. Gastroenterology 57:256, 1969.
5. White, B. V., Cobb, S., and Jones, C. M. Mucous

colitis. Psychosom. Med., Monograph Ser., No. 1, 1939.

6. Mendeloff, A. I., Monk, M., Siegel, C. I., et al. Illness experience and life stresses in patients with irritable colon and with ulcerative colitis. New Eng. J. Med. *282*:14, 1970.

7. Cannon, W. B. The movements of the intestines studied by means of the Roentgen rays. Amer. J. Physiol. *6*:251, 1902.

8. Wolf, S., and Wolff, H. G. Human Gastric Function. New York, Oxford University Press, 1943.

9. Almy, T. P. Experimental studies on the irritable colon. Amer. J. Med. *10*:60, 1951.

10. Grace, W. J., Wolf, S. G., and Wolff, H. G. The Human Colon. New York, Paul B. Hoeber, 1950.

11. Chaudhary, N. A., and Truelove, S. C. Human colonic motility: A comparative study of normal subjects, patients with ulcerative colitis, and patients with the irritable colon syndrome. III. Effects of emotions. Gastroenterology *40*:27, 1961.

12. Wangel, A. G., and Deller, D. J. Intestinal motility in man. Gastroenterology *48*:69, 1965.

13. Abbot, F. K., Mack, M., and Wolf, S. G. The relation of sustained contraction of the duodenum to nausea and vomiting. Gastroenterology *20*:238, 1952.

14. Wolf, S. G., and Almy, T. P. Experimental observations on cardiospasm in man. Gastroenterology *13*:401, 1949.

15. Menguy, R., and Masters, Y. F. Effect of cortisone on mucoprotein secretion by gastric antrum of dogs: Pathogenesis of steroid ulcers. Surgery *54*:19, 1963.

16. Kim, Y. S., Kerr, R., and Lipkin, M. Cell proliferation during the development of stress erosions in mouse stomach. Nature (London) *215*:1180, 1967.

17. Alexander, F. Psychological factors in gastrointestinal disturbances. *In* Studies in Psychosomatic Medicine, F. Alexander and T. M. French (eds.). New York, Ronald Press, 1948.

18. Weiss, E., and English, O. S. Psychosomatic Medicine. Philadelphia, W. B. Saunders Co., 1943.

19. Miller, N. E. Learning of visceral and glandular responses. Science *163*:434, 1969.

20. Stead, E. A., Jr. Meaning of human behavior to the physician of tomorrow. Arch. Intern. Med. *110*:409, 1962.

Chapter 2

Normal Gastrointestinal Function in Children up to Two Years of Age

Murray Davidson

MOUTH, PHARYNX, AND ESOPHAGUS

During feeding the neonate takes consecutive bursts of three to four sucks; after several days of life more efficient groupings of ten to thirty sucks may be observed.[1] Newborn sucking behavior is affected by medications given to the mother in labor, by the type of initial formula, and by individual differences in neonates.[2, 3] Normal babies of birth weights above 1500 g are endowed with a special integrated mechanism to prevent aspiration.[4-6] Since the oral cavity is relatively longer and the posterior aperture smaller in the neonate, separation of the mouth and pharynx is facilitated during certain stages of feeding by closure of the aperture by arching and elevation of the posterior portion of the tongue. The nipple is grasped between the front of the tongue and the hard palate and suction created by withdrawing the tongue from the hard palate, which fills the nipple with milk. Reapposition of the tongue against the palate squeezes the nipple empty and fills the mouth cavity. The infant breathes easily during this filling process, because the mouth is effectively separated from the respiratory tract. Deglutition is initiated when the tongue is lowered to refill the nipple and the contents of the mouth pass to the posterior pharynx and esophagus. This action is preceded by closing of the epiglottis to prevent aspiration of milk. However, as swallowing is begun, a variable amount of the air present in the posterior pharynx passes to the stomach before the bolus of milk. This explains why variable amounts of air are present in the gastrointestinal tract after each feeding and why burping of infants is necessary. Thus, air in the stomach is not the result of improper feeding techniques as often suggested. The coordinate breathing-feeding pattern gradually disappears, so that by the age of six to eight months it becomes necessary for the infant to take two or three sucks at a time with regular interruptions of the process to breathe as does the adult.

The young newborn is limited in his ability to distinguish the nipple from solid foods, and he treats all materials placed on the front of the tongue in similar fashion. If, as is popular, solid foods are offered too early, they tend simply to be "slurped" into the pharynx. By the age of three months the infant can distinguish between

13

the nipple and semi-solid food placed on the tongue. For the former the sucking process ensues. For the latter there is coordinated propulsion of the material to the back of the mouth and pharynx as in older individuals.

Study of esophageal and gastric motility by manometric techniques has revealed poor tone in the lower esophageal sphincter of the newborn.[7, 8] The resting sphincter pressure rises to adult values by one month of age, and the sphincter becomes elongated. Failure of these changes to occur in the face of the normal, gradual increase of the fundal to esophageal pressure gradient following birth is believed to account for persistent regurgitation in some infants.[8] Despite the fact that an abnormal pattern of esophageal motility may be seen in normal infants during the first days of life, there is generally no clinical difficulty with swallowing, and the motility records beyond the first week become normal.[7] In retarded infants, incoordinate esophageal peristaltic activity with a delayed and prolonged latent period may be observed for many weeks or months beyond birth.

Accurate measurements of the volume of saliva are not available in infants and children. The quantities of saliva and the titer of salivary amylase are relatively small for several months after birth, but these rise sharply after three months of age.[9] The composition of saliva has been studied in normals and in patients with cystic fibrosis of the pancreas.[10] Electrolyte levels of the salivary secretions are normally hypotonic to serum and rise with increased secretory rates. The parotid component of salivary secretions is relatively aqueous, whereas the submaxillary gland produces both an aqueous and a mucinous fraction. Electrolyte levels are somewhat higher in the newborn period. Protein content is mainly mucopolysaccharides and the enzyme amylase.

GASTRIC FUNCTION

Almost immediately after birth air can be demonstrated to have transversed the pylorus in the normal newborn. Adequate measurements of gastric emptying by double dilution techniques such as those used in adults have not been applied to young children. The primary methods of measurement have been radiographic, with contrast media or, in some cases, with aspiration following delayed intervals from measured intakes.[11, 12] The state of health of the infant, the degree of hunger at the time of the feeding, the types of meals, the psychic stimuli, the amount of handling during the feeding, whether the room is dark or light for the fluoroscopic studies, and the positions in which studies are performed and in which babies are fed are all important uncontrolled influences on differences in gastric motility,[13] even as measured by these relatively crude techniques. The amounts of air which are swallowed also seem to influence the emptying time. Thus, there is enormous variability in terms of the time at which the pylorus will open and the time at which an entire meal will have passed from the stomach, and the reports in this regard vary between one and one-half to 24 hours for infants.[14]

The same factors which influence gastric emptying in adults apply to children. Increase in the amount of saturated fat in the meal will delay gastric emptying, presumably via enterogastrone-like activity. The larger the curd of milk or chunks of solid food when these are taken, the slower is the emptying from the stomach. Low birth weight infants, i.e., those prematurely born or born small for gestational age, and sick older infants are particularly sensitive to the increased amounts of mucus elaborated by the stomach. The increased mucus production in these states is associated with delayed gastric emptying, in part caused by acidity which further inhibits gastric emptying.

Emptying is accelerated if the volume of a feeding is large, if carbohydrate content is high, if the food is chilled, and if the dietary protein is denatured and the particles are small. Relatively isosmotic material such as milk passes through the pylorus more readily than extremely hypotonic or hypertonic foods. The intervals usually employed in the feeding schedule are based upon the fact that the stomachs of most infants will be generally emptied by three to four hours after taking a milk feeding.[12]

Casein coagulation, usually attributed to

the enzyme rennin, is an important function of the stomach of the newborn. However, although this enzyme is readily recovered from calf gastric juice, it has never been demonstrated in the human infant, and it is possible that pepsin and/or gastric acidity are the major contributors to milk curdling in the newborn. The solubility of casein is minimal at its isoelectric point of pH 4.7.

Gastric acidity and the volume of gastric secretion appear to be at adult levels in the newborn premature and full term infant.[15] This may be related to the two- to threefold increase in parietal cell mass as compared to adults.[16] However, after maintaining these levels for a number of days, there is a rapid decrease in gastric juice production, and the acidity tends to remain depressed for a number of weeks to months, especially among low birth weight and malnourished infants. Because of this, low acidity conversion of pepsinogen to pepsin should be impeded in newborns. However, even with gastric pH, which is usually not below 4.0 and frequently is above 5.0 among bottle-fed infants, some gastric proteolysis occurs. Supplemental maternal corticosteroids may induce a higher output of pepsinogen to account for this process, because plasma pepsinogen levels among newborns have been shown to be higher than at a few months of age.[17] Another possibility to account for gastric proteolysis in the newborn is the presence of cathepsin.[18] Although a pure specimen of this enzyme has not been isolated, its activity has been shown to be distinct from that of pepsin, and to be effective over a wider pH range.

SMALL INTESTINE

Very few sophisticated studies of small intestinal motility have been carried out in infants. Radiographic follow-through with contrast material and measurements of total intestinal transit time with marker techniques have varied widely.[19] Children under one year of age display a clumping of contrast medium in the small intestine with a blunting of the normal feathery intestinal mucosal pattern. This simulation of the picture of celiac disease is presumably associated with increased mucus production and renders radiographic distinction of the condition impossible in the young infant.

Small intestinal protein hydrolysis is mainly accomplished by the peptidases of pancreatic juice which are secreted in inactive zymogen forms. They are activated by enterokinase from the duodenal mucosa which splits an isoleucine-lysine bond to activate carboxypeptidase and to convert trypsinogen to trypsin. Trypsin acts autocatalytically on trypsinogen and chymotrypsinogen to speed the elaboration of the active forms. Zymogen granules have been shown to be present in the pancreas of infants born up to four months prematurely.[20] The peptidases which have been demonstrated to be secreted in the newborn even among infants of very low birth weights are trypsin, chymotrypsin, and carboxypeptidase. Other enzymes which digest protein and which may be isolated from the pancreatic secretion of young children are pancreatic elastase, ribonuclease, and deoxoribonuclease. Failure of protein hydrolysis is not related to age or size of infants; it is seen only in those with congenital pancreatic exocrine insufficiency, usually because of cystic fibrosis of the pancreas. There are rare patients with congenital enterokinase insufficiency who may also be unable to activate trypsin from trypsinogen to initiate the autocatalytic process by which the pancreatic peptidases are converted to active forms.[21] Under normal circumstances, stools from infants may contain unsplit casein curds which form in the stomach. Inadequate mastication of solid foods may also lead to the appearance of undigested meat fibers in toddlers.

A number of authors have written about the possibility of whole protein absorption with subsequent formation of antibodies among infants with damaged intestinal mucosae.[22, 23] Some pediatricians advocate that after periods of acute infantile diarrhea, however brief, cow's milk be avoided and proteins from soybean or protein hydroysates be substituted in the immediate postdiarrheal refeeding period to avoid the possibility of antibody development and subsequent allergic phenomena.

Digestion of starch and glycogen by salivary and pancreatic amylase results in virtually quantitative splitting of the polysaccharides in all age groups. The commonly diagnosed entity of starch intolerance or starch malabsorption has little clinical and laboratory substantiation.[24] Salivary and pancreatic amylases have been shown to be delayed in development at birth and not to reach full activity until four to six months of age.[25] Hydrolysis and absorption of the disaccharides maltose and isomaltose from the polysaccharides and of the naturally occurring disaccharides lactose and sucrose are similar to these processes in adults and older children. Beta-glycosidase (lactase) develops very slowly in fetal life, and normal titers of activity are found only at the very end of gestation.[26] However, although prematurely born infants display a deficiency of lactase activity during the first three days of life, the birth process appears to induce the development of the enzyme. It is demonstrable after the first few days of life, even in these babies, at levels which are higher than in fetuses at the same gestational age.[27] Lactase activity in the newborn and young child remains at one-third to one-fifth the comparable activities for sucrase and isomaltase and approximately a fifth to a tenth of maltase activity.[28] Although there is normal loss of lactase activity with aging and decrease in titer of this enzyme as compared with the other disaccharidases, the differences from birth to two years of age are not profound, even among those ethnic groups with diminished activity in adulthood.

The child above one year of age digests and absorbs fat to the same extent as adults and balance studies normally yield coefficients of absorption above 90 per cent or more of ingested fat, but values above 80 per cent are accepted as normal until one year of age.[29] Most disease processes of infants which are associated with steatorrhea display much more profound depressions of fat absorption.

In the newborn period, especially among low birthweight infants, there may be difficulty with fat digestion and absorption. Steatorrhea occurs in many prematurely born infants and it improves only as they gain weight and mature.[30, 31] In these babies the degree of steatorrhea is usually related to the type of fat ingested. Small, prematurely born infants rarely absorb more than 50 per cent of a saturated fat diet such as that contained in whole cow's milk. Unsaturated fatty acids are better tolerated, absorption progressively increasing as the acids become more unsaturated. Virtually quantitative absorption results after the feeding of medium-chain triglycerides in even very small babies.[32] These studies suggest that one of the areas of difficulty may be insufficient secretion of bile salts to achieve the critical micellar levels.[33]

LARGE INTESTINE

Motility studies of the large intestine yield patterns approximating those of the adult. Both resting and propulsive patterns may be seen.[34]

The motor phenomenon least well studied in infants, disturbances of which ultimately result in symptoms, is defecation.[35] During the first weeks of life the infant usually has a bowel movement after each feeding from stimulation of the gastroileocolic reflex. By two months of age material may be propelled to the distal colon following feeding without resulting defecation. In the latter part of the first year children become aware of their control over defecation. Voluntary explusion of material from the rectum results from increase in intra-abdominal pressure via contraction of the rectus muscles and descent of the diaphragm. If this increased force is exerted while the lower segment is closed at the upper end via the pinching action of the pelvic sling muscles, stool is expelled. If, on the other hand, the rectum and sigmoid are not thus separated from more proximal colon, stool is retained in response to the Valsalva maneuver. In order that the sling muscles be pulled taut and forward to accomplish the separations of the colonic areas, it is necessary for the individual to assume a squatting position, with leverage being exerted by the feet on the floor.

INTESTINAL BACTERIA AND STOOL

The gastrointestinal tract is usually sterile at birth, but it is quickly invaded via both mouth and anus, and by the end of the first 24 hours an intestinal flora is firmly established.[36] The duodenum usually remains sterile, probably as a result of the discharge of acid from the stomach. Organisms are found in increasing number progressively cauded in the tract and are most abundant in the colon. The organisms are generally similar to those found in adults, i.e., aerobic cultures reveal the ever-present coliform organisms and many varieties of lactobacilli, streptococci, and staphylococci, but by far the most frequent organisms are various members of the anaerobic bacteroides group. Lactobacilli are always conspicuous, and a gram-positive flora predominates among breast-fed infants; in artificially fed infants the lower sugar and higher protein intakes favor growth of the coliform organisms. Passage of fatty acids to the colon tends to check the growth of a number of organisms, notably staphylococci.

Bacteria appear to be important for the synthesis of essential nutrients; the known B vitamins are all synthesized by the intestinal bacteria, as are folic acid and biotin, and there is evidence that synthesis in the intestine may be an important source of vitamin K in the early days of life.

Meconium, the initial discharge from the gastrointestinal tract following birth, is a dark brown-green, semisolid material high in mucopolysaccharides and bile and squamous epithelial cells swallowed in utero. Normal meconium contains representative amounts of pancreatic, amylolytic, tryptic, and lipolytic activity. Bacteria are usually absent from the first meconium, the colon only becoming colonized after a number of hours. The baby passes this material a number of times during the first 24 to 48 hours, prior to the appearance of normal stool from material ingested postnatally.

Stools of breast-fed infants are usually sour in odor with an acid reaction of pH 4.5 to 5.1. Stools of infants fed cow's milk are usually firmer and more homogeneous in appearance, with reaction ranging from pH 4.5 to 8.3. During the first year of life the number of stools decreases from the norm of five to six daily in the neonatal period to one to two per day by six months of age. The quantity of stool passed by healthy infants in the first weeks of life ranges between 30 and 45 g per day. This amount increases gradually, and the average output below five years of age is 100 to 150 g of stool per day. Water content varies from a low of 70 per cent in stools of constipated individuals to a high of 80 per cent in soft, semiformed stools.[37]

Bilirubin represents the major pigment of infants' stools. However, the reducing power of the infant's intestinal contents is quite variable and generally distinctly less than later in life, partly because of increased amounts of air swallowed by young children and partly because of the peculiar flora engendered by milk diets. Bilirubin, therefore, is often incompletely reduced to colorless stercobilin, and a variable amount is excreted unchanged. Pale stools which result from this artifact may be distinguished readily from acholic stools by virtue of the fact that they darken on standing. Bilirubin crystals may sometimes be identified in the stools on microscopic examination. This bilirubin is readily oxidized to biliverdin, and yellow stools therefore may become green on standing. Various vegetables and medications may add a predominating color to infant stools. Iron which is commonly prescribed may be passed as a sulfide, giving the stool a black color. Bacteria may also contribute to stool color, such as the red stools in diapers which result from *Bacteroides serratio.*

Microscopic examination of the stool yields little information that cannot be obtained by visual inspection. Chemical examination for fat may be useful, because the gross appearance is often deceptive and large fatty acid concentrations may not be apparent on inspection.[38] Impairment of fat assimilation cannot be accurately assessed by measuring the percentage of fat in individual stools, because this fecal fat varies considerably in children.

DIARRHEA

In most instances of acute or chronic diarrhea of young children in which balance studies have been carried out, little effect is demonstrable on protein digestion and assimilation unless the children become remarkably malnourished and secretion of peptidases by the pancreas is impaired.[39, 40] Variable defects in carbohydrate assimilation and absorption have been shown with diarrhea.[41] Fat digestion and absorption may be somewhat impaired; this defect may persist for longer periods than for other foodstuffs.

Acute diarrhea in the infant affects water and electrolyte balance much more than absorption of food. In fully grown individuals there is limited surface area of intestine for the large volume of cellular material and extracellular fluid contained by the body. In small infants there is a remarkably greater gut surface area over which fluid may be lost relative to the total fluid volume available. The loss of water and electrolytes in loose stools is promptly reflected by a reduction of blood volume and of interstitial fluid volume. Stool losses of water among children under two years of age with acute diarrhea may amount to ten to 15 times the normal, i.e., up to 500 ml or more. As stool water losses increase, electrolyte concentrations also increase and may approach values of ten times normal in the stool. Thus, milder degrees of dehydration are usually associated with more normal electrolyte and acid-base findings; severe dehydration is usually accompanied by severe hyponatremia, hypokalemia, and acidosis. Deficits of more than 15 per cent of the total body fluid are usually incompatible with life in the infant.

VOMITING

Vomiting caused by reverse peristalsis in children is seen only in pyloric obstruction, primarily hypertrophic pyloric stenosis. Such vomiting is usually projectile. In all other instances, as in adults, it results from pressure of reflexly contracted abdominal musculature and the diaphragm on an atonic stomach while the duodenum is in spasm.

Vomiting in the newborn period may be benign and self-limited and may result from irritating material which has been swallowed during birth. The presence of blood requires determination of the type of hemoglobin by alkaline denaturation to determine whether it is maternal in origin (from swallowing during passage through the parturient canal) or whether it arises from the infant's stomach.[42] Infectious processes and intracranial pathology may induce vomiting early in the newborn. A history of polyhydramnios in the mother or of the finding of a single umbilical artery at delivery increases the likelihood of a congenital anomaly of the gastrointestinal tract. Bile-stained or fecal vomiting usually indicates gastrointestinal obstruction. The diagnostic indications such as the timing and character of the vomitus or of the findings on abdominal exam are not different in the newborn infant from those in an adult with respect to the site of obstruction.

A very common form of vomiting in young infants results from distention of the stomach by overfeeding or swallowing of too much air. In these instances the infant may cry excessively from the discomfort of the distended stomach. He eats readily and vomits effortlessly within a few minutes after feeding. Persistent cases of such functional vomiting may respond to thickening of the liquid feedings with small amounts of infant cereals or to changes in formula to a milk containing vegetable oil as the source of fat. The less saturated vegetable oil may pass from the stomach to the small intestine more readily. At the least it results in a less malodorous vomitus in the event the child continues to regurgitate. The commonly prescribed sedatives and antispasmodics increase the degree of atonicity of the stomach and are, therefore, not only unphysiological but also ineffective.

Young infants also vomit easily during bouts of infections. This may be the result of greater delay in gastric emptying because of increased gastric mucus secretion and decrease in acidity and tonicity in the child under two with fever. As children grow older, vomiting caused by improper feeding techniques or respiratory infections decreases. However, some who have vomited repeatedly during the first year of life may discover the profound effect and anxiety induced in their parents by an episode of vomiting. This discovery may lead to habitual vomiting, which may pose a difficult diagnostic problem. If improperly handled it even may become a pernicious problem in children between one and two years of age.

REFERENCES

1. Gryboski, J. D.   The swallowing mechanism of the neonate. I. Esophageal and gastric motility. Pediatrics 35:445, 1965.
2. Kron, R. E., Stein, M., and Goddard, K. E.   Newborn sucking behavior affected by obstetric sedation. Pediatrics 37:1012, 1965.
3. Kron, R. E., Ipsen, J., and Goddard, K. E.   Consistent individual differences in the nutritive sucking behavior of the human newborn. Psychosomatic Med. 30:151, 1968.
4. Ardran, G. M., Kemp, F. H., and Lind, J.   A

cineradiographic study of bottle feeding. Brit. J. Radiol. *31*:156, 1958.

5. Ardran, G. M., Kemp, F. H., and Lind, J. A cineradiographic study of breast feeding. Brit. J. Radiol. *31*:156, 1958.

6. Adran, G. M., and Kemp, F. H. A correlation between sucking pressures and movements of the tongue. Acta Paediat. Scand. *48*:261, 1959.

7. Gryboski, J. D., Thayer, W. R., Jr., and Spiro, H. M. Esophageal motility in infants and children. Pediatrics *31*:382, 1963.

8. Strawczynski, H., Beck, I. T., McKenna, R. D., and Nickerson, G. H. The behavior of the lower esophageal sphincter in infants and its relationship to gastro-esophageal regurgitation. J. Pediat. *64*:17, 1964.

9. Lourie, R. S. Rate of secretion of the parotid glands in normal children. Amer. J. Dis. Child. *65*:455, 1943.

10. Barbero, G. J., and Chernick, W. Function of the salivary gland in cystic fibrosis of the pancreas. Pediatrics *22*:945, 1958.

11. Silverio, J. Gastric emptying time in the newborn and the nursling. Amer. J. Med. Sci. *247*:732, 1964.

12. Schell, N. B., Karelitz, S., and Epstein, B. S. Radiographic study of gastric emptying in premature infants. J. Pediat. *62*:342, 1963.

13. Hood, J. H. Effect of position on amount and distribution of gas in intestinal tract of infants and young children. Lancet. *2*:107, 1964.

14. Wolman, I J. Major motility patterns of the child's digestive tract: A review. Amer. J. Med. Sci. *207*:782, 1944.

15. Ames, M. D. Gastric acidity in the first ten days of life of the prematurely born baby. Amer. J. Dis. Child. *100*:252, 1960.

16. Polacek, M. A., and Ellison, E. H. Gastric acid secretion and parietal cell mass in stomach of a newborn infant. Amer. J. Surg. *111*:777, 1966.

17. Grayzel, H. G., Elkan, B., Moghazeh, M., Schneck, L., and Garza, S. Plasma pepsinogen levels in the newborn. Amer. J. Dis. Child. *103*:759, 1962.

18. Buchs, S., and Freudenberg, E. Die Rolle des Kathepsins bei der Eiweissverdauung. Ergebn. Inn. Med. Kinderheilk. *2*:544, 1951.

19. Tornwall, L., Lind, J., Peltonen, T., and Wegelius, C. The gastrointestinal tract of the newborn. I. Cineradiographic findings. Ann. Paediat. Fenn. *4*:209, 1958.

20. Mady, S., and Dancis, J. Proteolytic enzymes of the premature infant with special reference to his ability to digest unsplit protein food. Pediatrics *4*:177, 1949.

21. Hadorn, B., Tarlow, M. J., Lloyd, J. K., and Wolff, O. H. Intestinal enterokinase deficiency. Lancet *1*:812, 1969.

22. Schloss, O. M., and Worthen, T. W. The permeability of the gastroenteric tract of infants to undigested protein. Amer. J. Dis. Child. *11*:342, 1916.

23. Gryskay, F. L, and Cooke, R. E. The gastrointestinal absorption of unaltered protein in normal infants and in infants recovering from diarrhea. Pediatrics *16*:763, 1955.

24. Davidson, M., and Bauer, C. H. The value of microscopic examination of the stool for extracellular starch in the diagnosis of starch intolerance. Pediatrics *21*:565, 1958.

25. Andersen, D. H., and Di Sant'Agnese, P. A. Idiopathic celiac disease. Mode of onset and diagnosis. Pediatrics *11*:207, 1953.

26. Doell, R. G., and Kretchmer, N. Studies of small intestine during development. I. Distribution and activity of β-galactosidase. Biochim. et Biophys. Acta *62*:353, 1962.

27. Boellner, S. W., Beard, A. G., and Panos, T. C. Impairment of intestinal hydrolysis of lactose in newborn infants. Pediatrics *36*:542, 1965.

28. Auricchio, S., Rubino, A., Prader, A., Rey, J., Jos, J., Frezal, J., and Davidson, M. Intestinal glycosidase activities in congenital malabsorption of disaccharides. J. Pediat. *66*:555, 1965.

29. van de Kamer, J. H., ten Bokkel Huinink, H., and Weijers, H. A. Rapid method for the determination of fat in feces. J. Biol. Chem. *177*:347, 1949.

30. Gordon, H. H., Levine, S. Z., and McNamara, H. Feeding of premature infants: Comparison of human and cow's milk. Amer. J. Dis. Child. *73*:442, 1947.

31. Davidson, M. The feeding of prematurely born infants—a critique of current status. J. Pediat. *57*:604, 1960.

32. Snyderman, S. E., Morales, S., and Holt, L. E., Jr. The absorption of short-chain fats by premature infants. Arch. Dis. Child. *30*:83, 1955.

33. Lavy, U., Silverberg, M., and Davidson, M. Role of bile acids in fat absorption in low birth weight infants. Proceedings of the 81st Annual Meeting of the American Pediatric Society and the 41st Annual Meeting of the Society of Pediatric Research, 1971, p. 47.

34. Davidson, M., Sleisenger, M. H., Almy, T. P., and Levine, S. Z. Studies of distal colonic motility in children. I. Non-propulsive patterns in normal children. Pediatrics *17*:807, 1956.

35. Davidson, M. Constipation. *In* Ambulatory Pediatrics, M. Green and R. J. Haggerty. Philadelphia, W. B. Saunders Co., 1968, pp. 220–225.

36. Olsen, E. Studies on Intestinal Flora of Infants. Copenhagen, Munksgaard, 1949.

37. Lapin, J. Recurrent and chronic diarrhea in infancy and childhood. Amer. J. Dis. Child. *101*:454, 1961.

38. Weijers, J. A., and van de Kamer, J. H. Coeliac disease. I. Criticism of the various methods of investigation. Acta Paediat. *42*:24, 1953.

39. Bongstrom, B., Lindquist, B., Lundh, G. Digestive studies in children. Amer. J. Dis. Child. *101*:454, 1961.

40. Lindquist, B. Digestive studies in ulcerative colitis. Acta Paediat. *49*:512, 1960.

41. Sunshine, P., and Kretchmer, N. Studies of small intestine during development. III. Infantile diarrhea associated with intolerance to disaccharides. Pediatrics *34*:38, 1964.

42. Apt, L., and Downey, W., S., Jr. "Melena" neonatorum: The swallowed blood syndrome; a simple test for the differentiation of adult and fetal hemoglobin in bloody stools. J. Pediat. *47*:6, 1955.

Chapter 3

Nutrition and the Gastrointestinal Tract

Elliot Weser

BACKGROUND

In order to utilize the calories in food for energy balance, dietary nutrients must be appropriately digested and absorbed via the intestinal tract. It is not surprising, therefore, that nutrition has been intimately associated with all aspects of gut function. There are numerous psychological, physiological, and biochemical mechanisms which determine food preferences, actual intake, utilization, and excretion (bowel habit). Normal absorption and malabsorption are discussed on pages 250 to 289. We will review here only those factors affecting food intake which contribute to malnutrition.

The energy content of food, assuming normal digestion and absorption, must equal the expenditure in man if a steady state of energy balance is to be achieved. Some of our major health problems are caused by social, economic, or cultural events which alter the state of energy balance and produce either "undernutrition" or, equally important, "overnutrition" expressed as obesity. In many areas of the world, including the United States, large numbers of people receive insufficient food, either because there is not enough produced to meet the demands of an overexpanded population, or because adequate quantities of food cannot be pur-

chased for lack of money. In addition, the quality of food may be poor and deficient in essential nutrients. Thus a state of negative energy balance may occur and produce chronic undernutrition. At the other end of the spectrum, affluence is often accompanied by overindulgence of food intake and, at the same time, a significant reduction in energy expenditure because of diminished physical activity. This combination contributes to a high incidence of obesity which may be related to several other medical problems.

One of the important factors in maintaining energy balance is the mechanism by which food intake is regulated. The results of numerous studies in animals have indicated that the hypothalamus plays an important role. Unfortunately, relatively little of this complex subject is known with respect to man. However, it seems likely that some of the same mechanisms contribute to the control of food intake in man and may ultimately provide us with a better understanding of energy imbalances.

REGULATION OF FOOD INTAKE

It is important to define the sensations associated with food intake prior to any discussion of its regulation. *Hunger* is the clear awareness of the desire to eat food

20

when the body has been deprived of nutrients beyond a maintenance level, and is often accompanied by abdominal sensations of discomfort ("hunger pangs"), irritability, and food searching activity. It is a grouping of unpleasant sensations and is generally disagreeable. *Appetite*, on the other hand, represents a wish to ingest food and often remains present after sufficient food intake is achieved to abate hunger. It is strongly influenced by numerous psychological stimuli such as emotion, conditioning, and willful choice. *Satiety* is the loss of the desire to eat after the ingestion of food. *Anorexia* differs from satiety in that, despite all the physiological stimuli which would normally produce hunger, no desire to eat is present. Anorexia is common in many patients with organ diseases as well as in those with psychological conditions and therefore is an important but nonspecific symptom. It should be emphasized that nondigestive tract diseases commonly produce anorexia (i.e., renal disease, cancer, heart disease, etc.). Associated symptoms and signs such as abdominal pain, nausea, vomiting, diarrhea, melena, and clay-colored stools are necessary to implicate a gastrointestinal etiology.

CENTRAL NERVOUS CONTROL OF FOOD INTAKE

Abundant evidence obtained through animal experiments clearly indicates that the hypothalamus plays a major role in regulating the intake of food. A summary of the relationships between the hypothalamus, other areas of the central nervous system, and several physiological or biochemical mechanisms affecting these centers is shown in Figure 3–1. It has been well demonstrated in the rat that stereotaxic placement of symmetrical, bilateral lesions in the ventromedial nucleus of the hypothalamus will cause increased food intake (hyperphagia) and subsequent obesity.[1] These animals overeat only when food is readily available to them and not when they must obtain it under more complicated conditions. Furthermore, they appear less tolerant of unpleasantly flavored food and more prone to anorexia after anorexigenic drugs and diets containing excessive protein and unbalanced amino

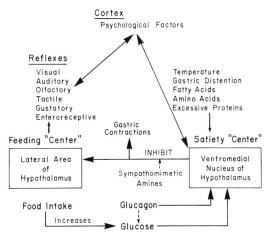

Figure 3–1. Schematic representation of hypothalamic regulations of food intake.

acid mixtures. This is of interest because studies in obese humans have shown similar behavior with respect to adjusting food intake according to nutrient value. Grossly obese adults seem incapable of regulating energy intake at the physiological level when the nutritive concentration of the diet is altered covertly.[2]

Additional studies have further shown that small lesions placed in the lateral area of the hypothalamus, at the same rostrocaudal plane as the ventromedial nucleus, will completely stop intake behavior. If animals were previously made hyperphagic by lesions placed in the ventromedial nuclei, the lateral lesions will offset the overeating activity and produce aphagia.

On the basis of these kinds of data a "satiety center" and "feeding center" in the hypothalamus have been proposed as the fundamental control-complex in regulating food intake. Stimulation of the satiety center inhibits the feeding center and, incidentally, gastric hunger contractions. The feeding center acts as an integrative station coordinating all the complex reflexes associated with food intake. It seems obvious that other parts of the central nervous system interact with the hypothalamus and play important, as yet undefined roles in food intake. The application of these findings to man is uncertain for want of experimental evidence. Nevertheless, hypothalamic injury or lesions in man have been associated with obesity, as have frontal lobotomy and bilateral frontal cortical lesions.[3]

Another interesting method of causing obesity in rats is by intraperitoneal or subcutaneous injection of gold thioglucose. This produces destructive lesions in the ventromedial nuclei in the hypothalamus and represents a chemically induced form of hypothalamic obesity. In general, the amount of gold concentration in the hypothalamus is proportional to the blood level of gold thioglucose shortly after injection. Other gold-carbohydrate compounds such as gold thiogalactose, gold thiosorbital, gold thiomalate, gold thioglycerol, gold thiocaprovate, and others do not damage the hypothalamus. Furthermore, the damage with gold thioglucose can be prevented by simultaneous administration of sodium thioglucose, suggesting competitive inhibition of the glucose moieties.

These findings suggest that the damage to the ventromedial nuclei is related to a special affinity for glucose, which is the basis for the glucostatic control theory of the satiety center. It has been suggested that the ventromedial nuclei may have special cells which act as glucose receptors capable of detecting rates of glucose utilization. The sensation of hunger appears when there is a small peripheral arteriovenous blood glucose difference. Satiety is accompanied by a large arteriovenous difference; i.e., high glucose utilization. Increased electrical activity of the satiety center has been found with elevated blood glucose concentrations, and just the opposite with low blood glucose levels.

Selective metabolic differences have also been found in the hypothalamic centers. It has been demonstrated that hungry rats preferentially take up P^{32} and C^{14}-labeled glucose in the feeding center compared with control areas. Unfortunately, the glucostatic hypothesis is not without question. Previous glucose loading in animals and man does not appreciably reduce spontaneous food intake. Also, fatty acid uptake and release by the fat depots may correlate better than glucose with the sensations of hunger and satiety. Although the specific ways in which the satiety center may be activated are not yet completely understood, the hypothesis

that the hypothalamus plays a key role in regulating food intake is attractive.

Glucagon has been shown to inhibit food intake and gastric hunger contractions in man and animals, probably through its action of stimulating hepatic glycogenolysis and increasing blood glucose concentrations. The increase in glucose concentration and subsequent glucose utilization is thought to stimulate the satiety center, because the effect of glucagon is significantly diminished in animals with lesions of the ventromedial nuclei. On the other hand, sympathomimetic amines, particularly amphetamines, are potent inhibitors of food intake even in animals with damaged ventromedial nuclei. In addition, they enhance weight loss by increasing spontaneous activity and probably mobilize fatty acids from adipose tissue.

Psychological factors override any subcortical mechanism for control of food intake. The attitudes toward food nurtured by cultural, emotional, and economic necessities will obviously affect eating habits. The reasons for compulsive eating, so common in our society, which produces obesity are not always clear. At this point, no morphological lesions of the hypothalamus in humans have been specifically correlated with excessive food intake. At the other end of the spectrum is the well known psychiatric disorder anorexia nervosa, which is discussed later in this chapter.

OVERNUTRITION

OBESITY

Although obesity is common in our society, its cause is still not clearly understood and, in general, diet therapy has not been very successful. Obesity is present when fat exceeds the normal fraction of total body weight. Actual measurements of total adipose tissue cannot be made directly. Therefore, the determination of skin fold thickness at standard sites, such as the triceps and subscapular areas, has been useful in quantitating obesity.[4] Although most grossly overweight individuals are also obese, the two terms are not synonymous. If the body weight exceeds standard values for ideal weight according to age, sex, and height, the excess pounds may be related to muscle, bone, or body fluid and not excess fat. Nevertheless, when the weight is 30 per cent greater than the ideal for height and age in moderately sedentary individuals, excess fat is usually the reason. It has been estimated that 25 to 40 per cent of the adult population in the United States over the age of 30 are more than 20 per cent overweight and that this is associated with an increased susceptibility to diabetes, as well as cardiovascular, respiratory, and biliary tract diseases.[5]

It has been proposed that obesity be classified as either regulatory, indicating a disturbance of regulation of food intake, or metabolic, suggesting an underlying metabolic defect as the cause of the fat accumulation. Unfortunately, no inherent metabolic abnormalities, antedating the obesity, have thus far been demonstrated in any group of obese subjects. Insulin insensitivity and abnormal glucose tolerance, well known to clinicians, represent adaptive changes to excess fat accumulation. Of course, "classic" endocrine abnormalities such as hyperadrenocorticism or hypothyroidism would represent instances of metabolic obesity. The role of the intestinal tract as an absorptive organ is normal and merely absorbs the food provided it. As will be discussed later, however, meal frequency may influence the accumulation of fat in adipose tissue.

Obesity results when caloric intake, particularly of fats and carbohydrates, exceeds the daily requirements for energy expenditure. Unused calories are converted to fatty acids and stored in adipose tissue cells. Many psychological and cultural factors determine how much we eat and the extent of our physical activity. There seems little doubt that with increased affluence a more sedentary mode of living has contributed to the high incidence of obesity in our society.

Recent studies have implicated the importance of the number of adipose cells in obesity. Rats that are exposed to increased food intake, particularly during their nursing period, increase their number of adipose cells, and this increase persists into adulthood. They have larger fat depots because of more fat in individual cells and

a greater total number of fat cells. The significance of these findings for human obesity is highlighted by similar observations in grossly obese individuals.[6] Neonatal feeding patterns may play an important role in predisposing to obesity. An adaptive increase in the number of adipose tissue cells may persist throughout the life of the individual and affect energy balance in adulthood. If the number of adipose cells is significantly increased in obese subjects, it may also explain the limited success of dietary therapy. Even if a reduction of adipose cell size to normal is achieved, a greater number of cells would remain and still contribute to an increased adipose tissue mass.

Another interesting and possibly important factor relating to human obesity may be the frequency or, more specifically, the infrequency of feedings. In numerous animal experiments, it has been shown that food ingested as large but infrequent feedings leads to increased fat storage compared with an isocaloric intake of food distributed as smaller, frequent feedings.[7] The major difference between the two types of feeding schedules is that an increased amount of nutrients must be absorbed from the intestinal tract and metabolized by various tissues per unit of time, whereas the intestinal tract remains empty for longer periods (fasting) between feedings. This type of eating pattern is associated with functional and morphological changes in the intestinal tract. Pancreatic and intestinal mucosal enzymes increase in activity, as does the rate of glucose absorption from the lumen. These changes may be related to the effects of feeding and fasting on epithelial cell renewal, resulting in mucosal hyperplasia. Of particular interest is the increase in lipogenic activity of adipose tissue which parallels an increase in enzymes involved in fat formation. There is a striking increase in the capability to make fat from carbohydrate precursors. Protein and nucleic acid synthesis in adipose tissue is also increased.

Similar changes occur in the liver, and this entire enteric response (to infrequent feedings) has been termed "adaptive hyperlipogenesis."[8] Periodic hyperinsulinemia after intermittent, high carbohydrate ingestion may play an important role in adaptive hyperlipogenesis, because under these circumstances adipose tissue may be more sensitive to lipogenic stimulation by insulin. In addition, animal experiments indicate that the periodic hyperinsulinemia may produce "functional exhaustion" of the pancreatic beta-cells and predispose to the development of diabetes.

Application of this information to man is still incomplete, but several studies suggest that infrequent feeding patterns may contribute to obesity and other problems. Serum lipids and cholesterol levels have been shown to be higher and related to reduced meal frequency.[7] Furthermore, epidemiologic studies have revealed a significant correlation between fewer meals and overweight, thicker skin folds, increased serum cholesterol, diminished glucose tolerance, and ischemic heart disease.[7] These relationships are summarized in Figure 3–2. In man, infrequent feeding schedules alone probably do not cause fat accumulation; but when associated with excessive caloric intake, insufficient physical activity, aging, and diet composition (high carbohydrates), adaptive hyperlipogenesis may be an important pathophysiological response in the production of obesity.

The role of heredity in human obesity is still obscure and thus of minimal clinical significance. Nevertheless, there is ample reason to believe that many important genetic factors are involved in the etiology of obesity. Several animal models exist in which specific genetic factors have been isolated. The best known example of ex-

perimental hereditary obesity is the obese-hyperglycemic strain of mice. These animals carry a recessive gene which expresses itself as obesity after the fourth week of life in one out of every four mice. The obesity is due in part to a combination of hyperphagia and hypoactivity. Even when food is restricted and the weight of these animals is kept in the range of normal mice, their carcasses will still yield three times as much fat as nonobese siblings. These animals are extremely resistant to insulin, and their blood glucose level is very sensitive to the hyperglycemic effect of growth hormone. They also exhibit pancreatic islet cell hypertrophy and extreme sensitivity to cold. The adipose tissue of these mice contains the enzyme glycerokinase, which is normally absent. Its activity permits the adipose tissue to form substantial amounts of α-glycerophosphate (the obligatory precursor of triglyceride glycerol) from noncarbohydrate sources. Triglyceride synthesis is continuously favored even under conditions which normally produce lipolysis. Thus, the metabolism of the adipose tissue is largely independent of carbohydrate and insulin metabolism; this abnormality is probably an important factor in the development of the obesity. In this regard the enzymes in the glycerolphosphate cycle from adipose tissue of obese patients have been shown to be about half as active as the enzymes in fat from normal individuals.[9] Although this probably represents an adaptive change, it would tend to salvage α-glycerolphosphate and in-

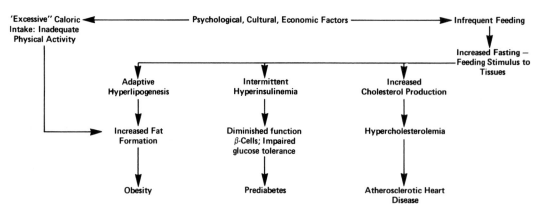

Figure 3–2.   Relationship of meal frequency to obesity and other associated conditions.

crease triglyceride glycerol synthesis and subsequently triglyceride formation.

Another strain of mice has been described which has a high incidence of obesity concurrent with ACTH-secreting tumors of the pituitary. Hypertrophy of the islets of Langerhans is a characteristic finding, and it has been postulated that the hyperadrenocorticism produces a secondary hyperinsulinism. Obesity may result because the corticosteroids fail to antagonize the lipogenesis-stimulating effect of the insulin in the adipose tissue. These observations are obviously of interest to man, because many patients with Cushing's disease and after castration become obese.

The comparative role of genetics in human obesity is difficult to assess because of the large number of cultural and environmental influences. In a recent review,[1] epidemiological data concerning familial occurrence, ethnic differences, studies of twins and adopted children, sex ratios, and somatotypes suggest that genetic factors very likely play a role in human obesity. However, at present our knowledge of genetic influences has no clear therapeutic value.

DIETS

The simple concept of persistently reducing caloric intake below expenditure follows the law of thermodynamics and should result in progressive weight loss. Energy expenditure may exceed intake by decreasing caloric ingestion, increasing physical activity, and possibly varying the efficiency of substrate oxidation. Whatever combination is chosen, there must be continued encouragement and psychological support from the physician.

A sound dietary approach aims at restricting calories while providing essential nutrients and a palatable, economically feasible regimen. The desired deficit of calories is determined by the fact that a pound of body fat is equal to 3500 calories. If a weight loss of two pounds a week is desired, then a daily calorie deficit of 1000 calories is planned. It is generally conceded that loss of two pounds a week is all that should safely be attempted by patients not under close medical scrutiny. More rapid weight loss, however, can be achieved initially if indications require it (such as impending surgery) by careful

metabolic and psychological supervision. After assessing the size (surface area) and activity pattern of the patient, an estimate of the calorie maintenance requirements can be made, usually between 2200 and 2500 calories daily. Since caloric intake below 1500 calories daily for men and 1000 calories daily for women is difficult to maintain, increased physical activity, such as walking, should be added to increase caloric requirements to justify the higher ranges of intake.

Adjustments of calorie intake should be made according to results of a trial period. Present evidence indicates that with reduction of calorie intake in obese patients, calorie expenditure is significantly reduced,[10] and therefore the expected rate of weight loss will be overestimated. Increasing exercise probably better provides a greater calorie deficit than severe calorie restriction.

A balanced diet containing 12 to 14 per cent protein, 35 per cent or less fat (with reduced saturated fats), and the remainder as carbohydrates (with sucrose limited to very low levels) is preferable to the numerous fad diets, which show no evidence of better, sustained weight reduction. For the obese patient, each new diet is likely to produce temporary weight loss followed by relapse to initial or even higher weight levels. Attempts at diet education may be extremely important for the individual patient. Spacing or lengthening the duration of meals may call more satiety factors into operation. There does not seem to be any benefit in using bulk agents such as methylcellulose. Natural bulk foods, raw carrots, apples, celery, and salads, which may become a lifelong pattern, serve the same purpose. They probably act more by slowing down the course of a meal than by distending the stomach. Formula diets are popular and of use in that they may provide an exact number of calories as replacement for one meal of the day. Too often they are supplemented by other food intake, so their value is lost. Moderate salt restriction may be required for many reducing obese subjects who tend to develop mild fluid retention. Diuretic agents used for this purpose should be discouraged. Above all, patients need continued encouragement and support for their motivation. To this end, various groups which

offer companionship of similarly motivated individuals have met with moderate success. In general, better results at
weight reduction are achieved by less
overweight individuals.

DRUGS

Use of amphetamines, which stimulate
the satiety center, should never replace
primary dietary management. Nevertheless, they may be helpful in the early
phase of weight reduction, particularly
when the patterns of satiety-hunger for the
individual patient are known. The dosages
and best timing of the drug will vary according to the patient. The effective duration of amphetamine treatment seems to
be about four to six weeks and is most successful in patients whose obesity is of
recent onset. This drug should be used
with caution in patients with cardiac disease because of its adrenergic effects on
the heart.

The therapeutic use of thyroid preparations is to be discouraged unless the patient is clearly hypothyroid by reliable
tests. Tri-iodothyronine may increase enzymes in the glycerolphosphate cycle of
adipose tissue and thereby reduce the efficiency of substrate oxidation and ATP formation. This activity may promote weight
loss, but no acceptable data supporting the
possibility are as yet available.

As suggested above, exercise is the most
significant variable in energy expenditure
and should be incorporated, more or less,
into any program of weight reduction. It
may be easier to increase daily caloric deficits by encouraging graded increases in
physical activity than by severe calorie restriction. Furthermore, exercise, up to certain limits, appears to reduce food intake.
Again, the degree of exercise should be
tailored to the life style and capabilities of
the patient. Initially, increased walking
is a good way to start, with gradual progression to more sustained and intense
activity.

SURGERY

Surgical bypass of the small intestine
has been used to bring about weight reduction in severely obese individuals. The
earlier procedure used was a jejunocolic
shunt with food bypassing most of the

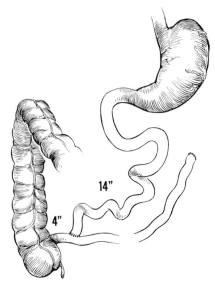

Figure 3–3. Jejunoileal bypass in the treatment of
extreme obesity. (Adapted from Scott, H. W., Jr.,
et al.: Ann. Surg. *171*:770, 1970.)

jejunum and the entire ileum.[11] More recently, a jejunoileal bypass has been preferred (Fig. 3–3). Obviously, a much reduced small bowel absorptive surface
causes severe steatorrhea and malabsorption. Other factors, such as the interruption
of the enterohepatic circulation of bile
salts (ultimately producing a deficiency of
conjugated bile salts) and inadequate mixing of digestive enzymes with food, also
contribute to the steatorrhea. These patients will all lose weight! These procedures are potentially dangerous, because
rapidly progressing metabolic deficiencies
may threaten the life of the patient. Severe
diarrhea, electrolyte losses, hypocalcemia,
and hypomagnesemia are common sequelae, particularly of the ileocolic procedure.[11] A peculiar type of polyarthritis has
also been noted after this type of shunt.[12]
Less severe deficiencies have been reported after jejunoileal bypass,[13,14] although fatty degeneration of the liver and
possible cirrhosis may occur.[15] This approach to the treatment of severe obesity
should generally be discouraged and reserved only for selected patients assured
of continuing close medical supervision.[14]

UNDERNUTRITION

There are numerous factors in the etiology of undernutrition which may be clas-

sified as primary or secondary reasons for insufficient food intake. Inadequate availability of food is most commonly associated with the economic inability to acquire it, either by self-production or by purchasing power. As a result, undernutrition related to insufficient food intake affects large numbers of people in the world, including some in the United States. Secondary factors such as ignorance, poor food habits, psychological or disease-related anorexia, primary intestinal diseases, and other illnesses frequently overlap with poverty and contribute significantly to diminished food intake.

In recent years, clinical studies have validated the prevalence of undernutrition in the United States, particularly among infants, preschool, and school age children from low income families.[16] The Food and Nutrition Board of the National Research Council has developed "Recommended Dietary Allowances" for various nutrients judged to be adequate for the maintenance of good nutrition in the population of the United States.[17] Although these allowances are useful only as guidelines for good nutrition, one might expect biochemical and clinical evidence of poor nutrition in populations receiving less than the recommended daily allowances. A recent study clearly associated deficiencies of several nutrients and hemoglobin levels with the lower poverty income ratios and minority group status.[11] Based on limited direct research data and indirect, but not necessarily invalid information, the Interim Report of the Select Committee on Nutrition and Human Needs, United States Senate,[18] has concluded that "coupled with other social and economic factors, hunger and malnutrition as found in this country can and does have a direct and major adverse effect on the normal physical and mental development of young children." Furthermore, the economic consequences of undernutrition to the United States are enormous.

Because of the close relationship between undernutrition and intestinal disease, it is essential to distinguish cause from effect and, when possible, to treat a primary intestinal disorder. Total caloric deprivation for periods up to 28 days will not significantly alter intestinal histology but will reduce protein concentration and disaccharidase activity.[19] Chronic protein malnutrition may, however, produce morphological and functional abnormalities in the small intestine.[20, 21] One of the difficult and confusing problems in assessing the primary role of nutrition on gut morphology or function is the high incidence of morphological abnormalities seen on intestinal biopsy in areas of the world where malnutrition is prevalent.[22] These changes in intestinal structure which are nonspecific but may resemble those found in celiac disease, may be present in asymptomatic individuals and be associated with varying degrees of malabsorption. Because these intestinal mucosal changes are too widespread in different tropical areas and may be acquired rapidly by North American residents of these areas,[23] a genetic etiology seems unlikely. It is unknown whether these changes are related to tropical sprue, food toxins, bacillary dysenteries, or parasitic infestation of the intestine. Undernourished populations, including those of the United States, frequently have bacterial and parasitic involvement of the intestinal tract which may produce diarrhea, anemia, and debility, and contribute to malabsorption.

The differential diagnosis of undernutrition should aim at separating a primary deficit of food intake from the numerous causes of anorexia and malabsorption. In some cases associated with poverty, the primary deficiency of food intake will be obvious. A good diet history is essential to appreciate the pattern of meal intake and the types of food eaten. This is particularly important in the elderly who may no longer desire or physically be able to prepare meals of sufficient variety and interest for themselves. If they live alone, the social aspects of dining in the company of a spouse or family no longer exist. To allay hunger, their diet may consist of frequent snacks of "tea and toast" at the expense of meat and vegetables, resulting in either a generally insufficient caloric intake or various nutrient deficiencies, including iron deficiency anemia.

Anorexia, nausea, and vomiting related to both intestinal and nonintestinal diseases may cause a significant reduction in caloric intake. Weight loss and undernutrition are well known clinical problems of chronic diseases, such as congestive heart failure, uremia, pulmonary disease, and, of course, malignancy. When undernutrition is associated with intestinal malabsorption, other symptoms are usually present (see pp. 250 to 289). In some instances, such as celiac disease, patients may have excellent appetite and consume more than their usual calories only to persist in losing weight. Significant weight loss under these circumstances is commonly accompanied by diarrhea and steatorrhea. Additional complaints of abdominal pain, cramping, borborygmi and distention implicate the gastrointestinal tract as the cause of the malnutrition. Radiological examination of the intestine may be helpful if a malabsorptive pattern is seen or other changes indicative of specific small bowel diseases such as granulomatous bowel disease are noted.

The physical signs of deficient nutrition are the same whether caused by inadequate food intake or inability to absorb ingested nutrients. Patients with undernutrition because of malabsorption may have stomatitis, cheilosis, glossitis, bleeding gums, peripheral edema, pellagrous dermatosis, pallor, ecchymoses, and other signs of vitamin and nutrient deficiencies. Similarly, biochemical determinations reflecting low levels of serum carotene, lipids, B-complex vitamins, fat-soluble vitamins, iron, and protein do not differentiate between primary and malabsorptive undernutrition. Only specific tests of intestinal digestive and absorptive function, including fecal fat determination, D-xylose and disaccharide tolerance tests, pancreatic secretin stimulation test, and several others can establish malabsorption as the cause of malnutrition. Peroral intestinal biopsy frequently provides a morphological diagnosis which may indicate specific therapy, including a selective diet.

ANOREXIA NERVOSA

This disease is most common in adolescent girls or young women and is characterized by anorexia, profound weight loss, and amenorrhea.[24] The anorexia results from severe psychological disturbances which relate to the normal intake of food. Although the classic form of the disorder is relatively rare, there are variants which may be chronic, unrecognized, and un-

diagnosed. Therefore, it is difficult to estimate accurately the incidence of this illness. It is not uncommon for the gastroenterologist to see a female patient with severe weight loss and no evidence for malabsorption. In such situations the diagnosis must be considered.

Clinical Picture. Usually an adolescent girl who may be overweight decides to reduce and goes on a "diet." Weight loss is initially rapid, and then slowly progresses to the point of wasting. Paradoxically, the patient often maintains an interest in food, particularly unusual kinds, or in gourmet cooking for others throughout the course. As time passes, the girl loses more and more weight, continually starving herself and insisting that she feels well. Outwardly, she is alert, quick, and usually unperturbed by her predicament. She may claim that she is hungry and that she is eating. It has been suggested that these patients experience hunger (and therefore "anorexia" per se need not be part of the syndrome) but that fantasies exist which make not eating more pleasurable. Some patients may even take amphetamines to reduce the discomfort of hunger. Often menses cease early in the course of the disease, sometimes even preceding the weight loss.

Other patients, either during adolescence or later in adulthood may present somewhat differently and be called "vomiting addicts." They alternate periods of anorexia with sessions of intense food cramming (or just have daily gorging periods), followed by secret vomiting. This obviously can be misleading to the patient's relatives or to the physician who focuses on the apparent adequate ingestion of food but is unaware of the patient's vomiting. The extent of clinical malnutrition may be less in these individuals but, if vomiting is persistent, they may present with a hypokalemic, hypochloremic alkalosis. Some patients may vary in that the vomiting is not secret and indeed may be the chief complaint.

Diagnosis. The diagnosis of anorexia nervosa should always be kept in mind when one is dealing with a young woman who has lost an extreme amount of weight. Often, denial by the patient that anything is really wrong should arouse suspicion that psychological factors may be related to the weight loss. In the typical case a careful history from the family must be obtained to exclude gastrointestinal symptoms which would suggest a primary intestinal disease. Malabsorption can cause significant weight loss but under these circumstances would likely be accompanied by diarrhea (steatorrhea), abdominal bloating, pain, or distention. The early stages of granulomatous bowel disease, in particular, may be very similar to anorexia nervosa. In a recent study,[25] three out of ten adolescent girls with anorexia and weight loss which clinically resembled anorexia nervosa were proved to have regional enteritis. It therefore seems justified always to obtain upper gastrointestinal, small bowel, and colon X-rays on all these patients. Abnormalities suggestive of a malabsorption pattern or specific changes of granulomatous bowel disease would indicate further studies for a specific intestinal disease diagnosis. Also, in patients who persistently vomit after ingesting large meals, a normal upper gastrointestinal series or endoscopy should help to exclude gastrointestinal pathology.

Malnutrition of moderate to severe degree, whether caused by malabsorption or reduced food intake, causes similar changes in blood chemistries. Serum proteins are likely to be reduced, although it is normal in many of these patients as is the blood cholesterol. Interestingly, the serum carotene may be elevated in some patients with anorexia nervosa possibly related to bizarre intake of high carotene foods. Vitamin deficiencies may be absent in the "ingestion-vomiting" variant of anorexia nervosa. In this instance, a hypokalemic, hypochloremic alkalosis should suggest the correct diagnosis. In the absence of malabsorption and steatorrhea, vitamin K deficiency is unusual. Probably both exogenously and endogenously derived vitamin K is lost significantly only when steatorrhea is present. In the final analysis, malabsorption can only be excluded by direct tests of absorption, such as quantitative fecal fat determination and D-xylose absorption. Intestinal biopsy may be helpful in establishing a tissue diagnosis. Although absorption may be somewhat impaired in severe protein deficiency states, it is unlikely that the changes would be as severe or indistinguishable from primary malabsorption.

In addition to bowel disease, endocrinological disorders must be differentiated from anorexia nervosa. A young woman with anorexia, weight loss bordering on cachexia, and amenorrhea, should bring to mind hypopituitarism or possibly hypoadrenocorticism. Patients with pituitary insufficiency who reach the stage of marked weight loss are usually lethargic, disinterested, and obviously chronically ill; they may have lost axillary and pubic hair. In contrast, patients with anorexia nervosa, despite a greater degree of cachexia, remain alert, quick, and active in their responses to the environment, frequently denying that they are ill at all.

The laboratory may be helpful in further differentiating these entities. In hypopituitarism serum levels of follicle-stimulating hormone and ACTH as well as thyroid function tests are usually sufficiently depressed to be diagnostic. In anorexia nervosa these tests may be only mildly to moderately depressed.

Treatment. Therapy consists of, first, restoring nutrition; second, arranging for psychiatric care; and third, maintaining a close follow-up. The patient should be hospitalized under the care of a physician and a psychiatrist. Tube feedings containing adequate amounts of protein should be instituted and weight gain monitored carefully. It should be made clear to the patient that if she does not progressively gain weight, tube feeding will readily be employed. As the patient begins to gain weight (and most do), psychotherapy may then be started.

A number of problems may be associated with initiation of the feeding program. If the malnutrition is severe, particularly protein deficiency, pancreatic enzyme function may be reduced as well as specific intestinal transport mechanisms. Digestive and absorptive functions may thus be sufficiently impaired to retard somewhat the rate of weight gain; some patients even develop diarrhea. Lactase deficiency secondary to protein malnutrition may prove particularly troublesome so that lactose may have to be restricted in the diet. In time, intestinal function, including lactase activity, will recover. If oral or tube feedings are very poorly tolerated because of impaired intestinal function, parenteral hyperalimentation may be necessary.

In general, patients can be expected to do reasonably well. Present fatality rates are judged to be about 5 per cent. It is difficult to find data which indicate long-term prognosis. Although many patients improve, they remain thin throughout life, possibly with some modified, chronic form of the disease. If a patient who has improved begins significantly to reduce her weight again, rehospitalization is indicated.

DIET THERAPY IN GASTROENTEROLOGY

Most patients have preconceived notions that certain foods regularly cause them to have distressing gastrointestinal symptoms. Superimposed may be beliefs that specific foods provide unusual health benefits either for the body generally or for a particular organ. Therefore patients expect dietary instructions from their physician. If not forthcoming, they will either adopt their own or seek another physician who will provide for their needs. Most dietary regulations are based on poorly substantiated information and tradition. Whenever diet therapy is prescribed it should provide for complete nutrition, be tailored to the patient as well as his disease, and avoid unsound restrictions which may alter the patient's general food intake and produce "dietary invalidism."

The diets that are of proved benefit or of theoretical value include (1) restriction of a specific sugar in various sugar intolerances, (2) gluten-free diet in celiac sprue, (3) fat restriction in symptomatic steatorrhea, (4) protein restriction in porta-systemic encephalopathy, (5) withdrawal of a specific food allergen, (6) reduction of osmotically active carbohydrates in the dumping syndrome, (7) "low roughage" or "low residue" diets in patients with a severely narrowed intestinal lumen, (8) fat restriction in symptomatic cholelithiasis and "chronic pancreatitis," and (9) avoidance of dietary gastric stimulants in peptic ulcer disease (Table 3–1).

Sugar Restriction. In conditions in which sugar absorption is impaired the unabsorbed sugar in the lumen of the intestine may produce gastrointestinal symptoms in several ways. The increased amount of sugar in the lumen of the small intestine causes a blood-to-lumen transfer of fluid which may distend the bowel and contribute to the formation of diarrhea. More important, the unabsorbed sugar enters the colon (which normally receives little if any dietary carbohydrate) and is metabolized by the colonic bacteria to form lactic, acetic, and pyruvic acids as well as hydrogen and carbon dioxide.[26] About 15 per cent of the hydrogen produced diffuses into the blood and is exhaled. The remaining 85 per cent is excreted as flatus. The acid metabolites of bacterial fermentation reduce the pH of colon fluid and may interfere with sodium and water reabsorption—all these factors contributing to flatulence, abdominal distention, cramping, or diarrhea.

TABLE 3–1.   DIET THERAPY IN GASTROINTESTINAL DYSFUNCTION

CONDITION	DIET
1. Sugar intolerance	
a. Lactase deficiency	Low lactose
b. Sucrase, isomaltose deficiency	Low sucrose, reduced starch
c. Glucose, galactose malabsorption	Low glucose, galactose, lactose; high fructose
d. Raffinose, stachyose malabsorption (shell bean ingestion)	Eliminate shell beans
e. Hepatic encephalopathy	Lactulose ingestion
2. Celiac sprue	Gluten-free
3. Steatorrhea	Low fat, medium-chain triglycerides
4. Hepatic encephalopathy	Low protein
5. Allergic gastroenteropathy	Eliminate specific allergen if known
6. Dumping syndrome	Low carbohydrate, dry meals
7. Intestinal narrowing	Low residue
8. Cholelithiasis, pancreatitis	Low fat
9. Peptic ulcer disease	Eliminate gastric secretagogues; frequent feedings?

There are a number of specific defects in sugar absorption. Intestinal lactase deficiency is probably the best known and occurs as an isolated defect in the adult or secondary to mucosal abnormalities in a variety of intestinal disorders. The isolated defect may be present in up to 20 per cent of Caucasians and 50 to 100 per cent in specific ethnic populations[27] (see p. 1019). In this case, lactose hydrolysis, required for normal absorption of its constituent monosaccharides, is impaired and excessive amounts of lactose pass into the colon. Impressive symptomatic improvement may be achieved by eliminating milk and restricting milk products from the diet.

A rare, genetically transmitted combined deficiency of intestinal sucrase and isomaltase occurs so that these patients are unable to tolerate sucrose or isomaltose. Withdrawal of table sugar (sucrose) from the diet is usually all that is necessary. Defects in the active transport of glucose and galactose, caused by an inherited defect in the intestinal carrier-transport system shared by these monosaccharides, also occurs, particularly in children.[28] These patients require withdrawal of dietary sources of glucose and galactose and substitution of fructose.

Some patients with a gastroenterostomy following ulcer surgery may deliver increased quantities of glucose rapidly into the small bowel and have such rapid transit through the small intestine that glucose absorption is incomplete. Increased amounts of glucose may therefore enter the colon and produce symptoms (see p. 822). Recently, it has also been shown that flatus, long known to follow shell bean ingestion, probably results from colonic bacterial metabolism of the poorly absorbed polysaccharides, raffinose and stachyose, which are contained in shell beans.[26]

Finally, ingestion of lactulose will produce the same results as unabsorbed lactose, because this disaccharide is not absorbed by the small intestine. Since metabolism of this sugar in the colon will reduce the pH of colon fluid, it has been used experimentally in the treatment of hepatic encephalopathy. Acidification of colon fluid reduces ammonia absorption by the colon and thus may prevent or improve hepatic encephalopathy. Re-

cently, it has been suggested that lactose be given to patients who have lactase deficiency and hepatic encephalopathy.[29]

Gluten-Free Diet. The benefit of dietary gluten restriction in celiac sprue is well documented and is reviewed on page 880. With strict adherence to this diet, it is usual for intestinal absorptive function to improve within a few weeks. Histological improvement is usually slower, and many months may pass before intestinal morphology reverts to normal. Of interest, instillation of gluten into the usually uninvolved ileum of patients with celiac sprue results in prompt and dramatic functional and histological changes.

Fat Restriction in Symptomatic Steatorrhea. Steatorrhea may occur in hepatobiliary diseases, pancreatic insufficiency, and primary intestinal malabsorption. Whether the pathophysiological mechanism is intraluminal and related to maldigestion of fat or secondary to impaired transport, excessive fat in the intestinal lumen enhances water and electrolyte losses. The amount of ingested fat which causes symptoms will vary from one patient to another, making fat tolerance an individual matter. When no specific treatment is available for the malabsorptive disease, the amount of fat in the diet should be adjusted to minimize symptoms and maintain weight and nutrition. Many of these patients may benefit from medium-chain triglyceride (MCT) therapy. MCT preparations contain triglycerides with fatty acid lengths varying from 6 to 12 carbon atoms and are readily hydrolyzed and less dependent on bile salts and pancreatic lipase for their absorption. They are transported away from the intestine via the portal vein and rapidly metabolized in the liver. MCT's are particularly useful in malabsorptive states involving maldigestion or lymphatic obstruction and in short bowel syndromes. Some preparations contain significant quantities of lactose which may worsen diarrhea in lactase-deficient subjects.

Protein Restriction in Hepatic Encephalopathy. This is a recognized dietary approach in patients with severe liver disease and portal hypertension. Dietary (and blood) protein acted on by bowel bacteria, particularly in the colon, produces ammonia and other nitrogenous compounds which are then absorbed and poorly metabolized by the liver. The association of ammonia and other nitrogen substances with hepatic encephalopathy is not well understood, but dietary protein restriction is helpful in many cases. The amount of protein tolerated in chronic encephalopathy varies and may be influenced by the administration of lactulose and neomycin.

Food Allergy. Some patients give such convincing histories for specific food allergies that withdrawal of the specific offender from the diet seems entirely justified. Newer techniques such as measurement of gastrointestinal protein loss, immunodiffusion assay, and intestinal biopsy have provided more than circumstantial evidence for allergic gastroenteropathies. Frequent offenders are milk protein, shellfish, and nuts. Several other food proteins, particularly those found in red meats, may cause protein-losing enteropathy, suggesting that many proteins may be capable of acting as intestinal antigens (see pp. 1066 to 1081).

Patients who relate intestinal symptoms to a large number of food items probably owe their symptoms to causes other than food allergy. Although we may not be able to attribute their symptoms to a specific mechanism at the present time, it is likely that mild mucosal metabolic defects will be found to exist in some of these individuals.

The Dumping Syndrome. Although the causes of this syndrome following gastrectomy are not completely known, the rapid entry of a hypertonic solution of chyme into the jejunum, resulting in excessive intestinal secretion and distention, certainly seems to play an important role. Diet therapy is aimed at avoiding osmotically active foods, such as carbohydrates, and omitting fluids at mealtimes. This approach should limit the volume of solutions of high osmolar content from rapidly entering the jejunum and thus reduce jejunal distention. Therefore diets low in disaccharides and starches but containing whole proteins and somewhat more than the usual amount of fat are prescribed (see pp. 822 to 824).

Low Residue Diets. These diets seem logical to use for patients who have intestinal stenosis or stricture, such as may occur in regional enteritis. Such patients should eliminate "roughage" or foods of high cellulose content, such as skins, chunky raw vegetables, and leafy vegetables. Patients with esophageal strictures should also eliminate solid foods that cannot be well chewed.

There does not seem to be any evidence that low bulk diets are useful in pyloric stenoses or any form of colonic disease. This is of interest in view of the widely held view that patients with diverticulosis, diverticulitis, irritable colon, and constipation should be treated with low residue diets. The contrary has even been suggested for the treatment of diverticular disease (see p. 1423).

Low Fat Diet in Gallbladder Disease and Pancreatitis. It seems logical that fat restriction should be of benefit in symptomatic cholelithiasis or cholecystitis. One reason is that fat-induced gallbladder contractions may have adverse effects in the presence of gallstones or inflammation, but this is entirely without supporting evidence. The therapy of choice, of course, is to remove the diseased organ in symptomatic gallbladder disease.

Similarly, even in the absence of pancreatic insufficiency, reduced fat ingestion in patients with inflammatory disease of the pancreas (between attacks) theoretically might be of benefit if this reduces pancreatic flow in a partially obstructed pancreatic duct. Ductal pressure may have some role in the genesis of pancreatitis. However, there is no evidence supporting the efficacy of low fat ingestion in "chronic symptomatic pancreatitis."

Diet Therapy in Peptic Ulcer Disease. No other gastrointestinal disease has had such attention or controversy concerning diet therapy as has peptic ulcer disease.[30, 31] Assuming that gastric acid secretion has something to do with peptic ulcer, the aims of diet therapy are to reduce acid secretion by (1) elimination of gastric secretagogues, (2) prevention of antral distention (and gastrin secretion) by small, frequent meal ingestion, (3) slowing of gastric motility by stimulating duodenal release of enterogastrone through high fat content of diet, and (4) prevention of "abrasive trauma" of the ulcer by eliminating high residue foods. Hence the familiar and wide use of milk and cream feedings in a patient with an active ulcer, and the subsequent use of a bland diet. Unfortunately, there is no evidence that this diet reduces gastric acidity or affects the rate of ulcer healing. Nor is there any support for "nonbland" diets being harmful to mucosa or an ulcer crater. Actually, the high fat content of a milk and cream regimen may cause significant weight gain and possibly increase the risk of coronary artery disease.

It therefore seems most practical to permit ulcer patients to eat what they like except for eliminating the gastric secretagogues alcohol and caffeine (in coffee, tea, and cocoa). Between-meal nourishment (without increasing total daily caloric intake) is also reasonable and has wide acceptance (see pp. 719 to 721).

PARENTERAL HYPERALIMENTATION

Total and prolonged parenteral nutrition is now both practical and useful with the development of intravenous hyperalimentation.[32] The indications for parenteral hyperalimentation are numerous and include both intestinal and nonintestinal disease states. It is particularly helpful in gastrointestinal disorders which eventually may be corrected or modified and in patients who require nutritional restoration prior to surgery.

The aim of parenteral nutrition should be to provide adequate calories, water, nitrogen, electrolytes, and vitamins to meet anabolic needs. Hypertonic solutions are necessary to do this, and therefore they must be administered in a high flow central vein at a consistent rate over a 24-hour period. This permits maximal utilization and minimal renal excretion.

The major source of calories in these solutions has thus far been provided by glucose. Infusion of 100 to 250 g of glucose daily results in the nitrogen-sparing effect, which reduces protein breakdown significantly. Emulsions of fat, which are potentially a more efficient source of calories, are not in general use at this time in the United States. Ethyl alcohol can also serve as a calorie source but is limited in amount because of its noxious pharmacological effects.

Nitrogen can be provided in the form of protein hydrolysates or the newer crystalline amino acid preparations. To achieve positive nitrogen balance intravenously, it is generally necessary to infuse between 80 and 160 gm. of protein equivalent per 24-hour period. A ratio of 150 to 250 calories to 1 g of nitrogen is necessary to utilize the nitrogen for tissue synthesis instead of energy. It is also important to provide appropriate amounts of essential and nonessential amino acids, although the optimal ratio for intravenous alimentation is not yet entirely known.

In addition to carbohydrate, nitrogen, and water, sufficient electrolytes and vitamins must be added to the solutions. For every 1000 calories infused, 40 to 50 mEq of sodium and 30 to 40 mEq of potassium should usually be provided. Other electrolytes such as magnesium, calcium, phosphorus, chloride, and sulfate plus trace elements are also included in long-term therapy. Fat-soluble and water-soluble vitamins added to the solutions or given intramuscularly complete the necessary requirements. There are several techniques by which these solutions may be readily prepared and monitored.[32]

The potential complications associated with parenteral hyperalimentation require careful attention: catheterization of the subclavian vein may produce vessel and thoracic perforations and thromboembolism; infection and sepsis may be associated with the catheter; and hyperosmolar hyperglycemic states may be associated with hypertonic glucose infusion.

The future would seem to include wider use of improved solutions for parenteral hyperalimentation. Greater availability of crystalline amino acid mixtures will simplify the preparation of solutions. The development and use of isotonic solutions, consisting of newer fat preparations and more efficient carbohydrate substrates such as maltose,[33] may permit the use of peripheral veins for infusion.

REFERENCES

1. Mayer, J.   Some aspects of the problem of regulation of food intake and obesity. New Eng. J. Med. 274:610, 662, 1966.
2. Campbell, R. G., Sami, A. H., and Van Italbe, T. B.   Studies of food-intake regulation in man. Responses to variations in nutritive density

in lean and obese subjects. New Eng. J. Med. 285:1402, 1971.

3. Mayer, J. Regulation of energy intake and body weight: Glucostatic theory and lipostatic hypothesis. Ann. New York Acad. Sci. 63:15, 1955.

4. Felzter, C. C., and Mayer, J. A. Simple criterion of obesity. Postgrad. Med. 38:101, 1965.

5. Marks, H. H. Influence of obesity on morbidity and mortality. Bull. New York Acad. Med. 36:296, 1960.

6. Bray, G. A. The myth of diet in the management of obesity. Amer. J. Clin. Nutr. 23:1141, 1970.

7. Fabry, P., and Tepperman, J. Meal frequency— a possible factor in human pathology. Amer. J. Clin. Nutr. 23:1059, 1970.

8. Tepperman, J., and Tepperman, H. M. Adaptive hyperlipogenesis—late 1964 model. Ann. New York Acad. Sci. 131:404, 1965.

9. Galton, D. J., and Bray, G. A. Metabolism of α-glycerolphosphate in human adipose tissue in obesity. J. Clin. Endocrinol. Metab. 27:1573, 1967.

10. Bray, G. A. The effect of caloric restriction on energy expenditure in obese patients. Lancet 2:397, 1969.

11. Lewis, L. A., Turnbull, R. B., Jr., and Page, H. Effects of jejunocolic shunt on obesity, serum lipoproteins, lipids, and electrolytes. Arch. Intern. Med. (Chicago) 117:4, 1966.

12. Shagrin, J. W., Frame, B., and Duncan, H. Polyarthritis in obese patients with intestinal bypass. Ann. Intern. Med. 75:377, 1971.

13. Payne, J. H., and DeWind, L. T. Surgical treatment of obesity. Amer. J. Surg. 118:141, 1969.

14. Scott, H. W., Jr., and Law, D. H., IV. Clinical appraisal of jejunoileal shunt in patients with morbid obesity. Amer. J. Surg. 117:246, 1969.

15. Drenick, E. J., and Simmons, F., and Murphy, J. F. Effect on hepatic morphology of treatment of obesity by fasting, reducing diets, and small bowel bypass. New Eng. J. Med. 282:829, 1970.

16. Ten-State Nutrition Survey in the United States, 1968–1970. Preliminary Report to the Congress—April 1971, 64 pp. U.S. Department of Health, Education and Welfare.

17. Recommended Dietary Allowances. A report of the Food and Nutrition Board, National Research Council. 101 pp. Washington, D.C., National Academy of Sciences, 1968.

18. The Food Gap: Poverty and Malnutrition in the United States. Interim Report together with supplemental, additional, and individual views prepared by the Select Committee on Nutrition and Human Needs, United States Senate. 48 pp. Washington, D.C., U.S. Government Printing Office, 1969.

19. Knudsen, K. B., Bradley, F. M., Lecocq, F. R., Bellamy, H. M., and Welsh, J. D. Effect of fasting and refeeding on the histology and disaccharidase activity of the human intestine. Gastroenterology 55:46, 1968.

20. Herskovic, T. The effect of protein malnutrition on the small intestine. Amer. J. Clin. Nutr. 22:300, 1969.

21. James, W. P. T. Intestinal absorption in protein calorie malnutrition. Lancet 1:333, 1968.

22. Editorial: The tropical intestine. Brit. Med. J. 1:2, 1972.

23. Lindenbaum, J., Kent. T. H., and Sprinz, H. Malabsorption and jejunitis in American Peace Corps volunteers in Pakistan. Ann. Intern. Med. 65:1201, 1966.

24. Bruch, H. Anorexia nervosa and its differential diagnosis. J. Nerv. Ment. Dis. 141:555, 1965.

25. Gryboski, J., Katz, J., Sangree, H., and Herskovic, T. Eleven adolescent girls with severe anorexia. Clin. Pediat. 7:684, 1968.

26. Levitt, M. D. Production and excretion of hydrogen in man. New Eng. J. Med. 281:122, 1969.

27. Welch, J. D. Isolated lactase deficiency in humans: Report of 100 patients. Medicine (Balt.) 49:257, 1970.

28. Meeuwisse, G. W., and Dahlqvist, A. Glucose-galactose malabsorption: A study with biopsy of the small intestinal mucosa. Acta Paediat. Scand. 57:273, 1968.

29. Welsh, J. D., and Langdon, D. E. Lactose to treat hepatic encephalopathy in patient with lactose malabsorption. New Eng. J. Med. 286:436, 1972.

30. Roth, J. L. A. The ulcer patient should watch his diet. In Controversy in Internal Medicine, F. J. Ingelfinger, A. Relman, and M. Finland (eds.). Philadelphia, W. B. Saunders Co., 1966, pp. 161–170.

31. Ingelfinger, F. J. Let the ulcer patient enjoy his food. In Controversy in Internal Medicine, F. J. Ingelfinger, A. Relman, and M. Finland, (eds.). Philadelphia, W. B. Saunders Co., 1966, pp. 171–179.

32. Dudrick, S. J., and Ruberg, R. L. Principles and practices of parenteral nutrition. Gastroenterology 61:901, 1971.

33. Young, J. M., and Wester, E. The metabolism of circulating maltose in man. J. Clin. Invest. 50:986, 1971.

Chapter 4

Protein Metabolism and Protein-Losing Enteropathy

Marvin H. Sleisenger, Graham H. Jeffries

PROTEIN METABOLISM AND PROTEIN-LOSING ENTEROPATHY

Leakage of plasma proteins into the gastrointestinal tract is a major cause of hypoproteinemia in many diseases and, indeed, may play an important part in the normal degradation of plasma proteins.[1-4] Early clinical studies described a syndrome of hypoproteinemia unexplained by decreased synthesis or external loss of plasma protein.[5, 6] Studies of I[131]-albumin turnover in patients with this syndrome showed an increase in albumin catabolism, but did not indicate the mechanism and site of this protein degradation.[6] Hydrolysis of plasma proteins entering the gastrointestinal lumen, with reabsorption of their amino acids, delayed the recognition of this site of plasma protein loss; thus the term "idiopathic hypercatabolic hypoproteinemia" included patients with unrecognized gastrointestinal lesions.

Hypoproteinemia with enteric loss of plasma protein was first recorded in 1957 in a patient with giant hypertrophic gastritis.[1] Since then excessive enteric protein loss has been described in association with a variety of gastrointestinal lesions, and the term "protein-losing gastroenteropathy" was introduced[1-10] (Table 4–1). The study of plasma protein metabolism in the gut was facilitated by the development of methods to identify plasma proteins in gastrointestinal secretions, and by the introduction of I[131]-labeled polyvinylpyrrolidone (PVP) and Cr[51]-labeled albumin. Sensitive techniques established that plasma proteins were normally present in gastrointestinal secretions, and that enteric losses usually accounted for up to 10 per cent of plasma protein degradation.[1-10]

The gut has been found to play other important roles in plasma protein metabolism. These functions include the absorption of intact protein, particularly immunoglobulin, during the neonatal period and the subsequent absorption of products of protein digestion that may be reutilized for plasma protein synthesis, including certain dipeptides as well as amino acids; and the intestinal synthesis of plasma proteins, particularly the immunoglobulin IgA, beta lipoproteins, and very low density lipoproteins (VLDL).

These functions of the gut will be discussed together with methods for study of the various aspects of plasma protein

35

TABLE 4–1.   CLASSIFICATION AND THERAPY OF DISEASES ASSOCIATED WITH ENTERIC LOSS OF PLASMA PROTEIN

DISEASE	THERAPY*
Mucosal ulceration	
Gastric carcinoma	
Gastric lymphoma	Surgical resection
Multiple gastric ulcers	
Colon cancer	
Granulomatous enteritis	
Diffuse nongranulomatous ileojejunitis	Corticosteroids
Mucosal disease without ulceration	
Rugal hypertrophy (Menetrier's, etc.)	Resection, if local
Celiac sprue disease	Gluten elimination
Tropical sprue	Antimicrobials; folic acid
Whipple's disease	Antimicrobials
Allergic gastroenteropathy	Elimination diet; steroids
Bacterial or parasitic enteritis	Antimicrobial drugs
Gastrocolic fistula	Resection
Villous adenoma of colon	Resection
Lymphatic abnormalities	
Capillaria philippinensis	Thiabendazole
Primary lymphangiectasia	Low-fat diet or MCT
Lymphenteric fistula	Resection
Lymphoma	Chemotherapy
Constrictive pericarditis	Pericardiectomy
Tricuspid valvular disease	Rx of heart failure

*Details of therapy may be found in chapters in Part II specifically dealing with these diseases.

metabolism in healthy individuals and in those with protein-losing enteropathy. Finally, the diseases underlying protein-losing enteropathy will be classified and the approach to therapy will be outlined.

PHYSIOLOGY OF ENTERIC METABOLISM OF PLASMA PROTEINS

ENTERIC PROTEIN ABSORPTION

The intestinal mucosa of neonatal animals has the capacity to absorb intact protein molecules.[11-13] This function has been studied experimentally by observing the incorporation of ferritin or fluorescein-labeled plasma proteins into vacuoles in the apical cytoplasm of intestinal epithelial cells after feeding these proteins (Fig. 4–1). Ultrastructural studies suggest that this transfer of protein into the epithelial cell is accomplished by microphagocytosis (pinocytosis).[12] This process, which persists for only a few days after birth, is selective; homologous gamma globulin is absorbed more readily than heterologous plasma proteins.

Recent studies have shown that gamma-A globulin (immunoglobulin A or IgA) is concentrated in colostrum; the maternal protein is conjugated with a "transfer protein" in the mammary gland.[14, 15] The absorption of specific antibodies from colostrum during the neonatal period is very important in providing immunological protection in some animals, but is probably less significant in the human infant, in whom the period of intestinal pinocytosis is brief and transplacental passage of material antibody to the fetus is of greater magnitude.[11]

Immunological studies in the adult animal have revealed that trace amounts of protein (antigenic peptide) may be absorbed from the gut; this has no known physiological significance but may occasionally be of pathological importance; e.g., botulism and other illnesses associated with endo- or exotoxins are due to partial absorption of protein.

Recent evidence indicates that unhydrolyzed dipeptides may be absorbed by the intestinal epithelium in man; this particularly applies to glycylglycine and glycylleucine.[16]

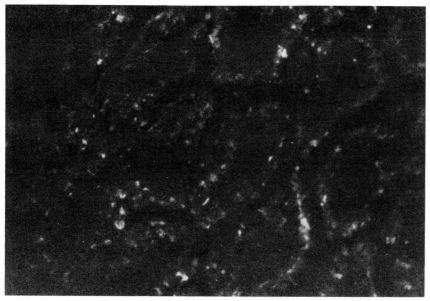

Figure 4–1. Intestinal absorption of gamma globulin in the neonatal rat. Fluorescein-labeled rabbit gamma globulin was fed by mouth to a three-day-old rat. Examination of a frozen section of the upper small intestine under ultraviolet illumination shows the presence of labeled protein in intestinal epithelial cells. Intestinal villi are sectioned transversely. (From Jeffries, G. H., and Sleisenger, M. H.: Secretion of plasma proteins into the digestive tract. *In* Handbook of Physiology, Section 6, Vol. V, 1968, p. 2776. Copyright 1968, The Williams and Wilkins Co., Baltimore.)

SYNTHESIS OF PLASMA PROTEINS

Most plasma proteins are synthesized by the liver parenchymal cells (albumin, alpha and beta globulins, and fibrinogen) and by plasma cells of the lymphoid system (immunoglobulins).[17] The liver synthesizes 16 to 18 g of albumin per day, or about 0.15 g per kilogram. As noted in Figure 4–5, this rate increased to 0.29 g per kilogram per day in a patient with protein-losing enteropathy. This degree of heightened synthesis—twice normal— is maximal for the liver. In this instance, it is possible for liver partially to compensate for abnormal catabolism, because the constituent amino acids of plasma proteins are absorbed by the small intestine and reutilized.

Two important plasma proteins relating to lipid transport are produced in the intestinal mucosa. Beta lipoprotein synthesized in the intestinal mucosal cell during lipid absorption appears necessary for the transfer of long-chain triglyceride as chylomicrons from vacuoles within the cell through the lateral cell membrane. In patients with abetalipoproteinemia (an inborn error of metabolism), and in animals treated with puromycin (an inhibitor of protein synthesis), triglyceride accumulates in large vacuoles in the cytoplasm of the epithelial cells, and chylomicrons do not appear in the lamina propria, the intestinal lymphatics, or the plasma after a fatty meal.[18] In addition to the function of chylomicrons during fat absorption, the small intestine also synthesizes lipoproteins during fasting (Fig. 4–2). Particles of VLDL (300 to 1000 A in size) are present in endoplasmic reticulum and Golgi apparatus as well as in intercellular spaces and lacteals of jejunal mucosa in the fasting state. In experimental animals these particles disappear when bile is diverted from the intestine, indicating that they are produced in the mucosa during the absorption of endogenous (biliary and epithelial cell) lipid.[19]

Although immunoglobulins are synthesized by mononuclear cells in the lamina propria of the mucosa, the lymphoid tissue of the gut differs from that of peripheral lymph nodes; whereas plasma cells in peripheral lymph nodes synthesize gamma-G globulin (IgG) predominantly (the number of cells staining with fluorescein-labeled antisera to the specific immunoglobulins, IgG, IgA, and IgM, is roughly proportional to the plasma con-

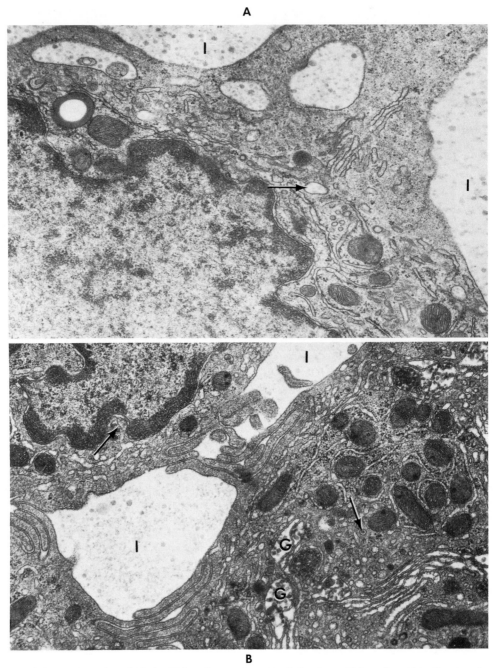

Figure 4–2. *A,* Jejunal epithelial cell from human intestine following a 40-hour fast. Note the abundance of lipoprotein particles within the endoplasmic reticulum and intracellular vacuoles as well as those in the intracellular space (I). Glutaraldehyde stained. × 38,500. *B,* Epithelial cells from human intestine, showing the large number of particles that can be observed normally in the Golgi apparatus (G) and endoplasmic reticulum (arrows) in human subjects who fasted for 40 hours. Glutaraldehyde stained. × 31,000. (From Jones, A. L., and Ockner, R. B.: J. Lipid Res. *12*:580, 1971.)

centration of these proteins), IgA is most prevalent in plasma cells infiltrating the lamina propria (Fig. 4–3).[20] IgA produced in the mucosa may contribute to the circulating pool of plasma protein but also has a specific protective function within the mucosa or on mucosal surfaces. Secretions from the nose, bronchi, salivary glands, stomach, and intestine contain IgA in excess of other immunoglobulins. In these

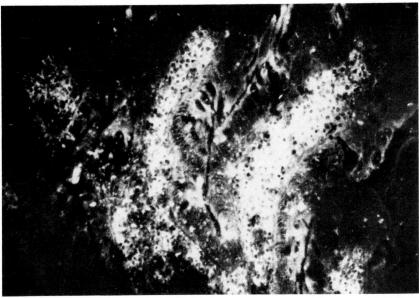

Figure 4–3. Distribution of plasma cells containing IgA in normal jejunal mucosa. A frozen section of human jejunal mucosa was incubated with fluorescein-labeled antibody to human IgA. The lamina propria is densely packed with mononuclear cells that contained IgA in their cytoplasm. Ultraviolet illustration. × 200. (From Jeffries, G. H., and Sleisenger, M. H.: Secretion of plasma proteins into the digestive tract. *In* Handbook of Physiology, Section 6, Vol. V, 1968, p. 2777. Copyright 1968, The Williams and Wilkins Co., Baltimore.)

secretions, as in colostrum, this immunoglobulin is combined with a "transfer protein" (secretory piece) which appears to be synthesized by the mucosal cells.[14, 15, 21] The protective role of secretory IgA is suggested from the studies on poliomyelitis immunization; oral vaccines lead to the appearance of specific IgA antibodies in the intestine. The gastrointestinal problems resulting from IgA deficiency are discussed on pages 51 to 68.

DEGRADATION OF PLASMA PROTEINS

Plasma proteins of all classes are present in low concentrations in saliva and gastrointestinal secretions from normal subjects.[4, 22, 23] These proteins may be detected by immunological methods (immunodiffusion and immunoelectrophoresis) when the secretions are collected and concentrated under conditions that prevent digestion of protein (Fig. 4–4). Normally, proteins that enter the lumen of the stomach or intestine are rapidly hydrolyzed to their constituent amino acids, which are reabsorbed in the intestine.

Two important aspects of the physiology of plasma protein degradation by the gut need clarification. One is the process by which plasma proteins pass through the mucosal or glandular epithelia, and the other is the quantitative significance of this phenomenon in relation to total plasma protein catabolism.

The answer to the question of how plasma proteins pass through the gastrointestinal mucosa is incomplete. With the exception of IgA, which appears to be actively secreted with a carrier molecule, there is no evidence that plasma proteins are actively transported across the mucosal epithelium from the lamina propria. Furthermore, the apical junctional complex between the lateral cell membranes of intestinal epithelial cells would appear to limit the passage of protein molecules between the cells. The most reasonable hypothesis, which still lacks experimental support, is that lymph escapes from the lamina propria at the apex of the intestinal villi with desquamating cells.

The exact amount of plasma protein lost into the gut per day is not known, but is normally less than 10 per cent of the total quantity of albumin catabolized daily. The final answer awaits the development of methods to measure accurately the quantities of specific plasma proteins that enter

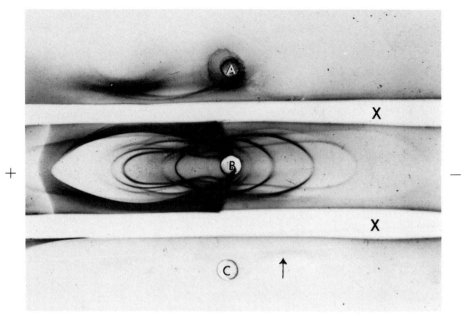

Figure 4–4. Immunoelectrophoretic analysis of plasma proteins in concentrated gastric juice and saliva. Wells *A*, *B*, and *C* contained concentrated gastric juice, serum, and concentrated saliva, respectively. The gastric juice had been neutralized by instilling phosphate buffer at *p*H 7 into the stomach. Both gastric juice and saliva were concentrated 50 times. After electrophoresis the troughs (X) were filled with antiserum to human plasma. Precipitin lines corresponding to albumin and several alpha and beta globulins indicated the presence of these proteins in the gastric juice. A single precipitin line (↑) demonstrated the presence of IgA in saliva. (From Jeffries, G. H., and Sleisenger, M. H.: Secretion of plasma proteins into the digestive tract. *In* Handbook of Physiology, Section 6, Vol. V, 1968, p. 2778. Copyright 1968, The Williams and Wilkins Co., Baltimore.)

the gut lumen each day, as well as the total amount of each protein that is catabolized daily.

Although a number of proteins and macromolecules labeled with radioisotopes have been used to study plasma protein turnover and enteric loss, none are ideal for this purpose. Waldmann has recently defined the characteristics of the labeled macromolecule that would be ideal for measuring enteric loss of plasma protein: "(a) The labeled serum protein should have a normal metabolic behavior, thus permitting the simultaneous determination of rates of endogenous protein catabolism, and intestinal protein loss. (b) There should be no absorption of the label from the intestinal tract after catabolism of the protein since this would result in an underestimation of the extent of the gastrointestinal protein loss. (c) There should be no excretion of the label into the gastrointestinal tract except when bound to protein. Such secretion of label . . . would result in overestimation of the magnitude of the gastrointestinal protein loss."[24]

METHODS FOR MEASURING GASTROINTESTINAL LOSS OF PLASMA PROTEIN

I[131]-Labeled Serum Proteins. Serum proteins carefully labeled with radioiodine (I[125], I[131]) exhibit normal metabolic behavior.[25-27] Thus, after an intravenous injection of radioiodinated albumin or gamma globulin the tracer protein is distributed throughout the intra- and extravascular pools of protein and is catabolized at the same rate as the recipient's protein. Under steady-rate conditions (when protein synthesis and degradation are equal) the plasma volume and intravascular and total protein pools can be calculated from the plasma protein concentration and the dilution of labeled protein after complete mixing in the intravascular and total pools, respectively.

After equilibration of the labeled protein in the intravascular and extravascular compartments (two to three days), the decline in plasma radioactivity corrected for radioactive decay reflects the degradation

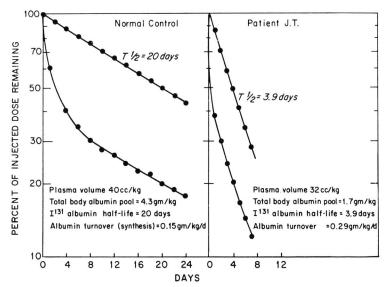

Figure 4–5. Turnover of I[131]-albumin in a normal subject and in a patient (J. T.) with gastrointestinal protein loss secondary to intestinal lymphangiectasia. Upper curves represent the decline in total body radioactivity with time. Lower curves represent the decline in plasma radioactivity. The total-body albumin pool was much reduced in patient J. T. The survival half-life of iodinated albumin was markedly shortened, and the albumin synthetic rate was slightly faster than normal. (From Waldmann, T. A.: Gastroenterology 50:422, 1966.)

of the protein and may be expressed as a percentage of the injected dose degraded daily or as grams of protein degraded per kilogram of body weight (Fig. 4–5).[25-27] The slope of the plasma decay curve after initial equilibration parallels the plot of the cumulative urinary excretion of radioiodine, i.e., that amount released from degraded protein (when uptake of radioiodine by the thyroid has been blocked by prior iodine therapy). The daily urinary excretion of radioiodine after initial equilibration has been shown to be a constant function of the plasma pool of labeled protein;[28] this supports the contention that plasma protein catabolism should thus be expressed as a percentage of the plasma pool, rather than of the total body pool.[27]

Nosslin has derived a formula for calculating plasma protein catabolism based on the assumption that newly synthesized protein is distributed initially in the plasma pool after its release from its site of synthesis and that the specific activity of labeled protein at the site of degradation is identical with that in plasma; it is assumed that the turnover and exchange between compartments can be described by exponential functions. The model is independent of the site of degradation and the number of extravascular pools.[29]

Although plasma proteins labeled with radioiodine are ideal for studying plasma protein kinetics, they are not suitable for measuring enteric loss. Iodine is concentrated and secreted by salivary glands and by gastric mucosa and is reabsorbed by the intestinal epithelium.

Plasma protein leakage into the gut has been estimated in experimental animals by collecting secretions from isolated segments of the intestine and by measuring their content of injected radioiodinated albumin or gamma globulin. These studies have suggested that between 40 and 60 per cent of plasma protein catabolism takes place in the gut.[30] This is difficult to reconcile with observations in eviscerated animals; removal of the gut prolonged the survival of injected iodinated albumin by less than 10 per cent.[31] Several factors may have contributed to an overestimation of enteric protein loss in animal studies; study periods were brief compared to the turnover time of the plasma protein, only short segments of the gut were used at one time, and operative injury to the gut may have caused excessive leakage of plasma or lymph.

In some patients with gastric mucosal disease, the measurement of albumin-bound I[131] in gastric juice collected after intragastric instillation of neutral buffer solution to prevent proteolysis has been of clinical value in demonstrating an excessive loss of plasma protein.[1] With this exception, radioiodinated albumin has not been of value in measuring gastrointestinal protein loss in man.

A technique in which an ion-exchange resin (Amberlite) was given orally in an attempt to chelate I^{131} that entered the gut after an intravenous injection of labeled protein did not provide a measure of enteric protein loss; radioiodine excreted with resin in the feces was derived not only from I^{131}-albumin leakage, but also from free iodide secreted by salivary glands and stomach.[32]

Cr^{51}-Labeled Albumin. Albumin labeled with $Cr^{51}Cl_3$ is unsuitable for measuring plasma protein kinetics; the half-life of the labeled protein is shortened by elution of chromium from the protein. The properties of the Cr^{51} label, however, make it ideal for enteric studies; chromium salts are neither secreted into nor absorbed from the gastrointestinal tract in significant amounts. Thus, Cr^{51}-albumin loss into the gut following an intravenous injection is reflected by excretion of Cr^{51} label in the stool.[24, 33]

When stools, uncontaminated with urine, are collected for a period of several days after an intravenous injection of Cr^{51}-albumin and the daily fecal radioactivity is related to the corresponding plasma radioactivity, the loss of albumin into the gut may be expressed as a fraction of the plasma pool or as milliliters of plasma excreted per day. This clearance of plasma albumin by the gut may be calculated from the following formula: gut loss of plasma albumin (milliliters of plasma per day) equals fecal radioactivity during the collection period per mean plasma radioactivity during the collection period times the number of days of collection. In normal subjects tested by this procedure, between 5 and 25 ml of plasma, or less than 1 per cent of the plasma albumin pool, was cleared daily by the gastrointestinal tract (Fig. 4–6).[24, 33] The evidence that Cr^{51} may exchange between albumin and other plasma proteins, particularly transferrin, reduces the value of this label in physiological studies, but does not detract from its value as a clinical tool.

Cu^{67}-Labeled Ceruloplasmin. Cu^{67}-labeled ceruloplasmin is an ideal labeled macromolecule for measuring enteric loss.[34] The copper is an integral part of the protein molecule, and the radioactive label is not absorbed from the gut. Calculations based on the excretion of Cu^{67} in the stools after an intravenous injection of Cu^{67}-ceruloplasmin in normal subjects indicated that about 2 per cent of the circulating protein was excreted daily. This accounted for only 10 per cent of the protein degradation, which corresponds to the fraction of catabolized plasma albumin that could be accounted for by enteric degradation in Cr^{51}-albumin studies. Major disadvantages of Cu^{67}-ceruloplasmin that preclude its use in routine studies are the very short half-life of the radioisotope and the expense of its preparation.

Other Labeled Macromolecules. I^{131}-labeled polyvinylpyrrolidone (I^{131}-PVP) has been used in clinical studies to diagnose excessive enteric loss of plasma protein.[35] Patients with excessive enteric loss of plasma protein excrete greater amounts of intravenously injected I^{131}-PVP than do normal subjects. However, studies with this labeled macromolecule do not yield physiological information. I^{131}-PVP is rapidly cleared from the plasma by the reticuloendothelial system and the kidneys, and instability of the iodine-PVP bond with release of free iodide permits both secretion and reabsorption of label in the gut.[24]

In summary, the evidence derived from the fecal secretion of intravenously injected Cr^{51}-albumin and Cu^{67}-ceruloplasmin indicates that no more than 10 per cent of the catabolism of albumin and ceruloplasmin can be accounted for by enteric loss of the proteins. These values are considerably lower than values estimated from studies of I^{131}-labeled plasma protein clearance in experimental animals, but they probably reflect the physiological state more accurately.

EXCESSIVE ENTERIC LEAKAGE OF PLASMA PROTEIN

PATHOPHYSIOLOGY

The common pathological bases for excessive enteric loss of plasma protein (protein-losing enteropathy) are disordered metabolism or turnover of epithelial cells (or both), mucosal ulceration, and lymphatic obstruction.[9, 24] Excessive loss of plasma protein may be due to increased mucosal permeability to protein because of impaired metabolism, inflammatory exudation through areas of ulceration, excessive cell desquamation, or direct leakage of lymph from obstructed lacteals.

In patients with protein-losing enteropathy, all serum proteins leak excessively into the gut. The change in concentration and total pool of individual plasma proteins that results from excessive enteric loss will depend on two compensatory mechanisms—increased synthesis and decreased endogenous (nonenteric) catabolism. Levels of proteins that normally have the longest survival (albumin and gamma globulins) tend to be more severely depressed than those of proteins with a relatively short survival (fibrinogen). Excessive enteric loss of protein is reflected by a shortening of the half-life of injected I^{131}-albumin, an increase in the fractional catabolic rate of this protein (percentage of plasma pool degraded daily), and an increased fecal excretion of injected Cr^{51}-albumin.

CLINICAL MANIFESTATIONS

Hypoproteinemia caused by excessive enteric loss of plasma protein may be manifested by dependent edema resulting from the lowered colloidal osmotic pressure of plasma with increased fluid transudation from the capillaries, and secondary hyperaldosteronism with sodium and water retention. Although losses of other plasma proteins may result in low plasma levels, these changes are usually not clinically apparent. Secondary hypogammaglobulinemia rarely gives rise to an increased incidence of infection. Analysis of the plasma proteins may show a decrease not only in albumin but also in gamma globulin, fibrinogen, lipoproteins, transferrin, and ceruloplasmin.[3, 4] In contrast to the hypoalbuminemia associated with the nephrotic syndrome, there is usually a low serum cholesterol value.

In many patients the manifestations of excessive plasma protein loss may be overshadowed by other manifestations of gastrointestinal disease. In some patients,

however, hypoalbuminemia with edema may be the only indication of a gastrointestinal lesion. The diagnosis of lesions causing excessive plasma protein loss will be based on radiological, endoscopic, histological and absorptive studies.

In patients with intestinal lymphatic obstruction, the transport of dietary longchain triglycerides as chylomicrons in the lymph may be impaired, and lymph containing both plasma proteins and lipids may be lost into the intestinal lumen, with variable steatorrhea.[6, 37] Of great interest, patients with lymphangiectasia and marked protein loss also lose immunologically competent lymphocytes into their gut, resulting in blunting of delayed hypersensitivity.[38]

DIAGNOSIS OF PROTEIN-LOSING ENTEROPATHY

Diagnosis is established clinically by use of Cr^{51} albumin injected intravenously and collection of stools for 96 hours. From plasma decay curve and stool counting, the quantity of albumin lost per day may be calculated as the percentage of plasma pool (see above; also see Figs. 4–5 and 4–6).

DISEASES ASSOCIATED WITH PROTEIN-LOSING ENTEROPATHY

As noted previously, the diseases that may be associated with excessive enteric loss of plasma protein fall into three categories: those diseases in which there is impaired metabolism or turnover of surface epithelial cells or both, those diseases in which there is mucosal ulceration, and those diseases in which there is obstruction to the flow of intestinal lymph (Table 4–1).

Impaired metabolism of surface epithelial cells or mucosal disease without ulceration, which may lead to a change in mucosal permeability to protein or to an increase in cell desquamation, is common to some diseases of the stomach or small intestine and, in the latter, is usually associated with intestinal malabsorption. Figures 4–7 and 4–8 are examples of two types of giant rugal hypertrophy of the stomach associated with protein-losing enteropathy.[1, 39] Diffuse disease of the intes-

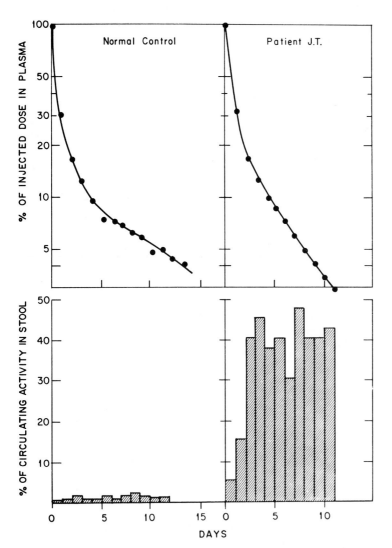

Figure 4–6. Fecal clearance of Cr^{51} after intravenous administration of Cr^{51}-albumin in a normal subject and a patient (J. T.) with gastrointestinal protein loss. The normal subject cleared 0.8 per cent of the plasma pool of labeled albumin into the gastrointestinal tract each day, whereas patient J. T. cleared more than 30 per cent of the plasma pool into the gastrointestinal tract each day, an indication of severe gastrointestinal protein loss. (From Waldmann, T. A.: Gastroenterology 50:422, 1966.)

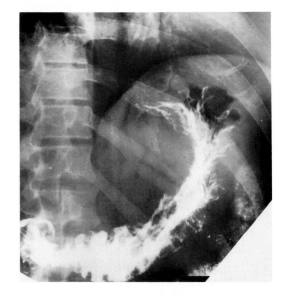

Figure 4–7. Menetrier's disease, as demonstrated by an upper gastrointestinal series in a patient with protein-losing enteropathy. These patients usually are hyposecretors of acid.

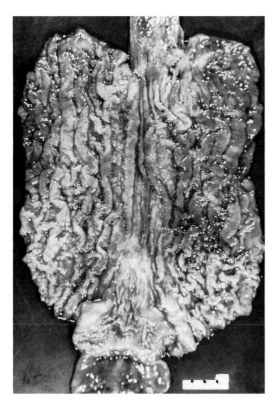

Figure 4–8. Gross surgical specimen of stomach in a patient with protein-losing enteropathy. Although the folds are enormous, mucous cell hyperplasia was not present and hypersecretion of acid was noted. Thus, it is not Menetrier's disease but hypertrophic, hypersecretory protein-losing gastropathy. (From Overholt, B. F., and Jeffries, G. H.: Gastroenterology 58:80, 1970.)

tinal mucosa may result from infection (viral, bacterial, or parasitic)[40-42] or a sensitivity to dietary substances (gliadin in celiac sprue disease, milk protein in allergic enteritis,[43, 44] or it may be unexplained (mucosal changes associated with defective synthesis of gamma globulin, particularly IgA).[45] It should be noted that hypogammaglobulinemia may be secondary to protein-losing enteropathy, or may be a primary problem with complicating protein-losing enteropathy.[45]

Mucosal ulceration may be localized or diffuse and may be associated with either benign or malignant conditions. The severity of the plasma protein leakage into the gut will depend on the extent of ulceration and the degree of associated inflammation or lymphatic obstruction. Copious amounts of these proteins are lost into the small intestine in acute, diffuse, nongranulomatous ileojejunitis (Figs. 4–9 and 4–10).[9]

Obstruction to lymphatic flow from the small intestine may be due to a congenital lymphatic malformation (intestinal lymphangiectasia associated with Milroy's disease),[37] to obstruction of lymphatic vessels by fibrosis or neoplastic infiltration (tuberculosis, lymphoma), or to an increase in the pressure in the superior vena cava (constrictive pericarditis, tricuspid

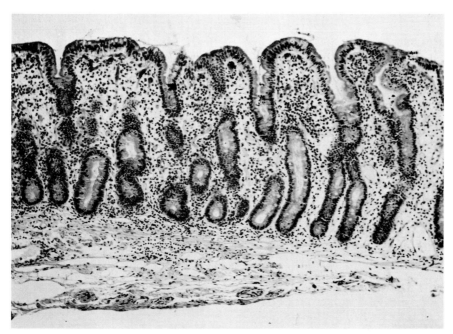

Figure 4–9. Fatal ileojejunitis with protein-losing enteropathy and hypoproteinemia. Jejunal biopsy before steroid therapy, showing partial atrophy of the villi.

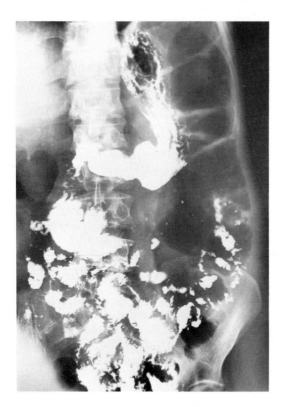

Figure 4–10. Small bowel series of patient with acute, diffuse, nongranulomatous ileojejunitis and marked protein-losing enteropathy. Note disordered pattern without proximal dilatation.

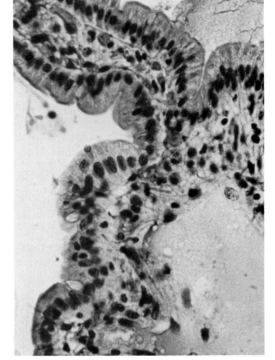

Figure 4–11. Jejunal biopsy of patient with lymphangiectasia and protein-losing enteropathy. Note very dilated lacteal at the base of the villus. Villous epithelium is normal. × 200.

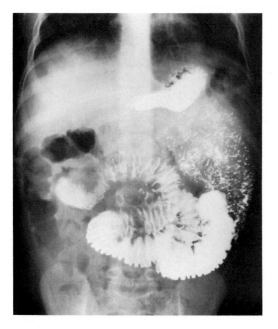

Figure 4–12. Small bowel series of patient with lymphangiectasia and protein-losing enteropathy. Note coarsened folds.

valvular disease, congestive heart failure.[46, 37] The histological picture of lymphangiectasia is demonstrated in Figure 4–11 and the corresponding abnormalities on X-ray in Figure 4–12.[36]

For further discussion of the clinical aspects of excessive enteric protein loss, the reader is referred to recent reviews.[9, 24, 48] The methods used to study protein loss in normal subjects have been applied extensively in studies of protein-losing enteropathy; in spite of their limitations for physiological studies, these methods have provided data that have increased understanding of the pathophysiology of derangements of plasma protein metabolism and have provided valuable aids to diagnosis.

TREATMENT

As Table 4–1 indicates, effective therapy for protein-losing enteropathy is available for a large number of underlying diseases. The reader is referred to other chapters of the text in which these specific diseases are discussed at length. It suffices here to demonstrate (Fig. 4–13) that the process is reversible to some degree, depending upon the disease and specificity of therapy. Plasma protein concentration rose significantly in patient K. S. in response to a very low fat diet.[36]

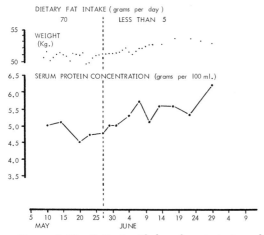

Figure 4–13. Patient with lymphangiectasia and protein-losing enteropathy. I[131]-Albumin turnover study also revealed diminution of enteric protein loss during low-fat diet. (From Jeffries, G. H., Chapman, A., and Sleisenger, M. H.: New Eng. J. Med. 270: 761, 1964.)

ALLERGIC GASTROENTEROPATHY WITH EDEMA IN INFANTS AND CHILDREN

Joyce D. Gryboski

From the data available it appears that allergic gastroenteropathy of infants and children may exist as one of two types: the acute, transient form, or the chronic form.

Acute, Transient Gastroenteropathy. This form is possibly related to hyperimmune mechanism and often follows an infectious gastroenteritis.[49-52] This is more common in children than the chronic form. The clinical picture is that of a child who after a nonspecific gastroenteritis develops generalized edema and occasionally ascites and pleural effusion (Fig. 4–14). This edema and associated hypoproteinemia may persist from two weeks to several months after the original gastrointestinal symptoms have subsided. The laboratory picture is characterized by hypoalbuminemia, hypogammaglobulinemia, and peripheral eosinophilia.[49, 51, 53] Proteinuria is absent, and hepatic and renal function are normal.

Although the stomach and small intestine are the usual catabolic sites for the plasma protein, the exact site of exudation in these transient enteropathies has not been defined. Protein loss itself is well demonstrated through stool radioisotope studies. In several patients reported, the stomach as well as the proximal small intestine was involved.[54] Radiologically the gastric changes simulate Menetrier's disease of giant hypertrophic gastritis in which hypoproteinemia results from loss of plasma proteins into the gastric juice.[1, 55] Gastric biopsy of the antrum in one patient revealed a mild mucosal edema and infiltration by lymphocytes and plasma cells.[54] In our own patient, biopsy from the fundus taken six weeks after the onset of hypoproteinemia showed tortuous glands compressed in their basal regions, mucosal edema, and a moderate infiltrate of eosinophils and mononuclear cells within the lamina propria.[56] Unlike true Menetrier's disease, these radiological and histological gastric abnormalities are self-limited and reversible, and the name should not be associated with this syndrome.

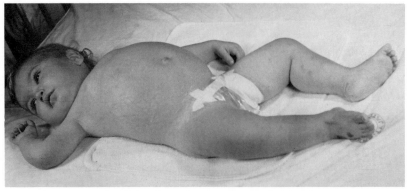

Figure 4–14. An 18 month-old female with acute transient protein-losing gastroenteropathy.

The proximal small bowel is involved and demonstrates thickened, edematous mucosal folds. The bowel lumen is slightly dilated and contains increased secretions. The history of the preceding allergy is not usually present in these patients nor is it remarkable in their families. One child, however, did have a mother with a history of angioneurotic edema.[57] As the disorder is self-limited, the treatment is symptomatic. A low salt diet may be used during the period of generalized edema. Reversal of the protein loss by use of a low fat diet during the acute state has been recommended.

Clinical Form. This picture differs somewhat from the chronic hypoproteinemia seen related to cow's milk. In those infants the edema is usually mild. An exudative enteropathy is demonstrated by shortened serum albumin half-life and excessive fecal excretion of Cr^{51} albumin. Radiologic examination of the small bowel may or may not show mucosal edema. Small bowel biopsy is normal except for infiltrate of the lamina propria by plasma cells and occasional eosinophils. The stools contain occult blood and Charcot-Leyden crystals.[58] Steroid therapy or institution of a milk-free diet will reverse these symptoms and the protein loss.

A very chronic form of allergic gastroenteropathy may be noted in children between two months and 2.5 years of age.[59] In this group the edema, hypoproteinemia, and eosinophilia are associated with growth retardation, anemia, and major allergies such as asthma or eczema. The duration of the edema may be over two years in the untreated patients, although it fluctuates in severity. The gastrointestinal symptoms are mild, and consist of intermittent diarrhea, vomiting after the ingestion of certain foods, or abdominal pains. The common food to which such children are intolerant is raw milk. The stools are positive for occult blood, and precipitating antibodies to milk are found in the serum. The rate of albumin synthesis is increased, and the half-time of survival is reduced. Excessive Cr^{51}-albumin is excreted in excess in the stool. Mucosal edema is noted in the small bowel on radiological examination, and biopsy of the jejunum reveals normal morphology and, in some, infiltration of the lamina propria by eosinophils. Amelioration of the clinical symptoms and reversal of the protein metabolism disorders follows steroid therapy or the dietary elimination of milk. For a more complete discussion of management, see page 1079.

see page 1079.

REFERENCES

1. Citrin, Y., Sterling, K., and Halsted, J. A. Mechanism of hypoproteinemia associated with giant hypertrophy of gastric mucosa. New Eng. J. Med. 257:906, 1957.
2. Schwartz, M., and Jarnum, S. Protein-losing gastroenteropathy: Hypoproteinemia due to gastrointestinal protein loss of varying aetiology, diagnosed by means of ^{131}I-albumin. Danish Med. Bull. 8:1, 1961.
3. Waldmann, T. A., Steinfeld, J. L., Dutcher, T. F., Davidson, J. D., and Gordon, R. S., Jr. Role of gastrointestinal system in "idiopathic hypoproteinemia." Gastroenterology 41:197, 1961.
4. Holman, H., Nickel, W. F., Jr., and Sleisenger, M.

H. Hypoproteinemia antedating intestinal lesions and possibly due to excessive serum protein loss into intestine. Amer. J. Med. 27:963, 1959.

5. Schwartz, M., and Thomsen, B. Idiopathic or hypercatabolic hypoproteinaemia: Case examined by ^{131}I-labelled albumin. Brit. Med. J. 1:14, 1957.

6. Albright, F., et al. Studies on fate of intravenously administered plasma proteins in idiopathic hypoproteinemia and osteoporosis. In Symposia on Nutrition of the Robert Gould Research Foundation, J. B. Youmans (ed.). Springfield, Ill., Charles C Thomas, 1950, Vol. 2, p. 352.

7. Gordon, R. S., Jr. Exudative enteropathy: Abnormal permeability of gastrointestinal tract demonstrable with labelled polyvinyl-pyrrolidone. Lancet 1:325, 1959.

8. Idiopathic hypoalbuminemias: Clinical staff conference at National Institutes of Health. Ann. Intern. Med. 51:553, 1959.

9. Jeffries, G. H., Holman, H. R., and Sleisenger, M. H. Plasma proteins and the gastrointestinal tract. New Eng. J. Med. 266:652, 1962.

10. Steinfeld, J. L., Davidson, J. D., Gordon, R. S., Jr., and Greene, F. E. Mechanism of hypoproteinemia in patients with regional enteritis and ulcerative colitis. Amer. J. Med. 29:405, 1960.

11. Brambell, F. W. R. The passive immunity of the young animal. Biol. Rev. 33:488, 1958.

12. Clark, S. L., Jr. The ingestion of proteins and colloidal materials by columnar absorptive cells of the small intestine in suckling rats and mice. J. Biophysic. Biochem. Cytol. 5:40, 1959.

13. Payne, L. C., and Marsh, C. L. Absorption of gamma globulin by the small intestine. Fed. Proc. 21:909, 1962.

14. South, M. A., Cooper, M. D., Wollheim, F. A., Hong, R., and Good, R. A. The IgA system. 1. Studies of the transport and immunochemistry of IgA in the saliva. J. Exp. Med. 123:615, 1966.

15. Tomasi, T. B., Tan, E. M., Solomon, A., and Predergast, R. A. Characteristics of an immune system common to certain external secretions. J. Exp. Med. 121:101, 1965.

16. Adibi, S. Intestinal transport of dipeptides in man: Relative importance of hydrolysis and intact absorption. J. Clin. Invest. 50:2266, 1971.

17. Miller, L. L., and Bale, W. F. Synthesis of all plasma protein fractions except gamma globulin by liver: Use of zone electrophoresis and lysine-ϵ-C^{14} to define plasma proteins by isolated perfused liver. J. Exp. Med. 99:125, 1954.

18. Dobbins, W. O. An ultrastructural study of the intestinal mucosa in congenital β-lipoprotein deficiency with particular emphasis upon the intestinal absorptive cell. Gastroenterology 50:195, 1966.

19. Jones, A. L., and Ockner, R. K. An electron microscopic study of endogenous very low density lipoprotein production in the intestine of rat and man. J. Lipid Res. 12:580, 1971.

20. Crabbé, P. A., and Heremans, J. F. The distribution of immunoglobulin-containing cells along the human gastrointestinal tract. Gastroenterology 51:305, 1966.

21. Bull, D. M., Bienenstock, J., and Tomasi, T. B., Jr. Studies on human intestinal immunoglobulin. Gastroenterology 60:370, 1971.

22. Gullberg, R., and Olhagen, B. Electrophoresis of human gastric juice. Nature 184:1848, 1959.

23. Soergel, K. H., and Ingelfinger, F. J. Proteins in serum and rectal mucus of patients with ulcerative colitis. Gastroenterology 40:37, 1961.

24. Waldmann, T. A. Protein-losing enteropathy. Gastroenterology 50:422, 1966.

25. Sterling, K. Turnover rate of serum albumin in man as measured by I^{131} tagged albumin. J. Clin. Invest. 30:1228, 1951.

26. Berson, S. A., Talow, R. S., Schreiver, S. S., and Post, J. Tracer experiments with I^{131} labeled human serum albumin: Distribution and degradation studies. J. Clin. Invest. 32:746, 1953.

27. MacFarlane, A. S. The behavior of I^{131}-labelled plasma proteins in vivo. Ann. New York Acad. Sci. 70:19, 1957.

28. Andersen, S. B. Intravascular or extravascular degradation of γ_{ss}-globulin. In Physiology and Pathophysiology of Plasma Protein Metabolism. Berne, Hans Huber, 1964, pp. 105–115.

29. Nosslin, B. Quoted by S. B. Andersen.[28]

30. Glenert, J., Jarnum, S., and Riemer, S. The albumin transfer from blood to gastro-intestinal tract in dogs. Acta Chir. Scand. 124:63, 1962.

31. Gitlin, D., Klinenberg, J. R., and Hughes, W. L. Site of catabolism of serum albumin. Nature 181:1064, 1958.

32. Jeejeebhoy, K. N., and Coghill, N. F. The measurement of gastrointestinal protein loss by a new method. Gut 2:123, 1961.

33. Waldmann, T. A. Gastrointestinal protein loss demonstrated by ^{51}Cr-labelled albumin. Lancet 2:121, 1961.

34. Waldmann, T. A., Morell, A. G., Wochner, R. D., and Sternlieb, I. Quantitation of gastrointestinal protein loss with copper^{67}-labeled ceruloplasmin. J. Clin. Invest. 44:1107, 1965.

35. Gordon, R. S., Jr. Exudative enteropathy: Abnormal permeability of the gastro-intestinal tract demonstrated with labelled polyvinyl-pyrrolidone. Lancet 1:325, 1959.

36. Jeffries, G. H., Chapman, A., and Sleisenger, M. H. Low-fat diet in intestinal lymphangiectasia: Its effect on albumin metabolism. New Eng. J. Med. 270:761, 1964.

37. Waldmann, T. A., Steinfeld, J. L., Dutcher, T. F., Davidson, J. D., and Gordon, R. S., Jr. The role of the gastrointestinal system in "idiopathic hypoproteinemia." Gastroenterology 41:197, 1961.

38. Strober, W., Wochner, R. D., Carbone, P. P., and Waldmann, T. A. Intestinal lymphangiectasia: A protein-losing enteropathy with hypogammaglobulinemia, lymphocytopenia and impaired homograft rejection. J. Clin. Invest. 46:1643, 1967.

39. Overholt, B. F., and Jeffries, G. H. Hypertrophic, hypersecretory protein-losing gastropathy. Gastroenterology 58:80, 1970.
40. Jeffries, G. H., and Sleisenger, M. H. Abnormal enteric loss of plasma protein in gastrointestinal diseases. Surg. Clin. N. Amer. 42:1125, 1962.
41. Laster, L., Waldmann, T. A., Fenster, L. F., and Singelton, J. W. Reversible enteric protein loss in Whipple's disease. Gastroenterology 42:762, 1962.
42. Whalen, G. E., Strickland, G. T., Cross, J. H., Uylangco, C., Rosenberg, E. B., Gutman, R. A., Watten, R. H., and Dizon, J. J. Intestinal capillariasis. A new disease in man. Lancet 1:13, 1969.
43. Gordon, R. S., Jr. Protein-losing enteropathy in the sprue syndrome. Lancet 1:55, 1961.
44. Wilson, J. F., Heiner, D. C., and Lahey, M. E. Milk-induced gastrointestinal bleeding in infants with hypochromic microcytic anemia. J.A.M.A., 189:568, 1964.
45. Waldmann, T. A., and Laster, L. Abnormalities of albumin metabolism in patients with hypogammaglobulinemia. J. Clin. Invest. 43:1025, 1964.
46. Petersen, V. P., and Hastrup, J. Protein-losing enteropathy in constrictive pericarditis. Acta Med. Scand. 173:401, 1963.
47. Davidson, J. D., Waldmann, T. A., Goodman, D. S., and Gordon, R. S., Jr. Protein-losing gastroenteropathy in congestive heart failure. Lancet 1:899, 1961.
48. Jarnum, S. Protein-Losing Gastroenteropathy. Oxford, Blackwell Publishing Co., 1963.
49. Collipp, P. J., and Dragutsky, D. Serum proteins in infant stools. New York State J. Med. 78:1965, 1968.
50. Degnan, T. J. Idiopathic hypoproteinemia. J. Pediat. 51:448, 1957.
51. Ulstrom, R. A., Smith, N. J., and Heimlich, E. M. Transient dysproteinemia in infants, a new syndrome. I. Clinical studies. Amer. J. Dis. Child. 92:219, 1956.
52. Wyngaarden, J. B., Crawford, J. D., Chamberlin, H. R., and Lever, W. F. Idiopathic hypoproteinemia: Report of a case with transient edema, depression of plasma albumin and gamma globulin and eosinophilia. Pediatrics 9:729, 1952.
53. Pittman, F., Harris, R., and Barker, H. Transient edema and hypoproteinemia. Amer. J. Dis. Child. 108:189, 1964.
54. Sandberg, D. Hypertrophic gastropathy in childhood. J. Pediat. 78:866, 1971.
55. Burns, B., and Gay, B. B. Menetrier's disease of the stomach in children. Amer. J. Roent. 103::300, 1968.
56. Herskovic, T., Spiro, H. M., and Gryboski, J. D. Acute transient gastrointestinal protein loss. Pediatrics 41:818, 1968.
57. Austen, K. F., and Sheffer, A. L. Detection of hereditary angioneurotic edema by demonstration of a reduction in the second component of human complement. New Eng. J. Med. 272:649, 1965.
58. Waldmann, T. A. The specific syndrome of intestinal lymphangiectasia. In Macromolecular Aspects of Protein Absorption and Excretion in the Mammalian Intestine. Columbus, Ohio, Ross Conference on Pediatric Research, 1965, p. 94.
59. Waldmann, T. A., Wochner, R. D., Laster, L., and Gordon, R. S. Allergic gastroenteropathy. A cause of excessive gastrointestinal protein loss. New Eng. J. Med. 276:761, 1967.

Chapter 5

Immunology and Disease of the Gastrointestinal Tract

James E. McGuigan

There is an increasing appreciation of the important relationships existing between immunology and diseases of the gastrointestinal tract. This intimacy of association has been facilitated by rapidly developing techniques in immunology, coupled with their recognition and application by clinicians and investigators concerned with disorders of the gastrointestinal tract.

Important relationships between immunology and gastroenterology may be placed in several broad categories. One category includes the development of our

TABLE 5–1. GASTROINTESTINAL DISEASES ASSOCIATED WITH IMMUNOLOGICAL ABNORMALITIES

CONDITION	IMMUNOLOGICAL OBSERVATIONS
Recurrent aphthous ulcers	? Reduced secretory IgA
Pernicious anemia	Parietal cell antibodies; binding and blocking antibodies to intrinsic factor; lymphocyte transformation
Gastric atrophy, atrophic gastritis	Parietal cell antibodies
Celiac sprue	Increased serum IgA; antibodies to milk protein; antigluten antibodies in serum and intestinal secretions
Ulcerative colitis	Serum antibodies against colonic epithelium and *E. coli* 0:14; lymphocytes cytotoxic against colon epithelial cells; antimilk antibodies
Regional enteritis	Serum antibodies against colonic epithelium; reduced responsiveness of lymphocyte transformation; lymphocytes cytotoxic against colon but not ileal epithelial cells
Whipple's disease	Hypogammaglobulinemia; lymphocyte depletion; anergy or decreased delayed hypersensitivity
Intestinal lymphectasia	Hypogammaglobulinemia; lymphocyte depletion; anergy or decreased delayed hypersensitivity
Milk allergy gastroenteropathy (infants)	Precipitins to whole milk in stool but not serum; α-lactalbumin binding by rectal immunocytes; hypogammaglobulinemia, eosinophilia, eczema, rhinitis
Mediterranean lymphoma	α-Heavy-chain protein in serum, urine, and saliva

understanding of the role of the gastrointestinal tract and its various components in the immune response. A second area of relationships between immunology and gastroenterology concerns the recognition and clarification of immune phenomena found in association with certain gastrointestinal diseases (Table 5–1). The appreciation of these associations has raised questions as to whether immunological mechanisms may be important in the initiation or perpetuation of certain gastrointestinal diseases. A third area relating immunology and gastroenterology includes the application of immunological methods to further understanding of gastrointestinal physiology and pathophysiology in those disorders which confront the physician caring for patients with gastrointestinal diseases.

THE GASTROINTESTINAL TRACT AND THE IMMUNE RESPONSE

LYMPHOID GUT COMPONENTS AND IMMUNE SYSTEMS

Evidence that the lymphoid components of the gastrointestinal tract play extremely important roles in various aspects of the immune response is increasing.[1] The major lymphoid elements of the gastrointestinal mucosa include the following: (1) Lymphoid follicles are located under the epithelial cell layer, in the mucosa as well as the submucosa. These lymphoid follicles may occur as isolated structures anywhere along the gut from the stomach to rectum and are most numerous and prominent in the adenoid tissue of the nasopharynx, ileum, and appendix. (2) Numerous lymphocytes and plasma cells are diffusely scattered in the mucosa of the stomach and intestine where they occupy interstitial locations beneath the epithelium and between adjacent glands. (3) Many small cells with morphological characteristics of lymphocytes may be identified between intestinal columnar cells of the gastrointestinal epithelium.

Plasma cells have been well defined as the major cellular sites of synthesis of those immunoglobulins conveying humoral immunity. The functions of small lymphocytes in the gastrointestinal tract, as well as in other sites, are less well understood, although they appear to play important roles in cellular immunity, including delayed hypersensitivity, and in graft and host relationships. In addition, some of these cells may be important in immunological memory. It is thought that a population of small lymphocytes, which may not be readily distinguished morphologically from others, may through progressive states of development evolve into antibody producing plasma cells (Fig. 5–1). Lymphoid components of the gastrointestinal tract, in some respects similar to other lymphoid tissues such as those contained in spleen and lymph nodes, serve as a peripheral lymphoid organ. In addition, it is possible that the gastrointestinal tract may serve what have been designated as central lymphoid functions. The central lymphoid tissues include the thymus and the avian bursa of Fabricius.[2] The central lymphoid organs contain lymphoepithelial components which, although not directly mediating immune responses, exert control over functions of peripheral lymphoid cells, particularly in areas of development of immunological capability. Experimental evidence indicates that central lymphoid tissues are most active in immediate prenatal and neonatal life.

The thymus, in man and in many lower species, exerts important control over peripheral lymphoid elements designated as the thymus-dependent system. Lymphoid elements of the thymus are derived from bone marrow cells. The thymus develops from the third and fourth pharyngeal pouches. Thymectomy at or near the time of birth induces defects in thymic-dependent immune function, including loss of homograft immunity, delayed hypersensitivity, and various graft-host reactions. However, the capacity of the animal to produce humoral antibody is not lost.[3]

In birds, the bursa of Fabricius, which, as well as the thymus, is a gut-derived lymphoepithelial structure, is the central lymphoid organ assigning immunological competence to peripheral lymphoid elements involved in the secretion of circulating antibodies.[2] The organ in man which serves this important function has not been identified. Lymphoid tissues suspected of serving bursal functions in the

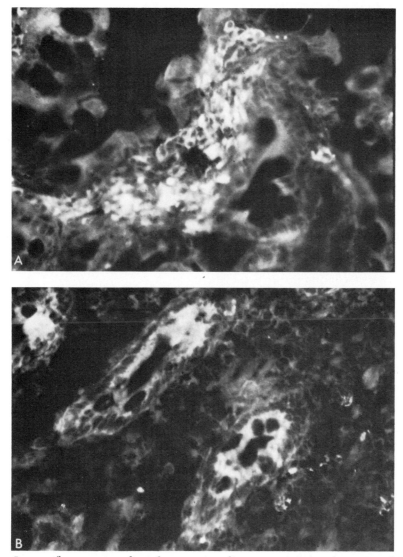

Figure 5–1. Immunofluorescent studies of mucosa in celiac sprue. *A*, IgA is demonstrated (as in normals) in plasma cells by fluoresceinated antibody to human IgA. *B*, Epithelial cells stained with fluoresceinated antigliadin antibody after washing with gliadin. Such binding is not seen in normal subject. × 375. (From Rubin, W., et al.: J. Clin. Invest. *44:*475, 1965.)

gastrointestinal tract include the tonsils, aggregated lymphoid tissues of the gastrointestinal tract, such as those found in the appendix and the Peyer patches of the intestine, and some nonaggregated lymphoid elements such as lymphocytes scattered about the lamina propria of the small intestine.

IMMUNOGLOBULINS AND THE GUT

Plasma cells of the mucosa of the small intestine are believed to synthesize and secrete antibodies with specificity against antigens present in the gut lumen. In man antibodies are contained in five classes of immunoglobulins, with classifications based on structural characteristics of their heavy (H) polypeptide chains; these classes are IgG, IgM, IgA, IgD, and IgE (also designated as γG, γM, γA, γD, and γE, respectively). Antibodies with specificity for each of these five immunoglobulin classes have been prepared and labeled with fluorescent dyes. Incubation of small intestinal biopsies with fluorescein-conjugated antibodies to one of the immunoglobulin classes, e.g., IgA, has been used to identify cells in lamina propria containing specific immunoglobulins in their cytoplasm.[4, 5] More than 80 per cent of plasma cells in the intestine contain IgA. Cells containing IgM in the cytoplasm are approximately one-sixth as common as those with IgA. IgG-containing plasma cells in the mucosa of the small intestine are relatively scarce. The prominence of IgA-containing plasma cells in the gastrointestinal mucosa is maintained in the stomach, small intestine, and large intestine. These results are in contrast to results with other peripheral lymphoid tissues such as spleen and lymph nodes. IgG, which is the predominant immunoglobulin in the peripheral circulation, is found most commonly in the cytoplasm of plasma cells in spleen and lymph nodes. The gut is by far the major source of IgA in the body. It is believed that the majority of IgA which is synthesized and secreted by intestinal plasma cells finds its way to the lumen of the gut. The relatively high concentrations of IgA in the gastrointestinal secretions can be easily explained on the basis of local IgA synthesis. Some IgA from the gut may find its way into the peripheral circulation.

The intestinal lymphoid tissue develops in response to exposure to antigen within the gut lumen. The fetal intestine, which has never been exposed to such antigens, does not have immunoglobulin-containing plasma cells; these cells, principally IgA-containing, are developed shortly after birth.

In the saliva, as well as in other exocrine secretions, IgA concentration is higher than IgG (a finding in reverse of that found in serum). In addition, secretory IgA, as found in gastrointestinal secretions, has a larger molecular weight than that of serum IgA (11S as opposed to 7S).[6] Secretory IgA molecules appear to be dimers of 7S IgA molecules. In addition, the secretory IgA dimer appears to contain an extra protein fragment of approximately 60,000 molecular weight which has been designated as the secretory piece (Fig. 5–2). Experimental evidence indicates that this secretory piece is contained within epithelial cells at exocrine locations, including the mucosa of the small intestine.[7] Secretory IgA, perhaps because of the di-

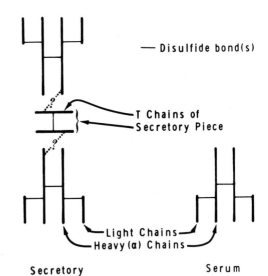

γA IMMUNOGLOBULIN

— Disulfide bond(s)

T Chains of Secretory Piece

Light Chains
Heavy (α) Chains

Secretory   Serum

Figure 5–2. Proposed model for IgA structure in secretions and serum, indicating so-called T-chains of the "secretory piece." (From Small, P. H., et al.: Characteristics of the secretory immunologic system. *In* Proceedings of the Conference on the Secretory Immunologic System, T. Tomasi (ed.). Washington, D.C., U. S. Department of Health, Education, and Welfare, 1969.)

meric configuration of the molecule, is relatively resistant to proteolytic digestion. The resistance of IgA to proteolysis would appear, of course, to provide a major advantage to the IgA molecule for excretion into, and expression of antibody activity within the enzyme-laden environment of, the gastrointestinal tract. That portion of the secretory IgA molecule which appears indistinguishable from serum IgA is synthesized within plasma cells in the lamina propria of the gastrointestinal mucosa. The secretory piece appears to be synthesized and, perhaps, attached to the dimeric IgA unit within the epithelial cells of the gastrointestinal tract.[7] Stimulation of IgA synthesis and secretion by antigen in the gut lumen, particularly by bacterial antigens, suggest that IgA antibody may have antibody activity against intestinal microbial flora. Antibody activity, in some instances identified as IgA, has been shown to be present in gastrointestinal secretions. Antibodies are directed against both normal and pathological microorganisms. IgA antibodies have been shown to be produced locally in the gut in response to fed protein materials such as ferritin.

The potential importance of the gastrointestinal IgA system can be exemplified by the following observations. Parenteral immunization of children with polio vaccines has been shown to produce high levels of serum antibodies to polio virus.[8] Parenteral immunizations did not produce secretory IgA antibodies to the polio virus in the gastrointestinal secretions. On the other hand, oral administration of live modified polio virus, an enterovirus, was associated with the presence of IgA antibodies to the polio virus in the gastrointestinal secretions, possibly secondary to local stimulation of immunoglobulin-producing sites in the gastrointestinal tract. Secretory IgA molecules have been shown to possess a variety of antibody activities, including isohemagglutination, virus neutralization, and other antiviral properties.[7, 9, 10] Immune complexes of secretory IgA antibodies and coliform organisms have been shown to fix complement in the presence of lysozyme, thereby effecting bacterial lysis.[11] Conversely, serum IgA antibody could not be shown to fix complement or to lyse bacteria.[12] These important observations appear to provide a mechanism by which secretory IgA, synthesized and released within the gastrointestinal tract, may provide protection against local gastrointestinal entry and infection.

Much is yet to be learned about the role of the secretory immunoglobulin system in the intestine and its relationship to both bacterial and other antigens, such as those contained in food to which the gut is constantly exposed.

IMMUNOLOGIC DEFICIENCY AND THE GUT

Immunological deficiency has been commonly recognized in association with certain diseases of the gastrointestinal tract, commonly with diarrhea and/or malabsorption (Table 5–2). The mechanism of production of malabsorption accompanied by immunological deficiency has not been defined; interrelationships between malabsorption and immunologic deficiency are probably multiple, and it is anticipated that with further immunological and gastrointestinal investigation these relationships will be clarified.

Inasmuch as IgA is the predominant immunoglobulin in those gastrointestinal cells synthesizing and secreting immunoglobulins, it comes as no surprise that the most common immunoglobulin defect associated with gastrointestinal abnormalities is that of IgA deficiency. In congenital primary agammaglobulinemia (or more precisely, profound hypogammaglobulinemia), immeasurable, or severely decreased, concentrations of IgA, IgM, and IgG are found in sera. These patients have markedly reduced, or absent, numbers of immunoglobulin-containing cells in lymph nodes and spleen. Small intestinal mucosal biopsies from these pa-

TABLE 5–2. IMMUNOLOGICAL DISEASES ASSOCIATED WITH DYSGAMMAGLOBULINEMIAS

DISEASE	GASTROINTESTINAL MANIFESTATIONS
Hypogammaglobulinemia (acquired)	Diarrhea and malabsorption in some; marked reduction to absent plasma cells in intestinal lamina propria; villi normal in most; flat mucosa in some (some respond to a gluten-free diet); may have *Giardia lamblia*
Nodular lymphoid hyperplasia (Dysgammaglobulinemia; IgA deficiency invariably)	Diarrhea and malabsorption frequent; hyperplastic germinal centers and scanty plasma cells in gut; villi normal except where distorted by nodules; *Giardia lamblia* infection very common
Selective IgA deficiency (1 in 500 healthy persons has deficient IgA)	Diarrhea and/or malabsorption; villi usually normal; mucosa may be flat (some respond to a gluten-free diet); normal to markedly decreased plasma cells; marked decrease in IgA-containing plasma cells; occasional marked increase in IgM-containing plasma cells; may have *Giardia lamblia*
Thymoma with hypogammaglobulinemia (adults >50)	Same as acquired hypogammaglobulinemia

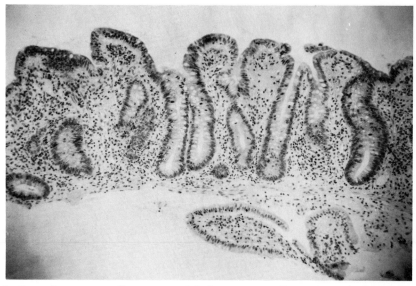

Figure 5–3. Jejunal mucosa in "hypogammaglobulinemic sprue." No plasma cells are seen in lamina propria—confirmed by higher power views. Hematoxylin and eosin stain. × 100. (Courtesy of L. L. Brandborg.)

tients show absent to markedly decreased numbers of plasma cells in the lamina propria (Fig. 5–3). Lymphoid follicles may be found in the intestinal mucosa of such patients, but these follicles are devoid of plasma cells.

Congenital hypogammaglobulinemia is characterized by recurrent pyogenic bacterial infections, usually with no detectable gastrointestinal malfunction. On the other hand, in the acquired primary form of agammaglobulinemia, with marked reductions in serum concentrations of IgG, IgM, and IgA, gastrointestinal abnormalities may be detected in 20 to 50 per cent of such patients.[13] The intestinal dysfunction may be associated with diarrhea without evidence of gross malabsorption or by the full-blown malabsorption syndrome identical to that observed in celiac sprue patients. Mucosal suction biopsy of the jejunum in patients with acquired agammaglobulinemia usually shows normal intestinal villi; however, in a few patients the intestinal mucosal morphological abnormalities characteristic of celiac sprue have been reported. Often these patients have no detectable plasma cells in the lamina propria of the jejunal mucosa, and a favorable response to a gluten-free diet, in respect to intestinal symptoms, has been variable.

A major physiological mechanism causing reduced serum immunoglobulins in patients with protein-losing enteropathy is excessive loss of immunoglobulins via the gastrointestinal tract. Protein-losing enteropathy may occur as a manifestation of a wide variety of gastrointestinal diseases, including, among others, intestinal lymphangiectasia, Whipple's disease, celiac sprue, giant gastric rugal hypertrophy, and allergic gastroenteropathy. Immunoglobulin metabolism has been studied in detail in a large group of patients with protein-losing enteropathy, hypoproteinemia, and edema.[14] Serum concentrations of IgG, IgA, and IgM are greatly reduced in patients with intestinal lymphangiectasia; rates of synthesis of these immunoglobulins have been found to be either normal or slightly increased. Lymphocytopenia has also been detected in patients with intestinal lymphangiectasia, with blood lymphocyte levels being one-third to one-fourth of those of normal individuals. Delayed hypersensitivity, an immune function of small lymphocytes, has been found to be defective in such individuals.[14, 15] The immunological disorders in patients with intestinal lymphangiectasia appear to result from loss of immunoglobulins and lymphocytes into the gastrointestinal tract secondary to disorders of the intestinal lymphatic channels. Lymphocyte depletion is believed to lead to the skin anergy and impaired homograft rejection which can be demonstrated in these patients.

Selective Immunoglobulin Deficiency. Deficiency of immunoglobulin synthesis may be restricted to one or two immunoglobulin classes; these disorders have been designated as dysgammaglobulinemias. Examples include the following:

IgA Deficiency with a Celiac Sprue-Like Lesion. Crabbé and Heremans have described patients with IgA deficiency who exhibited intestinal structural and functional abnormalities similar to those of celiac sprue.[16] They have designated this condition as "IgA-deficient sprue." IgA is absent or markedly decreased in sera and in exocrine secretions from these patients; IgG and IgM levels are either normal or slightly increased. Some of these patients' gastrointestinal symptoms responded favorably to gluten-free diets, which produced no increases in IgA levels. Jejunal mucosal biopsies revealed structural changes similar to celiac sprue and, in addition, a marked reduction or absence of IgA-containing plasma cells. There was an increase in plasma cells which contained IgM. IgG-containing cells were also increased in numbers. With a gluten-free diet intestinal mucosal structural abnormalities reverted to normal. In contrast, in most individuals with celiac sprue, serum levels of IgA are normal or increased, and in small intestinal mucosal biopsies IgA-containing plasma cells are abundant.[17]

Nodular Lymphoid Hyperplasia of the Small Intestine. Several groups of authors have identified immunological deficiencies associated with small intestinal nodular lymphoid hyperplasia, which is often sufficiently gross as to be identifiable radiographically.[18-20] Prominent lymphoid nodules, which do not contain plasma cells, are found in the intestinal mucosa (Fig. 5–4). Plasma cells in the lamina propria are reduced in numbers, but not absent. The mucosa is otherwise normal, without evidence of morphological abnormalities suggestive of celiac sprue. Serum IgA and IgM levels are usually reduced or undetectable, whereas IgG concentrations are usually normal. In some patients immunological deficiency has been restricted to IgA alone; and in yet others immunological deficiency of all major immunoglobulins (IgG, IgA, and IgM) has been found. The consistent ab-

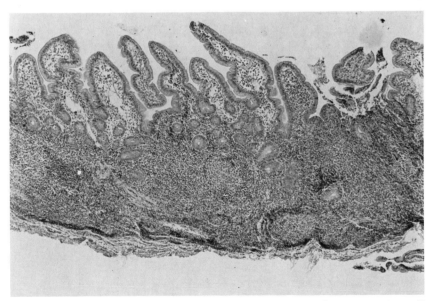

Figure 5–4. Jejunal mucosa in a patient with hypogammaglobulinemia, demonstrating so-called "nodular lymphoid hyperplasia." Hematoxylin and eosin stain. × 60. (Courtesy of L. L. Brandborg.)

normality in each of these groups of patients with intestinal nodular lymphoid hyperplasia is IgA deficiency. Diarrhea and malabsorption are frequently found in these patients and, when assiduously sought, *Giardia lamblia* can be isolated from stool specimens of most of them.

IMMUNOGLOBULIN DEFICIENCY IN ATAXIA TELANGIECTASIA. Ataxia telangiectasia is a disease transmitted as an autosomal recessive trait, its principal manifestations being cerebellar ataxia and oculocutaneous telangiectasia. Patients with ataxia telangiectasia have very low serum concentrations of IgA with either normal or high serum levels of IgM.[21] These patients, when compared with normal children, have been found to have marked reduction in IgA-containing plasma cells in the rectal mucosa. Increased IgM and decreased IgA concentrations have also been detected in external secretions from patients with this disease.

The Gastrointestinal Tract in IgA Heavy-Chain Disease. Gastrointestinal symptoms and morphological abnormalities have been identified in patients with a plasma cell dyscrasia identified as IgA heavy-chain (alpha-chain) disease.[22, 23] There is a lymphoma-like proliferation of abnormal plasma cells in the lamina propria of the small intestinal mucosa. These patients have chronic diarrhea, malabsorption, and progressive wasting. The symptoms are not responsive to a gluten-free diet. The abnormality was originally described in non-Ashkenazi Jews or Israeli Arabs; however, it has been described in other individuals as well. Genetic factors may be of major importance, although the disease is not restricted, as originally thought, to the Mediterranean population. Dietary and environmental factors may be important also.

With electron microscopy the abnormal plasma cells demonstrate an abundance of endoplasmic reticulum in whorl-like configurations. Studies of intestinal function indicate abnormalities in absorption of vitamin B_{12}, glucose, lactose, and fat. Barium examinations of the small intestine have shown thickened mucosal folds, segmentation, and dilated intestinal loops. Moderate osteoporosis, without destructive lesions, is found. Moderate increases in plasma cells are found in bone marrow as-

pirations. Examination of the serum by electrophoresis and other techniques reveals a marked increase in IgA heavy chains (alpha-chains).

With serum electrophoresis there is a broad peak in the beta and alpha-2 mobility range. The onset of symptoms may be either abrupt or gradual. The pathogenesis of IgA heavy-chain disease has not been defined.

Whipple's Disease. Immunological abnormalities have been detected in some patients with Whipple's disease. The most commonly observed abnormality is that of impaired delayed hypersensitivity, expressed as anergy in response to skin testing with a variety of common antigens. When studied, serum IgG and IgA levels in patients with Whipple's disease have been determined to be normal, whereas serum IgM levels in some patients have been found to be reduced.[24] Testing of lymphocyte responsiveness using phytohemagglutinin has demonstrated reduced responsiveness of lymphocytes in patients with Whipple's disease. These abnormalities have been noted in patients with Whipple's disease in remission following treatment with antibiotics. At present it is not certain whether these observed immunological abnormalities represent consequences of the disease or predispose to its occurrence. The nature of the immunological defect, or defects, in Whipple's disease is not clear. Possibilities include reduced lymphocyte activity associated with lymphopenia, possibly secondary to excessive losses of lymphocytes from the gastrointestinal tract, as appears to occur in intestinal lymphangiectasia. Another possibility is that macrophages, which are important in the processing of antigen for expressions of immune responsiveness, may be abnormal, either as a primary event accounting for the storage of bacterial breakdown products in Whipple's disease, or even possibly secondary to the accumulation of such products.

IMMUNOLOGICAL CONSIDERATIONS IN CELIAC SPRUE

Celiac sprue disease (discussed in detail on pp. 864 to 884) is characterized by malabsorption of a variety of nutrients in association with mucosal abnormalities of the small intestine. These include shortening and absence of intestinal villi and microvilli, an increase in depth of the intestinal crypts, and a prominence of mononuclear cells, principally lymphocytes and plasma cells, in the lamina propria of the small intestine. It is now well established that celiac sprue and its associated physiological and morphological abnormalities are consequences of intolerance to gliadin fractions from cereal glutens. Although gluten has been clearly implicated in the pathogenesis of celiac sprue, the mechanism or mechanisms by which gluten intolerance is expressed has escaped clarification. Major hypotheses concerning the etiology of gluten-associated enteropathy in celiac sprue include an enzyme defect or an immunological mechanism. It has been suggested that in patients with celiac sprue there may be a genetically determined or acquired absence of an enzyme required for hydrolysis of gluten to fragments which are not toxic to the small intestine. Patients with celiac sprue may lack this enzyme, resulting in the persistence of nonhydrolyzed gliadin fragments with the potential for exerting toxic effects on the mucosa of the small intestine.

The second pathogenetic mechanism considered in celiac sprue concerns potential immunological injury to the mucosa of the small intestine which may result from interaction of immune elements, such as antibody or sensitized lymphocytes, with small intestinal mucosal tissue or other substances, including products of partial gluten hydrolysis (Fig. 5–1). In addition, it is necessary to consider the possibility that gluten-associated damage to the small intestine in celiac sprue may be a combined abnormality, reflecting both enzymatic deficiency and immune events participating in development of the typical functional and morphological abnormalities. It is our purpose to indicate and consider some of the immunological abnormalities found in celiac sprue.

Serum Immunoglobulin Levels. Abnormal serum immunoglobulin levels have been reported in both children and adults with celiac sprue.[25, 26] Some have found increased serum IgA concentrations which decrease following withdrawal of gluten from the diet. The often-observed increase in serum IgA concentrations in patients with celiac sprue is of particular interest, because IgA is the principal immunoglobulin synthesized locally in the small intestinal mucosa. Serum IgA levels in patients with celiac sprue have also been noted to increase when the quantity of gluten ingested is increased. Gluten may provide an antigenic stimulus for IgA production. Patients with celiac sprue treated with a gluten-free diet have serum IgA levels not significantly different from those of control subjects. Progressive increases in serum IgA to relatively high levels in patients with celiac sprue have been associated with the development, or recognition, of intestinal lymphoma.[27] Serum IgM concentrations, although sometimes low, have usually been found to be within normal ranges.

Serum Antibodies to Milk Constituents. Circulating antibodies to milk protein antigens have been found in serum of patients with celiac sprue (as well as in other diseases of the gastrointestinal tract, including ulcerative colitis). A variety of explanations have been suggested for this observation: (1) Although no direct relationship has been established, it has been questioned whether these antibodies may be involved in the pathogenesis of the disorder. (2) The immune response in these individuals may be exaggerated. (3) These antibodies may merely represent normal immune responses to dietary antigenic protein, by virtue of mucosal intestinal damage in celiac sprue, permitted more than usual access to immunologically competent cells. Precipitating antibodies to milk protein in sera of tropical sprue patients suggests that these antibodies may result from antigenic stimulation permitted by small intestinal mucosal disruption. Intolerance to milk has been noted in some patients with celiac sprue; this probably is not an immune disorder but more likely reflects mucosal lactase deficiency. There is no clinical correlation between serum antibodies to milk proteins and clinical symptoms following milk ingestion.

Antibodies to Gluten in Celiac Sprue. Antibodies to gluten have been found in sera of 23 to 47 per cent of patients with celiac sprue; in contrast, gluten antibodies are not present in sera of tropical sprue patients. Differences in circulating gluten antibodies in patients with celiac and tropical sprue might be thought to provide evidence for a different immunological basis for these disorders. Alternatively, if an enzyme deficiency (perhaps glutaminase) is fundamental in celiac sprue, this enzyme absence might permit availability of antigens for stimulation of local and distant antibody production in patients with celiac sprue, but not in those with tropical sprue.

Antibodies to Gluten in Intestine and Intestinal Secretions. Antibodies to gluten components have been found in intestinal secretions from patients with celiac sprue.[28] The antibodies were demonstrable when the patients were ingesting gluten, and were detected in some patients six months after the elimination of gluten from the diet. Rates of synthesis of IgA by mucosal biopsies of patients with celiac sprue have been shown to be more rapid than those from normal individuals.[29] In addition, introduction of dietary gluten from patients with celiac sprue by small intestinal biopsy samples produces increased rates of synthesis of total protein, IgA, and IgM. These studies suggested that in patients with celiac sprue gluten challenge stimulates increased local intestinal immunoglobulin synthesis. It has been shown that in celiac sprue patients antibody to gluten is produced by small intestinal mucosal samples cultured in the presence of gluten.[30] Although gliadin may become attached to small bowel epithelial cells in this disease, an anti-autoimmune mechanism remains to be proved (Fig. 5–1).

Available studies examining immunological events in celiac sprue do not provide satisfactory explanations for these phenomena, nor do they answer the question of whether immunological mechanisms contribute to the pathogenesis of the disease. The need continues for further investigation of the potential contribution of immune mechanisms in the production of the celiac sprue lesion.

IMMUNOLOGICAL CONSIDERATIONS IN INFLAMMATORY BOWEL DISEASE

Major recognized forms of idiopathic inflammatory bowel disease include ulcerative colitis and granulomatous disease of the gastrointestinal tract (Crohn's disease). Although the causes of these diseases are not known, immunological phenomena have been detected in both, raising questions concerning the participation of immune responses in disease development.

Chronic Ulcerative Colitis. Extensive studies to identify bacterial or viral causes of chronic ulcerative colitis have been consistently negative. In many diseases of unknown cause autoimmunity has frequently been incriminated as a causative explanation. Laboratory studies have failed to establish autoimmunity as the cause of any disease, but have provided suggestive evidence in several diseases, including chronic ulcerative colitis.

In 1959 Broberger and Perlmann[31] identified, in the sera of some patients with ulcerative colitis, antibodies against an antigen contained in phenol-water extracts from colonic mucosal epithelial cells. Al-

TABLE 5–3. INCIDENCE OF ANTI-COLON ANTIBODIES*

AUTHOR	ULCERATIVE COLITIS No.	ULCERATIVE COLITIS per cent	REGIONAL ENTERITIS No.	REGIONAL ENTERITIS per cent	AUTOIMMUNE DISEASES† No.	AUTOIMMUNE DISEASES† per cent	NORMAL No.	NORMAL per cent	AMEBIC DYSENTERY No.	AMEBIC DYSENTERY per cent
Broberger et al.	28/30	93	—	—	5/32	16	0/38	0		
Asheron et al.	25/50	50	—	—	—	—	1/42	2		
Deodhar et al.‡	29/41	71	—	—	18/54	33	1/52	2		
Thayer et al.	25/55	46	6/15	40	—	—	2/34	6		
Lagercrantz et al.	52/101	52	12/18	66	—	—	6/45	13	5/15	33

*From Ginsberg, A. L.: Amer. J. Dig. Dis. 16:61, 1971.
†Nephritis, lupus, rheumatoid arthritis, thyroiditis, and pernicious anemia.
‡Titers of greater than 1:8 considered positive.

though the precise nature of the antigen to which these antibodies are directed is not known, it appears to be a polysaccharide similar to, but distinct from, polysaccharide ABO blood group substances. When carefully examined, many or most patients with ulcerative colitis are found to have circulating antibodies to the antigen, which is present in sterile fetal colon mucosa as well as in adult colon (Table 5–3). In contrast to patients with other gastrointestinal diseases or healthy control individuals, patients with ulcerative colitis often have elevated serum antibody titers to a polysaccharide found in the gram-negative *Escherichia coli* strain 014.[32] This *E. coli* strain is of particular interest because it possesses an antigen which is common for most E. Enterobacteriaceae but is more abundant, or more immunogenic, in 014 than in other *E. coli*. When tested with sera from patients with ulcerative colitis or from immunized rabbits, the colon antigen and the common bacterial antigen have been shown to represent cross-reacting antigens. Since gram-negative bacteria, which bear the colon-related antigen, are ever present in the contents of the large intestine, some have hypothesized that anti-colon antibodies in the sera of patients with ulcerative colitis result from stimulation with cross-reacting bacterial antigen.

The incidence and titer of anti-colon antibodies is higher in sera from children than adults with ulcerative colitis. The presence or titer of anti-colon antibodies does not relate to the severity or extent of ulcerative colitis. These colon antibodies, which are members of the IgG immunoglobulin class, have not been shown to be cytotoxic for cultured colon epithelial cells.[33] Most investigators view these circulating anti-colon antibodies in patients with ulcerative colitis as being secondary events, without established relevance as pathogenetic factors. Although they are not present in the sera of normal individuals, anti-colon antibodies have been found to occur with comparable frequency in sera of patients with ulcerative colitis and granulomatous disease of the gastrointestinal tract.

As in normal individuals, in the rectal mucosa of patients with ulcerative colitis IgA-containing plasma cells predominate over IgM-, IgG-, and IgD-containing cells; however, the absolute frequency of IgA-containing cells appears reduced when compared with those of normal control subjects. In rectal biopsies of patients with ulcerative colitis, IgA is frequently found in extracellular interstitial locations.

STUDIES OF LYMPHOCYTES IN ULCERATIVE COLITIS. Recent interest has centered on the potential role of sensitized lymphocytes in ulcerative colitis. As indicated previously, many small lymphocytes are believed to play important roles in cell-mediated hypersensitivity, transplantation immunity, and graft-host relationships. In contrast to circulating antibodies to colon, as cited above, circulating lymphocytes from patients with ulcerative colitis have been shown by several groups of investigators to be cytotoxic in vitro for cultured colon epithelial cells.[34-36] Certain features characterize this cytotoxicity for colon epithelial cells. (1) Cytotoxicity of lymphocytes for colon epithelial cells can be detected in virtually all patients with ulcerative colitis or Crohn's disease (regardless of its anatomic distribution). (2) Lymphocytes from patients with other inflammatory and neoplastic abnormalities of the gastrointestinal tract do not demonstrate this cytotoxicity. (3) Cytotoxicity appears to be specific for colon epithelial cells, inasmuch as there is no demonstrable toxicity for hepatic, renal, small intestinal, and gastric mucosal cells. (4) Cytotoxic effects are rapid, occurring within two hours. (Complement may be required, at least with use of intact lymphocytes.) (5) Cell-free extracts of lymphocytes from patients with ulcerative colitis have also been shown to be cytotoxic. (6) Cytotoxicity disappears shortly after removal of the inflammatory bowel disease. These results have suggested the possibility that ulcerative colitis may be a disease of delayed hypersensitivity in which small lymphocytes adversely affect colonic epithelium. It must be stressed, however, that the specificity of the cytotoxic reaction exhibited by lymphocytes from patients with inflammatory bowel disease remains to be proved. Antilymphocyte serum, which is capable of interfering with a variety of immunological reactions, including expressions of delayed hypersensitivity, has been shown to inhibit the cytotoxicity of lymphocytes from ulcerative colitis patients toward cultured colon epithelial cells.[36]

It remains to be proved whether the cytotoxicity expressed by lymphocytes from patients with inflammatory bowel disease on colon epithelial cells represents a true expression of delayed hypersensitivity. The rapidity of the in vitro effect and the apparent requirement for complement (a substance required for certain reactions mediated by humoral antibody but not by conventional delayed hypersensitivity reactions) argue against such an interpretation. In addition, the prompt disappearance of lymphocyte-mediated cytotoxicity following resection of diseased tissue would not be anticipated if the mechanism were genuinely that of delayed hypersensitivity. The nature of the cell-free material which is capable of inducing cytotoxic damage of colon epithelial cells is also not known.

Attempts have also been made to demonstrate delayed hypersensitivity of lymphocytes from ulcerative colitis patients against a variety of colon antigens by use of in vitro testing techniques, most commonly by testing for lymphocyte transformation. Lymphocyte transformation and macrophage inhibition have been viewed as in vitro correlates of delayed hypersensitivity. Cultured lymphocytes from patients with ulcerative colitis have been shown to be stimulated to the same degree as normal lymphocytes by immunologically specific agents, such as tuberculoprotein, and nonspecific agents, including phytohemagglutinin. Lymphocytes from patients with ulcerative colitis are not selectively stimulated by colon extract containing the antigen to which circulating antibodies have been demonstrated.[37] Others have demonstrated, in the presence of jejunal and colonic mucosa extracts, in vitro inhibition of macrophage migration by lymphocytes from patients with ulcerative colitis, but not Crohn's disease.[38] These data suggest possible delayed hypersensitivity of lymphocytes to antigens contained in these extracts.

Immunological Studies in Crohn's Disease. Increasing attention has been directed to the possibility that Crohn's disease may be associated with a disturbance in cell-mediated immunity. Reasons for such suspicion include the following: (1) The histological features of Crohn's disease, frequently with prominent granulomata, are not unlike those found in sarcoidosis. (2) Recognition of impairment of cell-mediated immunity in sarcoidosis. (3) The possibility, with no proof as yet, that Crohn's disease may be infectious in cause with prominent accompanying expressions of cell-mediated immunity. (4) The presence of antibodies in the sera of patients with Crohn's disease which cannot be distinguished from those of patients with ulcerative colitis.

Reduced responsiveness in lymphocyte transformation studies have been found in patients with Crohn's disease.[39] These results are similar to those with diseases of proved impaired cell-mediated immunity, including sarcoidosis, chronic lymphocytic leukemia, and Hodgkin's disease. Using in vitro techniques it has not been possible to demonstrate in patients with Crohn's disease any sensitivity of lymphocytes to a specific gastrointestinal antigen. Anergy, a customary accompaniment of depressed cellular immunity, has not been demonstrated in patients with Crohn's disease. The granulomatous histological reactions to mycobacteria and many fungi, which are in some ways similar to those of Crohn's disease, have long been interpreted as histological manifestations of delayed hypersensitivity. It is not possible to interpret the significance of demonstrated toxicity of lymphocytes from patients with Crohn's disease on colon epithelial cells but not on ileal cells. Until more precise information becomes available, it is perhaps useful to continue to consider the possibility that heretofore undefined infectious and perhaps immune processes may be involved in the development of Crohn's disease. Clearly, further investigation and understanding along both these lines are required.

IMMUNOLOGICAL STUDIES IN PERNICIOUS ANEMIA

Pernicious anemia, a disease of uncertain etiology, has been suspected to be of autoimmune nature because of a variety of factors. These include the nature of the histological lesion involving the gastric

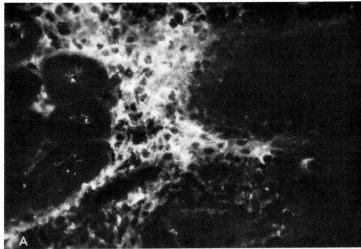
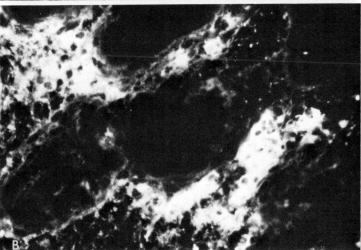

Figure 5–5. Immunoglobulins of gastric mucosa in pernicious anemia stained by fluoresceinated antibody to (*A*) human IgG and (*B*) human IgA. (From Jeffries, G. H., et al.: J. Clin. Invest., *44*:2021, 1965.)

mucosa, consisting of mucosal atrophy and prominence of lymphoid elements; the occurrence of a variety of immune phenomena, especially circulating antibodies to gastric mucosal cell constituents; and, certainly less specifically, morphological and functional improvement with the administration of glucocorticoids. An assortment of antibodies, not usually present in normal serum, have been detected in sera from patients with pernicious anemia. Some of these antibodies are less specific, occurring in other diseases, but others appear specific for pernicious anemia.

Antibodies to Parietal Cells. Antibodies which react with the cytoplasm of gastric parietal cells may be demonstrated in the sera of over 75 per cent of patients with pernicious anemia (Figs. 5–5 and 5–6). These antibodies are detected by complement fixation or immunofluorescence techniques.[40, 41] Most of these antibodies are IgG immunoglobulins. The antigen to which these antibodies are directed has not been precisely defined but is present in the microsomal faction of parietal cell cytoplasm. In addition, these antibodies may be found in patients with diabetes mellitus (especially if insulin-dependent), Addison's disease, iron deficiency anemia, assorted thyroid disorders, and in sera of patients with atrophy and inflammation of the gastric mucosa without pernicious anemia. These antibodies are also present in

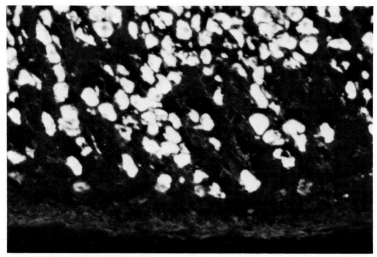

Figure 5–6. Human parietal cell antibody from pernicious anemia serum bound to rat gastric parietal cell and stained with fluoresceinated antibody to human IgG. × 375. (From Jeffries, G. H., et al.: J. Clin. Invest., 44:2021, 1965.)

increased frequency in the sera of relatives of patients with iron deficiency anemia, pernicious anemia, and thyroiditis. There is a high degree of correlation between the presence of serum antibodies to parietal cells and the presence of gastritis and gastric mucosal atrophy (Fig. 5–7). The greater the degree of histological change in the gastric mucosa, the greater the possibility that the patient will have circulating antibodies to parietal cells. When carefully examined, patients with circulating antibodies to parietal cells but without pernicious anemia will also have abnormal

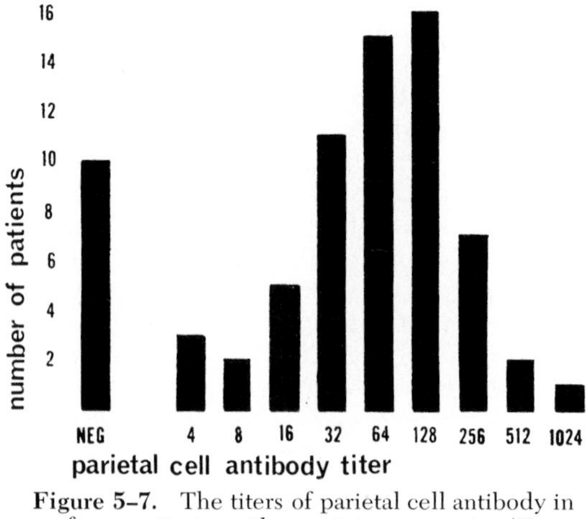

gastric mucosal histology. The overall incidence of antibodies to parietal cells increases with age, most likely reflective of the increase of gastric mucosal inflammatory and atrophic changes with increasing age. There is a general, but rather poor, correlation between the titer of the parietal cell antibody and the severity of the hypochlorhydria.

There is no correlation between the presence of antibodies to parietal cells and vitamin B_{12} absorption. The consequences of parietal cell antibodies and their relationships to disease are not known; there is no persuasive evidence that parietal cell antibodies are instrumental in the pathogenesis of the gastric inflammatory lesion. Most current thinking suggests that antibodies to parietal cells reflect rather than initiate or perpetuate the gastric inflammatory process. Inasmuch as antibodies to parietal cells are found in a variety of clinical states, their detection is of no diagnostic value in pernicious anemia.

Parietal cell antibodies have been demonstrated in the gastric juice of some subjects with circulating serum antibodies. Mononuclear cells have been demonstrated in gastric biopsies from patients with pernicious anemia which contain antibodies against two constituents of human gastric parietal cells. The first antibody is directed against the microsomal parietal cell component. The second population of

Figure 5–7. The titers of parietal cell antibody in sera from patients with pernicious anemia. (From Jeffries, G. H., et al.: J. Clin. Invest., 44:2021, 1965.)

antibodies reacts with gastric intrinsic factor.[42] In the gastric mucosa of patients with pernicious anemia IgA-containing cells have been found to be reduced to 10 per cent of normal, whereas IgG-containing cells were increased by 15 per cent. Despite these observations, levels of circulating serum immunoglobulins were normal. It has been suggested that in some patients with pernicious anemia reductions in gastric mucosal IgA-containing cells may be primary and predispose to the gastric atrophic lesion.

Antibodies to Intrinsic Factor. Many investigators have detected and described antibodies to gastric intrinsic factor in sera from patients with pernicious anemia.[43] These antibodies have been classified as "blocking" and "binding." Blocking antibodies are those which combine with intrinsic factor, inhibiting subsequent complex formation between vitamin B_{12} and intrinsic factor. Binding antibodies are those which bind intrinsic factor molecules before or following the complexing of intrinsic factor with vitamin B_{12}, but do not prevent formation of intrinsic factor–vitamin B_{12} complexes.

Antibodies to intrinsic factor, in contrast to antibodies to parietal cells, are specific for pernicious anemia and do not occur in patients with other diseases; for this reason the detection of antibodies to intrinsic factor may serve a useful, although usually adjunct, role in identifying patients with pernicious anemia. The frequency of detection of antibodies to intrinsic factor in patients with pernicious anemia has varied from 40 to 70 per cent. When antibodies are present, sera from patients with pernicious anemia usually contain both blocking and binding antibodies to intrinsic factor; however, although blocking antibody may be found alone, only rarely has binding antibody been found in the absence of blocking antibody. The significance of serum antibodies to intrinsic factor has not been established. These antibodies have not been proved to be important in interfering with vitamin B_{12} absorption in patients with pernicious anemia. Patients have been described with pernicious anemia and hypogammaglobulinemia with no serum antibodies to intrinsic factor or parietal cells.[44]

Both blocking and binding antibodies have been detected in gastric juice. Such antibodies are principally of the IgG class of immunoglobulins; however, in isolated instances secretory IgA antibody to intrinsic factor has been found in the gastric juice of patients with pernicious anemia.[45] It has been concluded that in certain patients with pernicious anemia immunologically competent cells of the gastric immune system may secrete IgA autoantibody to intrinsic factor.

To date there is no conclusive evidence to support the speculation that antibodies to intrinsic factor play an etiological role in the pathogenesis of the gastric atrophy which characterizes classic Addisonian pernicious anemia. No correlation has been established between the absence, presence, or levels of antibodies to intrinsic factor and the clinical course in patients with pernicious anemia. Although the precise role played by antibodies to gastric mucosal cell constituents has not been clarified, their detection continues to provide suggestive evidence that immune mechanisms may be important to the development of pernicious anemia.

The possibility that delayed-type hypersensitivity may participate in pernicious anemia on an autoimmune basis has been examined. Lymphocyte transformation studies have been performed on lymphocytes from patients with pernicious anemia.[46] Positive lymphocyte transformation has been observed in some patients with pernicious anemia when the lymphocytes are exposed to a variety of preparations, including the gastric mucosal homogenates, gastric juice, and intrinsic factor. Data from these lymphocyte transformation studies permit the consideration that cellular immunity may participate in the pathogenesis of pernicious anemia. Dogs have been immunized with gastric juice or gastric mucosal homogenates, producing degenerative and inflammatory changes in the gastric mucosa similar to those observed in pernicious anemia.[47, 48] In addition, these dogs developed antibodies to parietal cells, and the gastric mucosa was infiltrated with lymphocytes and plasma cells. Delayed skin reactions to antigens used in immunization were seen in most dogs, and were observed concurrently with the appearance of the inflammatory reaction involving the gastric mucosa.

ANTIGENS AND ANTIBODIES IN CARCINOMA OF THE GASTROINTESTINAL TRACT

A tumor antigen, perhaps antigens, has been demonstrated in many varieties of carcinomas arising from entodermal epithelium of the human digestive system.[49-52] The antigen has been demonstrated in gastrointestinal tumors, including those of the esophagus, stomach, duodenum, pancreas, colon, and rectum. Antigens, immunologically identical to those found in gastrointestinal carcinomas, have also been identified in gut, liver, and pancreatic fetal tissues prior to the seventh month of gestation. Recognition of the presence of these antigens in both gastrointestinal carcinoma and fetal tissues has led to the term "carcinoembryonic antigens of the human digestive system." The carcinoembryonic antigen appears to be a glycoprotein. It has been suspected that this antigen may reappear with the dedifferentiation of malignancy, perhaps by permitting production of these fetal antigens by the process of derepression. Both antigens and antibody to these antigens have been detected in sera from patients with gastrointestinal carcinoma, most prominently in colon cancer. The carcinoembryonic antigen has been detected in a large proportion (as great as 90 per cent) of patients with carcinoma of the colon. In addition, in some studies, patients with carcinoma of the pancreas have also been shown to contain the carcinoembryonic antigen in their sera. More recent studies suggest that the specificity of the carcinoembryonic antigen for malignant neoplasms of the gastrointestinal tract is not as great as originally suspected. The antigen has been detected in the sera of patients with a variety of nongastrointestinal neoplasms, including carcinomas of the lung, larynx, breast, and others.[52] It has been detected also in patients with reticulum cell sarcoma and multiple myeloma. The carcinoma embryonic antigen is present in the serum of approximately 50 per cent of patients with alcoholic liver disease. The antigen has also been detected in the sera of patients with other gastrointestinal diseases without known carcinoma; these have included ulcerative colitis and polyps. The carcinoembryonic antigen has also been detected in sera of patients with renal disease undergoing dialysis.

Accumulating evidence suggests the probability that more than one antigen has been detected in such studies by various groups of investigators, and that this antigen(s) is indeed probably a tumor antigen, though not necessarily specific for and restricted to gastrointestinal malignant neoplasms.

It is anticipated with further studies utilizing the carcinoembryonic antigen system that more detailed information will be obtained concerning the precise nature of the interacting antigens and antibodies. It is expected that from such studies valuable techniques will be evolved for the immunological identification of malignant neoplasms of the gastrointestinal tract, many of which may be recognized prior to the appearance of clinical symptoms.

RADIOIMMUNOASSAY IN GASTROENTEROLOGY

One of the most important immunological methods which has become available in the past decade is that of radioimmunoassay. Radioimmunoassay methods are now available for the sensitive and specific measurement of a variety of substances important in the study of diseases of the gastrointestinal tract. These methods have proved valuable in delineating the mechanisms and patterns of gastrointestinal hormone regulation. In addition the clinician can now take advantage of diagnostic usefulness of radioimmunoassay in evaluating disturbances of gastrointestinal hormone secretion. In particular, radioimmunoassay has been especially useful in measuring the gastrointestinal peptide hormones. Prior to the development of radioimmunoassay there were no uniform techniques available for satisfactory measurement of gastrointestinal peptide hormones in serum or plasma; only bioassay techniques were available. In general, available bioassay techniques, such as those for gastrin, did not combine sufficient specificity and sensitivity to be of clinical use in estimating gastrin concentrations in tissues or body fluids.

The techniques of radioimmunoassay involve the production of antibodies against the antigen to be measured, as, for example, the polypeptide hormone gastrin.[53, 54] Radioimmunoassay exploits the ability of an unlabeled hormone in serum, or other solutions, to compete with a radioactively labeled hormone for antibody binding sites, and thereby to inhibit antibody binding of the radiolabeled tracer hormone. As a result of this competitive inhibition, the ratio of antibody-bound to antibody-free radiolabeled hormone is decreased. Thus the concentration of the substance being measured in the unknown sample is obtained by comparing the inhibition observed in that sample with that produced by standard solutions containing known amounts of the hormone.

A variety of radioimmunoassay techniques have been developed for the sensitive and specific measurement of the gastrointestinal polypeptide hormone gastrin. Applications of these techniques have supplied substantial information concerning the physiological regulation and effects of the hormone gastrin both in man and in experimental animals. Radioimmunoassay has also provided important clinical information concerning gastrin. Marked elevations in fasting serum gastrin concentration have been demonstrated in patients with the Zollinger-Ellison syndrome.[55] Radioimmunoassay techniques for measurement of gastrin have provided the most sensitive and specific method for the diagnosis of the Zollinger-Ellison syndrome, i.e., detection of the fasting hypergastrinemia. Marked increases in fasting serum gastrin concentrations have also been detected in many patients with pernicious anemia.[56] The marked elevation of gastrin detected in patients with pernicious anemia results from the lack of gastric acid secretion, thereby permitting excess gastrin release.

Radioimmunoassay methods have also been developed for measurement of other important gastrointestinal hormones, including secretin and cholecystokinin-pancreozymin.[57, 58] With further development and availability of these techniques substantial information will be gained concerning the roles of these substances in normal and altered gastrointestinal physiology.

IMMUNOLOGY AND GASTROENTEROLOGY: THE FUTURE

It is certain that immunology, and the availability and application of immunological techniques, will contribute greatly to our understanding of the diagnosis and treatment of patients with gastrointestinal diseases. Perhaps no other area of scientific information and technology will contribute more importantly in the acquisition of knowledge in gastroenterology.

Reliable and specific serological methods will be available for the detection of neoplasms of the gastrointestinal tract. It is reasonable to expect that the identification of such patients with gastrointestinal malignancy may be possible prior to expression of clinical symptoms. The values of such techniques in diagnosis, detection of recurrence, determination of completeness of removal, and/or need for further surgery are enormous and obvious.

Radioimmunoassay of the gastrointestinal polypeptide hormones, as well as other small organic molecules mediating important physiological events in the normal and diseased gastrointestinal tract, is already making an important impact on our knowledge and decision-making in the care of patients with digestive diseases. It is anticipated that with further development of radioimmunoassay methods the chemical and pathophysiological bases of an assortment of diseases of the gastrointestinal tract will be clarified. Sensitive and specific radioimmunoassay measurements of gastrointestinal hormones, liberated in excess or in deficient quantities, will be readily available to the clinician.

Many gastrointestinal diseases of unknown cause have been suspected to be of autoimmune nature. One may expect that, with continued immunological investigation, the nature of the relationship of altered immune phenomena to these diseases will be clarified.

Enormous advances are currently underway in our understanding of basic immunological mechanisms and technical methodology related to organ transplantation and acceptance. It is anticipated that the acquisition of fundamental immunological information will provide the background for effective transplantation and acceptance of organs and tissues, including those of the gastrointestinal tract. Advances are being made which give promise to the future in respect to transplantation of organs such as the small intestine, liver, and pancreas.

Other applications of immunology in our understanding of human disease and our treatment of patients with gastrointestinal disease are obvious to the reader. There is left little doubt that immunology will contribute in most important ways to the rapidly increasing acquisition of knowledge relating to the diseases of the gastrointestinal tract.

REFERENCES

1. Good, R. A., Finstad, J., Gerwuz, H., Cooper, M. D., and Pollara, B. The development of immunological capacity in phylogenetic perspective. Amer. J. Dis. Child. 114:477, 1967.
2. Cooper, M. D., Gabrielson, A. E., and Good, R. A. Role of the thymus and other central lymphoid tissues in immunologic disease. Ann. Rev. Med. 18:113, 1967.
3. Cooper, M. D., Peterson, R. D. A., South, M. A., and Good, R. A. Functions of thymus system and bursa system in chickens. J. Exp. Med. 123:75, 1966.
4. Crabbé, P. A., Carbonara, A. O., and Heremans, J. F. The normal human intestinal mucosa as a major source of plasma cells containing gamma A-immunoglobulin. Lab. Invest. 14:235, 1965.
5. Crabbé, P. A., and Heremans, J. F. The distribution of immunoglobulin-containing cells along the gastrointestinal tract. Gastroenterology 51:305, 1966.
6. Tomasi, T. B., Jr. Human immunoglobulin A. New Eng. J. Med. 279:1327, 1968.
7. Tomasi, T. B., Jr., Tan, E. M., Soloman, A., and Prendergast, R. A. Characteristics of an immune system common to certain external secretions. J. Exp. Med. 121:101, 1965.
8. Ogra, P. L., Karzon, D. T., Righthand, F., and MacGillivray, M. Immunoglobulin response in serum and secretion after immunization with live and inactivated polio vaccine and natural infection. New Eng. J. Med. 279:893, 1968.
9. Berger, R., Ainbender, E., Hodes, H. L., Zepp, H. D., and Hevizy, M. M. Demonstration of IgA polioantibody in saliva, duodenal fluid and urine. Nature (London) 214:420, 1967.
10. Douglas, R. G., Rossen, R. D., Butler, W. T., and Couch, R. B. Rhinovirus neutralizing antibody in tears, parotid saliva, nasal secretions and serum. J. Immunol. 99:297, 1967.
11. Adinolfi, M., Glynn, A. A., Lindsay, M., and Malne, C. M. Serological properties of γA antibodies to Escherichia coli present in human colostrum. Immunology 10:517, 1966.
12. Ishizaka, T., Ishizaka, K., Boros, T., and Rapp, H. J. C'1 fixation of human isoagglutinins: Fixation of C'1 by gamma-G and gamma-M, but not by gamma-A antibody. J. Immunol. 97:716, 1966.
13. Good, R. A., Kelley, W. O., Rotstein, J., and Varco, R. L. Immunological deficiency diseases. Progr. Allergy 6:234, 1962.
14. Strober, W., Wochner, R. D., Carbone, P. P., and Waldmann, T. A. Intestinal lymphangiectasia: A protein-losing enteropathy with hypogammaglobulinemia, lymphocytopenia and impaired homograft rejection. J. Clin. Invest. 46:1643, 1967.
15. McGuigan, J. E., Purkerson, M. L., Trudeau, W. L., and Peterson, M. L. Studies of the immunologic defects associated with intestinal lymphangiectasia. Ann. Intern. Med. 68:398, 1968.
16. Crabbé, P. A., and Heremans, J. F. Selective IgA deficiency with steatorrhea: A new syndrome. Amer. J. Med. 42:319, 1967.
17. Rubin, W., Fauci, A. S., Sleisenger, M. H., and Jeffries, G. H. Immunofluorescent studies in adult coeliac disease. J. Clin. Invest. 44:475, 1965.
18. Hermans, P. E., Huizenga, K. A., Hoffman, H. N., II, Brown, A. L., Jr., and Markovitz, H. Dysgammaglobulinemia associated with nodular lymphoid hyperplasia of the small intestine. Amer. J. Med. 40:78, 1966.
19. Hermans, P. E. Nodular lymphoid hyperplasia of the small intestine and hypogammaglobulinemia: Theoretical and practical considerations. Fed. Proc. 26:1606, 1967.
20. Hodgson, J. R., Hoffman, H. N., and Huizenga, K. A. Roentgenologic features of lymphoid hyperplasia of the small intestine associated with dysgammaglobulinemia. Radiology 88:883, 1967.
21. Eidelman, S., and Davis, S. D. Immunoglobulin content of intestinal mucosal plasma-cells in ataxia telangiectasia. Lancet 1:884, 1968.
22. Rambaud, J. C., Bognel, C., Prost, A., Bernier, J. J., LeQuintrec, Y., Lambling, A., Danon, F., Hurez, D., and Seligmann, M. Clinicopathological study of a patient with "Mediterranean" type of abdominal lymphoma and a new type of IgA abnormality ("alpha-chain disease"). Digestion 1:321, 1968.
23. Seligmann, M., Danon, F., Hurez, D., Mihesco, E., and Preud'homme, J. L. Alpha-chain disease: A new immunoglobulin abnormality. Science 162:1396, 1968.
24. Martin, F. F., Velseck, J. R., Jr., Dobbins, W. O., III, et al. Immunologic defect in treated Whipple's disease. Gastroenterology 60:694, 1971.
25. Eidelman, S., Davis, S. D., and Rubin, C. E. The relationship between intestinal plasma cells and serum immunoglobulin A (IgA) in man. J. Clin. Invest. 45:1003, 1966.
26. Bletcher, T. E., Brzechwa-Adjukiewicz, A., McCarthy, C. F., and Read, A. E. Serum immunoglobulins and lymphocyte transforma-

tion studies in coeliac disease. Gut 10:57, 1969.

27. Asquith, P., Thompson, R. A., and Cooke, W. T. Serum immunoglobulins in adult coeliac disease. Lancet 2:129, 1969.

28. Katz, J., Kantor, F. S., and Herskovic, T. Intestinal antibodies to wheat fractions in celiac disease. Ann. Intern. Med. 69:1149, 1968.

29. Loeb, P. M., Strober, W., Falchuk, Z. M., and Laster, L. Incorporation of L-leveine-^{14}C into immunoglobulins by jejunal biopsies of patients with celiac-sprue and other gastrointestinal diseases. J. Clin. Invest. 50:559, 1971.

30. Falchuk, Z. M., Laster, L., and Strober, W. Gluten sensitive enteropathy: Intestinal synthesis of antigluten antibody in vitro. Clin. Res. 19:390, 1971.

31. Broberger, O., and Perlmann, P. Autoantibodies in human ulcerative colitis. J. Exp. Med. 110:657, 1959.

32. Perlmann, P., Hammarstrom, S., Lagercrantz, R., and Campbell, D. Autoantibodies to colon in rats and human ulcerative colitis: Cross-reactivity with Escherichia coli 0:14 antigen. Proc. Soc. Exp. Biol. Med. 125:975, 1967.

33. Broberger, O., and Perlmann, P. In vitro studies of ulcerative colitis. I. Reactions of patients' serum with fetal colon cells in tissue cultures. J. Exp. Med. 117:705, 1963.

34. Perlmann, P., and Broberger, O. In vitro studies of ulcerative colitis. II. Cytotoxic action of white blood cells from patients on human fetal cells. J. Exp. Med. 117:717, 1963.

35. Watson, D. W., Quigley, W. A., and Bolt, R. J. Effect of lymphocytes from patients with ulcerative colitis on human adult colon epithelial cells. Gastroenterology 51:985, 1966.

36. Shorter, R. G., Spencer, R. J., Huizenga, K. A., and Hallenbeck, G. A. Inhibition of in vitro cytotoxicity of lymphocytes from patients with ulcerative colitis and granulomatous colitis for allogenic colonic epithelial cells using horse anti-human thymus serum. Gastroenterology 54:227, 1968.

37. Hinz, C. F., Jr., Perlmann, P., and Hammarstrom, S. Reactivity in vitro migration of leukocytes in ulcerative colitis. J. Lab. Clin. Med. 70:752, 1967.

38. Bendixen, G. Specific inhibition of the in vitro migration of leukocytes in ulcerative colitis and Crohn's disease. Scand. J. Gastroenterol. 2:214, 1967.

39. Parent, K., Barrett, J., and Wilson, I. D. Investigation of the pathogenic mechanisms in regional enteritis with in vitro lymphocyte cultures. Gastroenterology 61:431, 1971.

40. Irvine, W. J., and Davies, S. H. Gastrin antibodies studied by fluorescence microscopy. Quart. J. Exp. Physiol. 48:427, 1963.

41. Jeffries, G. H., Sleisenger, M. H., and Margolis, S. Studies of parietal cell antibodies in pernicious anemia. J. Clin. Invest. 44:2021, 1965.

42. Baur, S., Fisher, J. M., Strickland, R. G., and Taylor, K. B. Autoantibody-containing cells in the gastric mucosa in pernicious anemia. Lancet 2:887, 1968.

43. Garrido-Pinson, G. C., Turner, M. D., Crookston, J. H., Samloff, I. M., Miller, L., and Segal, H. L. Studies of human intrinsic factor autoantibodies. J. Immunol. 97:897, 1966.

44. Twomey, J. J., Jordan, P. H., Retz, N. D., and Conn, H. O. The syndrome of immunoglobulin (Ig) deficiency and pernicious anemia (PA). Clin. Res. 16:457, 1968.

45. Goldberg, L. S., Shuster, J., and Fudenberg, H. Gastric autoimmunity in pernicious anemia. J. Lab. Clin. Med. 73:249, 1969.

46. Tai, C., and McGuigan, J. E. Immunologic studies in pernicious anemia. Blood 34:63, 1969.

47. Krohn, K. Experimental gastritis in the dog. I. Production of atrophic gastritis and antibodies to parietal cells. Ann. Med. Exp. Fenn. 46:249, 1968.

48. Krohn, K. Experimental gastritis in the dog. II. Production of antibodies to a gastric B$_{12}$-binding auto-antigen. Ann. Med. Exp. Fenn. 46:259, 1968.

49. Gold, P., and Freedman, S. O. Demonstration of tumor-specific antigens in human colon carcinomata by immunological tolerance and absorption techniques. J. Exp. Med. 121:439, 1965.

50. Gold, P., and Freedman, S. O. Specific carcinoembryonic antigens of the human digestive system. J. Exp. Med. 122:467, 1965.

51. LoGerfo, P., Krupey, J., and Hansen, H. J. Demonstration of an antigen common to several varieties of neoplasia: Assay using Zirconyl phosphate gel. New Eng. J. Med. 285:138, 1971.

52. Moore, T. L., Kupchick, H. Z., Macon, N., et al. Carcinoembryonic antigen assay in cancer of the colon and pancreas and other digestive tract disorders. Amer. J. Dig. Dis. 16:1, 1971.

53. McGuigan, J. E. Immunochemical studies with synthetic human gastrin. Gastroenterology 54:1005, 1968.

54. Yalow, R. S., and Berson, S. A. Radioimmunoassay of gastrin. Gastroenterology 58:1, 1970.

55. McGuigan, J. E., and Trudeau, W. L. Immunochemical measurement of elevated levels of gastrin in the serum of patients with pancreatic tumors of the Zollinger-Ellison variety. New Eng. J. Med. 278:1308, 1968.

56. McGuigan, J. E., and Trudeau, W. L. Serum gastrin concentrations in pernicious anemia. New Eng. J. Med. 282:358, 1970.

57. Young, J. D., Lazarus, L., and Chisholm, D. J. Radioimmunoassay of secretin in human serum. J. Nucl. Med. 9:641, 1968.

58. Young, J. D., Lararus, I., and Chisholm, D. J. Radioimmunoassay of pancreozymin-cholecystokinin in human serum. J. Nucl. Med. 10:743, 1969.

Chapter 6

The Relation of Enteric Bacterial Populations to Gastrointestinal Function and Disease

Robert M. Donaldson, Jr.

The bacterial populations present in the lumen of the alimentary canal constitute an important, if often forgotten, aspect of the host's environment, and the enteric flora profoundly influence a wide variety of processes in the healthy and diseased gastrointestinal tract. During the past ten to 15 years this long neglected subject has once again become a matter of intense interest. The prime importance of anaerobic microorganisms,[1] the effects of enteric microorganisms on the germ-free[2] and pathogen-free[3] host animal, the emphasis on methods for quantifying the microorganisms which populate the alimentary canal,[4] and the effects of enteric microorganisms on the metabolism of drugs[5] and a variety of nutrients have all stimulated an active reappraisal of the enteric flora. Interest has further intensified because of numerous studies which tend to implicate intestinal microorganisms in the pathophysiology of diverse human diseases ranging from hepatic coma to tropical sprue. This chapter will concern itself with the bacterial populations of the human alimentary canal, the factors which affect those populations, and the effects of indigenous microorganisms on intestinal morphology and function. Also considered is the role of the enteric flora in the pathogenesis of certain disease states with emphasis on the pathophysiological implications of small bowel bacterial overgrowth. Detailed reviews of these subjects are available.[6-10]

BACTERIAL POPULATIONS OF THE HUMAN ALIMENTARY CANAL

Knowledge concerning the kinds and numbers of microorganisms harbored within the alimentary canal continues to depend upon, and to be limited by, the methods available for the collection, isolation, culture, and enumeration of these microbes.[6, 9] Methodological problems have led to a diversity of techniques which makes comparison of results from different laboratories difficult. In general, microorganisms are cultured in various selective and nonselective media and are quantitated by serial tenfold dilutions of these media. Nonselective media provide conditions more favorable for overall microbial growth, but selective media are needed to prevent overgrowth of particularly fastidious species by more adaptable microorganisms. Results obviously depend upon the choice of media and the extent to which these media are serially diluted. Particularly important is rigorous attention to anaerobic techniques, including the use of media preserved in the oxygen-free state and provision of an anaerobic environment for inoculation and transfer of material.[11] Although a variety of methods for collecting gastrointestinal contents for bacterial culture have been proposed, most investigators currently agree that the easiest and probably most reliable technique is peroral intubation with a plastic tube.[12] This approach yields results comparable with other collection methods and has the advantage that samples from various levels of the alimentary canal can be obtained in the same subject.

In normal subjects the stomach and proximal small intestine contain relatively small numbers of bacteria; jejunal cultures fail to identify any bacterial growth in about one-third of healthy volunteers.[4] Characteristically present are gram-positive aerobes or facultative anaerobes such as lactobacilli and enterococci, usually present in concentrations of 10^1 to 10^4 viable organisms per gram of jejunal contents. Coliforms may be transiently present in the healthy jejunum, but rarely exceed 10^3 organisms per gram and probably represent ingested "contaminants" en route to the colon.[12] Anaerobic bacteroides are not found in the proximal small bowel.

Although the ileum harbors a similarly sparse flora in about one-third of healthy subjects, a distinct change in bacterial populations is observed in the distal small bowel of the majority of volunteers.[12] The total number of microbes remains relatively low, but concentrations approach 10^5 to 10^8 organisms per gram, clearly greater than the numbers seen in the proximal small bowel. In addition, gram-negative organisms, including coliforms and bacteroides, can be considered indigenous residents of the terminal ileum, which is distinctly not the case for the jejunum.

The enteric flora changes markedly across the ileocecal valve. The total number of microorganisms becomes enormously increased and usually approximates 10^9 to 10^{11} organisms per gram of colonic contents or feces. Particularly numerous are the more fastidious anaerobes, so that the large bowel flora is dominated by bacteroides, anaerobic lactobacilli, and clostridia. These microorganisms, although difficult to culture, actually outnumber aerobic and facultative organisms by as much as 10,000 to 1. Data concerning bacterial populations within the lumen of the colon remain scarce, but it would appear that the concentrations of bacteria in feces are probably 10 to 100 times those of colonic contents.

The alimentary canal of the host is sterile at birth, and animals raised in a germ-free environment harbor no microorganisms in the gut lumen.[2] Thus the enteric flora is derived exclusively from the environment. Although most of our information about the development of the bacterial populations of the intestine comes from studies in laboratory and domestic animals, it is clear from work in human infants that enteric bacteria colonize the gut in an oral-to-anal direction, and that oral contamination is the initial source of the development of the enteric flora.[7, 13] In newborn infants with complete intestinal obstruction, the bowel proximal to the site of obstruction is populated with large numbers of bacteria, whereas the distal bowel, including the colon and rectum, remains sterile. In a wide variety of animal species, including man, *Escherichia coli*, *Clostridium welchii*, and streptococci appear first and colonize the alimentary canal within a few hours of birth. Although coliforms are present in relatively high concentrations during the first one to three days of life, there occurs during the next seven to ten days a marked decrease in the numbers of these microorganisms, particularly in the small bowel. Anaerobic lactobacilli and enterococci become established at 24 hours and slowly increase in numbers during the next ten to 21 days, a period when the number of coliforms is decreasing. Bacteroides, destined to become the dominant constituent of the colonic flora, first make their appearance at ten days and rapidly proliferate during the next two weeks. Approximately three to four weeks after birth, the flora characteristic for the host is fairly well established and, except under unusual circumstances, does not change importantly thereafter.

Intestinal bacteria tend to adhere to the luminal surface of the bowel wall. Jejunal and ileal biopsies obtained from healthy human subjects have documented gram-positive organisms consisting mostly of lactobacilli and streptococci embedded in mucus on the epithelial surface.[14] In a similar fashion, bacteroides, fusiforms, enterococci, and coliforms adhere to large bowel mucosa. Although they tend to concentrate on the epithelial surface, enteric bacteria are found on the outer "fuzzy coat" of mucosal cells, and there is no evidence of penetration into microvilli, mucosal cytoplasm, or lamina propria.

FACTORS WHICH INFLUENCE THE ENTERIC FLORA

Although the bacterial populations of the gut may vary considerably from one animal species to another and even from one individual to another, the enteric flora in a given individual remains remarkably stable over long periods of time.[15] Although incompletely delineated, several factors determine the numbers and kinds of microorganisms present in the alimentary canal.[7] In the upper bowel, mechanisms appear to be directed at limiting bacterial proliferation so as to prevent uncontrolled overgrowth in those portions of the gut concerned with digestion and absorption of nutrients. The stomach serves as an important barrier to bacterial overgrowth. Gastric acid and perhaps other substances secreted into the gastric juice destroy most of the bacteria that are ingested with food. Gastric atrophy, as occurs in pernicious anemia, or surgical removal of the stomach allows increased numbers of viable microorganisms to pass into the small bowel. Bile is capable of inhibiting bacterial growth, a property which may be related to the presence of bile salts, but it is not at all clear whether bile, pancreatic juice, or the succus entericus has any specific influence on the numbers or kinds of microorganisms present in the intestinal lumen. The host factor most responsible for limiting bacterial proliferation in the small bowel appears to be the cleansing action of normal propulsive motility of the intestinal canal. In the relatively stagnant contents of the large bowel, bacterial growth is luxuriant, whereas microorganisms are rapidly cleared from the small intestine. Quantitative investigations have demonstrated that although microorganisms are destroyed in the acid contents of the stomach, those bacteria which survive and pass into the small bowel remain viable as they are swept into the colon at a relatively rapid rate. Mucus may aid in this mechanical process for removing bacteria, a possibility which is supported by the fact that microorganisms tend to concentrate in the mucous layer that lines the gastrointestinal mucosa.[15] In any event, the importance of this cleansing action of normal peristalsis is emphasized by the fact that whenever normal motility is slowed or interrupted, bacterial overgrowth rapidly ensues.

In addition to host factors, the environment in which the host exists undoubtedly influences the nature of his enteric flora.[16] Nevertheless, one cannot usually observe any striking effect on intestinal bacterial populations except when the environment is altered by extreme measures. Thus, for example, only when animals are rigorously raised in strict germ-free or pathogen-free environments does the habitat of the host seem to have any predictable effect on intestinal bacterial populations. Many have speculated that the enteric flora of humans living under poor sanitary conditions, particularly in the tropics, may develop an altered enteric flora which, in turn, influences intestinal function. Except for the finding of certain strains of coliforms in some patients with tropical diarrhea, however, no one has described any important yet consistent influence of geography or climate on the enteric flora. Although biomedical literature is replete with the effects of diet on intestinal microbial populations, most of the findings are conflicting; probably only extreme unphysiological alterations in diet influence the kinds and numbers of microorganisms which populate the intestinal canal.[6, 17] Thus, for example, diets extremely high in casein or meat protein may reduce the number of lactobacilli and increase the number of coliforms, but prolonged fasting or the ingestion of unusually large quantities of food probably affects the enteric flora more noticeably than does the specific kind of food one eats. Although it is widely held that ingestion of milk sugar increases the number of intestinal lactobacilli, one must ingest enormous quantities of lactose before the concentration of lactobacilli changes significantly. Since not only ingested material but also desquamated intestinal cells and various gastrointestinal secretions serve to nourish the microbial populations of the gut and since a large proportion of the diet is absorbed before ingested nutrients reach the bacteria-rich colon, it is not surprising that extreme changes in diet have only slight effects on colonic microorganisms. Certainly the fecal flora does not seem to be at all influenced by the kind of changes in diet that most individuals might reasonably expect to encounter in the ordinary course of their lives.[15]

Bacterial interactions within the gut lumen undoubtedly represent an important, if still poorly understood, determinant of the bacterial populations inhabiting the alimentary canal. Such interactions are numerous and complex and include (1) mutual competition for available nutrients, (2) alteration of intraluminal pH or redox potential, (3) production of toxic metabolites, (4) bowel synthesis of growth factors, (5) enzyme-sharing, and (6) transfer of antibiotic resistance. It is important to recognize, for example, that without the oxygen-utilizing aerobes such as coliforms and enterococci, the colon would not be sufficiently anaerobic to maintain the large populations of fastidious anaerobes such as the bacteroides.[7]

The stability of the colonic flora is undoubtedly related to the complex yet carefully balanced interactions between intestinal microorganisms. Attempts to infect the alimentary canal with specific serotypes of E. coli or with pathogens such as Salmonella, Shigella or Vibrio cholerae are usually unsuccessful except when rather large numbers of microorganisms are introduced. Furthermore, patients who are carriers of S. typhosa or V. cholerae may harbor these organisms in the gallbladder or small bowel at a time when fecal cultures are consistently negative. These organisms survive passage through the prox-

imal small bowel only to be destroyed within the colon by bacterially produced antibiotics such as the "colicines" and certain short-chain fatty acids.

Since antibiotics are widely used, not only as treatment for infections but also as additives in animal feed, one would like to understand the ways in which antibiotics influence the enteric flora. Unfortunately, meaningful generalizations are simply not possible concerning the effects of antibiotics on the microorganisms residing in the gut. The flora itself is extremely complex, and a variety of other factors, including dosage, route of administration, dietary intake, and season of the year, can markedly influence the results obtained with any given antibiotic.[6] Thus in general, it is unwise to base conclusions concerning the effects of the enteric flora on the host on the basis of studies in which the flora is altered by antibiotics. Such effects are much more readily interpreted when germ-free or pathogen-free animals are purposely contaminated with specific bacterial species and strains under controlled conditions.

EFFECTS OF ENTERIC FLORA ON INTESTINAL MORPHOLOGY AND FUNCTION

In many animal species the total absence of an enteric flora as occurs in the germ-free state is associated with marked reduction in the cellular infiltration of the lamina propria and an overall decrease in lymphatic and reticuloendothelial tissue in the intestinal wall.[18] Total intestinal mucosal thickness is reduced in the germ-free state, primarily because of the decreased depth of mucosal crypts. Villi are more slender and more regular in appearance than in conventionally reared healthy animals. The number of mitotic figures in the crypts is significantly reduced, and the rate of regeneration of the intestinal mucosa is clearly slowed in the absence of enteric microorganisms. The lamina propria consists of a sparse stroma containing only a few lymphocytes and mononuclear cells. Plasma cells are absent. Peyer's patches are reduced in size and number and show fewer reactive centers. Since many of these so-called normal characteristics of the mucosa fail to develop in the absence of a bacterial flora, the intestinal mucosa of conventionally reared animals and healthy subjects can be said to be in a state of "physiological inflammation."[18] When the germ-free animal is monocontaminated by cultures of one or another enteric microorganism, the intestinal mucosa rapidly assumes the "normal" appearance observed in conventionally reared animals. Villi become thicker, crypts deepen, and the lamina propria shows increased numbers of lymphocytes, histocytes, and macrophages. Plasma cells make their appearance.

In the total absence of intestinal microorganisms, there occurs a striking dilatation of the cecum associated with the accumulation of watery fluid. In some germ-free rodents, the cecum becomes large enough to account for half the animal's body weight.[19] The mechanism for this enlargement is not at all clear, but it is apparent that as soon as the gut becomes contaminated with *E. coli* or *L. acidophilus* or a mixture of aerobic microorganisms, there occurs a rapid reduction in cecal size. A biologically active peptide present in germ-free cecal contents may play a role in this dramatic cecal enlargement.

Compared with their effects on intestinal morphology, the influence of indigenous intestinal microorganisms on normal intestinal function is much less dramatic. When added to animal feed, antibiotics have a profound effect on nutrition, but the implication that this improved nutrition results from increased absorption of nutrients has in general not been substantiated. The germ-free animal appears to absorb xylose more efficiently than conventional animals, and antibiotics appear to increase the absorption of amino acids and calcium, but these differences are not quantitatively impressive, and except in the case of massive small bowel bacterial overgrowth the indigenous microflora does not seem to greatly affect the absorptive process.

There can be no question, however, that even in the healthy individual enteric microorganisms play an important, sometimes a critical, role in the intraluminal metabolism of a variety of substances.[7] Of particular importance is the effect of intestinal bacteria on the metabolism of various sterols and steroids, including bile acids. The primary bile acids synthesized by the liver (cholic and chenodeoxycholic acid) are conjugated with taurine or glycine, and these conjugates are excreted in the bile. In the absence of intestinal bacteria, hydrolysis of conjugated bile acids does not occur, whereas in the intestine of conventionally reared animals or man, bacterial conversion of conjugated to free bile acids is complete and can be demonstrated in vitro with pure cultures of a variety of microorganisms, including clostridia, enterococci, and bacteroides. Enteric microorganisms also remove the hydroxyl group at the 7 position of the primary bile acids. This results in conversion of cholic to deoxycholic acid while chenodeoxycholic is converted to lithocholic acid. The turnover of bile acids is slowed in absence of intestinal bacteria, and the total body pool is increased. These changes have been attributed to increased intestinal reabsorption and diminished fecal loss of bile salts. When bacteria are present in the lower intestinal tract, bile salt metabolites bind to enteric microorganisms so that these metabolites are not available for reabsorption. In addition to deconjugation and dehydroxylation, intestinal bacteria oxidize bile salts at C3, C7, and C12 to form a variety of keto acids which can subsequently be reduced to either alpha or beta hydroxyl groups. Finally bacterial action can result in the production of unsaturated derivatives of bile salts. Thus it is not surprising that a large number of bile salt metabolites are formed within the lumen of the distal bowel as a result of bacterial metabolism.

Little is known about the effects of the normal enteric flora upon the metabolism of unabsorbed lipids. It is clear, however, that bacterial lipase hydrolyzes glycerides within the lumen of the colon. Furthermore, bacteria synthesize lipids from simpler organic compounds such as acetate, and there is considerable evidence that fecal fatty acids differ from dietary fatty acids. The unusual branched and hydroxylated fatty acids recovered from feces result from bacterial synthesis. It is possible in vitro to demonstrate conversion of long-chain fatty acids to hydroxy fatty acids with pure cultures of a variety of microorganisms. Whether bacterially produced fatty acids, particularly the hydroxylated fatty acids, contribute to diarrhea is a subject under current consideration. Ricinoleic acid is a hydroxylated fatty acid which appears to be the active constituent of castor oil.

Bacterial metabolism of proteins and the other nitrogenous compounds has important physiological and clinical implications. Enteric bacteria degrade protein and urea within the intestinal lumen to produce ammonia. Ammonia production in antibiotic-treated or germ-free animals is markedly reduced. Although the implications of this ammonia production in health are not at all understood, the bacterial production becomes important when the body is unable to handle ammonia properly because of hepatic insufficiency or a primary metabolic defect in the urea cycle. It is apparent that the quantity of ammonia produced by enteric microorganisms depends not only on the kind and number of bacteria present but also upon the nature and quantity of substrate available to these bacteria. There is abundant clinical evidence to indicate that substantial reduction in the intestinal bacterial populations of man is associated with decreased serum and spinal fluid levels of ammonia and concomitant improvement in hepatic encephalopathy. This is most commonly accomplished by the administration of poorly absorbed, broad-spectrum antibiotics together with cathartics and enemas. Bacterial populations can also be effectively reduced when the colon is excised or bypassed, but this approach may be of limited value, because ultimately the ileum may dilate and become the site of profuse intestinal growth. The feeding of lactulose, a sugar which cannot be digested by intestinal disaccharidases and which is absorbed poorly if at all, results in diarrhea and diminished blood ammonia levels. Bacterial metabolism of the unabsorbed sugar results in the production of organic acids and lowered intraluminal pH which, in turn, prevents ammonia absorption. Although lactulose does increase the numbers of lactobacilli, the urea-splitting organisms such as the coliforms are by no means displaced by lactobacilli when lactulose is fed.

Other important substances subjected to bacterial metabolism within the intestinal lumen include pancreatic enzymes, bilirubin, mucus, and a variety of drugs. It should be emphasized that biologically active compounds other than ammonia may result from microbial action within the intestinal lumen. It has been suggested that a number of incompletely characterized organic substances produced by intestinal microorganisms accumulate in the blood when normal disposal is inadequate because of hepatic or renal failure.[20] There is experimental and clinical evidence to show that by reducing the amount of nitrogenous substrate available to the normal microflora, one can distinctly improve the course of hepatic or renal insufficiency. The nature of these bacterially produced enteric "toxins" remains poorly delineated, but there is considerable evidence that several aromatic compounds are derived from bacterial metabolism within the intestinal lumen.[6]

One source of these aromatic compounds is tryptophan, which is decarboxylated by bacteria to form a biologically active amine, tryptamine. Further bacterial metabolism of tryptophan and tryptamine results in the production of a variety of indolic compounds. Increased excretion of indolic substances, including indoxyl sulfate (indican), is observed in clinical and experimental disorders in which either bacteria are proliferating in the small bowel or the amount of unabsorbed nitrogenous substrate reaching the bacteria-rich colon is increased. Although an important biological effect of bacterially produced aromatic compounds has never been convincingly demonstrated, further investigations concerned with the possible pathophysiological implications of these substances are clearly indicated.

The role of the indigenous intestinal microflora in the intraluminal metabolism of sugars undoubtedly has important implications for the host. When a nonabsorbable sugar such as lactulose is ingested or when the host, because of disaccharidase deficiency or because of small bowel disease, is unable to absorb the usual dietary sugars, the unabsorbed carbohydrate is rapidly metabolized within the colon. Bacterial disaccharidases split dietary sugars such as maltose and lactose and metabolize the resulting monosaccharides to form lactate, acetate, butyrate, and other organic acids. Formation of these organic acids increases the osmolarity and reduces the pH of colonic contents, two factors which may contribute importantly to the pH production of diarrhea. Impaired absorption of carbohydrates and subsequent production of organic acids have been clearly implicated in the pathogenesis of nonspecific diarrhea in infancy.[21] Impaired glucose absorption, lowered stool pH, increased serum lactate, and a metabolic acidosis have been convincingly documented in infants with nonspecific diarrhea, with monosaccharide malabsorption, and with disaccharidase deficiency.

THE PATHOPHYSIOLOGICAL IMPLICATIONS OF SMALL BOWEL BACTERIAL OVERGROWTH

When the normal bacterial populations of the gut proliferate abnormally within the small bowel lumen, the metabolic consequences can be profound.[8, 10] Although there is at present no persuasive evidence that the presence of normal numbers of indigenous intestinal microorganisms impairs the absorptive capacity of the healthy host, malabsorption and consequent malnutrition often accompany an overgrowth of bacteria within the small bowel lumen.

Since, as outlined above, normal gastric secretion combined with the mechanical cleansing action of normal small bowel peristalsis constitutes the host's major defense against small bowel bacterial overgrowth, it is not surprising that bacterial proliferation within the small bowel lumen is most marked when, for whatever reason, there is stasis of small bowel contents, particularly when such stasis is combined with impaired or absent gastric acid secretion. The specific disorders known to be associated with small bowel bacterial overgrowth are discussed on pages 927 to 936, and it is necessary to state here only that any small bowel abnormality conducive to local stasis or recirculation of small bowel contents is likely to be accompanied by marked intraluminal proliferation of microorganisms. There is also considerable evidence that gastric atrophy and gastric surgery that effectively prevent gastric acid secretion also increase the number of microorganisms residing in the small bowel lumen. Although small bowel lesions conducive to stasis are clearly of primary importance in the pathogenesis of the so-called blind loop or stagnant syndrome, a contributory role for gastric achlorhydria must be seriously considered, because the syndrome occurs more frequently among elderly than among young patients and because gastric surgery with or without readily demonstrable concomitant small bowel stasis may be followed by clinically significant bacterial overgrowth.

The bacterial populations present in the small bowel lumen of patients or experimental animals with small bowel bacterial overgrowth are extremely complex.[4] The microorganisms cultured from the jejunum in this situation are those normally found in the colon, and in fact the small bowel flora closely resembles that observed in colonic contents or feces. The numbers of microorganisms present are often truly impressive, and it is not at all unusual to find 10^8 to 10^{10} viable microorganisms per gram of small bowel content. Bacteroides and anaerobic lactobacilli often predominate, but coliforms, enterococci, clostridia, and diphtheroids may also be present in high concentrations. Indeed, the most characteristic aspect of the microbiology of small bowel bacterial overgrowth is the complexity of the microbial populations present. When microbiological techniques are adequate, one can consistently find ten to twenty different bacterial species present in the small bowel contents of patients and experimental animals with metabolically significant small bowel bacterial overgrowth.

Vitamin B_{12} malabsorption regularly accompanies significant proliferation of bacteria within the small bowel. In fact, the most consistent feature of clinically significant small bowel bacterial overgrowth in patients and in experimental animals is abnormal vitamin B_{12} absorption which is not corrected by intrinsic factor. When the bacterial populations of the small bowel are definitely reduced, either by antibiotic therapy or by appropriate surgical correction of the small bowel lesion, absorption of the vitamin both in the clinical and in the experimental blind loop syndrome promptly returns to normal. Investigations to date have failed to demonstrate that bacteria produce an inhibitor capable of impairing any of the normal mechanisms for absorption of the vitamin, and it is apparent that malabsorption of vitamin B_{12} requires direct contact with the bacteria. There are, in addition, several observations which support the concept that enteric bacteria proliferating in the small bowel directly compete for dietary vitamin B_{12} and thus prevent absorption of the vitamin by the intestinal cell.[22] If one administers radioactive B_{12} to experimental animals or to patients with small bowel bacterial overgrowth, nearly all the radioactivity subsequently recovered from small bowel contents is firmly bound to enteric microorganisms. By injecting intrinsic factor–bound vitamin B_{12} directly into the blind pouch of an experimental animal, it is possible directly to demonstrate successful competition for the vitamin by bacteria within the bowel lumen.

Competitive uptake of the vitamin is particularly characteristic of gram-negative enteric microorganisms. Intrinsic factor effectively inhibits microbial uptake of vitamin B_{12}; nevertheless intestinal bacteria have a definite, although limited, capacity to bind the vitamin even when it is bound to intrinsic factor.[10, 22] When intrinsic factor is present, uptake of the vitamin by enteric microorganisms is slow, and consequently the extent of stasis in the small bowel lumen is probably an important factor in determining whether or not bacterial competition for the vitamin is successful. Further studies are required to determine whether enteric microorganisms alter the intrinsic factor–vitamin B_{12} complex in some way, preventing absorption of the vitamin by the intestinal cell and thus favoring bacterial uptake.

Enteric microorganisms proliferating in the small bowel also synthesize vitamin B_{12}, and thus are a rich source of this vitamin. Since the vitamin is contained within viable microorganisms, however, it is totally unavailable to the host. When vitamin B_{12} is bound to dead microorganisms and fed to rats, it is absorbed normally.[23] On the other hand, when the vitamin is bound to viable coliforms, it is poorly absorbed. The dead bacteria are digested and the vitamin becomes available for absorption by the host. Viable microorganisms, however, pass intact through the small bowel and into the colon, and any vitamin B_{12} taken up by these viable microorganisms never becomes available for use by the host. Thus in patients with small bowel bacterial overgrowth one is faced with a paradoxical situation: vitamin B_{12} deficiency develops in spite of the presence of large quantities of the vitamin in the small bowel lumen.

Enteric microorganisms synthesize not only vitamin B_{12} but also folic acid. In the case of folic acid, however, folate is released by the bacteria into the surrounding environment and thus becomes available for absorption by the host. Thus it is not surprising that folate deficiency is rare among patients with small bowel bacterial overgrowth and is most likely to occur in those patients with bacterial overgrowth associated with extremely complicated gastrointestinal disorders. Indeed bacterial production and release of folate in the lumen of the jejunum often lead to abnormally high rather than low serum folate levels.[24]

Since steatorrhea occurs in about one-third of patients with clinically significant small bowel overgrowth, and since this steatorrhea clearly does not result from endogenous overproduction of lipid, it is apparent that proliferation of enteric microorganisms within the small bowel lumen has a deleterious effect on normal fat absorption. Simple competition of bacteria for dietary lipid does not seem a plausible explanation. In the case of vitamin B_{12}, bacteria successfully compete for at most one or two micrograms of the vitamin. In the case of fat malabsorption, many grams of lipid are involved. Furthermore, unlike the situation with vitamin B_{12}, when radioactive triglyceride is administered to patients or to experimental animals with small bowel bacterial overgrowth, less than 1 per cent of radioactivity recovered from the small bowel lumen is bound to enteric microorganisms.[25] Similarly, it does not appear likely that bacteria proliferating within the lumen of the small intestine impair lipid absorption as a result of bacterial damage to the intestinal epithelium. Although in some patients there occurs a patchy inflammatory lesion of the small bowel mucosa in the presence of small bowel bacterial overgrowth, intestinal mucosal architecture does not appear to be consistently or severely damaged. Indeed, most reports indicate that the intestinal epithelial cell is normal by light and electron microscopy.[10] Although mild inflammatory changes in the mucosa may contribute to fat malabsorption in the blind loop syndrome, it seems unlikely that disturbances in mucosal structure play a quantitatively important role. Several investigators have demonstrated that intraluminal hydrolysis of dietary triglyceride proceeds normally in patients and experimental animals with small bowel bacterial overgrowth.[26] Thus it seems unlikely that bacterial destruction of pancreatic lipase is involved in blind loop steatorrhea.

At present there is general agreement that enteric bacteria proliferating within the proximal small bowel lumen have a profound effect upon bile salt metabolism and that altered bile salt metabolism is the major factor responsible for fat malabsorption and steatorrhea in the blind loop syndrome. As described above, enteric bacteria rapidly hydrolyze glycine and taurine conjugates of cholic, chenodeoxycholic, and deoxycholic acid. Fastidious anaerobes, normally present in the colon but also predominant when there is stasis of small bowel contents, are particularly active in deconjugation of the bile salts. There are several reasons for believing that bacterial conversion of conjugated bile salts to free bile acids leads to impaired fat absorption. At the pH of intestinal contents, conjugated bile salts exist as fully ionized, water-soluble bile salts capable of solubilizing the products of fat digestion in micellar solutions. These ionized bile salts are not readily reabsorbed from the proximal intestine and thus remain where they are needed within the small bowel lumen. In order to be reabsorbed, conjugated bile salts require a specific transport mechanism present only in the ileum.[27] Thus efficient reabsorption of conjugated bile salts occurs only from the distal small bowel. On the other hand, at the pH of intestinal contents free bile acids are present as protonated bile acids which are relatively insoluble in water and thus do not attain concentrations sufficient to form micelles. Ionized conjugated bile salts have a limited capacity to solubilize un-ionized free bile acids. It appears that four or five conjugated bile salt molecules

are required to hold one free bile acid molecule in micellar solution. Thus if the rate of bacterial hydrolysis in the proximal small bowel lumen is such that more than 20 per cent of the bile acids present are deconjugated, bile salt micelle formation is impaired. Any free bile acids formed are rapidly reabsorbed from the proximal intestine by passive nonionic diffusion. In additon, the free bile acid may precipitate from solution as bile acid crystals which, in some cases, may enlarge to form bile acid enteroliths. The overall result is a reduction in intestinal bile salt concentration below the level necessary for effective solubilization of monoglyceride and fatty acid formation during the digestion of dietary triglyceride. It is thus apparent that the severity of bile salt deficiency which develops in the presence of jejunal bacterial overgrowth will vary, depending upon the rate of bacterial hydrolysis, the pH of intestinal contents, and the rate of reabsorption of free bile acids.

There is considerable evidence to support the idea that relative deficiency of effective bile salts develops when intestinal bacteria proliferate within the proximal small bowel lumen.[28] Thus, for example, it has been possible to demonstrate diminished jejunal bile salt concentration and a decreased proportion of lipid present in an absorbable micellar phase in patients with the blind loop syndrome and in dogs with experimentally produced small bowel bacterial overgrowth and steatorrhea. Furthermore if such dogs are fed conjugated bile salts, fecal fat excretion is reduced.

Although accumulation of abnormal, "toxic" bile salts has been implicated in the pathogenesis of fat malabsorption, this appears to be a less likely mechanism. Because free bile acids, and particularly free deoxycholic acid, inhibit the uptake and esterification of fatty acids by intestinal tissue in vitro, it has been suggested that bacterial formation of deoxycholic acid within the small bowel might result in impaired intestinal mucosal function.[25] However, the in vitro effects of free bile acids are extremely nonspecific, are probably due to dissolution of cellular membranous elements as a result of unphysiological accumulation of free bile acids within the intestinal cell, have not been satisfactorily reproduced in intact animals, and are associated with morphologic alterations not found in patients or experimental animals with small bowel bacterial overgrowth and steatorrhea. At present there is no convincing evidence that "toxic" metabolites of bile salts accumulate as a result of bacterial overgrowth and cause direct harm to the host.

Although deficiency of normal rather than accumulation of abnormal bile salts appears to be responsible for steatorrhea in patients with the blind loop syndrome, the entire question of how indigenous microorganisms proliferating within the proximal small bowel lumen cause fat malabsorption is far from settled. A truly satisfactory evaluation of the effects of small bacterial overgrowth on bile salt metabolism requires determinations of pool, rate of recirculation, and turnover of individual bile salts in intact patients or animals with the blind loop syndrome, and such information is not yet available. Complete biliary diversion results in steatorrhea which is often much less severe than that observed in certain patients with small bowel bacterial overgrowth. Thus it seems unlikely that a relative deficiency of bile salts completely explains the fat malabsorption which develops in the blind loop syndrome. An important unanswered question is whether or not proliferation of microorganisms within the small bowel lumen produces lipid malabsorption over and above that brought about by complete biliary diversion. Further information is required concerning the role of bacterial hydroxylation of fatty acids and whether such hydroxylation contributes to lipid malabsorption. Since indigenous microorganisms present in the colon or those proliferating in the small bowel are capable of hydroxylation, studies are needed to determine the effects of hydroxy fatty acids on small bowel function. Also needed, of course, are investigations into the effects of bacteria upon dietary lipids in relation to fat malabsorption.

The effects of small bowel bacterial overgrowth on the metabolism and absorption of proteins and carbohydrates are not at all clear. Although low levels of serum proteins are a fairly regular feature of the clinical blind loop syndrome, little is known about the digestion, intraluminal metabolism, absorption, and enteric losses of protein in the presence of small bowel bacterial proliferation. One detailed study of protein metabolism in a patient with the blind loop syndrome demonstrated increased conversion of dietary protein to urea with a corresponding reduction in the formation of serum proteins.[24] These changes were most likely due to bacterial deamination of dietary amino acids within the small bowel lumen, but more detailed biochemical assessment of these phenomena is clearly needed. Abnormal xylose tolerance tests have been observed in some, but by no means all, patients with the blind loop syndrome.[30] Several enteric microorganisms are capable of metabolizing xylose, and it is possible that intraluminal destruction of xylose accounts for the abnormal xylose tolerance tests in some patients. Although, as described above, enteric microorganisms convert unabsorbed carbohydrate to organic acids and hydrogen, the extent to which this occurs in the clinical and experimental blind loop syndrome has not been delineated.

THE ROLE OF INDIGENOUS ENTERIC MICROORGANISMS IN DIARRHEAL DISORDERS

During an episode of acute diarrhea the enteric flora may be markedly altered.[4] When a pathogen can be clearly identified, the concentrations of the pathogen in feces may be very high and there may be concomitant reduction in the numbers of normal microorganisms. Thus, for example, during active diarrhea caused by V. cholerae, Shigella, Salmonella, or pathogenic E. coli, the concentration of the pathogen in feces is of the order of 10^7 to 10^9 viable organisms per milliliter. On the other hand, there usually occurs a simultaneous reduction in the concentration of anaerobes. Thus in patients with acute cholera or diarrhea associated with enteropathogenic E. coli the concentrations of anaerobes may decrease from 10^{10} to 10^{11} down to 10^5 organisms per milliliter. Since a similar decrease in the number of anaerobes can be demonstrated in experimentally induced catharsis, it seems likely that rapid passage through the bowel produces unfavorable conditions for maintenance and growth of fastidious anaerobes. Thus an "imbalance" of the normal enteric flora which occurs in any diarrheal disorder may have important pathophysiological consequences.

In general, there are three ways in which the indigenous microflora may contribute to the development of specific enteric infections. Since, as described above, the microbial populations of the gut tend to resist invasion by pathogenic bacteria, alteration of the "normal" intestinal flora may increase susceptibility to colonization by pathogens. Secondly, microorganisms often present in the healthy intestine may themselves become pathogenic and cause enteritis. Finally, since many of the enteric bacteria possess a "transfer factor" capable of transferring antibiotic resistance from one species or strain to another, the normal enteric flora may alter the susceptibility of pathogens to antibiotics.

There is considerable evidence to suggest that the indigenous microflora tends to suppress proliferation of enteropathogenic bacteria. Salmonellae, for example, do not ordinarily colonize mouse intestine, but certain strains of S. enteritidis proliferate readily when mice are pretreated with streptomycin. Similar studies have shown that antibiotics increase the susceptibility of mice to infection with S. typhimurium, of guinea pigs to Shigella and V. cholerae infection, and of mice to enteropathogenic strains of E. coli. Furthermore, germ-free mice and guinea pigs show an increased susceptibility to infection with Salmonella and Shigella. The normal microorganisms specifically responsible for resistance to invasion by pathogens have not been clearly delineated, but there is some evidence that Bacteroides and nonpathogenic E. coli play an important role.

In patients with so-called nonspecific diarrhea, proliferation of indigenous microorganisms such as Klebsiella, Aerobacter, Proteus, and Pseudomonas may be found in large numbers in fecal samples.[4] Although it is tempting to speculate that such microorganisms become pathogenic in cases of nonspecific diarrhea, the mere finding of increased numbers of these microorganisms does not by itself provide convincing evidence that they are in fact pathogenic. Nevertheless, the fact remains that many instances of so-called nonspe-

cific diarrhea occur in situations where one might expect marked alterations in the enteric flora. This is certainly the case in traveler's diarrhea in which an individual is exposed to a completely different environment and climate, in weanling diarrhea which occurs at a time when the infant is exposed to large numbers of microorganisms for the first time, and in the diarrhea which occurs following the administration of antibiotics.

Whether diarrhea in these situations truly results from the presence of one or more microorganisms which at that particular time becomes pathogenic for that particular host is an important question which remains to be settled. Unquestionably, however, there do exist enteropathogenic strains of E. coli which produce acute diarrhea, particularly in children. Enteropathogenic strains of E. coli are regularly cultured from the feces of infected individuals, and the disease can be reproduced by feeding these organisms to healthy volunteers. It would appear that for diarrhea to occur as a result of infection with enteropathogenic strains of E. coli, the organism must colonize the upper intestinal tract. Enteropathogenic strains of E. coli obtained from patients with diarrhea produce fluid accumulation and dilatation when placed in isolated loops of rabbit intestine. Further studies have shown that these strains elaborate a filterable exotoxin which stimulates secretion by rabbit small bowel.

Such toxin-producing strains of E. coli have recently been implicated in approximately 50 per cent of a group of patients with "undifferentiated" diarrhea occurring in the tropics.[17] Enteropathogenic strains were isolated not only from the feces but also from the small intestine, and broth filtrates from such strains produced fluid accumulation when tested in isolated rabbit intestinal loops. Furthermore, abnormal secretion of fluid and electrolytes by the jejunum and ileum could be demonstrated in these patients during their diarrheal illness. Although toxin-producing enteropathogenic strains of E. coli may exist in the colon of asymptomatic carriers, it would appear that conditions conducive to significant infection within the small bowel are required before diarrhea ensues.

Acute bacterial diarrhea can be induced

by at least two distinct mechanisms. First, the microorganisms may elaborate a filterable exotoxin which, perhaps by causing the accumulation of cyclic AMP, results in an abnormal secretion of salt and water by the intestinal epithelial cell. The microorganism does not penetrate the intestinal epithelium, and biopsy samples of the small bowel mucosa are normal. Diarrhea resulting from this mechanism is typically seen in patients with cholera and in those with enteropathogenic E. coli infections (see pp. 291 to 316). On the other hand, as appears to be the case with Salmonella and Shigella infections, the pathogen may penetrate the small or large intestine and, as a result of this penetration, produce mucosal alterations which result in increased secretion of fluid and electrolytes.

The normal microbial flora can also influence infectious diarrheas by directly affecting the sensitivity of the pathogen to antibiotics. Resistance to one or several antibiotics can be transferred from one enteric microorganism to another by means of self-replicating extrachromosomal genetic elements that resemble episomes and are called R factors.[31] The transfer of drug resistance from one bacterial cell to another is mediated by a portion of the R factor known as the "resistance transfer factor." Transferable resistance to penicillin, ampicillin, streptomycin, tetracycline, various sulfonamides, furazolidone, kanamycin, and neomycin or to any combination of these drugs has been demonstrated. In fact, an R factor conveying simultaneous resistance to seven antibiotics, all transferred at one time, has been described. The extent to which the transfer of antibiotic resistance from one strain to another is of clinical significance in acute diarrheal disorders remains questionable, but it is clear that indigenous Enterobacteriaceae resistant to one or several antibiotics can transfer this resistance to pathogenic microorganisms.

TROPICAL SPRUE

The possibility that tropical sprue results from an imbalance of the enteric flora or from infection by some pathogenic microorganism is supported by several obser-vations.[32] Tropical sprue often begins as an episode of acute gastroenteritis which then progresses to the more typical chronic malabsorption. Epidemics of tropical sprue have been described in prisoner-of-war camps and in villages in South India. The inflammatory changes observed in small bowel mucosal biopsy specimens from patients with tropical sprue are consistent with a bacterial effect. Impressive and lasting remissions consistently follow treatment with broad-spectrum antibiotics.

Although indirect evidence of this sort suggests a possible role for enteric microorganisms in the pathogenesis of tropical sprue, it is apparent that tropical sprue cannot merely be considered one of the disorders resulting from proliferation of bacteria within the small bowel lumen. There are in fact distinct differences between tropical sprue and the blind loop syndrome.[4, 7] Folate deficiency is rare in the blind loop syndrome but is a cardinal feature of the tropical sprue. Although administration of folate clearly benefits the tropical sprue patient, it has no such effect on the patient with the blind loop syndrome. Small bowel biopsies from patients with tropical sprue often show marked distortion of villous architecture not seen in the blind loop syndrome. Steatorrhea and vitamin B_{12} malabsorption in the blind loop syndrome can be corrected within a few days by appropriate administration of antibiotics. In patients with tropical sprue, however, meaningful response to antibiotics usually requires several weeks. Although the numbers of microorganisms present in the lumen of the small bowel may be slightly increased in tropical sprue patients, the massive bacterial overgrowth seen in those with the blind loop syndrome cannot be considered a feature of the patient with tropical sprue.

Since deficiencies of folate, vitamin B_{12}, or protein all favor the development of intestinal mucosal abnormalities, it is possible that even mild deficiencies of one or more of these nutrients might increase the mucosal susceptibility to injury by a microorganism which in the healthy host would be nonpathogenic. Certainly correction of folate deficiency followed by continued administration of folic acid produces prolonged remission in patients with tropical sprue. Acute diarrhea, particularly when it occurs in the tropics, can be associated with transient but definite inflammatory changes in the small bowel, vitamin B_{12} malabsorption, and steatorrhea. Thus, although far from proved, the disorder known as tropical sprue may in fact result from a combination of factors, including invasion by microorganisms which tend to flourish in the tropics, subclinical deficiency of critical nutrients, and pathophysiological alterations resulting from diarrhea (see pp. 978 to 987).

REFERENCES

1. Dubos, R. J., Schaedler, R. W., and Costello, R. L. Composition, alteration and effects of the intestinal flora. Fed. Proc. 22:1313, 1963.
2. Mickelsen, O. Nutrition: Germfree animal research. Ann. Rev. Biochem. 31:515, 1962.
3. Dubos, R., and Schaedler, R. W. Some biological effects of the digestive flora. Amer. J. Med. Sci. 244:265, 1962.
4. Gorbach, S. L. Intestinal microflora. Gastroenterology 60:1110, 1971.
5. Scheline, R. R. Drug metabolism by intestinal microorganisms. J. Pharm. Sci. 57:2021, 1968.
6. Donaldson, R. M. Normal bacterial populations of the intestine and their relation to intestinal function. New Eng. J. Med. 270:938, 994, 1050, 1964.
7. Donaldson, R. M. Role of indigenous enteric bacteria in intestinal function and disease. In Handbook of Physiology. Baltimore, Williams and Wilkins Co., 1968.
8. Donaldson, R. M. Small bowel bacterial overgrowth. Advan. Intern. Med. 16:191, 1970.
9. Gorbach, S. L., and Levitan, R. Intestinal flora in health and in gastrointestinal diseases. In Progress in Gastroenterology, Vol. 2, G. B. J. Glass (ed.). New York, Grune and Stratton, 1970.
10. Tabaqchali, S. The pathophysiological role of small intestinal bacterial flora. Scand. J. Gastroenterol. 5(Suppl. 6):139, 1970.
11. Savage, D. C., Dubos, R., and Schaedler, R. W. The gastrointestinal epithelium and its autochthonous bacterial flora. J. Exp. Med. 127:67, 1968.
12. Gorbach, S. L., Plaut, A. G., Nahas, L., et al. Studies of intestinal microflora. II. Microorganisms of the small intestine and their relations to oral and fecal flora. Gastroenterology 53:856, 1967.
13. Bishop, R. F., and Anderson, C. M. Bacterial flora of stomach and small intestine in children with intestinal obstruction. Arch Dis. Child. 35:487, 1960.
14. Gorbach, S. L., Nahas, J., and Weinstein, L. Studies of intestinal microflora. IX. The microflora of ileostomy effluent: A unique microbial ecology. Gastroenterology 53:874, 1967.
15. Gorbach, S. L., Nahas, L., and Lerner, P. I. Studies of intestinal microflora. I. Effects of diet, age and periodic sampling on numbers of fecal microorganisms in man. Gastroenterology 53:845, 1967.
16. Dubos, R. Indigenous, normal and autochthonous flora of the gastrointestinal tract. J. Exp. Med. 122:67, 1965.
17. Gorbach, S. L., Banwell, J. G., and Chatterjee, B. D. Acute undifferentiated diarrhea in the tropics. I. Alterations in intestinal microflora. J. Clin. Invest. 50:881, 1971.
18. Abrams, G. D., Bauer, H., and Sprinz, H. Influence of the normal flora on mucosal morphology and cellular renewal in the ileum. A comparison of germ-free and conventional mice. Lab. Invest. 12:355, 1963.
19. Gordon, H. A. Morphological and physiological characterization of germ-free life. Ann. New York Acad. Sci. 78:208, 1959.
20. Kramer, B., Seligson, H., Bathush, H., and Seligson, D. The isolation of several aromatic acids from hemodialysis fluids of uremia patients. Clin. Chim. Acta 11:363, 1965.
21. Torres-Pinedo, R., Lavastida, M., Rivera, C. L., Rodriquez, H., and Ortez, A. Studies on infant diarrhea. I. A comparison of the effects of milk feeding and intravenous therapy upon the composition and volume of the stool and urine. J. Clin. Invest. 45:469, 1966.
22. Donaldson, R. M., Corrigan, H., and Natsios, G. Malabsorption of Co^{60}-labeled cyanocobalamin in rats with intestinal diverticula. II. Studies on contents of the diverticula. Gastroenterology 43:282, 1962.
23. Booth, C. C., and Health, J. The effect of E. coli on the absorption of vitamin B_{12}. Gut 3:70, 1962.
24. Hoffbrand, A. V., Tabaqchali, S., and Mollin, D. High serum-folate levels in intestinal blind loop syndrome. Lancet 1:1339, 1966.
25. Donaldson, R. M. Studies on the pathogenesis of steatorrhea in the blind loop syndrome. J. Clin. Invest. 44:1815, 1965.
26. Donaldson, R. M. Intestinal bacterial and malabsorption. Ann. Intern. Med. 64:948, 1962.
27. Dietschy, J. M. Mechanisms for the intestinal absorption of bile acids. J. Lipid Res., 9:297, 1968.
28. Kim, Y. S., Spritz, N., Blum, M., Terz, J., and Sherlock, P. The role of altered bile acid metabolism in the steatorrhea of experimental blind loop. J. Clin. Invest. 45:956, 1966.
29. Jones, E. A., Craigie, A., Tavill, A. S., Franglen, G., and Rosenoer, V. M. Protein metabolism in the intestinal stagnant loop syndrome. Gut 9:466, 1968.
30. Donaldson, R. M. Role of enteric microorganisms in malabsorption. Fed. Proc. 26:1426, 1967.
31. Watanabe, T. Infectious drug resistance in enteric bacteria. New Eng. J. Med. 275:888, 1966.
32. Klipstein, F. A. Progress in gastroenterology: Tropical sprue. Gastroenterology 54:275, 1968.

THE ESOPHAGUS

Chapter 7

Physiology

Charles E. Pope II

Although the esophagus is not anatomically exciting, modern investigation of its transport functions and control has inspired new respect for this hitherto disregarded organ.[1] The description of its function must, of necessity, be highly dependent on the method, or methods, used to describe the events. In the description of esophageal physiology certain methods have been predominant. They include radiology with cinefluorography, intraluminal manometric studies, and measurement of electrical activity. Often these methods are mutually incompatible for simultaneous studies, and occasionally unwarranted assumptions have been made by combining the results of two different types of investigations without first making sure that in fact these observations were comparable.

Cineradiography is a technique which is becoming more available in many medical centers. High speed filming of the rapid events occurring during the transport of barium by the esophagus allows replay at slower speeds or frame-by-frame analysis. Transit time of barium can be analyzed and structural and volumetric relationships can be analyzed. However, muscular force of contraction cannot be measured and sphincters cannot be evaluated.

Intraluminal manometry has given great impetus to the study of mechanics of the gastrointestinal tract in general and has found greatest applicability to the description of peristaltic events in the esophagus. Early in manometric measurement, large balloons were used as sensing elements, and high-volume displacement pressure measuring devices were employed. The introduction of low-volume displacement transducers used in cardiac catheterization work has led to the use of fluid-filled end- or side-opening catheters. These catheters are often cemented together in a bundle so that the recording tip of each catheter is a known distance from the other tips. This allows recognition of peristalsis and the calculation of peristaltic velocity. If a constant infusion pump is connected to a side-arm on each catheter, then accurate estimates of sphincter strength and peristaltic force of closure can be obtained.

UPPER ESOPHAGEAL SPHINCTER AND PHARYNX

Combined cine-manometric studies have been essential in understanding the very rapid events that occur as swallowing is initiated.[2] When a manometric catheter is slowly advanced through the oral cavity, atmospheric pressure is recorded until the catheter approaches the bottom of the pharyngeal air column. Pressure is then observed to rise; it reaches a peak between the fifth and sixth cervical vertebrae. This high pressure zone extends over a length of approximately 2 cm. As the catheter passes beyond this zone of high pressure, the values recorded are slightly negative, respiratory variations are noted, and a swallow of barium demonstrates that the catheter tip is now in the upper portion of the cervical esophagus.

When a train of catheters is positioned along this pathway and a swallow of thin barium is given, several events are observed. The catheter tips proximal to the high pressure zone record an initial spike which is observed to correlate with elevation of the larynx. A secondary transitory spike is observed as the tongue thrusts the liquid bolus back in the retropharyngeal area, and the complex is terminated by a high monophasic pressure wave which occurs when a stripping pharyngeal wave passes through the retropharynx.

In the area of the high pressure zone there is an abrupt drop in recorded pressure at the moment of deglutition. This is maintained as the barium column passes through the area; most of the barium has cleared the zone before the high pressure zone is re-established. This sequence is the manometric evidence for a sphincter at the upper end of the esophagus (Fig. 7–1).

Resting pressure values in the upper esophageal sphincter are a function of the recording method. If balloons of different sizes are used, attached to a water-filled catheter and a pressure transducer, values of 41.8 mm, 153 mm, and 215 mm Hg are obtained for balloons 0.4 cm, 0.6 cm, and 0.8 cm in diameter, respectively.[3] If constant infusion is used, values ranging from 40 to 150 mm Hg are obtained. There is a great deal of variability from pull-through to pull-through and from tip to tip. It is not certain whether this represents intrinsically changing values of the sphincter or a problem in methodology. The latter possibility is the most likely. This marked variability makes studies of the upper esophageal sphincter somewhat difficult.

Factors influencing the tension of the upper esophageal sphincter have not been thoroughly investigated. If a balloon is distended in the esophagus below the upper sphincter, there is an increase in pressure recorded from the sphincter zone. This increase is present as long as balloon distention is maintained. It has been suggested that acid in the esophagus is a stimulus for increase in pressure in the upper esophageal sphincter.

A link between the control of upper and lower esophageal sphincter strength has been suggested. As the strength of the lower esophageal sphincter is caused to vary, there are corresponding alterations in the upper esophageal sphincter force of closure. More definitive studies of these relationships must await better methods of

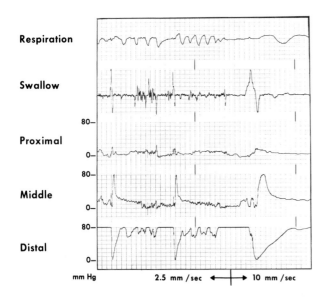

Figure 7–1.   Manometric tracing of upper esophageal sphincter. A catheter with three tips 1 cm apart was used. The distal tip was infused at 2.4 ml per min; the other tips were not infused. Respirations are shown in the top channel, inspiration producing a negative deflection. Deglutition is signaled by a spike appearing in the channel labeled Swallow. The proximal and middle tips are located in the pharyngeal cavity. The distal tip is in the upper esophageal sphincter and registers a pressure of 80 mm Hg. There is a drop in pressure to atmospheric level on deglutition. At a faster paper speed, it is seen that the pharyngeal pressure spike shown by the middle tip occurs while the sphincter is relaxed.

measuring upper esophageal sphincter strength.

BODY OF THE ESOPHAGUS

Events in the main portion of the esophagus are stimulated most commonly by deglutition. In normal man the lumen of the esophagus is obliterated by a wave which passes from the upper esophageal sphincter to the area of the lower esophageal sphincter. Radiologically, this is noted as a displacement of a barium bolus toward the stomach and a stripping of the barium from the lumen in a progressive manner. Manometrically, the deglutition complex can be comprised of several waves. In approximately one-third of the swallows in normal subjects there is a very brief negative wave which coincides with actual deglutition. Simultaneous measurements of intraesophageal and intrapleural pressure tracings reveal that this negative wave was only seen when a corresponding negative dip was recorded from the pleural space.[4] The most prominent manometric event is a monophasic positive wave caused by the obliteration of the lumen by peristalsis. When this primary peristaltic wave is triggered by a swallow of water, a rise in baseline esophageal pressure is observed which is then terminated by the high-amplitude wave produced by contraction of the esophagus on the pressure tip (Fig. 7–2). If multiple recording sites are used, it can be demonstrated that the third or peristaltic wave occurs sequentially along the length of the esophagus (Fig. 7–3). Occasionally, deglutition in normal subjects will cause a simultaneous pressure rise in three widely separated recording tips.

If the subject swallows repeatedly, as when sipping through a straw, a peristaltic wave will be inhibited until after the last swallow has occurred. The wave will then traverse the esophagus in the usual manner. This inhibition of peristalsis can be demonstrated in another interesting way. If the electrical activity in the esophagus is measured from an intraluminal site in humans, spike activity is observed after each swallow coincident with each peristaltic contraction. If, however, the subject swallows repeatedly, the electrical activity of the first swallow is inhibited by the swallows which follow it. When the swallowing sequence has been terminated, a final series of spikes is observed. [5]

A peristaltic wave can also be stimulated by material which has remained in the esophagus or which has been refluxed into the esophagus from the stomach. In this case no pharyngeal component to swallowing is observed and the upper esophageal sphincter remains closed. However, a peristaltic wave begins at or above the material which has been refluxed and continues down the length of the esophagus. This is known as *secondary peristalsis* in contrast to primary peristalsis which is initiated by deglutition. Experimentally, secondary peristalsis is most often initiated by distention of a balloon in the esophagus. In normal subjects transient balloon distention will stimulate secondary peristaltic wave in approximately 50 per cent of instances. Disease states such as diabetes and alcoholic neuropathy, as well as old age, decrease the frequency of such responses.

Figure 7–2. "Dry" and "wet" swallows. The proximal tip is located in the midesophagus. A dry swallow (D.S.) causes a monophasic wave. The second dry swallow shows no baseline elevation; there is a questionable elevation in the first dry swallow. In contrast, when the peristaltic wave is stimulated by a swallow of liquid (W.S.), the wet swallow produces a baseline elevation which lasts until the peristaltic wave reaches the tip.

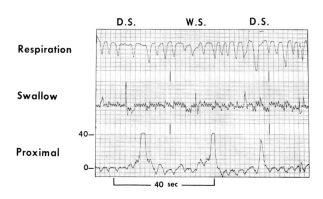

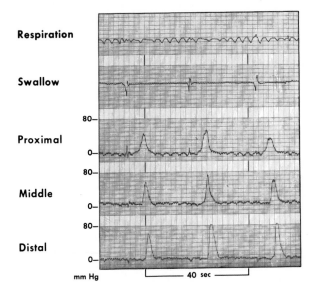

Figure 7–3. Normal peristalsis in the body of the esophagus. The three tips are located 5 cm apart and are infused at 2.4 ml per min. A swallow shown by the event marker in the second channel causes a high amplitude monophasic wave to be recorded sequentially by the three tips. Careful examination of the figure will show that the wave both begins and peaks at a slightly later point in time, if the middle tip is compared with the proximal tip, and the distal tip compared with the middle tip.

A larger balloon with prolonged distention elicits a different esophageal response, i.e., one which tends to displace the balloon toward the stomach and is not associated with peristaltic waves above the balloon.[6] This force, termed the esophageal propulsive force (EPF), is not observed after every trial of balloon distention. The EPF is rather large, sometimes reaching 100 g, and is adequate to propel the balloon if the restraining force on the distending balloon is temporarily relaxed. Experimental work using opossums suggests that the EPF might be mediated by the longitudinal muscle of the esophagus.

When the act of peristalsis is studied quantitatively, there are relatively few parameters to measure. One can measure the velocity of the wave as seen by cinefluorography, or by measuring the transit time between two pressure recording tips located in the esophagus. Velocity in the esophagus varies from 2 to 4 cm per second. It is slightly more rapid in the upper portion of the esophagus and can be varied by temperature. If a cold bolus is swallowed, the velocity is lowered; a warm bolus increases the velocity of the peristaltic wave.[7]

When the force with which the lumen is obliterated during a peristaltic wave ("squeeze") is investigated, it is found that there are several sources of variation in the normal individual. A recording tip which is maintained at the same level of the esophagus shows marked variation in the amplitude of the waves recorded from the same site on different swallows. This is true whether the swallow has been stimulated by a dry swallow or by ingestion of a measured quantity of fluid. The coefficient of variation of any one location is approximately 30 per cent. As the recording tip is moved from the lower esophageal sphincter to the upper esophageal sphincter, there is again a regional variation in the amount of squeeze. Squeeze values tend to be maximal in the lower portion of the esophagus, drop down and reach a low point in the upper one-third of the esophagus, and then rise again as the upper esophageal sphincter is approached. When the squeeze profiles of "normal" individuals are compared, marked differences are observed. However, when any one individual is studied repeatedly, his squeeze profile tends to remain constant over a period of at least four weeks.[8]

LOWER ESOPHAGEAL SPHINCTER

Since its manometric discovery in 1956, the lower esophageal sphincter has become more and more important in formulations of the explanation of gastroesophageal reflux.[9] If an anatomically demonstrable band of smooth muscle had been

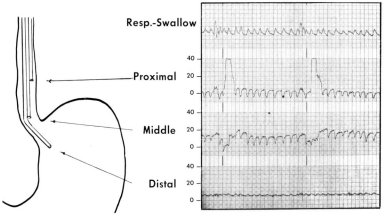

Figure 7–4.   Manometric evidence for the lower esophageal sphincter. The proximal tip is located in the body of the esophagus as shown by the wave inscribed after swallowing. The distal tip is in the stomach and is unaffected by deglutition. The middle tip is in the lower esophageal sphincter, and has a higher pressure than that recorded by the stomach or esophageal tip. This high pressure falls abruptly on deglutition and is not restored until the peristaltic wave has reached the sphincter area.

found in the lower esophagus, it would not have been difficult for the medical world to accept the concept of a lower esophageal sphincter.

The manometric characteristics of the sphincter are shown in Figures 7–4 and 7–

5. It can be seen that a zone of increased pressure is interposed between those pressures recorded from the stomach and from the esophagus. Deglutition or distention of a balloon in the esophagus causes an immediate drop in this area of high resting

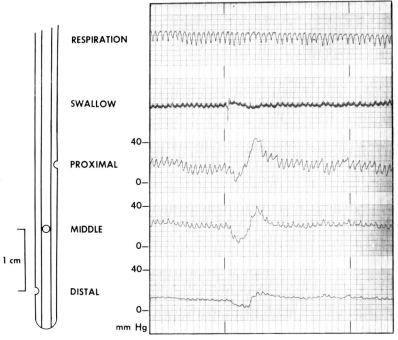

Figure 7–5.   Manometric characteristics of the lower esophageal sphincter. Three tips, 1 cm apart, are located in the lower esophageal sphincter. All tips respond to deglutition with a drop in pressure. Each tip records a different sphincter pressure, the middle tip recording the highest value. The proximal and middle tips record a contraction after the period of relaxation; this contraction is minimal in the distal tip.

pressure and the fall is maintained until the peristaltic wave reaches the high pressure zone. The high pressure, of course, merely reflects the fact that a portion of the lower end of the esophagus is closed tightly around the recording catheter. The fact that a pressure gradient exists from stomach to esophagus means that these two cavities have been separated by physical closure of the esophagus.

When measured by appropriate techniques the amplitude of the pressure in the lower esophageal sphincter serves as a guide to the strength of the lower esophageal sphincter. Normal and abnormal sphincters cannot be distinguished by measurement of sphincter pressure with fluid-filled catheters alone. However, when a slow constant infusion of fluid is added to the catheters through a side-arm, clear separation between the mean pressures of incompetent and competent sphincters is demonstrated.[10, 11]

Both mechanical and chemical factors have been shown to be important in the control of sphincter strength. The intra-abdominal location of the lower esophageal sphincter might aid in resisting increases in intra-abdominal pressure. Sphincter strength responds to increases in intra-abdominal pressure.[12] However, the rise in sphincter strength is considerably more than can be accounted for by merely passive transmission of the increase in intra-abdominal pressure through the walls of the sphincter.[13] Pressure rises in the sphincter in response to increased intra-abdominal pressure even if it is not located within the abdomen. Vagotomy, which does not interfere with the resting pressure of the sphincter, will, however, abolish this type of response.[14]

Hormonal effects can also be demonstrated on the lower esophageal sphincter. Maneuvers such as alkalinization of the antrum of the stomach or the feeding of a peptone broth, which would be expected to produce gastrin, will increase sphincter pressure. Acidification of the antrum, on the other hand, will cause an appropriate decrease. Direct administration of gastrin pentapeptide will cause elevations in sphincter pressure which are directly dose-dependent.[15] Other agents affecting sphincter strength are shown in Table 7–1.

Investigations of nervous control of the

TABLE 7–1. SOME AGENTS WHICH AFFECT SPHINCTER STRENGTH

Raise Sphincter Pressure	Lower Sphincter Pressure
1. Gastrin	1. Secretin
2. Metoclopramide	2. Essence of peppermint
3. Mecholyl (methacholine)	3. Anticholinergics
4. Urecholine (bethanechol)	4. Smoking
	5. Alcohol
	6. Vagotomy

lower esophageal sphincter raise certain questions. In the dog, radical sympathectomy has no effect on the tone and function of the sphincter. Vagotomy tends to decrease resting sphincter pressure and also interferes with relaxation following deglutition. Transection of the esophagus and even insertion of a prosthetic plastic device do not seem to interfere with sphincter function.[16]

In the guinea pig, when the esophagus is totally excised from the rest of the animal and suspended in a saline bath, the lower esophageal sphincter continues to function. Stimulation of the proximal end of the esophagus by a balloon will relax the sphincter. This effect must be transmitted through intramural channels, since transection of the esophagus between the stimulating balloon and lower esophagus sphincter abolishes the response.[17]

The question of sphincter control in man is less well settled. There are a few studies on patients with total sympathectomy and vagotomy. Occasionally there is clinical dysfunction of the sphincter area following vagotomy, but this would seem to be due to the mechanical effects of vagotomy rather than to loss of neural innervation. It has been shown that increase in sphincter strength associated with an increase in intra-abdominal pressure is abolished by vagotomy; presumably, the operation interferes with either the afferent or efferent limb of the reflex. Children with esophageal atresia who have an intact lower esophageal segment connected to the upper esophagus by a colon transplant retain sphincter relaxation on deglutition. It is possible that the sympathetic fibers accompanying the blood supply to this area may be important in its regulation in the intact human.

REFERENCES*

1. Ingelfinger, F. J. Esophageal motility. Physiol. Rev. 38:533, 1958.
2. Sokol, E. M., Heitmann, P., Wolf, B. S., and Cohen, B. R. Simultaneous cineradiographic and manometric study of the pharynx, hypopharynx, and cervical esophagus. Gastroenterology 51:960, 1966.
3. Rinaldo, J. A., Jr., and Levey, J. F. Correlation of several methods for recording esophageal sphincteral pressures. Amer. J. Dig. Dis. 13:882, 1968.
4. Vantrappen, G., and Hellemans, J. Studies on the normal deglutition complex. Amer. J. Dig. Dis. 12:255, 1967.
5. Hellemans, J., Vantrappen, G., Valembois, P., Janssens, J., and Vandenbroucke, J. Electrical activity of striated and smooth muscle of the esophagus. Amer. J. Dig. Dis. 13:320, 1968.
6. Winship, D. H., and Zboralske, F. F. The esophageal propulsive force: Esophageal response to acute obstruction. J. Clin. Invest. 46:1391, 1967.
7. Winship, D. H., Viegas de Andrade, S. R., and Zboralske, F. F. Influence of bolus temperature on human esophageal motor function. J. Clin. Invest. 49:243, 1970.
8. Pope, C. E., II. Effect of infusion on force of closure measurements in the human esophagus. Gastroenterology 58:616, 1970.
9. Fyke, F. E., Code, C. F., and Schlegel, J. F. The gastroesophageal sphincter in healthy human beings. Gastroenterologica 86:135, 1956.
10. Winans, C. S., and Harris, L. D. Quantitation of lower esophageal sphincter competence. Gastroenterology 52:773, 1967.
11. Pope, C. E., II. A dynamic test of sphincter strength: Its application to the lower esophageal sphincter. Gastroenterology 52:779, 1967.
12. Cohen, S., and Harris, L. D. Lower esophageal sphincter pressure as an index of lower esophageal sphincter strength. Gastroenterology 58:157, 1970.
13. Cohen, S., and Harris, L. D. Does hiatus hernia affect competence of the gastroesophageal sphincter? New Eng. J. Med. 284:1053, 1971.
14. Crispin, J. S., McIver, D. K., and Lind, J. F. Manometric study of the effect of vagotomy on the gastroesophageal sphincter. Canad. J. Surg. 10:299, 1967.
15. Castell, D. O., and Harris, L. D. Hormonal control of gastroesophageal sphincter strength. New Eng. J. Med. 282:886, 1970.
16. Greenwood, R. K., Schlegel, J. F., Code, C. F., and Ellis, F. H. The effect of sympathectomy, vagotomy and oesophageal interruption on the canine gastro-oesophageal sphincter. Thorax 17:310, 1962.
17. Mann, C. V., Code, C. F., Schlegel, J. F., and Ellis, F. H. Intrinsic mechanisms controlling the mammalian gastroesophageal sphincter derived of extrinsic nerve supply. Thorax 23:634, 1968.

---

*A general reference of significance to the physiology of the esophagus is Handbook of Physiology, Section 6, Alimentary Canal, Vol. IV, Motility. Washington, D.C., American Physiological Society, 1968.

Chapter 8

Motor Disorders

Charles E. Pope II

Motor disorders of the esophagus are those conditions in which the smooth coordination of the various components of the swallowing apparatus is disturbed by a defect in muscle function or nervous control, or both. Motor disorders have been recognized since the sixteenth century. Although some are quite well characterized in terms of pathology, course, and treatment, others are so recently recognized that course, prognosis, and methods of therapy have yet to be defined.

Clinical Picture. Symptomatically, motor disorders present usually with dysphagia or with esophageal colic. Dysphagia associated with motor disorders tends to be intermittent and to follow ingestion of either solids or liquids; it tends neither to be relentlessly progressive nor to be associated with signs of acute esophageal obstruction. Dysphagia caused by a bolus can usually be relieved by swallowing repeatedly, by drinking water, which acts as a hydrostatic ram to push the offending bolus downstream, or by merely waiting for the bolus to pass. The offending bolus is usually not regurgitated. Patients with motor disorders often report that their dysphagia is worse during times of emotional stress. Indeed, this tendency is so marked that it is quite common for the patient to be referred to a psychiatrist before the true nature of the problem has been appreciated.

Esophageal colic is felt below the sternum and radiates through to the back. Dis-

comfort tends to occur at night, waking the patient from a sound sleep. It is more common in younger patients with motor disorders. Confusion with angina pectoris caused by coronary artery disease is common, since the site of the pain is identical for these conditions. Unlike coronary disease, however, esophageal colic is not precipitated by exercise and responds only slowly, if at all, to nitroglycerin. It can be quite severe, requiring large doses of narcotics for relief. Radiation to the neck, jaw, and arms is less common than in angina pectoris, but may occur. The patient may notice difficulty in swallowing fluids during an attack. Esophageal colic is usually not produced by the ingestion of food; however, extremes in temperature may provoke distress.

Diagnosis and Differential Diagnosis. The diagnosis of a motor disorder of the esophagus, although suggested by the historical factors listed above, should be confirmed by methods which demonstrate motor abnormalities. Radiography and fluoroscopy certainly can often demonstrate the absence or impairment of peristalsis; however, they do not quantitatively measure muscular function. Since the motor abnormality may not involve the entire esophagus, it is conceivable that the fluoroscopist may miss abnormal motor function in only a portion of the esophagus. At present, measurement of intraluminal pressures by manometry is the accepted way of demonstrating and

90

quantitating motor abnormalities. Manometry effectively determines the presence or absence of peristalsis, as well as timing and correlating the rapid events of swallowing which take place at the inlet of the esophagus. Despite shortcomings which include missing some intermittent motor abnormalities and overinterpreting others, manometric study remains the most important method of documenting motor disorders of the esophagus. It is probable that other measurements of smooth muscle function will be developed to aid in the understanding and documentation of motor disorders.

DISORDERS OF STRIATED MUSCLE

The striated muscles of the pharynx and esophagus can be involved by systemic diseases, by neurologic lesions, or by diseases primarily affecting striated muscle. Most lesions in this area can be suspected if swallowing of fluids tends to lead to immediate aspiration. Occasionally, the patient states that it is difficult to initiate the downward progression of a bolus, or that liquids, when swallowed, cause either coughing or a sensation of fluid in the posterior nasopharynx.

PHARYNGEAL DISEASES

Although the pharyngeal muscles are not truly esophageal, lesions which affect them or their nerve supply will cause dysphagia. Malfunction of the pharyngeal musculature should be considered when dysphagia is the presenting clinical condition. In most cases, other manifestations of the underlying disease will overshadow the symptoms of dysphagia, thus making diagnosis considerably easier. Poliomyelitis, especially the bulbar form, has been demonstrated manometrically to interfere with the build-up of normal pharyngeal pressures.[1] Other lesions which interfere with nervous control of the pharynx, such as botulism and diphtheria, can also present with dysphagia. Bilateral cortical disease associated with signs of pseudobulbar palsy is also associated with dysphagia. Incoordination of the pharynx can be demonstrated by cineradiography, and abnormal

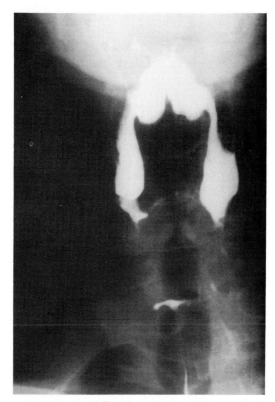

Figure 8–1. Vallecular pooling. This elderly male had difficulty in initiating deglutition. After a barium swallow, contrast material is seen to remain in the pyriform sinuses and valleculae. (Courtesy of Dr. F. E. Templeton.)

stasis of barium in the pyriform sinuses and valleculae can be demonstrated (Fig. 8–1). Relatively little attention has been paid to manometric documentations of these lesions. In a survey of various neuromuscular disorders, no consistent findings were discovered in patients with cerebral vascular disease, Parkinson's disease, amyotrophic lateral sclerosis, or multiple sclerosis.[2] Although some changes were found in these individuals, it would not seem outside the realm of possibility that similar findings would be noted in age- and sex-matched control subjects. Although both hyper- and hypothyroidism have been incriminated as causes of dysphagia by weakening esophageal striated muscle, documentation for this opinion is scanty.

CRICOPHARYNGEAL ACHALASIA

Motor disorder of the striated muscle has been termed cricopharyngeal achalasia.[3] This condition, which is often accompanied by a Zenker diverticulum, is usually manifested by the inability to initiate deglutition. Aspiration often occurs during attempted swallowing, so patients often avoid eating and thus lose much weight. The diagnosis may be suggested by the X-ray finding of a prominent ridge in the area of the cricopharyngeus muscle, by distention of the valleculae, and by aspiration of barium into the trachea. More definitive diagnosis can be provided manometrically if an incoordination is shown between the pharyngeal contraction and sphincteric relaxation.[4] The sphincter relaxes normally but closes before the pharynx has completed its contraction. Thus, achalasia is a misnomer for this condition in that the upper esophageal sphincter relaxes appropriately; it merely contracts before it should. The treatment for this condition is surgical and involves splitting the cricopharyngeus muscle. Although this does not improve the incoordination, it allows the pharyngeal muscle to propel fluid or solid material through the weakened cricopharyngeus muscle. If a Zenker diverticulum coexists with this lesion, often the diverticulum will disappear without any surgery aimed specifically at the pouch. Operative experience with this condition is not extensive; however, the reported results suggest that surgical therapy should be offered when this condition has been recognized and documented.

MYASTHENIA GRAVIS

This disease, which involves the motor end plate, affects the striated portion of the esophagus as well as other portions of the voluntary muscle system. Although dysphagia is usually overshadowed by other, more striking evidences of myasthenia, occasionally it is the presenting symptom. This disorder can be investigated using the Tensilon test, as follows: give 2 mg of edrophonium chloride (Tensilon) intravenously, followed by another 8 mg if the first dose is not successful. Swallowing function usually rapidly improves. Very little information exists as to manometric changes during this procedure, although one would expect to find improvement in the force of contraction of the pharyngeal muscles.

MYOTONIA DYSTROPHICA

This disease also clearly involves the esophageal striated muscle. It is a familial disease characterized by the "myopathic facies," swan neck, myotonia, muscle wasting, frontal baldness, testicular atrophy, and cataracts. Dysphagia is a common complaint, and manometric investigation of these individuals shows both a decrease in amplitude of pharyngeal and striated muscle contraction and an increased duration of the wave.[5, 6] In addition to the disturbances found in the striated muscle, there is decreased amplitude of smooth muscle contraction and a decrease in the number of peristaltic contractions following deglutition.

OTHER RARE SYNDROMES

Involvement of esophageal striated muscle characterizes several other diseases. Cineradiographic study of *dysautonomia* (Riley-Day syndrome) reveals pharyngeal incoordination with aspiration of barium.[7] Similar radiographic findings are reported in *dermatomyositis*.[8] Patients with the *oculopharyngeal syndrome,* a genetically transmitted syndrome manifested by ptosis and dysphagia, have been shown to aspirate barium, and have reduced amplitude of contraction in striated muscle of the esophagus.[9]

DISORDERS OF SMOOTH MUSCLE

ACHALASIA

Definition. Achalasia, or cardiospasm, was one of the first motor disorders of the esophagus to be recognized clinically. The changing names under which it has been known reflect the differing ideas of pathogenesis which have been present over the years since it was recognized. In this disease there is a double defect in esophageal function. The lower esophageal sphincter offers an impediment to the flow of liquid and solid material from the esophagus into the stomach. In addition, there is a failure of normal progressive peristalsis in the upper two-thirds or smoooth muscle portion of the esophagus. Although the smooth muscle can still contract (as it does in an aimless fashion or when stimulated pharmacologically), the progressive nature of peristalsis is lost. Thus, both the outflow tract and pumping mechanism of the esophagus are abnormal in achalasia.

Although in the past this diagnosis has been made on the basis of clinical history and confirmatory X-ray findings, it appears that more complete evaluation is necessary to be certain that classic achalasia is present. It would appear that there are variants of esophageal motor function which superficially resemble achalasia, and yet may not represent true achalasia. Clear diagnosis is vital for correct choice of therapy.

Historical Aspects. Although described quite well in 1682 by Thomas Willis, this disease did not attract much medical interest until the 1800's. Sporadic cases were reported in the two preceding centuries. Attention was first drawn to the huge, dilated esophagus found in autopsy material, and primary failure of esophageal musculature was assumed to be the cause. Later, obstruction at the lower end of the esophagus was postulated, either from the diaphragm or from adjacent organs such as the liver. After recognition of the fact that no organic obstruction was present, the concept of spasm at the lower esophageal sphincter, or cardiospasm, was developed. An alternative theory, that the cardia was normal but did not relax properly, has more recently been presented. It will be seen that perhaps both these interpretations are correct.

The lesion was recognized in the early 1900's, with the advent of X-ray contrast studies. Once the diagnosis became possible, both nonsurgical and surgical methods for therapy were developed. In 1912, Henry Plummer reported the hydrostatic dilatation of achalasia, a form of therapy still used. Surgically, the names of Wendel and Heller were attached to operations designed to disrupt the lower end of the esophagus and allow drainage.[10]

Etiology, Pathology, and Pathophysiology. The normal neural control of esophageal peristalsis is not so well understood that the defect or defects responsible for achalasia can be easily pinpointed. There is still no acceptable model of achalasia in animals and only one condition in which the etiology for achalasia in humans is known; that is, Chagas' disease caused by infection with *Trypanosoma cruzi*.[11] In this infection, symptoms and esophagrams classic for achalasia are seen. Clinical differences exist in that the megaloureter, megaduodenum, and megacolon are often associated with the esophageal lesion in Chagas' disease. There is a notable absence of Auerbach's ganglion cells, and the patients respond to stimulation with parasympathomimetic agents as do patients with achalasia.

The etiology of achalasia in North Americans is unknown. Pathological examination of specimens obtained at autopsy reveals muscular thickening, especially in the circular muscle of the lower esophagus. Changes of chronic stasis are often observed in the epithelial lining of the esophagus. One of the most controversial findings is that related to Auerbach's plexuses. Most observers agree that there are fewer ganglion cells in the body of the esophagus, and the ganglion cells present may be surrounded by chronic inflammatory cells. However, in the area of the lower esophageal sphincter, the number of ganglion cells has been reported as normal, reduced, or absent. Some observers have attributed the decrease in ganglion cells to the mechanical separation of the ganglion cells by esophageal dilatation. Nevertheless, autopsy studies in which serial circumferential sections of the esophagus were obtained seem to indicate that in most cases of achalasia the ganglion cells are markedly reduced in number.[12] A few cases have been reported in whom normal numbers of ganglion cells were seen. The diagnosis in these patients was usually made by clinical findings supplemented by X-ray examination. They may represent patients with a clinical variant of achalasia.

The smooth muscle cells in the lower end of the esophagus are described as normal by light microscopy. Electron microscopy shows detachment of myofilaments from the surface membranes and cellular atrophy.[12] It is not clear whether these changes are important in the pathogenesis of the disease, or merely represent a muscular adaptation to a primary nerve disorder.

The same investigators have described changes in the esophageal motor nerves. Although the vagus nerve was normal by light microscopy, degeneration of some of the myelin sheaths and breaks in the axon membranes were noted on electron microscopy, changes which resembled Wallerian degeneration. When the dorsal motor nucleus of the vagus was examined, many of the cells showed fragmentation and dissolution of the nuclear material. A significant reduction in the number of dorsal motor nuclear cells was noted in comparison with control specimens. It is of interest in the light of these findings in achalasia that experimentally produced lesions in the dorsal motor nucleus of cats caused aperistalsis.[13] However, in these animals there was no degeneration of Auerbach's plexuses and the sphincter relaxed in one-third of all swallows. Attempts to induce lesions in primates by high cervical vagectomy produced an occasional animal with a dilated esophagus and a positive Mecholyl test.[14] However, this was not a constant finding, and some of the animals seemed to have been quite ill from the surgical procedure.

There is pharmacological information which confirms the anatomic evidence of denervation. Muscle strips from the circular layer contract when exposed to acetylcholine, but not to nicotine.[15] This finding suggests that the ganglion cells were absent; the absence was histologically confirmed in the same muscle strips.

Both the esophageal body[16] and lower esophageal sphincter[17] react strongly when small amounts, 2.5 to 7.5 mg, of acetyl-β-methylcholine (Mecholyl) are injected subcutaneously. The heightened response to this synthetic acetylcholine has led many investigators to interpret this response as evidence of denervation hypersensitivity (Cannon's law).

Another fascinating pharmacological fact is that the sphincter in achalasia is hypersensitive to gastrin. It has been shown that suppression of endogenous gastrin causes the elevated sphincter pressures found in achalasia to drop to normal values. Serum gastrin levels in patients with achalasia are normal, and the addition of exogenous gastrin elevates sphincter pressure, indicating supersensitivity to exogenous gastrin.[18] It is not yet certain whether the supersensitivity to gastrin is a direct muscle characteristic in achalasia or secondary to denervation.

Any etiological theory must, therefore, explain the production of lesions in the ganglion cells and perhaps more central vagal lesions, the tendency of the disease to occur in young individuals, the lack of cluster cases in families or living units, and the apparent lack of exposure to chemical or biological agents.

Perhaps another analogy might be drawn between Chagas' disease and achalasia. The interval between acute infection with Chagas' disease and the esophageal, colonic, and ureteral lesions may be many years. Perhaps in achalasia the esophagus is exposed to a toxic substance or organism years before the disease becomes clinically manifest, making epidemiological investigation extremely difficult.

Clinical Picture. HISTORY. The histories of patients with achalasia vary widely.[19] Although the symptoms can be separated into esophageal and extraesophageal, dysphagia is the most common presenting symptom. (However, achalasia of long standing is not necessarily associated with dysphagia.) Dysphagia is caused by both solids and liquids and is worse during periods of emotional stress or when the patient is trying to eat rapidly. Certain postural maneuvers, such as throwing the shoulders back, lifting the neck, and performing a rapid Valsalva maneuver, help the material to pass into the stomach. The patient is occasionally conscious of gurgling during eating. An occasional patient states that alcohol is of benefit in helping the food to pass into the stomach. Alcohol has a direct effect on the sphincter of normal individuals;[20] in achalasia, whether this works directly on the sphincter or indirectly by way of the psyche, is not certain.

Odynophagia, or esophageal colic, is occasionally seen, most commonly at the beginning of the illness. However, when chest pain, whether or not associated with swallowing, continues for more than two to three years, it is likely that one of the variants of achalasia is the correct diagnosis.

Regurgitation of retained material is another common symptom provoked often by changes in position or by physical exercise. The material which is brought up from the esophagus is often recognized as food that has been eaten many hours previously. It tends not to have an acid taste. In fact, true heartburn is a very uncommon manifestation of achalasia, despite inflammatory changes in the epithelium owing to stasis of retained material. Regurgitation of material from the esophagus, whether or not appreciated by the patient, may lead to marked pulmonary changes. Frequent bouts of bronchopneumonia are always a strong indication for an esophagram to ascertain whether esophageal retention is the cause. Indeed, in some patients the bronchopulmonary manifestations or a mediastinal "mass"—dilated esophagus—found by routine chest X-ray, are the only clues to the diagnosis of this esophageal motor disorder (Fig. 8–2). Close questioning may fail to elicit evidence that the patient has noticed any esophageal symptoms during his lifetime.

PHYSICAL EXAMINATION. The physical examination of the patient is usually normal. Halitosis caused by retained esophageal material is sometimes present in advanced cases. Weight loss may be noted, particularly in advanced cases of esophageal stasis which are often associated with bronchopulmonary aspiration. Rarely, a widened area of mediastinal dullness may be percussed.

Diagnosis. It is uncommon to see air in the stomach, and occasionally retained food and fluid will be visible in the upright position either with or without contrast material added to the esophagus. Barium examination of the esophagus is the most common and easily available form of diagnostic aid. In the early case, when esophageal dilatation is not pronounced, the diagnosis may be missed. Often the pa-

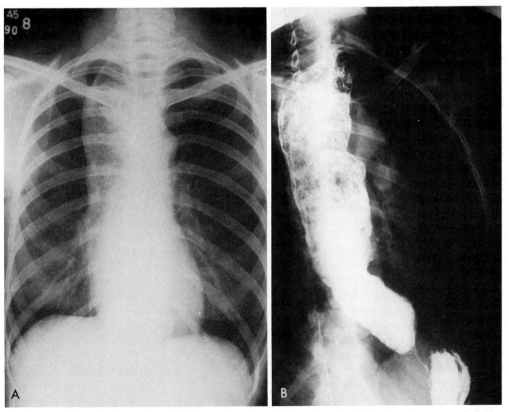

Figure 8–2. Achalasia seen on chest film. *A*, Occasionally the dilated, fluid-filled esophagus in achalasia can present as a mediastinal mass, as in this case. *B*, Confirmation of the identity of the mediastinal mass can be obtained by a barium swallow which shows the dilated esophagus of achalasia. (Courtesy of Dr. F. E. Templeton.)

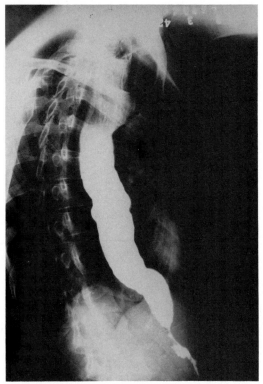

Figure 8–3. Achalasia of esophagus. This is the classic appearance of the dilated esophagus terminating in a narrowed segment. Fluid and mucus float on top of the more dense barium. (Courtesy of Dr. F. E. Templeton.)

three minutes, but then the strong contraction of the lower two-thirds will force barium down into the stomach and up, possibly spilling out over the observer!

Occasionally an epiphrenic diverticulum will be observed in the patient with achalasia (Fig. 8–5). This occurs immediately above the area of the lower esophageal sphincter, and usually extends to the right of the esophagus. Its main importance is that the endoscopist or those passing tubes be aware of its existence. In order to avoid perforating the diverticulum, it is often necessary to pass diagnostic or therapeutic tubes over a string which has been previously swallowed and allowed to anchor itself in the small bowel of such an individual.

MANOMETRY. Manometric study of a patient with achalasia reveals normal functioning of the upper esophageal sphincter and the presence of peristalsis in the uppermost portion of the esophagus. However, resting pressure in the body is usually elevated if the organ has not been previously emptied with a large bore tube. Simultaneous, low amplitude contractions which are not related to swallowing activ-

tient is examined in the upright position and the radiologist mistakes the effect of gravity for peristalsis. The patient should be examined in the supine position, so that gravity does not assist the passage of the barium. Special attention should be paid to the lower two-thirds of the esophagus, since the striated portion of the esophagus will demonstrate a peristaltic wave which usually terminates at the aortic arch. In the more marked case, esophageal dilatation is evident and the esophagus terminates in a "beak" (Figs. 8–3 and 8–4). Occasionally segmental contractions of the esophagus will be seen in the lower two-thirds. Again, in early cases these contractions are capable of obliterating the esophageal lumen. However, this is much less marked when dilatation is present. If methacholine (Mecholyl) is given when the esophagus is filled with barium, a slight increase in purposeless movements of the lower two-thirds will be observed after two or

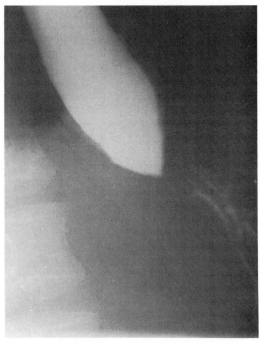

Figure 8–4. Esophageal "beak." A spot film from another patient with achalasia. The esophagus terminates in a beak or point.

ity are occasionally recorded. A swallow produces either no response or, more commonly, a low amplitude simultaneous rise of pressure in all tips (Fig. 8–6).

Manometric investigation of the lower esophageal sphincter with an uninfused tip will show no elevated pressure. From this finding some observers have deduced that no "cardiospasm" is present in this disease. However, when an infused tip is used, a high resting pressure is observed in the classic cases of achalasia. This resting pressure is usually about 40 mm Hg above gastric pressure.[21] As in the normal, swallowing is associated with a fall in this pressure, but rarely more than 10 to 20 mm Hg. Thus, even with swallowing, a high pressure zone is maintained (Fig. 8–7). This helps to explain why a patient with achalasia can support a column of barium in his esophagus when standing erect. It would be assumed that the height of a column that he is able to support would bear a direct relationship to the manometric pressure measured within his lower esophageal sphincter. When the manometric catheters are in the body of the esophagus, they will show an elevation, often dramatic, in resting pressure when Mecholyl is given to the patient. An increase in spontaneous activity will also be noted at this time.

The optimal way of recording the response of the esophagus to Mecholyl, however, is an oncometric determination. A 30-cc balloon can be placed in the body of the esophagus and connected to a micro-

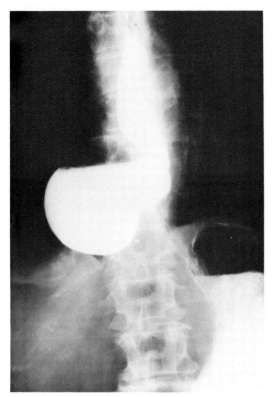

Figure 8–5. Epiphrenic diverticulum with achalasia. This patient, who presented with symptoms of pulmonary aspiration, had classic manometric findings of achalasia and a positive Mecholyl test. He responded well to bag dilation.

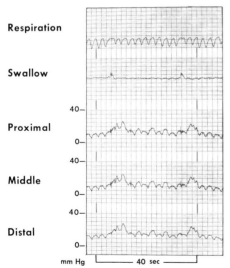

Figure 8–6. Motility of esophageal body in achalasia. In this tracing, three tips located 5 cm apart are in the body of the esophagus of a patient with achalasia. Note the elevated resting pressure of 10 mm Hg. Deglutition causes a broad, low amplitude simultaneous pressure wave to be seen in all three leads. No peristalsis is seen.

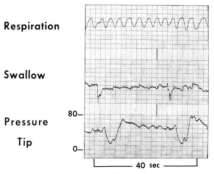

Figure 8–7. Lower esophageal sphincter in achalasia. With an infused catheter, this sphincter is found to have a pressure of 40 mm Hg. Deglutition causes a fall in pressure, but not to gastric levels. There is still a gradient maintained between sphincter and stomach.

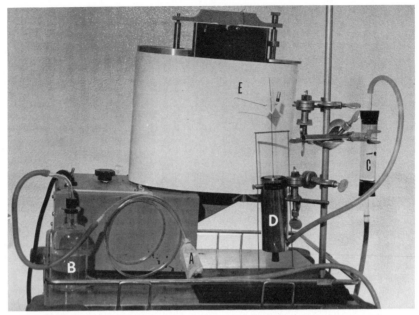

Figure 8–8. Esophageal oncometer for Mecholyl tests. The balloon (A) is placed so that it is in the lower two-thirds of the esophagus. When the lumen of the esophagus is obliterated either by a spontaneous contraction or by a tetanic response, air is displaced from balloon (A) to bottle (B). The increased air pressure in bottle (B) displaces water into cylinder (C). This displaced water in turn drives air into microrespirometer (D), which causes the inner cylinder of the microrespirometer to rise, carrying writing pen (E) with it. The record is inscribed on the kymograph. At the end of the esophageal contraction, the weight of the water in cylinder (C) causes air in bottle (B) to inflate balloon (A) and the cycle is complete.

respirometer. Displacement of air from the balloon is shown by a rise in the recording pointer of the microrespirometer (Fig. 8–8). Esophageal volume, not pressure, is being measured by this technique. With this device it is possible to record a positive esophageal response with very low doses of Mecholyl, thus avoiding the profound vasomotor and spastic response in the body of the esophagus seen with larger doses. Graded doses of Mecholyl should be used, starting with approximately 1 mg and increasing by 2-mg increments. With this technique, alarming results are rarely obtained. When the pulse is monitored, a rise in heartbeat is often noted even prior to a response recorded by the balloon. A positive response is shown by expulsion of

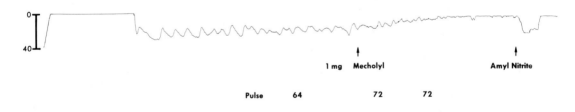

Figure 8–9. Positive Mecholyl test. The balloon was positioned in the lower two-thirds of the esophagus. When air is released into the balloon, it expands to a volume of 30 ml. The normal esophagus only allows a 10-ml volume to exist before contraction empties the balloon. Spontaneous rhythmic activity is observed. After subcutaneous injection of 1 mg of Mecholyl, pulse rises slightly and air is excluded from the balloon until the recording pen shows zero balloon volume. Temporary relaxation of the tightly contracted esophagus is caused by inhalation of amyl nitrite. Time is shown at the bottom of the tracing. Each small mark is 10 seconds; the larger marks are minutes.

all air from the esophageal balloon, thus producing a straight line record (Fig. 8–9). Failure to respond to Mecholyl is strong evidence against the diagnosis of achalasia. Unfortunately, subjects with achalasia are abnormally sensitive systemically to the effects of Mecholyl; thus they tend to develop tachycardia, flush markedly, and be troubled with salivation. The test is usually terminated by nausea and vomiting.

CYTOLOGY. Esophageal cytology can be helpful in differentiating achalasia from other causes of esophageal narrowing, and in detecting the presence of neoplasia in a well established case of achalasia. If the appearance of the lower end of the esophagus is at all questionable, or if the clinical picture is not that of pure achalasia, cytology is an extremely valuable way to exclude the possibility of an infiltrating fundal carcinoma. The question of whether patients with achalasia have an increase in incidence of carcinoma of the esophagus is not settled. However, when carcinoma is noted it is almost always in patients who have been known to have had achalasia for many years. Accurate esophageal cytology depends in these cases on prior emptying of the esophagus of all retained food particles and barium by intubation and lavage. In addition, the cytology tube should be placed under fluoroscopy to make sure that it has entered the stomach. Failure to enter the stomach often results in an inadequate specimen.

ENDOSCOPY. Esophagoscopy is rarely necessary for the establishment of diagnosis of achalasia. It is of value in discovering what the epithelial lining looks like, and some physicians feel that bag dilatation of the esophagus should not be performed if esophagoscopy reveals evidence of stasis esophagitis. When esophagoscopy is performed in patients with achalasia, a cavernous esophagus without peristaltic waves is seen. The esophagoscope can be felt to hesitate briefly at the lower esophageal sphincter before passing through easily into the stomach. If there is any suspicion of an invading fundal carcinoma, a fiber gastroscope can be passed into the stomach and then retroflexed in order to examine the gastroesophageal junction from below. Usually, however, the infiltrating tumor prevents passage of the gastroscope in this situation.

Differential Diagnosis. The main problem is in the differentiation of the dilated esophagus of achalasia from that caused by obstruction of a carcinoma or benign stricture (Fig. 8–10). There have been reports of positive Mecholyl tests in patients whose fundal carcinoma has infiltrated and destroyed the vagus nerve in the esophagus. The ability to pass a large bougie or esophagoscope through the cardia helps differentiate achalasia from other organic causes of esophageal obstruction.

Treatment. Theoretically, the optimal form of therapy for this disease would restore peristalsis and cause the lower esophageal sphincter to relax completely in response to a swallow. At present, no such therapy is available. Therefore, current forms of therapy are directed at weakening the lower esophageal sphincter so that

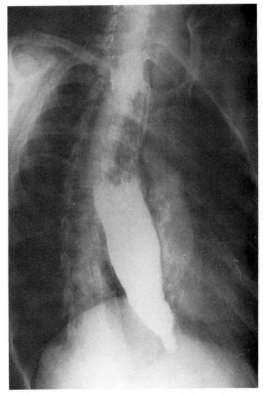

Figure 8–10. Simulation of achalasia by carcinoma. This patient's X-ray was first interpreted as achalasia. However, subsequent investigations showed an infiltrating fundal adenocarcinoma which had grown up into the lower esophagus.

gravity will empty the esophagus. Although attempts have been made to do so pharmacologically, no success has been reported. Therefore, mechanical means are currently employed.

In the original case report of achalasia, Dr. Willis presented a unique form of therapy. It consisted of a piece of whalebone tipped by a sponge which was used as a ramrod to propel the material through the lower esophageal sphincter into the stomach. Thus, bougienage was one of the earliest forms of therapy and is still used. Unfortunately, benefit from maximal dilatation, even with a No. 50 French dilator, is quite transient; i.e., symptoms are usually relieved for only two to three days, and self-bougienage is required for long-term therapy. This approach has been supplemented by more effective methods for mechanically disrupting the lower esophageal sphincter.

Several mechanical approaches to more forceful dilatation have been tried. The Starck dilator involves a metal basket arrangement which can be forcibly opened by a pull-wire. This instrument has been abandoned by most workers because of the high incidence of esophageal perforation attending its use.

Hydrostatic or pneumatic dilatation is the preferred form of mechanical interruption of the lower esophageal sphincter from within the lumen. Several forms of dilators are available: the Mosher bag, the Tucker mercury dilator, and the Browne-McHardy dilator; all these instruments depend on the forcible expansion of a balloon within the lower esophageal sphincter (Fig. 8–11). The Browne-McHardy bag contains a limiting nylon sack which restricts the maximal diameter of the dilatation to a predetermined diameter.

The procedure should be done on inpatients only. The patient is placed on a liquid diet on the night before dilatation, and, if necessary, the esophagus is emptied with an Ewald tube prior to passage of the instrument. Premedication with Demerol (50 to 100 mg given intramuscularly) is helpful in allaying anxiety. The dilator must be positioned under fluoroscopic control so that the bag extends across the area of the lower esophageal sphincter (Fig. 8–12). When the bag is in the correct position it is inflated to a pressure of at least 300 mm Hg and maintained in that position for a 10- to 15-second period. The patient usually complains of substernal pain. At this point it is well to observe the bag fluoroscopically and to take a spot film to confirm correct placement of the dilating instrument. Some authorities recommend two or three inflations of the balloon; I prefer to perform dilatation on another day if the first dilatation has not been satisfactory. When the balloon is

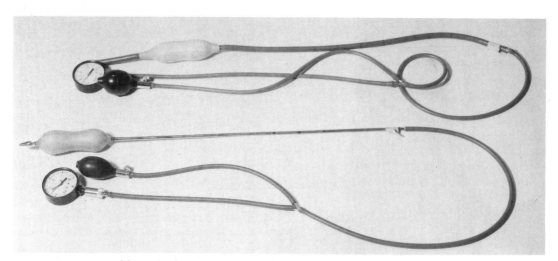

Figure 8–11. Bag dilators for the treatment of achalasia. The upper unit is the Browne-McHardy dilator. The dilating bag is at the distal end of a Hurst dilator. At the bottom, a Rider-Moeller dilator. Air is pumped into the balloons by the rubber hand bulbs and the pressure is monitored by the gauges.

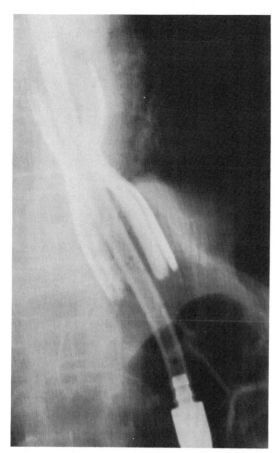

Figure 8–12. Bag dilator in position. Under fluoroscopy the dilator is positioned so that the bag crosses the lower esophageal sphincter zone. In this spot film, the indentation of the sphincter on the partially inflated bag is seen.

patient's ability to eat a normal diet without dysphagia and by decrease in retention of barium in the dilated esophagus. In several series, such results were obtained in 60 to 75 per cent of patients treated with one dilatation.[22] The number of satisfactory results following subsequent dilatation falls off rapidly, and it would seem unwise to offer more than two dilatations to a subject if symptomatic and X-ray relief is not obtained.

In the choice of subjects for dilatation it would seem best to avoid those with a tortuous sigmoid esophagus (Fig. 8–13). If thoracotomy is considered impossible because of co-existing pulmonary changes, relief may be attempted by swallowing the dilator over a guiding thread. However, such patients will probably not fare well with either medical or surgical therapy.

SURGICAL THERAPY. Surgical therapy is aimed at disruption of the lower esophageal sphincter from the outside of the

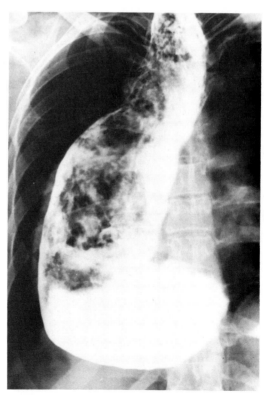

Figure 8–13. Sigmoid esophagus in achalasia. This film shows a large dilated tortuous esophagus. Introduction and successful dilatation of such a sigmoid esophagus is difficult indeed. (Courtesy of Dr. F. E. Templeton.)

withdrawn, it should be blood streaked if the stretching has been sufficiently forceful.

Food and fluids are then withheld for the next six hours and temperature and pulse are recorded hourly. If there is no severe pain or temperature elevation at the end of this period, clear liquids can be given and a normal diet resumed on the next day. Should fever or signs of perforation ensue, emergency thoracotomy is recommended after contrast study of the esophagus. Although some recommend a water-soluble, radiopaque dye, barium in the mediastinum can serve as a marker for the surgeon at time of laparotomy and does not lead to more severe mediastinitis than would be present ordinarily.

Satisfactory dilatation is signaled by the

esophagus. Early attempts to eliminate the effect of the lower esophageal sphincter by actually resecting it led to life-threatening esophagitis owing to massive reflux from the stomach. Patients unfortunate enough to have been offered this form of therapy will undoubtedly require a second, corrective anti-reflux operation, either jejunal interposition or a fundoplication-type operation.

Most modern forms of therapy are variations on an esophageal myotomy, first performed by Heller in 1913. This operation involves incising the circular muscle fibers down to the mucosa and allowing the mucosa to protrude through. Most of the current variations are related to the length of the myotomy. Classic achalasia does not require a long myotomy; some of the variants of the disease require a longer incision whose inferior margin should extend onto the gastric musculature and whose superior margin may reach as high as the aortic arch. In an attempt to forestall the reflux which sometimes occurs after a satisfactory esophageal myotomy, some workers now recommend that it be combined with fundoplication procedure.[23]

In the follow-up of the results of esophageal myotomy it appears that approximately 80 per cent of the patients undergoing this operation have a good clinical and radiological remission. The most common cause for dissatisfaction with this operation is the high incidence of postoperative reflux. Although this can be demonstrated in as many as half the subjects who have had esophageal myotomy, it causes symptoms and difficulties in a much smaller proportion of these individuals. It is not surprising that reflux occurs in the postoperative period, since the main barrier to such reflux has been surgically destroyed. In addition, the body of the esophagus no longer can empty the refluxed material by secondary peristalsis. It is of interest that postoperative difficulties are not more marked than they are. Certainly the benefits of an adequate myotomy, which include disappearance of dysphagia and, more important, cessation of overflow of reflux into the lungs, far outweigh difficulties with postoperative reflux which can be handled often by the same methods used in treatment of ordinary gastroesophageal reflux.

CHOICE OF THERAPY. Gastroenterologists recommend bag dilatation; surgeons suggest myotomy. The choice of therapy should be dictated by the skills of those caring for the patient and any unique problems of the patient. In uncomplicated achalasia, bag dilatation should be tried once or twice, for long lasting relief can be obtained easily and quickly without subjecting the patient to a thoracotomy. Lack of an individual skilled in bag dilatation, a tortuous esophagus which prevents easy intubation, failure of bag dilatation, or unresolved suspicion of malignancy at the gastroesophageal junction should lead to the choice of surgery as initial therapy for achalasia.

DIFFUSE SPASM

Definition. The term diffuse spasm has been used to represent a wide variety of clinical, radiological, and manometric findings. A collection of distinctive signs and symptoms merits recognition of this disorder as a separate entity. A patient with diffuse spasm will suffer from intermittent dysphagia and esophageal colic, and have an abnormal radiogram and abnormal manometric findings. Thus defined and with all criteria required to be present, it probably is not a common disease of the esophagus. Much more common are possible variants of the syndrome which are perhaps best classified as motor disorders of the esophagus. If too many variants are all lumped together and called diffuse spasm of the esophagus, it is difficult to evaluate clinical course and therapeutic results.

Pathophysiology and Etiology. As is true with many other motor disorders of the esophagus, the etiology and pathophysiology of diffuse spasm are not known. Even the pathological information is sparse, since this lesion rarely leads to death or even to an operation during which tissue may be obtained. The most striking pathological change reported grossly in the esophagus of those with diffuse spasm is diffuse muscular thickening, mainly of the lower two-thirds of the esophagus.[24] Thickening up to 2 cm has been reported in patients with clinical and manometric evidence of diffuse spasm. Unlike achalasia, ganglion cells are not reduced in number.

In one of the few thorough studies of patients with manometrically demonstrated diffuse spasm, operated upon because of symptoms, the esophageal muscle was shown to be essentially normal to light microscopy.[25] However, these patients exhibited changes in the vagus nerve which were much more diffuse than those reported for patients with achalasia. These consisted of fragmentation of neural filaments, increase in endoneural collagen, and fragmentation of mitochondria. Since these changes were seen diffusely in the vagus nerve, the authors concluded that they probably represented afferent fibers, because this type of fiber is a predominant one in the human vagus. However, there are no morphological criteria which allow classification of fibers as afferent or efferent in this nerve. No examination in the central nervous system in this disease has been reported, and it is not known whether there are changes in the dorsal motor nucleus of the vagus similar to those reported by the same authors in achalasia.

Clinical Manifestations. Diffuse spasm is said by some students to be a disease of later life. However, it may appear in the same age group afflicted by achalasia. The true incidence is unknown, and the interests of the referring physician often determine the incidence of the illness in a particular hospital or clinical setting. When all clinical, radiological, and manometric criteria are required to be present for diagnosis, I feel that this is a relatively uncommon disorder. In a personal series of over 600 patients, only three patients have been encountered who fit all the clinical, X-ray, and manometric criteria for the diagnosis of diffuse spasm. There is a much larger group who have some of the elements without the complete syndrome.

Chest pain is one of the most characteristic manifestations of this particular syndrome, especially in younger persons. The pain is located substernally and frequently radiates directly through to the back and shoulder blades. It characteristically awakens the sufferer from sleep at night and is often confused with angina pectoris. The pain can be quite severe, causing the patient to become ashen and perspire and, occasionally, to require relief with narcotics. The pain is not necessarily related to the act of deglutition. However, it can sometimes be triggered by the ingestion of either very hot or very cold liquids. During attacks of pain patients are usually unwilling to take any material by mouth, including therapeutic drugs.

Dysphagia is another common manifes-

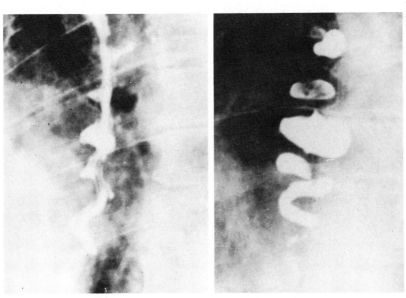

Figure 8–14. Diffuse spasm of the esophagus. Pronounced changes in the normal contour of the esophagus are shown. The sacculations and diverticula do not stay constant, but change in appearance from moment to moment. (Courtesy of Dr. F. E. Templeton.)

tation of diffuse spasm. It does not necessarily accompany chest pain, is felt with both solids and liquids, and seems to be most marked when the ingested material is either very hot or very cold. Occasionally, in the case of fluids, the patient is conscious of the fluid being forcefully ejected from the esophagus back into the nasopharynx. It is usually not necessary for the bolus to be regurgitated. The dysphagia is usually not progressive over time and remains episodic even after years of intermittent symptoms. Other manifestations of the condition, such as weight loss, are infrequent. There are no characteristic findings on physical examination.

X-Ray Examination. A plain film of the chest reveals no characteristic finding. When barium is swallowed a peristaltic wave is observed to travel as far as the aortic arch. Isolated, incoordinated movements of the lower two-thirds of the esophagus are sometimes seen which have elicited such descriptions as tertiary contractions, curling, corkscrew esophagus, sacculations, and pseudodiverticula (Figs. 8–14 and 8–15). All these synonyms refer to the incoordinated movements of the lower two-thirds of the esophagus. When the lumen of the esophagus is distended enough, the whole lower two-thirds of the esophagus contracts as a unit, propelling barium both retrogradely and into the stomach. No beaking is seen at the lower end of the esophagus.

Manometry. Manometric examinations reveal normal functioning of the upper esophageal sphincter and upper one-third of the esophagus. However, in the lower two-thirds the deglutition occasionally causes a normally progressive peristaltic wave, but, more frequently, a simultaneous contraction occurs (Fig. 8–16). The contractions in the lower two-thirds tend to be of higher amplitude, especially if an infused system or a small balloon is used as a recording device. Pressures as high as 500 cm H_2O have been recorded during such contractions. Contractions can be not only of large amplitude, but of abnormal duration, and occasionally patients will complain of their substernal discomfort at the same time that a high amplitude contraction is maintained over a period of ten to thirty seconds in the lower two-thirds of the esophagus. The lower esophageal sphincter occasionally contracts before the wave reaches this area. It also tends to maintain a higher resting pressure with values ranging from 30 to 40 mm Hg.

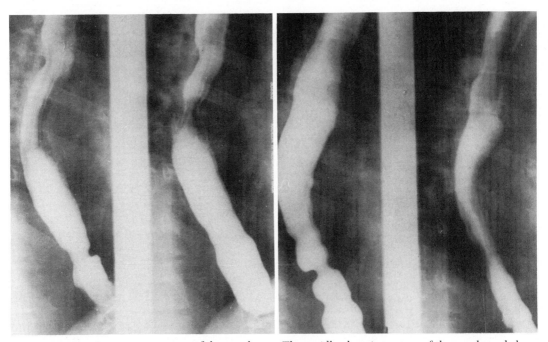

Figure 8–15. Tertiary contractions of the esophagus. The rapidly changing nature of the esophageal shape can be seen in these four films taken in rapid sequence. (Courtesy of Dr. F. E. Templeton.)

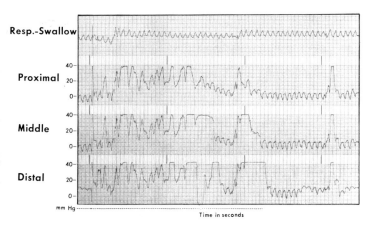

Figure 8–16. Manometric tracing of diffuse spasm. A deglutition has caused 3 tips 5 cm apart to record a prolonged (almost 60 sec) high amplitude contraction. A peristaltic wave is shown in the center of the record and a short simultaneous nonperistaltic contraction is shown on the right side of the record.

The response to subcutaneous Mecholyl may also contribute to the diagnosis. When the esophageal pressure is measured with an intraluminal balloon hooked to a kymograph, the resting tone of the esophagus in diffuse spasm is found to be normal or high in that a small balloon volume is maintained by frequent contractions of the esophagus. When patients with symptomatic diffuse spasm are stimulated with Mecholyl, positive responses are observed in most, but not all, of the subjects (Fig. 8–17). Slightly larger doses of subcutaneous Mecholyl (5.0 to 7.5 mg) are needed to produce a positive response in subjects with diffuse spasm as compared to those with achalasia. Asymptomatic subjects who also have tertiary contractions on X-ray usually respond negatively to Mecholyl.[26]

Therapy. The long-term course of diffuse spasm is still unclear. There have been interesting case reports that normal peristalsis has been restored after forceful balloon dilatation of the esophagus.[27] Con-versely, a single, well documented case of a transition from diffuse spasm to achalasia has also been presented.[28] In this case there is clear manometric evidence of the progression from diffuse spasm to classic achalasia. However, it would seem that both these transitions are uncommon events and that diffuse spasm is not merely a transient stage of another disease.

Pharmacological relief of the pain and dysphagia of diffuse spasm has been uniformly disappointing. Attempts to influence esophageal smooth muscle with anticholinergic agents and with muscle relaxants have not met with uniform success. Nitrites such as nitroglycerin have been used to give occasional relief, but the only effective pharmacological agents have been narcotics given to relieve severe pain.

Interest has been stimulated in the application of pneumatic dilatation of the lower esophageal sphincter to the treatment of this disease. One series presented nine patients who were dilated and sub-

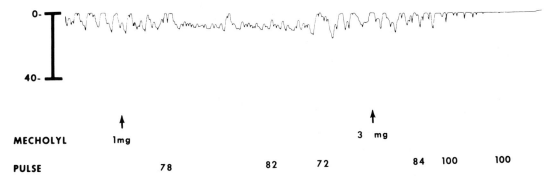

Figure 8–17. Positive Mecholyl test in diffuse spasm. The esophageal volume is low (about 6 to 8 cc) in contradistinction to the volume in achalasia (usually 25 to 35 cc). One milligram of Mecholyl causes no reaction, but 3 mg causes luminal obliteration, just as in achalasia.

sequently relieved.[29] It is difficult to see how attention to only the lower esophageal segment by forceful dilatation could assist a process which involves the entire two-thirds of the lower esophagus. Further trials of this technique for diffuse spasm will be necessary before balloon dilatation of the lower esophageal segment can be firmly recommended. At the moment, it certainly seems worth trying. It is of interest that frequent dilatations are necessary for relief in contrast to the usual experience in achalasia.

When dysphagia becomes truly severe and weight loss is evident, surgical relief has also been attempted. In such cases, a long myotomy extending from the gastric surface up as high as the aortic arch has been tried. The largest experience has been reported from the Mayo Clinic where 26 patients with diffuse spasm received such a long myotomy.[30] Approximately three-fourths of the patients developed marked relief of their symptoms of dysphagia and pain. However, only two-thirds of them had good or excellent results, which is a much poorer rate of success than is obtained with the same operation in achalasia.

VARIANTS OF DIFFUSE SPASM AND ACHALASIA

Some patients have combinations of symptoms, X-ray findings, and manometric test results which do not fit well into the category of either diffuse spasm or achalasia. These patients have been described under different headings; such terms as vigorous achalasia, dyschalasia, hypertensive sphincter, and hyper-reacting sphincter have been used to denote the most striking manifestations of their disease.

Vigorous achalasia is a term applied at the Mayo Clinic to patients who demonstrate features of both achalasia and diffuse spasm.[31] Pain and radiologic segmental spasm in these patients mimic diffuse spasm as their dysphagia and esophageal retention resemble achalasia. In contrast to the low amplitude simultaneous waves seen in classic achalasia, these patients demonstrate aperistaltic high amplitude esophageal contractions in the lower two-thirds of the esophagus (Fig. 8–18), have positive Mecholyl tests, and respond less well to bag dilation.

Even more puzzling were six patients who presented with dilated esophagi resembling achalasia and yet in whom primary peristalsis, secondary peristalsis, or sphincter relaxation could be demonstrated manometrically.[32] One patient was even so atypical as to have no ganglion cells on a full-thickness muscle biopsy, yet he was not responsive to Mecholyl.

It would seem well at the present time to gather all the clinical, X-ray, and manometric evidence on each patient presenting with a motor disorder of the esopha-

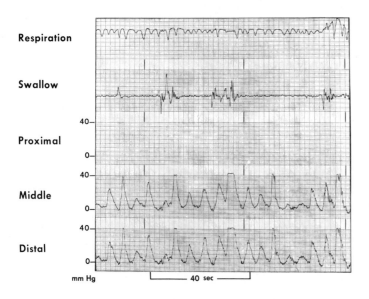

Figure 8–18. Manometric record of "active" achalasia. Numerous simultaneous contractions are seen in the middle and distal tips which are 5 cm apart. These are clearly not related to respiration. Deglutition often causes increase in the amplitude of the contractions, but no peristalsis is seen.

Respiration

Swallow

Proximal

Middle

Distal

mm Hg

40 sec

TABLE 8–1. SYMPTOMS AND SIGNS TO AID IN THE DIFFERENTIAL DIAGNOSIS OF ACHALASIA AND DIFFUSE SPASM

	ACHALASIA	DIFFUSE SPASM
Dysphagia	Yes	Usually
Esophageal colic	Occasionally early in disease	Yes
Regurgitation	Yes	No
Temperature sensitivity	No	Frequently
Dilatation on X-ray	Yes	No
"Breaking" on X-ray	Yes	No
Positive Mecholyl test	Yes	Almost always
Manometric peristalsis	No	Occasionally
Sphincter pressure	Elevated	Elevated
High amplitude contractions	No	Yes

gus. All information should point to either classic achalasia or diffuse spasm in order for these diagnoses to be made. A rough guide to the symptoms and signs of the two classic syndromes is given in Table 8–1. If some data are not consistent with either condition, the differences should be noted. Care in compiling information is essential for a classification of motor disorders which might allow recognition of significant variants and might eventually explain, for instance, the finding of ganglion cells in "achalasia." Recognition of significant variations from the classic pictures should lead also to more circumspect therapy and, perhaps, to better prognoses.

MOTOR DISORDERS AND SYSTEMIC ILLNESS

The esophagus can occasionally be involved by more generalized disease processes manifested primarily by derangement in motor function.

COLLAGEN VASCULAR DISORDERS

Scleroderma is the disease which clinically manifests the most pronounced abnormality of esophageal motor function. However, patients with other collagen diseases, especially when associated with Raynaud's phenomenon, can also have motor disorders of the esophagus.

Scleroderma often displays a double defect: aperistalsis in the lower two-thirds of the esophagus,[33] and lower esophageal sphincter insufficiency, leading to severe reflux.[34] Although it has been assumed that fibrosis affects the esophageal wall as it does the skin and thus leads to aperistalsis, correlative manometric-pathological studies suggest that the defect in peristalsis precedes significant pathological changes in the esophagus.[35] Signs of smooth muscle atrophy, but no striated muscle changes, are seen with this finding.

Often the other symptoms of scleroderma overshadow the esophageal manifestations. In one series,[34] dysphagia was found in 5 of 22 individuals. Heartburn tends to be relentless when it appears and is relatively unaffected by medical therapy directed against the reflux.

X-ray examination of the esophagus shows aperistalsis, retention of barium in the supine position, dilatation, and free gastroesophageal reflux. Often the normal "empty zone" between barium retained in the esophagus and in the stomach is not seen, and a common esophagogastric tube is seen. The esophagus will even contain air in the resting state.[36]

Manometry will show a lower esophageal sphincter with reduced strength (Fig. 8–19). Occasionally, there will be essentially no sphincter at all, and the normal change from an increase in pressure on inspiration in the stomach to a decrease in pressure on inspiration in the esophagus will not be found. This indicates that the stomach and esophagus are a common cavity, no longer separated by a lower

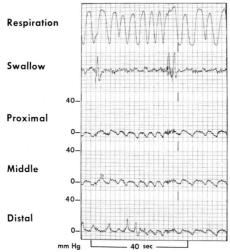

Respiration

Swallow

Proximal

Middle

Distal

mm Hg

40 sec

Figure 8–19. The lower esophageal sphincter in scleroderma. The proximal and middle tips are in the esophagus. The distal tip is in the stomach at the beginning of the tracing, as shown by the increase in pressure on inspiration. The assembly is then withdrawn until all tips are in the esophagus, as shown by a decrease in pressure on inspiration. Yet, no high pressure zone is detected by the infused catheter as it crosses from stomach into esophagus.

esophageal sphincter. Although peristalsis can still be demonstrated in the upper esophagus in scleroderma, the wave is not propagated into the lower portion of the diseased organ (Fig. 8–20).

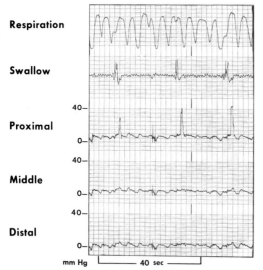

Respiration

Swallow

Proximal

Middle

Distal

mm Hg

40 sec

Figure 8–20. Aperistalsis in scleroderma. The proximal tip is located high in the esophagus and deglutition causes a normal contraction. However, the middle and distal tips, lying in the smooth muscle portion of the esophagus, show no propagation of a peristaltic wave.

There is no effective treatment for the patient whose esophagus is involved by scleroderma. Measures to restrict reflux, such as elevation of the head of the bed, can be tried. Vigorous antacid therapy, as in active duodenal ulcer disease (see p. 686), will be necessary, and in desperate circumstances a course of gastric radiation to induce achlorhydria can be tried. Theoretically, there is no reason why a fundoplication operation would not be of benefit (although not yet reported), but often the other manifestations of scleroderma render surgery impossible.

Other connective tissue disorders besides scleroderma can be associated with aperistalsis. Systemic lupus erythematosus, polymyositis, and other unclassified connective tissue disorders have been shown to demonstrate aperistalsis. The common denominator in these patients would seem to be the presence of Raynaud's phenomenon.[37] Patients suffering only from Raynaud's phenomenon without any other manifestation of a collagen disorder had an equally high incidence of aperistalsis. Reflux does not seem to be much of a problem in collagen disorders other than scleroderma, and the defect in peristalsis does not assume major clinical importance.

DIABETES MELLITUS

Defects in the motor function of the esophagus have been demonstrated by X-ray and manometry in diabetic patients suffering from neuropathy.[38] The defects were multiple and included decreased amplitude of contractions, a decrease in the number of peristaltic waves following deglutition, and a high incidence of tertiary contractions. These motor phenomena were not associated with clinical symptoms in a majority of the individuals tested. In some respects, these abnormalities were similar to manometric features of the aged esophagus.[39]

ALCOHOLIC NEUROPATHY

Another systemic disease associated with neuropathy and esophageal motor disorder is chronic alcoholism.[40] Alcoholics suffering from neuropathy have defects in esophageal function not found in alcoholics whose disease is of equal clinical severity but without neuropathy. A decrease in primary peristalsis and an increase in nonperistaltic contractions of the lower one-third of the esophagus are the outstanding defects in the neuropathic group. Secondary peristalsis stimulated by balloon distention is also markedly diminished in the neuropathic group. These defects are asymptomatic in these patients and require no therapy.

No other type of chronic neuropathy has yet been investigated manometrically, and it is not certain why neuropathy caused by alcoholism and diabetes should affect the esophagus. It seems very likely that other motor disorders will be described in the future, using manometry or other as yet undeveloped methods of testing esophageal motor function. Unfortunately, at present our methods of description are better than our methods of therapy.

REFERENCES

1. Kramer, P., Atkinson, M., Wyman, S. M., and Ingelfinger, F. J.   The dynamics of swallowing. II. Neuromuscular dysphagia of pharynx. J. Clin. Invest. 36:589, 1957.
2. Fischer, R. A., Ellison, G. W., Thayer, W. R., Spiro, H. M., and Glaser, G. H.   Esophageal motility in neuromuscular disorders. Ann. Intern. Med. 63:229, 1965.
3. Asherson, N.   Achalasia of the crico-pharyngeal sphincter. J. Laryngol. 64:747, 1950.
4. Ellis, F. H., Schlegel, J. F., Lynch, V. P., and Payne, W. S.   Cricopharyngeal myotomy for pharyngo-esophageal diverticulum. Ann. Surg. 170:340, 1969.
5. Siegel, C. I., Hendrix, T. R., and Harvey, J. C.   The swallowing disorder in myotonia dystrophica. Gastroenterology 50:541, 1966.
6. Garrett, J. M., DuBose, T. D., Jr., Jackson, J. E., and Norman, J. R.   Esophageal and pulmonary disturbances in myotonia dystrophica. Arch. Intern. Med. 123:26, 1969.
7. Margulies, S. I., Brunt, P. W., Donner, M. W., and Silbiger, M. L.   Familial dysautonomia. Radiology 90:107, 1968.
8. O'Hara, J. M., Szemes, G., and Lowman, R. M.   The esophageal lesions in dermatomyositis. Radiology 89:27, 1967.
9. Murphy, S. F., and Drachman, D. B.   The oculopharyngeal syndrome. J.A.M.A. 203:1003, 1968.
10. Ellis, F. H., and Olsen, A. M.   Achalasia of the Esophagus. Philadelphia, W. B. Saunders Co., 1969, p. 1–121.
11. Koberle, F.   Chagas' disease and Chagas' syndromes: The pathology of American trypanosomiasis. Advan. Parasitol. 6:63, 1968.
12. Cassella, R. R., Brown, A. L., Jr., Sayre, G. P., and

Ellis, F. H., Jr.   Achalasia of the esophagus: Pathologic and etiologic considerations. Ann. Surg. 160:474, 1964.
13. Higgs, B., Kerr, F. W. L., and Ellis, F. H., Jr.   The experimental production of esophageal achalasia by electrolytic lesions in the medulla. J. Thorac. Cardiov. Surg. 50:613, 1965.
14. Binder, H. J., Bloom, D. C., Stern, H., Solitare, G. B., Thayer, W. R., and Spiro, H. M.   The effect of cervical vagotomy on esophageal function in the monkey. Surgery 64:1075, 1968.
15. Misiewicz, J. J., Waller, S. L., Anthony, P. P., and Gummer, J. W. P.   Achalasia of the cardia: Pharmacology and histopathology of isolated cardiac sphincteric muscle from patients with and without achalasia. Quart. J. Med. 149:17, 1969.
16. Kramer, P., and Ingelfinger, F. J.   Esophageal sensitivity to Mecholyl in cardiospasm. Gastroenterology 19:242, 1951.
17. Heitmann, P., Espinoza, J., and Csendes, A.   Physiology of the distal esophagus in achalasia. Scand. J. Gastroenterol. 4:1, 1969.
18. Cohen, S., Lipshutz, W., and Hughes, W.   Role of gastrin supersensitivity in the pathogenesis of lower esophageal sphincter hypertension in achalasia. J. Clin. Invest. 150:1241, 1971.
19. Barrett, N. R.   Achalasia of the cardia: Reflections upon a clinical study of over 100 cases. Brit. Med. J. 1:1135, 1964.
20. Hogan, W. J., de Andrade, S. R. V., and Winship, D. H.   Ethanol-induced human esophageal motor dysfunction. Clin. Res. 18:383, 1970.
21. Cohen, S., and Lipshutz, W.   Lower esophageal dysfunction in achalasia. Gastroenterology 61:814, 1971.
22. Nanson, E. M.   Treatment of achalasia of the cardia. Gastroenterology 51:236, 1966.
23. Jekler, J., and Lhotka, J.   Modified Heller procedure to prevent postoperative reflux esophagitis in patients with achalasia. Amer. J. Surg. 113:251, 1967.
24. Gillies, M., Nicks, R., and Skyring, A.   Clinical, manometric and pathological studies in diffuse oesophageal spasm. Brit. Med. J. 2:527, 1967.
25. Cassella, R. R., Ellis, F. H., Jr., and Brown, A. L.   Diffuse spasm of the lower part of the esophagus. J.A.M.A. 191:107, 1965.
26. Kramer, P., Fleshler, B., McNally, E., and Harris, L. D.   Oesophageal sensitivity to Mecholyl in symptomatic diffuse spasm. Gut 8:120, 1967.
27. Bennett, J. R., Donner, M. W., and Hendrix, T. R.   Diffuse esophageal spasm; return to normality. Johns Hopkins Med. J. 126:217, 1970.
28. Kramer, P., Harris, L. D., and Donaldson, R. M.   Transition from symptomatic diffuse spasm to cardiospasm. Gut 8:115, 1967.
29. Rider, J. A., Moeller, H. C., Puletti, E. J., and Desai, D. C.   Diagnosis and treatment of diffuse esophageal spasm. Arch. Surg. 99:435, 1969.
30. Ellis, F. H., Olsen, A. M., Schlegel, J. F., and Code, C. F.   Surgical treatment of esophag-

eal hypermotility disturbances. J.A.M.A. *188*:862, 1964.

31. Sanderson, D. R., Ellis, F. H., Jr., Schlegel, J. F., and Olsen, A. M. Syndrome of vigorous achalasia: Clinical and physiologic observations. Dis. Chest *52*:508, 1967.

32. Hogan, W. J., Caflisch, C. R., and Winship, D. H. Unclassified oesophageal motor disorders simulating achalasia. Gut *10*:234, 1969.

33. Creamer, B., Andersen, H. A., and Code, C. F. Esophageal motility in patients with scleroderma and related diseases. Gastroenterologia *86*:763, 1956.

34. Atkinson, M., and Summerling, M. D. Oesophageal changes in systemic sclerosis. Gut *7*:402, 1966.

35. Treacy, W. L., Baggenstoss, A. H., Slocumb, C. H., and Code, C. F. Scleroderma of the esophagus. Ann. Intern. Med. *59*:351, 1963.

36. Dinsmore, R. E., Goodman, D., Dreyfuss, J. R. The air esophagram: A sign of sclero-

derma involving the esophagus. Radiology *87*:348, 1966.

37. Stevens, M. B., Hookman, P., Siegel, C. I., Esterly, J. R., Shulman, L. E., and Hendrix, T. R. Aperistalsis of the esophagus in patients with connective tissue disorders and Raynaud's phenomenon. New Eng. J. Med. *270*: 1218, 1964.

38. Mandelstam, P., Siegel, C. I., Lieber, A., and Siegel, M. The swallowing disorder in patients with diabetic neuropathy–gastroenteropathy. Gastroenterology *56*:1, 1969.

39. Soergel, K. H., Zboralski, F. F., and Amberg, J. R. Presbyesophagus: Esophageal motility in nonagenarians. J. Clin. Invest. *43*:1472, 1964.

40. Winship, D. H., Caflisch, C. R., Zboralske, F. F., and Hogan, W. J. Deterioration of esophageal peristalsis in patients with alcoholic neuropathy. Gastroenterology *55*:173, 1968.

Chapter 9

Symptomatology

Charles E. Pope II

Two symptoms are unique to the esophagus: dysphagia and heartburn or pyrosis. The esophagus also shares with other hollow viscera the capability of manifesting pain or bleeding. The medical history, gathered through careful and detailed interrogation of the patient, is frequently the most useful tool in unraveling and classifying esophageal malfunction. Eighty per cent of all esophageal problems can be diagnosed by history alone.

DYSPHAGIA

Dysphagia is a symptom which indicates an abnormality of esophageal structure or function. True dysphagia is never psychogenic, and the elicitation of this symptom from a patient should stimulate diagnostic and therapeutic attention from the physician confronted with it. The usual definition of dysphagia is "difficulty in swallowing." A more precise definition is somewhat difficult. Patients usually complain of food sticking, hesitating, or pausing. Normally, after swallowing has been initiated, the individual is unaware of the passage of the bolus down his esophagus. Dysphagia is the awareness that something has lodged in his esophagus. He may be quite accurate as to the location of the problem, or may refer the sensation to the suprasternal notch. Dysphagia is always associated with the act of swallowing. A similar sensation occurring in the absence

of food or fluid ingestion is not dysphagia. It is usually termed globus hystericus, the pathophysiology of which has not been defined.

The type of food usually producing dysphagia depends somewhat upon the abnormality causing the symptom. With organic obstruction of the esophagus, meat and spongy material such as potato or bread are the most likely offending materials. The presence of dysphagia for fluid, particularly of extreme temperature, as well as solids early in the course points to a muscular motor disorder more than to an organic obstruction of the esophagus.

Dysphagia itself does not imply pain, although marked discomfort may accompany impaction of food in the esophagus. The reader may be able to produce dysphagia by taking a large bolus of peanut butter and swallowing it intact after preliminary mastication. (Peanut butter dysphagia is a common symptom.) It is a benign manifestation of esophageal overload. Dainty eaters or those not addicted to peanut butter have probably not experienced this sensation.

The manner in which the patient seeks relief of dysphagia also offers diagnostic information. Regurgitation of a solid bolus strongly indicates a stricture or other organic narrowing of the esophagus. If it is possible to cause the bolus to pass by repeated swallowing, by ingestion of water, or by throwing back the shoulders and lifting the neck, a motor abnormality of the esophagus is more likely to be the cause.

HEARTBURN

Heartburn is the other unique esophageal symptom. The term is used commonly by both patients and physicians, although the former group tend to have a much broader concept of heartburn, using it as a synonym for indigestion or discomfort located almost anywhere in the chest or abdomen. It is necessary, therefore, that patient and physician have a common understanding of the symptom. Heartburn is usually a feeling of warmth or burning located in the substernal area which comes in waves and tends to rise toward the neck. The patient does not usually use the term "pain" to describe this sensation. "Burning" or "heat" is much more commonly used. When heartburn is severe, graphic descriptions of a "blowtorch" in the esophagus, or waves of "white-hot heat," are sometimes given. Although heartburn may be experienced in the neck, it is extremely unusual for it to be felt in the back or the arms. When prolonged, severe heartburn is described as a pain, usually located in the lower sternal area.

Heartburn may be accompanied by reflux of fluid into the mouth or nose. It can be produced by bending over, heavy lifting, or vigorous exercise. The tendency for heartburn to occur when the patient is supine at night is well recognized. Frequently the patient will report that lying on the right side produces the distress and lying on the left side relieves it. Some individuals complain of heartburn only after belching, and others only after a large meal. Excesses of alcohol or coffee seem to incite heartburn, as do meals which are high in fat or sugar, and fruit juices such as tomato and orange juice. Relief may follow by the swallowing or ingestion of water or antacids. Intermittent cigarette smokers often note heartburn soon after lighting up.

OTHER SYMPTOMS

Esophageal colic is a manifestation of disordered motor activity, just as it is further down in the gastrointestinal tract. Esophageal colic is usually perceived under the sternum; radiation through to the interscapular area is common. It tends to occur in the younger age population (between 20 and 40 years of age) and clinically is often confused with angina pectoris. It is described as a pressing, boring sensation, often of an intensity requiring narcotics for relief. It will occasionally radiate into the shoulders and down into the arms. During an attack patients are usually unwilling to attempt to swallow food or liquids. Ingestion of very cold fluids will relieve the symptoms in some patients and exacerbate them in others. If a barium swallow or a manometric study can be performed during the attack, abnormalities of motor function are usually demonstrated. During such an attack simultaneous contractions are seen, or prolonged high-amplitude contractions are recorded manometrically.

Odynophagia, or pain on swallowing, is the sensation of discomfort during the passage of food or fluid down the esophagus. Sometimes dysphagia, caused by an impacted bolus, can become odynophagia; more commonly pain on swallowing is caused by an irritated lesion of the esophagus either from a foreign body such as a chicken bone, or from inflammation resulting from reflux esophagitis or ingestion of caustic materials. Its intensity can vary from a sensation of food moving along the lower portion of the esophagus to intense pain requiring narcotics for relief.

Belching can be considered an esophageal symptom, although it usually does not denote the presence of esophageal disease. Ingestion of quantities of air along with fluid and solid foods often produces quantities of gas in the stomach. Less commonly, fermentation of material in the stomach will produce excess gas which is released by belching. Some patients have trained themselves to take quantities of air into the esophagus and then expel this gas audibly; the extreme example of this feat is esophageal speech. Under the fluoroscope a speaker will fill the entire esophagus or the upper portion of the esophagus only with gas and then expel this gas in a controlled manner while forming words with the lips and teeth. Theoretically, the esophageal speaker should be unable to produce any sound whatsoever. Distention of the esophagus should produce a secondary peristaltic wave which should carry the gas down into the stomach. The ability of the esophageal speaker to inhibit such secondary peristalsis remains unexplained.

Belching has been studied experimentally.[1] Infusion of air into the stomach results in reflux of air into the esophagus. This reflux triggers secondary peristalsis, and the air is returned to the stomach. The subject is unaware of this to-and-fro movement of air, although it can be demonstrated radiologically and manometrically. Occasionally, a spike in the gastric pressure associated with contraction of the abdominal muscles is observed and air is audibly expelled from the patient; of course, the patient is aware of this phenomenon. Therefore, experimentally at least, belching consists of both an "internal" and an "external" belch. It would seem logical to presume that the same dichotomy is present in the well fed, normal individual after a meal.

An uncommon symptom, but one which has attracted medical attention since the seventeenth century, is that of rumination.[2] Patients who tend to ruminate notice that 10 to 15 minutes after a meal their mouth suddenly fills with food and fluid which has been recently eaten. The food is usually chewed and reswallowed only to reappear in a relentless cycle. Some individuals have the ability to perform this act voluntarily; more commonly, it is involuntary and socially unacceptable. The food which is returned in this unexpected way usually does not taste acid to the individual. In fact, rumination often ceases 30 to 40 minutes after a meal when the material begins to take on an acid character. Such activity has even served as a basis for a rather astounding circus sideshow performance.[3] Ruminators, when questioned, are aware of an involuntary somatic movement of the abdominal muscles immediately preceding the arrival of food and fluid into the mouth.

Individuals with rumination seem to be unable to ruminate pure barium, so there are relatively few radiological studies of this phenomenon. Manometrically, during spontaneous rumination, one merely sees a rapid spike in the gastric pressure and esophageal pressure which is coincidental with the twitching of the abdominal muscles. In a patient who is able to ruminate voluntarily, manometric studies show voluntary relaxation of the lower esophageal sphincter maintained for up to three to four minutes (Fig. 9–1). It might be presumed that such relaxation, followed by a somatic twitch, would passively propel material from the stomach through the esophagus into the mouth. Reverse peristalsis has never been demonstrated in such individuals or, in fact, in the esophagus of any man, although four-legged ruminants which perform this action daily have been clearly shown to have reverse peristalsis.

Another esophageal symptom is that of

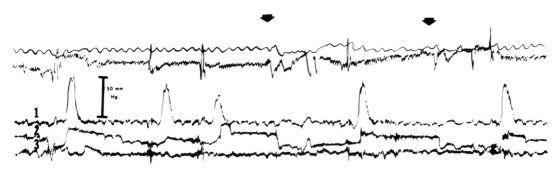

Figure 9–1. Manometric study of rumination. This record was obtained from a 32-year-old woman who could ruminate on command. The top tracing is respiration; the next signals swallowing. Three tips located 5 cm apart were placed so that tip 1 was in the esophagus, tip 2 in the lower esophageal sphincter, and tip 3 in the stomach. Notice the fall in sphincter pressure best shown by the first swallow. At the point marked by the first arrow, the sphincter pressure fell and remained down until the patient was asked to swallow. The period of sphincter relaxation lasted 30 seconds, far exceeding normal sphincter relaxation periods of 6 to 8 seconds. This same sequence was repeated at the second arrow.

water brash. Although sometimes this term is incorrectly used as a synonym for pyrosis or heartburn, it represents the sudden appearance of large quantities of clear fluid in the mouth, often to an extent requiring that the patient expectorate this material. It is usually described as salty, and the patient does not know whether it comes from the stomach, esophagus, or salivary glands. It appears to occur most commonly in people with severe esophagitis or peptic ulcer disease, and is usually an intermittent phenomenon.

REFERENCES

1. McNally, E. F., Kelly, J. E., Jr., and Ingelfinger, F. J.   Mechanism of belching: Effects of gastric distention with air. Gastroenterology 46:254, 1964.
2. Fabricius ab Aquapendente.   Tractatus de gula, ventriculo et intestinis. Padua, 1618.
3. Long, C. F.   Rumination in man. Amer. J. Med. Sci. 178:814, 1929.

THE STOMACH AND DUODENUM

Chapter 10

Motor Functions of the Stomach

Allan R. Cooke, James Christensen

The stomach receives and stores food, mixes it, reduces it to a slurry, and delivers it to the duodenum in a controlled manner. Storage of food occurs principally in the proximal stomach. Mixing, trituration, and regulated delivery are functions mainly of the distal part. Complex neural, muscular, and hormonal processes accomplish these processes.

ANATOMY[1]

The gross structure of the stomach varies greatly among mammals. In marsupials, the proximal stomach is enlarged. The proximal stomach is widened and extended into three chambers in ruminants. In most primates, rodents, and carnivora it is a single chamber. An enlarged proximal stomach containing chambers, sacculations, or diverticula appears to be an adaptation to a herbivorous diet. The langur, a wholly herbivorous monkey, has such a stomach in contrast to the simple stomach of omnivorous primates.[2]

The human stomach appears to hang from two fixed points at its poles, the esophagogastric and gastroduodenal junctions, because the organ is longer than the distance between the poles. Two borders join the poles, the lesser curvature on the right being shorter than the greater curvature on the left. The prevalent view of the division of the stomach into three parts (fundus, body, and antrum) is misleading, for it implies sharp distinctions among the three regions. These distinctions are vague. The terms proximal and distal stomach will be used here as much as possible, because they avoid the implication of sharp distinctions between regions. In terms of the muscular anatomy, the stomach is limited proximally by the esophagogastric sphincter (usually considered a part of the esophagus), and distally by the pylorus (commonly viewed as part of the stomach).

115

The *muscularis propria*, the main muscle coat of the stomach, contains outer longitudinal, middle circular, and inner oblique layers. The longitudinal and circular layers are continuous with those of the esophagus. The oblique layer is an extra layer, separate from both overlying coats of the stomach and from those of the esophagus and duodenum.

The outer longitudinal layer of muscle lies principally in two broad bands centered over the lesser and greater curvatures, respectively. The fibers of the middle circular layer lie at about 90 degrees to those of the longitudinal muscle, encircling the whole stomach except for a hiatus just to the left of the esophagogastric junction. The inner oblique layer lies over the apex of the stomach and extends down in two sheets which are thickest on the anterior and posterior surfaces of the stomach; it is thin along the greater curvature and very thin or absent along the lesser curvature. In the distal stomach the fibers of this layer tend to mingle with those of the circular layer. The circular muscle layer thickens along the antrum toward the pylorus. At the pylorus it reaches its greatest thickness to surround the gastroduodenal junction as the *anatomic* sphincter of the pylorus. The *physiological* sphincteric function of this region is questionable, as will be discussed later. The muscle of the pylorus contains prominent bands of connective tissue partially separating muscle fibers of the stomach from those of the duodenum. This separation is greater for the circular layer than for the longitudinal layer. Longitudinal fibers in part cross the sphincteric segment to join those of the corresponding layer of the duodenum and in part mingle with those of the circular layer at the sphincter.

The *muscularis mucosae* is a much thinner layer of muscle, distinct from the muscularis propria. Its fibers are divided into two indistinctly separated layers from which strands extend toward the lumen between the gastric glands.

The *intrinsic neural plexuses* of the stomach are generally like those of the small bowel and the esophagus.[3] The extrinsic nerves enter into the musculature to communicate with the subserous, myenteric submucosal and mucosal plexus. These apparently separate plexuses, named according to the stratum of the gut wall they principally occupy, are in fact interconnected. The plexuses, especially the myenteric plexus, are denser in the stomach than in other gastrointestinal viscera. As in other viscera, the cells of the plexuses exhibit morphological characteristics which suggest that the cells are not all of the same type. They probably constitute secondary parasympathetic ganglion cells, associative or internuncial cells and sensory cells. The task of assigning functions to specific cell types is difficult. The motor fibers within the plexuses probably also represent a variety of nerves. They include branches of secondary cholinergic neurons, adrenergic fibers, and, probably, nonadrenergic inhibitory nerves.[4] Others are certainly sensory in function. Some of these nerves can be distinguished by electron microscopy. The subject is so complex, however, that no detailed description of the distributions and interrelationships of all nerve types in the stomach is now possible.

The nerve plexuses of the gastric wall are connected to the central nervous system by way of the vagi and the splanchnic nerves and their plexuses.[5, 6] The vagi contain preganglionic parasympathetic fibers and other fibers which mediate sympathetic responses. In the cat, at least, the vagi may also contain fibers of the nonadrenergic inhibitory nervous system. All three types seem to be distributed to the gastric plexuses. The vagi also carry sensory fibers from the stomach. The splanchnic nerves and their plexuses constitute mainly sympathetic fibers and fibers of sensory function.

The central nervous system affects gastric movement. Despite its name, the autonomic nervous system in the gut is not autonomous. The two vagi contain (in the cat) about 31,000 nerve fibers, of which 90 per cent are sensory. At least some of these arise in the stomach wall, for stimulation of chemoreceptors or stretch receptors in the stomach excite vagal afferent fibers. Pain sensations arising from gastric distention are conveyed by way of splanchnic afferents which enter the spinal cord chiefly from the eighth to the thirteenth thoracic dorsal nerve roots.

Excitation of vagal motors fibers may cause either contraction or inhibition, suggesting two kinds of motor fibers. Those mediating inhibition require stronger electrical stimulation of the vagi than those which are excitatory. The inhibition is most prominent in the proximal stomach.

Excitation of sympathetic motor fibers may also produce either contraction or inhibition. The excitatory fibers have a lower threshold to electrical stimulation than do the inhibitory fibers. The former appear to be cholinergic, the latter, adrenergic.

The impulses traveling over sensory and motor fibers to and from the stomach are integrated within the central nervous system. Electrical stimulation at many levels within the brain and spinal cord have been observed to modify gastric movement.[7] These observations have led to the view that integration of gastric movement may involve a vast complex of neural circuits within the cortex, subcortex, midbrain, medulla oblongata, and spinal cord.

THE PHARMACOLOGY OF GASTRIC MUSCLE[8]

All nerves in the plexuses are presumed to exert their controls upon gastric movement by local release of neurotransmitter hormones from sites of storage within the nerve terminals. Other systemic hormones can affect gastric movements as well. An understanding of the effects of the nerves and systemic hormones on gastric movement requires an understanding of the actions of these specific substances upon the musculature. This subject, generally called the pharmacology of the gastric muscle, is made difficult by a number of uncertainties. In most studies, experiments assume the form of an examination of the responses of the muscle to exposure to the substances in question in a bath of physiological salt solution, or of the observation of responses of muscle to electrical stimulation of extrinsic or intrinsic nerves or to drug-induced excitation of nerves. Certain drug antagonists may be used to reach conclusions about mechanisms. The interpretation of such studies is difficult because of uncertainties about the anatomic and functional relationships among the several kinds of nerves, about the tissue (neural or muscular) upon which an agent is working, and about the degree of specificity of most antagonists.

The sympathetic innervation of the stomach is largely postganglionic, coming from neurons of the paravertebral ganglia, the prevertebral abdominal ganglia (principally the celiac ganglion), terminal ganglia lying near or in the stomach wall, and ganglia somewhere in the vagal system. A distribution of preganglionic fibers to the stomach through both vagal and splanchnic systems has not been excluded. The distal connections of sympathetic nerves are varied. Some postganglionic fibers synapse with cell bodies of the myenteric plexus, some enter the muscle layers, and others are distributed to the vasculature. The transmitters of the postganglionic sympathetic fibers are catecholamines.

The parasympathetic innervation of the stomach constitutes preganglionic fibers distributed by the vagi and their branches. The vagi are by no means "pure" nerves: they contain a mixture of various kinds of motor fibers and sensory fibers. The parasympathetic preganglionic fibers are the fibers usually meant when vagal functions are described. The transmitter of the parasympathetic postganglionic fibers is acetylcholine.

The nonadrenergic inhibitory innervation to the stomach arrives through the vagus nerves. Little is known of their anatomy: they can be identified only functionally and by electron microscopy. Their transmitter is not established.

The stomach is also affected by a variety of systemic neurohormones. Adrenal medullary catecholamines, gastrin, secretin, and cholecystokinin are the principal hormones considered of physiological importance.

Other physiological substances can affect the stomach muscle and may conceivably have some part in normal regulation of its movement. These include histamine, serotonin, angiotensin, vasopressin, and some prostaglandins.

The actions of real or putative hormones, local and systemic, cannot yet be synthesized into any total view of the control system. An attempt to do so requires the assumption of the existence of distinct types of receptors for agents of different classes. The possibility that drug receptors of different kinds exist is strengthened by the observation that certain agents which act alike share certain molecular configurations in common. Drug receptors are, by inference, like enzymes: the receptor-drug combination involves interaction of reactive groups in the drug molecule with active sites in the receptor structure. No receptors have been isolated, purified, or completely analyzed structurally. Still, the concept of specific receptors is useful.

Some kinds of receptors are reasonably well established. Others remain vague. The *cholinergic muscarinic receptor* is an active site mediating responses to acetylcholine and some of its analogues. Such receptors are more sensitive to acetyl-β-methacholine and acetylcholine than to carbamylcholine in the presence of cholinesterase inhibition. Responses are selectively antagonized by hyoscine and related agents, but not by nicotine or agents which act like nicotine. The *cholinergic nicotinic receptor* is an active site mediating responses to acetylcholine and its analogues in which carbamylcholine, acetylcholine, and nicotine are more potent than acetyl-β-methacholine in the presence of cholinesterase inhibition. Responses are selectively opposed by hexamethonium, *d*-tubocurarine, large doses of nicotine, and related agents. *Adrenergic alpha receptors* mediate responses to catecholamines in which norepinephrine and epinephrine are more potent than isopropyl-norepinephrine, and which are selectively opposed by dibenamine, tolazoline, phentolamine, and related antagonists. *Adrenergic beta receptors* mediate responses to catecholamines in which isopropylnorepinephrine and epinephrine are more potent than norepinephrine. Responses are selectively opposed by pronethalol, propranolol, and dichloroisopropylnorepinephrine.

In such a closely knit amalgam of neural, muscular, and secretory cells as the stomach wall, the site of action of any agent is difficult to determine precisely. Experimental evidence allows some statements of the localization of the four kinds of receptors described above. Muscarinic receptors are located in smooth muscle cells and in postganglionic sympathetic ganglion cells. Nicotinic receptors are located in postganglionic parasympathetic and sympathetic ganglion cells and in sensory nerve fibers. Alpha receptors are located both in smooth muscle cells and in cholinergic postganglionic nerves of the myenteric plexus. Beta receptors seem to be confined to smooth muscle cells.

Other kinds of receptors are less clearly defined. *Histamine receptors* mediate those responses to histamine which are selectively opposed by such agents as chlorpheniramine, and diphenhydramine. These receptors are located both in smooth muscle cells and in nerve tissue. *Serotonin receptors* mediate responses to serotonin and are antagonized selectively by serotonin antagonists. They seem to occur in both neural and smooth muscular tissues. *Gastrin and secretin receptors* have been postulated.

The effects of local and systemic hormones upon the net functions of the stomach, filling and emptying, may well be related to different actions of these agents on different parts of the stomach. Although the actions of particular receptor types upon gastric muscle in general have been described, it is possible that muscle from one part of the stomach may differ from that of another region in its responses to excitation of these receptors.

Activation of *muscarinic receptors* excites contractions in gastric muscle, as it does in all gastrointestinal muscle. There is no evidence that acetylcholine relaxes the pylorus or any sphincteric regions. Activation of *nicotinic receptors* may produce either excitation or inhibition of contractions. *Alpha receptor* activation usually inhibits contractions, but some studies suggest that such activation can also excite contractions, both in human stomach muscle and in stomach muscle from other species. Thus there seem to be two kinds of alpha receptors, inhibitory and excitatory. *Beta receptor* activation seems to be always inhibitory.

Histamine receptor activation may either excite or inhibit contractions. *Serotonin receptors* usually contract muscles from the proximal stomach and inhibit those of the distal stomach. *Gastrin* excites contractions of gastric muscle. *Secretin* is inhibitory, as are at least some preparations of *cholecystokinin-pancreozymin.*

One of the prostaglandins, E_2, is a very potent stimulant of gastric muscle and can be extracted from gastric mucosa.

The usual analysis of responses to agents in terms of contraction or inhibition of contraction is very difficult to apply to net gastric motor function. Net motor function of the stomach is probably much more closely related to the electrical slow wave of the antrum. Hormonal agents may alter gastric emptying at least as much through effects on this phenomenon as through effects on the contractions of the muscle.

FILLING[5, 6]

The filling of the stomach is probably not entirely a passive process, though it is not completely understood. It may be that, to a degree, the empty stomach simply unfolds to accommodate part of an ingested volume. However, this is probably not the whole process, considering the magnitude of the volume of the full stomach. Gastric muscle, in fact, seems to contract or relax to keep basal intragastric pressure quite constant over a wide range of volumes. This implies that tonic contraction of the whole stomach, or a part of it, is constantly regulated by a control system.

The control system appears, at least in part, to be a centrally mediated reflex. The response is called *receptive relaxation*. The reflex, first described many years ago, consists of an inhibition of tonic contraction of the proximal stomach in response to swallowing. This inhibition leads to an increase in volume such that there is no rise in intragastric pressure as a volume of ingesta enters the stomach. Both the sensory and motor pathways of this system are vagal. The motor fibers appear not to be either cholinergic or adrenergic. They may belong to the nonadrenergic nervous system.

EMPTYING[9]

The emptying of the stomach is regulated by many factors, yet the net result of their interaction is that gastric emptying occurs as a single exponential function. The factors involved with gastric emptying of meals include the volume of the meal and the composition of the meal acting through nervous reflexes and hormones to control the action of the muscle of the stomach.

Several methods are used to assess gastric emptying. (1) Gastric contents may be aspirated and the residual volume measured at fixed time intervals after a meal. The use of meals containing a nonabsorbable indicator (phenol red, polyethylene glycol, or Cr^{51}) allows correction for volume changes caused by absorption and secretion. Such methods are accurately quantitative but are restricted to liquid meals or to meals which are homogeneous. (2) Test meals may be made to contain radioactive isotopes (technetium, indium) and scanning techniques used to estimate residual volume at fixed time intervals after the meal. These techniques also are accurately quantitative, but they are limited to liquid and homogeneous meals and they require expensive equipment. (3) Residual gastric volume may be estimated by using radiopaque meals (barium sulfate, iodinated contrast media), photographing the stomach radiographically at fixed time intervals, and measuring the area of the opaque material on the radiographs. These methods are only very roughly quantitative, but they may be applied to nonhomogeneous meals.

In terms of emptying, the stomach is viewed classically as two functionally distinct areas; the proximal stomach (body and fundus) is a reservoir and the distal stomach (antrum) is a pump. The pump also accomplishes mixing and trituration.

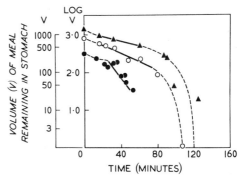

Figure 10–1. Gastric emptying of 1250 ml, 750 ml, and 330 ml of sucrose solution, 35 g per liter. Volumes of meals recovered, on a log scale plotted against time of recovery. (From Hunt, J. N. and MacDonald. I.: J. Physiol. [London]*126*:459, 1954.)

The rate of transfer of gastric contents is usually less than maximal, for the control mechanisms are nearly all inhibitory. The only known natural stimulus which accelerates emptying is gastric distention.

When a liquid meal is ingested and residual volume is measured at regular intervals, emptying is an exponential function (Fig. 10–1). This pattern, however, does not hold true at the very beginning and the very end of the process. When the data from Figure 10–1 are replotted against the square root of the residual volume, the fit is much better (Fig. 10–2). This suggests that the stomach can be viewed as a cylinder in which the radius is a function of the square root of volume.[10] It is obvious that the larger the volume of a meal, the greater will be the net rate of emptying. The general pattern of emptying is not affected by the nature of the meal and is true for meals of variable viscosity, meals containing fat, carbohydrate, or protein, and even for plastic spheres. This consistent pattern may be related to neural reflexes. There are mechanoreceptors in the gastric wall throughout the gastric body and antrum, and it is possible that these monitor gastric volume in some way and influence emptying by local or central reflex mechanisms.[11]

The composition of a meal is an important factor in regulating the rate of emptying (without changing the exponential pattern).

It has been known for decades that liquids leave the stomach faster than solids. Recent evidence confirms the old view that the distal part of the antrum acts to

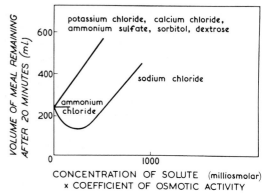

Figure 10–3. Effect of osmotic pressure of test meals on gastric emptying. Idealized representation of the relationship between volumes of 750 ml test meal recovered 20 minutes after instillation, and the milliosmolar concentration. (From Hunt, J. N., and Pathak, J. D.: J. Physiol. [London] *154*:254, 1960.)

prevent large solid particles from escaping the stomach; distal antrectomy accelerates emptying of solids but has little effect on emptying of liquids.

The osmolarity of the meal is critical. Over a wide range of concentrations of a variety of organic and inorganic solutes, Hunt and Pathak[12] found the common factor in rate of emptying to be the osmotic pressure (Fig. 10–3). To explain these results, they have proposed that the duodenal mucosa contains *osmoreceptors*. These are postulated to shrink or swell according to the osmotic pressure of the luminal fluid, exciting neural or hormonal mechanisms which influence emptying rate. Salts of potassium, calcium, sulfates, sorbitol, and glucose and very high concentrations of sodium, glycerol, urea, and ethanol are thought to penetrate slowly into the osmoreceptors and reduce the flux of water into them. The osmoreceptor shrinks, exciting an inhibitory mechanism. Ammonium chloride, in concentrations up to 200 milliosmols has no effect on emptying and thus is postulated to have no osmotic effect. Ammonium sulfate, however, is effective because of the effectiveness of the sulfate ion.

According to this hypothesis, if the osmoreceptor swells, the rate of gastric emptying should be increased. This could occur through active or facilitated transport of solute into the osmoreceptor. This may account for the increased rate of emp-

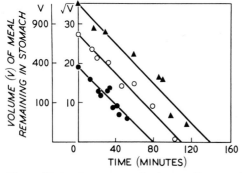

Figure 10–2. Square root of volumes of test meals recovered after various times. Data are the same as those shown in Figure 10-1. From Hopkins, A.:J. Physiol. [London] *182*:144, 1966.)

tying which occurs with meals containing low concentrations of sodium, glycerol, or urea. The emptying of meals of sodium chloride is maximal at concentrations of about 250 milliosmols, is equal to water at about 500 milliosmols, and is delayed progressively at higher concentrations. Concentrations of ethanol up to about 1300 milliosmols do not delay emptying.[13]

Studies of the effect of *amino acids* on the rate of emptying are consistent with the view that they act by way of the osmoreceptor mechanism.[14]

The osmoreceptors must be located beyond the plyorus, because isocaloric meals of starch and glucose empty at the same rate and more slowly than water. Since hydrolysis of starch occurs beyond the plyorus, the osmoreceptors must be there also. Studies of meals of disaccharides indicate that 1 mole of lactose or maltose is about equivalent to 2 moles of their hydrolysis products in their effectiveness in reducing the rate of emptying. Thus, hydrolysis of disaccharides by the brush border must occur before osmoreceptors can be affected by these sugars.

Thus, the osmoreceptors are not selective, but can respond to the osmotic effects of electrolytes, amino acids and carbohydrates.

Acids also slow gastric emptying by exciting a different duodenal receptor.[15] The receptor normally responds only to hydrochloric acid. Acids vary in their ability to retard emptying. For example, 45 mM hydrochloric acid is about as effective as 60 mM acetic acid or 120 mM citric acid. There is a direct relationship between the mean concentration of a variety of acids causing a fixed recovery of 450 ml of a 750 ml test meal and the square root of the molecular weight of the acid (Fig. 10–4). This suggests that the anions of the acids are important factors in the mechanism; the larger the anion of the acid, the greater the concentration of the acid required to be effective. The larger anion molecules may diffuse to the receptor more slowly than the smaller ones. Hydrogen ion must be present, however, because the substitution of sodium salts of these acids for the acids themselves at equivalent molar concentrations abolishes the effect; the sodium salts usually increase rate of empty-

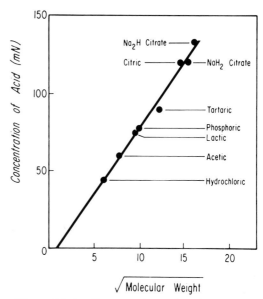

Figure 10–4. Concentrations of acids causing a fixed recovery of 450 ml of a 750 ml test meal plotted against the square root of the molecular weight of the acid. (From Hunt, J. N., and Knox, M. T.: Amer. J. Dig. Dis. *13*:372, 1968.)

ing over that of water. Further studies of this mechanism indicate that fat solubility and whether the acid is weak are not significant variables if the pK_a is less than 5.0.[15, 16] However, strong acids behave like hydrochloric acid because of the presence of chloride ion in duodenal contents and thus produce an environment of hydrochloric acid around the receptor.[16]

Fats have long been known to delay gastric emptying. Studies with sodium and potassium soaps of various fatty acids suggest that the chain length of the fatty acid is a critical factor.[17] The longer the chain of the fatty acid, the greater the effect in delaying gastric emptying. From acetic acid (2 carbons) to octanoic acid (8 carbons) there is little difference in the effect, but effectiveness increases above a carbon chain length of 8. Myristic acid (14 carbons) is the most effective.

The receptors which sense fatty acid concentrations, fat receptors, appear to be more sensitive than osmoreceptors and acid receptors. About 8 mM myristic acid has a retarding effect about equivalent to that of 45 mM hydrochloric acid and 500 mM glucose.

In summary, the rate of emptying of meals by the stomach varies with the volume of the meal, with the osmotic pressure of the meal (as affected by carbohydrates, amino acids, and electrolytes, with the concentration of acids in the meal, and with the fat content of the meal. The receptors sensing these properties of the meal are physiological entities, but no anatomical descriptions of their morphology or location in the duodenal wall exist.

The inhibitory mechanisms working to produce the effects described above are generally viewed as either neural or hormonal or both. Generally noxious stimuli, such as pain or distention of the intestine, will inhibit gastric emptying by way of the sympathetic motor innervation to the stomach. The inhibitory effects of osmotic solutions, fats, acids, and protein digestion products on gastric emptying appear to be served by *enterogastric reflexes.* These may in part be central, for vagotomy abolishes the inhibitory effect of hyperosomolar meals and the effects of fat meals on the electric slow waves of the antrum.[18] The newly described nonadrenergic nerves (which may act by release of purine compounds) may also be involved in these reflexes.[19]

Several of the enteric hormones are postulated as affecting gastric emptying. *Secretin* inhibits gastric emptying as well as gastric secretion in doses which are probably within usual physiological limits.[20] *Gastrin* and the synthetic pentapeptide (pentagastrin) inhibit gastrin emptying at doses considered physiological.[21, 22] *Cholecystokinin* (pancreozymin) also delays gastric emptying.[20] *Enterogastrone* is a postulated hormone not yet isolated in pure form. It refers to a substance liberated from the duodenum by fats which inhibits both gastric emptying and secretion. Its structure has been partly determined; it appears to be distinct from other gastrointestinal hormones.[23]

A fifth hormone, *motilin,* containing 22 amino acid residues, has been found to be released from the upper 1 meter of the small intestine by alkalinization of the lumen.[24] It causes increased motor activity of the fundal and antral pouches. Its possible role in modulating gastric emptying remains to be determined.

The movements of the antrum suggest that it is a peristaltic pump, and that the role of gastric emptying is a function of variations in output of this pump. The frequency of this pump is set at a maximum of three cycles per minute (in man) by the antral electrical slow wave, but the frequency may be less than that if action potentials (and therefore contractions) do not accompany all electrical slow wave cycles. If antral peristalsis is the sole factor in gastric emptying, then a reduction in frequency should reduce emptying. Obviously, emptying is also determined by stroke volume, a factor about which very little is known. It is not known, for example, whether a strong antral contraction is accompanied by a large stroke volume. Thus, if the pump hypothesis is true, force and frequency of antral contractions and stroke volume should all be interrelated variables in determining gastric emptying, but their interrelationships are not known.

The antrum appears to be much more complex than this, however, for recent evidence suggests that the antrum deals with liquid meals differently from solid meals. In situations in which the emptying of liquid meals was delayed physiologically, the force and frequency of antral contractions were either increased or decreased.[22] Furthermore, distal antrectomy does not affect the rate of emptying of liquid meals but does accelerate emptying of solids.[25] These studies suggest that the antrum acts mainly to mix chyme and to delay the passage of solid particles until they are reduced in size to some critical value. They indicate that the antrum may not be purely a peristaltic pump.

ELECTROMYOGRAPHY[26]

Electromyography of gastric muscle, like electromyography of all gastrointestinal smooth muscle, is a relatively new discipline, lagging many decades behind electromyography of cardiac and somatic muscle. This slowness of development is partly due to the fact that the techniques for smooth muscle electromyography are comparatively difficult. The relationships between myoelectrical events and motor functions of the stomach are slow to become clear because of the imprecision of our appreciation of patterns of contraction.

Electrical records from the wall of the distal stomach reveal two kinds of signals which are separate but related. One signal is a slow transient change in voltage, called the *electrical slow wave*. It is very like other such signals generated in small bowel and colon. Other synonyms used for this signal are the gastric pacesetter potential, pacemaking potential, antral control activity, and the basic electrical rhythm of the stomach. All these terms together suggest much of the nature and function of this phenomenon. It constitutes a slow electrical transient, stereotyped in configuration, occurring constantly at regular intervals of several seconds, whose function is to pace and integrate movements of the antral musculature. The second electrical signal detected in antral muscle is a much faster transient or group of transients. These signals are called action potentials, spike potentials, action spikes, a spike burst, or antral control activity. They are intermittent, occurring just before contractions and appearing to initiate them. They always occur with a fixed phase relationship to the electrical slow waves. The intermittent burst of action potentials is initiative of contractions: the constant slow wave is integrative, imposing a particular distribution of the action potentials (and their associated contractions) in time and space.

Slow waves appear to be generated by the outer longitudinal layer of muscle in the stomach and spread to the other layers of the gastric musculature. When they are recorded from a single muscle cell, using intracellular glass microelectrodes, they appear as partial depolarizations of the cell membrane. "Resting" transmembrane potential, of the order of 50 mv, is interrupted at intervals of 20 seconds or so by partial depolarizations of 25 to 30 mv. A rather rapid depolarization to a plateau lasting several seconds is followed by a slower repolarization to "resting" levels. The configuration of the event is very constant and its frequency is very regular, as biological phenomena go. The event is continuously repetitive and independent of contractions. These depolarizations seem clearly to reflect movements of ions across the gastric mucosa. Evidence suggests that sodium shifts are the principal ones.[27]

These slow waves can be recorded as well from needle electrodes implanted in the gastric wall. The recording is usually monopolar, the voltage difference being recorded between such a gastric electrode and a reference electrode implanted at a point remote from the stomach. Such a needle electrode must contact several hundred cells, yet it produces a record which is a unitary signal, usually having a configuration approximately a derivative of the waves of single-cell recording. The configuration of such needle electrode records varies with the geometry of the electrode-cell contact. When multiple needle electrodes are put along the stomach, slow waves appear at various points separated in time. Extensive studies have been made to map this apparent spread of slow waves through the antrum. These studies have revealed consistent patterns of slow wave spread.

Slow waves appear to spread away from a source, a pacemaking area, located high on the greater curvature of the stomach.[28] In this region they are very low-voltage signals. They cannot be detected above this region. They spread from this area toward the antrum. Their apparent velocity is very slow at first, but as they progress toward the antrum their voltage progressively increases and they seem to accelerate. In the terminal antrum, their velocity is so great that they are nearly synchronous over the last few centimenters of the antrum. The pacemaking region generates a new signal every 20 seconds in man (the frequency is slightly different in other species), and this frequency is remarkably constant. The frequency, velocity, and pattern of spread of the slow wave all seem so like the same characteristics of antral peristalsis that it has long been evident that they are related.

Slow waves do not themselves initiate contractions; they occur continuously even when the antrum is not moving. When contractions occur, however, they occur with slow waves. The electrical record then shows another kind of signal superimposed on the slow wave. In single-cell recordings, this may appear to be either a prolonged and greater depolarization, or a single or group of spikes, or both. With the spike configuration, these spikes are very rapid and very brief depolarizations rising from the period of maximal depolarization of the slow waves. Whatever their configuration, these signals precede and initiate contractions of the muscle mass. Significant contractions do not occur except in association with such signals. This phenomenon is called electrical response activity or the second potential. Since contractions are phase locked to second potentials, and second potentials are phase locked to slow waves, the effect of slow waves on contractions is clear.

The slow wave is like a carrier, pacing contractions and directing their distribution in time and space when other kinds of controls cause contractions to occur. The antrum is viewed as a pump which conveys fluid from a reservoir (the fundus) to a conduit (the duodenum). As a peristaltic pump, the antrum is functionally dependent upon the slow wave; changes in the slow wave mechanism should greatly influence the pumping of the antrum.

The antral slow wave is not immutable. Its frequency, though quite constant, is not locked. Acetylcholine can induce an extra cycle if it is given by close intra-arterial injection at a critical period in the slow wave cycle. Catecholamines induce a chaotic dysrhythmia. These are extreme stimuli; under physiological conditions, the variations in frequency are exceedingly small.

The patterns of spread of slow waves are probably more importantly susceptible to change. A variety of operative maneuvers have been shown to alter, at least transiently, the patterns of slow wave spread. Partial transection of the stomach along the greater curvature and vagotomy have both been reported to disturb slow wave spread. Pyloroplasty has also been reported to influence spread.

Since spreading patterns are susceptible to such operative maneuvers, it is important to understand the nature of slow wave spread. At first it was believed that slow waves spread through the stomach in a manner analogous to the spread of electric current through a cable, or in the manner of nerve impulses through an axon, being initiated repeatedly from a pacemaker. Such a view is probably not accurate for several reasons. For one, slow wave velocity is very slow compared with axonal conduction and varies systematically, increasing with distance from the pacemaking area. When the stomach is cut into small pieces, each muscle fragment continues to generate slow waves. These and other considerations long puzzled those who tried to understand the nature of slow waves.

A recent hypothesis seems to allow an explanation for the characteristics of slow waves and the basis of their spread.[29] This hypothesis, the coupled relaxation oscillator hypothesis, proposes that slow waves are independently generated by discrete units, relaxation oscillators, so called because of the configuration of the electrical wave-form they generate. It was first proposed for small bowel slow waves.[30] A single oscillator is probably composed of a cluster of no more than a few hundred adjacent cells. All the cells of the longitudinal layer are viewed as being organized into such oscillators, so that this layer is then composed of a matrix of hundreds of thousands of oscillators. These oscillators are electrically coupled bidirectionally, one being coupled to all its neighbors. This coupling is probably both resistive and capacitative. It is probably brought about through tight junctions seen to exist between adjacent smooth muscle cells. Each oscillator has an intrinsic frequency, the rate at which it generates signals when it is separated from its fellows. The intrinsic frequencies vary systematically over the stomach such that those with the highest frequency are proximal. When the oscillator matrix is intact, the coupling allows those oscillators with higher intrinsic frequencies to capture those with lower intrinsic frequencies and drive them at a rate faster than their intrinsic frequencies. Such a system allows a rational explanation of the characteristics of slow waves. Computer models of the antral oscillator matrix have been constructed. They respond to various perturbations of the matrix in the same way that the antral slow wave system responds to the same perturbations. Thus this hypothesis is an attractive and important advance. It may well allow a great expansion of our understanding of the effects of various physical disturbances upon antral function and gastric emptying.

AN OVERVIEW OF THE EMPTYING PROCESS

The stomach contains two functional units. The proximal stomach is a reservoir; the distal stomach is a peristaltic pump.

Gastric emptying is a consequence mainly of the antral pump. As in all cyclic pumps, the rate of pumping can vary with the frequency of the pump and the stroke output.

Pump frequency is established by a clock, the electrical slow wave. This signal also establishes the spatial integration of the pump. The clock is running constantly, whether or not the pump is working. For any single cycle of the clock, the pump may or may not respond; thus the frequency of the pump is a fraction of the frequency of the clock.

In each cycle of the clock, the choice of the muscle to contract or not to contract is determined by neural and hormonal controls. These controls, which appear to be autoregulatory, may determine whether or not the musculature responds to the slow wave and may determine the force or depth of the contractions. Thus they can produce gradations in stroke output.

These autoregulatory systems include local reflexes excited by duodenal chemoreceptors and mechanoreceptors and hormones liberated by the gastric and duodenal mucosa in response to excitants in contact with the mucosa. Despite the number and variety of the autoregulatory mechanisms, the net emptying of the stomach is uniexponential. This appears to represent a high degree of interaction among the several autoregulatory systems. The site (or sites) of this interaction is unknown.

GASTRIC EMPTYING IN DISEASE

A wide variety of conditions interfere with gastric emptying from time to time (e.g., uremia, diabetic ketoacidosis, migraine). The mechanism is unknown in such systemic diseases. In some patients with long-standing diabetes and, usually, many signs of diabetic polyneuropathy, gastric emptying may be delayed. This is attributed to autonomic neuropathy.

If they occur at the pylorus, local lesions may retard gastric emptying by mechanical means. These include carcinoma, duodenal or pyloric channel ulcer, and idiopathic hypertrophic plyoric stenosis (a condition which occurs rarely in adults, but more commonly in neonates).

Studies of patients with atrophic gastritis and gastric ulcer suggest that these lesions may be associated with delayed gastric emptying.[31] The mechanism is not clear, but it may be due in part to the elevation in serum gastrin concentration which occurs in these diseases. Gastrin delays gastric emptying.

Chronically delayed gastric emptying is probably not a benign process. It probably contributes to the difficulty in control of diabetes in those who have autonomic neuropathy. It has been postulated to be causative in at least some cases of gastric ulcer. In a significantly large proportion of patients with long-standing duodenal ulcer disease, gastric ulceration develops.[32] This has been attributed to gastric retention consequent to motor changes in the duodenal bulb. Conversely, some patients with active duodenal ulcer disease have been found to have more rapid gastric emptying than a group of control subjects.[33] Gastric hypersecretion combined with rapid gastric emptying may be causative in some cases of duodenal ulcer, but this is certainly not established.

REFERENCES

1. Schofield, G. C. Anatomy of muscular and neural tissues in the alimentary canal. *In* Handbook of Physiology, Sect. 6, Vol. IV, C. F. Code (ed.). Washington, D.C., American Physiological Society, 1968. pp. 1579–1627.
2. Bauchop, T., and Martucci, R. W. Ruminant-like digestion in the Langur monkey. Science *161*:698, 1968.
3. Pick, J. The Autonomic Nervous System. Morphological, Comparative, Clinical and Surgical Aspects. Philadelphia, J. B. Lippincott Co., 1970.
4. Burnstock, G. Evolution of the autonomic innervation of visceral and cardiovascular systems in vertebrates. Pharmacol. Rev. *21*:247, 1969.
5. Jansson, G. Extrinsic nervous control of gastric motility: An experimental study in the cat. Acta Physiol. Scand. (Suppl.) *326*:1, 1969.
6. Martinson, J. Studies on the efferent vagal control of the stomach. Acta Physiol. Scand. (Suppl) *255*:1, 1965.
7. Thomas, J. E., and Baldwin, M. V. Pathways and mechanisms of regulation of gastric motility. *In* Handbook of Physiology, Sect. 6, Vol. IV, C. F. Code (ed.). Washington, D.C., American Physiological Society, 1968, pp. 1937–1968.
8. Daniel, E. E. Pharmacology of the gastrointestinal tract. *In* Handbook of Physiology, Sect. 6, Vol. IV, C. F. Code (ed.). Washington,

D.C., American Physiological Society, 1968, pp. 2267-2324.

9. Hunt, J. N., and Knox M. T. Regulation of gastric emptying. *In* Handbook of Physiology, Sect. 6, Vol. IV, C. F. Code (ed.). Washington, D.C., American Physiological Society, 1968. pp. 1917-1935.

10. Hopkins, A. The pattern of gastric emptying: A new view of old results. J. Physiol. (London) *182*:144, 1966.

11. Paintal, A. S. A study of gastric stretch receptors. Their role in the peripheral mechanism of satiation of hunger and thirst. J. Physiol. (London) *126*:255, 1954.

12. Hunt, J. N., and Pathak, J. D. The osmotic effects of some simple molecules and ions on gastric emptying. J. Physiol. (London) *154*:254, 1960.

13. Cooke, A. R. The simultaneous emptying and absorption of ethanol from the human stomach. Amer. J. Dig. Dis. *15*:449, 1970.

14. Cooke, A. R., and Moulang, J. Control of gastric emptying by amino acids. Gastroenterology *62*:528, 1972.

15. Hunt, J. N., and Knox, M. T. The slowing of gastric emptying by nine acids. J. Physiol. (London) *201*:169, 1969.

16. Hunt J. N., and Knox, M. T. The slowing of gastric emptying by four strong acids and three weak acids. J. Physiol. (London) *222*:187, 1972.

17. Hunt, J. N., and Knox, M. T. A relation between the chain length of fatty acids and the slowing of gastric emptying. J. Physiol. (London) *194*:327, 1968.

18. Kelly, K. A., and Code, C. F. Effect of transthoracic vagotomy on canine gastric electrical activity. Gastroenterology *57*:51, 1969.

19. Burnstock, G., Campbell, G., Satchell, D., et al. Evidence that adenosine triphosphate or a related nucleotide is the transmitter substance released by non-adrenergic inhibitory nerves of the gut. Brit. J. Pharmacol. *40*:668, 1970.

20. Chey, W. Y., Hitanant, S., Hendricks, J., et al. Effect of secretin and cholecystokinin on gastric emptying and gastric secretion in man. Gastroenterology *58*:820, 1970.

21. Dozois, R. R. and Kelly, K. A. Effect of a gastrin pentapeptide on canine gastric emptying of liquids. Amer. J. Physiol. *221*:113, 1971.

22. Cooke, A. R., Chvasta, T. E., and Weisbrodt, N. W. Effect of pentagastrin on emptying and electrical and motor activity of the dog stomach. Amer. J. Physiol. *223*:934, 1972.

23. Brown, J. C., Mutt, V., and Pederson, R. A. Further purification of a polypeptide demonstrating enterogastrone activity. J. Physiol. (London) *209*:57, 1970.

24. Brown, J. C., Mutt, V., and Dryburgh, J. R. The further purification of motilin, a gastric motor activity stimulating polypeptide from the mucosa of the small intestine of hogs. Canad. J. Physiol. Pharmacol. *49*:399, 1971.

25. Dozois, R. R., Kelly, K. A., and Code, C. F. Effect of distal antrectomy on gastric emptying of liquids and solids. Gastroenterology *61*:675, 1971.

26. Daniel, E. E., and Irwin, J. Electrical activity of gastric musculature. *In* Handbook of Physiology, Sect. 6, Vol. IV, C. F. Code (ed.). Washington, D. C., American Physiological Society, 1968, pp. 1969–1984.

27. Papasova, M. P., Nagai, T., and Prosser, C. L. Two-component slow waves in smooth muscle of cat stomach. Amer. J. Physiol. *214*:695, 1968.

28. Kelly, K. A., and Code, C. F. Canine gastric pacemaker. Amer. J. Physiol. *220*:112, 1971.

29. Sarna, S. K., Daniel, E. E., and Kingma, Y. J. A simulation of the electric-control activity of the stomach by an array of relaxation oscillators. Amer. J. Dig. Dis. *17*:299, 1972.

30. Sarna, S. K., Daniel, E. E., and Kingma, Y. J. Simulation of slow-wave electrical activity of small intestine. Amer. J. Physiol. *221*:166, 1971.

31. Davies, W. T., Kirkpatrick, J. R., Owen, G. M., et al. Gastric emptying in atrophic gastritis and carcinoma of the stomach. Scand. J. Gastroenterol. *6*:297, 1971.

32. Rumball, J. M. Coexistent duodenal ulcer. Gastroenterology *61*:622, 1971.

33. Griffith, G. H., Owen, G. M., Campbell, H., et al. Gastric emptying in health and in gastroduodenal disease. Gastroenterology *54*:1, 1968.

Chapter 11

Vomiting

John S. Fordtran

Vomiting undoubtedly has some protective value, but its medical importance stems from the number of conditions which may cause or be associated with vomiting. Its frequency in such conditions as pregnancy, motion sickness, intestinal obstruction, psychoneurosis, drug toxicity, postgastrectomy states, and after anesthesia and the sometimes serious consequences (i.e., aspiration pneumonia, Mallory-Weiss syndrome, electrolyte depletion, and acid base imbalance) make vomiting one of man's most important symptoms.

NORMAL GASTRIC EMPTYING

Although the motor functions of the stomach are described in detail in Chapter 10, a brief review of normal gastric emptying will be useful in understanding vomiting. In making this summary, the author has relied heavily on an article by Thomas.[1]

Ingested food is usually a mixture of solids and liquids. The liquids in a meal tend to be emptied rapidly, whereas the solids are stored in the fundus until they are rendered into a liquid phase by digestion. The mechanisms whereby the stomach tends to empty liquids and retain solids are not entirely clear, although antral and pyloric contraction and possibly antiperistaltic waves may play a role. For whatever reason, the passage of gastric content through the pylorus is essentially a matter of the movement of fluid. Since gravity has little or no effect on gastric emptying, the problem is mainly reduced to a consideration of the pressure differentials developed by contraction and relaxation of the gastric and duodenal muscle and the resistance encountered at the pylorus.

The regularity of gastric peristalsis, particularly in the antrum, is remarkable. Peristaltic waves, beginning in the fundus and traveling to the prepyloric area, occur at a frequency of about three per minute. The waves deepen as they approach the pylorus. When the antral contraction reaches the prepyloric area, the antrum contracts very strongly, obliterating its lumen. At the same time the pyloric sphincter contracts and the proximal duodenum relaxes. A moment later the antrum relaxes and the duodenum regains its tone and rhythmic activity. The sphincter remains contracted momentarily, regurgitation is prevented, and the duodenal contents are propelled forward. The pylorus then relaxes.

Gastric emptying begins as soon as any considerable part of the gastric content becomes liquid enough to pass the pylorus, and once started it proceeds rhythmically, some fluid being emptied with each peristaltic cycle. Evacuation of gastric content begins as the antral wave approaches the pylorus, but before any elevation in antral pressure can be detected manometrically. Emptying ceases as bulbar and sphincteric contractions close the gastric outlet.

The gastroduodenal pressure, motility, and emptying cycle may be correlated as follows: A strong antral wave approaches the pylorus, and it finally obliterates the gastric lumen. Distal antral luminal pressure would rise if its contents were not free to escape via the pylorus. They do escape at first (relaxed sphincter and duodenum), hence there is initially no pressure rise. However, the sphincter soon begins to contract, its lumen narrows, resistance to emptying increases, and luminal pressure in the lower antrum increases. At first the pressure generated by antral contraction is sufficient to overcome resistance at the pylorus, and gastric emptying continues; but the rapidly contracting sphincter soon closes the pylorus and puts an end to this cycle of evacuation. The duodenum then regains its tone and empties, preparing itself for the next evacuation period.

The preceding is probably accurate for most normal foods. Liquid meals, however, may be emptied without rhythmic increases in pressure and in the absence of recognizable gastric peristalsis.

As noted in Chapter 10, gastric emptying is a *regulated* activity. Emptying rate is increased by increasing gastric volume (regulated by gastric receptors), and inhibited by a wide variety of the components of chyme (inhibition controlled entirely by duodenal receptors). Duodenal regulatory stimuli, listed in order of inhibitory potency when in the concentrations usually encountered, are fats, fatty acids, proteoses, peptones, amino acids, sugars and other osmotically active solutes, and hydrogen ions. Nonspecific irritants also inhibit emptying. The effect of these stimuli, mediated by duodenal hormones, osmoreceptors, and perhaps pH receptors, is to decrease the tone and peristaltic activity of the stomach, thus reducing the pressure gradient which develops with each gastric cycle (and thus reducing stroke volume). With more powerful inhibitors, such as fat, the gradient may be reversed, and duodenal contents will be regurgitated into stomach.

Although rhythmic contraction and relaxation of the pyloric sphincter are prerequisites to normal gastric emptying, and although sphincter contraction helps prevent duodenogastric reflux, there is no evidence that its function is important in regulating the overall rate of gastric emptying. The latter is more a function of the muscles on either side of the pylorus.

THE VOMITING ACT IN MAN[2-8]

Three stages are recognized: nausea, retching, and vomiting. Characteristic, but not invariable, changes in gastrointestinal motility have been recognized for each stage.

Nausea is a psychic experience of humans that defies precise definition. Although a variety of stimuli may produce nausea (labyrinthine stimulation, visceral pain, unpleasant memories), it is not known where the impulses originate. Nausea is usually associated with hypersalivation.

During nausea, gastric tone is reduced and peristalsis in the stomach is diminished or absent. In contrast, the tone of the duodenum and proximal jejunum tends to be increased, and reflux of duodenal contents into the stomach during nausea is frequent. Nausea is not caused by increased duodenal and jejunal tone, however, because these abnormalities are not always present in a nauseated person.

Retching consists of spasmodic and abortive respiratory movements with the glottis closed, during which time inspiratory movements of the chest wall and diaphragm are opposed by expiratory contractions of the abdominal musculature. Although the diaphragm moves violently downward, its range of motion is slight, and it remains in a high position through this stage. During retching, the pyloric end of the stomach contracts, whereas the upper part is relaxed. The mouth is closed.

Vomiting occurs as the gastric contents are forcefully brought up to and out of the mouth, which opens just prior to stomach evacuation. This occurs by virtue of a forceful sustained contraction of the abdominal muscles accompanied by descent of the diaphragm, at a time when the cardia of the stomach is raised and open and

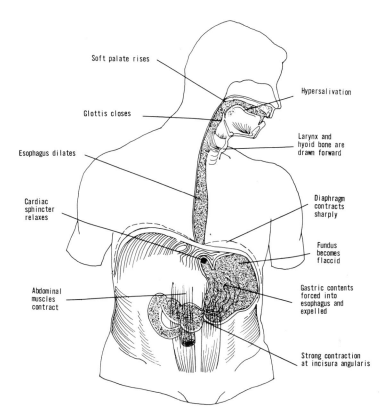

Soft palate rises

Glottis closes

Esophagus dilates

Cardiac
sphincter
relaxes

Abdominal
muscles
contract

Hypersalivation

Larynx and
hyoid bone are
drawn forward

Diaphragm
contracts
sharply

Fundus
becomes
flaccid

Gastric contents
forced into
esophagus and
expelled

Strong contraction
at incisura angularis

Figure 11–1. A summary of the act of vomiting in man. (From Searle: Research in the Service of Medicine 44:2, 1956.)

the pyloric stomach contracted (Fig. 11–1). Elevation of the cardia serves the purpose of eliminating the intra-abdominal portion of the esophagus, which if present would tend to prevent the high intragastric pressure from forcing gastric contents into the gullet. The cardia may be so high as to cause a temporary hiatal hernia. The mechanism by which the cardia opens during vomiting is not clear.

The gastrointestinal motor events may be summarized as follows. During nausea, gastric tone and peristalsis are decreased and duodenal tone is increased, with or without reflux of duodenal contents into the stomach. During retching, the upper stomach is relaxed and the antral portion contracts. During vomiting, the lower stomach remains contracted and the cardia rises and opens as gastric contents are forcefully expelled by high intra-abdominal pressure.

ASSOCIATED PHENOMENA

Hypersalivation. This is common and is probably due to the close proximity of

the medullary vomiting and salivary centers (see below).

Reverse Peristalsis. Intestinal contents are frequently present in vomited material, and some workers have implicated reverse peristalsis in the duodenum as the cause. Most workers do not accept reverse peristalsis as a proved occurrence during any stage of vomiting, and the vomiting act is not affected in animals whose gut has been denervated and even in animals in which the entire small bowel has been removed.[2] Obviously, the small bowel plays a minor role in the act of vomiting, although the intestine is a very important source of emetic impulses (see below).

The Heart. Nausea is usually accompanied by tachycardia, retching by bradycardia. Cardiac arrhythmias sometimes occur in animals made to vomit, and these may be prevented by pretreatment with atropine.

The Colon. Defecation often accompanies vomiting,[2] and it has been suggested that vomiting and defecation centers are acted on by essentially the same kind of stimuli, the response depending upon the state of the peripheral organs.

PATHOPHYSIOLOGY OF VOMITING

The mechanism of vomiting has been extensively studied by Borison and Wang, who summarized their ideas rather specifically in 1953.[2] Their concept appears to have been accepted by other pharmacologists and physiologists; at least, it has not been seriously challenged so far as this author is aware. Their experiments were carried out exclusively in animals, and naturally caution must be exercised in extrapolating these data to man. However, these experiments can never be repeated in intact human subjects, and what little is known about the pathophysiology of vomiting in man is compatible with the hypothesis of Borison and Wang.

The pathophysiology of vomiting can best be understood and appreciated by a brief review of five experimental observations:

1. Vomiting involves a complex and reproducible set of activities that suggests some central neurological control. This observation led to the concept of a vomiting center in 1865.

2. Vomiting can be induced by electrical stimulation of the medulla, especially in the area of the dorsal portion of the lateral reticular formation. No other portion of the brainstem yields such responses. Destruction of the electrically responsive region of the reticular formation, with implanted radon seeds, causes animals to become highly refractory to the emetic action of apomorphine and copper sulfate. This vomiting center is anatomically situated in close proximity with other centers of activity, such as those for salivation and respiration, and activities mediated by these centers are all involved in vomiting.

Although direct electrical stimulation of the vomiting center causes vomiting, it should not be inferred that any natural cause of vomiting directly stimulates this area of the medulla. Actually, there is no good evidence that any substance which causes vomiting does so by direct stimulation of the vomiting center. Rather, the center coordinates the activities of the other medullary structures to produce a patterned response.

3. Intravenously injected apomorphine induces vomiting. The emetic response to this drug is eliminated either by ablation of the vomiting center in the medulla or by ablation of the area postrema in the floor of the fourth ventricle. Direct application of apomorphine to an intact area postrema causes vomiting. From these observations it was concluded that apomorphine is a central emetic agent and has no peripheral activity. Its site of action is the area postrema in the floor of the fourth ventricle, which is named the *chemoreceptor trigger zone* (CTZ). In contrast to the vomiting center, the CTZ is not responsive to electrical stimulation. It is an afferent station related to the vomiting center, as illustrated in Figure 11–2.

4. Copper sulfate is a potent emetic when ingested orally. Interruption of the abdominal vagi and sympathetics makes animals highly refractory to oral copper sulfate. On the other hand, ablation of the chemoreceptor trigger zone, which makes animals completely resistant to apomorphine, has no effect on the sensitivity of animals to oral copper sulfate. These experiments were interpreted to mean that oral copper sulfate induces vomiting via afferent impulses that reach the medullary vomiting center directly, via the vagus and sympathetic nerves, without traversing the chemoreceptor trigger zone. This, also, is illustrated in Figure 11–2. Vomiting in response to a minimally effective oral dose of copper sulfate is probably a pure expression of gastrointestinal irritation mediated via visceral afferents in the vagus and sympathetic nerves.

5. Copper sulfate is also an effective emetic when injected intravenously. Ablation of the chemoreceptor trigger zone prevents vomiting in response to intravenous copper sulfate, whereas denervation of the gut is without effect. This evidence clearly indicates that intravenous copper sulfate is also a central emetic agent (like apomorphine) with its action on the chemoreceptor trigger zone.

These five observations indicate that the medullary emetic mechanism consists of two anatomically and functionally separate units: a vomiting center in the reticular formation, which is excited directly by vis-

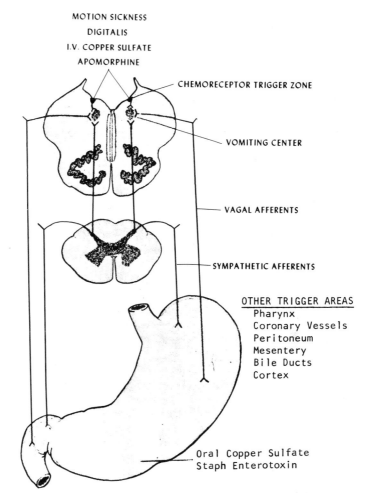

MOTION SICKNESS
DIGITALIS
I.V. COPPER SULFATE
APOMORPHINE

CHEMORECEPTOR TRIGGER ZONE

VOMITING CENTER

VAGAL AFFERENTS

SYMPATHETIC AFFERENTS

OTHER TRIGGER AREAS
Pharynx
Coronary Vessels
Peritoneum
Mesentery
Bile Ducts
Cortex

Oral Copper Sulfate
Staph Enterotoxin

Figure 11–2. The interrelation of the vomiting center, the chemoreceptor trigger zone and peripheral trigger areas. (Modified from Wang, S. C., and Borison, H. L.: Gastroenterology 22:1, 1952.)

ceral afferent impulses arising from the gastrointestinal tract, and a chemoreceptor trigger zone in the floor of the fourth ventricle, which is the site of emetic action of apomorphine and intravenously injected copper sulfate. The CTZ is not able to cause vomiting without the mediation of an intact vomiting center.

Cardiac glycosides act primarily on the chemoreceptor trigger zone; this zone is also important in mediating motion sickness as well as the nausea and vomiting associated with uremia and probably that due to other metabolic disturbances.

Borison and Wang have emphasized that their schema is in all likelihood an oversimplification, and to some extent incomplete. For instance, digitalis acts on unidentified receptors other than the CTZ, and vitrum alkaloids appear to act primarily on the nodose ganglion of the vagus nerve. Ipecac (Emitine and Cephaline) has a central action on the CTZ and a reflex action via the gastrointestinal mucosa, so that synergistic action is likely in some instances. Pilocarpine action originates in the frontal lobe.[9]

Whether the vomiting center is under the control of higher cortical and brainstem structures is debatable. Their importance has never been proved, and vomiting is known to occur in decerebrate animals and humans.

In summary, all emetic responses, as far as is known, are mediated via reflex arcs which pass through the vomiting center, regardless of whether these responses are initiated at peripheral or central sites. The central and peripheral trigger sites have been summarized in Figure 11–2.

NERVOUS PATHWAYS IN VOMITING

Efferent pathways are mainly somatic, presumably in the vagi, sympathetics, and phrenics and in the cranial supply to pharyngeal muscles. The spinal nerves supply the abdominal musculature. Since there is no essential difference in vomiting between intact and gut-denervated animals, it is assumed that visceral efferents are of little importance in the vomiting act.

In addition to the afferent pathways already discussed, many other receptor sites probably exist. There is fair to good evidence that such receptors may be located in the pharynx, coronary vessels and heart, peritoneum, mesenteric vasculature, and bile ducts. Presumably these peripheral receptors, like the gastrointestinal receptors stimulated by copper sulfate (Fig. 11–2), transmit afferent impulses directly to the vomiting center. With regard to receptors located in the gastrointestinal tract, it is of interest that distention of the pyloric end of the stomach (but not the fundus), duodenum, small bowel, colon, and biliary passages regularly leads to vomiting. Like that caused by irritation of the mucosa by copper sulfate or mustard, vomiting in response to distention is blocked by denervation of the organ in question. Obviously there are also corticobulbar afferents that mediate vomiting in response to some smells and tastes. These unknown supramedullary receptors may influence the reactivity of the vomiting center or the chemoreceptor trigger zone, and they may play a role in psychic vomiting.

CLINICAL FEATURES OF VOMITING

In marked contrast to pathophysiological experiments in animals, there has apparently never been a careful clinical study of vomiting in various diseases, and it is impossible to be certain of the accuracy or to trace the origin of statements handed down from generation to generation. For instance, the writer was unable to trace the origin of the idea that projectile vomiting without nausea is characteristic of increased intracranial pressure, and the timing of vomiting in relation to meals has not been studied by modern clinical techniques that would avoid the bias of preconceived notions. Much of this discussion should be taken in this light.

There is no doubt that a particular type of vomiting depends in large measure upon the amount and nature of the stomach contents, which determine the character of the vomitus and the character of any reflex impulses that are transmitted to centers (vomiting, respiratory, salivary) in the medulla.

Timing in Relation to Meals. Vomiting during or soon after a meal is common in patients with psychoneurotic vomiting and occasionally occurs in patients with peptic ulcer near the pyloric channel, presumably because of irritability, edema, and spasm. It has never been proved to the author's satisfaction that vomiting occurs owing to pylorospasm secondary to an ulcer elsewhere in the stomach or duodenum, although Crohn, in an excellent monograph published in 1927, considered this to be an accepted fact.[10] Delayed vomiting (more than one hour after eating), especially if it occurs repeatedly, is characteristic of gastric outlet obstruction or a motility disorder of the stomach, such as diabetic neuropathy or postvagectomy state. Repeated vomiting of material eaten 12 hours earlier is rarely, if ever, seen in patients with psychoneurotic vomiting, and is strong evidence for outlet obstruction or severe motor disorder of the stomach. Patients with this history will often have a succussion splash (clapotage).

Vomiting in the early morning, before breakfast, is characteristic of pregnant women and may be seen in patients with toxic states such as uremia and alcoholism and after gastric surgery. Vomiting caused by postnasal drip may also occur at this time.

Relief of Pain by Vomiting. Vomiting typically relieves pain associated with peptic disease, but not pain caused by pancreatic or biliary tract disease.

Projectile Vomiting. A clear definition of projectile vomiting is not generally available. Some use it simply to describe vomitus which is ejected forcefully from the mouth, whereas others define it as vomiting that occurs at the peak of maximum inspiration without the rhythmic hyperactivity of the respiratory muscles noted with retching. Used in the latter sense, it may be contrasted with the "dry heaves," characterized by repeated violent and explosive rhythmic respiratory activity, leading to fatigue but to little or no vomitus. The vomiting associated with raised intracranial pressure is often referred to as projectile, and is said to occur without nausea or retching. Like the headache, it may occur in the early morning and be precipitated by exertion or stooping. Frequently, however, vomiting caused by raised intracranial pressure is not forceful, and it is often preceded by nausea and retching.[11] It is a common experience to see forceful vomiting in many conditions other than those associated with disease of the central nervous system.

Content of the Vomitus. The significance of food has already been covered. Blood or "coffee grounds" in vomitus is of obvious importance. The presence of bile indicates an open connection between the proximal duodenum and the stomach. Bilious vomiting is common after gastric surgery, and is discussed more specifically under Specific Syndromes. Vomiting of undigested food suggests achylia gastrica or the possibility that the "vomitus" is from the esophagus (as in achalasia) or from an esophageal or pharyngeal diverticulum. Vomiting of pure gastric juice of high acidity suggests Zollinger-Ellison syndrome. In all instances, it is wise to test the gastric contents with pH paper to determine acidity.

Vomiting of mucus is occasionally noted, but its significance is not clear.

Odor of Vomitus. A fecal odor suggests intestinal obstruction, peritonitis with ileus, gastrocolic fistula, ischemic injury to the gut, or long-standing gastric outlet obstruction with bacterial overgrowth caused by stasis. Occasionally, fecal vomiting is seen in patients with bacterial overgrowth in the proximal small bowel.

Succussion and Visible Peristalsis. Patients with delayed vomiting often have a distended stomach and exhibit succussion. The latter is an extraordinarily important physical finding, and should be specifically sought in any patient with vomiting or in any patient liable to develop gastric outlet obstruction. In patients with delayed vomiting and/or with succussion, visible gastric peristaltic waves suggest pyloric obstruction, whereas absence of such waves suggests gastric atony.[12]

Other Considerations. The duration of vomiting, presence or absence of weight loss, abdominal mass, visible intestinal peristalsis, inguinal hernia, history of prior abdominal surgery, dysphagia, jaundice, and the presence of other diseases or conditions will weigh heavily in the initial diagnostic impression. Abdominal distention and the character of bowel sounds should be carefully evaluated in regard to the possibility of intestinal obstruction. Evidence of cardiovascular disease should suggest the possibility of mesenteric infarction.

CLINICAL SIGNIFICANCE

Although vomiting may not signify the presence of serious illness, it may be the first indication of an emergency, such as intestinal obstruction, peritonitis, acute abdomen, cholecystitis, pancreatitis, hypertensive crisis, Addisonian crisis, uremia, or drug overdosage. Vomiting can be an early symptom in patients with carcinoma of the stomach. Vomiting is frequent and may be distressing in pregnancy, motion sickness, after gastrectomy or radiation therapy, and during and after general anesthesia. Violent vomiting and collapse may occur in epidemics caused by food poisoning or (apparent) viral infection. Serious complications of vomiting include aspiration pneumonia (a function of acid in the aspirated material), severe hemorrhage caused by mucosal tears at the gastroesophageal junction (Mallory-Weiss syndrome), rupture of the esophagus (Boerhaave's syndrome), and electrolyte depletion and acid-base disturbance. As a consequence of metabolic derangements caused by vomiting, patients may become paralyzed[13] or develop renal failure.[14] Vomiting may cause fatal or near-fatal malnutrition in infants,[15] and is frequently present, albeit hidden, in patients with anorexia nervosa. Vomiting has been proposed as the cause of Reye's syndrome (encephalopathy and fatty accumulation in the viscera),[16] and it may be the cause of dental erosions in some patients.[17]

SPECIFIC SYNDROMES

PSYCHOGENIC VOMITING

Chronic and recurrent vomiting, especially in females, may be caused by underlying emotional disturbance. The latter is often related to sexual and marital conflicts, but apparently may also be caused by health problems and habits of relatives (e.g., alcoholism, aging, senility of parents), as well as by more deep-seated problems, such as loss of parental affection.

Psychogenic vomiting may be recognized by the following features:

1. The vomiting has usually been present for years. Frequently, history will reveal vomiting in childhood or while in high school when under emotional strain.

2. There is often a family history of vomiting.

3. The vomiting typically occurs soon after the meal has begun or just after it has been completed.

4. The actual vomiting act is often brought on by inserting the finger in the back of the throat.

5. Vomiting can be suppressed if necessary. Thus, although the patient may have to vomit after almost every meal, vomiting is suppressed until the patient reaches the bathroom. Rarely does vomiting occur in a public place, as on a bus or in a dining room.

6. The vomiting is of relatively little concern to the patient. It is usually the other members of the family who insist on the patient seeing a physician.

7. The patients are usually thin, but are rarely emaciated unless they also have anorexia nervosa.

Obviously, organic disease must be ruled out by appropriate tests, but the history in these patients is so typical that the diagnosis is usually strongly suspected prior to X-rays of the gastrointestinal tract or gallbladder. It is important that the correct diagnosis be made quickly and that the patient not be subjected to unnecessary and expensive diagnostic procedures or to abdominal surgery, which does not help and which may worsen and complicate the issue. It should also be recognized that patients with psychogenic vomiting may in time develop a second disease, and the physician should be alert for a change in the pattern of the illness that might indicate the presence of gastric cancer, cholecystitis, or pancreatitis.

Hill[13] studied 20 patients (15 female and five male) with psychogenic vomiting and compared them with 22 patients suffering from abdominal pain for which no cause could be found (the abdominal pain was apparently of psychogenic origin in the control subjects). In all patients the vomiting was worse at mealtimes, coming on during the meal or soon after. In all but one patient the vomiting was accompanied by nausea. Retching was not mentioned. Three of the patients had suffered from paralysis, probably caused by potassium deficiency. Ten had lost 14 pounds or more in weight. Only one of the patients had menstrual irregularity. Twelve of the 20 patients were living with a person to whom they were fundamentally antagonistic. The others experienced antagonism to other important people in their lives, but not in so striking a manner. Nine had lost a parent before reaching age 15, and three others had had a significant separation experience. In the control group, only two of 22 were involved in domestic situations comparable to 12 out of 20 in the vomiters. Only 3 of the control group had had a significant separation experience.

Ten of the vomiters gave a history of spells of vomiting during childhood, often at times of separation. In the control group, only one gave such a history. Nine of the vomiters gave a family history of functional or persistent organic vomiting, compared with none in the control group. Only one of the vomiters was thought to be significantly depressed.

Hill concluded that psychogenic vomiters are trapped in a hostile relationship, and especially significant is the fact that they shared the same house and ate with the source of their antagonism. (In the control group, in which the major somatic symptom of psychiatric disease was abdominal pain, hostile relationships were less common and, more important, were outside rather than inside the family unit, so that the patient did not have to eat with the source of his antipathy.) The much greater frequency of this disorder in women than in men may be due to the greater passivity of the female when faced with an unsatisfactory relationship. Thus none of the vomiters had ever taken active steps to break off an unsatisfactory relationship, whereas two in the control series had. The experience of a major loss in childhood may have made these patients reluctant to accept a further loss in later life.

In psychogenic vomiting it is not known whether the afferent impulses originate from within the gastrointestinal tract or centrally, and whether these afferents are hyperexcitable or whether the central vomiting mechanism is hypersensitive. The question might be settled by determining whether or not these patients vomit in response to a lower than normal dose of either apomorphine given intravenously or copper sulfate given orally.

It is apparently not known whether or not the patients with psychogenic vomiting improve with antiemetic drugs (no controlled studies were found). It is generally agreed that surgery (such as gastroenterostomy) is of no help in controlling the vomiting. It has been stated that such patients improve with verbal catharsis, but no proof was given for this assertion.[18]

RUMINATION IN ADULTS

Rumination in adults[19] consists of regurgitating food, one mouthful at a time, from the stomach to the mouth, chewing the food again, and reswallowing it. Regurgitation is usually involuntary, effortless, and not associated with abdominal pain or discomfort, heartburn, or nausea. Rumination usually begins 15 to 30 minutes after the meal, and lasts for about one hour. During this period the patient will ruminate up to 20 times. Rumination characteristically ceases when the food becomes acid to taste. It is apparently a pleasant sensation, but often embarrassing, so that patients tend to hide the fact that they reswallow their food. Rumination can be suppressed voluntarily, at least in some instances.

The cause and mechanism of rumination are unknown, although nearly all authors conclude that psychological factors are important. Physiological studies are difficult because the patients tend not to ruminate during X-ray or manometric experiments. Reverse esophageal peristalsis has never been demonstrated in these patients, but is known to occur in ruminant animals, such as sheep.[20] In some human cases a spastic contraction has separated the stomach into two compartments that simulate in some respect the stomach of ruminants.[19]

Although rumination in adults is rare, it is important to be aware of this entity so that needless surgery (such as hiatal hernia repair) can be avoided.

RUMINATION IN INFANTS

Rumination in infants is associated with failure to thrive, marasmus, and even death, if untreated. Typically, previously ingested food is regurgitated, rechewed, and reswallowed. The syndrome is believed to be caused by an abnormal mother-child relationship. The mothers of these infants tend to be immature and unable to develop a close and comfortable relationship with the baby. The rumination process is interpreted as an effort to recreate the gratification of the feeding process in an emotionally deprived infant. Hospitalization will often bring improvement, providing that hospital personnel can take on the role of a loving mother.[15, 21] In one instance in which rumination and vomiting were life threatening, an infant was treated by "conditioning therapy." Electric shock was given each time the baby ruminated, and within a few brief sessions vomiting and rumination ceased, and weight gain and other improvement were noted. This observation suggests that emesis and rumination in these children may be learned habits (i.e., a conditioned response).[22]

The differential diagnosis of apparent rumination[23] in infants includes gastroesophageal incompetence, hiatal hernia, drug reaction (including drugs given to the mother), diencephalic seizures, hypothalamic tumors, milk allergy, and metabolic disorders such as fructose intolerance, as well as many of the conditions mentioned on pages 139 to 140.

NAUSEA AND VOMITING IN PREGNANCY AND HYPEREMESIS GRAVIDARUM[24-30]

The term "nausea and vomiting of pregnancy" is generally restricted to a mild disorder of early pregnancy characterized especially by morning nausea and sometimes by vomiting. Although the nausea and vomiting may at times be quite distressing and persist throughout the day, by definition the patient does not develop fluid and electrolyte derangements or nutritional deficiency. The incidence is from 25 to 30 per cent of pregnancies, but many cases are mild. Symptoms typically begin early in pregnancy, usually shortly after the first missed menstrual period (rarely before), and disappear by the fourth month of pregnancy. Occasionally symptoms may last into the second half of pregnancy.[27] By definition, other causes of nausea and vomiting are not present. Treatment is antiemetic drugs such as the promazines, and supportive psychotherapy if indicated.

Hyperemesis gravidarum or pernicious vomiting of pregnancy refers to those patients who develop nutritional deficiency or fluid and electrolyte disturbances from intractable vomiting in early pregnancy. As in milder cases, the onset of symptoms tends to be soon after the first missed menstrual period, and almost always before the twentieth week of gestation. Classically the vomiting disappears during the third month, and rarely persists into the fourth month, although Guze and his colleagues reported that 60 per cent of their patients vomited during more than half of the pregnancy.[27]

The incidence of hyperemesis gravidarum varies considerably, with an average figure of 3.5 per 1000 deliveries. The incidence is not increased by parity, race, color, illegitimate pregnancy, or the desire for an abortion,[26] but is markedly decreased during wartime.[29] Patients with hyperemesis gravidarum do not have an increased incidence of toxemia of pregnancy or spontaneous abortion, and their babies are not underweight or deformed.

The cause of vomiting in pregnancy is not known. The mild form is common enough to be accepted as a normal or at least physiologically determined accompaniment of pregnancy.[25] The importance of psychic factors is controversial, some studies showing a high incidence of disturbed sexual functions, undue attachment to the mother, and a history of previous vomiting, whereas others reveal no significant differences between women with this disorder and a control group.[26] In one recent series, the incidence of sexual frigidity was not increased.[30] In hyperemesis gravidarum there is no longer any well founded support for a toxic etiology, and reflex vomiting secondary to uterine and cervical stimulation seems unlikely. Abnormalities in sex hormone secretion and concentration in body fluids have not been proved. The similarity of the symptoms to those of Addison's disease has suggested an insufficient stimulation of the adrenal gland, and, indeed, several reports attest to a striking decrease in vomiting with ACTH therapy.[31, 32]

No double-blind studies have been reported on the psychosomatic and psychiatric aspects of hyperemesis gravidarum. Several controlled but not double-blind studies have appeared, however. Guze et al.[27] conducted a careful follow-up study and found that hysteria occurred in 15 per cent of those who had hyperemesis gravidarum, compared with only 2 per cent of the controls. In other ways the vomiters were no different from the controls, and 41 per cent of the vomiters were without any psychological illness at the time of follow-up. Harvey and Sherfey[25] regularly obtained a clear-cut history of previous vomiting in response to emotional disturbances in 19 of their 20 patients. They also reported a strikingly high incidence of emotional immaturity, undue attachment to the mother figure, and sexual maladjustment in their cases. Fairweather[24] suggests that psychosomatic factors may be involved in 75 per cent of cases. The facts that hyperemesis gravidarum is seen only in humans, that it is treatable by hypnosis and other forms of suggestion, and that the incidence markedly decreases during wartime are further suggestive evidence of a psychosomatic etiology.

The metabolic consequences of hyperemesis gravidarum can be severe, and the mortality rate in untreated patients is high. Salt and water depletion and potassium deficiency (intracellular as well as extracellular) may be marked.

Treatment of hyperemesis gravidarum is mainly directed at fluid and electrolyte replacement and supportive psychotherapy. Antiemetic drugs are of relatively little value when the disorder has progressed to this stage.

CONCEALED VOMITING

Surreptitious vomiting[33-35] is not rare, and one needs a high index of suspicion and some ingenuity to make and confirm the correct diagnosis. Patients may become highly skilled in their ability to conceal vomiting. Most have no organic cause for the vomiting, although some patients with organic disease of the stomach deny vomiting, either for the enjoyment of the medical curiosity aroused by their metabolic disturbances or in order to prevent others from knowing of their illness. Concealed vomiting may lead to complicated metabolic derangements, suggesting the presence of serious organic disease. The differential diagnosis is discussed on pages 140 to 141.

CYCLIC VOMITING

Recurrent bouts of unexplained vomiting in children were described by Gee in 1882. The syndrome is characterized by recurring prolonged attacks of severe vomiting without apparent cause which may be associated with headache, abdominal pain, and fever. The onset is usually sudden, and the attack may last several days. Recovery is usually spontaneous, although the disease can threaten life by producing profound dehydration and alkalosis. The onset is usually before the age of six, and the episodes usually end at puberty. The frequency of attacks varies from more than one a month to three per year.[36] Many theories have been invoked to explain this syndrome, from chronic appendicitis to epilepsy. In the study of Hoyt and Stickler, headache was associated with vomiting in 36 per cent of the 44 patients when initially examined; 24 per cent of the 38 patients who could be traced for follow-up had recurrent headache after the vomiting had ceased. A family history of migraine was obtained in 25 per cent of the 44 patients. Many workers have con-

sidered the syndrome to be psychogenic in origin. On the other hand, Lang's studies[37] reviewed by Lorber,[38] suggest that perinatal and postnatal brain injury and lesions cause the disorder in a significant number of affected children.

The diagnosis can usually be made from history if numerous episodes of vomiting have occurred in the past. X-ray studies of the gastrointestinal tract as well as careful neurological examination will rule out the majority of organic lesions that may produce recurrent vomiting, such as malrotation of the midgut and intracranial tumors. It is important to reach a diagnosis early so as to avoid unnecessary laparotomy, which will only add to the confusion when future attacks of vomiting occur (adhesions, etc.). The physician must be alert to the possibility that an earlier diagnosis of cyclic vomiting was in error; frequent re-evaluation is necessary. One child originally included in a series of cyclic vomiting turned out to have an astrocytoma.[36]

BILIOUS VOMITING AFTER GASTRIC SURGERY[39-41]

Bilious vomiting is perhaps the most crippling long-term complication of the surgical treatment of peptic ulcer. This occurs most commonly on getting up in the morning, is accompanied by an unpleasant taste in the mouth, a burning substernal sensation, and intense nausea. In a severe case, within about 15 minutes after each meal the patient vomits clear bile-stained fluid which does not contain food.[41] This feature distinguishes it from outlet obstruction, in which the vomitus always contains food.

Although chronic bilious vomiting may be caused by mechanical derangements of the afferent loop (see p. 800), this is, in fact, quite rarely the true explanation. The pathogenesis in most cases is not clear, although some workers strongly implicate a chemical gastritis secondary to bile and pancreatic juice in the stomach or the gastric remnant.[41] It is proposed that such gastritis leads to abnormal sensitivity, and that the presence of bile in an irritable stomach causes vomiting. To the writer's knowledge, this has never been objectively proved by infusing bile and control solutions into the stomach of these patients. Nevertheless, Torrance and Watson report excellent relief of severe bilious vomiting in 17 patients by a surgical technique designed to prevent bile reflux into the stomach.[41]

Other workers have suggested that bilious vomiting after gastric surgery is related in some way to hiatal hernia, and reported excellent relief after correction of this anatomic abnormality.[40] Hiatal hernia appears to be especially high in this group of patients, and postulated reasons include damage to the phrenoesophageal ligament at the time of abdominal vagotomy[40] and recurrent vomiting itself.[41]

At present it would seem wise to maintain a skeptical attitude toward the idea that bile diversion and/or hiatal hernia repair will more or less uniformly relieve postgastrectomy bilious vomiting. However, when faced with severe bilious vomiting in a postgastrectomy patient, one or both of these operative procedures would be a reasonable approach, on the basis of current clinical evidence.

In some patients emotional factors may play a role in bilious vomiting after gastric surgery.[39] This would be suggested by a history of vomiting since childhood or adolescence, a tendency to car, motion, or emotional sickness, and a history of vomiting prior to gastric surgery without evidence of outlet obstruction. Management of such cases is extremely difficult. Antiemetic and antidepressant drugs are first employed, usually without benefit. Psychiatric referral is usually not helpful. When all else fails, and if the symptoms are intolerable, surgical procedures designed to prevent bile regurgitation, or hiatal surgery if appropriate, may be attempted. Admittedly, there is no proof that these procedures will help.

EPIDEMIC VOMITING[42, 43]

This has many synonyms, including nonbacterial gastroenteritis, epidemic nausea and vomiting, winter vomiting or disease, and epidemic collapse. The disease is characterized by sudden and explosive outbreaks of profuse vomiting which often begin in the early hours of the morning. The urge to vomit is so intense that vomiting often occurs before the pa-

tient can get out of bed.[43] Headaches, giddiness, muscular pains, sweating, and feverishness may also occur. Diarrhea may be a feature of some outbreaks, but not of the majority. Many cases are probably caused by viral infection, but attempts to identify a specific agent have been unsuccessful.[42] Chemical or bacterial food poisoning, especially staph enterotoxin, may cause a similar syndrome, in which case the incubation period rarely exceeds six hours and diarrhea (but not fever) is common.[42] In occasional instances, epidemic vomiting has apparently represented mass hysteria.

Rapid recovery is the rule, although the disorder may last up to ten days, and relapses may occur up to three weeks.

GASTRIC RETENTION WITHOUT OBSTRUCTION[12]

Vomiting of food eaten more than six hours earlier, a succussion splash that lasts longer than five hours after the last intake of food or water, or the presence of food in the stomach at the time of upper gastrointestinal series indicates gastric retention. Two misconceptions commonly lead to errors in the management of such patients. First, it is often assumed that gastric retention means gastric outlet obstruction; unnecessary and unhelpful surgery may be carried out. Second, if outlet obstruction is ruled out by X-ray, it may be assumed that the patient has nothing wrong with him. Such patients are often falsely accused of eating on the morning of the X-ray examination and are often misdiagnosed as psychoneurotics.

A classic example of gastric retention without obstruction is the diabetic with neuropathy. Diabetic gastric atony[44, 45] presents a radiological picture quite similar to a surgically vagectomized patient. The stomach is typically devoid of peristalsis and shows retained food and fluid, yet some barium can be manipulated to outline a patent pylorus and small bowel. No organic obstruction is present. Not all patients with delayed emptying vomit or have other symptoms related to the motor disturbance. Even in a patient who vomits, symptom-free intervals are common. Surgical intervention is generally said to be inadvisable, because it is gastric motor abnormality, not the gastric outlet, that causes retention. However, the number of reported cases is far too small to evaluate the risks and benefits of gastroenterostomy in this disorder.

Although vagal insufficiency has been suggested as the cause of diabetic gastric atony, Hollander tests apparently have not been performed in such patients. Other possible but unlikely etiological factors are hyperglycemia, a rising blood sugar, and elevated glucagon levels, all of which will reduce gastric contractions experimentally.

Presumably neuropathies of other causes might also produce similar abnormalities of gastric function, and gastric retention without obstruction has been noted at least occasionally in association with many diverse conditions,[12] from gallstones to menstruation. However, most of these patients apparently had transient episodes of gastric retention noted on an upper gastrointestinal X-ray, or had serious and usually obvious intra-abdominal disease such as pancreatitis or peritonitis.

Persistent delay in gastric emptying, unless adequately explained by a neuropathy or by drug therapy (such as anticholinergics), deserves a very careful work-up. Occasionally patients with gastric malignancy may present in this way, and delayed gastric emptying may occur after gastric surgery with vagotomy.

VOMITING IN INFANTS AND CHILDREN[46-48]

Vomiting is one of the most common problems encountered in infants. It may indicate anything from a minor feeding upset to complete intestinal obstruction,[46] and it can be a symptom of any disease system. A normal baby may vomit small amounts of food during or just after a meal; this may be associated with burping, which in the infant is often associated with regurgitation of milk or food. Posture has a marked effect on the tendency of a baby to vomit after a meal. In the supine position, the fundus and cardia are dependent and food accumulates there, tending to result in regurgitation. In the prone position or on the right side, food tends not to regurgitate because it is in the antrum. In these positions, gas rises to the cardia and burping tends to occur without food. The best way to hold the baby who regurgitates is obviously in the right antero-oblique position.[46]

Loss of weight, failure to gain weight, presence of bile (green or yellow color) in the vomitus, and abdominal distention in association with vomiting and regurgitation are definitely abnormal, and their presence demands a thorough evaluation. Various congenital lesions that are incompatible with life do not necessarily give symptoms immediately after birth. Diagnoses of pneumonia, vomiting caused by feeding difficulty, gastroenteritis, or "failure to thrive" in the first week of life may well be in error, with the symptoms caused in fact by congenital defects.[46]

If the vomiting has any suspicious features, including persistence, it is important to inquire about the passage of meconium, to perform a rectal examination, and to look carefully for evidence of abdominal distention. It should be recalled that renal lesions and disease of other organs (including intracranial birth injuries) may produce vomiting in infancy. Repeated physical examinations are necessary in order to make the correct diagnosis and to prevent a fatal outcome in some cases.

X-rays of the abdomen and in some instances of the gastrointestinal tract are of great value, especially in duodenal obstruction, atresia, fistulas, Hirschsprung's disease, meconium ileus, intussusception, and hiatal hernia.

Some of the serious causes of vomiting at different ages follow.

IN THE NEWBORN

Tracheoesophageal Fistula. These babies hypersalivate almost continuously, and feeding causes regurgitation associated with periods of cyanosis. Abdominal distention may occur from air forced into the intestine through the fistula.

Atresia and Stenosis. Some degree of abdominal distention is often present in addition to vomiting, and such infants may pass meconium.

Diaphragms Producing Obstruction. These may allow passage of gas and fluid, so that vomiting may not be associated with abdominal distention.

Duodenal Obstruction. Air fluid levels in the stomach and duodenum ("double bubble") should be looked for. Obviously, high small bowel obstructions produce vomiting without much abdominal distention.

Meconium Ileus. Rarely the cause of intestinal obstruction, when present it may signify cystic fibrosis of the pancreas.

Midgut Volvulus with Malrotation. The abdomen is scaphoid and vomiting is intermittent. Almost invariably, the vomitus is green. Bloody feces signify vascular damage and possibly fatal gangrene.

Hypertrophic Pyloric Stenosis. This disorder almost always occurs during the first seven weeks of life. These infants eat well at first and then progress from occasional regurgitation to forceful vomiting over a period of a few days to weeks. Bile is always absent. Gastric peristaltic waves and a pyloric tumor ("olive") just to the right of the midline are usually present.

IN INFANCY

Intussusception. Intussusception is characterized by intermittent colicky pain, a palpable mass, and "currant jelly" stool. Bloody stools may occur, indicating vascular damage.

IN CHILDHOOD

Appendicitis. Vomiting usually accompanies the initial symptoms. It is characteristic of these children to have continuous pain with exacerbation (but without complete relief). Patients usually do not have diarrhea, but they may, in which case gastroenteritis may be erroneously diagnosed. Vomiting may also occur later in the illness, especially at the time of perforation.

See page 1497 for the differential diagnosis in this disorder.

METABOLIC CONSEQUENCES OF VOMITING

These are depicted in Figure 11–3.*
Potassium deficiency results from de-

*Figure 11–3 is designed from information in references 33 to 35, 49, and a personal communication from D. W. Seldin.

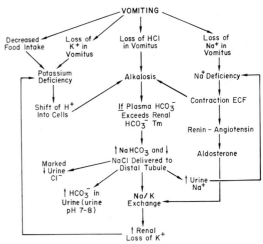

Figure 11–3.   Metabolic consequences of vomiting.

creased intake of food potassium, from loss of K^+ in the vomitus, and in some instances from renal potassium wasting. Alkalosis, if severe, is associated with a delivery of sodium bicarbonate to the kidneys, which exceeds the Tm for bicarbonate. Because of Na/K exchange in the distal tubule, renal K^+ loss will occur (as potassium bicarbonate). Sodium depletion may enhance this Na/K exchange via the renin-angiotensin and aldosterone pathway. The clinical features of potassium deficiency are muscle weakness, constipation, polydipsia, nocturia, and impaired urinary concentration. Renal biopsy typically reveals vacuolation of the tubular cells.

Alkalosis develops primarily because of loss of hydrogen ions in the vomitus, and secondarily because of contraction of the extracellular fluid (owing to salt depletion) without a commensurate loss of bicarbonate, and because of a shift of hydrogen ion into cells caused by potassium deficiency.

Sodium depletion develops because of loss of sodium in the vomitus and in some cases because of renal sodium loss in association with bicarbonate excretion (if the bicarbonate Tm is exceeded). The clinical features of sodium depletion are hyponatremia (not always present), hypotension, decreased blood volume, and high hematocrit. Plasma renin is raised, and the patients are insensitive to the pressor effects of angiotensin infusion. Plasma aldosterone levels are elevated. Creatinine clearance is reduced, and renal biopsy may show hyperplasia and increased granularity of the juxtaglomerular cells.

The urinary findings vary, depending upon whether or not the renal Tm for bicarbonate is exceeded (D. W. Seldin, personal communication). If the Tm is *not* exceeded, (1) the urine will not contain a high concentration of bicarbonate and the pH will vary within normal range, and (2) urinary levels of Na, K, and Cl will be low, correctly suggesting extrarenal loss of these ions. On the other hand, if the Tm for bicarbonate is exceeded, (1) urine Na and K will be high (even in the face of Na and K depletion), (2) urine chloride will be low, and (3) urine HCO_3 will be high, with alkaline pH.

Although the cause of these metabolic derangements will be obvious if there is a history of vomiting, great diagnostic difficulty will arise if vomiting is concealed. The following syndromes must be differentiated:

1. Bartter's syndrome.[50] Vomiting and Bartter's syndrome may present identical features, including elevated plasma renin levels, decreased response to angiotensin infusion, and hyperplasia of the juxtaglomerular apparatus.

2. Hyperaldosteronism. Hypotension, hyponatremia, and weight loss usually present in vomiting but not in aldosteronism. Plasma renin levels are high in vomiting, but not in aldosteronism.

3. Milk-alkali syndrome.

4. Welt's syndrome[51] (impaired renal conservation of potassium and magnesium). In addition to hypokalemia and hypomagnesemia, these patients have elevated plasma renin levels (aldosterone levels are normal).

5. Familial periodic paralysis.

ANTIEMETIC DRUGS

There is little doubt that some antiemetic drugs are helpful in preventing or treating nausea and vomiting. For example, Bonamine is 80 per cent more effective than a placebo against seasickness.[52]

These agents could theoretically work by depressing the vomiting center, the chemoreceptor trigger zone, the labyrinthine or vestibular apparatus, or the peripheral receptors. Unfortunately, it is usually not possible to definitely specify the mechanism of drug action. Thorazine, for instance, protects against the emetic action of apomorphine and digitalis, which act through the chemoreceptor trigger zone, but also against the emetic action of intragastric copper sulfate (which causes vomiting by a mechanism not involving the chemoreceptor trigger zone). Therefore a second site must be postulated for Thorazine activity, and this could be on the vomiting center itself or possibly on the peripheral receptors in the gastrointestinal tract. Some agents act both on the chemoreceptor trigger zone and on the vestibular apparatus (e.g., Dramamine, Marezine, and Bonamine). Others are believed to act strictly on the chemoreceptor trigger zone (e.g., Tigan).

As to which therapeutic agent to use, Moyer[52] made the suggestions shown in Table 11-1 in 1957. Unfortunately, a summary that includes more recently developed drugs is not available. Compazine would presumably be just as effective as Thorazine.

A review of the literature from 1960 to 1972 reveals only a few controlled and double-blind studies of antiemetic agents. Several of these are summarized below.

1. Compazine was better than Tigan when used intramuscularly for common causes of nausea and vomiting seen in office practice (acute gastroenteritis, flu-like states, etc.).[53] Actually, Tigan was no better than the placebo in this study. One other point of interest was that the placebo afforded complete relief in 45 per cent and some relief in 80 per cent of the patients who received it. Therefore, for self-limited illnesses, it is doubtful if one should risk the toxic effects of Compazine. (The extrapyramidal side effects of Compazine are especially important.) This has been emphasized by Anderson.[54]

2. In contrast to the previous study, Tigan was better than a placebo in patients with nausea and vomiting from a variety of causes—infection, gastrointestinal disturbances, allergy, hyperemesis gravidarum, and "toxicosis."[55] It produced no sedation and few side effects were noted.

3. Tigan, given intramuscularly, was very effective in controlling vomiting after tonsillectomy.[56]

TABLE 11-1. RECOMMENDATIONS FOR ANTIEMETIC THERAPY*

SOURCE OF EMESIS	RECOMMENDED AGENT
Drug-induced	
Digitalis	Thorazine
Antibiotics	Thorazine
Nitrogen mustard	Thorazine
Alcoholic states	Thorazine
Opiates	Bonamine, Marezine, or Dramamine
Infections	Thorazine
Toxicoses	
Diabetic acidosis	Thorazine
Uremia	Thorazine
Carcinomatosis	Thorazine
Radiation sickness	Thorazine
Other	Thorazine
Postoperative	
Prophylactic	Dramamine, Marezine, or Benadryl
Therapeutic	Thorazine
Pregnancy	Bonamine (with or without pyridoxine)
Motion sickness	
Air sickness	Scopolamine or Bonamine
Seasickness	Bonamine

*Moyer, J. H.: Med. Clin. N. Amer., March 1957, p. 405.

4. Neither Tigan nor Sinemet was better than a placebo in postoperative vomiting after abdominal surgery.[57]

5. Three hundred patients were observed during treatment with fluorouracil. Dartal and Compazine showed a statistically significant advantage over a placebo. Mornidine, Mitronal, and Tigan were progressively less effective, although each had some antiemetic effect.[58]

6. Quantril and prochlorperazine were both twice as effective as a placebo in the prophylaxis of postanesthetic vomiting.[59]

7. Prochlorperazine and metopimazine were no better than a placebo in treating radiation sickness.[60]

8. Metoclopramide was better than perphenazine when given intramuscularly at the end of surgery in preventing postoperative nausea and vomiting.[61]

REFERENCES

1. Thomas, J. E. Mechanics and regulation of gastric emptying. Physiol. Rev. 37:455, 2057.
2. Borison, H. L., and Wang, S. C. Physiology and pharmacology of vomiting. Pharmacol. Rev. 5:193, 1953.
3. Wang, S. C., and Borison, H. L. A new concept of organization of the central emetic mechanism: Recent studies on the sites of action of apomorphine, copper sulfate, and cardiac glycosides. Gastroenterology 22:1, 1952.
4. Lumsden, K., and Holden, W. S. The act of vomiting in man. Gut 10:173, 1969.
5. Ingelfinger, F. J., and Moss, R. E. The activity of the descending duodenum during nausea. Amer. J. Physiol. 136:561, 1942.
6. Johnson, H. D., and Laws, J. W. The cardia in swallowing, eructation and vomiting. Lancet 2:1268, 1966.
7. Abbot, F. K., Mack, M., and Wolf, S. The relation of sustained contraction of the duodenum to nausea and vomiting. Gastroenterology 20:238, 1952.
8. Wolf, S. Studies on nausea. Effects of ipecac and other emetics on the human stomach and duodenum. Gastroenterology 12:212, 1949.
9. Gupta, G. P., Dhawan, K. N., and Sinha, J. N. Evidence for absence of cholinergic mediation in central integration of vomiting. Japan. J. Pharmacol. 18:266, 1968.
10. Crohn, B. B. Affectations of the Stomach. Philadelphia, W. B. Saunders Co., 1927, p. 205.
11. Walshe, F. M. R. Diseases of the Nervous System. 10th ed. Baltimore, Williams & Wilkins Co., 1963.
12. Rimer, D. G. Gastric retention without mechanical obstruction. Arch. Intern. Med. 117:287, 1966.
13. Hill, O. W. Psychogenic vomiting. Gut 9:348, 1968.
14. Sigstad, H., and Jacobsen, C. D. Tertiary hyperparathyroidism. Acta Med. Scand. 188:337, 1970.
15. Menking, M., Wagnitz, J. G., Burton, J. J., Coddington, R. D., and Sotos, J. F. Rumination—a near fatal psychiatric disease of infancy. New Eng. J. Med. 280:802, 1969.
16. Brown, R. E., Madge, G. E., and Schiller, H. M. Observations on the pathogenesis of Reye's syndrome. South. Med. J. 64:942, 1971.
17. Allan, D. N. Dental erosions from vomiting. A case report. Brit. Dent. J. 126:311, 1969.
18. Leading Article. Psychogenic vomiting. Brit. Med. J. 4:344, 1968.
19. Brown, W. R. Rumination in the adult. A study of two cases. Gastroenterology 54:933, 1968.
20. Winship, D. H., Zboralske, F. F., Weber, W. N., and Soergel, K. H. Esophagus in rumination. Amer. J. Physiol. 207:1189, 1964.
21. Hollowell, J. G., and Gardner, L. I. Rumination and growth failure in male fraternal twin. Association with disturbed family environment. Pediatrics 36:565, 1965.
22. Lang, P. J., and Melamed, B. G. Avoidance conditioning therapy in an infant with chronic ruminative vomiting. J. Abnorm. Psychol. 74:1, 1969.
23. Affair of heart, cardia or toxic drug. New Eng. J. Med. 291:110, 1969.
24. Fairweather, D. V. I. Nausea and vomiting in pregnancy. Amer. J. Obstet. Gynec. 102:135, 1968.
25. Harvey, W. A., and Sherfey, M. J. Vomiting in pregnancy. A psychiatric study. Psychosomatic Med. 16:1, 1954.

26. Coppen, A. J. Vomiting of early pregnancy. Psychological factors and body build. Lancet 1:172, 1959.

27. Guze, S. B., DeLong, W. B., Majerus, P. W., and Robins, E. Association of clinical psychiatric disease with hyperemesis gravidarum. A three-and-a-half-year follow-up study of 48 patients and 45 controls. New Eng. J. Med. 261:1363, 1959.

28. Kroger, W. S., and De Lee, S. T. The psychosomatic treatment of hyperemesis gravidarum by hypnosis. Amer. J. Obstet. Gynec. 51:544, 1946.

29. Fitzgerald, J. P. B. Epidemiology of hyperemesis gravidarum. Lancet 1:660, 1956.

30. Semmens, J. P. Female sexuality and life situations. An etiologic psycho-socio-sexual profile of weight gain and nausea and vomiting in pregnancy. Obstet. Gynec. 38:555, 1971.

31. Carreras, B. B. Intravenous ACTH in the treatment of hyperemesis gravidarum. Obstet. Gynec. 3:50, 1954.

32. Youssef, A. F., and Staemmler, H.-J. Die Beziehung zwischen Allergie und Nebennierenrindenfunktion in ihrer Bedeutung für die Aetiologie der Hyperemesis gravidarum. Acta Endocrinol. 18:109, 1955.

33. Wallace, M., Richards, P., Chesser, E., and Wrong, O. Persistent alkalosis and hypokalemia caused by surreptitious vomiting. Quart. J. Med. 37:577, 1968.

34. Wolff, H. P., Vecsei, P., Kruck, F., Roscher, S., Brown, J. J., Dvsterdieck, G. O., Lever, A. F., and Robertson, J. I. S. Psychiatric disturbances leading to potassium depletion, sodium depletion, raised plasma renin concentration, and secondary hyperaldosteronism. Lancet 1:257, 1968.

35. Wrong, O., and Richards, P. Psychiatric disturbances and electrolyte depletion. Lancet 1:421, 1968.

36. Hoyt, C. S., and Stickler, G. B. A study of 44 children with the syndrome of recurrent (cyclic) vomiting. Pediatrics 25:775, 1960.

37. Lang, K. On the importance of central nervous damage in periodic vomiting in childhood (German). Mschr. Kindereilk. 111:161, 1963.

38. Lorber, J. Causes of cyclic vomiting. Develop. Med. Child. Neurol. 5:645, 1963.

39. Williams, J. A. Postgastrectomy problems – I. Brit. Med. J. 2:403, 1967.

40. Turner, F. P. Bilious vomiting after gastric surgery: A symptom of sliding hiatus hernia. Amer. J. Dig. Dis. 14:297, 1969.

41. Torrance, H. B., and Watson, A. Bilious vomiting after gastric surgery. Roy. Coll. Surg. (Edinburgh) 14:161, 1969.

42. Leading Article. Epidemic vomiting. Brit. Med. J. 2:327, 1969.

43. Leading Article. Winter vomiting disease. Brit. Med. J. 2:953, 1965.

44. Wooten, R. L., and Meriwether, T. W. Diabetic gastric atony: A clinical study. J.A.M.A. 176:1082, 1961.

45. Katz, L. A., and Spiro, H. M. Gastrointestinal manifestations of diabetes. New Eng. J. Med. 275:1350, 1966.

46. MacMahon, R. A., and Grattan-Smith, P. The baby who vomits. Med. J. Australia 2:543, 1966.

47. Greaney, E. M. Vomiting as a symptom of serious disease in infants and children. Calif. Med. 92:133, 1960.

48. Alcancia, E. Y., and Landor, J. H. Clinical experience with hypertrophic pyloric stenosis. Missouri Med. 63:719, 1966.

49. Burnett, C. H., Burrows, B. A., Commons, R. R., and Towery, B. T. Studies of alkalosis. II. Electrolyte abnormalities in alkalosis resulting from pyloric obstruction. J. Clin. Invest. 29:175, 1950.

50. Bartter, F. C., Pronove, P., Gill, J. R., and MacCardle, R. C. Hyperplasia of the juxtaglomerular complex with hyperaldosteronism and hypokalemic alkalosis. Amer. J. Med. 33:811, 1962.

51. Gitelman, H. J., Graham, J. B., and Welt, L. G. A new familial disorder characterized by hypokalemia and hypomagnesemia. Tr. Assn. Amer. Phys. 79:221, 1966.

52. Moyer, J. H. Effective antiemetic agents. Med. Clin. N. Amer. March 1957, p. 405.

53. Bordfeld, P. A. A controlled double-blind study of trimethobenzamide, prochlorperazine and placebo. J.A.M.A. 196:116, 1966.

54. Anderson, O. W. Antinauseant drugs in treatment of epidemic or virus gastritis. Pediatrics 46:319, 1970.

55. Kolodny, A. A controlled study of trimethobenzamide (Tigan), a specific antiemetic. Amer. J. Med. Sci. 239:682, 1960.

56. Marcus, P. S., and Ettenberg, M. Antiemetic prophylaxis in adenotonsillectomies. J.A.M.A. 189:695, 1964.

57. Doblem, A. B., Evers, W., and Israel, J. S. Double blind evaluation of metoclopramide (MK 745, Sinemet), trimethobenzamide (Tigan) and a placebo as postanaesthetic antiemetics following methoxyflurane anaesthesia. Canad. Anaest. Soc. J. 15:80, 1968.

58. Moertel, C. G., Reitemeier, R. J., and Gaye, R. P. A controlled clinical evaluation of antiemetic drugs. J.A.M.A. 186:116, 1963.

59. Finn, H., Vrbar, B. J., Thomas, J. S., and Steen, S. N. Antiemetic efficacy of benzquinamide. Controlled study. N.Y. State J. Med. 71:651, 1971.

60. Berry, G. H., Duncan, W., and Bowman, C. M. The prevention of radiation sickness. Report of a double blind random clinical trial using prochlorperazine and metopimazine. Clin. Radiol. 22:534, 1971.

61. Lind, B., and Breivik, H. Metoclopramide and perphenazine in the prevention of postoperational nausea and vomiting. A double-blind comparison. Brit. J. Anaesth. 42:614, 1970.

Chapter 12

Control of Gastric Secretion

John H. Walsh

INTRODUCTION

The human stomach secretes small ions and macromolecules into the gastric lumen and gastrin into the blood. These secretions are regulated by the functional capacity and integrity of the gastric mucosa and by neural and hormonal stimulants and inhibitors. Secretion can be subdivided into basal or interprandial and postprandial periods corresponding to the fasting and fed states. The volume and composition of gastric secretions are profoundly altered during the postprandial period. Unfortunately, the presence of food in the stomach and the loss of gastric contents into the intestine make the direct measurement of postprandial secretion in the intact stomach difficult. Consequently much experimental work has been carried out in dogs and other animals prepared with various gastric pouches and fistulas. For a variety of reasons these pouches may not reflect accurately the changes that occur in the intact human stomach following a meal. Since most of these studies have been carried out in dogs, species differences may lead to inaccurate conclusions when the results are applied to man. However, use of pouch preparations has permitted the demonstration of individual factors regulating gastric secretion, and many observations first made in animals subsequently have been confirmed in man. In this chapter the factors known to regu-

late human gastric secretion will be emphasized. However, results of animal experiments will be presented when similar studies have not been done in man.

FUNCTIONAL ANATOMY OF THE STOMACH

The stomach can be divided into three regions on the basis of the distribution of the gastric glands (see Figs. 38–1, 38–2, and 38–3, pp. 477 and 479. The cardiac gland area, located immediately below the gastroesophageal junction, is a narrow rim of mucoid glands. The mucosa of the remainder of the stomach can be divided into the oxyntic (acid-secreting) gland area, corresponding to the anatomic body and fundus, and the pyloric gland area, corresponding to the anatomic antrum and pylorus. Between the pyloric and oxyntic gland areas is a transitional zone in which there is intermingling of the two types of glands. In man the oxyntic glands secrete acid, pepsinogen, and intrinsic factor. Mucus is secreted by the entire gastric mucosa.

The surface of the gastric epithelium is lined by simple columnar surface mucosal cells which are the same throughout the stomach (see Figs. 38–4, 38–6, and 38–7, pp. 480 and 482. The mucosa contains numerous invaginations or gastric pits into which open one or more tubular glands

144

containing specialized secretory cells. The cardiac glands are mucous glands. The oxyntic glands are characterized by the presence of oxyntic (parietal) cells and peptic (chief) cells. Three to seven oxyntic glands open into each gastric pit. The neck of the oxyntic gland is lined with mucous cells, oxyntic cells are interspersed with mucous neck cells in the midportion, and peptic cells predominate at the base of the glands. The pyloric glands comprise 15 to 20 per cent of the mucosal area and are composed of surface mucous cells superficially and cells resembling mucous neck cells in the neck and base. Cells which contain the gastric secretory hormone gastrin are also found in the pyloric glands (see Fig. 38–8, p. 483).

Fine structural studies of the major glandular epithelial cell types have revealed specialized structures corresponding to the functions of the cells.[1,2] Surface mucous cells contain mucous granules tightly packed in the apical region of the cells. In the mucous neck cells, granules may be found in the base and perinuclear regions as well. Oxyntic cells have numerous long microvilli projecting into the glandular lumen and contain an extensive network of channels formed by the infolding of the luminal surface known as the secretory canaliculus also lined by microvilli and opening into the glandular lumen (see Fig. 38–5, p. 481). There is some evidence that the endoplasmic reticulum may be arranged in a tubular system and may be important in acid secretion. The oxyntic cells have also been identified as the site of intrinsic factor production in man.[3] The peptic cells contain numerous zymogen granules, containing pepsinogen, in their apical portions. Two immunochemically distinct types of pepsinogen have been identified in man.[4] The group I pepsinogens are found only in oxyntic gland mucosa. They have been localized by immunofluorescence to granules in the chief cells and in the mucous neck cells, which are felt to be the precursors of the chief cells. Group II pepsinogens are found in the same oxyntic gland cells but also in cells in the pyloric glands and in Brunner's glands in the duodenum. Gastrin immunofluorescence was localized by McGuigan[5] to cytoplasmic granules in endocrine cells predominantly located in the midportion of the pyloric glands.

INNERVATION AND BLOOD SUPPLY

The vagus nerve provides the parasympathetic innervation of the stomach through anterior and posterior trunks. Extragastric branches of the vagus nerve innervate the liver, gallbladder, pancreas, and intestine. About 90 per cent of the vagal fibers are afferent. Intrinsic nervous plexuses exist within the stomach. Preganglionic fibers of the vagus nerve synapse with cells of the intrinsic plexus, and postganglionic fibers go to secretory glands and to muscle. Only a small proportion of the ganglion cells in the intrinsic plexus have a direct relationship with the vagus. The vast majority are concerned with local reflexes, and some of these reflexes are probably related to secretion. It is important to note that interruption of the vagus nerve does not eliminate these local reflexes.

The sympathetic innervation of the stomach is via the thoracolumbar sympathetic nerves originating chiefly at T–7 and T–8. Efferent postganglionic fibers originate in the celiac ganglia. Afferent fibers do not synapse in the celiac ganglia. These afferent fibers are the principal pathways of visceral pain sensation.

The blood supply of the stomach forms a vascular submucosal plexus which provides extensive collateral circulation for all areas of the stomach except a small margin of the lesser curvature (see Fig. 51–1, p. 632). Three of the four major arterial branches can be ligated without producing ischemia. From the submucosal plexus, spiral muscular arteries penetrate to the mucosa and terminate in arteriolar capillaries which supply individual cells.

MUCOSAL BARRIERS TO SECRETION AND ABSORPTION

A continuous layer of gastric mucosal cells creates a barrier between the gastric lumen and the mucosal interstitial space. This barrier is composed of the apical cell walls and of tight junctions between adjacent cells. The cell membrane is composed of a lipid bilayer with a protein core. Ionized materials are poorly absorbed, but un-ionized lipid-soluble substances are absorbed. Under normal circumstances this barrier maintains a concentration gradient between hydrogen ions in the lumen and sodium ions in the mucosa.

The barrier can be damaged by a number of agents. In the damaged mucosa the net movement of sodium ions into the lumen and of hydrogen ions out of the lumen is enhanced, resulting in secretion of similar volumes of gastric juice with high sodium and low hydrogen concentration.[6] Even when the mucosal barrier is broken, the mucosa is capable of secreting acid in response to stimulation by histamine, which can be demonstrated by use of glycine buffer as a "trap" to retain secreted hydrogen ions in the lumen. With a strong enough insult the mucosal cells are destroyed, but it is possible to break the mucosal barrier reversibly. The net effect of breaking the barrier is that sodium, potassium, and some protein leak into the lumen and hydrogen enters the mucosa. Hydrogen entering the mucosa causes additional damage, partially through the release of tissue histamine. Substances which are un-ionized at acid pH and are lipid soluble readily penetrate the apical cell membrane. Once inside the cells, acidic substances with a pK less than the intracellular pH become ionized and are trapped in the cells where they may exert toxic effects. The model for this type of agent is aspirin, which has a pK_a of 3.5.[7] Following topical application of aspirin the lipid-protein layer on the cell surface and the tight junctions between cells are disrupted, causing desquamation of cells. The fluid leaked into the lumen after such damage is similar to interstitial fluid, including some plasma protein. If the damage is severe, blood cells also leak from the submucosal capillaries. The principal change noted is an increase in sodium and decrease in hydrogen ions in the lumen, with an increase in total volume of fluid in the lumen. Bleeding is exacerbated by cholinergic stimuli. This leakage of hydrogen into the mucosa and sodium into the lumen can cause misleading estimates of total acid secretion when the barrier is damaged. Other injurious agents include acetic acid, ethanol, and bile salts.

It should be emphasized that the gastric mucosal barrier is not the same as the "mucus barrier." The gastric mucosal cells are covered by a layer of adherent mucus with weak neutralizing capacity. This mucus is not an effective barrier for permeation of electrolytes and water and adds little to the barrier formed by the cell walls and intercellular tight junctions.

It should also be pointed out that the net fluxes of water and electrolytes are the algebraic sum of the movement into the mucosa and the movement out from the mucosa into the lumen. Even when there is no net flux, water molecules move bidirectionally. Flux from lumen to blood is around 50 per cent of the gastric water content every 30 minutes and is not affected by active secretion. During active secretion the flux into the lumen is increased while the flux into the mucosa remains the same, so the net flux into the lumen is increased and is reflected as an increase in gastric volume. Water flux varies little when the luminal contents are made hypo- or hypertonic to plasma. Sodium also has a bidirectional flux. Under normal circumstances there is little back diffusion of acid. Relative rates of insorption in the normal stomach expressed in per cent per minute are as follows: H_2O, 1.65; Na^+, 0.47; K^+, 0.10; and H^+, less than 0.10.[8] Thus the undamaged gastric mucosa is relatively impermeable to small ions.

ELECTRICAL POTENTIAL DIFFERENCE

The mucosal surface of the stomach is electrically negative when compared with the serosal surface. In man, the potential differences compared with blood (as reference for serosal surface) for various areas of mucosa were found to be (in millivolts):[9] esophagus, −15; gastric corpus, −44; gastric antrum, −35; duodenal bulb, −7; and postbulbar duodenum, +1.8. The potential appears to be generated primarily at the luminal cell border. The specific cell type responsible for generation of this potential has not been defined. Since the pyloric gland area maintains a negative potential, it is unlikely that the oxyntic cell is responsible entirely. The principal source of the potential difference is active transport of chloride ions from the intracellular space against both concentration and electrical gradients.[10] If the chloride in the serosal fluid bathing an isolated frog gastric mucosa is replaced by sulfate, an impermeable anion, the potential is abolished.[11]

During the secretion of acid, proton (hydrogen ion) secretion is coupled with secretion of an equivalent additional amount of chloride ions and the potential is not further increased. During stimulated secretion a positive potential can be produced by substituting sulfate for chloride in the serosal fluid. In this situation the secretion of protons continues and creates a positive charge on the mucosal surface. The basal membrane of the epithelial cell also contributes to the negative luminal potential. This membrane is highly permeable to chloride and less permeable to sodium. Since intracellular concentrations of chloride and sodium are lower than extracellular concentrations, both ions diffuse into the cell. Chloride diffuses more rapidly and causes build-up of a negative charge inside the cell. In addition, sodium is pumped out of the cell and potassium diffuses out. The net result is that the interior of the gastric mucosal cell is more negatively charged than the extracellular fluid, but the gastric lumen is even more negatively charged.

The practical applications of potential difference measurements in man have been limited. Measurement of potential difference is a very sensitive method for detecting damage to the gastric mucosal barrier.[12] Such measurements also offer a convenient method for determining the site of the gastroduodenal junction. They are not so useful in delineating the border between the oxyntic and pyloric gland mucosa, because the difference is not so great and in some individuals there is no clear zone of electrical change.[9]

CELL REPLICATION IN THE GASTRIC MUCOSA

Cells on the surface of the gastric mucosa are constantly being replaced by a process of desquamation and migration of new cells from the base to the surface of the crypts. The major cell type which undergoes mitosis is the mucous neck cell, which may be the precursor of the oxyntic and peptic cells as well as the mucous cells. The mitotic rate of the surface epithelial cells is 0.5 to 1 per cent and the mean generation time for the surface cells is in the order of two to six days. Cell turnover at the base of the glands is much slower, and the oxyntic and chief cells represent a much more stable population of cells.

Parietal cell hyperplasia in rats can be produced by prolonged administration of pentagastrin, a gastrin analogue.[13] This hyperplasia is associated with increased synthesis of protein[14] and RNA by the mucosa and results in an increase in maximal acid secretory capacity. Mucosal hyperplasia in response to pentagastrin can be partially prevented by the concurrent administration of secretin, a hormone which inhibits gastrin-stimulated acid secretion. The mucosal hyperplasia seen in the Zollinger-Ellison syndrome may be due to the prolonged hypergastrinemia found in this condition. In rats hypophysectomy causes a reduction in the volume of the gastric mucosa and in total numbers and concentrations of oxyntic and chief cells.

ACID SECRETION

PRODUCTION OF HYDROCHLORIC ACID

Hydrochloric acid is secreted into the gastric lumen by the oxyntic cells, also known as parietal cells. Hydrogen ion concentrations in the gastric juice are three million times greater than in the blood and tissues. The energy required to produce this concentration of hydrogen ions is generated in the oxyntic cells by aerobic metabolism and involves the production of high energy phosphate bonds.

For each hydrogen ion secreted a molecule of CO_2, derived from arterial blood or from mucosal metabolism, is converted to bicarbonate and ultimately enters the interstitial fluid. Oxyntic cells contain a high concentration of the enzyme carbonic anhydrase which catalyzes this conversion. The metabolic alkalosis produced by active acid secretion is known as the alkaline tide. The amount of bicarbonate entering the blood during secretion is directly proportional to the amount of acid secreted. The amount of excess bicarbonate entering the blood has been used to measure gastric acid secretion following a meal.[15]

The maximal concentration of hydrogen

ions found in the gastric juice is between 140 and 160 mN. The other principal cations are sodium and potassium. The principal anion is chloride. There is an inverse relationship between the concentrations of hydrogen and of sodium ions, whereas the concentrations of potassium remain within a fairly narrow range. There are two major theories regarding the source of sodium ions in human gastric juice. In the two-component theory, first proposed by Pavlov and Hollander, the assumption is made that the parietal cells secrete pure hydrochloride acid and the other electrolytes found in the gastric juice are secreted by cells other than the parietal cells. It is known that the parietal secretion is not pure HCl but also contains some potassium. The nonparietal secretion is slightly alkaline and contains sodium, bicarbonate, and other electrolytes. The maximal acidity which could theoretically be achieved by the stomach would correspond to pure parietal secretion. Variations in the composition of gastric juice depend on the proportion of parietal and nonparietal secretion. At low rates of secretion the non-parietal component constitutes a major fraction, whereas at high rates of secretion it is mainly the parietal component that increases, resulting in decreased concentration of sodium and increased concentrations of hydrogen, potassium, and chloride. Makhlouf and colleagues[16] have calculated by extrapolation that the parietal component of human gastric juice contains 166 mN Cl^-, 149 mN H^+, and 17 mN K^+. The calculated composition of the nonparietal component was similar to that of extracellular fluid and included 137 mN Na^+, 6 mN K^+, 117 mN Cl^-, and 25 mN HCO_3^-. Gastric juice also contains low concentrations of calcium, magnesium, and phosphate which probably also are derived from the nonparietal component.

The other theory, the Teorell hypothesis, also holds that the primary secretion of the parietal cells is a mixture of HCl and KCl. It differs from the two-component theory in that it accounts for the sodium in the gastric juice as originating by exchange for hydrogen ions across the mucosa. The two theories may not be mutually exclusive. This subject is discussed in detail elsewhere.[17]

RELATIONSHIP OF ACID SECRETION TO GASTRIC MUCOSAL BLOOD FLOW

Studies of total blood flow to the stomach during acid secretion have not shown consistent changes. This is not surprising when it is considered that much of the blood entering the stomach supplies the muscular layers and only a fraction perfuses the acid-secreting mucosa. Jacobson[18] has developed a method for measuring gastric mucosal blood flow and has used this method to clarify some of the conflicting data found in earlier studies. The technique is based on the permeability of the gastric mucosa to a weak base, aminopyrine. This substance is un-ionized at plasma pH and diffuses rapidly across the gastric mucosal barrier into the lumen. When exposed to acid in the lumen it becomes ionized and no longer able to diffuse across the mucosa. Since the capacity for diffusion of aminopyrine across the mucosa is far in excess of the amount presented to it, the rate-limiting factor is blood flow. Therefore aminopyrine accumulates in the gastric juice at a rate which is directly proportional to gastric mucosal blood flow. This method has been applied extensively to dogs but has not been used in man because of the toxicity of the agent.

In general, agents which stimulate acid secretion, such as food, histamine, and gastrin, also stimulate mucosal blood flow. For the same rate of acid secretion histamine increases mucosal blood flow more than gastrin does. However, an increase in blood flow may occur without an increase in acid secretion. This occurs, for example, with certain drugs such as isoproterenol. Blood flow has also been measured in the nonacid-secreting portion of the stomach by instilling acid into antral pouches. It was found that histamine also increased mucosal blood flow to areas of the stomach which do not secrete acid.[19] A stimulant of blood flow such as histamine could increase mucosal flow by several possible mechanisms, including a direct action on vascular smooth muscle, an increase in metabolic activity leading to the release of local vasodilator substances, or a redistribution of blood from the muscular to the mucosal area of the stomach. The current concept is that mucosal blood flow plays a permissive and supportive role in gastric secretory processes but blood flow per se is not the specific stimulant for acid secretion. This subject has been reviewed recently.[20]

BASAL ACID SECRETION

Normal gastric acid secretion in human subjects after an overnight fast ranges between 0 and 5 mEq per hour. When repeated tests are done in the same subject, considerable variations occur and periods of achlorhydria are not uncommon. A circadian rhythm of acid secretion has been found in fasting subjects, with the lowest output between 5 A.M. and 11 A.M. and the highest rate in the evening between 2 P.M. and 1 A.M.[21] The factors responsible for basal secretion are not known, but it is likely that tonic vagal stimulation and the constant release of small amounts of gastrin play significant roles. Basal acid secretion is decreased by vagotomy or by antrectomy. Although vagotomy obviously decreases vagal tone, it has not been possible to measure normal vagal tone with the vagus intact. It has been shown recently that vagotomy does not reduce fasting serum gastrin concentrations in man.[22] It would be desirable to be able to correlate fasting serum gastrin concentrations with basal acid output, but studies to date have shown no consistent relationship within the normal range. Antrectomy decreases both fasting gastrin concentrations and acid secretion.[22] Another factor which could play a part in regulation of basal acid secretion is the concentration of circulating inhibitors. It is known that duodenal acidification results in decreased acid secretion through the release of one or more inhibitory hormones from the intestine. Lack of methods for measuring intestinal inhibitors in the circulation has hampered research in this area. Finally, the secretory capacity of the stomach is important in regulation of basal secretion. Patients with decreased functional parietal cell mass as determined by low rates of stimulated secretion also have low rates of basal acid secretion.

STIMULATED ACID SECRETION

The major physiological stimulant to acid secretion in man is the ingestion of meals. The following paragraphs will consider the mechanisms which are known to stimulate and to modify the gastric acid response to feeding. For obvious technical reasons, it has been easier to measure acid responses to exogenous acid stimulants such as histamine and gastrin than to food. The doses of various stimulants required to produce maximal acid responses in man are given on pages 539 to 543. Rune[15] has calculated from measurement of bicarbonate released into the blood that the acid response to a meal in man is similar in magnitude to the maximal responses achieved by parenteral administration of gastrin or histamine. When the antrum is intact, central vagal stimulation by 2-deoxy-D-glucose (2-DG) in man and by sham feeding in dogs also can produce near maximal secretion.

Card and Marks[23] found that the maximal rate of acid secretion which can be achieved in man and in dogs is directly related to the number of parietal cells in the mucosa. They estimated that a maximal rate of acid secretion of 20 mEq per hour with histamine stimulation corresponded to a total parietal cell population of one billion cells. From this work arose the concept that maximal stimulated acid secretion provides a good estimate of the parietal cell mass. In general the parietal cell mass estimated in this way shows less variation with repeated testing than the basal acid secretion. This relationship between stimulated acid secretion and parietal cell mass does not hold under all circumstances. For example, vagotomy results in a prompt decrease in peak stimulated acid output in man without changing the parietal cell mass. Acid secretion can be restored to prevagotomy values by the administration of cholinomimetic drugs.[24]

NEUROHUMORAL CONTROL OF GASTRIC SECRETION

Discovery of gastrin by Edkins[25] made it necessary to modify Pavlov's view that gastric secretion was entirely under vagal control. This led to the idea that the cephalic phase was mediated by the vagus nerve and the gastric phase by the release of gastrin from the stomach. However Uvnäs[26] then showed that vagal stimulation had two effects, both a direct action on the oxyntic glands and an action on the pyloric glands leading to the release of gastrin. It is now known that the cephalic, gastric, and probably intestinal phases of acid secretion have dual nervous and hormonal components and that these components are closely related and potentiate each other. The division into cephalic, gastric, and intestinal phases provides a convenient way to identify the site at which stimulation is initiated. Following a meal the three phases of stimulation occur more or less simultaneously rather than sequentially. The subject of neurohumoral control of gastric secretion has been reviewed extensively by Grossman.[27]

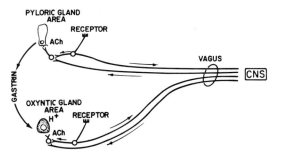

Figure 12–1. Pathways for cholinergic stimulation in the stomach. Vagal impulses arising during the cephalic phase release acetylcholine at the oxyntic cells and at the gastrin cells in the pyloric gland area. Release of acetylcholine also results from stimulation of receptors located in the gastric mucosa during the gastric phase, imitating both local intramural reflexes and vagal reflexes. (From Grossman, M. I.: Physiologist 6:349, 1963.)

ENDOGENOUS STIMULANTS OF ACID SECRETION

Three substances in the body are known to be capable of stimulating the oxyntic cell to produce hydrochloric acid. These are acetylcholine, gastrin, and histamine. The first two have been shown unequivocally to have important physiological roles. Although for a number of years histamine was felt to be the final common mediator of the activity of the other two substances, much evidence has been accumulated recently to suggest that endogenous histamine does not play an important physiological role in acid secretion. This evidence is summarized by Johnson.[28] Histamine remains an important agent for the exogenous stimulation of gastric secretion. It may someday prove to have a physiological role in gastric secretion, but it will not be considered further in this discussion.

ACETYLCHOLINE

Acetylcholine is the chemical substance which transmits excitation from preganglionic to postganglionic autonomic neurons. It is also released at the postganglionic nerve endings in the gastric mucosa. Cholinergic impulses are transmitted by the vagus nerve and by local intramural reflexes in the gastric wall. The principal

pathways for cholinergic stimulation in the stomach are illustrated in Figure 12–1. Receptors in the gastric mucosa may initiate vagal stimulation or may enter into local reflexes.[29] Vagal stimulation may also be initiated by central stimuli such as hypoglycemia. The result of either type of stimulation is the release of acetylcholine which either releases gastrin from the gastrin cell in the pyloric gland area or directly stimulates oxyntic cells to produce acid. Both these cholinergic effects can be prevented by the administration of sufficient doses of atropine, although there is evidence that the oxyntic cells may be more sensitive to the inhibitory effects of atropine than the gastrin cells.

GASTRIN

Gastrin is the peptide hormone released from the pyloric gland area which stimulates acid production by the oxyntic cells. The existence of such a hormone was first shown by Edkins in 1905.[25] In 1938 Komarov[30] showed that this stimulant was protein in nature and distinct from histamine. Gastrin was purified from antral mucosa by Gregory and Tracy,[31] its amino acid sequence was determined, and gastrins from several species were synthesized by Kenner and Sheppard.[32] Two molecular forms were isolated and were called gastrin I and gastrin II. Both were found to be heptadecapeptide amides with the structure shown in Figure 12-2, differ-

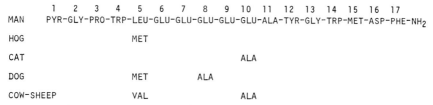

Figure 12-2. Structure of gastrin obtained from several species.

ing only in the sulfation of the tyrosine in gastrin II. Gastrins from different species are similar and differ by no more than two amino acid substitutions. The C-terminal tetrapeptide amide was found to possess all the biologic activities of the whole molecule but was less potent on a molar basis.[33] A synthetic derivative of the tetrapeptide in which β-alanine is substituted for glycine in the C-terminal pentapeptide, named pentagastrin, is more potent and has been used widely in testing gastric secretory function. Recently, Yalow and Berson[34] have reported that a significant portion of gastrin in the circulation is a larger molecule with a molecular weight of approximately 7000. This "big gastrin" seems to be composed of the heptadecapeptide amide (molecular weight 2100) covalently bound to a more basic peptide.

The tissue distribution of gastrin has been studied by bioassay and by radioimmunoassay[35] of tissue extracts and by immunofluorescent staining of tissue preparations.[5] The gastric antrum contains the greatest concentration and total amount of gastrin in the human, but considerable quantities are present in the proximal duodenum with diminishing quantities present in the remainder of the small intestine. Small amounts of gastrin are also found in the pancreas. The oxyntic mucosa contains very little. Heptadecapeptide gastrin predominates in extracts of antrum and pancreas. Higher proportions of big gastrin are found in the intestine. The gastrin cell was identified in the gastric antrum by McGuigan[5] by use of immunofluorescent staining. The cells were found predominantly in the middle third of the pyloric glands, bordering the lumen of the glands. Tumor cells from Zollinger-Ellison-type tumors and certain cells in normal human pancreatic islets also show immunofluorescence with antibody to gastrin.

Gastrin has a variety of physiological actions which can be demonstrated with endogenous release of the hormone or by infusion of small doses of exogenous gastrin.[36] In the stomach it is a strong stimulant of acid secretion, a moderate stimulant of pepsin secretion, and a stimulator of smooth muscle. It has a potent effect on the gastroesophageal sphincter, causing contraction. In dogs, gastrin also is a stimulant of pancreatic flow and bile flow. Other effects which have been found with the administration of exogenous gastrin include contraction of the gallbladder and small intestine smooth muscle, relaxation of the ileocecal valve and sphincter of Oddi, intestinal secretion of water and electrolytes, growth of gastric mucosa, and release of insulin, but it is uncertain whether these effects occur with physiological amounts of gastrin.

The half-life of gastrin in the circulation is between five and 15 minutes. Both the kidney and the small intestine can remove or inactivate circulating gastrin. The liver apparently does not metabolize gastrin but does inactivate gastrin tetrapeptide and pentagastrin. An enzyme has been found in liver tissue which causes deamidation of the tetrapeptide amide, converting it to a product devoid of biologic activity.[37]

Until recently, measurement of circulating gastrin was possible only by bioassay techniques which use acid secretion by gastric pouches to indicate gastrin activity. Such techniques are not sensitive enough to measure normal concentrations of gastrin in human plasma, but in some cases greatly increased amounts can be detected in the blood or urine of patients with Zollinger-Ellison syndrome. Radioimmunoassay techniques have now been developed which offer a sensitive and specific method for measuring gastrin in the blood.[38-41] By use of radioimmunoassay it has been possible to confirm many of the conclusions made by physiological experiments in animals and to apply some of these to man.

PHASES OF GASTRIC ACID SECRETION

CEPHALIC PHASE

The cephalic phase is mediated by the vagus nerve in response to stimulants acting in the region of the head. The precise areas in the brain which control vagal impulses have not been identified. Changes in acid secretion may be found when medullary, hypothalamic, limbic, or cortical areas of the brain are subjected to electrical stimulation.[42] There appear to be inhibitory as well as stimulatory centers.

The cephalic stimulation which occurs with eating is a result of the sight, taste, smell, and chewing and swallowing of palatable food. The cephalic phase can be studied as an isolated phenomenon when food is eaten but does not enter the stomach. In a few human subjects with esophageal fistulas resulting from cancer operations and gastric fistulas, eating food which then passes out through the esophagus has been found to elicit acid secretion in the stomach. The process has been studied in more detail in dogs equipped with esophageal fistulas and gastric pouches. Acid responses are greatly enhanced if the pyloric gland area is isolated from contact with gastric acid. Another type of cephalic stimulant is intracellular hypoglycemia which may be elicited by insulin or simulated by 2-deoxy-D-glucose.

Vagal release of gastrin can be demonstrated in dogs with vagally denervated pouches of oxyntic gland mucosa (Heidenhain pouches) and vagally innervated pyloric gland pouches. When cephalic stimulation is elicited by insulin hypoglycemia or by sham feeding, the Heidenhain pouches secrete acid. Gastrin release can also be demonstrated under these conditions by direct measurement of circulating gastrin. This stimulation is greatly reduced or abolished by resection or denervation of the pyloric pouch. Insulin also has an inhibitory effect on the Heidenhain pouch, making stimulation of acid secretion difficult to demonstrate.

Direct vagal stimulation of acid secretion can be shown by resection of the gastrin secreting areas of the stomach and intestine and leaving the remainder of the stomach as a vagally innervated pouch.[43] Under these conditions insulin hypoglycemia stimulates acid secretion, though the response is decreased. Uvnäs[26] obtained evidence that a synergism existed between vagal stimulation and gastrin by showing that antral resection greatly decreased the acid responses from vagally innervated oxyntic gland pouches (Pavlov pouches) with sham feeding but that the acid responses could be restored to preantrectomy levels by the infusion of very small doses of gastrin which did not produce acid secretion when given without concurrent vagal stimulation. Knutson and Olbe[44] found that antrectomy diminished but did not abolish sham feeding responses in man. In contrast to dogs, sham feeding responses in antrectomized duodenal ulcer subjects were not potentiated by threshold doses of exogenous gastrin. In addition, antrectomy in man also markedly reduced the maximal acid responses to exogenous gastrin or betazole.

Vagally mediated gastrin release can be prevented by acidification of the pyloric gland area. We have found that such acidification completely prevented an increase in immunoassayable gastrin with insulin stimulation but reduced Pavlov pouch acid output by only 60 per cent.

GASTRIC PHASE

The gastric phase is initiated by stimuli arising in the stomach and like the cephalic phase is mediated both by gastrin release and by direct cholinergic stimulation of acid secretion. It has already been pointed out (Fig. 12–1) that cholinergic stimulation can arise by activation of receptors in the oxyntic gland or the pyloric gland area and that the impulses may travel by way of long vagal reflexes or through local intramural nerve plexuses to stimulate the oxyntic cells or the gastrin cells.

Direct cholinergic stimulation of acid secretion in the gastric phase can be demonstrated by distention of vagally innervated or denervated oxyntic gland pouches.[27] Distention of the innervated pouch results in secretion of acid accompanied by a marked increase in pepsin output. There is good evidence that at least part of this response is mediated by long vagovagal reflexes. Distention of denervated pouches results in slight stimulation of acid secretion but produces marked augmentation of the acid response to small doses of gastrin and also produces marked stimulation of pepsin secretion. In the denervated pouch this stimulation is produced by local cholinergic reflexes. The possibilities that stimulation of cholinergic reflexes may be initiated by chemical stimuli in the oxyntic gland area or that distention of the vagally innervated oxyntic gland pouch may cause release of gastrin through vagovagal reflexes have not been tested.

Much work has been done to define the mechanisms by which gastrin is released from the gastrin cells in the pyloric gland area. The first conclusive proof that a gastric hormone was released from the antral region was obtained by Grossman et al. in 1948[45] when they showed that distention of transplanted pyloric pouches in dogs caused secretion of acid by the vagally innervated oxyntic gland mucosa.

It is now felt that the release of gastrin in response to mechanical distention and chemical stimuli is mediated by local reflexes in the pyloric gland area. Gastrin release by these forms of stimulation is not abolished by vagal denervation of antral pouches but is abolished by topical application of local anesthetics. Local anesthetics, however, do not prevent gastrin release caused by topical application of acetylcholine. This is taken as evidence that local anesthetics interfere with the neural pathways that release acetylcholine in the vicinity of the gastrin cell but do not interfere directly with gastrin release mediated by stimulation of the gastrin cell by acetylcholine. Topical application of anticholinergic agents such as atropine blocks the gastrin response to acetylcholine as well as to the other stimulants. Antral acidification to pH 1 prevents gastrin release by all forms of stimulation, including acetylcholine. The effect of acidification appears to be exerted directly on the gastrin cell. Until this inhibitory effect of acid on gastrin release was recognized, many physiological experiments designed to demonstrate gastrin release failed because of failure to maintain the antrum at sufficiently high pH.

The factors responsible for the gastric phase of gastrin release following meals are not well studied owing to the heterogeneous composition of foods. The protein component of food seems to be responsible for releasing gastrin. Liver, meat, and meat extracts are all potent stimulants. Amino acids, especially glycine, serine, and alanine, ethyl and propyl alcohols, and bile salts are effective gastrin releasing agents. The only known mechanical stimulant is distention. All these stimulants are pH dependent. The pH threshold for amino acids is about 3, and for distention, vagal stimulation, and alcohol is about 1.5.[46]

Thus the release of gastrin is dependent upon both vagal stimuli arising in the gastric phase and chemical and mechanical stimuli arising from the gastric phase. The chemical stimulants in food are not well characterized, but probably include amino acids and small peptides. The release of gastrin is regulated by the concentration of acid in the pyloric gland area which serves as a mechanism for autoregulation of acid secretion. Deacidification of the antrum alone does not appear to stimulate gastrin release. Protein and amino acids influence gastrin release by three mechanisms: distention, buffering acid, and chemical stimulation of gastrin release.

INTESTINAL PHASE

The intestine releases one or more hormones which stimulate acid secretion. Intestinal stimulation of gastric secretion has not been defined as well as have cephalic and gastric stimulation. The intestine also releases hormones which inhibit acid secretion. The intestinal hormone responsible for stimulating acid secretion has been called intestinal gastrin, but this does not imply that it is chemically identical with antral gastrin.

Sircus[47] demonstrated the hormonal nature of intestinal gastrin by showing that distention of the intestine stimulated acid secretion by Heidenhain pouches. Food introduced directly into the intestine also stimulates secretion from Heidenhain pouches when the remainder of the stomach is excised. The effects of hydrochloric acid on the intestinal phase depend on the portion of the intestine that is acidified.

When acid is introduced into the duodenum it usually inhibits acid secretion, but when acid is introduced into the jejunum it may stimulate acid secretion. There is some evidence that the release of intestinal gastrin may be neurally mediated, because the effects of distention and jejunal acidification are blocked by topical application of procaine to the mucosa.

It has not been established whether the intestinal stimulatory hormone is the same as antral gastrin. By immunochemical methods it has been possible to detect in extracts of intestinal mucosa a substance which reacts identically with antral gastrin.[35] The human duodenum contains high concentrations of this immunoreactive gastrin, whereas the distal duodenum and upper jejunum contain sharply decreasing concentrations. We have obtained evidence that feeding causes the release of human duodenal gastrin in patients with partial gastrectomy and gastroduodenal anastomosis.[48] The intestinal mucosa in dogs appears to contain much lower concentrations of immunoreactive gastrin than that in man. It has not been established whether the amounts of gastrin present in the dog intestine are sufficient to produce the acid responses that are seen after intestinal stimulation. There is some evidence to support the existence of another stimulatory hormone. The acid response of a denervated oxyntic gland pouch to feeding has a later peak and a longer duration than the serum gastrin response as measured by radioimmunoassay. Another point in favor of another intestinal stimulant is the observation that acid responses to feeding in the Heidenhain pouch dog are higher than the maximal responses that can be achieved by infusion of exogenous gastrin. If such a hormone exists, its chemical nature remains to be elucidated.

Acid secretion commonly increases following portacaval anastomosis in man and in dogs. In dogs stimulation of the jejunum by food or distention causes increased gastric acid secretion after portacaval shunt but food in the ileum or colon has little effect. Orloff and coworkers[49] have postulated the release of a hormone which, unlike gastrin, is normally inactivated by the liver. Such a hormone has not yet been identified.

Resection or isolation of segments of the intestine from intestinal continuity may result in acid hypersecretion. One possibility, that resection removes tissue necessary for gastrin catabolism, has not been borne out by serum gastrin measurements. Several patients with "short gut" have had normal to low gastrin values (unpublished observations). Other possibilities which remain to be explored include increased release or decreased inactivation of an acid-stimulating hormone other than gastrin or decreased release of an intestinal inhibitor of acid secretion.

OTHER STIMULANTS

Caffeine stimulates acid secretion when given alone and causes increased acid responses to submaximal doses of histamine and pentagastrin. It is not known whether caffeine releases gastrin or acts by some other mechanism such as activation of cyclic AMP.

Alcohol is a stimulant of gastric secretion and of gastrin release in the dog. In man alcohol seems to be a less effective stimulant of acid secretion, and increases in serum gastrin levels after the administration of ethanol have been difficult to demonstrate. Intravenous ethanol increases acid secretion in antrectomized dogs, suggesting a direct effect on the oxyntic cell. Alcohol can also damage the gastric mucosal barrier.

Calcium is a stimulant of acid secretion. Acute increases in serum calcium cause mild increases in acid secretion and in serum gastrin in normal subjects and subjects with peptic ulcer. In patients with Zollinger-Ellison syndrome, infusion of calcium may cause marked increases in serum gastrin and in acid secretion which differ significantly from the responses found in normal subjects. In general, patients with chronic hypercalcemia caused by hyperparathyroidism do not have marked acid hypersecretion unless they also have a gastrin-secreting tumor.

EFFECTS OF VAGOTOMY AND ANTRECTOMY

In man, vagotomy markedly decreases basal acid secretion and also decreases observed responses to ordinary so-called maximal doses of histamine and pentagastrin by about 65 per cent. Since the dose-response curves to these stimulants may be shifted to the right, it is possible that maximal responses are not actually diminished. These responses can be restored at least partially by concurrent administration of cholinergic agents. Complete vagotomy abolishes acid responses to cephalic stimuli such as insulin and sham feeding. About one-third of vagotomies in man have been found to be incomplete as judged by postoperative insulin tests. The gastric component of gastrin release is not prevented in man by vagotomy, and fasting serum gastrin concentrations and gastrin responses to feeding are the same or higher after vagotomy.

In dogs the effects of vagotomy can be studied by converting a vagally innervated Pavlov pouch to a vagally denervated Heidenhain pouch. Denervation decreases the submaximal and maximal responses to gastrin and the submaximal response to histamine. The maximal response to histamine is unchanged. The decreased responses to gastrin and low doses of histamine can be restored by administration of cholinomimetic drugs.[24] These findings are consistent with the idea that vagotomy decreases acetylcholine production in the oxyntic gland area which normally is maintained by tonic vagal stimulation. In dogs truncal or selective extragastric vagotomy also increases the maximal acid response of the Heidenhain pouch to stimulation by gastrin or feeding, possibly by decreasing the intestinal release of an inhibitor of gastrin-stimulated acid secretion.[50]

Antrectomy decreases basal and stimulated acid secretion in man. Broome and Olbe[51] performed sequential antrectomy and vagotomy in patients with duodenal ulcer disease. They found that antrectomy alone caused a 50 per cent decrease in maximal acid secretion, which could be accounted for only in part by resection of oxyntic gland mucosa and by losses of acid into the intestine. The decreased response to histamine could not be restored by exogenous administration of gastrin. An explanation for decreased acid secretion independent of the removal of gastrin is not apparent.

In dogs, antrectomy decreases the responses to cephalic stimulation, especially the response to sham feeding. As already discussed, these responses can be restored by administration of small doses of gastrin. Antrectomy increases the acid responses to gastrin by the innervated stomach in dogs and cats but not in man. The reason for this hypersensitivity to gastrin is not known.

Serum gastrin concentrations are decreased after vagotomy and antrectomy but not after vagotomy alone in man.[22] We have found after antrectomy in man that gastrin responses to feeding are not abolished when gastroduodenal anastomosis is performed but that feeding responses are greatly diminished or abolished when gastrojejunal anastomosis is done,[48] suggesting that duodenal gastrin may be released by feeding and may be quantitatively important. This observation may explain the higher recurrence rate with the Billroth I type resection than with Billroth II when vagotomy is not also performed.

ENDOGENOUS INHIBITORS OF ACID SECRETION

Several regulatory mechanisms have been demonstrated by which the acid secretory response to a meal may be modified. As already pointed out, acidification of the antrum inhibits gastrin release and thereby regulates the amount of gastrin released by cepahlic and gastric stimuli. For many years there has been speculation that a substance which inhibits acid secretion is released from the pyloric gland area in response to acidification. To date there is no convincing evidence that such a substance plays any physiologic role. The inhibition of secretion caused by antral acidification is probably due entirely to decreased release of gastrin. An inhibitor of gastric secretion, called gastrone, can be extracted from the mucous secretions of the stomach.[52] It is found in highest concentrations in patients with achlorhydria, and seems to be a large peptide or protein with chemical but not immunological similarity to the gamma globulins. It has not been established whether this material has any physiological role. Another inhibitory peptide, called urogastrone, has been found in the urine.

Ewald and Boas showed in 1886 that olive oil added to a test meal inhibited gastric emptying and decreased acid secretion. Subsequently it has been found that the presence of fat, acid, or hypertonic solutions in the duodenum releases humoral factors which inhibit gastric acid secretion. The term enterogastrone has been applied to a hormone released by fat, acid, or hypertonic solutions from the upper intestine which inhibits gastric acid secretion. This subject was reviewed recently.[53]

Two hormones known to be liberated from the small intestine by fat or acid are capable of causing inhibition of acid secretion. These are cholecystokinin (also known as pancreozymin) and secretin. Cholecystokinin (CCK) is liberated by fat, by some amino acids, and possibly by acid. Secretin is liberated by acid and possibly by fat. There has been considerable controversy about the role of each in the physiological inhibition of acid secretion.

Fat in the intestine inhibits acid secretion in man and in dogs but not in cats. In cats, cholecystokinin is a good stimulant of acid secretion and produces acid responses as great as those produced by gastrin or histamine. Therefore in the cat cholecystokinin administered exogenously or released by fat does not inhibit acid secretion. The structure of cholecystokinin has been determined by Jorpes and Mutt.[54] CCK, a peptide hormone composed of 33 amino acids, has the same C-terminal pentapeptide amide sequence as gastrin. Since this area of the molecule contains the active site for hormonal effects, it would be anticipated that CCK and gastrin might have common effects. This has been found to be the case, although there are differences in the magnitude of effects seen in different target organs and in different species. In man CCK is a strong stimulant of gallbladder contraction and pancreatic enzyme secretion but a very weak stimulant of acid secretion. When two hormones act on the same receptor site but one produces a maximal response that is less than the response to the other, the one with lesser response is said to be a partial agonist. In man and in the dog cholecystokinin is a partial agonist and competitive inhibitor of gastrin on acid secretion, but in the cat it is

a full agonist and does not inhibit. When a competitive inhibitor is administered, larger doses of full agonist (e.g., gastrin) are required to produce a half-maximal response (this dose is known as the D_{50}), but the maximal response which can be achieved with larger doses of stimulant is unchanged. Competitive kinetics have been shown for the inhibition of pentagastrin-stimulated acid secretion in the dog by cholecystokinin and by its C-terminal octapeptide, which has the same physiologic effects. In man, exogenous CCK inhibits only tiny doses of histamine, whereas fat in the intestine produces competitive kinetics, inhibiting all doses of histamine. Fat in the small intestine also inhibits pentagastrin-stimulated acid and pepsin secretion.[55] CCK inhibits acid but not pepsin secretion induced by pentagastrin in man. Fat in the intestine may release both CCK and another unidentified hormone which inhibits pepsin secretion and histamine-stimulated acid secretion.

The inhibitory effects of acid in the duodenum have been studied more extensively than the effects of fat. Many of these studies have been done in dogs. In man, Wormsley[56] found that duodenal acidification produced a transient decrease in pentagastrin-stimulated acid secretion followed by a tendency to a "rebound" increase. Johnston and Duthie[57] found evidence from cross-transfusion experiments in man that duodenal acidification inhibited histamine-stimulated acid secretion by a humoral mechanism.

Acidification of the duodenum in dogs produces decreased basal and gastrin-stimulated acid secretion from the innervated or denervated stomach. Secretin, the hormone which causes bicarbonate secretion by the pancreas, is an effective inhibitor of gastrin-stimulated acid secretion. The amino acid sequence of this 27 amino acid peptide was determined by Jorpes and Mutt.[54] It is released from the small intestine by acid. Duodenal acidification under conditions known to release secretin and to produce submaximal pancreatic bicarbonate secretion will also inhibit acid secretion, indicating a possible physiologic role of secretin. The question of whether secretin is the only enterogastrone released from the small intestine by acid has received much attention. The author's opinion is that it is at least one of the enterogastrones released by acid, but it may not be the only one. Andersson and colleagues[58] have localized the main site for acid inhibition in the dog to the duodenal bulb and feel that there may be a hormone other than secretin, which has been named bulbogastrone,[59] responsible for the inhibitory effect from this site. Histamine-stimulated secretion is not inhibited by acid in the duodenal bulb.

The effects of secretin in man differ from those in dogs or cats. In man secretin inhibits both pentagastrin and histamine-stimulated acid secretion, but it does not inhibit histamine-induced secretion in dogs or cats. Competitive kinetics were found for secretin-induced inhibition of pentagastrin-stimulated acid secretion in man.[60] In dogs the kinetics are noncompetitive. Secretin decreases basal acid secretion in man. Secretin may also decrease basal and stimulated serum gastrin concentrations. Intrajejunal acid releases secretin but does not inhibit basal acid secretion in man; it should be remembered that jejunal acidification may release both secretin and a stimulant of acid secretion.

Three other peptides which have structural similarities to secretin have been isolated from the upper intestine or pancreas: glucagon, gastric inhibitory peptide (GIP),[61] and vasoactive inhibitory peptide (VIP).[62] All three peptides are inhibitors of gastrin-stimulated gastric acid secretion. All three cause intestinal secretion of water and electrolytes. GIP also inhibits pepsin secretion and histamine-stimulated acid secretion. The factors regulating the release of GIP and VIP and their possible significance in the physiological inhibition of acid secretion have not been determined. The prostaglandins are long-chain, unsaturated fatty acids which occur widely in the body. One of the prostaglandins, E_1, inhibits both basal and stimulated acid secretion in man.[63] The physiological significance of this substance also remains to be determined.

It is possible that inadequate release of one or more of the enterogastrones may contribute to acid hypersecretion in patients with peptic ulcer disease, but no definite evidence for this hypothesis has been found.

PEPSIN SECRETION

Pepsins are the chief proteolytic enzymes found in human gastric juice. They are stored in an inactive form as pepsinogens in the peptic (chief) cells in the oxyntic gland area. In the presence of acid, pepsinogen with a molecular weight of 42,500 is converted autocatalytically to pepsin with a molecular weight of 35,000 by the cleavage of several small basic peptides. Pepsins are active at acid pH and are inactivated at neutral or slightly alkaline pH. There are two distinct pH optima for protein digestion in human gastric juice, one at pH 2 and one at pH 3.2.

It has been realized for some time that gastric pepsins could be subdivided into more than one type by chemical or immunological methods. The classification which will be used in this discussion is the one devised by Samloff.[4] By agar gel electrophoresis he separated eight distinct proteolytic fractions from human gastric mucosa. These could be divided into two immunologically unrelated groups: Group I (pepsinogens 1 to 5) and Group II (pepsinogens 6 and 7). The eighth proteolytic fraction was not inactivated by alkali and thus was not considered to be pepsin. Pepsinogens within each group are immunochemically similar. Pepsinogens in Group I are limited to oxyntic gland mucosa, whereas those in Group II are found in oxyntic, pyloric, and duodenal mucosa. Only Group I pepsinogens are found normally in the urine although both are found in the serum.

By immunofluorescent studies the Group I pepsinogens have been localized to the peptic and mucous neck cells in the oxyntic glands. Each of the seven electrophoretically distinct pepsinogens is converted by acidification to a distinct pepsin fraction. Group II pepsins are less resistant to heat, are more resistant to alkali, and have a higher pH optimum than the Group I pepsins. Group II pepsins do not hydrolyze the synthetic substrate N-acetyl-L-phenylalanyl-L-diiodotyrosine. This substrate is hydrolyzed by Group I pepsins and offers a chemical method for independent measurement of Group I activity. Since the two groups of pepsins are immunochemically distinct, it is likely that immunochemical methods for their independent measurement will be developed. In the past all measurement of pepsin activity has been based on determination of proteolytic activity at acid pH (see p. 545), and no distinction has been made between Group I which are localized to the oxyntic glands and Group II which are distributed more diffusely.

A genetic polymorphism has been reported for the pepsinogens in Group I.[64] Approximately 14 per cent of the white nonulcer-bearing population is deficient in pepsinogen 5, and this deficiency is inherited as a simple autosomal recessive trait. It has not been determined whether deficiency in this pepsinogen subtype is related to peptic ulcer disease.

Pepsinogen is secreted into the gastric lumen under basal conditions in man. Its secretion is increased in general by the same stimulants that increase acid secretion,[65] with the major exception that secretin inhibits acid secretion and stimulates pepsinogen secretion. It is not known whether the pepsinogen found in the blood is secreted by the peptic cells or is derived from degenerating cells. The general pattern of pepsinogen secretion after stimulation is an initial high rate of secretion caused by the release of pepsinogen from preformed granules, followed by a prolonged plateau of increased secretion at a lower level representing release of stored plus newly synthesized protein. The ratio of pepsin to acid secretion is thus higher during the initial phase of stimulation, because acid increases to a plateau without an initial high rate of secretion. In the remainder of this discussion the term pepsin secretion will be used interchangeably with pepsinogen secretion, because it is the pepsin derived from secreted pepsinogen which is assayed.

The strongest stimulants of pepsin secretion in man, as in other species, are the cholinergic stimulants. Cholinergic stimulants include the stimulants of vagal activity discussed in the section on cephalic stimulation of acid secretion, local cholinergic stimulation produced by gastric distention, and stable choline esters such as methacholine, bethanechol, and carbachol. Higher doses of insulin are required to produce maximal pepsin secretion than to produce maximal acid secretion in man.

Both histamine and gastrin (and gastrin-related peptides such as pentagastrin) stimulate pepsin secretion in man. The peak rates of pepsin secretion with histamine or gastrin are similar and range from two to four times basal secretion. On a molar basis gastrin is more potent than histamine, meaning that a lower dose is required to elicit maximal pepsin or acid secretion.

Secretin, which inhibits basal and gastrin stimulated acid secretion in man, is a strong stimulant of pepsin secretion whether administered exogenously by infusion or released endogenously by duodenal acidification.[66] The infusion of glucagon, which is a structurally related peptide, does not stimulate pepsin secretion, although it inhibits acid secretion. There is preliminary evidence that another related peptide, gastric inhibitory peptide, inhibits pepsin secretion.

The control of pepsin secretion has been studied extensively in dogs. The importance of cholinergic stimulation has been confirmed in numerous studies. It is difficult to compare gastrin and histamine stimulation in dogs unless full dose-response curves are done, because low doses of gastrin stimulate pepsin secretion but higher doses cause inhibition. Secretin is also a potent stimulant of pepsin secretion in dogs. Atropine is a potent inhibitor of vagal, pentagastrin, and histamine-stimulated pepsin secretion in man and dog.

The effects of vagotomy on pepsin secretion have been studied in man and dogs. In man vagotomy decreases basal pepsin output and abolishes the stimulation caused by insulin but not by meat extract.[67] This is similar to the effects of vagotomy on acid secretion and is consistent with the loss of direct vagal stimulation but not of gastrin-mediated stimulation. In dogs vagotomy abolishes pepsin responses to vagal stimulation but increases sensitivity to cholinergic drugs without changing the maximal response. As with acid secretion the dose-response curves to gastrin, pentagastrin, and histamine are shifted to the right and larger doses are therefore required to produce equivalent responses, but the maximal responses are not changed.

INTRINSIC FACTOR SECRETION

Intrinsic factor is a mucoprotein with a molecular weight of about 60,000 which interacts with vitamin B_{12} to form complexes which bind to specific receptors in the distal small intestine and facilitate intestinal absorption of B_{12}. Intrinsic factor deficiency was recognized by Castle as the cause of pernicious anemia. The biological activity of intrinsic factor, in the absence of intestinal malabsorption, can be measured by the absorption of radioisotopically labeled vitamin B_{12}. In vitro measurements are commonly carried out by radioimmunoassay methods. Intrinsic factor in the human gastric mucosa has been localized to the cytoplasm of the oxyntic cells by autoradiographic methods.[3]

In normal individuals, basal secretion of intrinsic factor greatly exceeds the amount required for normal vitamin B_{12} absorption. Stimulation of acid secretion by a number of agents results in a prompt increase in gastric intrinsic factor, followed by a decline to secretory rates that remain above baseline while acid secretion continues to increase. This pattern of secretion is similar to that found for pepsinogen. Vagal stimulation, cholinergic agents, histamine, and gastrin all have been shown capable of causing increased intrinsic factor secretion. The importance of stimulated intrinsic factor secretion is not known, because the basal secretion appears adequate for vitamin B_{12} absorption.

Other substances in the gastric juice will bind labeled vitamin B_{12} and are called nonspecific B_{12} binders. Binding of B_{12} to these substances is not blocked by antibodies to intrinsic factor. A nonparietal origin for these substances is suggested by the observation that betazole causes stimulation of intrinsic factor but not of nonspecific binders.

In general, secretion of acid and that of intrinsic factor are correlated, because both are secreted by the oxyntic cell. Patients with achlorhydria usually have low secretion of intrinsic factor. However, continued secretion of small amounts of intrinsic factor may be sufficient to prevent the development of pernicious anemia. Juvenile pernicious anemia is a condition in which there is normal acid production and specific deficiency of intrinsic factor secretion.[68] Circulating antibodies to parietal cells are found in the majority of patients with pernicious anemia and in many other patients with diffuse atrophic gastritis and achlorhydria or hypochlorhydria. The antral mucosa is usually not atrophic in patients with parietal cell antibodies, and serum gastrin concentrations are frequently markedly elevated, probably as a result of lack of normal inhibition of gastrin release by acid and possibly also because of hyperplasia of gastrin cells. Antibody directed against intrinsic factor is a more specific finding in pernicious anemia and is detected in the serum in about half the cases of this disease.

GASTRIC MUCUS SECRETION

The gastric mucosa is coated with a gelatinous material called gastric mucus which is composed of various macromolecules. These substances include proteins, glycoproteins, mucopolysaccharides, and the blood group substances. The glycoproteins are the principal constituents of gastric mucus. Mucus may exist in a gel form, dissolved in the gastric juice, or precipitated by acid as "visible mucus." The molecular composition of these three forms probably is the same.

The glycoproteins can be classified as acidic or neutral, based on the presence or absence of acidic sialic acid residues. Sulfated glycoproteins are found in saliva and esophageal secretions, but there is doubt that they are secreted by the gastric mucosa of adult man.[69] The principal glycoprotein of human gastric juice contains a carbohydrate component consisting of galactose, glucosamine, galactosamine, and fucose and a protein component composed chiefly of the amino acids serine, threonine, proline, and alanine.[70] Mucopolysaccharides with composition similar to that of chondroitin sulfate have been found in the gastric secretions and mucosa of dogs but only in negligible amounts in man.[71]

The glycoprotein macromolecules are long linear chains with numerous side-chains and charged end-groups and have a molecular weight of approximately 2×10^6.

The physical properties of mucus, such as viscosity and gel formation, result from noncovalent bonding between charged side-groups of adjacent chains. In the presence of high concentrations of hydrogen ions, binding between the chains is decreased and gel formation is impaired.

The mucoprotein substances in the gastric juice include the blood group substances A and B and another substance, H, which is the precursor of A and B substances. These substances are about 75 per cent carbohydrate and the remainder protein. About 78 per cent of individuals secrete these AB(H) substances into the gastric juice and are called "secretors." The relationships between secretor status and predilection for gastric cancer and peptic ulcer disease are discussed in other chapters.

Human gastric juice contains small amounts of normal serum proteins. Under certain conditions of mucosal injury the concentrations of serum proteins in the gastric juice may be greatly increased. Some examples are Menetrier's disease, gastric cancer, and topical application of agents which damage the gastric mucosal barrier.

The glycoproteins have been localized in man to the surface epithelium and mucous neck cells in the oxyntic gland area and to the cells of the pyloric glands. Under conditions of stimulation of mucus secretion this material is depleted from intracellular sites. When mucus secretion is stimulated by strong irritants the mucous cells are disrupted.

Studies of the physiological control of human mucus secretion have been hampered by the lack of specific uncomplicated methods for measuring mucus. Therefore studies done by different investigators have been performed with different methods and not unexpectedly have yielded conflicting results. The two major stimulants of mucus secretion which are reasonably well accepted are local mucosal irritation and cholinergic stimulation. Irritation by rubbing the mucosa, applying topical irritants, or local irrigation with HCl or strong solutions of NaCl causes outpouring of mucus. Cholinergic stimulation with cholinergic drugs or vagal stimulation is also effective. However, it has been easier to demonstrate

mucus secretion in response to vagal stimulation in dogs than in man. Infusions of gastrin or histamine either result in no stimulation or depress mucus secretion. Feeding appears to have no effect on mucus secretion. The control mechanisms for mucus secretion remain less well understood than for the other major gastric secretions.

The functions of mucus are also unclear. Because of its slimy nature it is assumed to have some lubricating function. The mucus barrier is not a complete physical barrier, and although it may offer some protection against surface injury by physical irritants it provides little impediment to the movement of water and electrolytes across the mucosal wall. The barrier to water and electrolyte movement is formed by the apical cell walls and intercellular tight junctions between the mucosal cells. Under basal conditions the buffering capacity of mucus is sufficient to provide some neutralization of acid, but under conditions of stimulated acid secretion this effect is probably negligible. Some components of mucus are inhibitors of pepsin activity, but they are not effective in the concentrations and pH ranges present in the normal stomach. The only strong pepsin inhibitors are sulfated, and those are absent from human stomach. At present more progress has been made in defining the chemical nature of mucus than in elucidating its functions and the factors responsible for its secretion.

REFERENCES

1. Ito, S. Anatomic structure of the gastric mucosa. In Handbook of Physiology, Vol. II, Sect. 6, C. F. Code (ed.). Washington, D.C., American Physiological Society, 1967, p. 705.
2. Lillibridge, C. B. The fine structure of normal human gastric mucosa. Gastroenterology 47:269, 1964.
3. Hoedmaeker, P. J., Abels, J., Wachters, J. J., Arends, A., and Nieweg, A. O. Investigations about the site of production of Castle's gastric intrinsic factor. Lab. Invest. 13:1394, 1964.
4. Samloff, I. M. Pepsinogens, pepsins, and pepsin inhibitors. Gastroenterology 60:586, 1971.
5. McGuigan, J. E. Gastric mucosal intracellular localization of gastrin by immuofluorescence. Gastroenterology 55:315, 1968.
6. Davenport, H. W., Warner, H. A., and Code, C. F.

Functional significance of gastric mucosal barrier to sodium. Gastroenterology 57:142, 1964.

7. Davenport, H. W. Salicylate damage to the gastric mucosal barrier. New Eng. J. Med. 276:1307, 1967.

8. Code, C. F., Higgens, J. A. Moll, J. C., Orvis, A. L., and Scholer, J. E. The influence of acid on the gastric absorption of water, sodium, and potassium. J. Physiol. (London) 166:110, 1963.

9. Andersson, S., and Grossman, M. I. Profile of pH, pressure and potential difference at gastroduodenal junction in man. Gastroenterology 49:364, 1965.

10. Durbin, R. P. Electrical potential difference of the gastric mucosa. In Handbook of Physiology, Vol. II, Sect. 6, C. F. Code (ed.). Washington, D. C., American Physiological Society, 1967, p. 879.

11. Davenport, H. W. Gastric secretion. In Physiology of the Digestive Tract. Chicago, Year Book Medical Publishers, 1966, p. 93.

12 Geall, M. G., Phillips, S. F., and Summerskill, W. H. J. Profile of gastric potential difference in man. Gastroenterology 58:437, 1970.

13. Crean, G. P., Marshall, M. W., and Rumsey, R. D. E. Parietal cell hyperplasia induced by the administration of pentagastrin (ICI 50, 123) to rats. Gastroenterology 57:147, 1969.

14. Johnson, L. R., Aures, D., and Yuen, L. Pentagastrin-induced stimulation of protein synthesis in the gastrointestinal tract. Amer. J. Physiol. 217:251, 1969.

15. Rune, S. J. Comparison of the rates of gastric acid secretion in man after ingestion of food and after maximal stimulation with histamine. Gut 7:344, 1966.

16. Makhlouf, G. M., McManus, J. P. A., and Card, W. I. A quantitative statement of the two-component hypothesis of gastric secretion. Gastroenterology 51:149, 1966.

17. Hunt, J. N., and Wan, B. Electrolytes of mammalian gastric juice. In Handbook of Physiology, Vol. II, Sect. 6, C. F. Code (ed.). Washington, D. C., American Physiological Society, 1967, p. 781.

18. Jacobson, E. D., Linford, R. H., and Grossman, M. I. Gastric secretion in relation to mucosal blood flow studied by a clearance technic. J. Clin. Invest. 45:1, 1966.

19. Rudick, J., Werther, J. L., and Chapman, M. L. Mucosal blood flow in canine antral and fundic pouches. Fed. Proc. 28:787, 1969.

20. Bynum, T. E., and Jacobson, E. D. Blood flow and gastrointestinal function. Gastroenterology 60:325, 1971.

21. Moore, J. G., and Englert, E. Circadian rhythm of gastric acid secretion in man. Nature 226:1261, 1970.

22. McGuigan, J. E., and Trudeau, W. L. Serum gastrin levels before and after vagotomy and pyloroplasty or vagotomy and antrectomy. New Eng. J. Med. 286:184, 1972.

23. Card, W. I., and Marks, I. N. The relationship between the acid output of the stomach following "maximal" histamine stimulation and the parietal cell mass. Clin. Sci. 19:147, 1960.

24. Payne, R. A., and Kay, A. W. The effect of vago-tomy on the maximal and secretory response to histamine in man. Clin. Sci. 22:373, 1962.

25. Edkins, J. S. The chemical mechanism of gastric secretion. J. Physiol. (London) 34:183, 1906.

26. Uvnäs, B. The part played by the pyloric region in the cephalic phase of gastric secretion. Acta Physiol. Scand. 4: Suppl. XIII, 1942.

27. Grossman, M. I. Neural and hormonal stimulation of gastric secretion of acid. In Handbook of Physiology, Vol. II, Sect. 6, C. F. Code (ed.) Washington, D.C., American Physiological Society, 1967, p. 835.

28. Johnson, L. R. Control of gastric secretion: No room for histamine? Gastroenterology 61:106, 1971.

29. Grossman, M. I. Integration of neural and hormonal control of gastric secretion. Physiologist 6:349, 1963.

30. Komarov, S. A. Gastrin. Proc. Soc. Exp. Biol. Med. 38:514, 1938.

31. Gregory, R. A., and Tracy, H. J. The constitution and properties of two gastrins extracted from hog antral mucosa. I. The isolation of two gastrins from hog antral mucosa. Gut 5:103, 1964.

32. Kenner, G. W., and Sheppard, R. C. Chemical studies of some mammalian gastrins. Proc. Roy. Soc. (Biol.) 170:89, 1968.

33. Morley, J. S., Tracy, H. J., and Gregory, R. A. Structure-function relationships in the active C-terminal tetrapeptide sequence of gastrin. Nature (London) 207:1356, 1965.

34. Yalow, R. S., and Berson, S. A. Size and charge distinctions between endogenous human plasma gastrin in peripheral blood and heptadecapeptide gastrins. Gastroenterology 58:609, 1970.

35. Nilsson, G., Yalow, R. S., and Berson, S. A. Distribution of gastrin in the gastrointestinal tract of human, dog, cat and hog. Nobel Symposium XVI: Frontiers in Gastrointestinal Hormone Research, Stockholm, July 20–21, 1970, in press.

36. Grossman, M. I. Physiological actions of gastrin. In Non-Insulin-Producing Tumors of the Pancreas, L. Demling and R. Ottenjann (eds.). Stuttgart, Georg Thieme Verlag, 1969, p. 1.

37. Laster, L., and Walsh, J. H. Enzymatic degradation of C-terminal tetrapeptide amide of gastrin by mammalian tissue extracts. Fed. Proc. 27:1328, 1968.

38. McGuigan, J. E. Immunochemical studies with synthetic human gastrin. Gastroenterology 54:1005, 1968.

39. Yalow, R. S., and Berson, S. A. Radioimmunoassay of gastrin. Gastroenterology 58:1, 1970.

40. Hansky, J., and Cain, M. D. Radioimmunoassay of gastrin in human serum. Lancet 2:1388, 1969.

41. Ganguli, P. C., and Hunter, W. M. Radio-immunoassay of gastrin in human plasma. J. Physiol. (London) 220:499, 1972.

42. Brooks, F. P. Central neural control of acid secretion. In Handbook of Physiology, Vol. II, Sect. 6, C. F. Code (ed.). Washington, D.C., American Physiological Society, 1967, p. 805.

43. Pevsner, L., and Grossman, M. I. The mechanism of vagal stimulation of gastric acid secretion. Gastroenterology 28:493, 1955.

44. Knutson, U., and Olbe, L. Significance of antrum in gastric acid response to sham feeding in duodenal ulcer patients. In Gastrointestinal Hormones and Other Subjects, E. H. Thaysen (ed.). Fifth Scandinavian Conference on Gastroenterology, Aalborg, Denmark, August 25–28, 1971. Copenhagen, Munksgaard, 1971, p. 25.

45. Grossman, M. I., Robertson, C. R., and Ivy, A. C. The proof of a hormonal mechanism for gastric secretion—the humoral transmission of the distention stimulus. Amer. J. Physiol. 153:1, 1948.

46. Elwin, C. E., and Uvnäs, B. Distribution and local release of gastrin. In Gastrin, M. I. Grossman (ed.). Los Angeles, University of California Press, 1966, p. 69.

47. Sircus, W. The intestinal phase of gastric secretion. Quart. J. Exp. Physiol. 38:91, 1953.

48. Stern, D. H., and Walsh, J. H. Release of duodenal gastrin in man. Clin. Res. 20:223, 1972.

49. Orloff, M. J., Abbott, A. G., and Rosen, H. Nature of the humoral agent responsible for portacaval shunt-related gastric hypersecretion in man. Amer. J. Surg. 120:237, 1970.

50. Andersson, S, and Grossman, M. I. Effect of vagal denervation of pouches on gastric secretion in dogs with intact or resected antrums. Gastroenterology 48:449, 1965.

51. Broome, A., and Olbe, L. Studies on the mechanism of the antrectomy-induced suppression of the maximal acid response to histamine in duodenal ulcer patients. Scand. J. Gastroenterol. 4:281, 1969.

52. Code, C. F. The recognition and assay of gastrone. In Gastric Secretion: Mechanism and Control, T. K. Shnitka, J. A. L. Gilbert, and R. C. Harrison (eds.). New York, Pergamon Press, 1965, p. 377.

53. Johnson, L. R., and Grossman, M. I. Intestinal hormones as inhibitors of gastric secretion. Gastroenterology 60:120, 1971.

54. Jorpes, J. E. Memorial Lecture: The isolation and chemistry of secretin and cholecystokinin. Gastroenterology 55:157, 1968.

55. Windsor, C. W. O., Cockel, R., and Lee, M. J. R. Inhibition of gastric secretion in man by intestinal fat infusion. Gut 10:135, 1969.

56. Wormsley, K. G. Response to duodenal acidification in man. II. Effects on the gastric secretory response to pentagastrin. Scand. J. Gastroenterol. 5:207, 1970.

57. Johnston, D., and Duthie, H. L. Inhibition of histamine-stimulated gastric secretion by acid in the duodenum in man. Gut 7:58, 1966.

58. Andersson, S., Nilsson, G., and Uvnäs, B. Effect of acid in proximal and distal duodenal pouches on gastric secretory responses to gastrin and histamine. Acta Physiol. Scand. 71:368, 1967.

59. Uvnäs, B. Role of duodenum in inhibition of gastric acid secretion. Scand. J. Gastroenterol. 6:113, 1971.

60. Berstad, A., and Petersen, H. Dose-response relationship of the effect of secretin on acid and pepsin secretion in man. Scand. J. Gastroenterol. 5:647, 1970.

61. Brown, J. C., and Dryburgh, J. R. A gastric inhibitory polypeptide II: The complete amino acid sequence. Canad. J. Biochem. 49:867, 1971.

62. Said, S. I., and Mutt, V. Polypeptide with broad biological activity: Isolation from small intestine. Science 169:1217, 1970.

63. Classen, M., Koch, H., Bickhardt, J., Topf, G., and Demling, L. The effect of prostaglandin E_1 on the pentagastrin-stimulated gastric secretion in man. Digestion 4:333, 1971.

64. Samloff, I. M., and Townes, P. L. Electrophoretic heterogeneity and relationships of pepsinogens in human urine, serum, and gastric mucosa. Gastroenterology 58:462, 1970.

65. Hirschowitz, B. I. Secretion of pepsinogen. In Handbook of Physiology, Vol. II, Sect. 6, C. F. Code (ed.). Washington, D.C., American Physiological Society, 1967, p. 889.

66. Brooks, A. M., Isenberg, J., and Grossman, M. I. The effect of secretin, glucagon, and duodenal acidification on pepsin secretion in man. Gastroenterology 57:159, 1969.

67. Tovey, F. I., Swaminathan, M., Parker, K., and Daniell, A. Effect of vagotomy on the gastric secretion of acid chloride and pepsin in response to antral stimulus and to insulin and maximal histamine stimulation. Gut 9:659, 1968.

68. Miller, D. R., Bloom, G. E., Streiff, R. R., LoBuglio, A. F., and Diamond, L. K. Juvenile "congenital" pernicious anemia. New Eng. J. Med. 275:978, 1966.

69. Lambert, R., Andre, C., and Berard, A. Origin of the sulfated glycoproteins in human gastric secretions. Digestion 4:234, 1971.

70. Schrager, J. The composition and some structural features of the principal gastric glycoprotein. Digestion 2:73, 1969.

71. Glass, G. B. J., Mori, H., and Pamer, T. Measurement of sulfated and non-sulfated glycoproteins in human gastric juice under fasting conditions and following stimulation with histamine, pentagastrin and insulin. Digestion 2:124, 1969.

Chapter 13

The Psychosomatic Theory of Peptic Ulcer

John S. Fordtran

DEFINITION, IMPLICATIONS, AND SIGNIFICANCE

There are three main suppositions to a general psychosomatic theory of the etiology of peptic ulcer: (A) Ulcer patients are exposed to long-standing psychic conflict, anxiety, and/or emotional tension. (B) This chronic emotional state predisposes to ulcer formation by stimulating acid-pepsin secretion or by reducing mucosal resistance. (Some have suggested that concomitant factors associated with emotional stress, such as fatigue, insomnia, long hours of work, and increased smoking, might actually be responsible for activating an ulcer rather than emotional tension per se.) Both A and B are present for long periods of time before the ulcer develops. (C) A precipitating event or situation occurs that accentuates A and B, and this is followed, usually in four to seven days, by the onset of an ulcer crater and ulcer symptoms.

The following points are made at this juncture in order to clarify the meaning and significance of the psychosomatic theory. First, the theory does not predict that everyone who has severe emotional tension of a type that affects gastric function will develop an ulcer. Such patients are predisposed to ulcer, but other factors, such as the level of mucosal resistance, the health, number, and reactivity of the parie-

tal cells, and the presence or absence of a precipitating event determine whether or not an ulcer will actually develop. Second, in the psychosomatic sense, stress means an event or situation which induces anxiety or depression. The death of a wife might not be stressful, whereas the death of a dog might be. Thus what is believed to be decisive in terms of ulcer pathogenesis is not the actual event or circumstance, but the way in which it is perceived and dealt with and the anxiety, fear, and irritation that are provoked. Third, the psychosomatic theory does not require that emotional tension be an important factor in all patients with ulcer. However, since the proof of its validity rests primarily upon the frequency of emotional tension in ulcer patients and control subjects, it would have to be a causative agent in many cases of ulcer in order for statistical methods to prove that it is correct. Fourth, according to the psychosomatic theory, the ulcer itself and the symptoms thereof have no primary or symbolic significance to the patient. This is in contrast to psychogenic diarrhea and vomiting, in which the symptoms supposedly have great psychological meaning. Fifth, if the psychosomatic theory is correct for a given group of patients, and if emotional tension predisposes to and precipitates an ulcer via vagal pathways, this implies that "vagal tone" is increased in this group of ulcer patients

163

and that vagotomy should cure the ulcer, but that cure of the ulcer should not influence the psychic disorder.

The following discussion is divided, somewhat arbitrarily, into five sections. The first deals with a general psychiatric description of ulcer patients. For the most part, this description is based on uncontrolled analysis of relatively few patients studied in great detail. The second and third sections describe studies which in one way or another are judged to stand as evidence for or against one of the three suppositions of the psychosomatic theory. The fourth section deals with some miscellaneous observations, and the fifth with the present writer's conclusions. Some overlap within the first four sections was unavoidable.

PSYCHIATRIC DESCRIPTION OF ULCER PATIENTS

Although many previous workers had suspected a causal relationship between emotion and peptic ulcer, the psychoanalytic studies reported by Alexander in 1934 constitute the beginning of a specific psychosomatic theory[1] as just outlined. Alexander and his coworkers analyzed a small number of ulcer patients in great detail, and contrary to popular opinion (then and now), they found no personality type or characteristic common to ulcer patients. Rather, ulcer patients were reported to have a typical "conflict situation," which developed in patients with many different personalities. The basic abnormality in ulcer patients was thought to be a marked *dependency*, and the wish to remain in the dependent infantile situation, to be loved and cared for, was supposedly in conflict with the adult ego's pride and aspiration for independence and accomplishment. Depending upon whether or not the patient gives in to his unconscious cravings for dependency, or overcompensates in his rejection of these cravings, he may outwardly appear as overtly dependent, demanding, and disgruntled, or efficient, productive, aggressive, ambitious, and willing to have others depend on him. In either case, it is the conflict resulting from the persistence of severe dependence that was considered basic to the character of peptic ulcer patients.

When dependency desires cannot find gratification in human relationships, Alexander proposed that a chronic emotional stimulus is created which results in acid secretion, increased gastric motility, and increased gastric mucosal blood flow. In psychosomatic terms, if the wish to receive, to be loved, and to depend on others is not gratified, then a regressive outlet for the dependency must be used. The wish to be loved is converted to the wish to be fed, and the stomach responds as if food were taken in or were about to be taken in. Onset of the illness occurs when the intensity of the patient's unsatisfied dependent cravings increases, either because of external deprivation or because the patient defends against his cravings by assuming increased responsibilities. The external deprivation often consists of the loss of a person upon whom the patient has been dependent, leaving home, or losing money or a position that had given the patient a sense of security. The increased responsibility may take the form of marriage, birth of a child, or assumption of a more responsible job or task.

For a number of years it appeared that a psychic conflict related to a dependency conflict was an almost universal finding in peptic ulcer patients — duodenal or gastric, male or female. The studies of Mittelmann and Wolff,[2] Kapp et al.,[3] Weisman,[4] and many others supported this view, with but minor modifications. Although all these studies were based on the study of relatively few patients, Stine and Ivy collected and reviewed over 300 cases that had been studied by psychoanalysts and psychiatrists, and found a virtually unanimous opinion that all patients had a serious conflict related to oral dependency.[5]

Critics failed to accept this notion for two related reasons. First, dependency traits of some degree can be found in practically all people, and, depending upon the psychiatrist's prejudice, can be emphasized or de-emphasized in a given individual. Second, there were virtually no control studies, and especially no control studies in which the analyst or psychiatrist did not know in advance which patients had ulcer.

In 1951, Alexander and his coworkers embarked on a momentous experiment to evaluate the frequency of oral dependent conflict in ulcer patients by a method that would hopefully avoid bias and prejudice.[6] Transcripts of interviews with patients with seven supposedly psychosomatic diseases (duodenal ulcer, asthma, rheumatoid arthritis, ulcerative colitis, essential hypertension, neurodermatitis, and thyrotoxicosis), each of whom was thought to have a characteristic psychic conflict or state, were carefully edited to remove clues and cues which might suggest the medical diagnosis. These edited records were then submitted to a panel of psychoanalysts and to a panel of internists. The latter were to serve as a control for clues that were inadvertently left in the record. With regard to the diagnosis of duodenal ulcer, the internists did as well as the analysts, so that, critically interpreted, this experiment does not support the hypothesis that ulcer patients have a specific conflict related to oral dependency. The authors felt, however, that the internists used clues that had been inadvertently left in the records, whereas the analysts used psychological data and disregarded the clues. Even if this is correct, the analysts were able to correctly diagnose only 34 per cent of the ulcer patients overall and 57 per cent of the male patients with ulcer. As already noted, the internists did just as well—31 per cent of the patients overall, and 56 per cent of the male patients. (Incidentally, the analysts did worse on duodenal ulcer than with the other diseases. For instance, the analysts were correct in 69 and 55 per cent of the patients with rheumatoid arthritis and ulcerative colitis, respectively, whereas the internists correctly diagnosed only 13 and 29 per cent of these patients correctly.)

Although these results cast grave doubt on the specificity of oral-dependent cravings in ulcer patients, they in no way invalidate the general psychosomatic concept. Even long before this study was published, some workers, notably Mahl,[7] had argued for an "anxiety" hypothesis, in which the underlying cause of anxiety (whether subconscious psychic conflict or conscious stress) was irrelevant.

It has been emphasized repeatedly that there is no characteristic ulcer personality. Even those who felt that the underlying conflict was specific made the point that the external personality façade varied greatly. Kapp and coworkers,[3] for instance, were able to divide their ulcer patients into three distinct groups:

Group A: These patients were outwardly independent, hard driving, and successful.

Group B: This group openly expressed dependent longings and were dependent on a mother or a mother substitute. The patients were fairly successful, but were outwardly meek, shy, and often effeminate.

Group C: Patients in this group represented a severe character disorder. Most were alcoholic, and many exhibited psychopathic traits such as gambling, delinquency, and inability to make a living. They had little or no guilt or socially acceptable defenses against selfish demanding impulses, and were openly parasitic on friends, spouses, and society.

It is not known what percentage of the overall ulcer population would fit into each of the aforementioned three groups. A given physician might see a gross preponderance of patients in any one of the three groups, depending upon the type of practice he has. A doctor who treats wealthy executives will have mainly type A patients; a doctor in a county or veterans hospital will have a quite different experience.

Most psychiatric and analytical studies in peptic ulcer have been in men, but Kezur et al. studied 25 women, four with gastric and 21 with duodenal ulcer.[8] In every patient there was evidence of a profound personality disturbance. Their personality façades varied from overt weakness and passivity to domination and aggressiveness. None of these women had a satisfactory sexual adjustment. Ulcer tended to develop when the patient was rejected by a meaningful person, nearly always the husband or father. In general these women adjusted poorly to their environment.

EVIDENCE SUPPORTING THE VALIDITY OF THE PSYCHOSOMATIC THEORY

SUPPOSITION A

This supposition states that ulcer patients have been exposed to long-standing psychic conflict, anxiety and/or emotional tension prior to the development of ulcer. Davies and Wilson found that their ulcer patients had much more pronounced emotional instability than did the inguinal hernia patients who served as a control group.[9] For instance, compulsive activity related to work was present in 58 of 100 ulcer patients and only 14 of 100 hernia patients. The results were apparently not analyzed "blind," and the data do not prove whether these emotional symptoms were the cause or the effect of the ulcer.

Hamilton studied 50 male patients in each of four groups: duodenal ulcer, gastric ulcer, nonulcer dyspeptics, and a control group having another chronic illness. Statistically significant differences among the groups were found with regard to the frequency of the presence of an anxiety state. In order of frequency: nonulcer dyspeptics > duodenal ulcer > gastric ulcer > control group.[10]

Højer-Pedersen studied 51 duodenal ulcer patients and 51 age-matched control subjects by means of a detailed questionnaire and by personal interview.[11] The dependent-independent type of character deviation was present in all 51 of the ulcer patients and in only 16 of the control subjects ($P < 0.001$). The frequency, intensity, extent, and duration of "conflict situations" in ulcer patients greatly surpassed similar findings in the control series. (P values for familial, educational, and occupational conflict situations were < 0.02, < 0.001, and < 0.001, respectively.) There was an abnormal parent-fixation in almost all ulcer patients, but in the control group about two-thirds also had abnormal parent-fixation. More than 30 other comparisons were made, and, in many, statistically significant differences in the ulcer and control groups were noted. The abnormal personality features noted in ulcer patients were judged to have been present since early life, and apparently remained unchanged with the onset of ulcer. The results were not analyzed blind.

Psychological tests and personal interviews were used by Eberhard to assess the personalities of 30 pairs of monozygous twins, at least one twin of whom had ulcer.[12] The tests were apparently interpreted without knowledge of which twin had ulcer. Although the author knew which twin had ulcer when he interviewed them, a second examiner, who did not, made a separate analysis of personality and stress factors from material submitted to him by the author. (It is doubtful if such records can be made free of clues or cues that give away, at least to some extent, which patient has ulcer. For example, see reference 6.) The results showed that the ulcer twins, or the twin with earlier onset of ulcer if both twins had ulcer, had a statistically significant higher sensitivity to stress and impaired defense mechanisms compared with the nonulcer twins or the twin with later onset of ulcer if both twins had ulcer. Nervous complaints were much more frequent in the ulcer than in the nonulcer group; this was due to increased sensitivity to stress, rather than to a greater amount of actual stress; i.e., actual stress was judged to be equal in the ulcer and nonulcer twins.

Many Rorschach and similar tests have been reported in ulcer patients. Poser[13] states that advantages of the Rorschach method are as follows: it is sensitive to a wide variety of personality factors which can be quantitatively expressed, it does not markedly distort the patient's usual reaction pattern, and it appears to the patient as a test of his imagination and he thus approaches it informally and unguardedly. Such studies have, in general, revealed abnormalities in ulcer patients compared with what is considered normal. However, in many instances control subjects were not studied, and in no instance were the results interpreted blind (except in one study in which there were only about 13 each in the patient and control groups, and statistics could not be applied).[14]

In a classic study, because it was prospective, Weiner et al.[15] and Mirsky[16] evaluated the entire psychosomatic concept. From a group of about 2000 draftees on whom serum pepsinogen levels had been determined, a group of hypersecretors and a group of hyposecretors (120 men in all) were selected for further study. A battery of psychological tests and an upper gastrointestinal X-ray series were done in each subject. The men were then sent to basic training camp. Subsequently, all but 13 of the men were again given the psychological tests and X-ray examination between the eighth and sixteenth weeks of basic training.

On the basis of the psychological tests alone, an attempt was made to pick out the men with high serum pepsinogen levels. In analyzing the psychological data, the authors looked especially for evidence of dependency, frustration, unexpressed anger, and hostility. They also tried to select the *hypo*secretors on the basis of psychological traits supposedly characteristic of hyposecretors—pseudomasculine defenses, paranoid trends, and so forth. To a degree, Weiner, Mirsky, and their colleagues were successful, in that a battery of 20 psychological tests separated the two groups to a statistically significant degree. However, no psychological test separated the two groups with a greater accuracy than 64 per cent (50 per cent separation would be expected by chance alone). Theoretically, what separation they did achieve could be the result of their accurate selection of some of the hyposecretors as well as some of the hypersecretors, so that this aspect of their study does not lend strong support to supposition A of the psychosomatic theory. The study would have been of much greater value, for present purposes at least, had they included a group of men with normal rates of gastric secretion.

A second aspect of the Weiner-Mirsky study was to see if it was possible to predict, on the basis of psychological tests, which men would develop ulcer under the stress of basic training camp. Looking for evidence of very intense dependency needs and anxiety, ten of the 120 men were selected as most likely to develop a duodenal ulcer. The X-ray studies revealed that seven of these ten subjects either had a duodenal ulcer on the first X-ray (two men) or developed one during basic training (five men). Of the three who did not develop a duodenal ulcer, two were hypersecretors and one was a hyposecretor Two other patients out of the total 120 men also developed a duodenal ulcer, and both were hypersecretors.

Thus nine of the 120 men who were studied had or developed a duodenal ulcer, and all were in the hypersecretor group. Seven of the nine men who developed a duodenal ulcer were in the top 8 per cent judged most likely to get an ulcer on the basis of psychological criteria. One of the men in the top 8 per cent of psychological data suggestive of ulcer was a hyposecretor, and he did not develop an ulcer.

The accuracy with which Weiner et al. were able, on the basis of psychological tests alone, to predict those patients most likely to develop an ulcer is statistically highly significant and most impressive. The interpretation of this aspect of their study is not marred greatly by their omission of a group of normal secretors, because they were able to pick out those most prone to ulcer even among a group containing a large number of hypersecretors. However, interpretation is limited by the fact that the authors gave no details of the clinical or X-ray manifestations of their patients with ulcer. It is implied but not specifically stated that the X-rays were interpreted blind. Whether or not the patients with X-ray evidence of duodenal ulcer had pain of an ulcer-like nature is not specified, and follow-up data on these patients were not described.

This study, taken at face value, lends strong support to certain aspects of the psychosomatic theory of ulcer pathogenesis in young men. It also suggests that hypersecretion may be, at least to some extent, independent of psychic conflict, and that psychic conflict, even if severe, will not cause an ulcer in a "hyposecretor." These studies are not immediately applicable to the etiology of ulcer in subjects who are not hypersecretors or to women or older patients with ulcer, and they have not been confirmed.

Rutter, in a prospective study, attempted to see to what extent psychosocial variables relate to the short-term outcome of duodenal and gastric ulcer.[17] It was found that psychiatric disability, mainly anxiety and depression, at the onset of the illness episode (by history taken in retrospect) correlated ($P < 0.05$) with a poor outcome six months later. Also, if anxiety or depression was present at the initial interview Rutter had with the patient, pain was much more likely to still be present six months later, as assessed by a separate physician ($P < 0.001$). Rutter concludes that, regardless of whether or not psychiatric and social factors cause peptic ulcer, anxiety and depression are very significant factors in precipitating complications and leading to intractability. Even mild symptoms of anxiety and depression were significant in predicting a poor outcome.

Although privation, fatigue, and mental anxiety have long been thought to coincide with the presence of gastric as well as duodenal ulcer, controlled studies devoted specifically to gastric ulcer are rare. Alp and colleagues recently studied the personality patterns and emotional state of 181 gastric ulcer patients by means of questionnaires, comparing the results with an age-matched control group.[18] The gastric ulcer group had a statistically significant higher incidence of domestic and financial stress and greater intake of aspirin, alcohol, and cigarettes than did the control group. By means of a neuroticism scale questionnaire, they concluded that a higher percentage of gastric ulcer patients are "tough minded," a trait believed to develop from early experience, and "submissive," a trait believed to be inherited. It was concluded that it is not possible to be certain whether these traits are the cause of or are caused by the gastric ulcer, and unfortunately no studies exist on subjects prior to development of a gastric ulcer. However, the "submissive" factor was very prominent, and this trait is so strongly genetic that the authors believe this trait, at least, must have preceded the gastric ulcer. Although controlled, the results of this study were apparently not analyzed blind.

SUPPOSITION B

This supposition states that a chronic emotional state predisposes to ulcer formation by stimulating acid-pepsin secretion or by reducing mucosal resistance in some way. Since there is no way to measure mucosal resistance, the supposition would not be disproved even if emotional tension were shown to have no effect on acid-pepsin secretion. If, on the other hand, anxiety and psychic tension could be shown to increase acid-pepsin secretion, supposition B would receive support.

Beaumont[19] and Wolf and Wolff[20] showed that *conscious* emotions can affect gastric secretion, motility, and mucosal blood flow in gastrostomy patients. (Although secretion, motility, and blood flow are often said to increase or decrease hand in hand, many workers have noted, and Margolin[21] stressed the fact, that these functions may vary independently of each other in response to various emotions.) Anxiety and aggressive feelings usually increased gastric activity, whereas fear and depressive states generally had the opposite effect. Margolin[21] studied the effects of *unconscious* emotion on the gastric function of a woman with a gastrostomy. On one occasion, intense unconscious oral cravings, in which the analyst was simply consumed cannibalistically, were associated with profuse gastric secretion. These workers noted that either increased or decreased secretion could occur with conscious emotions of anger, guilt, or anxiety, and state that the unconscious mental content determines the psychophysiological response.

Margolin claims to have been able, in all attempts, to accurately predict the response of the stomach from psychoanalytical data, and that this result was far beyond the statistical probability of chance. No data were given.

Højer-Pedersen[11] has discussed the difficulty inherent in the use of gastrostomy patients because of the intense meaning the gastrostomy has to the patient. In the patient reported by Margolin, the gastrostomy had become sexualized in the patient's mind. These unconscious attitudes and their interpretation led to marked changes in gastric function. Therefore, although the study of gastrostomy patients stimulated much interest in the psychosomatic theory of ulcer disease, particularly supposition B, results in these patients do not necessarily apply to patients who do not have gastrostomies.

Mittelmann and Wolff[2] analyzed the effects of various emotions on gastric secretion and motility in ulcer patients and in controls, using nasogastric intubation techniques. In the ulcer patients and in the control subjects, anxiety, frustration, resentment, and guilt were all associated with increased gastric acidity and motility. In general, the absolute changes in gastric secretion rate during emotional stress were modest, e.g., an increase from about 2 to 4 mEq per hour, and were caused mainly by an increase in acid concentration with little change in volume. For some reason, the volume of gastric secretion was not recorded in any of the charts of the duodenal ulcer patients.

Although some workers had suggested that *repressed* emotional tension was particularly likely to stimulate acid secretion, Szasz et al. reported a patient in whom *open* hostility appeared to enhance gastric secretion.[22] These workers also made the important observation that psychic tension stimulated acid secretion before but not after a vagotomy. This suggests that emotional tension stimulates acid secretion via the vagus nerve, and not by some other neuroendocrine mechanism. Apparently, this case study is the only experiment in which the effect of emotion on gastric secretion has been studied before and after vagotomy. Unfortunately, interpretation was complicated by the injection of enterogastrone during the experiment, and this second variable makes it difficult to be completely sure of the effect of the emotional tension.

Mirsky[16] reported one patient in whom gastric secretion was measured serially by means of urinary pepsinogen levels. Urinary pepsinogen increased impressively when the dependent relationship the patient had established with his wife was threatened. The patient did not develop an ulcer, but this case study suggests that emotional tension of a type seen commonly in ulcer patients may enhance gastric secretion.

Mahl measured gastric acidity in eight students in a control period and again on the morning of a difficult examination.[7] The sequence of testing (control versus examination day) was varied. During the control experiments the students were interviewed about their hobbies and other nonemotional topics. On the day of the examination they were interviewed about the significance of the examination and what it would mean if they failed it. An approximate measure of the anxiety level was made and recorded prior to the titration of the gastric juice, which was collected for 20 minutes. Six subjects were judged to have a high level of anxiety, and five of these showed a convincing rise in the hydrogen ion concentration of gastric juice (average increase of about 25 mEq per liter HCl). In two subjects who had no anxiety about the examination, gastric acidity did not increase. Unfortunately, only acid concentration, and not volume or total acid secretion, was reported in this study.

Crawshaw et al. showed that, after a latent period of 10 to 20 minutes, a definite increase in gastric acid secretion occurred when normal medical students thought about, saw or smelled an appetizing meal.[23] Teasing with food caused acid secretion to increase from less than 1 to about 3.5 mEq per hour. The latter value averaged about 11 per cent of the maximal response to pentagastrin, but one subject secreted at 30 per cent of his maximal rate in response to psychic stimulation by food. These results confirm in man what was previously well known from animal experiments; that is, psychic stimulation with food increases gastric acid secretion.

SUPPOSITION C

With regard to the event that supposedly precipitates an ulcer crater, Davies and Wilson found that 84 per cent of 205 ulcer patients (gastric and duodenal) gave a history of some stressful situation prior to the onset of dyspepsia.[9] The event usually occurred five or six days before the onset of ulcer symptoms. For a control group, they analyzed 100 patients with inguinal hernia. Only 22 per cent of this group had experienced a stressful situation prior to the symptoms produced by the hernia. In the ulcer group, the most common events were related to (1) a change in work—most common in patients under 25 years of age; (2) financial difficulties—most frequent in patients over 25 years of age; and (3) illness or misfortune in a member of the family. Sexual problems were conspicuous by their relative absence, and were present only when they were related to income and expenditure. Davies and Wilson stressed that these events were real, and not imaginary problems, and that they were largely concerned with responsibility, security, and independence. It is interesting that this study was reported in 1937, and stands as the only controlled study of the frequency with which an event precedes the onset of ulcer symptoms. Unfortunately, the study is not really conclusive, because Davies and Wilson knew which patients had ulcer and which had hernia prior to their assessment of whether or not an event preceded the onset of symptoms. Further, the patients themselves may have been prejudiced, because most lay people "know" that ulcer is brought about by emotional tension and "know" that hernia symptoms are not.

Several other workers, who did not analyze a control group, agree that severe emotional stress occurred shortly before or at the time of the onset of ulcer symptoms in about 85 per cent of the cases.[11, 24]

Mittelmann and Wolff[2] analyzed psychological and clinical data independently in a group of ulcer patients and then constructed life charts for each patient. Thus, although this is not a controlled study, it has perhaps more significance than if psychological and clinical data were obtained simultaneously. In each of their 30 patients it was possible to demonstrate a close association between the onset, recurrence, and course of ulcer symptoms and the occurrence of untoward emotional reactions. Situations that engendered sustained anxiety and conflict, feelings of being caught, resentment, guilt, self-denunciation, and helplessness were prominent inciting events. More sexual problems were present than in the series reported by Davies and Wilson. Further details of the type of event associated with the onset or with recurrences of ulcer are found in the papers by Mirsky,[16] Højer-Pedersen,[11] Myers,[24] and Weisman.[4]

The frequency of admissions to London hospitals for perforated ulcer increased from about 22 to about 35 cases per month during the air raid blitz in 1940 and 1941.[25] This was a statistically significant change, and suggests that severe stress may increase this complication of peptic ulcer, although environmental changes other than psychic stress obviously must have occurred during the blitz.

If one accepts the contention that precipitating events of an emotional nature are more frequently associated with recurrent ulcer disease than with recurrences of other diseases, it is obvious that in most cases there is nothing specific about these events; such problems are common to all people, whereas only a few of these develop a duodenal ulcer. Furthermore, patients destined to someday develop an ulcer have presumably undergone many such events without ulcer development in the past. The only inference that can be made is that the specific meaning of the event to the particular individual at a particular time determines whether or not the response is noxious. If the ulcer begins for the first time at age 60, the psychosomatic theory simply states that the event preceding the symptoms was outstanding, either in fact or as interpreted by the patient.

EVIDENCE AGAINST THE PSYCHOSOMATIC THEORY

The author is aware of no evidence that tends to disprove the psychosomatic theory as defined herein. Many critics have pointed out that various aspects of the theory, at least at the time of their writing, were unproved, but none of these critics presented negative evidence.

Several negative findings do need to be mentioned. Hamilton found that there was no correlation of ulcer disease with number of siblings, the patient's position in the family, the father's social group, marriage, and so forth.[10] Kellock compared 250 male duodenal ulcer patients with a similar number of control patients with other diseases.[26] There was no difference in the frequency of death, separation from or remarriage of one or both of the parents, place among siblings, number of siblings, and the like. Kessel and Munro reviewed these and other epidemiological studies and concluded that the evidence for an association with ulcer is inconclusive.[27] These studies show that actual stress as measured by these parameters is not increased in peptic ulcer patients. They do not rule out increased stress in the psychosomatic sense of the term or increased sensitivity to stress.

Roth has emphasized that there is no characteristic ulcer personality, as well as the limited and inadequate data upon which the oral-dependency conflict was based.[28] As already noted, the subsequent controlled study of Alexander et al. have showed that this specific conflict is present in at most one-third of ulcer patients.[6]

MISCELLANEOUS OBSERVATIONS

Few studies have correlated psychic tension and gastric secretory levels in groups of ulcer patients, most workers assuming their patients to be hypersecretors because they had duodenal ulcer. However, a significant number of duodenal ulcer patients are not hypersecretors, and some secrete amounts of acid well below the mean level for normal subjects. One wonders whether these relative hyposecretors with duodenal ulcer have the same level of psychic conflict and emotional tension that hypersecretors with duodenal ulcer supposedly have. Gundry and coworkers studied 25 male patients with proved duodenal ulcer and correlated psychic factors and acid secretion.[29] Unfortunately for present purposes, only one of their patients had a peak acid output of less than 20 mEq per hour (this patient had a peak output of about 15 mEq per hour) and could thus be classed as a relative hyposecretor. This patient had severe stress and severe marital conflict. Overall, these investigators found no correlation between emotional features and basal acid output, peak acid output (histamine), or the ratio of these values. All their patients regularly described unrepressed, intense emotion, which they periodically struggled to master.

If the psychosomatic theory is correct, and the ulcer is only an expression of psychic conflict and emotional tension, the conflict and tension would be expected to continue or perhaps even become worse after cure of the ulcer, for instance, by vagotomy. Szasz showed this to be true in a small and *selected* group of patients.[30, 31] Drug addiction, severe depression, memory impairment, anxiety attacks, hypersalivation, and phobias were some of the sequelae of ulcer cure after vagotomy. Others have shown that a high level of anxiety, deviant personality traits and disturbances of mood in ulcer patients portends a bad result from surgical treatment, even if the latter cures the ulcer disease.[32]

If psychic tension is important in the etiology of ulcer development, it would be interesting to know the personality structure of schizophrenic patients who have an ulcer. Generally speaking, the schizophrenic patient's personality is disorganized, and he deals with environmental problems by withdrawing from reality. Katz studied 30 patients with schizophrenia who developed an active peptic ulcer while institutionalized in veterans hospitals.[33] For comparison he studied a control group of schizophrenic patients who had no evidence of ulcer disease. The groups were well matched for age, education, and psychiatric diagnosis. The basic personality of each group was schizophrenic, and no "ulcer personality" was discernible. However, statistically significant different defense mechanisms were shown to be present. The nonulcer schizophrenic patients denied the external world, denied reality, and obeyed their emotional impulses. Thus they had no conflict. The ulcer schizophrenic patients, on the other hand, were more aware of the environment and reality. Reality thus broke through the schizophrenic's defense system; this led to a conflict of either dealing with environmental problems or regressing further into psychotic estrangement. The evidence suggested that the ulcer patients elected to deal with their environmental problems at the expense of visceral dysfunction, which eventuated in ulcer disease. From a psychiatric standpoint, the appearance of the ulcer was apparently a good prognostic sign.

Restrained monkeys which had learned to prevent an electric shock by pressing a lever at the correct time often developed ulcerations and erosions of the duodenum. By contrast, monkeys with a dummy lever, which would not prevent shock, lost interest in the lever, and did not develop gastrointestinal ulcerations, even though they received as many electric shocks as the experimental monkeys.[34] These studies became famous, mainly because the experimental monkey was referred to as the "executive monkey," based upon the unproved assumption that business executives are especially prone to develop ulcer.[35] It is not clear what relevance these or other methods of producing ulceration in animals have to chronic peptic ulcer in humans, because many such ulcerations are of the acute stress type, rather than chronic ulcers.

CONCLUSIONS

Supposition A. To prove supposition A it would be necessary to show that long-standing emotional tension is significantly more common in ulcer patients than in controls, and that this preceded rather than followed the ulcer. The evidence at hand strongly favors the validity of supposition A for duodenal ulcer, although this writer does not accept this as proved because (1) most of the controlled studies were not analyzed blind, (2) adequate follow-up data and X-ray data on the ulcer patients in the Weiner-Mirsky study were not provided, and (3) there has been no confirmation of the Weiner-Mirsky type prospective study. Very few controlled studies have been carried out in patients with gastric ulcer, but the data that are available support supposition A.

Supposition B. To prove supposition B it would be necessary to show that chronic emotional tension of a type which occurs frequently in ulcer patients leads to some derangement in gastric physiology that predisposes to ulcer formation. Uncontrolled studies suggested that certain emotional states, such as anxiety, were associated with increased secretion, whereas other emotional states, such as depression, were associated with decreased secretion. This is a classic set-up for self-deception. Given a little bias, some spontaneous variation in the rate of acid secretion, and considering the fact that anxiety and depression are very difficult to separate and define, one could get any result he wanted, unless the results are controlled, recorded blind and analyzed statistically. These criteria have almost never been met. The best study is that of Mahl,[7] who showed that anxiety over an examination enhanced gastric acidity. The data on motility are even less convincing than those on acid secretion, and the data on mucosal blood flow are limited to the study of gastrostomy patients. No study has shown that emotional tension produces more gastric activity in ulcer than in nonulcer patients, but supposition B does not state that this should necessarily be the case.

Supposition B should be regarded as inadequately studied but probably correct.

It should be noted again that it would be virtually impossible to *disprove* supposition B, because anxiety might predispose to ulcer by decreasing mucosal resistance, and there is, at present, no way to directly measure mucosal resistance.

Supposition C. To prove supposition C it would be necessary to show that the onset of ulcer development is more frequently preceded by a precipitating emotional event than the onset of other illnesses and that precipitating events (in the psychosomatic sense) are more common prior to ulcer development than at other times in a patient's life. These are very difficult things to prove. At least two major pieces of evidence are missing, one possible and the other probably impossible to obtain. With regard to the possible, we need to know the incidence with which severe emotional tension precedes ulcer development when the observer does not know whether or not the patient has an ulcer or is a control patient. With regard to the impossible, we need a comparable control group. The public "knows" that ulcer is caused by anxiety, and it "knows" that hernia symptoms are not. This could easily color the association between anxiety and symptoms as percieved by the patients, even if observer bias were carefully avoided by blind analysis of the data. An adequate control group for the testing of supposition C is seemingly nonexistent.

Other Conclusions. There is nothing specific about the stress that supposedly predisposes to ulcer, although the evidence at hand favors a role of anxiety in determining the course and prognosis of peptic ulcer as well as in its etiology.

It is likely that there are multiple etiological factors in peptic ulcer, and even if the psychosomatic theory were accepted as proved, this still would not tell us how important it is, quantitatively, in relation to other factors. To use tuberculosis to illustrate this point, we would not know whether anxiety played the role of the acid-fast bacillus or was analogous to a poor socioeconomic background. Obviously, psychosomatic factors might be much more important in the genesis of ulcer in some patients than in others. It is likely that further knowledge will come mainly from prospective studies.

REFERENCES

1. Alexander, F. Psychosomatic Medicine. New York, W. W. Norton & Co., 1950.
2. Mittelmann, B., and Wolff, H. G. Emotions and gastroduodenal function. Experimental studies on patients with gastritis, duodenitis and peptic ulcer. Psychosomatic Med. 4:5, 1942.
3. Kapp, F. T., Rosenbaum, M., and Romano, J. Psychological factors in men with peptic ulcers. Amer. J. Psychiatry 103:700, 1947.
4. Weisman, A. D. A study of the psychodynamics of duodenal ulcer exacerbations: With special reference to treatment and the problem of specificity. Psychosomatic Med. 18:2, 1956.
5. Stine, L. A., and Ivy, A. C. The effect of psychoanalysis on the course of peptic ulcer: A preliminary report. Gastroenterology 21:185, 1952.
6. Alexander, F., French, T. M., and Pollock, G. H. Psychosomatic Specificity, Vol. 1. Experimental Study and Results. Chicago, University of Chicago Press, 1968.
7. Mahl, G. F. Anxiety, HCl secretion, and peptic ulcer etiology. Psychosomatic Med. 12:158, 1950.
8. Kezur, E., Kapp, F. T., and Rosenbaum, M. Psychological factors in women with peptic ulcers. Amer. J. Psychiatry 108:368, 1951.
9. Davies, D. T., and Wilson, A. T. M. Observations on the life-history of chronic peptic ulcer. Lancet 2:1353, 1937.
10. Hamilton, M. The personality of dyspeptics. With special reference to gastric and duodenal ulcer. Brit. J. Med. Psychol. 23:182, 1950.
11. Højer-Pedersen, W. On the significance of psychic factors in the development of peptic ulcer. Acta Psychiat. Neurol. Scand. Suppl. 119, v. 33, 1958.
12. Eberhard, G. Peptic ulcer in twins. A study in personality, heredity, and environment. Acta Psychiat. Scand., Suppl. 205, v. 44, 1968.
13. Poser, E. G. Personality factors in patients with duodenal ulcer: A Rorschach study. J. Projective Tech. 15:131, 1951.
14. Marquis, D. P., Sinnett, E. R., and Winter, W. D. A psychological study of peptic ulcer patients. J. Clin. Psychol. 8:266, 1952.
15. Weiner, H., Thaler, M., Reiser, M. F., and Mirsky, I. A. Etiology of duodenal ulcer. I. Relation of specific psychological characteristics to rate of gastric secretion (serum pepsinogen). Psychosomatic Med. 19:1, 1957.
16. Mirsky, I. A. Physiologic, psychologic, and social determinants in the etiology of duodenal ulcer. Amer. J. Digest. Dis. 3:285, 1958.

17. Rutter, M. Psychosocial factors in the short-term prognosis of physical disease. I. Peptic ulcer. J. Psychosomatic Res. 7:45, 1963.
18. Alp, M. H., Court, J. H., and Grant, A. K. Personality pattern and emotional stress in the genesis of gastric ulcer. Gut 11:773, 1970.
19. Beaumont, W. Experiments and Observations on the Gastric Juice and the Physiology of Digestion. Plattsburgh, F. P. Allen, 1833.
20. Wolf, S., and Wolff, H. G. Human Gastric Function. New York, Oxford University Press, 1943.
21. Margolin, S. G. The behavior of the stomach during psychoanalysis. A contribution to a method of verifying psychoanalytic data. Psychoanalytic Quart. 20:349, 1951.
22. Szasz, T. S., Kirsner, J. B., Levin, E., and Palmer, W. L. The role of hostility in the pathogenesis of peptic ulcer: Theoretical considerations with the report of a case. Psychosomatic Med. 9:331, 1947.
23. Crawshaw, H. M., Fraser, D. M., and Warrender, T. S. Can psychic stimulation cause gastric acid secretion in man? Lancet 2:66, 1968.
24. Myers, T. M. Precipitating stresses in peptic ulcer. Stanford Med. Bull. 11:100, 1953.
25. Spicer, C. C., Stewart, D. N., and Winser, D. M. deR. Perforated peptic ulcer during the period of heavy air-raids. Lancet 1:14, 1944.
26. Kellock, T. D. Childhood factors in duodenal ulcer. Brit. Med. J. 2:1117, 1951.
27. Kessel, N., and Munro, A. Epidemiological studies in psychosomatic medicine. J. Psychosomatic Res. 8:67, 1964.
28. Roth, H. P. The peptic ulcer personality. Arch. Intern. Med. 96:32, 1955.
29. Gundry, R. K., Donaldson, R. M., Jr., Pinderhughes, C. A., and Barrabee, E. Patterns of gastric acid secretion in patients with duodenal ulcer: Correlations with clinical and personality features. Gastroenterology 52:176, 1967.
30. Szasz, T. S. Psychiatric aspects of vagotomy: A preliminary report. Ann. Intern. Med. 28:279, 1948.
31. Szasz, T. S. Psychiatric aspects of vagotomy. II. A psychiatric study of vagotomized ulcer patients with comments on prognosis. Psychosomatic Med. 11:187, 1949.
32. Leading Article. Mind and ulcer. Brit. Med. J. 3:374, 1969.
33. Katz, M. M. Psychodynamics of peptic ulcer pathogenesis in hospitalized schizophrenic patients. Psychosomatic Med. 16:47, 1954.
34. Porter, R. W., Brady, J. V., Conrad, D., Mason, J. W., Galambos, R., and Rioch, D. McK. Some experimental observations on gastrointestinal lesions in behaviorally conditioned monkeys. Psychosomatic Med. 20:379, 1958.
35. Brady, J. V. Ulcers in "executive" monkeys. Scientific American 199:95, 1958.

Chapter 14

Acid Secretion in Peptic Ulcer

John S. Fordtran

INTRODUCTION

The average rate of acid secretion in patients with duodenal ulcer is higher than in control subjects, no matter what the conditions of the study (basal, sham feeding, test meal, submaximal histamine, maximal histamine, etc.).[1, 2] By contrast, mean secretion rate in gastric ulcer patients tends to be lower than normal. Average secretion rate in patients who have both duodenal and gastric ulcers is similar to the average secretion rate in the duodenal ulcer group. Patients with prepyloric ulcer secrete acid at about the same rate as do normal individuals; that is, higher than those with ulcer in the body of the stomach, but not so high as those with duodenal ulcer. To a degree, the low secretion rate in some gastric ulcer patients may be due to gastritis, which usually surrounds an ulcer crater and diminishes the functional parietal cell mass.[3-5] Furthermore, the low secretion rates in gastric ulcer patients may be due to enhanced gastric permeability to hydrogen ions, so that secreted acid may diffuse across the gastric mucosa and not be collected in the sample of gastric juice.[6] There is some experimental evidence to support this hypothesis,[7] although the quantitative importance of this factor in relation to rates of acid secretion has not been established with certainty.

It should be emphasized that when patients and control subjects are selected at random, the overlap in secretory rates among the two groups is tremendous. This is illustrated in Figure 14–1, taken from the work of Wormsley and Grossman.[8] Such overlap is not particularly surprising, because (1) hypersecretors in the control group may be predisposed to, and later develop, an ulcer, (2) the secretory rates in an individual subject may dramatically increase or decrease with the passage of time, and (3) there are many predisposing causes of ulcer other than hypersecretion. (The evidence for [1] and [2] is direct, whereas the evidence for [3] is circular.)

Three statements are often made with regard to acid secretion and peptic ulcer which the author feels are not proved by the available evidence.

1. The peptic ulcer may heal in the absence of a change in gastric acidity. Although it is true that ulcers often heal without medical therapy, and that acid secretion may be the same before and after healing is induced by medical therapy,[9] this does not prove that gastric acidity remains constant during the healing process. With medical therapy, of course, acidity is deliberately reduced. Acidity during spontaneous healing has not been studied.

2. The occurrence and recurrence of peptic ulcer are not associated with increased gastric secretion. Most writers quote Brown and Dolkart[10] as they make this point, and these workers did conclude

174

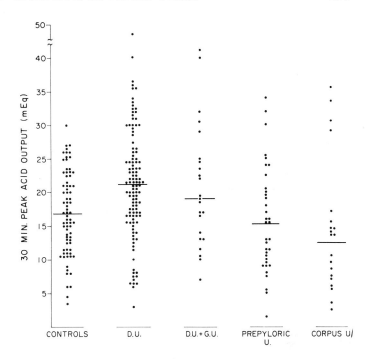

Figure 14–1. Distribution of values of peak 30-minute acid output, showing marked overlap of all groups, tendency of patients with duodenal ulcer to secrete more than the control subjects, and separation into two subgroups of patients with corpus ulcers. Histalog was the stimulus. (From Wormsley, K. G., and Grossman, M. I.: Gut 6:513, 1965.)

from repeated Ewald test meals that acid secretion did not change consistently as duodenal ulcer recurred. However, these data are inconclusive, because only infrequently was acid secretion measured during the few days preceding the recurrence of ulcer symptoms or during the first few days after ulcer symptoms began. Mirsky claimed that pepsinogen levels increased as ulcer disease became active, but that the increases were not usually statistically significant. No data were presented.[11] Littman[12] presented data suggesting that basal secretion is higher when the ulcer is active than when in remission, and Celestin found higher rates of acid secretion in response to broth irrigation of the antrum in patients with active duodenal ulcer than in control subjects or in duodenal ulcer patients in remission.[13] For various reasons, none of these studies is conclusive, and it seems necessary to conclude that the available evidence is conflicting and that the question has not been settled.

3. The high secretory rates seen in patients with duodenal ulcer are present for years before the ulcer develops. Most of the evidence is based on follow-up studies of doctors who had secretory studies performed while they were in medical school.

The most recent analysis of these data concluded that "there is an almost even probability that the differences shown could have been due to chance."[14] Mirsky, in a study that was still in progress at the time of his writing, stated that "a fairly large number of healthy hypersecretors (serum pepsinogen) who have been followed for several years developed typical signs and symptoms of duodenal ulcer that was subsequently established roentgenologically. In contrast, none of the individuals comprising the hyposecretor group have developed the ulcer syndrome."[11] Unfortunately, no data were presented. Roth said that some of his "normal subjects" who hypersecreted in response to a caffeine test meal later developed ulcer disease.[15] Blackman et al. make a similar statement with regard to the peak secretory response.[16] Thus the evidence suggests that hypersecretion precedes for some time the development of ulcer, but it is hardly conclusive.

NORMAL RATES OF ACID SECRETION

Estimates of the normal rate of acid secretion, and especially the upper limit of normal, have frequently been calculated statistically from data in control subjects without ulcer. For instance, the middle 80 per cent of control cases may be selected to represent the "normal zone." The remaining 10 per cent at either end seem likely to develop illness related to hypo- or hypersecretion, and thus are classified as abnormal.[2] This general approach is reasonable and consistent with the opinion already expressed that hypersecretors in control groups are predisposed to develop ulcer. However, the upper limit of normal calculated statistically changes drastically, depending upon the statistical criterion used. For instance, using the criterion that there be a 95 per cent probability of excluding *no more* than 5 per cent of normal subjects, Wormsley and Grossman calculated an upper limit of normal for basal secretion of 10.2 mEq per hour.[8] On the other hand, using a 97.5 probability that *more than* 5 per cent of the control population was excluded, Grossman calculated an upper limit of normal of 2.8 mEq per hour from a similar group of control subjects.[1] These examples make it clear that upper limits for acid secretion based on statistical analysis are quite arbitrary. (This has, of course, been well recognized by the investigators who have made these calculations.) Extensive and long-term follow-up of control subjects would be needed to decide on empirical grounds what is the cut-off between "normal" and levels of acid secretion which predispose to ulcer. Such data are not available, and therefore the upper limit of normal acid secretion is not known.

PEAK SECRETORY RESPONSE AND THE PARIETAL CELL MASS

The gastric secretory response to a maximum dose of histamine, Histalog, or gastrin is directly related to the number of parietal cells in the stomach. Since the average peak secretory response to these stimulants is higher in duodenal ulcer patients than in control subjects, it is generally agreed that duodenal ulcer patients have, on the average, an increased number of parietal cells, and that this, in turn, is at least one of the causes of increased

average rate of acid secretion in this group of patients.

What determines the parietal cell mass in a given individual is unknown. A genetic etiology is suggested by the strong influence of heredity on the development of peptic ulcer, but direct evidence on this point is meager and conflicting.[11, 17, 18]

Can the parietal cell mass be modified by environmental factors? There is good evidence that the peak histamine response is not reduced by prolonged anticholinergic therapy,[19] but that it can be increased by chronic hypergastrinemia, as seen in patients with the Zollinger-Ellison syndrome.[20] Experimentally, histamine, hypercalcemia (which may work through hypergastrinemia), and portacaval shunt increase the parietal cell mass,[21-24] although heavy coffee ingestion (caffeine stimulation) for three months in normal human subjects failed to increase the peak secretory response to histamine (my unpublished observations on five patients). It is not known whether or not basal hypersecretion caused by increased vagal activity can elevate the parietal cell mass.

With the exceptions just noted, there was, until recently, no evidence that the parietal cell mass fluctuated significantly in the usual group of patients with duodenal ulcer, and it was generally assumed that the parietal cell mass was fairly constant in a given individual. According to Sircus,[25] when tests were repeated on one or more occasions in 15 subjects over a two-year period, the coefficient of variation was only 9.7 per cent. However, in 1967, Weir reported a normal man who was studied three times in 1964, with less than 1.5 mEq per hour peak acid secretion on each occasion. When studied again one year later, he secreted greater than 20 mEq per hour on two occasions.[26] A transient gastritis at the time of the initial studies was postulated. Waterfall reported one normal and one duodenal ulcer patient who had a marked fall in their peak acid response to gastrin, which was given repeatedly. In the normal subject, parietal cell antibody and gastritis was demonstrated, possibly related to the pentagastrin injections.[27]

Norgaard and coworkers[19] studied the peak acid response to Histalog at three-month intervals over a one- to two-year

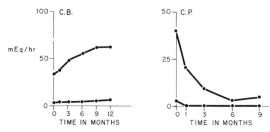

Figure 14–2. Sequential measurement of basal and peak Histalog response in two patients with duodenal ulcer. Basal secretion is shown in the lower lines, peak secretion in the upper lines. (Data from Norgaard et al.: Gastroenterology, 58:750, 1970.)

period in 33 unselected duodenal ulcer patients, none of whom had the Zollinger-Ellison syndrome or a related disease. Five (15 per cent) showed a convincing and significant sequential change in their parietal cell mass during the one- to one-and-one-half-year period of observation. Two of the most striking examples are shown in Figure 14–2. These results show that the functional parietal cell mass (as measured indirectly by the peak secretory response) can change markedly over the course of a relatively short period of time; although the cause is not known, the importance of this observation in terms of ulcer pathogenesis and treatment is obvious.

The pathophysiological significance of the peak secretory response, insofar as peptic ulcer is concerned, rests primarily on three points. First, the peak secretory response is an estimate of the number of functional parietal cells in a given patient at a particular time. Second, the peak response to histamine or gastrin is quantitatively very similar to the gastric secretory response to a steak and vegetable meal,[28, 29] and the results therefore give a fair estimate of how much acid a patient will secrete in response to normal food. Finally, there appears to be a peak secretion rate below which people do not develop an active duodenal ulcer. Baron, in a study of 70 patients, found this value to be 15 mEq per hour in males and 18 mEq per hour in females.[30, 31] Only two of 157 patients in two other large series had peak acid secretion rates below these levels.[32, 33] In Wormsley and Grossman's series of 152 duodenal ulcer patients, four had a peak response below 12 mEq per hour.[8] How-

ever, it should be noted that in all these series patients with inactive duodenal ulcer may have been included, and repeat tests to verify low results were not done, except in a few patients in the study of Wormsley and Grossman. In the latter series, half of their low results could possibly be explained by recent hemorrhage, perforation, or surgery. In our series of 69 duodenal ulcer patients,[19, 34] studied repeatedly and sequentially, we have never seen a peak response below 12 mEq per hour, except in patients with transient depression after bleeding or perforation, or in patients who initially had values greater than 12 mEq per hour but whose response fell sequentially as they were followed. When a fall in secretion rate below 12 mEq per hour was observed, the ulcer always became inactive. It seems likely that active (uncomplicated) duodenal ulcer requires a peak secretory capacity of greater than 12 to 15 mEq per hour. Exceptions to this rule must be rare.

Although the average peak secretory response is greater in duodenal ulcer patients than in control subjects, the degree of this difference is not great in all series,[8] and the overlap among individual results in the two groups is wide. Furthermore, the peak secretory response can be very high, yet the patient may not develop an ulcer; conversely, the secretion rate may be well below the mean secretion rate in normal subjects, yet the patient may have a duodenal ulcer. These latter observations simply mean that local mucosal resistance to ulceration is very variable in different people.

BASAL AND NOCTURNAL SECRETION

In the early 1930's, it was reported that ulcer patients secreted large amounts of gastric acid at night and that this could present a serious problem in ulcer management.[35, 36] Measurement of 12-hour nocturnal secretion soon became a popular test, and the results were thought to reflect the level of vagal tone. Winkelstein fractionated the 12-hour nocturnal secretion into hourly aliquots, and found that peak secretion occurred at 1:00 A.M.[37] More recently, Moore and Englert have studied basal secretion throughout the 24-hour period, and emphasize a circadian rhythm. Among a group made up of normal subjects, hospitalized patients without peptic disease, and duodenal ulcer patients, average secretion rate was higher in the evening than in the morning. The highest secretion rate occurred around 1:00 A.M.[38]

Some still prefer the 12-hour nocturnal secretion over other estimates of basal secretion. The advantages are that secretion is collected over a relatively long period of time and the results are less subject to errors caused by short-term fluctuations in secretion rate, and that during this test the subjects are usually asleep and therefore shielded from excitatory and inhibitory factors in the environment and from the usual stimuli for gastric secretion (thought of food at mealtime, for example).[35, 39] The disadvantages are that any discomfort from the nasogastric tube is prolonged, there is difficulty in adequately supervising such a long test, especially at night, and the test is not really basal because a meal is ingested three to four hours prior to starting the collection.

The popularity of the 12-hour test as a measure of basal secretion is decreasing in favor of a one- or two-hour test conducted in the morning after a 12-hour fast under close supervision. Most of the available evidence suggests that the results of basal secretion measured in this way correlate well with the results of nocturnal acid secretion. Ivy et al. found that the one-hour basal secretion gave almost exactly the same average results as the 12-hour nocturnal secretion.[2] Another study showed that a two- or four-hour basal collection during the day correlated well with the 12-hour nocturnal secretion, but that the one-hour basal secretion correlated poorly with the night secretion.[40] Still another study showed that the first hour of a basal study correlated well with acid secretion during a subsequent four-hour period.[41] To the writer's knowledge, the variability of the one- or two-hour basal secretion has not been compared with the variability of the 12-hour nocturnal test by repeat testing in the same patients.

Basal secretion, no matter how it is measured, is generally reported to be higher, on the average, in duodenal ulcer patients than in control subjects, although the scat-

ter is wide in both groups, and the degree to which basal secretion in duodenal ulcer patients exceeds that in the "normal" population varies markedly from series to series. For instance, Ivy et al.,[2] Baron,[30] and Correia and de Moura[42] found that average basal secretion in duodenal ulcer patients was about three times higher than in their control groups, whereas Wormsley and Grossman found that basal secretion in their normal subjects was 1.8 mEq per hour compared to 2.1 mEq per hour in their duodenal ulcer patients, a difference which was not statistically significant.[8] Dragstedt claims that 12-hour nocturnal gastric secretion rate is from three to 20 times higher in duodenal ulcer patients than in normal subjects,[35, 39] whereas Sandweiss and colleagues found nocturnal secretion to be the same in duodenal ulcer and normal subjects.[43] Obviously these discrepancies must somehow depend on the selection of the ulcer patients and the selection of the controls. Based on available evidence, it seems likely that if ulcer patients are selected at random (medical–surgical, inpatient–outpatient, severe–mild, in proportion to the incidence of these variables in the entire ulcer population), and if the control subjects are carefully matched in every way possible, most of patients in both groups will have relatively low basal secretion rates, with average secretion rates slightly higher in the duodenal ulcer group. On the other hand, if the patients are selected mainly from a surgical service, or from any unit interested in gastric hypersecretion, basal secretion will tend to be much higher in the ulcer patients than in the controls. There are three reasons why this might be the case. First, a high level of basal or nocturnal secretion is used by many as an indication for surgery, and such patients are therefore more apt to be referred to the surgical unit than are patients with low basal secretion. Second, it seems likely, but has not been proved, that duodenal ulcer patients with high basal secretory rates have a worse prognosis than do patients with low secretion rates, in which case they would tend to be admitted to the surgical ward. Finally, there is a tendency among all groups interested in acid secretion to save, keep track of, and repeatedly study ulcer patients who hypersecrete—such patients are inherently interesting and are valuable for drug evaluation studies. Ulcer patients with low secretion rates are of less interest and value in this regard and tend to be forgotten.

These same considerations probably explain the disagreement between Grossman[44] and Dragstedt[35, 39] on the question of whether or not basal secretion gives better separation of ulcer and control groups than stimulated secretion. If one is dealing with a high proportion of duodenal ulcer patients with basal hypersecretion, as Dragstedt obviously is, the basal secretion rate will separate the ulcer from the control patients to a much greater degree than the peak secretory response. The latter is only moderately higher in ulcer patients than in controls, regardless of the rate of basal secretion (the degree to which peak secretion can increase is limited, even when the stimulus to secretion is intense and prolonged). On the other hand, if a random population of ulcer patients and controls is studied, basal secretion does not separate the two groups any better than stimulated secretion, and neither does it very well.

RATIO OF BASAL TO PEAK SECRETION

The marked variation in the parietal cell mass (as measured by the peak secretory response) among different patients and normal individuals makes the absolute level of basal secretion difficult to interpret in terms of estimating the degree to which the parietal cells are active in the basal state. A basal secretion rate of 5 mEq per hour in a patient with a peak secretory capacity of 15 mEq per hour is quite different from a basal secretion rate of 5 mEq per hour in another patient with a peak secretory capacity of 100 mEq per hour. If basal secretion rate is expressed as the ratio of basal to peak secretory rate in response to maximum doses of histamine, Histalog, or gastrin, the result is a useful index of the degree to which the parietal cells of a given individual or group of patients are active in the basal state.

Is the ratio of basal to peak secretory response higher in duodenal ulcer patients than in control subjects? If it is higher,

then duodenal ulcer subjects must, as a group, have either a higher basal secretory drive or increased reactivity of the parietal cells to a normal level of "drive." (See section on control mechanisms below.) On the other hand, if the ratio of basal to peak secretion rates is the same in duodenal ulcer as in normal subjects, the entire increase in basal secretion noted in duodenal ulcer subjects can be attributed to an increase in the parietal cell mass.

Again, the data show great discrepancies, some studies showing the basal/peak secretion ratio to be the same in duodenal ulcer and in control groups, whereas others report markedly higher average ratios in duodenal ulcer than in normals. The method by which patients were selected for the control and for the ulcer group must explain this difference in results.

Several important aspects of basal secretion and the ratio of basal to peak secretion are illustrated in Figure 14–3. The ratio of basal to peak secretion rate is plotted against the basal secretion rate. Each subject shown in this figure was studied on at least four occasions, and the points are the average of all studies on a given individual. The data are thus highly reliable. Furthermore, none of the patients had Zollinger-Ellison or related syndromes, the blood gastrin and calcium levels were normal, and there was no effect of anticholinergic drugs. This figure shows that

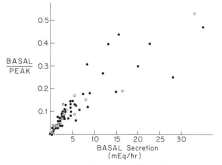

Figure 14–3. Correlation of basal secretion rate and the ratio of basal to peak histamine secretion rates. Each subject was studied on at least four occasions, and the symbols show the average result for each subject. Closed circles represent patients with duodenal ulcer. Open circles are subjects without evidence of gastrointestinal disease. (Data of Dr. Charles T. Richardson.)

the marked variation in basal secretion among different ulcer patients and among different control individuals cannot be explained, at least not entirely, by differences in the parietal cell mass (as measured by the peak secretory response to histamine, Histalog, or gastrin). If basal secretion were determined by the parietal cell mass (i.e., if a more or less constant fraction of the parietal cells were activated in the basal state), the data in Figure 14–3 would fit a horizontal line. However, the data clearly show that as basal secretion increases, the ratio of basal to peak secretion increases. Therefore, basal secretion rate is not determined, at least not entirely, by the parietal cell mass.

However, the question remains, do duodenal ulcer patients have a higher basal/peak ratio than normal people? The answer is (in the writer's opinion) that some of them do and most of them do not. Those who do fall in the right upper part of Figure 14–3. Those who do not fall in the left lower part of the figure.

To be sure, some people without ulcer may have a secretory pattern that places them in the right upper part of Figure 14–3. However, these are few in number, and they are probably predisposed to develop an ulcer and therefore not normal. Many of these individuals will have ulcer-like dyspepsia even though the X-ray fails to show an ulcer crater or ulcer deformity.

These conclusions differ from those in a consensus paper written by Hunt and colleagues.[45] These workers analyzed two large series of duodenal ulcer patients and a group of control subjects with regard to the percentage of the maximum secretory capacity activated by the stimuli of basal secretion. They concluded that there is no need to postulate any abnormal basal secretory drive in duodenal ulcer patients compared with people without duodenal ulcer. This widely quoted study, and especially the conclusions derived from it by the authors, is open to question, because for comparison with their duodenal ulcer subjects with high basal secretion, they *selected* a group of control subjects with equally high basal secretion rates. Since it is not known from their data what percentage of normal people have high basal secretion, compared with the percentage of duodenal ulcer patients who have basal

hypersecretion, their results do not argue against an average increase in the basal secretory drive in duodenal ulcer, and especially they do not disprove abnormal drive and/or sensitivity in ulcer patients or "normals" who have high rates of basal secretion.

TEST MEALS

A variety of test meals were widely used in the past. These included the Ewald carbohydrate,[46] the gruel,[2] the caffeine,[14] and the alcohol[2, 47] meals. These tests are carried out by taking a small sample of gastric content at multiple intervals after ingestion of the meal and determining hydrogen ion concentration. Alternatively, all the gastric content can be removed at a single time and total acid in the stomach calculated (concentration times volume). The results of these tests depend not only on acid secretion, but also on gastric emptying and neutralization of secreted acid by the test meal itself.

In a sense these tests are more "physiological" than basal or peak secretion, because they involve the response to a food stimulus similar to that which the patient receives under conditions of normal daily life. Presumably the stimulus of these meals is submaximal, although secretion rates in milliequivalents per unit time cannot be measured (except by the method of Rune[28, 29] which has not been used with these meals), because once the stomach is emptied the stimulus is removed.

Use of these tests has shown that duodenal ulcer patients have higher average acidity than normals, but the overlap is wide and the scatter great. Test meal results are less reproducible than the peak secretory response to histamine or gastrin, but whether they are less reproducible than basal secretion rate is not known. The Ewald meal response has a positive linear correlation with the peak response to histamine ($n = 0.78$), and in the patients studied by Marks and Shay, the Ewald meal was as good as the peak histamine response in predicting which patients had duodenal ulcer.[48]

Results of test meals can be analyzed in several different ways, but many workers have emphasized the tendency for duodenal ulcer patients to manifest a prolonged or "terminal" response to the Ewald type meal. All agree, however, that this characteristic response is not pathognomonic for duodenal ulcer, because it is encountered in some normal individuals.

Roth has reported that the caffeine test meal has greater specificity in separating duodenal ulcer patients from controls than the Ewald test meal, i.e., fewer false-positive and fewer false-negative results.[15] In addition to showing higher levels of acidity, the response of the ulcer group was sustained for longer periods of time after caffeine. He postulates that this may result from caffeine potentiation of the "higher level of interdigestive secretion" characteristic of duodenal ulcer patients. Littman et al. have confirmed that the caffeine test gives good separation of duodenal ulcer and control groups, but they made no comparison with other tests.[49] Musick et al.[50] claimed that the response to a caffeine test meal was greater during active duodenal ulcer disease than after the ulcer healed.

Although these data are often quoted as indicating that the caffeine test meal is superior to other methods of assessing gastric secretion in separating ulcer from nonulcer patients, the evidence is not convincing. For one thing, the point has been statistically examined only once, and this involved a comparison of the Ewald and caffeine meals, but not other tests. For another, in Roth's study the average basal secretion rate in the ulcer group was about 2.5 times the rate of basal secretion in the controls. The exaggerated response of the ulcer subjects to a caffeine stimulus is not, therefore, surprising. It has not been shown that the caffeine test would give a good separation of ulcer patients from controls in groups of patients who do not show marked differences in basal or peak secretory rate—for instance, in the patients reported by Wormsley and Grossman, where the control patients secreted 1.8 mEq per hour and the ulcer group secreted 2.1 mEq per hour in the basal state.[8]

INSULIN HYPOGLYCEMIA AND 2-DEOXY-D-GLUCOSE

Insulin hypoglycemia and intravenous injection of 2-deoxy-D-glucose are capable of strong vagal stimulation; the latter increases acid secretion by virtue of a direct effect on the parietal cells and secondarily by causing release of antral gastrin. Insulin hypoglycemia in man induces a peak secretory response approximately equal to or only slightly less than the peak histamine or Histalog response.[51, 52] It has been shown recently in dogs that continuous infusion of 2-deoxy-D-glucose stimulates acid secretion for at least 24 hours, without evidence of fatigue.[53] These results suggest that central nervous system activity, mediated by the vagus nerve, can stimulate gastric acid secretion continuously and at near maximum levels for relatively long periods of time. Thus, it is physiologically possible that increased vagal tone could cause prolonged basal hypersecretion. However, the response to insulin hypoglycemia or to 2-deoxy-D-glucose gives no indication of the level of vagal tone, at least insofar as these tests have been used in the past.

The gastric secretory response to insulin hypoglycemia or to 2-deoxy-D-glucose infusion is used clinically to test for the completeness of therapeutic vagotomy. The safety of these tests is in question, however.[54]

CONTROL MECHANISMS FOR THE RESPONSE TO SUBMAXIMAL STIMULATION

On purely theoretical grounds, *and assuming a constant parietal cell mass*, the rate of submaximal secretion is determined by the factors outlined in Figure 14–4.

The *secretory drive* is determined by the relative potency of stimulatory factors

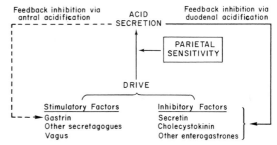

Figure 14–4. Control mechanisms of acid secretion.

(vagal tone and the blood level of secretagogues) and inhibitory factors (enterogastrones). The response of the parietal cells to a given level of drive is determined by the *parietal sensitivity*. Increased acid secretion tends to inhibit further secretion (feedback control) by two mechanisms. First, antral acidification inhibits further gastrin release. Second, duodenal acidification stimulates the release of greater amounts of the enterogastrones. Parietal sensitivity is probably influenced by several factors, among which may be vagal tone and the serum ionized calcium level.

According to this formulation, high rates of acid secretion (for a given parietal cell mass) could be caused by high vagal tone, high blood secretagogue level, low level of enterogastrone, or enhanced parietal cell sensitivity. There are, in turn, multiple reasons why a secretagogue or enterogastrone might be elevated or depressed. For instance, serum gastrin might be high because of some extragastric secretion, as in the Zollinger-Ellison syndrome, because of an increased number of gastrin-secreting cells, or because of a derangement in feedback control.

DEFECTS IN THE CONTROL MECHANISM THAT MIGHT EXPLAIN HIGHER AVERAGE SECRETION RATES IN DUODENAL ULCER PATIENTS

VAGAL TONE

For years it has been thought by many that duodenal ulcer patients have an abnormally high vagal tone. This idea originated from the observation that central nervous system lesions may cause gastric hypersecretion and ulcer disease (although the ulcers are usually stress ulcer rather than chronic peptic ulcer). Psychosomatic studies and theories and the observation that basal gastric secretion tends to be high in duodenal ulcer gave impetus to the hypothesis, and when vagotomy was found to markedly reduce basal hypersecretion and cure the ulcer diathesis, the evidence seemed complete. For good measure, it was found that the PR interval in the electrocardiogram is wider in male

duodenal ulcer patients than in males with gallbladder disease or hospital control patients,[55] suggesting increased vagal activity. Furthermore, increased rates of salivary flow (under parasympathetic but not vagal control) were reported to be correlated with the rate of gastric secretion,[56] and this is suggestive evidence that parasympathetic overactivity may be present in patients with gastric hypersecretion.[1] The supposedly greater gastric acid response to sham feeding in ulcer patients than in controls[37] and the rapid gastric emptying in some duodenal ulcer patients[57] were also used as evidence of increased vagal tone.

Recently, the concept of high vagal tone in duodenal ulcer patients has been seriously questioned on several grounds. First, the fact that vagotomy reduces basal secretion is not evidence for high vagal tone preoperatively, because vagotomy also reduces acid secretion in response to all stimuli, including histamine and gastrin.[1] Thus, an equally plausible interpretation of the vagotomy effect is that vagal tone modulates the responsiveness of the parietal cells to all stimuli. Second, it has not been shown that vagotomy reduces basal gastric secretion any more in duodenal patients than in patients who have vagotomy for other reasons. Third, vagal section reduces the response to histamine by approximately the same percentage as it reduces the basal secretion of acid, and this has been used as evidence against vagal hypertonicity as the cause of basal hypersecretion in duodenal ulcer patients.[58] Fourth, it has been reported that vagal block with hexamethonium bromide and atropine reduces basal secretion and peak histamine response to an equal extent in normal subjects and in patients with duodenal ulcer, and it was concluded that these results "negate the thesis of vagal hypertonicity to explain hypersecretion in duodenal ulcer patients."[59] Fifth, the results of some studies have failed to reveal an abnormally high ratio of basal to peak secretion rate.[8] If the ratio of basal to peak secretion rate is the same in ulcer patients as in others, all the higher basal secretory rate is explainable simply on the basis of higher parietal cell mass in ulcer patients. Sixth, one early study showed that the salivary response to pilocarpine was less in duodenal ulcer patients than in controls, which would argue against chronic overactivity of the parasympathetic nervous system in the ulcer group.[60] Finally, some recent studies suggest that, as a group, patients with duodenal ulcer do not have higher rates of gastric emptying than control groups.[58, 61]

In the absence of an independent and reliable method for measuring vagal tone, it must be concluded that the question of whether vagal tone is higher in ulcer patients than in controls, or even in an individual with severe basal hypersecretion, cannot be answered.

SERUM GASTRIN

One component of basal secretory drive, the serum gastrin level, can be measured directly by radioimmunoassay. Trudeau and McGuigan correlated the rate of acid secretion with the fasting serum gastrin levels in patients with gastric and duodenal ulcers and in a control group, and their data are summarized in Table 14–1.[62] These results reveal an inverse relation between the rate of basal acid secretion and the serum gastrin concentration in patients with duodenal ulcer, i.e., the highest rates of acid secretion are associated with the lowest serum gastrin level. This suggests that the antrum of duodenal ulcer patients responds to increasing acidity by a reduction in antral gastrin release, and that this feedback control loop is intact. However, because the serum gastrin level in the duodenal ulcer group as a whole did

not differ significantly from that of the control group, despite higher basal acid secretion in the ulcer group, Berson and Yalow suggested that the serum gastrin may be inappropriately high in these patients with duodenal ulcer. This would imply a relative failure of normal feedback inhibition of gastrin secretion.[63] Obviously, much more work needs to be done to decide whether or not feedback control of gastrin release is deranged in patients with duodenal ulcer, including the study of individual patients when antral acidity is systematically varied over a pH range of 1 to 5, and a study of the response of the serum gastrin to various test meals when antral acidity is also known.

In patients with gastric ulcer, Trudeau and McGuigan found the fasting serum gastrin level to be almost twice as high as in the control group, and the difference was statistically significant. Among the patients with gastric ulcer, there was an inverse correlation between serum gastrin level and the rate of acid secretion, suggesting that the higher gastrin level might be due to decreased inhibition of antral gastrin release because of higher antral pH. Other possibilities are that higher gastrin levels in these patients might be related to antral stasis or to antral gastritis. In any case, low acid secretion in gastric ulcer patients is associated with higher than normal levels of serum gastrin.

Many patients with gastric ulcer previously have had a duodenal ulcer.[3, 64–66] Johnson[67] and Dragstedt[68] have attributed the gastric ulcer in such cases to diminished gastric motility or to the development of pyloric stenosis and gastric retention. According to Dragstedt, antral distention releases gastrin, which stimulates acid secretion and causes the gastric ulcer to develop. A major weakness in this line of reasoning is that most of these patients do not have delayed gastric emptying. Mangold[64] noted delayed emptying by X-ray in only 19 per cent of 157 patients, and Capper[69] found stasis in only 7 per cent of 83 patients with combined ulcer disease. The ultimate proof of the hypothesis will be to see whether patients with both duodenal and gastric ulcers have higher gastrin levels than patients with ulcer in only a single location. This experiment has not been reported.

TABLE 14–1. CORRELATION OF FASTING SERUM GASTRIN CONCENTRATION AND GASTRIC ACID SECRETION RATE*

STUDY GROUP	BASAL SECRETION mEq/hr	PEAK SECRETION mEq/hr	SERUM GASTRIN pg/ml
Control subjects	2.0	17.4	85
Duodenal ulcer	4.6	26.2	78
Duodenal ulcer with high basal secretion	> 8.0	–	52
Gastric ulcer	1.5	16.4	159

*Data of Trudeau, W. L., and McGuigan, J. E.: New Eng. J. Med. 284:408, 1971.

INHIBITION OF ACID SECRETION

Fat or acid instilled into the duodenum or upper jejunum of normal subjects reduces the rate of stimulated gastric secretion and the rate of gastric emptying.[70] This effect is mediated by humoral enterogastrones, but the relative importance of secretin, cholecystokinin-pancreozymin, and other agents has not been established for humans. Neither secretin nor cholecystokinin-pancreozymin given intravenously mimics the effect of acid in the duodenum on histamine stimulated acid secretion,[71] but it is not known whether secretin and cholecystokinin-pancreozymin given together would inhibit secretion in this test model.

It is theoretically possible that the higher average rate of acid secretion in duodenal ulcer patients might be due to impaired release of enterogastrones or to some other defect in the inhibitory mechanism. Shay and colleagues in particular have emphasized this possibility, pointing out that the secretory response to an Ewald test meal is brief in many normals and relatively prolonged in many duodenal ulcer patients.[72] Failure of the normal inhibitory response to acid entering the duodenum might explain this sustained secretory response noted in many ulcer patients.

There is general agreement that fat instilled in the duodenum reduces Ewald meal and gastrin stimulated gastric acid secretion to the same extent in duodenal ulcer patients as in normal individuals.[72, 73] Furthermore, the data presented by Windsor and colleagues show that the degree to which fat inhibits acid secretion does not depend on the level of basal or peak secretion rate; i.e., fat inhibits secretion as well in the high secretors as in the low secretors in both the normal and the ulcer groups.[73]

With respect to acid inhibition, the results are not so clear cut. Shay et al. found that acid in the duodenum failed to inhibit Ewald meal stimulated acid secretion in three patients with duodenal ulcer. Acid also failed to inhibit emptying of the test meal in these three subjects.[72] Hunt found that six of 16 duodenal ulcer patients failed to show inhibition of acid secretion when acid was added to the test meal, whereas normally this procedure always inhibits

acid secretion.[74] Johnston and Duthie reported data in 1964 which suggested that duodenal ulcer patients had a defect in the inhibitory response to acid in the duodenum when histamine was the stimulus.[75] The results are very difficult to interpret, because the patients and control subjects received varying doses of histamine. In a later paper,[76] these authors used a standard dose of gastrin II as the stimulant and concluded that acid inhibition in duodenal ulcer was not impaired. However, they tested only two ulcer patients, and one of these had the lowest percentage inhibition of the entire study group of eight normal subjects and two duodenal ulcer patients. Furthermore, the two duodenal ulcer patients did not differ from the normal persons with respect to acid secretion, so their conclusion is not necessarily applicable to ulcer patients who hypersecrete in the basal state or in response to test meals.

Woodward and Shapiro showed that antral motility, measured by a transducer, was inhibited by acid in the duodenum equally well in duodenal ulcer patients and in normal individuals.[77] However, this does not prove that secretory inhibition by acid in the duodenum would have been the same in the two groups, because previously presented evidence suggested that it takes more duodenal acid to inhibit gastric secretion than to inhibit gastric emptying.[72]

No definite conclusion can be reached about whether the duodenal acid inhibitory effect is defective in duodenal ulcer. Repeated studies in individual patients are needed to assess the reproducibility of the test procedure, and then a correlation of the percentage inhibition with the secretory rates of the individual patients. Only then will we know whether a defect in inhibition can explain gastric hypersecretion in the basal state or in response to meals which elicit submaximal stimulation.

PARIETAL SENSITIVITY

Methods for specifically measuring parietal sensitivity have not been developed. Dose-response curves to gastrin or histamine, which at first sight might seem a simple way to estimate "sensitivity," are also influenced by "secretory drive."

Several dose-response studies in control subjects and duodenal ulcer patients have been performed, and the results are of great interest even though pathophysiological interpretation is difficult. Hunt and Kay[78] found no difference in the average results of dose-response curves to histamine between five normal subjects and five patients with duodenal ulcer. Wormsley and Mahoney[79] measured the ratio of the response to a small dose of gastrin to the response to a large dose of gastrin, and showed that this ratio was the same in normal medical students as in duodenal ulcer patients. In contrast to these negative results, Isenberg, Best, and Grossman have reported a shift to the left of the pentagastrin dose-response curves in duodenal ulcer.[80] They attribute this to a change in secretory drive (increased tone or decreased inhibition) rather than to an abnormal parietal sensitivity (see p. 546).

The explanation of these different results may be related to patient selection. In Hunt and Kay's study, the ratio of basal to peak stimulated secretion rate was the same in ulcer and control subjects, whereas in the study of Isenberg et al., basal secretion relative to peak stimulated secretion was higher in the ulcer than in the control subjects (J. Isenberg, personal communication to the author).

Dose-response studies are clearly of great interest and importance, because if the curve is shifted in duodenal ulcer compared with control subjects, as suggested by the results of Isenberg et al., this is further support for some abnormality in duodenal ulcer other than increased parietal cell mass.

CONTROL OF SUBMAXIMAL SECRETION IN INDIVIDUAL SUBJECTS

Although there is no compelling evidence that patients with duodenal ulcer as a group are under any special basal secretory drive (this has not been disproved either), it is clear that some people, most of them with ulcer disease, hypersecrete in the basal state compared with most other people. This fact is illustrated in Figure 14–3, in which the basal secretion rate is plotted against the ratio of the basal to the peak secretion rate.

Although there is a spectrum between very low and very high basal secretion rates, those who fall in the upper right part of the graph must in some way be different from those in the lower left. The high basal secretors must have increased stimuli for secretion, decreased inhibitory stimuli, or increased reactivity of the parietal cells to a normal basal secretory drive. It is also clear that most of the patients in the right upper section of this graph will have peptic ulcer, and those who do not are probably predisposed to ulcer.

In a detailed study of ten subjects with variable rates of basal secretion, it was shown that those with high ratios of basal to peak secretion required a much smaller dose of histamine to elicit a half maximal secretory response than those subjects with low ratios of basal to peak secretion.[81] Subjects with high basal to peak ratios also secreted a higher fraction of their maximal response to an Ewald meal than did subjects with a low ratio of basal to peak secretion. Although it is not certain from these results whether the basal hypersecretion is due to increased reactivity of the parietal cells to normal stimuli or due to increased basal secretory drive, the practical implications are clear. Patients with high ratios of basal secretion relative to their peak secretory capacity are primed to secrete briskly to small amounts of secretagogue or to test meals.

CAUSES OF BASAL HYPERSECRETION

There are three generally accepted causes of basal hypersecretion: hypergastrinemia caused by an islet cell tumor (Zollinger-Ellison syndrome), hypergastrinemia caused by a cuff of antrum left in contact with the afferent loop after Billroth II subtotal gastrectomy, and hypercalcemia.[82-84] (It is possible that hypercalcemia may also stimulate acid secretion *via* gastrin release.) On occasion basal hypersecretion has been reported with the following conditions: (1) portacaval shunts (possibly caused by histamine or a hormone liberated from the gut that bypasses the liver, escapes inactivation, and thus gains access to the parietal cells via the arterial circulation);[85-87] (2) small bowel resection (possibly caused by removal of inhibitory influence);[88-90] (3) malignant carcinoid syndrome originating in the foregut (probably caused by histamine secretion);[91, 92] (4) severe central nervous system trauma or disease (probably related to parasympathetic discharge);[93] (5) pyloric obstruction (possibly resulting from antral distention which causes gastrin release);[94] and (6) pancreatic disease (rare).[95, 96]

IDIOPATHIC BASAL HYPERSECRETION

In most patients with basal hypersecretion no specific cause can be found. These patients have basal secretion rates that amount to 20 to 60 per cent of their peak secretion rate, they usually have peptic ulcer, and they often have large rugal folds by X-ray. In addition, they may have diarrhea and steatorrhea, apparently caused by gastric hypersecretion. These patients thus mimic many features of the Zollinger-Ellison syndrome. However, they have low blood gastrin levels, rather than hypergastrinemia, and there is no evidence, even by angiogram or at exploratory laparotomy, of islet cell tumor. The cause of this syndrome is not known, but these patients presumably have some defect in the scheme outlined in Figure 14–4. When followed carefully over a period of months to years the degree of basal hypersecretion may fluctuate in these patients. Some may ultimately develop the Zollinger-Ellison syndrome; if so, the reason why gastrin levels were not elevated initially is obscure. See pages 542 and 543 for a discussion of meal, calcium, and secretin stimulation tests that may help separate idiopathic basal hypersecretion and Zollinger-Ellison syndrome without definite basal hypergastrinemia.

REFERENCES

1. Grossman, M. I. The pathologic physiology of peptic ulcer. Amer. J. Med. 29:748, 1960.
2. Ivy, A. C., Grossman, M. I., and Bachrach, W. H. Peptic Ulcer. Philadelphia, The Blakiston Company, 1950.
3. Marks, I. N., and Shay, H. Observations on the pathogenesis of gastric ulcer. Lancet 1:1107, 1959.
4. Mangus, H. A. In Modern Trends in Gastroenterology, 1st Series, F. Avery Jones (ed.). London, Appleton-Century-Crofts, 1952, p. 346.
5. Delaney, J. P., Cheng, J. W. B., Butler, B. A., and Ritchie, W. P., Jr. Gastric ulcer and regurgitation gastritis. Gut 11:715, 1970.
6. Davenport, H. W. Is the apparent hyposecretion of acid by patients with gastric ulcer a consequence of a broken barrier to diffusion of hydrogen ions into the gastric mucosa? Gut 6:513, 1965.
7. Ivey, K. J. Gastric mucosal barrier. Gastroenterology 61:247, 1971.
8. Wormsley, K. G., and Grossman, M. I. Maximal Histalog test in control subjects and patients with peptic ulcer. Gut 6:427, 1965.
9. Levin, E., Kirsner, J. B., and Palmer, W. L. Twelve-hour nocturnal gastric secretion in uncomplicated duodenal ulcer patients: Before and after healing. Proc. Soc. Exp. Biol. Med. 69:153, 1948.
10. Brown, C. F. G., and Dolkart, R. E. Gastric acid during recurrences and remissions of duodenal ulcer. Arch. Intern. Med. 60:680, 1937.
11. Mirsky, I. A. Physiologic, psychologic, and social determinants in the etiology of duodenal ulcer. Amer. J. Dig. Dis. 3:285, 1958.
12. Littman, A. Basal gastric secretion in patients with duodenal ulcer: A long-term study of variations in relation to ulcer activity. Gastroenterology 43:166, 1962.
13. Celestin, L. R. Antral activity and symptom periodicity in duodenal ulceration. Gut 8:318, 1967.
14. Baron, J. H. Gastric secretion in relation to subsequent duodenal ulcer and familial history. Gut 3:158, 1962.
15. Roth, J. L. A. Clinical evaluation of the caffeine gastric analysis in duodenal ulcer patients. Gastroenterology 19:199, 1951.
16. Blackman, A. H., Thayer, W. R., Jr., and Martin, H. F. In reply to Dr. Baron. Amer. J. Dig. Dis. 16:667, 1971.
17. Lander, F. P. L., and Maclagan, N. F. One hundred histamine test-meals on normal students. Lancet 2:1210, 1934.
18. Meyer, J., Maskin, M., and Necheles, H. Studies on constitution and ulcer. III. Gastric secretion in healthy members of "ulcer families." Amer. J. Dig. Dis. Nutr. 3:474, 1936.
19. Norgaard, R. P., Polter, D. E., Wheeler, J. W., Jr., and Fordtran, J. S. Effect of long term anticholinergic therapy on gastric acid secretion, with observations on the serial measurement of peak Histalog response. Gastroenterology 58:750, 1970.
20. Polacek, M. A., and Ellison, E. H. A comparative study of parietal cell mass and distribution in normal stomachs, in stomachs with duodenal ulcer and in stomachs of patients with pancreatic adenoma. Surg. Forum 14:313, 1963.
21. Marks, I. N. The effect of prolonged histamine stimulation on the parietal cell population and the secretory function of the guinea-pig stomach. Quart. J. Exp. Physiol. 42:180, 1957.
22. Neely, J. C., and Goldman, L. Effect of cal-

ciferol-induced chronic hypercalcemia on the gastric secretion from Heidenhain pouch. Ann. Surg. 155:406, 1962.

23. Ritchie, W. P., Jr., Delaney, J. D., Barzilai, A., Lande, A. J., and Wangensteen, O. H. Experimental alterations in gastric mucosal cellular population in dogs. J.A.M.A. 197:113, 1966.

24. Landor, J. H., Porterfield, J. F., and Wolff, W. S. The parietal cell response to chronic gastric secretory stimulation. Surg. Gynec. Obstet. 122:61, 1966.

25. Sircus, W. The application of the maximal histamine test of gastric secretion to problems of peptic ulcer surgery. J. Roy. Coll. Surg. Edinburgh 4:153, 1959.

26. Weir, D. G. Spontaneous recovery of gastric secretion. Brit. Med. J. 2:681, 1967.

27. Waterfall, W. Spontaneous decrease in gastric secretory response to humoral stimuli. Brit. Med. J. 4:459, 1969.

28. Rune, S. J. Comparison of the rates of gastric acid secretion in man after ingestion of food and after maximal stimulation with histamine. Gut 7:344, 1966.

29. Rune, S. J. Individual variation in secretory capacity of gastric acid stimulation with solid food and with histamine. Clin. Sci. 32:443, 1967.

30. Baron, J. H. An assessment of the augmented histamine test in the diagnosis of peptic ulcer. Gut 4:243, 1963.

31. Baron, J. H. The relationship between basal and maximum acid output in normal subjects and patients with duodenal ulcer. Clin. Sci. 24:357, 1963.

32. Kaye, M. D., Beck, P., Rhodes, J., and Sweetnam, P. M. Gastric acid secretion in patients with duodenal ulcer treated for one year with anticholinergic drugs. Gut 10:774, 1969.

33. Checketts, R. G., Gillespie, I. E., and Kay, A. W. Insulin potentiation of the augmented histamine response. Gut 9:683, 1968.

34. Rose, H., Fordtran, J. S., Harrell, R., and Friedman, B. A controlled study of gastric freezing for the treatment of duodenal ulcer. Gastroenterology 47:10, 1964.

35. Dragstedt, L. R. Gastric secretion tests. Gastroenterology 52:587, 1967.

36. Palmer, W. L. Fundamental difficulties in the treatment of peptic ulcer. J.A.M.A. 101:1604, 1933.

37. Winkelstein, A. A new therapy of peptic ulcer: Continuous alkalinized milk drip into the stomach. Amer. J. Med. Sci. 185:695, 1933.

38. Moore, J. G., and Englert, E. Circadian rhythm of gastric acid secretion in man. Nature (London) 226:1261, 1970.

39. Dragstedt, L. R. Reply to Dr. Grossman. Gastroenterology 54:322, 1968.

40. Dragstedt, L. R., II, and Lawson, L. J. Measurement of fasting gastric secretion. Arch. Surg. 88:287, 1964.

41. Sun, D. C. H., and Shay, H. Basal gastric secretion in duodenal ulcer patients: Its consideration in evaluation of gastric secretory inhibitants or stimulants. J. Appl. Physiol. 11:148, 1957.

42. Correia, J. P., and de Moura, M. C. Clinical experience with the augmented histamine test, with special emphasis on patients with gastrectomy. Gastroenterologica (Basel) 99:30, 1963.

43. Sandweiss, D. J., Friedman, M. H. F., Sugarman, M. H., and Podolsky, H. M. Nocturnal gastric secretion: Studies on normal subjects and patients with duodenal ulcer. Gastroenterology 7:38, 1946.

44. Grossman, M. I. Dragstedt's editorial on gastric secretion tests. Gastroenterology 53:681, 1967.

45. Hunt, J. N., Kay, A. W., Cord, W. I., and Sircus, W. The nature of basal hypersecretion in man with duodenal ulcer. In Skoryna, S. C., Pathophysiology of Peptic Ulcer. Philadelphia, J. B. Lippincott Co., 1963, p. 333.

46. Vanzant, F. R., Alvarez, W. C., Eusterman, G. B., Dunn, H. L., and Berkson, J. The normal range of gastric acidity from youth to old age. Arch. Intern. Med. 49:345, 1932.

47. Beazell, J. M., and Ivy, A. C. The influence of alcohol on the digestive tract. Quart. J. Stud. Alcohol 1:45, 1940.

48. Marks, I. N., and Shay, H. Augmented histamine test, Ewald test meal and Diagnex test. Amer. J. Dig. Dis. 5:1, 1960.

49. Littman, A., Fox, B. W., Kammerling, E. M., and Fox, N. I. A single aspiration caffeine gastric analysis in duodenal ulcer and control patients. Gastroenterology 28:953, 1955.

50. Musick, V. H., Avey, H. T., Hopps, H. C., and Hellbaum, A. A. Gastric secretion in duodenal ulcer in remission—response to the caffeine test meal. Gastroenterology 7:332, 1946.

51. Hubel, K. A. Insulin-induced gastric acid secretion in young men: Test reproducibility and correlation with the augmented histamine test. Gastroenterology 50:24, 1966.

52. Isenberg, J. I., Stening, G. F., Ward, S., and Grossman, M. I. Relation of gastric secretory response in man to dose of insulin. Gastroenterology 57:395, 1969.

53. Eisenberg, M. M., Chawla, R. C., and Sugawara, K. Sustained gastric secretion in response to 2-deoxy-D-glucose: Indefatigability of the vagal mechanisms. Gastroenterology 59:174, 1970.

54. Stempien, S. J. A note on the hazards of "maximal" insulin tests. Gastroenterology 60:345, 1971.

55. Draper, G., Bruenn, H. G., and Dupertuis, C. W. Changes in the electrocardiogram as criteria of individual constitution derived from its physiological panel. Amer. J. Med. Sci. 194:514, 1937.

56. Grossman, M. I. Inhibition of gastric and salivary secretion by Darbid. Gastroenterology 35:312, 1958.

57. Shay, H. The pathologic physiology of gastric and duodenal ulcer. Bull. N. Y. Acad. Med. 20:264, 1944.

58. Hunt, J. N. Some notes on the pathogenesis of duodenal ulcer. Amer. J. Dig. Dis. 2:445, 1957.

59. Singh, H., Goyal, R. K., Ahluwalia, D. S., and

Chuttani, H. K. Vagal influence in gastric acid secretion in normals and in duodenal ulcer patients. Gut 9:604, 1968.

60. Necheles, H., and Levitsky, P. Studies on constitution and peptic ulcer. IV. Salivary secretion test in peptic ulcer patients and normal subjects. J. Lab. Clin. Med. 22:624, 1937.

61. Brömster, D., Carlberger, G., and Lundh, G. Measurement of gastric emptying rate. Lancet 2:224, 1966.

62. Trudeau, W. L., and McGuigan, J. E. Relations between serum gastrin levels and rates of gastric hydrochloric acid secretion. New Eng. J. Med. 284:408, 1971.

63. Berson, S. A., and Yalow, R. S. Gastrin in duodenal ulcer. New Eng. J. Med. 284:445, 1971.

64. Mangold, R. Combined gastric and duodenal ulceration: A survey of 157 cases. Brit. Med. J. 2:1193, 1958.

65. Aagaard, P., Andreassen, M., and Kurz, L. Duodenal and gastric ulcer in the same patient. Lancet 1:1111, 1959.

66. Tanner, N. C. Surgery of peptic ulceration and its complications. Postgrad. Med. J. 30:448, 1954.

67. Johnson, H. D. The classification and principles of treatment of gastric ulcers. Lancet 2:518, 1957.

68. Dragstedt, L. R. Duodenal ulcer. Brit. Med. J. 1:1234, 1958.

69. Capper, quoted by Flint, F. J., and Grech, P. Gut 11:735, 1970.

70. Johnson, L. R., and Grossman, M. I. Intestinal hormones as inhibitors of gastric secretion. Gastroenterology 60:120, 1971.

71. Johnston, D., and Duthie, H. L. Inhibition of histamine-stimulated gastric secretion by acid in the duodenum in man. Gut 7:58, 1966.

72. Shay, H., Gershon-Cohen, J., and Fels, S. S. A self regulatory duodenal mechanism for gastric acid control and an explanation for the pathologic gastric physiology in uncomplicated duodenal ulcer. Amer. J. Dig. Dis. 9:124, 1942.

73. Windsor, C. W. O., Cockel, R., and Lee, M. J. R. Inhibition of gastric secretion in man by intestinal fat infusion. Gut 10:135, 1969.

74. Hunt, J. N. Influence of hydrochloric acid on gastric secretion and emptying in patients with duodenal ulcer. Brit. Med. J. 1:681, 1957.

75. Johnston, D., and Duthie, H. L. Effect of acid in the duodenum on histamine-stimulated secretion in man. Gut 5:573, 1964.

76. Johnston, D., and Duthie, H. L. Inhibition of gastrin secretion in the human stomach: Effect of acid in the duodenum. Lancet 2:1032, 1965.

77. Woodward, E. R., and Shapiro, H. Duodenal inhibitory mechanism in duodenal ulcer patients. J. Appl. Physiol. 12:55, 1958.

78. Hunt, J. N., and Kay, A. W. The nature of gastric hypersecretion of acid in patients with duodenal ulcer. Brit. Med. J. 2:1444, 1954.

79. Wormsley, K. G., and Mahoney, J. P. Parietal cell responsiveness in duodenal ulcer. Brit. Med. J. 1:278, 1967.

80. Isenberg, J. I., Best, W. R., and Grossman, M. I. The effect of graded doses of pentagastrin on gastric acid secretion in duodenal ulcer and non-duodenal ulcer subjects. Clin. Res. 20:222, 1972.

81. Richardson, C. T., and Fordtran, J. S. "Parietal sensitivity" as measured by histamine dose response curves—correlation with basal gastric secretion, Ewald meal response, serum gastrin and parotid salivary flow. Submitted for publication 1972.

82. Donegan, W. L., and Spiro, H. M. Parathyroids and gastric secretion. Gastroenterology 38:750, 1960.

83. Murphy, D. L., Goldstein, H., Boyle, J. D., and Ward, S. Hypercalcemia and gastric secretion in man. J. Appl. Physiol. 21:1607, 1966.

84. Barreras, R. F., and Donaldson, R. M., Jr. Gastric secretion during hypercalcemia in man. Gastroenterology 50:881, 1966.

85. Silen, W., and Eiseman, B. The nature and cause of gastric hypersecretion following portacaval shunts. Surgery 46:38, 1959.

86. Clarke, J. S., McKissock, P. K., and Cruze, K. Studies on the site of origin of the agent causing hypersecretion in dogs with portacaval shunt. Surgery 46:48, 1959.

87. Bendett, R. J., Fritz, H. L., and Donaldson, R. M., Jr. Gastric acid secretion after parenterally and intragastrically administered histamine in patients with portacaval shunt. New Eng. J. Med. 268:511, 1963.

88. Frederick, P. L., Sizer, J. S., and Osborne, M. P. Relation of massive bowel resection to gastric secretion. New Eng. J. Med. 272:509, 1965.

89. Reul, G. J., and Ellison, E. H. Effect of seventy-five per cent distal small bowel resection on gastric secretion. Amer. J. Surg. 111:772, 1966.

90. Osborne, M. P., Frederick, P. L., Sizer, J. S., Blair, D., Cole, P., and Thum, W. Mechanism of gastric hypersecretion following massive intestinal resection. Ann. Surg. 164:622, 1966.

91. Campbell, A. C. P., Gowenlock, A. H., Platt, D. S., and Snow, P. J. D. A β-hydroxy-tryptophan-secreting carcinoid tumour. Gut 4:61, 1963.

92. McGill, D. B., and Jones, H. R., Jr. Carcinoid syndrome with gastric hypersecretion and histaminuria. Arch. Intern. Med. 117:784, 1966.

93. Watts, C., and Clark, K. Effects of an anticholinergic drug on gastric acid secretion in the comatose patient. Surg. Gynec. Obstet. 130:61, 1970.

94. Sircus, W. Considerations on the effect of obstruction on gastric secretion. In Gastric Secretion: Mechanism and Control, T. K. Shnitka, J. A. L. Gilbert, and R. C. Harrison (eds.). New York, Pergamon Press, 1967, p. 293.

95. Mason, G. R., Eigenbrodt, E. H., Oberhelman, H. A., Jr., and Nelson, T. S. Gastric hypersecretion following pancreatitis. Surgery 54:604, 1963.

96. Hein, M. F., Silen, W., and Harper, H. A. Mechanism of canine gastric hypersecretion after pancreatic ductal obstruction. Amer. J. Physiol. 205:89, 1963.

Chapter 15

Pepsinogens and Pepsins in Peptic Ulcer

John S. Fordtran

INTRODUCTION

Pepsins may be defined as proteases which are active at low pH, coagulate milk protein, and are inactivated under neutral or slightly alkaline conditions.[1] Pepsins exist in the gastric mucosa and are secreted with the gastric juice in an inactive zymogen form (pepsinogen).

The proenzyme pepsinogen is completely inactive, i.e., it has absolutely no proteolytic activity, and it can be measured only by its protease activity after conversion to pepsin. In contrast to pepsin, pepsinogen is highly resistant to inactivation in an alkaline pH, being irreversibly denatured only when the pH is greater than 12.[2]

The conversion of pepsinogen to pepsin occurs spontaneously in solutions more acid than pH 6.0 by simple autocatalytic reaction; i.e., pepsin causes the destruction of pepsinogen with the formation of a new protein, pepsin. This process is extremely slow at pH 6.0, takes 12 hours at pH 4.6, and occurs almost instantaneously at pH 2.0.[2] In solutions more alkaline than pH 5.4, pepsin appears in combination with an inhibitor, which is part of the original pepsin molecule. Pepsin destroys this inhibitor, with a maximum rate at pH 3.5 to 4.0.[2]

DIFFERENT SPECIES OF PEPSINOGENS AND PEPSINS

Using electrophoretic and other separation techniques, up to eight separate pepsinogens can be identified,[3,4] and upon acidification these pepsinogens give rise to chromatographically and electrophoretically distinct pepsins.[1,4] These pepsins have somewhat different substrate specificities and differences in pH optimal values, but all fit the definition of a pepsin given here. None of these pepsins or their parent pepsinogens are homogeneous.[4]

Although there is uncertainty about the number of different human pepsinogens, all investigators agree that some fractions are limited to fundic mucosa, whereas others are found in fundic, antral, and proximal duodenal mucosa.[4] It has been suggested that those fractions limited to fundic mucosa be designated group I pepsinogens, and that the fractions which are also present in antral and duodenal mucosa be termed group II pepsinogens.[4]

CELLULAR ORIGIN OF THE PEPSINOGENS

The chief or peptic cells were first recognized in 1870, and from the outset it

189

was suspected that they were the source of pepsinogen secretion. This has subsequently been proved beyond any doubt. These cells possess characteristics which are common to zymogen secreting cells of other organs, such as the pancreas, stomach, and salivary glands. All contain granules of the respective proenzymes, all are arranged as part of tubular cell systems of which they occupy the base, and all are concerned with digestion of food and go through distinct histological cycles related to secretory activity.[5]

The limitation of group I pepsinogens to fundic mucosa suggests that these are synthesized mainly by the chief cells. Immunofluorescent studies have localized the synthesis of this group of pepsinogens to both chief and neck cells in fundic mucosa.[4] The cellular origin of group II has not been established,[4] although they presumably are synthesized by mucous neck cells in the antrum and possibly by Brunner's glands in the duodenum.

Although pepsinogen and acid are secreted by separate cells in man and other mammals, in lower species pepsinogen and acid are secreted by a single cell. In some species chief cells make intrinsic factor, but not in man, in whom intrinsic factor is made by parietal cells.[6]

Pepsinogen contained in the secretory granules of the chief cells represents a ready to be delivered stock of enzymes, but it is also possible for pepsinogen to be manufactured and secreted without going through a granule form when the cells are properly stimulated.[2] It has been suggested that pepsinogen storage in zymogen granules may involve a calcium-pepsinogen "polymerization," and that calcium may be involved in the release of zymogen from the membrane of the chief and other pepsinogen secreting cells.[7]

Although gastrin stimulates pepsinogen as well as acid secretion, Crean and co-workers have reported a selective increase in the parietal cell mass (but not the chief cell mass) in rats following chronic administration of pentagastrin.[8] Data in hypergastrinemic humans (Zollinger-Ellison syndrome) have apparently given contradictory results in this regard.[9] Duodenal obstruction in rats was shown to produce a significant increase in both the parietal and chief cell masses,[10] whereas vagotomy produced a decrease in the peptic cell mass but no significant change in the parietal cell mass.[11]

PEPTIC ACTIVITY

As already indicated, pepsin is active only in an acid environment, and in an acid environment peptic activity varies with pH levels. The pH optima of pepsins vary from about 1.8 to 3.5, depending on the species of pepsin, the ionic strength of the reaction mixture, and the type and concentration of substrate.[4]

The peptic activity of human pepsin(s) at different pH levels has been studied on numerous occasions, and the results of one recent study[12] illustrate some important physiological and clinical points. At pH 1.5 to 2.5 peptic activity was maximal. From pH 2.5 to 5.0, peptic activity persisted, but it decreased as pH 5 was approached. From pH 5 to 7, there was no peptic activity, but pepsin was stable at this pH level, as evidenced by complete restoration of activity when the mixture was adjusted to pH 2. Above pH 7.5, pepsin was irreversibly denatured, and a return to pH 2 did not restore any peptic activity.

Another interesting recent study compared hemoglobin and the cat esophagus as substrates for peptic activity of porcine pepsin.[13] As shown in Figure 15–1, with hemoglobin as the substrate, the pH optimum was 1.5 to 2.5, and peptic activity

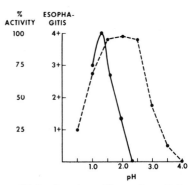

Figure 15–1. In vivo pH-pepsin activity curve, with esophageal proteins as substrate (———), is compared with that of an in vitro pH-pepsin activity curve utilizing hemoglobin as substrate (------). (From Goldberg, H. I., et al.: Gastroenterology 56:223, 1969.)

was not reduced to zero until the pH was 4.0. By contrast, with cat esophagitis as the endpoint, the pH optimum was approximately 1.2, and peptic activity became zero when the pH was raised above 2.3.

Although pepsin is irreversibly denatured in neutral or alkaline solutions, peptic activity is lost at only a very slow rate at pH 2.0. However, in solutions of pH 1 or less, pepsin digests itself, with more rapid loss of peptic activity.[2]

PEPSINOGEN SECRETION

Pepsinogen is secreted continuously in the resting or basal state in man. Secretion may occur independently of some of the other components of gastric juice, in part because synthesis is continuous and "overflow secretion" occurs when the peptic cells fill up with granules.[5] Thus, even when acid is absent, pepsinogen may be present in appreciable amounts in the gastric contents.[5]

Basal pepsinogen secretion is believed to result mainly from cholinergic stimulation, partly vagal and partly independent of the vagus nerve.[2, 5] The level of basal secretion presumably depends on the blood level of the various stimulants, the population of the pepsinogen secreting cells,[14] and the sensitivity of these cells. Basal secretion averages about 20 to 25 per cent of that after hypoglycemic stimulation with insulin.[5] Resting secretion is abolished or markedly reduced by atropine.[2]

In most species, including man, vagal and cholinergic mechanisms are the strongest stimuli of pepsinogen secretion,[15] and vagal tone increases the responsiveness of the peptic cells to other stimuli.[16] In man, hypoglycemic vagal stimulation enhances pepsinogen secretion from 10 to 20 per cent more strongly (relative to acid) than histamine.[5] Gastrin stimulates pepsinogen to about the same degree as histamine. For reasons that are apparently not understood, hyperventilation is a potent stimulus of pepsinogen secretion.[2, 15] Hypercalcemia induced by intravenous calcium infusion also increases pepsinogen secretion.[17]

Atropine inhibits pepsinogen secretion in response to vagal, hypercalcemic, and cholinergic stimulation, as well as that

response caused by histamine or gastrin.[15] In fact, atropine inhibits pepsinogen secretion even under conditions in which it does not reduce acid secretion, or inhibits acid secretion only slightly.[18] Magnesium will block the effect of hypercalcemia on pepsin (and acid) secretion.[17] Vagotomy diminishes pepsinogen secretion in response to most stimulants, but apparently not to antral irrigation with peptone broth.[19]

Although vagal stimulation, acetylcholine in small doses, hypercalcemia, gastrin, and histamine all stimulate the secretion of both acid and pepsinogen, there are a number of examples in which acid and pepsinogen secretion are affected differently. For instance, hyperventilation, Diamox, duodenal acidification, and secretin increase pepsinogen secretion and depress acid secretion.[2, 20] However, most stimulants of pepsin secretion stimulate all elements of gastric secretion, and acid and pepsinogen secretion rates usually go hand in hand when measured under most clinical and physiological circumstances.[15]

PEPSINOGEN SECRETION IN CLINICAL DISORDERS

By a variety of methods, most authors agree that patients with duodenal ulcer secrete more pepsinogen than normal subjects or than patients with gastric ulcer.[2] Since the concentration of pepsinogen is the same in gastric contents of the control and duodenal ulcer group, it has been suggested that the principal difference is higher volume of secretion in the duodenal ulcer group, resulting from increased mucosal mass (i.e., parallel increase in parietal and pepsinogen secreting cell masses).[15] Patients with pernicious anemia secrete only minute quantities of pepsinogen.[2]

Hunt[21] has reviewed data prior to 1957 on the relationship between acid and pepsinogen secretion, and concluded that both in normal subjects and in patients with peptic ulcer, the amount of pepsinogen secreted corresponds to the amount of acid secreted. This conclusion applied to basal secretion and to histamine, test meal, and hypoglycemia-stimulated secretion, but data on caffeine and cephalic stimulations were not available. Subsequently, it has been shown that acid and pepsinogen are secreted in equivalent amounts after stimulation by calcium infusion.[22]

Thus there is no evidence that gastric or duodenal ulcer is ever caused by a specific increase in pepsinogen secretion (out of proportion to the rate of acid secretion), and the low incidence of duodenal ulcer in women and the tendency of ulcer to heal during pregnancy cannot be accounted for by a drop in the secretion of pepsinogen without a drop in the concentration of acid.[21]

In spite of this general conclusion, which seems valid when all the available evidence is considered, there are several individual reports which suggest that pepsinogen output may be selectively increased in patients with duodenal ulcer. For instance, in a preliminary report it has been stated that pepsinogen secretion is increased in patients with active as compared with inactive duodenal ulcers, whereas acid secretion was apparently equal in the two groups.[23] It has sometimes been reported that acid secretion is higher in active than in inactive duodenal ulcer patients, but most studies do not confirm these impressions.

Methodological problems have made it difficult to measure pepsinogen secretion in disease states by the newer separation techniques. In a recent review,[4] Samloff concluded that there is no evidence at present for the existence of any abnormal proteases in patients with peptic ulcer, although Taylor[24] has reported that patients with both duodenal and gastric ulcer have a higher frequency and higher concentration of "pepsin I" (one of several group I pepsins) as measured by agar gel electrophoresis.

A few attempts have been made to estimate different pepsinogens and pepsins by indirect and less laborious techniques. In one study gastric juice was found to have two main peaks for optimal pH, 1.8 and 2.2.[25] Measurement of peptic activity at pH 2.2 was assumed to reflect pepsins originating in the fundic mucosa (group I pepsinogens), whereas peptic activity at pH 1.8 was assumed to represent pepsinogens originating in pyloric mucosa (group II pepsinogens). Control subjects and patients with duodenal ulcer had similar curves, with peptic activity greatest at pH 2.2. In patients with active gastric ulcer, peak peptic activity was at pH 1.8, whereas after healing, the pattern returned to normal. The authors suggest that in active gastric ulcer, the pyloric (group II) pepsinogens predominate. Obviously, these results need confirmation before they are accepted as generally valid.

PEPSIN: ACID RATIO

Recently several investigators have studied the ratio of pepsin to acid secretion in basal and stimulated gastric contents in control subjects and in patients with peptic ulcer.[9, 14, 26, 27] As shown in Figure 15–2, taken from Makhlouf,[9] pepsinogen secretion is proportional to acid secretion in the basal state and after stimulation with histamine or gastrin. However, the slopes of the regression lines are different, basal secretion containing about three times more pepsin relative to acid than the gastrin- or histamine-stimulated gastric juice. As predicted from this figure, patients with Zollinger-Ellison syndrome have low levels of pepsin in their basal gastric secretion, because hypersecretion of gastric juice in this disorder is mediated by high blood levels of gastrin, a strong stimulant of acid but a relatively weak stimulant of pepsin. This finding may aid

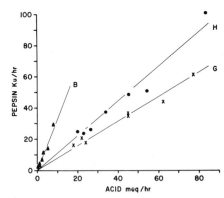

Figure 15–2. Relationship between acid and pepsin responses during the first hour following stimulation by gastrin II and histamine. B represents data during the basal hour. (From Makhlouf, G. M.: In Non-insulin Producing Tumors of the Pancreas, L. Demling and R. Ottenjann [eds.]. Stuttgart, Georg Thieme Verlag, 1969, p. 29.)

in the diagnosis of the Zollinger-Ellison syndrome.[9, 14, 26, 27]

In patients with common duodenal ulcer and in control subjects, the basal secretion shows considerable variation in the pepsin/acid ratio,[9, 14, 26, 27] but apparently no clinically or pathophysiologically important conclusions have been reached from the study of this ratio in this group of patients. Since stimulation by vagal pathways elicits a high pepsin response relative to acid secretion, the pepsin/acid ratio might be a good way to look for increased vagal tone in patients with gastric hypersecretion.

THE MUCOSAL BARRIER

It has recently been shown in canine fundic pouches that when the mucosal barrier to hydrogen diffusion is broken, pepsin output increases. It was suggested that this may be important in the pathogenesis of gastric ulceration.[28]

PEPSINOGEN IN BLOOD AND URINE

The serum contains proteolytic activity at low pH levels, and this is due to the presence in serum of pepsinogen, derived mainly from the chief cells in the stomach.[2] The serum pepsinogen level in any given healthy individual is relatively constant from day to day and does not change after eating or after injection of histamine or gastrin. It is believed that the serum pepsinogen level is related to the secretory capacity of the chief cells, although this has not been definitely proved.[2]

There is a fair correlation between serum pepsinogen level and the maximum concentration of pepsinogen in gastric juice when stimulated by histamine, but this correlation does not hold for basal conditions or after insulin stimulation. It is therefore not proper to speak in terms of gastric secretory activity if only the serum (or urinary) pepsinogen level is known.[2]

The concentration of pepsinogen in blood is elevated somewhat in patients with duodenal ulcer, implying a higher pepsinogen cell mass in the ulcer group.[2, 15] There is much overlap of values among control subjects and patients with duodenal ulcer, however.

Urinary pepsinogen also originates from the stomach,[2] and urinary excretion correlates roughly with gastric acid and pepsinogen secretion. Urinary pepsinogen level is, however, a poor index of gastric secretory function in an individual patient. The average urinary pepsinogen excretion is elevated in duodenal ulcer, normal in gastric ulcer, low in gastric cancer, and very low in pernicious anemia patients. Except in those with pernicious anemia, there is considerable overlap among patients in various disease groups.[2]

Both serum and urinary pepsinogen levels are raised in some patients with superficial gastritis,[1] presumably reflecting release of pepsinogen into blood from damaged pepsinogen secreting cells in the stomach.

Chromatographic studies have shown that both group I and group II pepsinogens are present in serum, whereas only group I pepsinogens are present in urine.[4] Group II pepsinogens are also found in seminal fluid, and theoretically might play a role in male fertility.[4] Group II pepsinogens are also present in esophageal mucosa.[4]

REFERENCES

1. Turner, M. D. Pepsinogens and pepsins. Gut 9:134, 1968.
2. Hirschowitz, B. I. Pepsinogen: Its origins, secretion and excretion. Physiol. Rev. 37:475, 1957.
3. Samloff, I. M. Slow moving protease and the seven pepsinogens. Electrophoretic demonstration of the existence of eight proteolytic fractions in human gastric mucosa. Gastroenterology 57:659, 1969.
4. Samloff, I. M. Pepsinogens, pepsins, and pepsin inhibitors. Gastroenterology 60:586, 1971.
5. Hirschowitz, B. I. In The Physiology of Pepsinogen in Pathophysiology of Peptic Ulcer, S. C. Skoryna (ed.). Philadelphia, J. B. Lippincott Co., 1963, p. 23.
6. Jeffries, G. H. Gastric secretion of intrinsic factor. Handbook of Physiology, Sect. 6, Vol. II, C. F. Code (ed.). Washington, D.C., American Physiological Society, 1967, p. 919.
7. Moore, E. W., and Makhlouf, G. M. Calcium in normal human gastric juice. A four-component model with speculation on the relation of calcium to pepsin secretion. Gastroenterology 55:465, 1968.
8. Crean, G. P., Marshall, M. W., and Rumsey, R. D.

E. Parietal cell hyperplasia induced by the administration of pentagastrin (ICI 50,123) to rats. Gastroenterology 57:147, 1969.

9. Makhlouf, G. M. Models for the pepsin response to gastrin and its derivatives in man. *In* Non-Insulin Producing Tumors of the Pancreas, L. Demling and R. Ottenjann (eds.). Stuttgart, Georg Thieme Verlag, 1969, p. 29.

10. Crean, G. P., Hogg, D. F., and Rumsey, R. D. E. Hyperplasia of the gastric mucosa produced by duodenal obstruction. Gastroenterology 56:193, 1969.

11. Crean, G. P., Gunn, A. A., and Rumsey, R. D. E. The effects of vagotomy on the gastric mucosa of the rat. Scand. J. Gastroenterol. 4:675, 1969.

12. Piper, D. W., and Fenton, B. H. *p*H stability and activity curves of pepsin with special reference to their clinical importance. Gut 6:506, 1965.

13. Goldberg, H. I., Dodds, W. J., Gee, S., Montgomery, C., and Zboralske, F. F. Role of acid and pepsin in acute experimental esophagitis. Gastroenterology 56:223, 1969.

14. Confils, S., and Lewin, M. More on models for the secretion of pepsin and other proteins. Gastroenterology 58:265, 1970.

15. Hirschowitz, B. I. Secretion of pepsinogen. *In* Handbook of Physiology, Sect. 6, Vol. II, C. F. Code (ed.). Washington, D.C., American Physiological Society, 1967, p. 889.

16. Emäs, S., and Grossman, M. I. Effect of truncal vagotomy on acid and pepsin responses to histamine and gastrin in dogs. Amer. J. Physiol. 212:1007, 1967.

17. Barreras, R. F., and Donaldson, R. M., Jr. Effects of induced hypercalcemia on human gastric secretion. Gastroenterology 52:670, 1967.

18. Rosato, E. F., Smith, G. P., and Brooks, F. P. Effect of atropine on acid and pepsin responses to histamine in conscious monkeys. Gastroenterology 55:68, 1968.

19. Tovey, F. I., Swaminathan, M., Parker, K., and Daniell, A. Effect of vagotomy on the gastric secretion of acid chloride and pepsin in response to antral stimulus and to insulin and maximal histamine stimulation. Gut 9:659, 1968.

20. Brooks, A. M., Isenberg, J., and Grossman, M. I. The effect of secretin, glucagon, and duodenal acidification on pepsin secretion in man. Gastroenterology 57:159, 1969.

21. Hunt, J. N. Some notes on the pathogenesis of duodenal ulcer. Amer. J. Dig. Dis. 2:445, 1957.

22. Smallwood, R. A. Effect of intravenous calcium administration on gastric secretion of acid and pepsin in man. Gut 8:592, 1967.

23. Venables, C. W. The relationship of pentagastrin-stimulated pepsin secretion to duodenal ulceration. Gut 10:1053, 1969.

24. Taylor, W. H. Pepsins of patients with peptic ulcer. Nature (London) 227:76, 1970.

25. Pritchard, M. H., and Connell, A. M. Peptic activity after the administration of pentagastrin and in gastroduodenal disease. Gut 10:303, 1969.

26. Makhlouf, G. M., Moore, E. W., and Blum, A. L. Models for the "secretion" of pepsin and other proteins by the human stomach. Gastroenterology 55:457, 1968.

27. Bader, J. P. Biological diagnosis of the Zollinger-Ellison syndrome. *In* Non-Insulin Producing Tumors of the Pancreas, L. Demling and R. Ottenjann (eds.). Stuttgart, Georg Thieme Verlag, 1969, p. 41.

28. Johnson, L. R. Pepsin output from the damaged canine Heidenhain pouch. Amer. J. Dig. Dis. 16:403, 1971.

Chapter 16

Gastrointestinal Bleeding

David H. Law, Daniel H. Gregory

INTRODUCTION

Gastrointestinal bleeding is not only one of the most common serious problems presented to the practicing physician; it is also one of the most vexing with regard to determining the specific cause and prescribing appropriate therapy. A correct approach to these problems requires early, close, and continuing cooperation among the primary care physician, surgeon, and radiologist.

Mortality for massive gastrointestinal bleeding is in the range of 5 to 50 per cent.[1-3] Major factors contributing to this high mortality include the failure to appreciate the problem as an emergent clinical situation and diagnostic errors in defining the source and site of bleeding.[4]

Since gastrointestinal bleeding is such a common clinical problem, it should be readily recognized. Bleeding may be profuse and manifested by *hematemesis* (vomiting of blood, either bright red or brown and precipitated, resembling coffee grounds), *melena* (the passage of tarry black, sticky stool with variable amounts of maroon or red blood interspersed), or *hematochezia* (the passage of fresh red blood per rectum). Bleeding, however, may be only *occult*, with normal appearing stools which, on chemical determination, are shown to contain blood. The significance of these varied manifestations will be discussed later, along with a presentation of the diagnostic and therapeutic approach to the patient with emergent or nonemergent gastrointestinal bleeding.

A series of general, nonlocalizing pathophysiological effects results from gastrointestinal blood loss, and these give rise to many of the symptoms and signs which have been shown to be of clinical importance in determining the presence and the severity of bleeding. There are, in addition, clinical and laboratory findings which indicate the probable site of bleeding and even the specific cause. There may be great difficulty in localizing the site of bleeding or establishing the nature of the bleeding lesion in a significant percentage of patients, especially during an initial episode.

PATHOPHYSIOLOGY OF GASTROINTESTINAL BLEEDING

The response of the patient to blood loss is, in large part, unrelated to the site or etiology of the lesion; rather it depends more upon the *rate* and *extent* of blood, fluid, and electrolyte loss and upon other factors such as the patient's age and associated medical problems (particularly cardiovascular). The effect of absorption of fluid and the degraded substances of blood is also important; however, the increased intestinal transit time associated with the presence of intraluminal blood initially minimizes this effect so that it does not greatly alter the initial response to acute gastrointestinal blood loss.

195

Bleeding may be categorized, arbitrarily, as *acute* or *chronic* and *massive* or *nonmassive.*

The most striking pathophysiological responses follow *acute massive* bleeding typified by loss of greater than 1500 ml of blood or 25 per cent of the circulating blood volume within a period of minutes to several hours. In this situation, as in the case of an equally large phlebotomy, a series of nonspecific cardiovascular responses ensues.[5,6] Cardiac output and systolic blood pressure decrease, followed by decreases in diastolic blood pressure, followed by tachycardia. Blood pressure responses are minimized with the patient in the horizontal position and may be noted first in the form of orthostatic hypotension. Indeed, using a tilt table device, or by cautiously comparing vital signs with the patient in the supine and sitting positions as a bedside evaluation, one can estimate the degree of blood loss by measuring blood pressure response to progressive elevation of the patient's head.

Pulse rate seems to be a far less accurate parameter and may be normal or even decreased during the early stages of bleeding, at a time when orthostatic hypotension is clearly evident to the point of syncope. There are compensatory vascular responses to the resultant decreased right atrial pressure and decreased cardiac output. Venous constriction maintains a higher percentage of the effective blood volume in the central circulation. Pulse rate usually does rise, and there is constriction of the arterial bed with skin pallor, decreased blood in the splanchnic arterial bed, and decreased renal blood flow with maintenance of blood flow to the cerebral and cardiopulmonary systems. If severe, this may be manifested by decreased urine flow or even anuria from acute tubular necrosis. Mesenteric vascular insufficiency may also result with bowel infarction and centrolobular necrosis of the liver as serious consequences. With continued acute blood loss, cerebral blood flow is embarrassed, reflected by electroencephalographic changes such as progressive generalized slowing of the pattern associated with clinical signs of confusion, progressing to obtundation. Blindness, which is rarely seen with acute hemorrhage and severe anemia, may result from severe retinal vessel spasm and retinal anoxia. Likewise, early electrocardiographic changes of T-wave flattening or inversion and possibly S-T segment depression document insufficiency of coronary blood flow. Most of these early, acute changes are responsive to replacement of the diminished plasma volume by blood transfusions or other plasma expanders such as electrolyte solutions (normal saline, Ringer's solution) or dextrans. If, however, loss continues unabated, the secondary effects of shock—increasing anoxia, cellular dysfunction, and acidosis—become evident and, if irreversible, lead to death.

More gradually after loss of blood volume, other compensatory physiological mechanisms such as release of antidiuretic hormone and aldosterone are initiated which act to re-establish intravascular volume at the expense of extravascular fluid. These fluid shifts are manifested by progressive dilution of plasma protein components, most notably a progressive drop in hematocrit or hemoglobin concentration.

Ebert et al. have shown that as much as one-third of this total effective plasma restoration may occur within the first two hours following a phlebotomy of about 1 liter, and up to half of the total compensation may occur within eight hours.[7] Clinically, considerable variation in this compensatory response is noted among individuals, depending upon their state of hydration, age, ability to resorb fluid lost into the gut, and the rate of both oral and parenteral fluid repletion. Thus the lowest hemoglobin levels and highest degree of plasma expansion may be noted as early as a few hours or as long as several days after an acute hemorrhage. The final plasma volume may be even greater than normal because of this compensatory mechanism. For these reasons hematocrit and hemoglobin concentration values may be difficult to interpret during acute bleeding episodes.

The hematopoietic system responds in a bimodal manner—first, with an abrupt increase in white blood cell count in response to the stress of bleeding, and then, frequently, with an outpouring of platelets into the peripheral circulation.

More sluggish responses to stimulation of the bone marrow include increase in red blood cell production, peripheral reticulocytosis, and gradual correction of hemoglobin concentration over a period of weeks, if adequate metabolic precursors (iron, folate, etc.) are available.

All these pathophysiological phenomena, especially those occurring abruptly, may be altered by a wide variety of factors peculiar to individual patients. Anticholinergic agents, ganglionic blocking agents, pitressin, and many other drugs which affect vascular tone may alter compensatory responses. The presence of preexisting oxygen unsaturation or dehydration and the level of blood volume or hematocrit at the onset of bleeding may also have a profound effect on the pathophysiological sequel. The age of the patient and the state of his vasculature, including the presence of severe arteriosclerotic disease, the level of plasma proteins, the presence of other disorders (spinal cord disease and neuropathy, liver failure, impaired renal function, endotoxic shock, congestive heart failure), and, finally, the rapidity with which the patient is treated all may alter these classic responses and must be considered when evaluating the clinical signs and symptoms which are the manifestations of the pathophysiological responses to acute blood loss. By recognizing these responses, the amount of reduction in blood volume can be immediately estimated and a logical sequence of diagnostic studies outlined to define the source and site of bleeding. The results of these studies will dictate appropriate management based upon whether the gastrointestinal bleeding is massive and emergent or less severe and/or chronic.

ESTIMATING BLOOD LOSS

Clearly, the volume of blood loss is the single most important parameter to be defined when one is initially confronted with a patient bleeding from the gastrointestinal tract. This information will establish the relative emergency of the problem and set the diagnostic and therapeutic pace to follow.

Although the clinical history is often nondiagnostic, it will provide valuable information in about one-third of patients and should be thoroughly evaluated. A single episode of hematemesis or melena should be distinguished from persistent hematemesis or melena and the latter estimated in terms of days or weeks. Qualitative characteristics of bleeding, such as the presence of clots and bright red, mahogany, and coffee ground material, have little quantitative significance but may help localize bleeding to a given area of the gastrointestinal tract.

Examination of the patient provides the best means of assessing blood loss. This can and should be done immediately and rapidly. The findings are based on the responses previously outlined. As a general rule, blood pressure less than 100 mm Hg or a pulse rate exceeding 100 per minute, in an otherwise normotensive patient, indicates a 20 per cent volume depletion.[8] Associated pallor and/or postural hypotension lend support to this estimate. Especially significant may be the loss of pink coloration in the palmar creases of the extended hand. A pulse rate increase of 20 per minute or blood pressure decreases of greater than 10 mm Hg in response to a postural change (i.e., sitting the patient up) further suggest acute blood loss in excess of 1000 cc. These parameters should be monitored at frequent intervals and sequential changes noted on a flow sheet at the patient's bedside. These sheets also should record transfusions, total fluid intake and output, and quantities of electrolytes as well as drugs administered (see Fig. 16–1).

Immediate *laboratory* evaluation should include a white blood cell count, hematocrit, hemoglobin, blood urea nitrogen, and prothrombin time. Bleeding diathesis should be evaluated. In all cases a nasogastric tube should be inserted and an estimate made of the amount of gross blood present, and guaiac tests performed on gastric contents. Stool guaiac test of rectal contents must also be done. Hemoglobin less than 11 g per 100 ml and a blood urea nitrogen (BUN) greater than 40 mg per 100 ml in an otherwise normal patient indicate a blood loss greater than 1000 cc, because the digestive products of blood in the upper intestine are resorbed and subsequently reflected in the BUN level. In the presence of a normal serum creatinine, a BUN above 40 mg per 100 ml thus

GASTROINTESTINAL BLEEDING:　　FLOW SHEET

Date: 4/17/73 Times:

CLINICAL:	AM	1³⁰	2³⁰				
Mental Status	CONFUSED		CLEAR				
Pulse	140	120	100				
Blood Pressure Supine	90/60	100/70	110/76				
Upright	—	70/50	100/70				
C.V.P.	1	2	6				
Gastric Lavage	bloody	bROWN	cLEAR				
Stool	bloody		500 cc blACk				
LABORATORY: Hg/Hct	7/20		8.5/25				
WBC	20,000	—	—				
BUN/ Creatinine	45/1.8						
Prothrombin (Sec.)	14	—					
Arterial pH & Gases							
Blood Electrolytes	NA 140 K 3.7						
DIAGNOSTIC: Note Endoscopy, Barium Studies angiography, string test, intubation, etc	ESOPHAGOSCOPY NEG.		X-RAY D.U.				
THERAPY: Blood Products	—	1500 whole BLOOD →					
Fluids (IV & PO)	1000 RiNGeRS						
Electrolytes	''						
Pharmacologic Rx	20 U. PITRESSIN						
Tamponade with pressure							
COMMENTS:							

NAME　　BLEEDER, G.I.

HOSP. NO. 000 000

Figure 16–1.

provides a valuable index of the extent of intestinal bleeding. Cessation of bleeding is accompanied by a rapid fall of the BUN (the level returning to normal within two to three days), and sequential determinations are as important as the initial measurement during the early stages of evaluation.[9] Blood volume measurements, when available, using Cr^{51}-tagged red blood cells or radioiodinated human serum albumin, may be a valuable adjunctive procedure to the other studies. This technique is especially valuable for patients in whom the assessment of bleeding is complicated by their inability to compensate normally owing to debility, associated infection, or serious cardiovascular disease. Although leukocytosis as high as 20,000 per mm^3 may be present with bleeding from the gastrointestinal tract, other causes must always be considered also.

When any of the aforementioned parameters indicate massive gastrointestinal hemorrhage, the clinical situation shall subsequently be termed emergent. This requires immediate management as outlined below.

MANAGEMENT OF THE PATIENT WITH EMERGENT BLEEDING

VOLUME REPLACEMENT

It is important to stress that management of patients with massive bleeding frequently does not permit the luxury of a thorough diagnostic search. Immediate steps must be taken to minimize the morbidity and potential mortality caused by the massive gastrointestinal hemorrhage per se.

The most important single aim in the management of emergent bleeding is the maintenance of an adequate blood volume. This first requires free flowing access to the intravascular space which can be achieved by either one or more large bore, 14 to 18 gauge needles placed securely in a large peripheral vein, or by an indwelling catheter of similar size advanced into a more central vein; indeed, with massive bleeding or shock two such access lines are desirable. Such central venous pressure measurement may be a valuable guide in determining the need for increasing or decreasing subsequent plasma expansion. Simultaneously with typing and cross matching of blood for transfusion, some form of plasma expander should be infused. Normal saline solution, Ringer's lactate solution, or even 5 per cent dextrose solution may be used initially, but dextran 6 per cent (molecular weight 60,000) or Plasmanate may be more effective while awaiting the arrival of whole blood. Currently the only practical means of re-establishing and maintaining adequate oxygen carrying capacity is through transfusion of whole blood or packed red blood cells.

GASTRIC LAVAGE

Following establishment of intravenous access, one should place an intragastric, large bore tube (ex. No. 30 F. Ewald or double-bore tube). Detection of blood in the gastric aspirate confirms a bleeding site proximal to the ligament of Treitz; however, the failure to find blood does not exclude this possibility. If blood is present, one should continuously lavage the stomach with ice water or saline until it is free of clots and returns are clear. The mechanisms by which this lavage controls hemorrhage are not certain but may include cold-induced vasoconstriction in the splanchnic bed and decreased local fibrinolytic activity. It may be of additional value by minimizing vomiting and providing continuous monitoring of the degree of bleeding. The tube should remain in the stomach for 24 hours following control of hemorrhage so that any further or recurrent bleeding may be detected.

The patient with suspected esophageal variceal hemorrhage constitutes a special problem and will be discussed separately in the section dealing with portal hypertension.

When gastrointestinal hemorrhage manifests as bright red rectal bleeding, early proctoscopy should be performed, because up to three-fourths of colonic disease occurs within reach of the 25 cm proctosigmoidoscope (vide infra).

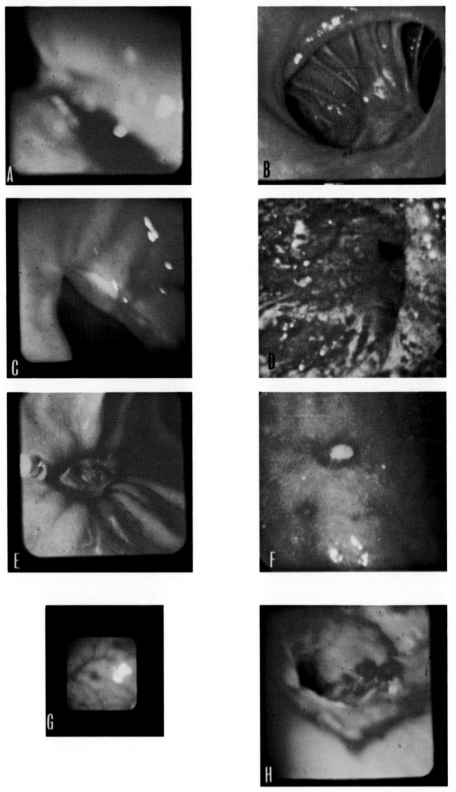

Figure 16–2. (Dr. George J. Brodmerkel, Jr., Allegheny General Hospital, Pittsburgh, Pa., contributed gastrophotographs *A, C, E, F* and *H*. Dr. Arnold Kaplan, Minneapolis Veterans Hospital, provided gastrophotographs *B* and *D*. The diagrams illustrating pertinent features of the color photographs were drawn by M. Norviel, University of New Mexico Department of Medical Illustration.)

Figure 16–2 continued on opposite page.

200

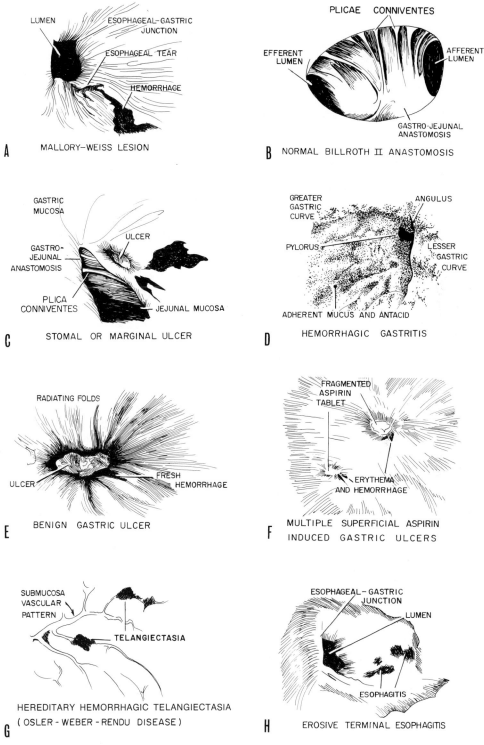

Figure 16–2 *Continued.*

PHARMACOLOGICAL AGENTS

The use of vasoconstrictor drugs is appropriate when the clinical situation is critical, but great care must be taken if the patient has evidence of hypertensive or arteriosclerotic cardiovascular disease. Rapid vasopressin infusion (20 units, diluted in 100 to 200 cc D5/w intravenously over 20 minutes) has been shown to be effective.[10] At times (vide infra), direct selective arterial infusion of vasoactive agents (Pitressin, epinephrine, or propranolol) may be directed at the bleeding lesion. Intravenous vitamin K (25 mg) is indicated when there is an abnormally prolonged prothrombin time. Other clotting defects should be defined and corrected (vide infra).

GENERAL APPROACH

Immediate documentation of the anatomic site of bleeding will help to determine whether the management is to be medical or surgical. In either case, an appropriate diagnostic and therapeutic plan outlined in advance will minimize operating and anesthesia time and permit optimal employment of specialized diagnostic procedures.

HISTORY AND EXAMINATION

In the acute situation, nine points of high diagnostic value may be investigated.

1. Presence of hematemesis indicates a bleeding site above the ligament of Treitz, whereas passage of red blood per rectum is most frequently associated with a bleeding site below the ligament of Treitz, usually from the colon.

2. Establishment of the temporal relationship of hematemesis to forceful vomiting suggests a Mallory-Weiss syndrome or esophageal rupture (Fig. 16–2) (see pp. 468 to 475).

3. The character of typical abdominal pain may suggest peptic ulcer or reflux esophagitis (see pp. 430 to 449 and 621 to 654).

4. Stress ulcers may occur hours to days following trauma, severe burns, or surgical procedures.

5. Associated and previous diseases may suggest the source of gastrointestinal hemorrhage; i.e., alcoholism is associated with gastritis and varices; arthritis is associated with salicylate and other drug ingestion which may cause gastritis; diverticulosis may bleed massively; emphysema carries an increased risk for development of peptic ulcer; cirrhosis and peptic ulcer suggest sources of blood loss.

6. Past surgical procedures may suggest a bleeding stomal ulcer (Fig. 16–2) or recurrent malignancy; an aortic aneurysm or prosthetic repair infrequently results in an intestinal vascular fistula.

7. Medications and toxins (analgesics, adrenocorticosteroids, antihypertensives, and alcohol) may be associated with gastritis or peptic ulcer (Fig. 16–2, D, E, and F) (see pp. 621 to 626 and 642 to 654).

8. The age and ethnic group of the patient can be important (e.g., duodenal ulcer is extremely rare in the American Indian).

9. Diarrhea, urgency, tenesmus, or abdominal cramps preceding passage of red blood per rectum may be indicative of colonic neoplasm or inflammatory bowel disease, including ulcerative colitis, regional enteritis, or amebic colitis (see pp. 1296 to 1367).

These nine clinical points should be considered along with the available statistical information from large series of cases in which the anatomic site of intestinal bleeding has been ascertained. The most common sources of upper and lower gastrointestinal hemorrhage are shown in Table 16–1.

The *physical examination* is of particular value in rapidly detecting associated disease which may be pertinent to gastrointestinal bleeding. In addition to changes in blood pressure, pulse rate, and skin pallor, one should focus particularly on the oral pharynx, skin changes of the upper trunk, hepatosplenomegaly, adenopathy, the presence of a rectal mass, and overt congenital anomalies. Bright red telangiectasias grouped about the mouth, lips, nose, and fingers are the lesions of the Osler-Weber-Rendu disease (Fig. 16–2). Buccal plus labial spots of brown pigmentation with similar lesions on the hands and fingers are characteristic of the Peutz-Jeghers syndrome with intestinal tumors

TABLE 16–1. SOURCES OF
GASTROINTESTINAL HEMORRHAGE

I. *Upper gastrointestinal bleeding*
  A. Inflammatory
    Duodenal ulcer
    Gastritis
    Gastric ulcer
    Esophagitis
    Stress ulcer
    Pancreatitis
  B. Mechanical
    Hiatus hernia
    Mallory-Weiss syndrome
    Hematobilia
  C. Vascular
    Esophageal or gastric varices
    Aortointestinal fistula
    Hemangioma
    Rendu-Osler-Weber syndrome
    Mesenteric vascular occlusion
    Blue nevus bleb
  D. Systemic
    Blood dyscrasias
    Collagen diseases
    Uremia
  E. Neoplasms
    Carcinoma
    Polyps—single, multiple, Peutz-Jeghers
      syndrome
    Leiomyoma
    Carcinoid
    Leukemia
    Sarcoma
II. *Lower gastrointestinal bleeding*
  A. Inflammatory
    Ulcerative colitis
    Diverticulitis
    Enterocolitis, regional (Crohn's disease)
    Enterocolitis, tuberculous
    Enterocolitis, radiation
    Enterocolitis, bacterial
    Enterocolitis, toxic
  B. Mechanical
    Diverticulosis
  C. Neoplasms
    Carcinoma
    Polyps—adenomatous and villous, familial
      polyposis, Peutz-Jeghers syndrome
    Leiomyoma
    Sarcoma
    Lipoma
    Metastatic (melanoma)
  D. Anomalies
    Meckel's diverticulum
  E. Vascular
    Hemorrhoids
    Aortoduodenal fistula
    Aortic aneurysm
    Hemangioma
    Mesenteric thrombosis
    Hereditary hemorrhagic telangiectasia
    Blue nevus bleb
  F. Systemic
    Blood dyscrasias
    Collagen diseases
    Uremia

(see pp. 1056 to 1057). A dark blue cutaneous bleb which collapses on compression and rapidly refills may be a clue to a similar bleeding intestinal lesion (blue rubber bleb nevus syndrome). Spider nevi scattered over the upper trunk associated with scleral icterus, palmar erythema, and hepatosplenomegaly are manifestations of cirrhosis with portal hypertension and varices. Malignancy and polyposis may manifest as adenopathy or be recognized on rectal exam. The triad of icterus, crampy right upper quadrant pain, and hematemesis may suggest hemobilia.

ENDOSCOPY VERSUS X-RAY

The clinical decision as to which of the two studies should be done first and when to do them requires judgment based on available information and the technical skills of the immediately available personnel. If peptic ulcer seems the most likely probability after considering all factors, a *barium-contrast study* of the esophagus, stomach, and upper intestine would be the procedure most likely to yield a diagnosis, while minimizing diagnostic risks. Conversely, evidence suggesting Mallory-Weiss syndrome, gastritis, or portal hypertension (vide infra) is an indication for *panendoscopy* as the *initial* diagnostic procedure. When skilled panendoscopy is not readily available and in the absence of any information upon which to make a decision, the barium-contrast examination would be the best choice, based on the statistical probability that the bleeding site would be a peptic ulcer of the duodenum.

PANENDOSCOPY

The availability of a wide selection of flexible fiberoptic instruments for direct visualization of the esophageal, gastric, and now the duodenal mucosa (Figs. 16–2 and 16–3) has greatly enhanced the contribution of endoscopy in detecting the precise location and lesion responsible for gastrointestinal bleeding. It is the most reliable procedure for diagnosing mucosal diseases of the esophagus, stomach, and duodenum. Although the choice of instrument will depend on the endoscopist,

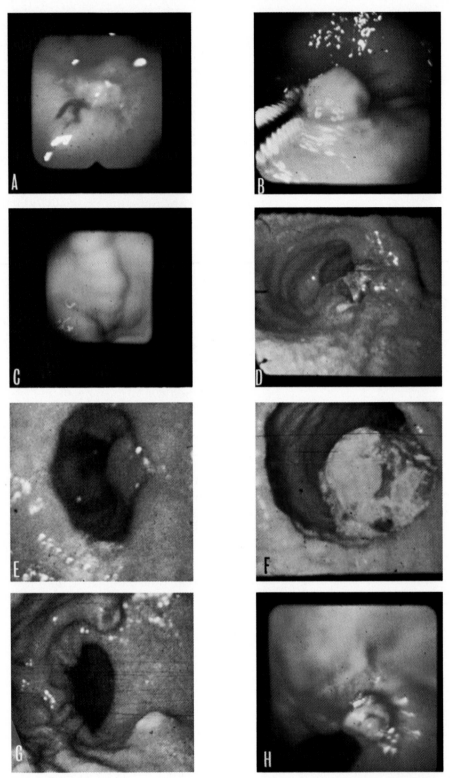

Figure 16–3. (Gastrophotographs *B* and *H* were contributed by Dr. George Brodmerkel, Jr., Allegheny General Hospital, Pittsburgh, Pa. *A* and *G* were provided by Dr. Jack Vennes, Minneapolis Veterans Hospital and University of Minnesota School of Medicine. The diagrams illustrating pertinent features of the color photographs were drawn by M. Norviel, University of New Mexico Department of Medical Illustration.)

Figure 16–3 continued on opposite page.

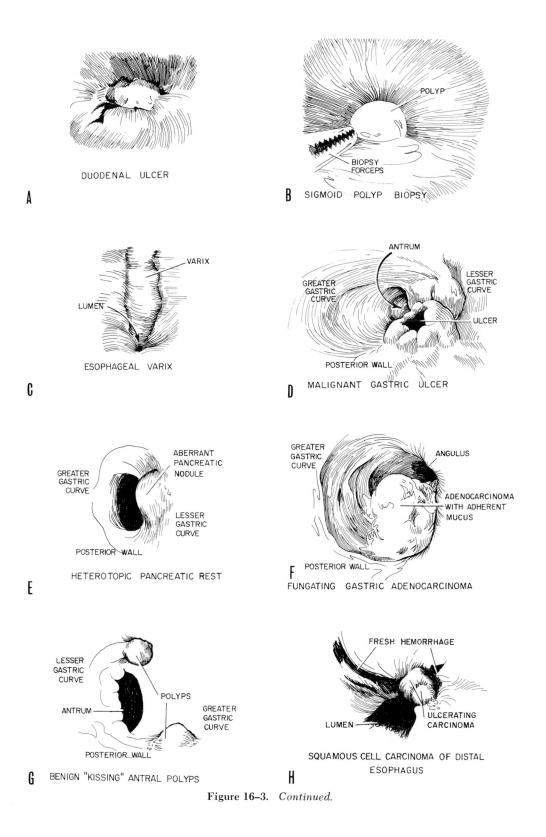

A DUODENAL ULCER

B SIGMOID POLYP BIOPSY

POLYP

BIOPSY FORCEPS

C ESOPHAGEAL VARIX

VARIX

LUMEN

D MALIGNANT GASTRIC ULCER

ANTRUM

GREATER GASTRIC CURVE

LESSER GASTRIC CURVE

ULCER

POSTERIOR WALL

E HETEROTOPIC PANCREATIC REST

ABERRANT PANCREATIC NODULE

GREATER GASTRIC CURVE

LESSER GASTRIC CURVE

POSTERIOR WALL

F FUNGATING GASTRIC ADENOCARCINOMA

GREATER GASTRIC CURVE

ANGULUS

ADENOCARCINOMA WITH ADHERENT MUCUS

POSTERIOR WALL

G BENIGN "KISSING" ANTRAL POLYPS

LESSER GASTRIC CURVE

ANTRUM

POLYPS

GREATER GASTRIC CURVE

POSTERIOR WALL

H SQUAMOUS CELL CARCINOMA OF DISTAL ESOPHAGUS

FRESH HEMORRHAGE

LUMEN

ULCERATING CARCINOMA

Figure 16–3. *Continued.*

we favor the 100 cm fiberoptic, forward viewing scope with wide angle vision and externally controlled, flexible tip. The capacity for photography provides a permanent record (Figs. 16–2 and 16–3), and the ability to obtain biopsy and cytological specimens further increases the diagnostic specificity of this instrument. Although skilled endoscopy in the emergent setting can be performed with minimum risk to the patient and provides vital diagnostic information, it should be emphasized that optimal visualization requires proper timing of the procedure, a clean stomach, and a relaxed, cooperative patient. These conditions are best accomplished when the patient's clinical situation is stable. Following the preparative ice water lavage previously mentioned, a topical pharyngeal gargle with 0.5 to 2.0 per cent Pontocaine is effective in suppressing the gag reflex, and the intravenous administration of a short-acting narcotic with atropine provides adequate relaxation and reduced pharyngeal secretions. (Diazepam [Valium] 5 to 15 mg given intravenously, or atropine, 0.6 mg mixed to volume with isotonic saline in a 20 cc syringe, is recommended). Sodium pentobarbital or meperidine is advocated by some endoscopists before administration of the topical anesthetic and diazepam. Nondiagnostic or technically poor endoscopy performed in the emergent situation may be repeated electively at a later date and will often confirm the initial diagnosis or contribute valuable follow-up information (see pp. 521 to 535).

X-RAY

Radiological evaluation is the procedure of choice when peptic ulceration is the most likely diagnosis. This procedure is least beneficial in acute esophagitis and gastritis (Fig. 16–2). It must be performed with close cooperation between the primary care physician and a well informed radiologist with preplanned course of action and special handling of the patient to avoid delays or untoward risks while the patient is away from his bed. A major disadvantage of the contrast barium exam is inability to associate an observed lesion with the bleeding site. Thus, in the presence of multiple lesions defined by X-ray, panendoscopy should be performed to establish which lesion is bleeding. Diagnostic accuracy of the upper gastrointestinal series therefore varies with the site of bleeding and should be considered complementary rather than supplmentary to panendoscopy. Cinefluoroscopy and hypotonic duodenography have increased the sensitivity of this procedure, but the latter rarely offers anything in the management of the patient with emergent bleeding.

NONDIAGNOSTIC X-RAY AND ENDOSCOPY

If panendoscopy and barium contrast studies are nondiagnostic and the rate of blood loss is >0.5 cc per minute, celiac and superior mesenteric angiography should be done while the patient is in the radiology unit. At this rate of bleeding, puddling may be noted within the lumen of the bowel. In addition, vascular malformations may occasionally be shown even when they are not bleeding actively. Although minimal risk is involved, the diagnostic reward in this setting makes this an acceptable procedure.[11] Since barium may interfere with angiographic visualization of the bleeding site, this study should probably be performed immediately after negative panendoscopy. In addition, when a bleeding lesion is identified, the catheter may be left in place and used in conjunction with a constant infusion pump to infuse vasoactive drugs such as Pitressin, propranolol, and epinephrine directly into the arterial system feeding the bleeding lesion. This approach is receiving growing support.[12, 13]

When all these studies are nondiagnostic and active bleeding persists, small intestine intubation with a 200-cm small-bore polyvinyl tube with sequential aspirations of the intestinal content may localize the bleeding site. Barium-contrast study should be performed through the tube to document a lesion at the site of bleeding. This test is most useful for locating obscure bleeding sites between the ligament of Treitz and the ileocecal valve, such as small bowel tumors, ulcers, Meckel's diverticula, or vascular anomalies.

EMERGENT LOWER GASTROINTESTINAL BLEEDING

Massive hemorrhage from lesions distal to the ileocecal valve is much less common than from the upper gastrointestinal tract. Nevertheless, when confronted by the patient in shock with profuse bright red bleeding from the rectum, the clinical setting is emergent. Blood volume must be restored, and the pertinent history acquired, as well as examination and laboratory procedures already outlined. The patient should then undergo immediate rectal examination and proctosigmoidoscopy without a cleansing preparation.

PROCTOSIGMOIDOSCOPY

Since rectal examination and proctosigmoidoscopy are most likely to detect the site and source of lower gastrointestinal bleeding, they should be done immediately in all patients suspected of lower bowel hemorrhage. The perianal region is scrutinized for the presence of fissures, fistulas, or hemorrhoids, and the rectal vault carefully palpated for tumor masses. The distal rectal mucosa should be adequately visualized for the presence of ulcers, strictures, edema, friability, inflammation, purulent discharges, tumors, and other active bleeding sites. Specimens should be aspirated for culture and examinations for parasites and cytology. A cotton swab should be employed to wipe off the mucous coat and evaluate the texture of the underlying mucosa for granularity and friability as may be seen in diffuse ulcerative colitis.

RADIOLOGICAL EVALUATION

If proctoscopy indicates blood coming from a point above the instrument, one of two radiological approaches should be considered. A barium enema may be performed and, if indicated, an air-contrast study which may outline polyps or small lesions not visualized in the barium-filled colon. Particular attention should be focused on the cecum for filling defects suggesting neoplasm. The terminal ileum is often seen with barium reflux and may

show terminal ileitis, an infrequent cause of massive gastrointestinal bleeding. Diverticula are increasingly frequent in older patients, but only rarely bleed and therefore cannot necessarily be implicated as the cause of bleeding merely by their presence. They do, however, constitute up to 70 per cent of the lower gastrointestinal lesions which bleed massively.[14]

The second possibility is to proceed initially and immediately to selective arteriographic studies in order to localize the bleeding site directly. This has been especially effective in patients with active bleeding from an obscure locus of diverticulosis and may save the surgeon great uncertainty if emergency operation is required.[13] In the patient with cirrhosis and portal hypertension, bleeding may occasionally occur from colonic varices.

COLONOSCOPY

Direct visualization of the entire colonic mucosa is now possible with the fiberoptic colonoscope.[15] Photography, biopsy, and cytology accessories are available with most instruments. Presently the cost and complexity of this instrument have restricted its use to a few medical centers in the United States. However, initial reports indicate that fiberoptic colonoscopy provides a valuable supplement to proctoscopy and barium enema for localizing colonic bleeding sites. Additionally, the capacity for obtaining biopsy specimens and cytological material increases the diagnostic usefulness of this instrument. In skilled hands, the midtransverse colon can be visualized in 70 per cent of patients. High diagnostic accuracy has been reported in detecting a wide spectrum of colonic lesions. Its use in massive bleeding is yet to be established and necessitates that the colon be clean. This may be accomplished by preparation with a liquid lunch and supper on the day prior to examination and oral administration of magnesium citrate (10 oz) and two or three Dulcolax tablets the night prior to study, followed by cleansing enemas prior to the examination. In patients with massive hemorrhage, however, this preparation is not feasible.

EMERGENCY SURGERY

Emergency surgical intervention must be considered for the patient with shock caused by uncontrollable massive hemorrhage with or without localization of the lesion. A number of specific situations associated with gastrointestinal bleeding have an increased mortality and suggest the need for early surgery, such as rebleeding while hospitalized with good medical management, and advanced age of patients (over 60 years). Time is usually critical in the management of such patients, and in this light the advisability of delaying surgery to perform diagnostic studies to localize the bleeding site must be carefully considered.

MANAGEMENT OF THE PATIENT WITH NONEMERGENT BLEEDING

In patients with nonemergent bleeding, a more deliberate plan involving detailed history, physical examination, and selected special studies, including endoscopy and complete radiological survey of the gastrointestinal tract, may be undertaken. Since bleeding may not be evident grossly, laboratory data may prove more important in establishing its existence and defining its source. Inspection and guaiac tests of fresh stool are important in assessing the presence and extent of nonemergent gastrointestinal bleeding.

Factors which influence the character of the stool include its volume, the action of digestive bacterial enzymes, and intestinal transit time. Blood pigments are considered the source of stool coloration. It has been demonstrated experimentally that the introduction of 100 ml of whole blood into the upper intestine may produce melena.[16] When 1000 ml of whole blood is placed in the upper intestine, melenic stools may persist for up to five days. It should be emphasized that any volume of blood over 100 ml placed in the upper intestine may initially result in a red stool if intestinal transit time is rapid.[16,17] The effect of bacterial action on stool color has been determined by observing red stools after placing 400 ml of whole blood in the upper intestine in subjects who had been pretreated with oral Neomycin.[18] Experiments in which peristalsis has been increased or decreased with pharmacological agents have shown that transit time from bleeding site to rectum is more important than volume of intraluminal blood or bacterial action in determining the appearance of the stool. Abnormal transit accounts for the clinical observations that, on the one hand, bright red rectal bleeding may result from a duodenal ulcer, and, on the other hand, melena is frequently associated with an obstructing neoplasm in the sigmoid colon. Black stools, of course, may occur as a result of ingested drugs such as bismuth compounds and iron.

A difficult problem with respect to localization of the bleeding site is encountered in the patient with normal appearing stools and a clinical history and examination suggesting gastrointestinal bleeding. This paradoxical combination of data indicates either that the bleeding has ceased or that the blood loss has not exceeded 100 ml per 24 hours.

STUDY OF OCCULT BLEEDING

GUAIAC

A number of laboratory tests are available to detect occult gastrointestinal bleeding.[19] Only the guaiac reagent has a range of reactivity most suitable for clinical use. Proper application of this test is based upon the assumption that the average adult daily stool bulk is 60 to 250 g and the normal daily fecal blood loss is less than 2.5 ml. If one accepts these physiological conditions, the adult with a hemoglobin of 18.3 g per 100 ml will have a stool hemoglobin concentration of 1.83 mg per ml. Whole blood diluted with isotonic saline to this concentration (Table 16–2) shows a 2+ guaiac reaction and 4+ benzidine reaction. Thus, guaiac reactions less than 3+ and all benzidine reactions are of questionable pathological significance and require correlation with daily stool bulk. Furthermore, interpretation of the guaiac test depends more upon the *rapidity* with which the color reaction develops than the intensity of color. A 4+ reaction develops in less than three seconds and a 3+ reaction appears within ten seconds. Robitussin

**TABLE 16–2. QUANTITATIVE
GUAIAC REACTION***

DILUTIONS	HEMOGLOBIN mg/ml	GUAIAC REACTION	BENZIDINE REACTION
Undil.	183	4+	4+
1:10	18.3	3+–4+	4+
1:100 †	1.83	2+	4+
1:500	0.9	1+	4+
1:1000	0.18	±	4+
1:5000	0.09	Neg.	4+
1:10,000	0.018	Neg.	4+

*J. Wheeler, unpublished data.
†*Calculation*: 2.5 ml of blood per 250 g of feces would equal 1.0 ml of blood per 100 g feces, and 1.0 ml blood is equivalent to 183 mg of hemoglobin if the hemoglobin concentration is 18.3 g per 100 ml of blood. 0.183 mg hemoglobin per 100 g of feces equals 1.83 mg hemoglobin per gram of feces or approximates 1.83 mg of hemoglobin per cubic centimeter of feces.

will give a positive guaiac reaction. Each laboratory should determine its own standards. The increasing scarcity of guaiac may necessitate substitute reagents with comparable sensitivity. Replacement of guaiac with orthotoluidine (0.2 per cent) and 0.3 per cent hydrogen peroxide rather than the standard 3.0 per cent hydrogen peroxide may be used in the same manner with approximately equal sensitivity. Vomitus, gastric, and small bowel aspirates should be tested for the presence of occult blood in patients suspected of bleeding also.

STRING TEST

An extension of this technique, the so-called string test, is used to localize a site of intestinal bleeding of submassive degree.[20] A flat, absorbent, commercially prepared, one-half inch umbilical tape (type II, manufactured by Advanced Laboratory Associates, Inc., 517 Miltown Road, North New Brunswick, N.J.), with longitudinally measured radiopaque markers and weighted, preferably by a mercury filled bag, should be passed orally to the ligament of Treitz (100 cm). Tape placement must be confirmed by radiologic evaluation of the abdomen (Fig. 16–4). While the patient is on the X-ray table, 20 cc (two ampules) of 5 per cent sodium fluorescite is

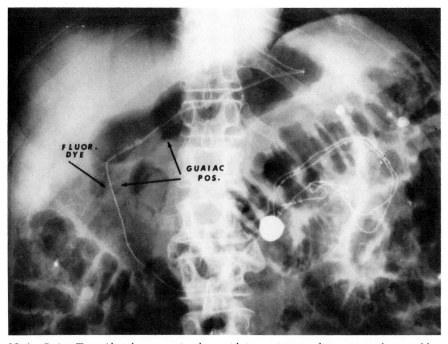

Figure 16–4. String Test. Absorbent tape in place with intermittent radiopaque markers visible to the level of the ligament of Trietz. Intravenous administration of sodium fluorescein dye may stain the string at the site of gastrointestinal hemorrhage and provide valuable diagnostic information in patients with occult gastrointestinal bleeding. (From Harrison, T. R.: Principles of Internal Medicine. 4th ed. New York, McGraw-Hill Book Co., 1962.)

administered intravenously over a two to three minute period. If this test is to yield valid results, careful attention should be focused on two details. First, sodium fluorescite readily contaminates everything it contacts. This necessitates the use of rubber gloves when withdrawing fluorescein from the vial. Gloves should be changed before intravenous administrations and again prior to withdrawing the tape from the patient. Second, the tape should not be left in place more than four minutes after fluorescein injection in order to prevent false-positive staining by hepatic secretion of fluorescein. Carefully extracting the string onto a towel held under the mouth will prevent autocontamination of fluorescein from one section of string to another. The presence of gross blood should be noted and testing with guaiac reagent performed. The location of yellow fluorescence under ultraviolet light with a Wood filter should be noted in a completely darkened room after soaking the string with alkaline alcohol at pH 7.8. Fluorescence will accurately localize the bleeding site.

SMALL BOWEL INTUBATION

When the aforementioned studies and routine radiography are nondiagnostic and persistent active bleeding is suspected, a small intestine aspiration study should be performed. The patient is intubated with a 200 cm small-bore polyvinyl weighted tip tube (PV-200) with sequential aspirations at 10 cm intervals. The intestinal aspirates are inspected for gross blood and tested for occult blood. When an aspirate is positive, barium or another contrast substance is instilled in order to outline the bleeding area. Prior to intubation, a specimen of the patient's red cells may be obtained and labeled with Cr^{51} and then administered intravenously, providing a sensitive marker for detecting the site of active bleeding from the intestine. This test is most useful for locating obscure bleeding sites between the ligament of Treitz and the ileocecal valve.[21] The combination of the string test and sequential aspiration techniques makes it possible to discriminate between an active bleeding site and the presence of stagnated old blood.

DIAGNOSTIC LAPAROTOMY

In approximately 10 to 20 per cent of patients with gastrointestinal bleeding the aforementioned sequence of diagnostic studies will fail to define the anatomic bleeding site or establish a diagnosis. Faced with the possibility of occult malignancy or recurrent bleeding, the question of exploratory laparotomy must be considered. Little information is available, however, regarding the diagnostic and therapeutic value of this procedure, although it has been reported to yield a positive or probable diagnosis in 47 per cent of cases when all other means have failed.[22] Further, on the basis of laparotomy findings, definite surgical therapy can prevent further bleeding in about one-third of these patients. There is no correlation between laparotomy findings, patient age, number of explorations, and duration of bleeding. The lesions most frequently found at laparotomy are peptic ulcer, malignancy, and diffuse intestinal disease. Gastrotomy is considered essential for detecting peptic ulcer, but gastrectomy is probably of no value when direct visualization of the gastric and duodenal mucosa is negative.

At this point in the diagnostic sequence, a few patients remain in whom all studies, including laparotomy, have been unrevealing. If bleeding recurs, the same diagnostic sequence should be repeated. Although even less data are available to support a decision for a repeat laparotomy, it may be valuable in selected cases *during* bleeding which requires multiple transfusions and in patients in whom the suspicion of occult malignancy is high.

SPECIAL PROBLEMS

PORTAL HYPERTENSION

Gastrointestinal hemorrhage from a ruptured gastric or esophageal varix (Figs. 16–3, C and 16–5) constitutes the most critical hazard to patients with portal hypertension. Approximately one-third of cirrhotic patients die from this complication. Although alcoholic liver disease with portal cirrhosis is the most common underlying intrahepatic lesion, postnecrotic cirrhosis resulting from viral hepatitis, biliary cir-

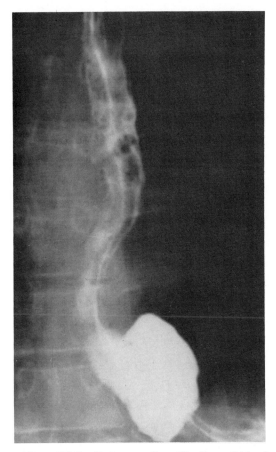

Figure 16–5. Barium swallow. The linear folds of the esophagus are interrupted by variceal distention. Gastric mucosa is displaced above the diaphragm. This combination of radiological findings constitutes a frequently seen diagnostic study associated with gastrointestinal hemorrhage. However, only endoscopy can determine whether or not this pathophysiological lesion is the site of bleeding.

rhosis, schistosomiasis, or intravascular obstruction of the hepatic or portal vein may also result in portal hypertension. Patients with bleeding from these latter conditions, in contradistinction to the cirrhotic group, are better operative candidates for decompression of the portal system and seem to tolerate individual bleeding episodes better.

When the patient with massive gastrointestinal bleeding also has portal hypertension, initial management should follow the guidelines noted for emergent bleeding.

Once it is determined that these measures will not control the hemorrhage, the gastric lavage tube should be withdrawn and panendoscopy performed to establish

that varices are, indeed, the site of blood loss, since up to one-fourth of the patients with varices who present with gastrointestinal hemorrhage may be bleeding from another source. When bleeding varices are not found, complete endoscopic visualization of stomach and duodenum is essential. Documentation of varices as the site of uncontrolled bleeding should be followed immediately with cardioesophageal tamponade and initiation of intravenous Pituitrin (20 units diluted in 100 cc isotonic saline or D5/w over a 20- to 30-minute period, repeated at two-hour intervals as indicated). Presently, tamponade may be adequately accomplished with the Sengstaken-Blakemore (SB) or Linton tube (Davol, Inc., Providence, R.I.).[23,24] Regardless of which tube is used, ultimate survival with minimal morbidity depends upon close supervision and strict attention to detail of the method. The immediate aim of therapy is to control hemorrhage, which is possible in the vast majority of cases. Ultimate therapy to prevent rebleeding is directed at elective surgical decompression of the portal system.

METHOD OF TAMPONADE

1. A new SB or Linton tube should be used, preceded by careful inspection of the balloons to check for air leaks. Both are triple-lumen tubes. The Linton tube is constructed with one lumen leading to a single 800 cc capacity intragastric balloon with the remaining two lumens serving as esophageal and gastric aspiration channels. By contrast, the SB tube has a single intragastric irrigating channel, a smaller 250 cc intragastric balloon, and an esophageal balloon that can be inflated to a pressure of 45 mm Hg. The large intragastric balloon and esophageal irrigation channel of the Linton tube are distinct advantages. The improved tamponade of intragastric veins achieved with this tube obviates the need for intraesophageal tamponade and minimizes erosion of esophageal mucosa. However, if the SB tube is used it should be modified by taping an accessory No. 18 French plastic nasogastric tube to it with the distal tip positioned at the top of the esophageal balloon, for esophageal aspiration.

2. The head of the bed should be ele-

vated 6 inches to help prevent reflux of gastric acid.

3. Intubation may be accomplished through the nose or mouth, using a well lubricated tube and constant suction on the esophageal irrigating channel. If difficulty is encountered during intubation, a flexible metal or fiberglass rod may be used as a stylet in order to pass the tube through the mouth much as one would pass a flexible gastroscope.

4. The gastric balloon should be inflated to capacity and snugged against the cardioesophageal junction and gastric fundus. Traction is best maintained using a traction helmet with $3/4$- to $1\frac{1}{4}$-lb constant spring load tension. (A small fish scale works well for monitoring traction pressure.)[25] The gastric irrigating channel should immediately be hooked to 50 to 90 mm Hg intermittent suction. Tube position should always be checked by X-ray. Gastric lavage with ice water is then continued and, following control of bleeding, this channel is utilized for instillation of neomycin, magnesium citrate, and antacids.

5. Failure to control bleeding by intragastric tamponade with the SB tube is an indication to inflate the esophageal balloon and may indicate that varices are not the source of bleeding.

6. When bleeding is controlled for 24 hours, the esophageal balloon is decompressed but suction is continued. If no further bleeding occurs in the next 24 hours, the intragastric balloon is deflated followed by tube removal when no additional bleeding is noted during another 24-hour period.

7. Rebleeding following balloon deflation or tube withdrawal is often controlled by repeat tamponade. However, at this time the decision for emergent surgical decompression must be considered.

SURGICAL DECOMPRESSION

Operative mortality approaches 70 per cent when emergent surgery is required to control variceal bleeding; therefore, prognosis for surgically decompressing the portal bed is optimal as an elective procedure.

The most important criteria for selecting successful surgical candidates are related to liver function and age. A serum albumin above 3.0 g per 100 ml, bilirubin of less than 3.0 mg per 100 ml, BSP retention of less than 20 per cent, the absence of ascites and liver biopsy showing only minimal fatty metamorphosis, and the absence of alcoholic hepatitis are the most important criteria to consider when selecting the ideal surgical candidate. Mortality and morbidity related to shunt surgery seem related directly to abnormalities of these parameters reflecting hepatic reserve. After the emergent gastrointestinal hemorrhage has been controlled, an intensive nutritional program, including protein, calories, vitamins, and cofactors, is essential to improve liver function. This may require up to three months to achieve maximum benefit.

SPLENOPORTOGRAPHY

When the patient with bleeding varices is considered a candidate for elective surgery, splenoportography yields valuable information. The presence and severity of esophageal varices can be defined, and the patency of the portal and splenic veins may be established. This procedure will also indicate the rate of portal venous flow, filling of intrahepatic vessels, and size of extrahepatic collaterals. When combined with intrasplenic manometry, portal pressure can be quantitated. Such data are of considerable value in predicting the effect of the shunt procedure on hepatic blood flow.[26]

LIVER BIOPSY AND INTRAHEPATIC MANOMETRY

The histological status of the liver and the level of portal pressure are important considerations in electing to perform a portosystemic shunt to prevent bleeding. Several techniques are available for assessing pressure, including percutaneous measurement of intrahepatic pressure with simultaneous liver biopsy, percutaneous splenic pulp pressure, and wedged hepatic vein pressure.[27] Intrahepatic pressure accurately reflects direct portal venous measurements and provides needed histological data. Since fatty metamorphosis has been associated with elevated portal pressure and its disappearance with a fall to normal, recovery of histological and functional integrity of the liver may obviate the need for a shunt procedure. Indeed, the detection of alcoholic hepatitis is reason for postponement of surgery to a time when the patient is a more favorable operative candidate. The optimal histological and manometric criteria are cirrhosis without fat or alcoholic hepatitis and an intrahepatic pressure above 30 mm Hg.

TYPE OF SHUNT

Shunting of blood from the portal to systemic circulation may be accomplished by a number of surgical procedures, including portacaval (end-to-side, side-to-side), splenorenal, and mesenteric caval anastomoses. The end-to-side portacaval shunt is technically the easiest to perform, provides the most effective reduction in portal pressure, the lowest incidence of recurrent hemorrhage (3 per cent) and the lowest incidence of shunt thrombosis, but the highest incidence of encephalopathy (25 per cent). By contrast, the splenorenal shunt is technically more difficult to perform, and is associated with a high incidence of recurrent hemorrhage (20 per cent) and a higher incidence of shunt thrombosis, but the lowest incidence of encephalopathy (12 per cent). The operative mortality for either procedure is not significantly different and the type of shunt employed does not seem to significantly influence the five-year cumulative survival rate of 22 per cent.[28] A combination of factors seems to favor long-term survival, including elective rather than emergent surgery, optimal hepatic function, younger age of the patient, and histological appearance, indicating a stable, noninflammatory status of liver disease.[29,30] Thus the ideal shunt candidate is one less than 55 years in whom variceal bleeding has been controlled by balloon tamponade, blood volume has been restored, and liver function has been improved, and whose surgical procedure is elective rather than emergent.

TABLE 16–3. DISORDERS POSSIBLY ASSOCIATED WITH GASTROINTESTINAL BLEEDING WHICH SHOULD BE CONSIDERED IN SELECTED CASES

Blood dyscrasias
    Leukemia
    Lymphoma
    Myeloid metaplasia
    Aplastic anemias
    Polycythemia vera
    Hemophilia
    Von Willebrand's disease
    Christmas disease
    Hypoprothrombinemia
    Specific clotting factor deficiencies
    Pernicious anemia
    Thrombocytopenic purpura
    Fibrinolytic syndromes
    Circulating anticoagulants

Vascular abnormalities
    Hereditary hemorrhagic telangiectasia
      (Osler-Weber-Rendu)
    Pseudoxanthoma Elasticum
    Turner's syndrome
    Blue rubber bleb nevus
    Scurvy
    Henoch-Schönlein purpura

Systemic diseases
    Hepatic failure
    Uremia
    Dysglobulenemias
      Multiple myeloma
      Macroglobulenemia
      Amyloidosis
    Periarteritis nodosa
    Disseminated lupus erythematosus

BLEEDING DIATHESIS

Although infrequently a cause of massive gastrointestinal hemorrhage, the patient with hematemesis or melena may have an associated blood dyscrasia, vascular abnormality, or multiple system disease with bleeding diathesis (Table 16–3). Therefore, when the history, physical examination, or clinical course suggests such a possibility, the sequence of diagnostic studies should include expert hematological consultation and the appropriate laboratory tests to detect these disorders.

COMPLICATIONS OF MANAGEMENT

Dangers to the patient are inherent in any active diagnostic or therapeutic approach to medical problems. In the management of massive gastrointestinal hemorrhage, volume replacement, specifically blood, is the most crucial need.

The dangers of transfusion therapy to the patient must always be remembered. Decisions made regarding quantity and rapidity of blood replacement are clinical judgments of the highest order. One must weigh the risks of mild hypotension and the sequelae of hypovolemia in terms of physiological status; i.e., the patient's ability to tolerate the anoxia resulting from red cell loss and volume depletion, plus the chances for continuing or worsening hemorrhage, against the known complications of whole blood transfusions. Adverse effects of transfusions are numerous and serious.[31] They include allergic or sensitivity reaction with skin lesions, asthmatic symptoms, febrile responses, mismatching of blood with resultant hemolysis and renal damage, overloading of plasma volume with precipitation of congestive heart failure and pulmonary edema, serum calcium depletion with repeated (greater than 5 units) transfusions, depletion of platelet and clotting factors if repeated (greater than 5 units stored blood) transfusions are required, and subsequent development of viral hepatitis.

In considering transfusion of blood, one should, when possible, prescribe only the components needed—plasma expanders or whole blood to treat massive acute blood loss; packed red blood cells when bleeding is more chronic and compensatory mechanisms have repleted much of the volume but hematocrit remains dangerously low; fresh whole blood when associated diseases or disorders deplete labile plasma clotting factors; and concentrated platelets when bleeding is mild and due to temporary platelet deficits.

Likewise, the use of intravenous Pitressin therapy may adversely affect the patient. The vascular response is not limited to the splanchnic vessels, and systemic hypertension may result. Angina pectoris, coronary insufficiency, and even myocardial infarction may follow. Induction of vomiting may result in aspiration pneumonia.

The dangers of gastroesophageal tamponade have been well documented.[32] If this procedure is used, rigid instructions must be followed compulsively to prevent asphyxiation, esophageal rupture, and aspiration pneumonia.[23]

The complications of endoscopy have been markedly diminished through the development of the flexible fiberoptic systems and cold lighting. Esophageal tears and ruptures, mucosal burns, and broken teeth are all much less frequent, but aspiration, anaphylactic reactions to premedication and trauma to the gastrointestinal tract may still occur. Angiographic studies may result in massive hematomas or thrombosis of major vessels.

Each drug and procedure carries inherent dangers of iatrogenic disease, and one must be familiar with the relative contraindications and possible sequelae prior to using them.

REFERENCES

1. Chander, G. N. Bleeding from the upper gastrointestinal tract. Brit. Med. J. 4:723, 1967.
2. Brick, I. B., and Jeghers, H. J. Gastrointestinal hemorrhage. New Eng. J. Med. 253:458, 511, 555, 1955.
3. Wilson, D. E., and Chalmers, T. C. Management of emergencies. XII. Acute hemorrhage from the upper gastrointestinal tract. New Eng. J. Med. 274:1368, 1966.
4. Berkowitz, D. Fatal gastrointestinal hemorrhage: Diagnostic implications from a study of 200 cases. Amer. J. Gastroenterol. 40: 372, 1963.
5. Wallace, J., and Sharpey-Schafer, E. P. Blood changes following controlled haemorrhage in man. Lancet 2:393, 1941.
6. Howarth, S., and Sharpey-Schafer, E. P. Low blood pressure phases following haemorrhage. Lancet 1:18, 1947.
7. Ebert, R. V., Stead, E. A., Jr., and Gibson, J. G., II. Response of normal subjects to acute blood loss, with special reference to the mechanism of restoration of blood volume. Arch. Intern. Med. (Chicago) 68:578, 1941.
8. Mailer, C., Goldberg, A., Harder, R., Grey-Thomas, I., and Burnett, W. Diagnosis of upper gastrointestinal bleeding. Brit. Med. J. 2:784, 1965.
9. Schiff, L., and Stevens, R. J. Elevation of urea nitrogen content of the blood following hematemesis or melena. Arch. Intern. Med. (Chicago) 64:1239, 1939.
10. Shaldon, S., and Sherlock, S. The use of vasopressin ('Pitressin') in the control of bleeding from oesophageal varices. Lancet 2:222, 1960.
11. Baum, S., Nusbaum, M., Clearfield, H. F., Kuroda, K., and Tumen, H. J. Angiography in the diagnosis of gastrointestinal bleeding. Arch. Int. Med. (Chicago) 119:16, 1967.
12. Rösch, J., Gray, R. K., Grollman, J. H., Jr., Ross, G., Steckel, R. J., and Weiner, M. Selective arterial drug infusions in the treatment of acute gastrointestinal bleeding: A preliminary report. Gastroenterology 59:341, 1970.

13. Baum, S., and Nusbaum, M.   The control of gastrointestinal hemorrhage by selective mesenteric arterial infusion of vasopressin. Radiology 98:497, 1971.

14. Noer, R. J., Hamilton, J. E., Williams, D. J., and Broughton, D. S.   Rectal hemorrhage: Moderate and severe. Ann. Surg. 155:794, 1962.

15. Wolff, W. I., and Shinya, H.   Colonofiberoscopy. J.A.M.A. 217:1509, 1971.

16. Schiff, L., Stevens, R. J., Shapiro, N., and Goodman, C.   Observations on oral administration of citrated blood in man: Effect on stools. Amer. J. Med. Sci. 203:409, 1942.

17. Hilsman, J. H.   The color of blood-containing feces following the instillation of citrated whole blood: At various levels of the small intestine. Gastroenterology 15:131, 1950.

18. Luke, R. G., Lees, W., and Rudick, J.   Appearances of the stools after the introduction of blood into caecum. Gut 5:77, 1964.

19. Irons, G. V., Jr., and Kirsner, J. B.   Routine chemical tests of the stool for occult blood: An evaluation. Amer. J. Med. Sci. 249:247, 1965.

20. Pittman, F. E.   The fluorescein string test: An analysis of its use and relationship to barium studies of the upper gastrointestinal tract in 122 cases of gastrointestinal tract hemorrhage. Ann. Intern. Med. 60:418, 1964.

21. Siemsen, J. K., Hill, L. D., Pillow, R. P., Ragen, P. A., and Tesluk, H.   The diagnosis of gastrointestinal bleeding site by the use of radiochromate-tagged red cells. Bull. Mason Clinic 13:111, 1959.

22. Retzlaff, J. A., Hagedorn, A. B., and Bartholomew, L. G.   Abdominal exploration for gastrointestinal bleeding of obscure origin. J.A.M.A. 177:104, 1961.

23. Pitcher, J. L.   Safety and effectiveness of the modified Sengstaken-Blakemore tube: A prospective study. Gastroenterology 61:291, 1971.

24. Linton, R. R.   The treatment of esophageal varices. Surg. Clin. N. Amer. 46:485, 1966.

25. Head, H. B., Kukral, J. C., and Preston, F. W.   Helmet-mounted constant traction spring for maintenance of position of Sengstaken tube. Amer. J. Surg. 112:465, 1966.

26. Warren, W. D., Restrepo, J. E., Respers, J. C., and Muller, W. H.   The importance of hemodynamic-studies in management of portal hypertension. Ann. Surg. 158:387, 1963.

27. Vennes, J. A.   Intrahepatic pressure: An accurate reflection of portal pressure. Medicine 45:445, 1966.

28. Portasystemic Shunts. Exhibit, American Gastroenterological Association Meeting, Philadelphia, 1968.

29. Hermann, R. E., Rodriguez, A. E., and McCormack, L. J.   Selection of patients for portalsystemic shunts. J.A.M.A. 196:1039, 1966.

30. Myers, R.T.   Bleeding esophageal varices: A study involving 100 consecutive cases. Amer. Surg. 33:919, 1967.

31. Grove-Rasmussen, M., Lesses, M. F., and Anstall, H. B.   Transfusion therapy. New Eng. J. Med. 264:1088, 1961.

32. Conn, H., and Simpson, J. A.   Excessive mortality associated with balloon tamponade of bleeding varices: A critical re-appraisal. J.A.M.A. 202:587, 1967.

THE SMALL AND LARGE INTESTINE

Chapter 17

Movements of the Small Intestine

James Christensen

INTRODUCTION

The small intestine is a tube of two concentric muscle layers, sheathed by the mucosa within and the serosa without. The muscle contracts in a complex way to stir the chyme and to move it from one end of the tube to the other. Mixing movements bring the chyme into optimal contact with the surface of the mucosa for absorption. Propulsive movements remove exhausted chyme.

These two processes, mixing and propulsion, are familiar enough, for they both occur in the flow of fluids in simple hydraulic systems. When fluids flow through passive conduits, propulsion is a consequence of a hydrostatic pressure difference between one end of the conduit and the other. Internal circulation or mixing comes from turbulence induced in the stream by several factors. The laminar or turbulent nature of the flow is determined by the size of the conduit, the velocity of flow, and the kinematic viscosity of the fluid.

The small intestine is very different from other hydraulic systems. The conduit is active: wall rigidity and conduit diameter vary with place and time. The forces inducing flow arise all along the conduit. Velocity of flow is continuously variable. The fluid volume is continuously changing along the conduit, and the viscosity of the fluid may be varying (viscosity of chyme is difficult to define, for the fluid is inhomogeneous and non-Newtonian). The small bowel, then, is an exceedingly complex hydraulic system, one for which no mechanical analogue is at hand.

Technical problems limit the study of this hydraulic system. When the small bowel is removed, its actions are altered from normal because of its isolation from such control systems as enteric hormones and the extrinsic innervation. To study the bowel in situ, one must put sensors in the lumen or sew them to the wall. Such sensors are hard to use, for the small bowel is difficult to reach without anesthesia. Drugs, emotions, and the sensors themselves may influence the movements of the wall and of the chyme because they may affect the control systems. Most techniques suffer from either poor resolution or inaccuracy in measurements. Nevertheless, the general nature of the system can now be seen, though many details remain obscure.

ANATOMY OF MOTOR MECHANISMS AND OF SOME OF THEIR CONTROLS[1-3]

THE MUSCLE

The muscle of the small bowel wall is smooth muscle, so called because the cells, viewed microscopically, lack the striations of cardiac and somatic muscle. There are two main muscle coats in the bowel wall. In the outer coat the cells are oriented with their long axes in the long axis of the bowel. In the inner coat they lie with their long axes at about 90 degrees from that, in the transverse axis or the circumference of the tube. Some say that the outer layer is a loosely wound helix and the inner layer a tight one.[4] Others deny this.[5] These two layers, apparently quite separate, may be joined together at intervals by small bundles of muscle crossing the intermuscular space,[6] though such bundles are not found by all. A third, thinner layer of muscle, the muscularis mucosae, lies within the circular muscle coat but separated from it by the thick submucosa. The cells of the muscularis mucosae, also smooth muscle, lie also in inner circular and outer longitudinal layers, but the two layers are mixed to a degree. Bundles of muscle cells extend from the muscularis mucosae into the valvulae conniventes and into villi where the bundles enclose lacteals.

Smooth muscle cells differ structurally from other kinds of muscle cells. Each elongated cylindrical or fusiform cell, about 5 μ in diameter and 100 to 200 μ long, contains one large central nucleus, 1 to 3 μ by 15 to 25 μ, ovoid in unshortened cells but spiral or folded in contraction. The fine nuclear chromatin is dispersed, with some clumping along the nuclear envelope. There are two to five nucleoli. The nuclear envelope contains two membranes, the inner thicker than the outer, fused together at scattered points. The cellular organelles, mostly perinuclear, include a centrosome, a rough-surfaced endoplasmic reticulum, and mitochrondria. Mitochrondria are small and sparse, occurring along the cell wall and in the perinuclear sarcoplasm. A smooth endoplasmic reticulum, or sarcoplasmic tubular system, radiates from the perinuclear region to ramify throughout the sarcoplasm and closely approach the sarcolemma.

The rest of the cell contains the fibrillar sarcoplasm made up of contractile protein filaments and matter between filaments. The major population of filaments, 50 to 70 Å in diameter, passes at intervals through dark bodies, regions of closely packed filaments, and ends in dark bodies along the sarcolemma. These filaments are actin. Myosin can be detected in smooth muscle, but its physical form and relationship to actin in the cell has been conjectural.[7] A second population of thicker filaments, found in some smooth muscles, may be myosin filaments,[8] but many structural details of these filaments and their relation to the actin filaments are unknown.

The sarcolemma contains two electron-opaque layers separated by an electron-lucent line. The full sarcolemmal thickness, 75 to 855 Å, is about equally divided into these three layers. Smooth muscle has many subsarcolemmal vesicles, pinocytotic vesicles or caveolae intracellulares, irregularly dispersed along the cell periphery. Some if not all of these communicate with the cell surface. Their distribution varies among cells, among tissues, and with techniques of fixation for electron microscopy. They seem to be separate from subsarcolemmal extensions of the smooth endoplasmic reticulum lying very close to these vesicles.[9]

The cells are separated by an intercellular space containing noncellular elements of connective tissues, but the muscle cells touch at frequent points. The cells have special structures at these points of contact. These contacts are of two general morphological types, nexuses and gap junctions.[2,10]

Nexuses are points where the sarcolemmas of adjacent cells partially fuse. The outer electron-opaque layers of the two triple-layered membranes fuse to produce a five-layered junction. Nexuses can be found only in specimens incubated in a physiological salt solution and fixed with permanganate. Although nexuses are found in many smooth muscles, in the small bowel (of the dog) they occur only in the circular muscle layer.

The longitudinal muscle layer (in the dog) shows a different kind of cell contact, the gap junction (the circular muscle layer also contains some gap junctions). Here the two adjacent cells do not actually touch, but their sarcolemmas lie parallel to each other for a short distance, separated by a gap of about 500 Å. The gap contains a condensation of intercellular material. The cytoplasm of both cells is condensed adjacent to the gap junction.

Both kinds of junction probably contribute to the mechanical continuity of the tissue, for they are resistant to mechanical separation, but they are not physically immutable. Their more important function is probably physiological; it is proposed that they permit electrical interaction among connected cells, accounting for the ability of intestinal smooth muscle to act as an electrical syncytium. This property of smooth muscle is described in more detail later in this chapter.

THE NERVES

The nerves of the small bowel are even more complex than early neuroanatomists found them to be when the classic descriptions were made at the end of the last century. Our understanding of the nerves to the bowel, their interconnection, and their connections to the muscle depends upon the proper interpretation of experiments using histological, physiological, and pharmacological methods. The techniques are sometimes imprecise and usually difficult. The present view will certainly be further modified.

The vagi contain far fewer motor fibers than sensory fibers. Most vagal motor fibers to the small bowel are parasympathetic preganglionic fibers coming from the brainstem vagal nuclei to connect with secondary parasympathetic cholinergic neurons of the local plexuses. Sympathetic fibers which enter the vagi through branches from the cervical sympathetic ganglia may also reach the small

bowel. The vagi probably also contain motor fibers of a third kind, nonadrenergic inhibitory nerves, or purinergic nerves.[11] These also may reach the small bowel. The peripheral connections of the vagal sensory nerves from the small bowel are obscure. Ultimately they are excited by sensory receptors in the bowel, mechanoreceptors, chemoreceptors, and osmoreceptors.

The splanchnic nerves carry both preganglionic and postganglionic sympathetic motor fibers to the abdominal sympathetic ganglia from which nerves pass to the small bowel alongside the arterial supply. The total number of fibers present in the vagi and splanchnic nerves is so small compared to the total number of nerve cells present in the walls of the abdominal viscera that it is clear that one motor fiber must ultimately contact thousands of cells in the plexuses. The sympathetic tracts also contain fibers sensory to pain (Fig. 24-2).

The fact that both motor and sensory nerves link the small bowel to the central nervous system implies a degree of central nervous influence on bowel movement. The small bowel certainly can show movement when isolated, but it is possible that the central nervous system influences the movement. The technique of operant conditioning has been used in rats to demonstrate a capacity for voluntary control of some functions controlled by the autonomic nervous system,[12] including movement of the colon, but this has not been shown for small bowel motility.

Nerve tissue in the bowel wall is roughly organized into laminar plexuses of unmyelinated nerve fiber bundles containing solitary and clustered nerve cell bodies. These nerves include secondary parasympathetic cells, internuncial or associative cells, and, probably, cells of sensory function. These types are hard to distinguish morphologically and physiologically. The plexuses, though named and often considered separately, are united by fasciculi connecting adjacent plexuses.

The *subserous plexus*, containing single and clustered cell bodies, is concentrated beneath the serosa along the mesenteric insertion. It connects to a similar ganglionated perivascular plexus in the mesentery.

The *myenteric plexus*, between the longitudinal and circular layers of the main muscle coat, consists of primary, secondary, and tertiary plexuses. The primary plexus is a gross irregular grid of large fiber bundles containing ganglia mostly at intersections of the grid. The ganglia vary in size and constitution. The secondary plexus, lying within the interstices of the grid of the primary plexus, is a closer web of smaller fiber bundles continuous with the primary plexus. It contains few cell bodies. The tertiary plexus is an even finer mesh of very small fiber bundles, without cell bodies, within the interstices of the secondary plexus but connected to it. A cell-free plexus within the circular muscle layer, the deep myenteric plexus or deep circular plexus, resembles the secondary and tertiary plexuses of the myenteric plexus with which it is closely connected.

The *submucous plexus*, less dense than the myenteric plexus, is a three-dimensional grid of small fiber bundles containing small ganglia.

The *mucous plexus* is a noncellular extension of very fine fiber bundles extending from the submucous plexus into the mucosa, where it appears to approach the epithelium.

The fine divisions of the myenteric and submucous plexuses give off fibers ramifying in the muscle layers. These fine elements to the muscle, and the branches of the mucous plexus to the epithelium, are too small to be seen well by light microscopy, so that the details of their destination are not clear. Within the muscle layers, they constitute an autonomic ground plexus whose elements are often seen in electron microscopic sections of the muscle. The approach of these fine terminals to the smooth muscle appears not to give rise to either neural or muscular specializations: the varicose nerve fibers simply wander among the cells.

The kinds of cells making up these plexuses, and their interconnections, remain incompletely understood. Classifications of cells on the basis of argyrophilia or morphology (the Dogiel classification) have not proved operationally useful. More functional significance attaches to the ability of cell bodies and fibers to take up stains for cholinesterase[13] or to be stained by fluorescence techniques to identify catecholamines.[14] These histochemical methods for light microscopy can identify some neural elements as cho-

linergic, others as adrenergic, and others as neither. With the electron microscope one can identify neurons as cholinergic, adrenergic, or purinergic on the basis of the size and granularity of the synaptic vesicles of the nerve fibers.

These techniques show interconnections, within the plexuses, between adrenergic and cholinergic elements. Adrenergic elements have been found to make extensive connections with cholinergic cell bodies through basket-like networks about the cells. Adrenergic elements are found principally in close relationship with blood vessels and cholinergic ganglion cells in the plexus; few seem to enter the main muscle layers.[15, 16]

A third kind of nerve fiber may exist in the small bowel, although it has been studied most extensively in other organs.[11] This neuron, the nonadrenergic inhibitory nerve or the purinergic nerve, cannot be distinguished by light microscopy, but is identifiable by electron microscopy on the basis of the morphology of the synaptic vesicles.[17] It has been most commonly identified in physiological studies. Electrical stimulation of these nerves produces inhibition of muscle, accompanied by hyperpolarization of the membrane of muscle cells, during the stimulus. Following the end of a period of stimulation, the membrane depolarizes and the muscle contracts. The transmitter liberated from such nerves is neither acetylcholine nor norepinephrine. The transmitter may be an adenosine nucleotide, hence the name purinergic.

At least one other kind of nerve may exist in the myenteric plexus, probably liberating serotonin.[18] The evidence for it rests on the demonstrated ability of myenteric plexus cells to synthesize and take up serotonin, and upon the ability of serotonin to induce contractions of small bowel muscle (in some conditions it is inhibitory). Such nerves may be internuncial neurons, but their actual connections are not known.

THE FUNCTIONS OF THE MOTOR NERVES

Neurohormonal Receptors.[19] The effects of neurohormones may be excitatory or inhibitory in muscle, depending upon the nature of the receptor sites upon which they act. These receptor sites are postulated configurations of organic molecules in cell membranes with special affinity for particular neurohormonal transmitters.

When a section of gut wall is exposed to acetylcholine or an acetylcholine analogue such as methacholine or carbachol, it contracts. This is interpreted as the consequence of the action of the drug, or *agonist*, either upon muscarinic receptors, lying in the muscle cell membranes, or upon nicotinic receptors, lying in the secondary parasympathetic ganglion cells. The two kinds of receptors can be distinguished by their relative susceptibility to such *antagonists* as hyoscine (acting on muscarinic receptors) and nicotine and hexamethonium (acting on the ganglionic nicotinic receptors). Acetylcholine and its analogues excite smooth muscle of the small bowel through both receptor types.

The two main kinds of receptors for catecholamines in the small bowel, adrenergic alpha and beta receptors, can be distinguished principally on the basis of the selectivity of the effects of such adrenergic antagonists as dibenzyline (acting on alpha receptors) and propranolol (acting on beta receptors). Subgroups can be distinguished on the basis of their susceptibility to certain other antagonists. Alpha receptors are more sensitive to epinephrine and norepinephrine than to isopropyl-norepinephrine; beta receptors are more sensitive to isopropylnorepinephrine than to the other two catecholamines. The small bowel muscle contains both beta receptors, which are inhibitory, and alpha receptors, some of which are inhibitory and others excitatory. Beta receptors appear to be located in the muscle cells; alpha receptors may exist chiefly in the muscle cells also, although there is the likelihood that some of them are in nerve tissue as well. The response of the muscle coats to norepinephrine is variable; excitation, inhibition, or no response may occur, depending upon the concentration of the agonist achieved in the neighborhood of the receptor and upon the kind of receptor mainly encountered by the neurohormone. The presence of synapses between adrenergic nerves and cholinergic ganglia suggests that some adrenergic effects on the gut may be the consequence of an effect of the adrenergic neurohormone on secondary parasympathetic ganglion cells of the myenteric plexus.

Serotonin receptors may be of several types, but, lacking sufficiently selective antagonists, they are not firmly classifiable. Available evidence suggests that they are mainly located in neurons, secondary parasympathetic ganglion cells, or their axons, from which they induce acetylcholine release.

THE NATURE OF THE MOVEMENTS OF THE SMALL BOWEL[20]

All the many methods used to observe movement in the small bowel suffer from limitations of one kind or another.

In *radiological methods*, one usually observes the movement of luminal content rather than movement of the walls. Such movements are difficult to quantify, the time of observation is usually short, and the radiopaque material used may influence the movement. *Direct observation* of the bowel in situ or in isolation is also difficult to report in quantitative terms, and the movements are probably altered by anesthesia, by opening the abdomen, by reflexes, by changes in temperature, and by the isolation of the gut from extrinsic controls. *Indirect methods* mainly use sensors of pressure or movement put into the small bowel perorally or sewn to the wall of the bowel. Intraluminal devices register pressure or volume changes in closed systems such as balloons of various sizes attached to water-filled rubber or plastic tubes, or open-tipped, perfused tubes. Telemetering capsules are miniature radio transmitters, built into small capsules, which continuously broadcast a radio signal as a function of pressure exerted on a window in the capsule. For the most part, such intraluminal devices can record events at only one or a few points in space, points which are hard to determine precisely or to maintain over time. The pressure changes such devices sense are probably entirely due to contractions of the wall, pressing on the sensitive part of the closed system. The sensors sewn to the wall of the gut are miniature strain-gauges. These certainly solve the problem of knowing the spatial localization of the activity being monitored, and their use allows prolonged observation without adverse effects of anesthesia. They are, however, rather difficult to make and, because they are rigid devices, they may limit the excursion of the bowel wall as it contracts, especially if they are closely spaced.

Despite these technical limitations, however, a reasonable picture of the movements of the bowel has emerged. There appear to be two types of movement: segmenting contractions and peristaltic contractions.

Segmentation refers to the occurrence of localized standing ring contractions spaced some distance apart, dividing the lumen and its contents into segments. In man, the contractions themselves are probably less than 1 to 2 cm long, last only a few seconds, and are spaced sometimes quite regularly 4 to 8 cm apart over a segment of the small bowel. When they disappear and re-form, the new ones sometimes appear to be located roughly equidistant between two old ones. They may, at times, occur quite regularly in time (rhythmic segmentation).

Peristalsis is a moving ring contraction 1 to 2 cm wide, moving aborad at a rate of a few centimeters per minute, over a distance of 4 to 5 cm. The velocity of peristalsis is faster in the proximal small bowel than in the ileum. Under abnormal conditions a *peristaltic rush* may occur, a moving ring contraction moving much more rapidly over much longer segments of the gut. Antiperistalsis, contraction rings moving orad, has been seen to occur in abnormal conditions of observation.

Intraluminal pressures recorded from small balloons or perfused catheters show two kinds of pressure waves. Type I waves are monophasic peaks, like isosceles triangles, mostly lasting three to seven seconds in the upper small bowel and around eight seconds in the ileum. The pressures recorded are mostly 15 to 60 cm H_2O above basal pressure. They occur 13 to 60 per cent of the time, the proportion probably varying with different conditions of feeding. Type III waves are rises in basal pressure, 5 to 20 cm H_2O high, lasting one to two minutes, upon which type I waves are often superimposed. A type IV wave,

30 to 40 cm H_2O high and lasting 25 to 50 seconds, may be a variant of the type III wave, described only in the terminal ileum.

The correlation of these manometrically recorded waves with net movements is conjectural. The pressure waves represent activity at one point in the bowel, whereas net flow is the consequence of action at many points. Type I waves seem to be the manometric correlate of segmentation; type III (and type IV) waves may or may not represent a different kind of movement to accomplish propulsion.

The distributions in time of type I waves appear to be random on gross inspection of records. Frequency seems to vary, but at times such contractions occur very regularly at about 11 per minute in the human duodenum, and about eight per minute in the ileum. Such a very regular occurrence of type I contractions is rare, however, and they usually occur with a lower frequency. When the frequency is examined in terms of the length of intercontractile periods, a clear pattern emerges.[21] The frequency distribution of the duration of intercontractile periods of type I waves, in the fed state in the human duodenum, shows a pattern with regular peaks and valleys (Fig. 17–1). The peaks occur at integral multiples of five seconds, the valleys halfway in between. This suggests the existence of a pacemaker in the duodenum, dividing time into five-second intervals; in each interval, a given point in the duodenum may exhibit either contraction or rest. The successive five-second intervals are electrical slow-wave cycles[22] (see below). Any slow-wave cycle, as the slow wave occurs over and over again at any point in the duodenum, may be a *contraction cycle* or a *rest cycle*. Based on this view, one may then compute the numbers of contraction cycles and rest cycles occurring sequentially in time at a single point in space. Most contractions occur as single events; that is, they are separated from other contraction cycles by a rest cycle. Most contractions (95 per cent) occur in groups of one to three. Most rest cycles are also single events; that is, they are separated from other rest cycles by one or more contraction cycles. Most rest cycles (95 per cent) occur in groups of one to 13. There is no gross correlation between the number

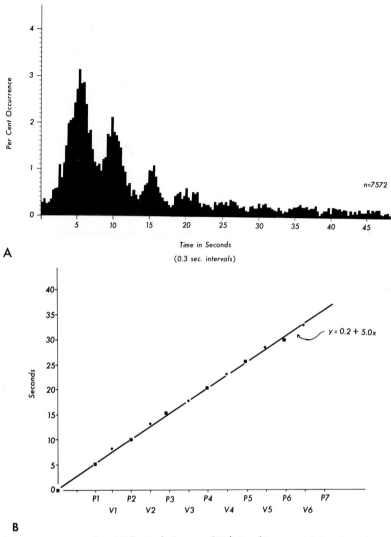

A

Time in Seconds

(0.3 sec. intervals)

B

Peaks and Valleys in the Frequency Distribution of Intercontractile Periods

Figure 17–1. The distribution of duodenal contractions in time. *A* is a frequency distribution of the lengths of time between successive contractions at a single point in the human duodenum. The horizontal axis shows time in 0.3-second intervals, marked at five-second intervals. The vertical axis shows the percentage of all inter-contractile periods whose lengths fall in each 0.3-second interval. The contractions, recorded manometrically, were all Type I contractions. The distribution shows peaks at five-second intervals, with valleys in between.

   B is a plot of the positions of these peaks and valleys in time. The horizontal axis shows successive peaks (P1, P2, . . .) and valleys (V1, V2, . . .) spaced evenly. The vertical axis shows time. Both peaks (squares) and valleys (circles) fall on a straight line whose slope, 5.0, indicates a five-second period for both the peaks and valleys, separately. (From Christensen, J., et al.: Amer. J. Physiol. *221*:1818, 1971.)

of contraction cycles in series and the number of subsequent rest cycles in series.

   Thus the electrical slow wave, the pacemaker for the type I waves, dictates the timing of type I contractions. Type I contractions cannot occur at a faster frequency than that of the electric slow wave. The electric slow wave is the most important of the basic control systems for type I contractions and, probably, for all movement in the small bowel.

CONTROL SYSTEMS FOR THE SMALL BOWEL

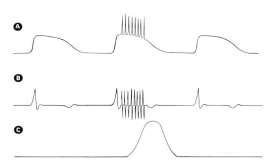

The Electrical Slow Waves.[23, 24] The slow wave, also called the basic electrical rhythm or pacesetter potential, is an electrical phenomenon arising in the muscle itself. Its function is to dictate the time of occurrence of type I contractions in time and space. A slow wave does not initiate contractions; it only sets the intervals, in time and space, when contractions can occur. When contractions occur, a different electrical phenomenon, a burst of action potentials (action spikes or a spike burst), marks the beginning of a contraction (Fig. 17–2). The spike burst is thus initiative of contractions; the slow wave is integrative.

The slow wave is a spontaneous depolarization of smooth muscle cells. In an intestinal smooth muscle cell, as in all smooth muscle, the electrical potential drop across the cell wall is quite variable, perhaps 40 to 80 mv, with the inside negative relative to the outside. In records from isolated strips of the longitudinal muscle layer, the resting membrane potential is interrupted by depolarizations. These occur at very regular intervals with a very uniform time-course. These depolarizations occur in adjacent cells of the longitudinal layer in synchrony. Thus they can be easily recorded from gross electrodes contacting many cells at once. Slow waves occur continuously, whether or not contractions are occurring. The action po-

Figure 17–2. Diagram of time relations between slow waves, spike bursts, and contractions. *A* represents the electromyogram of a single smooth muscle cell, recorded with an intracellular microelectrode. *B* represents the electromyogram recorded from several such cells by a large extracellular volume-recording electrode. *C* shows tension in the muscle mass. All three traces are drawn to a common time-base. In *A*, three slow waves appear as a monophasic depolarization from a stable maximal value, the resting membrane potential. Observe that the rate of depolarization is faster than the rate of repolarization. In *B*, the slow waves appear with two components, an initial biphasic spike which represents depolarization, and a secondary slower biphasic signal, representing repolarization. The trace shown in *B* approximates the second derivative of the trace shown in *A*. The second of the three slow waves bears a burst of spikes, appearing on the plateau of the slow wave. The tension record, in *C*, shows a contraction beginning during the spike burst, and apparently initiated by it. (From Christensen, J.: New Eng. J. Med. 285:85, 1971.)

tentials, a burst of one or more very rapid transients or spikes accompanying contractions, appear to rise from the peak of the depolarization in intracellular electrode records or from the corresponding part of the slow wave cycle in extracellular

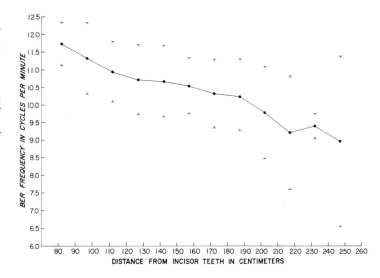

Figure 17–3. The slow wave frequency gradient in the normal human small bowel. The vertical axis shows slow wave frequency. The horizontal axis shows distance below the incisor teeth. Observe that this plot begins at 80 cm, about the ligament of Treitz. Frequency is constant to about that level, at an average of 11.7 cycles per minute. Below that point frequency declines. Dots connected by lines represent mean frequency derived from 12 normal subjects. Brackets indicate 2 SD from the mean. (From Christensen, J., Schedl, H. P., and Clifton, J. A.: Gastroenterology 50:309, 1966.)

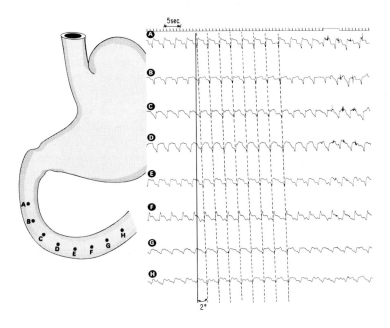

Figure 17-4. Slow waves recorded simultaneously from closely spaced electrodes in the unanesthetized cat. Eight monopolar AC-amplified records are shown as recorded from eight chronically implanted needle electrodes spaced uniformly 1 cm apart along the duodenum. Slow wave configuration is between that of the actual signal and its second derivative. The last few slow waves, at the right, carry spike bursts. Dashed lines are drawn through corresponding slow wave cycles from each record. The angle, 2 degrees, between these lines and the solid line, the common time-base, is a function of the apparent velocity of spread of slow waves and of the paper speed of the recording polygraph. (From Christensen, J.: New Eng. J. Med. 285:85, 1971.)

electrode records. The frequency of slow waves in the human duodenum is ten to 12 cycles per minute, declining to about eight in the terminal ileum (Fig. 17-3). Frequency is quite constant and is affected little by feeding, fasting, enteric hormones, and autonomic neurohormones.

When multiple electrodes are placed at close intervals along the duodenum, slow waves appear with a phase-lag in space, such that they appear to be migrating aborad along the bowel (Fig. 17-4). Phase-lock (a constant phase-lag) exists throughout the duodenum and well into the jejunum. Obviously, frequency must be constant throughout the segment of phase-lock. Beyond the proximal jejunum, frequency begins to decline. From here to the ileum, phase-lock must exist only over very short segments of the bowel, for the decline in frequency is quite gradual through this part of the bowel, without large steps in the frequency gradient (some investigators see steps, and others do not).

The distribution of the electrical slow wave in time and space along the bowel establishes the distribution of contractions along the bowel. The contractions, presumably type I contractions, must both mix and propel the chyme. The question of how the slow wave pattern influences movement of the chyme is unanswered. It may be that, in the duodenum and prox-

imal jejunum, the aborad vector of the phase-lag is the basis for propulsion. Further downstream, it may be the aborally declining frequency gradient, chyme tending to move away from a region of higher potential contraction frequency to a region of lower potential frequency.

The cellular mechanisms underlying the two elements of the electromyogram remain unknown. The resting membrane potential in smooth muscle must be the consequence of inequalities in ion distribution across the cell membrane. The actual distributions are not known with any certainty, but the intracellular potassium concentration in smooth muscle seems to be less than in other kinds of muscle, and resting membrane potential probably receives a significant contribution from differences in concentrations, across cell membranes, of other ions than potassium. The slow wave itself may represent the oscillatory performance of an electrogenic sodium pump. The action potentials are probably related to influx of calcium. It is proposed that action potentials represent movement of calcium ions from sites of storage in subsarcolemmal vesicles into the adjacent distal branches of the smooth endoplasmic reticulum, where they can initiate activation of the contractile apparatus. Thus the vesicles and the endoplasmic reticulum may be functionally analogous to the t-tubule system of striated muscle.

Although slow waves are clearly generated by the longitudinal layer of muscle, they are associated with contractions mainly of the underlying circular muscle. This can occur because slow waves invade the circular muscle from the longitudinal layer. The mechanism is not clear. Such spread may occur by way of muscular bridges between the two layers.[6] It appears to be electrotonic from muscle to muscle, not through neural or humoral connections. The action potentials which signal the initiation of contraction must arise mainly in the circular layer, but probably occur in the longitudinal layer as well. Thus, it appears that, in any single contraction, the two muscle layers must contract in phase. Some find this to be so on direct study, but others report that the two layers contract out of phase.

Since the patterns of spread of slow waves seem to be the major determinant of the patterns of spread of contractions, the nature of this spread is important. The fact that slow waves spread aborad along the duodenum suggests that slow waves are like nerve impulses, arising from a pacemaker and spreading like electric current through a cable. Two characteristics of slow waves makes this seem unlikely. First, wherever the bowel is transected the slow waves continue on both sides of the cut; frequency above the cut is unchanged, but frequency below the cut falls. Second, the velocity of slow waves in the duodenum, about 5 cm per second in man and no more than 20 cm per second in any species, is slower than nerve conduction velocities. An alternative hypothesis is that slow waves represent the action of a different kind of electrical mechanism, a chain of coupled relaxation oscillators.[24] This remains a hypothesis, although a chain of such oscillators has been made which can generate slow waves in patterns like those of the small bowel slow wave.

An oscillator is an electrical or mechanical device whose output is unsteady such that it alternately achieves maximal and minimal values. The term is usually applied to a device which finds such values at regular time intervals. Electrical generators of sine and square waves are familiar examples of electrical oscillators. Relax-ation oscillators are oscillators whose patterns of oscillation are defined by the Van der Pol equation. Relaxation oscillation describes a wide variety of biological oscillations, from the fluctuating population densities of various species to the oscillatory electrical signals of the gut.

The coupled relaxation oscillator hypothesis for small bowel slow waves proposes that slow waves are the output of a chain of such oscillators in which the oscillators are coupled together. Each electrical oscillator is coupled bidirectionally to the oscillators on each side. Each oscillator itself can be set to oscillate at any frequency, the intrinsic frequency of the oscillator. In the model, the oscillators are set to oscillate with intrinsic frequencies which decline from one end of the model to the other. These intrinsic frequencies are set at the intrinsic slow wave frequencies for the small bowel slow wave, the frequencies at which separate pieces of the small bowel produce slow waves when the bowel is cut into small parts. When the oscillators are then coupled bidirectionally, the whole system of oscillators generates slow waves in the same pattern in which they occur in vivo in the gut. Cutting the chain by uncoupling the oscillators at one point produces the same overall effect as cutting the bowel; raising the intrinsic frequency of one oscillator reproduces the effect of heating a segment of the bowel, a procedure which raises slow wave frequency in the heated segment. The fact that the model and the gut itself respond similarly to these and other perturbations suggests that the model, though vastly simplified, is appropriate. Further establishment of the validity of the model requires determinations, from the gut, of oscillator size, the nature of the coupling, and the length of the refractory period of the oscillators, among other characteristics of the system.

Reflexes in the Small Bowel.[25] A variety of reflex contractions can be demonstrated in the small bowel. These have been shown mainly in isolated preparations. Their role in normal movements of the bowel is not clear. Distention of the gut in vivo enhances contractions above the stimulus and inhibits contractions below it. This peristaltic reflex of Bayliss and Starling has long been cited as a major mechanism for propulsion in the small bowel, but the validity of this view remains to be established.

When an isolated segment of intestine is distended with water, only the longitudinal muscle layer contracts at low pressures (0.5 to 1.5 cm H_2O); at higher pressures (1.5 to 3.0 cm H_2O), there is further longitudinal contraction followed by a peristaltic contraction of circular muscle moving aborad. The responses of the two layers can be differentiated both by the strength of the stimulus and by drugs: cholinergic agents and histamine selectively block the response of the longitudinal layer; only the circular layer contraction is prevented by hexamethonium. These reflexes represent responses to deformation of mechanoreceptors in some layers of the wall deep to the mucosa. They are not pressure receptors. The receptors activate local reflexes. The reflex pathway to the longitudinal muscle does not contain a cholinergic synaptic interruption; that to the circular muscle layer does. The motor nerves in both reflexes are cholinergic, though part of the transmission to the longitudinal muscle layer is not.

There may also be mucosal receptors activating reflexes. Light mechanical stimulation of the mucosa and the application of various agents to the mucosa can cause excitation orad and inhibition aborad to the stimulus. These responses are opposed by hexamethonium. They do not involve the periarterial nerves.

The reflexes described above use intrinsic neural pathways. Extrinsic reflexes also exist. The location and morphology of the receptors for such reflexes using extrinsic neural pathways are not clear, but they appear to be in mucosal as well as muscular layers. The afferent and efferent links of these reflexes may be both in the vagal and in the periarterial-splanchnic nerve tracts. The principal reflex, the *intestino-intestinal inhibitory reflex*, is an inhibition of the whole small bowel in response to handling of the gut or to distention of one part. Both sensory and motor tracts may travel through the splanchnic nerves by way of the periarterial plexuses of the gut, and there is evidence to suggest that the central connections lie in the spinal cord below the sixth thoracic segment. A simi-

lar reflex inhibition of the whole small bowel to stimulation of the peritoneum may also be primarily sympathetic. Mechanoreceptors in the small bowel also activate vagal afferents, for cells of the nodose ganglion fire in response to distention of the small bowel, in patterns which indicate both rapidly and slowly adapting receptors.

SMALL BOWEL MOVEMENTS IN DISEASE

There is a widespread assumption that abnormal small bowel movement occurs in a wide variety of diseases associated with nausea, vomiting, diarrhea, constipation, and abdominal cramps. Such terms as hyperperistalsis imply quantitative changes in movement, whereas such terms as reverse peristalsis imply qualitative changes. In fact, very little can be said with certainty about the nature of movement in most such diseases, because the description of normal activity is still sketchy. The rate at which matter leaves the ileum relative to the rate at which matter enters the duodenum is a function of the rates of flow of material entering and leaving the lumen along its length, and the proportions of propulsive and resistive contractions all along the bowel. Furthermore, the reduction of volume by absorption from the lumen may be influenced by the nature of movements of the wall, to stir or circulate the luminal content or to affect the flow of lymph and blood through the vessels into which absorbed materials are transmitted (the relationship between motility and absorption remains one of the great challenges in gastrointestinal physiology). Net mechanical function of the bowel, then, is affected by so many different and interrelated variables that no single variable or set of linked variables can be entirely related to the symptoms usually attributed to small bowel motor malfunction.

Net motor function is frequently examined in man by looking at transit times for dye markers, timed from mouth to anus, or for radiopaque liquids, timed from duodenal entry to arrival at the cecum. Such determinations yield notoriously variable answers. This is not suprising in view of such sources of error as the independent transit times of stomach and colon, the possible effects of the markers themselves upon small bowel movement, and the possible effect of fasting upon the transit time.

In *ileus*, the movement of the entire small bowel is inhibited. A variety of things can produce ileus by activation of inhibitory reflexes, including severe somatic pain and pneumonia. Peritonitis, bowel obstruction and drug overdosage may act more directly. In ileus the bowel is sometimes not completely without movement. The remaining movements may or may not be qualitatively different from normal movements. The state has had little careful study. Such qualifying adjectives as adynamic, paralytic, primary, and secondary add little to our understanding of the pathogenesis of ileus.

Diabetic diarrhea[26, 27] is an occasional and troublesome complication of diabetes mellitus. It usually occurs in patients who are insulin-dependent and poorly controlled, and who have neuropathy. The diarrhea is usually intermittent and watery, although it may be steatorrheal. Fat absorption is sometimes impaired. Small bowel mucosal histology is normal. The mechanisms proposed include the overgrowth of bacteria in the small bowel, pancreatic exocrine deficiency, defects in absorptive processes, and autonomic neuropathy. Motor abnormalities are present, but they have not been well characterized.

Thyrotoxicosis[28] is often accompanied by an increased number of stools or by diarrhea. The nature of the movements in the bowel in thyrotoxicosis is unknown. The frequency of electrical slow waves is increased. In *myxedema*, in which constipation is the rule, slow wave frequency is diminished, but the nature of the abnormal movements of the small bowel is not clear.

Patients with *diffuse systemic sclerosis, dermatomyositis*, and similar diseases[29] may have intermittent watery diarrhea and constipation, abdominal cramping, and episodes of ileus or pseudo-obstruction. Because of the well known dysfunction of esophageal muscle in these disorders, it seems likely that changes in small bowel motor function arise from the same abnormality as the esophageal motor malfunction. The motor abnormality in the small bowel has not been studied well. It may be a consequence of both a vasculitis and fibrinoid degeneration in the smooth muscle. Bacterial overgrowth has been suggested also.

Some patients with *idiopathic diarrhea*[30] are found to have very rapid small-bowel transit; increased propulsive activity has been described in the jejunum in such patients and in patients after gastrectomy.

In occasional patients in whom it is desired to slow small bowel transit, segments of small bowel are reversed. Alternatively, a segment from the distal bowel may be interposed at a more proximal level. Such *reversed* or *interposed segments* slow net transit, taking advantage of the characteristics of the small bowel slow wave. After bowel transposition, the slow wave oscillators of the transposed bowel seem to retain their native intrinsic frequencies and native polarity of phase-lock even after complete healing has occurred. Presumably the retardation of flow is related to these fixed characteristics of the transposed segments.

REFERENCES

1. Pick, J. The Autonomic Nervous System: Morphological, Comparative, Clinical and Surgical Aspects. Philadelphia, J. B. Lippincott Co., 1970.
2. Dewey, M. M., and Barr, L. Structure of vertebrate intestinal smooth muscle. *In* Handbook of Physiology, Sect. 6, Vol. 4, C. F. Code (ed.). Washington, D.C., American Physiological Society, 1968, pp. 1629–1654.
3. Schofield, G. C. Anatomy of muscular and neural tissues in the alimentary canal. *In* Handbook of Physiology, Sect. 6, Vol. 4, C. F. Code (ed.). Washington, D.C., American Physiological Society, 1968, pp. 1579–1627.
4. Carey, E. J. Studies on the structure and function of the small intestine. Anat. Rec. *21*:189, 1921.
5. Elsen, J., and Arey, L. B. On spirality in the intestinal wall. Amer. J. Anat. *118*:11, 1966.
6. Kobayashi, M., Nagai, T., and Prosser, C. L. Electrical interactions between muscle layers of cat intestine. Amer. J. Physiol. *211*:1281, 1966.
7. Needham, D. M., and Shoenberg, C. F. Proteins of the contractile mechanism in vertebrate smooth muscle. *In* Handbook of Physiology, Sect. 6, Vol. 4, C. F. Code (ed.). Washington, D.C., American Physiological Society, 1968, pp. 1793–1810.
8. Rice, R. V., McManus, G. M., Devine, C. E., and Somlyo, A. P. Regular organization of thick

filaments in mammalian smooth muscle. Nature New Biology, *231*:242, 1971.

9. Gabella, G.   Caveolae intracellulares and sarcoplasmic reticulum in smooth muscle. J. Cell Sci. 8:601, 1971.

10. Henderson, R. M., Duchon, G., and Daniel, E. E. Cell contacts in duodenal smooth muscle layers. Amer. J. Physiol. *221*:564, 1971.

11. Burnstock, G., Campbell, G., Satchell, D., et al. Evidence that adenosine triphosphate or a related nucleotide is the transmitter released by non-adrenergic inhibitory nerves of the gut. Brit. J. Pharmacol. *40*:668, 1970.

12. Miller, N. E.   Learning of visceral and glandular responses. Science *163*:434, 1969.

13. Koelle, G. B.   Cytological and physiological functions of cholinesterases. Handbuch der experimentellen Pharmakologie, Vol. 15, D. Eichler and A. Farah (eds.). Berlin, Springer-Verlag, 1963, pp. 187–298.

14. Corrodi, H., and Jonsson, G.   The formaldehyde fluorescence method for the histochemical demonstration of biogenic amines: A review on the methodology. J. Histochem. Cytochem. *15*:65, 1967.

15. Jacobowitz, D.   Histochemical studies of the autonomic innervation of the gut. J. Pharmacol. Exp. Therap. *149*:358, 1965.

16. Norberg, K.-A.   Adrenergic innervation of the intestinal wall studied by fluorescence microscopy. Internat. J. Neuropharmacol. *3*:379, 1964.

17. Robinson, P. M., McLean, J. R., and Burnstock, G.   Ultrastructural identification of non-adrenergic inhibitory nerve fibers. J. Pharmacol. Exp. Therap. *179*:149, 1971.

18. Gershon, M.D., and Altman, R. F.   An analysis of the uptake of 5-hydroxytryptamine by the myenteric plexus of the small intestine of the guinea pig. J. Pharmacol. Exp. Therap. *179*:29, 1971.

19. Daniel, E. E.   Pharmacology of the gastrointestinal tract. *In* Handbook of Physiology, Sect. 6, Vol. 4, C. F. Code (ed.). Washington, D.C., American Physiological Society, 1968, pp. 2267–2324.

20. Hightower, N. C.   Motor actions of the small bowel. *In* Handbook of Physiology, Sect. 6, Vol. 4, C. F. Code (ed.). Washington, D.C.,

American Physiological Society, 1968, pp. 2001–2024.

21. Christensen, J., Glover, J. R., Macagno, E. O., Singerman, R. B., and Weisbrodt, N. W. Statistics of contractions at a point in the human duodenum. Amer. J. Physiol. *221*: 1818, 1971.

22. Prosser, C. L., and Bortoff, A.   Electrical activity of intestinal muscle under *in vitro* conditions. *In* Handbook of Physiology, Sect. 6, Vol. 4, C. F. Code (ed.). Washington, D.C., American Physiological Society, 1968, pp. 2025–2050.

23. Bass, P.   *In vivo* electrical activity of the small bowel. *In* Handbook of Physiology, Sect. 6, Vol. 4, C. F. Code (ed.). Washington, D.C., American Physiological Society, 1968, pp. 2051–2074.

24. Sarna, S. K., Daniel, E. E., and Kingma, Y. J. Simulation of slow-wave electrical activity of small intestine. Amer. J. Physiol. *221*:166, 1971.

25. Kosterlitz, H. W.   Intrinsic and extrinsic nervous control of motility of the stomach and intestines. *In* Handbook of Physiology, Sect. 6, Vol. 4, C. F. Code (ed.). Washington, D. C., American Physiological Society, 1968, pp. 2147–2171.

26. McNally, E. F., Reinhard, A. E., and Schwartz, P. E.   Small bowel motility in diabetics. Amer. J. Dig. Dis. *14*:163, 1969.

27. Whalen, G. E., Soergel, K. H., and Geenen, E. J. Diabetic diarrhea. A clinical and pathophysiological study. Gastroenterology 56: 1021, 1969.

28. Christensen, J., Schedl, H. P., and Clifton, J. A. The basic electrical rhythm of the human duodenum in normal subjects and patients with thyroid disease. J. Clin. Invest. *43*:1659, 1964.

29. Malkinson, F. D., and Rothman, S.   Changes in the gastrointestinal tract in scleroderma and other diffuse connective tissue diseases. Amer. J. Gastroenterol. *26*:414, 1956.

30. Ritchie, J. A., Salem, S. N.   Upper intestinal motility in ulcerative colitis, idiopathic steatorrhoea, and the irritable colon syndrome. Gut 6:325, 1965.

Chapter 18

Physiology of the Colon

Marvin H. Sleisenger

The main functions of the human colon are storage of intestinal content prior to discharge, absorption of water, electrolytes, and bile acids, and, to a minor extent, secretion. The last function mainly concerns mucus and electrolytes, particularly K+, but possibly HCO′3 also. Reservoir function and transit, of course, are closely linked.

ABSORPTION AND SECRETION

WATER AND ELECTROLYTES

An extremely important function of the human colon is absorption of sodium and water. This process proceeds through the length of this organ which averages about 135 cm (range 90 to 150) and has an area of 875 cm² (range 636 to 1613 cm²). Most absorption of water and electrolytes takes place in the right colon with progressively less activity caudad. This segment of the intestine receives fluid delivered to it, containing, per 24-hour period, 40 to 70 mEq of sodium, 3 to 6 mEq of potassium, 20 to 40 mEq of chloride, and 30 to 35 mEq of bicarbonate in a volume of about 500 to 600 ml. Analysis of stool water (100 to 150 ml per day) reveals sodium concentrations of 25 to 49 mEq per liter and potassium concentrations of 80 to 132 mEq per liter. Stool water thus has a high potassium and low sodium concentration, the ratio of so-

dium to potassium concentration being 0.3 in normal stool in contrast to 12 to 20:1 in terminal ileal fluid. The explanation appears to be a high transmembrane potential (PD) across colonic mucosa generated by active sodium transport, with potassium diffusing from blood to lumen down an electrochemical gradient.[1]

Fecal water contains about 15 mEq per liter of chloride, a concentration much lower than that in plasma. It is not certain whether chloride is actively absorbed, or whether all its absorption can be attributed to electrical PD generated by sodium transport. It is not clear whether there is a Cl′–HCO′3 exchange across colonic mucosa; thus the basis for the data on HCO′3 in Table 18–1 is uncertain. Since intraluminal chloride is essential for the secretion of bicarbonate, and since perfusion of saline solutions through the colon results in a decrease in chloride and a reciprocal increase in bicarbonate concentration, a coupled transport of these ions is suggested.

Considering the volume and electrolyte concentration of stool water, it is estimated that about 5 mEq of sodium, 5 to 15 mEq of potassium, and 2 mEq of chloride are excreted each day by the colon. Subtracting these values from the normal ileal effluent, it has been calculated that the colon absorbs about 400 ml of water, 55 mEq of sodium, and 28 mEq of chloride, and secretes 4 to 9 mEq of potassium per day (Table 18–1).[1, 2]

TABLE 18-1. COLON ABSORPTION AND SECRETION OF H_2O AND ELECTROLYTES

	H_2O (ml)	NA^+	K^+ (mEq)	C_L	HCO_3'
Terminal ileum	500–600	60	3–6	20–40	30–35
Stool	100–150	5	7–15	2	3
Net absorption or secretion	350–500	55	4–9	18–30	27–30°

° Mechanism unclear.

Studies of the colon by a perfusion technique in which isotonic sodium chloride solution without glucose is perfused indicate that the colon can absorb 2.5 liters of water, 403 mEq of sodium, and 562 mEq of chloride in the 24-hour period during which it would also secrete 45 mEq of potassium and 259 mEq of bicarbonate into the perfusion solution. Thus the colon has a capacity to absorb six to eight times more fluid than is delivered to it daily via normal ileal effluent.[3] Absorption in the right colon is greater than that in the transverse colon, which in turn is greater than that in the descending colon. The capacity in the rectum is relatively slight.

Under abnormal conditions such as sodium restriction in the diet or during periods of administration of salt-retaining hormones of the adrenal gland, the colon demonstrates its ability to increase absorption of sodium. Under these conditions, the ratio of sodium to potassium in stool water falls below 0.3. The potential difference (PD) of rectal mucosa increases, making the measurement a good clinical test of aldosteronism.

Adrenal hormones have a definite and consistent effect upon the movement of sodium and potassium in the colon. 9-α-Fluorohydrocortisone and aldosterone alter the concentration of these ions in stool water; thus 3 mg per day of 9-α-fluorohydrocortisone will result in mean sodium and potassium concentrations in stool water of 2 and 106 mEq per liter, respectively. The same effect is noted in normal subjects receiving aldosterone and may be observed in patients with primary hyperaldosteronism. Similar results have been obtained with perfusion techniques in which aldosterone has been shown in the normal human subject to increase colonic absorption of sodium from 24 to 40 mEq per hour.[4]

The concentration of sodium in colonic fluid influences the net rate of transfer of water. Thus no water absorption will take place when sodium concentration is below 20 mEq per liter. Neither will water or sodium absorption from isotonic test solutions be enhanced by the addition of glucose to the perfusion solution. Also, the rate of water and sodium absorption is markedly decreased when chloride is replaced by bicarbonate in a test solution. Water, however, can be absorbed from the colon when a lumen-to-blood osmotic gradient of as high as 50 milliosmols per kilogram exists. When the lumen-to-blood osmotic gradient, however, exceeds 150 milliosmols per kilogram, sodium and chloride enter the colonic lumen at a rate linearly related to that of water entrance.[3] Neither urea nor mannitol is absorbed in significant amounts from hypertonic solutions, suggesting a pore radius for the human colon epithelial cell which is smaller than the molecular radius of urea (2.3 Å).

Thus the colon's major role is concerned with water and electrolyte balance. The key is sodium absorption, an active process in turn influencing return of water from the lumen, which mechanism is therefore essentially passive. The colonic transport of chloride and bicarbonate is not clear, but an exchange is likely operative. Potassium appears to be secreted.

ABSORPTION OF BILE ACIDS

Bile acids are absorbed from the colon by nonionic (passive) diffusion. This mechanism is important in the absence of the distal small intestine, helping to maintain the total bile salt pool of the body. Ionic diffusion may also be responsible for some uptake by the mucosa.[5, 6] The process is important because only 300 to 600 mg of bile acids is excreted in man's stool daily.[7]

Estimates of the amount of bile acids absorbed by the human colon have been derived by measuring the concentration of unconjugated bile acids in rat portal blood, because deconjugation (as well as breakdown) of conjugated bile acids occurs primarily in the colon. Such estimates indicate that as much as 20 to 30 mg per day of bile acids may be absorbed from the rat colon. However, since some conjugated bile acids are hydrolyzed in the small intestine, this figure is probably high. On the basis of conversion of cholic acid to deoxycholic acid (since deoxycholic is the major metabolite of cholic and does not seem to be formed in the normal small intestine), the amount of bile acid absorbed from rat colon is estimated to be about 10 mg per day, or half the cholic acid pool. The corresponding figure in man would be about 600 to 650 mg per day. Injection of unconjugated C^{14}-labeled bile acids into the large intestine of rats and measurement of recovery in the bile indicate that about 50 per cent is recovered when the injected bile acid is unconjugated. From these studies, it was calculated that absorption from the large bowel of bile acids in the rat would be on the order of 5 mg per day, corresponding to about 300 to 350 mg in man per day. Granted that extrapolation of this information to man is hazardous, it is safe to assume that the magnitude of daily colonic absorption of bile acids from the colon is only 5 to 10 per cent of the total pool.[5] This contribution is further minimized in light of four to six enterohepatic circulations of this pool per 24 hours.

EFFECT OF BILE ACIDS ON TRANSPORT

Unconjugated bile acids affect the transport of water and electrolytes in the colon.[8, 9] The pertinent features of the enterohepatic circulation of conjugated and unconjugated bile acids are presented on pages 352 through 357. When conjugated bile acids are not normally absorbed in the distal small intestine, as, for example, following ileal resection or because of extensive ileal disease, these substances are hydrolyzed and metabolized by colonic bacteria; the products exert an effect on the function of the colonic mucosa. In man the diarrhea which results from such critical situations has been termed "cholereic enteropathy" and is due in part to the inhibition of electrolyte and water absorption from the colon by unconjugated dihydroxy bile acids, particularly the metabolite of cholic acid, deoxycholic acid.

The effect of these substances on absorption by normal colon in man and dog, although completely reversible, is clinically important with regard to water, sodium, chloride, and bicarbonate absorption; potassium secretion increases, but not in proportion to water and sodium (Fig. 18–1). Inhibition is not the exclusive property of unconjugated bile acids, because conjugated dihydroxy bile acids will also block water and electrolyte absorption (Fig. 18–2).[8, 9]

No evidence is at hand, however, that this adverse effect is due to a morphological change in the mucosal absorbing cells; in fact, studies in dogs indicate that perfusion of the colon with fluid isotonic to plasma at pH 8 to 8.2 containing 10 mM concentrations of cholic or chenodeoxycholic acids does not affect the gross and light or electron microscopic appearance of the colon epithelium; however, the amount of mucus found in colonic goblet cells on histological examination is reduced. It is likely that these substances

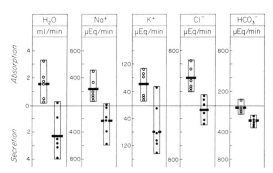

Figure 18–1. Effect of equimolar (10 mM total) mixtures of glycine or taurine conjugated bile acids on water and electrolyte transport. Each point represents a single study, that is, the mean of six sequential ten-minute periods. Open symbols represent control studies, and closed symbols represent bile acid studies. (From Mekhjian, H. S., et al.: J. Clin. Invest. 50:1569, 1971.)

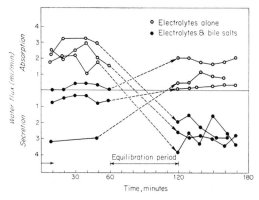

Figure 18–2. Influence of order of perfusion on net water transport during perfusion of control or 10 mM mixtures of conjugated bile acids, showing reversibility of induced secretion. Each point represents one ten-minute sample. (From Mekhjian, H. S., et al.: J. Clin. Invest. *50*:1569, 1971.)

stimulate discharge of mucus from the cells. Mucus depletion does not appear to be related to inhibition of absorption, because similar histological changes may be noted after perfusion with cholic acid (trihydroxy bile acid) which does not affect absorption of water and electrolytes in the dog.

These effects of bile acids are noted in man as well as dogs. Thus the human colon will secrete water, sodium, potassium, and bicarbonate when perfused with conjugated bile acids. The primary effect in man is thought to be stimulation of secretion of sodium which promotes secretion of water, and this in turn will "drag" other electrolytes into the lumen.[9] There appears to be some difference, not clearly understood, between the dog and man in

this regard, but the net effect is apparently the same. It does not appear to depend upon the degree of absorption of bile acid, because, as noted above, cholic acid has a nil effect; yet a greater amount of this bile acid is absorbed from 10 mM cholic acid perfusion solutions than from deoxycholic acid solutions of much lower concentration. Deoxycholic acid, which markedly inhibits water and sodium absorption, apparently acts independent of its degree of absorption; its effect appears to be related more to its intraluminal concentration and is most consistent at concentrations greater than its critical micellar concentration.[8, 9] The same is true for chenodeoxycholic acid in dogs; however, cholic acid is without effect even though present in micellar form.

Bacterial enzymes, in high concentrations in the colon, produce a large number of secondary fecal bile acids, particularly deoxycholic acid, via 7-α dehydroxylation.[5] Thus it is of great interest that deoxycholic acid, a metabolite of cholic acid and a bile acid which is found in significant concentrations in the stool normally, significantly inhibits water (and electrolyte) transport in the colon at lower concentrations than cholic and chenodeoxycholic acids (Fig. 18–3).[8, 9] One might speculate that a servomechanism exists here in which stasis leads to bacterial breakdown of a trihydroxy bile acid, cholic acid, to deoxycholic acid which inhibits transport of sodium and water, leading to a larger stool which stimulates propulsive activity and relief of stasis. The effect of the monohydroxy bile acid of chenodeoxycholic acid, lithocholic acid, is, how-

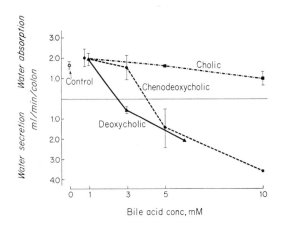

Figure 18–3. Effect of different concentrations of bile acids on absorption of water. Results from all studies with a given individual bile acid are included; mean ($\pm$ SE) has been calculated from perfusions with glycine and taurine conjugates, as well as unconjugated bile acid. (From Mekhjian, H. S., et al.: J. Clin. Invest. *50*:1569, 1971.)

ever, not known because its insolubility at body temperature has made testing in man impossible. Bacteria deconjugate bile acids quickly in man, behavior which makes their presence even more important in human disease.

WATER AND ELECTROLYTE ABSORPTION IN DISEASE OF THE COLON

In patients with chronic inflammatory disease of the bowel such as ulcerative colitis and Crohn's disease or granulomatous colitis, transport of water and electrolytes, particularly sodium, is significantly impaired. In Crohn's disease of the colon, net absorption of sodium, chloride, and water is decreased and potassium fluxes are not significantly altered. It is questionable whether this defect is correctable during periods of remission (see pp. 1296 to 1367).

OTHER FACTORS INFLUENCING WATER AND ELECTROLYTE TRANSPORT IN THE COLON

As would be expected, abnormal motility affects absorption of water and electrolytes by the colon. Any condition in which motility of the right colon is increased will shorten the time of contact between the mucosa and luminal contents. A multitude of conditions are characterized by excessive loss of fluid and electrolytes, particularly sodium, in the stool. In some of these conditions, an excessive quantity of water and electrolytes is presented to the colon, which, by virtue of the quantity of material involved, is unable to exert its usual "drying action." As the stool volume increases to large amounts, as noted particularly in cholera, the electrolyte composition approaches values close to those of plasma. In addition, there is a reversal of the normal ratio of stool sodium to potassium relating to the decreased contact time of intestinal contents with both ileal and colonic mucosae; thus the colon does not absorb sodium or secrete potassium normally. Not surprisingly, therefore, sodium loss is relatively greater than potassium loss.

MUCUS SECRETION

The goblet cells of the colon secrete mucopolysaccharides (glycoproteins) which serve to lubricate passage. Although immunoglobulins are also contained in colonic secretion, their site of origin is not known. Control mechanisms for synthesis of glycoprotein and, possibly, immunoglobulins are not known.

MOTOR TRANSPORT

MOTILITY OF THE COLON

The reservoir function of the colon is important, and depends upon the transport of intestinal contents, which process, for the most part, is a series of motor activities, some of which are clearly reflex responses. Generally, these components of colonic motility are due to smooth muscle contraction, either segmentally restricted or involving large portions. Transit time is slow, about 12 hours for passage from cecum to anus. It is affected by the gastroileal reflex, which probably initiates mass movements of the colon; local segmental contractions; and the defecation reflex. Although demonstration of pressure changes associated with these events is not satisfactory, some discussion of wave patterns is appropriate at this point.

COLONIC WAVES

The motor behavior of the colon has been studied intensively with many techniques for a number of years. Tubes with varying sized balloons, open-ended perfused tubes, radio telemetering capsules, and miniature balloons have all been utilized. The vast majority of studies have been confined to the rectum and rectosigmoid for obvious reasons; little information about the motor activity of the right colon is known. Because of its contact with the wall of the colon, the miniature balloon tends to be the most sensitive sensor of changes in intraluminal pressure—waves which are recorded by this method are generally of longer duration and higher pressure. Open-tipped tubes or tubes with lateral openings which are constantly perfused record true intraluminal

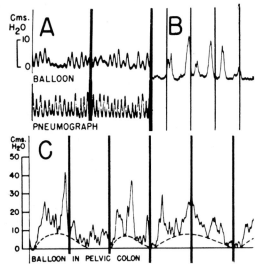

Figure 18–4. Wave forms recorded from the colon. *A*, Type I; *B*, type II; *C*, type III. (From Spriggs et al.: *Gastroenterology*, *19*:480, 1951.)

pressure with respect to atmospheric pressure. Most studies, however, have defined four wave types[10] as follows (see Fig. 18–4):

Type I. These local, phasic, i.e. intermittent, contractions are the most frequently noted; they last for five seconds on the average, and generate less than 10 cm of water pressure. They appear particularly in the rectum, but are also frequently seen in the cecum and sigmoid. They probably reflect contraction of the muscularis mucosae.

Type II. These waves are larger segmental contractions, generating more than 10 cm of water pressure, which are noted less frequently than Type I waves and are thought to be a response to resistance distal to the segment which is generating the contraction. These waves are obviously segmental, and define the "pockets" of the colonic lumen, the haustra; they move luminal contents minimally. They are seen in particular segments; however, the loci are not fixed. These contractions knead material, particularly in the sigmoid, for hours, disappearing and reappearing after variable intervals in other segments of the same part of the colon. These contractions serve to delay transit and promote maximum time for exposure of content to the

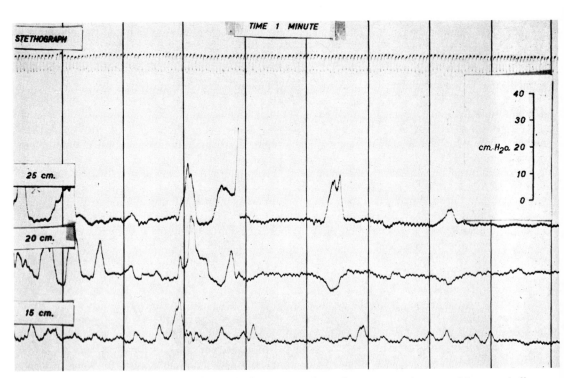

Figure 18–5. Record from a normal subject illustrating independent segmental activity. Miniature balloons at 25, 20, and 15 cm from the anus. Vertical lines, one-minute intervals. (From Connell, A. M.: *Gut* 2:175, 1961.)

mucosal surface for absorption of water and electrolytes (Fig. 18–5).

Type III. This infrequently observed wave represents a gradual elevation of baseline pressure, the significance of which is not clear.

Type IV. These are classic peristaltic waves. Peristaltic waves are a force which has been noted only very rarely in the normal colon but are occasionally seen in patients with diarrhea, particularly ulcerative colitis. Peristalsis appears to play no important role in the transit of material in the colon.

MASS MOVEMENTS

During the rapid transit of material from the right to the left colon, the haustra disappear. The left colon, following initial diminution in phasic activity, on receipt of the contents quickly begins to demonstrate segmental activity in an effort to delay further passage into the rectum. These movements are often stimulated by the gastroileal reflex (see below) which follows meals and propels material into the cecum. The so-called gastrocolic reflex is a mass movement.

THE GASTROILEAL REFLEX

Entry of food into the upper small bowel initiates a reflex response at the sphincter, perhaps mediated in part by gastrin, leading to passage of material from the distal small intestine into the cecum. Later, mass movements appear. That this response to food is dependent upon the release of gastrin or of secretin from the stomach is doubtful, because individuals who have undergone total gastrectomy have mass movements after meals.[11] Other hormones besides gastrin and secretin, particularly cholecystokinin-pancreozymin, may play a role in this integrated scheme; however, experimental evidence to support such a role for this hormone is not yet at hand. Neither does the response depend upon the vagus nerve, because it is present after either truncal or selective vagotomy. Whether it is dependent in some way on the rate of entry of food into the upper small intestine or upon the action of 5-hydroxytryptamine or prostaglandins remains to be determined also.

As noted, mass movement does not correlate with increased phasic activity; on the contrary, phasic activity of the left colon decreases or disappears as it shortens to receive material propelled into it from the proximal colon. After the material has arrived, phasic activity, initiating the "to-and-fro motion" which mixes contents and moves them slowly over very short distances, resumes. Thus they will be moved into the rectum which responds to distention by initiation of the defecation reflex (see below). Also the rectum may rapidly become distended as the result of mass movement of material into it from a more proximal location.

Recent measurements[12] indicate that mean pressure of phasic activity gradually rises from the distal rectum cephalad, being significantly higher proximal to the rectosigmoid. Similar results were obtained for mean duration of wave activity. Thus the index of motor activity, i.e., the product of mean duration and of mean pressure of activity, was higher at the rectosigmoid and just proximal to it than in the distal rectum. These findings are consistent with the gradual movement of material in the distal colon because this activity is *not* propulsive.

THE ILEOCECAL ZONE

The rapid movement of intestinal contents from the ileum into the cecum, the gastroileal reflex, most notable after eating, is the initiating event in mass transport of contents from the right to the left side of the colon. For many years there has been a question regarding the possibility of a sphincter at the ileocecal junction, a well defined anatomical structure, the function of which has been studied only rarely. Is it a valve or is it a sphincter? In studies of the motor activity of this segment of the intestine, first in dogs and then in man, by means of water-filled, constantly perfused, polyvinyl catheters, a zone of elevated pressure at the ileocecal junction was constantly recorded (Fig. 18–6).[13, 14] The zone measured 4 cm in length, and its pressure averaged about 20.3 mm Hg above mean colonic pressure. The re-

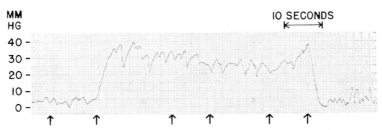

Figure 18–6. Pressure profile of human ileocecal junctional zone. Each arrow indicates a 1 cm movement of the recording tip from colon (left) across the ileocecal junction to ileum (right). (From Cohen, S., et al.: Gastroenterology 54:72, 1968.)

flex behavior of this zone may be tested by measuring its response to a sudden increase in pressure in the proximal ileum. In almost all instances, pressure discernibly decreases in the ileocecal junction, the magnitude of the drop varying between 20 and 100 per cent of mean pressure prior to distention. The duration of junctional zone relaxation correlates with the length of the balloon distention. Conversely, an increase in pressure in the colon distal to the junction is associated with a rise in pressure in the sphincter varying from 42 to 198 per cent above resting pressure, and the duration of the increase is directly correlated with the length of balloon distention.

Thus the ileocecal junction exhibits three necessary features for the definition of a sphincter: (1) it exhibits an intraluminal pressure greater than that found in the gut proximal and distal to it; (2) appropriate proximal stimulation is associated with a fall in this elevated pressure; and (3) distention distal to the area leads to a prompt rise in pressure within the area. Exactly how this sphincter works to control the rather slow flow of fluid from ileum into colon is not known; since proximal distention results in a fall of pressure in this area, it might have little, if any, influence on decreasing rate of flow. In the matter of prevention of retrograde flow, the function of the sphincter seems clear — it usually prevents reflux even in the presence of advanced distal obstruction of the colon. This behavior, however, could as well be attributed to a "flap valve" mechanism. Although reflux is freely seen on many barium enema X-ray examinations, the pressure generated during this procedure exceeds 90 cm H_2O, an exceedingly high level.

RELATIONSHIP OF MOTOR ACTIVITY TO COLON TRANSIT

Luminal contents of the colon are propelled principally by propulsive movements which manometrically and roentgenographically may not be considered peristalses. The so-called gastroileal reflex moves contents through the ileocecal sphincter into the cecum. There is a time lag of mass movement in the colon (the old "gastrocolic reflex") after eating, however, and this is likely due to the necessity for adequate distention of the cecum and right colon for initiation of mass movement. Thus the terminal small intestine is involved in a graded activity between it, the stomach, and cecum, facilitating passage of luminal contents into the right colon, and thence to the left colon. The effectiveness of the mass movement, it should be stressed, depends upon adequate volume of colonic content from which water has been reabsorbed. Mass movement is propulsive movement: contents may travel over the length of transverse and descending colons in a matter of seconds (Fig. 18–7).

Changes in segmental pressure of the colon are not correlated with propulsive activity; that is, increases in local pressure do not discernibly move material from one segment to another, but rather cause mixing (to-and-fro motion) within a segment (Fig. 18–8). Although propulsion of a radiotelemetering capsule in response to a meal from the cecal area to the splenic flexure is unaccompanied by a change in pressure, it must be moved by a gradient. It is not recorded because the capsule occupies a constant position within it.[15] Mass movements, however, have been only infrequently recorded; they have been noted

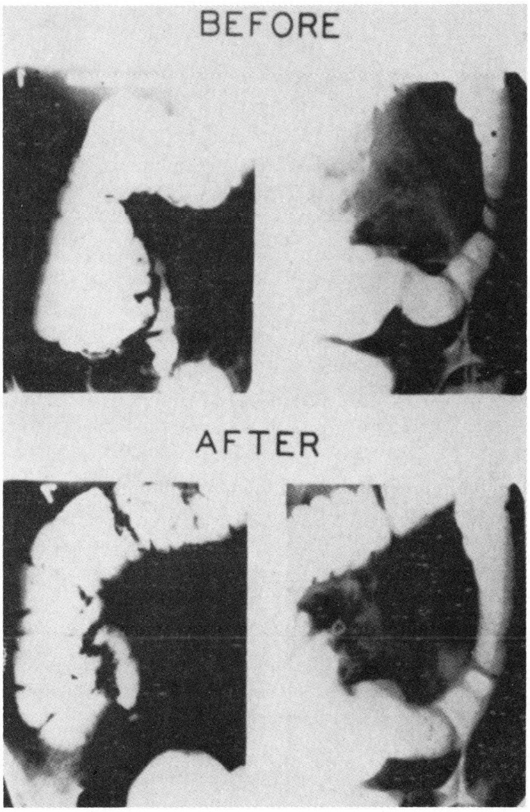

BEFORE

AFTER

Figure 18–7. Roentgenologic appearance of the right and left portions of the colon before infusion of acetylcholine and at the height of the effect of this agent. (From Kern, F., Jr., and Almy, T. P.: J. Clin. Invest. *31*:555, 1952.)

most commonly in patients with an irritable colon syndrome following meals. These individuals, more likely to have such mass movement in the colon on eating, also have more rapid than normal mouth-to-anus transit times (see pp. 1278 to 1294). If, however, propulsion is defined as movement of material over only a short distance (i.e., from 5 to 22 cm with an average of 10 cm), then such activity is

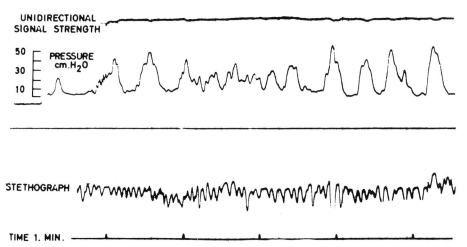

Figure 18–8. Record obtained from a pressure-sensitive radiotelemetering capsule in the sigmoid. Absence of changes in signal strength indicates little or no movement despite considerable pressure activity. (From Connell, A. M., et al.: Brit. Med. J. 2:771, 1963.)

commonly noted normally in parts of the colon following eating.

Techniques employed for measuring propulsion of material in the colon, whether ordinary propulsive activity or "mass movement," feature tracing of the progress of radiotelemetering capsules, of substances impregnated with radiopaque material (Cr^{51}-labeled capsules) by scintillation counter, or of free radioactive substances such as Cr^{51}. Combinations such as a radiotelemetering capsule which contains Cr^{51} simultaneously record changes in intraluminal pressure and propulsive activity.[15] The major difficulty with the radiotelemetering capsule, whether it includes a radioactive material or not, is that it will infrequently register the pressure within a segment of colon in which propulsion is taking place and only rarely during a mass movement of the colon.

Propulsive activity is motor change which moves material over variable distances of colon in contrast to segmentary contractions which underlie to-and-fro local motion. Mass movements are very rapid passage of material over both short and long segments, i.e., from proximal to distal colon. In any event, the motor pattern of propulsion, be it mass movement or not, is "wave-like" and sequential, but cannot be considered peristalsis because it is not preceded by a decrease in pressure.

ROLE OF AUTONOMIC NERVOUS SYSTEM

The anatomy of the autonomic innervation of the colon is described on page 1240. What is the role of the autonomic nervous system in colonic motor function? The answer is far from clear, and although both excitatory and inhibitory autonomic nerves are present, the main effect seems to be inhibitory, with some of this effect being mediated by adrenergic nerves. These are not particularly numerous in the distal colon. The relationship between the innervation and recently described electrical slow wave is not known; it is assumed, however, that such slow waves may be a pacemaker to which the autonomic system and, possibly, hormones respond. The parasympathetic system is thought to be excitatory; however, methacholine may inhibit muscular contraction and ganglionic blocking agents depress activity, an observation which supports the notion that the principal role of the nerves is inhibitory, particularly in the distal colon.[16, 17]

THE EFFECT OF EATING, EMOTION, AND EXERCISE ON COLON MOTILITY

The effect of eating upon the movement of material from the ileum into the colon and then its sudden transit by "mass movement" from right to left colon is pronounced and appears to be independent of the extrinsic innervation of the large bowel, as well as of longitudinal conduction of impulses in the spinal cord, because it is noted after transection of the cord. As noted, although gastrin may be involved, because eating is associated with the release of this hormone, mass movements are not abolished by total gastrectomy. Movement of contents into the cecum and diminution of pressure in the ileocecal valve, facilitated by reflex, somehow set off mass movement. Within three minutes of eating, the numbers of segmental contractions of the colon markedly increase, particularly in the sigmoid. The increase is about 25 per cent above the basal level in terms of numbers of contractions; however, the amplitude may also be greater (Fig. 18–9).[10, 14, 15, 18]

The effect of eating on the colon is normal, however, in patients with complete achlorhydria (pernicious anemia).[11] Since these patients probably do not stimulate normal release of secretin or cholecystokinin-pancreozymin, the role of these hormones in mass movement is presently unclear. No correlation with gastric acid output (and hence stimulation of upper intestinal hormone release) is found in patients with duodenal ulcer disease and acid hypersecretion. Perhaps the most important effects of small bowel activity upon colonic motor functions are mediated through release of 5-hydroxytryptamine, kinins, or prostaglandins.[19-21]

Emotion appears to play an important role in colon motility, although reports of this association have been conflicting (see pp. 3 to 11 and 1278 to 1288). In some ex-

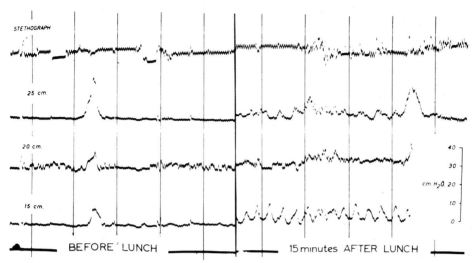

Figure 18–9. Stimulation of segmenting activity of the sigmoid by eating. Left, typical pre-lunch activity. Right, activity present 15 minutes after subject started to eat. Three miniature balloons record at 25, 20, and 15 cm from the anus. Vertical lines, one-minute intervals. (From Connell, A. M.: Gut 6:105, 1965.)

periments in which stress interviews were employed in patients with abnormal bowel habits, the evocation of certain emotional responses was associated with characteristic changes in motility patterns. For example, anger and hostility aroused thus in individuals might be associated with increased phasic activity and the appearance of higher waves; contrariwise, depression with weeping or feelings of resignation might be associated with abolition of all phasic activity in the left colon (Figs. 18–10 and 18–11).[22] Other investigators have not found a relationship between the emotional state of the patient and the motor activity of the left colon; in any event, it is difficult to interpret these experiments.[10] Clinically, emotion is thought to play an important role in the function of the colon during certain periods in the course of both ulcerative colitis and irritable colon.

Exercise has long been noted to affect bowel habit, being a recognized antidote in some for intermittent constipation. Motility studies in which telemetering capsules containing Cr^{51} were used indicate that physical activity increases colon motor activity, particularly propulsive movements after meals.[15]

Figure 18–10. Alteration in colonic motility during discussion of a stress-producing life situation. The gastric motility tracing provides a control on the effects of respiratory changes and altered intra-abdominal pressure. (From Almy, T. P., et al.: Gastroenterology *12*:425, 1949.)

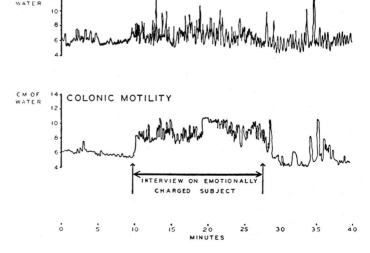

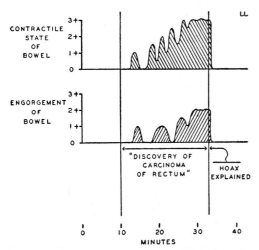

Figure 18–11. Sigmoidoscopic observations during a period of baseless fear in a healthy subject (see text). (From Almy, T. P., et al.: Gastroenterology *12*:425, 1949.)

EFFECT OF DRUGS ON MOTILITY

The effect of parenteral acetylcholine or methacholine on colon motor activity in normal subjects is to increase the pressure segmentally on the right side and, apparently, to reduce or abolish phasic activity on the left.[16] This effect has been interpreted to be a simulation of "mass movement" of material from right to left associated with the temporary disappearance of segmental contraction and haustra in the left colon (Figs. 18–7 and 18–12). Apparently, normal myenteric innervation is required for this effect on the left, be-

cause it is absent in approximately 50 per cent of the patients with congenital megacolon (Hirschsprung's disease) who have significant diminution or absence of ganglion cells of the myenteric plexuses of the rectum and proximal colon (see pp. 1463 to 1472).

Other drugs have a pronounced effect on the motor function and intraluminal pressure of the colon, for example, the opiates. Morphine given intravenously or intramuscularly will significantly increase intraluminal pressure, particularly in a segment of colon that may be abnormal, as in diverticulosis or in irritable colon.[23] The effect is characterized by increased phasic activity, beginning with a series of waves which reach a height of a few millimeters of mercury followed by a number of waves of equal duration—less than ten seconds—but of gradually increasing height, often achieving pressure greater than 40 mm Hg. This phenomenon gradually subsides after a period of 20 to 30 minutes, and the pressure returns to baseline levels. Intermittently thereafter, for a period of up to an hour or so, periodic phasic contractions would be noted in short sequences. When morphine is given intramuscularly or intravenously, it also raises the baseline pressure, superimposed on which appear the increased phasic contractions. The same effect, albeit less dramatic, may be noted after codeine is given parenterally. These phasic contractions in different parts of the colon bear no relationship to each other, and, as in the baseline recordings, seem to arise independently and often simultaneously.

Segments of colon involved with diverticula seem to over-respond with waves of average duration but with peaks often exceeding 50 mm Hg and, rarely, reaching 90 mm Hg. Although the number of such waves was not greater than in normal individuals given morphine, their height is significantly greater. This increase in phasic activity in the colon with significant rise in intraluminal segmental pressure following morphine is of some relevance in the consideration of management of a patient with diverticulosis (see pp. 1422 to 1424). Morphine, by increasing tonus of the colon, will increase its resistance to distention. The rate of accommodation to distention, however, is not altered.

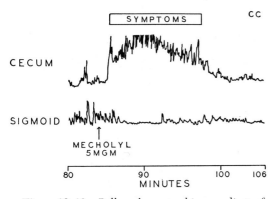

Figure 18–12. Balloon-kymographic recordings of motility of the cecum and sigmoid colon, showing coordinate action of methacholine on these regions of the bowel. (From Kern, F., Jr., and Almy, T. P.: J. Clin. Invest. *31*:555, 1952.)

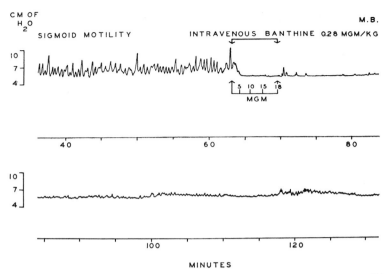

Figure 18–13. Intravenously administered Banthine promptly abolishes contractions of the sigmoid. This occurred after only 5 mg had been administered. (From Kern, F., Jr., et al.: Amer. J. Med. *11*:67, 1951.)

In contrast, meperidine (Demerol) does not cause the sigmoid colon to generate high pressures nor does it increase segmental pressure. Indeed, it diminishes the number of phasic contractions. Five milligrams of the meperidine analogue diphenoxylate (Lomotil) given orally or 2.5 mg given parenterally also has a decided inhibitory effect upon both mass movement and segmentary types of colonic activity. The clinical counterpart is the decided reduction in number of bowel movements in patients with diarrhea given this preparation.

Anticholinergic drugs such as Banthine and propantheline likewise abolish segmentary activity and reduce the effect of eating (Fig. 18–13). Of course, their action is atropine-like; however, in addition, a small degree of ganglionic blockade is thought to make it more potent at doses which less seriously disturb other parasympathetic mediated functions such as urinary bladder evacuation, etc.[25] In contrast to morphine, parenteral propantheline decreases the resistance of the colon to distention; like morphine, however, it does not affect the rate of accommodation to distention.[24]

Studies on the effect of 5-hydroxytryptamine (serotonin) on colon function indicate that this substance increases segmenting activity after intravenous injections. It also accelerates small bowel transit.[19]

Recent observations on the effect of prostaglandin E_1 on the colon indicate that when only 2.0 mg is given orally, propulsive activity in man increases with expulsion of gas and feces. It is not certain whether this effect was indirect and due to rapid transit in the small bowel or whether this substance affects the colon directly. Intravenous administration also produces an effect but only at higher doses, suggesting that a metabolite may be responsible for the diarrhea noted after oral administration.[21] Whether prostaglandin is responsible for diarrhea associated with certain tumors which secrete it, i.e., medullary carcinoma of the thyroid, remains to be determined. The fact that these drugs — meperidine, diphenoxylate, and anticholinergics — decrease phasic activity is not a criterion for routine use in patients with diarrhea. The management depends upon the underlying problem and is discussed in appropriate chapters in this book.

RECTAL CONTINENCE AND DEFECATION

The maintenance of continence of the internal and external anal sphincters is important and complicated. Small amounts of material in the rectum are not sufficiently stimulating to overcome the tonically contracted internal sphincter; the anal canal also remains closed when intra-abdominal pressure is increased except during a conscious attempt to defecate. Once, however, the internal anal sphincter relaxes — usually in response to rectal distention — material will pass into the anal canal; the mucosa therein will be stimulated, warning the individual of pending passage of material unless the external sphincter remains contracted. The voluntary contractions of the external sphincter therefore prevent defecation, and as pressure rises and the rectum adapts to its new volume of material which has moved cephalad, the anal stimulus for defecation is relieved.[26]

ANORECTAL SPHINCTERS

As with the gastrointestinal tract in general, the smooth muscle of the anorectal region is made up of a longitudinal layer (outer) and a circular layer (inner). The longitudinal muscles merge with the levator ani; deeper fibers are enmeshed in the internal and external anal sphincters, terminating near the mucocutaneous junction. Their contraction helps terminate defecation (see Fig. 97–14, p. 1246).

The sphincters are divided into the internal anal sphincter (see above) and the external anal sphincter. The internal anal sphincter is composed of circular smooth muscle. These muscle bundles form a wall which is three to four times thicker than the circular muscle of the colon itself. The external sphincter is made up of striated muscle located at various layers; the deeper one surrounds the internal sphincter, whereas the more superficial one lies caudad and surrounds the end of the anal canal. Both sphincters contribute to the proximal border of the anorectal ring which is composed posterolaterally of the puborectalis sling. The striated musculature involved in the defecation mechanism consists of an anorectal ring which is made up principally of the levatores ani, attached to the pubis anteriorly and the ischial spine posteriorly. Several muscle groups form slings within this ring, the most important one swinging from the posterior surface of the rectum and attaching to the pubis; its action moves the rectum forward and upward toward the pubis, providing a strong, sphincteric-like mecha-

nism at the anorectal junction. The other muscle group inserts into the fibrous thickening of the rectal sheath and binds the anal canal to the pelvic diaphragm; on contraction, it pulls the rectum upward and forward. Other muscle groups — the ileococcygeal portion of the levators — elevate the pelvic floor and provide some support for the abdominal viscera (Fig. 97–14, p. 1246).

INNERVATION OF THE ANORECTUM (see Fig. 97–10, p. 1240)

Sensation of the perineal skin and the anal margin is mediated by the same nerve fibers, with few organized endings, but with ample innervation of hair follicles. A profusion of nerve structures innervates the anal canal, mediating sensations of touch, cold, pressure, and friction. Proximal to the anal canal, the nerve endings are the same as those of the anal canal.

The rectal mucosa has no free nerve endings and few organized endings. Rather, it has both myelinated and nonmyelinated fibers. It also contains ganglion cells and processes of Meissner's plexuses which are easily identified in the submucosa.

The anus derives its normal cutaneous sensation from the branches of the pudendal nerve (S2, S3, S4); they provide to a lesser extent tactile sensation. The rectum, on the other hand, derives its sensory innervation from parasympathetic fibers passing through the same nerve trunks (S2, S3, S4) via the nervi erigentes. The fibers do not mediate ordinary painful stimuli, but are extremely sensitive to pressure.

Motor innervation is by way of the perineal and inferior hemorrhoidal branches of the pudendal nerve (S2, S3, S4) as well as from branches of the coccygeal plexus (S4, S5). The levator ani is supplied by branches both of the pudendal nerve and of the fourth sacral nerve.

Autonomic motor innervation of the internal anal sphincter is important because it plays such a major role in defecation (see pp. 1240 to 1241). Sympathetic supply is via the hypogastric nerves from the fifth lumbar segments, and the parasympathetic supply is via the nervi erigentes, from the first, second, and third sacral segments. The sympathetic nerve induces contraction of the sphincters, whereas the parasympathetic nerve provides an inhibitory action. On the other hand, the external sphincter receives only somatic pudendal innervation; its relaxation is due, therefore, to reduction in frequency of the existing motor impulses in the pudendal.

The rectum has an efferent sympathetic supply from the hypogastric plexus (L2, L3, L4) — distally and proximally from the inferior mesenteric plexus. Parasympathetic innervation is by the nervi erigentes (S2, S3, S4). The parasympathetics are motor for the rectum but inhibitory, as noted, for the internal anal sphincter. The sympathetic system is inhibitory for the rectum and motor for the internal anal sphincter.

MOTILITY STUDIES OF ANORECTUM

The resting rectal motility, as recorded by either balloons or open-tipped catheters, demonstrates phasic contractions of varying duration. The most accurate manner of recording appears to be by small open-tipped tubes or balloons which may be withdrawn from the sigmoid end of the rectum and anus. Tiny balloons record bands of increased pressure consistently in the rectum by this technique. They are thought to result from pressure applied to the balloon by bands or folds of the rectum as the balloon passes. A zone of elevated pressure representing the internal sphincter is found 3 to 7 cm proximal to the external anal margin. Although pressure varies from individual to individual, the range in this segment is 25 to 85 cm H_2O. For measurement of intrasphincter pressure, contributed to in major part by the internal sphincter, tiny balloons appear to be the most efficient sensor; however, they must be specially constructed in tandem so that simultaneous recordings may be made and so that the sensor will remain in place within the two sphincters. When so measured, these sphincters are found to be in a constant state of tonus; the internal sphincter has a higher resting pressure and is present in individuals with transection of the spinal cord, indicating its autonomic control.[26]

The external sphincter, although functioning at a lower baseline pressure, is also in a tonic state of contraction. Although its principal nerve supply is somatic and extrinsic, when separated from this nerve supply its muscular structure does not degenerate as do other voluntary muscles in such a situation. This sphincter, of course, responds to various changes of posture and activity, and any increase in intra-abdominal pressure is associated with evidence of increased external anal sphincter tone.

Of course, when increased intra-abdominal pressure is associated with defecation, the sphincter activity markedly diminishes; following defecation there is a rebound of increased sphincter activity, the so-called closing reflex. Micturition is also associated with inhibition of external anal sphincter activity. Dilatation of the anus, especially if sudden or forceful, will elicit a marked increase in sphincter tone. The external sphincter will also close in response to stimulation of the perianal skin.

The rectal sphincters are extremely responsive to sudden changes in intrarectal pressure above them; rectal distention

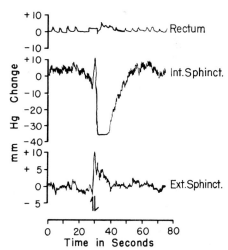

Figure 18–14. Transient distention of rectum. Internal sphincter relaxes and external sphincter contracts. Distention of the rectal balloon is indicated by an up-going arrow above the time scale, and deflation by a down-going arrow. Resting pressure recorded from each balloon is assigned a zero value. Increase in pressure above this level is termed positive and decrease below this level negative. (From Schuster et al.: Bull. Johns Hopkins Hosp. *116*:70, 1965.)

produces relaxation of the internal sphincter and contraction of the external sphincter (Fig. 18–14).[26] Relaxation of the internal sphincter is independent of peristalsis, although the internal sphincter will relax at the moment of rectosigmoid distention before the wave of contraction reaches mid-rectum. Rapid intermittent distention of the rectum will produce the same effect on the internal and external sphincters, only more pronounced; continuous and progressive distention, however, will be associated with a gradual return of pressure in both sphincters to prestimulus baseline levels. Studies of compliance of the rectosigmoid indicate that it may distend quickly with discomfort but not pain in response to the entrance of a large volume of material. This ability to stretch, provided intraluminal pressure is not suddenly increased *without* volume increase, initiates the defecation reflex.[26] Thus the internal sphincter responds mainly to rectal distention, whereas the external sphincter responds to a number of stimuli—voluntary effort, increased intra-abdominal pressure, anal dilatation, perianal stretch, and rectal distention.

CONTROL OF DEFECATION

Afferent and efferent pathways between the descending colon and rectum react to local stimulus resulting from the distention. Impulses are carried to the cortex which may then initiate the mechanism for voluntary defecation. This involves increased intra-abdominal pressure and relaxation of the pelvic floor and of the external anal sphincter. The cortex apparently also influences contraction of the muscles of the pelvic colon as they further aid in rapidly moving the contents caudally. However, much of the control is reflex, as attested by the control of defecation following transection of the spinal cord above the lumbosacral area. In this situation, the chief mediators of the efferent arc are the parasympathetic nerves from the sacral cord; stimulus originates in receptors for tension in the rectal musculature. Thus incontinence is controlled; however, defecation is inefficient in this situation, because contraction of the rectum and rectosigmoid is not normal, presumably because of the interruption of the pathways from the cortex which synapse with pelvic parasympathetics. Appropriate stimulus of the rectum, however, such as with enemata, will usually be sufficient to result in evacuation.

PHYSIOLOGICAL ASPECTS OF COLON PAIN

The relationship between stimulus intensity in the form of an acute distending force and its duration with onset of visceral pain is similar to cutaneous pain (Figs. 18–15 and 18–16). The duration to the threshold of pain in normal subjects when the intensity of stimulus is 100 cm H_2O averages 6.6 seconds with SD of 3.6 seconds (Fig. 18–17). The relationship of rate of distention to onset of pain is uncertain;

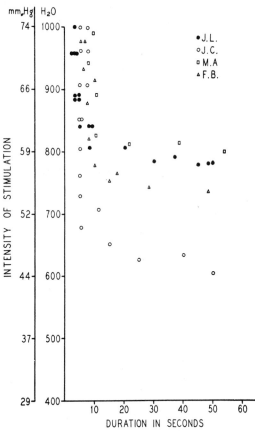

Figure 18–15. Relationship of intensity and duration of stimulus required to elicit pain following distention of the ileum. (From Lipkin, M., and Sleisenger, M. H.: J. Clin. Invest. 37:28, 1958.)

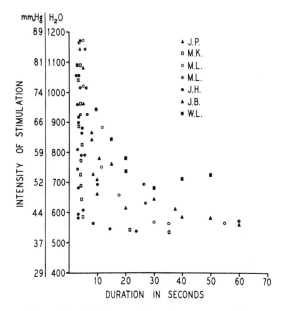

Figure 18–16. Relationship of intensity and duration of stimulus required to elicit pain following distention of the sigmoid colon. (From Lipkin, M., and Sleisenger, M. H.: J. Clin. Invest. 37:28, 1958.)

however, it is likely that a more intense stimulus, i.e., an increased rate of distention, lowers the pain threshold. On the other hand, increased intramural tension in the sigmoid associated with a decreased rate of distention might also result in an earlier onset of pain with correspondingly lowered threshold.[27]

The effect of drugs on colonic pain threshold and pressure to volume rela-

tionship is noteworthy. Morphine, 16 mg given subcutaneously, increases its resistance to distention, whereas an anticholinergic, propantheline, 15 mg given intravenously, decreases it. However, neither alters the rate of accommodation to distention. Correspondingly, visceral pain threshold is altered; it is noted only when the limit of distensibility of sigmoid is approached. The effect of morphine increasing the pressure to volume relationship is consistent with its "spastic" effect on colonic musculature.[24]

INTESTINAL GAS

COMPOSITION AND SOURCES

The major components of intestinal gas are nitrogen, oxygen, carbon dioxide, and methane. The total volume of gas in normal individuals ranges from 30 to 200 ml. Nitrogen is the predominant component, but has a wide range (26 to 88 per cent) in the postprandial state; oxygen concentration is low, averaging 0.69 per cent, with a standard deviation of 0.43 per cent. The total amount of oxygen and nitrogen is less than would be expected if swallowed air were the principal source of intestinal gas. About 19 per cent (±9.0 per cent) is methane, and 14.0 per cent (±7.0 per cent) is carbon dioxide. In such an analysis, in which a washout technique with inert

Figure 18–17. Frequency distribution of durations to pain threshold following distention of sigmoid colon, at a single intensity of applied stimulation. (From Lipkin, M., and Sleisenger, M. H.: J. Clin. Invest. 37:28, 1958.)

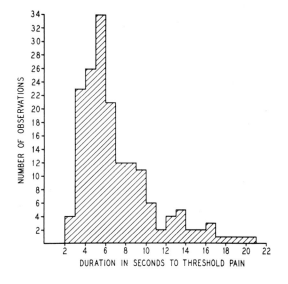

gases is used, an error is likely to be made only in the measurement of carbon dioxide, which is rapidly diffusible. Oxygen content could also be erroneously low owing to uptake by colonic bacteria.[28] Stomach gas normally contains a far lower proportion of carbon dioxide (4.0 per cent); it contains about 79 per cent nitrogen and 17 per cent oxygen. Hydrogen has been reported in stomach gas only occasionally, and then in trace amounts, and methane is present only under the most unusual pathological circumstances.

Human flatus is composed of 5 to 80 per cent carbon dioxide, zero to 10 per cent oxygen, zero to 54 per cent hydrogen and methane, and 17 to 88 per cent nitrogen. The concentration of hydrogen is lowest when flatus volume is large; that of carbon dioxide is high under the same circumstances.

Since carbon dioxide, hydrogen, and methane together comprise a large percentage of intestinal gas, and since they have low atmospheric concentrations, their appearance in intestinal gas must be due to intraluminal production. Thus it is likely that bacterial activity is the primary source of intraluminal gas. For example, 5 g of residual carbohydrates from a so-called low residue diet could yield as much as 975 ml of carbon dioxide, 375 ml of methane, and 200 ml of hydrogen, or about $1\frac{1}{2}$ liters of gas at body temperature. Further, conversion of lactic to butyric acid via bacterial action could release another $2\frac{1}{2}$ liters each of carbon dioxide and hydrogen from only 10 g of substrate.[29]

The principal source of hydrogen and methane is likely to be bacterial metabolism, because these gases are not present in the germ-free state. Bacteria also liberate carbon dioxide. The source of hydrogen is carbohydrate; i.e., nonabsorbable monosaccharides, raffinose, and stachyose contained in vegetables, particularly legumes. The source of methane production is unknown. The volume and composition of gas thus produced depend on both the substrate available and the type of enteric organism acting upon it. Thus, normal anaerobic, colonic organisms, bacteroides, and bifidobacteria produce carbon dioxide, methane, and hydrogen from sugars. These gases also evolve when amino acids are the primary substrate acted upon by the same organisms, with relatively more hydrogen and less carbon dioxide being formed with sugar as the substrate. Methane is present in only about one-fourth of normal human subjects in colon gas, a variation ascribed to cyclical change in the variety of organisms inhabiting the colon as well as present in diet. By and large, foods that are digested and absorbed slowly or not at all are the most likely to be the best medium for bacterial growth as well as for excessive production of gas.[29] The phenomenon is, of course, exaggerated in individuals with maldigestion and malabsorption, particularly those with the blind loop syndrome (see pp. 927 to 936). Foods that have a substantial content of essentially nondigestible sugars are the best substrates in normal subjects and in patients with malabsorption.

The pCO_2 of intestinal gas is twice that of venous blood; the principal sources are bicarbonate which has been split by hydrogen and bacterial action. Indeed, the pCO_2 of intestinal contents is at least 99 mm Hg; it is much higher after meals. The relative contributions to nitrogen content of intestinal gas via swallowing, bacterial action, and diffusion from blood are unknown. The partial pressure of carbon dioxide in the gut rises with increasing bicarbonate concentration in the presence of a relatively low pH of intestinal contents. High pCO_2 in the presence of bicarbonate concentrations, above 60 mEq per liter, helps maintain pH below 8; thus, carbon dioxide production may be regarded as an important contributor to the buffering mechanism for intestinal contents. Other evidence indicates that a higher secretion rate of acid as well as of bicarbonate will form more carbon dioxide in the gut. Carbon dioxide content is also affected by altitude; with progressive elevation larger percentages of carbon dioxide are found in rectal gas—from about 9 per cent on the average at ground level up to 60 per cent at 35,000 feet. Such an increase might be due to the absence of other diluting gases or from increased entry of carbon dioxide into the gut from endogenous sources.[9] The source of carbon dioxide in flatus is bacterial action, influenced by diet; it ranges from mean concentrations of

8 to 51 per cent (51 per cent with pork and beans!). The quantity of carbon dioxide in flatus parallels the rate of passage of hydrogen.[30]

Other mechanisms are also responsible for the presence of air in the gastrointestinal tract. Among these is swallowing of air, an invariable accompaniment of eating and drinking. Excessive swallowing of air, aerophagia, is more often associated with conditions in which swallowing is frequent and the mouth empty. These include hypersalivation, attempts to moisten an overly dry mouth, postnasal drip, gum chewing, and tobacco chewing. More air is swallowed with liquids than with solids; many foods contain air, either naturally or as a result of preparation or processing, and such added air may contribute substantially to the volume of the food.

Excessive amounts of air may be swallowed when it is inspired with the glottis closed because the large volume of air can easily pass through the patent gastroesophageal sphincter. This process is heightened when the esophagus is intubated, because the sphincter cannot close and the negative intrathoracic pressure of normal inspiration will carry large volumes of air into the stomach at an unusually rapid rate (about 40 mm per minute in man). In the patient with a nasogastric tube, air also enters the stomach with swallowing (2 to 3 ml per swallow); when added to the air entering with simple respiration, as much as $2^{1}/_{2}$ to 6 liters of air may theoretically enter the stomach, an amount which, actually, has never been measured.[29]

Atmospheric air thus contributes greatly to the accumulation of gas in the alimentary tract, and some authorities feel that it is the dominant source. Their case is based upon the observation of rapid accumulation of gas in the bowel during painful procedures, an accumulation which is prevented by nasogastric suction; further, the accumulation of gas proximal to small bowel obstruction may be reduced if simultaneously esophagostomy is performed and the distal end of the esophagus is closed. Finally, little gas is found to accumulate in a complete closed loop obstruction and none if the segment is emptied completely of air before it is experimentally closed.

DIFFUSION

The subject of diffusion of gas from the lumen of the intestinal tract into the blood is not clear. It is apparent, however, that gas diffuses into the circulation in accordance with physical laws of diffusion which relate primarily to rate and not direction of movement of these gases. Diffusion rates of oxygen, carbon dioxide, and nitrogen through the fluid layers of intestinal contents and across the intestinal membrane into the cells depend upon solubility and mass, and are directly proportional to the absorption coefficient of each gas divided by the square root of the density. Carbon dioxide moves out fastest because of its high absorption coefficient and because it is enzymatically assisted (carbonic anhydrase). The rate of diffusion also depends upon the differences in partial pressure on either side of the intestinal membrane; thus hydrogen, methane, and hydrogen sulfide, which have higher luminal concentrations, are instantly being removed.

Other important factors affecting the diffusion rate are the surface area and the membrane thickness. Rate of removal of gas is also influenced by blood flow to the particular segment of gut in which it is present. Finally, removal of gas from the alimentary tract is effected by perfusion of the lungs and, to a lesser extent, the skin. Hydrogen of intestinal contents passes into blood and thence into the breath; hydrogen from swallowed air tends to remain in the lumen; if large volumes of other gases are present in the gut, the partial pressure of nitrogen decreases and the diffusion gradient is favorable to influx of nitrogen from the tissues. Such diffusion of nitrogen from blood to lumen is noted after meals when pCO_2 is elevated and hydrogen and methane are produced. The relative contributions of swallowing and diffusion to total intestinal nitrogen are not known. These gases "trap" nitrogen, preventing its absorption, and favor its movement from blood to lumen. Nitrogen will shift out of the gut if its partial pressure with respect to the tissue is increased. Such an event follows breathing pure oxygen which increases threefold the rate of removal of nitrogen from a closed intestinal loop.[29, 30]

Oxygen in the upper gut usually moves away from the lumen because swallowed air is higher in oxygen content than are the blood and tissues. Lower in the gastrointestinal tract, the situation is reversed, for oxygen has been removed by diffusion, and by the active processes of the gut owing to its resident bacteria, and other gases have been added that serve to reduce further the partial pressure of oxygen. The gradient then favors movement of oxygen from blood to lumen.

Carbon dioxide moves out of the gut at a rate faster than any other gas because of its high absorption coefficient and because it is enzymatically assisted by carbonic anhydrase and has a rather specific transport mechanism in the blood. This movement of carbon dioxide is an important physiological mechanism for clearing the alimentary canal of its most dominant gas, carbon dioxide.

Nitrogen diffuses from blood to lumen because large gradients are noted in the upper gut after meals resulting from elevated pCO_2, and from the production of hydrogen and methane. However, the relative contributions of swallowing and diffusion to total intestinal nitrogen are not known. The trapping of swallowed nitrogen by lowering pN_2 probably causes diffusion of this gas from blood to lumen.[28]

REFERENCES

1. Fordtran, J. S., and Ingelfinger, F. J. Absorption of water, electrolytes and sugar from the human gut. In Handbook of Physiology, Sect. 6, Vol. III, C. F. Code and W. Heidel (eds.). Washington, D.C., American Physiological Society, 1968, p. 1465.
2. Wrong, O., and Metcalfe, G. The electrolyte content of faeces. Proc. Roy. Soc. Med. 58:1007, 1967.
3. Devroede, G. J., and Phillips, S. F. Conservation of sodium, chloride and water by the human colon. Gastroenterology 56:101, 1969.
4. Levitan, R., and Ingelfinger, F. J. Effect of aldosterone on salt and water absorption from intact human colon. J. Clin. Invest. 44:801, 1965.
5. Weiner, I. M., and Lack, L. Bile salt absorption, enterohepatic circulation. In Handbook of Physiology, Sect. 6, Vol. II, C. F. Code and W. Heidel (eds.). Washington, D.C., American Physiological Society, 1968, p. 1449.
6. Samuel, P. G., Saypol, M., Meilman, E., Mosbach, E. H., and Chafizadch, M. Absorption of bile acids from large bowel in man. J. Clin. Invest. 47:2070, 1968.
7. Danielsson, H. Present status of research on catabolism and excretion of cholesterol. Advan. Lipid Res. 1:335, 1963.
8. Mekhjian, H. S., and Phillips, S. F. Perfusion of the canine colon with unconjugated bile acids. Effect of water and electrolyte transport, morphology, and bile acid absorption. Gastroenterology 59:120, 1970.
9. Mekhjian, H. S., Phillips, S. F., and Hofmann, A. F. Colonic secretion of water and electrolytes induced by bile acids in man. J. Clin. Invest. 50:1569, 1971.
10. Connell, A. M. Motor action of the large bowel. In Handbook of Physiology, Sect. 6, Vol. IV, C. F. Code and W. Heidel (eds.). Washington, D.C., American Physiological Society, 1968, pp. 2075–2093.
11. Holdstock, D. J., and Misiweicz, J. J. Factors controlling colonic motility. Colonic pressures and transit after meals in patients with total gastrectomy, pernicious anemia or duodenal ulcer. Gut 11:100, 1970.
12. Ritchie, J. A., and Tuckey, M. S. Intraluminal pressure studies at different distances from the anus in normal subjects and in patients with irritable colon syndrome. Amer. J. Dig. Dis. 14:96, 1969.
13. Kelley, M. L., Jr., Gordon, E. A., and DeWeese, J. A. Pressure responses of canine ileocolonic junctional zone to intestinal distention. Amer. J. Physiol. 211:614, 1966.
14. Cohen, S., Harris, L. D., and Levitan, R. Manometric characteristics of the human ileocecal junctional zone. Gastroenterology 54:72, 1968.
15. Holdstock, D. J., Misiewicz, J. J., Smith, T., and Rowlands, E. N. Propulsion (mass movements) in the human colon and its relationship to meals and somatic activity. Gut 11:91, 1970.
16. Kern, F., Jr., and Almy, T. P. The effects of acetylcholine and methacholine upon the human colon. J. Clin. Invest. 31:555, 1952.
17. Christensen, J. The controls of gastrointestinal movement. New Eng. J. Med. 285:85, 1971.
18. Ritchie, J. A. Colonic motor activity and bowel function. I. Normal movement of contents. Gut 9:442, 1968.
19. Hendrix, T. R., Atkinson, M., Clifton, J. A., and Ingelfinger, F. J. The effect of 5-hydroxytryptamine on intestinal motor function in man. Amer. J. Med. 23:886, 1957.
20. Misiewicz, J. J., Waller, S. L., and Eiser, E. Motor responses of human gastrointestinal tract to 5-hydroxytryptamine in vivo and in vitro. Gut 7:208, 1966.
21. Misiewicz, J. J., Waller, S. L., and Kiley, N. Effect of oral protaglandin E₁ on intestinal transit in man. Lancet 1:648, 1969.
22. Almy, T. P., Kern, F., Jr., and Tulin, M. Alterations in colonic function in man under stress. II. Experimental production of sigmoid spasm in healthy persons. Gastroenterology 12:425, 1949.
23. Painter, N. S., and Truelove, S. E. The intraluminal pressure patterns in diverticula of the colon. Gut 5:201, 1964.

24. Lipkin, M., Almy, T. P., and Bell, B. M. Pressure volume characteristics of the human colon. J. Clin. Invest. *41*:1831, 1962.
25. Kern, F., Jr., and Almy, T. P. Effects of certain antispasmodic drugs on the intact human colon with special reference to Banthine. Amer. J. Med. *11*:67, 1951.
26. Schuster, M. M., and Mendeloff, A. I. Motor action of rectum and anal sphincters in continence and defecation. *In* Handbook of Physiology, Sect. 6, Vol. IV, C. F. Code and W. Heidel (eds.). Washington, D.C., American Physiological Society, 1968, pp. 2121–2146.
27. Lipkin, M., and Sleisenger, M. H. Studies of visceral pain. Measurements of stimulus intensity and duration associated with the onset of pain in esophagus, ileum and colon. J. Clin. Invest. *37*:28, 1958.
28. Levitt, M. D. Volume and composition of human intestinal gas determined by means of an intestinal washout technique. New Eng. J. Med. *284*:1394, 1971.
29. Calloway, D. H. Gas in the alimentary canal. *In* Handbook of Physiology, Sect. 6, Vol. V, C. F. Code and W. Heidel (eds.). Washington, D.C., American Physiological Society, 1968, pp. 2839–2860.
30. Levitt, M. D., and Bond, J. H., Jr. Volume, composition and source of intestinal gas. Gastroenterology *59*:921, 1971.

Chapter 19

Mechanisms of Digestion and Absorption of Food

Gary M. Gray

Traditionally the term malabsorption has been used to encompass both defective digestion and impaired absorption of food. In recent years, much new information about the processes of digestion and absorption has evolved, and it is now recognized that digestion of foods occurs sequentially at several different locations after ingestion. In order to identify the site of defective digestion and absorption, the overall process may be considered as a series of steps or phases. The principal processes occur either within the intestinal cavity or by action of the intestinal lining cell. Further, there are two different modes of exit from the intestinal cell, and only one of them is commonly affected in disease states. The stages of digestion and absorption are considered further on pages 259 to 277 in the discussion of maldigestion and malabsorption.

Although it is commonly believed that food is partially broken down in the stomach, little if any digestion occurs there. The initial phase of digestion occurs within the duodenal and jejunal lumen under the influence of secreted pancreatic enzymes and, in the case of dietary fat, by special solubilization with the aid of bile acids transported by the common bile duct. Further digestion of carbohydrate and protein then occurs on the intestinal

surface or within the intestinal cell yielding the final products for transport. The absorbed products of fat digestion are extensively modified within the cell. Careful consideration of the processes of fat, carbohydrate, and protein digestion will help the clinician develop a logical approach to the patient with maldigestion or malabsorption.

FAT DIGESTION AND ABSORPTION

INTRALUMINAL PHASE. LIPASE ACTION AND MICELLAR SOLUBILIZATION

Sixty to 100 g of fat is ingested daily by an adult in the Western world, and this fat is composed almost entirely of triglyceride containing three long-chain fatty acids on a glycerol backbone.[1] The typical structure and composition of fat in the diet are outlined in Figure 19–1.

The processes involved in fat digestion and absorption are diagrammed in Figure 19–2. Triglyceride is insoluble in the intraluminal intestinal water but is acted upon by secreted pancreatic lipase which functions at the oil-water interface to split off the two fatty acids from the α–positions

TRIGLYCERIDES

BASIC STRUCTURE	FATTY ACID COMPONENT	CHAIN LENGTH:SAT	FAT INTAKE
	PALMITIC	C16 : 0	
$H_2C-O-CO-R$	STEARIC	C18 : 0	
$HC-O-CO-R$			90 %
$H_2C-O-CO-R$	OLEIC	C18 : 1	
	LINOLEIC	C18 : 2	
	MCT	C:6 TO C:12	10 %

Figure 19–1. Structure and composition of dietary fat. Fatty acids on the glycerol backbone are represented by R. Note that long chain fatty acids make up 90 per cent of the diet. MCT, Medium chain triglyceride; SAT, degree of saturation or number of double bonded carbons in the fatty acid.

leaving the single fatty acid combined with the glycerol as a β–monoglyceride.[2] Neither the released long-chain fatty acids nor the monoglyceride are water soluble to any degree, but they are brought into the intraluminal solution by combining with secreted bile acids in a physicochemical complex called the micelle.[3]

The micelle forms because of the special property of bile acids which have both a polar and nonpolar region to their molecules. Molecules with such dual properties are called amphipaths or amphiphils.[3] At sufficient intraluminal concentration of secreted bile acids, the so-called critical micelle concentration (CMC), bile acids spontaneously become oriented to form a small sphere (5 mμ diameter, only one hundredth the size of an emulsion particle) with the water-soluble (polar) portion of each molecule at the exterior facing the

luminal water solution and the fat-soluble region located in the center of the sphere.[4] Fatty acids, monoglycerides, and the fat-soluble vitamins (A, D, E, and K) become included in the interior aliphatic region of the micelle and are effectively maintained in solution in the clear water phase of intestinal contents. Diglycerides and triglycerides remain in the oil phase and enter the bulk water phase via micelle solubilization only after hydrolysis by lipase to monoglyceride and fatty acids.

ABSORPTION OF FATTY ACIDS AND MONOGLYCERIDE

The micelle appears to disaggregate at the intestinal surface membrane, allowing the released monoglyceride and fatty acid to enter through the trilaminar lipoprotein membrane of the intestinal cell

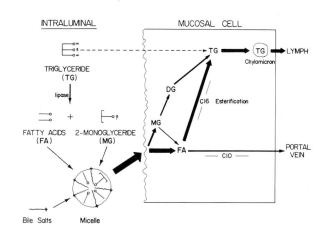

Figure 19–2. Fat digestion and absorption. Structures are represented diagrammatically as well as by name. C10 and C16 equals carbon chain length of fatty acids. See text for elaboration

by a process not requiring energy. Contrastingly, the bile acids remain within the intestinal lumen and enter into the formation of other micelles in jejunum and ileum.

BILE ACID REABSORPTION AND ENTEROHEPATIC CIRCULATION[*]

Bile acids are finally absorbed in the lower ileum by an active process which allows them to be transported against a concentration gradient. Only a small amount is unabsorbed and lost in feces. The absorbed bile acids are transported via the portal system to the liver parenchymal cells where they are taken up to be secreted again in the bile. This recirculation of bile acids occurs approximately six times in 24 hours and is commonly referred to as the enterohepatic circulation.[5] During a single recirculation, 95 per cent of bile acids are reabsorbed in ileum so that only 100 mg is lost into the colon and excreted in stool. Thus total bile acid losses are but 500 mg per day and the body pool is maintained by synthesis of this amount daily from cholesterol in the liver.

INTESTINAL CELLULAR ACTION ON ABSORBED FATTY ACID AND MONOGLYCERIDE

Once fatty acid and monoglyceride are absorbed, they are re-esterified to triglyceride by intracellular enzymes. Molecules of triglyceride then coalesce into a large particle (100 to 3500 mμ) of triglyceride which is coated with small amounts of protein,[6] cholesterol, and phospholipid (Fig. 19–2). This large particle, the chylomicron, has free exit out the base of the intestinal cell and preferentially enters the central lacteals of the villus, from which it moves via the thoracic duct to the venous system. Without the specialized coating to form the chylomicron, triglyceride is unable to leave the intestinal cell.

Overall assimilation of fat is more complex than for other nutrients, and it is notable that fat digestion and absorption require a specialized process at each intra-

luminal, cellular, and removal stage of digestion-absorption with the exception of entry at the brush border.

DIGESTION AND ABSORPTION OF MEDIUM-CHAIN TRIGLYCERIDES

Triglycerides composed of fatty acids of shorter chain length than the usual dietary long-chain fatty acids are called medium-chain triglycerides (MCT). These have been found to consist of C–6 to C–10 and have properties that are somewhat different from their longer chained counterparts.[7] The fate of MCT is shown schematically in Figure 19–3; it may be compared with that shown for LCT (Fig. 19–2). They can be absorbed intact in significant amounts (30 per cent of an oral dose). They are acted upon avidly by pancreatic lipase not only at the α-positions but also on the β-linked fatty acid yielding three molecules of medium-chain fatty acid (MCFA). These are more soluble in water than LCFA and appear to form micelles more readily with the bile acids. Once absorbed, the MCFA are not esterified in the intestinal cell but instead move across the cell and exit as fatty acids to be delivered via the capillary venous system and the portal vein.

The greater efficiency of handling of MCT at several stages of digestion-absorption has led to use of MCT-containing dietary preparations in patients with maldigestion or malabsorption. Therapy with MCT is discussed in detail in treatment of specific malabsorptive diseases (see pp. 259 to 277).

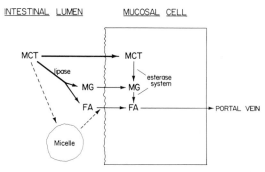

Figure 19–3. Fate of medium-chain triglyceride (MCT) in the intestine. Comparison with Figure 19–2 reveals that MCT has advantages over dietary fat (LCT) at each stage of digestion and absorption.

---

[*]The term "bile acid" is generically used to indicate either the protonated or unprotonated form of the molecule. "Bile salt" is the protonated form in the intestine.

CARBOHYDRATE DIGESTION AND ABSORPTION

Starch, sucrose, and lactose constitute the important carbohydrates in man's diet. All are inexpensive sources of food, and together they constitute the major source of calories when considered worldwide. In the Western world, about 400 g of carbohydrate are taken in daily, 60 per cent as starch, 30 per cent as sucrose as a sweetener, and 10 per cent as lactose. (Milk contains 50 g. of lactose per quart.)

Starch is a polysaccharide of molecular weight ranging from 100,000 to greater than 1 million with a straight chain of glucose molecules bridged by an oxygen between the first carbon (C–1) of one glucose unit and C–4 of its neighbor.[8] This type of starch is called amylose and makes up 20 per cent of starch in the diet. The glucose-to-glucose bridge is of the alpha type in contrast to the beta type which connects the glucose units in cellulose, an undigestible saccharide. About 80 per cent of starch that man ingests has branching points about every 25 molecules along the straight glucose chain. This starch is called amylopectin. These branches occur via an oxygen bridge between C–6 of the glucose on the straight chain and C–1 of the first glucose in the branched chain which then continues as another α–1–4 glucose-linked straight chain.

STARCH DIGESTION: AN INTRALUMINAL PROCESS

Salivary and pancreatic α–amylases have specificity for both types of starch, although little digestion occurs under influence of the oral enzyme because of the short exposure time before gastric acid stops the hydrolysis. Intraluminal digestion in the duodenum is extremely rapid because of tremendous amounts of secreted pancreatic amylase. Digestion to final products occurs by the time a meal reaches the distal duodenum. Some amylase becomes adherent to the intestinal surface and acts there by so-called "membrane digestion," but intraluminal amylase is ten times more active than necessary to explain the complete digestion occurring in duodenum[9] so that the physiological role of mucosal bound amylase is uncertain.

PRODUCTS OF α-AMYLASE ACTION ON STARCH

α-Amylase is an endo-enzyme that attacks the 1–4 α–glucose–glucose links at the interior of the starch molecule but is inactive against the outermost links and has little specificity for the 1–4 linkages adjacent to a 1–6 branching point. Further, it is completely incapable of splitting the α–1–6 glucose–glucose branching link. As can be ascertained from the specificity of amylase, the principal final products are maltotriose and maltose. When the starch is of the amylopectin type, the α–limit dextrins which contain one or more α–1–6 branching points are also formed. These branched saccharides are of varying size and contain an average of 8 glucose units. Maltose, maltotriose, and the α-limit dextrins are further digested by constitutive enzymes of the intestinal surface as outlined below. The overall process of carbohydrate digestion and absorption is diagrammed in Figure 19–4.

DIGESTION BY INTESTINAL SURFACE ENZYMES

Maltose, maltotriose, the α-limit dextrins, sucrose, and lactose are all hydrolyzed by enzymes integral to the intestinal brush border surface.[10] This intestinal surface digestion is followed by transport of the released monosaccharide products (Fig. 19–4).

TRANSPORT OF HEXOSE

The released six carbon sugars at the cell surface are of two types. The aldohexoses, glucose and galactose, are actively transported across the intestine by a process requiring energy and Na^+. It is likely but still unproved, that glucose binds to a specific protein (often called a carrier) in the brush border along with Na^+ and that the sugar and ion are thereby allowed entry across the membrane barrier of the cell.[8] Active pumping of Na^+ then occurs out the base and lateral sides of

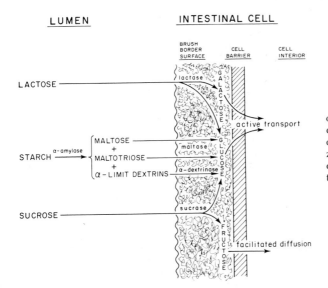

Figure 19–4. The digestion and absorption of carbohydrate. Note that only starch is digested in the lumen; other dietary saccharides are hydrolyzed by constitutive enzymes of the intestinal surface. The final monosaccharide products are then transported by their specific mechanisms.

the intestinal cell, thereby providing the driving force enabling glucose and galactose to be absorbed against a lumen-to-cell concentration gradient. Absorption of the high concentrations of glucose released from a carbohydrate meal at the cell surface probably occurs via carrier mediation but may be uphill only when luminal concentrations drop below those in blood. The active aspect of glucose-galactose transport permits the intestine to move these sugars actively when luminal concentrations decrease to those in blood, as occurs in the lower jejunum and ileum.

Fructose, the ketohexose released from hydrolysis of sucrose, is absorbed by a process called facilitated diffusion.[8] It appears to have a specific entry mechanism that is carrier mediated but energy independent, and it moves across the intestinal cell to capillaries by simple diffusion.

PROTEIN DIGESTION AND ABSORPTION

Knowledge of the assimilation of proteins has only recently begun to be elucidated.[11-12] Digestion of protein apparently begins in the stomach under the influence of pepsin. This lasts for one to two hours, because pH is lowered for that period by acid secretion stimulated by food. Most dietary protein, however, is hydrolyzed

initially in the duodenum and upper jejunal lumen under the influence of the pancreatic proteases which are secreted into proximal duodenum in inactive form.[11]

INTRALUMINAL DIGESTION BY PANCREATIC PROTEASES

Activation by a specific scission of each precursor peptidase is initially catalyzed by the duodenal mucosal surface enzyme, enterokinase, and finally by activated trypsin. Activation is essentially instantaneous in the first and second portions of the duodenal lumen. Intraluminal digestion of dietary protein occurs in the duodenum by sequential or essentially simultaneous action of pancreatic endopeptidases and exopeptidases. The endopeptidases, acting on peptide (CO–NH) bonds at the interior of the protein molecule, produce peptides that are ideal substrates for the exopeptidases which remove a single amino acid from the carboxyl terminal end of the peptide. The action of pancreatic proteases and the fate of the small peptides and amino acids released and presented to the intestinal cell are diagrammed in Figure 19–5. Actions by the endopeptidases (trypsin, elastase, chymotrypsin) yield oligopeptides that are further hydrolyzed by the pancreatic exopeptidases (carboxypeptidases) to yield neutral and basic amino

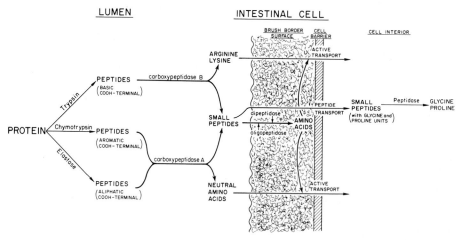

Figure 19–5. Diagram of digestion and absorption of dietary protein. Amino acid transport occurs principally by two independent mechanisms: one for neutral amino acids and the other for the basic amino acids (arginine, lysine).

acids and small peptides of two to six amino acid units.

There appears to be a tremendous overabundance of pancreatic peptidases secreted into the intestinal lumen under normal conditions in response to a meal. Thus, as noted for dietary carbohydrate, digestion and absorption of small peptides and amino acids by the intestinal cell are probably the rate-limiting processes in overall digestion and absorption of proteins.

CELLULAR DIGESTION OF PEPTIDES; SURFACE AND INTERIOR HYDROLYSIS

Small peptides released from pancreatic protease action must be handled by the intestinal epithelial cell. Oligopeptidases of the brush border are capable of hydrolyzing the residual di-, tri-, and tetrapeptides, particularly those containing neutral amino acids at the amino terminus of the peptide (Fig. 19–5).[13] However, peptides consisting primarily of glycine, proline, hydroxyproline, or dicarboxylic amino acids appear to be absorbed in peptide form when hydrolysis occurs in the cell cytoplasm.[14] The small fraction (10 per cent) of these glycine or proline peptides that are absorbed intact are not further hydrolyzed and exit from the intestinal cell in intact form to be presented to the kidney for filtration into the urine.

AMINO ACID ABSORPTION

Amino acids are taken into and transported across the intestinal cell by an active, Na^+-dependent process[12] analogous to that for glucose (see above). The neutral amino acid mechanism transports aromatic amino acids (e.g., phenylalanine, tyrosine, tryptophan) and aliphatic amino acids (e.g., leucine, valine, methionine) very rapidly. The basic amino acids (e.g., lysine, arginine) are absorbed by a separate and somewhat less efficient Na^+-dependent, active mechanism, but they are nevertheless transported rapidly. There are at least two other transport mechanisms in intestine, one for glycine, hydroxyproline, and proline and another for the dicarboxylic amino acids (aspartic and glutamic acids). However, small peptides containing these particular amino acids in abundance appear to be preferentially absorbed in intact form.

WATER AND ELECTROLYTE ABSORPTION

See pages 292 to 297.

IRON ABSORPTION

Ten to 20 mg of iron is ingested daily by an adult in the United States, and absorption from this is sufficient to prevent iron deficiency. In Asia, only 5 to 10 mg is provided in food, and iron deficiency anemia is very common.[15] However, it is difficult to establish that 10 mg is inadequate, because the Asian population also suffers from a high degree of malnutrition and parasitic disease that may predispose to gastrointestinal blood loss. Only 0.5 to 1.0 mg of iron is absorbed daily in healthy people; this increases several times to 3 to 4 mg when iron deficiency is present. Absorption of hemoglobin-iron (Hb–Fe) is most rapid, followed in order by ferrous ion (Fe^{++}) and ferric ion (Fe^{+++}).[15] Although absorption of organic iron (Hb–Fe) is not affected by chelators such as ascorbic acid, inorganic iron (Fe^{++} and Fe^{+++}) binds by chelation with ascorbate, dietary carbohydrates, or amino acids at acid pH in the stomach and upper duodenum to become soluble. This solubility is then maintained in the alkaline medium of more distal duodenum. Binding of inorganic iron with carbonates, oxylates, or phosphates evokes precipitation which makes iron unavailable for absorption. This precipitation may constitute a normal control mechanism to prevent hyperabsorption of iron[15] because patients with reduced intraduodenal bicarbonate resulting from pancreatic insufficiency may hyperabsorb iron.

Hemoglobin iron is hydrolyzed to heme and globin by intraduodenal proteases, the porphyrin ring then appearing to be absorbed intact to the interior of the intestinal cell where the heme is enzymatically split to release free inorganic iron.[16]

Absorption of inorganic iron (particularly Fe^{++}) in the diet occurs by a two-step process of *uptake* and *serosal transfer*.[17] Uptake occurs as a saturable process at low intraluminal concentrations of the iron and is an active process that requires energy by utilization of ATP. It is functional in all areas of the intestine. After mucosal uptake, the iron enters the ferrous pool where it either becomes stored as protein-bound Fe^{+++} or is transferred from the cell. The serosal transfer step is localized to the duodenum and appears to be rate-limiting for the overall absorption of iron.

Both these processes are regulated by the pre-existing amounts of iron in the intestine and in the body stores.[18] When these sites are saturated, absorption is markedly inhibited, and when there is iron deficiency, uptake and transfer are facilitated. Of the two steps, serosal transfer is most affected by the status of intestinal and other body stores and hence is probably the principal site of control.

CALCIUM ABSORPTION

Absorption of calcium occurs mainly in the duodenum; it appears to be an active process, different from that for iron, that is dependent upon an entry step perhaps followed by binding to a specific cytoplasmic protein (calcium binding protein),[19] followed by final transfer out the base of the intestinal cell. Recent evidence suggests that there is a bidirectional flux at both the luminal and serosal sides of the intestinal cell throughout the small intestine, but both entrance to and particularly exit from the cell are maximal in the duodenum,[20] making absorption most efficient at that level of intestine.

Vitamin D, via a metabolite, 1,25-dihydroxycholecalciferol, facilitates absorption of calcium by about four times the amount when there is deficiency of the vitamin.[21] Besides an increase in the amount of calcium-binding protein after vitamin D, there is suggestive evidence that the vitamin is capable of making the intestinal cell surface more permeable to calcium ion, probably by promoting synthesis of proteins that are playing either a catalytic or structural role in calcium absorption.[22]

ABSORPTION OF VITAMINS

Although thorough study of the mechanisms of absorption of many vitamins remains to be accomplished, most appear to be water soluble and their translocation across the intestine probably occurs by a passive mechanism. Absorption of two vitamins that are important for normal hematopoietic function appears to be unique and each is considered further below.

FOLIC ACID ABSORPTION

The primary food forms of folic acid are the polyglutamate conjugates of pteroylglutamic acid (PGA). Yeast and liver are the major sources for this vitamin, but appreciable amounts are also present in nuts and leafy green vegetables. On a regular diet 700 to 1500 μg of folate is ingested daily with 80 per cent in the conjugated form.[23]

Only PGA and the diglutamyl folate are physiologically active, so polyglutamates must be deconjugated prior to assimilation into the general body pool. There is strong evidence that intestinal γ–glutamyl peptidase activity in intestinal lysosomes[24] is responsible for cleaving the glutamic acid residues to yield the biologically active mono- and diglutamates. The intestinal hydrolysis of most natural polyglutamates yields the reduced dihydro- and tetrahydro-PGA rather than PGA itself, and these analogues are then quantitatively methylated within the intestinal mucosa. Methylated folates are the principal biologically active form circulating in the blood.[23]

Absorption of all folates is maximal in jejunum, and the small intestine capacity to handle the complex polyglutamates is nearly as great as it is for PGA itself.

VITAMIN B$_{12}$ ABSORPTION

Food in the usual Western diet contains 50 to 100 μg of vitamin B$_{12}$ per gram. A total of less than 2 μg of the vitamin is absorbed by an active, intrinsic factor-mediated process in the ileum.[25] A passive mechanism allows absorption of 1 per cent of very high intraluminal concentrations at all levels of small intestine; such large amounts of the vitamin are not available in the diet and cannot be economically administered as a supplement.

Intrinsic factor is a glycoprotein with molecular weight of about 50,000 to 60,000 that is secreted from gastric parietal cells.[26] Two molecules of intrinsic factor aggregate to form a 115,000 molecular weight dimer within the stomach, particularly when vitamin B$_{12}$ is present. Two molecules of the vitamin bind to the dimer, and the complex is carried with the intestinal contents to the ileum where it binds to a specific receptor protein.[27] The B$_{12}$ then appears to become disassociated and is absorbed. Although the intrinsic factor may remain bound to facilitate absorption of additional molecules of the vitamin, it does not appear to be absorbed, and its ultimate fate is not yet known.

In addition to the requirement for intrinsic factor, there is a substance in exocrine pancreatic secretions that appears to facilitate absorption of vitamin B$_{12}$ in some patients.[28] The mechanism of interaction has not yet been defined.

There has been an exponential increase in our knowledge of the physiology of digestive and absorptive processes in the last ten years, and fortunately much of this new information can be applied in the evaluation and treatment of patients. The purpose of this chapter is to provide a basic physiological background that will facilitate the clinician's approach to the patient with a defect in digestion or absorption.

REFERENCES

1. Mattson, F. H., and Volpenhein, R. A. The digestion and absorption of triglycerides. J. Biol. Chem. 239:2772, 1964.
2. Kayden, H. J., Senior, J. R., and Mattson, F. H. The monoglyceride pathway of fat absorption in man. J. Clin. Invest. 46:1695, 1967.
3. Hofmann, A. F., and Small, D. M. Detergent properties of bile salts: Correlation with physiological function. Ann. Rev. Med. 18:333, 1967.
4. Hofmann, A. F., and Borgström, B. Physico-chemical state of lipids in intestinal content during their digestion and absorption. Fed. Proc. 21:43, 1962.
5. Borgström, B., Lundh, G., and Hofmann, A. The site of absorption of conjugated bile salts in man. Gastroenterology 45:229, 1963.
6. Kay, D., and Robinson, D. S. The structure of chylomicra obtained from the thoracic duct of the rat. Quart. J. Exp. Physiol. 47:258, 1962.
7. Greenberger, N. J., and Skillman, T. G. Medium-chain triglycerides. Physiologic considerations and clinical implications. New Eng. J. Med. 280:1045, 1969.
8. Gray, G. M. Carbohydrate digestion and absorption. Gastroenterology 58:96, 1970.
9. Fogel, M. R., and Gray, G. M. Starch hydrolysis in normal and pancreatic insufficient man. Intraluminal process not requiring membrane digestion. Submitted for publication.
10. Miller, D., and Crane, R. K. The digestive function of the epithelium of the small intestine. II. Localization of disaccharide hydrolysis in the isolated brush border portion of intestinal epithelial cells. Biochim. Biophys. Acta 52:293, 1961.
11. Keller, P. J. Pancreatic proteolytic enzymes. In Handbook of Physiology, Sect. V, C. F. Code (ed.). Washington, D.C., American Physiological Society, 1968, p. 2605.
12. Gray, G. M., and Cooper, H. L. Protein digestion

and absorption. Gastroenterology *61*:535, 1971.

13. Kania, R. J., Santiago, N. A., and Gray, G. M. Intestinal cell surface peptidase: Potential role in protein digestion. Gastroenterology *62*:768, 1972.

14. Craft, I. L., Geddes, D., Hyde, C. W., Wise, I. J., and Matthews, D. M. Absorption and malabsorption of glycine and glycine peptides in man. Gut *9*:425, 1968.

15. Conrad, M. E. Intraluminal factors affecting iron absorption. Israel J. Med. Sci. *4*:917, 1968.

16. Weintraub, L. R., Weinstein, M. B., Huser, H.-J., and Rafal, S. Absorption of hemoglobin iron: The role of a heme-splitting substance in the intestinal mucosa. J. Clin. Invest. *47*:531, 1968.

17. Manis, J. G., and Schachter, D. Active transport of iron by intestine: Features of the two-step mechanism. Amer. J. Physiol. *203*:73, 1962.

18. Pinkerton, P. H. Control of iron absorption by the intestinal epithelial cell. Ann. Intern. Med. *70*:401, 1969.

19. Wasserman, R. H., and Taylor, A. N. Vitamin D_3 inhibition of radiocalcium binding by chick intestinal homogenates. Nature *198*:30, 1963.

20. Younoszai, M. K., and Schedl, H. P. Intestinal calcium transport: Comparison of duodenum and ileum *in vivo* in the rat. Gastroenterology *62*:565, 1972.

21. Taylor, A. N., and Wasserman, R. H. Correlations between the vitamin D-induced calcium binding protein and intestinal absorption of calcium. Fed. Proc. *28*:1834, 1969.

22. Adams, T. H., and Norman, A. W. Studies on the mechanism of action of calciferol. I. Basic parameters of vitamin D-mediated calcium transport. J. Biol. Chem. *245*:4421, 1970.

23. Rosenberg, I. H., and Godwin, H. A. The digestion and absorption of dietary folate. Gastroenterology *60*:445, 1971.

24. Hoffbrand, A. V., and Peters, T. J. The subcellular localization of pteroyl polyglutamate hydrolase and folate in guinea pig intestinal mucosa. Biochim. Biophys. Acta *192*:479, 1969.

25. Corcino, J. J., Waxman, S., and Herbert, V. Absorption and malabsorption of vitamin B_{12}. Amer. J. Med. *48*:562, 1970.

26. Fisher, J. M., and Taylor, K. B. The intracellular localization of Castle's intrinsic factor by an immunofluorescent technique using autoantibodies. Immunology *16*:779, 1969.

27. Donaldson, R. M., Jr., Mackenzie, I. L., and Trier, J. S. Intrinsic factor-mediated attachment of vitamin B_{12} to brush borders and microvillous membranes of hamster intestine. J. Clin. Invest. *46*:1215, 1967.

28. Toskes, P. P., Hansell, J., Cerda, J., and Deren, J. J. Vitamin B_{12} malabsorption in chronic pancreatic insufficiency. New Eng. J. Med. *284*:627, 1971.

Chapter 20

Maldigestion and Malabsorption: Clinical Manifestations and Specific Diagnosis

Gary M. Gray

The details of the normal processes of digestion and absorption of fat, carbohydrate, and protein are considered in depth on pages 250 to 257. Knowledge of these processes greatly facilitates the physician in his approach to patients with a defect in the assimilation of food. Digestion and absorption can be considered as a series of sequential stages or phases as outlined in Figure 20–1. In the broad sense, there are an *intraluminal phase*, an *intestinal phase*, and a *removal* or *delivery phase*. The removal phase simply indicates the vehicle used for carrying away the final products from the intestinal cell to other organs for storage or metabolism. Two of the three

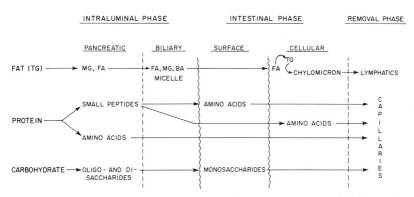

Figure 20–1. The phases of digestion and absorption of dietary constituents and the products released at each phase. Note that some phases are involved for each caloric source, whereas others are not; e.g., the biliary phase is essential only for fat, and the surface (brush border) phase is required only for digestion of carbohydrates and protein. (See pp. 250 to 257 for further details of digestion and absorption of fat, protein, and carbohydrate.)

major phases can be subdivided to allow precise localization of the defect or disease.

The *intraluminal phase* can be more precisely divided into two stages: the *secretory*, i.e., enzymes for digestion of all types of nutrients, and the *biliary*, because of the unique role that bile acids play in the solubilization of fat. The *intestinal phase* can be considered as the *surface* (or brush border) stage, because digestion of small carbohydrates and peptides occurs there, and the *cellular* stage, because transport or metabolism of the final digestive products takes place by specific action of the columnar lining cell. The five phases as related to digestion of fat, protein, and carbohydrate are shown in Figure 20–1.

Diseases that produce abnormal function of any phase of digestion and absorption can readily compromise man's ability to handle nutrients. Rather than attempting to memorize a list of diseases that produce malfunction based on the classic pathological categories such as inflammatory, vascular, and neoplastic disease, the author finds it much more logical to consider disease states that interfere with functioning of each individual stage of digestion and absorption.[1]

THE PATIENT WITH SUSPECTED DIGESTIVE-ABSORPTIVE DEFECT

Early Symptoms. Classic descriptions of malabsorption include massive weight loss with bulky, greasy, foul-smelling stools that float in the toilet. Unfortunately, such gross symptoms do not occur early in disease. Instead, patients often notice subtle changes such as alteration in the consistency or volume of the stool, something that they may not acknowledge as abnormal. Hence, the physician must carefully inquire about subtle changes in bowel habits occurring before the onset of weight loss, hyperphagia, pain, anorexia, or gross changes in bowel habits.

In intestinal or pancreatic disease, mild constitutional symptoms such as fatigue and disinterest in regular daily activities are often associated with passage of two or three soft stools per day long before the onset of classic symptoms. Such complaints can readily be passed over as being due to psychophysiological distress. At such a time, physical findings are usually absent, but smooth lateral margins of the tongue and hyperactive bowel sounds of normal quality may be noted in intestinal disease.

Late (Classic) Symptoms. If early complaints are overlooked, the patient progresses to a stage of malnutrition and cachexia. Deficiencies of the fat-soluble vitamins may produce hyperkeratosis of skin (vitamin A), ecchymosis and hematuria (vitamin K), and paresthesia, tetany, and bone pain (vitamin D). Malabsorption of the water-soluble vitamin B occurs in intestinal disease with complaints caused by glossitis, cheilosis, dermatitis, and peripheral neuropathy of the lower extremities. Anemia resulting from malabsorption of folic acid, vitamin B_{12}, or iron may produce pallor, fatigue, dizziness, or dyspnea, any of which can be the presenting symptom of the malabsorption.

Physical examination late in maldigestion-malabsorption reveals apathy, systolic blood pressures below 100 mm Hg, pallor, increased pigmentation of skin, hyperkeratosis, petechiae or ecchymosis, reddened, sore tongue with smooth lateral and anterior margins, positive signs for tetany (Chvostek, Trousseau), impaired touch and vibration sense of lower extremities, tender muscles, digital clubbing, and hyperactive bowel sounds often audible to others in the patient's room.

The clinical findings, supportive laboratory findings, and the alteration of function that explains these manifestations in maldigestion and malabsorption are outlined in Table 20–1.

CLINICAL TESTS OF DIGESTION AND ABSORPTION

A great many tests commonly used in clinical laboratories do not provide sufficient information on digestive and absorptive function to warrant the cost or the discomfort to the patient. Some of them are very popular, particularly the serum carotene test, which tends to be depressed in

TABLE 20-1.   CORRELATION OF DATA IN MALDIGESTION AND MALABSORPTION

CLINICAL FEATURES	LABORATORY FINDINGS	PATHOPHYSIOLOGY
Wasting, edema	↓ Serum albumin	↑ Albumin loss (gut), ↓ protein ingestion, ↓ protein absorption
Weight loss, oily bulky stools	↑ Stool fat excretion, ↓ serum carotene	↓ Ingestion and absorption fat, CHO, protein
Paresthesias, tetany	↓ Serum Ca^{++}, ↑ alkaline phosphatase, ↓ mineralization bones (X-ray), ↓ serum Mg^{++}	↓ Absorption Ca^{++}, vitamin D, Mg^{++}
Ecchymoses, petechiae, hematuria	↑ Prothrombin time	↓ Absorption vitamin K
Anemia	Macrocytosis, ↓ serum vitamin B_{12}, ↓ absorption vitamin B_{12} and/or folic acid, microcytosis, hypochromia, ↓ serum iron, no iron in marrow	↓ Absorption vitamin B_{12} and/or folic acid, ↓ Absorption iron
Glossitis	↓ Serum vitamin B_{12}, folic acid	↓ Absorption B vitamins
Abdominal distention, borborygmi, flatulence, watery stools	↓ Xylose absorption, ↓ disaccharidases in intestinal biopsy, fluid levels, small intestine (X-ray)	↓ Hydrolysis disaccharides and ↓ absorption, monosaccharides and amino acids

any patient with decreased intake of dietary fat as well as in intestinal defects, and the triolein-I_{131} absorption test, which is falsely negative in at least 20 per cent of patients with maldigestion and malabsorption, probably because available preparations of the radioactive triglyceride are impure.

Only a few tests have been substantiated to be of value in localizing the site of a digestive-absorptive defect. These include the quantitative fecal fat,[2] the D-xylose test,[3] pancreatic enzyme tests (secretin test[4] or Lundh test meal[5]), bile acid–C_{14} breath test,[6] vitamin B_{12} absorption test,[7] and the small intestinal biopsy.[8] In certain circumstances, it may be of value to assay the intestinal biopsy for digestive enzymes.[9] The quantitative stool nitrogen analysis is also of value but appears to be relatively less impaired in disease states than the fecal fat excretion and, like the fat test, does not permit localization of the defect to a particular phase of digestion and absorption.

QUANTITATIVE FECAL FAT

Despite being somewhat cumbersome for the patient and laboratory personnel, quantitative analysis of fecal fat[2] is the most sensitive test of overall digestive and absorptive function and is the first test to consider when a patient is suspected of having a defect in assimilation of nutrients. If no fat is taken in the diet, 1 to 3 g of fat is excreted per 24 hours because of daily loss of intestinal lining cells and bacterial lipids. When ingesting 60 to 100 g of fat per day, normal man excretes about 3 to 5 g of the fat ingested per 24 hours, and > 6 per day has been shown to be two standard deviations above the normal mean, usually indicating maldigestion or malabsorption, providing that the patient does not ingest large quantitites of undigestible fats such as castor oil.[1] The patient is placed on a 80 to 100 g fat diet, and completeness of fecal collection is assured by the use of stool softeners if necessary. Use of a pre-weighed gallon paint can is usually readily accepted by the patient for collection, because the container can be sealed and left in the bathroom during the collection period. Specimens can then be weighed and homogenized in a commercial paint shaker.

The classic Van de Kamer method of fat analysis[2] is based on extraction and neutralization of the long-chain fatty acids but is not totally accurate if a patient is taking medium-chain triglyceride supplements. However, the error is very small (about 10 per cent from the true value) even when all dietary fat is MCT, and modifications of Van de Kamer's methods can eliminate even this small error.[10, 11]

Since an abnormality at any state of digestion and absorption may cause increased excretion of fat, the test is a sensitive indicator but does not localize the lesion to one of the five stages. The other tests to be discussed are especially useful in defining the site of the defect once an increase in fecal fat excretion has been established.

PANCREATIC FUNCTION TESTS (PANCREATIC STAGE OF DIGESTION)

The secretin test[4] or the Lundh test meal[5] is used to measure secretory capacity of the exocrine pancreas. Duodenal luminal contents are aspirated via a tube positioned in the distal duodenum after stimulation of the pancreas by administration of secretin intravenously or by a peroral test meal. We use a small diameter (2 mm) polyvinyl tube with its sealed end covered by a latex rubber bag containing 1 ml of mercury. Collections are made by siphonage via three to six side-holes over the tube's terminal 6 inches. This method provides excellent specimens and is much easier for the patient to tolerate than the larger rubber or plastic small intestinal tubes. Aspirates are analyzed for HCO_3^- and pancreatic enzymes. Because of the tremendous reserve capacity of the pancreas, obstruction of the main pancreatic duct or extensive pancreatic disease is often required before aspirates are unequivocally abnormal. However, disease in the head of the pancreas may be discovered relatively early before other techniques such as radiographic studies reveal them. Technical difficulties are uncommon so long as the tube is placed properly and samples are chilled and analyzed within an hour or so after collection to avoid destruction of lipase, an unstable enzyme.

Normal values for enzyme concentration after secretin have been found to vary depending upon the laboratory but are reproducible in a particular laboratory. Bicarbonate concentration is normally 90 mEq per liter and tends to be diminished along with the enzyme concentrations uniformly in chronic pancreatitis and frequently in carcinoma of the head of the pancreas. Unfortunately, carcinoma of the body or tail of the pancreas is often associated with normal exocrine function of the organ (see pp. 1185 to 1197).

BILE ACID–BREATH TEST (BILIARY STAGE)

Although this test of bile acid function has only recently been described,[6] it is relatively simple to perform in any radioisotope laboratory and it permits a very sensitive measure of the fate of intraluminal conjugated bile acids. Since bile acids are secreted via the common duct in conjugated form, the use of a bile acid conjugated to glycine C^{14} or taurine C^{14} permits study of bile acid metabolism within the intestinal lumen. Under normal conditions, almost all the ingested radioactive conjugated bile acid is absorbed intact in ileum and recirculates back to the liver for re-excretion into the bile (see pp. 250 to 257); only a minute fraction of the conjugated bile acid–glycine C^{14} is lost into the colon, metabolized to $C^{14}O_2$, and excreted via the lungs. In contrast, whenever the bile acid–glycine C^{14} is exposed to large quantities of bacteria before absorption has occurred, deconjugation and metabolism of the released glycine C^{14} by bacterial enzymes produce appreciable amounts of $C^{14}O_2$ that then readily diffuse across the gut and are excreted via the breath.

The fate of orally ingested bile acid–glycine C^{14} in health and disease is outlined in Figure 20–2. Bacterial overgrowth in the small intestine and ileal dysfunction resulting from disease or surgical resection are the main causes of abnormal deconjugation of bile acids by bacteria. Small intestinal bacterial overgrowth will result in deconjugation and metabolism of the ingested bile acid–glycine C^{14} before it can arrive at the ileal site of active transport. The $C^{14}O_2$ released will readily diffuse across the intestine to be excreted in the breath. Similarly, ileal dysfunction prevents absorption of the bile salts, thereby allowing them to enter the colon where they are extensively metabolized. The pathological mechanisms leading to a ten-fold increase over normal in excretion of $C^{14}O_2$ in the breath in ileal disease or intestinal bacterial overgrowth are outlined in Figure 20–2.

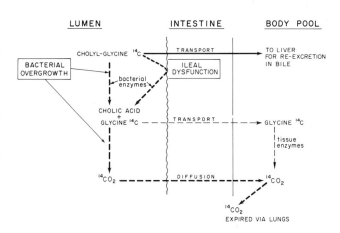

Figure 20–2. Outline of the fate of ingested cholyl-glycine-C^{14} in the bile salt–breath test. The solid line denotes ileal transport and normal recirculation. (See p. 252 for quantitative details of bile acid enterohepatic circulation.) The dashed lines represent alternate metabolism that is due either to small intestinal bacterial overgrowth or ileal dysfunction. Either condition produces release of $^{14}CO_2$ in the breath at concentrations ten times those found in normal man. (See text for detailed discussion.)

D-XYLOSE ABSORPTION-EXCRETION TEST[3] (INTESTINAL PHASES)

Xylose is a five-carbon sugar that is absorbed by the same transport mechanism as the hexoses glucose and galactose, but it has much less affinity for this mechanism and hence is relatively poorly absorbed. Assimilation of this sugar does not require the intraluminal pancreatic stage of digestion, and hence impairment of xylose absorption usually indicates small intestinal disease. When 25 g is ingested, only 50 per cent is absorbed in small intestine, and many individuals with a normal intestine have some diarrhea associated with the osmotic effect of both the residual intraintestinal xylose and the smaller fragments produced from bacterial action on the sugar. Of the xylose that is absorbed, only about half is excreted in the urine, the remainder being metabolized. As long as the subject does not vomit or have markedly delayed gastric emptying and providing that urinary output is maintained at about 60 ml per hour by oral hydration during the test, normal man excretes at least 4 g of the ingested xylose in the urine over a five-hour period.[3] Excretion decreases slightly after the age of 50 to 60 years, and in patients with renal disease; however, since intestinal absorption of the pentose remains normal, blood levels can be measured in these special circumstances at one and two hours after ingestion when the xylose concentration should be 20 mg per 100 ml. None of these pitfalls are common except poor hydration, which can be prevented by having the patient drink three to four glasses of water over the five-hour collection period. The xylose absorption test is simple and risk free for the patient, and laboratory analysis is relatively easy.[3] Overall, it is the most reliable test of the functional capacity of intestinal stages of digestion and absorption. Massive bacterial overgrowth sometimes produces an abnormal xylose test because of intraluminal metabolism of the sugar, but the test will return to normal after treatment with broad-spectrum antibiotics.

VITAMIN B_{12} ABSORPTION TEST (ILEAL INTESTINAL PHASE)

Orally ingested vitamin B_{12} combines with intrinsic factor in the lumen of the stomach and passes down the small intestine to bind as a complex to specific receptors on the ileal surface cells where the vitamin B_{12} is absorbed. In the conventional vitamin B_{12} absorption test an intramuscular injection of 1000 μg of the vitamin is given to ensure saturation of body stores so that an appreciable portion of the orally administered radioactive vitamin B_{12} will be excreted in urine after absorption. In most laboratories > 7 per cent of the radioactive vitamin B_{12} is excreted within 24 hours after ingestion of the isotope in normal subjects.

There are a few pitfalls that produce an erroneous test. Patients with pernicious anemia, stomach disease, or gastric surgery must have intrinsic factor given with the vitamin B_{12} dose in order to ensure that adequate B_{12}-intrinsic factor complex is presented to the ileum for absorption. As with the xylose test, adequate hydration and normally functioning kidneys are necessary to ensure excretion of the absorbed radioactive vitamin B_{12}. This test is useful in estimating ileal function, but may be abnormal in bacterial overgrowth because of binding of the vitamin B_{12} by organisms in the intestinal lumen. If massive bacterial growth in small intestine is responsible for diminished absorption of vitamin B^{12}, antibiotic therapy will return it to normal.

SMALL INTESTINAL BIOPSY
(INTESTINAL PHASES)

Suction biopsy of the small intestine can be safely carried out in older children and adults.[8] The procedure is more hazardous in infants and very young children; hence greater care in selection and execution is required.[12] The tube should be passed after an overnight fast; local pharyngeal rinse with 4 per cent lidocaine may be helpful. The patient should be placed on his right side after the tube enters the stomach and the tube slowly passed as one would intubate the small intestine for decompression. Position should be checked fluoroscopically before the sample is taken. (More details concerning the technique of suction biopsy, including illustrations of the instruments and procedure for mounting tissue may be found on pages 1501 to 1507).

When the biopsy is recovered, the muscularis mucosae at its base tends to contract, causing the tissue to assume a spherical shape with the villi pointing outward. The tissue can be easily reoriented by placing it on the index finger and rolling the muscularis outward with a small rod (e.g., the side of an 18-gauge needle). The villous surface will then adhere by surface tension as a sheet to the finger. The biopsy can then be touched to nylon mesh or filter paper so that the epithelial surface is upright and the muscularis mucosae is touching the supporting media. This special orientation allows serial sections to be cut from the base perpendicular to the long axis of the villi, a critical requirement for accurate histological interpretation.

Characteristic abnormalities are seen in a variety of diseases, but findings are closest to being specific in celiac sprue (nontropical sprue, celiac disease, gluten-sensitive enteropathy) because of the flattening of villi and morphological alteration of the digestive-absorptive surface cell from columnar to cuboidal type, as well as infiltration between these surface cells with round inflammatory cells. Whipple's disease, tropical sprue, amyloidosis, A-beta-lipoproteinemia, primary intestinal lymphoma, hypogammaglobulinemia, and nongranulomatous jejunoileitis may also be associated with characteristic changes in small intestinal morphology. Parasites (*Giardia lamblia*, coccidiosis) may also be discovered by biopsy (see pp. 989 to 1013).

ASSAY OF SMALL INTESTINAL
DIGESTIVE ENZYMES (SURFACE
STAGE)

Since the enzymes digesting oligo- and disaccharides are constituents of the brush border of the intestinal cell (see pp. 250 to 257), the small intestinal biopsy can also be analyzed for disaccharidase activity. Only a small portion (3 mg) of the biopsy is required for assay, the bulk being available for histological study. Normal values depend upon the laboratory but have been found to be remarkably similar throughout the world.[9] Generalized depression of these carbohydrases occurs very commonly secondary to small intestinal disease and usually constitutes as sensitive an indicator as intestinal histology of the status of the epithelial cells. A thorough discussion of disaccharidase deficiency is given on pages 1015 to 1019.

Oligopeptidases are also located in brush border, and specific assays have recently been developed. However, it is still premature to recommend intestinal peptidase assays, because specific deficiencies of these enzymes have not yet been identified, and the degree of their depression in generalized small intestinal disease is not yet known.

SMALL INTESTINAL X-RAYS[13]
(INTESTINAL AND DELIVERY
PHASE)

Barium sulfate contrast studies of the stomach and entire small intestine are

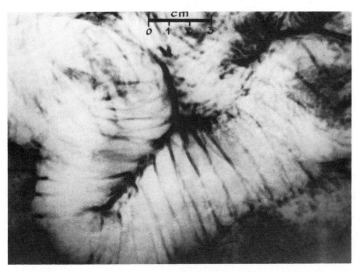

Figure 20–3. Barium contrast X-ray of the upper jejunum in a patient with celiac sprue. Note dilatation of folds but absence of thickening (compare with Fig. 20–5). (Used by the kind permission of the Honorary Editor of Clinical Radiology.)

most useful in defining anatomical defects (Diverticular pouches, congenital anomalies, postsurgical change) and primary disease of the small intestine. Findings in intestinal disease include dilatation of bowel lumen (see Figs. 20–3 and 20–4 for examples in celiac sprue and scleroderma), segmentation of barium to some bowel areas with only a thin line of contrast material in others, and dilution of barium because of increased intraluminal fluid. Transit time is frequently prolonged. Thickening of folds may occur owing to infiltration or edema; such thickening is seen in hypoproteinemia, Whipple's disease, amyloidosis (see Fig. 20–5), hypogammaglobulinemia, and radiation enteritis (Fig. 20–6). Intestinal lymphangiectasia may produce nodular filling defects, as demonstrated in Figure 20–7. Although often believed to be a finding in celiac sprue, thickening of folds is usually not found in patients with that disease (Fig. 20–3).

Pancreatic disease frequently produces abnormalities of the interior portion of the descending duodenum, with thickening and angulation of mucosal folds owing to inflammation of the adjacent pancreatic tissue. Pancreatic carcinoma frequently produces destruction of the duodenal mucosal folds caused by direct invasion.

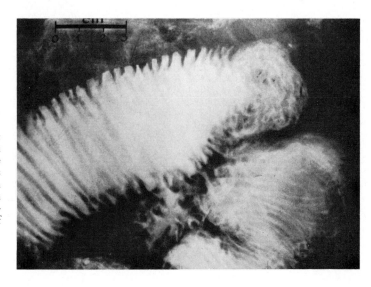

Figure 20–4. Barium contrast X-ray of jejunum in a patient with scleroderma. The mucosal folds are positioned closer together than is found with simple dilatation such as in celiac sprue (compare with Fig. 20–3). (Used by the kind permission of the Honorary Editor of Clinical Radiology.)

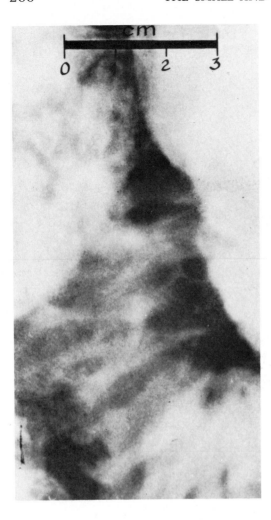

Figure 20–5. Barium contrast X-ray of jejunum in a patient with proved amyloidosis involving smooth muscle and blood vessels of intestinal wall. The mucosal folds are typically thickened and tortuous owing to the infiltrative disease. (Used by the kind permission of the Honorary Editor of Clinical Radiology.)

Figure 20–6. Barium contrast X-ray of upper and mid-jejunum in a patient with radiation enteritis. The folds are thickened (> 2 mm) and their perpendicular relationship to the lumen has been lost. The arrows indicate folds that are "tacked-down" at angles. (Used by the kind permission of the Honorary Editor of Clinical Radiology.)

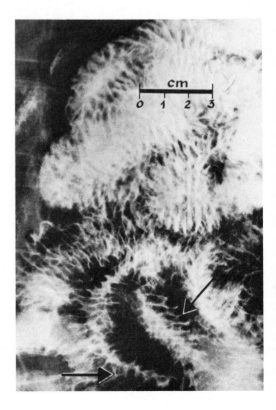

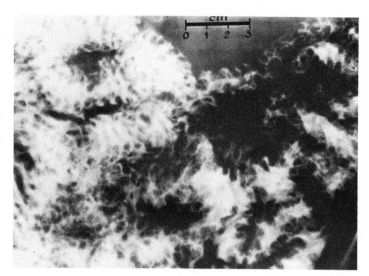

Figure 20-7. Barium contrast X-ray of jejunum of patient with severe lymphangiectasia proved at surgery. Note the multiple nodules with areas of thickening and irregularity of folds. (Used by the kind permission of the Honorary Editor of Clinical Radiology.)

Any patient with clinical and laboratory evidence of maldigestion and malabsorption should have upper gastrointestinal and small bowel barium X-ray studies.

SELECTION OF TESTS FOR MALDIGESTION AND MALABSORPTION

The physician should attempt to restrict the use of laboratory tests to those that establish the presence of impaired assimilation of food and to define the defect to a particular phase of the overall process. Even with these selections, there are still many worthwhile laboratory tests and procedures available, and a rational approach to the sequence of testing is most important to avoid needless discomfort and expense to the patient.

The approach to the sequential use of laboratory tools is diagrammed in Figure 20-8. In general, any patient suspected of having inadequate digestion and absorption of food should have a quantitative measure of fecal fat. If normal, selective malabsorption is still possible (pp. 280 to 289). If fecal fat excretion is elevated, a small intestinal x-ray and the xylose test should then be performed to determine the state of small intestinal structure and function. If xylose absorption is depressed, a small intestinal biopsy should be performed. If histology is abnormal, then attempts should be made to characterize the bowel disease (see discus-

sions of specific entities below). If histology is normal, bacterial overgrowth may be the cause of the abnormal fecal fat and xylose test. In such a case, special tests of ileal function (bile acid–breath test and vitamin B_{12} absorption test) can be carried out. If possible, intestinal aspirates, usually jejunal, should be cultured for anaerobic organisms. When the small intestinal X-ray reveals an abnormal jejunum, there is additional reason to biopsy the intestine. Evidence of diverticula, blind surgical pouches, or an abnormal ileum should prompt consideration of bacterial overgrowth or ileal dysfunction and calls for measurement of bile acid and vitamin B_{12} absorption as well as culture of aspirates. Finally, when a small intestinal biopsy is taken from a patient having carbohydrate intolerance as a major symptom, the disaccharidase assay can be carried out

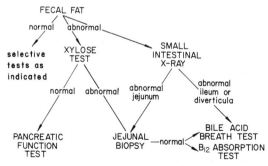

Figure 20-8. Diagram of the way in which specific tests can be sequentially chosen to evaluate a patient with suspected maldigestion and malabsorption.

on a small portion of the biopsy, the remainder being used for histological study.

DISEASES PRODUCING DEFECTS AT A SPECIFIC STAGE OF DIGESTION AND ABSORPTION

The diseases producing maldigestion and malabsorption according to major site of defective function, along with typical results of the digestive and absorptive

tests used are listed in Table 20–2. Figure 20–1 and Table 20–2 will serve as a reference for the discussion below on disease states and on the site of the defect. More detailed discussions of these conditions will be found on pages 864 to 1081.

PANCREATIC STAGE: DEFICIENT INTRALUMINAL PANCREATIC ENZYMES

Digestion of fat, protein, and carbohydrate requires pancreatic enzymes, and

TABLE 20–2. TYPICAL LABORATORY FINDINGS IN DISEASES CAUSING MALDIGESTION-MALABSORPTION

CATEGORY OF DEFECT/DISORDER (Normal Values)	FECAL FAT <6 gm/24 hr	XYLOSE TEST° >4 gm/5 hr	VITAMIN B$_{12}$ ABSORPTION° >7.0%/24 hr	SMALL BOWEL BIOPSY°
1. *Deficient intraluminal pancreatic enzymes (pancreatic phase)*				
Chronic pancreatitis	40	NL		NL
Pancreatic resection	40	NL		NL
Pancreatic carcinoma	40	NL	NL	NL
Cystic fibrosis of pancreas	25			
2. *Deficient intraluminal bile acids (biliary phase)*				
Biliary obstruction with jaundice	16	NL	NL	NL
without jaundice	19	NL	NL	NL
Jejunal bacterial overgrowth†	17	2.0–3.5	0.9	See Ref. 20
Ileal resection†	24	NL	3.0	
Ileitis (Crohn's disease)†	15	NL		
3. *Small intestine disease (surface phase)*				
Disaccharidase deficiencies	NL	NL	NL	Abnormal enzyme assay
4. *Small intestinal disease (cellular and delivery phases)‡*				
Massive resection	40	1.0–3.0	1.0	
Radiation enteritis	30	2.5–3.5	3.0	ABN
Intestinal ischemia	15	1.5–2.5	NL or ABN	
Celiac sprue	30	1.5–2.5	NL or ABN	ABN
Collagenous sprue				
Tropical sprue	15	1.0–3.0	ABN	ABN
Whipple's disease	35	3.0–4.0	NL	ABN
Primary intestinal lymphoma	40	1.5–2.5	ABN	ABN
Lymphangiectasia	20	NL		ABN
Hypogammaglobulinemia	20	2.5–5.0	NL	ABN
Dermatitis herpetiformis	10	2.5–3.5	NL	ABN
Eosinophilic gastroenteritis	15	1.5–3.0	3.0	ABN
Food allergy	15			
Nongranulomatous jejunitis	30	2.5–4.5	2.0	ABN
Amyloidosis	15	2.0		ABN
Parasitoses	15	1.0–4.0		NL or ABN
5. *Defects of multiple stages of digestion-absorption*				
Postgastrectomy	15	2.5–3.5	3.0	NL
Diabetes mellitus	25	3.5–4.5	NL or ABN	NL
Endocrinopathies	20	NL or ABN	NL or ABN	NL
Scleroderma	15	2.5–3.5	NL or ABN	NL
6. *Drugs producing maldigestion and malabsorption*				
Cholestyramine 12 g/day	7			
24–36 g/day	15			
Cathartics	10	NL		
Cholchicine	10	3.5	NL	ABN
Neomycin 2–6 g/day	10	3.0	NL	ABN
8–12 g/day	20	2.0		ABN

°NL, normal; ABN, abnormal.

†Bile acid breath test usually abnormal; xylose test and vitamin B$_{12}$ absorption return to normal after antibiotic treatment of bacterial overgrowth.

‡See Table 20–3 for comparison of histological changes in small intestinal disorders.

diseases of the pancreas may produce marked increase of fecal fat excretion (typically >35 g per day). In contrast, the xylose test is usually completely normal. The vitamin B_{12} absorption may be borderline (7 per cent) perhaps because of some facilitation of vitamin B_{12} absorption by a factor in pancreatic secretion, but it is never as low as in defects of small intestinal function (zero to 2 per cent). X-rays of small intestine may show abnormalities of the descending duodenum (see description above). If a small intestinal biopsy is obtained, it will be found to be completely normal.

In the Western world, chronic pancreatitis,[14] usually associated with alcoholism, is by far the most common cause of deficient pancreatic secretion of digestive enzymes. Pancreatic resection[15] for chronic pancreatitis probably now represents the second most common cause of defective pancreatic exocrine function. Pancreatic carcinoma,[16] although less common, is a devastating disease in which a rare opportunity for early diagnosis may stem from symptoms of maldigestion produced by a lesion in the head of the pancreas involving the main pancreatic duct. Cystic fibrosis is the most frequent cause of pancreatic maldigestion in children (see pp. 1206 to 1224).

BILIARY STAGE; DEFICIENT INTRALUMINAL BILE ACID CONCENTRATION

Fat maldigestion producing excretion of 15 to 20 g of fat daily may occur in extrahepatic biliary obstruction,[17] in intrahepatic biliary tract disease[18] with or without jaundice, after ileal resection, and in jejunal bacterial overgrowth[19] owing to intestinal stasis or after ileal resection. In each case, the excretion, intraluminal functioning, or ileal reabsorption of the conjugated bile acids is abnormal so that recirculation of bile acids is no longer efficient. Occasionally development of a cholecystocolonic fistula will also shunt bile acids and produce mild steatorrhea (approximately 15 g per day).

As noted, in jejunal bacterial overgrowth or ileal disease, increased excretion of fat will be accompanied by an abnormal bile acid C_{14} breath test. However, digestion and absorption of other nutrients do not require bile acid action, and the small intestinal histology is characteristically normal, although recent careful electron microscopic studies suggest that bacteria may invade and alter the epithelium.[20]

Intestinal stasis caused by multiple strictures such as those seen in extensive regional enteritis, multiple jejunal diverticula, surgical blind loops, intestinal diabetic neuropathy, or scleroderma gives rise to massive bacterial overgrowth in the duodenum and jejunum. The bacteria are capable of deconjugating and metabolizing bile salts[21] so they can no longer participate efficiently in micellar solubilization of lipid. In addition, the massively overgrowing bacteria frequently bind the vitamin B_{12}–intrinsic factor complex and thereby prevent vitamin B_{12} absorption.[22] The bacteria may also metabolize the bulk of xylose ingested before the pentose can be transported across the intestine. Hence, besides the expected mild increase in fat excretion, intestinal stasis is very often associated with a markedly depressed vitamin B_{12} absorption test (< 2 per cent per 24 hours) and a borderline or abnormal xylose test, all of which usually return to normal after administration of the appropriate antibiotic to reduce the overgrowing bacteria. This beneficial response to antibiotic therapy may be critical in establishing the diagnosis of the intestinal stasis syndrome (see pp. 927 to 936).

Of particular note in the biliary stage of absorption is the fact that the major defect is in the solubilization of fat. Pancreatic enzyme secretion and small intestinal function are both normal except in the intestinal stasis syndrome, in which massive bacterial action on vitamin B_{12} and sugars may prevent their assimilation and minor secondary intestinal anatomical changes may result from bacterial invasion of the intestinal epithelium.

SMALL INTESTINAL DISEASE; SURFACE PHASE

Disaccharidase Deficiencies.[23] These enzymes are confined to the brush border of the intestinal cell, and hence analysis of an intestinal biopsy will yield valuable information on the status of the digestive surface (see pp. 253 and 1015 to 1028). In general, disaccharidases are depressed in proportion to the severity of the intestinal cellular disease, and their activity correlates well with the histological status of the epithelium.

SMALL INTESTINAL DISEASE; CELLULAR AND DELIVERY PHASES OF DIGESTION AND ABSORPTION

Defects of small intestinal brush border surface or of the lining cells are associated with a mild to moderately increased excretion of fat in the stool, but the steatorrhea is not usually as severe as that seen in pancreatic disease (Table 20–2). However, xylose absorption is markedly abnormal, and the vitamin B$_{12}$ absorption test is frequently defective as well if there is significant involvement of the ileal mucosa.

Only a limited number of small intestinal diseases cause villous flattening of varying degrees. The histological abnormalities in the small intestinal diseases which affect villi and have characteristic alterations are detailed in Table 20–3. Notably, many diseases produce at least a partial flattening of the intestinal mucosa, and these include celiac sprue, tropical sprue, granulomatous and nongranulomatous jejunitis, primary intestinal lymphoma, hypogammaglobulinemia with giardiasis, and certain skin diseases such as dermatitis herpetiformis. Usually they can be differentiated by subtle differences in clinical features and histological changes. Other causes of malabsorption resulting from intestinal disease which can be identified by peroral biopsy are Whipple's disease, A-beta-lipoproteinemia, amyloidosis, and mast cell disease.

The classic disease of malabsorption is celiac sprue (nontropical sprue, gluten-sensitive enteropathy),[24] a disease associated with total flattening of the intestinal villi and stunting of the digestive-absorptive surface cells in the proximal small intestine. The most common causes of small intestinal malabsorption are iatrogenic, i.e., massive small intestinal resections in inflammatory and ischemic small bowel disease and high voltage X-irradiation for treating intra-abdominal malignancies. Maldigestion and malabsorption caused by either extensive *small*

intestinal resection[25] or *radiation enteritis*[26] are associated with fecal fat excretion of 30 to 50 g per day, depending upon the extent of the small intestine involved. Another entity causing increasingly more frequent malabsorption is arteriosclerotic *ischemic disease*[27] of the small intestine.

Celiac sprue[24] is the most frequently considered small intestinal disease producing malabsorption of all nutrients because of an inflammation and flattening of the intestinal surface epithelium. The cause is unknown, but family studies suggest that it may be genetic because of the presence of abnormal intestinal mucosa in asymptomatic relatives. The jejunum is involved extensively, but the ileum is often spared so that steatorrhea is moderate (25 to 30 g per day) and the xylose test abnormal, but vitamin B$_{12}$ absorption is often normal. Removal of the gluten from the diet is highly effective in reversing the intestinal lesion. The characteristic intestinal lesion is described in Table 20–3 and shown in Figure 20–9. (See also pp. 864 to 884.)

Tropical sprue[28] (see pp. 978 to 987) is associated with mild to moderate malabsorption (15 to 25 g per day) but accounts for more disease the world over than does celiac sprue. With the development of more rapid and inexpensive means of world travel, this disease is now being seen in the United States in people who may return to this country after having been asymptomatic when living in another land, such as Vietnam or Puerto Rico, where tropical sprue is sometimes endemic.

Collagenous sprue[29] is a newly recognized type of idiopathic sprue in which there is a dense band of collagen immediately beneath the epithelial cell layer. There is no response to a gluten-free diet, nor is there an association with ischemic or collagen vascular disease. The typical intestinal lesion in this disorder is shown in Figure 20–10. Comparison with Figure 20–9 reveals obvious differences from the morphological defect in celiac sprue.

Whipple's disease[30] has been of interest for many years because of the unusual macrophages beneath the lining epithelium of the intestine (Fig. 20–11) and the finding of bacillary bodies in electron micrographs of intestinal biopsies.[31] Steatorrhea is appreciable in this disease, but

TABLE 20-3. HISTOLOGY IN SMALL INTESTINAL DISEASE

DISEASE	VILLI	CRYPTS	EPITHELIUM	LAMINA PROPRIA
Normal	Tall	Villus: crypt = 4:1	Columnar; rare round cell infiltrating	Few plasma cells, histiocytes, lymphocytes, eosinophils
Celiac sprue (see Fig. 20–9)	Flat	Marked ↑ depth; villus:crypt = 3:1 or less	Cuboidal; plasma cell infiltrate	Loaded plasma cells
Collagenous sprue (see Fig. 20–10)	Flat		Cuboidal, round cell infiltrate	Collagen deposition immediately beneath epithelial cell layer, round cell infiltrate
Tropical sprue	Semi-flat	Moderate ↑ depth; villus:crypt = 3:1	Columnar to cuboidal; lymphocyte infiltrate	Loaded lymphocytes
Primary lymphoma	Semi-flat	Decreased in number	Columnar to cuboidal; inconsistent lymphocyte or histiocyte infiltrate	Malignant histiocytes or packing with lymphocytes in sheets infiltrating muscularis
Whipple's disease (see Fig. 20–11)	Broad; semi-flat	Usually normal	Columnar (normal)	Foamy macrophages that are periodic acid–Schiff positive; bacteria-like structures with electron microscopy
Dermatitis herpetiformis	Similar to celiac sprue; sometimes villous flattening and inflammation are less severe			
Lymphangiectasia (see Fig. 20–12)	Broad; dilated lymphatics	Normal	Normal	Dilated lymph channels
Regional enteritis	Shortened or normal		Normal to slightly cuboidal	Round cell infiltration; non-caseating granulomas
Hypogammaglobulinemia	May be similar to celiac sprue	Normal	Normal to cuboidal; giardia may be present	Lymphoid nodular hyperplasia may be present; reduced number to absent plasma cells
Parasitoses	Normal to flat	Normal	Normal to slightly cuboidal	Increased plasma cells, lymphocytes, and occasionally eosinophils
Nongranulomatous jejunitis	May be shortened or flattened – patchy	Normal or crypt abscesses	Normal to cuboidal, patchy ulceration	Increased polymorphonuclear leukocytes and round cells
Radiation enteritis	Shortened or flattened – patchy	Diminished mitoses; crypt abscesses	Normal to cuboidal; patchy ulceration	Increased polymorphonuclear leukocytes and round cells

Note: Amyloidosis affects vessels primarily; A-β-lipoproteinemia affects the cell only. Eosinophilic gastroenteritis may have only an eosinophilic infiltrate of the lamina propria. For details see relevant chapters in Section 11.

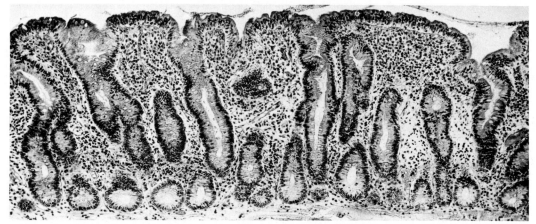

Figure 20–9. Small intestinal biopsy taken near the duodenojejunal junction from a patient with celiac sprue, showing the typical flat lesion with increased inflammatory cells in both the lamina propria and epithelial layer. Hematoxylin and eosin stain. ×120. (Courtesy of M. E. Ament and C. E. Rubin.)

xylose absorption is borderline or moderately reduced (Table 20–2) (See pp. 938 to 948).

Small intestinal resection or bypass[25, 32] produces a varied reduction in absorptive capacity, depending on the extent of resection or bypass. Jejunal resection produces very mild fat malabsorption (approximately 10 g per day) and no impairment of xylose or vitamin B_{12} absorption, probably because the ileum undergoes hyperplasia to take over the jejunal loss. Perhaps partly because the jejunum cannot compensate for loss of ileum which has a special role in bile salt reabsorption, extensive ileal resection or disease is associated not only with appreciable malabsorption of fat, but also with malabsorption of vitamin B_{12} and bile salts (see pp. 971 to 977). Xylose can be handled adequately by the jejunum, and hence the xylose test is usually normal in patients after ileal resection or with ileal disease.

Primary intestinal lymphoma[33] (see pp. 950 to 958) has been particularly identified in non-European Jews, but it is now being described in Mexicans living in the United States.[34] It is frequently confused with celiac sprue, but the intestinal surface cells are normal and the underlying lamina propria is loaded with lymphocytes which invade the muscle layers or with his-

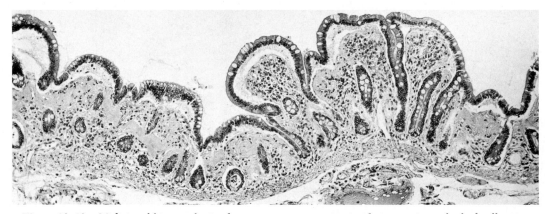

Figure 20–10. Midjejunal biopsy obtained at postmortem examination from a patient who had collagenous sprue. The intestine is severely altered. Surface epithelial cells are columnar in shape and have basally oriented nuclei as found in normal intestine. However, dense collagen has replaced the loose connective tissue normally found in the lamina propria. The lamina propria is hypocellular because of the displacement of mononuclear cells by collagen. Hematoxylin and eosin stain. ×120. (Courtesy of W. F. Weinstein and C. E. Rubin.)

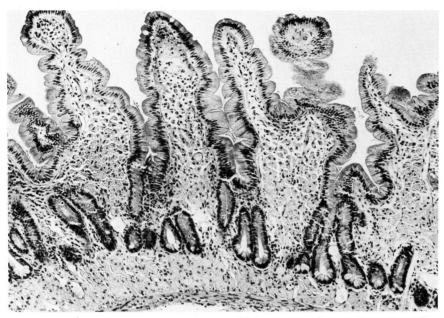

Figure 20–11. Proximal jejunal biopsy taken from a patient with Whipple's disease. The lamina propria is filled with histiocytes with finely granular cytoplasm. The muscularis mucosae, which normally lies against the base of the crypts, is separated from them by a band of histiocytes. Hematoxylin and eosin stain. × 120. (Courtesy of M. E. Ament and C. E. Rubin.)

tiocytes showing malignant cytological characteristics. Interference with the delivery phase of absorption is extreme, and fecal fats may reach 50 to 100 g per day. Symptoms are similar to those in celiac sprue, except that abdominal pain is a hallmark of the disease and there is no response to a gluten-free diet. Unlike celiac sprue, which spares the ileum, primary intestinal lymphoma usually involves the entire small intestine, and absorption of vitamin B_{12} is abnormal. Diagnosis is most difficult, and multiple exploratory laparotomies may reveal only a nonspecific lymphoproliferative pattern in intestine and mesentery which is probably a prelymphoma. Patients live many years but eventually die from local intestinal involvement and toxicity and the associated malnutrition. Intestinal perforation is common late in the disease. One of our patients who was near death responded dramatically to radiation therapy and is alive without recurrent disease three years after treatment. It is important to differentiate this disease from celiac sprue, because treatment and prognosis are very different and the disease appears to be more common than was previously believed.

Intestinal lymphangiectasia,[35] a disease of the structure of the lymphatics, has not been well characterized, but the lymph channels beneath the intestinal layer are dilated and functionally obstructed so that they do not readily accept chylomicrons (see pp. 250 to 257). Intestinal biopsies frequently show the lymphatics to contain macrophages loaded with lipid; additionally, chylomicrons, usually not seen in biopsy specimens, appear between intestinal cells and at extracellular sites in the lamina propria. Notably this disease is almost unique in interfering nearly exclusively with the delivery phase of absorption. The severe distortion of villous architecture that is produced by the marked dilatation of the central lacteals is demonstrated in Figure 20–12.

In *A-β-lipoproteinemia,*[36] mild steatorrhea occurs in patients with an inability to make the protein-phospholipid-cholesterol coating of the chylomicron. Intestinal surface cells are laden with triglyceride even when the patient is fasting. Since chylomicron formation is important only for fat absorption, the xylose test and vitamin B_{12} absorption test are normal (see pp. 1046 to 1049).

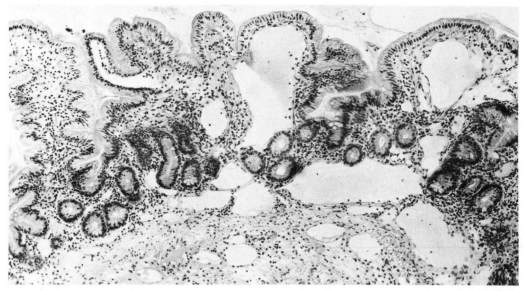

Figure 20–12. Proximal jejunal biopsy from a patient with intestinal lymphangiectasia. The biopsy is diagnostic, with abnormally dilated lacteals distorting the villous architecture. For comparison, a single normal villus is present at the left margin. Hematoxylin and eosin stain. × 120. (Courtesy of M. E. Ament and C. E. Rubin.)

In *hypogammaglobulinemia*,[37, 38] depressed serum globulins, whether congenital or acquired, are frequently associated with malabsorption. Recently, giardiasis has been found to be present in many of these patients. Flattened villi have also been found on small intestinal biopsy.[38] Appropriate treatment for the parasite may revert the intestinal histology to normal and eliminate the malabsorption in some patients. In others a gluten-free diet may lead to clinical remission and return of villi to normal. It is probable that absence of an immunoglobulin allows minor pathogens to overgrow in the intestine, producing chronic but reversible damage to the integrity of the mucosal barrier. It is likely that more syndromes of generalized intestinal disease associated with various types of immune deficiency states will be identified (see pp. 51 to 68 and 384 to 405).

Small intestinal ischemia[27, 39] is becoming an ever-increasing cause of small intestinal malabsorption, perhaps because treatment of many diseases has made it possible for patients to live longer until abdominal arteriosclerotic disease results in an inadequate blood supply to the small intestine. Occasionally patients with *polycythemia vera* or *vasculitis* related to the collagen diseases develop vessel narrowing and consequent ischemia. Fecal fat is mildly elevated (approximately 15 g per day), and xylose absorption is definitely abnormal. Pancreatic function tests are frequently normal but may also be reduced owing to ischemia to this organ.

Eosinophilic gastroenteritis and apparent allergy to foods[40, 41] have some qualities of true allergic reactions. Although both entities are associated with mild steatorrhea (10 to 15 g per day), the exact cause of those entities and their relationship to each other are unknown (see pp. 1066 to 1081).

Skin diseases,[42] such as dermatitis herpetiformis, are not infrequently associated with an intestinal histological lesion similar to celiac sprue (Tables 20–2 and 20–3). However, not all patients have malabsorption, and the clinical status of the skin lesion does not correlate well with intestinal histology. Patients with skin diseases and a suggestive history of malabsorption should be suspected of having abnormalities of both these rapidly replicating surface epithelia (see pp. 864 to 884).

Regional enteritis[43] although most commonly found in the ileum, may extensively involve jejunum. It is manifested by histological changes of surface epithelium similar in many respects to celiac sprue. However, granuloma can frequently be seen in the lamina propria and muscularis mucosae on small intestinal biopsy (Table 20–3) (see pp. 886 to 908).

Nongranulomatous jejunitis[44] may be a variant of celiac sprue or an early stage of primary intestinal lymphoma; it is manifested by jejunal ulcerations and flattened villi without signs of granulomatous change.

Amyloidosis,[45] both primary and secondary, may cause malabsorption because of vascular involvement of the submucosa. However, mucosal biopsies are usually normal until late in the disease, and the diagnosis may be very difficult to make from the small intestine. Rectal biopsies are known to be reliable in diagnosis of this disease (see pp. 1061 to 1065).

Parasitoses (see pp. 989 to 1013) can be associated with partial flattening of intestinal villi and malabsorption. Those particularly noteworthy are hookworm,[46] strongyloidiasis,[47] coccidiosis,[48] capillariasis,[49] and giardiasis.[50] However, malabsorption is usually mild (15 g per day), and patients with massive infestations often suffer from chronic malnutrition or have become compromised hosts so that there may be a variety of abnormalities that in the aggregate produce the malabsorption. It is often not possible to implicate the parasite as the sole cause of the malabsorption.

DEFECTS OF MULTIPLE STAGES OF DIGESTION AND ABSORPTION

Postgastrectomy[51] (see pp. 822 to 827): The interruption of the integrity of the pyloric sphincter and the intricate interrelationship of stomach emptying to pancreatic and biliary secretion is particularly important after a Billroth II resection, but some interference with normal function follows even a pyloroplasty and vagotomy. The principal reasons appear to be failure of maximal stimulus of pancreatobiliary secretion and, particularly, inadequate mixing of food with these secretions. In a Billroth II gastrectomy, food typically moves ahead of the bulk of these solubilizing and digestive secretions. Rapid intestinal transit may also contribute to the malabsorption by reducing the contact time of food with the intestinal surface, but anticholinergics usually do not eliminate the malabsorption. An occasional patient will have sufficient stasis, especially in the afferent loop of a Billroth II anastomosis, to produce a genuine intestinal stasis syndrome with bacterial overgrowth.

Although malabsorption is mild (approximately 15 g of fat per day), postgastrectomy is a very common condition and malabsorption resulting from this iatrogenic cause probably accounts for more cases of steatorrhea than any other.

Diabetes mellitus[52] may be associated with malabsorption in patients requiring insulin for longer than two years, although the malabsorption may occasionally antedate gross clinical evidence of diabetes. Most patients have watery stools before malabsorption can be documented, with a tendency to awaken to pass several stools after bedtime. A few patients have been found to have a flat intestinal biopsy or exocrine pancreatic insufficiency, but in most diabetics, intestinal histology and pancreatic function are normal. Small intestinal X-rays frequently show marked dilatation of small intestinal loops, suggesting a motility disturbance. Because of this and since a peripheral neuropathy with an associated autonomic insufficiency as manifested by postural hypotension and a depressed capacity to sweat is present in a majority of patients, the steatorrhea is probably at least partially related to an enteric neuropathy. Secondary bacterial overgrowth and intestinal stasis are found in some patients, although this cause of malabsorption appears to be surprisingly uncommon. Fecal fat excretion is mild to moderate (15 to 30 g per day), and xylose absorption is usually slightly impaired. Vitamin B_{12} absorption is normal unless there is massive bacterial overgrowth.

Scleroderma,[53] a collagen disease, frequently involves the small intestinal mucosa with fibrosis of the submucosal and muscle layers, resulting in dilatation of bowel loops and decreased capacity to propel intestinal contents. Bacterial overgrowth is a common concomitant because of the intestinal stasis, and the moderate malabsorption produced can often be at least partially eliminated by treatment with broad-spectrum antibiotics.

TABLE 20–4. REPRESENTATIVE DOSAGES FOR AGENTS USED IN MANAGEMENT OF PATIENTS WITH THE MALABSORPTION SYNDROME*

1. CALCIUM
   Oral: Calcium gluconate (91 mg Ca^{++}/gram), 1 to 5 g three times daily
   Intravenous: Calcium gluconate injection, U.S.P. 10 per cent solution (9.1 mg Ca^{++}/ml), 10 to 30 ml administered slowly intravenously depending upon response
2. MAGNESIUM
   Oral: Magnesium sulfate (8 mEq/gram), 1.0 to 6.0 g daily in divided dosage
   Intramuscular: (20% sol.) 10 ml two or three times daily
   Intravenous: Magnesium sulfate, 0.5 per cent solution, up to 1000 ml at a rate not faster than 1.0 mEq/minute
3. IRON
   Oral: Ferrous gluconate, 0.6 g three times daily
   Intramuscular: (Imferon). Must be calculated according to severity of anemia. Detailed instructions accompany preparation.
4. FAT-SOLUBLE VITAMINS
   a. VITAMIN A
      Oleovitamin A capsules, U.S.P. (25,000 units per capsule), 100,000 to 200,000 units daily in severe deficiencies; maintenance, 25,000 to 50,000 units daily.
   b. VITAMIN D
      Synthetic oleovitamin D, U.S.P. (10,000 U.S.P. units vitamin D/gram), 30,000 units daily; increase dosage as necessary to raise serum calcium to normal. Dosage varies considerably depending on response as determined by level of serum calcium and urinary calcium.
   c. COMBINATION A AND D VITAMINS
      Concentrated oleovitamins A and D, U.S.P. (50,000 to 65,000 U.S.P. A units and 10,000 to 13,000 U.S.P. D units/gram) may be used rather than separate preparations.
   d. VITAMIN K
      Oral: Menadione, U.S.P., 4 to 12 mg daily. Vitamin K_1 tablets (Mephyton), 5 to 10 mg daily.
      Intravenous: (Bleeding episodes – acute situations.) Vitamin K_1 (Mephyton), 50 mg ampule. Administer 50 mg slowly over 10-minute period. Repeat in 8 to 12 hours if prothrombin time has not returned to normal.
5. FOLIC ACID, U.S.P. (5 mg tablets)
   Dose: Initial, 10 to 20 mg daily
   Maintenance, 5 to 10 mg daily
6. VITAMIN B_{12} INJECTION, U.S.P. (15 mcg/ml)
   Dose: Initial, 30 to 60 mcg daily for two to three weeks
   Maintenance, 30 to 100 mcg monthly
   If combined system disease is present, a more intensive program is indicated.
7. VITAMIN B COMPLEX
   Any multivitamin preparation that contains daily requirements (thiamine 1.6 mg, riboflavin 1.8 mg and niacin 20 mg). Use two or three tablets daily. Intramuscular preparations are available for severe deficiencies.
8. PANCREATIC SUPPLEMENTS, ORAL
   Recently these agents have been shown to be more effective when given at 6 to 12 regular intervals during the day rather than at meal times.
   a. *Pancreatin,* U.S.P. (0.3 g tablet), 6 to 18 g daily.
   b. *Viokase* (0.3 g tablet), 4 to 12 g daily in divided doses at meals or hourly per day.
   c. *Cotazym* (0.3 g capsule), 4.0 to 12.0 g daily, divided doses at meals or hourly per day.
9. BROAD-SPECTRUM ANTIMICROBIALS
   Oral: Chloramphenicol, tetracycline, or oxytetracycline (0.25 g), 1.0 g per day in divided doses for 10 to 14 days; ampicillin (0.25 g), 2.0 to 4.0 g per day in divided doses; kanamycin (0.5 g), 2.0 to 4.0 g per day in divided doses; sulfisoxazole (0.5 g), 1.0 to 2.0 g daily in divided doses; lincomycin (0.25 g), 1.0 to 2.0 g daily. Repeated courses often necessary or administration for three to four days each week indefinitely.
10. HUMAN ALBUMIN, SALT POOR (0.25 g/ml)
    Intravenous administration of 50 to 100 g each day for three to seven days to elevate a severely depressed serum albumin level
11. GLOBULIN, IMMUNE SERUM (0.165 g/ml)
    Intramuscular injection of 0.05 ml/kg each three to four weeks in patients with hypogammaglobulinemia and recurrent infection.
12. CORTICOTROPHIN AND ADRENOCORTICOSTEROIDS
    a. Corticotrophin, 30 to 40 units intravenously each day, 10 to 21 days or longer for severely ill patients.
    b. Prednisolone or prednisone, 30 to 60 mg orally each day as needed; 5.0 to 15.0 mg maintenance dose.
13. ANTIDIARRHEAL AGENTS
    Oral: Diphenoxylate hydrochloride (2.5 mg), 5.0 mg twice or three times daily. Deodorized tincture opium, 10 drops twice to three times per day. Propantheline (15.0 mg), 30 mg twice or three times daily.
14. CHOLESTYRAMINE, ORAL RESIN
    4.0-g dose, three to six times daily, before feedings.
15. CALORIC SUPPLEMENTATION
    Oral: (a) Medium: chain triglyceride (MCT). "Home or Hospital Mix" (MCT: 45 per cent calories; caseinate, 15 per cent; dextrose, 40 per cent). Ingredients homogenized with H_2O to one liter (MCT: 75 ml; caseinate, 60 g; dextrose 160 g). Keep at 20°C for one year. Defrost day's formula each morning; give three ounces at meals; gradually increase between-meal feedings to six ounces. Portagen (MCT: 45.0 g fat/quart; 30 cal/oz; 10 per cent carbohydrate). Formula mix. Prepare according to instructions. Give 16 oz every day.
    (b) Vivonex, 80 g = 300 cal: 90.8% CHO; 0.7% fat; 8.5% aminoacids, plus minerals and electrolytes. Dissolve in 100 ml water. Feed up to 480 gm q.d.
    Intravenous: Prepare solution of approx. 0.9 cal/ml.: 20% dextrose and 3½% fibrin hydrolysate (w/v). Give 1500–3000 ml q.d. Increase amounts cautiously.

*Modified from Sleisenger, M. H.: Diseases of malabsorption. *In* Textbook of Medicine, 13th ed., P. B. Beeson and W. McDermott (eds.). Philadelphia, W. B. Saunders Co., 1971.

Endocrine disease: A few cases of hyperthyroidism,[54] hypoadrenalism,[55] hypoparathyroidism,[56] and pseudohypoparathyroidism[57] have been associated with an increased secretion of fecal fat, but the cause of the malabsorption is unknown. Presumably the affected hormones play an important role in some stage of digestion or absorption.

DRUGS INTERFERING WITH DIGESTION AND ABSORPTION

Although it is not certain at exactly what stage the several drugs causing maldigestion and malabsorption play their pathological role, it is important to note those that can produce significant interference with assimilation of foods.

Cholestyramine[58] is an ion exchange resin which binds bile acids in the intestinal lumen so that they are not available for micellar solubilization. The extent of steatorrhea depends on the dose utilized; with 12 g of drug per day fat excretion is just above normal, but with 24 to 36 g per day fat excretion reaches 15 g daily.

Cathartics[59] of various types produce diarrhea, excessive albumin loss, and mild steatorrhea (10 g per day) when used in excess. Those implicated include bisacodyl, colocynth, jalap, and podophyllin. The cause has not been well defined, but is probably related to hastened intestinal motility and the resulting decreased contact time for nutrients.

Colchicine[60] is still used widely for the treatment of gout and has an appreciable effect on intestinal epithelial cell function. It is capable both of inhibiting epithelial crypt cell division (at high doses) and of increasing the rate of cell migration up the intestinal villi (at moderate doses). Mild steatorrhea (10 g per day) and an abnormal xylose test are frequently found during therapy with this drug.

Neomycin[61] is widely used perorally to alter intestinal bacterial flora that might produce ammonia and thereby contribute to encephalopathy in patients with hepatic disease. This antibiotic produces flattening of the intestinal villi and inhibition of lipase action on triglyceride and precipitation of bile salts. Fat excretion reaches 10 g per day and xylose excretion falls to 3 g per five hours when 2 to 5 g of neomycin is taken; with 8 to 12 g per day, the values are about 20 g per day and 2 g per five hours, respectively.

REPLACEMENT THERAPY FOR MALABSORPTION SYNDROME

Often the physician must prescribe medications to replete losses of calories, minerals, or vitamins suffered by patients with malabsorption syndrome. For aid in such therapy, the reader is referred to Table 20–4. Specific details concerning each category are presented in appropriate chapters in the text.

COMMENT

This chapter takes a physiological approach to maldigestion and malabsorption by considering the particular phase or stage of the overall process that is defective. Normal digestion and absorption are considered in detail on pages 250 to 257 and serve as the basis for the pathophysiology. Although such an approach is a departure from the traditional listing of disease category, the great increase in our knowledge of biochemical and physiological mechanisms over the last 20 years has brought forth information that is of direct help to the practicing physician in his approach to the patient.

Although the incidence of such well recognized diseases as celiac sprue or Whipple's disease may not have changed in recent years, treatment of intra-abdominal conditions with irradiation or surgical resection now accounts for an increasing proportion of maldigestive and malabsorptive disease. Indeed, iatrogenic steatorrhea will undoubtedly continue to increase in ensuing years as advances continue to be made in surgical technique and irradiation therapy.

REFERENCES

1. Wilson, F. A., and Dietschy, J. M. Differential diagnostic approach to clinical problems of malabsorption. Gastroenterology *61*:911, 1971.
2. Van de Kamer, J. H., Huinink, H. T. B., and Weyers, H. A. Rapid method for the determination of fat in feces. J. Biol. Chem. *177*:347, 1949.

3. Finlay, J. M., Hogarth, J., and Wightman, K. J. R. A clinical evaluation of the d-xylose tolerance test. Ann. Intern. Med. *61*:411, 1964.

4. Dreiling, D. A., and Janowitz, H. D. The measurement of pancreatic secretory function. *In* The Exocrine Pancreas, Ciba Foundation Symposium, A. V. S. de Reuck and M. P. Cameron (eds.). London, Churchill, 1962, pp. 225–258.

5. Lundh, G. Pancreatic exocrine function in neoplastic and inflammatory disease: a simple and reliable new test. Gastroenterology *42*:275, 1962.

6. Fromm, H., and Hofmann, A. F. Breath test for altered bile-acid metabolism. Lancet *2*:621, 1971.

7. Schilling, R. F. Intrinsic factor studies. II. The effect of gastric juice on the urinary excretion of radioactivity after the oral administration of radioactive vitamin B_{12}. J. Lab. Clin. Med. *42*:860, 1953.

8. Rubin, C. E., and Dobbins, W. O., III. Peroral biopsy of the small intestine. A review of its diagnostic usefulness. Gastroenterology *49*:676, 1965.

9. Dahlqvist, A. Assay of intestinal disaccharidases. Anal. Biochem. *22*:99, 1968.

10. Saunders, D. R. Medium-chain triglycerides and the Van de Kamer method. Gastroenterology *52*:135, 1967.

11. Braddock, L. R. I., Fleisher, D. R., and Barbero, G. J. A physical chemical study of the Van de Kamer method for fecal fat analysis. Gastroenterology *55*:165, 1968.

12. Partin, J. C., and Schubert, W. K. Precautionary note on the use of the intestinal biopsy capsule in infants and emaciated children. New Eng. J. Med. *274*:94, 1966.

13. Marshak, R. H., and Lindner, A. E. Malabsorption syndrome. Sem. Roentgenol. *1*:138, 1966.

14. Cerda, J. J., and Brooks, F. P. Relationships between steatorrhea and an insufficiency of pancreatic secretion in the duodenum in patients with chronic pancreatitis. Amer. J. Med. Sci. *253*:38, 1967.

15. Kalser, M. H., Leite, C. A., and Warren, W. D. Fat assimilation after massive distal pancreatectomy. New Eng. J. Med. *279*:570, 1968.

16. Rastogi, H., and Brown, C. H. Carcinoma of the pancreas. A review of one hundred cases. Cleveland Clin. Quart. *34*:243, 1967.

17. Atkinson, M., Nordin, B. E. C., and Sherlock, S. Malabsorption and bone disease in prolonged obstructive jaundice. Quart. J. Med. *25*:299, 1956.

18. Marin, G. A., Clark, M. L., and Senior, J. R. Studies of malabsorption occurring in patients with Laennec's cirrhosis. Gastroenterology *56*:727, 1969.

19. Rosenberg, I. H., Hardison, W. G., and Bull, D. M. Abnormal bile-salt patterns and intestinal bacterial overgrowth associated with malabsorption. New Eng. J. Med. *276*:1391, 1967.

20. Ament, M., Shimoda, S., Saunders, D., and Rubin, C. The pathogenesis of steatorrhea in three cases of small intestinal stasis syndrome. Gastroenterology *63*:728, 1972.

21. Donaldson, R. M., Jr. Studies on the pathogenesis of steatorrhea in the blind loop syndrome. J. Clin. Invest. *44*:1815, 1965.

22. Giannella, R. A., Broitman, S. A., and Zamcheck, N. Competition between bacteria and intrinsic factor for vitamin B_{12}: Implications for vitamin B_{12} malabsorption in intestinal bacterial overgrowth. Gastroenterology *62*: 255, 1972.

23. Gray, G. M. Intestinal digestion and maldigestion of dietary carbohydrates. Ann. Rev. Med. *22*:391, 1971.

24. Benson, G. D., Kowlessar, O. D., and Sleisenger, M. H. Adult celiac disease with emphasis upon response to the gluten-free diet. Medicine *43*:1, 1964.

25. Kalser, M. H., Roth, J. L. A., Tumen, H., and Johnson, T. A. Relation of small bowel resection to nutrition in man. Gastroenterology *38*:605, 1960.

26. Tankel, H. I., Clark, D. H., and Lee, F. D. Radiation enteritis with malabsorption. Gut *6*:560, 1965.

27. Carron, D. B., and Douglas, A. P. Steatorrhea in vascular insufficiency of the small intestine. Quart. J. Med. *34*:331, 1965.

28. Sheehy, T. W., Baggs, B., Perez-Santiago, E., and Floch, M. H. Prognosis of tropical sprue. A study of the effect of folic acid on the intestinal aspects of acute and chronic sprue. Ann. Intern. Med. *57*:892, 1962.

29. Weinstein, W. M., Saunders, D. R., Tytgat, G. N., and Rubin, C. E. Collagenous sprue—an unrecognized type of malabsorption. New Eng. J. Med. *283*:1297, 1970.

30. Gross, J. B., Wollaeger, E. E., Sauer, W. G., Huizenga, K. A., Dahlin, D. C., and Power, M. H. Whipple's disease. Report of four cases including two in brothers, with observations on pathologic physiology, diagnosis, and treatment. Gastroenterology *36*:65, 1959.

31. Chears, W. C., Jr., and Ashworth, C. T. Electron microscopic study of the intestinal mucosa in Whipple's disease. Demonstration of encapsulated bacilliform bodies in the lesion. Gastroenterology *41*:129, 1961.

32. Hardison, W. G., and Rosenberg, I. H. Bile-salt deficiency in the steatorrhea following resection of the ileum and proximal colon. New Eng. J. Med. *277*:337, 1967.

33. Eidelman, S., Parkins, R. A., and Rubin, C. E. Abdominal lymphoma presenting as malabsorption. A clinico-pathologic study of nine cases in Israel and a review of the literature. Medicine *45*:111, 1966.

34. Yamashiro, K. M., and Gray, G. M. Primary intestinal lymphoma: Response to radiotherapy. Clin. Res. *20*:183, 1972.

35. Waldmann, T. A., Steinfeld, J. L., Dutcher, T. F., Davidson, J. D., and Gordon, R. S., Jr. The role of the gastrointestinal system in "idiopathic hypoproteinemia." Gastroenterology *41*:197, 1961.

36. Isselbacher, K. J., Scheig, R., Plotkin, G. R., and Caulfield, J. B. Congenital β-lipoprotein and transport of lipids. Medicine *43*:347, 1964.

37. Johnson, R. L., VanArsdel, P. P., Jr., Tobe, A. D., and Ching, Y. Adult hypogammaglobulinemia with malabsorption and iron deficiency anemia. Amer. J. Med. 43:935, 1967.

38. Ament, M. E., and Rubin, C. E. Relation of giardiasis to abnormal intestinal structure and function in gastrointestinal immunodeficiency syndromes. Gastroenterology 62:216, 1972.

39. Birchir, J., Bartholomew, L. G., Cain, J. C., and Adson, M. A. Syndrome of intestinal arterial insufficiency ("abdominal angina"). Arch. Intern. Med. 117:632, 1966.

40. Leinbach, G. E., and Rubin, C. E. Eosinophilic gastroenteritis: A simple reaction to food allergens? Gastroenterology 59:874, 1970.

41. Klein, N. C., Hargrove, R. L., Sleisenger, M. H., and Jeffries, G. H. Eosinophilic gastroenteritis. Medicine 49:299, 1970.

42. Brow, J. R., Parker, F., Weinstein, W. M., and Rubin, C. E. The small intestinal mucosa in dermatitis herpetiformis. I. Severity and distribution of the small intestinal lesion and associated malabsorption. Gastroenterology 60:355, 1971.

43. Hermos, J. A., Cooper, H. L., Kramer, P., and Trier, J. S. Histological diagnosis by peroral biopsy of Crohn's disease of the proximal intestine. Gastroenterology 59:868, 1970.

44. Jeffries, G. H., Steinberg, H., and Sleisenger, M. H. Chronic ulcerative (nongranulomatous) jejunitis. Amer. J. Med. 44:47, 1968.

45. Gilat, T., Revach, M., and Sohar, E. Deposition of amyloid in the gastrointestinal tract. Gut 10:98, 1969.

46. Sheehy, T. W., Meroney, W. H., Cox, R. S., Jr., and Soler, J. E. Hookworm disease and malabsorption. Gastroenterology 42:148, 1962.

47. Milner, P. F., Irvine, R. A., Barton, C. J., Bras, C., and Richards, R. Intestinal malabsorption in Strongyloides stercoralis infestation. Gut 6:574, 1965.

48. Brandborg, L. L., Goldberg, S. B., and Breidenbach, W. C. Human coccidiosis—A possible cause of malabsorption. New Eng. J. Med. 283:1306, 1970.

49. Whalen, G. E., Rosenberg, E. B., Strickland, G. T., Gutman, R. A., Cross, J. H., and Watten, R. H. Intestinal capillariasis. A new disease in man. Lancet 1:13, 1969.

50. Hoskins, L. C., Winawer, S. J., Broitman, S. A., Gottlieb, L. S., and Zamcheck, N. Clinical giardiasis and intestinal malabsorption. Gastroenterology 53:265, 1967.

51. Corsini, G., Gandolfi, E., Bonechi, I., and Cerri, B. Postgastrectomy malabsorption. Gastroenterology 50:358, 1966.

52. Wruble, L. D., and Kalser, M. H. Diabetic steatorrhea: A distinct entity. Amer. J. Med. 37:118, 1964.

53. Kahn, I. J., Jeffries, G. H., and Sleisenger, M. H. Malabsorption in intestinal scleroderma. Correction by antibiotics. New Eng. J. Med. 274:1339, 1966.

54. Crane, C. W., and Evans, D. W. Thyrotoxic steatorrhoea. Brit. Med. J. 2:1575, 1966.

55. Guarini, G., and Macaluso, M. Steatorrhoea in Addison's disease. Lancet 1:955, 1963.

56. Clarkson, B., Kowlessar, O. D., Horwith, M., and Sleisenger, M. H. Clinical and metabolic study of a patient with malabsorption and hypoparathyroidism. Metabolism 9:1093, 1960.

57. Jackson, W. P. U., Hoffenberg, R., Linder, G. C., and Irwin, L. Syndrome of steatorrhea, pseudohypoparathyroidism and amenorrhea. Observations on the calcium infusion test, and the effect of probenecid on calcium and phosphorus metabolism. J. Clin. Endocr. 16:1043, 1956.

58. Zurier, R. B., Hashim, S. A., and Van Itallie, T. B. Effect of medium chain triglyceride on cholestyramine-induced steatorrhea in man. Gastroenterology 49:490, 1965.

59. Heizer, W. D., Warshaw, A. L., Waldmann, T. A., and Laster, L. Protein-losing gastroenteropathy and malabsorption associated with factitious diarrhea. Ann. Intern. Med. 68:839, 1968.

60. Race, T. F., Paes, I. C., and Faloon, W. W. Intestinal malabsorption induced by oral colchicine. Comparison with neomycin and cathartic agents. Amer. J. Med. Sci. 259:32, 1970.

61. Rogers, A. I., Vloedman, D. A., Bloom, E. C., and Kalser, M. H. Neomycin-induced steatorrhea. J.A.M.A. 197:185, 1966.

Chapter 21

Malabsorption in Children

J. R. Hamilton

Diseases causing malabsorption are relatively rare in children. The diagnostician must keep in mind conditions seldom, if ever, encountered in adults.[1-3] Recently, knowledge of normal digestive and absorptive processes has grown rapidly. These advances have been complemented by the elucidation of several newly recognized defects of digestion and absorption. The clinical manifestations of some of these defects do not fit the classic description of malabsorption given in 1888 by Samuel Gee: ". . . the faeces, being loose, not formed, but not watery, more bulky than the food taken would seem to account for; pale in colour, yeasty, frothy, stinking . . . the patient wastes more in the limbs than in the face."[4] This chapter will consider malabsorptive diseases in a wide context, including conditions which differ from this typical clinical pattern, and some in which there may be no gastrointestinal symptoms.

ETIOLOGY

The diseases and conditions that may produce malabsorption in childhood are listed in Table 21-1.[1,2] Congenital anatomical or metabolic anomalies must be given particular consideration in the diagnostic appraisal of a malabsorptive problem in children. Since reliable incidence data are available for only a few conditions, the diseases have been grouped arbitrarily into common and less common. The crude estimate of relative frequency is based on experience in North America and may not be applicable to populations in other regions, particularly in the tropics. Emphasis in discussion will be given to those malabsorptive disorders occurring mainly in children and not described elsewhere in this text and to the pediatric aspects of certain other disorders.

CLINICAL ASSESSMENT

Three basic processes coalesce to produce the clinical manifestations of malabsorption disorders. Accumulation of nutrients and their metabolites within the intestinal lumen may produce bowel distention, diarrhea, vomiting, and excessive gas. Failure of a single or several nutrients to cross the absorptive membranes and reach metabolic pools may lead to undernutrition. The additional clinical features of a particular disease may be superimposed upon these two processes.

In assessing the pediatric patient one must have a clear concept of the diagnostic possibilities in this age group and a thorough understanding of certain characteristics of pediatric patients and the way in which they react to malabsorptive illness.

The child may be too young to speak for himself. Much historical information has to be obtained from parents, and the clinician must judge its validity carefully.

Because congenital disorders are important in the etiology of childhood malabsorption, genetic factors and the history of the pregnancy, particularly with respect to illness or drug ingestion in the first trimester, are important. Maternal hydramnios suggests that the baby may have an obstructive lesion in the intestine or a congenital transport defect.

The clinical manifestations of undernutrition, dehydration, and electrolyte and acid-base imbalance occur earlier and are more severe in children than in adults. The child has proportionately smaller nutritional reserves and a larger extracellular fluid volume, and in young infants the renal compensatory mechanisms may be immature.

The normal processes of growth and maturation in children may be retarded by malnutrition because of malabsorption. Growth can only be assessed in relation to previous body measurements and charts of normal growth patterns. Although the progress of maturation can be gauged by the eruption of teeth and the onset of signs of puberty, observations must be interpreted in the light of family and racial patterns.

Since so many of the clinical manifestations of malabsorption are those of undernutrition, an accurate account of food intake is essential. Particular care must be taken to elicit this information about the small child who neither feeds himself nor chooses what he eats. His physician or parent may have unduly restricted the food intake to control gastrointestinal symptoms.

At the physical examination the condition of the buccal mucosa and tongue may be overlooked in the rush to see the pharynx and tonsils, particularly if the tongue is covered with a wooden depressor. A smooth tongue or ulcerated mucosa may be early signs of undernutrition caused by malabsorption. A rectal examination is essential, particularly in a young infant who may pool water and stool in the gut early in malabsorptive disease, making the description of the type and number of stools misleading. Rectal examination also usually provides a fresh stool specimen for microscopic and biochemical tests.

LABORATORY ASSESSMENT

For patients who are small or incontinent, specialized facilities are required for detailed assessment of absorptive function. Therefore complex laboratory investigations should be reserved for those patients in whom the clinical examination signals malabsorption.

BIOCHEMICAL STUDIES

ABSORPTIVE FUNCTION

Fecal Fat Excretion. This test is the best method for detecting steatorrhea and the only practical method for measuring absorptive function of the small intestine quantitatively. The child should be consuming an adequate amount of fat before and during the stool collection. The fat excreted is measured in stools excreted over a minimum of 72 hours and should not exceed 4.5 g per day. Excretion is better expressed as a percentage of fat intake. Less than 15 per cent is normal for infants up to six months of age and 10 per cent after that.[1] If the diet contains medium-chain triglycerides, the usual technique for fat assay is inadequate.[5]

Unfortunately, fecal fat excretion is not measured in many pediatric centers because it requires, in addition to experienced personnel, a specialized collection area with adequate ventilation and refrigeration and a laboratory with a large fume cupboard and disposal equipment.[6] In diaper-age children a plastic-coated liner for the diaper is usually adequate for collection, but if the stools are fluid a metabolic frame may be necessary (Fig. 21–1).

So-Called Screening Tests for Steatorrhea. Because quantitative fat measurement in stools is difficult in children, many short-term loading tests have been devised, but they are unreliable. These tests include fasting serum carotene, vitamin A absorption, serum turbidity measurements after a load of dietary fat, I-labeled triolein, and oleic acid excretion. Lipoidal excretion shows a strong positive correlation with fat excretion, and fasting serum-carotene concentration is relatively simple to measure. However, none of these tests are quantitative. Provided that the patient is eating fat and lubricant has

TABLE 21–1. ETIOLOGY OF CHILDHOOD MALABSORPTION*

	MORE COMMON	LESS COMMON
I. INTESTINAL DISEASE		
A. Anatomical abnormalities		
1. Stasis of small bowel contents		
Blind loop syndrome		
a. Congenital	*Intestinal malrotation*	*Web*
	Atresia (postoperative)	*Stenosis*
		Duplication
b. Acquired	*Fibrous adhesions*	*Faulty anastomosis*
		Inflammatory disease
2. Loss of absorptive surface		
a. Congenital		*Short small bowel*
b. Acquired	*Massive resection*	
3. Obstructed drainage		
a. Lymph	*Lymphangiectasia*	*Neoplasia-lymphoma*
	Pericarditis	
b. Blood		
B. Inflammation		
1. Chronic infestations		
a. Bacteria	*E. coli*	Tuberculosis
	Salmonella	
b. Parasites	*Giardia lamblia*	*Coccidiosis, hookworm*
c. Others		Whipple's disease
2. Allergy	Milk	Other foods
3. Nonspecific inflammation		Crohn's disease
C. Metabolic defects		
	Celiac disease	
	Disaccharide intolerance	
	Secondary disaccharidase	Primary lactase deficiency
	deficiency	Sucrase – isomaltase deficiency
		Glucose-galactose malabsorption
		Amino acid disorders
		Cystinuria
		Hartnup disease
		Methionine malabsorption
		"Blue diaper" syndrome
		Iminoglycinuria
		Familial protein intolerance
		Lysine malabsorption
		Oculocerebrorenal syndrome of
		Lowe
		Enterokinase deficiency
		A-β-lipoproteinemia
		Chloride-losing diarrhea
		Immune deficiency states
		Humoral
		Cellular

*Conditions shown in *italics* may cause steatorrhea.

TABLE 21-1. ETIOLOGY OF CHILDHOOD MALABSORPTION (*Continued*)

	More Common	Less Common
		Vitamin B_{12} malabsorption
		Pernicious anemia
		Imerslund's
		Folic acid malabsorption
		Primary hypomagnesemia
		Vitamin D dependent rickets
D. Iatrogenic		Medications — *calcium, neomycin* (massive), *paregoric*
		Postoperative (see A1 and A2)
E. Nutrition		Undernutrition
F. Neoplasm		
1. involving bowel		Lymphoma (see A3)
2. functioning		
a. neural crest		*Ganglioneuroma, neuroblastoma*
b. pancreas		Delta cell (Zollinger-Ellison)
c. bowel		Carcinoid
G. Endocrine		*Adrenal insufficiency*
		Hypoparathyroidism
H. Miscellaneous		*Tropical sprue*
		Acrodermatitis enteropathica
		Dermatitis herpetiformis
		Familial dysautonomia (Riley-Day syndrome)
II. PANCREATIC INSUFFICIENCY	*Cystic fibrosis*	*Hypoplasia with neutropenia*
		Chronic pancreatitis
		Traumatic
		Familial
		With aminoaciduria
		Without aminoaciduria
		Hyperlipemia
		Hyperparathyroidism
		Malnutrition
		Isolated enzyme deficiencies
		Trypsinogen deficiency
		Lipase
		Amylase
		Enterokinase deficiency (see 1C)
III. LIVER DISEASE		
A. Biliary obstruction, congenital	*Biliary atresia*	
	"*Neonatal hepatitis*"	
B. Hepatocellular damage	*Cirrhosis*	
	Hepatitis	

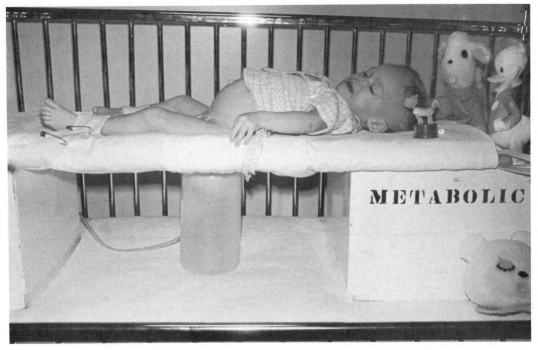

Figure 21–1.　Infant on a metabolic frame for collection of stools and urine.

not been used on a rectal thermometer or an examining finger, microscopic examination of unstained stool is a rapid, simple, and useful technique for detecting excess fat in stool. It may be no more accurate than the tests listed above, but it is at least as good. Furthermore, an experienced observer can distinguish between droplets of neutral fat and crystalline aggregates of fatty acid.

Fecal Sugar Concentration. If a patient has sugar malabsorption, fresh stools will usually be acid, but a more reliable index is the presence of sugar in the stools. A useful office test for sugar is to add Clinitest tablets to fresh stool diluted five drops to ten of water and read the color. More than a trace of reducing sugar is excessive. If sucrose is suspected in stool, the specimen must be first hydrolyzed with dilute hydrochloric acid before the tablet is added (see pp. 1015 to 1028).[7]

D-Xylose Excretion. Excretion in the urine over a five-hour period of less than 15 per cent of an oral dose of D-xylose indicates malabsorption in the upper gut. Excretion of greater than 25 per cent is normal. The meaning of intermediate values is equivocal. In children, collection may be difficult. Unfortunately, the correlation between an abnormal test and the diagnosis of celiac disease, an important cause of damage to the upper gut, is poor.[8]

Oral Carbohydrate Tolerance Curves. Oral glucose tolerance, widely used as a test for glucose absorption, is influenced by many factors other than intestinal absorption. It is even less reliable in children than in adults because of the variability in the time for gastric emptying associated with emotional reaction to the test. In children the specific disaccharide to which the child may be intolerant can be given and the blood sugar measured, but these disaccharide tolerance tests are subject to all the same variations as the glucose tolerance test.

Indirect Measurements of Absorptive Function. In general, these are measurements of nutritional status as reflected in plasma concentrations of various nutrients, proteins, iron, vitamins, coagulation factors, calcium, phosphorus, and magnesium, for example. How relevant the results are to absorption depends upon recent dietary intake.

PANCREATIC FUNCTION

The same techniques used in the assessment of pancreatic function in adults may be employed safely in children.[9] Pancreatic enzymes and bicarbonate can be measured quantitatively in duodenal juice before and after the exocrine pancreas has been stimulated by secretin and pancreozymin, using a marker perfusion technique. Because the procedure is arduous for children, attempts have been made to develop simpler screening tests. Pancreatic trypsin and chymotrypsin can be measured in stools using specific substrates. This test must be done on a timed collection, preferably of at least three days' duration, and the results are best expressed as total output of the particular enzyme activity in stool over a stated period.

ROENTGENOGRAPHIC STUDIES

Plain films of the abdomen may show a gas pattern indicative of some degree of intestinal obstruction or the calcification associated with neural crest tumors, gallstones, or pancreatitis. The main use of barium studies of the small intestine is to identify localized lesions.

For infants micropulverized barium can be fed through a nipple with a large opening. Adequate immobilization of the patient, palatable barium, proper shielding of regions not examined, and a nasogastric tube for the recalcitrant patient are essentials. The variation in rate of gastric emptying and intestinal transit necessitates frequent fluoroscopy to observe the progress of the barium so that films can be taken at appropriate times to demonstrate each region of the small bowel.

SMALL INTESTINAL BIOPSY

Peroral biopsy of the small bowel provides viable samples of the highly complex mucosa for morphological and biochemical measurements. The instruments are scaled-down versions of those used for adults, except that instruments retrieving multiple specimens are not generally used in small children (pp. 259 to 277). Some centers report an alarming incidence of complications, such as perforation and hemorrhage, but most record that peroral biopsy of the small bowel is safe, providing that proper precautions are taken. The most important of these is to limit the number of people in an institution allowed to do the procedure. The child is lightly sedated and immobilized with a blanket. A sheath or nipple over the biopsy tube protects it from the teeth. The full potential of metabolic studies on biopsy specimens has not yet been realized.

MICROBIOLOGY

The techniques are identical to those used in adults. Pathogenic organisms are not always excreted uniformly in stools, and a significant infection may go undetected unless more than one stool specimen is examined. Intubation techniques can provide representative samples of small bowel contents, but at present culture techniques are inadequate to find a complete picture of the bacterial content of such samples. Occasionally *Giardia lamblia* can be seen as mobile organisms in an unstained, unconcentrated sample of very fresh, warm duodenal juice when they cannot be found in stools.

SWEAT TEST

See pages 1219 to 1220.

TREATMENT

Obviously specific treatment depends on the diagnosis. Most children with malabsorption will require long-term, if not lifelong therapy. The physician must be prepared to arrange a program of continuing care that includes various members of the health care team. At least for the young child, that team should include the parents or others responsible for him. As the child grows up responsibility for his care will shift to a new team experienced with adults. Such simple and logical measures are easily forgotten in the rush to prescribe a newly discovered drug.

SPECIFIC DISEASES

CELIAC DISEASE IN CHILDHOOD

The disease in children seems to be identical to that in adults (see pp. 864 to 884). It occurs more frequently in relatives of patients than in the general population, and the mode of inheritance appears to be multifactorial. Among relatives, the incidence of clinical disease is lower than the incidence of the mucosal lesion. As in adults the minimal criteria for diagnosis should be the histological finding of villous atrophy in the mucosa of the proximal intestine and proof of improvement after the removal of gluten from the diet.[10-14]

Symptoms begin after wheat-containing foods are introduced into the diet, usually in the second year of life, rarely in later childhood, and apparently never in adolescence for reasons that are not known. The recent rise in numbers of cases presenting in the first year of life can perhaps be attributed to the contemporary practice of introducing solid foods into the diet in the early weeks of life. Many patients are irritable and anorexic and have chronic diarrhea, in keeping with the traditional concept of this disease. It is clear, however, that significant numbers of patients are neither anorexic nor irritable and may even be constipated. Diagnostic attention has tended to focus on patients with chronic diarrhea, when probably those who fail to thrive, with or without diarrhea, would yield proportionately more cases.

The impact of the disease in children differs from that seen in adults, probably because children are growing when the diagnosis is made. Growth retardation is an important sign of malabsorption, tend-

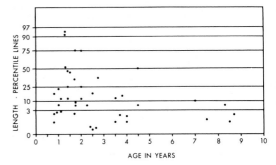

Figure 21–2. Forty-two cases of celiac disease. Height in relation to standard percentiles at times of diagnosis.

ing to occur in older children after weight gain has diminished (Figs. 21–2 and 21–3). The muscles of the upper arms and thighs are wasted; abdominal distention is usually gaseous, but occasionally there is ascites. Clubbing of the fingers, if present, is not severe. Rickets is rare, probably because growth is retarded and because vitamin supplements are used widely. Neither peripheral neuropathy nor severe encephalopathy has been reported. Rectal prolapse may occur, although it is usually associated with cystic fibrosis rather than celiac disease.

Diagnosis rests on light microscopy of a correctly oriented, fixed, and sectioned mucosal biopsy. The typical lesion seen in children is indistinguishable from that seen in adult patients. For practical purposes, in temperate climates, and in the absence of enteric infection, panhypogammaglobulinemia, dermatitis herpetiformis, and soybean sensitivity, villous atrophy means gluten intolerance. Additional disease entities in which similar lesions occur probably will be defined in the future.

Evidence is accumulating that all patients with celiac disease by modern diagnostic criteria must eat restricted diets for years, if not for a lifetime. It is clear that many children with celiac disease can tolerate oats. Milk restriction is rarely necessary in the early stages of treatment, although lactase activity is invariably decreased in the duodenal mucosa.

Within a week the patient starts to gain weight, and in two to three weeks the steatorrhea disappears. If treatment is adequate, the morphology of the mucosa of the small intestine returns to normal, usually within six to twelve months. This seemingly simple treatment imposes a

TABLE 21–2. SYMPTOMS IN 42 PATIENTS WITH ACTIVE CELIAC DISEASE*

Failure to gain or grow	36
Diarrhea	30
Irritability	30
Vomiting	24
Anorexia	24
Foul, bulky stools	21
Abdominal pain	8
Excessive appetite	6
Rectal prolapse	3

*Hospital for Sick Children, Toronto, Canada.

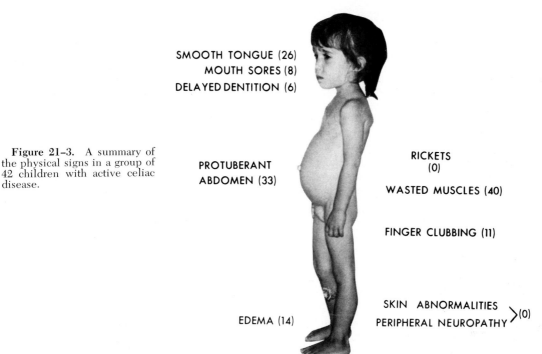

SMOOTH TONGUE (26)
MOUTH SORES (8)
DELAYED DENTITION (6)

Figure 21–3. A summary of the physical signs in a group of 42 children with active celiac disease.

PROTUBERANT
ABDOMEN (33)

RICKETS
(0)

WASTED MUSCLES (40)

FINGER CLUBBING (11)

SKIN ABNORMALITIES
PERIPHERAL NEUROPATHY ⟩(0)

EDEMA (14)

heavy burden upon patient and family. If treatment is to succeed, the attending physician must be certain that the diagnosis is firmly established and that dietary information is available to and understood by the patient and his family. He must also be certain that continuing care is available throughout childhood.

CONGENITAL CHLORIDE-LOSING DIARRHEA

The devastating sequelae of severe, isolated, congenital impairment of intestinal chloride transport are impressive. The basic defect appears to be confined to the lower bowel where the bicarbonate-chloride exchange acts in reverse, in the direction of chloride secretion.[15, 16] Loss of chloride leads to loss of potassium and water and to hypovolemia (see p. 307).

The mode of transmission of this familial disorder is unknown. Although cases are reported from several countries, more than half have been found in Finland. The severity of the clinical disturbance varies between patients for reasons unknown. Usually a severe watery diarrhea begins in early infancy. It persists and may kill the

baby. The abdomen is distended, the patient is lethargic, and growth and motor development are retarded. Apparently diarrhea may even begin in utero, because maternal hydramnios is a frequent associated finding.

The unusual findings of systemic alkalosis, profound hypokalemia with hyponatremia and hypochloridemia are important clues to the diagnosis. Chloride concentration in the stool may be as high as 150 mEq per liter, and exceeds the sum of the concentrations of sodium and potassium. Lesions are described in the kidney typical of hypertensive angiopathy, but the blood pressure is normal.

Specific treatment is not available. No pharmacological agents have been found that improve the patient's condition. Early recognition and aggressive supportive measures are crucial to survival of severely affected babies. Massive potassium supplements must be supplied throughout childhood. Restriction of dietary chloride seems to diminish fecal water and potassium loss, but care must be taken not to induce profound chloride depletion by this means. General health and even the diarrhea may improve in later childhood, presumably because the patient is better able to compensate for the defect.

NEURAL CREST TUMORS

Functioning neural crest tumors may cause severe, intractable, watery diarrhea. The cause is unknown. The tumors secrete catecholamines, but none of these substances or their metabolites or the prostaglandins found recently in the tumor tissue have been identified as the cause of the diarrhea. Usually the tumor is a benign ganglioneuroma, but occasionally it is malignant. Neuroblastoma, a malignant tumor, may also cause diarrhea, but the clinical state is dominated early by the effect of its spread to the liver.[17-19]

Typically, clinical symptoms begin in infancy with watery diarrhea, perhaps intermittent at first, but becoming constant and massive. Systemic manifestations can be attributed to losses of water and electrolyte, particularly potassium from the intestine. Mild steatorrhea has been reported. Blood pressure is normal. Because the tumor is located in the adrenal gland or along the sympathetic chain, a mass is rarely palpable, even under anesthesia.

In addition to the clinical findings, the severe hypokalemia is a useful clue to the diagnosis. The existence of a secreting neural crest tumor is usually confirmed by measuring catecholamines or their metabolite vanillylmandelic acid (VMA) in the urine. Normal (VMA) excretion does not preclude the diagnosis. Individual catecholamines may have to be assayed. The tumor may show on a plain roentgenogram of the abdomen if there is calcification or on a chest roentgenogram if the tumor is in the posterior mediastinum. The usual site is the adrenal gland, where it may displace a kidney seen by pyelography. If all these findings are normal and the diagnosis still seems likely, arteriography or even laparotomy may be required to find the tumor. Removal of the tumor, if it is benign, cures the diarrhea (Fig. 21–4).

VITAMIN B₁₂ MALABSORPTION

This rare familial disorder is characterized by an intestinal defect selectively affecting vitamin B_{12} absorption. Intrinsic factor secretion is normal, there are no antibodies to intrinsic factor or parietal cells in serum, and exogenous intrinsic factor fails to correct the vitamin B_{12} malabsorption. All other absorptive functions of the small bowel that have been measured and the structure of the gastric and intestinal mucosa are normal.[20, 21]

The patient develops megaloblastic ane-

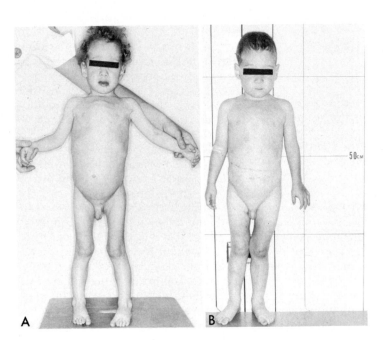

Figure 21–4. Two-year-old boy. A, Before operation to remove a functioning adrenal ganglioneuroma. Patient had voluminous diarrhea and marked muscle wasting. B, Six months postoperative. Diarrhea ceased immediately following surgery. (From Hamilton, J. R., et al.: Amer. J. Med. 44:453, 1968.)

mia with typical features in the blood and bone marrow, usually after the first year of life. Anemia is corrected by the administration of parenteral vitamin B_{12} and controlled by regular supplements by this route. The patient has no gastrointestinal symptoms, but has proteinuria and an increased incidence of urinary tract anomalies—in particular, duplication of the collecting system. The proteinuria is mild, probably of glomerular origin, and not accompanied by progressive renal disease.

DISORDERS OF AMINO ACID METABOLISM

Among this varied but rare group of congenital disorders, there are several in which defective intestinal transport of particular amino acids has been described. The intestinal defect is seldom of major clinical concern. It may be that, in the future, detailed study of intestinal tissue from patients with these diseases will shed new light on basic disease mechanisms.

Cystinuria is the amino acid disorder in which the small intestine has been studied in the most detail. Amino acid uptake by mucosal biopsies in vitro has been characterized for the different forms of cystinuria, although none of the patients have intestinal symptoms.[22, 23]

In Hartnup disease there is malabsorption of several amino acids: tryptophan, causing nicotinamide deficiency and the clinical manifestations of cerebellar ataxia, skin rash, and intellectual deterioration; phenylalanine, leading to formation of indoles which can be detected in urine; and l-histidine.[24, 25]

Methionine malabsorption is associated with episodes of diarrhea. Patients are fair, blue eyed, retarded, and subject to seizures; their urine has a characteristic sweet smell and contains excessive alpha-hydroxybutyric acid.[26]

In children with familial protein intolerance, ingestion of large quantities of protein causes diarrhea, vomiting, and increased blood ammonia. Renal clearance of dibasic amino acids, particularly lysine, is altered, and plasma levels of arginine, lysine, leucine, and tyrosine are low. Whether a specific defect in intestinal transport of these amino acids underlies this defect is unclear.[27, 28]

REFERENCES*

1. Anderson, C. M. Intestinal malabsorption in childhood. Arch. Dis. Child. 41:571, 1966.
2. Shmerling, D. H., Berger, H., and Prader, A. (eds.) Intestinal absorption and malabsorption. In Modern Problems in Pediatrics. Basel, S. Karger, 1968, Vol. II.
3. Hamilton, J. R. Diarrhea in infants. Modern Med. 38:131, 1970.
4. Gee, S. On the coeliac affection. St. Bartholomew's Hosp. Report (London) 24:17, 1888.
5. Jeejeebhoy, K. N., Ahmad, S., and Kozak, G. Determination of fecal fats containing both medium and long chain triglycerides and fatty acids. Clin. Biochem. 3:157, 1970.
6. Shmerling, D. H., Forrer, J. C. W., and Prader, A. Fecal fat and nitrogen in healthy children and in children with malabsorption or maldigestion. Pediatrics 46:690, 1970.
7. Burke, V., Kerry, K. R., and Anderson, C. M. The relationship of dietary lactose to refractory diarrhoea in infancy. Aust. Pediat. J. 1:147, 1965.
8. Hubble, D., and Littlejohn, S. The d-xylose excretion test in coeliac disease in childhood. Arch. Dis. Child. 38:476, 1963.
9. Hadorn, B., Zoppi, G., Shmerling, D. H., Prader, A., McIntyre, I., and Anderson, C. M. Quantitative assessment of exocrine pancreatic function in infants and children. J. Pediat. 73:39, 1968.
10. Hamilton, J. R., Lynch, J. J., and Reilly, B. J. Active coeliac disease in childhood. Quart. J. Med. 38:135, 1969.
11. Young, W. F., and Pringle, E. M. 110 children with coeliac disease 1950–1969. Arch. Dis. Child. 46:421, 1971.
12. Visakorpi, J. K., Kuitunen, P., and Savilahti, E. Frequency and nature of relapses in children suffering from the malabsorption syndrome with gluten intolerance. Acta. Pediat. Scand. 59:481, 1970.
13. Sheldon, W. Prognosis in early adult life of coeliac children treated with a gluten-free diet. Brit. Med. J. 2:401, 1969.
14. McCrae, W. M. The inheritance of coeliac disease. In Coeliac Disease, Booth, C. C., and Dowling, R. H. (eds.). Proceedings of an international conference held at the Royal Postgraduate Medical School, London, 1969. Edinburgh, Churchill, Livingstone, 1970, pp. 55-61.
15. Launiala, K., Perheentupa, J., et al. Familial chloride diarrhea–chloride malabsorption. In Symposium on Intestinal Absorption and Malabsorption, Zurich, 1967, D. H. Shmerling (ed.). Basel and New York, S. Karger, 1968. pp. 137–149.
16. Turnberg, L. A. Abnormalities in intestinal electrolyte transport in congenital chloridorrhoea. Gut 12:544, 1971.
17. Stickler, G. B., Hallenbeck, G. A., Flock, E. V., and Rosevear, J. W. Catecholamines and

*A complete bibliography may be obtained from Dr. Hamilton on request.

diarrhea in ganglioneuroblastoma. Amer. J. Dis. Child. *104*:598, 1962.

18. Voorhess, M. L., Pickett, L. K., and Gardner, L. I. Functioning tumors of neural crest origin in childhood. Amer. J. Surg. *106*:33, 1963.

19. Hamilton, J. R., Radde, I. C., and Johnson, G. Diarrhea associated with adrenal ganglioneuroma. New findings related to the pathogenesis of diarrhea. Am. J. Med. *44*:453, 1968.

20. Imerslund, O., and Bjornstad, P. Familial vitamin B_{12} malabsorption. Acta Haematol. *30*:1, 1963.

21. Mohamed, S. D., McKay, E., and Galloway, W. H. Juvenile familial megaloblastic anemia due to selective malabsorption of vitamin B_{12}: a family study and a review of the literature. Quart. J. Med. 35:433, 1966.

22. Morin, C. L., Thompson, M. W., Jackson, S. H., and Sass-Kortsak, A. Biochemical and genetic studies in cystinuria; Observations on double heterozygotes of genotype I/II. J. Clin. Invest. 50:1961, 1971.

23. Rosenberg, L. E., Downing, S., Durant, J. L., and Segal, S. Cystinuria: Biochemical evidence for three genetically distinct diseases. J. Clin. Invest. *45*:365, 1966.

24. Navab, F., and Asatoor, A. M. Studies on intestinal absorption of amino acids and a dipeptide in a case of Hartnup disease. Gut *11*:373, 1970.

25. Milne, M. D. Hartnup disease. *In* Proceedings of the Biochemical Society, the 488th meeting, Nov. 21–22, 1968. Biochem. J. *111*:3P, 1969.

26. Hooft, C., Carton, D., Snoeck, J., Timmermans, J., Antener, I., van den Hende, C., and Oyaert, W. Further investigations in the methionine malabsorption syndrome. Helv. Paediat. Acta *23*:334, 1968.

27. Kekomäki, M., Visakorpi, J. K., Perheentupa, J., and Saxen, L. Familial protein intolerance with deficient transport of basic amino acids: An analysis of 10 patients. Acta. Pediat. Scand. 56:617, 1967.

28. Perheentupa, J., and Visakorpi, J. K. Protein intolerance with deficient transport of basic aminoacids. Another inborn error metabolism. Lancet 2:813, 1965.

Chapter 22

Diarrhea

John S. Fordtran

Diarrhea may be caused, at least theoretically, by five mechanisms: (1) the presence in the gut lumen of unusual amounts of poorly absorbable, osmotically active substances (osmotic diarrhea); (2) intestinal secretion (secretory diarrhea); (3) deletion or inhibition of a normal active ion absorptive mechanism; (4) abnormal mucosal permeability; or (5) deranged intestinal motility.[1] In a given disease or condition it may not be possible, owing to lack of data, to specify which of these derangements is the cause of diarrhea, but it is likely that all diseases and disorders that produce diarrhea do so by one or more of them. These mechanisms are not mutually exclusive, and osmotic, secretory, permeability, transport deletion, and motility components may all play a role in the same patient.

The volume and composition of diarrheal fluid depends upon which of these factors initiates the diarrhea and upon the specific region or regions of the gut that are involved. In addition, the character of the diarrheal process is influenced by bacteria residing in the intestinal lumen. Plasma, interstitial fluid, and intracellular volume and composition often become deranged during diarrhea, and sometimes these systemic effects may secondarily affect gastrointestinal transport, permeability, or motility, and be responsible for continuing diarrhea after the primary cause has disappeared.

Since an understanding of normal physiology is essential to an understanding of diarrhea, the normal handling of water and electrolytes by the gut will first be described.

NORMAL PHYSIOLOGY

FUNCTIONAL ANATOMY

The intestinal content is functionally separated from the rest of the body fluids by the various membranes of the mucosal cells (Fig. 22–1, *A*). The brush border membrane faces the luminal content, and substances that enter the epithelial cells during their absorption must somehow permeate this barrier. The cells also have a lateral and serosal cell membrane, and a substance must also penetrate one of these barriers in order to complete the absorptive process across the mucosal cells. Individual cells are joined near their apex by a "tight junction," and it is very likely that many small solutes, ions, and water traverse this "shunt pathway" during passive intestinal absorption or secretion. Thus there are two routes of absorption across the intestinal mucosa—transcellular and intercellular. Both pathways are probably used by some substances, whereas the movement of other substances is probably restricted to a single pathway. During absorption of fluid the intercellular spaces become dilated, as illustrated in Figure 22–1, *B*.

291

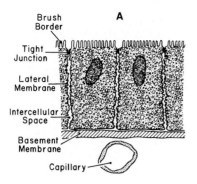
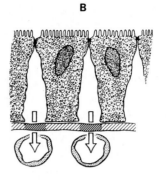

Figure 22–1. Functional anatomy of intestinal mucosal cells. *A*, Resting state. *B*, During rapid fluid absorption.

Thus absorption or secretion involves the movement of solutes and water across a complex barrier made up of several different membranes and/or a shunt pathway. The cells that line the villi and crypts are not uniform, but probably have specialized functions in the absorptive and secretory activities of the intestinal mucosa; however, it has so far been impossible to study absorption or secretion of individual cells, and all experimental methods actually record the net result of the different activities of the various cells which make up the mucosa. Even the activity of the crypts and villi has not been studied separately, but this may become possible by the use of methods similar to those used for micropuncture of the kidney tubule.

MECHANISM AND DETERMINANTS OF WATER AND ELECTROLYTE MOVEMENT

The rate and direction of water and electrolyte movement across the intestinal mucosa depends primarily on three factors: the passive permeability characteristics of the mucosa, the effective osmotic pressure gradient across the mucosa, and the active and facilitated transport systems within the membrane. There are important differences in permeability and transport mechanisms at different levels of the gastrointestinal tract.

Permeability Characteristics. It is generally believed that intestinal cell membranes, like all other cell membranes, are basically lipoidal in nature. Nonlipid substances, like water, electrolytes, and glucose, can penetrate in only two ways: first, by passing through the aqueous channels, or "pores," which are believed to be present in the membrane; or second, for some electrolytes and nonelectrolytes, by movement via a membrane carrier; i.e., facilitated diffusion or active transport. There are no carriers for water, so the movement of water occurs exclusively through aqueous channels.[2]

The forces which cause passive movement of water or ions through pores in the membrane are electrochemical gradients, osmotic pressure gradients, and solvent drag; e.g., movement of water secondary to active solute transport or osmotic pressure gradients can carry small solutes through the aqueous channels, even against adverse electrochemical gradients.[2]

The anatomical location of pores within the intestinal mucosa is not known. They may reside in the cell membranes proper, although more recent evidence suggests that they are located in between two adjacent cells at the tight junctions.[3] Functional pores may, of course, be present at both sites.

An interesting feature of the pores of the intestinal mucosa concerns their effect on transmucosal potential difference (PD). When balanced electrolyte solutions are perfused through either the upper or lower part of the small intestine, the PD is near zero. However, if sodium chloride in the perfusing solution is replaced by mannitol, the luminal side of the mucosa becomes positively charged, relative to the serosal side. This PD is caused by the more rapid passive diffusion of cations than anions through the pores of the mucosa. This effect is possibly due to fixed negative charges which are believed to line the intestinal pores, and thereby facilitate cation and retard anion movement.

Although the jejunum and ileum are alike in their higher permeability to cations than to anions, there are other marked differences in the permeability of these two regions of the human small intestine. The "effective pore radius" of the jejunal mucosa is approximately two and a half times larger than that of the ileal mucosa,[1] and there are several practical consequences of this difference in permeability of the upper and lower small bowel. (1) Hypertonic luminal solutions elicit marked secretion of water and ions from plasma into the jejunal lumen, but not into the ileal lumen. (2) Sodium chloride may be passively absorbed or secreted at rapid rates in the jejunum but not in the ileum. (3) Water absorption secondary to active glucose and amino acid transport is an important mechanism (solvent drag) for ion absorption in the jejunum but not in the ileum. (4) Active ion absorption is relatively inefficient in the jejunum, because transported ions tend to diffuse back across the leaky membrane; in the ileum active transport is efficient, because a transported ion leaks back at a very slow rate. Consequently impressive electrochemical gradients can be established and maintained across ileal but not jejunal mucosa.[4]

Recent experiments suggest that the colon is similar to the ileum with regard to its permeability characteristics; i.e., it is a "tight" membrane.[5]

Water Transport. All water transport is passive secondary to osmotic pressure gradients. Such gradients can be externally imposed, as when hypotonic or hypertonic fluids are ingested, or they can be generated by active solute transfer. In the latter instance, the linkage between net solute and net water transport is such that an approximately isotonic solution is absorbed or secreted.[2]

Although water movement is passive, water absorption can occur against a water concentration gradient, i.e., water absorption may continue even though luminal contents have a higher osmolality than plasma. This apparent paradox is explained by the serial membrane hypothesis,[6] as illustrated in Figure 22–2. Active transport of solute (NaCl, for example) from the intestinal lumen occurs across Barrier A, which is a tight membrane. NaCl accumulates in the restricted compartment, and the osmolality in this compartment rises to a level higher than that in the gut lumen. Water flows passively from the lumen into the restricted compartment, raising the hydrostatic pressure. This rise in pressure causes fluid to flow from the restricted compartment across Barrier B, which is a "leaky" membrane. Significant backflow into the lumen is prevented by the small size of pores in Barrier A. This model explains net water movement against adverse osmotic pressure gradients without the necessity of invoking active water transport. For instance, during absorption of a NaCl solution, osmolality in the lumen might be 400, in the middle compartment 700, and on the serosal side 300; water absorption is still passive, even though water is moving from the lumen to the serosa against an adverse osmotic pressure gradient.

As shown in Figure 22–2, the anatomical counterpart of the middle compartment is probably the intercellular spaces, as first proposed by Whitlock and Wheeler.[8] Barrier A is presumably the lateral cell membranes, and Barrier B is presumably the basement membrane, the blood and lymph capillaries, or a combination of these.

Facilitated and Active Transport Characteristics. Facilitated and active transport are believed to result from the action of membrane "carriers." The nature of these carriers is not understood, but they are characterized by their ability to move water-soluble solutes across the membrane at rates considerably higher than

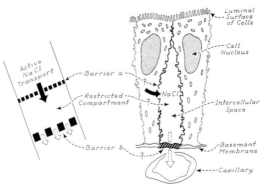

Figure 22–2. Correlation of the three-compartment model of Curran and anatomical structures of transporting epithelia. (From Dietschy, J. M.: Gastroenterology 50:263, 1966.)

would be expected by passive diffusion. For example, glucose and mannitol have approximately the same molecular radius, and their rate of passive diffusion through pores should be equal. In fact, glucose is absorbed much more rapidly than mannitol, owing to a carrier in the membrane with a high affinity for glucose. This carrier not only causes glucose absorption to be rapid, but also can transport glucose against steep concentration gradients. This is, by definition, an example of carrier-mediated active transport. Facilitated transport is also carrier mediated, but in this instance the carrier cannot effect absorption or secretion against a concentration (or electrochemical) gradient. An example is fructose absorption. Fructose is absorbed as rapidly as glucose when both are present in the lumen in high concentration, but only glucose can be absorbed against a concentration gradient. The glucose carrier has a high affinity for D-glucose and D-galactose and a low affinity for D-xylose, but the fructose carrier is, so far as is known, specific for fructose. The small bowel probably has other carriers for nonelectrolytes. The colon, on the other hand, has no known carriers for nonelectrolytes.

Special mechanisms (carriers) have also been postulated for sodium, hydrogen, bicarbonate, and chloride, and these are different in the proximal and lower small intestine. As shown in Figure 22–3, transport in the ileum is visualized as occurring by two double exchange carriers: sodium absorption for hydrogen secretion, and chloride absorption for bicarbonate secretion.[9, 10] If the exchanges work at the same rate, hydrogen and bicarbonate are secreted in the same amounts; they react chemically with each other in the gut lumen with the formation of CO_2 and water, both of which are free to diffuse across the ileal mucosa. Under this condition sodium and chloride are absorbed at equal rates, and there is no absorption or secretion of bicarbonate. If the anion exchange works faster than the cation exchange, the rate of chloride absorption will exceed that of sodium absorption, and bicarbonate will be secreted (because bicarbonate secretion via the anion exchange is occurring faster than hydrogen secretion via the cation exchange). If the cation exchange works faster than the anion exchange, sodium absorption exceeds chloride absorption, and bicarbonate is absorbed.

In the jejunum there is good suggestive evidence that a sodium-hydrogen exchange exists, but no evidence for a chloride-bicarbonate exchange. Perhaps not by coincidence, an adequate supply of bicarbonate in the proximal intestine is assured by pancreatic secretion. Functionally, jejunal sodium-hydrogen exchange, in the absence of chloride-bicarbonate exchange, results in sodium bicarbonate absorption from the lumen.

In neither area of the small bowel are these exchange carriers believed to generate an electrical charge, because each results in an exchange of one ion species for another of the same charge. Hence absorption via this model is non-electrogenic.

This model explains most of the known facts about active electrolyte absorption in the normal human small intestine in vivo (which does not, of course, prove its validity), and some of these are listed below.

1. The jejunum equilibrates its contents at a pH of about 6.0 owing to the unopposed Na:H exchange.

2. Ileal fluid has a pH of about 7.8, and the ileum is often observed to secrete bicarbonate; these facts are explained by more rapid anion than cation exchange

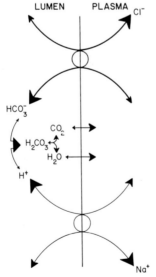

Figure 22–3. A double-exchange model for ion transport in the ileum. (From Turnberg, L. A., et al.: J. Clin. Invest. 49:557, 1970.)

under most physiological circumstances.

3. The PD across the small bowel is near zero when the small bowel content is a physiological solution, even though sodium, chloride, and bicarbonate may be transported against steep electrochemical gradients. This is explained by the fact that both exchange carriers are nonelectrogenic.

4. When chloride in ileal fluid is replaced by a poorly absorbed anion, such as sulfate, the ileum secretes acid. This is explained by the continued operation of the cation exchange (hydrogen secretion in exchange for sodium absorption) while the anion exchange ceases owing to the absence of chloride in the lumen.

5. Bicarbonate cannot be secreted unless chloride is absorbed.[11]

6. Acetazolamide inhibits sodium and chloride absorption. This is explained by postulating that hydrogen and bicarbonate availability for exchange depends on carbonic anhydrase.

7. Bicarbonate added to jejunal fluid enhances sodium absorption. This is because luminal bicarbonate reduces hydrogen ion concentration and favors Na-H exchange.

It should be noted that the location of the postulated anion and cation carriers is not specified. They might be located on either the brush border membrane or on the lateral or serosal membrane, and there is, at present, no reason to suggest that they must both be located on the same membrane. It has also not been proved that the two exchange processes are actually mediated by carriers as opposed to passive exchange driven by electrochemical gradients across the individual cell membranes.

In vitro studies in the small bowel of various laboratory animals have markedly increased our knowledge of transport physiology in general, but unfortunately the results of in vitro studies differ in at least four fundamental respects from the results of experiments carried out in vivo. First, in vitro preparations have revealed no evidence for an important role for solvent drag, yet there is no doubt that this is important in the human jejunum. Second, active chloride absorption in the ileum is either absent or very difficult to demonstrate in vitro, but strikingly apparent in vivo. Third, bicarbonate and hydrogen movements are not observed in vitro, but are clearly present in vivo. Fourth, the PD across the in vitro ileum is always positive on the serosal side, yet there is no consistent PD across the human ileum in vivo. Last, the Km for ileal glucose absorption is about 15 mM in vivo, but only 1 to 2 mM in vitro.

In contrast to the double exchange model proposed for ileal transport in vivo, in vitro studies have suggested that a sodium pump is responsible for ion and water absorption.[12, 13] In order to explain the serosal positive potential difference, this pump is considered to be electrogenic. Because of the fact that the lateral membranes give a positive reaction for Na-K dependent ATPase, and because of the association of this enzyme with a sodium pump in other tissues, the pump is postulated to be on the lateral membrane of the mucosal cell. This would be in accord with the three-compartment model for water transport shown in Figure 22–2, and with the fact that ouabain (a Na-K dependent ATPase inhibitor) stops ion transport when applied to the serosal but not the mucosal surface of the intestine. In addition, a sodium pump located at this point would explain the low intracellular sodium concentration characteristic of intestinal cells. If the pump extrudes three sodium ions in exchange for two potassium ions, the high intracellular potassium concentration, the low intracellular sodium, and the potential difference across the mucosa are all explained.

Why in vivo and in vitro experiments yield such different results is not clear at present. It is likely that these discrepancies will be resolved by further study, but for the moment a complete description of ion transport in the intestine cannot be given.

Coupling of Electrolyte and Nonelectrolyte Transport in the Small Intestine. Effect of Sodium on Active Glucose Transport. In vitro the intestine cannot absorb glucose unless sodium is present in the gut lumen. Furthermore, inhibitors of sodium pump systems, such as the cardiac glycoside, also inhibit glucose transport. These observations formed the basis for Crane's sodium gradient hypothesis.[14] There are two main features of this model: first, the affinity of a mobile carrier for glucose, located in the brush border membrane of the epithelial cells, is directly proportional to sodium concentration; second, the sodium concentration within the absorbing cells is maintained at a low level by an outwardly directed sodium pump. Because the sodium concentration in the gut lumen is higher than that inside the cell, the affinity for glucose at the luminal surface of the brush border membrane is higher than at the intracellular surface. This differential affinity results in net movement of glucose from the gut lumen into the cell. Once inside the cell, glucose diffuses passively across the serosal membrane to complete the absorptive process. In this model, the driving force for glucose transport against a concentration gradient is the gradient of sodium ion across the membrane which contains the glucose carrier. A similar theory is postulated for active amino acid transport.

Much evidence has been accumulated, mainly from a study of in vitro systems, to support the validity of this model.[15] Only rarely have in vitro studies been interpreted as not favoring this hypothesis, and the concept is widely accepted. It should be noted, however, that in vivo the human small bowel absorbs glucose as well, or almost as well, in the near absence of sodium as when lumen sodium concentration is 140 mEq per liter.[16, 17] The cause of this discrepancy between in vivo and in vitro studies is not entirely clear.

EFFECT OF GLUCOSE ON SODIUM ABSORPTION. Glucose in the lumen stimulates sodium absorption and causes a potential difference across the intestinal mucosa (mucosal side negative). That this effect is related to glucose transport and not to metabolism of glucose by the cell is shown by the fact that 3-methylglucose, which is actively absorbed but not metabolizable, has the same effect. There are two possible mechanisms for this phenomenon. One theory, derived mainly from in vitro studies, is that glucose stimulates sodium entry into the cell across the mucosal membrane (via the carrier postulated in the previous section), and that this increases the availability of sodium for pumping at the lateral membrane, which in turn stimulates electrogenic sodium transport.[12] Another theory, derived from in vivo studies, is that glucose stimulates water ab-

sorption and that sodium absorption is stimulated by solvent drag.[4] In the latter instance, the PD change is attributed to a diffusion potential (i.e., sodium diffuses more rapidly than chloride through aqueous channels).

Whatever the mechanism by which glucose stimulates sodium absorption, in the human this effect is mainly noted in the duodenum and jejunum. In these areas, glucose markedly increases the rate of sodium chloride absorption as well as the gradient against which these ions can be absorbed. The glucose effect on sodium chloride absorption in the human ileum is relatively trivial, although the potential difference response to glucose is prominent.[4]

Actively absorbed amino acids also stimulate sodium absorption from the small intestine.

Passive Ion Transport in the Small Bowel. Currently available evidence suggests that potassium absorption or secretion in the small intestine is entirely a passive process.[18] Although there are special mechanisms for active sodium and chloride absorption, it should be remembered that passive absorption or secretion of these ions is also quantitatively very important in the proximal small bowel.

Ion Transport in the Colon. The colonic membranes are tight,[5] and thus capable of sustaining steep electrical and chemical gradients. In contrast to the small bowel, which has no significant PD in vivo when perfused with physiological solutions, the colonic lumen is electrically negative with respect to the serosal surface, usually by about 30 mv. The origin of this colonic PD is not known, although many workers have ascribed it to electrogenic sodium transport. Since sodium is absorbed against concentration gradients, even though the lumen PD is negative, sodium transport must be ascribed to some active process. Aldosterone markedly stimulates the rate of colonic sodium absorption and also increases the lumen negative PD.[19, 20]

Most colonic perfusion studies have suggested that potassium movement is passive.[19, 20] This has been somewhat difficult to reconcile with the very high concentration of potassium in fecal dialysate, which increases even further with aldosterone treatment. To a degree, high lumen potassium concentration can be explained by the lumen negative colonic PD, although it seems unlikely that this factor alone can explain potassium concentrations of 100 to 120 mEq per liter, which are commonly noted in fecal dialysates (it would require a PD of about 85 mv to explain this concentration gradient between colonic lumen and blood, and PD values of this magnitude have not been reported). Needed are simultaneous measurements of ion concentration and PD at different levels of the colon. Another factor that might cause potassium concentration to become so elevated in fecal water is more rapid water than potassium absorption, with resulting concentration of the potassium remaining in the colon. Also, colonic mucus might play a role.[19] Finally, active potassium secretion has not been conclusively ruled out.

Chloride is absorbed against steep concentration gradients but in the direction favored by the electrical gradient. Fecal dialysates often contain chloride in concentrations as low as 10 mEq per liter, which would require an electrical gradient of about 63 mv, lumen negative, which has rarely if ever been reported. Low chloride concentrations obviously cannot be explained by rapid water absorption, because chloride concentrations fall as the colon absorbs fluid. Active chloride absorption seems likely, but simultaneous perfusion and PD studies have not clearly established the point.

Perfusion studies have demonstrated that the colon secretes bicarbonate against electrochemical gradients, strongly suggesting active bicarbonate secretion (or active hydrogen absorption).[21] If the bicarbonate concentration is raised high enough, the colon absorbs bicarbonate passively.

As in the small intestine, there is suggestive evidence that the colonic absorption of chloride and secretion of bicarbonate are linked in some manner. For instance, it has been shown that bicarbonate secretion is enhanced by the presence of chloride in the lumen.[21] This suggests the possibility of chloride-bicarbonate exchange.

In summary, sodium, chloride, and bicarbonate are probably actively transported in the colon, whereas potassium movement is probably passive. The colon avidly absorbs sodium and chloride, and can continue to absorb both these ions until their luminal concentration becomes lower than 25 mEq per liter. (For comparison, the ileum absorbs sodium down to a concentration of about 35 mEq per liter, and chloride down to concentrations of about 5 mEq per liter; the duodenum and jejunum cannot maintain gradients anywhere near this magnitude.) The colon responds to aldosterone administration by enhancing its rate of sodium chloride absorption, whereas the small bowel responds equivocally to such treatment. During passage of fluid through the colon, potassium and bicarbonate concentrations rise; the rise in potassium is probably a secondary phenomenon caused by rapid water absorption, electrical gradients, and mucus, and the rise in bicarbonate concentrations is most likely due to active secretion, linked in some manner to chloride absorption.

NORMAL INTESTINAL SECRETION

When the normal human small intestine is perfused with physiological solutions, the net effect of its diverse transport processes is usually absorption of the luminal fluid. Occasionally an apparently normal subject will secrete fluid into the intestinal lumen, even though there are no physical factors (such as osmotic pressure gradients) to explain this secretion. In some experimental animals, notably the guinea pig, small bowel secretion is the rule, rather than the exception,[22] and the vermiform appendix normally secretes fluid. This raises the possibility that the small bowel may always secrete fluid normally, but that this is masked by higher rates of normal intestinal absorption. In particular, it has been suggested that cells in the crypts secrete whereas cells on the villi absorb.[23, 24] Such a fluid circuit was suggested as long ago as 1940 by Wright et al.[25] This suggestion was and is based on histological evidence of crypt secretion, on the fact that fat and glucose are absorbed primarily by the villous cells, and on experimental data in disease states (celiac sprue and cholera) which suggest that the crypts are the source of intestinal secretion. Although preferential fat and glucose absorption from the villi may reflect special absorptive capacities of these cells, this observation could also be explained by the unstirred water layer which may form a significant diffusion barrier and limit fat and glucose absorption in cells far removed from the villous tips (J. M. Dietschy, personal communication).

The physiological and clinical importance of the hypothetical normal small bowel secretion is not known. It is generally agreed that loops of jejunum or ileum in conscious dogs show no increase in secretion following a meal, and this suggests that the intestinal secretory cells are not under neural and hormonal control in the sense of the gastric and pancreatic glands.[23] This does not preclude the possible importance of individual gastrointestinal hormones regulating the rate of intestinal absorption and secretion, but the combined effect of the various hormones and nervous impulses released after a meal appear not to stimulate secretion by small bowel mucosal cells, at least not in the dog. On the other hand, there is evidence to suggest that the dog small bowel does secrete at a slow rate in response to local chemical and mechanical stimuli,[23] but the mechanism of this secretion and its significance are not clear. To some extent such secretion might result from osmotic pressure gradients.

On the basis of present evidence it seems likely that normally there is a component of small intestinal secretion that is masked by more potent absorptive transport mechanisms. How large this hypothetical secretory component is and whether its accentuation is responsible for secretory diarrhea are not known. Better methods for studying components of the small bowel mucosa must be developed to further extend knowledge in this area.

Three clarifying points should be made. First, intestinal secretion *cannot* be equated with the unidirectional flux of water, sodium, or other electrolytes from blood to lumen as measured by radioisotope data. Second, bicarbonate and hydrogen secretion shown in Figure 22–3 is part of the normal absorptive process, and not a mechanism for the secretion of salt

solution. It is possible, of course, that reversal of the two exchange carriers (sodium secretion in exchange for hydrogen absorption and chloride secretion in exchange for bicarbonate absorption) could result in sodium chloride or sodium bicarbonate secretion, but this is quite a different explanation for small bowel secretion from that of two separate and competing transport processes, such as crypt secretion and villous absorption. Third, the fluid circuit model[4] proposed to explain the effect of glucose on sodium and urea absorption does not represent competing absorptive and secretory transport processes. Rather, the fluid moving into the intestine in this model is in response to an osmotic pressure gradient— in the absence of such a gradient, the fluid moves only in the absorptive direction, driven by active solute transport.

PATTERN OF WATER AND ELECTROLYTE MOVEMENT IN THE GASTROINTESTINAL TRACT AFTER EATING

The normal human intestinal tract contains almost no fluid in the fasting state. However, following the ingestion of meals, relatively large amounts of fluid, both from ingested food and from digestive secretions, are presented to the small bowel for absorption. That the normal intestine can tolerate and absorb the diverse meals which man ingests is truly remarkable. The complexity of the job it does with such apparent ease can be appreciated by considering the osmotic, fluid, and electrolyte problems associated with total parenteral alimentation.

Man is able to ingest foods without causing osmotic disequilibrium of the body fluids for five main reasons. First, the stomach mucosa is relatively impermeable to bulk water flow,[26] so that hypertonic fluids in the stomach (pineapple juice has an osmolality of 900 milliosmols per kilogram) elicit hardly any water movement from plasma into the stomach lumen. Second, stomach emptying is closely regulated by osmoreceptors located in the duodenum (see p. 120), and hypertonic solutions are emptied slowly into the proximal small bowel (which in contrast to the stomach is highly permeable to bulk water flow in response to osmotic pressure gradients). Third, the nutrients of the meal are to a large extent presented to the small bowel as macromolecules (starches, disaccharides, peptides, etc.) rather than molecules of monosaccharides and amino acids, and thus the caloric value of chyme is great, whereas its osmolality is relatively low. Fourth, as macromolecules are digested the component monosaccharides and amino acids are absorbed very rapidly by either active transport or facilitated diffusion; the result is that the effective osmotic pressure of chyme is much lower than it would be across a mucosa not endowed with special transport carriers. Finally, the small bowel can absorb fat, and fat does not contribute to the effective osmotic pressure of chyme.

When a person ingests a steak, about 2 liters of fluid is delivered to the proximal duodenum. Absorption of this fluid is rapid, and only about 750 ml of the meal remains as it reaches the ligament of Treitz, and the volume of fluid reaching the lower ileum is less than 200 ml. By contrast, when milk and doughnuts are ingested, the volume of water and amount of sodium chloride increase as the meal travels through the proximal small intestine. Absorption then commences in the mid-jejunum and continues through the rest of the small intestine, and about 250 ml remains unabsorbed as the meal reaches the lower ileum.[26] The difference in the pattern of net water and electrolyte movement in the proximal small bowel after these two meals is caused primarily by their different osmolality—the steak meal is hypotonic, whereas the milk and doughnut meal is very hypertonic. Other

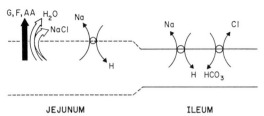

Figure 22–5. Major mechanisms of absorption in the human jejunum and ileum after eating. G, Glucose; F, fructose; AA, amino acids. In the jejunum, NaCl absorption is mainly passive, linked to active nonelectrolyte transport via solvent drag. Sodium bicarbonate absorption is accomplished by sodium-hydrogen exchange. The ileum absorbs mainly an electrolyte solution by a double ion exchange, the efficiency of which is great owing to the tight nature of the ileal mucosal membranes (which limits back diffusion of transported ions).

factors which determine the pattern of water and electrolyte movement in the intestine after a meal are the rate of its digestion (which determines the rate at which osmotically active solutes are added to the small bowel contents) and the relative concentration of actively and rapidly absorbed versus slowly or nonabsorbable solutes in the meal or in its digestive products.

As summarized in Figures 22–4 and 22–5, the major features of the proximal small bowel mucosa are its high degree of permeability to water and to sodium chloride, a sodium-hydrogen exchange mechanism, and a tremendous capacity to rapidly absorb glucose, galactose, fructose, disaccharides, and amino acids. Thus the proximal small bowel rapidly adjusts the osmolality of ingested meals to values near those of plasma,[26] absorbs pancreatic bicarbonate (via the Na:H exchange), and absorbs sodium chloride rapidly and without the expenditure of energy by coupling its movement to the active transport of dietary glucose and amino acids via solvent drag. It is also possible that glucose and amino acids stimulate sodium absorption more directly (see p. 292), but the major effect of active nonelectrolyte absorption on sodium chloride absorption in the proximal small bowel of humans after eating is via solvent drag.

Most of the carbohydrate and protein products of a meal are absorbed as chyme traverses the jejunum, and the fluid which reaches the ileum is mainly an electrolyte solution having an osmolality of about 290 milliosmols per kiligram, a sodium con-

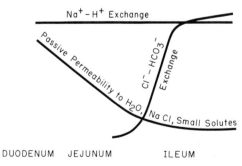

Figure 22–4. Differences in active ion transport mechanisms and permeability characteristics in different regions of the human small intestine.

centration of about 135 mEq per liter, a potassium concentration of about 8 mEq per liter, a chloride concentration of about 120 mEq per liter, and a bicarbonate concentration of about 15 mEq per liter. The anion gap is made up of bile acids. Unabsorbed nutrients in the lower small bowel are relatively small in amount and contribute negligibly to the osmolality of ileal fluid. The ileum is designed to absorb this electrolyte solution by virtue of the anion and cation exchange mechanisms and the tightness of its mucosa (which prevents actively transported ions from leaking back into the ileal lumen) as illustrated in Figures 22–3, 22–4 and 22–5. Probably because the anion exchange operates more rapidly than the cation exchange, ileal chyme develops a high concentration of bicarbonate and a low concentration of chloride (as low as 30 mEq per liter). The sodium concentration remains close to that of plasma unless nonabsorbable solutes are present in the ileal lumen, in which case water absorption is retarded and sodium concentration falls. The potassium concentration remains slightly higher than that in plasma, probably because ileal PD is negative on the lumen side after meals (owing to the active absorption of the small amount of amino acids and sugars that were not absorbed by higher regions of the small bowel).

The average volume and ionic makeup of fluid delivered to the colon from the small intestine (derived mainly from the study of ileostomy subjects) and the average volume and electrolyte concentration of stool are shown in Table 22–1. By subtracting fecal output from ileal inflow,

it can be calculated that the normal colon absorbs about 500 ml of water, about 71 mEq of sodium and about 34 mEq of chloride, and secretes 4 mEq of potassium per day. (Varying levels of dietary sodium have relatively little effect on the amount of sodium delivered to the colon, and the small bowel is relatively insensitive to variations in serum concentrations of adrenal and other hormones, so that these estimates are probably valid even in disease states.) This represents only about 20 per cent of the colon's capacity to absorb water and electrolytes,[27] and if ileal delivery rate were steady and the colon's function were normal, over 2 liters of fluid would have to be delivered to the colon per day before diarrhea would ensue. This estimate assumes delivery to the colon of normal ileal fluid without an excess concentration of nonabsorbable solutes. Looked at from another viewpoint, the almost complete reabsorption of sodium chloride by the normal colon, which occurs even in the presence of cation exchange resins, and the ability of the colon to increase sodium absorption in response to adrenal hormones, probably accounts for the ability of normal man to tolerate very low sodium diets for long periods of time without ill effects. Removal of the colon clearly limits man's adaptability to such diets and to any environmental situation requiring conservation of sodium chloride and water.

In a preliminary report, it has been claimed that the ileum of normal subjects delivers much larger volumes of fluid to the colon than the ileostomy data suggest.[28] If true, the colon absorbs more water, sodium, and chloride under normal

TABLE 22–1. COMPARISON OF APPROXIMATE DAILY WATER AND ELECTROLYTES DELIVERED TO AND FROM THE NORMAL COLON°

| | FLUID DELIVERED TO COLON† | | FLUID DELIVERED TO STOOL | |
	Amount	Concentration, mEq/liter	Amount	Concentration, mEq/liter
Water	600 ml		100 ml	
Sodium	75 mEq	125	4 mEq	40
Potassium	5 mEq	9	9 mEq	90
Chloride	36 mEq	60	2 mEq	15
Bicarbonate	44 mEq	74	3 mEq	30

°From Fordtran, J. S.: Fed. Proc. 26:1405, 1967.
†Based on patients with ileostomy.

conditions than previously suspected and absorbs rather than secretes potassium, and the ileum must adapt to an ileostomy by increased absorption of electrolytes and water. Furthermore, the degree to which delivery of small bowel contents could increase before the absorbing capacity of the colon was overwhelmed would be less than predicted in the peceding paragraph.

From the average concentration of electrolytes in ileal fluid and in stool (see Table 22–1), it is obvious that the colon drastically alters the ionic makeup of fluid passing through it. Note that the concentration of sodium in stool is 40 mEq per liter, much lower than plasma sodium concentration. This is a result of the ability of the colon to absorb sodium very efficiently and against high concentration gradients. The nonabsorbable solutes in normal food are highly concentrated in stool water; this inhibits water absorption, and sodium concentration falls. Also note that the potassium concentration of stool water is 90 mEq per liter, much higher than plasma. This is probably due to rapid water absorption with concentration of unabsorbed potassium, to passive potassium secretion down an electrical gradient, to colonic mucus, and possibly to active potassium secretion.

The chloride concentration of stool water is very low, 15 mEq per liter; this probably results from an exchange of lumen chloride with plasma bicarbonate. Therefore, a very high bicarbonate concentration would be expected. However, the bicarbonate concentration of stool water is only about 30 mEq per liter, and there is an anion gap of 85 mEq per liter. The remaining anions in stool water are made up of organic anions such as propionate, butyrate, and the like, that result from bacterial fermentation of unabsorbed carbohydrates.[29] The chemical reaction of these organic acids with bicarbonate lowers the concentration of bicarbonate in stool water.[1]

The osmolality of stool water is usually somewhat higher than that of plasma, about 350 milliosmols per kilogram. This, too, is related to colonic bacteria. Presumably bacteria split one sugar molecule into two or three smaller solutes at a rate which exceeds the capacity of the colon to equilibrate its contents osmotically with plasma.

If antibiotics are given to normal subjects, stool osmolality is the same as that of plasma.[30]

WATER AND ELECTROLYTE CHANGES IN STOOL DURING DIARRHEA

CATIONS

As previously noted, normal stool water contains a higher concentration of potassium than of sodium. However, as stool volumes increase during diarrhea, there is a progressive rise in the sodium and chloride concentration and a corresponding fall in potassium concentration. If the diarrhea is very severe, with stool volumes of 3 liters per day or more, the electrolyte composition of stools approaches values close to those of plasma. The explanation of the reversal of the normal ratio of stool sodium to potassium concentration in diarrhea is probably related to the fact that in diarrhea large volumes of fluid are moving through the colon and active sodium reabsorption and passive and possibly active potassium secretion are incomplete owing to decreased contact time of any given amount of intestinal contents with colonic mucosa.[1] In some diseases, defective active sodium transport in the colon and/or colonic secretion might also be responsible for this reversal. Persistence of the normal high concentration of potassium in small volume diarrhea is an indication of normal colonic function.

In all diarrheal diseases, sodium loss increases in direct proportion to the severity of the diarrhea, as gauged by stool volume. Potassium loss, on the other hand, is increased less dramatically with increasingly severe diarrhea. This is but another way of saying that there is a progressive rise in sodium and decrease in potassium concentrations in stool water as the severity of the diarrhea increases, and that sodium and potassium losses in diarrhea are to a large degree flow dependent.

These points are summarized diagrammatically in Figure 22–6. It appears, admittedly on the basis of very few clinical studies (summarized in reference 1), that sodium loss relative to stool water is ap-

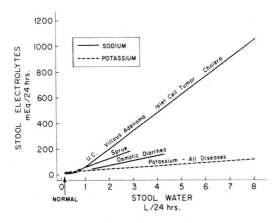

Figure 22–6. Relationship of stool volume to stool sodium and potassium losses in various diarrheal diseases. (From Fordtran, J. S.: Fed. Proc. 26:1405, 1967.)

proximately the same in patients with cholera, ulcerative colitis, islet cell adenoma, and villous adenoma of the rectum even though actual losses of water and electrolytes are remarkably different in these disease processes. By contrast, in those with celiac sprue and with pure osmotic diarrhea, sodium loss for a given rate of water loss is lower. Although sodium relative to water loss varies with different diseases, potassium relative to water loss seems more or less fixed, regardless of the disease process.[1]

Sodium absorption in the colon, and perhaps to a lesser extent in the small intestine, is stimulated by high blood levels of adrenal hormones and by salt depletion. One might expect that as a diarrheal disease progressed from an acute to a chronic state, with consequent salt depletion and high plasma levels of aldosterone, an effect on sodium and potassium losses would be evident. Specifically, net sodium losses would be expected to be lower and net potassium losses higher in chronic compared with acute diarrhea, provided salt depletion had developed in the former. However, such an event has apparently not been described in diarrheal disorders of man.

ANIONS

In cholera, infantile gastroenteritis, ulcerative colitis, laxative diarrhea, carcinoid syndrome, and diarrhea associated with islet cell tumor of the pancreas, the sum of the concentrations of sodium plus potassium invariably exceeded that of chloride. In contrast, in "congenital chloridorrhoea" and in "acquired chloridorrhoea" fecal chloride concentrations exceed the sum of sodium plus potassium.[31]

As in normal stools, organic acids of bacterial origin may react with the bicarbonate of intestinal contents to form the sodium salt of the organic acid. This reaction may cause bicarbonate to completely disappear from stool water, its place being taken by acetate, propionate, butyrate, etc.[32] These organic anions of bacterial origin are present in large amounts only when patients ingest carbohydrates, so that, in general, diarrheal stools will have a high bicarbonate concentration if patients fast and a low bicarbonate concentration if patients eat. For example, cholera patients are usually studied under fasting conditions, and the bicarbonate concentration in their stools is relatively high. On the other hand, in most chronic diarrheal diseases, stools are usually collected while patients are eating, and the bicarbonate concentration in stools is relatively low (see p. 303 for a discussion of the significance of measured stool bicarbonate concentration).

OSMOLALITY OF DIARRHEAL STOOLS

The osmolality of diarrheal stool has been reported rarely, and some of the data that do exist are difficult to understand.[1] For instance, the osmolality of stool in patients with cholera is somewhat hypotonic to plasma, and in infants with diarrhea stool osmolality is occasionally as low as 160 milliosmols per kilogram (approximately half the osmolality of plasma).[33] One possible explanation of these interesting observations is an abnormal jejunal permeability (specifically a decrease in effective pore size) or marked loss of jejunal surface area, or very rapid small bowel transit, coupled with oral ingestion of hypotonic fluid, such as water. Under these circumstances, osmotic equilibration, a prime function of the normal jejunum, might not be complete, and ingested hypotonic fluid could travel through the entire gastrointestinal tract, causing stool to be hypotonic to plasma.

Hyperosmotic stools have been reported in congenital chloridorrhoea[31] and in nonspecific infant diarrhea.[32] In infant diarrhea, hypertonic stools were present only when patients were on oral carbohydrate feedings. Other studies in these patients suggested that hyperosmolality of stools in diarrheal states is secondary to the production of organic acids from bacterial fermentation of orally ingested carbohydrates that escaped absorption in the small bowel. This implies that bacterial fermentation adds osmotically active solutes to intestinal water at a rate that exceeds the rate at which osmotic equilibration across colonic mucosa can occur. These considerations may explain the beneficial effects of antibiotics in apparently noninfectious diarrheal diseases.

In some reports of stool electrolytes in diarrhea, the value of $([Na^+] + [K^+]) \times 2$ has accounted for practically all the osmolality of stool water, whereas in other cases this value is much less than the measured osmolality.[1] The explanation for this difference probably relates to whether the patient has osmotic or some other form of diarrhea and whether the patient has recently eaten or not. For instance, if ingested food is incompletely absorbed in the small bowel, a significant fraction of stool osmolality will consist of hydrolyzed dietary products.

SYSTEMIC EFFECTS OF DIARRHEA

SALT AND WATER DEPLETION

When salt and water are lost in isotonic proportions, a contraction of the extracellular fluid compartment occurs and hemoconcentration develops. The serum sodium is normal and the intracellular compartment is not significantly reduced. If such patients take salt-poor fluids or water orally or intravenously, water may be retained, owing principally to increased secretion of antidiuretic hormone. Hyponatremia (and consequently a decreased effective osmotic pressure of the extracellular fluid) therefore commonly results. The retained water is distributed throughout the total body water, with only a small amount being retained in the extracellular compartment. In "osmotic diarrhea," water loss is proportionately greater than that of sodium. Dehydration, with hypernatremia, therefore results. The effective osmotic pressure of the extracellular fluid is thereby increased, and this causes a shift of fluid from the intracellular to the extracellular compartment. Severe thirst is characteristic of this form of salt and water depletion. Loss of water in excess of salt also occurs in sweat. This may be an important contributing cause of hypernatremia, especially in patients who are salt depleted (aldosterone) and who have fever.

Thus diarrhea with water and salt depletion may be associated with a normal, low, or high serum sodium concentration, depending upon the nature of the diarrhea and upon the type of fluid ingested.

POTASSIUM DEPLETION

Potassium, salt, and water depletion may develop with any severe diarrhea, but of particular interest is the occurrence of isolated potassium depletion. This is most likely to occur in long-standing mild diarrheal states, such as chronic laxative abuse.[34] Under these conditions there is adequate contact time of intestinal fluid with colonic mucosa, and potassium diffusion into the lumen of the gut reaches near equilibrium, resulting in stool water with relatively high potassium concentrations. (This assumes normal colonic function.) Another factor predisposing to isolated potassium depletion with mild diarrhea is the fact that mild salt depletion is associated with complete reabsorption of filtered sodium by the kidneys, whereas renal potassium losses usually continue even after potassium depletion has developed.

ACID-BASE DISTURBANCES

For practical purposes, the effect of diarrhea on acid-base balance can be ascertained from sodium, potassium, and chloride measurements of stool. If the sum of sodium plus potassium minus chloride is greater than the plasma concentration of bicarbonate, the patient must be losing bicarbonate or its equivalent, and the result is to acidify body fluids. On the other hand, if the sum of sodium plus potassium minus chloride is less than plasma bicarbonate, acid in some form is being lost, and this tends to produce alkalosis.

Stool pH and the direct determination of bicarbonate concentration in stool water are of no help in determining the effect of diarrhea on acid-base balance, and indirect measurements of bicarbonate loss (Na + K − Cl) are of much greater clinical value. For instance, organic acids of bacterial origin may react with the bicarbonate of intestinal contents to form the sodium salt of the organic acid and CO_2 and cause bicarbonate to decrease in or disappear from stool water. However, organic anions of bacterial origin in stool water are equivalent, in terms of acid-base balance, to sodium bicarbonate. Thus, although the diarrheal stools have a low pH and a low bicarbonate concentration, the patient may be sustaining a loss of base from the body and develop a systemic acidosis.

In addition to the primary effects of stool losses, secondary effects caused by hypokalemia, starvation, shock, and renal impairment are very important in determining the exact acid-base picture that will be encountered in a given patient. For instance, alkalosis may result not only from acid loss in stools, but also from contraction of the extracellular fluid without a commensurate loss of bicarbonate (contraction alkalosis) and potassium deficiency. Similarly, acidosis may result not only from loss of bicarbonate or its equivalent in stools, but also as a consequence of renal failure or from lactic acid acidosis secondary to shock. The entire spectrum of acid-base disturbance may be seen in different patients with the same disease, and in the same patient at different times.

PATHOGENESIS OF DIARRHEA

OSMOTIC DIARRHEA

Osmotic diarrhea is caused by retardation of water and electrolyte absorption secondary to accumulation of nonabsorbable solutes in the gut lumen.[1] There are three subtypes: (1) ingestion of poorly absorbed solutes such as some laxatives, (2) maldigestion of ingested food, and (3) failure to transport a solute which is normally absorbed by a special mechanism.

The presence of nonabsorbable solutes in the intestine retards water absorption secondary to active solute transport and by its osmotic effect tends to cause a net water movement from plasma to gut lumen. This is because the *effective* osmotic pressure of luminal contents containing nonabsorbable solutes is higher than that of plasma, even though the osmolality of luminal contents may be less than or equal to plasma. If jejunal permeability is normal, sodium and chloride also move into the jejunal lumen because of both solvent drag and concentration gradients between plasma and luminal contents. This passive secretion of sodium chloride takes place almost exclusively in the proximal small bowel, because in the ileum solvent flow and concentration gradients have relatively little effect on sodium chloride movement.

When osmotic diarrhea is caused by failure to transport nonelectrolytes which are normally actively absorbed (as in glucose-galactose malabsorption), the ability of the small intestine, especially the proximal part, to absorb sodium chloride is impaired (see pp. 295 to 296). Both the rate of sodium chloride absorption and the gradient against which absorption can take place are reduced. This is, in addition to the osmotic effect of unabsorbed solutes, a contributing factor in causing diarrhea.

In osmotic diarrhea, sodium concentration in the stool is lower than that in plasma, because both the ileum and colon can absorb sodium against large concentration gradients; the nonabsorbable solutes retard water movement and the concentration of sodium in stool water falls. There is therefore a tendency for hypernatremia. In sprue, accumulation of nonabsorbable solutes is only one factor causing diarrhea—active jejunal secretion and abnormal jejunal permeability are also involved, and thus the relation of sodium to water loss is not the same as with a pure osmotic diarrhea.

Clinically, osmotic diarrhea is distinguished by the fact that diarrhea stops when the patient fasts, and by the fact that the osmolality of stool water is higher than the sum of the electrolyte concentrations (in most diarrheal diseases the latter can be estimated by [Na + K] × 2).

SECRETORY DIARRHEA

With the exception of the Zollinger-Ellison syndrome (see pp. 743 to 750), all known secretory diarrheas are of small or large intestinal origin. It is, of course, possible that hypersecretion by the pancreas or hepatobiliary system might produce diarrhea, but no such entities have been described.

On a priori grounds, there are three possible causes of intestinal secretion: (1) passive secretion caused by increased hydrostatic and tissue pressure; (2) decreased intestinal absorption, unmasking a high rate of normal intestinal secretion; and (3) stimulation of active ion secretion by the mucosal cells.

Increased hydrostatic and tissue pressure is the probable cause of intestinal secretion in experimental animals who are volume expanded.[35, 36] The route of secretion may be via widening of the tight junctions between epithelial cells; some increase in mucosal permeability is an absolute prerequisite for high rates of intestinal secretion by this mechanism.[1] Increased tissue and hydrostatic pressure is a possible explanation of the secretory diarrhea associated with intestinal inflammation, such as salmonellosis,[37] and perhaps in chronic inflammatory bowel diseases.

Decreased absorption, unmasking a high normal secretory process, is a theoretical possibility, but there is no evidence to suggest that this is an important mechanism of intestinal secretion. It is a possibility that has not been excluded.

Intestinal secretion secondary to active ion secretion by the small intestine is probably the most important cause of secretory diarrhea. Knowledge in the area of active small bowel secretion has advanced rapidly in the past few years, primarily owing to studies with cholera toxin.[24, 38–41]

It is now generally agreed that the diarrhea of cholera is due to active intestinal secretion by the small bowel, and that this is primarily due to stimulation of active anion secretion by an enterotoxin elaborated by *Vibrio cholerae*. This response to cholera toxin is not associated with any inflammation or other evidence of histological damage to the small bowel mucosa, and although cholera toxin alters permeability in other tissues, there is at present no firm evidence that altered mucosal permeability plays a role in the cholera secretion.[24, 38, 39] Active intestinal glucose and amino acid absorption remain normal, perhaps because the cholera secretion originates in the crypts whereas absorptive processes are mainly a villous function.[24] It is also possible that active ion absorption processes are normal during cholera, although identification of normal electrolyte absorption in the face of a superimposed electrolyte secretion is difficult, if not impossible, by current experimental methods.

The mediator of intestinal secretion in cholera appears to be high intracellular concentration of cyclic AMP, secondary to stimulation of adenyl cyclase by the cholera toxin. Cyclic AMP and agents which raise cyclic AMP, such as theophylline and prostaglandins, mimic the action of cholera toxin on the small bowel.[24, 38, 40, 41]

Some features of the stimulation of secretion in experimental animals by cholera toxin are of interest: (1) Only brief exposure of the intestinal mucosa to toxin results in a steady increase in the rate of small bowel secretion, and once the secretion has started it cannot be reversed by washing the toxin off of the mucosal surface. (2) The entire length of the small bowel secretes in response to cholera toxin, but not the colon. (3) Cholera toxin induces secretion when applied to the mucosal but not the serosal surface of the small intestine. (4) There is a characteristic delay in the action of cholera toxin, which may be from 15 to 60 minutes in various preparations. (5) Adenylcyclase in the mucosal cells is present in the basal and lateral membranes, and not in the brush border; therefore the toxin exerts its action on the opposite side of the cells to which it is applied.[41] (6) The secretion is due mainly to active anion secretion. In vivo, bicarbonate is the ion transported most obviously against electrochemical gradients,[39] and this agrees with the well known high bicarbonate concentration in the secreted fluid. Chloride is also secreted against an electrochemical gradient, but all sodium and most potassium secretion can be explained passively, secondary to electrochemical gradients.[39] In the short-circuited in vitro system, chloride is the ion most obviously secreted against an electrochemical gradient, whereas bicarbonate movement is apparently not affected.[40] Although most studies have failed to show active sodium secretion, active sodium absorption is usually depressed by cholera toxin in vitro.

Secretory diarrhea mediated by cyclic AMP is also probably caused by toxins of *Clostridium welchii* and enteropathogenic *Escherichia coli* (colonization of the small bowel with these and related organisms is the probable cause of many cases of acute nonspecific diarrheal diseases,[42, 43] and the toxins of these bacteria are also responsible for some outbreaks of food poisoning[43]) and by prostaglandin secreting tumors (medullary carcinoma of the thyroid.[44]) This raises the possibility that the cyclic AMP system is a general mechanism for other secretory diarrheas. Sharp and coworkers[41] note three mechanisms for cyclic AMP-induced intestinal secretion: (1) stimulation of adenylcyclase, either irreversibly as in cholera or transiently as with prostaglandins; (2) inhibition of phosphodiesterase (the enzyme which destroys cyclic AMP); and (3) potentiation of cyclic AMP-dependent protein kinase activity. They point out that each of these steps is theoretically susceptible to pharmacological blockade, although safe and effective blocking agents have not as yet been developed.

A large number of other diseases and conditions are associated with intestinal secretion, but the mechanism of secretion is not clear in most instances. These include pancreatic cholera (islet cell adenoma without gastric hypersecretion), villous adenoma of the rectum, celiac and tropical sprue,[45, 46] and in some instances the effect of unconjugated bile salts on the colonic mucosa. There is clinical evidence to suggest that the colon secretes fluid, and that this contributes to the diarrhea in some patients with ulcerative colitis;[1] other mechanisms for diarrhea, such as decreased absorption by the colon, sec-

ondary disaccharidase deficiency, motility changes in the colon, and possibly decreased absorption by the small bowel must also contribute to the diarrhea of this condition. Experimentally, nematode infection, X-ray damage, and colchicine treatment in rats; niacin deficiency, hemorrhagic shock, and intestinal obstruction in dogs; and shigella enterotoxin in rabbits produce intestinal secretion (see references 22 and 24 for specific references). Antidiuretic hormone induces small bowel secretion in human subjects,[48] and pharmacological amounts of various gastrointestinal hormones, either alone or in combination, may elicit intestinal secretion.[49] Section of the nerves to an intestinal loop is followed by copious but temporary intestinal secretion ("paralytic secretion").[23] In these conditions it is not known whether the intestinal secretion is due to active ion secretion, to increased tissue and hydrostatic pressure, to inflammation, to decreased normal absorption, or possibly even to other unknown mechanisms of secretion. Furthermore, in most instances the ionic makeup of the secreted fluid is not known. The intestinal secretion induced by cholinergic drugs is apparently due to active chloride secretion.[50]

The diarrhea of the Zollinger-Ellison syndrome is a special instance of diarrhea caused by secretion of intestinal fluid; in this case the site of secretion is in the stomach and the fluid secreted is hydrochloric acid. Data on the relationships of sodium and water losses in this disease have apparently not been reported. The diarrhea of this disease is probably due to multiple factors — steatorrhea related to inhibition of bile salt and pancreatic enzyme activity, acid-induced jejunitis, and inhibition of sodium absorption because of the high acidity of jejunal contents. Specifically, the high hydrogen ion concentration of jejunal contents would inhibit the active component of sodium absorption that is linked to hydrogen secretion.

The major clinical features of a pure secretory diarrhea are that the diarrhea persists even when the patient fasts, that stool volumes may be and often are very large, and that the stool osmolality is almost entirely acccounted for by electrolytes (i.e., $[Na + K] \times 2 = $ stool osmolality). The relationship of sodium and potassium losses relative to fecal water loss in some secretory diarrheas is shown in Figure 22-6. As stool volume increases, sodium concentration rises and potassium concentration in stool water falls.

It is of interest to note that although potassium secretory states have been postulated, in such conditions the stool potassium concentration would be expected to increase rather than decrease with increasing stool volume. Such a phenomenon has not been reported, and there is, at present, no evidence that potassium secretory states ever occur as a cause for diarrhea. As already noted, the persistence of relatively high fecal potassium concentrations in patients with small volume diarrheas is indicative of normal colonic function.

DELETION OR INHIBITION OF A NORMAL ACTIVE ION ABSORPTIVE MECHANISM

The classic example is congenital chloridorrhea.[31, 51, 52] In this disease the patient is unable to absorb chloride actively, yet passive absorption or secretion of chloride in response to electrochemical gradients readily occurs.[52] The disease is probably due to a defect in the normal ileal (and probably also the normal colonic) anion exchange described in Figure 22-3. The sodium-hydrogen exchange is normal, but the chloride-bicarbonate exchange is not able to transport anions against electrochemical gradients. Sodium absorption is accomplished at the expense of acidification of the luminal contents, owing to the fact that secreted hydrogen in exchange for sodium is not balanced by secreted bicarbonate in exchange for chloride. The net result of this defect is reduced rate of fluid absorption, acidification of the luminal contents, and a high chloride concentration in the unabsorbed fluid remaining in the lumen of the ileum and colon. This is expressed clinically by a diarrheal fluid with a chloride concentration greater than the sum of the sodium and potassium concentration and by systemic alkalosis.

Quite likely there are other conditions in which a specific deletion of normal active ion transport causes diarrhea. For instance, some of the fatal congenital diarrheas that are not due to monosaccharide malabsorption or to congenital chloridorrhea are probably due to the deletion of other normal active ion transport processes. There are, in addition, several acquired conditions in which defects in normal active ion transport probably cause diarrhea. Acquired chloridorrhea,[53] diarrhea associated with bile acid malabsorption[47] and diarrhea caused by fatty acids[54, 55] are possible examples.

ABNORMAL MUCOSAL PERMEABILITY

Permeability to water and electrolytes may be altered by changes in surface area, or by specific abnormalities in mucosal cell membranes. In celiac sprue there is a marked loss of surface area, and a gross decrease in permeability to water and electrolytes must obviously be present in this disease, even assuming that the remaining mucosa retains the permeability characteristics of normal jejunal cells. Recent studies have shown, however, that the permeability of the remaining mucosal cells is not normal; rather, the effective pore size of sprue jejunal mucosa is markedly decreased, to levels lower than that seen in the normal ileum.[45] As a result, water flow in response to osmotic pressure gradients is markedly decreased, passive absorption of sodium chloride and other small water-soluble solutes is impossible, and net water movement has lost its effect on sodium chloride movement. Paradoxically, these abnormalities are probably protective, because the abnormal osmotic load (caused by malabsorption of digested food) presented to the proximal small bowel cannot result in massive passive secretion of water and sodium chloride that would occur if the jejunal permeability were normal. Patients with tropical sprue appear to have the same defect in permeability as do those with celiac sprue.[45] Patients with these diseases also secrete fluid into the proximal small bowel, but of course the diarrhea is probably due mainly to the osmotic effect of unabsorbed solutes.

In contrast to the situation in sprue, in which decreased jejunal permeability probably reduces the severity of diarrhea, permeability defects in other situations might reduce the rate of fluid absorption or even lead to fluid secretion, and thus contribute to diarrhea. For instance, reduced jejunal permeability in instances in which active nonelectrolyte transport is normal would markedly reduce the rate of passive sodium chloride absorption. On the other hand, if permeability were markedly increased, hydrostatic and tissue pressure could result in intestinal secretion. This is the probable mechanism whereby plasma volume overload results in intestinal secretion, possibly via widened tight junctions.[35] Experimentally, some bile salts increase intestinal permeability.[56]

DERANGED INTESTINAL MOTILITY

In some cases diarrhea is probably caused by abnormalities in intestinal motility. Decreased motility promotes stasis and bacterial overgrowth, whereas increased motility produces rapid transit of food and chyme and thus inadequate contact time for normal absorption of luminal contents. Hyperserotonemia, irritable colon syndrome, most instances of diabetic diarrhea, and postvagotomy diarrhea are at present best classified under this heading. Abnormal motility also plays a role in diarrheas of other primary causes. For instance, in osmotic diarrhea luminal volumes are high, stimulating peristalsis and rapid transit; this reduces contact time, compounding the osmotic component of the diarrhea. Also, inflamed bowel is irritable and empties its contents prematurely, and some types of prostaglandins stimulate motility rather than intestinal secretion.[57] In spite of its obvious importance, the interrelationship of motility and absorption has been little studied.

DIAGNOSIS OF CHRONIC AND RECURRENT DIARRHEA

INITIAL EVALUATION

In evaluating patients with diarrhea, the history is of great importance in suggesting the probable location and nature of the disease process.[58] The location of the underlying disorder within the bowel is suggested by the character of the stools and by the location and quality of any accompanying pain. It is helpful to distinguish between large stool and small stool diarrhea. When the stools are consistently large, the underlying disorder or disease is likely to be in the small bowel or the proximal colon. Such stools are likely to be light in color; to be watery, frothy, soupy, or greasy; to be foul; to be free of gross blood; and to contain undigested food particles. When pain accompanies this large stool diarrhea, it is likely to be periumbilical or localized to the right lower quadrant. These areas have been recognized as zones of pain reference from the mesenteric small intestine and the cecum. The pain in such instances is often intermittent, cramp-like, and accompanied by audible borborygmi.[58]

In small stool diarrhea the patient frequently has urges to defecate but passes small quantities of feces. In its extreme form he may, despite a great sense of urgency, pass only flatus or a small quantity of mucus. This syndrome is likely to be associated with disease or disorder of the left colon and rectum. The increase in irritability of that section results in the premature discharge of a quantity of stool otherwise insufficient to trigger a defecation reflex. When fecal matter in any quantity is passed, it is mushy or jelly-like, and in some diseases it is often mixed with visible mucus or blood. It is usually dark in color and rarely excessively foul. Pain, when present, is likely to be in the hypogastrium or in the left or right lower quadrant, or in the sacral region, reflecting the established zones of pain reference from the colon and rectum. It is usually griping, aching, or with a quality of tenesmus. It may be continuous, but it is usually relieved to some extent by an enema, a bowel movement, or even the passage of flatus.[58]

These two patterns of diarrhea are, of course, not mutually exclusive. With widespread inflammation or dysfunction of the intestines the two mechanisms may occur in the same patient, and even on the same day.

The history also usually provides valuable information about the nature of the disorder or disease process. Passage of blood indicates an inflammatory, infectious, or neoplastic disease, and rules out psychogenic diarrhea. (Of course, it is possible that hemorrhoidal or vaginal bleeding may occur in someone with irritable colon and confuse the issue, but bleeding from these sources can usually be distinguished from bleeding from the intestine by history alone.) Passage of pus or exudate in the stools indicates inflammation or infection, although exudate is often incorrectly assumed to be mucus. Lack of odor and presence of blood-tinged mucus is characteristic of shigellosis, whereas green, slimy "pea soup" stools are usually associated with Salmonella (and in infants, with enteropathogenic *Escherichia coli*).[59] Passage of nonbloody mucus is suggestive of irritable colon syndrome. Mushy stools that are frothy or contain oil suggest malabsorption. Intermittent diarrhea and constipation suggest irritable colon syndrome, especially if the stools are pellet-like during the constipation phase. Intermittent diarrhea and constipation are also frequent in diabetic autonomic neuropathy. Diarrhea which persists during fasting and is voluminous suggests a secretory diarrhea. Diarrhea that stops when the patient fasts suggests osmotic diarrhea. Diarrhea at night favors organic disease over irritable colon snydrome, but this is not always specific. Complaints of nocturnal diarrhea and fecal soiling are especially frequent in patients with neurological problems and those with diabetic autonomic dysfunction. The occurrence currently or in the past of a perianal fistula or abscess is suggestive of Crohn's disease.

The family history of any diarrheal disease is very helpful. The probability of exposure to infectious agents must be estimated, and the duration of the symptoms, their mode of onset, and variable occurrence or progression in severity, and the age of the patient when the symptoms began should be taken into account. Any correlation with diet, especially milk, should be noted.

The temporal association of diarrhea and emotional conflict should be searched for, as discussed on pages 1278 to 1288. Much information can be obtained as the patient reviews her complaints (most patients with psychogenic diarrhea are women), provided she is allowed to tell the story in her own way. Facial expressions, blushing, weeping, or unwillingness to discuss certain events may indicate the nature and causes of emotional conflict. It is also wise to include in the initial history gentle but systematic inquiry into the more important interpersonal relationships of the patient's life: those with parents, siblings, schoolmates, teachers, employers and coworkers, sexual and marital partners, children, and in-laws.[58] Interpersonal problems in the home are especially important in women; problems at work are more important in men.[60] In many instances the anxiety may be related to relatively trivial problems, but the stress to the patient may be severe. It is very important to find out why the patient is seeking medical help—whether she is worried about what might be causing her symptoms or is primarily interested in relief of her symptoms. (An irritable colon-like syndrome sometimes appears to follow an episode of dysentery,[60] so not all are necessarily psychogenic in origin.)

A complete physical examination will often reveal important clues to the cause of diarrhea. The importance of an abdominal mass, abdominal bruit, anemia, fever, edema, postural hypotension, lymphadenopathy, hyperpigmentation, skin lesions, purpura, neuropathy, cataracts, lipomas, goiter, clubbing of the fingers, liver enlargement, ascites, gaseous abdominal distention, a rectal mass or impaction, or decreased anal sphincter tone is obvious. The finding of perianal fistula or abscess suggests Crohn's disease. The nutritional status of the patient and any evidence of fluid and electrolyte depletion should be carefully noted.

It is clear that the history and physical examination may, in a patient with diarrhea, suggest the most probable diagnostic possibilities. For instance, the association of arthritis with diarrhea suggests ulcerative colitis, Crohn's disease, or Whipple's disease. Liver disease and diarrhea suggest ulcerative colitis, Crohn's disease, or bowel malignancy with metastasis to the liver. Fever and chronic diarrhea suggest inflammatory bowel disease, amebiasis, lymphoma, and, more rarely, chronic infectious diseases such as tuberculosis. Diarrhea with marked weight loss suggests malabsorption syndrome, inflammatory bowel disease, and cancer. Diarrhea and eosinophilia suggest eosinophilic gastroenteritis and strongyloidiasis. Diarrhea and lymphadenopathy suggest Whipple's disease and lymphoma. Diarrhea and neuropathy suggest diabetic diarrhea and amyloidosis. Diarrhea and postural hypotension suggest diabetic diarrhea, Addison's disease, and idiopathic orthostatic hypotension. Diarrhea with loud bowel sounds, flushing, a heart murmur, or attacks of wheezing suggests malignant carcinoid syndrome. Diarrhea and nephrotic syndrome suggest amyloidosis. Diarrhea and any collagen disease suggest mesenteric arteritis. Diarrhea and a large liver suggest malignant carcinoid syndrome. Diarrhea and ulcer-like dyspepsia suggest Zollinger-Ellison syndrome. Diarrhea (steatorrhea) and chronic lung disease suggest cystic fibrosis, even in adults. Diarrhea and heart disease or atherosclerotic disease of large vessels suggest ischemic injury to the gut. Diarrhea and susceptibility to bacterial infection suggest immunoglobulin deficiency. Diarrhea and vomiting suggest diabetic autonomic neuropathy. Diarrhea with a history of passage of air in the urine or air from the vagina suggests regional enteritis with fistula formation. Diarrhea and a past history of attacks of severe abdominal pain suggest pancreatic insufficiency. Diarrhea that in the past has responded to adrenal steroid therapy suggests ulcerative colitis, Crohn's disease, Whipple's disease, celiac sprue, islet cell adenoma (pancreatic cholera), and eosinophilic gastroenteritis. Chronic diarrhea that has in the past responded to antibiotic therapy suggests blind loop syndrome, tropical sprue, and Whipple's disease. Diarrhea with any symptom or physical finding of hyperthyroidism suggests thyrotoxicosis. Diarrhea with hyperpigmentation suggests Whipple's disease, celiac disease, or Addison's disease. It is imperative that adrenal insufficiency be recognized promptly, because such patients may die during a work-up for diarrhea.

Proctosigmoidoscopy. This is a very important aspect of the examination in most patients with chronic and recurrent diarrhea. It will not be helpful in most patients with malabsorption syndrome.

In the work-up of the patient with diarrhea, it is important that proctosigmoidoscopy be done without cleansing enemas, which distort the mucosa and wash away mucosal exudate. In most instances the small amounts of fecal matter encountered can be easily got around, and since most abnormalities are diffuse, fecal matter does not greatly interfere with proctosigmoidoscopy in the absence of enemas. Specimens of stool can be promptly obtained for gross inspection and special tests, as discussed in the next section.

As emphasized by Anthonisen and Riis,[61] rectal and sigmoid mucosal smears for pus are of tremendous importance (Fig. 22–7). Pus is encountered in inflammatory bowel disease and in shigellosis and Salmonella infection, but not in viral diarrhea or in irritable colon syndrome. The latter should not be diagnosed without a negative mucosal smear. The importance of mucosal smear is enhanced by the fact that in mild ulcerative colitis the smear is grossly abnormal, even when the mucosa may look normal to the naked eye of an expert sigmoidoscopist and is not friable. Smears are preferable to biopsy, especially initially, because they can be taken from multiple areas, never produce serious bleeding, and will not delay barium enema examination. In the author's opinion, mucosal smears should be a routine procedure in the evaluation of any patient with diarrhea.

During proctoscopy, the mucosa should be carefully examined for ulceration, friability, crypt abscesses, polyps, and tumors (secretory villous adenomas of the rectum are often missed for surprisingly long periods of time). The anal region can also be well visualized with the sigmoidoscope

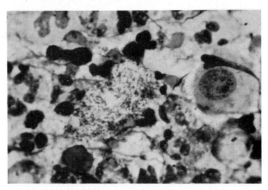

Figure 22–7. Mucosal smear from a patient with mild ulcerative colitis, stained with Wright's stain. Such smears are obtained with a metal rod without the use of suction.

as it is withdrawn. The specific findings in ulcerative colitis, granulomatous colitis, and amebic colitis by proctoscopy are covered in detail on pages 1305, 1356, and 1389. Briefly, ulcerative colitis is a diffuse process with large amounts of pus, whereas amebic proctitis typically causes discrete, flask-shaped ulcers with normal intervening mucosa and relatively few pus cells in the exudate. Shigellosis and occasionally salmonellosis may mimic exactly the sigmoidoscopic findings of ulcerative colitis. A rare disease, lymphopathia venereum proctitis, also mimics ulcerative colitis at proctosigmoidoscopy, as may gonococcal proctitis. The findings in Crohn's proctitis as differentiated from ulcerative proctitis are discussed in detail on page 1506.

Stool Examination. Every patient with diarrhea should have his stool examined for blood by gross inspection and by the guaiac reaction. In addition, every patient with diarrhea should have his stool examined by inspection for oil droplets (which are especially common in pancreatic insufficiency) and microscopically for fat droplets after Sudan stain. The presence of meat fibers can be determined microscopically as the Sudan-stained specimen is examined. The following tests are indicated initially in many cases, depending on the nature of the diarrhea: bacterial culture for ova and parasites, warm stage examination for *E. histolytica*, Wright's stain for pus, gram stain for staphylococci and monilia overgrowth, and pH (an acid pH suggests carbohydrate malabsorption of any type). Although rarely indicated initially, stool osmolality and electrolyte concentrations and determinations of 24-hour stool weight and volume are very useful in difficult cases.

PLANNING ADDITIONAL STUDIES

After the history, physical examination, proctosigmoidoscopy, examination of the rectal mucosal smear, initial examination of a stool specimen for blood (guaiac reaction) and fat (Sudan stain), complete blood count, and a routine battery of laboratory values by autoanalysis (including calcium, blood urea nitrogen, bilirubin, alkaline phosphatase, and serum electrolytes), the clinician usually has a good idea of the na-

ture of the problem, and a plan for additional studies is formulated to reach a specific diagnosis as rapidly as possible. Of course, X-ray studies should not be done if there is any chance of pregnancy. In some instances treatment of acid-base imbalance and salt and water depletion is of more importance initially than reaching a specific diagnosis.

If irritable colon syndrome (psychogenic diarrhea) seems most likely, it is important to begin therapy during the initial visit with the patient, as discussed on page 1285. Gastrointestinal X-rays are usually not required for diagnosis in children and young adults, but they may be advisable in that negative X-rays afford added assurance that organic disease is not present. In older patients, such X-rays are necessary to rule out organic disease before the diagnosis can be accepted. Stool cultures, stool pH, a further search for *E. histolytica*, and disaccharide tolerance tests may be indicated in some but not all patients.

If an acute infectious cause seems most likely (pp. 1369 to 1404), initial efforts will be toward examination and culture of the stool, mucosal exudate, and perhaps blood and urine cultures. Barium contrast X-rays should be delayed until after these are completed, because such X-rays interfere with the identification of *E. histolytica* and other parasites for periods of up to several weeks. It should be recalled that arsenic and cadmium poisoning may cause acute and often bloody diarrhea, and that several members of a family may become ill at the same time, suggesting an infectious cause.

If the patient has recently traveled to a foreign country, the differential diagnosis will be between tourista or travelers' diarrhea (which in some instances at least is probably due to colonization of the small bowel with specific strains of *E. coli*,[62] amebiasis, giardiasis, salmonellosis, shigellosis, and other infectious and parasitic agents). Diarrhea lasting longer than ten days is probably not tourista.[63]

If the patient has been taking antibiotics, the stool and/or mucosal exudate should be stained and searched for staphylococcal and monilial overgrowth, and stool cultures for these organisms should be carried out even though they are only rarely the cause of post-antibiotic diarrhea.[64, 65] In addition, the stool culture should be evaluated to see whether it contains normal flora, as well as lacking pathogens. Lincomycin may produce a colitis similar in some respects to ulcerative colitis.[66] Neomycin may induce a mild malabsorption syndrome. The mechanism of diarrhea after tetracycline is usually not clear.

If the patient has steatorrhea or other evidence of malabsorption, xylose and vitamin B_{12} absorption tests, quantitative stool analysis for fat, abdominal X-ray for pancreatic calcification, small bowel X-ray series, mucosal biopsy, tests for disaccharidase deficiency, and small bowel cultures may be indicated, but frequently a specific diagnosis can be reached with only a few of these procedures. Barium studies of the small bowel should follow

collection of stool.for quantitative fat analysis (if this is deemed necessary), but precede mucosal biopsy.

If the patient has gaseous abdominal distention, early abdominal X-rays are strongly advisable in order to help decide on the presence of ileus, obstruction, pseudo-obstruction, or toxic megacolon; if the patient has ascites, a diagnostic paracentesis is often of help.

If neoplasm or inflammatory bowel diseases are suspected, barium contrast X-ray studies are used initially (unless the patient is too ill to be submitted to such X-ray study) to confirm or refute the diagnosis, and to determine the extent and location of the disease in the small and large intestine. In patients with ulcerative colitis (known from proctoscopy), the radiologist

TABLE 22-2.
CHRONIC DIARRHEA IN INFANCY

UNKNOWN CAUSE	GI CAUSES			EXTRA-GI CAUSES

	INFLAMMATORY	FUNCTIONAL	ANATOMIC	Occult infection
				Neural crest tumor
				Hypoparathyroidism
				Hyperthyroidism
				Adrenocortical
				  insufficiency
				Galactosemia
				Immunological deficiency
				  syndromes
				Acrodermatitis
				  enteropathica
				Pellagra
				Folic acid deficiency
				Copper deficiency
				Magnesium deficiency
				Chronic heavy metal
				  poisoning
				Familial dysautonomia
				Orotic aciduria
				Lipidosis with adrenal
				  calcification
				Hereditary angioneurotic
				  edema

	Shigella
	Salmonella
	Candida
	Related vibrios
	Parasites
	Ulcerative colitis
	Regional enteritis
	Tuberculosis
		Drugs -- direct toxic effect
		  - alteration of normal GI flora
		Dietary - starvation
		  overeating
		  food intolerance
		  food allergy
		Irritable colon syndrome
		Congenital chloridorrhea
		Fructose intolerance
		Malabsorption syndromes
		  celiac syndromes
		  cystic fibrosis
		  disaccharidase deficiency
		  glucose-galactose malabsorption
		  pancreatic lipase deficiency
		  pancreatic deficiency with
		    pancytopenia
		  abetalipoproteinemia
		  methionine malabsorption
		  selective malabsorption of vitamin
		    B_{12} with proteinuria
			Congenital aganglionic
			  colon and other
			  causes of fecal
			  impaction
			Fistulae
			Blind loops
			Ileal stenosis
			Malrotation
			Intestinal
			  lymphangiectasia
			Lymphosarcoma of
			  small bowel
			Surgical resection of
			  small bowel (short
			  gut syndrome)	

NOTES: 1. Work-up should be orderly rather than shot-gun; follow-up clues from history, physical and routine lab.
2. For "Extra GI" group:
   a. all can be suspected from history and physical examination if one asks the correct questions and looks for the appropriate things and/or from abnormalities in routine laboratory work.
   b. specific diagnostic tests as indicated based upon the clues uncovered.
3. For "GI" group:
   a. detailed history; observe character and volume of stools.
   b. initial laboratory tests of stools: culture, ova and parasites, pH, reducing substance, guaiac, trypsin, qualitative fat.
   c. initial blood tests: culture, CBC, BUN, electrolytes, serum proteins.
   d. sweat chloride.
   e. supine and upright x-ray of abdomen.
   f. work-up for malabsorption syndromes:
      (1) stool and urine pH and reducing substance
      (2) quantitative stool fat
      (3) lactose tolerance test, including measure of urine sugar
      (4) sucrose tolerance test (as control for LTT or for diagnosis)
      (5) glucose or glucose/galactose tolerance test
      (6) small bowel biopsy for morphology, enzyme assay and giardiasis
   g. further diagnostic tests such as dye contrast x-rays, proctoscopy, serum cholesterol, etc., as indicated.
4. Diarrhea may or may not be a sign of protein-losing enteropathies which may be secondary to renal, cardiac or gastrointestinal disease.

Table prepared by Dr. John D. Nelson, Department of Pediatrics, University of Texas Southwestern Medical School at Dallas.

should be warned of mucosal friability and air contrast should not be used because of the danger of perforation. As already noted, barium enema should not be done for ten days following a rectal biopsy. It is wise to search carefully for amebiasis in every case diagnosed as ulcerative colitis, because occasionally amebiasis may look like ulcerative proctitis at sigmoidoscopy and because steroid therapy may cause severe exacerbation of amebiasis.

In the infant with diarrhea,[59, 67, 68] the following disorders should be considered: bacterial and viral infections, including cytomegalic inclusion disease; Hirschsprung's disease; partial intestinal obstruction (bands, intussusception); ulcerative colitis; monosaccharide malabsorption and primary and secondary disaccharide deficiency (acid stools); congenital chloridorrhea; cystic fibrosis (sweat chloride); pancreatic hypoplasia (neutropenia); allergy to milk protein; and tumors such as neuroblastoma and ganglioneuroma. Of course, systemic infections and severe undernutrition are important causes of diarrhea in infants. Celiac disease does not usually begin until after one year of age. Galactosemia may present with diarrhea. The causes of chronic diarrhea in infants and a suggested diagnostic approach are listed in Table 22–2 (see pp. 280 to 289).

CHRONIC AND RECURRENT DIARRHEA THAT IS NOT DIAGNOSED BY INITIAL WORK-UP

It is well recognized that chronic diarrhea may be a manifestation of an enormous number of diseases. In some instances these are perfectly obvious, and there is no diagnostic problem. In the following discussion it is assumed that the patient has had a reasonable work-up; that psychogenic diarrhea (irritable colon syndrome) seems unlikely; and that uremia, cavitary tuberculosis, gastrocolic and other fistulas, radiation injury, cancer of the stomach, colon, and pancreas, and diarrhea around a fecal impaction have been excluded. It is further assumed that the easily diagnosed malabsorption diseases (celiac sprue, Whipple's disease, pancreatic insufficiency), regional enteritis, ulcerative colitis, and pernicious anemia have been ruled out, and that the patient has not

had abdominal surgery known to be associated with diarrhea (e.g., vagotomy, gastric resection, small bowel resection). Factitious diarrhea caused by laxatives has been adequately stressed, and there is no need to review the importance of a careful examination of the stool to rule out parasitic infections, especially E. histolytica.

Even after such obvious diseases and problems have been excluded, chronic diarrhea often remains unexplained. This, coupled with inadequate measures to control the symptom, often leads to severe disability.

Diarrhea in the face of a negative initial work-up raises the possibility that it is functional or psychogenic in origin, even though initially this seemed unlikely. At this point it is well to review in one's mind the characteristics of the diarrhea in these conditions. First, the diarrhea is usually intermittent and associated with pain, but it may be constant and painless. Second, the stools are usually small in volume by history (although admittedly the range of stool volumes in this disease has not been documented). Third, the stools are not excessively foul. Fourth, the history, physical examination, and special tests should reveal no evidence of organic disease. Specifically, the X-rays should be negative, the stools should be negative for blood, the rectal mucosal smear should be negative for E. histolytica and pus cells, the stool cultures should contain normal flora and no pathogens, and steatorrhea should be absent. Fifth, the onset and/or recurrence of diarrhea theoretically should be associated with stress, although at times this correlation may not be readily apparent. As already noted, the irritable colon syndrome sometimes follows and is apparently caused by an episode of dysentery.

A negative work-up in a patient with chronic diarrhea that does not, for one reason or another, fit the irritable colon syndrome constitutes a major clinical problem. In these instances, a pathophysiological approach to the diagnosis may prove very helpful, and it is wise at this point to determine whether or not the diarrhea persists when the patient fasts for 24 hours, and to measure the stool volume, osmolality, and electrolyte concentrations. These procedures usually help in determining whether the patient has a secretory or an osmotic diarrhea. The more classic approach to the diagnosis, looking by specific test for a specific disease, is also helpful, and both approaches are usually necessary. It may be necessary to take an investigative approach and perform perfusion, permeability, and motility studies, special absorption procedures, and analysis of blood for hormones and other substances that may only be available in only a few research centers. The possibility of laxative use, especially phenolphthalein, should be specifically ruled out.

The following diagnoses should be considered in patients with chronic and recurrent "idiopathic" diarrhea which does not fit the irritable colon syndrome.

Reconsideration of Inflammatory Bowel Disease. X-rays are sometimes negative on initial study in patients with both regional enteritis and ulcerative colitis. It should be ensured that rectal mucosal smear and/or biopsy were done and were negative.

Secretory Diarrheas. ZOLLINGER-ELLISON SYNDROME. These patients usually have steatorrhea as well as diarrhea. Diarrhea may be present without peptic ulcer in 7 per cent of cases.[69] The stomach usually has excess fluid on upper gastrointestinal X-ray series. Diagnosis is made by gastric analysis and serum gastrin.

CHRONIC DIARRHEA AND MEDULLARY CARCINOMA OF THE THYROID. The diarrhea is probably secretory, cuased by prostaglandin secretion by the tumor.[44] The diarrhea disappears if tumor is resected. It may occur in association with pheochromocytoma, although patients with pheochromocytoma alone rarely have diarrhea.[70]

GANGLIONEUROMA.[71-74] This massive watery diarrhea with or without steatorrhea may respond favorably to adrenal steroids. Diarrhea will be cured by removal of the tumor. Hypertension, flushing and fever may be absent, with diarrhea the only manifestation. Abnormal catecholamine excretion is usually but not invariably present, and laparotomy may be necessary for diagnosis. The cause of the diarrhea is probably some substance secreted by the tumor other than catecholamines, because the latter do not produce diarrhea when infused into patients, and patients with pheochromocytoma usually do not have diarrhea (p. 288).

PANCREATIC CHOLERA CAUSED BY ISLET CELL TUMOR (see pp. 365 to 375). Watery diarrhea occurs usually without steatorrhea. Hypokalemia is prominent. There is no gastric hypersecretion and such patients are often achlorhydric. The adenoma probably secretes a hormone which causes intestinal secretion. Patients may respond to steroid therapy. The diagnosis is made by angiography and laparotomy.

Osmotic Diarrheas. Disaccharidase deficiency, monosaccharide malabsorption and some laxatives are major causes. The stool osmolality is greater than twice the sum of sodium and potassium concentrations, and stool pH is acid with carbohydrate malabsorption. Tolerance tests are indicated. Disaccharidase assay of small bowel mucosa is available in some centers.

Diarrhea and Bacteria. BLIND LOOP SYNDROME. Patients usually have evidence of stasis by X-ray, a disease known to be associated with stasis (scleroderma, diabetes, etc.), or previous gastrointestinal surgery. The disorder is diagnosed by small bowel culture and colony count and by the Schilling test with and without antibiotics (see pp. 927 to 936).

ABNORMAL BACTERIAL FLORA. The patient will present with a history of travel, antibiotic therapy, immunological defects, or tropical sprue. It must be ensured that stool cultures have normal flora as well as "no pathogens." A small bowel culture and colony count should be performed to rule out colonization by bacterial strains generally not considered as pathogens, but which may produce a secretory diarrhea.

SCLERODERMA. Scleroderma may involve the gut primarily, but esophageal motility by X-ray and manometry will almost always be abnormal if scleroderma is the cause of diarrhea or malabsorption. In some cases, steatorrhea is due to bacterial overgrowth in the small bowel, and either antibiotics or resection of dilated segments of small bowel may result in dramatic improvement.[75-77]

Endocrine Disease. ADDISON'S DISEASE.[78, 79] Diarrhea may be a serious symptom, although its cause is uncertain.

It may be associated with steatorrhea, which is common in patients with Addison's disease, and may be an important cause for weight loss in these patients. Stool fat may be as high as 32 g per day. Appropriate treatment of Addison's disease reverses the steatorrhea completely. Pituitary deficiency may also be associated with diarrhea. If the nature of the endocrine problem is not recognized, the patient may die during work-up for the diarrheal problem.

THYROTOXICOSIS.[78] This causes diarrhea in 20 per cent of cases. In masked hyperthyroidism, severe diarrhea and weight loss may dominate the picture. The mechanism is not known, and no well studied cases from the gastrointestinal standpoint are available.

HYPOPARATHYROIDISM.[78, 80-82] Diarrhea is an occasional symptom. It may be a direct effect of hypocalcemia on the bowel. Cramps, steatorrhea, and tetany may be present, and there may be a history of previous thyroidectomy (a common cause of hypoparathyroidism). The serum inorganic phosphorus is raised in patients with hypoparathyroidism, and normal or low in those with most malabsorption syndromes (see pp. 384 to 405).

Drugs. Lincomycin ("colitis"),[67] neomycin (malabsorption), tetracycline (altered flora), some antacids, antihypertensive agents, digitalis, and colchicine may cause diarrhea. Osmotic laxatives produce osmotic diarrhea, whereas "irritant" laxatives produce diarrhea by causing intestinal secretion and/or inhibiting normal active ion absorption.

Tumors. ABDOMINAL LYMPHOMA.[83-85] This may masquerade initially as celiac disease, but a gluten-free diet will not alter its course. It may be a complication of celiac disease which previously was well controlled by a gluten-free diet. The diagnosis may be suspected from small bowel X-ray or biopsy, but laparotomy is usually required.

MALIGNANT CARCINOID SYNDROME. These patients almost always have a large liver. Diagnosis is confirmed by high urinary 5HIAA. (Celiac sprue patients also have mild elevation of urinary 5HIAA.)

Immunoglobulin Deficiency. Diarrhea with or without steatorrhea, with or without sprue-like jejunal biopsy abnormalities, and with or without thymoma may be associated with a wide spectrum of immunoglobulin deficiencies, especially IgA deficiency. Severe and resistant giardial infestation is common, and is probably the cause of diarrhea in many instances. On jejunal biopsy plasma cells are absent from the lamina propria. See pages 51 to 68 and 384 to 405.

Infections. GIARDIASIS. Giardiasis is frequently present with IgA deficiency. In some patients giardiasis appears to be the only cause of diarrhea, with or without malabsorption. Cysts may not be present in stool, and diagnosis by jejunal aspirate or jejunal biopsy may be necessary. The presence of Giardia does not necessarily mean that this parasite is causing the diarrhea. Response to specific therapy is confirmatory. See pages 384 to 405 and 909 to 925 for further discussion of giardiasis and other infectious diarrheas.

Neurogenic. DIABETIC DIARRHEA. This may occur with or without steatorrhea. All patients have peripheral neuropathy, but manifestations may be mild. Impotence and postural hypotension are especially common. If steatorrhea is present without neuropathy, steatorrhea is probably due to another problem, such as celiac disease or pancreatic insufficiency.

AMYLOIDOSIS.[86, 87] Diarrhea with or without steatorrhea occurs in about 15 per cent of patients. Its mechanism is unknown. Amyloidosis should be suspected when diarrhea is associated with peripheral neuropathy and/or autonomic dysfunction in a nondiabetic and when diarrhea is superimposed on other chronic diseases. Proteinuria is common.

OTHER "NEUROGENIC DIARRHEAS.[88] These include tabes dorsalis, multiple sclerosis, myelitis, encephalitis, heat stroke, lead poisoning, Charcot-Marie-Tooth disease, orthostatic hypotension, and dystrophica myotonia.

Miscellaneous. PARADOXICAL DIARRHEA WITH OPIATES. Chronic diarrhea can result from the use of opiates.[89] Attempts to reduce the dose may make diarrhea worse for several days to a week. Only complete withdrawal cures diarrhea.

SPURIOUS STEATORRHEA DUE TO INGESTION OF OIL OR NUTS.[90]

ALLERGY. Allergy has not been established as a cause of diarrhea in adults except in those with Henoch-Schönlein syndrome and, possibly, with eosinophilic gastroenteritis. Allergy to milk protein is the likely cause of diarrhea in some children. Skin tests are an unreliable index of gastrointestinal allergy.

CIRRHOSIS. Severe unexplained diarrhea may be the chief complaint of patients with cirrhosis, especially that associated with alcoholism. The exact cause can rarely be pinpointed. Malabsorption caused by bile salt deficiency or associated pancreatic insufficiency is often incriminated if steatorrhea.is present. Passive congestion of the gut or disaccharidase deficiency (caused by protein malnutrition) is blamed if there is no or little steatorrhea. Diarrhea usually abates after several weeks in hospital.

DIARRHEA AND MALABSORPTION IN SYSTEMIC MAST CELL DISEASE.[91, 92] Its cause is unknown. Jejunal mucosa is either normal or may contain mast cells. Skin pigmentation occurs in this disease as well as in sprue; this may cause confusion.

COLONIC DIVERTICULA. See pages 1415 to 1430. If diverticula are found in a patient being worked up for diarrhea, a cause-and-effect relationship should be accepted with caution unless the diarrhea is definitely associated with flare-ups of diverticulitis. It may be difficult to decide whether a patient has mild diverticulitis or irritable colon syndrome. Diarrhea caused by diverticulitis is usually a small stool diarrhea.

EXCESSIVE BILE SALTS IN COLON. Abnormally high concentrations of some bile salts either inhibit normal colonic absorption or stimulate colonic secretion. Diarrhea associated with ileal resection or disease is probably mediated in part by this mechanism.[47] In most instances the diagnosis is obvious, because the patient will have ileal disease by X-ray or a history of ileal resection. It is possible that ileal malabsorption of bile salts could cause diarrhea in the absence of abnormal ileal X-rays. Indirectly this might be suggested by an abnormal Schilling test or by a good response to cholestyramine therapy. Direct assessment of this possible cause of diarrhea would require special tests of bile acid absorption that are available in only a few centers (see pp. 971 to 977).

EOSINOPHILIC GASTROENTERITIS. See pages 1068 to 1075.

CHRONIC NONGRANULOMATOUS JEJUNITIS AND ILEITIS. See pages 922 to 924.

ACQUIRED OR CONGENITAL CHLORIDORRHEA. See page 307.

A-BETA-LIPOPROTEINEMIA. This disorder is associated with acanthocytosis on wet peripheral blood smear from a finger stick. Fasting jejunal cells (mucosal biopsy) contain fat.

FOLIC ACID DEFICIENCY. In some patients with tropical sprue, diarrhea and malabsorption are corrected by folic acid therapy, suggesting that the intestinal disorder was due to folic acid deficiency. In some instances these patients had never been in the tropics, and in others the time since residence in the tropics is very long.[93–95] The author has seen two patients with chronic diarrhea and intermittent steatorrhea of unknown cause with normal jejunal histology who (apparently) responded dramatically to therapy with oral folic acid. It is recommended that serum folate be measured and a therapeutic trial with folic acid be considered in patients with idiopathic chronic diarrhea, even in those who have not resided in the tropics.

ADULT FORMIMINOTRANSFERASE DEFICIENCY AND FAILURE OF ADAPTATION OF GLYCOLYTIC ENZYMES. This may be a cause of diarrhea, although the causes are not yet fully documented.[96]

MAGNESIUM DEFICIENCY.[97]

REFERENCES

1. Fordtran, J. S. Speculations on the pathogenesis of diarrhea. Fed. Proc. 26:1405, 1967.
2. Fordtran, J. S., and Dietschy, J. M. Water and electrolyte movement in the intestine. Gastroenterology 50:263, 1966.
3. Frömter, E., and Diamond, J. Route of passive ion permeation in epithelia. Nature (New Biology) 235:9, 1972.
4. Fordtran, J. S., Rector, F. C., Jr., and Carter, N. W. The mechanisms of sodium absorption in the human small intestine. J. Clin. Invest. 47:884, 1968.
5. Billich, C. O., and Levitan, R. Effects of sodium concentration and osmolality on water and electrolyte absorption from the intact human colon. J. Clin. Invest. 48:1336, 1969.
6. Curran, P. F., Sodium chloride and water transport by rat ileum in vitro. J. Gen. Physiol. 43:1137, 1960.
7. Dietschy, J. M. Recent developments in solute and water transport across the gallbladder epithelium. Gastroenterology 50:692, 1966.
8. Whitlock, R. T., and Wheeler, H. O. Coupled transport of solute and water across rabbit gallbladder epithelium. J. Clin. Invest. 43:2249, 1964.

9. Turnberg, L. A., Fordtran, J. S., Carter, N. W., and Rector, F. C., Jr. Mechanism of bicarbonate absorption and its relationship to sodium transport in the human jejunum. J. Clin. Invest. 49:548, 1970.

10. Turnberg, L. A., Bieberdorf, F. A., Morawski, S. G., and Fordtran, J. S. Interrelationships of chloride, bicarbonate, sodium, and hydrogen transport in the human ileum. J. Clin. Invest. 49:557, 1970.

11. Hubel, K. A. Bicarbonate secretion in rat ileum and its dependence on intraluminal chloride. Amer. J. Physiol. 213:1409, 1967.

12. Schultz, S. G., and Curran, P. F. Intestinal absorption of sodium chloride and water. In Handbook of Physiology, Sect. 6, Vol. III, C. F. Code (ed.). Washington, D.C., American Physiological Society, 1968, p. 1245.

13. Schultz, S. G., and Frizzell, R. A. An overview of intestinal absorptive and secretory processes. Gastroenterology 63:161, 1972.

14. Crane, R. K. Hypothesis for mechanism of intestinal active transport of sugars. Fed. Proc. 21:891, 1962.

15. Schultz, S. G., and Curran, P. F. Coupled transport of sodium and organic solutes. Physiol. Rev. 50:637, 1970.

16. Olsen, W. A., and Ingelfinger, F. J. The role of sodium in intestinal glucose absorption in man. J. Clin. Invest. 47:1133, 1968.

17. Saltzman, D. A., Rector, F. C., Jr., and Fordtran, J. S. The role of intraluminal sodium in glucose absorption in vivo. J. Clin. Invest. 51:876, 1972.

18. Turnberg, L. A. Potassium transport in the human small bowel. Gut 12:811, 1971.

19. Phillips, S. F. Absorption and secretion by the colon. Gastroenterology 56:966, 1969.

20. Turnberg, L. A. Electrolyte absorption from the colon. Gut 11:1049, 1970.

21. Phillips, S. F., and Schmalz, P. F. Bicarbonate secretion by the rat colon: Effect of intraluminal chloride and acetazolamide. Proc. Soc. Exp. Biol. Med. 135:116, 1970.

22. Powell, D. W., Malawer, S. J., and Plotkin, G. R. Secretion of electrolytes and water by the guinea pig small intestine in vivo. Amer. J. Physiol. 215:1226, 1968.

23. Gregory, R. A. Secretory Mechanisms of the Gastro-intestinal Tract. London, Edward Arnold Ltd., 1962.

24. Hendrix, T. R., and Bayless, T. M. Digestion: Intestinal secretion. Ann. Rev. Physiol. 32:139, 1970.

25. Wright, R. D., Jennings, M. A., Florey, H. W., and Lium, R. The influence of nerves and drugs on secretion by the small intestine and an investigation of the enzymes in intestinal juice. Quart. J. Exp. Physiol. 30:73, 1940.

26. Fordtran, J. S., and Locklear, T. W. Ionic constituents and osmolality of gastric and small-intestinal fluids after eating. Amer. J. Dig. Dis. 11:503, 1966.

27. Levitan, R., Fordtran, J. S., Burrows, B. A., and Ingelfinger, F. J. Water and salt absorption in the human colon. J. Clin. Invest. 41:1754, 1962.

28. Giller, J., and Phillips, S. F. Colonic absorption of electrolytes and water in man: A comparison of 24-hour ileal content and feces. Gastroenterology 58:951, 1970.

29. Wrong, O., Metcalfe-Gibson, A., Morrison, R. B. I., Ng, S. T., and Howard, A. V. In vivo dialysis of faeces as a method of stool analysis. I. Technique and results in normal subjects. Clin. Sci. 28:357, 1965.

30. Wrong, O., and Metcalfe-Gibson, A. The electrolyte content of faeces. Proc. Roy. Soc. Med. 58:1007, 1965.

31. Evanson, J. M., and Stanbury, S. W. Congenital chloridorrhoea or so-called congenital alkalosis with diarrhoea. Gut 6:29, 1965.

32. Torres-Pinedo, R., Lavastida, R. M., Rivera, C. L., Rodriguez, H., and Ortiz, A. Studies on infant diarrhea. I. A comparison of the effects of milk feeding and intravenous therapy upon the composition and volume of the stool and urine. J. Clin. Invest. 45:469, 1966.

33. Teree, T. M., Mirabal-Font, E., Ortiz, A., and Wallace, W. M. Stool losses and acidosis in diarrheal disease in infancy. Pediatrics 36:704, 1965.

34. Schwartz, W. B., and Relman, A. S. Metabolic and renal studies in chronic potassium depletion resulting from overuse of laxatives. J. Clin. Invest. 32:258, 1953.

35. Humphreys, M. H., and Earley, L. E. The mechanism of decreased intestinal sodium and water absorption after acute volume expansion in the rat. J. Clin. Invest. 50:2355 1971.

36. Higgins, J. T., Jr., and Blair, N. P. Intestinal transport of water and electrolytes during extracellular volume expansion in dogs. J. Clin. Invest. 50:2569, 1971.

37. Powell, D. W., Plotkin, G. R., Maenza, R. M., Solberg, L. I., Catlin, D. H., and Formal, S. B. Experimental diarrhea. I. Intestinal water and electrolyte transport in rat salmonella enterocolitis. Gastroenterology. 60:1053, 1971.

38. Carpenter, C. J. C. Cholera enterotoxin: Recent investigations yield insights into transport processes. Amer. J. Med. 50:1, 1971.

39. Moore, W. L., Jr., Bieberdorf, F. A., Morawski, S. G., Finkelstein, R. A., and Fordtran, J. S. Ion transport during cholera-induced ileal secretion in the dog. J. Clin. Invest. 50:312, 1971.

40. Field, M. Intestinal secretion: Effect of cyclic AMP and its role in cholera. New Eng. J. Med. 284:1137, 1971.

41. Chen, L. C., Rohde, J. E., and Sharp, G. W. G. Properties of adenyl cyclase from human jejunal mucosa during naturally acquired cholera and convalescence. J. Clin. Invest. 51:731, 1972.

42. Cohen, R., Kalser, M. H., Arteaga, I., Yawn, E., Frazier, D., Leite, C. A., Ahearn, D. G., and Roth, F. Microbial intestinal flora in acute diarrheal disease. J.A.M.A. 201:835, 1967.

43. Gorbach, S. L. Acute diarrhea—a "toxin" disease? New Eng. J. Med. 283:44, 1970.

44. Williams, E. D., Karim, S. M. M., and Sandler, M. Prostaglandin secretion by medullary carcinoma of the thyroid. Lancet 1:22, 1968.

45. Fordtran, J. S., Rector, F. C., Locklear, T. W., and Ewton, M. F. Water and solute movement

in the small intestine of patients with sprue. J. Clin. Invest. 46:287, 1967.

46. Banwell, J. G., Gorbach, S. L., Mitra, R., Cassells, J. S., Mazumder, D. N. G., Thomas, J., and Yardley, J. H. Tropical sprue and malnutrition in West Bengal. II. Fluid and electrolyte transport in the small intestine. Amer. J. Clin. Nutr. 23:1559, 1970.

47. Mekhjian, H. S., Phillips, S. F., and Hofmann, A. F. Colonic secretion of water and electrolytes induced by bile acids: Perfusion studies in man. J. Clin. Invest. 50:1569, 1971.

48. Soergel, K. H., Whalen, G. E., Harris, J. A., and Green, J. E. Effect of antidiuretic hormone on human small intestinal water and solute transport. J. Clin. Invest. 47:1071, 1968.

49. Barbezat, G. O., and Grossman, M. I. Effect of glucagon on water and electrolyte movement in jejunum and ileum of dog. Gastroenterology 60:762, 1971.

50. Tidball, C. S. Active chloride transport during intestinal secretion. Amer. J. Physiol. 200:309, 1961.

51. Turnberg, L. A. Abnormalities in intestinal electrolyte transport in congenital chloridorrhoea. Gut 12:544, 1971.

52. Bieberdorf, F. A., Gorden, P., and Fordtran, J. S. Pathogenesis of congenital alkalosis and diarrhea. Implications for the physiology of normal ileal absorption and secretion. J. Clin. Invest. 51:1958, 1972.

53. Leading article. Diarrhea and acid-base disturbances. Lancet 1:1305, 1966.

54. Ammon, H. V., and Phillips, S. F. Fatty acids inhibit intestinal water absorption in man: Fatty acid diarrhea? Gastroenterology 62:717, 1972.

55. Bright-Asare, P., and Binder, H. J. Hydroxy fatty acids (OHFA) stimulate colonic secretion of water and electrolytes. Gastroenterology 62:727, 1972.

56. Feldman, S., and Gibaldi, M. Bile salt-induced permeability changes in the isolated rat intestine. Proc. Soc. Exp. Biol. Med. 132:1031, 1969.

57. Misiewicz, J. J., Waller, S. L., Kiley, N., and Horton, E. W. Effect of oral prostaglandin E₁ on intestinal transit in man. Lancet 1:648, 1969.

58. Almy, T. P. Chronic and recurrent diarrhea. Disease-a-Month, October 1955.

59. Nelson, J. D., and Haltalin, K. C. Accuracy of diagnosis of bacterial diarrheal disease by clinical features. J. Pediat. 78:519, 1971.

60. Chaudhary, N. A., and Truelove, S. C. The irritable colon syndrome: A study of the clinical features, predisposing causes and prognosis in 130 cases. Quart. J. Med. 31:307, 1962.

61. Anthonisen, P., and Riis, P. A new diagnostic approach to mucosal inflammation in proctocolitis. Lancet 2:81, 1961.

62. Rowe, B., Taylor, J., and Bettelheim, K. A. An investigation of travellers' diarrhoea. Lancet 1:1, 1970.

63. Kean, B. H. The diarrhea of travelers to Mexico. Summary of five-year study. Ann. Intern. Med. 59:605, 1963.

64. Angel, J. H., and Lacey, B. W. Comparison of side-effects of tetracycline and tetracycline plus nystatin. Brit. Med. J. 4:411, 1968.

65. Leading article. Tetracycline diarrhoea. Brit. Med. J. 4:402, 1968.

66. Pittman, F. E., and Pittman, J. C. Lincomycin colitis. Clin. Res. 20:626, 1972.

67. Hamilton, J. R. Diarrhea in infants. Modern Med. 131, 1970.

68. Lloyd, A. V. C., and Shwachman, H. Diarrhea in children. New Eng. J. Med. 267:1081, 1962.

69. Ellison, E. H., and Wilson, S. D. The Zollinger-Ellison syndrome: Reappraisal and evaluation of 260 registered cases. Ann. Surg. 160:512, 1964.

70. Williams, E. D. A case of diarrhoea and goitre (demonstrated at the Royal Postgraduate Medical School). Brit. Med. J. 3:295, 1967.

71. Cameron, D. G., Warner, H. A., and Szabo, H. A. Chronic diarrhea in an adult with hypokalemic nephropathy and osteomalacia due to a functioning ganglioneuroblastoma. Amer. J. Med. Sci. 253:417, 1967.

72. Peterson, H. D., and Collins, O. D. Chronic diarrhea and failure to thrive secondary to ganglioneuroma. Arch. Surg. 95:934, 1967.

73. Hamilton, J. R., Radde, I. C., and Johnson, G. Diarrhea associated with adrenal ganglioneuroma. Amer. J. Med. 44:453, 1968.

74. Hunt, T. C. Carotid body tumour associated with diarrhea and abdominal pain. Proc. Roy. Soc. Med. 54:227, 1961.

75. Hoskins, L. C., Norris, H. T., Gottlieb, L. S., and Zamcheck, W. Functional and morphologic alterations of the gastrointestinal tract in progressive systemic scleroderma. Amer. J. Med. 33:459, 1962.

76. Heinz, E. R., Steinberg, E. R., and Sackner, M. A. Roentgenographic and pathologic aspects of intestinal scleroderma. Ann. Intern. Med. 59:822, 1963.

77. Salen, G., Goldstein, F., and Wirts, C. W. Malabsorption in intestinal scleroderma. Relation to bacterial flora and treatment with antibiotics. Ann. Intern. Med. 64:834, 1966.

78. Welbourn, R. B. Endocrine causes of diarrhea. Proc. Roy. Soc. Med. 56:1080, 1963.

79. McBrien, D., Jones, R. V., and Creamer, B. Steatorrhea in Addison's disease. Lancet 1:25, 1963.

80. Jackson, W. P. U., Hoffenberg, R., Linder, G. C., and Irwin, L. Syndrome of steatorrhea, pseudohypoparathyroidism, and amenorrhea. J. Clin. Endocrinol. 16:1043, 1956.

81. Snodgrass, R. W., and Mellinkoff, S. M. Idiopathic hypoparathyroidism and small-bowel X-ray features of sprue, without steatorrhea. Amer. J. Dig. Dis. 7:273, 1962.

82. Russell, R. I. Hypoparathyroidism and malabsorption. Brit. Med. J. 3:781, 1967.

83. Seijffers, M. J., Levy, M., and Hermann, G. Intractable watery diarrhea, hypokalemia, and malabsorption in a patient with Mediterranean type of abdominal lymphoma. Gastroenterology 55:118, 1968.

84. Eidelman, S., Parkins, R. A., and Rubin, C. E. Abdominal lymphoma presenting as malabsorption. Medicine 45:111, 1966.

85. Austad, W. I., Cornes, J. S., Gough, K. R., McCarthy, C. F., and Read, A. E. Steatorrhea and malignant lymphoma: The relationship

of malignant tumors of lymphoid tissue and celiac disease. Amer. J. Dig. Dis. *12*:475, 1967.

86. French, J. M., Hall, G., Parish, D. J., and Smith, W. T. Peripheral and autonomic nerve involvement in primary amyloidosis associated with uncontrollable diarrhoea and steatorrhoea. Amer. J. Med. *39*:277, 1965.

87. Kyle, R. A., Spencer, R. J., and Dahlin, D. C. Value of rectal biopsy in diagnosis of primary systemic amyloidosis. Amer. J. Med. Sci. *251*:501, 1966.

88. Wilson, S. A. K. Neurology, Vol. 1., Baltimore, Williams & Wilkins Co., 1941.

89. Cohen, R. A., and Pope, M. A. Paradoxical diarrhea with opiates. J.A.M.A. *205*:802, 1968.

90. Bamforth, J., Murray, P. J. S., and Roberts, A. H. Spurious steatorrhea. Brit. Med. J. *2*:682, 1967.

91. Bank, S., and Marks, I. N. Malabsorption in systemic mast cell disease. Gastroenterology *45*:535, 1963.

92. Jarnum, S., and Zachariae, H. Mastocytosis (urticaria pigmentosa) of skin, stomach and gut with malabsorption. Gut 8:64, 1967.

93. Veeger, W., Ten Thije, O. J., Hellemans, N., Mandema, E., and Nieweg, H. O. Sprue with a characteristic lesion of the small intestine associated with folic acid deficiency. Acta Med. Scand. *177*:493, 1965.

94. Klipstein, F. A., Samloff, I. M., Smarth, G., and Schenk, E. A. Treatment of overt and subclinical malabsorption in Haiti. Gut *10*:315, 1969.

95. Goldstein, F., Dammin, G. J., Mandle, R. J., and Wirts, C. W. Clinical syndrome resembling tropical sprue in lifelong rsidents of temperate zone. Amer. J. Dig. Dis. *17*:407, 1972.

96. Rosensweig, N. S., Herman, R. H., Stifel, F. B., Herman, Y. F., Dreskin, A., and Chipman, D. Effect of folic acid on jejunal glycolytic enzyme activity in tropical sprue. Gastroenterology 56:1261, 1969.

97. Woodward, J. C., Webster, P. D., and Carr, A. A. Primary hypomagnesemia with secondary hypocalcemia, diarrhea and insensitivity to parathyroid hormone. Amer. J. Dig. Dis. *17*:612, 1972.

Chapter 23

Constipation

Thomas P. Almy

Constipation may be defined objectively as the passage of excessively *dry* stools, of stools of *insufficient size* (less than 50 g per day), or of *infrequent* stools (less often than every other day). To many patients, however, the important features of this complaint are the associated subjective sensations of incomplete emptying of the rectum, bloating, passage of flatus, lower abdominal discomfort, anorexia, malaise, headache, weakness, and giddiness. The relationship of these symptoms to the disordered evacuation of the distal colon is inferred from the common clinical observation that they are promptly relieved by purgation or by an enema, and from their experimental production by distention of the rectum and sigmoid colon.

As constipation is readily recognized by the layman and self-treatment is widely sanctioned, the physician may assume at once in all but a few patients that the disorder has been complicated by the use or abuse of laxatives. In some cases of cathartic addiction the stools have, indeed, been kept frequent and loose in the effort to relieve the subjective complaints referred to above.

PATHOGENESIS

The factors determining the volume, composition, and time of appearance of the normal stool have been discussed in detail on pages 229 to 248. In brief review,

oriented toward the conditions which may lead to constipation, these may be conveniently divided into those affecting the *filling* and the *emptying* of the rectum.

The *filling* of the rectum is the end result of a series of events, affecting the colon as a whole, which are under neural (autonomic) and humoral control. Under normal conditions the efficiency of absorption of water and sodium by the colon is high, although this process is inhibited by deoxycholic and other deconjugated, secondary bile acids. Although the oral use of ox bile has long been advocated as a cathartic measure, there is no evidence that excessive absorption of water, resulting from deficiency of bile acids, is a significant cause of constipation. The drying of the stools is, however, a function of *stasis* in the colon caused by weak, infrequent, or ineffective propulsive motility. In most instances, this results from exaggeration and persistence of segmental nonpropulsive motility, particularly in the distal colon. In other words, there is interference with the initiation or propagation of propulsive contractions, owing to inadequate filling of the right colon or impairment of smooth muscle contractility. More rarely, mechanical obstruction of the lumen is present. The various causes are outlined below:

1. Lesion within the lumen or the intestinal wall.
   a. Benign or malignant tumor, intrinsic or extrinsic.

b. Inflammatory disease of the bowel — usually a granuloma, such as Crohn's disease, scleroderma, tuberculosis, or lymphogranuloma venereum; but some cases of idiopathic ulcerative colitis are included.

c. Diverticulitis with cicatrizing obstruction — but a primary motor disorder is the more usual mechanism of stasis in this condition.

d. Chronic amebiasis.

2. Systemic disorder or disease affecting function of the intestine.

a. Pregnancy(!) — in the later stages of which irritability of smooth muscle is generally diminished, apparently as the result of the action of progesterone.

b. Hypothyroidism.

c. Hyperparathyroidism, and other hypercalcemic states.

d. Lead poisoning.

3. Untoward effects of medication — opiates, anticholinergic agents, ganglionic blockers, antidepressants, some nonabsorbable antacids (calcium and aluminum compounds).

4. Disorders of central and peripheral integrative mechanisms.

a. Psychotic depression.

b. Irritable colon (spastic constipation).

c. Congenital aganglionic megacolon (Hirschsprung's disease).

d. Impaired gastroileal reflex — for example, in gastric disease caused by infiltrating carcinoma, or gastroparesis of diabetics.

The *emptying* of the rectum, on the other hand, is the result of the defecation reflex, the action of which largely involves the somatic musculature. The passage of feces from the sigmoid to the normally empty rectum stimulates pressure receptors in the muscular walls of the rectum and initiates this reflex, giving rise to dull pain in the anal region and the sacrum. The rectum accommodates more slowly than the sigmoid to distention from within,[1] thus sustaining the period of high pressure and of the accompanying sensations. By way of a center in the sacral portion of the spinal cord the internal anal sphincter is relaxed, the diaphragm descends, the muscles of the abdominal wall contract, the lumbosacral spine is flexed, and by these means as well as a Valsalva maneuver the intra-abdominal pressure is greatly increased, leading to expulsion of the rectal contents. The muscles of the pelvic floor at first bulge outward, but finally their elevation completes the act, in effect pulling the anus upward over the fecal mass. The primitive squatting position assumed by both man and animals while defecating offers a mechanical advantage in increasing intra-abdominal pressure and aligning rectum and lower sigmoid more nearly in the vertical axis of the body.

Thus the segmental apparatus for defecation is largely somatic, and its activity can be interfered with at several points. Damage to the afferent or efferent fibers or to the sacral cord is fortunately rare, but the threshold of pressure for the perception of rectal distention and the initiation of the reflex rises significantly with age.[2] This is probably significant in the genesis of constipation in the aged. The relaxation of the internal anal sphincter may be prevented by defective innervation (as in congenital megacolon)[3,4] or by local disease such as an anal ulcer or thrombosed hemorrhoid. The effector muscles of the abdominal wall and back may be weakened by multiple pregnancies, obesity, or neuromuscular disease. Departure from the squatting posture, the result of high toilet seats or bedpans, may impair the mechanical efficiency of defecation. The movement of the pelvic floor may be reduced as the result of damage during parturition. Lastly, a tumor or benign stricture of the anal canal or the lower rectum may physically obstruct the passage.

The defecation reflex is, however, subject to suprasegmental influences, or conditioning. Through the processes of toilet training, now understood in terms of the neurophysiology of reward or goal-seeking behavior, the child learns to respond to the stimulus of intrarectal pressure by the additional mechanism of strong contraction of the external anal sphincter,[5] accompanied by the inhibition of abdominal muscle contraction and of the Valsalva maneuver, until such time as defecation is socially acceptable. Under optimal conditions, the child is equally rewarded for achieving continence by inhibiting the reflex at certain times and for achieving regularity of bowel evacuation by reinforcing the reflex at others. In the mature adult the inhibition of the reflex is so rigidly and regularly expected that its release is possible only under the influence of strong and often complex conditioning. Thus a ritual which specifies the time of day, the nature of the preceding meal, a particular toilet, and often a cigarette or other added factor is apparently necessary in many individuals to achieve regularity of the bowel movements. Under ideal conditions, this ritual is practiced at a time when the segmental reflex is most active, i.e., when propulsive movements in the colon, usually generated by a gastroileal reflex, have moved feces into the rectum and abruptly increased its intraluminal pressure. In most individuals, this occurs within one hour after breakfast.

The disruption of these highly conditioned mechanisms is seen, with resulting constipation, in many psychotic or demented individuals, including those with eminently treatable conditions such as subdural hematoma, myxedema, or pernicious anemia. At times it is the presenting complaint in such cases.

Much more often—indeed, it is certainly the most common cause of constipation—the disruption is due to changes in the pattern of living. Going away to college, working on the night shift, going on a trip, and becoming a commuter after years of walking to work are examples of such altered patterns. Hospitalization for an operation or intercurrent illness may account for the onset of persistent constipation. Some patients cannot defecate readily within sight or sound of others, as in a locker room or a military barracks.

The vast majority of such persons, on their own initiative or on the prescription of a physician, will soon resort to laxatives. Although affording temporary relief, these agents may postpone the return of normal habits by too complete emptying of the bowel or by stimulating the defecation reflex at unfamiliar times. In many patients, anxiety aroused by the original change in life pattern is compounded by the fear of ill effects from retention of feces, and later by the short-lived symptomatic relief from laxatives. In this way

the phenomena of "spastic constipation" often become intermingled with "habitual" or "rectal" constipation (see pp. 1278 to 1288).

Impaction, the result of prolonged retention and excessive dehydration of feces, may occur at times in the rectum and rarely in the sigmoid colon. This may be accompanied at first by persistent sacral ache and more obstinate constipation, and often later by lower abdominal cramps and *diarrhea*, as liquid feces are propelled around the inspissated mass. Rarely, and apparently through ischemia of the mucosa produced by pressure of this mass, a *stercoral ulcer* results and may lead to severe bleeding. Such complications are exceedingly rare except in bedridden, debilitated patients.

As indicated previously, the debility and bodily discomfort popularly attributed to constipation and exploited in the advertising of proprietary remedies are largely the result of reflex phenomena resulting from intestinal distention. The ancient doctrine of autointoxication need not be invoked; and stasis in the colon appears to lead to none of the biochemical mischief resulting from stasis and bacterial overgrowth in the small bowel. On the contrary, the absorptive capacity of the colon and the extraordinary adaptability of the colonic flora in disposing of food residues, including cellulose, enables an otherwise healthy man to remain vigorous for weeks at a time without a bowel movement.

DIFFERENTIAL DIAGNOSIS

With the mechanisms mentioned above in mind, a *modus operandi* for diagnostic study begins with a painstaking history to disclose signs of relevant systemic diseases or the use of constipating medications. The presence of cramping colonic pain suggests an obstructive process owing to muscle spasm or a tumor. The characteristic size and consistency of individual fecal masses is important. In disorders of defecation the size of the stool may not be much reduced, whereas in spastic constipation (irritable colon) the stool is passed in small pellets, often invested in mucus. (These features should, of course, be confirmed by direct inspection of the stool by the physician.) The natural history of the disorder should be carefully defined—the duration, changes in intensity, and temporal relationship to stressful situations (see pp. 1278 to 1283) and changes in habits of living offer valuable diagnostic clues.

Aside from signs indicative of systemic diseases and from noting the degree, if any, of abdominal distention, the major dividends from physical diagnosis relate to the rectal examination. The significance of thrombosed hemorrhoids, anal ulcer, other perianal disease, or of weakness or laceration of the perineal muscles, either as primary or secondary factors, has already been emphasized. The most important finding on digital examination is a carcinoma; up to 50 per cent of all colonic cancers can be felt with the index finger. But the most regularly useful finding is the presence or absence of stool in the rectum. The absence of stool in a patient currently constipated places the point of obstruction at the rectosigmoid or above, and makes a disorder of defecation unlikely as a primary mechanism.

Although the technique of rectal examination is fully discussed in texts of physical diagnosis and of proctology, only a few points will be emphasized here. The unsanitary finger cot is a thing of the past, as disposable plastic or neoprene gloves encourage more thorough palpation. The proper position of the patient is *anything but* the head down or knee-chest positions, because these allow lesions in the pelvis to fall away by gravity from the examining finger, and because bimanual palpation is impossible. The patient must be coached to bear down as in a Valsalva maneuver: Before insertion of the finger, this brings the mucosa of the anal canal into view, and sometimes prolapses internal hemorrhoids; during insertion of the finger, this maneuver causes reflex relaxation of the external sphincter, permits deeper and less painful penetration of the anus, and forces pelvic lesions toward the examining finger.

Unless the rectum is packed with feces, immediate anoscopy and proctoscopy (without preparation) are indicated, mainly for the purpose of collecting stool or exudate from the rectal wall for culture, microscopic examination for amebas and other parasites, and tests for occult blood. These tests are then repeated on submitted stool specimens, usually once or twice, before cleansing the colon for further examination. Sigmoidoscopy is then performed in the knee-chest position, most conveniently about one hour following use of a prepackaged, hypertonic enema preparation (e.g., Travad, Fleet's, Clyserol), followed by barium enema *on another day*—otherwise, gas admitted to the lumen during sigmoidoscopy may distort the barium outline of the colon. The barium enema X-rays should include spot films of early filling of the sigmoid and of the ileocecal region. In many instances an upper gastrointestinal series with small bowel films is required. In many instances, multiple factors productive of constipation are disclosed; thus the discovery of a single adequate cause should not terminate the orderly study of the patient for additional mechanisms. As emphasized elsewhere in this volume, the irritable colon can coexist with any disease of the bowel, and the regularity of laxative abuse by constipated persons complicates virtually every other mechanism.

TREATMENT

The following suggestions for treatment of constipation as a symptom are directed primarily to the relief of habitual or rectal constipation (dyschezia, laxative abuse). Treatment of the many other underlying diseases and disorders is discussed elsewhere in this and in other textbooks. Because nearly all patients require retraining in toilet habits, it is appropriate to begin this regimen before the diagnostic study is completed.

The secondary consequences of prolonged constipation, if any, need first be corrected. *Fecal impactions* may be eliminated with a single large (1 liter or more) enema of mild soap suds. The majority, however, will require preliminary fragmentation by digital pressure against the posterior surface of the rectum, with manual removal and/or a retention enema of dioctyl sodium sulfosuccinate (e.g., Colace or Doxinate, 5 ml of 1 per cent solution diluted to 100 ml in water), or of warm cottonseed oil (150 ml), prior to the cleansing enema. *Thrombosed hemorrhoids* and *anal ulcers* should be treated by mineral oil (liquid petrolatum, U.S.P.) 30 to 60 ml, or dioctyl sodium sulfosuccinate, 100 to 200 mg orally each night; hot sitz baths for 15 to 30 minutes before each attempted bowel movement; and lidocaine (Xylocaine) or ethylaminobenzoate (e.g., Medicone) suppositories after each movement.

Both the segmental and the suprasegmental elements in the defecation reflex should thus be reinforced. On the effector side, the aforementioned measures to relieve local irritation of the anal sphincter should be adopted, and the support of weakened abdominal muscles by corsets or otherwise and the surgical repair of hernias or cystoceles which dissipate intra-abdominal pressure should be undertaken. The mechanical advantage of the squatting position in defecation should be regained, for example, by placing a footstool before the commode.

The stimulus to defecation is strengthened by increasing the indigestible residue of the diet by larger feedings of fruits and vegetables, or by the regular use of a hydrophilic colloid preparation such as psyllium seed or agar (e.g., Metamucil, or Konsyl, 1 to 2 rounded teaspoons stirred into 200 ml water and quickly swallowed, at bedtime and on arising). The gastroileal reflex is augmented by eating a large breakfast, including fruit juice, stewed fruit, cereal with milk and sugar, toast with preserves, and coffee. This is expected to produce rapid emptying of the stomach, an increase in the filling of the cecum with ileal contents, and more forceful movement of upper colonic contents into the sigmoid and rectum. The volume of fluid ingested at other times of the day has little effect on the regularity of defecation.

For positive reinforcement or conditioning of the defecation reflex, the patient is required to visit the toilet *each day*, with or without the urge to defecate, at a specified time, judged to be that of maximal spontaneous propulsive colonic motility—for most persons, this is 15 to 60 minutes after breakfast. The patient should remain on the toilet at least ten minutes, if need be, without interruption (the telephone, for example, may have to be disconnected). Distraction should be provided (and the conditioning reinforced)

by some ritual such as a crossword puzzle, the newspaper, a seed catalog, or a magazine—the choice matters little, so long as the ritual is held constant. Laxatives are forbidden.

Patients who have been severely constipated or laxative-dependent must be warned that their subjective discomfort is likely to increase temporarily in the early stages of this regimen, and that regular spontaneous bowel movements may not be expected in less than four to six weeks. They should be strongly reassured that their discomfort does not reflect any potential harm to themselves, and that long periods without bowel movements are compatible with health. Instructed to call the physician by telephone after two, three, or more days for advice in case of severe discomfort, they are then advised to take an enema of at least 1 liter of lukewarm tapwater, preferably one hour or more after breakfast, and after the day's regular toilet visit. The patient should assume the left lateral or knee-chest position, place the enema bag not more than 2 feet above the anus, and control the inflow by pressure of his fingers on the tubing. He should be instructed to halt the inflow periodically for any rectal or abdominal discomfort, but to continue when the pain disappears until the entire contents of the bag are instilled. Only in this way can most or all of the distal colon be evacuated without irritation.

This procedure can usually be depended upon for prompt relief of the associated symptoms, and can be repeated at increasing intervals until spontaneous bowel movements appear and the symptoms subside. The hydrophilic colloids and rectal medications should then be withdrawn one by one, and the patient should be urged to maintain his retrained toilet habit and breakfast menu indefinitely, with special care at times of unavoidable breaks in routine (travel, intercurrent illness, etc.).

The aforementioned regimen, designed for the ambulatory patient, can also be applied in principle to the invalid or the temporarily bedfast patient. Because inactivity suppresses both appetite and gastrointestinal motility in general, mild laxatives should be temporarily used (e.g., milk of magnesia, 30 ml, and/or fluid extract of cascara 5 ml h.s., two nights out of three). Special attention should be given to avoidance of concurrent constipating medication (e.g., one should substitute meperidine for opiates as analgesic agent) and to rapid elimination of barium residues from intestinal X-ray examinations. The bedpan should be replaced by the bedside commode as soon as possible: studies of the metabolic work of defecation under these two conditions confirm that the commode is far less exhausting, and even the patient with a myocardial infarction can usually make the change by the seventh to the tenth day. In earlier stages of acute illness bowel regularity can be first ignored, then treated with enemas alone, often conveniently by use of the packaged hypertonic solutions (Fleet's, Clyserol, Travad, etc.). The use of the bedpan or commode in nonprivate hospital rooms often presents psychological problems for sensitive patients, and importuni-ties to move the bowels daily, coming from routine-minded medical and nursing staff, may be self-defeating.

REFERENCES

1. Lipkin, M., Almy, T., and Bell, B. Pressure-volume characteristics of the human colon. J. Clin. Invest. *41*:1831, 1962. Lipkin, M., et al. Unpublished data.
2. Roth, H. P., Fein, S. B., and Sturman, J. F. The mechanisms responsible for the urge to defecate. Gastroenterology *32*:717, 1957.
3. Tobon, F., Reid, N. W. R. W., Talbert, J. L., and Schuster, M. M. Nonsurgical test for the diagnosis of Hirschsprung's disease. New Eng. J. Med. *278*:188, 1968.
4. Ustach, T. J., Tobon, F., and Schuster, M. M. Simplified method for diagnosis of Hirschsprung's disease. Arch. Dis. Child. *44*:694, 1969.
5. Schuster, M. M., Hookman, P., Hendrix, T. R., and Mendeloff, A. I. Simultaneous manometric recording of internal and external anal sphincteric reflexes. Bull. Johns Hopkins Hosp. *116*:79, 1965.

Chapter 24

Abdominal Pain

Lawrence W. Way

Pain is a subjective sensation resulting from central transmission of peripherally received noxious stimuli. It is usually a harbinger of tissue damage unless the stimulus is removed. The type of pain that is experienced is partly due to factors other than intensity of the initial stimulus.

The word pain is derived from the Latin *poena*, or punishment. Punishment is usually painful, and pain, from whatever cause, may be interpreted psychologically as a form of punishment. However, pain may act as the stimulus that brings the ailing patient to his physician, and a careful analysis of the pain may help the physician to determine its cause and to outline appropriate treatment. Clinically, when pain has outlived its useful purpose, it should be allayed by drugs, specific treatment, or, occasionally, palliative neurosurgical techniques.

The general factors involved in the production of abdominal pain will be presented so that origins of symptoms and signs of clinical syndromes can be understood. The general principles of the management of patients with abdominal pain will also be discussed.

ANATOMY AND PHYSIOLOGY[1-3]

There are no specific pain receptors. Whether the stimulus affects skin, muscle, or viscera, it is detected by free nerve endings which in some cases may also subserve sensations other than pain.

The transmission of pain in the peripheral nervous system is performed by two types of fibers, small myelinated A-delta fibers, and small unmyelinated C fibers. It seems doubtful that these fibers are reserved solely for carrying pain sensations. The quality of the sensation carried by A-delta and C fibers differs. The A-delta fibers, 3 to 4 μ in diameter, are distributed principally to skin and muscle. They mediate the sharp, sudden, well localized pain that follows an acute injury (epicritic pain). The C fibers are found in muscle, periosteum, parietal peritoneum, and viscera. The sensory afferents which convey intraperitoneal abdominal pain are of this type. The sensation transmitted by C fibers tends to be dull, sickening, poorly localized, and of more gradual onset and longer duration (protopathic pain).

The vagi do not transmit pain from the gut despite the fact that 90 per cent of their nerve fibers are sensory, and the ability to feel pain from the abdominal viscera is unaltered after vagotomy.

Pain from the esophagus is transmitted to the spinal cord by afferents in small, unnamed sympathetic nerves. Visceral afferents from the capsule of the liver, the hepatic ligaments, the central portion of the diaphragm, the splenic capsule, and the pericardium are derived from dermatomes C3 to C5 and reach the central nervous system via the phrenic nerve. The fibers from the periphery of the diaphragm, gallbladder, stomach, pancreas, and small intestine travel through the celiac plexus and the greater splanchnic nerves, and enter the spinal cord from T6 to T9 (Fig. 24–1).

Stimuli from the colon, appendix, and pelvic viscera enter the tenth and eleventh thoracic segments by way of the mesenteric plexus and lesser splanchnic nerves.

The sigmoid, rectum, renal pelvis and capsule, ureter, and testes are innervated by fibers which reach the T11 to L1 segments through the lowest splanchnic nerve. The bladder and rectosigmoid send afferents through the hypogastric plexus to enter the cord from S2 to S4.

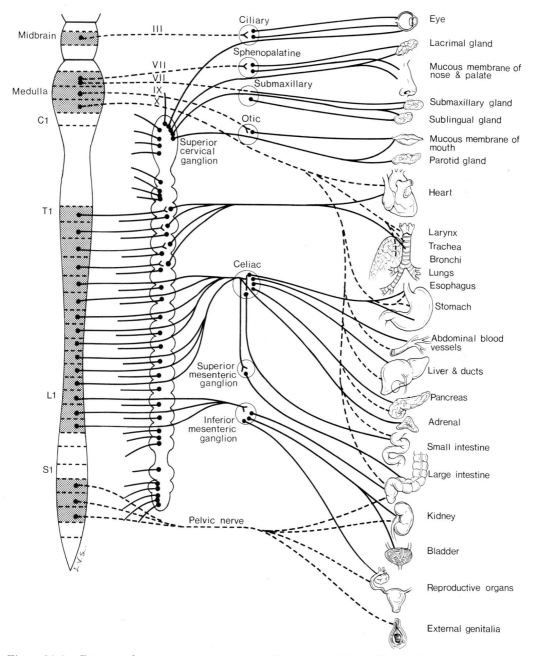

Figure 24–1.   Diagram of autonomic nervous system. The visceral afferent fibers mediating pain travel with the sympathetic nerves, except for those from the pelvic organs which follow the parasympathetics of the pelvic nerve. Sympathetics are represented here by solid lines; parasympathetics by dashed lines.

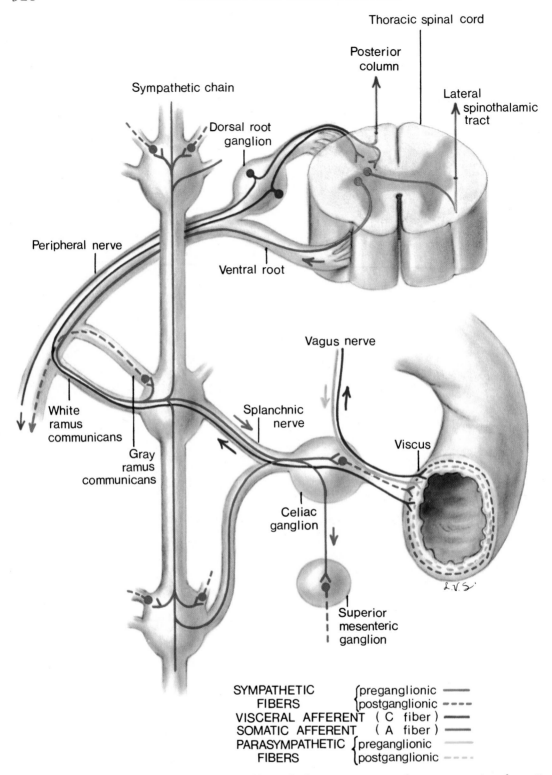

Figure 24–2. Relationship of visceral afferent fibers which transmit pain impulses to autonomic and somatic afferent fibers. The visceral afferents for pain pass through the splanchnic ganglia, reach the sympathetic chain in the splanchnic nerves, and enter the dorsal root via the white ramus communicans. They synapse with cell bodies in the dorsal horn which send impulses toward the brain in the lateral spinothalamic tract. These relays may be inhibited by sensory impulses which enter in large afferents from the periphery (A fibers). The connections undoubtedly are much more complex than shown here. (Adapted from Netter.)

The cell bodies of the visceral afferent neurons are located in the dorsal root ganglia (Fig. 24–2). The fibers in the splanchnic nerves join the sympathetic chains and reach the dorsal roots via the white rami communicantes. After entering the spinal cord their fibers send branches directly into the posterior horn and others through the tract of Lissauer cranially and caudally for several segments before terminating on dorsal horn cells. The visceral afferent neurons synapse with cells in the marginal zone of the posterior horn, in the substantia gelatinosa, and at the base of the horn. Relays and additional connections within the dorsal horn form a network which modulates the transmission of pain. For example, large myelinated afferent neurons (A-alpha fibers) which mediate touch, vibration, and proprioception send branches into the substantia gelatinosa before ascending in the dorsal column. Impulses arriving in these fibers inhibit the transmission of pain entering in C fibers. Other fibers which reach the dorsal horn from higher centers may facilitate or inhibit pain. Additional networks located at other levels of the central nervous system modify the sensation before it is perceived in the cerebral cortex. Cells in the base of the dorsal horn send axons which cross through the anterior commissure, ascend in the lateral spinothalamic tracts, and end in the reticular formation of the medulla and midbrain. Other fibers in the lateral spinothalamic tracts do not terminate until they reach thalamic nuclei. In either case the cerebral terminations receive fibers from both sides of the body. The cells in the thalamic nuclei relay the pain impulses to the postcentral gyrus of the cerebral cortex, at which point conscious sensation is perceived.

STIMULI FOR ABDOMINAL PAIN[1, 3-5]

Abdominal viscera are ordinarily insensitive to many stimuli which, when applied to the skin, evoke severe pain. Cutting, tearing, or crushing of viscera does not result in a perceptible sensation. The principal forces to which visceral pain fibers are sensitive are stretching or tension in the wall of the gut. This can be the result of traction on the peritoneum (neoplasm), distention of a hollow viscus (biliary colic), or forceful muscular contractions (intestinal obstruction). The nerve endings of pain fibers in the hollow viscera (gut, gallbladder, and urinary bladder) are located in the muscular walls. Those in the solid viscera, such as the liver and kidney, supply the capsule and respond to stretching of the capsule from parenchymal swelling. The mesentery, parietal peritoneum, and peritoneal covering of the posterior abdomen are sensitive to pain, but the parietal peritoneum and greater omentum are insensitive. The rate at which tension develops must be fairly rapid for pain to be produced. Gradual distention, such as that in malignant biliary obstruction, may be painless.

Inflammation, whether of bacterial or chemical etiology, may also produce visceral pain. Moreover, inflammation and tissue congestion sensitize the nerve endings and lower the threshold to pain from other stimuli. Action on nerve endings by the tissue hormones, bradykinin, serotonin, histamine, or prostaglandin has been postulated as the mechanism by which inflammation produces pain.

Ischemia causes abdominal pain by increasing the concentration of tissue metabolites in the region of the sensory nerves. Ischemia also lowers the threshold to other noxious stimuli. Since the adventitia of mesenteric blood vessels are also supplied with pain fibers, traction on blood vessels may cause pain.

Intra-abdominal pain can also be caused by involvement of sensory nerves by neoplasms. This is the mechanism for pain produced by some retroperitoneal tumors such as pancreatic carcinoma. Malignant invasion of the walls of viscera is painless unless obstruction or ulceration develops.

TYPES OF ABDOMINAL PAIN[3, 6]

Classically, abdominal pain is separated into three categories: visceral pain, parietal (somatic) pain, and referred pain. Although neurophysiological differences between them are slight, the distinctions possess value for understanding patterns of clinical pain.

Visceral Pain (Fig. 24–3). Visceral pain is felt in the abdomen when noxious stimuli affect an abdominal viscus. The pain is usually dull and poorly localized in the epigastrium, periumbilical region, or lower mid-abdomen. Visceral pain is felt near the midline because, with few exceptions, the abdominal organs receive sensory afferents from both sides of the spinal cord. The site where the pain is felt corresponds roughly to the dermatomes from which the diseased organ receives its innervation. The diffuseness of the localization derives from the overlapping multisegmental innervation of most viscera plus the relative paucity of nerve endings in viscera compared with skin. The quality is generally crampy, burning, or gnawing. Secondary autonomic effects such as sweating, restlessness, nausea, emesis, perspiration, and pallor often accompany visceral pain. The patient may move about in a vain attempt to relieve the discomfort.

Parietal (Somatic) Pain. Pain sensations which arise from noxious stimulation of the parietal peritoneum are generally more intense and more precisely localized to the site of the lesion than visceral pain. An example is the localized pain in acute appendicitis produced by inflammatory involvement of the peritoneum at McBurney's point. Parietal pain is usually aggra-

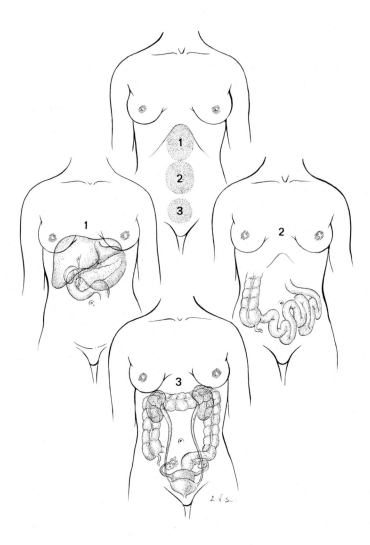

Figure 24–3. Sites where visceral pain is felt. Pain arising from organs depicted in 1, 2, and 3 is felt in the epigastrium, midabdomen, or hypogastrium respectively.

vated by movement or coughing. The nerve impulses travel in C fibers within somatic sensory nerves. The nerve endings activated by stimulation of the parietal peritoneum are distributed in the areolar connective tissue beneath, rather than in, the mesothelium. The fibers reach the spinal cord in the peripheral nerves corresponding to the cutaneous dermatomes from T6 to L1. Lateralization of the discomfort of parietal pain is possible because at any given point the parietal peritoneum obtains innervation from only one side of the nervous system.

Pain elicited by traction on the mesentery or posterior abdominal peritoneum has the characteristics of visceral pain and is carried in splanchnic nerves.[7]

Referred Pain.[3, 6, 8] Referred pain is felt in remote areas supplied by the same neurosegment as the diseased organ because of shared central pathways by afferent neurons from different sites. Referred pain may be felt in skin or deeper tissues but is usually fairly well localized, much as the somatic sensory nerves themselves. As a rule, referred pain appears when the noxious visceral stimulus becomes more intense. For example, pain produced experimentally by distention of a balloon within the intestine is first entirely visceral and is then accompanied by referred pain in the back as distention is increased. In some cases referred pain may exist in the absence of visceral pain, but this is unusual.

Hyperesthesia of skin and hyperalgesia of muscle may develop in the distribution of the referred pain. When hyperesthesia and hyperalgesia are present, infiltration of the spinal nerves to that area will abolish the heightened sensitivity and may also reduce or eliminate the referred pain itself.[5]

PERCEPTION OF PAIN

Melzack and Wall[9] proposed a theory of pain which reconciled many seemingly contradictory observations in the older specificity and pattern theories. The specificity theory had postulated that pain was the result of activation of a special subsection of the nervous system in which pain was conceived as involving specific receptors, peripheral fibers, and central tracts. In such a system one might suppose that any given stimulus would elicit a predictable reproducible response.

Alternatively, the pattern theory postulated that there were no specialized neural structures or centers for pain. The sensation was thought to be a result of activation of general receptors and fibers in a special pattern coded for pain which was deciphered as such by the cerebral cortex. This theory ignored the increasing evidence for at least some specialization in transmission of pain impulses. Both theories overlooked the substantial variations in an individual's pain perception owing to factors other than the intensity and nature of the noxious stimulus.

Melzack and Wall proposed what they called a "gate theory" to account for the observed phenomena. Central to their hypothesis was a complex neural system in the dorsal horn of the spinal cord which could integrate central and other peripheral impulses with the incoming ones for pain. Augmentation or inhibition of the pain impulses was possible before they reached consciousness in the cerebral cortex. Although details of this mechanism have been shown to be incorrect, the authors synthesized a large body of data into a comprehensive system and provided a more sophisticated model than had been previously available. The fundamental concept of substantial modulation before central perception remains valid.

Sternbach[10] emphasized that pain should be considered a single entity, at times divisible into neural, psychological, and secondary autonomic effects for analytical purposes, but ultimately involving all three in every case. Failure to appreciate the critical role of the psychological component in every painful event would be shortsighted and likely to impair clinical interpretations and management of pain. The tendency to maintain a duality of thinking regarding physiological and psychological pain is widespread and is based upon a misconception of pain mechanisms.

Beecher[11, 12] observed that soldiers wounded in battle often denied feeling any pain at all in their wounds. This he interpreted to be the result of anticipation by the soldier of increased safety after evacuation from the front lines plus other psychological effects related to a battlefield situation. Once reaching the hospital the same soldier might complain of discomfort from an inept venipuncture. In either case the patient actually did or did not experience true pain. Another important observation[13] was that placebo injections can alleviate pain from an organic injury in about one-third of patients. Both the pain and relief by the placebo are real. Inexperienced clinicians, frustrated in their attempts to discover the cause of abdominal pain in a difficult patient, are sometimes tempted to assign a psychological origin for the symptom when the patient responds to a placebo injection. This disregards the inevitable interaction of organic stimulus and psychological modification in pain which makes predictions of etiology impossible by this technique.

The principal psychological factors which modify pain perception[14] are the interpretation of the consequences of the stimulus (injury), previous experience (conditioning), psychological stability, personality, and cultural background. Heightened anxiety lowers the pain threshold, and relief of anxiety or depression, by any means, generally raises tolerance to pain.

PAIN FROM SPECIFIC ORGANS[6]

Numerous observations have been made on experimental pain produced by stimulation of abdominal organs or the splanchnic nerves. These experimental observations have been compared with clinical pain patterns, and generalizations have emerged concerning the location and quality of pain from different segments of the gut.

Esophagus. Lesions of the esophagus usually produce substernal discomfort near the disease. Balloon distention at various levels has demonstrated the ability of the subject to indicate accurately the site of the stimulus in this organ. Upper esophageal stimulation produces pain in the neck, and stimulation in the lower third is felt near the xiphoid process. In some subjects a low esophageal stimulus is felt high in the esophagus, but the opposite pattern is uncommon. More severe stimulation produces referred pain in the middle of the back.

Stomach and Duodenum. Experimental stimulation or spontaneous visceral pain from the stomach and duodenum causes pain in the midline of the epigastrium. Disease of the duodenal bulb may cause discomfort somewhat to the right side of the upper abdomen. Farther down the duodenum the pain is experienced gradually lower in the epigastrium. Radiation to the back is fairly common in experimental subjects and clinical patients.

Small Intestine. Pain originating from jejunum to distal ileum is located in the mid-abdomen about the umbilicus. Referred pain may appear in the middle of the back if the stimulus is of sufficient intensity or if the individual's threshold is relatively low.

Ileum. Disease or other stimuli in this area usually cause pain near the umbilicus, but sometimes in the lower abdomen or to the right of the midline.

Colon. Pain from the colon is poorly localized to the lower midabdomen. Stimulation of the rectum usually creates discomfort felt posteriorly over the sacrum.

Gallbladder and Common Bile Duct.[8, 15] Experimental dilatation of either of these structures causes pain in the midepigastrium or right upper quadrant. Both may be associated with referred pain in the back between the scapulae or to one side of the midline. The biliary system is supplied with fibers from T6 to T10, but most originate from the T9 dermatome. Although the innervation is bilateral, most of the fibers reach the cord through the right splanchnic nerves.

Pancreas. Pain from the pancreas is felt in the midline or left side of the epigastrium. The nerves arise from segments T8 to T10. Pancreatic disease is often accompanied by referred pain in the middle of the back. Somatic pain felt in the left shoulder may result from activation of pain fibers in the left diaphragm by an adjacent inflammatory process in the tail of the pancreas.

Pelvic Organs.[16] Pain sensation from the uterus passes in fibers derived from segments S2 to S4 through the hypogastric plexus. The uterus becomes painful in response to obstruction, distention, or severe contraction, much like other hollow viscera.

In contrast to other solid organs, the

ovary is insensitive to most stimuli because it does not have a capsule. Ovarian inflammation or tumors are usually silent unless there is strangulation by torsion or rupture of a cyst.

CLINICAL MANAGEMENT[3, 5, 17]

When abdominal pain is the presenting complaint it must be evaluated by the usual process of obtaining historical, physical, and laboratory data which usually suggest diagnostic hypotheses and therapeutic plans. The acuteness of the illness is a major factor in determining the clinical approach to abdominal pain. If symptoms have been present for weeks or months without recent exacerbation, the work-up may be slow and deliberate, aimed at achieving an exact diagnosis. In patients with acute illness, however, the principal goal is to determine whether they require prompt surgical care as indicated by local or diffuse peritonitis or intestinal obstruction. A tentative diagnosis is usually available for acute pain, but it is secondary in importance.

HISTORY

The common innervation of many abdominal organs, the low concentration of nerve endings in the viscera, the patient's lack of previous experience with sensations arising from these organs, and the often nonspecific localization of the pain all interact to complicate the diagnostic process. The patient must be questioned carefully regarding his pain. The following dimensions of a complaint of abdominal pain must be explored.

Location. The site of the pain and the extent to which it is localized must be determined. Significant radiation of pain may be present such as the sensation of pain in the thigh with disease in the ureter or testicle. Pain in the shoulder may signify diaphragmatic involvement. The pain in biliary, duodenal, or pancreatic disease is often referred to the back. Visceral pain tends to be poorly localized, but pain produced by irritation of the parietal peritoneum is confined to the area involved by disease.

Intensity and Character. The severity of the pain is loosely related to the magnitude of the noxious stimulus. Acute perforated duodenal ulcer or mesenteric occlusion, for example, evokes excruciating pain, and the obvious intensity of the symptom is of diagnostic value. On the other hand, estimates of severity are at times unreliable because of the interaction of the various factors which determine the response. As might be expected, the significance of the amount of pain is more obvious at the extremes of severity than in between.

Certain diseases produce pain with distinct qualities. Well known examples are the burning or gnawing pain of duodenal ulcer or the crampy pain of intestinal obstruction. Melzack and Torgerson[18] suggested that a systematic study of the taxonomy of pain may lead to a better understanding of its production. They point out the wide range of adjectives used to describe different kinds of pain and their significance in support of a pattern concept of pain production.

Chronology. The quantity and quality of pain in relationship to time are often clues as to its cause. Acute abdominal pain which has persisted for more than six hours usually indicates a surgical problem. Chronic pain of duodenal ulcer rarely occurs before breakfast but appears later in the interprandial period. Acute appendicitis evolves steadily over 12 hours without remission. Intestinal obstruction is associated with crampy pain, separated by pain-free intervals. Steady pain is produced by ischemia from strangulation obstruction.

Setting. What are the circumstances in which the pain appears? Heartburn may only be experienced when abdominal pressure is increased. Emotional tension may aggravate peptic ulcer pain or that associated with the irritable colon syndrome.

Aggravating or Alleviating Factors. Numerous important diagnostic clues are discovered in this category such as the response of peptic ulcer pain to antacids. In fact, therapeutic trials of antacids, antispasmodics, or diets are sometimes prescribed with the aim of obtaining diagnostic data as well as relieving the patient.

Associated Signs and Symptoms. Information should be obtained regarding changes in gastric function (anorexia, nausea, emesis), evacuation (diarrhea, constipation), weight, renal function, gynecological function, and the like. Diarrhea may signify pain from gastroenteritis, whereas obstipation suggests intestinal obstruction. Bloody urine may be seen with ureteral colic caused by a ureteral stone. Jaundice can direct attention to the biliary tree in cases of upper abdominal pain.

PHYSICAL EXAMINATION

The clinical history often provides only enough information to suggest that the diagnosis is one of several possibilities. The physical examination must be carried out systematically to uncover unsuspected abnormalities as well as to test specific hypotheses formed from symptom analysis. A thorough physical examination is essential, because it may provide the answer in many a puzzling case. The examination begins with a general inspection and includes the head, neck, extremities, and chest as well as the abdomen.

The patient's appearance may provide a clue to the nature of his disease. Tachycardia, fever, and perspiration suggest sepsis from peritonitis, cholangitis, pyelonephritis, or severe bacterial enteritis. The patient with pure visceral pain may change position frequently, but if localized or general peritonitis is present he avoids movement.

The abdomen should be inspected for distention from intestinal obstruction or ascites. All potential hernial sites must be carefully examined in every case. Incarceration of a segment of bowel in a small femoral hernia can be easily missed if not specifically looked for. Hyperperistalsis may be audible with the stethoscope in intestinal obstruction or enteritis. Generalized peritonitis causes decreased or absent peristalsis. Vascular bruits may be clues to an aortic or splenic artery aneurysm.

Palpation of the abdomen should be performed with a mental picture of its contents. It should be especially gentle at first and started at a distance from the painful area. Otherwise the patient may lose confidence in the examiner and become so guarded that an accurate examination is impossible.

Abdominal rigidity or involuntary guarding may be the result of adjacent peritonitis. The most classic example is the board-like upper abdominal rigidity which occurs early in perforated peptic ulcer. Lesser degrees of guarding or rigidity develop over the area of an acutely inflamed gallbladder or appendix or in acute diverticulitis. If the abdomen is examined when the patient's knees are drawn up, this may provide just enough relaxation to facilitate an examination which was otherwise impossible because of guarding. An abnormal mass may be produced by enlargement of a diseased organ, tumors, or inflammatory processes.

Pure visceral pain is usually unaccompanied by tenderness. When tenderness is present the most important question is the extent of its localization. Generalized peritonitis is suggested by severe diffuse tenderness with rigidity and clinical toxicity. However, mild general tenderness without toxicity is more compatible with acute gastroenteritis, salpingitis, or some other nonsurgical condition. The early uncomplicated stage of acute cholecystitis, appendicitis, or diverticulitis is characterized by tenderness which can usually be well localized to a small area. The key to determining localization is gentle palpation with one finger until the tender area has been thoroughly mapped out. Localized tenderness over McBurney's point is by far the most important finding when making the diagnosis of acute appendicitis. Regardless of the remainder of the history, if tenderness is confined to a spot a few centimeters in diameter, acute appendicitis will nearly always be present.

Rebound pain is produced by pressing slowly and deeply over a tender area and then suddenly releasing the hand. This maneuver merely confirms the presence of peritonitis of the parietal peritoneum. Since the same information can be obtained by light percussion over the tender spot, the quest for rebound tenderness is usually unnecessary.

Hyperesthesia in response to gently touching the skin may appear in the dermatome affected by intraperitoneal parietal pain. If present, this finding is useful, but it is often absent even though significant localized peritonitis exists.

Genital, rectal, and pelvic examinations

are part of the evaluation of every patient with abdominal pain. Acute pelvic inflammation or a twisted ovarian cyst or uterine fibroid may be found, or rectal examination may reveal a tumor, abscess, or occult blood in the feces.

LABORATORY FINDINGS

Routine hematological studies should include a complete blood count and a serum creatinine. Other tests should be ordered according to clinical clues derived from symptoms and signs.

Gastrointestinal X-ray examination with barium is often required to establish the proper diagnosis. Oral or intravenous cholecystography may be indicated to verify biliary disease. Selective mesenteric angiography may reveal mesenteric arterial stenosis in patients suspected of suffering from intestinal angina. Endoscopy via the upper or lower gut orifices is increasingly of diagnostic value. Esophageal manometry is clinically useful in the differential diagnosis of substernal pain, and manometry may eventually earn a place in the evaluation of colonic or other intestinal disorders.

DIAGNOSIS

The history, physical examination and laboratory findings generally result in a correct diagnosis and treatment plan (Table 24–1). In some cases, however, the etiology of recurrent or persistent abdominal pain cannot be further defined. In this situation one must consider the long list of rare causes of pain and perform special tests if the complaint truly appears to be of clinical significance.

Prospective analyses[19, 20] of symptom reliability in the diagnosis of chronic upper abdominal pain have shown that in the average case an accurate diagnosis is not possible without the help of X-rays and sometimes endoscopy. In some patients the story of peptic ulcer is so typical that the X-rays are merely confirmatory. However, the pain patterns of gallstone disease, duodenal and gastric ulcer, gastritis, esophagitis, and cancer overlap greatly.

Chronic recurrent undiagnosed abdominal pain is a significant clinical problem which often has led to repeated laparotomies.[21-23] It is more common in women than men. The usual patient has had recurrent attacks for years without developing weight loss or signs of morbidity other than the pain. Barium X-ray studies of the upper and lower gastrointestinal tract may be normal or may show questionable abnormal findings in the duodenal bulb, leading to gastrectomy. Other patients have had appendectomy for "chronic appendicitis," hiatal hernia repair for undocumented esophagitis, or cholecystectomy for postprandial pain despite a normal cholecystogram.

Many of these patients are psychologically unstable, and follow-up examination usually fails to reveal an organic source of the symptom.[24] However, it has recently been shown that in some cases functional disturbances characterized by spasm of the gut are responsible for pain.[25] For example, increased intraluminal pressures coincident with pain have been found in patients with the irritable colon syndrome.[26] The common syndrome of chronic episodic pain in the right lower quadrant may have a similar explanation, but no simple techniques are suitable for studying cecal peristalsis.

A method has been developed for estimation of painful gallbladder dysfunction.[27] The gallbladder is opacified by tyropanoate, and cholecystokinin is injected during fluoroscopy. If the resulting gallbladder contraction does not empty the organ promptly or causes pain, the test suggests dysfunction (cystic duct syndrome, biliary dyskinesia) and the possibility of symptomatic relief by cholecystectomy. Controlled trials are being conducted to determine the reliability of cholecystokinin cholecystography.

Perhaps other methods will be developed to study the relation of spasm to chronic abdominal pain. In any event the diagnosis of chronic appendicitis to account for intermittent abdominal pain has been seriously challenged. Unless findings are fairly specific, appendectomy is unlikely to eliminate the complaint.

In perplexing cases, a question arises as to the value of diagnostic laparotomy. If there are no objective findings (fever, jaundice, mass, X-ray abnormality), laparotomy is usually negative.[28, 29] On the other hand,

TABLE 24-1. CAUSES OF ABDOMINAL PAIN

I. Intra-abdominal
  A. Generalized peritonitis
    1. Perforated viscus: peptic ulcer, gallbladder, colonic diverticulum
    2. Primary bacterial peritonitis: pneumococcal, streptococcal, enteric bacillus, tuberculous
    3. Nonbacterial peritonitis: ruptured ovarian cyst, ruptured follicle cyst
    4. Familial Mediterranean fever (familial periodic peritonitis)
  B. Localized peritonitis: many types of local peritonitis may become generalized by rupture into the free peritoneal cavity
    1. Appendicitis
    2. Cholecystitis
    3. Peptic ulcer
    4. Meckel's diverticulitis
    5. Regional enteritis
    6. Acute colonic diverticulitis
    7. Colitis: ulcerative, amebic, bacterial
    8. Abdominal abscess: postoperative, hepatic, pancreatic, splenic, diverticular, tubo-ovarian
    9. Gastroenteritis
    10. Pancreatitis
    11. Hepatitis: viral, toxic
    12. Pelvic inflammatory disease, gonococcal perihepatitis (Fitz-Hugh and Curtis syndrome)
    13. Endometritis
    14. Lymphadenitis
  C. Pain from increased tension in viscera
    1. Intestinal obstruction: adhesions, hernia, tumor, volvulus, fecal impaction, intussusception
    2. Intestinal hypermotility: irritable colon, gastroenteritis
    3. Biliary obstruction: gallstone, stricture, tumor, parasites, hemobilia
    4. Ureteral obstruction: calculi

    5. Hepatic capsule distention: acute hepatitis (toxic or viral), common duct obstruction, Budd-Chiari syndrome
    6. Renal capsule distention: pyelonephritis, ureteral obstruction
    7. Uterine obstruction: neoplasm, childbirth
    8. Aortic aneurysm
  D. Ischemia
    1. Intestinal angina or infarction: arterial stenosis, embolism, polyarteritis
    2. Splenic infarction
    3. Torsion: gallbladder, spleen, ovarian cyst, testicle, omentum, appendix epiploica
    4. Hepatic infarction: toxemia
    5. Tumor necrosis: hepatoma, uterine fibroid
  E. Retroperitoneal neoplasms
II. Extra-abdominal
  A. Thoracic
    1. Pneumonitis
    2. Pulmonary embolism
    3. Empyema
    4. Myocardial ischemia
    5. Myocarditis, endocarditis
    6. Esophagitis, esophageal spasm
    7. Esophageal rupture
  B. Neurogenic
    1. Radiculitis: spinal cord or peripheral nerve tumors, degenerative arthritis of spine, herpes zoster
    2. Tabes dorsalis
    3. Abdominal epilepsy
  C. Metabolic
    1. Uremia
    2. Diabetes mellitus
    3. Porphyria
    4. Acute adrenal insufficiency
  D. Toxins
    1. Hypersensitivity reactions: insect bites, reptile venoms
    2. Drugs: lead poisoning, etc.
  E. Miscellaneous
    1. Muscular contusion, hematoma, or tumor

---

in the presence of at least one objective finding, diagnostic laparotomy will frequently solve the puzzle.[30-32]

TREATMENT

The principal objective is to find a specific treatment such as antacids for peptic ulcer or cholecystectomy for gallstones. Even the use of anticholinergic agents in the irritable colon syndrome has a sound pathophysiological rationale.

In patients with acute abdominal pain, one may not be able to define the condition more precisely than "acute surgical peritonitis." Laparotomy is indicated be-

cause of the protean nature of common problems such as acute appendicitis and the much greater morbidity if it is allowed to become complicated by perforation.

Some patients with chronic abdominal pain require chronic administration of analgesics for relief.[33] Unless the pain is caused by an untreatable progressive disease, such as an incurable malignant tumor, narcotics must be avoided because of possible addiction or tolerance.

Neurosurgical measures may be required for some chronically painful conditions. Unfortunately, resection of the splanchnic nerves which carry the visceral afferent fibers provides only short-term benefit. Chronic pain from the abdomen has been difficult to control permanently with any of the ablative procedures (rhizotomy, cordotomy, thalamotomy).[34] Prefrontal lobotomy does not eliminate pain but alters the patient's concern over it. Recently electroanalgesia[35] has been introduced to block transmission of pain physiologically by exciting inhibitory fibers in the dorsal column of the spinal cord. Preliminary results with dorsal column stimulation have been quite promising in patients with visceral pain.

REFERENCES

1. Sweet, W. H. Pain. *In* Handbook of Physiology, Sect. 1, Vol. I, C. F. Code (ed.), Washington, D.C., American Physiological Society, 1959, pp. 459–506.
2. Mullen, S. The transmission and central projection of pain. Med. Clin. N. Amer. 52:15, 1968.
3. Almy, T. P. Basic considerations in the study of abdominal pain. *In* The Differential Diagnosis of Abdominal Pain, S. M. Mellinkoff (ed.). New York, McGraw-Hill Book Co. 1959.
4. Menacker, G. J. The physiology and mechanism of acute abdominal pain. Surg. Clin. N. Amer. 42:241, 1962.
5. Wolff, H. G., and Wolf, S. Pain. 2nd ed. Springfield, Ill., Charles C Thomas, 1958.
6. Jones, C. M. Digestive Tract Pain. New York, The Macmillan Company, 1938.
7. Doran, F. S. A. Observations on referred pain from the posterior abdominal wall and pelvis. Brit. J. Surg. 49:376, 1962.
8. Doran, F. S. A. The sites to which pain is referred from the common bile duct in man and its implication for the theory of referred pain. Brit. J. Surg. 54:599 1967.
9. Melzack, R., and Wall, P. D. Pain mechanisms: A new theory. Science 150:971, 1965.
10. Sternbach, R. A. Pain. A Psychophysiological Analysis. New York, Academic Press, 1968.
11. Beecher, H. K. Relationship of significance of wound to pain experienced. J.A.M.A. 161:1609, 1956.
12. Beecher, H. K. Pain in men wounded in battle. Ann. Surg. 123:96, 1946.
13. Beecher, H. K. The use of chemical agents in the control of pain. *In* Pain, Henry Ford Hospital International Symposium, R. S. Knighton and P. R. Dumke (eds.). Boston, Little, Brown Co., 1964, Chapter 15.
14. Melzack, R. The perception of pain. Scientific American 204:41, 1961.
15. Schrager, V. L., and Ivy, A. C. Symptoms produced by distention of the gallbladder and biliary ducts. Surg. Gynec. Obstet. 47:1, 1928.
16. Jeffcoate, T. N. A. Pelvic pain. Brit. Med. J. 3:431, 1969.
17. Cope, Z. The Early Diagnosis of the Acute Abdomen. 13th Ed., New York, Oxford University Press, 1968.
18. Melzack, R., and Torgerson, W. S. On the language of pain. Anesthesiology 34:50, 1971.
19. Rinaldo, J. A., Jr., Scheinok, P., and Rupe, C. E. Symptom diagnosis. A mathematical analysis of epigastric pain. Ann. Intern. Med. 59:145, 1963.
20. Edwards, F. C., and Coghill, N. F. Clinical manifestations in patients with chronic atrophic gastritis, gastric ulcer, and duodenal ulcer. Quart. J. Med. 37:337, 1968.
21. Ingram, P. W., and Evans, G. Right iliac fossa pain in young women. Brit. Med. J. 2:149, 1965.
22. Stone, R. T., and Barbero, G. J. Recurrent abdominal pain in childhood. Pediatrics 45:732, 1970.
23. Rang, E. H., Fairbairn, A. S., and Acheson, E. D. An enquiry into the incidence and prognosis of undiagnosed abdominal pain treated in hospital. Brit. J. Prev. Soc. Med. 24:47, 1970.
24. Hill, O. W., and Blendis, L. Physical and psychological evaluation of "nonorganic" abdominal pain. Gut 8:221, 1967.
25. Chaudhary, N. A., and Truelove, S. C. The irritable colon syndrome. Quart. J. Med. 31:307, 1962.
26. Holdstock, D. J., Misiewicz, J. J., and Waller, S. L. Observations on the mechanism of abdominal pain. Gut 10:19, 1969.
27. Nathan, M. H., Newman, A., Murray, D. J., and Camponovo, R. Cholecystokinin cholecystography. Amer. J. Roent. 110:240, 1970.
28. Devor, D., and Knauft, R. D. Exploratory laparotomy for abdominal pain of unknown etiology. Arch. Surg. 96:836, 1968.
29. Hubbard, T. B., and Harris, R. A. Diagnostic laparotomy. Amer. J. Surg. 33:258, 1967.
30. Scott, P. J., Hill, R. S., Fook, A. L. S., and Bensley, K. E. Benefits and hazards of laparotomy for medical patients. Lancet 2:941, 1970.
31. Keller, J. W., and Williams, R. D. Laparotomy for unexplained fever. Arch. Surg. 90:494; 1965.
32. Bourke, J. B., Cannon, P., and Ritchie, H. D. Laparotomy for jaundice. Lancet 2:52l, 1967.
33. Wang, R. I. H. Pain and principles for its relief. Mod. Treatment 5:1083, 1968.
34. Rosonoff, H.L. Neurosurgical control of pain. Ann. Rev. Med. 20:189, 1969.
35. Shealy, C. N., Mortimer, J. T., and Hagfors, N. R. Dorsal column electroanalgesia. J. Neurosurg. 32:560, 1970.

Chapter 25

An Approach to the Acute Abdomen and Intestinal Obstruction

R. Scott Jones

The term "acute abdomen" designates a clinical situation in which the patient has an intra-abdominal disease which may be treated best by a surgical operation. It is the reason for a large number of hospital admissions and may affect the very young, the very old, either sex, and all socioeconomic groups. Many diseases, some of which do not require surgery, produce this syndrome (Table 25–1). Acute appendicitis is the most common cause of the acute abdomen requiring surgical treatment. In evaluating the patient with abdominal pain, it is frequently impossible to make a definitive diagnosis. In such cases, the important decision that must be made is: should an operation be performed? This decision must be made after careful evaluation of the patient's history, physical findings, laboratory data, and X-rays.[1]

GENERAL CLINICAL FEATURES

The most prominent symptom of the patient with the acute abdomen is abdominal pain. Pain of sudden onset is generally characteristic of a perforated viscus or occlusion of the blood supply to an organ; oc-

casionally the distress of acute bowel obstruction, particularly in the upper small intestine, is quite sudden. Pain of more gradual onset suggests an inflammatory lesion. Poorly localized or generalized abdominal pain is characteristic of inflammation, particularly bowel disease in which the process is confined to the bowel and its serosa. When the parietal peritoneum becomes involved, pain is usually localized to that portion of the abdomen in which the peritoneum is inflamed.

The radiation of abdominal pain may assist in the diagnosis. For example, irritation of the diaphragm frequently causes pain referred to the shoulders. The pain of gallbladder disease may be referred to the back or to the shoulder, particularly to the scapular area. The pain of a ureteral stone may be referred to the genitalia or to the groin. Steady, continuous pain usually denotes an inflammatory process in an abdominal organ, whereas intermittent or crampy pain is characteristic of obstruction of a hollow viscus such as the gallbladder or the intestine.[2]

Vomiting may be a symptom of the acute abdomen and is quite characteristic of acute cholecystitis as well as acute pan-

338

TABLE 25–1. DIFFERENTIAL DIAGNOSIS OF SEVERE ABDOMINAL PAIN

Alimentary
  Stomach and duodenum
    Peptic ulcer
  Small bowel
    Perforation
    Obstruction
    Inflammatory disease (Crohn's disease, gastroenteritis, regional enteritis)
  Appendix
    Appendicitis
  Colon
    Inflammatory disease (Crohn's disease, diverticulitis, ulcerative colitis)
    Tumor
    Obstruction
  Pancreas
    Pancreatitis
    Pancreatic tumor
  Liver
    Hepatitis
  Gallbladder and bile ducts
    Acute cholecystitis
    Cholangitis
Vascular
  Abdominal aortic aneurysm
  Mesenteric thrombosis or embolism
Gynecologic
  Pelvic inflammatory disease
  Mittelschmerz
  Ovarian cyst (rupture, torsion)
  Ectopic pregnancy
  Complications of uterine instrumentation
Urologic
  Stone
  Infection
  Obstruction
  Tumor
Other
  Spleen (rupture, marked splenomegaly, e.g., lymphoma)
  Sickle cell disease
  Lead poisoning
  Acute porphyria
  Heat exhaustion
  Black widow spider bite
  Herpes zoster

creatitis; however, it may result from any intra-abdominal inflammatory lesion which produces ileus. The presence of blood in the vomitus suggests a mucosal lesion; bile-stained vomitus indicates at least partial patency of the bile ducts and pylorus. Vomiting will temporarily relieve the pain of gastric outlet obstruction, but not the pain of inflammatory lesions.

Anorexia and nausea are important symptoms in the patient with the acute abdomen. The patient who has abdominal pain but maintains a good appetite is unlikely to have serious gastrointestinal disease.

PHYSICAL EXAMINATION

The vital signs may be important in assessing patients with abdominal pain. The temperature is usually normal early in most diseases causing the "surgical abdomen." However, if tissue necrosis occurs in the abdomen, the temperature can rise to the range of approximately 101° F. In the later stages of diseases associated with intestinal gangrene or perforation, the temperature may be subnormal. Patients with fever in the range of 104° F are more likely to have urinary tract or pulmonary infection than an acute surgical abdomen.

The pulse rate is also usually normal early in acute abdominal pain. Some elevation of pulse in such patients may be due, in part, to apprehension or fever. A pulse rate rising progressively during the course of an illness may suggest intra-abdominal gangrene, perforation, or both. Alterations in pulse or temperature are unreliable signs in patients receiving large doses of corticosteroid hormone or in elderly, debilitated patients.

The patient with the acute abdomen generally looks ill. If he is lying quietly on the examining table and resists movement and change in position, it is likely that he has peritonitis. Sudden or jarring movements accentuate the pain of early peritonitis. The patient who is hyperactive, tending to move about frequently, changing his position, probably has an obstructed hollow organ, such as a ureter. The abdomen should be inspected carefully for the presence of scars, indicating a previous surgical procedure which may have an important relationship to the present illness. The umbilicus and the groin should be inspected carefully for the presence of hernias, and visible abdominal masses should be sought. Abdominal palpation is probably the most important step in evaluating the acute abdomen. The patient, as well as the examiner, should be positioned as comfortably as possible. It is frequently helpful for the doctor to examine the abdomen from a sitting position.

The patient complaining of abdominal pain should be examined very gently. Palpation of the abdomen should begin in that portion farther away from the pain, reserving examination of the tender or painful area until last. Direct tenderness is present when palpation elicits pain in an area. Rebound tenderness is present when the sudden release of deep palpation accentuates the pain. Tenderness, particularly rebound tenderness, is an important sign of peritonitis. Guarding is increased resistance of the abdominal musculature in response to palpation; it may be voluntary, in which case the patient consciously contracts the abdominal musculature, usually to avoid the pain associated with palpation. Involuntary guarding, on the other hand, is a result of reflex muscle spasm caused by underlying peritoneal irritation and is a very important physical finding of peritonitis. In its extreme form, involuntary guarding may be present as abdominal rigidity, producing the board-like abdomen classically caused by perforated duodenal ulcers.

In examining the abdomen of a patient complaining of abdominal pain, one should ascertain where the pain is located and whether tenderness is localized to this area. If direct and rebound tenderness associated with guarding is localized to an area of the abdomen, it is probable that the patient has a disease requiring surgery. An abdominal mass in a patient with abdominal pain may suggest a tumor, an abscess, or a ruptured aortic aneurysm. Abdominal percussion will suggest whether or not an excessive amount of intra-abdominal gas is present, and loss of the area of dullness over the anterior aspect of the liver suggests free intraperitoneal air. Abdominal auscultation should be performed for several minutes to characterize the bowel sounds. Quantitatively they may be absent, as in generalized peritonitis, or hyperactive, as in gastroenteritis. The quality of bowel sounds may be normal, or the pitch of the sounds heard upon abdominal auscultation may be increased, suggesting distention of intestinal loops. Bruits should also be sought on abdominal auscultation.

Rectal examination is an integral part of the physical examination of the patient with acute abdominal pain. Particular note should be made of the location of tenderness and of the presence or absence of both feces and a mass. A sample of feces must always be tested for the presence of occult blood. In females, a pelvic examination is essential to ascertain the presence or absence of masses and tenderness of uterus or the adnexae.[3] Careful gynecological history is crucial in many women because their acute lower abdominal pain may be due to acute pelvic inflammatory disease, particularly gonococcal.

LABORATORY EXAMINATION

Although there are many laboratory tests available today, most of these are not particularly helpful in establishing the diagnosis in a patient with an acute abdomen. The white blood cell count is a very useful adjunct to the physical findings; leukocytosis in the patient with abdominal pain substantiates the presence of inflammation. The hematocrit determination may be very useful; a low hematocrit suggests a lesion or disorder which tends also to bleed as well as cause pain, e.g., peptic ulceration, intestinal carcinoma, or ruptured aneurysm. An elevated hematocrit indicates dehydration, particularly if the patient has been vomiting or has signs of intestinal obstruction.

Urinalysis. The presence of numerous white blood cells in a urine specimen suggests an inflammatory lesion of the urinary tract, such as pyelonephritis or cystitis. The presence of red blood cells in the urine may indicate the presence of tumor or injury to the urinary tract. Hematuria is a very frequent finding in patients with urinary stones. This procedure is essential to evaluation of the acute abdomen.

Blood Chemistries. Serum electrolytes, sodium, potassium, chloride, and carbon dioxide levels are helpful in the assessment of patients who may have a history of vomiting and the physical findings of dehydration. In addition to documenting the nature of electrolyte imbalances, it is helpful to obtain these determinations serially to document restoration of normal fluid and electrolyte balance. Blood urea nitrogen and creatinine afford information about the state of hydration as well as renal function. Other blood tests may be of help; for example, serum and urinary amylase levels are usually elevated in patients with acute pancreatitis. Unfortunately the amylase measurement is not a specific test, and it may be elevated in patients with other diseases such as perforated ulcers, strangulated obstruction, and acute cholecystitis.

X-RAY EXAMINATION

Radiological examination of the patient with acute abdominal pain usually provides helpful adjunctive information. The most frequently performed X-ray is the plain survey film of the abdomen. Osseous and soft tissue densities are inspected first. The presence and location of gas should then be noted carefully (Figs. 25–1, 25–2, and 25–3); free air in the peritoneal cavity is frequently associated with perforation of a hollow viscus, the most common being perforated duodenal ulcer. (Of course, recent abdominal surgery will allow free air in the peritoneal cavity, which may persist for a week postoperatively.) Normally, gas may be seen in the stomach and colon, but the amount of gas in the small bowel is scant. Gas outlining the biliary tree may be

present with the following conditions: surgical anastomoses between the alimentary tube and the biliary ductal system, a spontaneous internal biliary fistula, or an infection of the biliary system with gas-producing organisms. The presence of gas has been reported rarely in the portal vein and is an ominous finding. If gas is present in the alimentary tract, the quantity should be noted. Large quantities of gas may be present in the small bowel and colon as the result of either mechanical obstruction or the ileus associated with inflammatory disease or mesenteric ischemia. Air-fluid levels are commonly noted in the stomach and are not abnormal; however, such levels in the small bowel or colon are abnormal and indicate either obstruction or ileus or both. The finding of an air-fluid level at a site other than in the bowel strongly supports the diagnosis of an abscess.

Soft tissue masses, for example, a large ovarian cyst, can frequently be ascertained on plain films in the abdomen. The presence or absence of calcification should be sought. Pancreatic calcification is almost pathognomonic of chronic pancreatitis. Renal calculi are usually radiopaque and

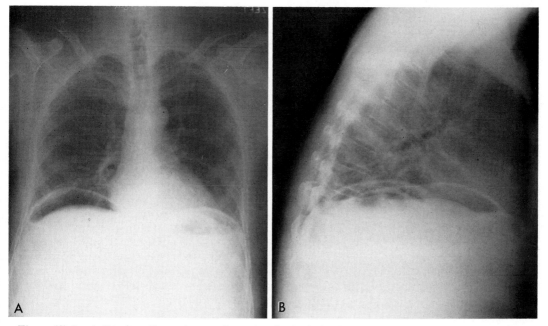

Figure 25–1. A, PA chest X-ray, showing free air under both diaphragms. B, Lateral chest X-ray, confirming the presence of free air under the diaphragm.

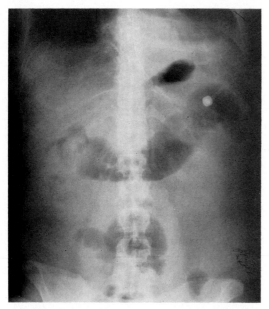

Figure 25-2. This plain abdominal X-ray was taken in a patient who developed postoperative pancreatitis. Note the ileus pattern with gas in the stomach, small bowel, and colon. Also note the sentinel loop of small intestine in the midabdomen.

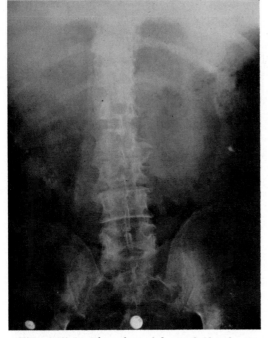

Figure 25-3. This plain abdominal film depicts retroperitoneal gas around the pancreas in a patient with acute pancreatitis, fever, and leukocytosis.

can be seen on plain films. Opaque biliary calculi are infrequent, but nonetheless may occur. Fecaliths may become calcified, as may intra-abdominal lymph nodes. Vascular calcifications, particularly in the abdominal aorta, are noteworthy. The gynecological organs may be a site of calcium deposits, as in leiomyomata of the uterus or ovarian tumors, particularly teratomas.

A routine chest X-ray is a most helpful examination for revealing free intraperitoneal air under the diaphragms (Fig. 25-1). In addition, there are intra-abdominal diseases which may produce abnormalities on the chest X-ray. For example, acute pancreatitis is frequently associated with left pleural effusion. Subphrenic abscesses may cause elevation and immobility of the diaphragms with inflammation in the overlying lung, probably with pleural effusion. Patients with upper abdominal inflammatory disease may splint respiration and develop atelectasis of the lower lobes. Conversely, there are intrathoracic diseases which may be diagnosed on chest X-ray which may contribute to the findings of the acute abdomen. For example, lower lobe pneumonia may produce upper abdominal pain; acute congestive heart failure, associated with distention of the liver capsule, may also produce right upper quadrant abdominal pain.

The majority of patients with acute abdominal pain can be evaluated satisfactorily by history, physical examination, laboratory studies, and plain X-ray examination of the chest and abdomen. If the patient is then believed to have an acute surgical abdomen, further studies probably should not be undertaken and appropriate therapy should be employed. Under special circumstances, more specialized radiographic tests may be indicated. An intravenous cholangiogram may assist in the evaluation of a patient believed to have acute cholecystitis, because cholangiographic visualization of the gallbladder makes a diagnosis of acute cholecystitis very unlikely. Upper gastrointestinal series may help in evaluating patients with severe upper abdominal pain and may reveal the presence of a gastric or duodenal ulcer. A gastrointestinal series may help in the diagnosis of acute pancreatitis, for this disease will often enlarge the duodenal

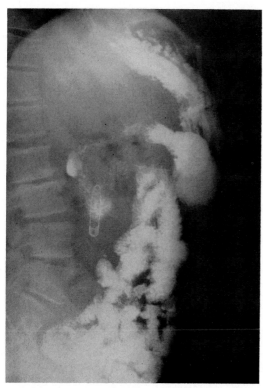

Figure 25–4. This upper gastrointestinal series was obtained on a patient during the course of acute pancreatitis. Note the anterior displacement of the stomach, the narrowing of the second portion of the duodenum, and the presence of retroperitoneal gas around the pancreas.

loop, displace the stomach, or, in some instances, deform the duodenum (Fig. 25–4). A barium enema may be helpful in certain instances to exclude the possibility of a colonic tumor or to reveal the presence of diverticula of the colon. Barium enema should be avoided in patients believed to be having an exacerbation of ulcerative colitis.

THE NONSURGICAL ACUTE ABDOMEN – DIFFERENTIAL DIAGNOSIS

Many diseases causing abdominal pain do not require surgical therapy. Clues to these diagnoses are found in the history and physical examination. Thus diseases which may affect the pleura, such as pneumonia or pulmonary infarction, often have a component of pleuritic inflammation affecting the chest as well as the upper abdomen. Areas of lung consolidation, rubs, and bloody or purulent sputum are crucial in diagnosis, as is an adequate chest film and lung scan. Acute pericarditis may cause epigastric pain, as may myocardial infarction. The patient with pericarditis will be much more comfortable sitting than lying; a rub or signs of tamponade may be present. Acute congestive heart failure may occasionally cause abdominal pain, presumably owing to stretching of Glisson's capsule by a congested liver. Disorders of the gastrointestinal system such as acute gastroenteritis or hepatitis, occasionally produce syndromes of abdominal pain difficult to distinguish from diseases requiring surgical therapy. Indeed, the pain of hepatitis may closely simulate that of acute cholecystitis; however, an enlarged tender liver will be felt, the white blood count is normal or low, and the serum glutamic oxaloacetic transaminase will be markedly elevated. Sickle cell disease causes crises of abdominal pain mimicking acute abdomen. Thus all black patients must have adequate rapid hematological evaluation. Acute intermittent porphyria, a rare disease, produces episodes simulating the acute abdomen. The diagnosis of this condition may be suggested by a history of repeated attacks for which previous surgery had futilely been performed, and by finding of dark urine or urine which is positive for porphobilinogen (Watson-Schwartz). Intoxications, such as lead poisoning, may produce abdominal pain. Other diseases which cause pain but which are rarely confused with an acute surgical abdomen are the abdominal "crises" of diabetic neuropathy and of tabes dorsalis. Black widow spider bites have been reported to be a cause of severe abdominal pain, and a good history helps clarify this picture. Infrequently, the patient with herpes zoster may have pain in a dermatome distribution over the abdomen, which may simulate the acute abdomen until vesicles appear. Withdrawal from opiates may also cause abdominal pain with nausea and vomiting. Acute pancreatitis often presents as an acute abdomen with signs and symptoms suggesting that the patient requires surgery. Epigastric tenderness may give way to diffuse tenderness, both direct and on rebound. Diagnosis is made on the basis of a high index of suspicion (e.g., alcoholism, evidence of biliary tract disease, use of certain drugs) and a marked elevation of plasma (within 48 hours of onset) and urinary amylase (up to five or so days after onset).

THE DECISION TO OPERATE

The main problem in the management of the patient with abdominal pain is to decide whether or not the patient's signs and symptoms are indicative of an acute abdominal disease requiring surgery. This decision is more difficult when dealing with patients at the extremes of age. The infant simply lacks the ability to communicate. Thus diseases producing the acute abdomen in infants are frequently not diagnosed until paralytic ileus or intestinal obstruction supervenes. Likewise, in the geriatric population, abdominal symptoms may go unrecognized and unheeded until the disease has advanced to a late stage. The problem here is partly communication and partly that geriatric patients are less responsive to pain than are younger age groups.

Anti-inflammatory drugs, such as corticosteroids, in any age group may inhibit the usual inflammatory responses or defense mechanisms to inflammatory processes and in addition may mask the symptoms and physical findings in patients with an acute abdomen. The situation is further complicated by a euphoria sometimes noted in patients taking these drugs.

An initial examination which indicates the possibility that a patient may have an acute abdomen requires immediate consultation with a surgeon. Promptness of operation may be vital for the life and health of patients with disease causing acute abdomen. If the surgeon has sufficient doubt that an acute abdominal disease exists, the patient should be examined several hours later and laboratory tests should be repeated. Evidence of a progressing intra-abdominal process may then be conclusive. Thus direct and rebound abdominal tenderness may become unequivocal or may be unquestionably localized in a given area. Likewise, the white blood cell count may continue to rise.

The decision as to whether to admit such a patient to the hospital initially will depend upon several factors, including the facilities available for holding patients for periods of observation without hospitalization, the degree of suspicion that an acute abdomen requiring surgery exists, and the estimate of reliability of the patient to follow instructions carefully. Some patients with persisting abdominal pain but minimal abdominal findings may be sent home to return again for re-examination in several hours.

In many instances, the diagnostic criteria for acute abdomen are obvious and it is clear that the patient will need an operation. In some cases, such as perforated duodenal ulcer of long duration, loss of plasma volume may be sufficient to justify a brief period of resuscitation prior to induction of anesthesia. Such preoperative preparation is necessary to allow safe operation on critically ill patients. In patients who are suspected of having other disease processes, such as pre-existing heart disease, pneumonia, pulmonary diseases, or renal disease, an evaluation of these organ systems is necessary before the patient is subjected to surgery. This information can ordinarily be gathered in a very brief period of time so that operation is not unduly delayed. Patients with abdominal pain caused by rupture of an abdominal aortic aneurysm should be operated upon as promptly as possible.

The successful management of an acute abdomen is one of the more gratifying experiences in surgery, because prompt diagnosis and appropriate surgical therapy will often result in complete reversal and cure of what otherwise would have been a fatal disease.

INTESTINAL OBSTRUCTION

Intestinal obstruction exists when there is any pathological impediment to the aboral progression of intestinal luminal content. It may be produced by occlusion of the bowel lumen, mechanical obstruction, or by paralysis of the intestinal muscle, paralytic ileus.

MECHANICAL OBSTRUCTION

There are three categories of abnormalities responsible for mechanical bowel obstruction.

Obturation Obstruction. Obturation obstruction may be caused by polypoid bowel tumors, intussusception, large gallstones, meconium, or bezoars.

Intrinsic Bowel Lesions. Intrinsic bowel lesions associated with bowel obstruction are often congenital, such as atresia or stenosis, and are usually seen in infants and children. The usual acquired intrinsic bowel lesions producing intestinal obstruction are benign or malignant strictures.

Extrinsic Bowel Lesions. Extrinsic bowel lesions are probably the most frequent cause of intestinal obstruction. Occlusion of the intestine by adhesions from previous surgery is the leading extrinsic cause of small intestinal obstruction. External hernias are the second most frequent cause of mechanical small bowel obstruction. Extrinsic masses, such as neoplasms and abscesses, may also obstruct the bowel. A volvulus is usually associated with either an abnormality in the development of the mesenteric relationships of the bowel or the presence of adhesions.

PARALYTIC ILEUS

Paralytic ileus occurs to some extent in most patients undergoing abdominal surgery. This abnormality is caused by neural, humoral, and metabolic factors. Distention of organs such as the intestines or the ureter causes reflex inhibition of intestinal motility. A humoral factor in paralytic ileus has been suggested. Clinically, peritonitis is associated with paralytic ileus. Electrolyte imbalances, particularly hypokalemia, contribute to this abnormality. Ischemia of the intestine also rapidly inhibits motility.

PATHOGENESIS OF BOWEL OBSTRUCTION

Simple mechanical obstruction of the small intestine results in accumulation of fluid and gas proximal to the obstruction, causing intestinal distention by ingested fluid, digestive secretions, and intestinal gas. Swallowed air is the most important source of gas in patients with acute intestinal obstruction. One of the most important pathophysiological events during simple mechanical bowel obstruction is diminution of plasma volume contributed to by vomiting, decreased absorption from the lumen of the small bowel, and increased secretion of water and electrolytes in the obstructed segment.

Proximal small bowel obstruction causes relatively greater vomiting and less intestinal distention than distal small bowel obstruction. Proximal obstruction is associated with losses of sodium chloride, hydrogen ion, and potassium, producing dehydration, hypochloremia, hypokalemia, and metabolic alkalosis. Distal small bowel obstruction may entail loss of fluid into the bowel; however, the abnormalities of serum electrolytes are less dramatic. Oliguria, azotemia, and hemoconcentration may accompany the dehydration of bowel obstruction. If dehydration persists, circulatory changes, such as tachycardia, low central venous pressure, and reduced cardiac output, may lead to hypotension and hypovolemic shock.

Another important pathophysiological event occurring in intestinal obstruction is the rapid proliferation of intestinal bacteria. During small intestinal stasis, whatever the cause, bacteria proliferate rapidly, producing the feculent small intestinal content noticed during small bowel obstruction. Normally the colon, which functions as a reservoir, contains large numbers of bacteria even in the absence of obstruction. Bacteria in the small intestine probably play no particular role in the ill effects of simple mechanical upper small bowel obstruction, as bacteria and bacterial toxins probably do not cross normal intestinal mucosa.[4]

STRANGULATION OBSTRUCTION

Strangulation exists when the circulation to the obstructed intestine is impaired. Such impairment of circulation may be caused by sustained increase in intraluminal pressure or by pressure necrosis from unyielding adhesive bands or hernial rings. In addition, the mesenteric blood vessels can be occluded by deformity or twisting of the mesentery as in volvulus or intussusception. A closed-loop obstruction exists when the bowel lumen is occluded at two points along its length.

Patients with strangulation obstruction suffer vastly more ill effects than those with simple obstruction alone. The strangulated segment bleeds and "weeps" plasma as well; if unattended, strangulation leads to gangrene and peritonitis with its dire sequelae. Indeed, the compromised segment of bowel may perforate with devastating effects. In addition to the loss of blood and plasma, the effect of toxic material released from a strangulated loop is extremely important. Bacteria and necrotic tissue are necessary for the development of this toxic fluid. Apparently, the lethal factors are formed in the lumen of the strangulated intestine and pass through the intestinal wall which is injured by distention, vascular compromise, and bacterial invasion.[5]

CLINICAL PICTURE

Intestinal obstruction is characterized by abdominal pain, vomiting, obstipation, abdominal distention, and failure to pass flatus. The pain of intestinal obstruction is typically crampy, with paroxysms occurring every four to five minutes in proximal obstruction and less frequently in distal obstruction. After a long period of mechanical obstruction, the crampy pain may subside because intestinal motility may be inhibited by bowel distention. If crampy abdominal pain is replaced by continuous pain, strangulation obstruction should be suspected. Proximal intestinal obstruction may produce profuse vomiting unassociated with abdominal distention. Distal bowel obstruction produces less frequent vomiting; however, the character of the vomiting may be feculent because of the large bacterial population of the intestinal content. Obstipation and failure to pass gas from the rectum are characteristics of complete bowel obstruction, but are noted only when the bowel distal to the obstruction has been evacuated. Increasing abdominal girth owing to the accumulation of fluid and gas in the intestine often accompanies mechanical obstruction or paralytic ileus.

PHYSICAL EXAMINATION

Particular attention should be given to certain points in the physical examination. Tachycardia and hypotension may indicate dehydration, peritonitis, or both, whereas fever suggests the possibility of strangulation. Mucous membranes and skin should be examined to evaluate the status of hydration. The patient's abdomen is usually distended; peristaltic waves, characteristic of small bowel obstruction, are sometimes visible through the abdominal wall of thin patients with long-standing obstruction. Surgical scars should be noted because of the etiological implications of previous surgery; for example, the presence of adhesions or cancer. Incarcerated hernias may be obscure, particularly in obese patients, but should always be sought. Abdominal masses may suggest intra-abdominal neoplasm, intussusception, or an abscess. Abdominal tenderness is usually noticed in patients with intestinal obstruction; however, localized tenderness, rebound tenderness, and guarding suggest peritonitis, indicating the likelihood of strangulation. Abdominal auscultation in patients with mechanical bowel obstruction will reveal periods of increasing bowel sounds separated by relatively quiet periods. The quality of bowel sounds in intestinal obstruction is usually high pitched or musical in character. Rectal examination should be done to detect rectal masses, the presence or absence of feces should be noted, and the fecal examination for occult blood should be done. Blood in the feces suggests an alimentary mucosal lesion, such as may occur in neoplasm, intussusception, or infarction. Sigmoidoscopy is indicated if colonic obstruction is suspected. Any patient having crampy abdominal pain, vomiting, obstipation, abdominal distention, abdominal tenderness, and peristaltic rushes should be diagnosed as having intestinal obstruction until that diagnosis can be excluded with confidence.

RADIOLOGICAL EXAMINATION

X-rays are important to confirm the clinical diagnosis of intestinal obstruction and to locate more accurately the site of the obstruction. The outstanding characteristic of an abdominal X-ray examination of patients with intestinal obstruction is an excessively large quantity of bowel gas.

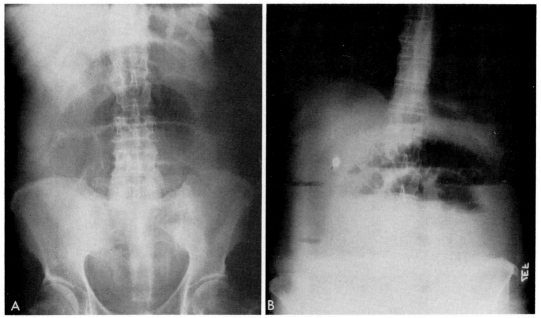

Figure 25-5. *A,* This plain X-ray was taken with the patient in the supine position. Note the excessive amount of gas in the small intestine. The small intestine is identified in this film by its central location in the abdomen and the presence of valvulae conniventes. There is little or no colon gas seen on this film. *B,* An upright film, showing air-fluid levels in the small intestine. The films in *A* and *B* were obtained on a 61-year-old man with a history of crampy abdominal pain, vomiting, obstipation, failure to pass gas, and abdominal distention. After a period of fluid replacement, surgical exploration revealed complete mechanical obstruction of the ileum caused by Crohn's disease with infarction of a segment of bowel proximal to the point of obstruction. This patient had an uncomplicated recovery following resection of the involved bowel.

Plain films will usually demonstrate whether the small intestine, colon, or both are distended (Fig. 25-5, 25-6, 25-7, *A,* and 25-9). Gas in the small bowel outlines the valvulae conniventes, which usually occupy the entire transverse diameter of the bowel image. Colonic haustral markings, on the other hand, occupy only a portion of the transverse diameter of the bowel. Typically, the small intestinal pattern occupies a more central location in the abdomen, whereas the colonic shadow is usually on the periphery or in the pelvis. Patients with mechanical small intestinal obstruction usually have minimal colonic gas. Patients with colonic obstruction and an incompetent ileocecal valve usually have radiographic evidence of small intestinal and colonic obstruction. Upright or lateral decubitus films on patients with mechanical obstruction usually show multiple gas-fluid levels. Occasionally, plain X-ray films fail to discriminate colonic from small intestinal obstruction, and additional

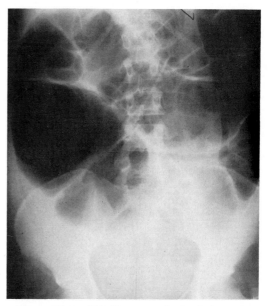

Figure 25-6. This X-ray was obtained on a patient with a mechanical obstruction of the sigmoid colon with a competent ileocecal valve. Note the marked distention of the colon and the paucity of small bowel gas.

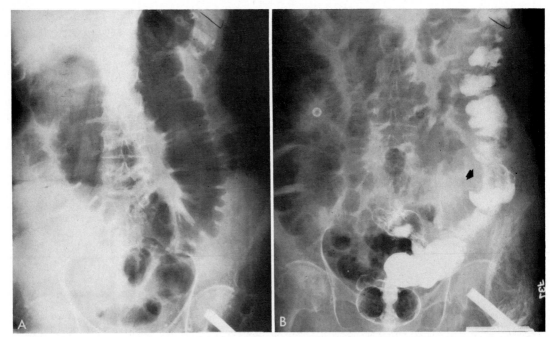

Figure 25–7. *A*, A plain abdominal film on a 71-year-old woman with a several-day history of increasing abdominal distention and failure to pass gas or feces from the rectum. The presence of a large quantity of gas in the transverse and descending colon and a small amount of small intestinal gas suggests the diagnosis of obstruction of the descending colon. *B*, Barium enema on the same patient, revealing an obstructing carcinoma of the descending colon. Note the presence of small bowel gas on this film, compatible with incompetent ileocecal valve. Note the haustral markings on the colon in both *A* and *B*. This patient was treated by right transverse colostomy. After she recovered from the effects of the episode of obstruction, she was reoperated upon and underwent a left colectomy and colocolostomy. After recovery from that procedure, her colostomy was closed.

studies may be necessary. Probably the safest and quickest way to distinguish colonic from small intestinal obstruction preoperatively is by a carefully performed barium enema (Figs. 25–7, *B*, 25–8, and 25–10).

It is often difficult to distinguish paralytic ileus from mechanical obstruction radiographically. One radiographic feature of ileus is that the gaseous distention occurs somewhat uniformly in stomach, small bowel, and colon. Gas-fluid levels may also be seen in paralytic ileus. Examination with the oral administration of a contrast material may assist in distinguishing between paralytic ileus and mechanical obstruction, but should be avoided if colonic obstruction cannot be excluded.

LABORATORY STUDIES

Patients suspected of having intestinal obstruction should have laboratory mea-

surements of serum sodium, chloride, potassium, bicarbonate, and creatinine, in addition to hematocrit and white blood cell count. These values should be obtained serially to assess the adequacy of therapy.

TREATMENT

OBSTRUCTION

In most circumstances, the appropriate treatment for intestinal obstruction is surgical relief of the obstruction. However, optimal timing is crucial and requires careful judgment. The decision must be individualized, based upon three factors: the severity of fluid and electrolyte imbalances; whether or not vital organ function can be improved preoperatively, e.g., rapid digitalization for those in early or unequivocal heart failure or suffering rapid atrial fibrillation; and consideration

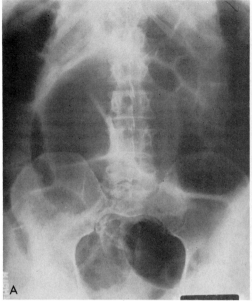

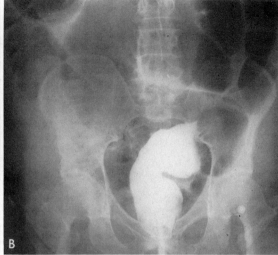

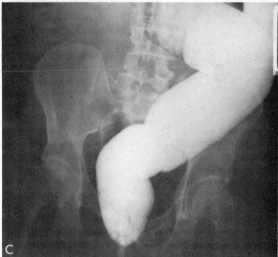

Figure 25-8. *A,* A plain abdominal X-ray obtained on a patient who developed marked abdominal distention, abdominal pain, and tenderness, while convalescing from a neurosurgical operation. *B,* Barium enema performed on this patient, illustrating the typical "bird's beak" picture of sigmoid volvulus. This patient was treated by passing a fiberoptic colonoscope through the narrowed area and decompressing the colon. *C,* A barium enema performed on the day following reduction of the sigmoid volvulus.

of the risk of strangulation. Intestinal gangrene greatly magnifies the mortality rate in patients with bowel obstruction. Since there is no reliable way to detect strangulation preoperatively, operation should be performed as soon as feasible when it is suspected. Patients with symptoms of short duration with minimal metabolic disturbance and no clinically significant pulmonary, cardiac, or renal disease can be operated upon shortly after the diagnosis is made. An elderly patient with fluid and electrolyte imbalance after several days of illness may benefit from 18 to 24 hours of preoperative preparation. Patients with bowel obstruction are usually depleted of water, sodium, chloride, and potassium, so that intravenous therapy should usually

begin with intravenous isotonic sodium chloride solution. For patients in congestive failure or with minor cardiac disease, 0.45 per cent NaCl may be safer than the 0.9 per cent solution. With adequate urine flow (60 to 100 ml per hour), potassium chloride should be added to the infusion and sufficient fluids administered to elevate the central venous pressure to normal. The administration of blood or plasma should be considered if the patient is in shock and if strangulation obstruction is suspected. If marked hemoconcentration and severe electrolyte imbalance were present initially, laboratory studies should be repeated, and if the values are returning to normal, the patient should be operated upon. Broad-spectrum antibiotics

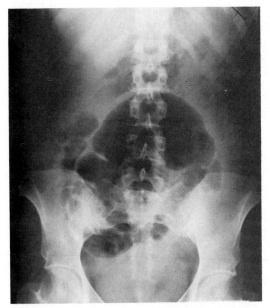

Figure 25-9. Plain X-ray obtained on a patient who developed severe abdominal pain and distention. This film shows a large amount of gas which appears to be in the cecum situated in the mid-abdomen; there is a paucity of gas in the transverse, descending, and sigmoid colon, and in the rectum. This patient had a cecal volvulus.

should be given during this period of resuscitation, particularly if strangulation is suspected (e.g., "high dose" penicillin, 20×10^6 units, and gentamicin, 15 mg per kilogram intravenously, daily, or ampicillin, 4.0 g intravenously, and kanamycin, 4 mg per kilogram intramuscularly, daily).

In addition to fluid therapy, another important adjunct in the supportive care of patients with intestinal obstruction is nasogastric or intestinal suction. Nasogastric suction with a Levin tube will empty the stomach, reducing the hazard of pulmonary aspiration of vomitus as well as minimizing further intestinal distention from swallowed air during the preoperative period. A nasogastric tube is ineffective in decompressing the distended intestine. A long intestinal tube, such as the Miller-Abbott tube, may be passed; usually it is necessary to position the tip in the antrum fluoroscopically in order to facilitate intubation of the small intestine. When the small bowel is successfully intubated, the

tube should be allowed to pass distally on suction to deflate the bowel. The principal hazard of the use of the long intestinal tube in small bowel obstruction is that it may delay operative treatment in patients with unsuspected strangulation obstruction. Operation for intestinal obstruction should generally not be delayed if the bowel is not successfully intubated or decompressed preoperatively.[6]

Operation may be delayed reasonably safely under the following circumstances: (1) Patients with pyloric obstruction may delay being operated upon until fluid and electrolyte imbalance is corrected. (2) Patients with intestinal obstruction in the immediate postoperative period of an abdominal operation may initially be treated

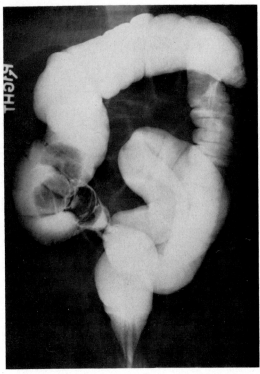

Figure 25-10. Barium enema on a young child with severe abdominal pain and the passage of dark bloody material from the rectum. The radiolucent filling defect in the cecum and ascending colon with a pattern suggestive of mucosa and failure to reflux barium into the small bowel are the typical findings of an ileocecal intussusception. Because this intussusception could not be reduced hydrostatically with the barium enema, the patient was operated upon and underwent resection of the terminal ileum.

conservatively with a Miller-Abbott tube, care being taken not to overlook strangulation. (3) Patients with obstruction caused by disseminated intra-abdominal cancer may be treated with a Miller-Abbott tube. (4) Infants with ileocecal intussusception (Fig. 25–10) may be managed by hydrostatic reduction of the intussusception, which may avoid operation entirely; adults with intussusception should be operated upon, because frequently there is an underlying cause for the intussusception, such as Meckel's diverticulum or small bowel tumor. (5) Patients with sigmoid volvulus may instead have decompression performed with a sigmoidoscope; however, elective operation should be considered later to avoid a recurrence of the volvulus (Fig. 25–8, A and B).

The operative approach to the relief of intestinal obstruction is determined by the nature of the obstruction. Simple intestinal obstruction can frequently be treated by local correction of the obstruction at its site. An example of such treatment is the reduction of an incarcerated inguinal hernia or the division of peritoneal adhesions or of a constricting band. Obstruction may also be corrected by the creation of an intestinal bypass. An example of this type of therapy is ileotransverse colon anastomosis for an obstructing lesion in the ileum. As another alternative, an enterocutaneous fistula such as a colostomy may be placed proximal to an obstruction – this procedure is a standard form of therapy. Finally, the lesion may be excised and intestinal continuity restored by anastomosis. This approach is used frequently. An example is excision of the right colon with an ileotransverse colon anastomosis for obstructing carcinoma of the cecum. Generally, operations for intestinal obstruction should be performed under general anesthesia administered with an endotracheal tube, because one of the risks in operating on such patients is vomiting with tracheal aspiration of the vomitus.

The operative approach to colon obstruction may be somewhat different from that of small bowel obstruction. The classic method of treating obstruction of the left colon entails three operative steps: relief of gaseous distention by colostomy proximal to the obstruction; removal of the diseased segment of colon and anastomosis, leaving the colostomy intact; and closure of the colostomy when healing of the anastomosis is complete. In the elderly poor-risk patient with extensive colon distention, a tube cecostomy inserted under local anesthesia may be performed in selected instances. Obstructive lesions of the cecum and right colon are managed differently, and one usually has to choose between a right colectomy and an ileotransverse colonic anastomosis or a bypassing operation, ileotransverse colostomy, to relieve the obstruction with the intention of later resecting the right colon. The bypass operation should be reserved for poor-risk patients.

PARALYTIC ILEUS

Paralytic ileus is treated by nasogastric suction and intravenous fluid administration. Correction of electrolyte imbalance, especially hypokalemia, is particularly important in managing this disorder. In some patients with paralytic ileus, particularly those with extreme distention, passage of a Miller-Abbott tube into the intestine should be tried, because this method of suction provides superior intestinal decompression. Most often, ileus develops after abdominal surgery and is transient, lasting two or three days. When ileus persists or recurs without obvious etiology, one should endeavor to rule out mechanical obstruction or intra-abdominal sepsis, and in some instances a laparotomy may be necessary to exclude confidently these possibilities.

REFERENCES

1. Cope, Z.   The Early Diagnosis of the Acute Abdomen. New York, Oxford Univ. Press, 1957.
2. Botsford, T. W., and Wilson, R. E.   The Acute Abdomen. Philadelphia, W. B. Saunders Co., 1969.
3. Dunphy, J. E., and Botsford, T. W.   Physical Examination of the Surgical Patient. Philadelphia, W. B. Saunders Co., 1959.
4. Schwartz, S. I.   Principles of Surgery. New York, McGraw-Hill Book Co., 1969, pp. 843-855.
5. Miller, L. D., Mackie, J. A., and Rhoads, J. E.   The pathophysiology and management of intestinal obstruction. Surg. Clin. N. Amer. 42:1285, 1962.
6. Moore, F. D.   Metabolic Care of the Surgical Patient. Philadelphia, W. B. Saunders Co., 1959.

Section 5

THE GALLBLADDER AND PANCREAS

Chapter 26

Bile Formation and Biliary Tract Function

William Admirand, Lawrence W. Way

BILE FORMATION

In many ways hepatic bile is similar to plasma. It is isosmotic, containing 300 milliosmoles per liter, and its predominant cation is sodium, present in a concentration of 170 mEq per liter. The major difference between hepatic bile and plasma is the concentration of anions; bile contains approximately 90 mEq per liter of chloride (less than plasma) and 70 mEq per liter of bicarbonate (more than plasma). As a result of the excess bicarbonate, hepatic bile is alkaline, with the pH ranging from 7.5 to 9.5. In addition, bile contains an abundance of organic anions such as bilirubin and bile salts. The apparent discrepancy between cation concentrations in bile and total osmolality is due to trapping of cation within multimolecular aggregates of bile salts, micelles which are osmotically less active. The major lipids in bile are cholesterol and lecithin. Only trace amounts of fatty acids and protein are present.

The mechanism by which bile is excreted from the hepatocyte has not been definitely established. Hydrostatic pressure is unlikely to be the driving force, because livers perfused under controlled conditions in vitro secrete bile even when hydrostatic pressure in the common bile duct exceeds perfusion pressure.[1] Since the Golgi apparatus is located close to the cholangiole, the possibility has been raised that bile is excreted by reversed pinocytosis. However, no direct evidence has appeared in support of secretion through the Golgi apparatus into a ductal network.

In fact, numerous studies indicate that the mechanism for bile formation consists of energy-requiring transport of solute from the hepatocyte into the bile capillary. Bile salts, which represent 70 to 80 per cent of the total solids in bile, are transported actively, whereas cations and water follow passively, rendering the bile electrically neutral and isosmotic.[2] Active transport of other solutes from the hepatocyte also contribute to the secretion of bile. When bile salts are depleted experimentally, increased excretion of other organic anions can increase bile flow. Thus this fraction of bile excretion is inde-

352

pendent of bile salts, but quantitatively it is minimal compared with the bile salt-dependent fraction.

The ductal epithelium is thought to contribute a second component to bile in a manner dissimilar to that in the hepatocyte.[3] Bicarbonate and sodium are actively secreted into the lumen by a coupled pump which generates a negative electrical potential on the mucosal surface. This mechanism is under the influence of the hormones secretin, cholecystokinin, and gastrin, all of which increase biliary flow and bicarbonate concentration. In addition, vagal impulses enhance the hormonal effects. Water diffuses into the lumen along the osmotic gradient, and passive exchange of Cl^- and HCO_3^- may take place across the epithelium as the bile flows along the ducts. Potassium diffuses to achieve electrochemical equilibrium. Thus bile emerging from the liver is the pooled product of at least two sources governed by different regulatory controls.

BILE SALT METABOLISM

Bile salts are the 24-carbon steroid compounds which are synthesized in the liver from cholesterol. The first step in bile salt synthesis is the addition of a hydroxyl group in the alpha position at the 7-carbon of the steroid nucleus. This step is under feedback regulation and is rate-limiting for the entire synthetic process.[4] In the synthesis of cholate an additional alpha hydroxyl group is added at the 12-carbon position. Subsequently, the double bond is saturated, and the β-hydroxyl at the 3-carbon position is converted to a ketone and then to an α-hydroxyl group. In the final step, the cholesterol side-chain is broken by the formation of a terminal carboxyl at the 24-carbon position (Fig. 26–1).

It has recently been shown in man that 26-hydroxycholesterol serves as a precursor for bile salt synthesis.[5] In this pathway, the 24-carbon is converted to a carboxyl prior to changes in the steroid nucleus. The quantitative importance of this second pathway has not yet been determined. One of the minor metabolites of 26-hydroxycholesterol is 3-β-hydroxy-5-cholanoate. The latter compound has been shown to produce cholestasis in animals.[6] The finding of large amounts of this substance in the urine of patients with intrahepatic biliary atresia[7] suggests the possibility that synthesis of monohydroxy-bile salts from 26-hydroxycholesterol might contribute to the cholestasis in certain forms of liver disease.

In man the two primary bile salts synthesized in the liver are cholate (3α,7α, 12α-trihydroxy-5β cholanoate) and chenodeoxycholate (3α,7α-dihydroxy-5β cholanoate) (see Fig. 26–1). The normal rate of bile salt synthesis is 200 to 500 mg per 24 hours. This represents one of the major routes by which cholesterol is eliminated from the body.

Bile salts are conjugated in the liver with glycine or taurine. The amino acids are linked to the 24-carbon of the bile salts by an amino bond. Normally, 60 per cent of bile salts in bile are conjugated with glycine and 40 per cent with taurine. Conjugation lowers the pKa of bile salts. Thus, the pKa of free bile salts is pH 6, whereas the pKa of glycine-conjugated bile salts is pH 4 and that of taurine-conjugated bile salts, pH 2.

The pH of the intestine often approaches pH 6. Therefore failure of conjugation would lead to the accumulation of large amounts of unconjugated, unionized, protonated bile acids within the intestinal lumen. These protonated bile acids have limited water solubility, and the small amount that is soluble can be absorbed in the upper small intestine by a process of passive nonionic diffusion.[8] Both these mechanisms would lower the concentration of bile salts in the upper intestine where they are needed to solubilize fatty acids and monoglycerides. Thus conjugation of bile salts with taurine or glycine not only prevents the formation of protonated bile acids but also provides concentrations of ionized bile salts adequate to assure normal fat absorption.

Conjugated bile salts are absorbed from the intestine in the terminal ileum by an extremely efficient active transport process which requires energy and a specific carrier.[9, 10] Approximately 90 to 95 per cent of bile salts are absorbed in a single passage of the intestine (Fig. 26–2). The remaining 5 per cent enter the colon where anaerobic bacteria, mainly Bacteroides, split

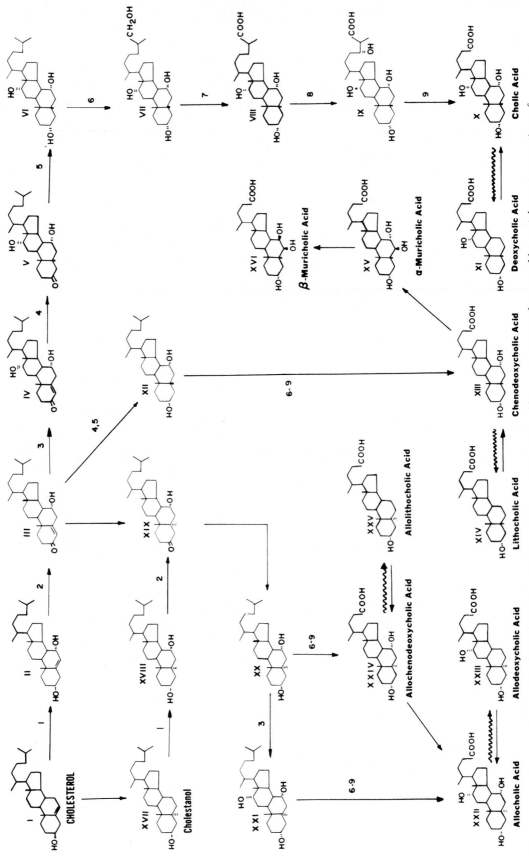

Figure 26–1. Biosynthesis of bile acids from cholesterol. Reactions of liver enzymes are designated by straight arrows; reactions of intestinal microorganisms are designated by wavy arrows. (From Elliott, W. H., and Hyde, P. M.: Amer. J. Med. 51:568, 1971.)

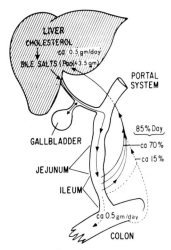

Figure 26–2. Schematic representation of the enterohepatic circulation of bile salts. The solid lines entering the portal system represent conjugated bile salt absorbed via ileal transport. The broken lines represent unconjugated bile salts resulting from bacterial action. (From Tyor, M. P., Garbutt, J. T., and Lack, L.: Amer. J. Med. 51:614, 1971.)

off the amino acid from the side-chain and remove the 7α hydroxyl group from steroid nucleus. Thus cholate ($3\alpha,7\alpha,12\alpha$-trihydroxy-5β cholanoate) is converted to deoxycholate ($3\alpha,12\alpha$-dihydroxy-5β cholanoate), and chenodeoxycholate ($3\alpha, 7\alpha$-dihydroxy-5β cholanoic acid) is converted to lithocholate (3α hydroxy-5β cholanoate). Lithocholate is almost completely insoluble at body temperature, and therefore most of it is excreted in the stool.[11] A small quantity of lithocholate is absorbed, probably by being solubilized in micelles of the other bile salts. The other secondary bile salt, deoxycholate, is water soluble, and much of it is absorbed from the cecum or by reflux into the terminal ileum. Normal bile in humans contains approximately 50 per cent cholate, 30 per cent chenodeoxycholate, 15 per cent deoxycholate, and 5 per cent lithocholate.

Once bile salts are absorbed from the bowel, they are transported to the liver via the portal circulation bound to plasma proteins. The bile salts are almost completely extracted from the portal blood in a single passage through the liver. Thus the concentration of bile salts in peripheral blood rarely exceeds 2 μg per milliliter. In the liver the bile salts are reconjugated, if necessary, and re-excreted into the bile.

The normal rate of bile salt synthesis in man is 0.2 to 0.5 g per 24 hours, which in the steady state equals fecal excretion. Only trace amounts of bile salts are excreted in the urine. The bile salt pool is 2.5 to 4.5 g, but this entire pool passes through the enterohepatic circulation approximately twice during the course of a single meal. This rapid recycling of bile salts is essential to normal fat absorption. Anything that interrupts the enterohepatic circulation, such as resection of the terminal ileum or obstructive liver disease, can result in severe malabsorption of fat and fat-soluble vitamins.

GALLBLADDER FUNCTION

The major functions of the gallbladder are to concentrate and store bile and then to deliver concentrated bile to the duodenum during meals. The importance of the latter function is somewhat debatable, because its absence in man and in numerous other species does not alter digestion significantly.

In the gallbladder, hepatic bile is concentrated to the extent that 90 per cent of the water is removed as an isotonic solution composed principally of sodium, chloride, and bicarbonate.[12] The absorption of water and inorganic ions results in a markedly increased concentration of bile salts and sodium within the lumen of the gallbladder. Since the bile salts exist as multimolecular aggregates, or micelles, sodium concentration is the major determinant of osmotic activity in concentrated gallbladder bile just as in hepatic bile.

Isotonic fluid is absorbed rapidly from the gallbladder; indeed, intact rabbit gallbladder absorbs fluid at a rate of 30 per cent of the gallbladder volume per hour.[13] Histological study of the gallbladder has revealed the presence of large intercellular spaces which became dilated with fluid during the process of absorption. The exact mechanism by which fluid and electrolytes are absorbed by the gallbladder mucosa has not been definitely established; it is not simple active transport of solute with passive movement of water.

Two theories have been proposed to explain absorption from the gallbladder lumen. The first suggests that the luminal surface of the gallbladder epithelium serves as a semipermeable membrane between the lumen and the intercellular spaces.[14] Solutes are actively transported across this membrane, and water follows passively to maintain osmotic equilibrium. The theory is based upon the concept that the distal portions of the intercellular spaces are bounded by a nonselective barrier. Thus the hydrostatic pressure developed within the intercellular spaces serves to drive solution out through the basal portion of the gallbladder mucosa (Fig. 26–3). A second theory to explain absorption in the gallbladder is based on the principle of local osmosis, and proposes that solute is actively transported into the fluid-filled intracellular spaces of the gallbladder wall.[15] Since the channels are unstirred, osmotic equilibrium is achieved as the fluid passes toward the basal end of the cell. Thus there is always an osmotic gradient in the luminal portion of the intracellular spaces, whereas the fluid transported out of the gallbladder is isotonic (Fig. 26–4).

The degree of absorption of larger organic compounds by the gallbladder is based upon their lipid solubility. Lipid-soluble compounds easily penetrate the gallbladder wall and are absorbed; compounds which are predominantly water soluble are poorly absorbed. Thus unconjugated bile acids, which are relatively lipid soluble, can be absorbed from the gallbladder. In contrast, conjugated bile salts which are water soluble are not absorbed.[16]

BILIARY DYNAMICS

The physiological regulation of the flow of bile into the duodenum can be thought of as the result of a balance between two types of pumps and one major resistance.[17] The active transport mechanisms of the hepatocytes can generate hydrostatic pressure which will support a column of bile 30 to 35 cm high in an otherwise occluded ductal system. This pressure actually represents an equilibrium between active secretory forces and the tendency for bile to leak from the biliary tree into interstitial areas or the bloodstream. That the leakiness of the collecting system is of physiological significance has been demon-

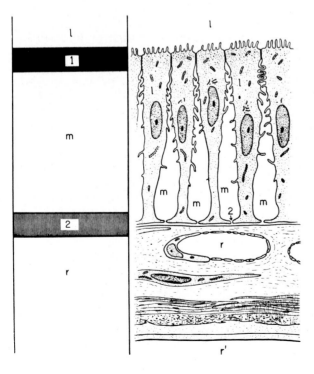

Figure 26–3. Representation of the Curran serial membrane model (left) and the gallbladder wall (right). The Curran model is composed of three compartments (l, m, r) separated by a semipermeable membrane (1) and a nonselective barrier (2). Active solute transport across barrier 1 from l to m would create an osmotic gradient which would cause water to move from l to m. The resulting hydrostatic pressure in m would drive the fluid across nonselective barrier 2. This system will "pump" solution from l to r even if the osmolality in l is greater than that in r. In the gallbladder epithelium it is postulated that the lateral intercellular compartment is analogous to m. The basal clefts and lamina propria are analogous to barrier 2 (including the entire wall in in vitro systems). Active solute transport across the lateral cell walls into compartment m could accomplish net fluid movement despite an adverse osmotic gradient across the wall and would normally cause transport of a virtually isotonic fluid. (From Kaye, G. I., et al.: J. Cell Biol. 30:237, 1966.)

Chapter 27

Pancreatic Physiology

Lloyd L. Brandborg

NATURE OF PANCREATIC SECRETION

ENZYMES

The pancreas is a veritable factory for the synthesis of proteins for export, mostly enzymes. The following enzymes were identified in pure pancreatic secretion from two human subjects:[1] amylase, lipase, ribonuclease, deoxyribonuclease, proelastase, procarboxypeptidases A and B, chymotrypsinogen, trypsinogen, and trypsin inhibitor. Proelastase was present in unfractionated human pancreatic juice, but not in lyophilized material. Collagenase and lysozyme were not detected. Cholesterol esterase, phosphatidase, and phosphatase had been observed by other investigators. The determination of individual pancreatic enzymes is time consuming, and for clinical purposes the total protein content of the juice is a reasonable approximation of enzyme content. Only small amounts of serum protein are contained in the pancreatic juice, and they do not significantly add to the total protein secreted by the gland.

The proteolytic enzymes are secreted into the pancreatic duct as inactive zymogens. On contact with enterokinase in the presence of calcium in the duodenum, trypsin is activated. Until trypsin is activated, it is in balance with trypsin inhibitor. On activation, trypsin activates chymotrypsinogen, elastase, and phospholipase, and trypsin inhibitor is inactivated. Once these reactions are initiated, they become autocatalytic. Pancreatic kallikrein, which is not secreted in pancreatic juice, is also activated by trypsin and inhibited by trypsin inhibitor.

Amylase is secreted as the active enzyme, and lipase appears to require bile acids, at least in part, for activation. Pancreatic amylase is an alpha amylase; i.e., it is an endoamylase that randomly hydrolyzes the inner 1-4 alpha-glycosidic linkages of starch and glycogen. Whether pancreatic isoamylases occur is still being investigated. Trypsin and chymotrypsin are endopeptidases splitting peptide bonds within large protein molecules, whereas the carboxypeptidases act only on terminal peptide bonds. Ribonuclease and deoxyribonuclease split nuclear proteins in the diet. Lipase is necessary for the hydrolysis of triglyceride in the gut to fatty acids and monoglyceride.

Basic trypsin inhibitor from the pancreas appears to be identical to inhibitors of other trypsin-like proteases; e.g., thrombin and plasmin. Bovine pancreatic trypsin inhibitor has been found to be identical to kallikrein inhibitor from bovine lung and parotid gland.[2] It also inhibits chymotrypsin and bacterial fibrinolysin.

FLUID AND ELECTROLYTES

The pancreas of man can secrete fluid isosmotic with plasma at rates of flow up to 4.7 ml per minute.[3] The electrolyte con-

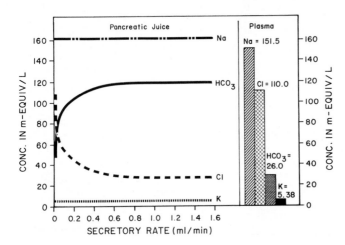

Figure 27-1. Relationship of pancreatic secretion and concentration of electrolytes. (Adapted from Bro-Rasmussen, F., Kilman, S. A., and Thaysen, J. H.: Acta Physiol. Scand. 37:97, 1956.)

tent of this fluid is unique in that bicarbonate concentration may reach 150 mEq per liter. Sodium and potassium concentrations in the juice approximate those of plasma water and are not related to the rate of flow. The concentration of sodium varies between 139 and 143 mEq per liter, and that of potassium between 6 and 9 mEq per liter.[4] Calcium is present in a much lower concentration than in plasma, and magnesium is present in small quantities.

The principal anions in pancreatic secretions are bicarbonate and chloride. Bicarbonate concentration ranges from 25 to 150 mEq per liter and is directly related to the rate of flow. Chloride concentration is reciprocally related to bicarbonate concentration, and their sum remains constant. These relationships have been determined by stimulation with either exogenous secretin or endogenous secretin released by physiological stimulants introduced into the gut (Fig. 27–1).

FUNCTION OF ACINAR CELLS

ENZYME SYNTHESIS AND TRANSPORT

The current concepts of enzyme synthesis and transport within acinar cells are derived from morphological, ultrastructural, biochemical, autoradiographic, and isotope labeling studies.[5] Animal studies have shown that injected labeled amino acids are first found in proteins associated with the ribosomes. These newly synthesized enzymes are transported across the membranes of the rough endoplasmic reticulum. They accumulate in this region and are then transported to the region of the Golgi complex where they acquire a smooth-surfaced membrane and become visible by electron microscopy. As these membrane-enveloped granules migrate toward the apex of the cell, they develop into fully mature zymogen granules, perhaps through the aggregation of small particles or through the exclusion of water (Fig. 27–2).

It is not entirely clear whether the newly synthesized enzyme passes first into the cell sap or whether it is transported directly from the rough endoplasmic reticulum to the Golgi complex. The earliest labeling of enzyme after the injection of radioactive amino acids in several species occurs in the cell sap or soluble fraction, with relatively little labeling of the zymogen granules. Because of the high activity of newly synthesized enzyme in the soluble fraction, it is probable that two routes exist which enzymes may take between their sites of synthesis and the storage form, the zymogen granule. One route is probably direct transfer of newly synthesized enzyme across the rough-surfaced endoplasmic reticulum with accumulation in this site. The smooth membrane may be derived from the rough membrane. The other mechanism is the release of newly synthesized enzyme from the ribosome into the cell sap and its trans-

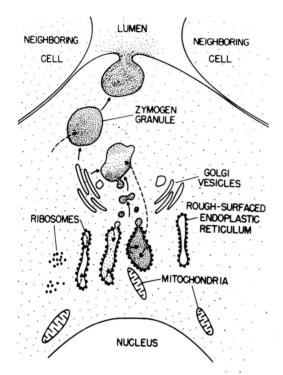

Figure 27–2.   Route of intracellular secretory protein (enzyme) transport. Secretory proteins are synthesized on the ribosomes. They are then transferred to and accumulate within the rough-surfaced endoplasmic reticulum. Smooth membranes bud from the ends of the rough-surfaced cisternae in the region of the Golgi complex. The small vesicles which contain the newly synthesized enzyme coalesce to form immature zymogen granules. Mature zymogen granules result from extrusion of water, by transport of additional enzyme across the zymogen membrane, or by both mechanisms. Solid arrows indicate migration of membrane; dashed arrows, transmembrane transport of enzyme; and dots, secretory protein. (Reprinted with permission of Dr. L. E. Hokin and the American Physiological Society.[5])

port into the region of the Golgi complex where it receives its smooth membrane. With prolonged stimulation enzyme secretion occurs at a high level without zymogen granule formation. It is likely that no synthesis occurs in the Golgi region.

Synthesis of enzymes by the pancreas is very rapid and requires only one to two minutes after the amino acid precursor reaches the acinar cell. Approximately one hour is required for newly synthesized enzyme to make its appearance in the pancreatic juice.

Another related, but independent, phenomenon occurs during enzyme synthesis and secretion. This is a marked stimulation of phospholipid synthesis, particularly of phosphatidylinositol and, to a lesser extent, phosphatidylethanolamine. These phospholipids have been shown to be incorporated in about equal distributions into the smooth and rough membrane fractions with localization primarily in the intracellular membranes, including the membrane surrounding the zymogen granule. The current morphological data show that the smooth membrane of the zymogen granule and the apical plasma membrane fuse on contact. There is a separation at the luminal aspect of the acinus, a reverse pinocytosis, with a discharge of the zymogen granule into the duct. Little or no phospholipid appears in pancreatic juice. Its fate is not known, but it may serve as a precursor for new membrane or it may be a source of cell energy.

CONTROL MECHANISMS

Control of protein synthesis is complex. DNA-directed synthesis of messenger RNA is one of the required steps. Yet, despite the very high RNA content of pancreatic acinar cells, protein synthesis and RNA synthesis are not parallel. Stimulated enzyme synthesis in vivo and in vitro is not accompanied by increases in RNA or in increased incorporation of P^{32} into RNA. Two explanations for this apparent discrepancy have been advanced. One is that the rate of RNA synthesis in the pancreas is so rapid that the formation of messenger RNA is not detected. The other possibility is that messenger RNA in the pancreas is stable and is replenished very slowly This explanation would assume that each RNA molecule is repeatedly utilized for synthesis of many protein molecules.[5]

The kind and content of protein in the diet influence pancreatic synthetic function.[6] With total starvation the pancreas undergoes atrophy which is confined to the acinar cells and is reversible on refeeding a complete diet. Inadequate protein, or protein lacking essential amino acids, e.g., zein which lacks lysine, in the presence of sufficient carbohydrate and fat calories, leads to kwashiorkor, which is characterized by pancreatic insufficiency. The pancreatic lesion consists of loss of acinar cytoplasm, disruption of acini, necrosis, vacuolization, and ultimately fibrosis. Cystic dilatation and epithelial metaplasia of the ducts may also be present. Fatty liver, which is a classic feature of kwashiorkor, follows the pancreatic damage. If the diagnosis is established early enough, pancreatic damage is reversible on feeding protein containing all the essential amino acids.

In experimentally developed kwashiorkor, lipase disappears from pancreatic secretion first, followed by trypsin, ribonuclease, esterase, and chymotrypsin. Amylase is reduced by 50 per cent but never completely vanishes. Adaptation occurs in response to composition of the diet in some species but not in others. In rats, a diet high in starch results in a marked increase in amylase synthesis.[7] A diet rich in protein significantly increases synthesis of chymotrypsinogen. Trypsinogen remains constant. Lipase is not influenced by the lipid content of the diet, but is depressed by high protein intake.

FUNCTION OF DUCTULAR EPITHELIUM

BICARBONATE SECRETION

The consensus holds that the intercalated ducts and the centroacinar cells are the probable site of water and the electrolyte secretion.[3, 5] The supporting evidence is indirect. Ethionine pancreatitis in dogs which damages the acinar cells more than the ductules leads to decreased secretion of water, trypsinogen, and trypsin inhibitor. Water secretion is less impaired than protein.[8] DL-Ethionine which affects ductular cells decreases bicarbonate secretion.[3] Alloxan which causes a morphological change in the duct cell raises the threshold to secretin stimulation.

Carbonic anhydrase, by histochemical techniques, is present only in the ductular epithelium.[9] It is intimately involved in bicarbonate secretion through the reversible reaction $H_2O + CO_2 \rightleftarrows HCO_3^- + H^+$. Acetazolamide which inhibits carbonic anhydrase depresses water and bicarbonate secretion but does not abolish them. In secretin-stimulated juice the high bicarbonate concentration tends to be preserved in the presence of acetazolamide.

Most of the bicarbonate is derived from carbon dioxide from the blood and part from metabolism of the cell. Metabolic alkalosis results in a secretion of an increased bicarbonate concentration, and metabolic and respiratory acidosis hinder bicarbonate secretion. If carbon dioxide is omitted from the bathing fluid, the in vitro rabbit pancreas is only able to secrete bicarbonate at 10 per cent of control value.

Apical "blebs" have been observed by electron microscopy at the surface of the intralobular duct cells during secretin-stimulated secretion.[10] These may contain water and electrolytes.

CHLORIDE-BICARBONATE "EXCHANGE"

Several theories exist to explain the electrolyte composition of pancreatic juice.[3] One postulate is that the electrolyte secretion consists of a mixture of three different fluids: one, a neutral chloride at a concentration of 174 mEq per liter; another, bicarbonate of equal concentration; and a third, containing enzymes, mucus, and acid chloride. The final composition is considered to be due to admixture of varying quantities of the three. Another hypothesis is that the centroacinar and ductal cells secrete an isotonic solution of bicarbonate which is altered as it traverses the collecting ducts by an exchange of bicarbonate and chloride with interstitial fluid. The third concept is that a single cell type secretes these ions at varying ratios. This scheme supposes an active transport of sodium and accumulation of potassium in the cell which have not been proved. The only feature of bicarbonate secretion about which there is universal agreement is that it is an energy-requiring process. Water flow is determined by electrolyte secretion. The exact mechanism is unknown, but it is almost certainly passive and regulated by the secretion of electrolyte.

The micropuncture technique has been applied to investigation of electrolyte composition of pancreatic fluid.[11] In the rabbit pancreas concentrations of bicarbonate and chloride in the interlobular duct and the main duct are the same, and briefly occluding the duct does not produce a change. Flow rates in in vivo specimens range between 240 and 800 μliters per hour in unstimulated glands. Under this experimental condition a bicarbonate-chloride exchange does not occur in the interlobular or the main pancreatic duct. Such an exchange in the intralobular ducts or the centroacinar cell cannot be excluded.

CONTROL OF PANCREATIC SECRETION

Control of pancreatic secretion under physiological conditions is through complex neurohumoral mechanisms.[12-15] Pancreatic secretion in man is stimulated by the presence of food in the stomach and by acid and food in the small intestine. The hormones which have been found to be physiologically important in control of exocrine pancreatic secretion are gastrin, secretin, and cholecystokinin. Pancreozymin and cholecystokinin are the same hormone.

Gastrin is localized largely to the pyloroantral mucosa of the stomach. Secretin and cholecystokinin are contained in the mucosa of the small intestine with the highest concentrations in the more proximal intestine. Some activity is found in the ileum.

Human gastrins I and II have been analyzed, their amino acid sequences identified, and the hormones synthesized. Porcine secretin has been isolated and its structure determined. Synthesis has been achieved. Cholecystokinin has been fully characterized but not synthesized.[16] The cellular origin of these hormones is not conclusively known.

With the availability of the pure hormones it has become apparent that they interact with each other and have common target organs, and that each affects many functions.[16] Gastrin, which is under cholinergic control, is a potent stimulant of gastric acid and a weak stimulant of water and bicarbonate from the pancreas; it has a potent cholecystokinetic affect on the pancreas. Cholecystokinin is a weak stimulant of both gastric acid and pancreatic bicarbonate and water, but a potent stimulant of pancreatic enzymes. Secretin inhibits gastrin-stimulated gastric acid secretin; it is a potent stimulant of pancreatic bicarbonate and a weak stimulant of pancreatic enzymes.

Electrical stimulation of the vagus nerves has led to conflicting results on pancreatic function.[14] Species differences exist as they do with exogenous hormone administration. The use of anesthetized or unanesthetized animals also results in different responses. Agreement exists that vagal stimulation when superimposed on secretin infusion results in a marked increase in the output of enzymes by the pancreas. Cholinergic drugs have been shown to be potent stimulants of enzyme secretion with little effect on volume of pancreatic juice. Pancreatic volume response to small doses of secretin is augmented by cholinergic drugs. The response of the pancreas to vagotomy has been puzzling. In man vagotomy does not affect volume response to stimulation with exogenous secretin. The response to endogenously released secretin is depressed. Although vagotomy might conceivably reduce pancreatic response to secretin, the normal response to exogenous secretin suggests that reduced secretin release is the more important effect of vagotomy.

Anticholinergic drugs markedly decrease the pancreatic response to exogenous secretin in man. Anticholinergic drugs also inhibit the response of the pancreas to peptones and other substances in the intestine. Volume and enzyme secretion are both depressed. A gastropancreatic reflex, resulting in increased volume and enzyme secretion, produced by distention of the fundus of the stomach has been demonstrated. It is only temporarily abolished by the sections of the vagus and splanchnic nerves and is blocked by atropine. A cephalic phase of pancreatic secretion has been demonstrated in man in response to sham feeding.[17] Both bicarbonate and enzyme secretion are increased.

The relative importance of the various mechanisms controlling pancreatic secretion in man is not known. Optimal pancreatic secretion requires a complex neurohumoral mechanism.

ABNORMAL PANCREATIC SECRETION

Abnormal pancreatic secretion is observed primarily in patients with diseases of the gland itself. These include cystic fibrosis; kwashiorkor; acute, relapsing, and chronic pancreatitis; and tumors.[18] In cystic fibrosis, enzyme and bicarbonate secretions are depressed. The pancreatic juice is very low in volume and very viscous and does not increase after secretin administration. In kwashiorkor, bicarbonate and enzyme secretions are depressed but, interestingly, amylase persists after trypsin, chymotrypsin, or lipase is no longer detectable.[6] In individuals with tumors of the pancreas the volume of pancreatic secretion in response to secretin is decreased, but the bicarbonate concentration usually remains normal. This depends upon the location of the tumor, the amount of pancreatic tissue destroyed or obstructed, and whether pre-existing pancreatic disease is present. Abnormalities in the secretin test in pancreatitis depend on the stage of the disease at which the patient is examined. Most patients with chronic pancreatitis have a depressed volume and bicarbonate. The response in acute and acute relapsing pancreatitis is often normal. Excessively large secretion of water with low bicarbonate concentrations has been found in patients with cirrhosis of the liver and in those with hemochromatosis.

Stimulation with cholecystokinin has not been so widely applied, clinically, as the secretin test, but by using increasing doses of cholecystokinin, normal subjects may be separated from patients with pancreatic disease on the basis of protein (enzyme) secretion. For clinical purposes the secretin and cholecystokinin tests are of considerable value in separating normal from abnormal. They are of little use in differentiating different diseases. One must take into consideration the significant fluid and bicarbonate contribution by the liver and perhaps by the small intestinal mucosa. Gastric acid must be prevented from entering the small intestine in these clinical studies.

REFERENCES

1. Keller, P. J., and Allan, B. J. The protein composition of human pancreatic juice. J. Biol. Chem. 242:281, 1967.
2. Greene, L. J., and Giordano, J. S., Jr. The structure of the bovine pancreatic trypsin inhibitor. Kazal's inhibitor. I. The amino acid sequences of the tryptic peptide from reduced aminoethylated inhibitor. J. Biol. Chem. 244:285, 1969.
3. Janowitz, H. D. Pancreatic Secretion of Fluid and Electrolytes. In Handbook of Physiology, Sect. 6, Vol. II, C. F. Code (ed.). Washington, D.C. American Physiological Society, 1967.
4. Dreiling, D. A., and Janowitz, H. D. The secretion of electrolytes by the human pancreas. Gastroenterology 30:382, 1956.
5. Hokin, L. E. Metabolic aspects and energetics of pancreatic secretion. In Handbook of Physiology, Sect. 6, Vol. II, C. F. Code (ed.). Washington, D.C., American Physiological Society, 1967.
6. Veghelyi, P. V., and Kemeny, T. T. Protein metabolism and pancreatic function. In The Exocrine Pancreas, A. V. S. de Reuck and M. P. Cameron (eds.). Boston, Little, Brown, and Co., 1961.
7. Desnuelle, P., Reboud, J. P., and Ben Abdeljlil, A. Diet and enzyme content of pancreas. In The Exocrine Pancreas, A. V. S. de Reuck and M. P. Cameron (eds.). Boston, Little, Brown, and Co., 1962.
8. Kalser, M. H., and Grossman, M. I. Pancreatic secretion in dogs with ethionine-induced pancreatitis. Gastroenterology 26:189, 1954.
9. Becker, V. Histochemistry of the exocrine pancreas. In The Exocrine Pancreas, A. V. S. de Reuck and M. P. Cameron (eds.). Boston, Little, Brown and Co., 1962.
10. Ekholm, R. T., Zelander, T., and Edlund, Y. The ultrastructural organization of the rat exocrine pancreas. II. Centroacinar cells, intercalary and intralobular ducts. J. Ultrastruct. Res. 7:73, 1962.
11. Reber, H. A., and Wolf, C. J. Micropuncture study of pancreatic electrolyte secretion. Amer. J. Physiol. 215:34, 1968.
12. Thomas, J. E. Neural regulation of pancreatic secretion. In Handbook of Physiology, Sect. 6, Vols. I, II, C. F. Code (ed.). Washington, D.C., American Physiological Society, 1967.
13. Harper, A. A. Hormonal control of pancreatic secretion. In Handbook of Physiology, Sect. 6, Vol. II, C. F. Code (ed.). Washington, D.C., American Physiological Society, 1967.
14. Preshaw, R. M. Integration of nervous and hormonal mechanisms for external pancreatic secretion. In Handbook of Physiology, Sect. 6, Vol. II, C. F. Code (ed.). Washington, D.C., American Physiological Society, 1967.
15. Dupré, J. Regulation of the secretions of the pancreas. In Annual Review of Medicine, Vol. 21, A. C. DeGraff, and W. P. Creger (eds.). Palo Alto, Annual Reviews, Inc., 1970.
16. Grossman, M. I. Gastrointestinal hormones. Viewpoints on Digestive Disease, 2: No. 3, May, 1970.
17. Sarles, H., Dain, R., Prezelin, G., Souville, C., and Figarella, G. Cephalic phase of pancreatic secretion in Man. Gut 9:214, 1968.
18. Lagerlöf, H. O. Pancreatic secretion: Pathophysiology. In Handbook of Physiology, Sect. 6, Vol. II, C. F. Code (ed.). Washington, D.C., American Physiological Society, 1967.

Chapter 28

Syndromes Caused by Functioning Islet Cell Tumors

John H. Walsh, Marvin H. Sleisenger

The Zollinger-Ellison syndrome (see pp. 743 to 750) is only one of the clinical conditions caused by functioning islet cell tumors. Insulin-secreting tumors have been recognized as a cause of hypoglycemia since 1927. Another type of pancreatic tumor secretes a diarrhea-producing hormone which has not yet been identified with certainty. The clinical manifestations of all these tumors are due to the elaboration of peptide hormones under circumstances in which normal homeostatic mechanisms are not operative. The tumors themselves are usually small and seldom produce local tumor symptoms. Instead they must be diagnosed by recognition of the effects of hormone overproduction in the patient, by awareness that pancreatic tumors can be responsible for the observed findings, by bioassay or radioimmunoassay demonstration of increased hormone secretion, and, finally, by direct demonstration of the tumor.

For convenience, although not correct etymologically, islet cell tumors are commonly named according to the hormone they produce, e.g., insulinoma, glucagonoma, gastrinoma. In the case of the syndrome of severe watery diarrhea and hypokalemia, or pancreatic cholera, the causative hormone is as yet unknown (Fig. 28–1). A single pancreatic tumor may occasionally produce more than one hormone, or two different tumors producing different hormones may coexist in the same pancreas. Functioning adenomas of other endocrine glands, especially parathyroids, are found in about 10 per cent of patients with islet cell tumors. A familial polyendocrine syndrome with tumors and hyperplasia of endocrine glands, inherited by a dominant form of genetic transmission, involves primarily the pancreas and parathyroid glands. This chapter will consider the spectrum of syndromes of endocrine overproduction, other than the Zollinger-Ellison syndrome, caused by pancreatic islet cell tumors.

PANCREATIC CHOLERA

As pointed out on page 748, diarrhea is a common manifestation of the Zollinger-Ellison syndrome. This diarrhea is due to the entry of large amounts of highly acid gastric juice into the upper small intestine and possibly also to a direct effect of gastrin upon small bowel secretion of water and electrolytes. Usually there is associated steatorrhea which results from inactivation of pancreatic lipase and pre-

365

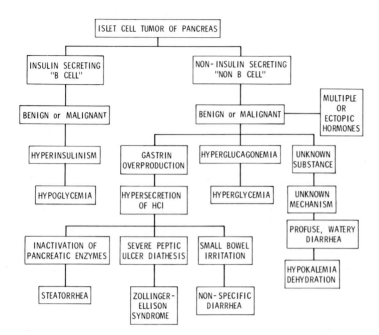

Figure 28-1. Classification of functioning pancreatic islet cell tumors relating clinical manifestations to hormone overproduction. (From Matsumoto, K. K., et al.: Gastroenterology 50:231, 1966.)

cipitation of bile salts in the intestinal lumen at acid pH in the intestine. Potassium loss is not a prominent feature, and aspiration of gastric contents typically results in temporary amelioration of the diarrhea.

In contrast to these patients, almost three dozen cases have been reported of another diarrheal syndrome distinguished from Zollinger-Ellison syndrome by the absence of acid hypersecretion. This syndrome was described first in 1958 by Verner and Morrison.[1] They reported two patients with profuse watery diarrhea, severe hypokalemia, shock, and dehydration in whom benign pancreatic islet cell tumors were found at autopsy. In the first papers written on this syndrome, histamine-fast achlorhydria was considered essential for the diagnosis and the name WDHA syndrome (watery diarrhea, hypokalemia, achlorhydria) was applied.[2] Subsequently it has become apparent that many patients with this disease have only moderately decreased or normal acid secretion. The term pancreatic cholera describes the clinical feature of massive watery diarrhea and recognizes the pancreatic etiology of the disease.[3] The clinical and laboratory findings in this syndrome have been considered in several reviews.[2-7]

CLINICAL PICTURE

The predominant clinical feature of pancreatic cholera is prolonged massive watery diarrhea, usually associated with symptoms of hypokalemia and dehydration. Females are affected slightly more commonly than males, and the average age at the time of diagnosis is 44 years with a reported range of 19 to 67 years. Symptoms have usually been noted for months to years before the diagnosis is first made.

Periods of fulminant diarrhea frequently alternate with periods in which the stool volume is less, and the stools may be semiliquid. Episodes of severe diarrhea tend to increase in frequency and severity with the passage of time. During exacerbations, symptoms of dehydration and hypokalemia are prominent. Lethargy, muscular weakness, nausea and vomiting, and crampy abdominal pain are frequent complaints. Acute weight loss of up to several kilograms is common during these attacks. This weight loss can be accounted for by the average daily stool volume of nearly 6 liters. During these exacerbations the stool has the appearance of weak tea, and fecal fluid losses in excess of 10 liters per day have been reported. The stool contains high concentrations of potassium and sodium, leading to electrolyte depletion. Inadequate replacement of fluid and electrolytes during diarrheal episodes has resulted in the death of at least seven patients with this disease.

Peptic ulcer is not a feature of this syndrome, although occasional patients may have a remote history of previous peptic ulcer or may develop gastric ulceration while receiving steroids. During attacks of diarrhea, several patients have had symptoms of flushing of the face and trunk resembling carcinoid syndrome.[7-9] Serum and urine examination failed to reveal increased amounts of serotonin or serotonin metabolites, and these symptoms remain unexplained. Skin pigmentation has been described in a few cases.

LABORATORY FINDINGS

The serum electrolytes reflect fecal losses of potassium, bicarbonate, and water. The serum potassium may be less than 2 mEq per liter and is invariably less than 3 mEq per liter until potassium replacement is given. Serum bicarbonate is usually moderately depressed, reflecting metabolic acidosis resulting from fecal bicarbonate losses. Serum sodium and chloride may be normal. Dehydration may lead to increased blood urea nitrogen and serum creatinine. Usually these are corrected by adequate fluid and electrolyte replacement, but they may persist on account of hypokalemic nephropathy.

Fecal water losses average 5 liters per day during acute diarrhea. Potassium losses in the stool are generally in the order of 200 to 400 mEq per day.[6] Potassium content of the stool is inversely related to stool volume. The sum of sodium and potassium is relatively constant.[7] Stoker and Wynn compared duodenal and fecal electrolyte concentrations in one patient with pancreatic cholera and found the pH of both was 8.1, but that fecal potassium and carbon dioxide levels were higher and sodium and chloride levels were lower.[7] Espiner and Beaven administered K^{42} to a patient with the disease. The amount recovered in the stool was three times greater than in a patient with active ulcerative colitis, and was the same whether the isotope was administered orally or intravenously.[10] Stool fat excretion is usually normal or very slightly increased. Examinations for ova and parasites and stool cultures are unrevealing.

About half the patients with this disorder have decreased glucose tolerance. This might be explainable on the basis of chronic hypokalemia or might be due in part to an effect of the diarrheagenic hormone. In one patient an increase in blood sugar was noted during dissection of the tumor.[10] Glucose tolerance has returned to normal after tumor resection in several patients. In these patients both factors, hypokalemia and abnormal hormone secretion, were corrected.

Hypercalcemia is another frequent laboratory finding, occurring in about half the patients and becoming more marked during episodes of severe diarrhea.[6] Parathyroid adenomas have been found only occasionally, but the hypercalcemia has abated in several patients after successful resection of the pancreatic tumor. It has been suggested that the tumor secretes a parathyroid-like hormone or indirectly stimulates the release of parathyroid hormone from the parathyroid glands. Balance studies in these patients have revealed negative calcium balance and have suggested that the calcium originates from bone.[11]

Gastric secretory studies reveal normal to histamine-fast achlorhydric values. Hypersecretion of acid is not compatible with the diagnosis as the disease is presently defined. However, diarrhea and hypokalemia are found in some patients with Zollinger-Ellison syndrome. It is possible that these patients secrete both gastrin and another hormone responsible for the diarrhea. In patients with pancreatic cholera, resection of the tumor usually results in some increase in gastric acid secretion. Gastric biopsies in several of these patients, including those with achlorhydria, have been normal.[2, 6, 12] These findings are compatible with the idea that a gastric inhibitory hormone is released by the tumors. Some improvement in acid secretion has been observed following potassium replacement in one patient,[13] but most patients with low acid secretion continued to have diminished acid despite normal serum potassium until a tumor was removed. Andersson and colleagues also found decreased gastric secretions of pepsin and intrinsic factor which were corrected by tumor resection.[13] Renal function abnormalities reflect prolonged hypokalemia and dehydration. Loss of concentrating ability is the most prominent early abnormality. Azotemia frequently responds to fluid replacement, but progressive renal failure may occur in patients with severe hypokalemic nephropathy. Urinary tract infections have been reported in several patients.

Gastrointestinal X-rays are not especially helpful. Pancreatic function tests have been reported in two patients.[2, 12] Basal volume and bicarbonate output and stimulated output following the administration of secretin were normal.

DIFFERENTIAL DIAGNOSIS

The diagnosis of pancreatic cholera is made by exclusion of other known causes of severe chronic diarrhea with hypokalemia and by demonstration of a pancreatic islet cell tumor. Unfortunately no biological or immunological tests currently available permit the identification of the hormone circulating in excess.

Chronic overadministration of laxatives must be excluded by history and by observation. Villous adenoma of the colon, usually found in the rectum, may produce a similar picture of massive diarrhea with electrolyte depletion.[14] These tumors are usually readily accessible to the sigmoidoscope and should present no diagnostic difficulty. Other chronic diarrheal states usually do not produce the same degree of hypokalemia and may be excluded by usual diagnostic methods. The distinction of pancreatic cholera from gastrinoma can be made by measuring gastric acid secretion and by determining serum gastrin concentrations. Malignant carcinoid syndrome may be suspected in some of these patients. The tumors are similar histologically, and some patients with pancreatic cholera have flushing episodes. In patients with the carcinoid syndrome, serum potassium is not severely depressed and serum and urinary concentrations of serotonin or its metabolites, 5-hydroxytryptophan and 5-hydroxytryptamine, are abnormal.

PATHOGENESIS

Thus it would appear that pancreatic cholera is caused by the secretion of one or more hormones by pancreatic islet cell tumors. This conclusion is borne out by the reversal of all abnormalities following successful tumor resection. However, the exact nature of the hormone or hormones responsible for this syndrome has not been established.

It appears almost certain that the hormone in question has a major effect on intestinal water and electrolyte transport and inhibits gastric acid secretion. Other hormonal effects which are less completely established are a hypercalcemic action, a hyperglycemic action, inhibition of gastric pepsin and intrinsic factor secretion, and liberation of a substance causing facial flushing.

No known gastrointestinal hormone has all the actions described above. Zollinger and colleagues have suggested that the responsible hormone might be secretin.[15] This speculation was based on the findings of distended gallbladder filled with diluted bile, inhibition of acid secretion, and diarrhea. However, it has been difficult to demonstrate diarrhea after prolonged administration of high doses of secretin to man or dogs. Zollinger et al. were able to demonstrate a secretin-like activity in extracts from hepatic metastases of one tumor, but not from extracts of the pancreatic tumor in the same patient or from hepatic or pancreatic tumor tissue obtained from another patient.[15] Normal pancreatic function tests with normal responses to exogenous secretin found in two other patients[2, 12] are further evidence against secretin as the responsible hormone. Extracts of other tumors have given negative or inconclusive results when tested for secretin-like activity. However, most of these have been prepared in saline or water, and hormone activity might have been destroyed by tissue enzyme activity.

Tumor extracts have been tested for other types of activity. Gardner and Cerda found that an aqueous tumor extract, but not serum from the same patient, inhibited sodium, chloride, and water transfer in the hamster ileum.[16] Semb et al. reported a gastrone-like effect in a saline tumor extract which caused inhibition of both histamine- and pentagastrin-stimulated acid secretion.[17] Andersson et al. found no prostaglandins and no kallikrein activity but slight secretin-like activity in another tumor.[13] Several of these tumors have been assayed for gastrin activity, always with negative results. One tumor contained no glucagon.[17]

Of the known gastrointestinal hormones which might be responsible for this syndrome, gastrin has been eliminated as a possibility. Barbezat and Grossman found that several other gastrointestinal hormones were capable of stimulating water and electrolyte secretion by the dog jejunum and ileum.[18] Three of these hormones, glucagon, gastric inhibitory peptide (GIP),[19] and vasoactive inhibitory peptide (VIP),[20] are structurally related to secretin (Fig. 28-2). Secretin, however, did not cause small intestine secretion in the dog. However, other workers have found that secretin may stimulate intestinal secretion in the rat[21] and in man.[22] By comparison of the structures of the four hormones, it was found that the 9-Asp, 10-Tyr residues were common to the three which stimulated canine intestinal secretion and may therefore be part of the active site for this effect. Pentagastrin also stimulated secretion, but the active C-terminal portion of cholecystokinin did not. Prostaglandins also cause secretion of small bowel fluid in the dog[23] and inhibit gastric acid secretion.

Further identification of the hormone responsible for pancreatic cholera awaits isolation of the hormone from tumors or identification of increased concentrations of circulating hormone in the blood. Bioassays and immunoassays for glucagon have been unsuccessful in a few cases. Glucagon is a good theoretical candidate, because it stimulates intestinal secretion, inhibits gastric acid secretion, and increases the blood sugar. However, glucagon could not account for hypercalcemia, because it decreases the serum calcium.[24] Less is known of the biological actions of GIP and VIP. GIP is known to inhibit gastric acid pepsin and acid secretion after stimulation by pentagastrin, histamine, or insulin.[19] VIP increases peripheral and mesenteric blood flow and is about one-third as effective as glucagon in increasing blood sugar.[20]

The clinical picture and nature of the diarrheal stool in pancreatic and bacterial cholera are similar. It is not known whether intestinal secretion is stimulated through similar mechanisms in the two conditions. There is some evidence that cholera toxin releases a substance into the circulation, possibly an intestinal hormone, which stimulates intestinal secretion.[25] There is also evidence that cholera toxin ultimately stimulates intestinal adenosine cyclic monophosphate.[26] Glucagon acts in other tissues by stimulation of cyclic AMP and possibly has the same effect in the intestine. The effects of GIP and

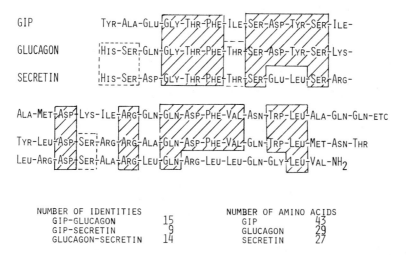

NUMBER OF IDENTITIES		NUMBER OF AMINO ACIDS	
GIP-GLUCAGON	15	GIP	43
GIP-SECRETIN	9	GLUCAGON	29
GLUCAGON-SECRETIN	14	SECRETIN	27

Figure 28-2. Structural similarity of three peptide hormones extracted from pancreas or upper intestine. GIP: Gastric inhibitory polypeptide of Pederson and Brown.[19] Vasoactive inhibitory polypeptide of Said and Mutt[20] resembles these three hormones, but the complete amino acid sequence has not yet been published.

VIP on cyclic AMP have not yet been reported. Fecal losses of potassium in bacterial cholera are similar to those found in pancreatic cholera. Hypokalemia is not so severe in bacterial cholera because of the short duration of the disease. Moore and coworkers obtained evidence in the dog that cholera toxin causes active secretion of chloride and bicarbonate and probably of potassium in the ileum against concentration and electrical gradients.[27]

PATHOLOGY

Of the 33 patients reviewed by Verner, 14 had malignant tumors, 17 had benign adenomas, and two had islet hyperplasia.[1] These tumors tend to be somewhat larger than gastrin- or insulin-secreting islet cell tumors. Histologically they are identical to the nonalpha, nonbeta cell tumors found in patients with Zollinger-Ellison syndrome, but they do not contain gastrin. They may contain more necrotic and hyalinized material than the smaller tumors. In two patients these tumors have been demonstrated by angiography before surgery,[13] but usually they are not vascular enough to permit detection. A typical tumor is illustrated in Figure 28–3.

THERAPY

Initial therapy must be directed at adequate fluid and electrolyte replacement. It may be difficult or impossible to correct hypokalemia completely during active diarrhea. The preoperative evaluation may be highly suggestive of pancreatic cholera, but definitive diagnosis is made only by surgical exploration and histological examination of the pancreatic tumor. Complete cures can result from resection of benign adenomas, and temporary remissions have been reported after resection of primary malignant tumors which later recurred. Tumor resection usually results in restoration of elevated serum calcium to normal values. If increased serum calcium persists after operation, parathyroid adenoma may also be present. When complete resection of the tumor is impossible and severe diarrhea continues, steroid therapy should be instituted. Doses of 20 mg of prednisone or greater per day have been effective in controlling diarrhea in six of ten patients so treated.[5] One reported complication of steroid treatment has been the development of gastric acid hypersecretion and peptic ulceration.[2] Successful chemotherapy and X-ray therapy for metastatic disease have not been reported.

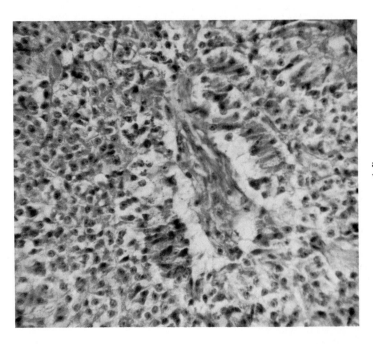

Figure 28–3. Section of pancreatic tumor resected from a patient with pancreatic cholera. × 450.

INSULINOMA

Although patients with insulinoma are seen by the gastroenterologist less frequently than patients with gastrinoma, these tumors are probably the most common type of functioning islet cell tumor. The association between fasting hypoglycemia and islet cell tumors has been recognized for nearly half a century; over 1000 cases have been reported in the world literature. Insulinoma is the most common cause of fasting hypoglycemia in adults. A complete discussion of the hypoglycemic syndromes is beyond the scope of this chapter. The subject has been reviewed in an excellent monograph by Marks and Rose,[28] and hypoglycemic tumors have recently been reviewed by Laurent and colleague.[29]

CLINICAL PICTURE

The symptoms produced by insulinomas are caused by chronic and episodic hypoglycemia. They are frequently present for months to years before the diagnosis is recognized. Symptoms produced by malignant insulinomas may be more rapidly progressive and therefore may lead to earlier diagnosis.

Two general types of symptoms are found in patients with insulinoma. The first type occurs during rapid decrease in blood sugar. Symptoms usually do not develop until the true blood glucose concentration falls below 40 to 50 mg per 100 ml, but the threshold varies considerably among patients. Typical complaints include trembling, nervousness, sweating, palpitations, and apprehension.

More frequently, in patients with insulinoma, symptoms arise after a gradual onset of hypoglycemia. These symptoms are due to cerebral dysfunction caused by a lack of the glucose substrate necessary to maintain normal brain metabolism, and resemble the changes which occur with cerebral anoxia. Behavioral and neurological symptoms predominate. Thus patients with insulinoma are likely to be seen first by a psychiatrist or neurologist. Members of the family or friends of the patient may note erratic behavior, memory loss, or inability of the patient to perform tasks. Such patients often receive incorrect diagnoses of psychiatric disorders such as schizophrenia, hysteria, or manic psychosis, or of neurological disorders such as epilepsy, cerebrovascular disease, or brain tumor.

Gastrointestinal complaints are not especially noteworthy. Sensations of hunger are common but not invariable early symptoms. Associated duodenal ulcer probably occurs no more often than would be expected in the general population. Occasionally insulinoma and gastrinoma are found in the same patients; usually these are patients with pluriglandular syndrome.

Attacks of symptomatic hypoglycemia may be separated by symptom-free periods of up to several months. Initially symptoms are likely to occur later in the day, especially after missing a meal and following strenuous exercise. However, the patient frequently fails to make any association between eating and relief of symptoms. Later in the course of the disease symptoms are more frequent and are more likely to occur in the morning before breakfast. Clinical suspicion of symptomatic hypoglycemia can be confirmed during an attack by observing Whipple's triad: (1) blood sugar level of less than 40 mg per 100 ml; (2) symptoms of hypoglycemia; and (3) dramatic and immediate relief of symptoms upon intravenous administration of glucose. Following severe, prolonged hypoglycemia some of the neurological findings may not be reversed by glucose, indicating permanent brain damage. Demonstration of symptomatic hypoglycemia does not establish the diagnosis of insulinoma, because this condition can be produced by a number of other diseases.

Insulinomas occur in all age groups, including infants, but are more common in middle adult years and are slightly more common in females. No increased racial incidence has been demonstrated. Like gastrinomas, these tumors are especially common in patients with the familial pluriglandular syndrome.

LABORATORY FINDINGS

Clinical manifestations of insulinoma are produced by the inappropriate elaboration of insulin by the tumor. Most of this insulin appears to be identical to normal

pancreatic insulin, but a variable fraction—usually no greater than 10 per
cent—may be a larger molecule which is
fully immunoreactive in the insulin radioimmunoassay and corresponds closely
to proinsulin.[30] The most reliable diagnostic tests for insulinoma are based on the
findings of inappropriately elevated
plasma insulin concentrations in the setting of hypoglycemia, or plasma insulin
hyperresponses following intravenous injection of insulin-releasing agents. Glucose is the most effective stimulant of insulin release from the normal pancreas,
whereas tolbutamide, glucagon, and leucine are usually more effective than glucose in releasing insulin from tumor tissue.

The two major laboratory abnormalities
found in patients with insulinoma are hypoglycemia and inappropriate elevation of
plasma insulin concentration. For measurement of blood sugar, glucose oxidase
methods are preferable, because they
measure true glucose and are more accurate in the hypoglycemic range. Values
less than 40 mg per 100 ml are indicative
of hypoglycemia. Plasma insulin concentrations are determined by the radioimmunoassay method of Yalow and Berson or
by one of the modifications of this
method.[31]

Demonstration of fasting hypoglycemia
eliminates some of the most common
causes of hypoglycemia in the adult including idiopathic "reactive" hypoglycemia. It may be necessary to prolong fasting
for 48 to 72 hours to demonstrate hypoglycemia, and even then a period of exercise
may be necessary. However, in most instances an 18 to 24 hour fast is sufficient.
Because fasting may lead to severe symptoms, patients should be observed in the
hospital. Blood should be obtained at least
every eight hours for determination of
blood sugar and plasma insulin.

An alternative test for insulinoma is the
tolbutamide test. This test should not be
performed in the patient who is already
hypoglycemic, but it is useful for screening out questionable patients. When combined with insulin measurements, it is
probably the most specific test for insulinoma. A positive test is obtained when the
blood sugar shows prolonged depression
and the plasma insulin becomes markedly

elevated within the first few minutes after
injection of 1 g tolbutamide intravenously.
Similar degrees of insulin hypersecretion
may be produced by intravenous glucagon
and, in about half the patients with insulinoma, by leucine. The specific details of
these tests are given elsewhere.[32, 33]

Glucose tolerance tests are not very
helpful in establishing the diagnosis of
insulinoma. The glucose curve may be
normal or diabetic in the early phases,
and may or may not reveal a hypoglycemic
"rebound" three to six hours after glucose.

Since the tumors are small, routine
gastrointestinal X-rays and hypotonic
duodenography are not particularly helpful in demonstrating the tumor. Selective
celiac axis arteriography has been successful in localizing these vascular
tumors in up to half the reported attempts.[34] Pancreatic scanning procedures
have yielded disappointing results.

DIFFERENTIAL DIAGNOSIS

Insulinoma must be differentiated from
other conditions which cause fasting hypoglycemia in the adult. The combination
of fasting hypoglycemia and increased
plasma insulin concentration is not found
in any other condition except exogenous
administration of insulin. This possibility
must be excluded by observation of the patient. Repeated injections of insulin lead
to development of insulin antibodies,
usually within six to eight weeks after
beginning repeated injections, and these
antibodies can be detected by radioimmunoassay methods. Hypoglycemia may
also result from administration of oral hypoglycemic agents, alcohol, and other
drugs and poisons. Other common hypoglycemic conditions, including essential
reactive hypoglycemia, postgastrectomy
hypoglycemia, and hypoglycemia associated with early diabetes, occur only
after carbohydrate ingestion and are not
found in the fasting state.

The major causes of fasting hypoglycemia in the adult are listed in Table 28–1.
Hypoglycemia is not a common complication of severe hepatocellular disease. It
has been reported as an occasional complication of a diverse group of liver diseases,
including cirrhosis, metastatic carcinoma,

TABLE 28–1. CLASSIFICATION OF FASTING HYPOGLYCEMIA IN ADULTS

Pancreatic beta cell tumor
  Carcinoma
  Adenoma
  Microadenomatosis

Nonpancreatic tumor
  Mesenchymal
  Hepatic
  Adrenal
  Epithelial

Liver disease
  Hepatocellular
  Biliary
  Congenital: glycogen storage disease,
    galactosemia

Endocrine deficiency
  Anterior pituitary
  Adrenal cortex
  Pancreatic alpha cell
  Thyroid

Starvation

Factitious
  Exogenous hypoglycemic agents
  Ethanol

ascending cholangitis, hepatic abscess, and passive congestion. The pathogenesis is obscure in these cases.

Deficiency of insulin-antagonizing hormones is another cause of hypoglycemia. The most common extrapancreatic endocrine disorder in which this occurs is adrenal insufficiency which may be due to primary adrenal failure, ACTH deficiency, or adrenogenital syndrome. Deficiency of cortisol leads to diminished gluconeogenesis and glycogenesis as well as enhanced peripheral effects of insulin and decreased antagonism by epinephrine and glucagon. Hypoglycemia is found in about 10 per cent of patients with pituitary insufficiency, especially with growth hormone deficiency. Growth hormone impedes glucose uptake by muscle and activates lipolysis, providing glycerol and fatty acids for metabolism. One case of fasting hypoglycemia caused by primary glucagon deficiency has been reported.[32]

After the aforementioned diagnostic considerations have been excluded by appropriate tests, the differential diagnosis includes insulinoma and nonpancreatic neoplasms. The nonpancreatic neoplasms can be further subdivided into mesenchymal and nonmesenchymal tumors. The mesenchymal tumors are composed predominantly of spindle cells of fibroblastic origin. They have been found in approximately equal distribution in intra-abdominal, intrathoracic, and retroperitoneal sites.[29] They are invariably large, usually 10 to 20 cm in diameter and weighing 1 to 5 kg, and occur in an older age group than insulinomas as a rule. Of the nonmesenchymal tumors, hepatoma and adrenocortical carcinoma are most commonly associated with hypoglycemia. About 40 patients with hypoglycemia associated with hepatoma have been reported.[29] Hypoglycemia usually occurs within the first three months of the onset of tumor symptoms. About 80 per cent have been reported in men. The blood sugar effects are apparently not due to parenchymal liver destruction, because similar involvement of the liver with metastatic carcinoma seldom causes hypoglycemia. In the eight reported cases of adrenocortical tumors with hypoglycemia, fasting hypoglycemia usually occurs late in the disease and is accompanied by signs of adrenocortical hyperactivity. A heterogeneous group of metastatic epithelial tumors producing similar symptoms has included primary carcinomas of the stomach, esophagus, colon, urinary bladder, bronchus, testicle, and ovary.[29]

The mechanism of hypoglycemia in these tumors is not completely understood. Some tumors appear to produce substances with insulin-like activity but which are immunochemically distinct from insulin and are not measured by the insulin radioimmunoassay.[35] These tumors are thus distinguished from insulinomas by the lack of increased plasma insulin concentrations. The tumors are large, and metabolism of glucose by the tumors may play an important role. They may also interfere in some way with gluconeogenesis and glycogenolysis.[36, 37] Resection of the whole tumor or even of a major portion usually ameliorates the hypoglycemic attacks.

PATHOLOGY

Insulinomas are derived from pancreatic beta cells. The tumors are usually small, averaging 1 to 2 cm in diameter and rarely exceeding 5 cm. About 10 to 15 per cent produce metastases, and a similar proportion of patients have two or more pancreatic adenomas. Islet cell hyperplasia alone is not a well recognized cause of hyperinsulinism. Distribution of insulinomas in the pancreas corresponds to the distribution of normal islet tissue. Microscopically the tumors resemble the other islet cell tumors but tend to be more vascular. Beta granules can usually be demonstrated by electron microscopy or by special staining techniques, but tumor cells frequently contain fewer granules than normal beta cells.

THERAPY

Once the diagnosis of insulinoma has been made, the tumor should be surgically removed as soon as possible. Delay increases the chances of permanent brain damage caused by profound hypoglycemia. Complete mobilization of the pancreas is essential, with careful exploration to exclude the possibility of multiple adenomas. Successful excision of the tumor should result in prompt increase in blood sugar. If no tumor is found, subtotal pancreatectomy is usually performed. Blind resection of the distal two-thirds of the pancreas is likely to be curative in about 60 per cent of patients in whom no tumor is found.[38] Usually there is a period of hyperglycemia in the postoperative period until normal beta cell function is re-established.

In patients with metastatic insulinoma or in whom surgical removal of the tumor is not otherwise possible, management is a difficult problem. Insulin antagonists such as steroids, growth hormone, and long-acting glucagon have been tried with limited success. Frequent carbohydrate feedings are used as supplementary therapy. Diazoxide, a nondiuretic benzothiadiazine with hyperglycemic properties, has been prescribed successfully in several patients with islet cell carcinoma.[32, 39] It appears to act both by lowering the plasma insulin concentration and by extrapancreatic effects. Since diazoxide causes salt and water retention, thiazide diuretics usually are administered also. These diuretics also appear to potentiate the hyperglycemic effects of diazoxide by depletion of potassium and may also minimize gastrointestinal side effects of the drug.

Another promising agent for management of metastatic insulinoma is streptozotocin, an antibiotic derived from *Streptomyces acromogenes*, which produces beta cell damage in animals. Several patients have responded favorably to this agent, given in doses of 1 to 4 g with total doses up to 20 mg.[40, 41] Renal toxicity appears to be the major side effect.

GLUCAGONOMA

Malignant islet cell tumors have been described in two patients with hyperglycemia and markedly elevated plasma glucagon concentrations.[43, 43] The tumors were found to be composed of alpha cells by histochemical and electron microscopical examination. Immunoreactive and biologically active glucagon was extracted from hepatic metastases in one patient.[42] No additional patients have been described in the past several years, except one whose tumor apparently produced insulin, gastrin, and glucagon.[40] The clinical course of these patients does not support the idea that glucagon hypersecretion causes the pancreatic cholera syndrome, as neither patient had diarrhea or hypokalemia. Recently a patient with a glucagon-producing renal tumor was reported.[44] This patient had steatorrhea without diarrhea, abnormal small bowel X-rays, and marked hypertrophy of intestinal villi. After successful tumor resection the patient regained normal bowel function. Until more patients with glucagon-producing tumors are discovered, it is impossible to predict the probable clinical manifestations other than hyperglycemia.

MULTIPLE AND ECTOPIC HORMONE SECRETION

Occasionally a single islet cell tumor may produce more than one peptide hormone or may secrete a hormone not known to be produced by normal islet cells. The carcinoid syndrome may occasionally be produced by islet cell tumors. Since the normal pancreas contains a few argentaffin cells, this is probably not an example of ectopic hormone secretion. Secretion of ACTH is a better example and has been found several times. Some examples of multiple hormone secretion by single tumors include the secretion of gastrin, ACTH, and MSH; insulin and gastrin; insulin and ACTH; ACTH and MSH; insulin and serotonin; and insulin, gastrin, and glucagon. Production of hypercalcemia in patients with pancreatic cholera may reflect secretion of a parathyroid-like hormone from these tumors, but such a substance has not yet been extracted.

TABLE 28–2. FEATURES OF FAMILIAL POLYENDOCRINE DISEASE

Organs Involved		Clinical Features	
Parathyroid	88%	Hyperparathyroidism	87%
Pancreas	81%	Peptic ulcer disease	56%
Pituitary	65%	Hypoglycemia	36%
Adrenals	19%	Chromophobe adenoma	28%
Thyroid	19%	Acromegaly	19%
		Diarrhea	13%
		Lipomas	13%
		Cushing's syndrome	2%
		Hyperthyroidism	2%

ASSOCIATION OF ISLET CELL TUMORS WITH OTHER ENDOCRINE TUMORS

Tumors of nonpancreatic endocrine tissues are found in about 20 per cent of patients with Zollinger-Ellison syndrome and in about 5 per cent of patients with insulinoma or pancreatic cholera. Hyperparathyroidism is the most common associated endocrine abnormality. Pituitary tumors are also common. The pathological abnormality in the endocrine glands may consist of carcinomas, single or multiple adenomas, or diffuse hyperplasia. Because of the diverse endocrine pathology, the term pluriglandular syndrome would seem preferable to multiple endocrine adenomatosis.

A familial incidence of pluriglandular syndrome was described by Wermer in 1954.[45] Subsequently, several other families have been discovered with a similar syndrome,[46] also called multiple endocrine neoplasia, type I.[47] Another disease, called multiple endocrine neoplasia, type II, is characterized by the association of pheochromocytoma, medullary carcinoma of the thyroid, and hyperparathyroidism, but is not associated with pancreatic tumors.[48] In the familial form, pluriglandular syndrome is inherited as an autosomal dominant with high but variable expressivity. The distribution of organ involvement and most common clinical features are listed in Table 28–2, compiled from 85 patients reviewed by Ballard et al.[46] Pluriglandular syndrome is also found in patients with no apparent familial endocrinopathy, especially patients with Zollinger-Ellison syndrome and hyperparathyroidism.

The most common causes of death in patients with pluriglandular syndrome are complications of peptic ulcer and hypoglycemia. Patients with this syndrome are much more likely to have multiple parathyroid adenomas or diffuse hyperplasia of all four parathyroid glands than are patients with uncomplicated hyperparathyroidism. Multiple adenomas and diffuse hyperplasia of the pancreas and pituitary are also common.

All patients with islet cell tumors should have determinations of serum calcium and X-rays of the sella turcica as screening procedures for associated endocrine tumors. When pluriglandular syndrome is discovered or when two or more members of a single family are discovered to have islet cell or parathyroid tumors, the remaining family members should be examined. Hyperparathyroidism is the most common asymptomatic endocrine tumor in this syndrome, and it can usually be detected by serum calcium determinations. Patients with Zollinger-Ellison syndrome, insulinoma, or pancreatic cholera are usually symptomatic. Family members with symptoms of peptic ulcer, hypoglycemia, or diarrhea should be investigated more extensively. It has not yet been established whether all patients with single functioning islet cell tumors represent variants of the familial pluriglandular syndrome with differing clinical manifestations.

REFERENCES

1. Verner, J. V., and Morrison, A. B. Islet cell tumor and a syndrome of refractory watery diarrhea and hypokalemia. Amer. J. Med. 25:374, 1958.
2. Marks, I. N., Bank, S., and Louw, J. H. Islet cell tumor of the pancreas with reversible watery diarrhea and achlorhydria. Gastroenterology 52:695, 1967.
3. Matsumoto, K. K., Peter, J. B., Schultze, R. G., Hakim, A. A., and Franck, P. T. Watery diarrhea and hypokalemia associated with pancreatic islet cell adenoma. Gastroenterology 50:231, 1966.
4. Walsh, J. H., and Sleisenger, M. H. Clinical syndromes associated with tumors of the pancreas. In Disease-a-Month, H. F. Dowling (ed.). Chicago, Year Book Medical Publishers, Inc., 1967.
5. Verner, J. V. Clinical syndromes associated with non-insulin producing tumors of the pancreatic islets. In Non-Insulin-Producing Tumors of the Pancreas, International Symposium at Erlangen, July 16–17, 1968, L. Demling and R. Ottenjann (eds.). Stuttgart, Georg Thieme Verlag, 1968, p. 125.
6. Kraft, A. R., Tompkins, R. K., and Zollinger, R. M. Recognition and management of the diarrheal syndrome caused by nonbeta islet cell tumors of the pancreas. Amer. J. Surg. 119:163, 1970.
7. Stoker, D. J., and Wynn, V. Pancreatic islet cell tumour with watery diarrhoea and hypokalaemia. Gut 11:911, 1970.
8. Murray, J. S., Paton, R. R., and Pope, C. E., II. Pancreatic tumor associated with flushing and diarrhea. New Eng. J. Med. 264:436, 1961.
9. Shafer, W. H., McCormack, L. J., and Hoerr, S. O. Non-beta islet-cell carcinoma of the pancreas, with flushing attacks and diarrhea. Cleveland Clin. Quart. 32:13, 1965.
10. Espiner, E. A., and Beaven, D. W. Non-specific islet-cell tumour of the pancreas with diarrhoea. Quart. J. Med. 31:447, 1962.
11. Kofstad, J., Frøyshov, I., Gjone, E., and Blix, S. Pancreatic tumor with intractable watery diarrhea, hypokalemia and hypercalcemia electrolyte balance studies. Scand. J. Gastroenterol. 2:246, 1967.
12. Gjone, E., Fretheim, B., Nordöy, A., Jacobsen, C. D., and Elgjo, K. Intractable watery diarrhoea, hypokalaemia, and achlorhydria associated with pancreatic tumour containing gastric secretory inhibitor. Scand. J. Gastroenterol. 5:401, 1970.
13. Andersson, H., Dotevall, G., Fagerberg, G., Raotma, H., Walan, A., and Zederfeldt, B. Pancreatic tumour with diarrhoea, hypokalemia and hypochlorhydria. Acta Chir. Scand. 138:102, 1972.
14. DaCruz, G. M. G., Gardner, J. D., and Peskin, G. W. Mechanism of diarrhea of villous adenomas. Amer. J. Surg. 115:203, 1968.
15. Zollinger, R. M., Tompkins, R. K., Amerson, J. R., Endahl, G. L., Kraft, A. R., and Moore, F. T. Identification of the diarrheogenic hormone associated with non-beta islet cell tumors of the pancreas. Ann. Surg. 168:502, 1968.
16. Gardner, J. D., and Cerda, J. J. In vitro inhibition of intestinal fluid and electrolyte transfer by a non-beta islet cell tumor. Proc. Soc. Exp. Biol. Med. 123:361, 1966.
17. Semb, L. S., Gjone, E., and Rosenthal, W. S. Bioassay for gastric secretory inhibitor in extract of pancreatic tumor from patient with WDHA-syndrome. Scand. J. Gastroenterol. 5:409, 1970.
18. Barbezat, G. O., and Grossman, M. I. Intestinal secretion: Stimulation by peptides. Science 174:422, 1971.
19. Pederson, R. A., and Brown, J. C. Inhibition of histamine-, pentagastrin-, and insulin-stimulated canine gastric secretion by pure "gastric inhibitory polypeptide." Gastroenterology 62:393, 1972.
20. Said, S. I., and Mutt, V. Polypeptide with broad biological activity: Isolation from small intestine. Science 169:1217, 1970.
21. Hubel, K. A. Effects of secretin and glucagon on intestinal transport of ions and water in the rat. Proc. Soc. Exp. Biol. Med. 139:656, 1972.
22. Mekhjian, H., King, D., Sanzenbacher, L., and Zollinger, R. Glucagon (Gl) and secretin (Se) inhibit water and electrolyte transport in the human jejunum. Gastroenterology 62:782, 1972.
23. Pierce, N. F., Carpenter, C. C. J., Elliott, H. L., and Greenough, W. B., III. Effects of prostaglandins, theophylline, and cholera exotoxin upon transmucosal water and electrolyte movement in the canine jejunum. Gastroenterology 60:22, 1971.
24. Birge, S. J., and Avioli, L. V. Glucagon-induced hypocalcemia in man. J. Clin. Endocrinol. 29:213, 1969.
25. Serebro, H. A., McGonagle, T., Iber, F. I., Royall, R., and Hendrix, T. R. An effect of cholera toxin on small intestine without direct mucosal contact. Johns Hopkins Med. J. 123:229, 1968.
26. Field, M. Intestinal secretion: Effect of cyclic AMP and its role in cholera. New Eng. J. Med. 284:1137, 1971.
27. Moore, W. L., Jr., Bieberdorf, F. A., Morawski, S. G., Finkelstein, R. A., and Fordtran, J. S. Ion transport during cholera-induced ileal secretion in the dog. J. Clin. Invest. 50:312, 1971.
28. Marks, V., and Rose, F. C. Hypoglycemia. Oxford, Blackwell Scientific Publications, 1965.
29. Laurent, J., Debry, G., and Floquet, J. Hypoglycaemic Tumours. Amsterdam, Excerpta Medica, 1971.
30. Goldsmith, S. J., Yalow, R. S., and Berson, S. A. Significance of human plasma insulin sephadex fractions. Diabetes 18:834, 1969.
31. Yalow, R. S., and Berson, S. A. Immunoassay of endogenous plasma insulin in man. J. Clin. Invest. 39:1157, 1960.
32. Bleicher, S. J. Hypoglycemia. In Diabetes Mellitus: Theory and Practice, M. Ellenberg and H. Rifkin (eds.). New York, McGraw-Hill Book Company, 1970.
33. Marks, V. Progress report: Diagnosis of insulinoma. Gut 12:835, 1971.
34. Dunn, D. C. Pancreatic islet cell tumour demonstrated by aortography. Proc. Roy. Soc. Med. 61:957, 1968.

35. Yalow, R. S., and Berson, S. A. Dynamics of insulin secretion in hypoglycemia. Diabetes *14*:341, 1965.

36. Unger, R. H. The riddle of tumor hypoglycemia. Amer. J. Med. *40*:325, 1966.

37. Chandalia, H. B., and Boshell, B. R. Hypoglycemia associated with extrapancreatic tumors: Report of two cases with studies on its pathogenesis. Arch. Intern. Med. *129*:447, 1972.

38. Moss, N. H., and Rhoads, J. E. Hyperinsulinism and islet cell tumors of the pancreas. *In* Surgical Diseases of the Pancreas, J. M. Howard and G. L. Jordan (eds.). Philadelphia, J. B. Lippincott Company, 1960, p. 321.

39. Marks, V., Rose, F. C., and Samols, E. Hyperinsulinism due to metastasizing insulinoma: Treatment with diazoxide. Proc. Roy Soc. Med. *58*:577, 1965.

40. Murray-Lyon, I. M., Eddleston, A. L. W. F., Williams, R., Brown, M., Hogbin, B. M., Bennett, A., Edwards, J. C., and Taylor, K. W. Treatment of multiple-hormone-producing malignant islet-cell tumour with streptozotocin. Lancet *2*:895, 1968.

41. Blackard, W. G., Garcia, A. R., and Brown, C. L., Jr. Effect of streptozotocin on qualitative aspects of plasma insulin in a patient with a malignant islet cell tumor. J. Clin. Endocrinol. *31*:214, 1970.

42. McGavran, M. H., Unger, R. H., Recant, L., Polk, H. C., Kilo, C., and Levin, M. E. A glucagon-secreting alpha-cell carcinoma of the pancreas. New Eng. J. Med. *274*:1408, 1966.

43. Yoshinaga, T., Okuna, G., Shinji, Y., Tsujii, T., and Nishikawa, M. Pancreatic A-cell tumor associated with severe diabetes mellitus. Diabetes *15*:709, 1966.

44. Gleeson, M. H., Bloom, S. R., Polak, J. M., Henry, K., and Dowling, R. H. Endocrine tumour in kidney affecting small bowel structure, motility, and absorptive function. Gut *12*:773, 1971.

45. Wermer, P. Genetic aspects of adenomatosis of endocrine glands. Amer. J. Med. *16*:363, 1954.

46. Ballard, H. S., Frame, B., and Hartsock, R. J. Familial multiple endocrine adenoma-peptic ulcer complex. Medicine *43*:481, 1964.

47. Craven, D. E., Goodman, A. D., and Carter, J. H. Familial multiple endocrine adenomatosis: Multiple endocrine neoplasia, type I. Arch. Intern. Med. *129*:567, 1972.

48. Steiner, A. L., Goodman, A. D., and Powers, S. R. Study of a kindred with pheochromocytoma, medullary thyroid carcinoma, hyperparathyroidism and Cushing's disease: Multiple endocrine neoplasia, type II. Medicine *47*:371, 1968.

Chapter 29

Blood Supply of the Gut and Pathophysiology of Ischemia

Robert K. Ockner

In the past decade, advances in angiography and vascular surgery and in the management of problems of nutrition and fluid balance after intestinal resection have led to an increased understanding and awareness of various vascular syndromes of the gastrointestinal tract.[1, 2] As a result, although a number of these syndromes continue to carry a grave prognosis, it is now possible to approach them more vigorously, with the expectation that, in certain situations, early diagnosis and treatment may significantly improve the outlook.

ANATOMY OF THE SPLANCHNIC CIRCULATION

The intra-abdominal portions of the digestive tract are nourished almost entirely by three major unpaired arterial trunks arising from the ventral aspect of the abdominal aorta, including the celiac axis, superior mesenteric artery, and inferior mesenteric artery. The anatomy of these vessels, including their anastomotic interrelationships and potential for collateral formation, determines the consequences of acute or chronic vascular occlusion and, therefore, is important not only to an understanding of the pathogenesis of intestinal ischemia, but also as the basis for a sound approach to its clinical diagnosis and management.

Celiac Axis. This large vessel usually originates at a level between the twelfth thoracic and first lumbar vertebrae, passes next to the median arcuate ligament of the diaphragm, and almost immediately gives rise to three major branches: the splenic, left gastric, and hepatic arteries (Fig. 29–1). All three branches contribute to the blood supply of the stomach. The splenic artery supplies the greater curvature via the short gastric and left gastroepiploic branches. The left gastric artery supplies primarily the lesser curvature of the stomach, and may anastomose with the right gastric branch of the hepatic artery. The hepatic artery also gives rise to the gastroduodenal artery; this vessel in turn divides into the right gastroepiploic and superior pancreaticoduodenal arteries. Because of this rich, interconnecting network about both the greater and the lesser curvatures of the stomach, ischemic infarction of this organ as an isolated event is most unusual.[3]

Of particular importance are the smaller vessels, derived from the hepatic artery, which supply the pancreas and duodenum. As noted, the gastroduodenal artery gives rise to the *superior* pancreaticoduodenal arteries (anterior and posterior), and these in turn form a series of anastomotic connections about the second, third, and fourth portions of the duodenum, designated the pancreaticoduodenal arcades. The important contribution to these arcades by branches of the *inferior* pancreaticoduodenal arteries (derived from the superior mesenteric

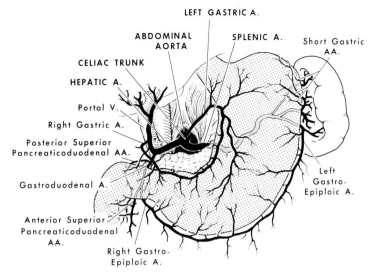

Figure 29-1. Blood supply to the stomach and duodenum. Each of the three major branches of the celiac axis supplying the stomach and the anastomotic connections to the superior mesenteric artery near the duodenum are illustrated.

artery) constitutes an anastomotic connection of major importance between the celiac and the superior mesenteric arteries (Figs. 29–1 and 29–2).

Superior Mesenteric Artery. This vessel (Fig. 29–2) originates behind the pancreas at the level of the first lumbar vertebra, just caudal to the celiac axis. It emerges from behind the lower border of the body of the pancreas, and passes anterior to the uncinate process of the pancreas and the third portion of the duodenum. Distal to the origin of the inferior pancreaticoduodenal artery, the superior

mesenteric artery gives rise to three major branches, the middle colic, right colic, and ileocolic arteries, and also to a series of smaller intestinal branches which nourish the jejunum and ileum. The intestinal branches form a series of three or four arcades before entering the wall of the intestine as the arteriae rectae. Although there is considerable potential for collateral flow within the primary and secondary arcades, the arteriae rectae appear to represent end arteries, and few, if any, important anastomotic connections are present within the bowel wall itself. Accordingly,

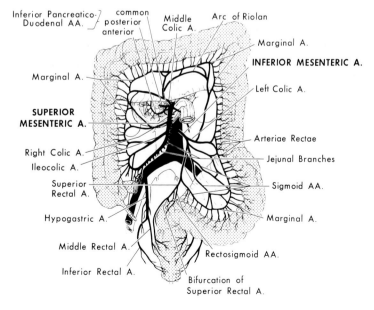

Figure 29-2. Blood supply to the small and large intestines. Anastomotic connections to the celiac axis in the region of the duodenum are shown, as are those between the superior and inferior mesenteric arteries. Illustrated here are those branches of the left and middle colic arteries which in a number of patients connect directly (and apart from the marginal artery) to form the arc of Riolan, or "meandering mesenteric" artery.

occlusion of these distal vessels may lead to local areas of infarction. The ileocolic artery anastomoses in the vicinity of the cecum with the continuation of the main trunk of the superior mesenteric and supplies the terminal ileum, cecum, and proximal ascending colon. The right colic artery (which may arise directly from the middle colic artery itself) is responsible primarily for supplying the ascending colon and hepatic flexure, whereas the middle colic artery supplies the proximal portion of the transverse colon. Anastomotic connections of major clinical importance exist between the middle colic artery and branches of the inferior mesenteric artery, as noted below.

Inferior Mesenteric Artery. This vessel, smaller in caliber than the celiac and superior mesenteric, originates at the level of the third lumbar vertebra and carries blood to the distal transverse colon, the descending and sigmoid colon, and the proximal portions of the rectum (Fig. 29–2). The left colic branch supplies the distal transverse and descending colon and may, in addition, anastomose directly with the middle colic artery through the arc of Riolan, or "meandering mesenteric" artery (Fig. 29–3).[4, 5] The inferior mesenteric artery also gives rise to two or three sigmoid arteries and finally terminates as the superior rectal artery. In addition to the meandering mesenteric artery, the adjacent branches of the sigmoidal, left colic, middle colic, right colic, and ileocolic arteries form a continuous arterial channel paralleling the course of the large intestine along its mesenteric aspect. This channel, the marginal artery of Drummond, gives rise to arteriae rectae which enter the wall of the colon itself. In some individuals, this channel is of adequate caliber to function as a route for collateral supply in the event that one of the larger vessels from which it is derived is occluded. In many, however, it is the meandering mesenteric artery that serves as the major collateral route between superior and inferior mesenteric arterial systems.[4]

The distal portions of the rectum are supplied primarily by the middle rectal and inferior rectal arteries, derived from the hypogastric (internal iliac) arteries.

General Anatomical Considerations. From this brief review of the

splanchnic vascular anatomy, it is evident that the blood supply to the intra-abdominal portion of the gastrointestinal tract is richly endowed with several anastomotic interconnections which help protect against the consequences of occlusive vascular disease. These anastomotic interconnections, including the pancreaticoduodenal arcades, the meandering mesenteric artery, and the marginal artery of Drummond, are normally sufficiently developed to permit collateral flow. Thus it is theoretically possible for *all* the intra-abdominal viscera to be adequately supplied by only one of the three major aortic branches, and, indeed, this circumstance has been documented.[6]

Conversely, it is equally apparent that the arterial supply to the digestive organs possesses certain areas of particular vul-

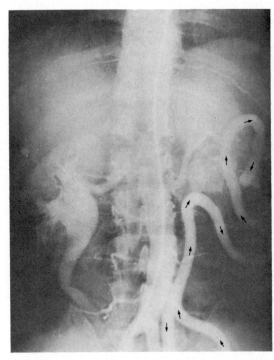

Figure 29–3. Arteriographic demonstration of the meandering mesenteric artery. In this patient with extensive splanchnic arterial disease, the inferior mesenteric artery and the meandering mesenteric artery (arrows) play a major role in the blood supply to the entire intra-abdominal gastrointestinal tract via anastomotic connections with the superior mesenteric artery. (From Sachs, R. P., Sheft, D. J., and Freeman, J. H.: Amer. J. Roent. Radium Ther. Nuc. Med. *102*:418, 1968.)

nerability, at which collateral supply may be of only marginal adequacy. These areas include the arteriae rectae as they enter the wall of the small intestine, and the "water-shed" areas in the distal transverse colon and splenic flexure and at the junction of the superior and middle portions of the rectum, where branches of the inferior mesenteric artery anastomose with branches of the superior mesenteric and hypogastric arteries, respectively.

Venous Circulation. In general, veins parallel arteries in the smaller branches and for portions of the main mesenteric trunks. However, rather than entering the vena cava, the superior mesenteric and splenic veins join to form the portal vein which enters the liver, after receiving additional blood from the gastric circulation via the coronary vein. The inferior mesenteric vein drains into the splenic vein.

REGULATION OF SPLANCHNIC BLOOD FLOW

In addition to its dependence on adequate vascular channels, the flow of blood to the abdominal viscera is subject to modification by a wide variety of physiological factors.[7, 8] These factors operate primarily by regulating the degree of constriction or dilatation at the arteriolar level. Thus, small intestinal blood flow and mucosal oxygen consumption are increased by the presence of nutrients in the intestinal lumen, as well as by certain hormones, including gastrin, secretin, and cholecystokinin. In addition, as in other structures, metabolites produced during muscular activity may exert a local vasodilatory effect. Sympathomimetic amines affect splanchnic arteriolar muscle in a predictable manner: alpha-adrenergic stimulators cause vasoconstriction, whereas beta-stimulators cause dilatation. In this way isoproterenol, almost exclusively a beta-stimulator, causes increased splanchnic blood flow. It should be noted, however, that the overall effect of autonomic activity on *blood flow* is complex, and reflects not only arteriolar tone, but also concomitant effects on smooth muscle and intraluminal pressure. Regulation of splanchnic blood flow is further complicated by the phenomenon of autoregulation, by which variations in systemic arterial pressure are compensated for by changes in arteriolar tone, so as to maintain a relatively constant capillary flow.[9]

Factors which cause a decrease in intestinal blood flow include physical exercise, marked increases in intraluminal pressure, angiotensin II, and alpha-stimulating sympathomimetic amines, including epinephrine and norepinephrine. There is evidence suggesting that adrenergic stimuli have a relatively more pronounced effect on mucosal blood flow than on flow to the remainder of the gut wall.[10] In addition, there is evidence that cardiac glycosides also cause mesenteric arteriolar constriction and a decreased splanchnic blood flow.[9]

PATHOPHYSIOLOGICAL CONSIDERATIONS

The state of the visceral circulation, including such phenomena as local or widespread changes in blood flow and the extent, severity, and possible reversibility of any ischemic manifestations, will be the result of several factors. These factors may be temporal, anatomical, or physiological, and each must be evaluated for a proper understanding of the pathophysiology of ischemic vascular disease.

Temporal Factors. Slowly progressive occlusion of a large vessel may permit the development of adequate collaterals so that, although the major vessel itself may become completely occluded, collateral flow tends to minimize or prevent ischemia. This phenomenon, well recognized in the coronary and cerebral circulations, also applies to the splanchnic circulation. In contrast, a similar or even lesser degree of occlusion of the same vessel which occurs abruptly, or over a period of time too short for development of adequate collaterals, is more likely to cause ischemic necrosis. A classic example of this situation is that of the acute arterial embolus to the superior mesenteric artery in a young person with mitral stenosis but with relatively normal arteries. Undue delay in recognition and treatment of this event may result in intestinal infarction even though only one major vessel is occluded and collateral channels *in theory* are present.

In contrast, chronic occlusive disease ordinarily does not cause symptoms or signs of ischemia unless two or more major vessels are affected, because of the large number of potentially available collateral channels interconnecting the major arterial trunks. Thus, in the absence of some acute superimposed episode (e.g., embolization of an atherosclerotic plaque, hypotension, or anoxia), it would be unusual for a patient with chronic atherosclerotic disease to develop symptoms of intestinal ischemia without significant involvement of at least two major arterial trunks. An apparent exception to this generalization, however, is the fact that chronic occlusive disease of the celiac axis alone has been well documented as a cause of recurrent abdominal pain in some patients without evidence of other splanchnic arterial disease (see pp. 1563 to 1564).

Anatomical Factors. Disease processes (such as certain forms of vasculitis) which affect smaller vessels, particularly the arteriae rectae and/or the intramural arteries and arterioles, may cause segmental intestinal infarction, because anastomotic connections between these vessels are limited. Arterial emboli to the viscera almost always lodge in the superior mesenteric artery, probably because of its relatively large caliber and the obliquity of its take-off from the aorta. In contrast, the celiac axis, although large in caliber, originates at nearly a right angle to the aorta, whereas the inferior mesenteric artery, although oblique in its take-off, is relatively small in caliber. As a result, neither of these latter vessels is a frequent site of arterial embolization.

Physiological Factors. The foregoing temporal and anatomical considerations have dealt only with the factors that may affect the patency of a conduit for the flow of blood. It is clear that the amount of blood which actually flows through that conduit and the oxygen content of that blood are equally important in determining the adequacy of tissue oxygenation. As noted, arteriolar resistance is affected by a wide variety of local and systemic (including pharmacological) factors, any of which may enhance or reduce the blood supply to the organ in question. Moreover, blood which is poorly oxygenated, either because of reduced gas exchange in the pulmonary capillaries or because of stagnation and poor tissue perfusion, will predispose to ischemia. In this connection, a countercurrent exchange of oxygen in the arterioles and venules of intestinal villi

has been postulated.[9] In states of reduced blood flow, diffusion of oxygen from arteriole to venule (resulting in a lower arteriolar oxygen tension) becomes increasingly significant and may contribute to mucosal ischemia.

Another important factor is the oxygen requirement of the tissue at any given time. Thus increased oxygen consumption by the viscera during digestion of a meal is presumably the basis for the syndrome of abdominal angina, an uncommon but well described syndrome of postprandial abdominal pain in patients with diffuse splanchnic occlusive vascular disease.

An extreme example of the importance of physiological factors in determining the oxygen supply to the intestine is represented by the syndrome of nonthrombotic intestinal infarction. In ths disorder, widespread ischemic necrosis of the small intestine may occur in patients with anoxia and congestive heart failure or hypotension, but with no evidence of splanchnic vascular occlusion.

In the final analysis, adequate oxygenation of the abdominal viscera is a function of many factors, including patency of the major arterial trunks, arteriolar resistance, adequacy of perfusion pressure, arterial oxygen saturation, and the oxygen requirement of the tissues themselves. Any or all of these factors may change gradually or abruptly, depending upon the clinical circumstances, and may result in visceral ischemia.

HISTOPATHOLOGICAL AND FUNCTIONAL SEQUELAE OF VISCERAL ISCHEMIA

Acute ischemic necrosis is characterized by phenomena which reflect loss of capillary integrity, i.e., submucosal edema and hemorrhage. The epithelial layer is most sensitive to oxygen deprivation, and, experimentally, within five to ten minutes after occlusion of the superior mesenteric artery, ultrastructural changes are evident with the absorptive cells.[11] Subsequently, it undergoes necrosis and ulceration, and a variable inflammatory cell infiltrate appears (particularly in the colon), presumably in response both to tissue necrosis and to secondary bacterial invasion. The muscular layers of the bowel are more resistant to oxygen deprivation; only with more prolonged or severe ischemia do they undergo necrosis.

Viewed in the context of these histopathological events, certain of the clinical phenomena associated with bowel ischemia are readily understandable. For example, submucosal edema and hemorrhage are the basis for the so-called thumbprint pattern seen radiographically in patients with ischemic disease. Later, the tremendous outpouring of protein-rich fluid (and ultimately bleeding) into the lumen of the bowel reflects extensive loss of vascular and epithelial integrity. The development of peritonitis is a late manifestation, suggesting that even the relatively resistant muscular layers have become necrotic and that perforation has occurred or is imminent. In those ischemic episodes which are self-limited (i.e., those which do not perforate or require resection), the resolution of the acute inflammatory reaction is accompanied by granulation tissue, fibrosis, and, finally, the scar and stricture typical of this process.

GENERAL DIAGNOSTIC CONSIDERATIONS

Clinical diagnosis of visceral ischemic syndromes may be extremely difficult. The symptoms with which the patient may present are usually quite nonspecific, and often are classified mistakenly as unexplained abdominal pain, intestinal obstruction, or some other disease process which causes mucosal ulceration, bleeding, and edema. Moreover, routine radiographic procedures (plain films and barium contrast studies) are often not helpful, except when they can definitely exclude other more obvious disease processes. Furthermore, even the angiographic demonstration of stenosis, narrowing, or occlusion of a major vessel does not establish ischemia as the cause of the patient's symptoms, because such anatomic abnormalities are frequently noted in asymptomatic individuals. Indeed, Dick et al., in a detailed angiographic and clinical study of mesenteric vascular disease, could show only a relatively poor correlation between vessel size and clinical symptoms in the individual patient.[12] Conversely, the demonstration of patent vessels by arteriography does not exclude

ischemic disease, because of the critical dependence of mesenteric blood flow on circulatory, hormonal, and metabolic factors. Evidence for collateral circulation, e.g., angiographic visualization of the meandering mesenteric artery, suggests the presence of arterial occlusive disease, but does not establish it as a cause of symptoms. Moreover, disease of the smaller intramural vessels, such as may occur in certain forms of vasculitis, may or may not be demonstrable by selective angiography. Accordingly, the diagnosis of visceral ischemic syndromes requires not only a high index of suspicion but a careful evaluation of all available clinical, laboratory, and radiographic information. *No single clinical, laboratory, or radiographic finding, by itself, is either necessary or sufficient to establish the diagnosis of visceral ischemia.*

REFERENCES

1. Boley, S. J. (ed.). Vascular Disorders of the Intestine. New York, Appleton-Century-Crofts, 1971.
2. Williams, L. F., Jr. Vascular insufficiency of the intestine. Gastroenterology 61:757, 1971.
3. Cohen, E. B. Infarction of the stomach: Report of three cases of fatal gastric infarction and one case of partial infarction. Amer. J. Med. 11:645, 1951.
4. Moskowitz, M., Zimmerman, H., and Felson, B. The meandering mesenteric artery of the colon. Amer. J. Roent. 92:1088, 1964.
5. Gonzales, L. L., and Jaffe, M. S. Mesenteric arterial insufficiency following abdominal aortic resection. Arch. Surg. 93:10, 1966.
6. Reiner, L. Mesenteric arterial insufficiency and abdominal angina. Arch. Intern. Med. 114:765, 1964.
7. Bynum, T. E., and Jacobson, E. D. Blood flow and gastrointestinal function. Gastroenterology 60:325, 1971.
8. Jacobson, E. D. The gastrointestinal circulation. Ann. Rev. Med. 19:133, 1968.
9. Price, W. E., Rohrer, G. V., and Jacobson, E. D. Mesenteric vascular diseases. Gastroenterology 57:599, 1969.
10. Folkow, B., Lewis, D., Lindgren, O., Mellander, S., and Wallentin, I. The effect of the sympathetic vasoconstrictor fibers on the distribution of the capillary blood flow in the intestine. Acta Physiol. Scand. 61:458, 1964.
11. Brown, R. A., Chiv, C., Scott, H. J., and Gurd, F. N. Ultrastructural changes in the canine mucosal cell after mesenteric arterial occlusion. Arch. Surg. 101:290, 1970.
12. Dick, A. P., Gruff, R., and Gregg, D. An arteriographic study of mesenteric arterial disease. Gut 8:206, 1967.

Chapter 30

Systemic Disease and the Gut

David M. Roseman, Marvin H. Sleisenger

The gastrointestinal tract is affected to varying degrees by systemic diseases. Indeed, the most compelling clinical manifestations may originate in this organ system. The opportunity for diagnosis of systemic disease may likewise be in analysis of gut fluid or tissue. The extent of this involvement is discussed in the following pages, although much of this material is covered in greater detail in Part II.

ENDOCRINE DISEASES

DIABETES

Esophageal motor disturbances are more common in diabetes than is generally realized; they have recently been studied with both manometric and cineradiographic techniques.[1] Although depressed contraction of the posterior pharyngeal musculature is noted occasionally, dysfunction of the cricopharyngeal sphincter is unusual. Primary peristalsis in the cervical esophagus, or striated muscle segment, is often weak or absent. Incoordinated segmental contractions are common in the thoracic esophagus, or smooth muscle segment, and the primary peristaltic wave in this segment is likewise weak or absent. Depressed lower esophageal sphincter pressure is a common finding. The gastroesophageal sphincter frequently fails to relax fully in response to swallowing, or contracts prematurely. Although these motor alterations

delay esophageal emptying, clinical dysphagia is infrequent, and clinical symptoms of gastroesophageal reflux are rare. Esophageal dysfunction does not correlate with age or duration of diabetes or the presence of autonomic neuropathy. Cineradiographic studies confirm absent or diminished primary peristaltic waves, delayed esophageal emptying, and frequent tertiary contractions in many diabetic persons. These alterations may be a result of vagal neuropathy in the esophagus secondary to diabetes.

As seen radiographically, delayed emptying of the stomach is common in diabetes, occasionally leading to marked gastric retention. However, these changes are rarely associated with clinical symptoms. Basal and augmented acid secretions are lower than normal in the diabetic; in one study 17 per cent of diabetics secreted no acid after histamine.[2] The decrease in gastric secretion may explain the reported low incidence of duodenal ulcer in diabetics. Gastric ulcers occur with the usual frequency. The gastric mucosa in diabetics becomes atrophic at an earlier age and more commonly than in nondiabetics. As high as 65 per cent of diabetic subjects may have partial or complete atrophy of gastric mucosa. Studies indicate good correlation between impaired gastric secretion and histological mucosal abnormalities. Gastric parietal cell antibodies are increased in diabetics compared with control subjects, especially in young, female, insulin-dependent diabetics.[3] The duration of diabetes is apparently not an important factor in the production of parietal cell antibodies. Studies also indicate an increased incidence of intrinsic factor antibody in middle-aged and elderly female diabetics, with equal distribution between insulin-dependent and insulin-independent diabetic subjects. Most patients of this group with intrinsic factor antibody have achlorhydria and an abnormal Schilling test but not necessarily depleted body stores of vitamin B_{12}. Latent pernicious anemia appears to be more common in middle-aged and elderly diabetics, and is perhaps as high as 5 per cent in females in this age group. The association between problems of autoimmunity and insulin-dependent diabetes is probably due to a common genetic mechanism. Therapeutically, periodic testing of gastric secretion and/or a Schilling test seem indicated in middle-aged diabetics; if achlorhydria or malabsorption of Vitamin B_{12} is detected, monthly vitamin B_{12} administration by the parenteral route seems advisable for life.

Differentiation should be made between diarrhea and steatorrhea complicating diabetes. Diabetic diarrhea is found predominantly in insulin-dependent, young male diabetics (ages 20 to 40 years), often in association with retinopathy, nephropathy, and, most constantly, diabetic neuropathy.[4] The last is manifested by peripheral neuropathy and features of autonomic dysfunction, including impotence, defective sweating, pupillary abnormalities, orthostatic hypotension, impaired bladder emptying, and retrograde ejaculation. In diabetic diarrhea, bowel movements are profuse, watery, sometimes urgent, often preceded by abdominal cramps, and most frequent at night. The nocturnal bowel movements are a troublesome feature, often occurring unnoted during sleep. Daytime incontinence is also common. Unexplained and unexpected remissions and exacerbations of diarrhea are the rule. The impaired perception of rectal distention and subsequent defecation suggests a defect in afferent impulses. Measurement of anal sphincter strength, including pressures generated by maximal voluntary contraction, indicates no difference between normal subjects and diabetic patients. Radiographic features of diabetic diarrhea are those of diabetic autonomic neuropathy and include delayed gastric emptying, prolonged transit time, dilated bowel loops, segmentation, and coarsening of mucosal folds. Studies by more refined techniques show considerable variability in intestinal transit time, which may be shortened or unduly prolonged. Autonomic neuropathy appears to play a crucial but poorly understood role in the genesis of diabetic diarrhea, perhaps analogous to the disordered gastric and small bowel motility common in postvagotomy patients. The only significant autonomic lesions reported in patients with diabetes, whether diarrhea is present or not, have been nonspecific dendritic swellings in the sympathetic prevertebral and paravertebral ganglia. Ganglion cells of the plexuses of Auerbach and Meissner have been normal. Therapeutic avenues are limited. Probably most useful is strict control of diabetes with carefully regulated insulin dosage. Ice drinks should be restricted. Psyllium hydrophilic mucilloid (Metamucil) powder and diphenoxylate hydrochloride with atropine sulfate (Lomotil) may be tried.

Steatorrhea[5] may complicate diabetic diarrhea, and, if severe, should be evaluated by specific tests of malabsorption, as outlined on pages 260 to 268. The mechanism of steatorrhea in diabetes is unexplained, but in a small number of patients it may be due to (1) defective pancreatic exocrine function; (2) bacterial overgrowth complicating motility disturbances; or (3) concomitant adult celiac disease (see Table 30–1). Subacute and chronic pancreatitis may be associated with diabetes, and in some patients is causal. Clinical studies have found that 20 to 70 per cent of unselected diabetic patients, including juvenile diabetics, have abnormalities in the standardized secretin test, usually low volume and/or low amylase. Gross pancreatic exocrine deficiency, however, is a rare sequel of the diabetic state. Pancreatic enzyme replacement therapy usually does not ameliorate the steatorrhea even when abnormalities are detected in the secretin test. Attempts to demonstrate bacterial overgrowth in diabetic steatorrhea have been largely unrewarding. However, a small number of patients appear to have excessive bacterial flora in the proximal

TABLE 30–1. DIABETES WITH ADULT
CELIAC DISEASE*

DETERMINATIONS	RESULTS
Stool fat	40.0 g/24 hr
5HIAA	13.4 mg/24 hr
IAA	54.3 mg/24 hr
Indican	167.0 mg/24 hr
D-Xylose	1.3 g/5 hr
Small bowel series	Malabsorption pattern
Pancreatic drainage	Vol. 160 cc;
	$HCO_3 = 104$ mEq/liter
Jejunal biopsy	Villous atrophy

*This patient had slightly depressed serum choles-
terol and was losing weight despite good control of
diabetes. Diarrhea was not nocturnal.

small intestine.[6] Theoretically, in such patients, deconjugation of bile salts by enteric anaerobic bacteria may lead to defective micellar formation and fat malabsorption. Deconjugated bile salts may act
directly on intestinal mucosal cells to impair absorption of long-chain fatty acids.
Such patients may respond to broad-spectrum antibiotics, such as ampicillin or
tetracycline. The dose and duration of
therapy should be individualized.

Diabetes and adult celiac disease may
coexist. Clinical studies are contradictory
as to whether these two diseases are
associated more commonly than might
be expected by chance alone. Gluten
enteropathy should be suspected if
steatorrhea is severe and antedates the
diabetic state. In such patients, the D-
xylose absorption test is abnormal, serum
albumin is low, hypoprothrombinemia is
present, and often hypocalcemia with osteomalacia complicates the picture. The
peroral jejunal biopsy specimen is characteristic and shows varying grades of villous
atrophy, cellular infiltrates in the lamina
propria, and hyperplasia of cells in the
basal portions of the crypts of Lieberkühn.
Response to a gluten-free diet is usually favorable and reasonably specific (see pp.
880 to 882).

Carcinoma of the pancreas is more common in diabetic patients than in control
subjects, representing 5 to 33 per cent of
all malignancies occurring in diabetic patients in various studies. Dental caries and
periodontal infections are more common
in diabetics and actually may be helpful in
detecting latent diabetes.

Gallbladder contractility in diabetes is
often impaired, probably another manifestation of autonomic neuropathy. The incidence of gallstones is significantly increased in diabetic patients. In one
autopsy study, 38.5 per cent of white diabetic females had gallstones, compared to
21.7 per cent in nondiabetic females; the
incidence was 17.9 per cent in white diabetic males, compared to 8.7 per cent in
nondiabetic males.[7] Acute cholecystitis in
diabetics carries a formidable mortality
rate of 19 to 22 per cent and a high incidence of postoperative complications.[8]
The incidence of emphysematous cholecystitis is increased, a complication related
to gas-forming bacteria in the gallbladder
wall. Thus elective cholecystectomy is
strongly recommended in acceptable risk
diabetic patients with asymptomatic gallstones.

THYROID DISEASES

Hyperthyroidism is frequently associated with histological gastritis and diminished acid output,[9] abnormalities
which return toward normal as thyrotoxicosis is controlled. Studies are contradictory as to whether peptic ulcer disease is
increased. Radiological investigations
suggest that "intestinal hurry" is common,
presumably related to smooth muscle hyperactivity.[10] Clinically, diarrhea and steatorrhea are more frequent than is generally
appreciated, the daily fat excretion exceeding 7g in perhaps 25 per cent of patients. Rapid gastric emptying and intestinal hypermotility may contribute to the
malabsorption; however, D-glucose absorption is increased and D-xylose absorption is normal.[11] Fecal calcium excretion is
increased and may contribute to the negative calcium balance often found in hyperthyroidism. Occasionally patients with
thyrotoxicosis present with severe anorexia, persistent nausea and vomiting, or
frank malabsorption as the initial manifestation of their disease.[12]

HYPOTHYROIDISM

Histamine-fast achlorhydria is increased
in patients with spontaneous hypothyroidism, often accompanied by varying stages
of gastritis. Since at least 20 per cent of

patients with primary myxedema show antibodies to gastric mucosa, an immunological mechanism may be inferred.[13] The known clinical association between spontaneous hypothyroidism and pernicious anemia may be explained by the overlap of antibodies to gastric mucosa and thyroid tissue found in these two diseases. Gastric emptying is often prolonged.

Obstinate constipation is common in myxedema and may lead to fecal impaction and rectal prolapse. Sigmoid volvulus is also noted. Myxedematous and inflammatory cell infiltration of the bowel wall at times causes extreme distention of small bowel and colon. Indeed, these patients may have megacolon with obstipation (see pp. 1463 to 1480). The small bowel may also be atonic, obstruct, and cause death.[14] Motility studies indicate markedly reduced amplitude and frequency of rhythmic motor waves in both the small intestine and colon.[15] In some patients, there is no increase in colon motility following injection of the parasympathomimetic agent bethanechol (Urecholine), probably signifying irreversible muscle degeneration. Ascites of unknown cause may be the presenting feature of myxedema. The ascitic fluid tends to have a high protein content similar to that of the pleural and pericardial effusions of this disease. Cardiac failure is usually not responsible; the ascites regresses as appropriate replacement therapy is given. Patients with spontaneous or postoperative hypothyroidism may have clinical signs and laboratory confirmation of malabsorption, including steatorrhea. Intestinal mucosal biopsy specimens in such patients usually show subtotal villous atrophy. The malabsorption improves as thyroid replacement is given.

TUMORS OF THE THYROID GLAND

Medullary carcinoma of the thyroid gland is a solid, amyloid-containing tumor of neuroectodermal origin, often familial, that secretes calcitonin.[16] Frequently a pheochromocytoma of the adrenal medulla, Cushing's syndrome, multiple mucosal neuromas, and hyperparathyroidism coexist. About one-third of patients have watery diarrhea with stools characteristically consisting of 85 to 95 per cent water with increased sodium and potassium content, and weighing 500 to 700 g per 24 hours. The diarrhea is often explosive, preceded by abdominal cramps. Intestinal peristaltic waves are increased, and intestinal transit time is usually shortened; however, steatorrhea is minimal and infrequent. Peroral small bowel biopsy usually shows normal structure, but occasional partial villous atrophy is demonstrated. Excision of the medullary carcinoma causes prompt remission of the diarrhea, a result that points to a humoral mechanism, possibly secretion of a prostaglandin or serotonin. Serum assays for various substances, however, have been inconclusive, and calcitonin itself does not directly stimulate gut motility. Mucosal neuromas may also be found in the lips and throughout the intestinal mucosa, and are formed by bundles of nerves and ganglioneuromatous proliferation. Therapy consists of total thyroidectomy with block dissection of lymph nodes.

PARATHYROID DISEASE

Hyperparathyroidism is often associated with anorexia, nausea, vomiting, abdominal pains, constipation, and/or diarrhea.[17] The gastrointestinal manifestations of hyperthyroidism are probably due to (1) hypercalcemia per se, (2) associated peptic ulcer disease, (3) associated pancreatitis, and (4) associated malabsorption. Hypercalcemia frequently produces nausea and vomiting, as well as mental obtundation, readily reversible with reduction of the serum calcium level. Duodenal ulcer disease is increased in association with hyperparathyroidism, being as high as 15 per cent in some series. The incidence of gastric ulcer disease, however, is not increased. Experimentally, in both man and animals, intravenous infusions of calcium increase basal secretion of hydrochloric acid.

There is occasional association of acute and chronic pancreatitis with hyperparathyroidism. Although pain may be absent, the usual manifestations of chronic pancreatitis are present, including vomiting, weight loss, steatorrhea, and diabetes. In patients with acute pancreatitis, the previously elevated calcium may fall to normal range, thus obscuring the underlying hyperparathyroidism. Elevated calcium levels rather than parathormone seem to be responsible for the pancreatitis. Pancreatic calcification has been noted in some of these patients. A small number of patients with parathyroid adenoma and hyperparathyroidism have malabsorption.[18] Studies of intestinal mucosa are not available on such patients, and the mechanism of steatorrhea has not been defined. One hypothesis holds that osteomalacia, which develops as a consequence of malabsorption, stimulates replication of sensitive cells in the parathyroid glands which eventually develop into autonomous hyperplastic nodules. However, in some cases, the parathyroid hyperplasia is reversible by vitamin D therapy.

Primary hypoparathyroidism may be associated with steatorrhea and malabsorption, as well as hypoadrenalism, pernicious anemia, and chronic cutaneous moniliasis.[19] Only a few studies in depth have been done, and these indicate absence of morphological change in the intestinal epithelium; the mechanism of

steatorrhea is undefined. Correction of the hypoparathyroidism with either parathormone or vitamin D_2 corrects the malabsorptive stage (Fig. 30–1).

SKIN DISEASES

Steatorrhea may complicate extensive skin disease, especially eczema and psoriasis. Besides fat malabsorption, vitamin B_{12} and folate malabsorption have been reported. Peroral biopsy usually reveals normal jejunal mucosa. The cause of the steatorrhea is not known, but it usually remits as the skin eruption clears. Some have termed this entity dermatogenic enteropathy.[20]

DERMATITIS HERPETIFORMIS

This disease is characterized by crops of bilateral symmetrical pruritic vesicles and papules involving extensor surfaces of the body; it is readily suppressed by sulfapyridine and dapsone. Two-thirds of pa-

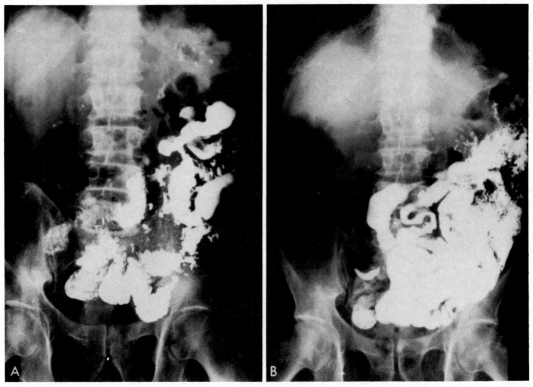

Figure 30–1. Small bowel series in a patient with hypoparathyroidism and malabsorption. Before therapy with vitamin D (A); after therapy (B). (From Clarkson, B. O., et al.: Metabolism 9:1053, 1960.)

tients with dermatitis herpetiformis have structural abnormalities in the small intestinal mucosa. Changes range from "flat" jejunal biopsies identical to the lesion of untreated celiac sprue through a spectrum of subtotal villous atrophy to normal.[21] Maximal mucosal abnormalities are found at the duodenojejunal juncture with improvement as one proceeds from the proximal to the distal small bowel. In some cases the distribution of mucosal lesions is patchy. Most patients lack laboratory evidence of malabsorption. Only a few have frank steatorrhea or protein-losing enteropathy. Following institution of a gluten-free diet, villous architecture improves, as in celiac sprue. Fecal fat excretion diminishes in those patients with significant steatorrhea. Dietary gluten withdrawal, however, appears to play no role in clearing the skin eruption. Thus a gluten-free diet does not seem indicated in dermatitis herpetiformis, except in those cases with significant steatorrhea. Similarly, the enteropathy of dermatitis herpetiformis does not respond to specific treatment of the rash with sulfapyridine or dapsone.

Available evidence strongly favors the concept that most patients with dermatitis herpetiformis who also have significant malabsorption have coexistent celiac sprue.[22] It is of interest that there is an increased incidence of celiac sprue in relatives of patients with dermatitis herpetiformis. Many patients with dermatitis herpetiformis have a high incidence of autoantibodies, and, in addition, deposition of IgA has been found at the dermoepidermal junction. Management of patients with dermatitis herpetiformis should include periodic screening for clinical or laboratory evidence of malabsorption. Routine jejunal biopsy and institution of a gluten-free diet do not seem indicated except in those patients with significant steatorrhea.

DYSGAMMAGLOBULINEMIAS AND THE GUT

Although our understanding of those diseased states characterized by underproduction or disordered production of gamma globulins is rudimentary, a suggested classification of the dysgammaglobulinemias that are associated with abnormalities in the gastrointestinal tract is presented in Tables 5–1 and 5–2 (pp. 51 and 55).

CONGENITAL SEX-LINKED HYPOGAMMAGLOBULINEMIA

This is a congenitally determined deficiency of serum and secretory IgA manifest in the first years of life. In such infants, cellular immunity remains intact. Diarrhea is frequent, and occasionally steatorrhea is present. The jejunal mucosa is invariably normal in biopsy. Isolated lactose deficiency may occur in about 40 per cent of patients. A nonspecific granuloma of the intestine may be found (Fig. 30–2).

IMMUNOGLOBULIN DEFICIENCIES WITH MALABSORPTION

Malabsorption is usually associated with acquired hypogammaglobulinemia which may become manifest in childhood, adolescence, or young adulthood.[23] Paradoxically, malabsorption is rarely associated with the congenital hypogammaglobulinemias. The common patterns found in the acquired form are (1) depression of all immunoglobulins of variable extent; (2) selective IgA deficiency; and (3) deficiency of IgA and IgM, but normal IgG.

It has been estimated that malabsorption may complicate 20 to 50 per cent of patients with acquired hypogammaglobulinemia. Many cases are associated with nodular lymphoid hyperplasia.[24, 25] Associated findings that have been described in patients with hypogammaglobulinemia include (1) steatorrhea and other features of malabsorption; (2) protein-losing enteropathy; (3) pancreatic insufficiency, usually defined by abnormal bicarbonate concentration following secretin stimulation; (4) giardiasis; (5) gastric achlorhydria; (6) intestinal bacterial overgrowth; and (7) increased incidence of autoimmune syndromes, including rheumatoid arthritis, dermatomyositis, and lupus erythematosus. Clinically, diarrhea may be severe, with grossly fatty malodorous stools. Sometimes

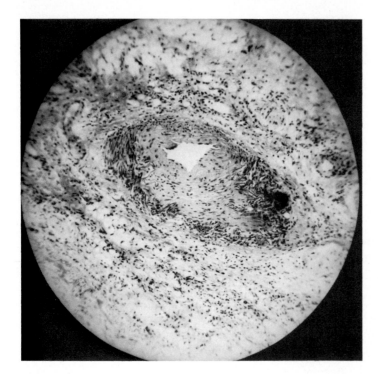

Figure 30–2. Nonspecific granulomatous lesion in ileum of a patient with congenital hypogammaglobulinemia. × 250.

the diarrhea has a profuse watery character and is intractable, leading to dehydration and electrolyte depletion. Intestinal hemorrhage has also been described. Isolated lactase deficiency may occur. Since patients with this syndrome have significant depletion of one or more immunoglobulins, recurrent bacterial infections, especially pneumonia, may be a prominent feature.

Radiologic study often shows segmentation and flocculation of barium in the small intestine. Multiple radiolucent defects have been described when nodular lymphoid hyperplasia is present (Fig. 30–3). In many patients, however, gastrointestinal X-ray survey is entirely normal. Laboratory studies often reveal significant anemia, which may be related to depletion of iron, folic acid, or vitamin B_{12}. Thus serum iron, folic acid, and/or vitamin B_{12} levels may be depressed. The prothrombin time may be slightly elevated. Three-day stool fat collection on a 100-g fat diet usually reveals significant steatorrhea. The D-xylose absorption test is abnormal, and low vitamin E levels and elevated urine 5-hydroxyindoleacetic acid have been reported. Study of serum immunoglobulin levels reveals depression of one or more of the immunoglobulins IgA, IgG, or IgM. The serum albumin is often low. Frequently no plasma cells are found in marrow specimens.

Jejunal biopsy may show total or subto-

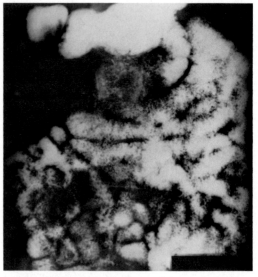

Figure 30–3. Small intestinal roentgenogram in nodular lymphoid hyperplasia. Note the multiple radiolucent defects throughout the entire small bowel. (From Hughes, W. R., et al.: Ann. Intern. Med. 74:903, 1971.)

tal villous atrophy, or may be normal (see Figs. 30–4 and 30–5). Increased round cell infiltration of the lamina propria has been reported, but plasma cells are dramatically reduced or absent. Nodular lymphoid hyperplasia in the lamina propria is a frequent finding. In some cases subjected to open intestinal biopsy, gross subepithelial lymphoid nodules have been described, 3 to 5 mm in diameter, giving a hobnail appearance to the intestinal mucosa. Intestinal mucus should be smeared and examined for *Giardia lamblia* if a nodular lymphoid hyperplasia is present.[26] In some instances, Salmonella, Shigella, or overgrowth of staphylococci is found in the stool culture.

Since humoral or circulating antibodies are depressed, there is often an impaired skin reaction of the immediate variety to pollens, molds, and house dust. In addition, active immunization with typhoid vaccine fails to induce appropriate anti-O or anti-H antibodies. There may also be reduced antibody response to red blood cell isoagglutinins. Delayed or cellular immunity is usually intact, although occasionally this system is also involved. Cellular immunity may be evaluated by determining skin reactions of the delayed type to tuberculin, histoplasmin, mumps, or DCNB. It may also be tested by evaluating lymphocyte transformation in the presence of phytohemagglutinin.

The primary defect of this syndrome may be impaired production of one or more immunoglobulins on a genetic basis but with delayed expression related to environmental factors. In support of this thesis is the finding that family members of affected patients are frequently found to have immunoglobulin deficiencies. Affected patients probably have a defective secretory IgA system in the lamina propria, thus permitting bacteria to penetrate the intestinal epithelial cell and cause malabsorption, perhaps analogous to the pathogenesis of Whipple's disease or tropical sprue. Other factors may contribute to the malabsorption, such as bacterial overgrowth in the intestinal lumen, gastric achlorhydria, pancreatic insufficiency, and invasive giardiasis. The nodular lymphoid hyperplasia may be a compensatory reaction to the immunoglobulin deficiency and/or bacterial proliferation.

Various therapeutic maneuvers have been tried with some measure of success. Gamma globulin injections have been helpful in some cases. However, since gamma globulin does not contain IgA or IgM, infusions of fresh frozen plasma

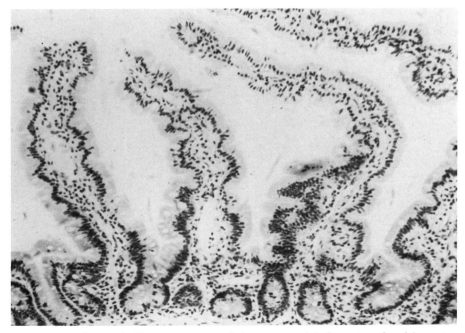

Figure 30–4. Normal jejunal villi in a patient with hypogammaglobulinemia and malabsorption. Plasma cells are absent, however. × 200.

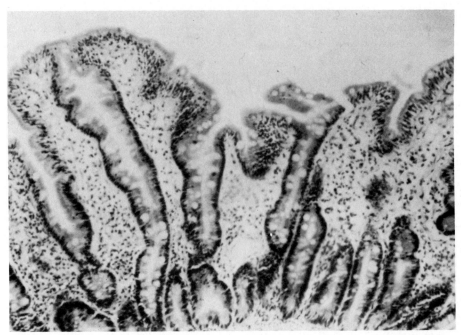

Figure 30–5. Partial villous atrophy in hypogammaglobulinemia and malabsorption. Plasma cells are absent. × 200.

which contains all immunoglobulins seem more logical. Broad-spectrum antibiotics may be tried if malabsorption is severe. It is not always possible to accurately quantitate bacterial overgrowth; however, recent studies indicate that bacterial overgrowth of the upper small bowel is not an important cause of malabsorption in these patients.[27, 28] In some patients, especially those in whom jejunal biopsy has indicated subtotal villous atrophy, a gluten-free diet is warranted. If giardiasis is found, a course of quinacrine or metronidazole is indicated and has been shown not only to ameliorate diarrhea and malabsorption, but also to improve the histological picture (Tables 30–2 and 30–3). However, many cases have not remit-

TABLE 30–2.   HISTOLOGICAL CHANGES IN PATIENTS WITH HYPOGAMMAGLOBULINEMIA AND DIARRHEA*

Group	Patient	Age	Sex	Diarrhea	Duration	γ-Globulin	Prior Therapy	Immunoglobulin† IgG	IgM	IgA
								mg/100 ml		
Mixed lesions	1	50	M	Watery	14 mo	40 cc/mo	Quinacrine; dihydroxyquinoline	200	0	0
	2	37	F	Watery	2 years	40 cc/mo	Tetracycline	110	0	0
	3	24	F	Intermittent	4 years	40 cc/mo	Tetracycline	110	6.5	0
Nodular lymphoid hyperplasia	4	24	F	None‡		None	Antiemetics	50	15	0
	5	42	M	Loose stools	6 years	None	None	500	70	13
Hypogammaglobulinemic sprue	6	46	M	Intermittent	6 years	40 cc/mo	Corticosteroids	475	50	7
	7	46	M	Watery	12 years	None	Gluten-free diet; corticosteroids for 10 years	550	10	11
	8§	37	F	Watery	10 years	40 cc/mo	Gluten-free diet	100	15	0

*From Ament, M. E., and Rubin, C. E.: Gastroenterology 62:216, 1972.
†Normal values in milligrams per 100 ml: IgG, 770 to 1130; IgM, 90 to 170; IgA, 80 to 200.
‡Vomiting was this patient's main symptom; she had steatorrhea but no diarrhea.
§Not infected with *Giardia lamblia.*

TABLE 30–3. CLINICAL AND LABORATORY IMPROVEMENT IN PATIENTS WITH HYPOGAMMAGLOBULINEMIA TREATED FOR GIARDIASIS*

Group	Patient	Weight		Fecal Fat (Normal, <6.0 g/day)		Carotene (Normal, 50–250 μg per 100 ml)		Folate (Normal, >5 mμg/ml)		Protein Loss (Normal, <50 ml/day)		B₁₂ Urinary Excretion (Normal, >15%)	
		Before	After	Before	After	Before	After	Before	After	Before	After	Before	After
		kg		g/day		μg/100 ml		mμg/ml		ml/day		%	
Mixed lesions	1	68.0	76.0	10	3	50	155	3.3	18.6	150	12	9.7	30.0
	2	30.9	41.3	11	5	40	90	6.3	17.5			<1.0	<1.0
	3	51.7	51.9	3		152	164	29.0	16.0			10.6	22.0
Nodular lymphoid hyperplasia	4	29.9	34.1	10	3	79	114	3.3	10.5	300		7.1	13.0
	5	70.3	70.4	4		70	76	4.8	7.8			8.4	9.3
Hypogammaglobulinemic sprue	6	60.0	63.0			27	75	1.3	7.0				
	7	43.0	55.0	24	1	10	70		6.7			0.1	9.0
	8†	50.6	47.8	19	16	27	48	1.6	1.0			16.0	9.0

*From Ament, M. E., and Rubin, C. E.: Gastroenterology 62:216, 1972.
†Only patient without giardiasis.

ted even though *Giardia lamblia* has been successfully eliminated.[27, 28] If there is overgrowth of the stool with known enteric pathogens, such as Salmonella or Shigella, a course of chloramphenicol or ampicillin might be considered. Cholestyramine has recently been used successfully in a patient with this syndrome and incapacitating diarrhea and electrolyte depletion. It prevents "choleraic enteropathy" by binding dihydroxy bile salts found in large quantity as a result of excessive bacterial dehydroxylation of primary bile salts.

SELECTIVE IgA DEFICIENCY WITH CELIAC SPRUE

IgA is the major immunoglobulin of most human exocrine secretions, including the respiratory tract and gastrointestinal tract. It is the predominant immunoglobulin found in plasma cells in the lamina propria of the gastrointestinal epithelium. The secretory IgA molecule consists of two 7S IgA molecules plus a nonimmunoglobulin glycoprotein called secretory component which has a molecular weight of about 60,000. Thus secretory IgA is an 11S immunoglobulin of 385,000 mol wt, compared with serum IgA, which is a 7S immunoglobulin of 170,000 mol

wt. Secretory IgA is strongly resistant to proteolytic enzymes.

A small number of patients have been described with complete absence of IgA in association with the usual changes of celiac sprue.[30] Malabsorption may be severe, and the jejunal mucosal biopsy is flat (Fig. 30–6). Response to gluten deprivation is excellent in some, with correction of the malabsorption parameters. However, in these patients the deficiency of IgA persists despite clinical remission on a gluten-free diet. This had led to the hypothesis that the deficiency of IgA is a primary event.[31] Patients with selective IgA deficiency have also been shown to have an increased incidence of milk precipitins. This has led to the postulate that IgA is important in preventing intestinal absorption of dietary antigens. In addition, a high incidence of antibodies to basement membrane has been detected in patients with selective IgA deficiency. However, this group of patients may simply represent another variant of dysproteinemia complicating celiac sprue.

CELIAC SPRUE AND DYSPROTEINEMIA

Serum IgA levels are often elevated in patients with celiac sprue on normal diets,

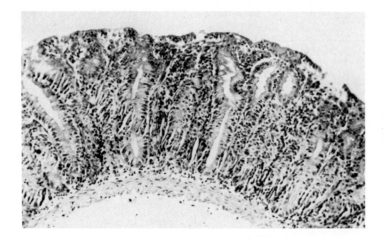

Figure 30–6. Villous atrophy and inflammatory cell infiltration. Jejunal mucosa in IgA deficiency with malabsorption. × 60.

and tend to fall to normal when a gluten-free diet is instituted. A possible but unproved explanation is that gluten provides an antigenic stimulus which invokes antibody response to IgA. There is some indication that a rise in IgA in a patient with celiac sprue on a strict gluten-free diet may herald a gastrointestinal lymphoma. (As noted, occasional patients with isolated IgA deficiency will have celiac sprue, and their response to a gluten-free diet is satisfactory.) In the jejunum of most patients with celiac sprue, absolute counts of IgA-containing plasma cells and levels of 11S IgA in jejunal secretions are normal.

Serum IgM levels, which are low in about one-third of patients with untreated celiac sprue, usually return to normal with institution of a gluten-free diet.[32] It seems likely that decreased synthesis is responsible for IgM deficiency in these patients, probably owing to depression of lymphoreticular function resulting from gluten-induced injury. It is of interest that absolute numbers of IgM-containing plasma cells and IgM levels in jejunal secretions are commonly raised in celiac sprue. Abnormally high or abnormally low serum IgG levels have been reported in a minority of cases with celiac sprue but cannot be related directly to the activity or extent of the disease. One theory holds that

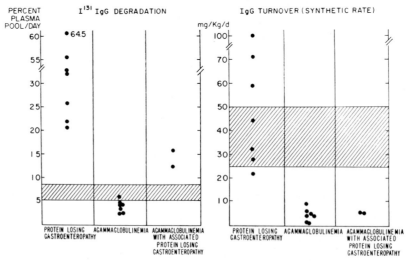

Figure 30–7. The IgG catabolic and synthetic rates in patients with gastrointestinal protein loss, agammaglobulinemia, and combined disorders. Range of normal values is cross-hatched. (From Waldmann, T. A., and Schwab, P. J.: J. Clin. Invest. 44:1523, 1965.)

qualitative impairment of IgA response to antigenic stimulus is impaired in celiac sprue and, as a result, there is local over-production of 19S IgM which mediates Arthus-type reactions.

DYSPROTEINEMIA AND PROTEIN-LOSING ENTEROPATHY

As discussed on page 35, protein-losing enteropathy may be a feature of many primary bowel diseases, including regional enteritis, celiac sprue, Whipple's disease, allergic gastroenteropathy, and intestinal lymphangiectasias. However, it may also complicate extraintestinal disorders such as constrictive pericarditis and tricuspid insufficiency. Secondary immunological defects may result from loss of serum im-munoglobulins and lymphocytes into the lumen of the bowel.[33] This causes depres-sion of both humoral and cellular immu-nity with lymphocytopenia and a relative state of anergy. Occasionally, diseases of the small bowel associated with hypogam-maglobulinemia may be associated with protein-losing enteropathy. In such in-stances measurement of catabolic and syn-thetic rates of IgG serve to distinguish con-genital and acquired agammaglobulinemia from agammaglobulinemia caused by pro-tein-losing enteropathy (Fig. 30–7). The latter condition, of course, will also be characterized by hypoalbuminemia with its characteristically associated catabolism and increased synthesis. In cases of ac-quired agammaglobulinemia complicated by protein-losing enteropathy, plasma gamma globulin remains low despite the increase of albumin which follows suc-cessful therapy.

INCREASED IgE WITH PARASITIC DISEASES

Parasitic disorders may be associated with elevated IgE levels, especially as-cariasis, visceral larva migrans, and human intestinal capillariasis.[35] IgE mediates the Prausnitz-Küstner reaction and is known as reagin or skin-sensitizing antibody. Ca-pillariasis may be associated with severe malabsorption, including enteric protein loss, and may incite IgE serum levels up to nineteen times normal. Simultaneously,

other immunoglobulin levels, especially IgA, may be depressed owing to enteric protein loss. With successful treatment of the underlying parasitic infestation, the elevated IgE levels return toward normal.

ATROPHIC GASTRITIS AND PERNICIOUS ANEMIA

Immunological deficiency states, includ-ing IgG, IgA and IgM, may be found in as-sociation with atrophic gastritis and per-nicious anemia.[36] The gastric lesion in these patients differs from that of classic pernicious anemia in that (1) it tends to de-velop at a younger age; (2) no plasma cells are found in gastric mucosal infiltrates; (3) parietal cell, intrinsic factor, and thy-roid antibodies are not demonstrable; and (4) serum gastrin levels are not elevated. The normal serum gastrin level in these patients may indicate that, in contrast to the gastric lesion of primary pernicious anemia, the gastric lesion in immunologic deficiency states involves the gastrin-producing cells of the gastric antrum as well as the parietal cells of the gastric body and fundus. There is a high inci-dence of diarrhea, giardiasis, and associ-ated autoimmune disorders. Although not proved, atrophic gastritis may be a direct consequence of immunoglobulin deficien-cies, especially IgA, because this would render the gastric mucosa more suscepti-ble to injury by infectious agents. In those patients with pernicious anemia and asso-ciated immunoglobulin deficiencies, it is important to note that both stages of the Schilling test may be abnormal. Because of the frequent association of intestinal dysfunction with immunoglobulin de-ficiency, there may not be significantly enhanced absorption of vitamin B_{12} when intrinsic factor is added. In addition to atrophic gastritis and pernicious anemia, there appears to be an increased incidence of carcinoma of the stomach in late-onset immunoglobulin deficiency states. Car-cinoma of the stomach may develop whether or not atrophic gastritis is present.

Therapy consists of monthly vitamin B_{12} injections. If the immunoglobulin defi-ciency is severe and recurrent secondary infection a problem, periodic gamma glob-ulin injections are indicated.

COLLAGEN VASCULAR DISEASES

SCLERODERMA

Scleroderma (progressive systemic sclerosis) is characterized by proliferation of fibrous connective tissue as well as vasculitis. The skin and multiple organ systems may be involved.

Oral Cavity Involvement. The skin around the mouth may become atrophic and fibrotic, restricting opening of the mouth. Hypertrophy of the periodontal ligament causes characteristic X-ray changes around dental roots. Gingivae may become indurated and friable, later undergoing atrophy. In advanced cases, the buccal mucosa becomes thinned and tongue papillae atrophy. Taste and touch perception may be severely impaired.

Esophagus. Esophageal involvement is common in scleroderma. An incidence of 80 per cent has been found when sensitive manometric techniques are employed. Viscera, including esophagus, may be involved in the absence of skin changes. Uncoordinated motor pattern is the earliest change in esophageal motility with simultaneous or repetitive contractions of reduced amplitude.[37] The lower esophageal sphincter frequently fails to relax with swallowing, and esophageal emptying is severely impaired. Eventually, complete motor paralysis may result. These changes reflect progressive atrophy of the smooth muscle in the distal two-thirds of the esophagus. Submucosal sclerosis is also present. The proximal esophagus comprised of skeletal (striated) muscle is spared, as is the pharyngoesophageal sphincter. The lower esophageal sphincter, however, is progressively weakened and eventually destroyed with loss of the protective high-pressure zone. As a result, reflux of acid-peptic gastric secretions into the lower esophagus is common, leading to esophagitis and, occasionally, to stricture. Thus patients with scleroderma frequently experience lower substernal burning discomfort, indicating esophagitis, which may later change to progressive dysphagia as stricture develops. Studies indicate a 50 per cent occurrence of hiatal hernia when esophageal involvement is severe. A small number of patients with scleroderma experience diffuse spasm, which clinically is associated with intermittent rather than progressive substernal pain and dysphagia. In at least 50 per cent of patients esophageal involvement does not progress in concert with skin and visceral changes of scleroderma.[38] Radiographic findings include impaired motility in the distal esophagus, dilatation, gastroesophageal reflux, hiatus hernia, and stricture. Esophageal involvement is best documented by fluoroscopy or cineradiography with the patient in the prone position. Treatment consists of measures designed to minimize gastroesophageal reflux, which include a head-up bed and frequent administration of antacids. Anticholinergic medication is best avoided. In the presence of esophageal stricture, a soft or even liquid diet may be necessary. Meat, in particular, should be thoroughly masticated—advice that is not always practical in view of the high incidence of oral cavity, gum, and dental involvement in this disease. Nuts, beans, shrimp, and the like should be avoided.

Stomach. Gastric involvement occasionally occurs in patients with scleroderma.[39] Radiologic study often shows retention of small amounts of barium for many hours despite initial prompt emptying. Antral mucosal nodularity and thickening have been noted on gastroscopy. Pyloric stenosis with obstruction has been reported, as has gastric ulceration with fatal hemorrhage.

Small Intestine. When sought radiologically, small bowel involvement has been reported in 57 per cent of scleroderma patients. Clinical symptoms are frequent but do not invariably accompany X-ray changes. Extensive small bowel involvement is possible with minimal skin involvement. The duodenum is characteristically dilated, often with retention of barium for hours after most of the barium meal has reached the cecum.[40] Dilatation may occur throughout the small bowel, although the changes are usually more apparent in the proximal jejunun. The valvulae conniventes are typically thickened and prominent, giving rise to a characteristic appearance (see Fig. 30–8). Pseudodiverticula, i.e., small outpouchings with broad necks, are also a feature. Reduced peristalsis, flocculation, and segmentation

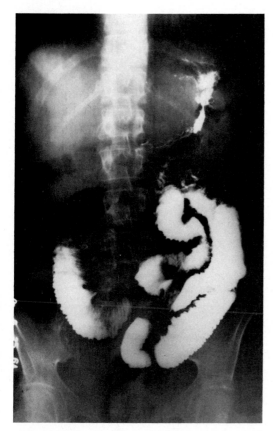

Figure 30-8. Small bowel series in a patient with scleroderma. Note some dilatation of loops and "spiculation."

of barium are also common features. The pathological changes of intestinal scleroderma include variable smooth muscle atrophy and patchy deposition of collagenous tissue in submucosal, muscular, and serosal layers. The mucosa is spared except for scant infiltration of the lamina propria with chronic inflammatory cells. Clinical symptoms include abdominal discomfort, bloating, distention, borborygmi after meals, anorexia, nausea, and vomiting. Weight loss is very common. Intermittent diarrhea sometimes alternates with constipation. Acute or chronic "pseudo-obstruction" complete with persistent vomiting, abdominal distention, and dilated intestinal loops with fluid levels may lead to surgical exploration.[41] Dilated and atonic small bowel is generally found without organic obstruction. Infarction of ileum and colon with fatal peritonitis has been reported owing to thrombosis of the celiac and superior mesenteric arteries.

Pneumatosis cystoides intestinalis is a rare complication of scleroderma and may coexist with pseudo-obstruction and pneumoperitoneum.[42] The radiologic features include multiple radiologic cysts or linear streaks of gas within the bowel wall or mesentery.

Malabsorption with steatorrhea complicates about 50 per cent of cases with small bowel involvement.[43] Fecal fat is increased, and D-xylose and vitamin B_{12}–intrinsic factor complex absorption are impaired. Bacterial colonization of the small bowel has been well documented in such patients. Stasis of intestinal contents in wide hypomotile loops or pseudodiverticula favors massive bacterial overgrowth. Significant deconjugation and dehydroxylation of bile acids result. Steatorrhea may relate to decreased concentration of conjugated bile acids which impair the micellar phase of fat absorption. Bacteria also bind vitamin B_{12}–intrinsic factor complex, thus preventing its absorption, and may also metabolize xylose. Peroral biopsies of intestinal mucosa in such cases usually reveal normal villous structure with increased numbers of chronic inflammatory cells in the lamina propria (Fig. 30–9). The defect in fat absorption is usually mild in these cases of the intestinal stasis syndrome, but occasionally therapy is warranted. Broad-spectrum antibiotics such as tetracycline, 1 g daily, or ampicillin, 2 g daily, inhibit bacterial overgrowth in the intestinal lumen. Characteristically, abnormal values for fecal fat and vitamin B_{12} absorption return to normal within a few days. Intermittent antibiotic therapy for an indefinite period is probably indicated in these patients.

Colon. Colonic involvement in scleroderma usually occurs in association with small bowel involvement. Radiological features include wide neck pseudodiverticula, especially on the antimesenteric border of the transverse and descending colon, with areas of rigidity between these sacculations. Loss of haustrations also occurs. As the disease progresses, generalized dilatation of the colon occurs (see p. 1477). Clinically, severe constipation is common, at times leading to large bowel obstruction secondary to impaction. On sigmoidoscopy the rectal wall may appear pale, dry, and rigid. Deep rectal biopsy

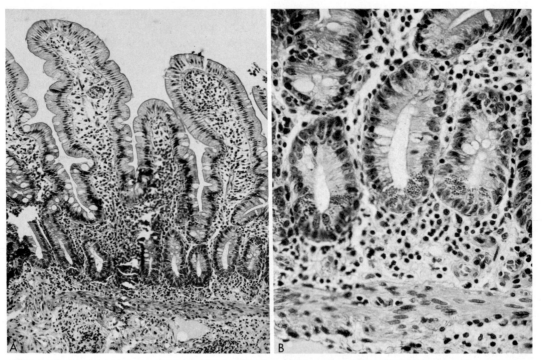

Figure 30–9. Jejunal mucosa in a patient with scleroderma and malabsorption. Normal villi with inflammatory cells infiltrating the lamina propria (A); higher magnification shows the cells to be mononuclear (B). (From Kahn, I. J., et al.: New Eng. J. Med. *274*:1339, 1966.)

may show the typical sclerodermatous changes. Manometric studies of the anorectal segment have demonstrated selective impairment of smooth muscle function.[44] The internal sphincter (smooth muscle) fails to relax with rectal distention, whereas the external sphincter (striated muscle) contracts in normal fashion.

DERMATOMYOSITIS

Stomatitis may complicate dermatomyositis, and feeding problems may be compounded by weakness of facial musculature. In contrast to scleroderma, the striated muscles of the hypopharynx and cervical esophagus are often involved, leading to problems of deglutition and, not infrequently, tracheal aspiration.[45] Regurgitation of barium through the nose may occur. Barium retention in the hypopharyngeal vallecula is common. Dysphagia may also be related to motor disturbances involving the smooth musculature of the mid- and lower esophagus. Peris-

talsis may be diminished and poorly coordinated. The esophagus may become moderately dilated. In contrast to scleroderma, however, reflux esophagitis, stricture and hiatus hernia are not significant problems.

Gastric atony with delayed emptying is found. The small bowel may exhibit varying degrees of dilatation and segmentation, with hypomotility and delayed transit time. The colon may also show dilatation, sacculation with pseudodiverticula, and incomplete evacuation. Manometric studies of the anorectal segment have shown selective involvement of striated musculature. Thus in response to rectal distention, the external sphincter (striated muscle) response is absent (fails to contract), whereas the internal sphincter (smooth muscle) responds in a normal manner (by relaxing). As might be anticipated, clinical manifestations include abdominal discomfort, distention, bloating, and constipation.

Gastric hemorrhage from mucosal ulcerations is another complication. Gross pathological features include thickening and edema of the bowel wall. Often multiple mucosal ulcerations are present. Histological features include edema of the submucosa, atrophy and fibrosis of the muscular layer, and infiltration with lymphocytes and plasma cells.

SJÖGREN'S AND BEHÇET'S SYNDROMES AND OTHER PROBLEMS

Sjögren's syndrome is an autoimmune disorder characterized by keratoconjunctivitis sicca, xerostomia, and connective tissue disease. Rheumatoid arthritis is present in about half the patients. Oral findings consist of dry mouth, lip fissures, dental caries, and decreased salivary flow.[46] Patients experience difficulty chewing. The parotid glands are frequently enlarged, and lymphoma and macroglobulinemia may develop.

In Behçet's syndrome, painful multiple ulceration of the oral cavity is a constant feature. The genitalia may be similarly involved. Uveitis, arthritis, and nonulcerating skin lesions are frequently associated. Diarrhea caused by inflammation of the colon, either segmental or universal, may complicate this disorder.

In disseminated lupus erythematosus, oral lesions occur in 20 per cent of cases, including shallow painful ulcers, petechiae, lip fissuring, gingivitis, and parotitis.

Reiter's syndrome is a triad of conjunctivitis, urethritis, and arthritis occurring in young men. Oral lesions occur in up to 40 per cent of cases and characteristically consist of painless, shallow, clean-based ulcers with smooth margins affecting the palate, buccal mucosa, lips, and tongue.

SYSTEMIC LUPUS ERYTHEMATOSUS

Systemic lupus erythematosus may be complicated by gastrointestinal ulceration and hemorrhage usually related to underlying vasculitis.[47] Most patients have been on steroid therapy. Intestinal infarction, perforation, and obstruction, sometimes recurrent, have been reported. Abdominal pain has also been related to perihepatitis, perisplenitis, peritonitis, and pancreatitis.[48] At times, recurrent abdominal pain may be troublesome but unexplained. A few cases of malabsorption associated with subtotal villous atrophy

have been reported.[49] Systemic lupus erythematosus may also coexist with ulcerative colitis or granulomatous (Crohn's) colitis.[50]

RHEUMATOID ARTHRITIS

In rheumatoid arthritis, temporomandibular joint involvement is noted in 85 per cent of patients, leading to tenderness, swelling, and crepitation at this site. Mastication may be impaired. Abdominal vasculitis is a complication reported in steroid-treated patients, leading to bowel infarction, perforation, and peritonitis.[51, 52] In some cases, parameters of malabsorption may be abnormal. Selective lactase deficiency has been reported, and intestinal amyloidosis is a rare complication.

RENAL DISEASE

Nausea and vomiting are common manifestations of uremia, related to the blood urea level and possibly resulting from mucosal irritation by ammonia.[53] Intractable hiccups may be a problem. Stomatitis, an uncommon manifestation of uremia, is probably due to ammonia liberated from salivary urea by the action of ureases found in oral bacterial flora.[54] A white, thick membrane often envelops the floor of the mouth and buccal mucosa with unpleasant taste and painful mastication. Xerostomia is a frequent associated complication. Acute parotitis may also occur. Gingival bleeding may be brisk and difficult to control, reflecting the generalized hemorrhagic tendency of the uremic state. In treatment of the stomatitis, an acid mouthwash, such as half-strength hydrogen peroxide, is used, along with dental scaling and topical steroids in a protective paste. Correction of the uremia by dialysis is curative.

In 60 per cent of patients with uremia, mucosal abnormalities occur throughout the gastrointestinal tract from the esophagus to the rectum.[55] Hemorrhagic lesions predominate, varying from petechiae and ecchymoses to marked mucosal and submucosal hemorrhages. Multiple, acute ulcers are relatively common; they are usually located in the stomach and duodenum, but they are also found in the small and large bowel. Focal pseudomembranous necrotic lesions are also common.

Mucosal bleeding frequently complicates the uremic state and has a dual origin: mucosal abnormalities, including focal ulcers, and the generalized hemorrhagic tendency. The latter is due to platelet dysfunction, primarily defective platelet factor III activation by ADP, causing impaired platelet adhesiveness.[56, 57] These platelet abnormalities are probably related to the high concentration of guanidinosuccinic acid, an intermediary of urea metabolism, found in uremic serum. Often gastrointestinal bleeding is due to diffuse mucosal oozing rather than a specific lesion. Secondary or tertiary hyperparathyroidism may predispose to peptic ulceration.

The pathogenesis of uremic enterocolitis is uncertain. Urea diffuses freely from the blood into the gut lumen where it is converted into ammonia and carbon dioxide by the enzyme urease derived from intestinal bacterial flora. Ammonia may have a direct toxic effect upon bowel mucosa. In some cases, uremic vasculitis may lead to focal ischemia with secondary necrosis and ulceration. It has also been shown that the gastric mucosal barrier can be disrupted by urea, permitting back diffusion of acid.[58] This mucolytic property of urea may initiate dissolution of the protective mucous layer throughout the gut as a prelude to uremic lesions. The most effective therapy is correction of the uremic state and its associated biochemical abnormalities by peritoneal and hemodialysis. In a few patients with uncontrolled bleeding, resection of involved bowel segments has been successfully performed, but this approach is seldom indicated.

Gastrointestinal complications also appear after renal transplantation. These include esophagitis, peptic ulceration, hemorrhagic gastritis, ileal perforation, and intestinal obstruction.[59] Immunosuppressive therapy, which usually includes steroids and azathioprine, may predispose to some of these conditions. Both the basal and maximal acid outputs are increased after renal transplantation and may play a role in the development of post-transplant peptic ulcers. Hyperparathyroidism has also been thought to underlie these ulcers. Pancreatitis complicates about 2 per cent of renal allograft recipients;[60] both oral steroids and vasculitis have been implicated as possible causes.

NEUROHUMORAL DISEASES

MASTOCYTOSIS

Systemic mastocytosis is characterized by mast cell proliferation in skin (urticaria pigmentosa), bones, lymph nodes, and parenchymal organs. Symptoms are due to episodic release of histamine from mast cells, and include pruritus, flushing, tachycardia, asthma, and headaches.[61] Gastrointestinal manifestations, present in almost 50 per cent of cases, include nausea, vomiting, abdominal pain, and diarrhea and, in some patients, symptoms of peptic ulcer. One case has been reported of chronic gastric ulcer associated with high basal and stimulated gastric acid secretion, presumably owing to the elevated blood histamine levels found.[62] In most patients, however, gastric acid secretion has been within normal limits. Radiological findings include thickened mucosal folds in the stomach and duodenum and disordered motor pattern in the small bowel. Malabsorption is an uncommon finding in systemic mastocytosis.[63] Such cases may be associated with steatorrhea, impaired D-xylose and lactose absorption, hypocalcemic tetany, and failure to absorb vitamin B_{12}. Jejunal biopsy has shown large numbers of mast cells in the lamina propria, muscularis mucosae, and submucosa, but intact villous architecture.[64] Jejunal gastric biopsies have shown increased histamine content. Pancreatic function tests remain normal. The cause of the malabsorption is unexplained, but it may be due in part to histamine-induced hypermotility. Degradation products of histamine may also play a role. Therapeutically, a gluten-free diet may be helpful. Restriction of fats and supplements of medium chain triglycerides may provide symptomatic relief.

PHEOCHROMOCYTOMA

Pheochromocytomas are tumors arising from chromaffin tissue, usually within the adrenal medulla, but occasionally in extraadrenal sites. These tumors release catecholamines, either paroxysmally or constantly, and are thus responsible for a rare form of secondary hypertension. Gastrointestinal manifestations include nausea, vomiting, abdominal pain, and, less frequently, diarrhea and gastrointestinal bleeding.[65] Obstipation and megacolon have been reported with improvement following resection of the tumor.[66] Paralytic ileus is an unusual complication associated with a poor prognosis, probably related to the inhibitory effect of epinephrine and norepinephrine on the smooth musculature of the gastrointestinal tract.[67] Ischemic enterocolitis is a rare complication, probably caused by vasoconstriction and veno-occlusive disease related to high circulatory levels of catecholamines.[68]

HERITABLE CONNECTIVE TISSUE DISORDERS

EHLERS-DANLOS SYNDROME

The Ehlers-Danlos syndrome is characterized by hypermobility of joints, hyperextensibility and fragility of skin, and thin, wide scars overlying bony prominences. Patients are at risk from a variety of gastrointestinal complications, including spontaneous intestinal perforation in association with hemorrhage.[69] Fragility of both intestinal tissue and blood vessel walls, in association with a coagulation defect, predisposes to alimentary bleeding. The nature of the coagulopathy has not been well defined but may reside in abnormalities of platelet ultrastructure and aggregation. Spontaneous arterial rupture is not uncommon and, among other things, may lead to retroperitoneal hemorrhage. Diverticula are present throughout the gastrointestinal tract, probably related to hyperelasticity of mucous membranes. Eventration of the diaphragm, rectal prolapse, hiatus hernia, external hernias, gastric atony, megaesophagus, and megacolon have been found. Abdominal surgery in such patients is made difficult by fragility of tissues, leading to tearing out of sutures and wound dehiscence.

PSEUDOXANTHOMA ELASTICUM

This disease is associated with widespread degeneration of elastic fibers. Char-

acteristic yellowish macules are found in skin folds and angioid streaks in the optic fundi. Occlusive vascular disease is common. Abdominal pain may relate to visceral ischemia. Recurrent unexplained gastrointestinal bleeding is common, probably caused by hemorrhage from small submucosal vessels. Severe hematemesis may occur. Visceral arteries are thickened and tortuous with intimal sclerosis common and occasional microaneurysms.[70] Angiomatous malformations also occur. On gastroscopy, raised yellowish nodular submucosal lesions have been observed throughout the stomach.

NEUROLOGIC AND MYOPATHIC DISEASES

MYOTONIA DYSTROPHICA

Myotonia dystrophica is a heredofamilial disorder characterized by myotonia, characteristic facies, wasting of sternomastoid and shoulder girdle musculature, myocardial involvement, cataracts, and mental degeneration. Dysphagia is not uncommon. Striated musculature of the tongue, pharynx, and upper esophagus is involved, as well as smooth muscle of the lower half of the esophagus.[71] Degenerative changes include atrophy and edema of myofibers, increase of connective tissue, and lymphocytic infiltration.[72] Myotonic distortion may involve the musculature, suspending the tongue and hyoid bone and thus impairing the normal sequence of deglutition. Intraluminal manometric studies have further elucidated the physiologic basis of the dysphagia.[73] Amplitude of peristaltic contractions of the pharynx is significantly reduced. Resting pressure within the upper esophageal sphincter (cricopharyngeus) is reduced. Likewise esophageal contraction waves are weak both in the upper (striated muscle) and lower (smooth muscle) esophagus. In occasional patients, esophageal peristaltic waves are absent completely. Resting pressure within the lower esophageal sphincter remains normal.

Similar smooth muscle abnormalities have also been reported in the stomach, intestinal tract, and rectum, although the intrinsic nerve plexuses of Auerbach and

Meissner remain normal. Abdominal pain, vomiting, diarrhea, and troublesome constipation with recurrent impactions have been reported, probably related to motor abnormalities. Obstipation may be associated with megacolon. Malabsorption with steatorrhea has not been noted, but occasionally the motor disorder leads to abnormal D-xylose absorption. Radiologic studies also demonstrated impaired deglutition of the barium bolus with pooling of the barium in the pharynx, poor peristalsis, and occasional dilatation of the esophagus. Manometric studies of the enterocolonic segment have shown characteristic responses. Although digital examination reveals weak anal sphincters, balloon rectal distention induces strong contraction of high amplitude and prolonged duration in both the internal and external sphincter.[74]

STIFF MAN SYNDROME

The stiff man syndrome consists of symmetrical progressive stiffness and painful spasm of axial musculature; it affects men in middle life. Dysphagia has been reported in a few cases, apparently caused by acute pharyngeal muscle spasm inducted by chewing and swallowing. A case of complete esophageal obstruction has been reported, apparently caused by spasm of the striated muscle of the cricopharyngeus and upper cervical esophagus, with normal peristalsis in the nonstriated musculature below this level.[75]

CARDIAC DISEASE

A variety of cardiac disorders cause protein-losing enteropathy, including constrictive pericarditis, cardiomyopathies, tricuspid regurgitation, interatrial septal defect, and pulmonary stenosis. Low serum albumin is a common feature which may exacerbate interstitial edema. Peroral biopsy usually shows dilated intestinal lymphatics. Lymphocytopenia results from excessive loss of lymphocyte-rich lymphatic fluid into the bowel lumen. Skin tests that define cellular mediated immunity, such as purified protein derivative, DNCB, *Candida albicans*, and mumps antigen, are nonreactive. Cardiac hemodynamics are similar in these patients, in that

right heart failure is present with elevation of right atrial and central venous pressure. The venous hypertension apparently causes functional obstruction to normal lymph drainage and, in some cases, an increase in lymph production as well.[76] Congestion of the lymphatic system leads to dilated intestinal lymphatics which are morphologically similar to those found in patients with intestinal lymphangiectasia.

Successful surgical correction of the cardiac defect, with return of central venous pressure to normal, usually ameliorates the abnormal protein loss in the gut.[77] Serum albumin, absolute lymphocyte count, small bowel biopsy, and immunological defects often return to normal. In refractory cases, supportive measures include a low-fat diet and supplements of medium-chain triglycerides.

HEMATOLOGIC DISEASES

In systemic disorders of coagulation, spontaneous or post-traumatic gastrointestinal bleeding may complicate the clinical picture. In hemophilia, for example, 19 per cent of all hemorrhages originate in the gastrointestinal tract.[78] In coagulopathies, intraluminal bleeding is often brisk, but on occasion it may be slow and protracted. Bleeding into the bowel wall, more common in the small intestine, produces a varied pattern of pain, at times mimicking an acute surgical abdomen. Intestinal obstruction is an infrequent complication. If improved hemostasis can be achieved by medical means, nonoperative management is usually successful. Radiological features of intramural bleeding include thickened mucosal folds, rigidity, and luminal narrowing. When gastrointestinal bleeding complicates anticoagulant therapy, and coagulation values are in the therapeutic range, peptic ulcer, polyps, or large bowel malignancy should be considered. (Spontaneous bleeding without cause, of course, may result when either prothrombin or coagulation times are markedly prolonged). The effects of coumarin derivatives on blood coagulation may be promptly counteracted by the parenteral administration of vitamin K_1 oxide (Mephyton).

Patients with chronic iron deficiency anemia have a higher incidence of achlorhydria and gastritis than do healthy control subjects. In addition, as many as 10 per cent of patients with chronic iron deficiency may have a postcricoid web when sought by cinefluorography during barium swallow. There is an increased frequency of edentia, angular stomatitis, and glossitis in patients with webs, as well as an unexplained association with thyroid disease (with increased thyroid antibodies), pernicious anemia, rheumatoid disease, Sjögren's syndrome, ulcerative colitis, and malignancy of the upper gastrointestinal tract.[79]

Esophageal involvement has been reported in 40 per cent of patients with acute leukemia and 20 per cent of those with chronic leukemia.[80] Leukemic infiltration is found most commonly in the lamina propria, usually in association with widespread leukemic infiltration of other organs. Leukemic plugging of blood vessels, often with perivascular infiltrates, occurs less frequently. Esophageal erosions occur in 34 per cent of patients, usually an aftermath of agranulocytosis complicating chemotherapy or extensive bone marrow replacement by leukemic cells. Esophageal moniliasis is found in 33 per cent of patients with esophageal erosions, most of whom had received antibiotics or chemotherapy. A small number of patients have monilial ulcers in the stomach and small intestine as well. Clinically, dysphagia is only occasionally found. Rarely complete esophageal obstruction results from extensive leukemic overgrowth. In acute leukemia, esophageal erosions may occasionally be extensive and serve as the portal of entry for fatal bacteremia or the site of massive hemorrhage.

INFILTRATIVE DISEASES

SYSTEMIC AMYLOIDOSIS

Systemic amyloidosis is a multisystemic disorder, characterized by diffuse tissue deposition of an amorphous eosinophilic extracellular protein-polysaccharide complex. Blood vessels, connective tissue, muscles, skin, mucous membranes, and the parenchyma of many organs may be infiltrated. All levels of the gastrointestinal tract may be involved, the chief sites of amyloid deposition being the walls of blood vessels, mucous membrane, muscularis mucosae, and outer muscular coats.[81] The diagnosis is often established by direct gingival, gastric, intestinal, or rectal biopsy. Congo red stain reveals sites of amyloid deposition, clarified further by birefringent staining under polarized light. Patients have now been reported in whom stomach involvement has been confirmed by fiberoptic gastroscopy.

Gastrointestinal manifestations are varied but directly related to amyloid deposition in blood vessel walls, epithelial surfaces, muscular coats, or submucosal and myenteric ganglia.[82] The following complications of amyloidosis have been recognized.

Motility Disturbances. These have been related to autonomic neuropathy and muscle layer infiltration.[83] Physiological abnormalities have included delayed gastric emptying, prolonged small bowel transit time, and segmental dilatation of small bowel loops. Esophageal motility studies have indicated marked impairment or absence of motor activity in the distal two-thirds of the esophagus, and megaesophagus has been reported. Clinically, intractable diarrhea may be present, although occasionally constipation is the presenting manifestation.

Malabsorption. Steatorrhea has been found in some patients.[84] Fecal fat may be as high as 25 g daily, with an abnormal D-xylose test and low serum carotene and serum albumin levels. Immunoglobulins may also be low. Radiological study often reveals nonspecific dilatation of small intestine with coarsening of mucosal folds. The definitive mechanism of malabsorption has not been elucidated. Contributing factors include the following: (1) mucosal infiltration, especially with villous involvement; (2) motility disorder with secondary stasis and bacterial overgrowth; (3) exocrine pancreatic insufficiency related to infiltration of acinar elements with amyloid; and (4) mesenteric vascular insufficiency caused by vessel wall involvement (see pp. 1061 to 1065).

Gastrointestinal Ulceration. This is probably of ischemic origin and related to amyloid blood vessel disease. Ulcers have been reported in both the stomach and colon.

Mesenteric Ischemic Attacks. These are characterized by recurrent abdominal pain.

Gastrointestinal Bleeding. This is often severe and is probably due to ischemic necrosis or disruption of local blood vessel integrity by impingement of amyloid deposits. Muscoal friability is commonly found at sites of amyloid infiltration.[85]

Gastric Outlet Obstruction. This is often associated with antral deformity and prominent folds detected by both endoscopy and radiologic study. Flattening of mucosal folds with absent antral peristalsis and focal white infiltrates has also been found on gastroscopy.

Protein-Losing Enteropathy. This phenomenon has been reported in association with gastrointestinal amyloidosis.[86] The mechanism is probably not lymphatic obstruction but amyloid deposition in mucosal blood vessel walls, altering capillary permeability to plasma proteins. Inflammatory bowel disease of long duration may also be complicated by systemic amyloidosis, especially if sepsis and fistulas have been prominent features.

There is no effective therapy for systemic amyloidosis. However, broad-spectrum antibiotics, such as ampicillin or tetracycline, may prove useful in malabsorption syndromes if stasis with bacterial overgrowth is suspected. Coexistent clinical signs of autonomic neuropathy should raise the suspicion of this form of malabsorption.

SARCOIDOSIS

Occasionally granulomatous infiltration of the stomach is noted in association with disseminated sarcoidosis.[87] Such patients often present with clinical symptoms of pyloric obstruction. Thickened folds are noted on X-ray with antral narrowing simulating gastric neoplasm. Similar granulomatous pathology may be seen in patients with regional enteritis; a few patients with isolated granulomatous gastritis have also been reported. Because of clinical symptoms and the similarity to carcinoma, partial gastric resection is usually carried out. The effect of steroid therapy is not known.

LIPID STORAGE DISEASE

Congenital β-Lipoprotein Deficiency. In this disease the underlying defect is the inability to form β-lipoprotein molecules. The disease is transmitted as an autosomal recessive disorder. Its characteristics are spiny appearance of red cells (acanthocytes); serum lipid abnormalities, which include low to absent β-lipoproteins, reduced α-lipoproteins, low cholesterol and phospholipids, and very low triglycerides; steatorrhea with onset during the first two years of life; neurological disorder resembling Friedreich's ataxia and reflecting involvement of the cerebellum, basal ganglia, posterior columns, and peripheral nerves; and atypical retinitis pigmentosa.[88] The intestinal villi of patients with β-lipoprotein deficiency are normal in length and configuration. The characteristic feature is the presence of lipid droplets in the mucosal epithelial cells.[89] By contrast, the submucosa and lamina propria show practically no fat droplets, and the villous lymphatics are empty. Studies indicate that mucosal esterification of fatty acids and monoglycerides to triglycerides is normal. The diminished fat absorption is due to impaired transport of triglyceride out of the mucosal cell (exit block), as a result of impaired chylomicron synthesis. Since steatorrhea is not severe, the portal route probably serves as a major pathway of long-chain fatty acid transport from the intestine. A striking feature in this disease is the reduction in blood and tissues of the essential fatty acid, lineoleic acid. The cause of the multiple neurological defects in not known. In management, the use of medium-chain triglycerides to replace conventional dietary long-chain fatty acids may improve nutrition and reduce steatorrhea (see pp. 1046 to 1049).

Tangier Disease. In this disease, esterified cholesterol accumulates in macrophages, whereas plasma cholesterol is low because of absence or near absence of high density lipoproteins (α 1-lipoprotein). Clinical features may include yellow-streaked tonsils, hepatomegaly, splenomegaly, diarrhea, and peripheral neuropathy. Inheritance is probably autosomal recessive. Large collections of pale, cholesterol-containing macrophages are found in tonsils, thymus, lymph nodes, marrow, liver, and intestinal tract.[90] Mucosal elevations, 1 to 2 mm in size, may be found in the small bowel, colon, and rectum, which represent collections of lipid-containing macrophages. Numerous macrophages may be found in the lamina propria of the colon and rectum and are also found in the submucosa of the jejunum and at the base of lymphoid tissue in the small intestine. Steatorrhea is not a feature, probably because α-lipoproteins are not important constituents of chylomicrons.

Wolman's Disease. There is also prominent cholesterol storage in lymphoid tissues and intestinal mucosa in this disease. However, calcified adrenal glands and marked hepatosplenomegaly are distinctive features.[91]

PULMONARY DISEASE

Both acute and chronic gastric and duodenal ulcers have been reported to have an increased incidence in chronic obstructive pulmonary disease. Acute ulcers, commonly found at autopsy, might relate to the stresses of terminal illness. Chronic duodenal ulcers have been found in up to 30 per cent of males with chronic pulmonary disease in the sixth decade of life.[92] Possible causal factors might include the frequent use of adrenal steroids and the physiological effects of hypoxia and hypercapnia. However, clinical and laboratory studies are contradictory as to whether elevation of blood carbon dioxide, and/or systemic hypoxia, increases gastric acid secretion.[93] Whatever the mechanism, the association between chronic peptic ulcers and chronic obstructive pulmonary disease is important, because both emergency and elective surgery in such patients involves significant risk.[94]

REFERENCES

1. Vela, A. R., and Balart, L. Esophageal motor manifestations in diabetes mellitus. Amer. J. Surg. *119*:21, 1970.
2. Katz, L. A., and Spiro, H. M. Gastrointestinal manifestations of diabetes. New Eng. J. Med. *275*:1350, 1966.
3. Irvine, W. J., Scarth, L., Clarke, B. F., et al. Thyroid and gastric autoimmunity in patients with diabetes mellitus. Lancet *2*:163, 1970.
4. Malins, J. M., and Mayne, N. Diabetic diarrhea. A study of 13 patients with jejunal biopsy. Diabetes *18*:858, 1969.
5. Wruble, L. D., and Kalser, M. H. Diabetic steatorrhea: A distinct entity. Amer. J. Med. *37*:118, 1964.
6. Goldstein, F., Wirts, C. W., and Kowlessar, O. D. Diabetic diarrhea and steatorrhea. Microbiologic and clinical observations. Ann. Intern. Med. *72*:215, 1970.
7. Katz, L. A., and Spiro, H. M. Gastrointestinal manifestations of diabetes. New Eng. J. Med. *275*:1350, 1966.
8. Grodski, M., Mazurkiewicz-Rozynska, E., Czyzyk, A., et al. Diabetic cholecystopathy. Diabetologia *4*:345, 1968.
9. Middleton, W. R. Thyroid hormones in the gut. Gut *12*:172, 1971.
10. Hellesen, C., Friis, T., Larsen, E., et al. Small intestinal histology, radiology, and absorption in hyperthyroidism. Scand. J. Gastroenterol. *4*:169, 1969.
11. Broitman, S. A., Bondy, D. C., Yachnin, I., et al. Absorption and disposition of D-xylose in thyrotoxicosis and myxedema. New Eng. J. Med. *270*:333, 1964.
12. Chapman, E. M., and Maloof, F. Bizarre clinical manifestations of hyperthyroidism. New Eng. J. Med. *254*:1, 1956.
13. Siurala, M., Varis, K., Lambert, B. A., et al. Intestinal absorption and auto-immunity in endocrine disorders. Acta Med. Scand. *184*:53, 1968.
14. Chadha, J. S., Ashby, D. W., Cowan, W. D., et al. Fatal intestinal atony in myxedema. Brit. Med. J. *3*:398, 1969.
15. Duret, R. L., and Bastenie, P. A. Intestinal disorders in hypothyroidism. Clinical and manometric study. Amer. J. Dig. Dis. *16*:723, 1971.
16. Kaplan, E. L., and Peskin, G. W. Physiologic implications of medullary carcinoma of the thyroid gland. Surg. Clin. N. Amer. *51*:125, 1971.
17. Eversmann, J. J., Farmer, R. G., Brown, C. H., et al. Gastrointestinal manifestations of hyperparathyroidism. Arch. Intern. Med. *119*:605, 1967.
18. Smith, J. F. Parathyroid adenomas associated with the malabsorption syndrome and chronic renal disease. J. Clin. Path. *23*:362, 1970.
19. Morse, W. I., Cochrane, W. A., Landrigan, P., et al. Familial hypoparathyroidism with pernicious anemia, steatorrhea, and adrenocortical insufficiency. N. Eng. J. Med. *264*:1021, 1961.
20. Marks, J., and Shuster, S. Intestinal malabsorption and the skin. Gut *12*:938, 1971.
21. Brow, J. R., Parker, F., Weinstein, W. M., et al. The small intestinal mucosa in dermatitis herpetiformis. I. Severity and distribution of the small intestinal lesion and associated malabsorption Gastroenterology *60*:355, 1971.
22. Weinstein, W. M., Brow, J. R., Parker, F., et al. The small intestinal mucosa in dermatitis herpetiformis. II. Relationship of the small intestinal lesion to gluten. Gastroenterology *60*:362, 1971.
23. Hughes, W. S., Cerda, J. J., Holtzapple, P., et al. Primary hypogammaglobulinemia and malabsorption. Ann. Intern. Med. *74*:903, 1971.

24. Hermans, P. E., Huizenga, K. A., Hoffman, H. N., et al. Dysgammaglobulinemia associated with nodular lymphoid hyperplasia of the small intestine. Amer. J. Med. 40:78, 1966.

25. Kirkpatrick, C. H., Waxman, D., Smith, O. D., et al. Hypogammaglobulinemia with nodular lymphoid hyperplasia of the small bowel. Arch. Intern. Med. 121:273, 1968.

26. Hoskins, L. C., Winawer, S. J., Broitman, S. A., et al. Clinical giardiasis and intestinal malabsorption. Gastroenterology 53:265, 1967.

27. Brown, W. R., Savage, D. C., Dubois, R. S., Alp, M. H., Mallory, A., and Kern, F., Jr. Intestinal microflora of immunoglobulin-deficient and normal human subjects. Gastroenterology 62:1143, 1972.

28. Parkin, D. M., McClelland, D. B. L., O'Moore, R. R., et al. Intestinal bacterial flora and bile salt studies in hypogammaglobulinemia. Gut 13:182, 1972.

29. Ament, M. E., and Rubin, C. E. Relation of giardiasis to abnormal intestinal structure and function in gastrointestinal immunodeficiency syndrome. Gastroenterology 62:216, 1972.

30. Bjernulf, A., Johansson, S. G., Parrow, A., et al. Immunoglobulin studies in gastrointestinal dysfunction with special reference to IgA deficiency. Acta Med. Scand. 190:71, 1971.

31. Crabbé, P. A., and Heremans, J. F. Selective IgA deficiency with steatorrhea. Amer. J. Med. 42:319, 1967.

32. Asquith, P., Thompson, R. A., Cooke, W. T., et al. Serum-immunoglobulins in adult coeliac disease. Lancet 2:129, 1969.

33. Eisner, J. W., and Bralow, S. P. Intestinal lymphangiectasia with immunoglobulin deficiency. Amer. J. Dig. Dis. 13:1055, 1968.

34. Waldmann, T. A., and Schwab, P. J. IgG metabolism in hypogammaglobulinemia. J. Clin. Invest. 44:1523, 1965.

35. Twomey, J. J., Jordan, P. H., Jarrold, T., et al. The syndrome of immunoglobulin deficiency and pernicious anemia. Amer. J. Med. 47:340, 1969.

36. Rosenberg, E. B., Whalen, G. E., Bennich, H., et al. Increased circulating IgE in a new parasitic disease — human intestinal capillariasis. New Eng. J. Med. 283:1148, 1970.

37. Neschis, M., Siegelman, S. S., Rotstein, J., et al. The esophagus in progressive systemic sclerosis: A manometric and radiographic correlation. Amer. J. Dig. Dis. 15:443, 1970.

38. Carrett, J. M., Winkelmann, R. K., Schegel, J. F., et al. Esophageal deterioration in scleroderma. Mayo Clin. Proc. 46:92, 1971.

39. Peachey, R. D. G., Creamer, B., Pierce, J. W., et al. Sclerodermatous involvement of the stomach and the small and large bowel. Gut 10:285, 1969.

40. Bluestone, R., Macmahon, M., Dawson, J. M., et al. Systemic sclerosis and small bowel involvement. Gut 10:185, 1969.

41. Matolo, N. M., and Albo, D., Jr. Gastrointestinal complications of collagen vascular diseases. Surgical implications. Amer. J. Surg. 122:678, 1971.

42. Miercort, R. D., and Merril, F. G. Pneumatosis

43. Kahn, I. J., Jeffries, G. H., and Sleisenger, M. H. Malabsorption in intestinal scleroderma. Correction by antibiotics. New Eng. J. Med. 274:1339, 1966.

44. Schuster, M. M. Clinical significance of motor disturbances of the enterocolonic segment. Amer. J. Dig. Dis. 11:320, 1966.

45. Feldman, F., and Marshak, R. H. Dermatomyositis with significant involvement of the gastrointestinal tract. Amer. J. Roent. 90:746, 1963.

46. Cummings, N. A. Oral manifestations of connective tissue disease. Postgrad. Med. 49:134, 1971.

47. Brown, C. H., Shirey, E. K., and Haserick, J. R. Gastrointestinal manifestations of systemic lupus erythematosus. Gastroenterology 31:649, 1956.

48. Pollack, V. E., Grove, W. J., Kark, R. M., et al. Systemic lupus erythematosus simulating acute surgical condition of the abdomen. New Eng. J. Med. 259:258, 1958.

49. Bazinet, P., and Marin, G. A. Malabsorption in systemic lupus erythematosus. Amer. J. Dig. Dis. 16:460, 1971.

50. Kurlander, D. J., and Kirsner, J. B. Association of chronic "nonspecific" inflammatory bowel disease with lupus erythematosus. Ann. Intern. Med. 119:359, 1967.

51. Bienenstock, H., Minick, C. R., and Rogoff, B. Mesenteric arteritis and intestinal infarction in rheumatoid disease. Arch. Intern. Med. 119:359, 1967.

52. Russell, P. S., and Castleman, B. Abdominal pain in patients with rheumatoid arthritis. New Eng. J. Med. 268:438, 1963.

53. Merrill, J. P., and Hampers, C. L. Uremia. I. New Eng. J. Med. 282:953, 1970.

54. Gruskin, S. E., Tolman, D. E., Wagoner, R. D., et al. Oral manifestations of uremia. Minn. Med. 53:495, 1970.

55. Mason, E. E. Gastrointestinal lesions occurring in uremia. Ann. Intern. Med. 37:96, 1952.

56. Stewart, J. H., and Castaldi, P. R. Uraemic bleeding: A reversible platelet defect. Quart. J. Med. 36:409, 1967.

57. Bayer, W. L., Szeto, I. L., Domm, B. L., et al. Uremic bleeding. Penna. Med. 72:65, 1969.

58. Davenport, H. W. Destruction of the gastric mucosal barrier by detergents and urea. Gastroenterology 54:175, 1968.

59. Hadjiyannakis, E. J., Smellie, W. A., Evans, D. B., et al. Gastrointestinal complications after renal transplantation. Lancet 2:781, 1971.

60. Woods, J. E. Pancreatitis in renal allografted patients. Mayo Clin. Proc. 47:193, 1972.

61. Burgoon, C. F., Jr., Grahan, J. G., McCaffree, D. L., et al. Mast cell disease. A cutaneous variant with multisystem involvement. Arch. Dermatol. 98:590, 1968.

62. Keller, R. T., and Roth, H. P. Hyperchlorhydria and hyperhistaminemia in a patient with systemic mastocytosis. New Eng. J. Med. 283:1449, 1970.

63. Broitman, S. A., McCray, R. S., May, J. C., et al.

and pseudo-obstruction in scleroderma. Radiology 92:359, 1969.

Mastocytosis and intestinal malabsorption. Amer. J. Med. 48:382, 1970.

64. Jarnum, S., and Zachariae, H. Mastocytoses (urticaria pigmentosa) of skin, stomach, and gut with malabsorption Gut 8:64, 1967.

65. Huston, J. R., and Stewart, W. R. C. Hemorrhagic pheochromocytoma with shock and abdominal pain. Amer. J. Med. 39:502, 1965.

66. Duffy, T. J., Erickson, E. E., Jordan, G. L., Jr., et al. Megacolon and bilateral pheochromocytoma. Amer. J. Gastroent. 38:555, 1962.

67. Cruz, S. R., and Colwell, J. A. Pheochromocytoma and ileus. J.A.M.A. 219:1050, 1972.

68. Rosati, L. A., and Augur, N. A., Jr. Ischemic enterocolitis in pheochromocytoma. Gastroenterology 60:581, 1971.

68. Beighton, P. H., Murdoch, J. L., and Votteler, T. Gastrointestinal complications of the Ehlers-Danlos syndrome. Gut 10:1004, 1969.

70. Bardsley, J. L., and Koehler, P. R. Pseudoxanthoma elasticum; angiographic manifestations in abdominal vessels. Radiology 93:559, 1969.

71. Bosma, J. F. Progressive motor disabilities. Postgrad. Med. 49:162, 1971.

72. Huvos, A. G., and Pruzanski, W. Smooth muscle involvement in primary muscle disease. II. Progressive muscular dystrophy. Arch. Path. 83:234, 1967.

73. Siegel, C. I., Hendrix, T. R., and Harvey, J. C. The swallowing disorder in myotonia dystrophica. Gastroenterology 50:541, 1966.

74. Schuster, M. M. Clinical significance of motor disturbances of the enterocolonic segment. Amer. J. Dig. Dis. 11:320, 1966.

75. Sulway, M. J., Baume, P. E., and Davis, E. Stiffman syndrome presenting with complete esophageal obstruction. Amer. J. Dig. Dis. 15:79, 1970.

76. Strober, W., Cohen, L. S., Waldmann, T. A., et al. Tricuspid regurgitation. A newly recognized cause of protein-losing enteropathy, lymphocytopenia, and immunologic deficiency. Amer. J. Med. 44:842, 1968.

77. Wilkinson, P., Pinto, B., and Senior, J. R. Reversible protein-losing enteropathy with intestinal lymphangiectasia secondary to chronic constrictive pericarditis. New Eng. J. Med. 273:1178, 1965.

78. Dodds, W. J., Spitzer, R. M., Friedland, G. W., et al. Gastrointestinal roentgenographic manifestations of hemophilia. Am. J. Roent. 110:412, 1970.

79. Chisholm, M., Ardran, G. M., Callender, S. T., et al. Iron deficiency in auto-immunity and post-cricoid webs. Quart. J. Med. 40:421, 1971.

80. Givler, R. L. Esophageal lesions in leukemia and lymphoma. Amer. J. Dig. Dis. 15:31, 1970.

81. Gilat, T., Revach, M., and Sohar, E. Deposition of amyloid in the gastrointestinal tract. Gut 10:98, 1969.

82. Gilat, T., and Spiro, H. M. Amyloidosis and the gut. Amer. J. Dig. Dis. 13:619, 1968.

83. French, J. M., Hall, G., Parrish, D. J., et al. Peripheral and autonomic nerve involvement in primary amyloidosis associated with uncontrollable diarrhea and steatorrhoea. Amer. J. Med. 39:277, 1965.

84. Levinson, G. C., and Kirsner, J. B. Infiltrative diseases of the small bowel and malabsorption. Amer. J. Dig. Dis. 15:741, 1970.

85. Amir, J., Kessler, E., and de Vries, A. Skin and mucosal hemorrhage of prolonged duration in systemic amyloidosis. Blood 35:530, 1971.

86. Jarnum, S. Gastrointestinal haemorrhage and protein loss in primary amyloidosis. Gut 6:14, 1965.

87. Fahimi, H. D., Deren, J. J., Gottlieb, L. S., et al. Isolated granulomatous gastritis: Its relationship to disseminated sarcoidosis and regional enteritis. Gastroenterology 45:161, 1963.

88. Isselbacher, K. J., Scheig, R., Plotkin, G. R., et al. Congenital β-lipoprotein deficiency: An hereditary disorder involving a defect in the absorption and transport of lipids. Medicine 43:347, 1964.

89. Dobbins, W. O. III. An ultrastructural study of the intestinal mucosa in congenital β-lipoprotein deficiency with particular emphasis upon the intestinal absorptive cell. Gastroenterology 50:195, 1966.

90. Bale, P. M., Clifton-Blight, P., Benjamin, B. N. P., et al. Pathology of Tangier disease. J. Clin. Path. 24:609, 1971.

91. Lough, J., Fawcett, J., Wiegensberg, B., et al. Wolman's disease. An electron microscopic, histochemical, and biochemical study. Arch. Path. 89:103, 1970.

92. Ellison, L. T., Ellison, R. G., Carter, C. H., et al. The role of hypercapnia and hypoxia in the etiology of peptic ulceration in patients with chronic obstructive pulmonary emphysema. Amer. Rev. Resp. Dis. 89:909, 1964.

93. Glick, D. L., and Kern, F., Jr. Peptic ulcer in chronic obstructive bronchopulmonary disease. A prospective clinical study of prevalence. Gastroenterology 47:143, 1964.

94. Okinaka, A. J. Surgery for peptic ulcer in patients with chronic lung disease. Amer. J. Surg. 113:545, 1967.

Chapter 31

Clinical Pharmacology

Marvin H. Sleisenger

In this chapter we will review briefly the types of therapeutic agents used for common gastrointestinal symptoms and disorders. Rather than discussing in depth the basic pharmacological action of these drugs, we will consider their use in terms of the gastrointestinal problems for which they are prescribed. Included also will be a brief reference to dietotherapy; although it is not strictly a pharmacological topic, its historical role in gastroenterology justifies reference to it. Drugs, particularly those which are effective for infections, as well as diets which are specific for a few gastrointestinal disorders, are discussed in greater detail in the various chapters in Part II of this volume.

IMPORTANCE OF THE GUT IN ABSORPTION AND SECRETION OF DRUGS

The way in which drugs are absorbed and the height of blood levels achieved depend to a large extent upon the rate of gastric emptying, small bowel mucosal integrity, and adequate surface area for absorption. Thus a patient who is partially obstructed or who has gastric atony for other reasons will not absorb drugs normally, nor will those who have small bowel disease or who have undergone massive resection. At the other extreme, increased small intestinal peristalsis may decrease absorption by reducing the critical time required for exposure to the mu-

408

cosal membrane. Gastric acid will play a role in the reduction of potency of certain preparations used in gastrointestinal disease, particularly pancreatic enzymes and, perhaps, administered bile salts. Absence of gastric acid impairs normal absorption of iron. Absence of the terminal ileum will ensure that neither vitamin B_{12} nor conjugated bile salts will be absorbed.

Cholestyramine given to reduce the level of blood and tissue bile acids and thus help alleviate pruritus may, by binding these substances in the gut, contribute to an existing steatorrhea and malabsorption. A delicate balance has to be struck between relieving onerous symptoms and increasing debility as a result of heightened steatorrhea. Antacid gels may adsorb drugs, especially tetracycline.

A cause of malabsorption which has received great publicity is the administration of neomycin, albeit in large doses (8 to 12 per day for weeks or months). The role of the intestinal flora is extremely important in the catabolic fate of drugs, and little is known about their behavior in this regard except for their ability to deconjugate bile salts, take up vitamin B_{12}, and interfere with synthesis by other organisms of vitamin K. A more complete discussion of drugs causing malabsorption will be found on page 277.

ANTIDIARRHEAL COMPOUNDS

The types of antidiarrheal drugs range from adsorbent substances (binders of gases, bacteria, and other noxious substances) such as kaolin, a hydrated aluminum silicate (usually combined with pectin: kaolin [20 per cent], pectin [1 per cent], to opiates (tincture of opium or paregoric) with marked motor inhibitory action on intestinal smooth muscle.

Regardless of mode of action, antidiarrheal compounds are employed for relief of a symptom and only temporarily affect the underlying pathology or pathophysiological mechanism.

ADSORBENTS

Adsorbing substances such as kaolin are relatively ineffective for severe diarrhea, but are harmless. Other adsorbents include bismuth subcarbonate and activated charcoal, neither of which is pharmacologically potent.

ANTICHOLINERGICS

Drugs such as the belladonna alkaloids (atropine and tincture of belladonna) or synthetic substitutes, particularly the quaternary amine compounds such as propantheline, are commonly used for diarrhea. They are particularly helpful in patients with diarrhea of irritable colon and, occasionally, in patients with acute diverticulitis and loose stools. Their efficacy appears very limited in severe enteric infections (amebiasis, salmonellosis, or shigellosis) or inflammatory diseases such as ulcerative colitis and regional enteritis.

DIPHENOXYLATE

Intermediate in its potency between anticholinergics and the opiates is Lomotil, a combination of 2.5 mg diphenoxylate and 0.6 mg atropine. Diphenoxylate is a meperidine derivative which has been shown to be essentially nonaddictive and to act directly on gastrointestinal smooth muscle, inhibiting propulsive movement and reducing diarrhea. It is an effective agent in doses of 5.0 mg two or three times daily, but extreme caution must be exercised, as with the opiates, in treating the diarrhea in the acutely ill individual with ulcerative

colitis, because toxic megacolon may result from their injudicious use.

OPIATES

Opiates are potent antidiarrheal agents. Their mode of action appears to be directly on the smooth muscle or on the myenteric plexus; regardless, their effect is to inhibit propulsive activity and to raise tonus intrasegmentally in both the small and large intestine. Part of the beneficial effect, of course, is due to their analgesic properties. Although extremely good for diarrhea, their use should be limited to conditions which are likely to be short lived, because they are addictive. Traditionally, tincture of opium (0.5 to 1.0 ml), paregoric (4 ml), or codeine (30 to 60 mg) is the preparation of choice, because these oral doses are effective for diarrhea without providing significant analgesia. Merperidine (Demerol) and its derivatives are used as well as opiates. These synthetic agents also diminish propulsive activity and increase pressure; in addition, some are addictive.

CATHARTICS

A common symptom which must be treated by the physician is constipation. The necessity to have a bowel movement daily is ingrained in the folklore of most cultures in western society. Cathartics are classified according to their basic mode cf action, which in many instances is not well understood. These are *lubricant, bulk forming, saline,* and *stimulant.* The most benign and commonly used cathartics belong to the lubricant and bulk laxative categories.

LUBRICANTS

The lubricants include mineral oil and dioctyl sodium sulfosuccinate. These compounds soften and thus facilitate passage of stools in those patients who have hard, dry feces and painful movements owing to inspissated stool or rectal and anal inflammation (hemorrhoids, fissures, etc.).

Although cautionary notes have been sounded about the use of mineral oil, on the basis of its interference with vitamin A absorption and reports of lipoid pneumonia caused by aspiration, it remains a highly valuable agent. Proper use dictates that it be given between meals, that it never be given to infants or to those with impaired gag reflex, and that it not be given to the elderly at bedtime. Within these limitations, evidence indicates that mineral oil is relatively harmless. If given excessively, soiling will result.

BULK FORMERS

These cathartics include natural and semisynthetic polysaccharide and cellulose derivatives which contain residues that reflexly stimulate peristalsis and evacuation. They also have some lubricant property, because they swell in the luminal water to form viscous solutions. Examples of compounds in this group are methylcellulose, carboxymethylcellulose (Metamucil), plantago seed, agar, and bran. If patients receive instructions in good toilet training and have sufficient bulk in their diet, indications for such preparations will be minimized.

SALINE LAXATIVES

The so-called saline laxatives, salts which are slowly absorbed from the small bowel, include magnesium salts as well as sulfates and tartrates. Some contain high concentrations of sodium. These substances act by drawing water from blood to lumen owing to the gradient of osmolar concentrations. Increased volume of intraluminal fluid stimulates peristaltic activity and flow of a large volume of fluid into the colon which can absorb only a fraction of it, resulting in passage of loose stools. The usual preparations are magnesium sulfate (5.0 g), magnesium citrate (200 ml), milk of magnesia (15.0 ml), sodium sulfate (15.0 g), or sodium phosphate (4.0 g). Dangers include hypermagnesemia with coma and death in patients with renal insufficiency; congestive heart failure may be precipitated in susceptible individuals by indiscriminate or chronic use of sodium salts as cathartics.

In either congenital or acquired megacolon, lubricant and saline agents are employed, particularly in congenital aganglionosis (Hirschsprung's disease). The treatment of constipation is further discussed on pages 1285 to 1288.

IRRITANTS

The most potent cathartics belong to the group of irritant laxatives, comprised of such compounds as cascara segrada, phenolphthalein, acetphenolisatin, and castor oil. The mode of irritant action of cascara and phenolphthalein is not well understood; however, they appear to inhibit the movement of water and sodium from lumen to blood in the colon; they also stimulate increased mucus secretion. Melanosis coli may result from phenolphthalein and cascara usage. Castor oil acts on the small intestine. Its potency depends on release of ricinoleic acid after hydrolysis. Ricinoleic acid may also block transport of water and electrolytes from lumen to blood. Hepatitis caused by oxyphenisatin has been reported; fortunately, it appears to be reversible when the agent is withdrawn.[1]

Habitual use of these compounds may be hazardous. They may be associated with dehydration, serious hypokalemia (including nephropathy), anatomic changes in the colon resembling ulcerative colitis (so-called cathartic colon), or even megacolon on barium enema. The loss of mucus rich in plasma proteins may be sufficient also to lower plasma proteins.[2]

The use of irritant cathartics constitutes misdirected therapy. The physician should attempt to diminish preoccupation with frequent bowel movements and to help the patient achieve normal bowel habit by sympathetic support and careful instruction. Mineral oil or even some saline cathartics may be used in patients with obstipation without megacolon.

DRUGS AND AGENTS TO NEUTRALIZE ACID (PEPTIC ULCER)

ALUMINUM HYDROXIDE AND CALCIUM CARBONATE

Intensive medical therapy is required for the treatment of peptic ulcer disease, particularly duodenal ulcer (see pp. 665 to 688). The goal is to achieve as complete neutralization of acid-peptic activity as possible in these individuals, particularly since eating stimulates the secretion of gastric acid. Agents are used which can neutralize acid, are relatively safe (provided they are administered properly), and are inexpensive.[3]

Two neutralizers are commonly emphasized: aluminum hydroxide preparations and carbonates, particularly calcium carbonate. A detailed consideration of the pharmacology and relative merits of non-absorbable aluminum hydroxide compounds and absorbable calcium carbonate antacid preparations is presented on pages 410 to 411. Both medications should be used with the knowledge that frequent administration is necessary, that the patient with peptic ulcer disease must be treated even after his ulcer is healed and that these agents have some undesirable and even toxic side effects.

Some of the toxic effects of these various agents will be briefly mentioned. The aluminum hydroxide compounds tend to constipate patients and therefore are often mixed with magnesium compounds, either hydroxide or trisilicate. Calcium carbonate (2 to 4 per dose) in some individuals may lead to hypercalcemia, particularly in those with renal disease, in whom its use is contraindicated. Increased absorption of calcium promotes alkalosis, because the net loss of hydrogen ions in the stomach is no longer balanced by the binding of bicarbonate in the upper small intestine by unabsorbed calcium. In reality, however, careful scrutiny of large numbers of patients receiving 2 to 4 g of calcium carbonate every hour daily will reveal very few or no instances of hypercalcemia or of renal lithiasis or of symptoms commonly identified with the so-called milk alkali syndrome. Hypermagnesemia may result in patients with severe renal disease given Al-Mg antacids for ulcer disease. Aluminum hydroxide gels may also bind phosphorus in the gut and reduce blood phosphate. Whether or not significant bone dimineralization may result from their long-term use is conjectural.

MILK

Milk is not a useful therapeutic agent for the treatment of peptic ulcer disease. It is a poor buffer, contains a high content of lipid which is not desirable for individuals in their middle years (or even in young adulthood) and, further, is somewhat constipating. Epidemiologically, patients treated with large amounts of milk and cream have an increased incidence of fatal myocardial infarction at earlier ages than matched controls.[4]

ANTICHOLINERGICS

Anticholinergics are the major antisecretory drugs in treatment of peptic ulcer and are discussed separately on pages 418 to 419.

OTHER AGENTS
Pepsin inhibitors and gastrin antagonists have also been used in the treatment of peptic ulcer. The results of such therapy are not clear at present, and judgment awaits further controlled clinical trials. Carbenoxolone sodium, synthesized from glycyrrhizinic acid, has also been reported to accelerate the rate of healing of peptic ulcer, particularly gastric ulcer in nonhospitalized but not in hospitalized patients.[5] It must be considered a strange effect. The mode of action is unknown. Side effects, related to an aldosterone-like action, however, may be serious. Whether a deglycyrrhizinated preparation will be effective is unknown. See page 700 for a description of clinical trials with this agent.

REPLACEMENT THERAPY IN GASTROINTESTINAL DISEASE

Replacement therapy is extremely important in patients with gastrointestinal disease, particularly in those with malabsorption. Table 20–4 (p. 276) indicates the agents which may be used as replacement therapy in malabsorption. The reader is also referred to the discussions of nutrition, absorption, and malabsorption elsewhere in this volume.

CALORIES

Daily requirements for calories may be achieved in some individuals with malnutrition by supplementing the diet with medium-chain triglycerides (MCT), which are mixtures of neutral fat containing fatty acids with chain lengths of eight to twelve carbons. This material requires appreciably less hydrolysis than triglycerides with longer chain fatty acids for uptake by the mucosa. Indeed, they may be taken up unsplit and passed directly through the cell into the portal system. Fatty acids which are liberated in the lumen are rapidly taken up by the mucosa and also pass directly into the portal venous system.

This material may be given in an olive oil medium or as the commercial product Portagen, which also contains protein and some carbohydrate. It should be given as supplemental feedings between meals; patient acceptance varies; some complain of nausea and diarrhea after ingestion. It seems particularly helpful in patients who have had massive small bowel resection and in children with malabsorption. The carbohydrate in the commercial preparation containing MCT also has lactose which may aggravate diarrhea in those individuals who have lactase deficiency associated with mucosal disease of the small bowel or after intestinal resection.

More recently a preparation entitled Vivonex has been introduced to supplement caloric intake. This material is a mixture of essential nutrients, provides total nourishment, and has little, if any, residue. It is well accepted by patients, and is increasingly being used in the treatment of a variety of gastrointestinal diseases in which supplemental intake is indicated. Details of intravenous alimentation for those seriously ill or postoperatively is discussed on page 33. These products are indicated only as caloric supplements and have little use in treatable intestinal disease such as celiac sprue and Whipple's disease.

MINERALS

The major cations which require replacement in malabsorption are calcium, magnesium, and iron. When these are not absorbed normally, serious consequences result—in the instance of calcium and magnesium, paresthesias, tetany, hyperexcitability, tremors, irritability, abnormal behavior, and, in some instances, seizures. It is often necessary to replace magnesium before hypocalcemia can be corrected, be-

cause magnesium appears to be essential for the parathyroid mechanism required to help correct hypocalcemia.[6] Further, if calcium supplements are given without correcting the magnesium deficiency, the symptoms caused by the latter may be increased by aggravating the loss of magnesium in the stool as a result of its competition for a common carrier mechanism with calcium.

The dosage for calcium in hypocalcemic states is outlined in Table 20–4 (p. 276). Whether supplemental calcium must be given for a protracted or indefinite period of time depends to a large extent upon whether an accompanying vitamin D deficiency has been corrected. In some instances both substances must be given simultaneously until the plasma calcium level is normal; if it cannot be maintained by an adequate diet, then the relative amounts of calcium and vitamin D required should be determined empirically.

WATER-SOLUBLE VITAMINS

Supplementation of the water-soluble B complex vitamins as well as ascorbic acid is required for a large number of diseases associated with malnutrition and for the ravages of alcohol.

FAT-SOLUBLE VITAMINS

Vitamins A, D, and K are required for patients with malabsorption in whom steatorrhea is prominent and in whom absorption of these substances is subnormal. The dosages are presented in Table 20–4. Vitamin K should be given parenterally initially to those with severe hypoprothrombinemia or bleeding as a result of vitamin K deficiency. If liver function is normal, parenteral injection of 10 mg of vitamin K will correct the deficiency within 24 to 36 hours. Thereafter, a water-soluble form of the preparation may be given orally, the amount and frequency to be determined by the response of the prothrombin activity as measured by serial determinations.

Vitamin D. Vitamin D_2 and cholecalciferol, vitamin D_3, are the precursors of the substance essential for absorption of calcium. Cholecalciferol is converted in the gut to 25-OH-cholecalciferol and later, in the kidney, to 1,25-dihydroxycholecalciferol.[7] Both substances are active in the absorption of calcium. Vitamin D therefore, 5000 or more units every day, must often be prescribed for patients with steatorrhea; often it must be given along with calcium supplementation. However, care must be taken to avoid vitamin D intoxication, which is manifested by the symptoms of hypercalcemia, a serious and potentially fatal condition. It is manifested by anorexia, nausea, vomiting, constipation, epigastric pain resembling ulcer pain, polyuria, increasing stupor, and, finally, coma and death. Chronic intoxication leads to nephrocalcinosis and metastatic calcification in various tissues of the body, including the cornea.

Vitamin A. Vitamin A is an alcohol found in fish liver oils and in green vegetables. Its precursor, carotene, is converted in the intestine to vitamin A. Carotene is a lipid-soluble substance, as are vitamins D_2 and D_3, and vitamin K. Deficiency will result from prolonged steatorrhea. Vitamin A deficiency may be reflected more by low serum carotene than by common signs and symptoms. The dosage of vitamin A is listed in Table 20–4, and should be given to those individuals who have evidence of deficiency of this substance.

HEMATINICS

Iron, folic acid, vitamin B_{12}, and pyridoxine are the major hematinics required for red cell synthesis.

Iron. Iron deficiency is commonly found in patients with malabsorption and subtotal gastrectomy, particularly those who have undergone gastrojejunostomy (Billroth II). It is also, of course, commonly due to chronic blood loss. The mechanism for normal iron absorption is described on page 256. Iron may be replaced via oral or parenteral routes. The latter is preferable for individuals who have difficulty taking iron, who would benefit from rapid repletion of iron stores, or who are in sufficiently serious condition that oral medications cannot be used. Imferon may be given intravenously in 10 ml doses weekly for three to six weeks, depending upon the state of depletion of the iron stores.

Oral iron therapy is usually in the form of ferrous compounds—0.6 to 1.2 g ferrous gluconate or ferrous sulfate per day. A chelating agent such as ascorbic acid is recommended for those individuals who have had subtotal gastrectomy and have low or absent acid production, because chelation facilitates absorption in the duodenum and jejunum. Ascorbic acid (as well as amino acids and other substances) maintains iron in a soluble form over a pH range of 2 to 11. An acid pH is essential for the solubilization of ferric iron, and because this is unlikely in patients with subtotal gastrectomy, ferrous salts should be used.

Folic Acid. Folic acid requirements are easily met even by a diet marginally adequate in nutrition. In extreme instances such as patients with alcoholism or those who are not eating at all, folate deficiency may result. It is also seen in patients with malabsorption, particularly in those with severe proximal intestinal disease and tropical sprue. Replacement with 5 to 10 mg orally per day over a period of several weeks will correct the evidence of deficiency such as megaloblastic anemia.

Vitamin B_{12}. Absorption of vitamin B_{12} by the ileum is essential for normal hematopoiesis. It requires binding with intrinsic factor, an important glycoprotein secreted by the stomach (probably by the parietal cells). Deficiency of vitamin B_{12} therefore is noted in patients with pernicious anemia, total gastrectomy, resection of a long segment of terminal ileum (12 to 18 inches), selective malabsorption of vitamin B_{12}, pancreatic insufficiency (rare), and the so-called blind loop syndrome. Replacement of vitamin B_{12} is easily accomplished: 30 μg given intramuscularly monthly for life to patients whose underlying condition cannot be corrected (pernicious anemia, hereditary defect in the normal binding site of the ileum for vitamin B_{12} intrinsic factor complex, uncorrectable blind loop syndrome, resection of the terminal ileum). In patients with bacterial overgrowth (blind loop syndrome), which is correctable, vitamin B_{12} absorption will be restored to normal and injections will no longer be required. Rarely, pancreatic insufficiency may also be associated with vitamin B_{12} malabsorption; in some of these patients, administration of pancreatic extract restores uptake of the vitamin to normal.

FLUID AND ELECTROLYTES

Fluid and electrolyte replacement is extremely important in a number of serious gastrointestinal diseases, particularly those associated with profuse diarrhea or severe vomiting. In these situations, an individual may rapidly lose as much or more than 10 per cent of body weight (for example, cholera or Salmonella infection). Massive intravenous therapy must be given to those with obvious signs of dehydration, markedly diminished renal perfusion, and hypotension. As many as 10 to 15 liters of fluid may be required intravenously, and the replacement should be monitored by continuously measuring central venous pressure with an appropriately placed line in the vena cava. Another good index for adequate full replacement of fluid is a urinary output of 100 ml per hour. Intravenous fluid should contain ample amounts of saline (either normal or half normal in concentration) to replete sodium loss. Hypokalemia is another common and serious deficit noted in such individuals, and potassium replacement must proceed as soon as urinary output is adequate. Paradoxically, in such individuals hypokalemia may coexist with acidosis, because large amounts of bicarbonate are lost with profuse diarrhea. A normal serum K^+ in severe acidosis may reflect marked K^+ depletion, and K^+ levels must always be considered in light of the actual pH. Care must be taken to replace the potassium at the same time the acidosis is being corrected, because a rising intravascular pH may displace plasma potassium further unless the electrolyte is being adequately replaced. In many instances, these patients can be given liquids which contain potassium—broth or orange juice, for example. Calcium and magnesium may be seriously depleted quickly in individuals with chronic diarrhea and must be repleted. If acidosis is particularly severe, small amounts of bicarbonate solution should also be given intravenously, but not before replacement of potassium has been initiated.

PANCREATIC EXTRACTS

In patients with pancreatic insufficiency or in those with subtotal gastrectomy (Billroth II), there is clear evidence for inadequate concentrations of proteolytic enzymes in the jejunum. In addition, the luminal contents are deficient in lipase; as a result, the patient has significant steatorrhea and creatorrhea. This dual problem may be effectively managed in many instances by the administration of potent pancreatic extracts in dosages recommended in Table 20–4. Debate continues as to the frequency of administration of these compounds; at the moment it seems that administration of two or three capsules of Cotazym before meals, three capsules with meals, and two capsules within an hour after completion of a meal is a satisfactory program (see Table 20–4 and pp. 1195 to 1196).

BILE SALTS

Recently evidence has appeared that administration of conjugated bile salts, particularly chenodeoxycholic acid, may cause gallstones to disappear.[8] In addition, evidence indicates that the administration of taurine-conjugated bile acids will cause disappearance of oxalate stones in the kidney which are noted following massive resection of the distal small bowel.[9] Confirmation of both therapeutic developments is awaited, as is proof that neither therapy is toxic.

IMMUNOGLOBULINS

Presently, patients with immunoglobulin deficiencies may be treated with periodic injections of purified human immunogamma globulin intramuscularly or fresh frozen plasma intravenously. The efficacy of such management in allaying gastrointestinal manifestations of these disorders remains to be proved (see Table 20–4).

ANTIMICROBIAL AGENTS FOR INFECTION

SPECIFIC INFECTIONS

The intestine is prone to infection by protozoans, viruses, and bacteria. Effective therapy, for example, is available for a number of bacterial and protozoan infections, including Whipple's disease, tuberculosis, gonorrhea, shigellosis, lymphogranuloma venereum, amebiasis, schistosomiasis, flat worms, tapeworms, and giardiasis. Such therapy is also discussed in detail in the appropriate chapters in Part II.

Therapy for some bacterial infections of the intestine, e.g., the enteric form of salmonellosis, may be effective but not always indicated. Chloramphenicol has been the agent of choice for those patients with obvious septicemia and systemic involvement by this organism. Antibiotic treatment alone is not recommended for those who are Salmonella carriers. Whipple's disease is an entity for which antimicrobial therapy is specific. Tropical sprue is a disease of unknown etiology; however, ample evidence exists that it may be, in part, due to an enteric infection which is responsive to antimicrobial therapy.

Specific therapy for enteric tuberculosis is available with streptomycin (1.0 g intramuscularly daily); isoniazid (INH, 100 mg orally three times a day); and para-aminosalicylic acid (PAS, 6.0 to 12.0 g daily), along with pyridoxine (50 to 100 mg orally per day) to prevent peripheral neuropathy. INH may cause hepatic injury, central nervous system symptoms, and peripheral neuropathy. PAS may cause diarrhea, allergic reactions, hepatic and renal damage, and blood dyscrasias, as well as malabsorption. Ethambutol (400 mg three times daily, orally), a newer anti-tuberculosis agent, has replaced PAS in many hospitals. Its major side effects include optic neuritis with decreased visual acuity, central scotomata, and loss of red-green perception. The changes are usually reversible if the drug is discontinued.

Broad-spectrum antimicrobial agents decrease the severity of infection with enteropathic *Escherichia coli* or cholera and make early oral feedings feasible. Even with such drugs, however, substitution therapy in the form of massive infusion of fluids and electrolytes, particularly for cholera, is required. Glucose solution should be given orally as soon as tolerated, because glucose uptake is not impaired. Broth containing a high content of sodium chloride should be offered as well, because glucose absorption will bring sodium with it across the intestinal mucosal cell barrier.

THE BLIND LOOP SYNDROME

A number of disorders are characterized by overgrowth of anaerobic bacteria, particularly Bacteroides and *Clostridium perfringens*. The effect of these organisms is to cause steatorrhea and vitamin B_2 malabsorption. If overgrowth results from conditions which are not amenable to surgical correction, then chronic administration of broad-spectrum antimicrobial drugs is in order. These include tetracycline, chloramphenicol, kanamycin, lincomycin, gentamicin, and sulfonamides. These drugs should be given according to the results of standardized in vitro susceptibility tests; often it is necessary to rotate them for periods of six to eight weeks or longer, as resistant strains emerge. Bacteroides is often resistant to kanamycin and gentamicin.

GASTROINTESTINAL TOXICITY ASSOCIATED WITH ANTIMICROBIAL AGENTS

The toxicity of broad-spectrum antimicrobials includes diarrhea (rarely with minimal superficial inflammation of the colon) and superimposed staphylococcal or fungal infections (usually in debilitated patients or those who have recently undergone major abdominal surgery with an episode of hypotension). These drugs have many adverse effects, ranging from rashes caused by sulfonamides (including Azulfidine) and penicillin and derivatives, to nephrotoxicity caused by kanamycin and fatal depression of the bone marrow caused by chloramphenicol. The practitioner treating gastrointestinal or intra-abdominal bacterial infection must be aware of the potential dangers of these drugs, weighing the indications for use against them. In the area of prophylaxis, for example, the weight of evidence is against the use of antimicrobial drugs to sterilize the gut before major gastrointestinal surgery, except in ulcerative colitis, and routinely in the treatment of acute pancreatitis to prevent secondary infection.

INTRA-ABDOMINAL SEPSIS

The principal conditions for which antimicrobial therapy is indicated include complications of acute cholecystitis and choledocholithiasis, diverticulitis, perforation of the bowel associated with peptic ulcer disease, abscess caused by granulomatous disease of the bowel, appendicitis with perforation, and toxic dilatation of the colon in ulcerative or granulomatous colitis.

The regimen used depends upon the experience of the individual and his colleagues interested in clinical microbiology. For septic disease of the bilary tract, perforation of the intestine, bacterial peritonitis, appendicitis with rupture, diverticulitis, or intra-abdominal abscess, a combination of drugs which covers the major organisms is indicated. One such regimen recommended is high-dose penicillin, 20 million units intravenously per day, and gentamicin 3.0 to 5.0 mg per kilogram intramuscularly per day. Another is ampicillin, 4 to 8 g intravenously, and kanamycin, 15 mg per kilogram intramuscularly or intravenously per day. These infections require surgical drainage; antimicrobial drugs alone are rarely curative.

Some authorities would add either tetracycline (1.0 to 1.5 g intravenously) if the patient is only moderately sick, or chloramphenicol (2.0 g intravenously) if he is very ill. The evidence is accumulating to favor clindamycin (intravenously, when available) or possibly metronidazole. These are all better agents than penicillin G or ampicillin against *Bacteroides fragilis*.

ANTI-INFLAMMATORY AND ANTIPYRETIC AGENTS

The principal anti-inflammatory agents in use in clinical gastroenterology are adrenocorticosteroids, salicylates, phenylbutazone, and the so-called immunosuppressive agents such as azathioprine (Imuran).

CORTICOSTEROIDS

Corticosteroids are used primarily in acute and chronic inflammatory diseases of the gastrointestinal tract which have no clear cause; for example, ulcerative colitis, granulomatous enteritis or colitis, acute nongranulomatous ileojejunitis, nonbacterial sclerosing cholangitis, and eosinophilic gastroenteritis. Dosages for these agents vary according to the severity of the condition, usually being highest in those patients with ulcerative colitis (60 to 80 mg per day at onset of therapy, with gradual tapering of dosage). The rationale for the use of these agents is that they are antipyretic and anti-inflammatory, increase appetite and the sense of well-being, and may combat abnormal immune mechanisms. Whether or not these agents influence the natural history of any of these diseases is not known; however, they are of clear benefit in managing acute flare-ups of these disorders.

The undesirable side effects of chronic corticosteroid therapy are well known and include acne; cushingoid facies; susceptibility to infection, myopathy, hypertension, tuberculosis, diabetes (particularly in those with a hereditary tendency to the disease), and skeletal demineralization; and an apparent risk of upper gastrointestinal ulceration and bleeding. Topical steroids in the form of enemas and other infusible solutions are commonly used in ulcerative colitis, particularly when the disease is predominantly distal. Side effects are rare, although chronic administration causes many serious effects (see pp. 1314 to 1318).

SALICYLATES

These drugs are frequently used for fever in patients with gastrointestinal disease whether caused by the underlying disorder or caused by a superimposed problem (flu, colds, headache). They also have a beneficial effect upon the myalgia and arthralgia (as well as occasionally for arthritis with effusion and erythema nodosum) associated with ulcerative colitis or granulomatous disease. The basis for their anti-inflammatory and antipyretic properties is unclear, and discussion of this topic is beyond the purpose of this text. The toxic effects of salicylates on the stomach and duodenum are discussed on page 646. It must also be remembered that salicylates in excess may interfere with normal clotting as well as causing serious acidosis or alkalosis and hypokalemia.[10]

PHENYLBUTAZONE

This drug is used for treatment of spondylitis and sacroiliitis, more common in patients with chronic inflammatory disease of the small bowel and colon than in the general population. Its mechanism of action is unknown, but complications of therapy are found in 20 to 40 per cent of cases, the most serious being hematopoietic (particularly dangerous in patients with inflammatory disease of the gut), including agranulocytosis and possibly gastrointestinal (ulcer) bleeding.

AZATHIOPRINE

Recently some evidence has accumulated that other immunosuppressive agents, particularly azathioprine (Imuran), may be useful in the treatment of chronic inflammatory diseases of the intestinal tract, especially granulomatous disease of the small bowel and colon. The drug is converted to 6-mercaptopurine in vivo and acts by interfering with the multiplication and transformation of cells engaged in antibody synthesis. Suppression of normal immune function is the major toxic effect. Controlled studies in a double-blind fashion are under way in the United Kingdom to ascertain the validity of this suggestion.

X-RADIATION AND CYTOTOXIC AGENTS

These modes of therapy are directed toward malignancies of the gastrointestinal tract, particularly carcinoma with metastases, either local or hepatic, and lymphoma. Most carcinomas are radioinsensitive, but some lymphomas, including lymphosarcoma, may respond to such therapy. In addition, courses of chlorambucil may be given for lymphoma of the bowel and 5-fluorouracil (5FU) for metastatic carcinoma. Nausea, anorexia, and leukopenia are the principal toxic effects. Discussions of radiation effect will be found on pages 1406 to 1413 and of toxicity of 5FU on page 1459.

DIETOTHERAPY IN GASTROINTESTINAL DISEASE

Along with the folklore concerning the necessity for "regular bowel habits" is the equally destructive and mythical concept that certain diets must be employed to treat certain gastrointestinal diseases. Actually, the number of diseases for which diet is specific is limited. The reader is referred to specific chapters in Part II dealing with these entities.

CELIAC SPRUE

The efficacy of a diet in which gluten has been eliminated by interdiction of foods containing wheat, rice, and barley has proved to be specific in most patients with this disease. Some individuals with flat jejunal mucosa and gluten sensitivity who have hypogammoglobulinemia also respond to gluten withdrawal. This regimen has not been of any benefit in any other gastrointestinal disease.

EOSINOPHILIC GASTROENTERITIS

An occasional patient with this syndrome will respond to withdrawal of an offending agent from the diet—possibly milk, meat, and, in some rare instances, fruits. In the majority of patients, however, corticosteroids must be used to control the symptoms of the disease.

MILK SENSITIVITY

Some individuals develop serious, even debilitating symptoms following the ingestion of milk and milk products. Most prominent among these is profuse watery diarrhea. Such a reaction may be due either to lactase deficiency of the intestinal brush borders of jejunal cells or to an allergy of undefined nature to one or more milk proteins. Withdrawal of milk from these individuals will very often result in dramatic disappearance of the symptoms. Awareness of lactase deficiency in adults may occasionally lead to cure of individuals who had been thought to have irritable colon.

SOYBEAN ALLERGY

Rarely, infants who have been fed formulas which contain soy proteins rather than milk may develop abdominal discomfort, diarrhea, dehydration, and wasting. The jejunum may demonstrate a flat mucosa which reverts to normal when soy protein has been removed from the diet.

DIET IN PEPTIC ULCER DISEASE

Here the power of folklore still flourishes and holds many medical practitioners in its grip. They still prescribe bland diets, baby food diets, milk diets, and combinations of baby food and milk diets for this disease. In reality, the only foods which must be interdicted in patients with peptic ulcer disease are known stimulants of gastric acid secretion without any buffering capacity, namely, coffee and alcohol. It is probably also well to forbid smoking, because there is a significant correlation between smoking and active peptic ulcer, particularly in the stomach. Frequent feeding as an effective method for neutralizing acid is a myth, because food in the stomach triggers antral stimulation of acid secretion. Although milk has been touted for years as the magic food for treatment of peptic ulcer, it has, in fact, a very low buffering capacity. (Also, everybody does *not* need milk, particularly adults.) There is no evidence that so called spicy foods are bad for patients with peptic ulcer disease except on an individual, idiosyncratic basis.

COLONIC DIVERTICULA

The defense of a low residue diet in the treatment of diverticula of the colon is weak. Theoretical considerations and epidemiological observations combine to indicate that a diet high in roughage is perhaps preferable, at least to prevent further formation of diverticula. The use of low roughage diets for patients with vague dyspepsia, irritable colon or "gas problems" is also unfounded. Low residue diets are of value only in patients with small bowel strictures. Likewise, the efficacy for a low-fat diet in cholelithiasis, other than idiosyncratically, is unfounded.

DRUGS FOR "SPASM"

Much of gastrointestinal pain is due directly to "spasm" (markedly increased seg-

mental pressure) or indirectly to the stretching of bowel proximal to the functional obstruction. Accordingly, drugs which diminish pressure are antispasmodic. This term has been applied to the belladonna alkaloids (atropine), quaternary amine anticholinergics (propantheline) and smooth muscle relaxants which act directly (Trasentine, Bentyl) which are prescribed for the cramping abdominal discomfort usually associated with irritable colon. Perhaps interruption of bowel reflexes regulating tone and motility is the basis for their antispasmodic action.

Most drugs used for relief of abdominal discomfort belong to the former group of compounds — their anticholinergic properties result both in diminished reflex activity and in fall of intrasegmental pressure (see below). Combinations of such drugs with sedatives or tranquilizers should be avoided, not only as a violation of basic clinical pharmacological principles, but also because it appears likely that tranquilization is more important than "antispasmodic effect" in treating many patients with distress caused by spasm of smooth muscle. When spasm is extreme, as in biliary tract colic or small intestinal obstruction (after key steps in diagnosis are underway), it should be treated with meperidine, not with antispasmodics or tranquilizers. Since anticholinergics are important drugs for this problem as well as in treatment of other common gastrointestinal problems, they will now be discussed separately.

ANTICHOLINERGIC AGENTS

This group of compounds, represented clinically by the belladonna alkaloids (atropine) and in recent years by quaternary amine compounds (propantheline, etc.), inhibits the propulsive activity of the gastrointestinal tract and, to a limited extent, the secretory activity of the stomach and pancreas. Their mode of action is by blocking the effect of acetylcholine at the termini of the parasympathetic fibers acting on smooth muscle and secretory glands. Thus, pharmacological doses which delay gastric emptying and reduce the effect of stimuli on propulsive activity of the small and large bowel will also affect the function of the heart, urinary bladder, eyes, and salivary glands. The desired effect on the gastrointestinal tract with agents such as atropine and propantheline is not achieved unless the patient has a dry mouth and slight tachycardia. The more serious side effects are blurring of vision and impairment of bladder emptying; thus individuals who have increased intraocular tension or a history of glaucoma, as well as males with prostatic problems, should be given such medication either with great care or, preferably, not at all.

An additional pharmacological action of the quaternary compounds is ganglionic blockade. This demonstrated behavior is the reason that they are preferred to atropine; in addition, most clinicians feel that these drugs are more effective than atropine.

CLINICAL INDICATIONS

Anticholinergic drugs are used in treatment of diarrhea, the "spasm" of irritable colon, peptic ulcer, and acute pancreatitis. It must be emphasized here that, although the anticholinergic agents depress the vagal mediated or "cephalic phase" of gastric secretion, their antisecretory effect in patients who are eating three to six meals per day is offset by prolonged antral stimulation caused by delayed emptying. Unquestionably, however, they reduce motor activity of the stomach (and probably of the duodenum as well), allaying pain. Relief of distress may also be due in fact to prolonged retention of antacids. These drugs thereby contribute to the clinical improvement of the patient. Although some evidence is presented that daily, prolonged therapy with anticholinergic drugs benefits peptic ulcer, confirmation is required.[11] At present, the clearest indication for use is at bedtime (propantheline 30.0 mg orally) in order to reduce nocturnal gastric acid output. The patient should be instructed to elevate the head of the bed on 8 inch blocks because these agents reduce or abolish lower esophageal sphincter pressure, leading to reflux.

The evidence that anticholinergic drugs affect the immediate clinical condition and prognosis of acute pancreatitis is highly debatable, despite experimental evidence that their antivagal effect reduces total volume and enzyme output basally and after stimulation with hormones.[12] It is not likely, however, that anticholinergics significantly reduce the level of pancreatic secretion achieved by efficient and continuous nasogastric suction. The disadvantages and dangers of this type of medication in acute pancreatitis are clear: inhibition of gastrointestinal motor activity contributing to ileus, further confusing evaluation of a difficult and serious clinical problem; bladder atony, often necessitating catheterization of elderly males with the great danger of infection; increase in pulse rate, which may be readily misinterpreted in patients with an acute abdomen and fever; and glaucoma in the elderly or those with heightened intraocular tension.

IRRITABLE COLON

Anticholinergic drugs can be very effective in alleviating spasm of the irritable colon syndrome as well as in reducing the frequency of bowel movements in those who have diarrhea as a major symptom of this disorder. When taken before meals they reduce the magnitude of the so-called gastroileocolic reflex, a combination of events which is at least in part dependent on parasympathomimetic activity of the bowel. However, other active circulating substances are undoubtedly involved in this mechanism (perhaps the prostaglandins, serotonin, and possibly the kinins), so that anticholinergics are not specific for treatment of this disorder.[13]

SEDATION

Very often the potent agent which the physician has in the treatment of a patient with gastrointestinal disease or disorder is a sedative or tranquilizer. Certainly, patients with peptic ulcer disease or anxiety about their immediate and long-term fate, or those with chronic inflammatory disease of the gut as well as irritable colon, and a large group of patients who suffer from vague symptoms of one sort or another, classified as dyspepsia, benefit from the judicious prescription of such agents. There is no doubt that the interest of the physician in the patient's problems and the psychodynamics of the personal situation are of utmost importance in successful management as well (see pp. 3 to 11).

The barbiturates are still very effective drugs for allaying anxiety and tension. Phenobarbital, 32 to 64 mg two or three times a day, and Seconal, 0.1 at night, are often extremely helpful during periods of exacerbation of these diseases or during periods of tension which are known to often precede a flow of symptoms. More recently other tranquilizing drugs have been rising rapidly in popularity. These include diazepam (Valium) and chlordiazepoxide (Librium). The dosage of these drugs is 2.5 to 10 mg two to three times a day, respectively, for functional gastrointestinal distress related to anxiety. Whether diazepam and chlordiazepoxide have some direct effect upon the colon is not clear. Thus the potency of these drugs in the treatment of irritable colon characterized either by diarrhea or discomfort caused by spasm is attributable to their depressant effects upon the central nervous system.

ANALGESIA

Alleviation of pain originating in the gut is a very important part of treatment in gastroenterology. Severe pain caused by biliary tract or small bowel obstruction is well relieved by adequate doses of morphine or meperidine (Demerol); however, since morphine increases interluminal pressure, meperidine, 100 mg intramuscularly (or intravenously if necessary), is preferred. The minimum dose required for relief should be used, and in no case should these agents be given more than once in patients who may possibly have conditions requiring early surgery. Narcotics must not be given except for short-term or expected short-term problems, because addiction is a real hazard, especially in an emotionally unstable patient with long-standing complaints.

Cramping abdominal pain associated with acute diarrhea may be best treated with codeine, 30 to 60 mg intramuscularly. The use of anticholinergic drugs as well as other antispasmodics has been discussed. Sedatives and tranquilizers should not be given primarily for pain.

REFERENCES

1. Reynolds, T. B., Peters, R. L., and Yamada, S. Chronic active and lupoid hepatitis caused by a laxative, oxyphenisatin. New Eng. J. Med. 285:813, 1971.
2. Heizer, W. D., Warshaw, A. L., Waldmann, T. A., and Laster, L. Protein-losing gastroenteropathy and malabsorption associated with factitious diarrhea. Ann. Intern. Med. 68:839, 1968.
3. Fordtran, J. S., and Collyns, J. A. H. Antacid pharmacology in duodenal ulcer—effect of antacids on postcibal gastric acidity and peptic activity. New Eng. J. Med. 274:921, 1968.
4. Sandweiss, D. J. The Sippy treatment for peptic ulcer—fifty years later. Amer. J. Dig. Dis. 6:929, 1961.
5. McHardy, G. What is carbenoxolone sodium? Gastroenterology 56:818, 1969.
6. Muldowney, F. P., McKenna, T. J., Kyle, L. H., Freaney, R., and Swan, M. Parathormone-like effect of magnesium replenishment in steatorrhea. New Eng. J. Med. 281:61, 1970.
7. Tanaka, Y., DeLuca, H. F., Omdahl, J., and Holick, M. F. Mechanism of action of 1,25-dihydroxycholecalciferol in intestinal calcium transport. Proc. Nat. Acad. Sci. USA 68:1286, 1971.
8. Danzinger, R. G., Hofmann, A. F., Schoenfield, L. J., and Thistle, J. L. Dissolution of cholesterol gall stones by chenodeoxycholic acid. New Eng. J. Med. 286:1, 1972.
9. Admirand, W. H., Earnest, D. L., and Williams, H. E. Hyperoxaluria and bowel disease. Trans. Assn. Amer. Phys. 84:307, 1971.
10. Melman, K. L., and Morrelli, H. F. Clinical Pharmacology. New York, Macmillan Co., 1972, pp. 94-96.
11. Sun, D. C. H. Longer term anticholinergic therapy for prevention of recurrences of duodenal ulcer. Amer. J. Dig. Dis. 9:706, 1964.
12. Dreiling, D. A., and Janowitz, H. D. Inhibitory effect of newer anticholinergics on the basal and secretin stimulated pancreatic secretion. Amer. J. Dig. Dis. 5:639, 1960.
13. Holdstock, D. J., and Misiewicz, J. J. Factors controlling colonic motility: Colonic pressures and transit after meals in patients with total gastrectomy, pernicious anaemia or duodenal ulcer. Gut 11:100, 1970.

Part II

Diagnosis and Management

THE ESOPHAGUS

Chapter 32

Anatomy and Developmental Anomalies

Charles E. Pope II

ANATOMY

The esophagus is a hollow tube composed of both striated and smooth muscle, extending from the pharynx to the stomach. Its length, as measured in the cadaver, ranges from 25 to 35 cm in the adult. When measured by endoscope or with a manometric catheter, the transition from esophagus to stomach is found approximately 40 cm from the teeth. In its resting state the esophagus is collapsed; however, it is capable of distending to accommodate fluid and solid material. It is approximately 30 mm in lateral diameter and 19 mm in anteroposterior diameter. Both ends of the esophagus are specially modified to maintain closure under resting conditions. Only the upper portion has a clearly defined anatomical structure which marks this point of closure.

The esophagus begins as the apex of a funnel formed by the pharyngeal constrictors. When viewed from above, the mouth of the esophagus appears to be a slit running in a transverse direction. On either side of this slit are the pyriform sinuses

(Fig. 32–1). This anatomic fact explains why it is important to keep a tube centered in the midline so that the tip of the tube does not stray into, and perhaps perforate,

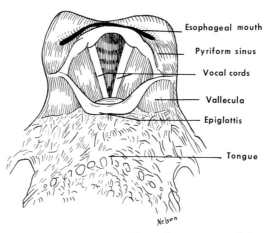

Figure 32–1. View of hypopharynx. Beyond the tongue is the epiglottis, in this view pulled forward to show the larynx. The valleculae are depressions at the base of the epiglottis. Behind the larynx is the opening of the esophagus, which appears as a crescentic slit. The pyriform sinuses are lateral to the esophageal opening.

one of the laterally located pyriform sinuses.

The fibers of the cricopharyngeus muscle, traditionally considered to represent the upper esophageal sphincter, are transversely oriented and insert on the cricoid cartilage at the level of the sixth or seventh cervical vertebra. Two areas exist between the cricopharyngeus and the fibers of the inferior constrictor superiorly and the esophageal fibers inferiorly in which the muscle is attenuated and in which it is possible for diverticula to form.

Once the esophagus leaves this point of fixation, it is relatively mobile as it passes through the posterior mediastinum. It lies immediately posterior to the trachea and then close by the left main stem bronchus (Fig. 32–2). However, it can be displaced relatively easily by enlargement or deviation of any of the structures. The esophagus swings slightly to the left of the mediastinum as it passes behind the heart and leaves the thorax through the diaphragmatic hiatus. During this course through the mediastinum, impingement on the esophagus by osteophytes, an enlarged thyroid gland, an aortic aneurysm, a dilated left atrium, or hyperplastic carinal lymph nodes can be recognized during fluoroscopy by characteristic impressions on the barium-filled esophagus.

The area of the diaphragmatic hiatus has intrigued anatomists, as well as members of the other disciplines, and the names and subdivisions of this controversial 3- to 4-cm segment are indeed numerous. Many of the supposed anatomic features are an attempt to blend radiological features with the prosector's imagination. A composite drawing of many of the supposed anatomic features of this area is shown in Figure 32–3.

In its passage from the thoracic cavity to the abdominal cavity, the esophagus passes from a low pressure area to a high pressure area. How is this pressure differential maintained? A tight muscular seal of the diaphragm around the esophagus might lead to inability of large boluses to pass down the esophagus into the stomach. The problem is met by allowing the diaphragm opening to be relatively large and to be filled with loose areolar tissue. The pressure seal is maintained by the phrenoesophageal membrane, a condensation of the transversalis fascia, which rises on the under portion of the diaphragm and extends up in a fibrous cone to insert on the esophagus 2 to 3 cm above the diaphragmatic opening. This phrenoesophageal ligament is in itself a source of surgical disagreement. Some surgeons feel that this ligament offers a firm anchor for sutures placed to reduce a hiatus hernia; other equally competent investigators find this wispy film of fibrous tissue difficult to find, much less to utilize. When dissections of this area are made en bloc, there seems to be little question that in fact such a fibrous membrane does exist.[1,2]

Much effort has been expended in searching for the muscular equivalent of the pyloric sphincter at the lower end of the esophagus. Although a few enthusiasts remain, most workers now believe that there is no anatomic evidence of a specialized muscular sphincter in the lower esophagus. The fibers of the lower esophageal segment blend imperceptibly with those of the stomach.

The esophagus is lined with squamous mucosa, and the demarcation between esophageal and gastric mucosa can be easily seen as an irregular line, the ora serrata. As the esophagus is distended, this wavy

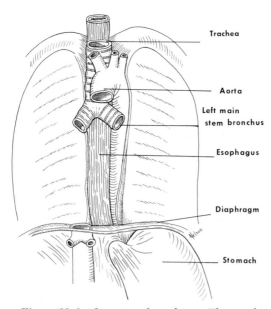

Trachea

Aorta

Left main
stem bronchus

Esophagus

Diaphragm

Stomach

Figure 32–2. Location of esophagus. The esophagus is located behind the trachea and close to the aorta. It swings to the left before penetrating the diaphragm.

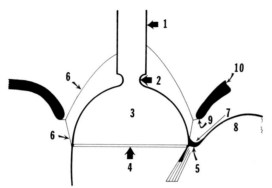

Figure 32-3. Simplified diagrammatic representation of lower esophageal anatomy. Terms used in this report are in italics below. Synonyms frequently used for each area follow, with the name of the author (if known) responsible for introducing or popularizing each term.

1. *Lower Esophagus*

   supra ampullary esophagus (Botha, 1962)
   tubular esophagus (Wolf, 1967)

2. *Inferior Esophageal Sphincter* (Lerche, 1950)

   constriction caused by hiatus (Luschka, 1857)
   narrowing of Laimer (1883)
   sphincter-like inferior esophageal constriction
     (Strecker, 1905)
   constrictor cardiae (Gould and Barnhard, 1957)
   sub-ampullary constriction of Hacker
     (Turano, 1959)
   Ring A (Wolf, 1967)
   tubulo-vestibular sphincter (Wolf, 1967)

3. *Vestibule* (Lerche, 1950) *or Lower Esophageal Sphincter*

   cardia (Sommering, 1796)
   cardiac antrum (Arnold, 1838)
   esophageal ampulla (Barclay, 1915)
   epicardia (Ackerlund, 1929)
   cardiac sphincter (Abel, 1929)
   phrenic ampulla (Templeton, 1944)
     the term "phrenic ampulla" was first suggested
     by Waterson (1905) to describe hiatal hernia and
     has been used indiscriminately by radiologists
     for many years
   epiphrenic ampulla (Hillemand, Beau and Ber-
     nard, 1953), inferior esophageal sphincter

4. *Transverse Mucosal Fold* (TMF)

   lower esophageal ring (Schatzki, 1953)
   Schatzki ring
   lower esophageal web
   lower esophageal diaphragm
   Ring B (Wolf, 1967)
   cardia (originally used by Thucydides—423

B.C.—and Hippocrates—430 B.C.—to denote cardiac end of the stomach)

5. *Sling Fibers of Stomach*

   A thick muscle band lying within the other gastric muscle layers which also marks the esoph-
   ago-gastric junction at its left lateral margin.
   A smaller muscle band, the constrictor cardiae,
   arises above it and encircles the esophagogastric junction.
   sling fibers of Willis (Willis, 1674)
   muscle of Verheyen (1699)
   oblique fibers of stomach (Helvetius, 1719)
   collar of Helvetius
   Swiss cravat
   bundle of His (His, 1903)

6. *Phreno-Esophageal Membrane*

   ligaments of Galen (Galen, A.D. 200)
   hiatal aponeurosis (Blandin, 1826)
   diaphragmatico-esophageal elastic membrane
     (Treitz, 1853)
   Laimer's membrane (Laimer, 1883)
   phrenico-esophageal diaphragm (Jonnesco, 1895)
   phreno-esophageal fascia (Le Double, 1897)
   phreno-esophageal fascial tube (Favera, 1906)

7. *Cardiac Notch*

   incisura cardiae (His, 1903)

8. *Fundus of Stomach*

   apex of stomach

9. *Margin of Esophageal Hiatus in Diaphragm*

10. *Diaphragm*

   (From Zboralske, F. F., and Friedland, G. W.:
   Calif. Med. *112*:33-51, Jan. 1970. Reprinted by permission.)

line tends to straighten and become a simple circle. When viewed through an esophagoscope, the mucosa is fairly featureless, a glistening pink surface, without prominent blood vessels. At autopsy or at thoracotomy the mucosa is not firmly bound down to the underlying muscle. This leads to difficulties in precise localization of mucosal features and their relationship to other, more fixed structures.

The esophagus receives its blood supply mainly from small branches of the thoracic descending aorta. The uppermost portion of the esophagus is supplied by branches from the inferior thyroid artery. The lower portion of the esophagus is supplied from the left gastric artery. There is little overlap in the esophageal territory supplied by the left gastric artery and branches of the descending aorta, so that ischemia can be a problem in reconstructive surgery.

The venous drainage of the esophagus is also split into three portions. The upper third drains into the superior vena cava, the middle third into the azygos system, and the lower third into the portal vein via the gastric veins. All three systems have anastomotic connections which allow blood to be diverted if any one is blocked by disease processes. The most common manifestation of such blockage is esophageal varices resulting from portal hypertension. However, "upside down" varices can also be formed by blockage of the superior vena cava and dilatation of the anastomotic veins by the diverted venous flow.

The motor nerve supply to the esophagus rises in the dorsal motor nucleus of the vagus nerve and in the nucleus of the spinal accessory nerve. The latter innervates the high cervical portion of the esophagus; the vagus supplies most of the rest of the esophageal musculature. Fibers from the vagus anastomose in Auerbach's plexuses with short postganglionic fibers which are distributed to the individual groups of muscle cells. The vagus nerve also carries afferent fibers; however, precise details of the afferent nervous supply of the esophagus are not well known. The esophagus receives sympathetic fibers from cervical sympathetic ganglia and from the ganglia in the thoracic sympathetic chain.

The lymphatics of the esophagus form a highly interconnected system, the upper third of the esophagus draining to the cervical nodes, the middle third to the mediastinal nodes, and the lower third to the celiac and gastric lymph nodes. The wide distribution and interconnection of the system help explain why tumors of the esophagus rarely remain localized.

Microscopic Anatomy. The esophagus is lined with stratified squamous epithelium and consists of a basal layer of two to three cells containing dark nuclei and a series of layers of squamous cells heaped upon one another (Fig. 32–4). The nuclei of these cells become pyknotic and eventually disappear before the luminal border is reached. There is no specialized structure on the free border of the squamous epithelium. Into it protrude extensions of the lamina propria, the dermal pegs. These extend less than one-half the way to the free luminal border. The dermal pegs often contain capillaries which are filled with erythrocytes. The lamina propria itself consists of loose connective tissue containing mononuclear cells, lymphocytes, and an occasional plasma cell. These cells may be scattered or occasionally organized into lymphoid nodules. Polymorphonuclear leukocytes are not normally seen. There are well organized mucus-producing glands, especially at the upper and lower ends of the esophagus. Ducts lead from the glands and empty on the surface of the epithelium. A thin band of smooth muscle, the muscularis mucosa, separates the lamina propria from the underlying submucosa. The submucosa consists of loose connective tissue with fibrous and elastic elements as well as blood vessels and nerve fibers.

Underlying the submucosa are the outer muscular layers. The upper one-quarter to one-third of the esophagus consists of striated muscle and the lower two-thirds consists of smooth muscle; the transition between these types is gradual. The muscle bands are arranged like coiled springs; the inner bands are horizontally wound and the outer bands have a steeper pitch, giving more of a longitudinal orientation. Between the two external muscle coats one finds the intramuscular nerve plexuses named after Auerbach. Interconnections between the different plexuses form a local nerve network in the body of the esophagus. Presumably, this allows a cer-

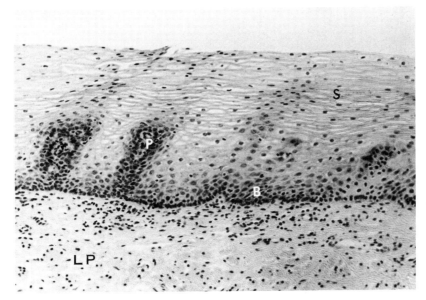

Figure 32–4. Normal esophageal mucosal biopsy. The basal layer (B) is approximately 10 per cent of the total epithelial thickness. The dermal pegs (P) extend approximately one-half the distance to the epithelial surface. The lamina propria (LP) contains scattered round cells. The stratified squamous cells (S) blend with the basal layer. × 170.

tain degree of autonomy and allows integration of muscular activity in the esophagus without the necessity of connections with higher centers.

Unlike most of the rest of the gastrointestinal tract, the esophagus is not surrounded by serosa. This makes the surgeon's job more difficult when he is constructing an anastomosis in the esophagus and may contribute to the more rapid spread of tumor cells outside the anatomic boundaries of the esophagus. The only serosal covering is the insertion of the phrenicoesophageal ligament which arises from the abdomen and inserts into the lower one-quarter of the esophagus.

DEVELOPMENTAL ANOMALIES

FISTULAS

In embryological development, the gut and respiratory tract start out as a single tube. However, they soon divide, so that by the second month the esophagus is in a dorsal position and the trachea and lung buds lie ventrally. It is, therefore, easy to see that the failure of these two important structures to separate completely might

lead to difficulties at birth or soon thereafter. The most common abnormality is the tracheoesophageal fistula. In the most common type of tracheoesophageal fistula, the upper end of the esophagus ends in a blind sac and the lower end of the esophagus inserts posteriorly into the trachea (Fig. 32–5, A). A child born with this abnormality will soon demonstrate overflow of mucus from the blind proximal pouch and will be troubled with aspiration. An X-ray of the abdomen will show the presence of air in the bowel since it will enter freely from the connection to the trachea. This is the most common lesion and is found in from 85 to 90 per cent of tracheoesophageal fistulas presenting in the neonatal period. In the next most common lesion (Fig. 32–5, B), the proximal portion of the esophagus is connected directly to the trachea and the distal portion of the esophagus ends as a pouch from the stomach. Those afflicted with this condition will suffer immediately from aspiration, and films of the abdomen will show no air in the bowel since there is no pathway for air to enter the bowel. A much more uncommon type, when both trachea and esophagus are intact but connected by a fistulous tract, is the so-called H-

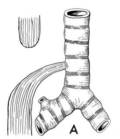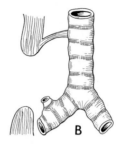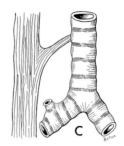

Figure 32–5.   Types of tracheoesophageal fistulas. A, The upper end of the esophagus ends in a blind sac; the lower end joins the trachea. B, The proximal esophagus joins the trachea; there is no connection of esophagus or trachea to the distal end of the esophagus. C, The trachea and esophagus are attached by a short connection, thus creating an H-fistula.

type fistula (Fig. 32–5, *C*). In childhood this presents with repeated bouts of pulmonary infection and abdominal distention, since crying causes air to be forced from the trachea to the esophagus. Such a lesion can become manifest in adulthood and usually presents with repeated pulmonary infections.

Diagnosis.   Diagnosis is usually easy when neonatal infants have difficulty in handling secretions and/or when feeding provokes cyanotic coughing spells or other evidence of aspiration. A lipidol swallow with cine filming is the most helpful diagnostic maneuver. Occasionally, endoscopy will demonstrate the fistulous opening, but such openings are small and easily overlooked. Even in experienced hands, the correct classification of the type of anomaly is only made at surgery.[3]

Therapy.   Surgical correction is the only adequate form of therapy, but timing and approach are important. In the fistulas depicted in Figure 32–5, *A* and *C*, constant aspiration is not so great a problem as the existence of a fistula between the upper pouch and trachea. Therefore, a feeding gastrostomy can be performed and the procedure delayed for four to eight weeks. This allows the infant to gain weight and become more stable. Mercury bougies can be used to elongate the proximal pouch. With successful elongation, it is unnecessary to interpose a length of colon between upper and lower segments of the esophagus. In the case of an H-type fistula, or if an unrecognized second fistula is discovered after primary anastomosis, it is possible to divide the fistula by utilizing a cervical incision.[3]

Surgical results are affected by the type of anomaly present, by other congenital lesions, and by the age of the infant. The mortality rate is about 25 per cent for the more common types of fistula, but may approach 50 per cent for the less common types.[4]

Even if a satisfactory primary anastomosis is performed, problems may persist. Approximately 33 per cent of individuals surviving anastomosis will have postoperative swallowing difficulties.[5] Often a narrowing of the anastomotic site can be demonstrated at fluoroscopy, and dilatation seems to offer relief. This may not represent a purely mechanical obstruction, however. Studies have demonstrated aperistaltic segments of esophagus in these individuals, and the area of aperistalsis may extend even above the site of anastomosis.[6] This suggests a pre-existing disturbance of motility in these patients and helps to explain why dysphagia may persist even after an adequate lumen has been restored by dilatation.

Other Abnormalities.   A much less common form of tracheoesophageal abnormality is a congenital bronchopulmonary foregut malformation.[7] These lesions are collections of pulmonary tissue which lie either within the lung substance or separated from the lung by another pleural covering and which, in addition, have a highly organized connection to the gut, usually to the lower end of the esophagus. Such patients commonly present either with a mediastinal mass or with repeated pulmonary infection. These lesions presumably arise as the result of imperfect separation of the pulmonary and esophageal anlage.

Another result of a developmental quirk usually presenting in the neonatal period, but occasionally at an older age, is vascular compression of the esophagus by an aberrant artery. This lesion presents with dysphagia, and has been dignified with the special title of dysphagia lusoria. This term is usually applied to an aberrant right subclavian artery springing from the descending aorta, but many other vascular abnormalities are possible. In embryologic life the aortic arch has both a right and left arch. Failure of the normal resorption of the right arch may lead to other vascular abnormalities. Diagnosis is usually made by the demonstration of an indentation on the column of barium high in the thorax. Esophagoscopy may show indentation of the esophagus, but is not necessary for the diagnosis. Often such vascular abnormalities are associated with other cardiovascular abnormalities, and the prognosis of the patient is often dependent on the extent of the associated anomalies. Although aortic arch contrast injections can be performed, overlap of vessels sometimes makes interpretation difficult. Occasionally, the full extent of the abnormality is found only at the time of thoracotomy.[8]

A more controversial congenital lesion is that of a web or ring located elsewhere than in the terminal portion of the esophagus or in the cricopharyngeal region. Such rings or webs usually present with dysphagia, consist of squamous epithelium, are not associated with esophagitis, and can be treated by various forms of bougienage. These lesions are unusual and present most commonly during the first six years of life. They are not to be confused with the lower esophageal ring or with the cervical web associated with iron deficiency.[9, 10]

REFERENCES

1. Strasberg, S. M., and Silver, M. D. The phren-oesophageal membrane. Surg. Forum *19*:294, 1968.
2. Friedland, G. W., Melcher, D. H., Berridge, F. R., and Gresham, G. A. Debatable points in the anatomy of the lower esophagus. Thorax *21*:487, 1966.
3. Hays, D. M., Woolley, M. M., and Snyder, W. H., Jr. Esophageal atresia and tracheoesophageal fistula: Management of the uncommon types. Pediat. Surg. *1*:240, 1966.
4. Cozzi, F., and Wilkinson, A. W. Oesophageal atresia. Lancet 2:1222, 1967.
5. Livaditis, A., Okmian, L., and Eklöf, O. Esophageal atresia. Scand. J. Thor. Cardiovasc. Surg. 2:151, 1968.
6. Burgess, J. N., Carlson, H. C., and Ellis, F. M., Jr. Esophageal function after successful repair of esophageal atresia and tracheoesophageal fistula. J. Thor. Cardiovasc. Surg. 56:667, 1968.
7. Gerle, R. D., Jaretzki, A., III, Ashby, C. A., and Barne, A. S. Congenital bronchopulmonary foregut malformations. New Eng. J. Med. 278:1413, 1968.
8. Lincoln, J. C. R., Deverall, P. B., Stark, J., Aberdeen, E., and Waterston, D. J. Vascular anomalies compressing the oesophagus and trachea. Thorax 24:295, 1969.
9. Bluestone, C. D., Kerry, R., and Seiber, W. K. Congenital esophageal stenosis. J. Laryngol. 79:1095, 1969.
10. Adler, R. H. Congenital esophageal webs. J. Thor. Cardiovasc. Surg. *45*:175, 1963.

Chapter 33

Reflux Esophagitis

Charles E. Pope II

Definition. An accurate definition of terms is essential in considering the problem of reflux into the esophagus, as reflux esophagitis may be interpreted by various disciplines in separate ways. To the clinician, esophagitis is a combination of heartburn and hematemesis. The endoscopist would have to see punctate hemorrhage and mucosal friability before he would diagnose it. The pathologist looks for classic signs of inflammation with polymorphonuclear leukocyte infiltration, or fibrosis in the submucosa. Patients suffering the consequences of reflux do not necessarily manifest all these characteristics. Therefore a series of definitions seems in order.

REFLUX. This would seem to be the least controversial term to define. Reflux occurs when gastric or duodenal contents escape into the esophagus without associated belching or vomiting. This process may or may not produce symptoms. It does not necessarily produce pathological changes, and may not apparently indispose the individual concerned.

REGURGITATION. This term implies that the patient has become aware of reflux which has passed not only the lower esophageal sphincter, but also the upper esophageal sphincter. It may manifest itself by the appearance of fluid on the pillow at night, by filling of the mouth with fluid, or by aspiration and coughing.

HIATUS HERNIA. The terms hiatus hernia and esophageal reflux are often incorrectly considered synonyms. If this were so, then reflux could not occur without a hiatus hernia being present, and a hiatus hernia would always be accompanied by reflux. Current evidence refutes this rigid association. Although a hiatus hernia and reflux may coexist in many patients, primary attention should be focused on the esophageal reflux and not upon the hernia. Failure to do so may lead to unnecessary therapy for those with the anatomical structure, a hiatus hernia, but whose symptoms are caused by problems other than reflux.

REFLUX ESOPHAGITIS. Broadly defined, reflux esophagitis is the constellation of symptoms and/or consequences to the esophagus which results from contact of gastric or intestinal contents with the esophageal mucosa.

Etiology and Pathogenesis. Esophageal reflux must occur and tissue damage must result in order for reflux esophagitis to exist. To understand this disorder, it is therefore necessary to examine each of the components of the illness. How does reflux occur? What are the factors that determine tissue damage? What defenses does the esophagus possess?

The primary barrier to reflux is the lower esophageal sphincter. Many other structures, both real and fanciful, have been invoked to explain why gastric contents re-

430

main in the stomach. Structures such as the diaphragm, the phrenicoesophageal ligament, the collar of Helvetius, and the mucosal rosette, each in its turn, have been extolled as the most important guardian against reflux. Experimental work in dogs can usually be marshaled to support the importance of each of these structures. It is never certain, however, that the experimental procedure devised to destroy the structure under question does not also damage the lower esophageal sphincter.

What evidence exists that the lower esophageal sphincter is in fact the primary barrier to reflux? Manometric studies provide the most convincing evidence. If completely normal subjects are compared with subjects demonstrating radiological reflux, clear separation of the sphincter pressures of the two groups is possible.[1] If subjects are divided on the basis of whether or not heartburn is present, there is still a statistical relationship, but overlap is much more marked. If reflux with a pH electrode is demonstrated, there is better separation in sphincter pressures between those with and without pH probe proved reflux, but overlap still exists (Fig. 33–1).[2] It must be realized that the lower esophageal sphincter is not static, but rather varies in response to physical and hormonal influences. Therefore it is not surprising that the correlation between sphincter pressure and the presence or absence of reflux may not be 100 per cent. A sphincter being studied manometrically may react differently from a sphincter which is experiencing its ordinary daily life stresses. If the lower esophageal sphincter is resected, or a myotomy performed, reflux invariably results.

Is the presence of a hiatus hernia necessary or even important in the pathogenesis of esophageal reflux? Certainly reflux can occur without a demonstrable hiatus hernia, and large hiatus hernias can be present for a number of years without reflux. Perhaps even the high correlation between symptomatic reflux and a hiatus hernia is an artifact caused by the radiologist's desire to please the clinician by demonstrating some small pouch at the lower end of the esophagus. In most normal subjects, such a pouch can be produced by having the subject hold his breath as the barium column approaches the stomach.

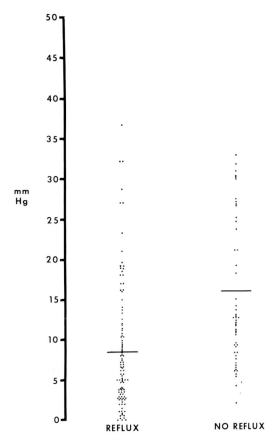

Figure 33–1. Sphincter pressures and esophageal reflux. Each dot represents the mean sphincter pressure in millimeters of mercury above gastric pressure of one individual. Separation into groups was made by demonstrating the presence or absence of reflux with an intraesophageal electrode after loading the stomach with 300 ml of 0.1 N HCl. Although the means of the two groups are statistically significant, $P < 0.001$, there is a fair amount of overlap.

The importance of a hiatus hernia in the production of reflux has been attributed to the displacement of the lower esophageal sphincter into the chest. It is felt that this displacement removes the esophagus from the buttressing effect of intra-abdominal pressure applied externally to the lower esophageal sphincter. Although passive increase in tension might be produced in this manner, active reflex increases in sphincter strength are undoubtedly much more important in allowing the sphincter to withstand the onslaught of increased intragastric pressure. A competent sphincter has the ability to increase its tension whether or not it is located within the abdominal cavity.[3, 4]

It has also been suggested that the creation of a hiatus hernia changes the insertion of the phrenicoesophageal membrane so that it tends to interfere mechanically with the functioning of the lower esophageal sphincter. This is an attractive hypothesis, but very difficult to confirm or refute, since tension in the phrenicoesophageal ligament cannot be directly measured in either the normal or the abnormal situation.[5]

Another possibility is that the small hernial sac might possibly act as a pump to force material through the lower esophageal sphincter. If the hernial sac were small and the diaphragmatic hiatus able to close off the lower end of the hernial sac, transient elevations in pressure in the hernia loculus might be high enough to force material through the sphincter. Combined pressure measurement and radiological studies during actual reflux have suggested that there is an elevation of pressure in such a small sac which allows reflux when the lower esophageal sphincter relaxes in response to a swallow. If the hernial sac is reduced, a sphincter with the same capability would not then have to resist the stress of the high pressure in the loculus.[6]

Other factors are undoubtedly important in the pathogenesis of reflux, but are less well understood. One example is obesity. Many subjects report that reflux becomes severe after pronounced weight gain. Weight reduction is often recommended but rarely attained in the treatment of esophageal reflux. An increase in the abdominal pressure caused by obesity has not been demonstrated; thus the association is unexplained. Pregnancy is another, more self-limited cause for weight gain with a clear association with reflux. Although the fact that reflux is associated with pregnancy has been attributed to an increase in intra-abdominal pressure, recent work shows that there is only a minimal increase in intra-abdominal pressure during pregnancy, and the increase is similar in women with and without reflux.[7] A more attractive hypothesis is that in some women the sphincter responds to the altered hormonal environment present during pregnancy. Most of these women will lose their heartburn after delivery. Of course, both mechanical and hormonal factors change with delivery.

Another important factor in reflux is the quantity of gastric or intestinal content available for reflux. For example, in outflow blockage of the stomach owing to either mechanical or muscular dysfunction, symptoms of reflux are often persistent and relatively refractory to medical therapy. Whether retained gastric acid turns off gastrin and thus lowers sphincter strength, or whether the physical presence of increased fluid leads to more reflux is not clear. Increased levels of gastric acid output have been felt to be important in whether reflux occurs, but hypersecretion has not always been found in those suffering from symptoms of reflux.

The esophagus defends itself against reflux in several ways. Obviously it can do so effectively, for under experimental conditions over 50 per cent of control subjects have transient bursts of reflux. If a large amount of food or fluid enters the esophagus, secondary peristalsis is stimulated through distention of the esophageal wall. Manometrically, this can be seen in patients suffering from free reflux. Pressure in the esophagus suddenly rises, and a wave is triggered off without an accompanying swallow.

When reflux is not in such massive quantities, but is rather a trickle, other mechanisms are brought into play. If a quantity of acid is placed in the esophagus, the normal individual can restore esophageal pH to 6 or above within eight to nine swallows; however, individuals suffering from symptoms of reflux have a great deal more difficulty in "clearing" the acid from the esophagus and some cannot do it at all.[8] Normally, when a pH electrode is withdrawn from the stomach into the esophagus, the pH will rise from a level of 1 to 2 up to 6 even without swallowing; in subjects with symptoms of reflux, often the pH will remain at a low level. It is necessary to infuse fluids through the catheter or have the patient swallow water in order to bring the pH up to 6. Perhaps the normal esophagus has an intrinsic capability to neutralize small quantities of acid, whereas this ability has been destroyed in the esophagus damaged by repeated reflux.

An additional esophageal defense may be mucus production in response to reflux. Patients suffering from severe reflux often complain of excess mucus which is often all too evident during the passage of tubes in such subjects. Whether this is an effective method of protection remains to be demonstrated. The resistance of the epithelium to digestion must also be important. As is true of the stomach, it is easier to state this belief than to document it. The fragmentary work mentioned earlier suggests that the epithelial turnover time of the esophagus is much more prolonged than that of the small bowel further downstream. It is conceivable that some individuals with reflux esophagitis have a defect in this normal turnover time; however, since no clinically applicable methods for study of this function are available at present, this hypothesis cannot be tested.

The character of the fluid which has been refluxed into the esophagus is another important variable which determines the amount of damage that will ensue. Experimental work in cats has shown that both pepsin and acid are important in the production of esophagitis and that these two substances have an additive effect. A solution of 0.1 N hydrochloric acid will produce a lesion in cats, but the concentration of acid necessary for damage can be reduced if pepsin is added to the perfusing solution. Conversely, if this solution is neutralized so that pepsin is no longer active, the esophagus will not be injured by it.[9] Most medical therapy of reflux esophagitis is aimed at the interference with acid and pepsin through antacids.

Another type of fluid, however, must be considered. Patients repeatedly state that the material refluxed is bitter and occasionally describe its color as green or brown. It seems quite likely that these individuals are refluxing duodenal contents, containing both bile salts and proteolytic enzymes from the pancreas. These substances might be injurious to the mucosa of the esophagus. Certainly, individuals with subtotal gastrectomies can suffer from reflux of intestinal contents, and it may be the reflux of duodenal contents which produces heartburn in patients with pernicious anemia, an oft-quoted but rarely seen phenomenon.

Natural History and Clinical Picture. The most common clinical manifestation of reflux is heartburn. Heartburn is a word used by many with the same connotations as indigestion. It is well for the physician and the patient to settle on the exact meaning of the term. Heartburn is usually not described as a pain, but rather as an uncomfortable burning sensation located below the sternum, tending to move up into the neck, waxing and waning in intensity. Often the patient's hand will describe an up and down movement over the sternum. Statements such as, "It feels like I'm on fire," "Hot rolling," and "It feels as if fire is going to come out of my mouth," are common from those with heartburn. Heartburn is more common when the patient is recumbent or when bending over; occasionally vigorous exercise, such as running in place while doing the Royal Canadian Air Force exercises, will cause it. Heartburn tends to occur approximately one hour after meals, and can be induced by ingestion of citrus juices. Citrus juice sensitivity is especially interesting, since pH measurements of the juice indicate that its acid content is insufficient to stimulate the esophagus.

The incidence of heartburn is extremely difficult to obtain. Many individuals consider this sensation normal and do not seek medical attention. Discussion of esophageal function with medical audiences indicates that from 30 to 50 per cent of the medical profession have suffered heartburn at some time. From the annual sale of over-the-counter antacid preparations and their high-priced advertising, it must be assumed that heartburn is common, indeed. Although the statement has been made that its incidence in patients with duodenal ulceration is high, this allegation has not been satisfactorily substantiated.

A response to therapy can be useful in trying to determine whether a symptom represents heartburn or not. As most individuals have discovered, ingestion of antacids usually alleviates the symptoms of heartburn within three to five minutes, and self-medication is extremely common. Long-term sufferers from heartburn prefer baking soda to most other forms of commercially available antacid.

An unequivocal symptom of esophageal reflux is the regurgitation of fluid into the mouth, usually at night, or upon bending over. The patient may state that he wakes up coughing and strangling, or that he wakes up with a mouth full of fluid. Mucus, bile, or gastric acid may be found on the pillow. Regurgitation reflects rather severe reflux. If it is accompanied by pulmonary symptoms, a vigorous attempt to correct the condition should be made.

A less common manifestation of reflux esophagitis is painful swallowing, or odynophagia. Some individuals seem to blend symptoms of heartburn and odynophagia. Usually the latter, however, is seen only when severe reflux has been present for some time. When it occurs, the patient is aware of a dull substernal ache which is intensified by swallowing fluids or liquid. Such distress is usually felt in the anterior chest. This symptom responds less promptly to antacids than does heartburn.

Dysphagia may indicate esophageal damage caused by reflux, although it does not necessarily indicate an organic stricture of the esophagus. In fact, when endoscoped, many patients with reflux esophagitis and dysphagia have a normal intraluminal diameter. Dysphagia is usually for solid foods only, and arrest of the bolus is usually transitory. The sensation of dysphagia is not usually referred to the suprasternal notch, and often repeated swallows will cause the bolus to pass down. In addition to bolus arrest, the patient is occasionally aware of the food moving down the esophagus and can indicate and follow this sensation quite accurately with his finger. The accuracy of this sensation may be tested by giving a marshmallow dusted with barium to the subject and watching his bony finger on the X-ray screen follow the radiopaque marshmallow in its course down the esophagus. It is uncommon for an arrested bolus to be regurgitated; if the bolus will not move with a couple of swallows, a swallow of water can usually make it pass into the stomach.

Another manifestation of esophageal reflux is hemorrhage. When one looks at a suction biopsy of a normal esophagus and notes the abundant bed of capillaries present in the epithelial layer, it is difficult to understand why hemorrhage is not more common. However, bleeding certainly results from reflux esophagitis; it can occasionally be extremely vigorous and necessitate emergency surgery. The bleeding is usually either bright red or coffee ground in nature. Although the patient may give a preceding history of other symptoms of reflux esophagitis, it is not uncommon for bleeding to be the first clinical manifestation of reflux esophagitis. It would seem that patients without the early warning system of heartburn are those in whom bleeding is a manifestation of this particular illness.

Another more uncommon symptom of esophageal reflux is "water brash." Although some individuals use this term synonymously with heartburn or pyrosis, it actually refers to the filling of the mouth suddenly with a clear, slightly salty fluid which comes in extremely large quantities. Sometimes the flow of fluid is so great that the individual must expectorate it. It seems unlikely that this material is brought up from the esophagus or from the stomach. The fluid appears to be secreted by the salivary glands. It tends to be more marked with periods of other symptoms of reflux, and usually is not a persistent symptom.

As is true with many other esophageal conditions, physical examination is unrewarding in the diagnosis of reflux esophagitis. The complications of reflux esophagitis such as repeated pulmonary aspiration and stricture of the esophagus may produce the appropriate changes in the lung and changes of weight loss. A rim of caked antacid around the mouth of one taking hourly antacids is often the only physical sign of the presence of reflux.

Pediatric Manifestations. Esophageal reflux is extremely common in the neonatal period, and it is not yet certain at what point in life it can be considered abnormal. Studies of sphincter function have shown that adult values of sphincter pressure are usually attained within two months of birth.[10] Reflux esophagitis in the very young is extremely difficult to recognize. It may present merely as a failure to thrive, or as bronchopneumonia, or, much more rarely, with hemorrhage.

Less fulminant cases will present as refractory iron deficiency anemia. As in adults, radiological examination will show hiatus hernia in some but not all individuals undergoing studies. Diagnostic techniques are much more difficult in infants and small children, and therapy is often offered on an empiric basis. The surgical results in small children seem to be less satisfactory than in adults and may reflect the more advanced stage of the disease necessary to attract clinical attention in the pediatric age group.[11]

Diagnosis and Differential Diagnosis. There are several different diagnostic maneuvers available to answer specific questions about esophageal reflux. However, the questions must be carefully formulated and the tests are not interchangeable.

BARIUM STUDY. The first question that might be asked is, is reflux occurring? The most common way of answering this question is by obtaining a barium study. However, it is the experience of most radiologists that reflux of barium is noted in only a small proportion, perhaps 15 to 20 per cent of the patients who have a good clinical history of esophageal reflux. Thus, a common situation is the following: A patient, complaining of reflux, visits a physician and a barium study is obtained. However, no reflux is observed, and the patient's complaints are dismissed. A possible reason for failure to demonstrate the phenomenon in a higher percentage of cases is that the high density of the barium makes it unsuitable for a demonstration of reflux. When radiological evidence of reflux of barium is observed, the patient usually has fairly marked symptoms and reflux can be confirmed by other methods of study quite easily.

A modification of the standard barium examination, however, leads to the other extreme. This test, the water siphon test, involves giving a large quantity of barium to the patient, placing him in a head-down position, and having him sip water.[12] A positive test is recorded when barium is observed to reflux into the esophagus. Since the constant sipping of water is a very effective stimulus for sphincter relaxation, a positive examination should be obtainable in every subject.

MANOMETRY. Reflux can also be demonstrated by continuous aspiration of small indwelling tubes located in the esophagus. However, a more practical method involves the use of a pH electrode placed in the esophagus under manometric control.[13] In this test a pH electrode (Beckman No. 39402) is cemented to a manometric catheter (Fig. 33–2). The assembly is swallowed into the stomach and then withdrawn until the manometric catheter senses the lower esophageal sphincter. Then the catheter assembly is withdrawn until the tip of the pH electrode is 2 cm above the upper extent of the lower esophageal sphincter. As can be seen from Figure 33–3, at this point the pH rises promptly to 6 and remains at this level. After waiting for three minutes, the patient is instructed to perform a Valsalva maneuver, to lift his legs, and to sniff

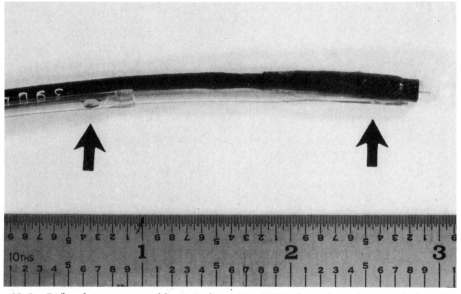

Figure 33–2. Reflux-detecting assembly. A Beckman No. 39042 electrode is shown with the pH-sensitive glass tip to the right. Two manometric catheters are cemented to the electrode; the arrows indicate the side openings.

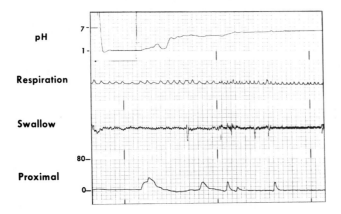

Figure 33–3. Negative reflux test. The top channel records *p*H. At the beginning of the tracing, the *p*H is 1. The proximal pressure tip is pulled through the lower esophageal sphincter, the first pressure hump. The *p*H rises abruptly to 4, and several swallows cause it to reach a level of 6.

vigorously three or four times. If no reflux is demonstrated, the assembly is returned to the stomach and 300 ml of 0.1 N HCl is placed in the stomach through the manometric catheter. Again the catheter is withdrawn to the same location as before, and a period of observation followed by maneuvers is again carried out. Reflux is demonstrated to occur when the *p*H drops to 2 after having attained a level of 6 (Fig. 33–4).

Occasionally, the esophageal *p*H does not spontaneously rise to 6 when the catheter is withdrawn into the esophagus. Although in the original description of this test this result is interpreted as a positive test, it is better to raise the *p*H of the esophagus to 6, either by infusing more water through the manometric catheter or by having the subject drink two or three swallows of water.

A classification of the *p*H reflux test is given in Table 33–1. It would be logical to assume that the farther down the list a test result is found, the worse the reflux from which the patient suffers. Although most patients who report a history of heartburn can be demonstrated to have reflux through this technique, there remain 15 to 20 per cent of individuals expected to have reflux in whom this particular test is negative. Conversely, there are "normal" individuals who never complain of reflux symptoms who will have an occasional burst of reflux during this examination.

BERNSTEIN TEST. Another question one might ask is: Do the patient's symptoms result from reflux esophagitis? The

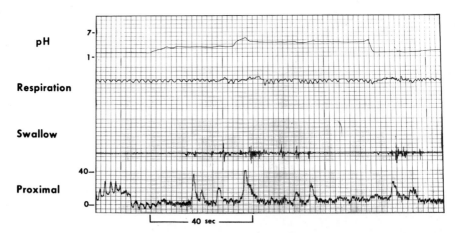

Figure 33–4. Positive reflux test. The pressure tip (Proximal) is pulled through the sphincter at the left of the tracing. The *p*H rises to 3. Then repeated swallows elevate the level to 5. However, there is a sudden precipitous fall to 2. Careful examination of the tracing will show a slight rise in the baseline pressure value and a peristaltic wave which was not triggered by a swallow. The second spike on the pressure tracing was caused by deglutition, as shown by the swallow marker.

TABLE 33-1. REFLUX TEST GRADING

GRADE

0	No reflux under any circumstances.
1	Reflux observed only after loading the stomach with 300 ml 0.1 N HCl and with provocative maneuvers.
2	Reflux observed after loading the stomach.
3	Reflux induced by maneuvers without loading the stomach.
4	Reflux occurring spontaneously.
5	Constant reflux, often with associated secondary peristaltic waves.

answer to this query can be obtained by performing acid perfusion of the esophagus (Bernstein test).[14] A tube is positioned in the upper one-third of the esophagus with its opening 30 cm from the teeth. The other end of the tube is connected to a Y-tube, which in turn is connected to both 0.1 N HCl and saline reservoirs. A three-way stopcock allows rapid change from one solution to the other without the patient's knowledge. The patient is placed in an upright position and instructed to indicate whether or not the drip produces new or old complaints. After an initial five-minute drip of saline, 100 to 120 drops per minute for ten minutes or until symptoms appear, flow is switched to 0.1 N HCl at the same rate. The acid is allowed to flow until symptoms appear or until thirty minutes have elapsed. If the patient's usual symptoms are reproduced, the drip is switched back to saline. If symptoms vanish within three or four minutes, redripping the acid will turn them on rapidly if they are due to an esophageal lesion.

If after an initial period of acid perfusion the patient complains of symptoms, despite switching to saline, it is possible that the acid in the stomach is inciting the patient's discomfort. To clarify this situation, acid perfusion with the tube in the stomach should be done at a later time; if pain is not reproduced, then an esophageal origin for the distress can be assumed. Occasionally the patient complains of an entirely new sensation either during the saline drip or during the acid drip. This result is inconclusive.

It is rarely necessary to perform this test when the patient gives a classic description of heartburn, as the correlation is almost 100 per cent. Although the test is simple and requires little equipment, it is not always easy to interpret. Often the patient's statements are vague or inconclusive, and much time may be required before the examiner can evaluate the test as positive, negative, or inconclusive. It should be stressed that this is not a test for reflux esophagitis. A Bernstein test can be negative in a patient whose reflux has led to bleeding or to stricture formation without previous discomfort. Its value is in its ability to reproduce the symptoms of the patient, providing evidence of the esophageal origin of the patient's complaints.

ESOPHAGOSCOPY. Endoscopy, the principal method of visually examining the entire mucosal surface of the esophagus, has become a practical procedure since the advent of flexible endoscopes (Fig. 33-5). Endoscopy is worthwhile for seeking a source of gastrointestinal bleeding, or discovering whether symptoms of reflux are associated with visible changes in the mucosa of the esophagus. With the flexible endoscope, the procedure can be performed in almost all patients, but it should not be done in a totally uncooperative patient, a patient with fever, or one with a recent myocardial infarction.

After an initial injection of 50 mg of Demerol, the patient's throat is anesthetized with 25 per cent tetracaine. The procedure is explained to the patient, for a reassured and cooperative patient is much more important than the amount of sedation given. After pharyngeal anesthesia is checked with the finger, the patient is placed in the left lateral decubitus position. Diazepam is administered slowly by vein until the jaw becomes slack and the patient's voice is slurred. The dose required is 8 to 20 mg, but may be as high as 30 mg. Hiccups are common, and care is necessary to avoid oversedation and apnea.

After checking the endoscope to make sure that light, air insufflation, and suction are in order, the tip of the esophagoscope is guided into the midline of the pharynx with the left forefinger. The patient is instructed to swallow, and during the period of swallowing the endoscope is slipped into the esophagus. Once through the cricopharyngeus, the instrument is advanced under direct vision. Most new instruments have a flexible tip that can be controlled by

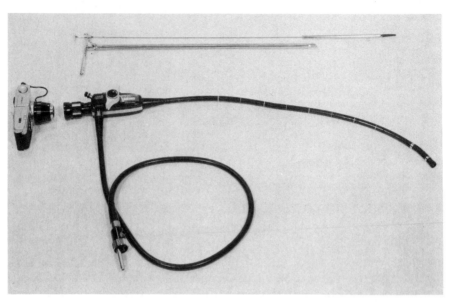

Figure 33–5. Semi-rigid and flexible esophagoscopes. The Eder-Hufford semiflexible esophagoscope is pictured at the top. The rubber-tipped obturator has a flexible end which acts as a lumen-finder. Once introduced, the obturator is withdrawn. Illumination is provided by a distal light bulb. The fiberoptic Olympus esophagoscope shown below transmits light into the esophagus through the fiber bundle curled at the bottom of the illustration. The tip is controlled by the white handle. Provisions are made for air insufflation and suction. Photographs may be obtained by placing a camera at the eyepiece.

the operator, allowing inspection of the entire mucosa. Small amounts of air can be insufflated to distend the esophagus for better viewing. The instrument is passed down into the stomach and withdrawn again. Normally, there is a sharp transition zone between gastric and esophageal epithelium. This sharp distinction tends to vanish when reflux esophagitis has been present. The normal esophageal mucosa is fairly featureless and has a light salmon-pink color. Blood vessels and petechiae are not seen.

The earliest change of reflux esophagitis is hyperemia, a subjective impression at best. Next, patches resembling leukoplakia are observed. If these patches are carefully scrutinized, they will be found to have a thin rim of hyperemic mucosa around them. If the tip of the endoscope is used to disturb one of these patches, friability of the mucosa can be observed. These patches may become confluent, tend to run in linear streaks in a longitudinal direction, and probably represent small superficial mucosal ulcerations. As the process becomes more marked, hemorrhage and denudation of the mucosa are more easily seen.

Strictures can also be seen during esophagoscopy. In their early stages they usually present as a crescent of white tissue; in more advanced stages a stricture may involve the entire circumference of the lumen. Biopsies can be taken through the suction channel of the endoscope; however, the specimens obtained are small and difficult to orient, and usually are not helpful in the understanding of reflux esophagitis.

At the termination of the procedure, the patient is instructed not to eat or drink anything for a one-hour period. The patient then swallows a glass of water. If no coughing ensues, the pharyngeal anesthesia has vanished and the patient may eat. If the patient suffers from a sore throat during the afternoon, anesthetic lozenges may help. The procedure is usually done on an inpatient basis, and temperatures are followed every two hours until late in the evening.

The reported incidence of complication with this instrument has been quite low — three perforations in 3211 procedures.[15] However, if the patient complains of unusual distress or discomfort, it is wise to take a lateral soft tissue view of the cervical region and a chest film. If a perforation is suspected, the patient should then be given barium or water-soluble contrast material to swallow. The dangers of barium in esophageal perforation have been overemphasized. Unlike perforation of the colon, in which the mixture of barium and feces can produce a very large tissue reaction, barium in the mediastinum can actually serve as a signpost to the surgeon who is exploring the mediastinum searching for the rent in the esophagus.

SUCTION BIOPSY. Abnormal mucosal findings are seen in approximately two-thirds of all subjects seeking attention for symptoms of reflux. It is sometimes frustrating to obtain a history strong enough to induce symptoms in the interviewer and yet to see a pale, glistening, apparently normal mucosa. A negative endoscopic examination certainly does not rule out the possibility that reflux has been occurring or that histological changes might not be found. Visible lesions, on the other hand, are definite evidence of reflux. Unquestionably, patients having them will require some form of therapy.

For many years the correlation between biopsies obtained through an endoscope and the clinical, radiological, and endoscopic appearance of the patient has been poor. Normal biopsies have been obtained from patients with gross evidence of esophagitis on endoscopy, and conversely "esophagitis" has been diagnosed from biopsies of individuals with perfectly normal-appearing esophagi. Part of this confusion might well have been that no biopsies were obtained from completely normal individuals, since such people are usually not endoscoped. This difficulty can now be obviated by the use of suction biopsy.

In contrast to the normal biopsy appearance of the esophageal mucosa shown on page 427, a biopsy specimen obtained from a patient with clinical symptoms of reflux in whom reflux has been demonstrated by a pH electrode has a thickened basal layer, constituting over 15 per cent of the entire epithelial thickness (Fig. 33–6). Although there are more mitotic figures, the ratio of mitotic figures to nuclei is actually decreased because of the large increase in number of basal cells. The dermal pegs reach toward, or actually reach, the luminal surface. In approximately 20 per cent of the biopsies taken from individuals with reflux, polymorphonuclear leukocytes are seen in the lamina propria.[16]

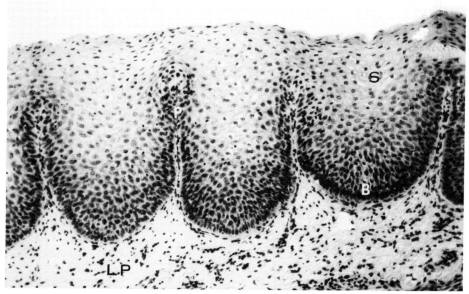

Figure 33–6. Esophageal mucosal biopsy of a patient with reflux. The basal layer (B) is thickened and is more than 15 per cent of the mucosal thickness. The stratified squamous cells (S) seem less vacuolated. The dermal pegs (P) extend almost to the free surface. The lamina propria (LP) contains round cells as do biopsies from normal individuals.

These changes are not uniform but are distributed randomly. If two biopsies are taken from the same location in an individual with reflux, the chance that both would be classified abnormal is only about 40 per cent. However, one of the two would be abnormal in 80 per cent of reflux patients biopsied. If more samples are taken from the esophagus, this change is observed in over at least a 10-cm level, with the odds of an abnormal biopsy at any level being approximately 50 per cent. The changes described in the abnormal biopsies will revert toward normal in some subjects in whom reflux has been corrected by surgical means.

Other methods may be used to study the effects of reflux. Manometric measurement of the sphincter can be done, and, as previously pointed out, pressure will tend to be low in the subjects who are having reflux. However, this is truer in terms of groups than it is in the individual, since overlapping values exist between subjects with and without reflux. Manometric evidence of disturbed peristalsis can also be sought. Although heartburn may be associated with disturbances in peristalsis, normal manometric records can be obtained during a period when a subject is suffering rather intense heartburn. Further efforts to study reflux-associated motor abnormalities have been done with acidified barium. Although peristalsis is replaced by disordered simultaneous contractions when acid-barium is ingested by a patient with reflux, some normal individuals have the same response.[17]

Another change in the esophagus affected by reflux is its response to instilled acid.[8] When 15 cc of 0.1 N HCl is instilled into the esophagus of a control subject, the intraesophageal pH is returned to 6 by ten or fewer swallows. In contrast, subjects suffering from reflux require as many as 30 swallows before raising the esophageal pH to pre-instillation values. This occurs even if the presence of acid does not cause disorders of peristalsis as measured manometrically.

Diagnosis of Hiatus Hernia. Although the primary emphasis in this discussion has been placed on determining the presence or absence of reflux and its consequences, a discussion of hiatus hernia is still necessary. The presence of a gastric loculus in the chest cavity has long been noted by radiologists investigating patients with heartburn or endoscopic evidence of esophagitis. Since radiological reflux was uncommon, the radiologist was impressed by the good association between symptoms and the structural abnormality of hiatus hernia. It was overlooked that some hiatus hernias are totally asymptomatic and that severe signs and symptoms of reflux are noted without hernia. Gradually somehow, hiatus hernia, a structural definition, and reflux, a physiological condition, were equated. Many physicians still hold so tightly to this belief that a patient with reflux symptoms in whom no hernia is demonstrated is returned to the radiologist with the admonition to search harder for it. Radiologists, on the other hand, have admitted to minimizing a small hernia in their report, fearing possible surgery for the patient.

Even granting that the presence or absence of a hiatus hernia might be important per se, there is still difficulty in setting up a precise criterion for its presence. Both the exact location of the diaphragmatic opening and the junction between the esophagus and stomach need to be located precisely before a hernia can be defined, and finding both sites can be difficult.

Radiology is the most frequently used method of diagnosis. Can the diaphragmatic opening be recognized by X-ray? Not easily, because clips placed on the edge of the diaphragmatic opening are seen on X-ray well above, at, or below the dome of the diaphragm.[18]

Neither the mucosal nor the gross morphological junction between the esophagus and stomach can be readily defined radiologically. Certainly when a large portion of the stomach is displaced into the chest (Fig. 33–7), there is no doubt as to the presence or absence of a hiatus hernia. The major and most common problem is the recognition of the small hiatus hernia. Some radiologists would interpret Figure 33–8 as a phrenic ampulla; other equally competent radiologists would unequivocally call this a small hiatus hernia. Many factors have been used as indications for the presence or absence of a hernia. The presence of gastric folds, a mucosal notch, a supradiaphragmatic (sic!) pouch without peristalsis and not in a line with the body of the esophagus have all been recommended as diagnostic aids.[19] It is easy to see how the reported radiological in- cidence of hiatus hernia varies between 3 and 75 per cent. In addition to the varying criteria used by different radiologists, it is likely that some variation exists in the same observer from examination to exami- nation.

Intraluminal manometry has also been suggested as a method for detecting the presence or absence of hiatus hernia. A double respiratory reversal (a change from positive to negative deflection on inspira- tion), a double peak of pressure in the junctional zone and an increased length of the junctional zone, and a plateau of pres- sure all have been mentioned as mano- metric signs of a hiatus hernia.[20] Since the radiological criteria of a hiatus hernia are in doubt, it is very difficult to find a stan- dard against which to check these observa- tions. Manometry has been helpful when combined with cinefluorography in dem- onstrating that many small pouches which have been interpreted as small hiatus her-

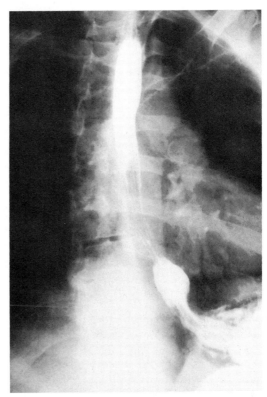

Figure 33–8. Small hiatus hernia. A pouch at the end of the esophagus is seen. A phrenic ampulla? A small hiatus hernia? Opinions of radiologists vary.

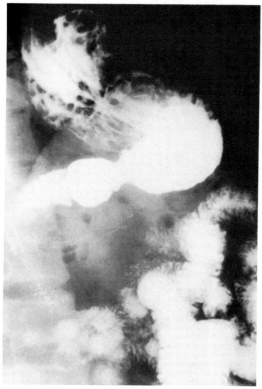

Figure 33–7. Large hiatus hernia. Extending up from the barium-filled body of the stomach is an air and barium contrast view of the fundus of the stom- ach well up into the thoracic cavity. (Courtesy of Dr. F. E. Templeton.)

nias are in fact located above the lower esophageal sphincter and hence are not hernias at all.[21]

Since he can recognize the mucosal junction and can detect the edge of the diaphragm indenting the esophageal well, the endoscopist is theoretically in the best position to evaluate whether or not a hiatus hernia is present. However, even this ability can be influenced by the type of instrument; e.g., in one study, the stan- dard Eder-Hufford esophagoscope was able to identify hiatus hernias in only 27 per cent of the patients in whom the flexi- ble fibergastric endoscopes demonstrated hernias.[22] This difference might be due to the ability of the latter instrument to in- flate the esophagus and thus make the diaphragmatic impression more visible. Further correlation of the endoscopist's hiatus hernia with the hernia of the radi- ologist or the manometrist suffers from too many uncertainties.

Gastroscopy can also be used to determine the presence or absence of hiatal herniation. The semi-rigid Eder-Palmer gastroscope can be used by watching for the mucosal junction while insufflating air during withdrawal into the esophagus. If gastric mucosa can be seen both below and above the impression of the diaphragm, a hiatus hernia is present. In the absence of a gastric pouch, the esophageal mucosa usually collapses over the viewing part of the endoscope and no image at all is seen.

With the flexible gastroscopes, the viewing head can be turned so that the gastroesophageal junction can be viewed from below. Normally, this junction surrounds the tube of the endoscope quite tightly. When a hernia is present, the body of the endoscope vanishes into a wide lax pouch and the point of closure of the gastroesophageal junction around the endoscope can no longer be seen.

Thus there are several different methods of diagnosing a hiatus hernia. The question of how often esophageal reflux is associated with hiatus hernia will have to wait uniform agreement as to the best method of determining whether or not a hiatus hernia is present. The argument will probably continue to be an unproductive quarrel. A hiatus hernia is not an illness; it is an anatomic condition. The main thrust of our activity must focus on the diagnosis and treatment of reflux, not hiatus hernia.

The foregoing remarks apply to the axial or "sliding" hiatus hernia. A much different clinical and radiological appearance is presented by the less common paraesophageal hernia (Fig. 33–9). Careful radiology will demonstrate that the gastroesophageal junction is below the diaphragm; reflux is not a clinical problem in paraesophageal hernias. A feeling of fullness and discomfort after eating is the usual presenting symptom, and strangulation and infarction or ulceration of the herniated stomach are the feared complications. So devastating are these latter complications that some authorities recommend surgical reductions of all paraesophageal hiatus hernias when discovered.[23]

DIFFERENTIAL DIAGNOSIS. The entities with which reflux esophagitis may be confused depend upon the response of the esophagus to reflux. Heartburn itself is a classic symptom of reflux, but occasionally it is localized to the epigastric area. It thus

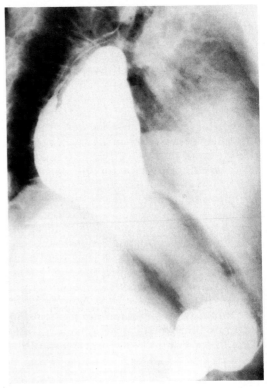

Figure 33–9. Paraesophageal hernia. A large paraesophageal hernia with the esophagus entering the stomach at the side instead of at the top of the herniated stomach. (Courtesy of Dr. F. E. Templeton.)

may be confused with the discomfort arising from a duodenal or gastric ulcer. A normal upper gastrointestinal series and a positive Bernstein test will help resolve this confusion.

Much attention has been paid to problems of differentiating pain of cardiac and esophageal origins. Although esophageal motor abnormalities are more easily confused with coronary artery disease, occasionally the discomfort caused by reflux esophagitis will become so marked as to mimic heart disease. The Bernstein test and response to antacid therapy can be used to point toward reflux esophagitis as the cause for pain. A positive exercise tolerance test with electrocardiographic monitoring will point toward a cardiac cause of discomfort. The possibility of the coexistence of the two diseases must be kept in mind, but patients with both ailments can usually distinguish the two symptom complexes from one another.

Viral infections of the esophagus can present as heartburn and odynophagia. This type of infection can also produce a hemorrhagic esophageal mucosa which resembles severe reflux esophagitis. The abrupt onset, vesicular lesions in the mouth and pharynx, and self-limited course will help in this differential diagnosis.

Complications. Reflux esophagitis is usually a disease of the mucosa and lamina propria. Many of its manifestations may be understood if it is assumed that only these two layers of the esophagus are involved by the reflux process. However, if the changes induced by reflux extend below this level, fibrous tissue formation may be stimulated and a stricture may result. Strictures are most commonly located in the lower portion of the esophagus near the lower esophageal sphincter. They may be very short or may extend up to the aortic arch. Some strictures may involve only a portion of the esophageal lumen when viewed from above through an esophagoscope. More advanced strictures are circumferential. If the stricture has been present for a long time, there is dilatation of the esophagus above the stricture (Fig. 33–10).

Dysphagia is the most common clinical presentation of an esophageal stricture. Unlike the dysphagia of uncomplicated reflux esophagitis, dysphagia caused by a stricture is usually progressive, in both frequency of occurrence and decrease in the size of the bolus which can be passed through the stricture. When a piece of food is arrested by the stricture, it usually must be regurgitated. Gradually the patient changes his diet so that he avoids solid foods and, eventually, semisolid foods. This transition may take place so slowly that the patient is not too concerned about his change in diet. Only careful questioning can bring out the fact that a change in diet has prevented recurrent dysphagia. Although an antecedent history of heartburn is usually obtained, occasionally the dysphagia will be the presenting symptom of stricture, causing concern about cancer.

When dysphagia signals the possibility of a stricture, several diagnostic maneuvers can be of use. It is necessary that the patient drink sufficient barium to distend the esophageal lumen fully. If the patient

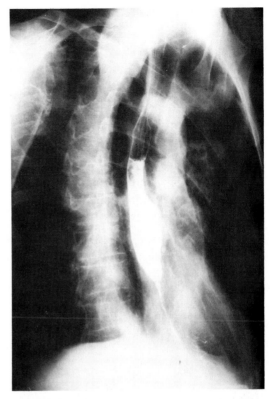

Figure 33–10. Benign peptic stricture. A narrowing is noted at the lower end of the esophagus in a patient with a history of many years of symptomatic reflux. Note dilatation of esophagus above the stricture. Differentiation on radiological grounds from a malignancy is difficult.

is unwilling or unable to do so, the narrowing caused by a stricture might be missed. In the radiographic evaluation of the length of the stricture, it is helpful to allow barium to pass the stricture, place the patient in the Trendelenburg position, and note whether refluxed barium distends the uninvolved esophagus below the stricture. Without such a maneuver, the length of strictures tends to be overestimated.

Giving a marshmallow or a piece of bread with the barium is also extremely useful in detecting the presence of a stricture. The bolus is taken into the mouth along with a sip of barium, chewed two or three times, and then immediately swallowed. Prolonged chewing will fragment the bolus and destroy its diagnostic effectiveness.

If a suspected area of narrowing is identified on X-ray examination, either endoscopy or blind passage of a large bougie can confirm whether or not the lumen is compromised. Only a positive cytology or an endoscopy with cancer-positive biopsy can define the exact nature of a stricture; X-ray criteria are not sufficiently precise.

Another uncommon complication of reflux esophagitis is an esophageal ulcer. Although many patients with reflux esophagitis will have endoscopic evidence of superficial ulceration, a very small percentage progress to deeper ulceration involving the muscular layers of the esophagus. Occasionally these ulcers perforate through the esophageal wall into adjacent structures. Esophageal ulceration is usually manifested by a rather intense continuous pain and may present with very brisk, even life-threatening, hematemesis. The esophageal ulcer is usually seen as a defect on a barium swallow (Fig. 33–11) and, as in the case of esophageal stricture, represents a complicated form of reflux esophagitis.

A third complication of reflux esoph-

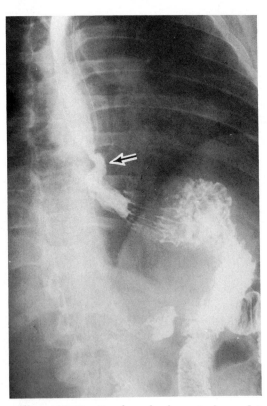

Figure 33–11. Esophageal ulcer. A large flat ulcer is shown (arrow). This ulcer was confirmed by endoscopy. (Courtesy of Dr. F. E. Templeton.)

agitis is the replacement of the normal squamous epithelium with a metaplastic epithelium, the so-called Barrett epithelium.[23] Although first thought to be a congenital lesion, these metaplastic epithelial changes have been shown to be most common in subjects with severe and continuous reflux esophagitis. An actual progression of the lesion from squamous epithelium to the metaplastic epithelium has been demonstrated in several individuals on serial biopsy. The squamous epithelium is replaced by metaplastic epithelium which resembles absorptive intestinal cell morphologically, and numerous mucous glands are observed (Fig. 33–12). Parietal cells are seen in some specimens of this type of epithelium, and it is possible that they may function. Usually at the transition zone between the metaplastic epithelium and the squamous epithelium there is a narrowing. On endoscopy one sees first normal esophagus, then inflamed esophagus, a stricture, and then epithelium which again is intact, although slightly more red in color than normal.

Another complication is that of esophageal overflow and pulmonary aspiration. This sequence of events is easy to suspect but difficult to prove. It should be considered whenever recurrent, unexplained bouts of pneumonitis are seen in either child or adult. Symptoms of reflux may or may not be prominent. Since pulmonary disease, especially in the aged, is common and so is reflux, it is tempting to draw a causal relationship between these two events; however, it is difficult to prove unless the patient wakes up coughing gastric contents at night. It seems likely that there are some cases of adult onset "asthma" which are due to unrecognized repeated bouts of nocturnal aspiration.

Treatment and Prognosis. Medical therapy is directed toward prevention of reflux by gravity and by alteration of the material which refluxes. At present there are no acceptable methods of pharmacologically strengthening the lower esophageal sphincter so that it is better able to resist reflux. Therefore it is necessary to use other techniques. Elevation of the head of the bed on 8-inch concrete building blocks is a very effective way of preventing reflux at night. With a certain

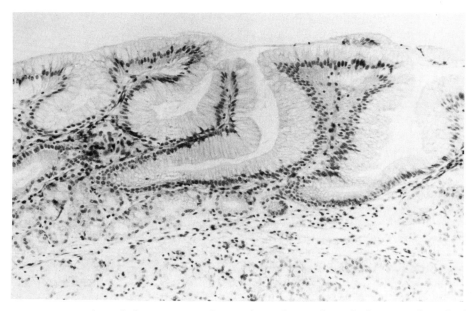

Figure 33–12. Barrett's epithelium. A suction biopsy obtained 8 cm above the lower esophageal sphincter. The normal squamous epithelium has been replaced by tall columnar epithelium. There are glands present in the lamina propria. In this biopsy specimen there are occasional cells with centrally located nuclei which resemble parietal cells. × 170.

amount of cooperation from the spouse, this minor change in life pattern is not disruptive and occasionally affords tremendous relief. It should definitely be included in the management of those who are aspirating. Propping up the patient on pillows is a much less effective way of taking advantage of gravity. It is also probably well to avoid tight belts and garments that might increase intra-abdominal pressure. However, we are no longer living in the wasp-waisted 1890's, and casual styles of modern dress fit in well with the acceptable method of caring for reflux. The patient may be instructed to eat a diet of his own choosing, with the exception that he avoid food for at least four hours before retiring, since an empty stomach will reduce the amount of material available for reflux. If symptoms are severe, it is probably well also for him to avoid alcohol and coffee.

The mainstay of therapy of reflux esophagitis at present is the vigorous use of antacids during the symptomatic period. Since antacids leave the stomach rapidly, hourly ingestion is mandatory for intensive therapy. The hospitalized patient may be treated with 30 cc of liquid aluminum hydroxide – magnesium hydroxide antacid hourly. Care must be paid to the effect of

these preparations on the colon. If diarrhea ensues, more calcium carbonate (2 g per hour) or pure liquid aluminum hydroxide in 30-cc doses must be used. For constipation, increasing the amount of magnesium hydroxide to 30 cc per hour is helpful.

For the ambulatory patient who finds it difficult to transport liquid antacid, several tablet preparations containing calcium carbonate are available. Several come in rolls of various flavors and can be easily obtained and carried about. Tablet forms of the aluminum hydroxide preparation are much less satisfactory. Anticholinergic agents should be avoided, since they tend to retard gastric emptying and to weaken the lower esophageal sphincter.

When severe symptoms or complications of reflux are present and do not respond to the measures mentioned previously, a more vigorous approach must be taken. In the individual who is not a candidate for surgical therapy because of coexisting disease, gastric radiation might be considered. This therapy is aimed at reducing acid-pepsin output by selective damage of the stomach's secretory epithelium. Sixteen hundred rads is delivered to the stomach over a ten-day period.[24] Relatively little formal evaluation of this form of therapy is available, but it does seem to offer relief in selected individuals.

TREATMENT OF COMPLICATIONS. In dealing with the complications of reflux esophagitis, one may use bougienage to increase the esophageal lumen when a stricture has formed. Several types of dilators are available (Fig. 33–13). The Maloney or tapered dilator is a good device to use when a long stricture occurs, since the pointed end of the dilator tends to serve as a lumen-finder. The blunt end of the Hurst dilators is sometimes equally effective. Each stricture seems to have its own preference as to the type of dilator most easily accepted. When the lumen is very small or extremely tortuous, it is better to perform the bougienage under better control with a lumen-finder. Either olives can be introduced over a previously swallowed string, or a device such as the Peustow dilator, which consists of a small wire terminating in a flexible string which can be introduced through the stricture under fluoroscopic control, can be used. Once it is safely in the stomach, olive dilators can be passed over the wire. Since the dilators will follow the string or wire, there is

much less chance of straying from the esophageal lumen.

The patient is made comfortable and the procedure explained. Sometimes 15 cc of viscous 2 per cent lidocaine taken five minutes prior to the procedure helps both pharyngeal anesthesia and the passage of the esophageal dilators. The dilator is passed down until resistance is met, and then gentle pressure is applied until the dilator passes or no progress is made. It is wise to start with the largest dilator used during the preceding dilatation. Fluoroscopy can be of great help, not only with the Peustow dilator, but also with the Maloney and Hurst dilators, since it is sometimes difficult to tell by calibration marks or by the patient's sensations whether or not the dilator has actually passed into the stomach. Fluoroscopy should always be used in doubtful instances as an adjunct in dilatation. Different patients vary in their capability to tolerate dilatation, and at least two dilators should be passed at every session. Small amounts of blood streaking on the dilator should not be a cause for tremendous alarm, but its appearance usually terminates the procedure for that particular day. It is wise to continue the series of

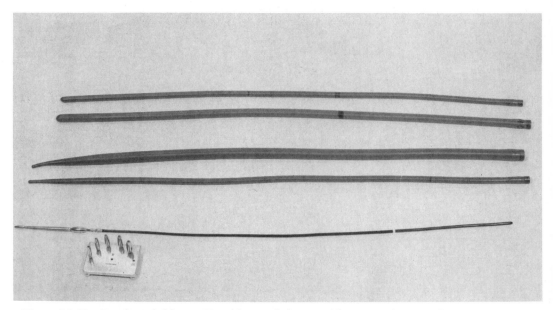

Figure 33–13. Esophageal dilators. Two blunt-ended Hurst dilators are shown at the top. Two tapered Maloney dilators are in the middle of the picture. A Plummer dilator with olives of graduated size is at the bottom. The whalebone rod has a threaded end to which the olives are attached. The flexible tip is pierced so that it can be threaded over a previously introduced string.

dilatation until a No. 45 French dilator will pass through the stricture zone. As the stricture is dilated, hourly antacids should be prescribed, since the stricture may have been protecting the esophagus above it from esophageal reflux. Once the stricture is dilated, the patient should be seen at frequent intervals and sounded with an appropriate-sized dilator to make sure that maximal patency of lumen is being maintained. Gradually the intervals between dilatation can be increased if the patient is instructed to present himself at any time dysphagia recurs. Some individuals can be sufficiently dilated not to require further treatment for years. However, it is more common for the patient to need dilatation at variable intervals. Self-dilatation is feasible only if the stricture is easily dilated and the patient is intelligent and dextrous.

SURGICAL THERAPY. When medical treatment has not controlled the complications of reflux esophagitis, surgical therapy should be employed. Significant bleeding, continued aspiration, and luminal narrowing in which meat is impacted are prime indications for corrective surgery. Symptoms unresponsive to vigorous medical measures are another indication, but the decision for surgery requires very careful evaluation by the physician. Unfortunately, too many patients are operated upon without adequate medical attempts to control their symptoms of reflux. Resistance to dilatation by either stricture or patient also calls for surgical correction.

Surgical approaches to the problems of reflux have been varied. For a number of years the main surgical thrust has been directed toward the anatomic correction of a hiatal hernia.[25] This approach implicitly assumed that reflux and hernia were interrelated or, in fact, synonymous. Results of surgery were evaluated in terms of patient satisfaction and whether or not anatomic recurrence of the hernia could be demonstrated. No comment was usually made about reflux, and no specialized procedures to evaluate its presence or absence were employed.

Another surgical approach was to attempt to decrease acid output by performing vagotomy and antrostomy or other drainage procedure. The goal was to reduce the amount of fluid available for reflux and to decrease the concentration of acid and pepsin in the refluxed fluid. Vagotomy would be expected to interfere with lower esophageal sphincter function, and some patients who have had vagotomy for treatment of peptic ulcer disease report symptoms of reflux for the first time after vagotomy.

In recent years, attention has been turning to providing a valve-like mechanism to prevent reflux. In many cases, a coincidental hiatus hernia may be repaired, but the operation usually done below the diaphragm can be done in the chest, thus actually creating a hernia. The principal operations involve invagination of the esophagus into itself (Belsey operation), or the creation of a gastric wrap-around pouch (Nissen and Hill procedures) (Fig. 33–14). In animals and in cadaver studies, these procedures have been shown effectively to prevent reflux. Clinical results of these procedures over five- to ten-year follow-up periods are encouraging. In contradistinction to results after hiatus hernia repair by the Allison technique and subsequent modifications, objective measurements before and after surgery point to improvement after anti-reflux operations.[27] Many more such objective studies must be done on different types of patient populations in order to define the good and bad effects of such surgery. The current procedures require much skill and judgment, and it is likely that further modifications of technique will be employed in the future.

The anti-reflux operations seem to fail more commonly in alcoholic subjects and in those with previous partial gastric resections. Often patients are unable to expel air from their stomachs, although esophageal burping is still possible. In some in whom eructation has become a way of life, the inability to belch causes great unhappiness. Perhaps more serious problems are faced by the alcoholic who is unable to vomit and thus loses one important safety valve. Postoperative dysphagia is common and usually transitory; if it persists, it can be corrected by one dilatation with a large bougie.

The anti-reflux operations will prevent reflux even when no lower esophageal sphincter is present at all. In one patient with achalasia who had unfortunately had the gastroesophageal junction resected, pre- and postoperative studies demon-

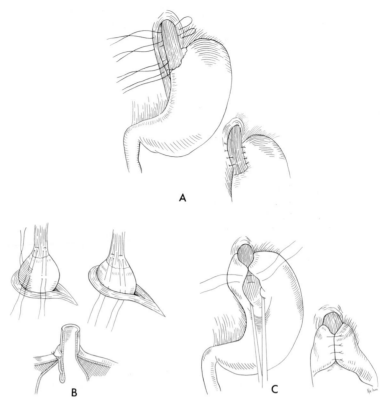

Figure 33–14. Anti-reflux operations. *A*, Hill repair. The posterior phrenicoesophageal ligament is sutured to the median arcuate ligament. The fundus is also approximated around the terminal esophagus. *B*, Belsey repair. The esophagus is essentially invaginated into the stomach by traction on the sutures shown. This repair can be done above or below the diaphragm. *C*, Nissen repair. The fundus of the stomach is wrapped around the terminal esophagus and held with sutures. All these operations end up with a variable portion of the stomach surrounding the lower esophagus.

strated no high pressure zone, but a *p*H probe demonstrated no postoperative reflux, and the patient was free from symptoms for the first time in 15 years.

Whether a vagotomy and pyloroplasty should be done in conjunction with the anti-reflux operation depends upon the clinical situation. If there is associated peptic ulcer disease, the additional procedure is indicated. However, to perform the vagotomy and drainage operation as "insurance" is not a good idea, because vagotomy is unnecessary in the prevention of reflux and may leave the patient with unpleasant side effects.

If fundoplication is not feasible, or if the extent of the esophageal damage is too great, it is better to consider interposition of a segment of colon or jejunum in place of the damaged esophagus. Interposition is a fairly formidable operation, especially when the individual's nutrition is marginal. Preliminary gastrostomy with tube feedings may be necessary to build up the patient enough to tolerate surgery. Operative mortality for the procedure varies from 10 to 15 per cent, but the clinical state of those who successfully survive the operation is really quite good. Most of them have some occasional residual dysphagia, but the major problems of reflux are solved by the operation.

PROGNOSIS. The prognosis of reflux esophagitis varies tremendously and is dependent on the manifestations. Many subjects with occasional heartburn will require neither medical nor surgical therapy. A much smaller number of individuals will require antacids occasionally to control the symptoms of heartburn. A still smaller group will be so troubled by the symptoms of heartburn as to require a vigorous medical management. Persistence of symptoms in spite of optimal medical therapy, serious bleeding episodes, or problems of aspiration will require corrective surgical therapy. It is very difficult to obtain meaningful incidence figures of the size of these groups with complication exclusive of stricture. One clue is afforded by the experience of a thoracic surgeon who finds it necessary to operate on 15 to 20 per cent of all individuals coming to him for help in the management of reflux symptoms.[28] It is even more difficult to know what will be found to be the case in the pediatric group. Although several large series quote unsatisfactory results in as many as 25 per cent of the patients operated upon, there is no doubt that the correction of reflux in selected pediatric patients will allow resumption of normal growth and disappearance of bronchopulmonary signs. The prognosis of the adult or older age individual suffering from bronchopulmonary disease with associated reflux is uncertain.

REFERENCES

1. Winans, C. S., and Harris, L. D. Quantitation of lower esophageal sphincter competence. Gastroenterology 52:773, 1967.
2. Pope, C. E. II. A dynamic test of sphincter strength: Its application to the lower esophageal sphincter. Gastroenterology 52:779, 1967.
3. Lind, J. F., Warrian, W. G., and Wankling, W. S. Responses of the gastroesophageal junctional zone to increases in abdominal pressure. Canad. J. Surg. 9:32, 1966.
4. Cohen, S., and Harris, L. D. Does hiatus hernia affect competence of the gastroesophageal sphincter? New Eng. J. Med. 284:1053, 1971.
5. Dillard, D. H., and Anderson, H. N. A new concept of the mechanism of sphincter failure in sliding esophageal hiatus hernia. Surg. Gynec. Obstet. 122:1030, 1966.
6. Longhi, E. H., and Jordan, P. H. Pressure relationships responsible for reflux in patients with hiatal hernia. Surg. Gynec. Obstet. 129:734, 1969.
7. Lind, J. F., Smith, A. M., and McIver, D. K. Heartburn in pregnancy—a manometric study. Canad. Med. Assoc. J. 98:571, 1968.
8. Booth, D. J., Kemmerer, W. T., and Skinner, D. B. Acid cleaning from the distal esophagus. Arch. Surg. (Chicago) 96:731, 1968.
9. Goldberg, H. I., Dodds, W. J., and Gee, S. Role of acid and pepsin in acute experimental esophagitis. Gastroenterology 56:223, 1969.
10. Strawczynski, H., Beck, I. T., and McKenna, R. D. The behavior of the lower esophageal

11. Cahill, J. L., Aberdeen, E., and Waterston, D. J. Results of surgical treatment of esophageal hiatal hernia in infancy and childhood. Surgery 66:579, 1969.
12. Crummy, A. F. The water test in the evaluation of gastroesophageal reflux: Its correlation with pyrosis. Radiology 87:501, 1966.
13. Tuttle, S. G., and Grossman, M. I. Detection of gastroesophageal reflux by simultaneous measurement of intraluminal pressure and pH. Proc. Soc. Exp. Biol. Med. 98:225, 1958.
14. Bernstein, L. M., and Baker, L. A. A clinical test for esophagitis. Gastroenterology 34:760, 1958.
15. Katz, D. Morbidity and mortality in standard and flexible gastrointestinal endoscopy. Gastrointest. Endosc. 15:134, 1969.
16. Ismail-Beigi, F., Horton, P. F., and Pope, C. E. II. Histological consequences of gastroesophageal reflux in man. Gastroenterology 58:163, 1970.
17. Donner, M. W., Silberger, M. L., Hookman, P., and Hendrix, T. R. Acid-barium swallows in the radiographic evaluation of clinical esophagitis. Radiology 87:220, 1966.
18. Botha, G. S. M. Radiological localization of the diaphragmatic hiatus. Lancet 1:662, 1957.
19. Wolf, B. S., and Guglielmo, J. Method for roentgen demonstration of minimal hiatal herniation. J. Mt. Sinai Hosp. N.Y. 23:738, 1956.
20. Code, C. F., Kelley, M. L., Schlegel, J. F., and Olsen, F. M. Detection of hiatal hernia during esophageal motility tests. Gastroenterology 43:521, 1962.
21. Fleshler, B., and Roth, H. P. Concomitant manometric and radiologic observations in apparent hiatal herniae. J. Lab. Clin. Med. 60:320, 1962.
22. Trujillo, N. P., Slaughter, R. L., and Boyce, H. W. Endoscopic diagnosis of sliding type diaphragmatic hiatal herniae. Amer. J. Dig. Dis. 13:855, 1968.
23. Hill, L. D., and Tobias, J. A. Para-esophageal hernia. Arch. Surg. (Chicago) 96:735, 1968.
24. Barrett, N. R. Chronic peptic ulcer of the esophagus and "esophagitis." Brit. J. Surg. 38:175, 1950.
25. Cooper, J. N., Gelzayd, E. A., and Kirsner, J. B. Mild gastric fundal irradiation in the treatment of peptic esophagitis. Gastrointest. Endosc. 14:222, 1968.
26. Allison, P. R. Reflux esophagitis, sliding hiatal hernia and the anatomy of repair. Surg. Gynec. Obstet. 92:419, 1951.
27. Hill, L. D. An effective operation for hiatal hernia: An eight year appraisal. Ann. Surg. 166:681, 1967.
28. Silber, W. Late results of the treatment of hiatal herniae; an analysis of 200 cases. Amer. J. Dig. Dis. 13:252, 1968.

Chapter 34

Rings and Webs

Charles E. Pope II

Definition. Although in the literature the terms ring and web have been used interchangeably, the term esophageal web will be restricted to a thin (2 mm) mucosal luminal obstruction located in the upper one-third of the esophagus. The lower esophageal ring is defined as a thin, circumferential structure, consisting of both gastric and esophageal mucosa, located in the lower esophagus. Other rings will be individually defined.

Etiology and Pathogenesis. With the exception of congenital rings (see previous discussion), both webs and rings usually become manifest in middle or late life, raising the question as to whether these structures represent congenital or acquired mucosal lesions. The association of cervical webs with iron deficiency and other mucosal changes in the oropharynx lends some credence to the idea that these lesions are acquired as the result of mucosal change.[1, 2] However, identical webs have been described in asymptomatic individuals without iron deficiency anemia or mucosal changes. Therefore mucosal change may not play an exclusive pathogenetic role.[3]

The same reasoning can be applied to discussions of the etiology of the lower esophageal ring. Although most often found when symptoms cause this portion of the gastrointestinal tract to be carefully examined, this abnormality can be found with careful X-ray examination of asymptomatic individuals.[4] It is difficult to know whether these rings have been present since birth or whether they are acquired later. Pathological examination usually reveals the upper esophageal surface to be lined by squamous epithelium and the lower by gastric epithelium.[5, 6] There is minimal smooth muscle tissue underlying the mucosa, most of the space being filled by lamina propria. Evidence of inflammation is usually lacking. Rarely, rings have been described which consist entirely of squamous epithelium, and one ring is described as being lined totally with gastric epithelium. These probably represent rare congenital lesions and not the more common lower esophageal ring.

Perhaps the intermittent nature of the symptoms of a ring and their late appearance are more related to loss of propulsive activity of the esophagus than to the appearance of stenosis of the ring. Dysphagia caused by a ring is probably related to a combination of a large bolus and a peristaltic wave which develops much less force. The force of swallowing varies from swallow to swallow, and perhaps it is the combination of a large piece of food and a relatively weak peristaltic wave which leads to obstruction at the site of the lower esophageal ring.

Natural History and Clinical Picture. Esophageal webs usually present with intermittent dysphagia, mostly for solid food. When a patient with such complaints and a web is found to have iron deficiency anemia, the title of Plummer-Vinson syn-

450

drome, or Paterson-Kelly syndrome, is usually applied. Such patients will often demonstrate leukoplakia in the mucosal membranes of the oropharynx and will also demonstrate spooning of the nails and physical signs of anemia. An association between hypopharyngeal cancers and webs has also been noted.

The clinical presentation of a lower esophageal ring is often sufficiently distinctive to make the diagnosis. Classically, the patient suffers from intermittent dysphagia. During meals a bolus of meat or bread may become impacted; the patient will regurgitate the offending bolus and then will be able to continue eating without further dysphagia. This event usually happens intermittently and often slowly increases in frequency over a number of years. Dysphagia that occurs every day is very unlikely to be caused by a lower esophageal ring. These patients do not often suffer from symptoms of esophageal reflux and have no other manifestations of systemic illness.

Another classic presentation of lower esophageal ring is sudden, total esophageal obstruction caused by meat impaction. A barium swallow taken at this time will often show a foreign body lodged in the lower portion of the esophagus. The patient is then esophagoscoped and the piece of meat is removed; the endoscopist usually comments that the esophagus appears normal. A follow-up barium swallow is interpreted as normal and the patient is discharged with the diagnosis of hysterical dysphagia (sic). This sequence is often repeated two or three times before the correct diagnosis is made. Of course, physical examination provides no clues to the diagnosis; it usually reveals only normal-appearing patients who are usually in the fifth to seventh decades of life at the onset of their symptoms. Frequently, however, a history of intermittent dysphagia of a more transitory nature for several decades can be elicited.

Diagnosis and Differential Diagnosis. Radiology is the best method for diagnosis of both webs and lower esophageal rings. Since the early phases of deglutition proceed so rapidly, it is unlikely that conventional spot films will demonstrate webs frequently. Hence, cineradiography will detect webs more often. The webs are usually located on the anterior surface of the esophagus; lateral and oblique films are necessary to demonstrate them. Occasionally, the web may be visible on a straight anteroposterior view of the upper esophagus (Fig. 34–1).

The lower esophageal ring is best demonstrated when the lower segment of the esophagus is distended. The patient takes a deep breath and holds it as the peristaltic wave approaches the area of the diaphragm. This maneuver causes the lower esophageal segment to balloon out and makes the ring visible (Figs. 34–2 and 34–3). If the segment is not adequately filled, no statement can be made as to whether or not a ring is present. An ancillary measure is the administration of a bolus which can be arrested in the area of the ring, thus calling special attention to this particular area. Bread or marshmallows soaked in barium are the most easily available bolus materials. Theoretically, it is possible to calibrate the lumen of the ring by giving barium tablets of known size. Practically, however, since the ring only produces intermittent dysphagia, arrest of the bolus cannot always be demonstrated unless the ring diameter is very small.

Endoscopy is a less satisfactory method of identifying webs and rings. Upper esophageal webs are very close to the cricopharyngeus opening, and it seems likely that many webs inadvertently rupture while they are being sought endoscopically, since dysphagia often disappears after the procedure. When seen, they appear as thin mucosal webs which can be easily moved with the tip of the instrument.

Endoscopy is not so efficient as radiology in demonstrating the lower esophageal ring. One possible explanation is that the esophagoscope is usually only 12 mm in diameter and can pass through a ring without detection. With the newer fiberoptic instruments, the esophagus can be distended ahead of the instrument by air insufflation. As in radiological investigation, distention causes the ring to become prominent and more easily seen. The lower esophageal ring at endoscopy appears to be a thin, pliant membrane, usually with a hole in the center. It can be easily moved by the tip of the esophagoscope. Associated changes of esophagitis

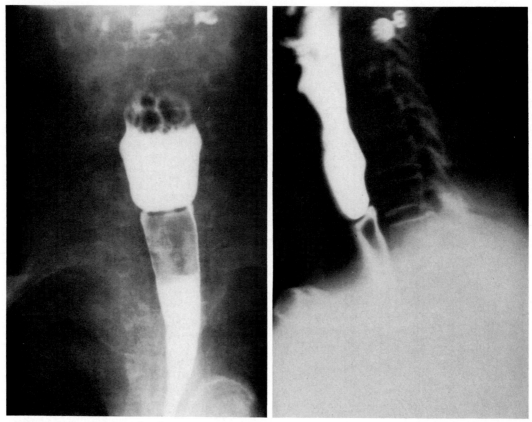

Figure 34-1. Esophageal web. Anteroposterior and lateral views of an upper esophageal web in a 62-year-old woman with iron deficiency anemia and dysphagia. It is unusual to obtain this clear a definition in the anteroposterior plane; the lateral view is usually more productive. (Courtesy of Dr. F. E. Templeton.)

are usually not seen at the time of endoscopy.

The differential diagnosis of both webs and rings takes in the whole gamut of diseases and disorders which cause dysphagia. The intermittency of dysphagia for only solid foods makes necessary the most thorough consideration of carcinoma and benign stricture in the differential diagnosis. Radiology and endoscopy are the simplest way of ruling out these conditions. In questionable cases, cytology must be used for added assurance that squamous cancer is not being overlooked. As mentioned earlier, hysteria or psychogenic problems should never be considered in the differential diagnosis of these lesions, since dysphagia always represents a mechanical difficulty in structure or function of the swallowing apparatus.

Treatment. Esophageal webs are best managed with dilatation either endo-scopically or with a bougie. Webs associated with iron deficiency anemia seem to disappear spontaneously when the iron deficiency is treated. This statement is difficult to document, but it has been my own personal experience in two cases. Esophagoscopy with rupture of the web or bougienage can also be useful.

Therapy directed at the lower esophageal ring depends in part on the frequency and intensity of the patients' complaints. Demonstration and explanation of the problem often will convince the patient to eat more slowly and to chew his food more thoroughly. This advice may give complete relief. If symptoms are more troublesome, mechanical methods of alleviating the obstruction must be found. Bougienage with large dilators has been recommended. If this form of therapy is to be used, it is wise to use a large dilator, such as a No. 50 French, without progres-

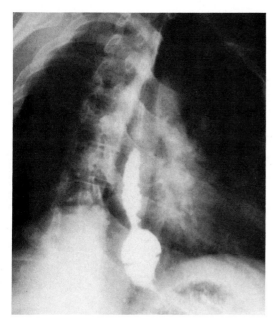

Figure 34–2. Lower esophageal ring. The patient has performed a Valsalva maneuver after drinking barium. This balloons out the lower segment of the esophagus, allowing the ring to be demonstrated.

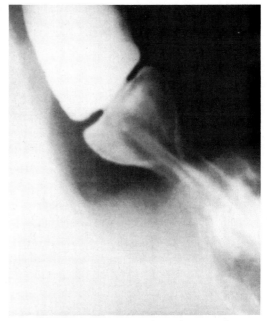

Figure 34–3. Lower esophageal ring. Close-up view of a lower esophageal ring. Note the impression of the ring on the column of barium as well as the notches formed by seeing the ring from the side.

sively stretching the ring with dilators of smaller caliber. If relief is not obtained after one dilatation, it might be repeated under fluoroscopic control to make sure that the dilator has indeed passed through the ring. Occasionally this form of therapy will not produce good results. It is then necessary to use a pneumatic dilator, preferably a 4-inch bag. The technique is similar to that used in the dilatation of a patient with achalasia, and fluoroscopic localization of the dilating bag is essential. One dilatation should cure the condition permanently. Although the ring may still be demonstrated radiologically after this procedure, the patient will not complain of recurring bouts of dysphagia (pp. 90 to 109).

Nonendoscopic treatment of meat impaction is also helpful. If a bolus of meat becomes impacted, the esophagus should first be emptied with a nasogastric tube. Then 15 to 30 cc of a solution made by crushing ten tablets of Papase in 50 cc of water should be instilled through the tube and the patient kept in an upright position. If Papase is not available, commercial meat tenderizer may be used instead. Thirty cubic centimeters of solution should be sipped every half hour. Usually the meat bolus will pass within two to three hours. This material will not harm the esophageal wall. It should not be used if preliminary radiographs demonstrate spicules of bone within the lodged meat.

Surgical attempts to remove this lesion have also been recommended. These include fracture of the ring digitally through a gastrostomy opening, or actual segmental removal of portions of the ring. Repair of associated hiatus hernias has also been employed in treatment of symptomatic rings, but occasionally the patient will still complain of intermittent dysphagia even though the ring structure has been reduced to a position below the diaphragm. It would seem that surgical therapy for this lesion alone would not be warranted, since intraluminal therapy with a dilator will frequently give good relief in these patients for whom instruction about the nature of the condition is inadequate.

REFERENCES

1. Chisholm, M., Ardran, G. M., Callender, S. T., and Wright, R. Iron deficiency and autoimmunity in post-cricoid webs. Quart. J. Med. 40:421, 1971.

2. Chisholm, M., Ardran, G. M., Callender, S. T., and
   Wright, R. A follow-up study of patients
   with post-cricoid webs. Quart. J. Med. *40*:409,
   1971.
3. Seaman, W. B. The significance of webs in the
   hypopharynx and upper esophagus. Radiology
   89:32, 1967.
4. Kramer, P. Frequency of the asymptomatic lower

esophageal contractile ring. New Eng. J. Med.
   254:692, 1956.
5. MacMahon, H. E., Schatzki, R., and Gary, J. E.
   Pathology of a lower esophageal ring. New
   Eng. J. Med. *259*:1, 1958.
6. Goyal, R. K., Clancy, J. J., and Spiro, H. M. Lower
   esophageal ring. New Eng. J. Med. *282*:1298,
   1970.

Chapter 35

Tumors

Charles E. Pope II

The esophagus is the site for both benign and malignant tumors. For all practical purposes, only malignant tumors of the esophagus are important. Benign tumors of the esophagus are usually an incidental finding at autopsy and rarely cause any major clinical manifestations. Certain striking exceptions to this statement will be presented later in this chapter. Of the malignant tumors, epidermoid carcinoma is the predominant type; if extension of gastric carcinoma into the distal esophagus is eliminated from consideration, adenocarcinoma of the esophageal mucosa is quite rare.

BENIGN TUMORS OF THE ESOPHAGUS

Of the benign tumors of the esophagus, leiomyomas are the most common type. This type of tumor is much less common than carcinoma of the esophagus. There does not seem to be any characteristic clinical presentation of leiomyomas; over half of them are discovered incidentally at autopsy. Unlike gastric leiomyomas, bleeding is a very unusual presentation.

The diagnosis is usually made in life by X-ray. A filling defect with sharp margins is seen, and the mass is often mobile (Fig. 35–1). Endoscopy can usually demonstrate elevation of the mucosa over the lesion. Endoscopic biopsy is not recommended because of the inability to obtain a diagnostic biopsy and the possible hazard of perforation of a deep biopsy. Surgical therapy consists of enucleation of the tumor

through an appropriately placed thoracic or abdominal incision. The size and location of the lesion, the inability to differentiate a filling defect from carcinoma, and

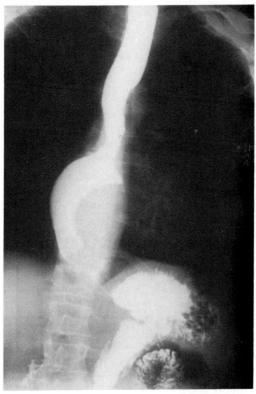

Figure 35–1. Leiomyoma of esophagus. This large filling defect was found in a patient with no esophageal symptoms who was having an upper gastrointestinal series for other reasons. Note the sharp edge of the filling defect. The leiomyoma was successfully removed. (Courtesy of Dr. F. E. Templeton).

455

the general condition of the patient will determine whether or not surgery is offered.

A much less common tumor is a fibrovascular polyp. Composed of adipose cells, connective tissue, and vascular elements, this tumor can grow to a very large size without producing clinical symptoms. Since most of them are located in the upper one-third of the esophagus and are pedunculated, regurgitation of the polyp with subsequent asphyxiation is a truly dramatic clinical presentation. If found in time, these tumors can be removed intraluminally. Hemangiomas and other rare tumors are occasionally found in the esophagus.[1]

CANCER OF THE ESOPHAGUS

As is true of most other human cancers, cancer of the esophagus has no definite etiology. However, certain associated conditions should be considered in the discussion of etiology of epidermoid carcinoma. The first important factor is chronic irritation. The incidence of carcinoma in esophagi damaged by lye is high and has been estimated to be one thousand times as great as in a sex- and age-matched control group.[2] It might equally well be supposed that incidence of cancer would be much higher in subjects with reflux esophagitis. Documentation of this supposition is difficult, although many case reports have mentioned the association of hiatus hernia with carcinoma of the esophagus. A prospective study, however, has failed to reveal such an association.[3]

The use of cigarettes and alcohol is also clinically correlated with development of esophageal carcinoma.[4] It would not seem unreasonable that both bronchial and esophageal epithelium might be exposed to the same toxic material in cigarette smoke. Examination of the esophageal epithelium of smokers by Auerbach has revealed many foci of atypia.[5] From his findings it is surprising that cancer of the esophagus is not even more common. It is more difficult to understand the etiological role of alcohol.

Another example of chronic irritation leading to cancer of the esophagus is the recognized association between achalasia and squamous carcinoma of the esophagus.[6] The reported incidence ranges from 2 to 19 per cent of all patients with achalasia—the incidence seems to rise as the number of years following diagnosis of achalasia increases. The incidence of leukoplakia and papillomata is also increased. It is logical to assume that all these lesions might result from increased irritation owing to stagnation of esophageal contents. If so, bag dilatation or myotomy should eliminate stagnation and decrease the incidence of carcinoma. Report of a long-term follow-up of a large number of such patients is not yet available.

Other material which has been ingested must influence the incidence of carcinoma of the esophagus. The differences in adjusted incidence of carcinoma of the esophagus in different countries are so striking that local environmental factors in these areas must have a role in the production of the lesion. The incidence of cancer of the esophagus in the United States is approximately 5.8 cases annually per 100,000 Caucasians.[7] In Southern Rhodesia it is 157 cases per 100,000. In the Transkei in South Africa, it rises to 357 cases per 100,000, and to 547 cases per 100,000 in Kazakhstan, Asia. Such marked increases in local incidence have caused dietary habits to be examined in these locations. Many individuals living in these areas consume large quantities of hot beverages throughout their lives. However, genetic differences or chemicals included in the diet certainly cannot be eliminated as possible etiological agents.

Another association exists between Plummer-Vinson syndrome and esophageal cancer. Plummer-Vinson syndrome, esophageal webs, and other mucous membrane abnormalities associated with iron deficiency and vitamin deficiencies are not common in the United States (see p. 450). In Scandinavia, the syndrome has been recognized much more frequently, and an increased incidence of esophageal cancer has been reported in women suffering from it.[8] Another genetically linked syndrome with which esophageal cancer has been linked is tylosis (thickened skin of hands and feet).[9]

Experimentally, aniline dyes can be used to produce tumors in rats; however, the lesions do not resemble those of the human type.[10] A much better animal model has been produced by long-term irradiation of the esophagus by implanting cobalt 60 wires near the esophagus.[11] However, radiation exposure does not seem to be a significant factor in the production of the disease in humans.

Natural History and Clinical Picture. Carcinomas of the esophagus represent about 4 per cent of all fatal cancers of the human. In the United States the incidence is 5.8 per 100,000 white persons annually; the incidence figure for nonwhites is 20.5 per 100,000. Esophageal cancer is unusual up to the age of 40 and rises to a peak incidence in the decade between ages 60 and 70.

History. Progressive dysphagia is the most common clinical presentation of carcinoma of the esophagus. Dysphagia in an individual over 40 years of age should always be assumed to be due to cancer until proved otherwise. Usually the dysphagia is progressive, first being produced by meat, potatoes, and bread, and then advancing so that semi-solid foods and liquids give difficulty. Pain is also a manifestation of cancer of the esophagus and represents an unfavorable sign since it usually signifies the extension of a lesion beyond the confines of the wall. The pain is usually steady, located substernally or occasionally in the back.

Systemic symptoms are usually present by the time the patient presents himself to the physician, and consist principally of anorexia and weight loss. Sometimes it is difficult to decide whether anorexia is caused by difficulty in swallowing or results from the presence of the tumor per se.

Brisk hemorrhage is an unusual presenting symptom, occurring in approximately 5 per cent of all cases. It is more common for the subject to suffer from slow blood loss manifested by symptoms of iron deficiency anemia. Other rare symptoms are hoarseness caused by the involvement of the recurrent laryngeal nerve, and cough caused either by overflow of retained material in the esophagus or by the formation of a tracheoesophageal fistula. Physical examination may give evidence of weight loss; occasionally, supraclavicular lymphadenopathy or an enlarged liver, caused by the deposits of tumor, may be felt. Physical

findings are usually not striking in this disease.

The distribution of the tumor depends on whether clinical findings or autopsy staging is employed. In the main, lack of a serosal layer leads to early contiguous spread of the lesion, regardless of the location. Lesions of the upper one-third tend to metastasize to the cervical lymph nodes; of the middle one-third to the tracheobronchial lymph nodes; and of the lower one-third to the gastric and celiac lymph node groups. In terms of visceral metastasis, the liver and lungs are the most common sites, but the tumor also spreads to the kidney, stomach, pleura, thyroid, trachea, and diaphragm.

The most common complication of the tumor is aspiration pneumonitis, which results from obstruction of the lumen. This complication produces difficult problems in management, since the patient will

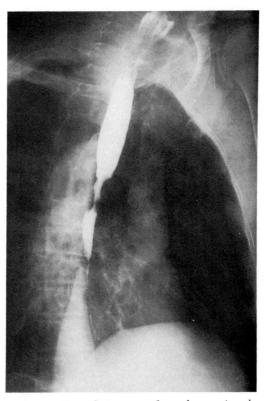

Figure 35–2. Carcinoma of esophagus. An obliterating circumferential lesion is seen in the mid-third of the esophagus. There is a suggestion of a shelf at the upper margin of the tumor. No marked dilatation of the proximal esophagus exists.

aspirate saliva despite discontinuance of oral alimentation and construction of gastrostomy. At autopsy, bronchopneumonia is found in approximately one-half of all patients with cancer of the esophagus.

Involvement of contiguous organs is the second most common type of complication with tracheoesophageal fistula at the top of the list. Esophagobronchial fistulas or esophagopleural fistulas can also form. These fistulas are usually manifest as recurrent pneumonia or pulmonary abscess. A much less common but more dramatic form of fistulization is erosion of the tumor into the nearby aorta with rapid exsanguination.

Diagnosis and Differential Diagnosis. X-ray continues to be the main method of diagnosis of tumors of the esophagus. Malignant tumors of the esophagus usually demonstrate luminal encroachment (Fig. 35–2), but may present as merely a diffuse thickening of one wall of the esophagus (Fig. 35–3). Often a ridge or shelf is noted

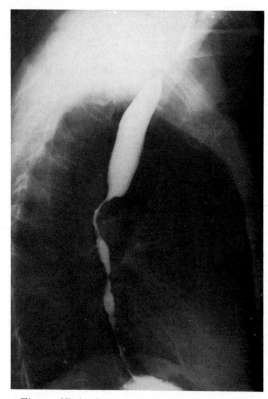

Figure 35–4. Stricture or cancer? The smooth tapering upper margin and esophageal dilatation might lead to a diagnosis of benign stricture. Cytology demonstrated this lesion to be a squamous carcinoma.

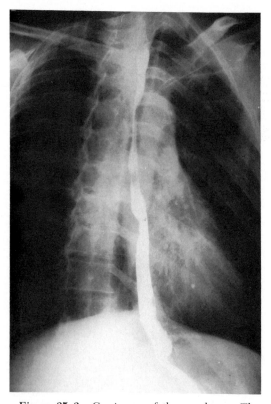

Figure 35–3. Carcinoma of the esophagus. The minimal luminal encroachment on the right side of the esophageal wall in the middle third might be easily overlooked. This patient had no dysphagia because the lesion was not circumferential.

at the superior portion of the tumor. The tumor can present as merely a smooth narrowing, and differentiation of a tumor from a benign stricture can be extremely difficult radiologically (Fig. 35–4). Dilatation of the esophagus is not common above a malignant stenosing lesion. Rarely, it is possible to delineate a soft tissue swelling in the mediastinum caused by involvement of the entire thickness of the esophagus by tumor growth.

If the patient complains of dysphagia as a manifestation of the tumor, it is also helpful to use a bolus diagnostically during X-ray examination. Either a marshmallow sprinkled with barium or a piece of bread dipped in a barium mixture will serve as a satisfactory bolus. After evaluation of the esophagus by a conventional barium swallow, the patient is instructed to chew the bolus as few times as possible and then swallow the piece of bread or marsh-

mallow before it has become too frag-
mented. The arrest of the bolus at a particular location is important, since mucosal
abnormalities may become much more noticeable when attention is drawn to a specific area.

More refined esophageal radiological
techniques will occasionally be of benefit.
Cineradiography will occasionally allow
attention to be drawn to an area which
is not as pliable as the rest of the esophagus.
There has also been interest in the use
of pneumomediastinography.[12] Air is injected through a needle inserted through
the left mainstem bronchus during bron-
choscopy. This technique allows enlarged
nodes to be visualized and the extent of
the swelling caused by tumor to be evaluated.

One of the most valuable diagnostic
techniques available for the diagnosis of
cancer of the esophagus is esophageal exfoliative cytology. Unfortunately, the technique is valuable only when specimens
are selected with care and evaluated meticulously. Its diagnostic accuracy in
trained hands is very high, approaching
the limits of any biological test. For instance, in individuals with proved cancer
of the esophagus, cytology detected abnormal cells in 94 per cent of the patients
evaluated. Conversely, in another group
who had lesions mimicking carcinoma,
there were no false-positive results in 94
cases thus examined.[13]

The technique for the examination involves the insertion of a radiopaque nasogastric tube through the area of interest
under radiological control. The fasting
specimen of gastric contents is taken and
spun down, and a smear of the sediment is
made and stained. Sips of water are then
taken by the patient, and aspiration is performed below the lesion. Finally, the lesion itself is directly washed by injecting
fluid forcibly through the nasogastric tube.
All washings are immediately spun down.
The sediment is spread on the slide, fixed
in alcohol, and stained by Papanicolaou
methods. If it is impossible to pass the
tube through the lesion, washings may be
obtained from above it. In this case, if no
abnormal cells are seen, the test must be
considered inadequate. Only cytological
preparations in which gastric columnar
cells are seen should be used for interpre-

tation, since the presence of gastric cells
demonstrates passage of the tube through
the entire esophagus.

A positive cytology report has not always
been accepted as unequivocal proof of
malignancy. Some workers feel that a histological biopsy is more certain. However,
a cytological preparation represents a total
mucosal biopsy, and it is often easier to obtain a positive cytology than a positive
biopsy from a person with demonstrated
carcinoma of the esophagus. In a small
personal series, 23 subjects, who were
later shown to have a cancer by surgery or
autopsy, were investigated by both endoscopy with biopsy and cytology; a positive
diagnosis was made in all but one patient
by cytology. Positive biopsies were obtained in only 15 of the 23 subjects undergoing endoscopy with biopsy, a diagnostic accuracy of 65 per cent. Moreover,
seven of the subjects had more than one
endoscopy, and multiple biopsies were
taken at each endoscopy.

Error is possible when the patient has
both a benign stricture of the esophagus
and an epidermoid cancer in either lung or
nasopharynx. Cells exfoliated from the
lung or pharyngeal lesion which have
been swallowed will be recovered from
the stomach and assumed to be from the
benign lesion. Fortunately, this combination of events is rare.

Esophagoscopy with biopsy allows both
for evaluation of the extent of the esophageal lesion and for its direct sampling
if cytology cannot be performed adequately. Many epidermoid cancers stimulate
fibrous tissue reaction at the advancing
margins. It is not uncommon to see a lesion which grossly resembles cancer and
yet to find only chronic inflammatory tissue on biopsies taken from what would
seem to be an obvious cancer. Bronchos-
copy is a valuable form of endoscopy in the
total evaluation of the patient with a
cancer of the esophagus. It will allow recognition of involvement of the tracheobronchial tree by expanding carcinoma,
and may well demonstrate unresectability
without thoracotomy.

DIFFERENTIAL DIAGNOSIS. Benign
stricture of the esophagus, presumably of
acid peptic origin, can clinically mimic carcinoma very closely. It may occur in a patient in the 50 to 60 year age group who

has not previously complained of symptoms of reflux and may present with increasing dysphagia. Radiological differentiation may be difficult indeed, and the frequency of negative biopsies in cases of esophageal cancer may lead to additional confusion. In such instances, exfoliative cytology is the clearest method of differentiating between the two lesions. If an inadequate cytological specimen is obtained because the stricture is tight, then cautious dilatation with repeat cytology when the lumen is larger may allow an adequate specimen to be obtained.

Fundal adenocarcinoma of the stomach has a propensity to grow upward and invade the esophagus, producing symptoms of an esophageal tumor. It is very difficult to differentiate these two tumors on a clinical basis. Careful X-ray examination with insufflation of the gastric fundus with Seidlitz powders or Coca-Cola will occasionally show a mass high in the gastric fundus (Fig. 35–5). The fundus is a difficult area to examine, and occasionally in patients without dysphagia a roentgenographic abnormality near the gastroesophageal junction will be seen. A workable rule is that a fundal mass associated with dysphagia represents carcinoma; a similar appearing mass without dysphagia is a benign anatomic abnormality. Differentiation is aided by visualizing a fundal lesion upon retroflexing the gastroscope after it has been passed into the stomach. However, the onset of dysphagia usually means that passage of the instrument will be impossible. It is of more than academic interest to differentiate between fundal lesions and cancer of the esophagus, since a fundal lesion is an adenocarcinoma and will not respond as well to radiation as will a squamous cell cancer of the esophagus.

Achalasia of the esophagus may present with symptoms of dysphagia, and the esophagram may now show a markedly dilated esophagus. If the radiologist is not perceptive, he may mistake the influence of gravity for the presence of peristalsis and thus may not recognize the motor abnormality of achalasia. Differentiation can be made by obtaining a negative cytology test and also by the easy passage of a large bougie or an esophagoscope through the area which appears narrow on X-ray exam-

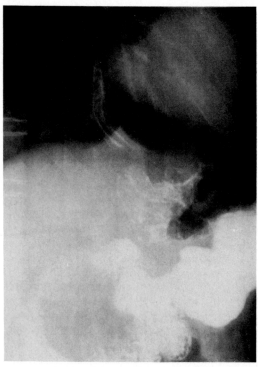

Figure 35–5. Fundal adenocarcinoma involving the esophagus. In this patient complaining of dysphagia, a mass was seen in the gastric fundus. Often the demonstration of such a mass by X-ray technique is quite difficult.

ination. Manometry and a positive Mecholyl test may point toward achalasia, but positive Mecholyl tests have been reported owing to vagal involvement by carcinoma[14] (see pp. 90 to 109).

Therapy. The ideal treatment of carcinoma of the esophagus has not yet been determined. Most reported series come from either surgeons or X-ray therapists who treat all their patients by the method with which they are the most familiar. A controlled random trial of therapy is urgently needed. It is clear that both forms of therapy will occasionally produce cure, and guidelines for the selection of the method of therapy are badly needed. It should also be carefully distinguished whether eradication or palliation is the aim of therapy.

SURGERY. The nature of esophageal cancer brings the patient to medical attention relatively late in the course of the disease. Although there is a certain amount of self-flagellation in the literature about doctor-delay interfering with adequate therapy, it is necessary for the tumor to involve most of the circumference of the esophagus before symptoms bring the patient to medical attention. That only 50 per cent of the patients presenting at the Mayo Clinic for medical or surgical therapy are operative candidates is startling proof of this grim fact; the remaining half already have far distant metastases. Further, of these subjected to thoracotomy, approximately half cannot have a curative procedure. Therefore, only a small number, approximately 20 per cent, are candidates for surgical cure of their disease.[15] Even a more recent series from the same institution shows that over half of all the patients are not candidates for resection, even of a palliative nature.[16]

The decision for operation must also be related to the position of the lesion. Carcinomas in the lower third of the esophagus below the aortic arch offer the best chance for surgical resection. Technical problems in the middle of the esophagus lead to an unacceptably high incidence of anastomotic leaks. Surgery can be performed in the upper third and cervical portion of the esophagus, but this site is more frequently felt to be the province of the radiotherapist.

Three- and five-year survival rates following surgery for carcinoma of the esophagus can be calculated, therefore, in many ways. If all cancers of the esophagus are considered and operative deaths are included, then approximately 15 per cent of operable patients will survive for five years. The range is from 7 per cent for upper thoracic to 28 per cent for lower thoracic levels of the esophagus. On the other hand, patients who are resected for cure and in whom no lymph node invasion is found in the pathological specimen, may have five-year survival rates as high as 54 per cent. It should be emphasized, however, that this group is highly selected and cannot be recognized prior to surgery.[16] Reports from the Mayo Clinic indicate that there is slight improvement in mortality in the period 1956 to the present when compared with 1946 to 1956. The most common cause of death was an anastomotic rupture.

If surgical therapy for cure seems undesirable, certainly surgical palliation is worthy of consideration. This approach involves either placement of a tube through the lesion or resection of the lesion with an anastomosis between the esophagus and the stomach. Rarely, an interposed loop of colon or small bowel is used in the palliation of malignant disease, but the complexity and stress of this operative procedure render its use uncommon.

Palliation with an indwelling tube allows a passage to be opened and maintained through the tumor growth. Representative types of tubes are shown in Figure 35–6. Tubes are available that can be inserted from above through an esophagoscope without the necessity of performing a gastrostomy. A Celestin tube requires fixation through a gastrostomy. These tubes, although offering a clear passage for saliva and liquid foods, can easily be blocked by an attempt to swallow more solid fare. In addition, all these tubes have a propensity to erode through the tumor mass and either obstruct the bowel farther down or wander into the mediastinum.

Surgical palliation, which is most effective in the lower one-third of the esophagus, allows re-establishment of continuity of the gastrointestinal tract and good palliation of swallowing. Survival for over one year after such a procedure is unusual, although five-year survivals after palliative resection are occasionally recorded.

A special problem exists when a tracheoesophageal fistula has resulted from an extension of an esophageal cancer. Attempts to remove such a lesion have not been successful. In an experience with both benign and malignant causes for tracheoesophageal fistula, two patients were apparently well palliated with a transplanted segment of bowel serving as a conduit.[17] In most cases of tracheoesophageal fistula, it is recommended that a gastrostomy be performed so that alimentation through the esophagus can cease. However, most patients with tracheoesophageal fistula caused by malignancy are dead within three months.

ROENTGEN THERAPY. The enthusiasm for radiation therapy of squamous carcinoma as opposed to surgical extirpation has waxed and waned. In the years prior to effective surgical therapy, radiation therapy, either with orthovoltage machinery or by local radium implants, offered the best form of palliation and an occasional cure.

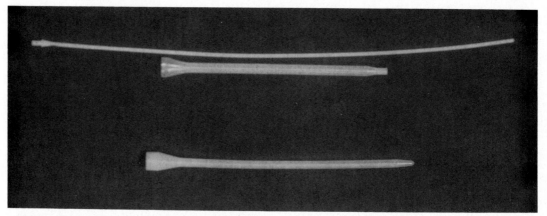

Figure 35–6. Tubes for palliation of esophageal obstruction. The upper tube is a Celestin tube with its lumen finder. These two tubes can be screwed together, then traction applied to the lumen finder through a gastrotomy until the flange of the tube engages the upper margin of the tumor. The excess tube is then cut off. The lower tube is a Hurwitz tube.

However, as thoracic surgery improved, radiation was restricted to palliative purposes. As the failure of surgical therapy to cure many patients has become apparent, enthusiasm again swings toward curative radiotherapy bolstered by the appearance of therapy units which are able to deliver much higher doses to the lesion.

In terms of five-year cure, figures usually range from 8 to 15 per cent. In Edinburgh, megavoltage radiation is being tried for squamous carcinoma, and they report that 20 out of 99 selected patients are alive five years after radiation.[18] Each patient has a normal stomach and voice, the only problem having been an occasional stricture in the area of the radiated carcinoma which usually responds well to therapy. Certainly these results compare favorably with those for surgical extirpation of squamous cell lesions. When surgical and radiation therapy were compared, the relative survival curves after five years were the same. However, there were fewer deaths from radiation therapy in the first year after therapy, reflecting the absence of operative and postoperative mortality. These workers now feel that all squamous cell cancers of the esophagus should receive megavoltage therapy regardless of location.

Combined therapy also has its advocates. The most exciting results of preoperative radiation followed by surgical extirpation have been reported from Japan.[19] This institution has a large experience with carcinoma of the esophagus, as measured by a reported operative mortality of 7.4 per cent in contrast to rates of 20 to 50 per cent reported from other centers. This clinic now prefers to do a gastrostomy and celiotomy, and to give 2500 rads to the lesion over a two-week period, using cobalt teleotherapy. After two weeks, the esophagus is removed and continuity is restored between the esophagus and the stomach by use of an external rubber tube. One year later, if there has been no evidence of recurrence, an esophagogastrostomy is performed. Nakayama reports survival rates of 19.1 per cent for squamous cell cancer for five years in patients treated without radiation, and 37.5 per cent of patients who received preoperative radiation. There is undoubtedly a tremendous selection, since only patients who survive 12 months after the first two stages receive the third stage of the operation. It is difficult to tell whether this 37.5 per cent cure rate represents a selected segment of the total patient population, or whether it represents a more generalized experience.

This dichotomy of opinion and varying cure rates with apparently similar procedures urgently calls for an accomplished medical center to set up a randomized trial of the different modalities of therapy. Until this is done, it will be extremely difficult to decide whether surgery, radiation, or a combination of the two forms of therapy offers the best hope to a patient with squamous cell carcinoma of the esophagus.

Current decisions will be made on the availability of these different forms of therapy and local experience.

TREATMENT OF ADENOCARCINOMA. In the treatment of adenocarcinoma of the gastroesophageal junction, the physician is not offered a choice of therapy, but must rely on surgical extirpation for palliation and cure. Some authors do not separate histological types when considering surgical results; an 8.8 per cent five-year cure rate with an operative mortality of 11 per cent is typical.[20] An intriguing experience is reported from Scandinavia: in 46 patients with adenocarcinoma who were operated upon, operative mortality was 28 per cent, but the five-year survival rate was 22 per cent.[21] None of 17 patients who had a resection of the esophagus and partial gastrectomy survived; however, 10 patients who had a distal esophagectomy plus total gastrectomy lived more than five years. This experience would seem to indicate that a more radical operation would perhaps offer a better chance to the individual with adenocarcinoma of the gastroesophageal junction. It must again be emphasized that such cure rates represent a selected portion of the population whose tumors have not spread to an extent which would preclude operative intervention.

REFERENCES

1. Watson, R. R., O'Connor, T. M., and Weisel, W. Solid benign tumors of the esophagus. Amer. Thor. Surg. 4:80, 1967.
2. Lansing, P. B., Ferrante, W. A., and Ochsner, J. L. Carcinoma of the esophagus at the site of lye stricture. Amer. J. Surg. 118:108, 1969.
3. Michel, J. O., Olsen, A. M., and Dockerty, M. B. The association of diaphagmatic hiatal hernia and gastroesophageal carcinoma. Surg. Gynec. Obstet. 124:583, 1967.
4. Wynder, E. L., and Bross, I. J. A study of etiological factors in cancer of the esophagus. Cancer 14:389, 1961.
5. Auerbach, O., Stout, A. P., Hammond, E. C., and Garfinkel, L. Histologic changes in esophagus in relation to smoking habits. Arch. Environ. Health 11:4, 1965.
6. Just-Viera, J. O., and Haight, C. Achalasia and carcinoma of the esophagus. Surg. Gynec. Obstet. 128:1081, 1969.
7. Doll, R. The geographical distribution of cancer. Brit. J. Cancer 23:1, 1969.
8. Wynder, E. L., Hultberg, S., Jacobsson, F., and Bross, I. J. Environmental factors in cancer of upper alimentary tract; Swedish study with special reference to Plummer-Vinson (Patterson-Kelly) syndromes. Cancer 10:470, 1957.
9. Howel-Evans, W., McConnell, R. B., Clarke, C. A., and Sheppard, P. M. Carcinoma of the esophagus with keratosis palmaris et plantaris (tylosis). Quart. J. Med. 27:413, 1958.
10. Napalkov, N. P., and Pozharisski, K. M. Morphogenesis of experimental tumors of the esophagus. J. Nat. Cancer Inst. 42:927, 1969.
11. Gates, O., and Warren, S. Radiation-induced experimental cancer of the esophagus. Amer. J. Path. 53:667, 1968.
12. Holub, E., and Simeček, C. Pneumomediastinography in carcinoma of the oesophagus. Thorax 23:77, 1968.
13. MacDonald, W. C., Brandborg, L. L., Taniguchi, L., and Rubin, C. E. Ann. Intern. Med. 59:332, 1963.
14. Kolodny, M., Schrader, Z. R., Rubin, W., Hochman, R., and Sleisenger, M. H. Esophageal achalasia probably due to gastric carcinoma. Ann. Intern. Med. 69:569, 1968.
15. Ellis, F. H., Jr., Jackson, R. C., Krueger, J. T., Jr., Moersch, H. J., Clagett, O. T., and Gage, R. P. Carcinoma of the esophagus and cardia; results of treatment 1946 to 1956. New Eng. J. Med. 260:351, 1959.
16. Gunnlangsson, G. H., Wychulis, A R., Roland, C., and Ellis, F. H., Jr. Analysis of the records of 1,657 patients with carcinoma of the esophagus and cardia of the stomach. Surg. Gynec. Obstet. 130:997, 1970.
17. Petrovsky, B. V., Perelman, M. I., Vantsian, E. N., and Bagirov, D. M. Palliative and radical operations for acquired esophagotracheal and esophagobronchial fistulas. Surgery 66:463, 1969.
18. Pearson, J. G. The value of radiotherapy in the management of esophageal cancer. Amer. J. Roent. Radium Ther. & Muc. Med. 105:500, 1969.
19. Nakayama, K., Orihata, H., and Yamaguchi, K. Surgical treatment combined with preoperative concentrated irradiation for esophageal cancer. Cancer 20:778, 1967.
20. Magill, T. G., and Simmons, R. L. Resection of cardio-esophageal carcinoma. Arch. Surg. (Chicago) 94:865, 1967.
21. Kock, N. G., Lewin, E., and Pettersson, S. Partial or total gastrectomy for adenocarcinoma of the cardia. Acta Chir. Scand. 135:340, 1969.

Chapter 36

Diverticula

Charles E. Pope II

Definition. Esophageal diverticula are outpouchings of one or more layers of the esophageal wall. These outpouchings occur in three main areas: (1) immediately above the upper esophageal sphincter (Zenker's diverticulum), (2) near the mid-point of the esophagus (traction diverticulum), and (3) immediately above the lower esophageal sphincter (epiphrenic diverticulum).

Etiology and Pathogenesis. Although esophageal diverticula have been described in infants and children,[1] they are usually discovered in later life. This late appearance is undoubtedly dictated by the factors which produce diverticula. It is commonly stated that Zenker's diverticula and epiphrenic diverticula may result from motor abnormalities of the esophagus, and that the mid-esophageal or traction diverticulum is a response to scarring and traction on the walls of the esophagus by external inflammatory processes. This latter explanation is probably incorrect, as the mid-esophageal diverticulum may well represent an expression of abnormal motor activity of the esophagus.

The evidence that Zenker's diverticulum is associated with motor abnormalities has already been discussed on page 92. To summarize briefly, manometric studies show that the upper esophageal sphincter relaxes appropriately in response to the swallow, but restores its high resting pressure before the pharyngeal pressure wave reaches the

area.[2] Thus, the area above the sphincter is subject to repeated periods of elevated pressure occurring with each swallow. Although the force of the pharyngeal contraction is adequate to push the swallowed bolus through the sphincter in most cases, the repeated elevations of pressure eventually cause an outpouching of the esophageal wall posteriorly. The sac consists mostly of mucosa and submucosa, although a few muscle fibers are often seen on the outside of the sac.

The pathogenesis of the mid-esophageal diverticulum remains less certain. Although fibrous adhesions from tuberculous mediastinal nodes are felt to produce diverticula, the actual demonstration of such adhesions is rare in autopsy material. Manometric changes consisting of high amplitude, prolonged contractions in upper and lower esophagus have been described,[3] but it is not certain how often these changes are found in patients with mid-esophageal diverticula. No large number of individuals with mid-esophageal diverticula have received manometric attention. However, a motility disturbance can be implicated by other observations. A mid-esophageal diverticulum with a bolus of meat stuck well below the diverticulum is shown in Figure 36–1. Subsequent esophagoscopy and repeated barium swallow revealed no organic obstruction in this area. At autopsy seven years later no evidence of luminal compromise or adhesion of fibrous bands was found. However, the

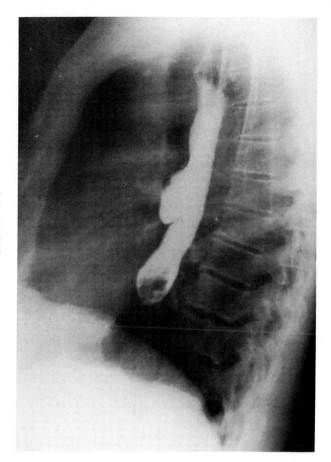

Figure 36–1. Mid-esophageal diverticulum. A large mid-esophageal diverticulum is seen in the mid-thoracic area. Below this is an impacted bolus of meat, causing esophageal obstruction. Subsequent films after the bolus was removed showed no narrowing at the site where the bolus arrested.

esophageal muscular wall was thickened. These findings are certainly consistent with a disturbance in motor function, although they do not prove it.

All diverticula in the middle of the esophagus may not be due to motor activity. A diverticulum which is much closer to the lower esophageal sphincter and seems to have a different appearance is shown in Figure 36–2. This patient was totally asymptomatic, so it is difficult to implicate a motor disorder.

Epiphrenic diverticula can also be shown to be associated with motor abnormalities of the esophagus. As with Zenker's diverticulum, incoordination of sphincteric relaxation and esophageal peristalsis might occur. The lower esophageal segment would then be subject to increasing amounts of pressure. A high (65 to 70 per cent) incidence of motor abnormalities of the esophagus has been reported.[4] Motor incoordination must be postulated until an adequate number of subjects with epiphrenic diverticula have been studied manometrically.

Symptoms. Zenker's diverticulum presents the most classic group of symptoms. Transient dysphagia may be noted early in the course. However, when the pharyngeal sac becomes large enough to retain contents, the patient may complain of pulmonary aspiration, gurgling in the throat, appearance of a mass in the neck, or regurgitation of food into the mouth. Some patients develop a series of maneuvers used to empty the pouch which consists of pressure on the neck and repeated coughing and clearing of the throat. The sac may become so large that its retained contents may push anteriorly on the esophagus and completely obstruct it.

The mid-esophageal diverticula are much more likely to be found in a totally

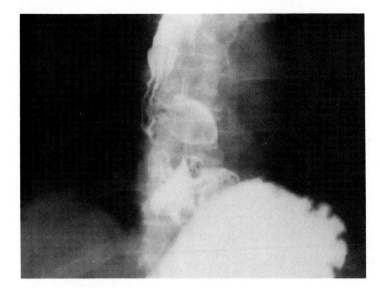

Figure 36–2. Mid-esophageal diverticulum. A diverticulum resembling a duodenal diverticulum is shown in a totally asymptomatic patient.

asymptomatic patient. However, occasional patients with such diverticula will complain of dysphagia or, rarely, of esophageal obstruction owing to a retained bolus.

It is difficult to tell whether the symptoms of an epiphrenic diverticulum are caused by the presence of the diverticulum itself, or by the associated motor abnormalities in the esophagus. As previously noted, many motor abnormalities are described as achalasia or diffuse spasm (see pp. 90 to 109). One symptom seems to be fairly unique to the presence of the diverticulum: the regurgitation of massive amounts of fluid, usually occurring at night. Presumably, this fluid has been stored in the diverticulum during waking hours and regurgitated during periods of recumbency.

Diagnosis and Differential Diagnosis. These diverticula are most often discovered during X-ray examination of the esophagus (Fig. 36–3). Small diverticula can be superimposed on the shadow of the barium-filled esophagus and may be missed unless the patient is rotated during the examination. It is very difficult to confuse these structures with any other abnormalities. The only possibility of confusion lies in an esophagus undergoing tertiary contractions which may give a temporary appearance of numerous diverticula in the lower esophagus. However, the changing pattern on subsequent swallows soon eliminates this possibility.

It is not necessary to perform endoscopy in order to investigate esophageal diverticula. In fact, the procedure may represent a hazard to the patient, since it is dif-

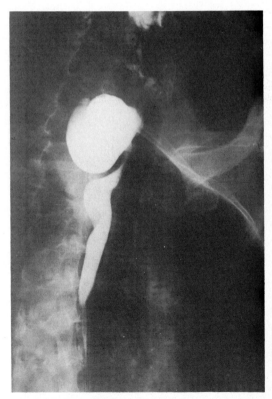

Figure 36–3. Zenker's diverticulum. This diverticulum is large enough to cause esophageal obstruction when it fills with contents.

ficult to avoid entering the pharyngeal esophageal diverticulum with the tip of the instrument. Therefore, when it is known that a Zenker diverticulum exists, an endoscopic procedure necessary for other reasons should always be performed under direct vision. Manometric examination will not be clinically helpful, although it may throw light on the pathogenesis of these structures.

Treatment. The main method of treatment, of course, is surgical. There are three methods of surgical correction of a Zenker diverticulum: (1) a two-stage operation involving mobilization of the diverticulum and excision subsequently when granulation tissue has formed around the diverticulum; (2) excision of the diverticulum in one step; and (3) a cricopharyngeal myotomy, leaving the diverticulum unmolested.[2] The recurrence rate with simple resection is extremely high, approaching 85 per cent in one series,[5] presumably because the motor abnormality has not been corrected. Cricopharyngeal myotomy is relatively new, and large experience has not been gained with this method. Theoretically, it has the advantage that it eliminates the causal reason for the diverticulum and presumably would help to guard against recurrence.

Mid-esophageal diverticula usually do not require any form of therapy. The diverticula tend to be small and not to retain material. It is conceivable that if an associated motor abnormality becomes too troublesome, a long myotomy might be offered to the individual.

Simple excision of epiphrenic diverticula would seem to have an unacceptably high mortality and morbidity rate.[4] However, when attention is directed to the associated motor condition, be it achalasia or diffuse spasm, and a myotomy performed in the lower esophageal wall, better results have been reported.[4] The need for surgical therapy is dictated by the clinical manifestations of the epiphrenic diverticulum.

REFERENCES

1. Meadows, J. A., Jr. Esophageal diverticula in infants and children. Southern Med. J. 63:691, 1970.
2. Ellis, F. H., Schlegel, J. F., Lynch, V. P., and Payne, W. S. Cricopharyngeal myotomy for pharyngo-esophageal diverticulum. Ann. Surg. 170:340, 1969.
3. Cross, F. S., Johnson, G. F., and Gerein, A. N. Esophageal diverticula. Arch. Surg. (Chicago) 83:525, 1961.
4. Allen, T. H., and Clagett, O. T. Changing concepts in the surgical treatment of pulsion diverticula of the lower esophagus. J. Thor. Cardiov. Surg. 50:455, 1965.
5. Einarsson, S., and Hallén, O. On the treatment of esophageal diverticula. Acta Otolaryngol. 64:30, 1967.

Chapter 37

Involvement of the Esophagus by Infections, Systemic Illnesses, and Physical Agents

Charles E. Pope II

INFECTIOUS DISEASE

Older textbooks on the esophagus mention that bacterial infections, especially diphtheria, occasionally involve the esophagus,[1] with an extension of the pseudomembrane from the oropharynx. Treatment of this condition is the same as for the diphtheria itself. Modern therapy has made it a rarity.

Tuberculosis of the esophagus is very rare and is, for practical purposes, never an isolated infection. More commonly, the esophagus is affected along with other organs, usually by direct extension, either from a laryngeal focus or from contiguous tuberculosis nodes. Even when tuberculosis was much more prevalent than it is today, esophageal involvement occurred in only 1 per cent of the cases. Treatment is the same as for pulmonary tuberculosis.

Involvement of the esophagus by syphilis is also rare. Usually presenting as a stenosing process, involvement of the upper and middle esophagus seems more common in contradistinction to peptic in-

volvement which favors the lower third.[2] Biopsy reveals perivascular round cell infiltration, and the lesion responds to antisyphilitic therapy with penicillin.

The esophagus may also be involved by acute viral illness. Herpes simplex, which attacks mucous membranes, has been implicated as a self-limited disease of the esophagus.[3] A similar clinical picture associated with aphthous ulcers without herpes virus has also been described.[4] The patient will have a history of an acute febrile illness and will complain of intense dysphagia and odynophagia. Swallowing is so painful that no nutrients can be taken. Inspection of the oropharynx will show numerous vesicles which tend to break, leaving a raw, denuded surface. Endoscopy demonstrates the same lesions of the mucous membranes of the esophagus as well. This illness is usually of short duration, lasting about three or four days. No specific therapy is available, but the patient can be treated with viscous 2 per cent lidocaine, 5 cc every four hours, for relief of pain and a clear liquid diet. This infection has no known sequelae.

468

MONILIASIS

Moniliasis of the esophageal mucosa is caused either acutely or chronically by *Candida albicans*. This yeast, which is widely distributed in nature, usually attacks only individuals whose resistance has been lowered by systemic infection, neoplasia, or chemotherapy.[5] One special condition in which the disease takes a chronic form is hypoparathyroidism, in which the Candida infection can linger for a number of years.[6]

The symptoms of this infection are dysphagia and odynophagia, usually of short duration. The dysphagia and odynophagia are intense, and most patients are able to tolerate only liquids. Less frequently the symptoms of the infection are due to localized stricture of the esophagus. Physical examination may or may not reveal the lesions of oral moniliasis. Diagnosis depends on radiology and endoscopy. An esophagogram shows either a shaggy mucosa or numerous round filling defects. Endoscopically, a white membrane may be seen; more commonly, the mucosa is friable and edematous, with overlying whitish plaques. As noted, a stricture may be identified. Biopsy obtained through the esophagoscope will show hyphae and yeast forms as well as acute and chronic inflammation in the biopsy material (Fig. 37–1).

Treatment consists of nystatin (Mycostatin), 250,000 units suspended in water, to be swallowed every two hours. If the patient is receiving antibiotics, it is well to discontinue them, if possible. When the infection is chronic it is well to suspend the nystatin in a 0.5 per cent methylcellulose–0.7 per cent carboxymethylcellulose vehicle.[6] This technique allows more prolonged contact of the nystatin with the involved mucosa. This drug should cure the infection; however, the patient's prognosis is essentially determined by the severity of the underlying disease which predisposed the patient to moniliasis.

SYSTEMIC ILLNESS

PEMPHIGOID AND EPIDERMOLYSIS BULLOSA

The squamous epithelium of the esophagus shares with the external skin some of the manifestations of severe epithelial injury. Two good examples of this are pem-

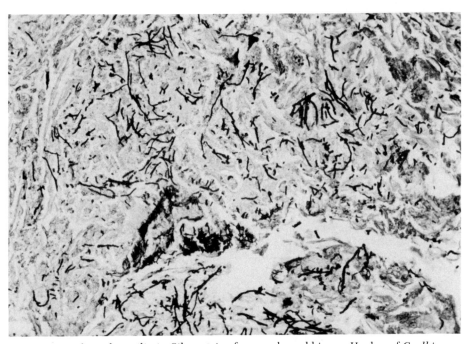

Figure 37–1. Esophageal moniliasis. Silver stain of an esophageal biopsy. Hyphae of *C. albicans* are seen. Routine hematoxylin and eosin staining of the same biopsy demonstrated these structures very poorly, if at all. ×480.

phigoid and epidermolysis bullosa, both presenting as bullous lesions of the external skin and of the mucosa of the esophagus. The pathogenesis and etiology are not understood, but it must be noted that the clinical manifestations of pemphigoid and epidermolysis bullosa are related to the fact that the epidermis separates very freely from the dermis in both conditions.

Natural History and Clinical Picture. Involvement of the esophagus in epidermolysis bullosa has been reported more frequently than involvement with pemphigoid. Epidermolysis bullosa itself has two clinical forms, simplex and dystrophic. In the simplex form, the bullae heal without scarring and the disease usually ceases at puberty. The dystrophic form, in which esophageal damage has been described, involves the skin, nails, and teeth, and usually progresses to involve all organs which are lined with squamous epithelium or which are derivatives of this layer. In addition to the obvious external forms of the disease involving the skin and nails, patients with esophageal involvement will describe dysphagia and odynophagia. The bullae will come in crops and will progress from tense, fluid-filled bullae to exuding ulcers. At first the esophagus is merely involved by these bullae, but scarring and stricture formation eventually result.

Pemphigoid is another bullous disease which occurs relatively late in life and is not associated with extensive scarring of the skin or esophagus. Biopsy of the skin shows subepithelial bullae. These tend to involve the esophageal mucosa as well, but the clinical manifestations are less striking. One exception to this rule was a man who vomited up a cast of his entire esophagus.[7] Serial studies revealed regeneration of the esophageal mucosa.

Treatment. Steroid therapy will occasionally help in the management of the bullous phase of epidermolysis bullosa. An initial oral dose of 75 to 80 mg of prednisolone a day is recommended, tapering to between 10 and 20 mg of the steroid per day after the desired effect has been maintained. Cautious tapering off of the steroids after prolonged periods of remission is worthwhile. Occasionally, if the scarring and contractions of the esophagus become so marked as to interfere with nutrition, a colonic interposition has been recommended. Standard dilatation and even esophagoscopy are not recommended in these conditions because of the possibility of damage to the esophageal mucosa.

PHYSICAL AGENTS

LACERATIONS AND PERFORATIONS OF THE ESOPHAGUS

Esophageal lacerations, intramural dissections, and perforations occur as the result of trauma. The most common form of trauma is laceration during the act of vomiting. External trauma to the body, usually in the form of high-speed automobile accidents, can also result in transection or perforation of the esophagus. Instrumentation by the physician may also damage the esophagus.

Etiology and Pathogenesis. The most amazing fact about emetic injury of the esophagus is that it is not more common. Vomiting is an act associated with rapid changes in the thoracic and intra-abdominal pressure. Although manometric study of the act of vomiting is very difficult, transient rises in esophageal pressure as high as 250 to 300 mm Hg have been observed during episodes of retching. When cineradiograms are taken of vomiting, the diaphragm is observed to descend very rapidly, and a large cone of stomach is forced up through the hiatus. At least transiently, the X-ray appearance is one of a large hiatus hernia with marked distention. The change in caliber of the gastroesophageal junction is quite marked, and it is difficult to see why vomiting is not always associated with esophageal injury. Two main types of injury are observed. A mucosal tear can occur which usually begins in gastric epithelium and crosses over the gastroesophageal junction. A through-and-through perforation usually involves the esophagus at the lower end and only very rarely involves the stomach.

It is postulated, but not proved, that emetic rupture of the esophagus is more likely when the upper esophageal sphincter does not relax during vomiting. It is easy to conceive of a situation in which a rapid downward thrust of the diaphragm associated with abdominal wall contractions will greatly increase pressure in the stomach and esophagus. If the upper end of the esophagus does not immediately relax to allow this material to exit, it is possible that the rapid rise of pressure in the esophagus would rupture it at its weakest point, which is the posterolateral aspect of the esophagus. Most of the esophageal rents are longitudinal rather than transverse.

Natural History and Clinical Picture. The extent of esophageal injury determines the clinical presentation. If, as a result of the trauma of vomiting, the mucosa has been lacerated, hematemesis is the most common manifestation. First described by Mallory and Weiss in 1929,[8] the mucosal tear as a result of vomiting has been recognized more frequently in later years as a cause for upper gastrointestinal hemorrhage. Although the classic presentation demands that a previously healthy individual vomit forcibly, first bringing up clear material and then blood in the vomitus, this sequence of events is not always observed. Frequently the patient will complain of pre-existing gastric distress, and blood may become visible on the first episode of emesis.

Diagnosis and Differential Diagnosis. The actual incidence of mucosal laceration will be a function of the accuracy and the method for recognizing the lesion. It is a relatively infrequent finding at autopsy, since many of the lesions will not cause death. Laparotomy in a case of an unexplained bleeding will have a higher incidence, although it is possible to miss a short mucosal tear because of inadequate exposure. (Hopefully the patient will not reach the operating room before endoscopy has been performed to rule out this lesion.) At surgery packing of the stomach and identification of blood coming from the cardioesophageal region will lead to a correct diagnosis. X-ray is an inadequate method of demonstrating the lesions, as they are not sufficiently deep to be filled with barium.

The diagnosis basically rests on clinical suspicion and demonstration of the tear at endoscopy. The advent of the new fiberoptic instruments and the capability of inspecting the fundus of the stomach with a retroflexed fibergastroscope should increase recognition of this lesion. In 170 patients endoscoped soon after recognition of upper gastrointestinal hemorrhage, this lesion was found in 25.[9] Of the patients thus diagnosed, only 5 of the 25 required surgery in order to control hemorrhage. If this ratio is confirmed in other series, then it is clear that many of these lesions stop bleeding without therapy.

PERFORATION

Perforation of the esophagus, first described by Boerhaave in 1749,[10] occurs most frequently in males and usually follows a heavy meal. Vomiting is followed by pain in the epigastrium which may radiate through between the shoulder blades. The patient becomes dyspneic, cyanotic, and diaphoretic, and appears gravely ill. On examination, he is pale and sweaty, has a tachycardia, and may be in shock. The epigastric discomfort may lead to an incorrect diagnosis of acute pancreatitis or perforated peptic ulcer. Dullness at the left base can be demonstrated, and in a matter of a few hours signs of mediastinal air will be apparent. These may take the form of palpable crepitation on the chest wall, neck, or supraclavicular fossae, or a mediastinal crunch synchronous with heartbeat may be detected.

The same changes may be observed when the perforation is the result of an automobile or endoscopic accident. Instrumental perforations usually do not manifest themselves until an hour or so has elapsed. Recognizing esophageal perforation as the result of automobile trauma may be very difficult, since an accident severe enough to produce esophageal rupture has most likely caused splenic rupture, pneumothorax, or other overwhelming clinical conditions which overshadow the manifestations of esophageal rupture.

Diagnosis and Differential Diagnosis. An upright chest film will be helpful in the initial evaluation of someone suspected of esophageal rupture. Absence of free air under the diaphragm will aid in the differential diagnosis between this condition and a perforated intra-abdominal viscus. A pleural effusion may be seen and mediastinal air may be detected.

Confirmation of a perforation is possible with a swallow of radiopaque contrast material (Fig. 37–2). Although barium is

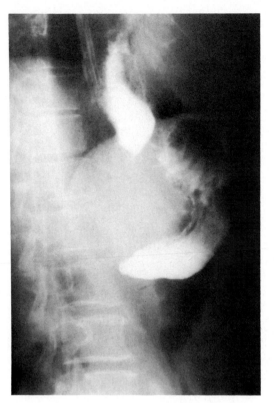

Figure 37–2. Esophageal perforation. Extravasation of barium is seen from a perforation caused by attempted dilation of a stricture.

confused with other clinical conditions. Penetration of a peptic ulcer is the most common condition which is confused with rupture. Approximately 25 per cent of the patients with esophageal ruptures will undergo laparotomy with the mistaken diagnosis of perforated intra-abdominal viscus. Although this approach may be used to suture the lesion if the perforation is low lying enough, and may aid in the evacuation of material which has spilled, it may also be ineffective for adequate repair of lesion and subjects the patient to an unnecessary procedure.

Acute pancreatitis may also mimic this condition, since elevated amylase values have been recorded in esophageal rupture. Signs of subcutaneous emphysema should help in the differential diagnosis, since this is not observed in acute pancreatitis. Other conditions such as dissecting aneurysm and spontaneous pneumothorax may produce the pain. But the combination of pain, subcutaneous emphysema, and fluid at the lung base is usually specific for esophageal rupture.

Treatment. A mucosal laceration with hemorrhage may spontaneously cease bleeding; however, if arterial hemorrhage continues, then laparotomy with oversewing of the arterial bleeding site is imperative. In such patients, previous endoscopy and localization of the lesion facilitate surgical cure. Therapy of perforation of the esophagus depends on the stage of this complication at which the patient is first seen. If perforation has occurred as the result of instrumentation, the patient should be taken immediately to surgery and the rent in the esophagus closed. If this instrumental perforation occurred in the process of evaluating a diseased esophagus, e.g., one with a stricture or carcinoma, excision of the esophagus with replacement by gastric tube or colonic transplant is recommended.[11] Such recommendation, of course, will be tempered by the clinical status of the patient.

Emetogenic rupture of the esophagus will require closure of the esophageal rent and adequate drainage of the mediastinum. Empyema and atelectasis will usually follow such a procedure. Rarely, when the lesion is more than three to four days old and seems to have been satisfactorily sealed off, drainage of mediastinal

thought to be dangerous in this condition, some authorities use it if a large collection of fluid is not present in the mediastinum, since barium staining of the mediastinum at time of thoracotomy may draw attention to the exact location of an esophageal perforation. If a large collection of fluid exists, then it might be wiser to use a water-soluble contrast material. Extravasation of contrast materials may not always be demonstrable, since the perforation may have become sealed. In cases in which the diagnosis is entertained, aspiration of fluid from the thorax may provide definitive evidence of the presence of a perforation, since recovery of gastric acid or food particles from the thorax proves that a communication exists or has recently existed.

The differential diagnosis of this condition includes most catastrophic thoracic and abdominal conditions. Perforations following instrumentation are usually easily recognized; "spontaneous" perforations following vomiting are more often collections without repair of the esophagus has been recommended.[12] However, those electing to treat perforation of the esophagus in this way are assuming a major risk. Whenever possible, an attempt should always be made to seal the defect surgically. The prognosis of perforations and lacerations is good if the primary process can be controlled. Rarely, a patient will suffer from more than one mucosal laceration. Even more rarely, an individual will perforate more than once.

CHEMICAL INJURY TO THE ESOPHAGUS

Chemical injury to the esophagus usually results from the ingestion of lye or other strong alkali agents normally used in the home for cleaning. The ingestion may be accidental, as in the case of children, or with suicidal intent. Less commonly, the esophagus can be badly injured by the ingestion of strong acids, usually with suicidal intent. Such injuries are the result of exposure of the esophageal mucosa to a strong chemical agent. Experimentally, only brief contact by either acids or alkali with the esophageal mucosa is required for irreparable damage. Thus, a ten-second period of contact with strong sodium hydroxide will cause a through-and-through lesion in the esophagus.[13] Chemically, strong alkalis will dissolve the squamous epithelium and fat and cause muscle necrosis.

Natural History and Clinical Picture. Soon after the ingestion of a caustic substance, the patient will complain of intense pain in the mouth and chest. He will be unable to swallow saliva or any other material, will appear to be in considerable distress with tachycardia, and will be spitting out large amounts of frothy mucus. If the damage has been severe, he may retch, vomit, and bring up quantities of blood and esophageal tissue. If the entire esophagus has been digested, the patient will be tachypneic and will show signs of esophageal perforation and mediastinitis. More commonly, within three to four days, the acute distress of the episode will fade and the patient will be able to ingest fluid and solid material. This period of improvement will then be followed by renewed symptoms of dysphagia secondary to stricture formation.

Physical examination during the acute phase will show evidence of oropharyngeal burns, with white membranes and edema of the soft palate and uvula. Absence of all burns makes the possibility of esophageal damage unlikely. However, severe burns do not necessarily indicate the effect of damage of the esophagus; the patient may well not have ingested much caustic material after the initial burns in the pharynx.

Diagnosis and Differential Diagnosis. The history and characteristic oropharyngeal burns usually establish the diagnosis, but the extent of the injury must be ascertained in order to plan further therapy. X-ray and barium swallow will occasionally show evidence of segmental spasm, but mucosal injury will not always be demonstrated by this method. In the later stages of caustic injury, when stricture has appeared, a barium examination is essential for delineating the anatomic extent and degree of disarrangement (Fig. 37–3).

Esophagoscopy within the first 24 hours of caustic ingestion is essential for delineating the extent of esophageal injury. If esophagoscopy reveals a normal mucosa, no therapy is indicated and the patient can be saved prolonged hospitalization and treatment with potentially dangerous forms of therapy. If superficial damage of the esophagus is identified at endoscopy, the patient should be considered a candidate for therapy and very careful follow-up. If the endoscope reveals a circumferential or deep burn, endoscopy should be terminated without passage of the instrument below this area, and therapy should be instituted immediately.

Therapy. Several forms of therapy are available for the patient with caustic burns. In spite of interest in the subject for a number of years, and some investigation in experimental animals, no adequate controlled trial of different forms of therapy has been reported. Thus it is very difficult to be certain of the relative efficacy of the different forms of therapy.

Bougienage has a place in managing the esophageal stricture when it is formed, and it was therefore logical to attempt to prevent stricture formation by early bougienage. This has a theoretical and practical risk of perforation in the esopha-

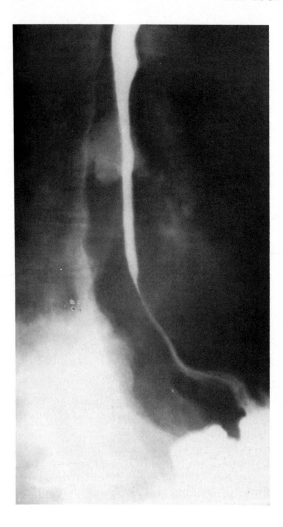

Figure 37–3. Lye stricture of the esophagus. A long stricture of the esophagus beginning at the thoracic inlet and terminating in the stomach. This resulted from the ingestion of lye three years before the film was taken. (Courtesy of Dr. F. E. Templeton.)

gus which has been severely damaged by caustics. In the superficially damaged esophagus, bougienage will probably not lead to unwarranted consequences. If bougienage is to be used, it probably should not be begun before five or six days have elapsed. Because no evidence exists that routine bougienage is helpful, it probably should be withheld until radiological evidence of a compromised esophageal lumen is present.

Another mechanical aid to avoid stricture formation is the introduction of a nasogastric tube or a larger plastic tube to serve as a splint.[14] Although this has the theoretical advantage of maintaining an open lumen, it also has the disadvantage of serving as an irritating focus which may enhance scar formation. If such a tube is used, suction should be applied so that gastric acid is not using the indwelling tube as a wick, thus further compounding the problem of esophageal tissue healing.

In an attempt to inhibit fibrosis, steroids have been used in large doses. Although in the human the correct form of dosage and length of treatment have not been established, work in experimental animals indicates that steroid therapy should begin soon after caustic damage has occurred. Treatment in relatively high doses, 40 mg of prednisone intramuscularly daily, is recommended for the first week. Opinion is divided as to whether steroids should be gradually decreased and terminated within three weeks or should be maintained at lower levels for approximately two months.

Experimental work in animals has suggested that when high doses of steroids are used they should be accompanied by antimicrobial agents. If used, a wide-spectrum drug such as tetracycline, 250 mg four times a day, or ampicillin, 500 mg four times a day, should be administered parenterally. There is no evidence that such agents by themselves offer any significant advantage in the treatment of caustic burns.

Another maneuver of unproved utility is to have the patient with demonstrated esophageal damage swallow a weighted string to serve as a guide for future dilatations. When multiple strictures occur, such a guideline can be very useful. However, its utility must be balanced against the discomfort of maintaining such a string for three to four weeks.

In the late treatment of caustic ingestion, attention is focused on maintenance of an adequate esophageal lumen. If the stricture that forms is limited in duration, dilatation by weighted mercury bougies should be adequate to open and maintain an esophageal lumen. However, it is more common to have severe or multiple strictures which present a very difficult problem in dilatation. If such a problem should occur, esophageal interposition with a colon transplant should be considered.

REFERENCES

1. Terracol, J., and Sweet, R. H. Diseases of the Esophagus. Philadelphia, W. B. Saunders Co., 1958.
2. Stone, J., and Friedberg, S. A. Obstructive syphilitic esophagitis. J.A.M.A., 177:711, 1961.
3. Moses, H. L., and Cheatham, W. J. The frequency and significance of human herpetic esophagitis. Lab. Invest. 12:663, 1963.
4. Collins, W. J., and Wells, R. F. Aphthous esophagitis. Gastrointest. Endosc. 17:115, 1971.
5. Holt, J. M. Candida infection of the oesophagus. Gut 9:227, 1968.
6. Kantrowitz, P. A., Fleischli, D. J., and Butler, W. T. Successful treatment of chronic esophageal moniliasis with a viscous suspension of nystatin. Gastroenterology 57:424, 1969.
7. Foroozan, P., Enta, T., Winship, D. H., and Trier, J. S. Loss and regeneration of the esophageal mucosa in pemphigoid. Gastroenterology 52:548, 1967.
8. Mallory, G. K., and Weiss, S. Hemorrhages from lacerations of the cardiac orifice of the stomach due to vomiting. Amer. J. Med. Sci. 178:506, 1929.
9. Wells, R. F. A common cause of upper gastrointestinal bleeding—the Mallory-Weiss syndrome. Southern Med. J. 60:1197, 1967.
10. Boerhaave, H. Atrocis, nee descripti prius, morbi historia. Secundum medicae artis leges conscripta. Lugduni Batavorum, Boutesteniana, 1724.
11. Kaiser, G. A., Bowman, F. O., and Wylie, R. H. Definitive surgery for the treatment of esophageal perforation with distal obstruction. Ann. Thor. Surg. 8:75, 1969.
12. O'Connell, N. D. Spontaneous rupture of the esophagus. Amer. J. Roentgen. 99:186, 1967.
13. Krey, H. On treatment of corrosive lesions in the esophagus. (Experimental study.) Acta Otolaryngol. Suppl. 102:1, 1952.
14. Dafoe, C. S., and Ross, C. A. Acute corrosive oesophagitis. Thorax 24:291, 1969.

Section 10

THE STOMACH AND DUODENUM

Chapter 38

Anatomy

James E. McGuigan

THE STOMACH

GENERAL ANATOMICAL CONSIDERATIONS

The stomach is that portion of the gastrointestinal tract located between the esophagus superiorly and the initial portion of the duodenum inferiorly. The stomach (gaster) is the most dilated portion of the gastrointestinal tract, although in the empty state it may assume an almost tubular shape. The contour of the stomach may assume many forms, depending upon the body habitus of the individual, the volume of its contents, and the position of the patient upon whom the examination is performed. In general, the stomach is approximately 10 to 12 inches in length, with its maximum transverse diameter approximating 4 to 5 inches. In the erect position the greater curvature descends to a position inferior to the umbilicus, whereas in the supine position the greater curvature is an inch or greater above the umbilicus. The capacity of the adult stomach is variable, but is usually about 1 liter or somewhat greater. The stomach is attached in-

feriorly to the proximal duodenum. The stomach and proximal duodenum are attached to the lesser omentum (hepatoduodenal ligament) and greater omentum and, in contrast to the distal duodenum, are freely mobile. The long axis of the stomach passes downward, forward, to the right, and finally backward and slightly upward.

The convex anterior surface of the stomach is directed both upward and forward, and, in great part, is shielded by the right and left lobes of the liver. Downward and to the left the anterior surface of the stomach rests against the inner surface of the anterior abdominal wall. In the left hypochondrium the stomach is covered not only by the ribs but also by the left lung, pleural cavity and diaphragm. The posterior surface of the stomach constitutes a large portion of the anterior wall of the lesser peritoneal sac (omental bursa). The greater curvature of the stomach is located immediately above and anterior to the transverse colon, with the adjoining posterior gastric surface resting on the transverse mesocolon. Above the transverse mesocolon the stomach is in direct contact with the anterior surface of the pancreas and higher yet with the superior portion of the left kidney and adrenal. The fundus of the stomach rests in part against the spleen and is in direct contact with the concavity of the left diaphragm. The stomach is an intraperitoneal organ, because the peritoneum covers all gastric surfaces. Along the lower portion of the greater curvature the two layers of peritoneum pass downward as the greater omentum; on the left they attach to the spleen as the gastrosplenic ligament. The greater curvature is more freely movable than the lesser curvature, and its position alters as the stomach becomes full or empty, contracted or relaxed.

ANATOMICAL REGIONS OF THE STOMACH

The stomach has been separated into various different portions (Fig. 38–1). That region of the stomach immediately adjacent to the entrance of the esophagus into the stomach has been designated the cardiac portion (cardia) of the stomach. The cardia is fixed to the diaphragm and is located about 1 inch to the left of the midline at the level of the ninth thoracic vertebra. That portion of the stomach which is located to the left of the esophagus and is cephalad to the entry of the esophagus into the stomach has been designated the fundus of the stomach. The pyloric sphincter is the most caudad portion of the stomach and contains the pyloric channel, which is surrounded by the greatly thickened circular mus-

cle which demarcates this termination of the stomach proper. That portion of the stomach distal to the *incisura angularis* has often been referred to as the pyloric portion of the stomach and by some authors as the antrum. This region has been demarcated inferiorly by the distal extent of the pyloric sphincter and proximally by the incisura angularis. The incisura angularis is an indentation on the lesser curvature of the stomach most easily recognized during barium examination of the upper gastrointestinal tract (Fig. 38–2). The incisura angularis is usually located at a point approximately two-thirds of the way down the lesser curvature of the stomach and often at the point at which the vertical portion of the stomach meets the more distal horizontal portion. Although often readily identified by roentgen examination, at the operating table the incisura angularis often cannot be found or can only be vaguely located. The opening of the pylorus to the first portion of the duo-

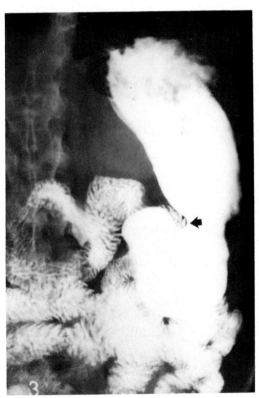

Figure 38–2. Upper gastrointestinal series, in which incisura angularis is demonstrated (arrow).

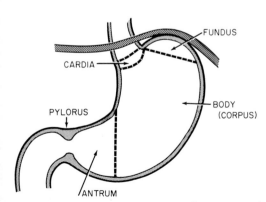

Figure 38–1. Diagram indicating the anatomical regions of the stomach.

denum is located 1 inch to the right of the midline at the level of the first lumbar vertebra. The pylorus is located immediately posterior to the quadrate lobe of the liver and immediately anterior to the neck of the pancreas.

The body of the stomach has been designated as that portion of the stomach between the pylorus and the cardiac and fundal regions. The shorter and (for the most part) superior gastric curvature is called the lesser curvature and the inferior and longer one, the greater curvature.

The antral portion of the stomach may not be identified with precision by gross anatomical landmarks. The antrum can be more readily identified by the functional and histological characteristics of its mucosal cells. The antrum includes the pyloric region of the stomach and extends somewhat further proximally, although variably, along the lesser curvature of the stomach than along the greater gastric curvature. The antral mucosa is relatively free of parietal cells, contains the pyloric glands, and is the site of residence of the hormone gastrin. The oxyntic portion of the stomach, which bears parietal cells, is located cephalad to the antrum (excluding the gastric cardia).

TISSUE LAYERS OF THE STOMACH

The stomach, as most other portions of the gastrointestinal tract, is composed of four tissue layers: the mucosa, submucosa, muscularis propria, and serosa.

The mucosa lining the interior of the stomach in man during life is grayish pink, except for paler regions at the cardia and the pylorus. In the partially empty or partially contracted state the gastric mucosa forms numerous principally longitudinal folds or rugae. In the filled stomach the mucosa may be stretched evenly and smoothly. These differences result from the loose consistency of the submucosa layer and perhaps, to some degree, to contraction by muscularis mucosae components. Numerous, barely visible gastric pits (foveolae gastricae) may be seen to invaginate the gastric mucosa.[1]

The thicker muscular portion of the gastric wall (muscularis propria) is comprised of three muscle layers: outer longitudinal,

middle circular, and inner oblique layers. The oblique muscle sheets in the anterior and posterior walls of the stomach parallel the lesser curvature and are united across the lesser curvature by circular muscle bundles.[2] The three major muscle layers are fused together, and are easily separable from the underlying submucosa and mucosa. The pyloric sphincter is primarily a localized thickening of the middle circular muscle component of the muscularis propria. This pyloric sphincter muscle thickening commences gradually on the gastric side and terminates abruptly at the duodenal limit of the sphincter. The pyloric sphincter may be further divided into two loops of circular muscle; the proximal muscle loop obliquely surrounds the cephalad portion of the pyloric canal, and the distal loop marks the entry into the duodenum from the stomach.[3]

ARTERIAL BLOOD SUPPLY AND VENOUS AND LYMPHATIC DRAINAGE OF THE STOMACH

The arterial blood supply to the stomach is derived principally from branches of the celiac axis and to a lesser extent from the branches arising from the superior mesenteric artery. The lymphatic drainage of the stomach is parallel to, but in reverse to, that of the arterial blood supply.[4] The gastric arterial supply and venous and lymphatic drainage are described in detail on pages 378 to 381.

INNERVATION OF THE STOMACH

The stomach is innervated by both sympathetic and parasympathetic components of the autonomic nervous system. The sympathetic innervation of the stomach is supplied by postganglionic fibers arising in the celiac ganglia. The afferent sensory innervation of the stomach parallels that of the sympathetic distribution. The stomach and duodenum receive most of their sympathetic innervation from the seventh and eighth thoracic spinal segments.[5] Pain associated with peptic ulcer disease is therefore most commonly appreciated in the seventh and eighth thoracic dermatomes which include the region of the epigastrium. Patients treated with thoracolumbar sympathetectomy for hypertension may therefore not perceive pain associated with peptic ulcer disease and may only appreciate discomfort following perforation when symptoms occur following the development of peritonitis. Parasympathetic innervation of the stomach is supplied by the vagus nerves. The anterior and posterior vagal trunks are formed distal to the complexity of the vagal plexus which is located adjacent to the esophagus. The anterior gastric division of the anterior trunk of the vagus nerves supplies the anterior wall of the stomach, and the posterior gastric division of the posterior vagal trunk supplies the posterior gastric wall. The hepatic division which arises from the anterior trunk of the vagal nerve supplies the proximal duodenum.

MICROSCOPIC ANATOMY OF THE GASTRIC MUCOSA

The gastric glands, which are of several types, extend deeply from the bottoms of the gastric pits (foveolae gastricae) (Figs. 38-3 and 38-4). The epithelium which lines the foveolae gastricae and the intervening free mucosal surface is uniform; however, the differences in the gastric glands permit histological identification of three principal gastric regions. The first region, which is 1.5 to 3 cm in length, contains the cardiac glands and corresponds with the gastric cardia. The second region (the oxyntic portion of the stomach) constitutes the fundus and body, including the proximal two-thirds of the stomach, and contains the oxyntic (or fundic) glands. The third portion of the stomach is characterized by the presence of the pyloric glands, corresponds with the antrum of the stomach, includes the distal portion of the stomach, including all that has been previously identified as pylorus, and extends farther superiorly along the lesser than the greater curvature of the stomach (Fig. 38-3).

The Surface Epithelium. Tall columnar epithelial cells, 20 to 40 μ in height, comprise the surface of the gastric ridges and pits. This columnar epithelium commences abruptly at the cardia with the termination of the stratified squamous epithelium of the esophagus. These cells have

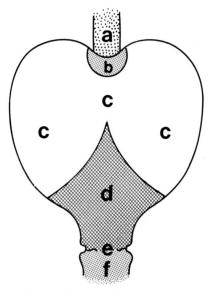

Figure 38-3. Diagram showing the microscopic anatomy of the gastric mucosa (stomach opened along the greater curvature). a, Squamous epithelium; b, cardiac epithelium; c, chief and parietal cell area; d, antral gland area; e, pylorus; and f, duodenal mucosa.

basally located nuclei with large supranuclear portions which are occupied in part by mucigen-containing granules. This mucigen may be stained with mucicarmine as well as the periodic acid–Schiff reaction which stains mucus. When discharged, these granules produce a layer of mucus which lubricates the gastric mucosa. These cells may extend into the necks of the glands. They appear to originate in the deeper portions of the foveolae and in the necks of the glands, and then migrate upward, replacing those lost by desquamation at the surface. These surface mucus cells appear to be completely renewed approximately every one to three days.[7-9]

Gastric Glands. The oxyntic (parietal) glands are simple branched epithelial tubular glands, about 50 μ in outside diameter, which are closely packed and oriented in a perpendicular fashion to the gastric mucosal surface (Fig. 38-4). In the superficial two-thirds of their length these tubes are nearly straight, but they are tortuous in their deepest third.[10] They extend from 0.3 to 1.5 mm in length, averaging approximately 1.2 mm. One or more glands enter through a slight constriction, which has been designated the neck of the gland, to the deepest portion of each foveola. The

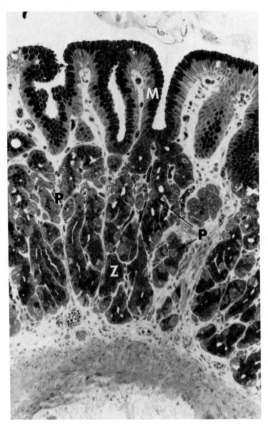

Figure 38–4. Photomicrograph of normal human gastric mucosa (parietal cell region). Mucous cells (M) line the foveolae. Large, oval, light-staining parietal cells (P) are seen in the midportion of the glands. In the base of the glands dark-staining zymogen cells (Z) may be seen. × 250. (Courtesy of Dr. Clinton B. Lillibridge.)

average foveola, which is entirely lined by mucous cells, is approximately 70 μ wide and 200 μ deep. At least four types of cells have been identified as constituents of the oxyntic glands, including (1) zymogen or chief cells, (2) oxyntic or parietal cells, (3) mucous neck cells, and (4) endocrine or endocrine-like cells.

The *chief (zymogen) cells* are present in greatest number in the deepest portions of the glands, lining the glandular lumen in the lower half to one-third of the glandular tubule. Zymogen cells appear as irregularly truncated pyramids approximately 7 by 16 μ. The apical cytoplasm of these cells is packed with large, highly refractile zymogen granules, which range in diameter from 1 to 3 μ. Following stimulation with subsequent secretion, these

cells appear smaller with substantial reduction in their granular content. The granules contain pepsinogens, the zymogenic precursors of pepsins. The fine structure of the zymogen cells, discernible by electron microscopy, is similar to that of other cell types secreting proteolytic enzymes such as the pancreatic acinar cells. Large oval or round granules of relatively low density are found in the apical cytoplasm. The supranuclear region contains a well developed Golgi apparatus. Granular endoplasmic reticulum, especially concentrated in the basal portion of the cells, is found throughout the cytoplasm. The basophilic staining characteristics of these cells are accounted for by the presence of abundant ribosomes both free in the cytoplasm and attached to reticulum membranes.

Parietal (oxyntic) cells are interspersed, usually singly, among the zymogen cells, and together they constitute the oxyntic glands (Fig. 38–4). The oxyntic cells, which are usually wedged between their zymogen cell neighbors, are large (20 to 35 μ) and are either spheroidal or pyramidal in shape. Their tapered apical ends usually face the tubular glandular lumen, with their broader basal surfaces placed against the basement membrane of the glands. The parietal cell nucleus is large and round, and the cytoplasm is strongly eosinophilic. Oxyntic cells are found most commonly in the mid-region of the glands. Numerous rod-shaped or spherical mitochondria are found in the cytoplasm of the oxyntic cell. In contrast to the zymogen cell, there are no secretory granules in the cytoplasm of the oxyntic cell. The electron microscopy of the oxyntic cells reveals them to be packed with oval mitochondria (Fig. 38–5).[10] The most conspicuous morphological feature of the oxyntic cell is the presence of a secretory canalicular system. This intracellular canalicular system forms a loose network surrounding the oxyntic cell nucleus and opens into the lumen of the gastric gland. The intracellular canaliculi are lined with microvilli. Between the mitochondria and canaliculi there are fine tubules. Cytoplasmic vacuoles are abundant in oxyntic cells, especially in those cells found in the neck region of the glands. Endoplasmic reticulum is scant and is dispersed throughout the cy-

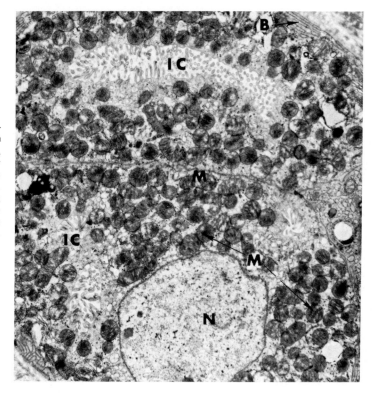

Figure 38–5. Electron micrograph of a parietal cell. Between numerous oval mitochondria (M), parts of the intracellular secretory canaliculus (IC), lined by numerous slender microvilli, may be seen. Basal infoldings (B) of the plasma membranes are located at the edge of the cell. The nucleus (N) appears in the lower portion of the micrograph. × 9000. (Courtesy of Dr. Clinton B. Lillibridge.)

toplasm. Parietal cells are responsible for the secretion of hydrochloric acid. In man these cells also contain intrinsic factor.[11] The cytoplasm of the oxyntic cell near the secretory canaliculus contains an extensive system of minute tubules which appear to communicate with the cell surface. The Golgi complex, which in most epithelial cells is located in a supranuclear position, in the oxyntic cell is located between the base of the cell and the nucleus. With stimulation, as with Histalog (betazole), the cytoplasmic vesicles are greatly reduced in number, the canalicular system becomes enlarged, and there is a decrease in the number and size of microvilli located in the canalicular system.

The mucous neck cells are relatively few in number and are located between the parietal cells in the neck regions of the glands. The granules which fill the apical cytoplasm are deeply stained by periodic acid–Schiff or mucicarmine. The mucous secretory product of these cells may be somewhat different from that of the surface mucous cells. By electron microscopy the apical regions of the cells are seen to contain numerous dense granules of spheroid,

discoid, or ovoid shape. Each mucus droplet has a characteristic stippled appearance; however, the stippling of the mucous granules is most apparent in cells of the surface epithelium, being less so in mucous cells of the neck region. There is a generous supranuclear Golgi complex.

A variety of *endocrine cells* are present in the mucosa of the gastric epithelium. These cells are scattered, usually singly, between the basement lamina and the zymogenic cells. These endocrine cells are rounded and are sometimes pyramidal in shape. Their cytoplasm is filled with small granules which in many instances may be stained with silver or chromium salts. One group of endocrine cells may be identified as argentaffin cells; the granules in these cells reduce silver salt without special pretreatment.[12-14] These cells have been shown to contain serotonin (5-hydroxytryptamine).[15] Other endocrine cells require exposure to a reducing substance before their granules will react with silver; they have been designated as argyrophil cells.[12] The explanations for affinity for metallic salts exhibited by these cells and for the differences in the staining proper-

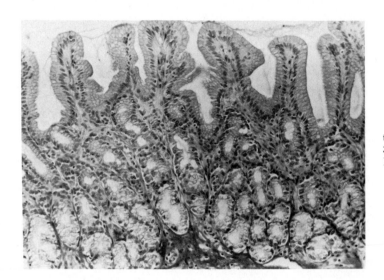

Figure 38–6.   Human gastric antrum. Hematoxylin and eosin. × 300. (Courtesy of Dr. Clinton B. Lillibridge.)

ties of these two populations of cells have not been elucidated.

It appears that these endocrine cells are heterogeneous in nature. Various populations of these or structurally related cells probably synthesize and release those hormonal agents originating in the stomach.

In the pyloric, or antral, mucosal portion of the stomach the foveolae gastricae (gastric pits) are much deeper than in other regions of the stomach (Figs. 38–6 and 38–7). The glands, which are usually designated as pyloric glands, are simple, branched, and extensively coiled tubular glands. Most of the cells lining the gland lumens have pale cytoplasm, with their nuclei located adjacent to basement membranes, and appear similar to mucous neck cells and to the cells of duodenal Brunner's glands. Argentaffin and argyrophil cells are also interspersed singly or in small clusters along the course of the antral pyloric glands.

Gastrin has been shown to be contained in or on cytoplasmic granules of a population of endocrine cells (Fig. 38–8). The gastrin-containing cells are interspersed along the course of the antral pyloric glands.[16] The gastrin cells are found most frequently in the mid-portions of the glands and to some extent in the neck region. They are least commonly found in the depths of the antral pyloric glands. The gastrin cells have not been demonstrated conclusively to stain positively with either argentaffin or argyrophilic staining procedures.

The lamina propria is the connective tissue portion of the gastric mucosa adjacent to the gastric mucosal epithelium. The muscularis mucosae, a delicate muscle layer, comprises the deepest layer of the mucosa. Immediately deep to the mucosa is the submucosa, a connective tissue layer

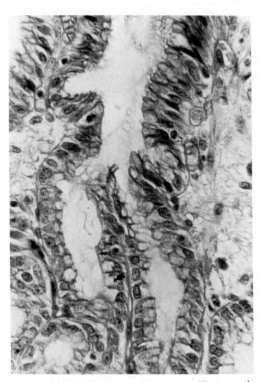

Figure 38–7.   Human gastric antrum. Hematoxylin and eosin. × 900. (Courtesy of Dr. Clinton B. Lillibridge.)

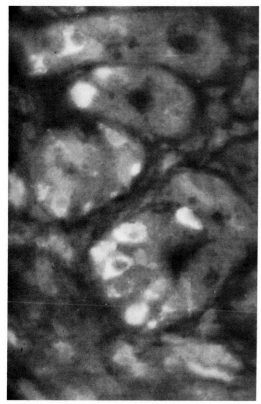

Figure 38–8. Human antral mucosal gastrin cells, which appear white, are identified using direct immunofluorescence techniques with fluorescein-labeled antibodies to human gastrin I. × 900.

containing small arteries and veins, lymphoid elements including lymphocytes and plasma cells, and the submucosal neural plexuses.

THE DUODENUM

The duodenum is a tubular organ, approximately 12 inches in length, which is in continuity with the stomach and for the most part is located retroperitoneally. It is shaped approximately in the form of the letter C with the cavity toward the left and the head of the pancreas residing in this concavity. The first portion of the duodenum, which is attached to the pylorus of the stomach, is approximately 2 inches in length. It is readily movable. It passes slightly posteriorly and to the right. The second portion of the duodenum, or descending portion, is approximately 3 inches in length. The third portion of the duodenum, or horizontal portion, which is approximately 4 inches long, crosses transversely anterior to the inferior vena cava and aorta. The fourth portion of the duodenum, which is about 2 inches in length, ascends along the left side of the aorta and then descends abruptly at the ligament of Treitz to become the jejunum. The first part of the duodenum is intraperitoneal; the remaining three portions are retroperitoneal.

The duodenum, which is a muscular tube with outer longitudinal and inner circular smooth muscle layers, is lined by mucosa and in many respects is structurally similar to other portions of the small intestine which will be described in detail elsewhere. Although there are minor gross and microscopical differences between the duodenum and the other portions of the small intestine, the jejunum and ileum, the portions of the small intestine have the same general organization, and transitions between the three portions are gradual.

Just inferior to the midportion of the descending duodenum is the ampulla of Vater, at which site the major pancreatic and common bile duct gain entry into the intestinal lumen. The accessory pancreatic duct may enter 2 cm superior to the ampulla of Vater.

The duodenal glands, or Brunner's glands, begin in the vicinity of the gastric mucosa of the pylorus and are usually present, in gradually diminishing numbers, in the proximal two-thirds of the duodenum. They are not usually found in the jejunum or ileum. They are generously branched and coiled tubular glands arranged in lobules approximately 0.5 to 1.0 mm in diameter, penetrating the mucosa and located for the most part in the submucosa. Brunner's gland ducts empty into the crypts of Lieberkühn. The secretory product of Brunner's glands is clear in appearance, viscous, and alkaline (pH 8.2 to 9.3). It has been proposed that the principal role of the alkaline Brunner's gland secretion is to protect the duodenal mucosa against erosion by acid gastric secretion.[17]

REFERENCES

1. Bloom, W., and Fawcett, D. W. A Textbook of Histology. Philadelphia, W. B. Saunders Co., 1968, p. 547.
2. Oi, M., Tanaka, Y., Yoshida, K., and Yoshikawa, K. Dual control of peptic ulcers by both the gastric mucosa and musculature. Rev. Surg. 23:373, 1966.
3. Torgersen, J. Muscular build and movements of stomach and duodenal bulb: Especially with regard to problems of segmental divisions of stomach in light of comparative anatomy and embryology. Acta Radiol. (Suppl.) 45:1, 1942.
4. Coller, F. A., Kay, E. B., and McIntyre, R. S. Regional lymphatic metastases of carcinoma of the stomach. Arch. Surg. 43:748, 1941.
5. Kimura, C. Visceral sensation. Acta Neuroveg. 28:405, 1966.
6. Griffith, C. A. Anatomy. In Surgery of the Stomach and Duodenum, H. N. Harkins and L. M. Nyhus (eds.). Boston, Little, Brown and Co., 1969, pp. 25–52.
7. Baker, B. L. Cell replacement in the stomach. Gastroenterology 46:202, 1964.
8. Lipkin, M. P., Sherlock, P., and Bell, B. Cell proliferation kinetics in the gastrointestinal tract of man. II. Cell renewal in stomach, ileum, colon, and rectum. Gastroenterology 45:721, 1963.
9. MacDonald, W. C., Trier, J. S., and Everett, N. B. Cell proliferation in the stomach, duodenum, and rectum of man. Gastroenterology 46:405, 1964.
10. Lillibridge, C. B. The fine structure of normal human gastric mucosa. Gastroenterology 47:269, 1964.
11. Hoedemaeker, P. J., Abels, J., Wachters, J. J., Arends, A., and Nieweg, N. O. Investigations about the site of production of Castle's gastric intrinsic factor. Lab. Invest. 13:1394, 1964.
12. Dawson, A. B. Argentophile and argentaffin cells in the gastric mucosa of the rat. Anat. Rec. 100:319, 1948.
13. Holcenberg, J., and Benditt, E. P. A new histochemical technique for demonstration of enterochromaffin cells. J. Histochem. Cytochem. 7:303, 1959.
14. Holcenberg, J., and Benditt, E. P. A new color reaction for tryptamine derivatives. Histochemical applications to enterochromaffin cells. Lab. Invest. 10:144, 1961.
15. Pentilla, A. Histochemical reactions of the enterochromaffin cells and the 5-hydroxytryptamine content of the mammalian duodenum. Acta Physiol. Scand. 69, Suppl. 281:7, 1966.
16. McGuigan, J. E. Gastric mucosal intracellular localization of gastrin by immunofluorescence. Gastroenterology 55:315, 1968.
17. Grossman, M. I. The glands of Brunner. Physiol. Rev. 38:675, 1958.

Chapter 39

Embryology and Developmental Anomalies

James E. McGuigan

EMBRYOLOGICAL DEVELOPMENT OF THE STOMACH AND DUODENUM

In the fifth week of embryological development the stomach first emerges as a fusiform dilatation of the foregut. During the following weeks a variety of changes occur secondary to the rotation of the stomach on two axes—a longitudinal axis and an anteroposterior axis.[1, 2] By clockwise rotation on the longitudinal axis for 90 degrees, that which was the left side of the stomach in the early embyro becomes the anterior gastric surface, and that which was the right side becomes the gastric posterior surface. During this period of rotation, that which was originally the posterior portion of the stomach grows more rapidly than the anterior portion, accounting for the formation of the greater curvature, which exceeds in length that of the lesser curvature of the stomach. Originally the cephalic and caudal portions of the stomach are located in the midline; however, during development the caudal (pyloric) portion migrates upward and to the right, and the cephalic (cardiac) portion migrates downward and to the left.

The duodenum is formed by the terminal portion of the embyronic foregut and the cephalic portion of the midgut. The posi-

tion at which these two embryonic portions of the primitive gut meet is located immediately distal to that which will become the ampulla of Vater. During gastric rotation the duodenum also rotates to the right, approximating the shape of a U in its retroperitoneal position. During the second month of embryonic development the duodenal lumen may be temporarily obliterated; however, the channel becomes reestablished.

The dorsal mesentery in the 8-mm embryo extends from the terminal portion of the esophagus to the cloaca. The ventral mesentery is present only in the most distal portion of the esophagus, stomach, and upper duodenum. During gastric rotation the liver extends into the ventral mesentery. Therefore eventually the ventral mesentery extends from the lesser curvature of the stomach as the lesser omentum to, and encasing, the liver and then further extends as the falciform ligament to the ventral abdominal wall. That portion of the dorsal mesentery which suspends the primitive foregut is designated the dorsal mesogastrium and extends to the left in the form of a large sac, the omental bursa. That which originally was the right peritoneal surface of the dorsal mesogastrium becomes the lining of the interior of this sac; that which was the left surface of the dorsal mesogastrium constitutes the exterior of the omental bursa. The anterior wall of this sac envelops the spleen and attaches to the greater gastric curvature. The posterior surface of this sac is pressed against the dorsal body wall and covers the pancreas.

CONGENITAL ABNORMALITIES OF THE STOMACH AND DUODENUM

HYPERTROPHIC PYLORIC STENOSIS

Definition. Hypertrophic pyloric stenosis, as its name so vividly describes, is a congenital obstructing lesion involving the gastric outlet at the level of the pylorus.[3] This abnormality is by no means rare, occurring in from approximately one in 300 to one in 900 live births,[4,5] and is the most common event requiring abdominal surgery during the first six months of life. It may be less common among black than white infants.[5]

Etiology and Pathogenesis. The etiology of hypertrophic pyloric stenosis has not been defined. It is congenital in nature, sometimes occurring in members of the same family, or in family clusters. The accepted genetic mode of transmission of the congenital form of hypertrophic pyloric stenosis is that of multifactorial inheritance.[6-8] Studies of twins have revealed a higher rate of concordance in monozygotic and dizygotic twins.[9-11] First-degree relatives of male index patients with hypertrophic stenosis have been found to be affected in the proportion of 4.6 per cent for males and 2.3 per cent for females; these incidences, respectively, are 10 times and 25 times those of the general population.[6-7] In relatives of female index patients with hypertrophic pyloric stenosis, 15.4 per cent of males and 9.8 per cent of females are affected; these values are 30 and 100 times higher than the anticipated values for the general population. The pathological anatomy is that of hypertrophy and hyperplasia of the circular muscle of the muscularis propria of the pylorus. With time inflammatory changes may develop; these include edema and mononuclear cell infiltration which are often particularly conspicuous in the mucosa. Congenital hypertrophic pyloric stenosis has been detected rarely in infants at birth, including those following premature delivery.[4]

Clinical Features and Diagnosis. A family history of pyloric stenosis may be helpful in suspecting the diagnosis. Hypertrophic pyloric stenosis is more commonly found in the male, with a ratio of 3 or 4 to 1 over its incidence in the female.[6,7]

Infants with hypertrophic pyloric stenosis are usually well during the first week of life, with the development of vomiting most commonly during the third week. At first gastric contents are lost by regurgitation and later by vigorous and sometimes projectile vomiting. The vomitus may contain blood, but seldom contains bile. Constipation results from vomiting and decreased oral intake; dehydration causes diminished urinary output.

Examination of the infant with hypertrophic pyloric stenosis may show varying degrees of fluid depletion. Inspection of the abdomen following feeding will usually reveal visible peristaltic contractions. The mass resulting from the hypertrophic pyloric stenosis can usually be palpated in the epigastrium.[12,13] The mass is smooth, very firm, ovoid, and only 1 to 2 cm in diameter; it is located just to the right of the midline in the epigastrium. Repeated, careful, and prolonged gentle examination may be required for detection and appreciation of the mass. An optimal time to examine for it is immediately after vomiting, when the previously overdistended stomach may no longer interfere with examination. In patients with hypertrophic pyloric stenosis, barium examination of the stomach demonstrates the pyloric channel to be elongated and narrowed (Fig. 39–1). In addition, as a result of the presence of the hypertrophic muscle mass, the duodenum may be circumferentially indented around the entry of the pylorus into the first part of the duodenum.

Hypertrophic pyloric stenosis must be differentiated from gastroesophageal reflux, which is common in infants. The latter is usually associated with regurgitation, but seldom with genuine vomiting. The distinction between these two entities should be readily made by barium examination of the upper gastrointestinal tract.

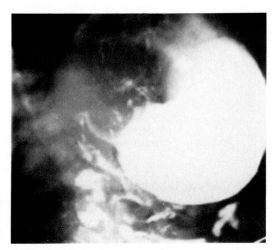

Figure 39–1. Congenital hypertrophic pyloric stenosis in an infant.

Projectile vomiting associated with intracranial abnormalities must, of course, be differentiated from that associated with hypertrophic pyloric stenosis. The presence of bile in vomitus from persistently vomiting children should suggest the possibility of duodenal obstruction rather than hypertrophic pyloric stenosis.

Treatment. The treatment of infants with hypertrophic pyloric stenosis is surgical. Dehydration and fluid and electrolyte disturbances, commonly metabolic alkalosis with hypokalemia, which result from vomiting must be corrected by appropriate infusions, prior to surgery for the hypertrophic pyloric stenosis. In some infants blood transfusion may also be required preoperatively. The preferred surgical procedure is the Ramstedt pyloromyotomy,[14] in which a longitudinal incision is made on the anterior surface of the pylorus through the serosa down to the submucosa, resulting in a division of the ring of pyloric muscle.

Prognosis. Surgical treatment will relieve the persistent vomiting of hypertrophic pyloric stenosis;[15] failure to do so may indicate incompleteness of pyloromyotomy.[12, 15] The serosa will eventually become continuous; however, the muscular ring does not reunite. Gradually the mass of hypertrophic pyloric muscle will disappear. It is interesting that in patients previously treated by a diverting procedure such as gastroenterostomy, without

pyloromyotomy, the hypertrophic pyloric muscle mass persists.

PREPYLORIC MEMBRANE (CONGENITAL PREPYLORIC ATRESIA)

Depending upon its completeness, a prepyloric membrane, or diaphragm, may be noted in the stomach over a wide age range—from newborn infants to adulthood.[16–18] The gastrointestinal symptoms are largely due to upper gastrointestinal tract obstruction.

Etiology and Pathogenesis. Membranous obstruction in the prepyloric area may be either complete or incomplete (Figs. 39–2 and 39–3). The etiology of this abnormality, which is interpreted as representing failure of recanalization of this portion of the primitive foregut, is not known. This abnormality may manifest itself as a single diaphragmatic membrane, a double membrane,[19] or even a localized segment of aplasia in the prepyloric region of the stomach.

Clinical Features and Diagnosis. If obstruction is complete, the newborn infant vomits, salivates excessively, and often has dyspnea and cyanosis, associated with the

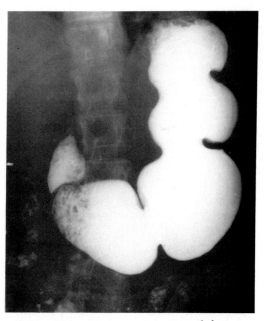

Figure 39–2. Barium examination of the upper gastrointestinal tract, demonstrating membranous obstruction of the prepyloric area of the stomach.

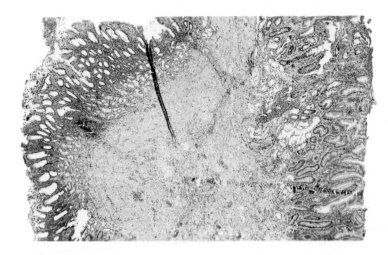

Figure 39–3. Histological section of pyloric diaphragm in an adult. × 60. (From Shartsis, J. M., and Fox, T. A.: Gastroenterology 56:580, 1969.)

failure to cope with gastric and salivary secretions.

Incomplete membranous obstruction may become manifest even in adulthood,[20] with vague or cramping abdominal discomfort or sometimes with vomiting caused by incomplete prepyloric obstruction. The diagnosis of complete obstruction may be made in the newborn infant by the persistence and severity of symptoms and the collection of air in the stomach. The absence of a mass distinguishes it from congenital hypertrophic pyloric stenosis. Preoperative diagnosis of complete prepyloric obstruction, usually does not require confirmation by barium examination of the upper gastrointestinal tract. Older infants, children, and adults have some degree of luminal patency; the diagnosis is usually made by an upper gastrointestinal series performed for symptoms suggesting gastric obstruction.

Treatment and Prognosis. When possible, surgical excision of the membrane is preferable to diverting procedures such as gastroenterostomy.[16, 18, 19] Successful excision of the obstructing diaphragm is usually associated with relief of symptoms.[20]

DUODENAL STENOSIS AND ATRESIA

Definition. A variety of congenital abnormalities may result in partial or complete obstruction of the gastrointestinal tract at the level of the duodenum. Principal among these are duodenal stenosis, duodenal atresia, and the presence of an annular pancreas. The term duodenal atresia usually denotes complete obliteration of the lumen of the intestine at the level of the duodenum, whereas stenosis indicates partial obstruction. Congenital stenosis and atresia of the duodenum arise, presumably, on the same, or a similar, basis and have been observed in from one in 16,000 to one in 20,000 live births.[21, 22] In the neonatal infant intrinsic obstruction of the duodenum is more commonly due to duodenal atresia than stenosis.[23] The duodenal obstruction may be present in any one of several forms; the lumen may be entirely discontinuous with no evidence of any remnant of the intestinal channel, a membranous ring may be present in the duodenum, the duodenum may terminate in a dilated blind end with a fibrous core running to the distal undilated bowel, or diaphragmatic obstruction of the duodenum may be relatively complete with only a tiny lumen.

Etiology and Pathogenesis. The etiology of the duodenal atresia and stenosis has not been defined. Two possible explanations have been proposed. In the sixth or seventh week of embryonic development epithelial proliferation in the duodenum occludes its lumen; however, in normal embryological development this transient obstruction is shortly relieved by recanalization owing to vacuolization. Thus it has been suggested that duodenal atresia or stenosis may result from partial or complete failure of recanalization of the duodenal lumen.[21] Others have proposed that duodenal stenosis and atresia result from ischemia caused by vascular defects in the embryo.[24, 25]

Although in most instances a single area of stenosis or atresia is present, there are cases with more than one area of atresia. The site of stenosis or atresia in the duodenum is usually distal to the ampulla of Vater. Approximately 70 per cent of patients with duodenal atresia or stenosis have some other variety of congenital malformation.[23] These abnormalities may involve other areas of the gastrointestinal tract, as well as the central nervous, genitourinary, or respiratory systems. Prematurity and mongolism are also common in this group.

Clinical Features and Diagnosis. In newborn infants with complete obstruction, i.e., duodenal atresia, vomiting, which usually begins on the first day of life, is relentless. The vomitus usually, but not invariably, contains bile. The presence of bile in the vomitus may serve as an aid to distinguish this abnormality from congenital hypertrophic pyloric stenosis and prepyloric membrane. Abdominal distention, when present, is usually restricted to the epigastrium, and stools are dry, scanty, and grayish green. During the first several days of life the danger is great that the blind sac proximal to the level of atresia will perforate, because the obstructed sac rarely tolerates distention beyond 72 hours. In this situation fever and clinical evidence of peritonitis herald proximal rupture.

With severe duodenal stenosis the symptoms are indistinguishable from those of duodenal atresia. When stenosis is less complete, vomiting may not appear until later infancy or childhood. Rarely, this anomaly may appear in adults (Fig. 39–4). In addition, the child may show crucial evidences of chronic illness, including poor appetite and failure to gain weight normally.

The clinical features associated with duodenal atresia or stenosis are usually sufficient to establish the diagnosis; however, radiographic examination may be used to confirm the level of obstruction. Plain films of the abdomen usually show distention of the stomach and duodenum proximal to the level of obstruction. Rarely will contrast media be required to establish the diagnosis of duodenal atresia; however, when deemed necessary, contrast agents other than barium (for example, Gastrografin) are probably desirable for localization and definition of obstruction.

Associated congenital abnormalities substantially increase the mortality rate in infants with congenital stenosis or atresia and obstruction.[23] For example, esophageal atresia and intestinal abnormalities, especially intestinal volvulus, are commonly found. In fact, malrotation of

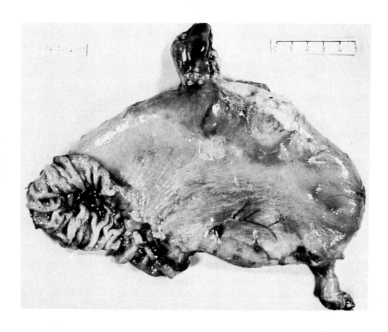

Figure 39–4. Operative specimen of hypoplastic duodenum. (From Lubbers, E. J. C., and Rijnders, W. P. H. A.: Gastroenterology 57:574, 1969.)

the midgut loop and annular pancreas each occur in approximately one-third of these infants with duodenal obstruction caused by stenosis or atresia.[23] Jaundice, from a variety of causes, is found in almost half of those infants with intrinsic duodenal obstruction. Congenital abnormalities of the cardiovascular system are also commonly noted; in one study, 27 per cent of these patients were mongoloid.[23] The urinary tract and skeletal system may also have an assortment of abnormalities.

Treatment. The substantial mortality of duodenal atresia and severe stenosis in the early days of life could be reduced by earlier surgical correction, which is mandatory.[26] Surgical correction may be achieved by duodenoduodenostomy or by isoperistaltic duodenojejunostomy.[26] In premature infants, and in infants with atresia of the first portion of the duodenum, gastrojejunostomy may be a necessary alternative. During exploration, examination of the remaining portions of the small and large intestine for other sites of atresia, and for the presence of malrotation which sometimes accompanies duodenal atresia and stenosis, is mandatory.[23, 26, 27] It is not usually possible to resect localized duodenal diaphragms or stenotic atretic segments; therefore it appears preferable to utilize a bypass procedure.

Prognosis and Complications. The mortality rate associated with surgical correction of duodenal stenosis or atresia in early infancy has ranged from 12 to 53.8 per cent. The lowest mortality rates are in infants with an early diagnosis and correction before perforation and peritonitis.

MALROTATION WITH DUODENAL OBSTRUCTION

The most common cause of duodenal obstruction in children is intestinal malrotation.

Etiology and Pathogenesis. The failure of attachment of the mesentery to the posterior abdominal wall results in an incompletely rotated or highly mobile cecum. When the cecum is not completely rotated, the second portion of the duodenum may be obstructed by peritoneal bands extending from the cecum to the right posterior-lateral abdominal wall. With nonrotation of the cecum the initial portion of the small intestine, the right side of the transverse colon, and the superior mesenteric vessels are encased together by a peritoneal attachment; therefore the small intestine may twist on this single central attachment. Volvulus occurs commonly with malrotation of the intestine. When volvulus develops it is usually clockwise in rotation. Malrotation accounts for approximately 50 per cent of cases of duodenal obstruction. Volvulus obstructs the intestinal lumen, and, more serious, possibly the superior mesenteric vessels as well, causing ischemia and infarction of the intestine.

Occasionally, duodenal bands, commonly found in the third portion of the duodenum, may obstruct the intestine. Obstructive symptoms resulting from volvulus and/or duodenal bands are usually found in small infants; however, they may appear in later childhood and in adulthood.[28, 29]

Clinical Features and Diagnosis. The most common cause of intestinal obstruction in the newborn is intestinal malrotation. The infant vomits severely; older children and adults differ, having recurrent episodes of nausea, vomiting, and abdominal pain. The flat film of abdomen will demonstrate dilatation of the proximal duodenum and the stomach and, in the small infant with severe obstruction, the absence of air in the intestine. Barium examination not only delineates the site of obstruction, but also reveals the malrotation by demonstrating the cecum in the right upper abdomen.

Treatment. The treatment of midgut volvulus with duodenal obstruction is surgical, because it is likely to result in ischemic necrosis of the bowel. Infarction of the intestine necessitates resection of the involved intestine. The corrective surgical procedure consists of division of obstructing bands and relief of the volvulus; stabilization of the cecum may be necessary to avoid recurrent episodes of volvulus.[30]

Prognosis and Complications. The mortality rate of infants and children operated upon for malrotation is 15 to 20 per cent.[26] Patients with recurrent episodes of volvulus caused by malrotation are usually relieved by stabilization of the cecum. Resection of ischemic small intestine is often followed by malabsorption, requiring specific medical treatment (see pp. 259 to 289).

DUPLICATION OF THE STOMACH AND DUODENUM

Duplication of the intestinal tract is most common in the ileum, but it also affects the stomach and duodenum.[31, 32]

Etiology and Pathogenesis. Duplications of the stomach and duodenum arise from a primordial anlage which has the potential to develop this organ unit. The cause for this maldevelopment is unknown. The gastric or duodenal duplication may be elongated, ovoid, or spherical; it may be attached to the normal portion of the gastrointestinal tract, and approximately 20 per cent communicate with the lumen of the stomach or duodenum. The duplications are lined by duodenal or gastric mucosa and contain smooth muscle in their walls, which are usually attached to the smooth muscle walls of the normal organ. The duplications may contain the secretory product of the mucosa of the respective organ; e.g., gastric juice in the duplicated stomach.

Clinical Features and Diagnosis. Duplication of the stomach may occur without symptoms and be detected only during incidental barium examinations of the upper gastrointestinal tract. Although duplications of the stomach and duodenum are more commonly found in infancy and childhood, they may also be recognized during adulthood. The clinical manifestations of duodenal or gastric duplication may be comprised of an expanding cystic intra-abdominal mass, possibly secreting the common product of the involved organ. Necrosis of the mucosa may result. In some patients peptic ulceration may develop within the duplication or in the adjacent small intestinal mucosa.[33, 34] Obstruction may occur at the level of the pylorus or duodenum secondary to the progressively increasing size of the duplication.

Diagnosis is usually made by barium examination of the upper gastrointestinal tract or, commonly, during surgical exploration for a mass in the region of the stomach or duodenum, whose presence has been signaled by its smooth impingement on the barium-filled lumen of the stomach or duodenum.

Treatment. The treatment of duplication of the duodenum or stomach is surgical resection; it is usually possible in the stomach, but not in the duodenum. For duodenal duplication, therefore, the usual surgical procedure is anastomosis with the normal duodenum.

Prognosis and Complications. The mortality rate for adults operated upon with duplication of the duodenum and stomach is less than 10 per cent; however, it is substantially higher for infants. Patients with gastric and duodenal duplications who survive surgery are generally relieved of their symptoms.

GASTRIC NECROSIS AND RUPTURE IN THE NEWBORN

Acute necrosis and rupture of the stomach in the newborn infant can no longer be considered rare.[35] Only with early recognition of this abnormality and subsequent early surgical correction will the high degree of infant mortality be reversed.

Etiology and Pathogenesis. In early reports it was suspected that the most common cause of gastric rupture of the newborn infant was underlying peptic ulcer disease; however, in only a small portion of these patients does perforation appear to result from peptic ulcer. Associated phenomena such as distal gastric obstruction and external trauma, perhaps during birth, may also play a role in some cases.[36, 37] In isolated instances diverticula of the stomach rupture. Although the precise cause for most instances of acute gastric necrosis and rupture in the infant has not been clarified, it has been proposed that rupture occurs at sites of weakness in the muscular wall of the stomach.[35, 38] In autopsy studies of the gastric wall in 15 infants whose deaths were unrelated to gastric rupture or to disease of the stomach,[38] the wall was thinnest in precisely those areas in which rupture and perforation are known to occur, i. e., along the greater curvature, on the anterior surface of the stomach, and in the region of the cardia. In half the infants no oblique muscle fibers could be demonstrated, and in almost all infants there were numerous gaps in the circular muscle layer. Conceivably these muscle defects, associated with ill-defined precipitating causes, may predispose to this catastrophic event.

Clinical Features and Diagnosis. In almost all infants symptoms begin within the first seven days of life, with a peak incidence at three days both among premature and full-term infants.[35] Slightly more than half of the infants with acute gastric necrosis and perforation are premature; indeed, this event is approximately 12 times as common in premature as in full-term infants. Seventy per cent of the reported instances of gastric necrosis and perforation have been in black infants, strongly suggesting a racial predilection. Approximately two-thirds of the affected infants are male. Signs and symptoms may include vomiting, cyanosis, respiratory distress, fever, jaundice, and blood in the stool. Abdominal distention, although not an early sign, is almost invariably present. Vomiting is a relatively early symptom in approximately half the infants. Flat film of the abdomen reveals free air in the abdominal cavity. Barium examination of the gastrointestinal tract is not necessary for diagnosis, and is interdicted in infants with suspected acute gastric necrosis and perforation.

Treatment. The treatment is surgical, requiring early closure of the gastric perforation. Two-thirds of patients reported in the literature have died. Slightly over half of the full-term infants operated upon for acute gastric necrosis with perforation have survived. Mortality is substantially higher among premature infants.[35] In certain instances extensive necrosis may require gastrectomy.[37]

Prognosis. Children surviving the catastrophic event and the surgical correction usually do not have further difficulties related to the gastric disease.

ADULT HYPERTROPHIC PYLORIC STENOSIS

Rarely, adults may suffer the symptoms of congenital hypertrophic pyloric stenosis.[39–41]

Etiology and Pathogenesis. The incidence of congenital hypertrophic pyloric stenosis is five per 1000 males and one per 1000 female births in the general population in England.[6] The incidence of adult hypertrophic pyloric stenosis is not known

and is most difficult to ascertain. There is substantial variability not only of its awareness but also in the diagnostic criteria of the adult form. In addition, differences in classification make the true incidence difficult to assess.

Two principal positions are espoused concerning the etiology of hypertrophic pyloric stenosis in the adult. Some investigators hold that this condition is secondary to local disease[42, 43] such as pyloric ulcer disease, cancer, gastritis, and rarely, prolonged pyloric spasm which may lead to hypertrophy of the circular pyloric muscle bundles.[44] Others state that hypertrophic pyloric stenosis in the adult is the same entity as that observed in infants and children, but is milder later in its clinical appearance.[4, 39, 45, 46] Several families with well documented interoccurrence of both infantile and adult congenital hypertrophic pyloric stenosis have been described.[4, 47, 48] Individuals with adult hypertrophic pyloric stenosis may experience symptoms from infancy or childhood. In these patients with the adult variety of the disease the obstructing lesion is obviously not sufficiently severe to cause symptoms in infancy. The histological and anatomical abnormalities in adult hypertrophic pyloric stenosis are indistinguishable from the infantile form. The absence of documented associated local disease and the demonstration of the family interoccurrence of infantile congenital hypertrophic pyloric stenosis with the adult form would appear to support, at least in some instances, the genetic predisposition to the development of adult hypertrophic pyloric stenosis.[4]

Clinical Features and Diagnosis. In some individuals, but not in most, symptoms may extend back to infancy. Symptoms in the adult usually include nausea and vomiting, some degree of epigastric distress (often with early satiety), weight loss, and anorexia. The symptoms may be either persistent or episodic. In some instances the patient is asymptomatic or if symptoms are present, they are minimal.

The lesion is demonstrated by barium examination of the upper gastrointestinal tract. Unlike infants with congenital hypertrophic pyloric stenosis, an abdominal mass is not palpable. This difference almost surely reflects the difficulty in appre-

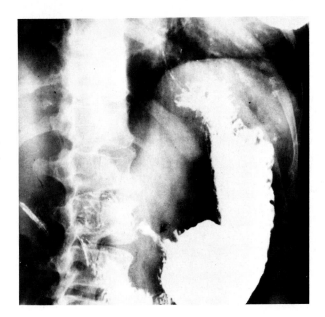

Figure 39–5. Congenital hypertrophic pyloric stenosis in an adult. (Courtesy of Dr. M. H. Sleisenger.)

ciating a small mass in the adult. The diagnosis is usually strongly suspected, or established, by barium examination of the upper gastrointestinal tract. The pyloric channel is demonstrated to be substantially elongated and narrowed, often with circumferential indentation around the pyloric opening into the first part of the duodenum, owing to the hypertrophic pyloric sphincter muscle (Fig. 39–5). Emptying of barium from the stomach is usually delayed. In the adult, hypertrophic pyloric stenosis must be differentiated from a variety of other abnormalities, including pyloric channel peptic ulcer disease and gastric carcinoma involving this portion of the stomach.[49]

Treatment. Surgical treatment is required for alleviation of the symptoms associated with adult hypertrophic pyloric stenosis. Surgical correction may be achieved either by pyloromyotomy, as is performed in infants, or with local resection to include the region of the involved pylorus. The need for certain diagnosis and, particularly, for excluding localized carcinoma in this region of the pylorus often dictates resection with its attendant histological diagnosis.

ANNULAR PANCREAS

Rarely, obstruction at the level of the duodenum is secondary to an anomalous ring of pancreatic tissue which encircles the second portion of the duodenum. Although commonly discussed, this lesion is relatively rare.[50]

Etiology and Pathogenesis. Both the hepatic and pancreatic buds develop from primitive endoderm and represent primordia of the duodenum. The pancreas develops from two outpouching buds from opposing sides of the duodenum. Growing more rapidly within the omental bursa, the dorsal pancreas extends into the dorsal mesentery. The smaller ventral pancreatic bud migrates dorsally to a position below and behind the dorsal pancreas. Later the parenchymal and duct systems of the dorsal and ventral pancreatic buds fuse in the formation of the pancreas. Under normal conditions the ventral pancreatic bud rotates around the duodenum in such a manner that it comes to lie beneath the dorsal pancreatic bud. Occasionally this event fails to occur; rather, a portion of the ventral bud migrates along its normal route, and an additional portion migrates in the opposite direction. In this way the duodenum becomes encircled by pancreatic tissue forming the annular pancreas.

Clinical Features. Clinical abnormalities result from the extrinsic pancreatic obstruction of the intestine at the level of the second portion of the duodenum. Occasionally atresia is concomitant with intrinsic duodenal obstruction at the level of the pancreatic ring. In some instances the distal portion of the common bile duct passes through the posterior part of the annular pancreas, resulting in its obstruction by sharp angulation or by constriction. Thus the patient with an annular pancreas may suffer bouts of pancreatitis or biliary tract obstruction, in addition to gastrointestinal tract obstruction at the level of the duodenum.

When the annular pancreas produces a high degree of impingement on the duodenal lumen, evidence of duodenal obstruction appears shortly after birth. Despite its congenital origin, the clinical expression of annular pancreas may be greatly delayed, even into adulthood, with patients developing symptoms including anorexia, nausea, vomiting, growth failure, and malnutrition.[51] The diagnosis is suspected when barium examination of the upper gastrointestinal tract, performed for suspicion of obstruction, reveals compression in the region of the second portion of the duodenum.

In the infant with complete obstruction, barium examination is unnecessary and the stomach and duodenum are seen to be distended with air. Little or no air is seen in the intestine distal to the obstruction.

Treatment. The treatment of annular pancreas is surgical, with the diagnosis usually established at the time of laparotomy. It is usually not possible to resect or transect the constricting ring of pancreatic tissue. The customary procedure is a bypass, diverting the gastrointestinal tract by means of a retrocolic duodenojejunostomy. The surgeon should avoid cutting into or through the pancreas because of the possible development of a pancreatic fistula.

Prognosis. Mongolism has been found in approximately 30 per cent of individuals with annular pancreas. Following surgical relief of the obstruction imposed by the annular pancreas, patients are generally asymptomatic.

REFERENCES

1. Dankmeyer, J., and Miete, M. Le développement précoce de l'ectomac chez l'embryon humain. Compt. Rend. Assn. Anat. 103:341, 1958.
2. Langman, J. Medical Embryology, Baltimore, Williams and Wilkins Co., 1969, p. 257.
3. Hirschsprung, H. Fälle von angeborener Pylorusstenose; Beobachtungen bei Säuglingen. Jahrb. f. Kinderhlk. 28:61, 1888.
4. Pollack, W. F., Norris, W. J., and Gordon, H. E. The management of hypertrophic pyloric stenosis at the Los Angeles Children's Hospital (a review of 1422 cases). Amer. J. Surg. 94:335, 1957.
5. Laron, Z., and Horne, L. M. The incidence of infantile pyloric stenosis. A.M.A. J. Dis. Child. 94:151, 1957.
6. Carter, C. O. The inheritance of congenital pyloric stenosis. Brit. Med. Bull. 17:251, 1961.
7. Carter, C. O. The inheritance of common congenital malformations. In Progress in Medical Genetics, Vol. IV, A.C. Steinberg and A. G. Bearn (eds.). London, Heinemann, 1965.
8. Zavala, C., Bolio, A., Montalvo, R., and Lisker, R. Hypertrophic pyloric stenosis: Adult and congenital types occurring in the same family. J. Med. Genet. 6:126, 1969.
9. Powell, B. W., and Carter, C. O. Pyloric stenosis in twins. Arch. Dis. Child. 26:45, 1951.
10. Metrakos, J. D. Congenital hypertrophic pyloric stenosis in twins. Arch. Dis. Child. 28:351, 1953.
11. MacMahon, B., and McKeown, T. Infantile hypertrophic pyloric stenosis: Data on 81 pairs of twins. Acta Genet. Med. 4:320, 1955.
12. Donovan, E. J., and Stanley-Brow, E. G. Congenital hypertrophic pyloric stenosis. Surg. Gynec. Obstet. 115:403, 1962.
13. Toyama, W. M. Infantile hypertrophic pyloric stenosis. An improved technic for diagnosis. Amer. J. Surg. 117:650, 1969.
14. Ramstedt, C. Zur Operation der angeborenen Pylorusstenose. Med. Klin. 8:1702, 1912.
15. Benson, C. D., and Warden, M. J. 707 cases of congenital hypertrophic pyloric stenosis. Surg. Gynec. Obstet. 105:348, 1957.
16. Touroff, A. S. W., and Sussman, R. M. Congenital prepyloric membranous obstruction in a premature infant. Surgery 8:739, 1940.
17. Berman, J. K., and Ballenger, F. Prepyloric membranous obstruction. Quart. Bull. Indiana Univ. Med. Center 4:14, 1948.
18. Brown, R. P., and Hertzler, J. H. Congenital prepyloric gastric atresia. A.M.A. J. Dis. Child. 97:857, 1959.
19. Metz, A. R., Householder, R., and DuPree, J. F. Obstruction of the stomach due to a congenital double septum with cyst formation. Tr. West. S. A. 50:242, 1951.
20. Benson, C. D., Mustard, W. T., Ravitch, M. M., Snyder, W. H., and Welch, K. J. Pediatric Surgery. Chicago, Yearbook Medical Publishers, Inc., 1962, p. 660.
21. Ernst, N. P. A case of congenital atresia of the duodenum treated successfully by operation. Brit. Med. J. 1:644, 1916.
22. White, C. S., and Collins, J. L. Congenital duodenal obstruction. Arch. Surg. 43:858, 1941.
23. Young, D. G., and Wilkinson, A. W. Abnormalities associated with neonatal duodenal obstruction. Surgery 63:832, 1968.
24. Taillens, J. P. Atresie congenitale de duodenum. Rev. Med. Suisse Rom. 23:168, 1903.
25. Bernard, C. M. The genesis of intestinal atresia. Surg. Forum 7:393, 1956.

26. Jones, T. W. Pediatric diseases of the stomach and duodenum. *In* Surgery of the Stomach and Duodenum, H. N. Harkins and L. M. Nyhus (eds.). Boston, Little, Brown and Co., 1969, p. 333.

27. Webb, C. H., and Wangensteen, O. H. Congenital intestinal atresia. A.M.A. J. Dis. Child. *41*:262, 1931.

28. Findlay, C. W., Jr., and Humphreys, G. H., II. Congenital anomalies of intestinal rotation in the adult. Surg. Gynec. Obstet. *103*:417, 1956.

29. Wang, C. A., and Welch, C. E. Anomalies of intestinal rotation in adolescents and adults. Surgery *54*:839, 1963.

30. Bill, A. H., Jr., and Gauman, D. Rationale and technic for stabilization of the mesentery in cases of nonrotation of the midgut. J. Pediat. Surg. *1*:127, 1966.

31. Lewis, P. L., Holder, T., and Feldman, M. Duplication of the stomach. Arch. Surg. *82*:634, 1961.

32. Jelenko, C. Duplication of the duodenum: A review and report of a case. Amer. Surg. *28*:120, 1962.

33. Sieber, W. K. Alimentary tract duplications. Arch. Surg. *73*:383, 1956.

34. Kieseweter, W. B. Duplication of the stomach. Ann. Surg. *146*:990, 1957.

35. Saracli, T., Mann, M., French, D. M., Booker, C. R., and Scott, R. B. Rupture of the stomach in the newborn infant. Report of three cases and review of the world literature. Clin. Pediat. *6*:583, 1967.

36. Inouye, W. Y., and Evans, G. Neonatal gastric perforation: A report of six cases and a review of 143 cases. Arch. Surg. *88*:471, 1964.

37. Rees, J. R., and Redo, S. F. Neonatal gastric necrosis and perforation treated by gastrectomy and esophagogastric anastomosis. Surgery *64*:472, 1968.

38. Kneiszl, F. Some data on the aetiology of gastric rupture in the newborn. Biol. Neonat. *4*:201, 1962.

39. MacCann, J. C., and Dean, M. A. Hypertrophy of pyloric muscle in the adult. Experiences with conservative and radical surgical treatment. Surg. Gynec. Obstet. *90*:535, 1950.

40. Lumsden, K., and Truelove, S. C. Primary hypertrophic pyloric stenosis in the adult. Brit. J. Radiol. *31*:261, 1958.

41. Hiebert, B. W., and Farris, J. M. Hypertrophic pyloric stenosis in the adult. Review of 22 cases. Amer. Surg. *32*:712, 1966.

42. Horwitz, A., Alvarez, W. C., and Ascanio, H. The normal thickness of the pyloric muscle and the influence on it of ulcer, gastroenterostomy and carcinoma. Ann. Surg. *89*:521, 1929.

43. Raffensberger, E. C. Time required for the development of pyloric muscle hypertrophy in the adult. Gastroenterology *28*:458, 1955.

44. Atkinson, M., Edwards, D.A.W., Honour, A. J., and Rowlands, E. N. Comparison of cardiac and pyloric sphincters: A manometric study. Lancet *2*:918, 1957.

45. Keynes, W. M. Simple and complicated hypertrophic pyloric stenosis in the adult. Gut *6*:240, 1965.

46. McConnell, R. B. The Genetics of Gastrointestinal Disorders. London, Oxford University Press, 1966.

47. Fenwick, T. Familial hypertrophic pyloric stenosis. Brit. Med. J. *2*:12, 1953.

48. Woo-Ming, M. Familial relationship between adult and infantile hypertrophic pyloric stenosis. Brit. Med. J. *1*:476, 1961.

49. DuPlessis, D. J. Primary hypertrophic pyloric stenosis in the adult. Brit. J. Surg. *53*:485, 1966.

50. Gross, R. E. The Surgery of Infancy and Childhood. Philadelphia, W. B. Saunders Co., 1953.

51. Ravitch, M. M. Pediatric Surgery. *In* Principles and Practice of Surgery, J. G. Allen, H. N. Harkins, C. A. Moyer, and J. E. Rhoads (eds.). Philadelphia, J. B. Lippincott Co., 1957, Chapter 20.

Chapter 40

Roentgen Diagnosis of Ulcerative Diseases

Henry I. Goldberg

GASTRIC ULCERS

ROENTGENOGRAPHIC TECHNIQUE

The successful roentgenographic detection of gastric ulcers depends upon strict attention to proper roentgenographic technique. The optimal technique includes (1) use of small amounts (30 to 60 ml) of slightly viscous barium sulfate suspensions to coat the mucosa, without flooding the stomach with a dense barium mixture; (2) positioning of the patient so that the fundus, anterior gastric wall, and greater and lesser curvatures are all shown in profile and en face; and (3) air-barium contrast of the contour of the gastric wall and pattern of mucosal folds to aid in the detection of small or shallow ulcers.

Special techniques may be employed to interpret the nature of an ulcer, once it is discovered. Inducement of hypermotility in the stomach may aid in the determination of whether areas adjacent to an ulcer transmit peristalsis or are fixed and rigid, suggesting malignant invasion. Morphine may be administered for this purpose.[1] By means of parietography the extent and degree of mass and gastric wall thickening associated with ulcers may be ascertained. This technique requires the production of a pneumoperitoneum and use of gastric tomography.[2] Recently, celiac angiography, after histamine stimulation, has been combined with parietography to provide excellent opacification of the gastric wall.[3]

ROENTGENOGRAPHIC CRITERIA OF BENIGN AND MALIGNANT GASTRIC ULCERS

Profile Features of Benign Ulcers. A benign ulcer often has a flat, broad, or conical crater with smooth margins. The ulcer projects abruptly from the gastric wall and penetrates beyond the expected course of the gastric lumen (Fig. 40-1, A). The luminal margin of the ulcer may be demarcated by a thin, sharply defined line, called Hampton's line, which parallels the lumen (Fig. 40-1, B). This line represents overhanging edges of the mucosa. Although typical for benign ulcer, Hampton's line is not often demonstrated. Those ulcers that induce edema and inflammation in surrounding submucosa may be accompanied by an ulcer collar. An ulcer collar[4, 5] is a thicker lucent band of tissue that projects across the opening of the ulcer. This thickened rim of tissue represents edema and cellular infiltrate of gastric mucosa and submucosa and forms the ulcer margin. The collar appears smooth,

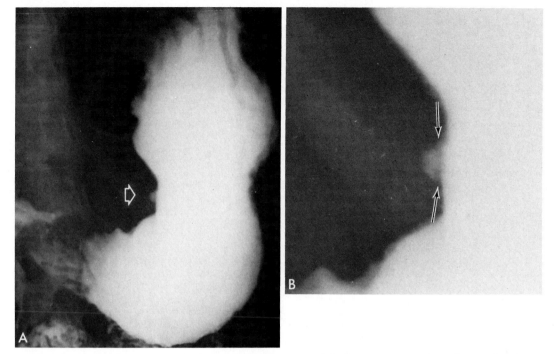

Figure 40–1. *A,* A small, sharply demarcated ulcer crater of the lesser curvature (arrow). *B,* A thin, lucent band at the ulcer orifice – Hampton's line – represents the mucosal edge of ulcer in this magnified view (arrows).

and radiating folds do not traverse it (Figs. 40–2 and 40–29). More extensive edema and infiltrate of the ulcer margin result in considerable thickening of gastric mucosa and submucosa adjacent to the ulcer. This circumferential inflammatory response produces a smooth mound of tissue that projects into the gastric lumen. When viewed in profile, the ulcer sometimes appears not to project beyond the expected course of the gastric lumen because the surrounding inflammatory reaction has produced an intraluminal mass. The benign ulcer is symmetrically placed in the center of this smooth mound. The angle that the mound forms with the gastric wall is obtuse rather than acute (Fig. 40–3).

En Face Features of Benign Ulcers. Radiating gastric folds converge on the benign ulcer (Fig. 40–4). These folds are best shown with the air-barium contrast technique, or by compression of the stomach. In those sharply punched out ulcers with only a thin overhanging margin (Hampton's line in profile), the folds radiate from the margin of the ulcer crater.

This appearance is the best single roentgen sign of benignancy.[6]

When an ulcer collar or mound is present, the radiating gastric folds do not originate at the ulcer margin but from the circle of edematous mucosa around the ulcer. An ulcer mound may produce a broad, smooth, circumferential lucent halo (Fig. 40–5). The smooth contour of the mound, the central location of the ulcer, and the undisturbed mucosal pattern adjacent to the mound are indicative of a benign ulcer. The ulcer crater itself is smooth margined and round or oval (Fig. 40–6).

An area of spasm of circular muscle may form a deep indentation of the gastric wall opposite the ulcer. This incisura usually points to the ulcer (Fig. 40–7).

Malignant Ulcers. In profile, the malignant ulcer may appear irregular, with fissure-like extensions from its base and a nodular contour to the base (Fig. 40–8). Hampton's line is not present. The crater is in a mass and does not project beyond the margin of the gastric lumen. The outer margins of the mass may form acute angles

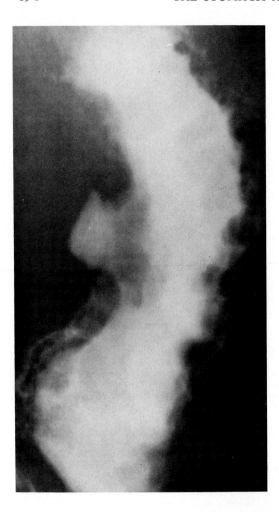

Figure 40–2. A benign ulcer of the lesser curvature is surrounded by an ulcer collar—the broad lucent band resulting from edema at the ulcer orifice. Gastric mucosal folds radiate from this mass of edema.

Figure 40–3. A lucent area surrounds the orifice of the benign ulcer of the lesser curvature. A mound of edema produces this lucency. The ulcer is in the center of the mound. The tissue mound blends smoothly with the gastric wall at its margins (arrows), producing obtuse angles.

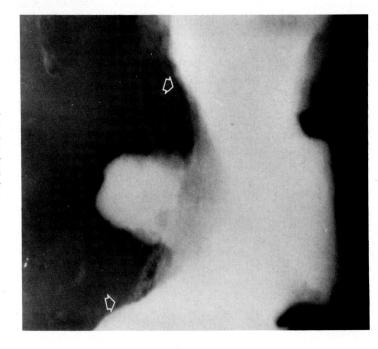

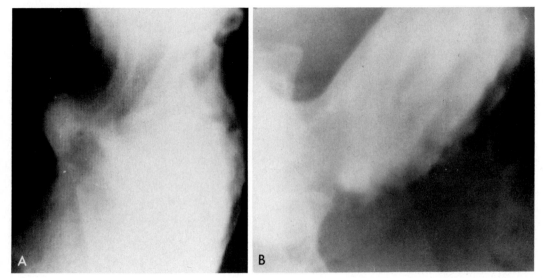

Figure 40–4. *A,* Gastric folds radiate from the margin of this benign ulcer of the lesser curvature. *B,* Gastric folds radiate from the margin of a benign gastric ulcer of the posterior wall. This pattern of folds was best demonstrated by compression of the body of the stomach during the fluoroscopic examination.

with the gastric wall, in contrast to the obtuse angle produced by an edematous ulcer mound of a benign ulcer (Fig. 40–9).

When a malignant ulcer is seen en face, its nodular, thickened, and irregular margins are in contrast to the smooth mound or collar of a benign ulcer (Fig. 40–10). The ulcer is eccentrically situated in the tumor, and its shape, as well as the surface of the mass itself, is irregular. Because of tumor infiltration of the gastric wall, radiating folds are usually absent; if seen, they appear asymmetric and nodular.

Occasionally, large antral, ulcerating

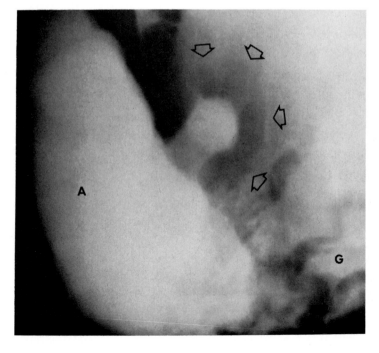

Figure 40–5. An ulcer mound surrounds a crater situated on the lesser curvature of the stomach. The stomach is in an oblique position so that the ulcer is seen en face. A mound of edema surrounds the crater, forming a lucent "halo" (arrows). A, Antrum; G, greater curvature.

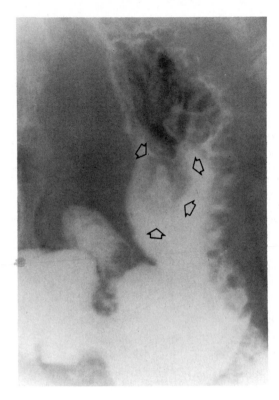

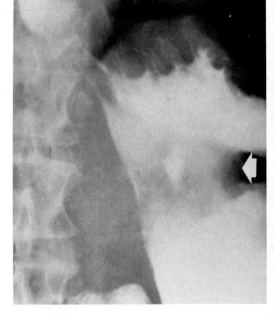

Figure 40–6. The ulcer collar with smooth margins (arrows), viewed en face, circumferentially surrounds the ulcer crater. This benign ulcer was situated on the posterior gastric wall. The ulcer crater is oval shaped.

Figure 40–7. An oval ulcer crater on the proximal lesser curvature of the posterior wall of the stomach is demonstrated en face. An incisura, or indentation, attributed to circular muscle spasm, points toward the ulcer from the greater curvature (arrow).

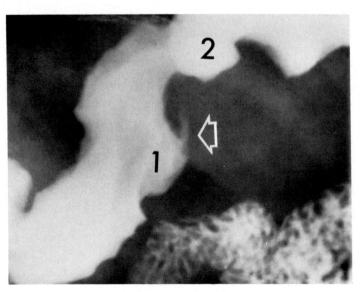

Figure 40–8. Two ulcer craters are demonstrated on the greater curvature (1 and 2). A fissure extends from the base of one ulcer into the adjacent mound of tissue (arrow). Such fissures are noted in malignant ulcers.

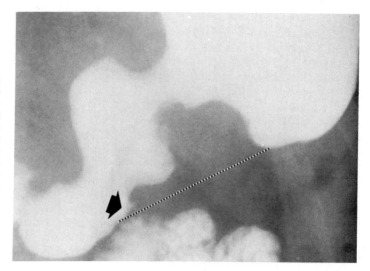

Figure 40–9. An ulcer crater is situated eccentrically within a large gastric mass on the greater curvature. The crater does not project beyond the expected course of the gastric wall (dotted line). The mass of tissue that surrounds the ulcer produces an acute angle with the gastric wall (arrow). The roentgenographic features are those of a malignant ulcer seen in profile.

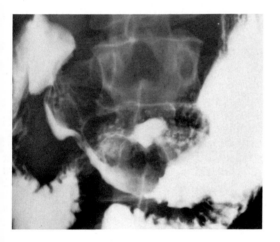

Figure 40–10. A malignant ulcer of the lesser curvature is situated within an irregular lobulated mass.

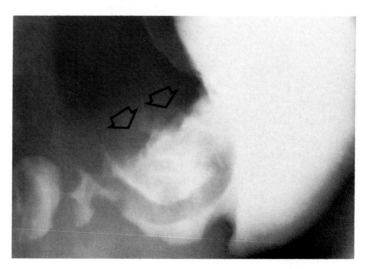

Figure 40–11. A crescentic rim of tumor separates the barium trapped in this antral ulcer of the lesser curvature from the barium in the lumen of the antrum. The ulcer base is ragged and irregular (arrows) (Carman's ulcer or Carman's meniscus sign).

neoplasms of the lesser curvature produce a form of ulcer termed Carman's ulcer, characterized by a "meniscus sign." Much confusion exists about the nature of this finding. The barium, which is trapped in the ulcer crater when the antrum is compressed, is separated from the main column of barium by a broad crescentic rim of tumor with irregular nodular margins. The border of the ulcer is convex toward the lumen and indicates malignant ulcer in a tumor (Fig. 40–11); this finding, however, is not common.[5, 7] Furthermore, large necrotic benign ulcers may produce roentgenographic findings similar to Carman's ulcer.

Considerations of Size, Depth, and Location. The size of an ulcer crater does not aid in the roentgenographic determination of malignancy. Malignant ulcers may be only a few millimeters wide, whereas benign ulcers may measure 10 to 20 cm.[8] In about 5 per cent of benign ulcers the diameter is more than 4 cm.[9] Giant gastric ulcers, 10 cm and larger in diameter, may not be detected by examiners who do not recognize large irregularities that represent ulcers (Fig. 40–12). Although the initial size of the ulcer does not aid in the distinction between benign and

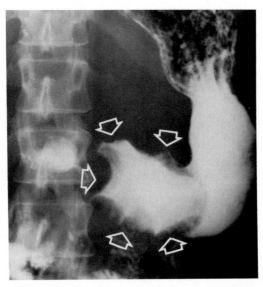

Figure 40–12. A benign, giant gastric ulcer is situated in the antrum (arrows). The ulcer crater is so large and irregular that roentgenographically it was incorrectly diagnosed as a malignant ulcer.

malignant ulcer, the change in size after medical therapy is started is most helpful. Partial healing over a two- to three-week period often results in disappearance of edema so that the roentgenographic characteristics of the ulcer become more evident. An ulcer originally diagnosed roentgenographically as indeterminate, i.e., with both benign and malignant features, may subsequently appear as clearly benign in roentgenograms (Fig. 40–13). Complete healing by roentgenographic criteria is evidence for a benign ulcer, although, occasionally, malignant ulcers may also heal completely. Gastric deformity, however, may be the residuum of healing in the form of persistent folds that radiate to a scarred or flattened area at the site of previous ulcer.[6] Noteworthy, however, is the recurrence several weeks to months later of apparently healed malignant ulcers.[10] Thus follow-up roentgenographic evaluation of patients with "healed" gastric ulcer is important.

In general, its location does not indicate whether the ulcer is benign or malignant, except that ulcers in the cardia or in the fundic area are more likely to be malignant.[11, 12] Thus ulcers situated in this area, regardless of roentgenographic features, should be considered malignant until proved otherwise by endoscopic and cytologic examinations (pp. 523 and 589). In addition, a recent study of ulcers of the greater curvature, carried out in Japan as part of a national survey on gastric cancer, revealed that approximately 95 per cent of the greater curvature ulcers were malignant (H. Ichikawa, personal communication). These statements do not apply to the high ulcers in the lesser curvature of geriatric patients;[13] in these patients, 42 per cent of benign ulcers are seen high on the lesser curvature or in the cardia. Collections of barium in the typical location of simple gastric diverticula (the lesser curvature–cardia junction) must be differentiated from benign and malignant ulcers. Diverticula, unlike ulcers at this site, change shape during roentgenographic examination and are not associated with overhanging edges of mucosa at the base, or with marginal edema.[14] Carefully obtained spot films may demonstrate mucosa within these lesions.

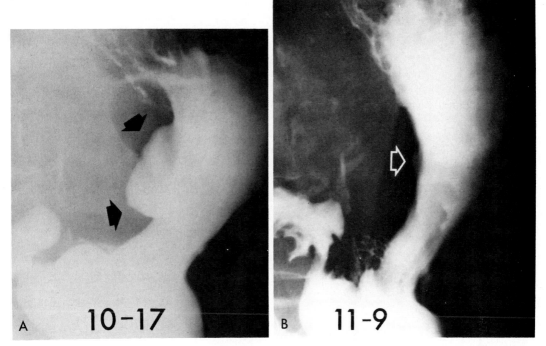

Figure 40–13.   *A*, October 17, 1967. A large benign ulcer of the lesser curvature (arrows) in a patient who was hospitalized and received hourly antacid therapy. *B*, November 9, 1967. A second upper gastrointestinal series was obtained. During the 23-day interval, the size of the ulcer crater had diminished greatly (arrow denotes crater).

ACCURACY OF ROENTGEN DIAGNOSIS AND PITFALLS IN DIAGNOSIS

When all roentgen criteria indicate a benign ulcer, this diagnosis is accurate in 96 to 98 per cent of patients.[15] Ulcers of the distal antrum and those of the fundus and cardia are often classified roentgenographically as indeterminate. The ability to detect gastric ulcers by roentgenographic means and to classify them as benign or malignant is influenced by many factors. These include the presence of blood clot, mucus, or food filling an ulcer crater; edematous mucosal folds or an ulcer collar that occludes the ulcer orifice; excessive fatty tissue of an obese patient and consequent difficulty in technique and in detection of small ulcers; shallowness of ulcers (a few millimeters in depth), whose roentgenographic detection is impossible in from 5 to 10 per cent of gastric ulcers;[15] spasm in the antrum and prepylorus, which alters the lumen and fold pattern so that a mass surrounding the ulcer may be difficult to see (Fig. 40–14); and, finally,

segmental spasm of circular musculature associated with ulcers of the greater curvature, which retracts the niche toward the lesser curvature so that the ulcer appears to be situated in an intraluminal mass (Fig. 40–15).[16]

Although detection of a gastric lesion is the major goal of the radiologist, classification of an ulcer is equally important. In most patients, cytological gastric studies and gastroscopy are not obtained because the techniques are not always available. Furthermore, human skill and technical factors greatly influence the reliability of these techniques. Thus the roentgenographic diagnosis often determines the therapy. The radiologist must therefore attempt to distinguish between a benign or malignant ulcer, if the roentgenographic features warrant it. This responsibility must not be abdicated to the cytologist or endoscopist.

PYLORIC CHANNEL ULCERS

Clinical and roentgenographic abnormalities produced by ulcers of the pyloric

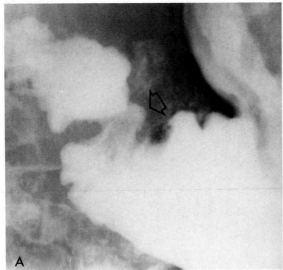
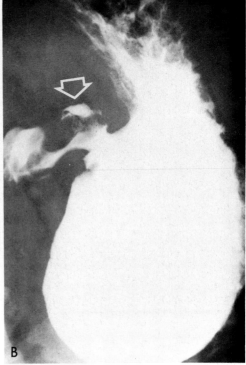

Figure 40–14. *A,* Some of the roentgenographic criteria of a benign antral ulcer (arrow) (sharply punched out crater with radiating folds). *B,* The antrum of the lesser curvature is foreshortened, and the antrum and the base of the duodenal bulb are narrowed, the result of edema and spasm induced by an antral ulcer (arrow). Because of the pronounced antral deformity, detection of the roentgenographic criteria for the diagnosis of benign ulcer is difficult. This benign antral ulcer has caused partial obstruction of the gastric outlet.

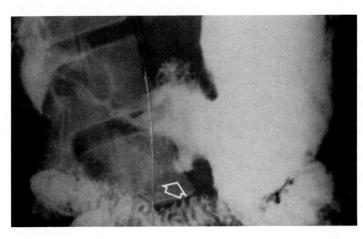

Figure 40–15. A benign ulcer of the greater curvature is retracted toward the lesser curvature so that it appears to be situated within an intraluminal mass (arrow). This retraction may be misinterpreted as evidence of a malignant change. The central location of the ulcer and the smooth contour of the mass are not features of malignancy, however.

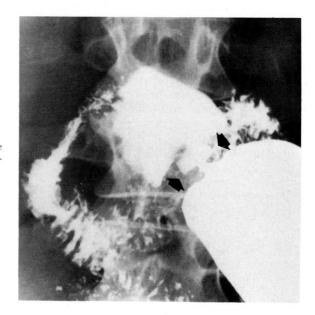

Figure 40–16. A large benign ulcer of the pyloric channel (arrows) has not produced pyloric obstruction.

channel may differ from both gastric and duodenal bulb ulcers because of the location and caliber of the pylorus.[17, 18] Although symptoms may be the same as in duodenal ulcer, they are often atypical; i.e., nausea and vomiting, midepigastric pain immediately after meals unrelieved by antacids, and weight loss. These symptoms characterize the pyloric channel syndrome (see pp. 677 to 678).[17, 18]

Typical channel ulcers are smaller than 1 cm. They are shallow and project beyond the lumen as a tent-shaped or nipple-like outpouching. When channel ulcers are small, a surrounding ring of edema may not be identifiable roentgenographically. Ulcers of the pyloric channel induce longitudinal and circular muscle spasm, which frequently foreshortens or angulates the pylorus toward the lesser curvature of the stomach. The pylorus is often, but not invariably, narrowed.[17] Folds radiating from the ulcer are seen rarely.

Roentgenographic evidence of obstruction of the gastric outlet is often not present with small (less than 1 cm) pyloric ulcers, although with larger ulcers the frequency is higher. Clinical findings of the pyloric channel syndrome are not correlated with the width of the pyloric channel (Fig. 40–16).[17]

A roentgenographically identifiable zone of edema surrounds the large pyloric ulcers (greater than 1 cm) and results in deformity of the base of the duodenal bulb and of the prepyloric gastric antrum (Fig. 40–17). The contour of these large ulcers may be irregularly angled. Differentiation therefore between large, benign pyloric ulcers and malignant ulcers in the mucosa at the antral end of the pylorus may be difficult on the basis of roentgenographic features alone.

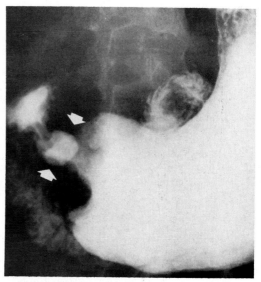

Figure 40–17. A large ulcer of the pyloric channel (arrows) has deformed the gastric antrum and base of the duodenal bulb. The gastric outlet was obstructed partially. (From Glickman, M. G., et al.: Amer. J. Roent. Radium Ther. Nuc. Med. *113*:147, 1971.)

Ulcers of the pyloric channel may be situated at the antral or duodenal end of the pylorus as well as in the center. Fibrosis and scar formation, which take place with healing of pyloric ulcers, result in abnormal angulation of the pyloric channel. In addition, deformity of the opposite end of the pylorus may result from healing. Histological examination of specimens of these healing ulcers shows that longitudinal tracts of fibrosis have foreshortened a portion of the pyloric channel and thereby produced a roentgenographic appearance of ulcer migration.[17]

DUODENAL ULCERS

The roentgenographic diagnosis of duodenal ulcers depends upon detection of an ulcer crater. Without roentgenographic demonstration of a crater, the radiologist can report only secondary signs of peptic ulcer; hence the frequent phrase: "Evidence of peptic ulcer disease without demonstration of an ulcer." In either instance, detection of abnormalities of the duodenal bulb depends upon attention to careful roentgenographic technique.

ROENTGENOGRAPHIC TECHNIQUES

Distention of the duodenal bulb with barium sulfate is essential for information about the size, shape, and contour of the lumen. The bulb is frequently filled by gravity and by the action of antral contraction when the patient is placed in the prone right anterior oblique position. Manual compression of the antrum, however, is often necessary for the bulb to fill in the upright position. Compression of the barium-filled duodenal bulb is an important maneuver that enables ulcers of the posterior wall to be detected en face (Fig. 40–18). The posterior wall of the duodenal bulb, the most common site of duodenal ulcers,[19] is best seen in profile when the patient is in the prone left anterior oblique position. This position, along with the supine left posterior oblique, is essential for the detection of posterior duodenal ulcers. Anterior ulcers are demonstrated best in views obtained in the prone oblique position and with bulb compression. Ulcers on the superior and inferior surfaces of the bulb are best seen in profile in prone, supine, steep oblique, or lateral views. In some instances, contraction of the duodenal bulb is so frequent, or spasm so severe, that bulbar filling and roentgenography are impossible. In these situations, administration of 30 to 60 mg of propantheline intramuscularly to induce hypotonia is recommended. A more transient hypotonia may be produced by an intramuscular injection of 1 mg of glucagon.

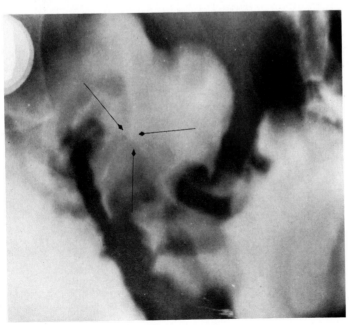

Figure 40–18. Edematous folds radiate from a pinpoint ulcer of the posterior duodenal wall (arrows). Compression of the duodenal bulb by the radiologist produced the best roentgenographic demonstration of this ulcer.

ROENTGENOGRAPHIC APPEARANCE OF DUODENAL ULCERS

The ulcer crater in the duodenal bulb is more often round or oval. Rarely is Hampton's line demonstrated, as in gastric ulcers. Frequently, a mound of edema surrounds the ulcer and produces a mass that projects into the lumen (Fig. 40–19). Most posterior ulcers are demonstrated en face with a mound of edematous folds surrounding them (Fig. 40–20). When the folds are entirely effaced by edema, the mound may be smooth. A lobulated contour to the ulcer mound results from incomplete effacement of edematous folds. Folds radiating from the ulcer margin may be seen, particularly as the ulcer heals.[20] The ulcer crater is often conical, although, because of marginal edema, it may appear wider at the base than at its orifice. The ulcer base may contain blood or debris, which produces an irregular contour.

An ulcer crater may elude roentgenographic detection because of overhanging edematous folds, which prevent filling with barium; bulbar spasm, which expels barium; shallowness of the crater; and failure to obtain roentgenograms in multiple positions.

Sometimes the presence of an ulcer may be suspected by certain secondary signs, even though the ulcer is not demonstrated

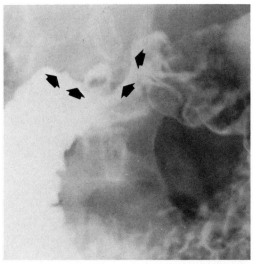

Figure 40–19. The mound of edema that surrounds the ulcer crater on the superior portion of the duodenal bulb has produced a mass that projects into the lumen (arrows).

roentgenographically. The principal sign is deformity of the bulb, but its degree does not appear to be related to ulcer size. Small ulcers may produce a large deformity, and huge ulcers may produce little deformity. Deformity may be caused either by spasm and edema in the presence of an ulcer that eluded detection or by scarring of a healed ulcer. Deformity may be manifested by flattening of superior or inferior

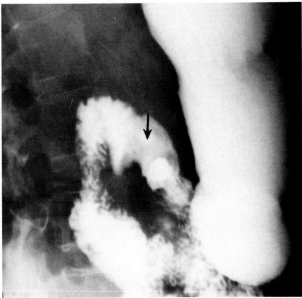

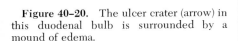

Figure 40–20. The ulcer crater (arrow) in this duodenal bulb is surrounded by a mound of edema.

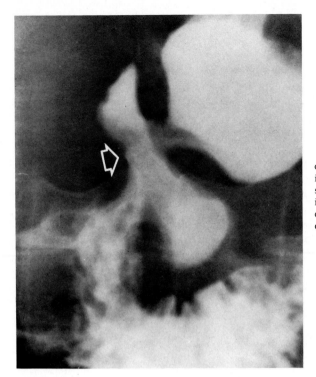

Figure 40–21.   A small ulcer (arrow) has produced deformity of the duodenal bulb. Flattening of the superior surface of the bulb has resulted from edema and spasm. The superior and inferior recesses of the base of the bulb appear as diverticular outpouchings, so-called pseudo-diverticula.

Figure 40–22.   The arrows outline an oval-shaped, irregular barium collection at the site of the duodenal bulb. Serial roentgenograms demonstrated the same unchanging configuration. A giant duodenal ulcer occupied the entire bulb in the surgical specimen.

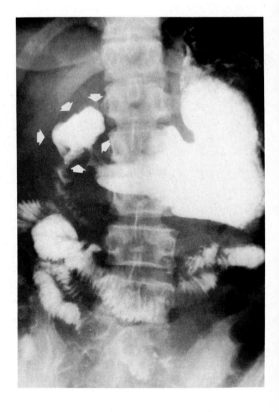

recesses and surfaces of the bulb, eccentricity of the pyloric entrance into the bulb, flattening and narrowing of the bulb, or pseudodiverticula or exaggerated outpouching of recesses at the base of the bulb. This last-mentioned type of deformity results from narrowing of the area that contains the ulcer and from spasm of circular muscle opposite the ulcer, similar to that of an incisura opposite a gastric ulcer (Fig. 40–21).

Edematous folds may produce a scalloped contour of the bulb and a roentgenographic appearance of streaks of barium separated by thick folds. Enlarged duodenal folds represent a nonspecific roentgenographic finding.

Bulbar spasm without a demonstrated ulcer may be noted. This nonspecific finding may be so severe as to result in transient, incomplete filling of the bulb, or it may persist as segmental circular muscle spasm and narrow a portion of the bulb. An important but infrequent secondary roentgen sign of duodenal ulcer is gastric outlet obstruction from edema and spasm that narrow the pylorus.

On occasion, the entire duodenal bulb may be ulcerated. The only clue to giant duodenal ulceration may be the constancy of an oval or irregularly shaped bulb on multiple supine, prone, and upright views (Fig. 40–22). Frequently, also, the lumen of the bowel will be narrowed proximal and distal to these ulcers (Fig. 40–22).[21] Rarely, an ulcerating lymphosarcoma or carcinoma may produce a giant duodenal ulcer.

ROENTGENOGRAPHIC EVIDENCE OF PENETRATION AND PERFORATION OF GASTRIC AND DUODENAL ULCER

The presence of a pneumoperitoneum on abdominal roentgenograms in the absence of recent surgery is evidence of a perforated viscus. Most commonly the pneumoperitoneum is caused by perforation of a duodenal or gastric ulcer. With proper positioning of the patient and the correct sequence of roentgenograms, as little as 5 ml of free air in the abdomen may be detected.[22]

In instances of suspected perforation (clinical signs and symptoms of acute ab-

dominal and shoulder pain), air may be injected through a nasogastric tube. If possible, roentgenograms of the abdomen should be obtained in the supine, cross-table lateral decubitus, and erect positions. The patient should first lie on the left side. This position allows air to rise to the right margin of the abdominal wall between the parietal peritoneum and liver. After the patient has remained on the left side for ten minutes, an erect roentgenogram of the diaphragmatic region can be obtained. If the clinical state of the patient interdicts the erect position, then roentgenography in the left lateral decubitus position may be employed to demonstrate free air in the peritoneal cavity.

Gastric ulcers of the posterior wall perforate into the region of the lesser peritoneal sac. Consequently, air may be trapped in a retrogastric location; evidence of air is frequently seen superimposed over the spine. Perforations of the posterior wall of the gastric antrum and duodenal bulb are nearly always walled off in the pancreatic bed or retroperitoneal strictures, so that a pneumoperitoneum usually does not develop.

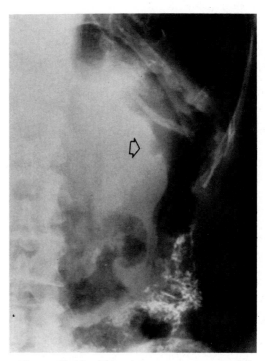

Figure 40–23. This plain roentgenogram of the supine abdomen demonstrates an air-filled stomach and an ulcer of the lesser curvature (arrow).

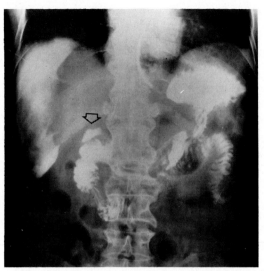

Figure 40-24. This 45-year-old woman experienced abdominal pain three days before upper gastrointestinal roentgenography, but was pain free on the day of the examination. The roentgenogram demonstrates the results of perforation of a duodenal ulcer. Water-soluble contrast material has extravasated into the peritoneal cavity. Most of this material is in the right upper quadrant where it surrounds the liver and outlines the undersurface of the diaphragm. A small amount (arrow) has collected at the site of perforation of the duodenal bulb.

The exact location of the perforated ulcer may be outlined occasionally by air on the plain roentgenogram (Fig. 40–23). The site of perforation is best shown by means of water-soluble contrast material such as diatrizoate methylglucamine (Gastrografin) (Fig. 40–24).[23]

A routine upper gastrointestinal series may demonstrate a deeply penetrating ulcer crater. Craters deeper than 5 mm may be expected to reach serosa. Often, local inflammation of the head of the pancreas results from a penetrating ulcer that is walled off by retroduodenal tissue. This effect may be manifested on serial roentgenograms of the upper gastrointestinal tract by nodular defects and areas of picket-fence-like irregularity along the medial aspect of the second portion of the duodenum, the result of inflammatory response and edema. Duodenal ulcers occasionally perforate into the common bile duct or gallbladder and cause cholecystoduodenal fistula. Such a fistula is demonstrated on plain roentgenograms of the abdomen by air that outlines the biliary tract.

Most perforated gastric ulcers are walled off by granulation tissue around the ulcer crater. This tissue may not only deform the ulcer crater but may also simulate malignant growth, because on barium study it projects into the gastric lumen as a mass. For this reason, the roentgenographic exclusion of malignant tumor in a perforated gastric ulcer is difficult.

POSTBULBAR ULCERS

Postbulbar ulcerations, which account for only a small percentage of all duodenal ulcers, are often difficult to diagnose clinically and equally difficult to detect roentgenographically.[24-26] Their recognition is important, because they may be the source of obstruction, pancreatitis, gastrointestinal hemorrhage and pain whose distribution and frequency are atypical for duodenal bulbar ulcers. They often elude detection by fiberoptic endoscopy. The major cause of difficulty in demonstrating postbulbar ulcers is the severe spasm of the duodenum in the area of ulceration. Spasm with narrowing and deformity of the duodenal lumen often prevents barium from filling an ulcer crater (Figs. 40–25 and 40–26). The observation of a narrowed postbulbar area during a routine upper gastrointestinal series warrants further attempts to demonstrate an ulcer by hypotonic duodenography.[24, 27] After intramuscular or intravenous injection of atropine (0.5 mg) or propantheline (15 to 30 mg), roentgenograms of the duodenum obtained with barium and air frequently demonstrate reversal of narrowing and deformity that are caused by an ulcer.

The ulcer crater may appear as a shallow, flattened niche on the medial portion of the second duodenum. Although mucosal folds may radiate from the ulcer, they are not common, and a mound of edema may surround the ulcer. Frequently, an incisura or indentation is present on the wall opposite the ulcer (Fig. 40–27). This incisura, produced by spasm, points toward the ulcer crater and causes eccentric narrowing of the lumen. In chronic ulceration, or after healing of a postbulbar ulcer, the site of incisura may persist as a stricture and produce a ring-like narrowing of the duodenum, 1.5 to 2 cm in diameter[24] (Fig. 40–28). The narrowing, however,

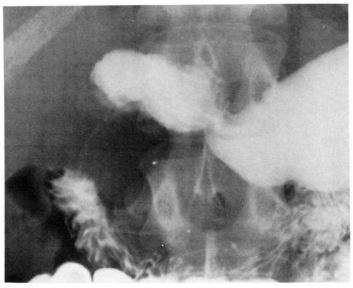

Figure 40-25. A thin, straight tract of barium outlines the lumen of a markedly narrowed portion of the descending duodenum. At surgery, a postbulbar peptic ulcer was found in the center of the narrowing. The roentgenographic appearance simulates that of a malignant constriction.

does not often cause significant dilatation of the duodenal bulb and stomach. When the ulcer is situated on the posterior wall of the duodenum, compression of the barium-filled duodenum and air-barium hypotonic duodenography are necessary to detect the ulcer. The mucosal folds may be thickened for a few centimeters above and below the ulcer.

Penetration into the pancreas may be detected because of nodular contour defects on the medial aspect of the barium-filled second duodenum. These nodular indentations, widening of the duodenal curve, and spike-like projections of barium perpendicular to the lumen all reflect an adjacent pancreatitis.

Occasionally a healed postbulbar ulcer adjacent to the ampulla of Vater may produce deformity and insufficiency of the ampulla. These changes result in reflux of barium and air into the common bile duct or pancreatic ducts (Fig. 40-28).

Not all postbulbar craters are peptic ul-

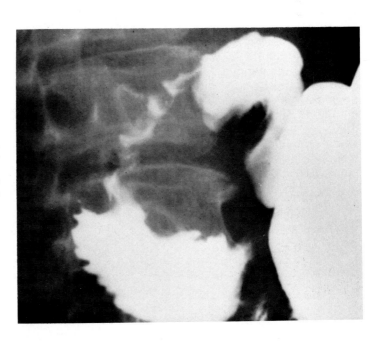

Figure 40-26. Edema and spasm have caused postbulbar duodenal narrowing and irregularity. At surgery, two postbulbar ulcers were found. A Zollinger-Ellison syndrome was diagnosed.

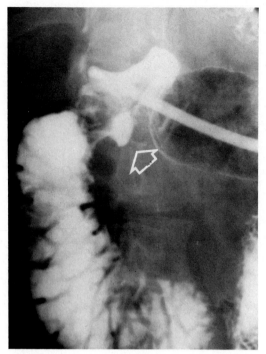

Figure 40–27. A postbulbar ulcer crater (arrow) is surrounded by a zone of lucency, resulting from duodenal mucosal edema. This duodenogram was obtained after the intramuscular injection of 60 mg of propantheline, which resulted in hypotonicity of the duodenum. This technique demonstrates not only the ulcer, but also the incisura, or indentation, opposite the ulcer.

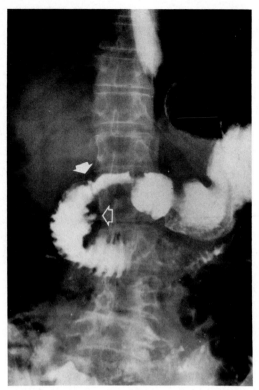

Figure 40–28. A postbulbar ulcer is present just distal to the apex of the duodenal bulb (solid arrow). The bulb has been narrowed by an old peptic ulcer. The healing postbulbar ulcer is smaller than on a roentgenographic study one month earlier. A ring-like narrowing is present at the level of the ulcer. Barium has refluxed into the ampulla of Vater (open arrow) because healing of postbulbar inflammatory disease has caused scarring and deformity of the orifice of the ampulla.

cerations. Occasionally, a small diverticulum of the second duodenum may be misinterpreted as an ulcer. Within these diverticula, however, mucosa is usually identifiable; they change shape during the roentgen examination and are not associated with luminal narrowing. Carcinoma of the head of the pancreas may erode into the second portion of the duodenum, producing ulceration. Primary duodenal adenocarcinoma may narrow and ulcerate the duodenal sweep. The detection of an ulcer crater with an incisura opposite it, however, is strong roentgenographic evidence of benign peptic ulcer.

ULCERS IN ZOLLINGER-ELLISON SYNDROME

Ulcerogenic endocrinopathy caused by gastrin-secreting tumors, more often in the pancreas, may produce gastric or duodenal ulcers. Such ulcers may occur simultaneously in patients with the Zollinger-

Ellison syndrome and may be single or multiple in either location. The appearance of the ulcers, their number and locations, and the appearance of the stomach and small bowel mucosa all provide information that leads to the specific roentgenographic diagnosis of the Zollinger-Ellison syndrome.[28]

In the Zollinger-Ellison syndrome, ulcers are most commonly situated in the duodenal bulb. About 75 per cent of peptic ulcers in patients with the Zollinger-Ellison syndrome develop in the base, body, or apex of the duodenal bulb.[28] The 25 per cent of ulcers situated elsewhere should alert the radiologist to the possibility of the Zollinger-Ellison syndrome, particularly because most of these are postbulbar, in the second and third portions of the duodenum. Jejunal ulcers are particularly suggestive of the Zollinger-Ellison syndrome. Occasionally gastric ulcers, which develop in 10 per cent of these patients, may be present without concomitant duodenal ulcers.[29] Roentgenographic evidence of a healing ulcer in one location and development or extension of an ulcer at another site in a patient given medical therapy are highly suggestive of the Zollinger-Ellison syndrome. Recurrence of ulcer, gastric, stomal, or jejunal, after surgery for peptic ulcer is also typical of an unrecognized Zollinger-Ellison syndrome. Such recurrence has been reported in 55 per cent of patients with the Zollinger-Ellison syndrome in whom total gastrectomy was not performed.[30]

The roentgenographic features of the ulcers themselves are not sufficiently different from those of ordinary peptic ulcers to allow a diagnosis on the basis of the ulcer alone (Fig. 40–29). Multiple ulcers, particularly those that involve different areas of the duodenum or stomach and duodenum,[28, 29] are suggestive of the Zollinger-Ellison syndrome. Ulcers in this syndrome may penetrate into the pancreas and produce acute pancreatitis.

Megaduodenum is a frequent accompaniment of multiple duodenal ulcers in the

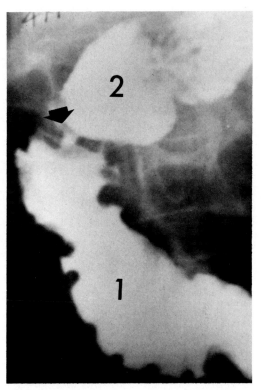

Figure 40–30. The descending duodenum (1) is enlarged. The mucosal folds are thickened and have produced nodular indentations in the barium column. A postbulbar ulcer (arrow) is present. The duodenal bulb (2) appears normal. A gastrin-secreting pancreatic neoplasm was found at surgery, and a total gastrectomy was performed.

Zollinger-Ellison syndrome. Coarse, thick folds are present in this dilated, hypotonic duodenum. Inflammation and edema of the duodenum, the result of a chemical enteritis brought on by the onslaught of large volumes of gastric acid, first cause spasm and later hypotonia or atony (Fig. 40–30).[28] The motility of the jejunum and ileum, however, may be normal or slightly increased.

Thickened, edematous valvulae conniventes or mucosal folds in the jejunum, associated with increased intraluminal fluid that dilutes the barium in the presence of a gastric, duodenal, or jejunal ulcer, suggest a gastrin-secreting lesion. Likewise, markedly thickened gastric rugae in a patient with retained gastric fluid and a peptic ulcer also suggest the Zollinger-Ellison syndrome. Often, all the various roentgen manifestations of the Zollinger-Ellison syndrome are present; i.e., giant gastric rugae with retained gastric

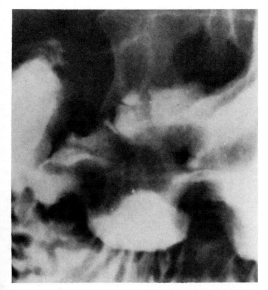

Figure 40–29. A large ulcer situated in the antrum on the greater curvature is surrounded by a mound of edema, which has produced a broad, lucent band at the mouth of the ulcer and a mass that projects into the lumen. Enlarged folds radiate from the ulcer mound. The patient with this benign gastric ulcer had the Zollinger-Ellison syndrome.

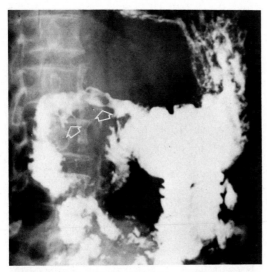

Figure 40–31. Enlarged gastric rugal folds, along with increased gastric secretions, have produced a mottled appearance of the barium in the stomach. Two duodenal ulcers are present (open arrows). Thickened mucosal folds are present in the second portion of the duodenum and in the jejunum. The patient had the Zollinger-Ellison syndrome.

secretion; single or multiple ulcers of the duodenum, jejunum or stomach; megaduodenum; edematous small bowel with hypermotility; and increased fluid (Fig. 40–31). With this extensive array of roentgenographic abnormalities, the Zollinger-Ellison syndrome may be diagnosed with a high degree of accuracy (see also p. 746).

MARGINAL OR ANASTOMOTIC ULCERS AFTER GASTRIC SURGERY

Ulcers at or adjacent to an anastomosis between stomach and small bowel are due to multiple causes. They are situated either at the margin of the anastomosis or on the small bowel side within a few centimeters of the anastomosis. Almost never are they found on the gastric side.[31]

Retained gastric antrum after gastric resections and Billroth II anastomosis results in continued gastrin production and subsequent acid-pepsin hypersecretion, as does incomplete vagotomy in association with antrectomy. Placement of a gastroenterostomy stoma too far to the left or too high on the gastric remnant may lead to inadequate gastric emptying, antral distention, and continued gastrin release. Un-

derlying gastrin-secreting pancreatic lesions (Zollinger-Ellison syndrome), as previously noted, may also cause postgastrectomy anastomotic ulcers.

The incidence of marginal ulcers depends upon the type of operation performed for gastric or duodenal ulcer and the underlying pathophysiological state.[31] The frequency of marginal ulcers after Billroth I and II gastrectomies is similar (5 to 10 per cent).[32] Surgical procedures associated with a high incidence of postsurgical anastomotic ulcers are antral exclusion (40 per cent), gastroenterostomy (30 per cent),[31] and retained antrum after Billroth II (30 to 50 per cent).[33] Less than total gastrectomy in patients with an underlying Zollinger-Ellison syndrome is followed by marginal ulcers in 55 per cent of patients.[30] In general, marginal ulcers follow surgery for gastric ulcer less frequently than for duodenal ulcer.

For various reasons, approximately 50 per cent of marginal ulcers are not detected roentgenographically.[34] Frequently, marginal ulcerations are too superficial or shallow to be detected. At times, barium may become trapped between converging gastric or jejunal folds about an anastomotic site, simulating an ulcer. Conversely, identification of an ulcer in the midst of overlapping jejunal mucosal folds may be extremely difficult. The variety of surgically produced pouches, outpouchings, and irregularities at the anastomotic site also causes difficulty in the diagnosis of marginal ulcers.

Roentgenographic detection of marginal ulcers depends to a great extent upon the persistence of the radiologist. Omission of certain techniques is an important reason that ulcers are not demonstrated. On roentgen examination of an anastomosis in the upright position with large amounts of barium, the anastomotic site and the small bowel pattern adjacent to the anastomosis are often obscured. Proper technique requires first that the patient be examined in the supine and prone positions with small amounts of relatively thick barium to obtain good mucosal coating. In these positions, air normally present in the gastric pouch is maneuvered into the stoma and anastomotic small bowel. If air is insufficient, it must be introduced into the stomach by means of effervescent

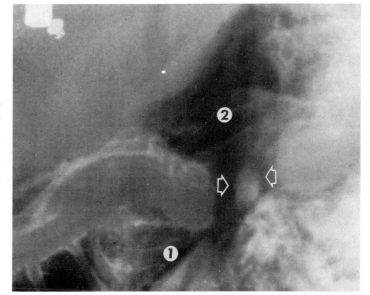

Figure 40–32. By means of the air-barium contrast technique, an ulcer at the margin of the jejunal (1) gastric (2) anastomosis was demonstrated en face (open arrows). The jejunum is narrowed near the site of anastomosis toward which jejunal folds radiate.

powders. This air-barium contrast technique is essential in the examination for postgastrectomy and anastomotic ulcers (Fig. 40–32).[35] Recently, injection of air and barium through a nasogastric tube whose tip is in the stoma has been proposed for roentgenographic examination of the patient who has been given 30 to 60 mg of propantheline and whose anastomotic small bowel is atonic.[36]

An ulcer of the anastomotic site is usually the most easily detected. It tends to penetrate deeply; it may be tent shaped and conical, its base irregular, and its size several centimeters. Ulcers at the margin of the anastomosis or in the small bowel also tend to penetrate into adjacent structures. Walled-off retroperitoneal abscesses and penetrations into the left lobe of the liver, the transverse colon, and the lesser sac have been reported.[32]

When secondary signs of marginal ulcer similar to those of duodenal ulcer are present, the degree of roentgenographic detection reaches 80 per cent, because these secondary signs usually alert the

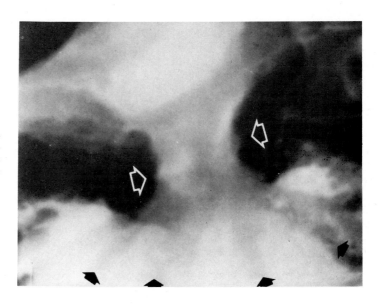

Figure 40–33. Thickened, edematous jejunal folds (solid arrows) radiate to a narrowed, irregular anastomosis. Two small ulcers are present at the margin of the anastomosis (open arrows).

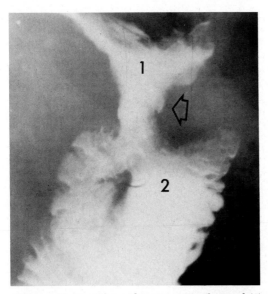

Figure 40-34. The wide separation of jejunal (2) from gastric (1) segments, and effacement and flattening of jejunum adjacent to the anastomotic site are secondary signs of marginal ulceration. An ulcer crater is also seen at the margin of the anastomosis (arrow).

radiologist to the diagnosis. These signs include edema of the duodenal or jejunal folds at the anastomotic site and flattening and rigidity of the jejunum adjacent to the ulcer.[37] Frequently narrowing and thickening of the stoma with edema surround the anastomotic site and efface adjacent jejunum, and occasionally markedly thickened gastric folds may radiate from the site of the ulcer (Figs. 40–33 and 40–34).

MISCELLANEOUS ULCERATIONS

Steroid ulcers have been common in this era of liberal steroid administration. Their development appears to be related to steroid dose (see p. 644).[38] In patients with healing duodenal ulcers, corticosteroid medication may cause exacerbation of clinical symptoms with growth and extension of an ulcer, or it may produce ulcers de novo. Steroid ulcers are not limited to the duodenum, but arise frequently in the stomach. Often they are shallow, but they may penetrate without significant surrounding inflammation so that ulcer collars or mounds may not be present.[20] Deep extension of steroid ulcers may produce

edema in the gastric wall. Multiple gastric ulcers are common in long-term or high-dose steroid therapy; as many as eight ulcers have been seen in the antrum alone (H. J. Burhenne, personal communication). Curling's ulcers after burns or severe trauma may produce discrete gastric ulcerations.[39] These, like steroid-induced ulcers, are often shallow and may evade roentgenographic detection. Stress ulcers have been described as more common in the antral area[40] and in the fundus.[41] In either case, they are rarely detected roentgenographically unless they progress to perforation (see pp. 657 to 662).

No distinctive roentgenographic features separate ulcers induced by such drugs as aspirin, phenylbutazone, reserpine, histamine, cincophen, and 5-fluorouracil from other benign gastric ulcers (see pp. 642 to 654).

Ulcers caused by granulomatous disease (tuberculosis, Crohn's disease) may be ragged, irregular lesions eccentrically situated in a segment of gastric or duodenal wall, which is thickened and rigid. The roentgen features suggest a malignant lesion. Granulomatous lesions do not generally cause discrete ulcerations.[42] Although ulcers may appear in the duodenum, they are not the typical, discrete ulcers of peptic disease. Ulceration may be present in any portion of the duodenum associated with irregular narrowing of the lumen that results from spasm or transmural infiltrate (Fig. 40–35). The roentgen diagnosis should be suspected when atypical duodenal ulcers are associated with disease of the small bowel or colon.

Discrete gastric or duodenal ulcers may appear in various benign and malignant neoplasms. Most of these ulcers, however, are contained within a mass of neoplastic tissue and therefore may be differentiated from benign peptic ulcers. Surrounding gastric or duodenal inflammatory response is not elicited in ulcerations associated with aberrant pancreas in the gastric antrum or duodenum, ulcerating leiomyoma, or other connective tissue tumor, such as neurofibromas, adenomyomas, lipomas, glomus tumors, and lymphangiomas.[43] Consequently, radiating folds and muscle spasm are rarely present. These discrete ulcers develop in the center of smooth, mound-like masses of submucosal tissue of

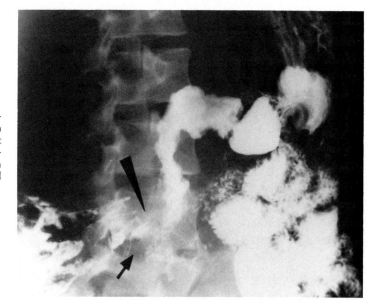

Figure 40–35. The arrows delineate a fistula from the duodenum to the transverse colon in a patient with Crohn's disease of the duodenum. The entire second portion of the duodenum is narrowed and its contour irregular.

benign tumors (Fig. 40–36). The shape of the ulcer may vary from shallow or conical to flask shaped with a wide base extending into necrotic tissue.[44] Carcinoid tumors situated in gastric antrum or duodenum may contain a discrete ulcer (Fig. 40–37).[45] The roentgen features of the ulcer and tumor are not characteristic. Single ulcers with surrounding collars which give a halo effect en face may be seen in metastatic melanoma.[46] Profile views, however, show these lesions to be mucosal or submucosal masses that protrude into the lumen.

Pancreatic carcinoma that extends into the greater curvature of the stomach or into the duodenum is perhaps the most common extragastric neoplasm to invade these areas. A single gastric ulcer caused by invasive extragastric cancer has characteristic features of a malignant neoplasm. Whether such invasive ulcers are the result of primary adenocarcinoma or pancreatic carcinoma is often difficult to determine roentgenographically.

Discrete ulceration has been reported in primary lymphoma that involves the stomach, although it is relatively rare. More often, lymphoma infiltrates widely and produces multiple irregular ulcerations (Fig. 40–38). Discrete ulcers, when seen, are within an infiltrative mass and simulate adenocarcinoma. Leiomyosarcomas may also ulcerate; large, irregular craters

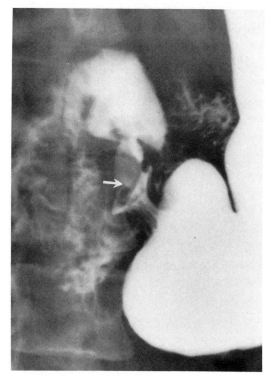

Figure 40–36. A smooth, oval mass projects into the antrum of the stomach. Within this mass is a small ulcer (arrow). No radiating folds are seen. This lesion originated in the submucosa. It was classified histologically as an adenomyoma, or myoepithelial hamartoma. (From Goldberg, H. I., and Margulis, A. R.: Amer. J. Roent. Radium Ther. Nuc. Med. 96: 382, 1966.)

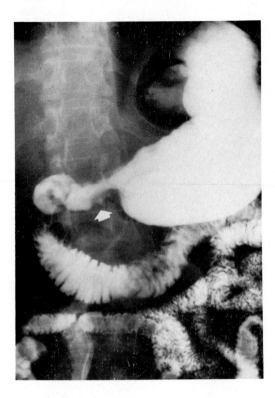

Figure 40–37. An ulcer is seen within a mass that projects into the gastric lumen from the greater curvature of the antrum. The contour of the mass is smooth, and the mass blends smoothly with the gastric wall. No radiating folds were present. The lesion was a gastric carcinoid, originating in the submucosa. A discrete surface ulceration was present (arrow).

Figure 40–38. Two ragged, irregular ulcers are present on the greater curvature of the stomach (arrows). The ulcers appear to undercut the rigid gastric wall. These discrete malignant ulcers developed within a lymphomatous infiltrate in a patient with Hodgkin's disease.

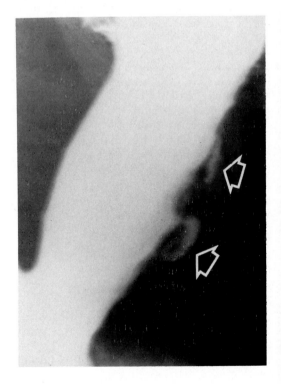

result, often extending into a large exogastric cavity that represents the center of
necrotic tumor (see p. 599).[44, 47]

REFERENCES

1. Silbiger, M. L., and Donner, M. W. Morphine
   in the evaluation of gastrointestinal disease;
   a cineradiographic study. Radiology 90:1090,
   1968.
2. Frimann-Dahl, J., and Traetteberg, K. Parietography of the stomach. Brit. J. Radiol.
   35:249, 1962.
3. Taylor, D. A., Macken, K. L., Bachman, A. L., and
   Seaman, W. B. A new method for visualization of the gastric wall; a preliminary report.
   Radiology 84:351, 1965.
4. Wolf, B. S., and Marshak, R. H. Profile features
   of benign gastric niches on roentgen examination. J. Mount Sinai Hosp. N.Y. 24:604,
   1957.
5. Zboralske, F. F. Gastric ulcer. In Alimentary
   Tract Roentgenology, Vol. 1, A. R. Margulis
   and H. J. Burhenne (eds.). St. Louis, C. V.
   Mosby Co., 1967, p. 475.
6. Keller, R. J., Wolf, B. S., and Khilnani, M. T.
   Roentgen features of healing and healed benign gastric ulcers. Radiology 97:353, 1970.
7. Nelson, S. W. The discovery of gastric ulcers
   and the differential diagnosis between benignancy and malignancy. Radiol. Clin. N.
   Amer. 7:5, 1969.
8. Zaterka, S., Bettarello, A., Meireles Filho, J. de
   S., Montenegro, M. R., and Pontes, J. F.
   Giant gastric ulcer; report of 27 cases. Amer.
   J. Dig. Dis. 7:236, 1962.
9. Turner, J. C., Jr., Dockerty, M. B., Priestley, J. T.,
   and Comfort, M. W. A clinicopathologic
   study of large benign gastric ulcers. Surg.
   Gynec. Obstet. 104:746, 1957.
10. Sakita, T., Oguro, Y., Takasu, S., Fukutomi, H.,
    Miwa, T., and Yoshimori, M. Observations
    on the healing of ulcerations in early gastric
    cancer. Gastroenterology 60:835, 1971.
11. Bryk, D. Penetrated ulcer near the cardia of the
    stomach. Amer. J. Dig. Dis. 11:728, 1966.
12. Wohl, G. T., and Shore, L. Lesions of the car-
    diac end of the stomach simulating car-
    cinoma. Amer. J. Roent. 82:1048, 1959.
13. Amberg, J. R., and Zboralske, F. F. Gastric
    ulcers after 70. Amer. J. Roent. 96:393, 1966.
14. Wilson, J. W., and Wilson, B. J. Pseudo-ulcera-
    tion of the stomach and duodenum produced
    by traction diverticula. Amer. J. Roent.
    75:297, 1956.
15. Stein, G., and Finkelstein, A. Roentgenologic
    classification of ulcerating gastric lesions. In
    Gastroenterology, Vol. 1, H. L. Bockus (ed.).
    2nd ed. Philadelphia, W. B. Saunders Co.,
    1963, pp. 517–518.
16. Zboralske, F. F., and Stargardter, F. L.
    Roentgenographic characteristics of benign
    greater curvature gastric ulcers. Presented at
    the Annual Meeting of the Radiological Soci-
    ety of North America, Chicago, November
    1968.
17. Glickman, M. G., Szemes, G., Loeb, P., and
    Margulis, A. R. Peptic ulcer of the pyloric
    region. Amer. J. Roent. 113:147, 1971.
18. Texter, E. C., Jr., Smith, H. W., Bundesen, W. E.,
    and Barlorka, C. J. The syndrome py-
    lorique; clinical and physiologic observa-
    tions. Gastroenterology 36:573, 1959.
19. Shanks, S. C., and Kerley, P. A Text-Book of X-
    ray Diagnosis, Vol. 4. Philadelphia, W. B.
    Saunders Co., 1969, pp. 202-217.
20. Prévôt, R. Roentgenology of the duodenum. In
    Alimentary Tract Roentgenology, Vol. 1, A.
    R. Margulis and H. J. Burhenne (eds.). St.
    Louis, C. V. Mosby Co., 1967, pp. 522-545.
21. Mistilis, S. P., Wiot, J. F., and Nedelman, S. H.
    Giant duodenal ulcer. Ann. Intern. Med.
    59:155, 1963.
22. Miller, R. E., and Nelson, S. W. The roentgeno-
    logic demonstration of tiny amounts of free
    intraperitoneal gas; experimental and clini-
    cal studies. Amer. J. Roent. 112:574, 1971.
23. Jacobson, G., Berne, C. J., Meyers, H. I., and
    Rosoff, L. The examination of patients with
    suspected perforated ulcer using a water-
    soluble contrast medium. Amer. J. Roent.
    86:37, 1961.
24. Bilbao, M. K., Frische, L. H., Rösch, J., Benson, J.
    A., Jr., and Dotter, C. T. Postbulbar duo-
    denal ulcer and ring-stricture; cause and ef-
    fect. Radiology 100:27, 1971.
25. Golden, R., Cimmino, C. V., Collins, L. C.,
    Dreyfuss, J. R., and Janower, M. L. In
    Golden's Diagnostic Radiology, Sect. 5,
    L. L. Robbins (ed.). Baltimore, Williams
    and Wilkins Co., 1969.
26. Hyman, S., Steigmann, F., and Schorsch, H.
    Postbulbar ulcer; a growing diagnostic and
    therapeutic program. Amer. J. Gastroent.
    40:255, 1963.
27. Tréheux, A., Fays, J., and Velut, A. Apport de la
    duodénographie hypotonique dans le diag-
    nostic des ulcères post-bulbaires. Ann. Ra-
    diol. 12:451, 1969.
28. Zboralske, F. F., and Amberg, J. R. Detection of
    the Zollinger-Ellison syndrome: The radiol-
    ogist's responsibility. Amer. J. Roent. 104:
    529, 1968.
29. Marshak, R. H., and Lindner, A. E. The Zol-
    linger-Ellison syndrome. In Radiology of the
    Small Intestine. Philadelphia, W. B.
    Saunders Co., 1970, pp. 88-98.
30. Wilson, S. D., and Ellison, E. H. Survival in pa-
    tients with the Zollinger-Ellison syndrome
    treated by total gastrectomy. Amer. J. Surg.
    111:787, 1966.
31. Burhenne, H. J. The postoperative stomach.
    In Alimentary Tract Roentgenology, Vol. 1,
    A. R. Margulis and H. J. Burhenne (eds.). St.
    Louis, C. V. Mosby Co., 1967, pp. 546-586.
32. Kiefer, E. D., and Sedgwick, C. E. Marginal
    ulcer following partial or subtotal gastrec-
    tomy. Surg. Clin. N. Amer. 44:641, 1964.
33. Kay, A. W. The pyloric antrum and peptic ulcer-
    ation. Gastroenterologia 89:282, 1958.

34. Wychulis, A. R., Priestley, J. T., and Foulk, W. T. A study of 360 patients with gastrojejunal ulceration. Surg. Gynec. Obstet. 122:89, 1966.

35. Samuel, E. The radiology of the stomach after gastrectomy. Brit. J. Radiol. 27:151, 1954.

36. Shields, J. B., and Holtz, S. Method of examination of gastroenterostomy stomas. Invest. Radiol. 4:104, 1969.

37. Schatzki, R. The significance of rigidity of the jejunum in the diagnosis of postoperative jejunal ulcers. Amer. J. Roent. 103:330, 1968.

38. Kirsner, J. B. Peptic ulcer; a review of the recent literature on various clinical aspects. Gastroenterology 54:611, 1968.

39. O'Neill, J. A., Jr., Pruitt, B. A., Jr., Moncrief, J. A., and Switzer, W. E. Studies related to the pathogenesis of Curling's ulcer. J. Trauma 7:275, 1967.

40. Pincus, I. J., and Horowitz, R. E. The acute stress ulcer. In The Stomach, C. Thompson, D. Berkowitz, and E. Polish (eds.). New York, Grune and Stratton, 1967, pp. 314-320.

41. Skillman, J. J., and Silen, W. Acute gastroduodenal "stress" ulceration: Barrier disruption of varied pathogenesis? Gastroenterology 59:478, 1970

42. Marshak, R. H., and Lindner, A. E. Regional enteritis. In Radiology of the Small Intestine. Philadelphia, W. B. Saunders Co., 1970, pp. 158-222.

43. Goldberg, H. I., and Margulis, A. R. Adenomyoma of the stomach; report of a case. Amer. J. Roent. 96:382, 1966.

44. Davis, J. G., and Adams, D. B. The roentgen findings in gastric leiomyomas and leiomyosarcomas. Radiology 67:67, 1956.

45. Siegelman, S. S., Gold, J. A., Simon, M., and Soifer, I. Ulceration of intramural gastric neoplasms. Amer. J. Dig. Dis. 14:127, 1969.

46. Potchen, E. J., Khung, C. L., and Yatsuhashi, M. X-ray diagnosis of gastric melanoma. New Eng. J. Med. 271:133, 1964.

47. Phillips, J. C., Lindsay, J. W., and Kendall, J. A. Gastric leiomyosarcoma; roentgenologic and clinical findings. Amer. J. Dig. Dis. 15:239, 1970.

Chapter 41

Gastroscopy and Duodenoscopy

Joseph P. Belber

GASTROSCOPY AND ESOPHAGOSCOPY

HISTORICAL BACKGROUND AND INSTRUMENT DEVELOPMENT

The goals of upper gastrointestinal endoscopy are to visualize all portions of the esophagus, stomach, and duodenum without blind spots; to be able to perform biopsy where desired; and to be able to perform the procedure without significant discomfort or risk to the patient and with relative ease by the endoscopist. Current instrumentation has virtually enabled us to achieve these goals and is responsible for making upper gastrointestinal endoscopy the definitive procedure it has become.

Rudolph Schindler introduced the first useful semiflexible gastroscope in 1932.[1] It was a side-viewing instrument, employing multiple lenses in its flexible distal half and rigid proximal half. The patient was examined lying on his left side, and his head was held in extension by an assistant. Unfortunately, sizable portions of the stomach were too frequently not seen, including the prepyloric lesser curvature, the pylorus, the mid-greater curvature, the upper posterior wall against which the instrument rested, and the fundus. Although a large body of knowledge was ac-

cumulated and, in selected cases, it provided valuable information not furnished by X-ray, nevertheless its major visual blind spots kept gastroscopy from becoming more than a supplementary procedure.

The first fully flexible gastroscopes were introduced by Hirschowitz and coworkers in 1958.[2] They were side-viewing instruments, employing a fiberoptic bundle for image transmission and subsequently also for light transmission, and were a major advance. The patient no longer had to be held with extended head, the antrum and pylorus became more uniformly accessible, and some proximal duodenal visualization was actually achieved in selected cases.[3-5] However, the upper posterior wall, mid-greater curvature, and fundus were still not regularly seen, and gastroscopy remained a supplementary procedure. In 1963 a forward-viewing instrument was introduced by Hirschowitz[6] for use in the esophagus; it was modified by LoPresti and Hilmi.[7] Although its potentiality as a gastroscope was appreciated, it was of limited use because the lens could not be brought to bear on large portions of the gastric wall.

Technical improvements of both forward-viewing and side-viewing instruments came at an ever increasing rate — in fact, came so rapidly that many in-

521

struments of intermediate design became obsolete overnight but continued to remain in use because of budgetary limitations. Statistical comparisons between X-ray and endoscopy or analyses of causes of upper gastrointestinal bleeding only a few years old are no longer valid, as endoscopes have become the highly efficient instruments they now are. To summarize the improvements, fields of view have been widened from 35 degrees in the original fiberscope to 70 degrees in modern instruments, both increasing the view and simplifying orientation. A controllable deflecting segment at the distal end of the instrument was incorporated in a side-viewing instrument to permit it to look back on itself and see the fundus. The tip was too long, and the deflection somewhat limited, but it led to the development of short-tipped instruments which now can be deflected up to a full 180 degrees in any direction, permitting a forward-viewing instrument to look back on itself. Instruments were lengthened enough to reach the ligament of Treitz. Channels were incorporated to permit passage of biopsy forceps, cytology brushes, irrigating or injecting cannulas, and even snares and cautery for additional operative procedures. Fingertip controls for employment of air inflation, water injection to wash lenses, and suction have reduced the burden upon the endoscopist and considerably shortened examination time.

The modern forward-viewing endoscope with omnidirectional tip deflection of 180 degrees rapidly visualizes the average esophagus, stomach, and duodenum without significant blind areas, although supplementation with a side-viewing instrument may be of help in about 10 per cent of cases to see into certain deep pockets in deformed duodenal bulbs or, rarely, to visualize some portions of a grossly distorted stomach. Orientation is easier to learn with the forward viewer; in fact, the whole procedure of gastroduodenoscopy is simplified. Biopsy with the forward viewer is usually readily accomplished, but in an occasional case if the view is highly tangential a side viewer may be advantageous. It is our policy to use the forward viewer as the routine instrument and to use a side viewer only when there is a specific need for it. There is one consistent exception: visualization and cannulation of the papilla of Vater at present require a side viewer, and in general we prefer a side-viewing duodenoscope for visualization beyond the superior flexure of the duodenum.

INDICATIONS AND CONTRAINDICATIONS

Although the indications for esophagoscopy have been discussed elsewhere, the interrelationship between diseases of the esophagus, stomach, and duodenum is so great that we include the symptoms of disease in the esophagus as an indication for examination of the stomach and duodenum and always perform esophagoscopy when gastroduodenoscopy is indicated. This applies particularly to peptic disease, the gastrointestinal effects of alcohol, upper gastrointestinal bleeding, and hiatus hernia.

Indications are really so broad that we could summarize by saying that whenever we suspect the upper gastrointestinal tract may be the site of disease, symptomatic or nonsymptomatic, we feel it is advisable to have a look.

We tabulate the indications as follows:

1. Unexplained chest or abdominal pain, even in the absence of X-ray abnormalities.

2. Upper gastrointestinal bleeding, whether overt, as manifested by hematemesis or melena, or cryptic, as suggested by iron deficiency anemia or occult blood in the stool.

3. Certain definite X-ray abnormalities, including hiatus hernia; gastric ulcer; neoplasm of the esophagus, stomach, or duodenum; and gastric outlet obstruction.

4. Indeterminate X-ray abnormalities, including suspicion of ulcer or neoplasm, and in particular the deformed duodenal bulb.

5. Evaluation prior to upper gastrointestinal tract surgery.

6. Evaluation of symptoms in the stomach postoperatively, including hiatus hernia repair, gastric resection, gastrojejunostomy, and pyloroplasty.

7. Transduodenal pancreatography and cholangiography.

Upper gastrointestinal endoscopy is absolutely contraindicated under the following circumstances:

1. The patient is uncooperative or unwilling.
2. The probability of a perforated viscus exists.
3. The patient is in shock.

It is not wise to perform the examination in patients with serious associated illness such as myocardial infarction, pneumonia, or thoracic aneurysm, unless immediate endoscopic diagnosis is absolutely necessary for the institution of life-saving therapy.

THE EXAMINATION

Although upper gastrointestinal endoscopy can be performed with virtually no premedication, we firmly believe in adequate sedation and analgesia unless there is a specific contraindication. We employ sodium pentobarbital (100 mg), meperidine (100 mg), and atropine (0.6 mg) prior to arrival at the endoscopy room to allay anxiety. Pontocaine, 2 per cent, is used topically for pharyngeal anesthesia, an antifoaming agent is administered, and then the patient is slowly titrated with intravenous diazepam until he begins to doze. The average dose is 15 mg, considerably less in the elderly. We insert a wedge-shaped bite block. We examine the esophagus, but defer biopsy until later. The stomach is surveyed rapidly, but biopsy and retroversion inspection of the fundus are deferred. The duodenal bulb is examined completely before the descending duodenum is entered. However, if the procedure is being performed to cannulate the papilla of Vater, the instrument is passed as rapidly as possible into the descending duodenum. Occasionally propantheline hydrobromide (30 mg) is administered intravenously to aid in duodenal examination. Details of the mechanics of the procedure are described elsewhere.[8]

GASTRIC ULCER VERSUS CARCINOMA

One of the prime indications for gastroscopy is the evaluation of gastric ulcer in the hope of discovering early gastric carcinoma. Experience in Japan suggests that a five-year survival rate of approximately 95 per cent may be achieved in early gastric carcinoma involving only the mucosa or submucosa,[9] based on the classification established in 1962 by the Japanese Gastroenterological Endoscopy Society. A discussion of this classification was presented to the American Society for Gastrointestinal Endoscopy in 1969 and subsequently published.[10] In the United States, however, with the possible exception of Hawaii, the incidence of gastric carcinoma is significantly lower than in Japan, and the discovery of a small early carcinoma in an American endoscopic clinic is an uncommon experience. The classic, sharply demarcated ulceration whose walls and surrounding mucosa show no suggestion of nodularity or infiltration may be classified as benign by an experienced endoscopist with surprising accuracy (Fig. 41-1). Morrissey and Koizumi found that only one of a group of approximately 300 such typical ulcers was subsequently found to have a malignant focus.[11] In our own experience over a period of 25 years, an ulcer classically benign by gastroscopic criteria has never subsequently been found to be malignant. However, it is required that the ulcer have smooth sharp margins and no suggestion of surrounding nodularity, or thickened walls. Folds should radiate all the way to the ulcer margin without clubbing at the ulcer edge. No nodules should be present in its base. Ten to 20 per cent of ulcers do not meet these rigid criteria, and in this group malignancy is best suspected until it has been definitely ruled out. Questionable ulcers are checked with repeated biopsy or cytologic study with brush or washing techniques until their true nature is clarified; if significant doubt still exists, the lesion is excised for more thorough pathological study. In some of these lesions malignancy has subsequently been found, by either endoscopic or surgical biopsy.

Modern endoscopes permit biopsy or brush cytology with comparative ease. Multiple biopsies are advisable in all questionable cases and, although usually satisfactory, may not always be deep enough if the lesion in question is infiltrating submucosally beneath normal mucosa.[11]

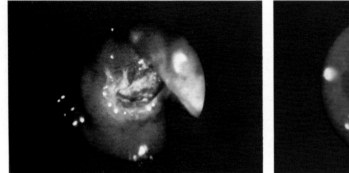

Figure 41-1   Figure 41-2

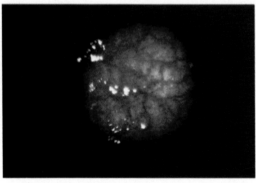

Figure 41-3

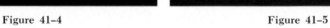

Figure 41-4   Figure 41-5

Figure 41-1.   Three-cm benign gastric ulcer on lesser curvature at angulus.

Figure 41-2.   Five-cm ulcerating carcinoma in fundus.

Figure 41-3.   Five-cm primary, solitary lymphosarcoma in midportion of stomach.

Figure 41-4.   Gastric atrophy, showing network of fine vessels.

Figure 41-5.   Erosive antral gastritis – hyperemic patches with small central erosions.

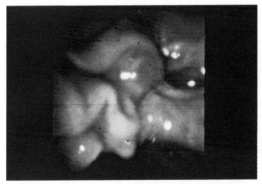

Figure 41-6

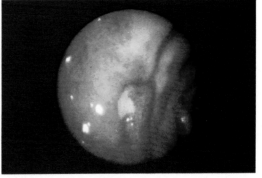

Figure 41-7

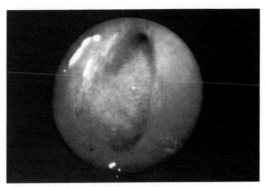

Figure 41-8

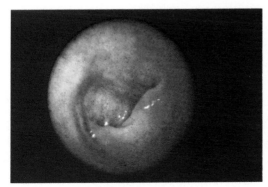

Figure 41-9

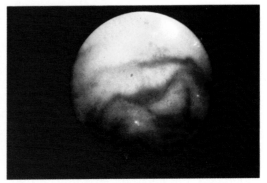

Figure 41-10

Figure 41-6. Papilla of Vater, just above center of picture. It is partially covered by a hood.

Figure 41-7. Small, 6-mm superficial duodenal ulcer with associated duodenitis.

Figure 41-8. Midbulb constriction deformity without ulcer, showing proximal hyperemia.

Figure 41-9. "Superficial" duodenitis at apex of bulb.

Figure 41-10. "Nodal" duodenitis, showing hyperemia on nodular prominences.

Modern upper gastrointestinal endoscopes permit visual and biopsy access to any part of the stomach; an ulcer of any size anywhere in the stomach should be demonstrable and biopsiable by a competent endoscopist unless there is extreme distortion or proximal stricturing. This has certainly been our experience in recent years. Furthermore, the endoscopist discovers a significant number of ulcers not identified radiologically, particularly shallow lesions some distance from the major curvatures, or small prepyloric ulcers which may readily become concealed in prominent folds, particularly if there is associated gastritis. The Veterans Administration Cooperative Study on Gastric Ulcer,[12] which included only ulcers demonstrable by X-ray and excluded those diagnosed only by endoscopy, indicated that 95 per cent of the ulcers were on or near the lesser curvature; that ulcers were rather evenly distributed over the distal 9 cm of the stomach, with somewhat higher percentages adjacent to the pylorus; that 69 per cent of the ulcers were 6 to 20 mm wide, with 13 per cent smaller and 18 per cent larger; and that the larger ulcers tended to be located further from the pylorus and were more likely to be malignant. Studies of comparative size employing endoscopy with the newer instruments are not yet available, but there is no reason to believe that they would significantly disagree with the overall concept of gastric ulcer as set forth in that report. However, although the Veterans Administration Cooperative Study provides an excellent survey of the incidence, distribution, and behavior of gastric ulcer, we must take exception to the inclusion of the chapter on gastroscopy, which is utterly unrealistic by modern endoscopic standards. All the endoscopic examinations reported in that study were performed with instruments obsolete at the time of publication of the study. It is unfortunate that such an archaic résumé of endoscopy should become part of a study on gastric ulcer which in other respects is highly commendable and may well become a classic.

MORE ABOUT NEOPLASMS

The overwhelming majority of ulcerating carcinomas seen endoscopically (Fig. 41–2) are readily distinguished from benign ulcers. They obviously look like malignancies which are ulcerated. Identification of polypoid neoplasms presents little difficulty. Adenomatous polyps are much less common in the stomach than in the large bowel; but, as in the colon, the possibility of malignancy increases if lesions are multiple or are more than 2 cm in diameter.[13]

Submucous neoplasms are occasionally encountered, the most common being leiomyomas, fibromas, and lipomas. Biopsy of submucosal lesions is often not helpful, because the normal overlying mucosa is often avulsed from atop the lesion and the lesion itself will not be caught in the biopsy forceps. Submucosal tumors have a tendency to undergo central necrosis with umbilication or actual ulceration, and may be responsible for gross bleeding. This occurs not only with primary neoplasms but also with metastatic tumors, of which melanoma is a well recognized example.[14]

All the varieties of lymphoma may occur in the stomach or duodenum and may be quite polymorphic, masquerading as giant folds, multiple erosions or ulcers, or frank tumors. Diagnosis may be established by endoscopic biopsy, because many lymphomatous processes infiltrate into the surface epithelium. Primary isolated lymphosarcoma (Fig. 41–3) or Hodgkin's disease may also occur in either the stomach or duodenum; both diseases have been diagnosed by endoscopic biopsy in our clinic.

Endoscopy is useful not only in the evaluation of definite neoplasms, but also in clarifying X-ray abnormalities which only suggest the possibility of neoplasm. Not infrequently, these prove to be abnormal fold patterns secondary to old scarring, or even inflammatory reactions around small benign ulcers out of proportion to the size of the ulcer.

The individual with unexplained chest or abdominal pain is a proper candidate for as thorough an exploration of the body orifices as possible. Hiatus hernia with significant esophagitis, unsuspected carcinoma of the esophagus or stomach, gastric or duodenal ulcer, and even carcinoma of the pancreas involving the stomach or duodenum have been encountered. The percentage of such positive findings is small in the face of thorough and negative

X-ray studies, but statistics have little bearing upon the individual case. Suffice it to say that if there is a serious possibility that a lesion may be present, or if there is any doubt about the findings of another diagnostic modality, endoscopy is indicated.

GASTRITIS AND RELATED STATES

All that passes for gastritis is not necessarily inflammatory, and the correlation between endoscopic diagnosis and pathological diagnosis has not always been good. There are explanations for some of the discrepancies. Gastritis is often a patchy disease, and the past reliance upon blind biopsy techniques may have led to errors. Now that biopsies may be obtained transendoscopically under direct vision, correlation may improve. However, endoscopic biopsies may be too shallow to allow accurate diagnosis of some thick lesions such as giant hypertrophic gastritis. Another problem is the difficulty for the pathologist in setting the limits of normal, because elements of inflammatory reaction, including round cells and eosinophils, normally reside in the lamina propria.[15] How many are too many? A problem faced by the endoscopist is the tendency for the pathologist to consider that vascular engorgement, intramural hemorrhage, or even edema is an artifact of the biopsy, even when the endoscopist saw visible congestion and intramural hemorrhage and took the biopsy for that specific reason.

As indicated in the opening statement, not all that has been called gastritis is necessarily inflammatory. Some of it is just a variation in the physiognomy of the stomach. The normal mucosa should be pliable, pink, and mildly textured, and should contain folds most prominent along the greater curvature of the body. Occasionally, sizable vessels may be seen in the upper third of the stomach, particularly with a retroversion view. The general appearance may vary, depending upon the degree of inflation of the stomach, muscle tone, or the hemoglobin level, but the overall characteristics do not change significantly.

At one end of the spectrum is gastric atrophy. The endoscopist encounters an unusually pallid, thin, transparent mucosa of grayish hue in which the submucosal network of fine vessels is readily seen. Sizable veins may also be noted in the upper two-thirds of the stomach. We shall not encroach on the pathologists' prerogative and discuss whether this abnormal mucosa is atrophic gastritis or gastric atrophy, but from the visual point of view the term gastric atrophy is more appropriate unless there are other evidences of gastritis. Although termed atrophic, this mucosa may be associated with hyperplastic nodules or even true polyp formation and an increased incidence of malignancy. Advanced degrees of atrophy as seen endoscopically (Fig. 41–4) are usually associated with achlorhydria and are characteristic of adult pernicious anemia, but some mucosae, suggesting milder degrees of atrophy, may still produce enough acid to be associated with duodenal ulcer.

On the opposite end of the spectrum, Schindler described a lush, florid mucosa, showing cobblestoning or mamillation between the folds in the acid-bearing portion of the stomach and called it hypertrophic gastritis. This has been demonstrated to be normal mucosa by the pathologists. However, this mucosa is commonly associated with a large parietal cell mass and high acid output and is the "hypertrophic hypersecretory gastropathy" described by Stempien and others.[16, 17]

Yet another variation of appearance is the presence of large rugal folds which may result from underinflation but may persist with full inflation. If these folds appear otherwise normal endoscopically, they are probably of no significance and should cause no concern. If there is any question, biopsy may readily be obtained.

True gastritis may not only be a patchy disease, but may also be sharply limited to only a single portion of the stomach. The distal antrum is an area commonly involved, as is the upper midportion. Occasionally the entire stomach may be involved. We arbitrarily divide true gastritis into two types: superficial, which shows little alteration of the X-ray pattern; and hyperplastic, which may be accompanied by coarse folds radiologically, particularly in the antrum.

Superficial gastritis (Fig. 41–5) is manifested endoscopically by localized vascular engorgement, intramural hemorrhage and erosions covered with fibrin or hemorrhagic eschars, or a mixture of the two. Erosions vary in size from a few millimeters to more than 1 cm. In patients with alcoholic gastritis, erosions just a few millimeters wide and several centimeters long have been encountered, resembling Mallory-Weiss lacerations in appearance, but usually located in the mid-zone of the stomach. Similar lesions may be encountered in those with stress gastritis. Aspirin also produces superficial gastritis, although we have not encountered the markedly elongated erosions.

A more nodular appearing form of gastritis is also encountered, most commonly in the antrum. It is characterized by lesions 5 to 7 mm in diameter which project a few millimeters into the lumen. They are usually hyperemic, and may have small central erosions or umbilications. When seen on folds, they resemble elongated beads or nodes on the folds, and as peristalsis passes through them they show some degree of stiffness. There may be just a few lesions present in the distal antrum, or there may be scores scattered throughout the stomach. They may be responsible for large antral folds radiologically, and may help conceal peptic ulcer. Biopsies of these lesions have indicated true gastritis but do not differ significantly from "superficial" gastritis.

Giant hypertrophic gastritis or Menetrier's disease[18] is a more specific lesion than the gastritis previously described. Space does not permit a detailed discussion of its pathology. Endoscopically it may be suspected if large, stiff, somewhat nodular folds are seen, either generally or in a localized patch. There may be large amounts of thick mucus present. Biopsy is advisable. The biopsy will usually not be deep enough to establish the diagnosis but can be helpful in ruling out lymphoma or carcinoma. Carcinoma has been reported in the presence of Menetrier's disease.

Rare forms of specific gastritis and other generalized conditions affecting the gastric wall, including sarcoid, tuberculosis, eosinophilic gastritis, hemochromatosis, or amyloidosis, may be encountered and may be diagnosed by biopsy if fortune smiles; they will not otherwise be discussed here.

The endoscopist must be aware of iatrogenic artifacts. A nasogastric suction tube may result in intramural hemorrhage, petechiae, and erosions. A gastric analysis with histamine or histalog is particularly likely to produce hemorrhagic or erosive lesions, so it is well to remember that endoscopy should be performed before gastric analysis or 12-hour overnight collections if at all possible.

The Mallory-Weiss lesion is a laceration of varying length and depth close to the gastroesophageal junction, presumably caused by the stress of vomiting; it is usually associated with hiatus hernia. Similar lesions occur in the lower esophagus or more distally in the stomach, particularly where the diaphragm pinches the hiatus hernia. To single out this lesion as the only one produced by the stress of vomiting is not being entirely realistic. The orientation of some lesions of superficial gastritis or duodenitis in the long axis of the alimentary tract, arranged around the lumen like corset stays, suggests that muscular stress may have played a significant role in their formation as well.

THE POSTOPERATIVE STOMACH

The patients who are commonly examined endoscopically after operation are those who have had gastric resection with either gastrojejunostomy or gastroduodenostomy, simple gastrojejunostomy, and pyloroplasty. The creation of a surgical anastomosis or pyloroplasty may result in sufficient distortion to render X-ray interpretation of morphology difficult and create special problems in identifying small or superficial ulcerations. Even larger ulcerations may occasionally escape detection. Most ulcerations occur at the anastomosis or within a few centimeters of the stoma, usually on the jejunal or duodenal side, but may be several centimeters distal. Modern endoscopes have little difficulty in visualizing these lesions or passing well into the small bowel if necessary.

The adequacy of the gastric outlet can be readily determined and the existence of obstruction often recognized. Partial obstruction may be due to an unusually small stoma or subsequent scarring and distortion caused by ulceration or severe stomatitis. But it may also be due to severe degrees of gastritis with the production of enlarged edematous hyperemic folds which may permit passage of the endoscope but may not permit adequate emptying following a meal. We have encountered several such instances following Billroth I antrectomy and vagotomy of the Schoemaker type. We have also encountered instances of stenosis distal to the anastomosis secondary to high degrees of jejunitis or duodenitis with or without associated ulcer. Following vagotomy and gastric resection, emptying may be poor, and food bezoars may form even in the presence of a widely patent stoma and no organic obstruction. This situation is readily identified endoscopically.

Ideally, neither the gastric mucosa nor the adjacent small bowel mucosa should show any evidence of inflammation, but some degree of postoperative gastritis is often present following anastomotic procedures and even after some pyloroplasties. This is assumed to be due to reflux of bile and enzyme containing pancreatic juices. It may be quite severe and may be associated with pain and refractory bilious vomiting after meals. Most often it is associated with low or no acid output and may require surgical correction by a diversionary procedure such as the Roux-Tanner 19, the Roux-en-y, or an enteroenterostomy. It should be recognized that such diversionary procedures are ulcerogenic unless acid output is low and vagotomy is performed. We have rehabilitated several gastric cripples by correcting this most disturbing complication, and others have had similar success.[19] On the other hand, the presence of stomal inflammation associated with jejunitis or duodenitis or ulceration at or beyond the stoma suggests that acid output is still too high and that surgery has not accomplished the physiological purpose for which it was intended.

In the process of making an anastomosis or in closing a portion of the resected stomach, an exuberant collection of tissue, called a plication defect, may remain within the lumen. Occasionally this pseudopolypoid conglomeration must be differentiated from neoplasm by endoscopy. However, we have seen true adenomatous polyps develop on either side of a gastro jejunostomy stoma. One such jejunal polyp was actually responsible for upper gastrointestinal bleeding.

It is not unusual to see retained sutures in the mucosa, even years after the original surgical procedure. These are usually innocent, but they may cause foreign body ulceration. Years ago we encountered a single suture which had transfixed an artery and for many months had acted as a wick which led to severe chronic blood loss until it was discovered and removed surgically.

UPPER GASTROINTESTINAL HEMORRHAGE

One of the special uses of upper gastrointestinal endoscopy is the early identification of the source of upper gastrointestinal bleeding. Endoscopy is preferred to X-ray, because it can identify lesions which are too superficial or too small to be accurately diagnosed radiologically (selective angiography excepted). Included in this group are such commonplace lesions as esophagitis, gastritis, Mallory-Weiss lesions, and small superficial ulcers in the esophagus, stomach, or duodenum. Even when X-ray demonstrates a lesion such as esophageal varices, it does not establish the fact that the lesion is the source of bleeding, although it is often presumed. A particular problem is created when two or more diverse lesions are identified radiologically and an attempt is made to assess which is the more important (see pp. 195 to 214).

If it is elected to employ both X-ray and endoscopy, endoscopy should be performed first; if it is not definitive, other diagnostic means should be undertaken. It has become common practice in many clinics to stabilize the patient's vital signs, with transfusions if necessary, and then, using a large bore tube, to irrigate the stomach with copious amounts of ice water until clots are removed and the irrigating fluid is either clear or light pink. At that time an endoscope is passed for direct inspection of the upper gastrointestinal tract. In most instances this is quite satisfactory; but if the stomach is not adequately cleared of small clots or if bleeding continues briskly, small lesions, especially those close to the gastroesophageal junction, may be overlooked, owing to puddling of blood or reflux back into the esophagus. A scattering of small clots over the gastric or duodenal mucosa may conceal ulcers up to 1 cm in diameter, or even suggest a diagnosis of hemorrhagic gastritis which may not be present. There is usually no difficulty even under these adverse circumstances in identifying esophageal varices, hiatus hernia, severe esophagitis, or other lesions of sufficient size—for example, ulcers or tumors 2 cm in diameter; but even in the presence of variceal bleeding, the actual point of bleeding may be difficult to identify or to attribute absolutely to the varix.

We prefer to examine the patient during a lull in the bleeding or just after the bleeding has ceased. This cannot always be achieved; if a diagnosis is critically required, we do not hesitate to perform endoscopy during massive bleeding. We use a polydirectional forward-viewing endoscope to examine the esophagus, stomach, and duodenum. It permits a direct diagnosis of duodenal ulcer, whereas in the past the duodenum was only implicated indirectly as the source of bleeding if blood was seen refluxing back through the pylorus, or if the endoscopist saw nothing significant and subsequent X-ray showed a deformed bulb.

We are concerned about the use of tubes prior to endoscopy; although we acknowl-edge their importance in the overall management of the patient, we wonder how much artifact results from suction and forceful irrigation and how much "hemorrhagic gastritis" is created.

During 1971, endoscopy was performed on 400 patients in our clinic, of whom 88 were acute upper gastrointestinal bleeders. Because of a high incidence of cirrhosis and esophageal varices, alcoholics were tabulated separately. Of the 400 patients, 83 were alcoholic, 41 of whom were examined because of acute upper gastrointestinal bleeding; of the 317 nonalcoholics, only 47 were examined for acute bleeding. Seventeen of the alcoholics had esophageal varices, of whom only ten were bleeding from their varices and seven were bleeding from other sources. There were no nonalcoholics with varices in this series.

The causes of hemorrhage in the alcoholics and nonalcoholics are given in Table 41-1. Although the series is small, several conclusions may be drawn:

1. The mere presence of esophageal varices does not mean that they are the source of the bleeding.

2. Alcoholics are prone to bleed from esophagitis. Incidentally, all cases of esophagitis in this series were associated with hiatus hernias.

3. Mallory-Weiss lacerations are a common cause of upper gastrointestinal bleeding, particularly in the alcoholic.

TABLE 41-1. CAUSES OF BLEEDING IN 88 PATIENTS WITH
ACUTE UPPER GASTROINTESTINAL HEMORRHAGE

	TOTAL ALCOHOLICS	ALCOHOLICS WITH ESOPHAGEAL VARICES	NON- ALCOHOLICS	TOTAL
Esophagitis	7	(1)	5	12
Esophageal varices	10	(10)	0	10
Mallory-Weiss lacerations	8	(0)	1	9
Gastritis	3	(1)	1	4
Stress gastritis	0	(0)	1	1
Gastric ulcer	7	(4)	11	18
Duodenal ulcer	2	(0)	19	21
Stomal ulcer	2	(1)	3	5
Carcinoma of stomach	0	(0)	1	1
Carcinoma invading stomach (from gallbladder)	0	(0)	1	1
Unknown	2	(0)	4	6
Total	41	(17)	47	88

4. Gastritis as a cause of upper gastrointestinal bleeding may not be so common as some have suggested[20] (refer to conclusion number 6).

5. Peptic ulcer remains the most common cause of upper gastrointestinal hemorrhage.

6. The composition of one's clientele may have a profound influence on causes of upper gastrointestinal bleeding.

Patients with cryptic upper gastrointestinal bleeding, suspected because of guaiac positive stools or iron deficiency anemia, are routinely endoscoped. We have encountered several gastric malignancies, severe esophagitis with hiatus hernia, virtually asymptomatic gastric or duodenal ulcers, and even salicylate erosions. We invariably survey the entire gastrointestinal tract even if upper gastrointestinal endoscopy has discovered a lesion which may have bled. We strongly emphasize that the mere presence of a hiatus hernia with chronic esophagitis, or a partially healed peptic ulcer, does not excuse us from looking for the oozing cecal carcinoma or other lesion which may be the real culprit.

DUODENOSCOPY

HISTORY AND INSTRUMENTATION

The importance of duodenal ulcer as a major cause of disability is well recognized. In the past objective diagnosis has depended upon radiology, which is helpful if a crater is demonstrated but is not a reliable indicator of active disease in the absence of crater. The radiologically deformed duodenal bulb presents a special problem, because it not infrequently persists unchanging while the patient undergoes a series of clinical exacerbations and remissions.

With the initial introduction of the fiberoptic gastroduodenoscope by Hirschowitz and coworkers in 1958,[2] it was hoped that endoscopy would be a valuable adjunct in the management of duodenal ulcer disease. Neither the original instrument nor its early modifications lived up to expectations, although some endoscopists were ultimately able to enter the duodenum in from 20 to 35 per cent of cases by relying on hand manipulation of the instrument through the abdominal wall or by altering the patient's position on the table.[21] This was small reward for a sometimes difficult technique, but it did establish the potential usefulness of duodenoscopy for the evaluation of peptic disease if it could be accomplished easily and consistently. The rapid development of duodenoscopes during the period from 1968 to 1971 resulted in steadily increasing effectiveness.[21] In the author's 1970 series,[8] using a 77-cm forward-viewing endoscope now obsolete, the duodenal bulb was entered in 91 per cent of cases. Of 70 active ulcers positively identified, endoscopy visualized 66 (94 per cent), compared with 45 (64 per cent) discovered by X-ray. In addition, X-ray diagnosed ten false-positives compared with no false-positive results for endoscopy. With instruments currently available the duodenal bulb can be entered in virtually every patient in whom the lumen can be dilated to the diameter of the endoscope, unless there is extreme distortion proximally.

At present, the Machida Manufacturing Company and the Olympus Optical Company produce side-viewing instruments which provide excellent visualization in the entire duodenum and permit cannulation of the papilla of Vater or biopsy wherever indicated. These instruments are widely used in Japan and are now in use in several centers in the United States. In the United States, the American Cystoscope Makers, Inc., pioneered the development of a practical, wide-angled forward-viewing endoscope useful in the esophagus, stomach, and duodenum. A comparable instrument is now also manufactured by the Olympus Optical Company. Although the forward-viewing endoscopes are useful for visualizing the descending duodenum, the papilla of Vater is often concealed behind its hood and cannot be cannulated. In about 10 per cent of patients, supplementation of either a forward viewer or a side viewer by the other may be required for maximal visualization or biopsy in difficult situations.

THE NORMAL DUODENUM

Terminology applied to the proximal duodenum varies widely, so it is appropriate to define terms. From the endoscopist's point of view the terms duodenal bulb, duodenal cap, first portion, and superior portion are used interchangeably. The duodenal bulb is a tubular structure, 3 to 7 cm long, which tapers very gently if at all. It terminates at its apex, which is synonymous with the superior flexure of the duodenum, the curve leading into the descending or second portion of the duodenum. The internal angle of that curve is the superior duodenal angle, and it is used as a primary landmark in duodenoscopy. The degree of angulation is subject to considerable variation in different patients and may vary with change in body position. We prefer using the designations "superior and inferior walls or quadrants" rather than "greater or lesser curvatures of the bulb," because the latter terms are often reversed, depending upon whether one bases the terms on continuity with the adjacent gastric curvature or applies them to the actual curvature taken by the first portion of the duodenum.

In appearance, the mucosa of the duodenum is paler than the gastric mucosa and is more beige. It may appear velvety or shaggy, owing to the existence of villi, although at times it may appear smooth and translucent. The walls of the duodenal bulb are generally smooth, with an occasional low mamillation. There may be occasional longitudinal, circular, or cross-hatched folds. True Kerckring's folds usually start just beyond the superior flexure, although they may be found in an occasional bulb. The papilla of Vater (Fig. 41–6) is somewhat variable in size and shape, and is usually rougher in texture and darker in color than the adjacent duodenal mucosa. Proximally it is covered by a hood, and there is a horizontal fold or frenulum extending distally which acts as a landmark. The inferior flexure and angle are less prominent than the superior, and are not difficult to negotiate.

Duodenal motility differs from that of the stomach in that it is faster, may move in both directions, and lacks the slow, stripping, type II wave seen in the stomach.

DUODENAL ULCER AND RELATED ABNORMALITIES

The major disorder encountered in the duodenum is duodenal ulcer and its two handmaidens, duodenal deformity and duodenitis. The three conditions so often coexist that they will be discussed as a unit. However, duodenitis in some settings has its own special implications and will also be discussed separately.

Most duodenal ulcers occur within 3 cm of the pylorus, but about 10 per cent occur at the superior flexure or beyond. They are fairly uniformly distributed around the circumference of the lumen, except that fewer are seen in the inferior quadrant. The average duodenal ulcer is small (Fig. 41–7). In our experience, roughly 70 per cent are between 3 and 7 mm in diameter, 15 per cent are between 8 and 10 mm and 15 per cent are over 1 cm. Less than 5 per cent are over 2 cm. Larger ulcers tend to be round or oval and of considerable depth. The smaller lesions are more often superficial and may be more irregular in shape. Triangular, stellate, or spindle shapes are not uncommon. Healing may be quite rapid, and shape and depth may alter as healing progresses.

In the presence of ulcer some degree of duodenitis is invariably present, at times confined to the area surrounding the ulcer, but at other times, widespread and intense, suggesting that ulceration is only a small part of the whole inflammatory process. It may be found in the complete absence of ulceration and may be associated with peptic symptoms. It may persist for months after an ulcer has healed, suggesting that the pathological process is continuing.

If there are sufficient edema and inflammatory infiltrate around an ulcer, there may be formation of an obvious tumor mass which may resemble malignancy if it displays intense hyperemia and superficial erosion. A lesion so severely inflamed is rarely seen in the stomach.

Some ulcers which may acutely distort the bulb may resolve with little residue. However, many duodenal bulbs become permanently deformed as a result of fibrosis and contracture into contours which remain surprisingly consistent over the years.

The most common deformity associated with duodenal ulcer is the midbulb constriction deformity which occurs 2 to 3 cm distal to the pylorus (Fig. 41–8). In its mildest form there may be a persistent incisura which endoscopically appears as a semilunar fold. When more advanced, there may be a full contraction ring. Large pseudodiverticula may be formed between the constriction deformity and the pylorus, usually superiorly or inferiorly. When both are present, the cloverleaf bulb results. Recurrent ulcers tend to occur on the crest of the constriction or proximal to it and are usually not located in the pseudodiverticula. It is in this deformity that radiologists overlook the greatest number of ulcers, which tend to be small and superficial and disproportionate in size to the degree of deformity. Commonly, there is diffuse duodenitis as manifested by intense hyperemia and occasional erosion formation proximal to the constriction deformity, even in the absence of ulcer. Distal to the constriction there may be no inflammation at all, or very little, suggesting that the deformity, although exposing the proximal bulb to insult, has protected that portion beyond the deformity. As one sees the recurrent ulcers which occur in many of these bulbs, one is struck by their small size and superficial nature and questions whether these are the same types of lesions which resulted in the deformity, or whether the deformity itself has altered the pattern of disease and in some instances now becomes responsible for the recurrences. Although in most cases the constriction deformity can be readily passed by the endoscope, it is at this level that obstructing stenosis usually occurs.

Another common deformity results from the pyloroduodenal, pyloric channel, or juxtapyloric ulcer. Although some of these ulcers are purely gastric, most of them are wholly or in part within the duodenum. These ulcerations, usually situated superiorly, lead to longitudinal contraction which results in flattening or loss of the superior recess of the duodenal bulb, eccentricity of the pylorus, and proximal displacement of the superior recess, so that a duodenal ulcer may radiologically appear to be in the stomach. The lower quadrants of the involved segment become redundant and may project into the lumen as prominent pseudopolyps. Although pyloric stenosis may occasionally develop, it occurs less frequently than a casual glance at the X-ray would suggest. There is a strong tendency for recurrence of pyloro-

duodenal ulcers, and the X-ray may not be entirely reliable in differentiating scar from recurrent ulcer, particularly if the ulcer is less than 7 mm in diameter. Endoscopically, on the other hand, one has little difficulty in exploring the involved area.

Some duodenal bulbs are so grossly deformed that they become hard to classify. This may result from a combination of simple deformities, external adhesions, or other miscellaneous influences. In this situation both the radiologist and the endoscopist may have problems. Endoscopy is particularly difficult if an ulcer is located behind large pseudopolyps which virtually fill the lumen, beyond long areas of stenosis, or beyond sharp kinks.

MORE ABOUT DUODENITIS

The association of duodenitis with duodenal ulcer disease has already been discussed and should not be a subject for controversy, but further words on the subject of duodenitis are in order. Duodenitis is considered to be present endoscopically if there is obvious mucosal abnormality manifested by gross hyperemia, intramural hemorrhage, and/or superficial erosion. Microscopically, it is characterized by vascular engorgement, edema, and varying numbers of round cells, eosinophils, and polymorphonuclear leukocytes, depending upon the acuteness, severity, or duration of the process. Mucosal erosion may or may not be present. The borderline between normal or excessive numbers of round cells and eosinophils is a tenuous one, and may lead to disagreement among pathologists; there is a tendency for pathologists to view vascular engorgement or red cell extravasation as artifacts produced by the biopsy forceps. Although it might be more accurate to label these lesions "hemorrhagic mucosal lesions with or without erosion," it is simpler to use the shorter term "duodenitis."

Two broad types of duodenitis are generally seen. The first shows little distortion of mucosal contour, and for this reason it is referred to as superficial duodenitis (Fig. 41–9). It is not usually recognizable radiologically. The modifying terms hemorrhagic or erosive may be added when these features are striking. Aspirin and alcohol may be responsible for some lesions of this type. The second type is associated with localized swellings, which appear as hyperemic mamillations when located on smooth mucosa or as reddened beads or nodes when seen on folds (Fig. 41–10). Superficial erosion may also be present on some of these lesions. This type of abnormality is loosely referred to as "nodal" and is usually visible radiologically as an enlargement of folds. However, not all radiologically enlarged folds are an indication of duodenitis.

Occasionally the endoscopist encounters multiple flat nodules or beads, many showing marked hyperemia on their apices. Radiologically these are readily demonstrated; they are often referred to as hypertrophy of Brunner's glands. Perhaps they are. Endoscopic biopsy in several of these cases has shown an inflammatory infiltrate descending into the Brunner gland zone, indicating that more might be going on than simple hypertrophy. Full-thickness surgical biopsy might be helpful in further elucidating this problem.

DUODENAL NEOPLASMS

The duodenum may occasionally be the site of neoplasms, both benign and malignant, including most of the varieties found elsewhere in the gastrointestinal tract. Those lesions which involve the mucosa may be diagnosed by biopsy; but submucosal neoplasms may escape identification, because the small biopsy forceps now in use may only avulse normal mucosa from the surface of the neoplasm.

Of the benign neoplasms, adenomas are the most common. They may be composed of mucosal cells or the cells of Brunner's glands. Lipomas and leiomyomas are the most common of the wide variety of submucous neoplasms which may occur.[22] Pancreatic cell rests and gastric mucosal cell rests may also be encountered.[23, 24]

Primary malignancies are rare; they include adenocarcinoma, the lymphoblastomas, sarcomas of various types, and carcinoid. Malignancy in adjacent structures may invade the duodenum and may ulcerate and bleed. We have encountered primary lesions extending from the right kidney, gallbladder, and pancreas. Metastatic malignancy rarely occurs and usually involves the submucosa, invading the mucosa by extension.[25] Central necrosis with ulceration and hemorrhage may ensue. Melanoma is among the most common.[14] Radiologically these lesions may resemble a bull's-eye owing to the mass with central umbilication or ulceration.

Not everything that resembles neoplasm radiologically is actually neoplastic. Abnormal fold patterns or associated inflammatory reaction may result in the formation of pseudotumors either in the bulb or elsewhere in the duodenum. Endoscopy can be helpful in ruling out neoplasm and avoiding unnecessary surgery.

MISCELLANEOUS STATES

Any of the wide variety of pathological processes involving the duodenum may be encountered and may require biopsy for identification. Unfortunately, the small size and superficial nature of the specimens obtainable may not always yield sufficiently specific information. Those malabsorptive states with diffuse mucosal involvement such as Whipple's disease may be identified, but the superiority of suction biopsy specimens makes them more suitable for diagnosis so long as pinpoint accuracy is not required.

Diverticula may be encountered; they are best inspected with a lateral viewing instrument. True diverticula of the bulb are rare. It should be possible to obtain cultures directly from diverticula if these are deemed to serve any useful purpose in a given situation.

THE DESCENDING DUODENUM, INCLUDING PANCREATOGRAPHY AND CHOLANGIOGRAPHY

Endoscopy beyond the duodenal bulb as far as the ligament of Treitz is now a practical procedure, and it can be expected to furnish more specific information than hypotonic duodenography. The detection of postbulbar ulcers and mucosal diaphragms,[26] inspection of diverticula, and identification and biopsy of neoplasms have all been accomplished. Its most spectacular use, however, is to visualize the papilla of Vater both for purposes of biopsy and for cannulation of the pancreatic and biliary ducts in order to obtain contrast radiography.

Extensive research and development in Japan by the Machida Manufacturing Company and the Olympus Optical Company in cooperation with a number of endoscopists, including Oi, Shindo, Soma, and Niwa and their colleagues, culminated in the production of practical duodenoscopes[27-30] and the successful cannulation of the papilla of Vater in 1969. In 1970, Oi summarized his experiences at the annual meeting of the American Society for Gastrointestinal Endoscopy. This detailed presentation, subsequently published,[31] described the technique of the procedure and some of the significant findings, including the diagnosis of pancreatic neoplasms, biliary tract neoplasms, and calculi in both the common duct and the gallbladder. The procedure is now widely practiced in Japan and is coming into use in the United States and other parts of the world as instruments become available. Its true usefulness in comparison with transhepatic cholangiography, selective arteriography, and scanning techniques has not yet been fully evaluated, but it would seem to have much to offer in safety and in the nature of the information to be obtained.

REFERENCES

1. Schindler, R. Ein völlig ungefährliches flexibles Gastroskop. München Med. Wchnschr. 79:1268, 1932.
2. Hirschowitz, B. I., Curtiss, L. E., and Peters, C. W. Demonstration of a new gastroscope, the "fiberscope." Gastroenterology 35:50, 1958.
3. Hirschowitz, B. I. Endoscopic examination of the stomach and duodenal cap with the fiberscope. Lancet 1:1074, 1961.
4. Burnett, W. An evaluation of the gastroduodenal fiberscope. Gut 3:361, 1962.
5. Belber, J. P. Intraduodenal cinematography in normal and pathologic duodenal bulbs. Gastrointest. Endoscop. 15:160, 1969.
6. Hirschowitz, B. I. A fibreoptic flexible oesophagoscope. Lancet 2:388, 1963.
7. LoPresti, P. A., and Hilmi, O. M. Clinical experience with a new Foroblique fiberoptic esophagoscope. Amer. J. Dig. Dis. 9:690, 1964.
8. Belber, J. P. Endoscopic examination of the duodenal bulb. A comparison with X-ray. Gastroenterology 61:55, 1971.
9. Hayashida, T., and Kidokoro, T. End results of early gastric cancer collected from 22 institutions. Stomach Intest. 4:1077, 1969.
10. Kobayashi, S., Prolla, J. C., Yagi, M., et al. Gastroscopic diagnosis of early gastric carcinoma based on Japanese classification. Gastrointest. Endoscop. 16:92, 1969.
11. Morrissey, J. F., and Koizumi, H. The endoscopic diagnosis of gastric cancer. Proc. Nat. Cancer Conf. 46:433, 1968.
12. Veterans Administration Cooperative Study of Gastric Ulcer. Gastroenterology 64:433, 1968.
13. Monaco, A. P., Roth, S. I., Castleman, B., et al. Adenomatous polyps of the stomach. A clinical and pathological study of 153 cases. Cancer 15:456, 1962.
14. Belber, J. P. Malignant melanoma metastatic to the stomach, gastroscopic observations. Gastrointest. Endoscop. 8:20, 1961.
15. MacDonald, W. C., and Rubin, C. E. Gastric biopsy—a critical evaluation. Gastroenterology 58:143, 1967.
16. Stempien, S. J., Dagradi, A. E., Reingold, I. M., et al. Hypertrophic hypersecretory gastropathy. Amer. J. Dig. Dis. 9:471, 1964.
17. Silvis, S. E., Blackwood, W. M., and Vennes, J. The selection of gastric hypersecretory patients by blind gastroscopic film review. Gastrointest. Endoscop. 18:116, 1972.
18. Palmer, E. D. What Menetrier really said. Gastrointest. Endoscop. 15:83, 1968.
19. Mackman, S., Lemmer, K. E., and Morrissey, J. F. Postoperative reflux alkali gastritis and esophagitis. Amer. J. Surg. 121:694, 1971.
20. Amer-Ahmadi, H., McCray, R. S., Martin, F., et al. Reassessment of massive upper gastrointestinal hemorrhage on the wards of the Boston City Hospital. Surg. Clin. N. Amer. 49:715, 1969.
21. Belber, J. P. Duodenal bulb visualization with the Hirschowitz gastroduodenal fiberscope and the Hirschowitz gastroduodenal fiberscope with deflecting tip: A comparative study. Gastrointest. Endoscop. 17:34, 1970.
22. River, L., Silverstein, J., and Tope, J. W. Benign neoplasms of the small intestine. A critical comprehensive review with reports of 20 new cases. Internat. Abstr. Surg. 102:1, 1956.
23. Belber, J. P., and Musick, R. Ectopic gastric mucosa in the duodenum. Annual meeting of the American Society for Gastrointestinal Endoscopy, Boston, Massachusetts, May 20, 1971 (abstract).
24. James, A. H. Gastric epithelium in the duodenum. Gut 5:285, 1964.
25. Willis, R. A. The Spread of Tumours in the Human Body. 2nd ed. London, Butterworth, 1952, pp. 212, 216.
26. Ahmed, M. Y., Kepkay, D. L., Beck, I. T., et al. Congenital duodenal diaphragm in an adult. Diagnosis by duodenoscopy. Gastrointest. Endoscop. 18:120, 1972.
27. Oi, I. Additional report on study of duodenofiberscope. Endoscopy 10:420, 1968.
28. Ogoshi, K., Tobita, Y., and Hara, Y. Endoscopic observation of the duodenum and pancreatocholedochography using duodenal fiberscope under direct vision. Gastroenterol. Endoscop. 12:83, 1970.
29. Shindo, S., Kanki, K., and Yanagisawa, F. Duodenofiberscopy. Gastroenterol. Endoscop. 12:70, 1970.
30. Soma, S., Fujita, R., and Kidokoro, T. Clinical application of duodenofiberscope. Gastroenterol. Endoscop. 12:97, 1970.
31. Oi, I. Fiberduodenoscopy and endoscopic pancreatocholangiography. Gastrointest. Endoscop. 17:59, 1970.

Chapter 42

Gastric Secretory Testing

Jon I. Isenberg

The greatest body of data relating gastric secretory tests to gastrointestinal disease concerns gastric acid secretion. In certain diseases, however, there may be alteration of other gastric secretory constituents (see below). Gastric acid secretion will be reviewed in some detail, and the other constituents of gastric juice will be briefly discussed.

HISTORY

On June 6, 1822, William Beaumont began caring for his famous patient Alexis St. Martin. Over the succeeding 11 years, Beaumont conducted and meticulously recorded his classic series of experiments on gastric secretion.[1] These series of well designed and conducted experiments initiated gastric secretory testing in man.

In 1876, Leube studied the effect of a standard meal on gastric secretion aspirated with a large orogastric tube seven hours after the meal. In the latter part of the last century and the early part of this century, Ewald and Boas,[2] Ehrenreich,[3] and Rehfuss[4] reported their results of taking samples of gastric juice at frequent intervals after a standard meal. This test became known as the "fractional test meal."

In the 1920's resting, or basal, gastric acid secretion was measured. Basal secretion was interpreted as being secondary to "psychic" factors.[5] In 1932, Henning and

Norjsoth reported that the amount of gastric juice aspirated overnight in patients with duodenal ulcer disease was greater than in normal subjects.[6] Dragstedt confirmed this observation, and he introduced the 12-hour overnight gastric aspiration test for evaluation of patients with peptic ulcer disease.[7]

In the 1930's Ihre[8] and Polland and Bloomfield[9] measured the effect of 0.01 mg per kilogram of histamine dihydrochloride on human gastric acid secretion. In 1953 Kay reported that the dose of 0.04 mg per kilogram of histamine acid phosphate produced "maximal acid output" in man.[10] This test became known as the augmented histamine test. Kay proposed that there might be a correlation between "maximal acid output" and parietal cell mass in man. Card and Marks later demonstrated that there is indeed a strong correlation between parietal cell mass and "maximal acid output."[11]

METHODS

PATIENT SELECTION

Gastric secretory testing can be arbitrarily divided into two main categories: (1) clinical secretory testing, and (2) investigative or research-oriented testing. In hospitals which have a secretory laboratory, gastric secretion is usually measured in patients in whom alteration of gastric acid secretion is suspected (e.g., increased acid secretion in patients with duodenal ulcer disease, or decreased acid secretion in patients with gastric ulcer, gastric cancer, or pernicious anemia). At present a difficult question to answer is: What is the role of gastric secretory testing in the diagnosis and management of patients with gastrointestinal disease? Only in rare instances do secretory results directly influence the diagnosis or treatment of a specific patient (see below).

It is our opinion that secretory testing should be performed in the following cases:

1. In patients in whom the diagnosis of Zollinger-Ellison syndrome (see pp. 743 to 750) is clinically suspected. The great majority of these patients have an increased basal and stimulated gastric acid secretion,[12] but a small percentage may have normal secretory studies.[13]

2. In those preoperative patients in whom an acid-reducing surgical procedure is being considered for the treatment of peptic ulcer disease. In these patients, both pre- and postoperative secretory testing should be performed in order to measure the effect of surgery on gastric acid secretion.

3. In patients with duodenal ulcer disease. Gastric secretory testing should probably be performed at least once in these circumstances. Some subjects with Zollinger-Ellison syndrome will have a clinical picture indistinguishable from uncomplicated duodenal ulcer disease, and these patients may be diagnosed by secretory testing.

4. In patients who have had an acid-reducing operation for peptic ulcer disease and who develop symptoms which suggest recurrent ulceration. Some of these patients may have the Zollinger-Ellison syndrome or a retained gastric antrum (see pp. 829 to 839), or may be achlorhydric. This latter finding makes the clinical diagnosis of recurrent ulceration extremely unlikely.

5. In patients with gastric ulcer. Acid secretion should be measured in these patients to be certain that they are capable of secreting acid. The combination of achlorhydria (i.e., the inability of the gastric pH to decrease to less than 6.0 with a maximal stimulatory dose of a gastric secretagogue capable of producing maximal gastric acid secretion) with benign gastric ulcer is exceedingly rare,[14] and suggests that the gastric lesion is malignant (see p. 587).

6. In patients in whom the diagnosis of Menetrier's disease[15] (see pp. 528 and 570), gastritis,[16] or gastric atrophy[17] (see pp. 566 to 570) is suspected. In addition to measuring gastric acid secretion in these subjects, measurement of gastric electrolyte and protein secretion may be of clinical value.

7. In postvagotomy subjects to test for the completeness of vagotomy.

8. In patients with pernicious anemia to demonstrate achlorhydria and to rule out other causes of vitamin B_{12} deficiency (e.g., terminal ileal disease).

There are a number of investigative gastric secretory tests. Until their clinical value becomes apparent, their role in the diagnosis or management of gastrointestinal disease remains to be determined.

PATIENT PREPARATION

Subjects should fast for approximately ten to 12 hours before secretory testing. In subjects with delayed gastric emptying of solids (e.g., post-truncal vagotomy, gastric antral ulcer, or gastric antral carcinoma), it may be necessary to place the patient on a clear liquid diet for a day or so before secretory testing. If there is retained food in the stomach on the morning of testing, the patient's stomach should be lavaged clear with water. He should be instructed to ingest only clear liquids that day, and return the next day for testing. Gastric secretory testing should not be performed in a subject with retained food in the stomach. Since food within the stomach is a potent stimulus for gastric acid secretion and since food is a potent buffer of acid secretion, secretory testing under these conditions will be inaccurate.

All medications which might affect gastric secretion should be discontinued at least 24 hours prior to testing. The patient should be questioned specifically regarding certain drugs which have been shown to alter gastric secretion, such as cholinergic drugs,[18] anticholinergic drugs,[19] some tranquilizers (e.g., diazepam),[20] and carbonic anhydrase inhibitors.[21]

In some series, patients have been instructed to expectorate their saliva during secretory testing.[22] In other series no efforts have been made to separate salivary secretion from gastric secretion.[23] There have been no studies to determine the advantage or disadvantage of expectorating saliva on the measurement of gastric acid secretion. Although the presence of a nasogastric or orogastric tube may stimulate salivary secretion, there appears to be no appreciable advantage in separating salivary secretion from gastric secretion.

GASTRIC TUBES AND TUBE POSITION

A number of nasogastric and orogastric tubes are available for gastric secretory testing. Recently a plastic tube with a second, smaller side sump tube for an air-bleed to improve gastric aspiration has been introduced to collect gastric juice.[24] At present, no one type of tube has been convincingly shown to be superior to another. Since fluoroscopic tube placement may improve the accuracy of collection,[25] it is advisable that the tube be radiopaque.

At fluoroscopy, the tip of the tube should rest in the middle of gastric antrum. At the time of fluoroscopy it is not uncommon to find the tip of the tube coiled in the gastric fundus, the esophagus, or even the tracheobronchial tree.[26] If fluoroscopic placement is not readily available, the tube can be passed so that the tip is approximately 55 to 60 cm from the nares. After aspiration of the gastric residual, a known quantity (30 to 60 ml) of water may be rapidly instilled via the tube. If the tube is correctly placed, immediate aspiration of the instilled water should yield the instilled amount. If less than 90 per cent of the instilled volume returns, the tube should be adjusted so that the instilled volume is easily aspirated. By showing that the instilled volume can be readily recovered before starting testing, information can be obtained as to whether the tube is properly placed and accurate secretory testing can be performed.[27]

PATIENT POSITION

During secretory testing the patient should be in a comfortable position. There is some evidence to suggest that positioning the patient in a recumbent position, on his left side with feet elevated, may be better than having him in a sitting position.[28] If convenient, it is advisable to have the patient supine during secretory testing, particularly when using a secretagogue which may produce hypotension (e.g., histamine or betazole) or hypoglycemia (e.g., insulin). If it is not possible to have the patient supine, the sitting position is adequate for clinical testing.[27]

NONABSORBABLE MARKERS

Infusion of nonabsorbable markers (e.g., phenol red, $Cr^{51} Cl_3$) into the stomach during collection of gastric juice in order to improve the accuracy of collection has been studied.[29] At present there is no evidence that infusion of any marker significantly improves the accuracy of measuring acid secretion.[30] Markers need not be used for routine gastric secretory testing.

GASTRIC ASPIRATION

Gastric juice may be collected either by manual suction or with a pump with negative pressure (approximately 50 mm Hg). Both methods are effective, but the former is more tedious and requires more personnel when performing many studies on a single day. When using a suction pump, it is important that the suction be broken at approximately two- to three-minute intervals and the tube manually lavaged with air to ensure tube potency. Air lavage need not be performed as frequently when using a tube with an air vent.

TUBELESS TESTS

Small radiotelemetry capsules have been used to record intragastric pH.[31] These capsules are capable of transmitting a radio signal to a receiver placed on the patient's abdomen. The signal is then converted into pH and may be recorded on a standard recorder. These capsules are capable of accurately recording both in vitro and in vivo pH from 1.5 to 9.0. Tests have been devised in an attempt to measure basal and stimulated acid secretion by using the pH capsule and having the patient swallow known quantities of bicarbonate.[32] This method, however, lacks accuracy when compared with the standard method involving collection of gastric juice. The pH capsule is of little value in accurately measuring the quantity of gastric juice secreted. It is useful, however, in measuring the intravisceral pH of other areas within the gut (e.g., esophagus and small intestine).

Azur-A resin (Diagnex Blue) is an exchange resin which, in the presence of acid, dissociates and is absorbed from the gut.[33] The absorbed dye is then excreted via the kidneys, coloring the urine blue. Although some studies have found adequate correlation between the Diagnex Blue test and acid secretion, a recent review of 420 patients disclosed a high incidence of false-negative tests, as well as some false-positive tests.[34] Since this test is not quantitative, it should not be used as a method for measuring gastric acid secretion. It may be of value in screening large numbers of subjects for decreased acid secretion to aid in the detection of gastric carcinoma.[35]

Recently, technetium (^{99m}Tc-pertechnetate) has been reported to be secreted by the stomach and salivary glands as is iodide. It was evaluated as a potential method of measuring gastric acid secretion. Since technetium can be secreted by the achlorhydric stomach, and since there is a poor correlation between ^{99m}Tc gastric uptake and acid secretion, it is of no value in measuring gastric acid secretion.[36]

BASAL SECRETION

After ensuring proper tube position and making the subject comfortable, the stomach should be completely emptied. Since this gastric sample is frequently diluted with swallowed water and saliva during passage of the tube, it is usually discarded. In patients in whom excessively large volumes, greater than 500 ml, are aspirated just after tube placement, the volume should be recorded. This finding suggests gastric retention, and further evaluation is indicated.

Gastric juice is then collected in ten- or 15-minute periods for one hour. The volume obtained during each collection period is recorded, and titratable acid mea-

sured (see below). The acid secretory rate obtained during this hour is referred to as the basal secretion.

STIMULANTS OF GASTRIC ACID SECRETION

A number of stimulants have been used to produce gastric secretion in man. Histamine, betazole, and the antral hormone gastrin or one of its analogues are the most commonly used agents in routine clinical testing. Insulin or other glucocytopenic agents are used in testing for completeness of vagotomy. The effects of caffeine,[37] alcohol,[38] food,[39] and intravenous calcium[40] have also been studied.

HISTAMINE AND BETAZOLE

At present, the principal stimulus used in gastric acid secretory testing in the United States is histamine (3-β-aminoethylimidazole) or its analogue betazole (3-β-aminoethylpyrazole). Histamine and betazole have many untoward side effects.[41-42] The major side effect of each is hypotension with shock. In addition, each agent may produce pain at the injection site, dizziness, nausea, palpitations, abdominal cramps, headache, and flushing. The administration of an antihistaminic drug prior to histamine administration decreases the severity of the side effects without altering the effect of histamine on gastric secretion.[43] Since betazole has fewer side effects than histamine, an antihistamine need not be given before betazole injection. The incidence of betazole-induced hypotension (2 mg per kilogram subcutaneously) has been estimated at approximately 2.5 per cent.)[42] In the vast majority of subjects, betazole produces pain at the injection site and a flushed sensation without other untoward effects. Histamine has been used for gastric secretory testing in patients with pulmonary disease without altering pulmonary function.[44]

Since the introduction of the augmented histamine test by Kay, the standard dose of histamine acid phosphate has been 40 μg per kilogram, injected either intramuscularly or subcutaneously (Table

TABLE 42–1. DOSE, ROUTE, AND TIMING OF PEAK ACID SECRETORY RESPONSE TO VARIOUS STIMULI

	Dose	Route	Timing of Peak Response
Histamine			
HAP	40 μg/kg	SC	20–60 min
Hdi HCl	50 μg/kg	SC	30–45 min
HAP	40 μg/kg/hr	IV	30–45 min
Betazole	1.5 μg/kg	SC	30–90 min
	2.0 μg/kg	SC	45–90 min
	100 mg	IM	45–75 min
	200 mg	SC	45–90 min
Gastrin	2 μg/kg	SC and IM	30–40 min
	1 μg/kg	IM	
	0.8 μg/kg/hr	IV	20–60 min
Pentagastrin	6 μg/kg	SC	15–45 min
	1 mg q 10 min	Snuff	15–45 min
	6 μg/kg	IM	10–30 min
	6 μg/kg/hr	IV infusion	5–20 min
Tetragastrin	10 μg/kg	IM	
	20 μg/kg	IM	15–45 min
Insulin	0.2 units/kg	IV	30–90 min

42–1). The dose usually required for maximal acid secretion when given as an intravenous infusion is 40 μg per kilogram per hour.[10] In patients weighing less than 60 kg, the dose of histamine acid phosphate required for maximal acid secretion is somewhat greater than 40 μg per kilogram.[45] Histamine is available either as histamine acid phosphate or as histamine dihydrochloride (2.75 mg histamine acid phosphate = 1.66 mg histamine dihydrochloride = 1 mg histamine base).[46] After histamine acid phosphate injection, the peak secretory effect usually occurs during the first postinjection hour.[47]

The dose of betazole (Histalog) required for maximal acid secretion is approximately 1.5 to 2.0 mg per kilogram injected intramuscularly or subcutaneously.[48] The incidence of side effects is slightly greater with the 2.0 mg per kilogram dose. Betazole usually produces its peak effect during the second postinjection hour (Fig. 42–1).[49] Therefore in order to measure maximal acid secretion with betazole, it is necessary to collect gastric juice for two hours after injection. Betazole, 2 mg per kilogram given subcutaneously, produces a slightly greater peak acid output than histamine dihydrochloride, 50 μg per kilogram subcutaneously, but there is a highly significant correlation between the secretory responses produced by the two agents (r = 0.89; see Fig. 42–2).[50]

In summary, both betazole and histamine are potent stimulants of gastric acid secretion. Since histamine requires antihistamine premedication and may have more frequent side effects, betazole is preferable. The recommended dose is 1.5 mg per kilogram, and gastric juice should

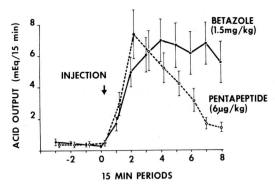

Figure 42–1. Gastric acid output before and after betazole (1.5 mg per kilogram subcutaneously) or pentagastrin (6 μg per kilogram subcutaneously) in 20 patients with various gastrointestinal diseases. Each patient was studied once with each drug. Each point represents the mean of 20 studies, and the vertical lines represent standard error of mean. (From Isenberg, J. I., Brooks, A. M., and Grossman, M. I.: J.A.M.A. 206:2897, 1968.)

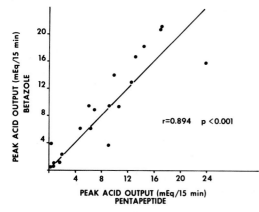

Figure 42–2. Comparison of peak gastric acid output (milliequivalents per 15 minute period with pentagastrin (6 μg per kilogram subcutaneously) and betazole (1.5 mg per kilogram subcutaneously) as stimulants. Each point is result of two tests in one subject. Line is the line of identity; all points would fall on it if all responses of two agents were equal. (From Isenberg, J. I., Brooks, A. M., and Grossman, M. I.: J.A.M.A. *206*:2897, 1968.)

be collected for two hours after injection. Because betazole may infrequently produce potentially life-threatening side effects, the patient should be carefully attended throughout the test. In addition, sterile intravenous tubing, sterile saline, and vasopressors should be readily available in the event of hypotension and shock.

GASTRIN, TETRAGASTRIN, AND PENTAGASTRIN

Pure gastrin I and gastrin II have been chemically characterized, and gastrin I has been synthesized.[51] Gastrin II has been used as a gastric secretory stimulant in investigative studies in man,[52] but it is not readily available. Although pure gastrin has not been studied in large series of patients, it does not appear to have significant side effects.[52]

The C-terminal tetrapeptide amide of gastrin (Trp-Met-Asp-Phe-NH$_2$) possesses all the physiological actions of the parent molecule, heptadecapeptide gastrin.[53] The synthetic tetrapeptide amide (tetragastrin) has been used in secretory testing, and produces maximal gastric acid secretory response which is comparable to the max-

imal response produced by histamine acid phosphate.[54] Tetragastrin also produces minimal side effects.

More recently, pentagastrin (N-tertiary butyloxycarbonyl-β-Ala-Trp-Met-Asp-Phe-NH$_2$: Peptavalon) has been used for gastric secretory testing in man.[55] It is effective when given intravenously as a continuous infusion or as an intramuscular or subcutaneous injection. It has also been shown to be effective when given as intranasal snuff.[56] Pentagastrin is capable of producing peak rates of gastric acid secretion which are similar to peak responses produced by histamine, betazole, or gastrin II.[55-57] The dose of pentagastrin required for maximal acid secretion in man is approximately 1 to 6 μg per kilogram when injected intramuscularly or subcutaneously, or 1 to 6 μg per kilogram per hour when given by continuous infusion (Table 42–1).[55] The timing of the peak response to pentagastrin is rapid, occurring within the first 45 to 60 minutes after injection (Fig. 42–1).[55]

Gastrin, tetragastrin, and pentagastrin are all capable of producing untoward side effects. The side effects for the most part are minor, consisting of nausea, sweating, abdominal and lower chest cramps, faintness, and infrequent hypotension.[55] The frequency of side effects increases with increasing dose, and in our experience is more common with rapid (30-second) intravenous injection (as has been used to measure the effect of pentagastrin on lower esophageal sphincter pressure).[58] When compared with histamine or betazole, pentagastrin has two major advantages: it has considerably fewer side effects, and it produces an earlier peak response than betazole.

Unfortunately, at present, pentagastrin, tetragastrin, and gastrin are not approved by the U.S. Food and Drug Administration for routine clinical use in the United States.

In summary, for routine gastric secretory testing, pentagastrin is the agent of choice in those countries in which it is approved for clinical use. After measuring basal secretion, pentagastrin (6 μg per kilogram) is then given either intramuscularly or subcutaneously. Gastric juice should be collected for four to six 15-minute postinjection periods.

INSULIN, TOLBUTAMIDE, 2-DEOXY-D-GLUCOSE

Hypoglycemia is an effective method for inducing vagal-stimulated gastric acid secretion (pp 152 and 181).[59] Vagotomy, with drainage procedure or antrectomy, is a commonly performed operation in patients with peptic ulcer (see pp. 779 to 787). In order to test for the completeness of vagotomy, three agents which produce a decrease in intracellular glucose concentration have been used: insulin, tolbutamide, and 2-deoxy-D-glucose (2DG).

Graded doses of insulin have been shown to produce graded gastric acid secretory responses in normal subjects and in subjects with an incomplete vagotomy.[60-62] The dose of insulin which produced peak acid secretory rates in both groups was 0.2 unit per kilogram given as a rapid intravenous injection. After insulin injection, gastric juice should be collected in 10- or 15-minute periods for two hours. The major side effect of insulin is hypoglycemia, resulting in seizures, coma, and even death.[63] It is of critical importance that a physician be in attendance throughout insulin testing. In addition, 50-ml ampules of 50 per cent glucose solution with 50-ml syringes and needles should be readily available in the event that the patient demonstrates signs of marked hypoglycemia. The insulin test need not be terminated if the patient develops diaphoresis, nervousness, or the sensation of hunger, because these are signs of effective hypoglycemia. If the patient is sleepy and not arousable, the test should be terminated and the patient should be given 50 per cent glucose intravenously and other necessary supportive measures.

Some laboratories collect venous blood samples for glucose measurement at one or more intervals (30 and 45 minutes) after insulin injection;[64] others do not.[65] The nadir in blood sugar occurs approximately 30 minutes after insulin injection.[66] If a patient develops symptoms of hypoglycemia (i.e., diaphoresis, nervousness, hunger, somnolence) and has a good secretory response to insulin, blood sugar measurement is not necessary.[65] If, however, there is no insulin-induced secretory response even in the presence of symptoms of hypoglycemia, it is important to be certain that the blood sugar decreased to less than approximately 50 mg per 100 ml. Since blood sugar determination is readily available and is an accurate laboratory measurement, it is advisable to measure blood sugar 30 minutes after insulin injection.

Tolbutamide has been used instead of insulin to induce hypoglycemia to test for vagal innervation of the stomach.[67] The dose used is 1 mg intravenously. There is no apparent clinical advantage to using tolbutamide instead of insulin in testing for completeness of vagotomy. It is not known whether or not untoward side effects are any less frequent with tolbutamide than with insulin.

Recently 2DG has been used instead of insulin to produce glucocytopenia.[68] 2DG is converted into 2-DG-6-phosphate, which is not metabolizable and thereby produces glucocytopenia. The side effects are similar to those of insulin. Since intravenous glucose injection probably does not immediately correct 2DG-induced glucocytopenia, 2DG is potentially more dangerous than insulin. 2DG therefore should not be used for routine postvagotomy clinical testing.

CALCIUM

Calcium infused intravenously is an effective stimulus of gastric acid secretion.[40] Calcium (4 mg per kilogram per hour) increases gastric acid secretion to approximately 30 per cent of maximally stimulated acid secretion as produced by histamine (4 μg per kilogram). The effect of calcium infusion is gradual, and the peak effect is seen during the second or third hour after starting the infusion. The stimulatory effect of calcium can be abolished by atropine, pentolinium, and magnesium.[40] Reeder and coworkers have reported a moderate, approximately two-fold increase in serum gastrin during calcium infusion.[69]

Passaro et al. have reported that calcium infusion (4 mg. per kilogram per hour) produces a marked increase in gastric acid secretion and serum gastrin in patients with Zollinger-Ellison syndrome. They have proposed that the calcium infusion test may be of value in differentiating patients with Zollinger-Ellison syndrome from non-Zollinger-Ellison syndrome hypersecretors.[70]

TEST MEALS

The effect of a number of test meals on gastric acid secretion has been studied (see p. 180). Rune quantitated the amount of gastric acid secretion after a meal of meat, potatoes, and vegetables.[71] He measured arterial pH and pCO_2 at frequent intervals, and calculated the base excess. He concluded that the response to the meal was comparable to maximal stimulated gastric acid secretion as produced with histamine acid phosphate infusion (40 μg per kilogram per hour).

The effect of other test meals (e.g., caffeine, carbohydrate, protein, and alcohol) on gastric acid secretion has also been studied.[2, 37-39] At intervals after meals, a small aliquot can be aspirated and hydrogen ion concentration measured.[39] If a liquid meal plus a nonabsorbable marker is injected, the amount of meal which has left the stomach can be calculated as well as the amount of gastric acid secretion.[72]

Since these tests are not well standardized, and are time consuming, they are not commonly used in the routine measuring of gastric acid secretion.

CHOLINERGIC AGENTS

Cholinergic agents increase gastric secretion in man.[18] These agents, however, do not increase gastric acid secretion to maximal levels of secretion with clinically tolerable doses. Also, they have not been systematically studied in large groups of patients. Therefore they are not of clinical value at present.

INHIBITORS OF GASTRIC ACID SECRETION

There are a number of hormones and drugs which are capable of inhibiting gastric acid secretion. These include secretin,[73] cholecystokinin,[74] prostaglandins,[75] glucagon,[76] and probably other yet unidentified "enterogastrones." Drugs such as anticholinergics, carbonic anhydrase inhibitors, and diazepam also decrease gastric acid secretion.[19-21] At present, there is little information on the effect of these inhibitors on gastric acid secretion in various disease states.

ANALYSIS OF GASTRIC JUICE

After proper tube placement, gastric juice should be collected for at least one hour to determine basal gastric acid secretion. In past years, an overnight collection of gastric juice was obtained to measure nocturnal (i.e., basal) gastric acid secretion. It has been noted that there is a good correlation between a well performed one-hour basal collection and basal secretion as measured by overnight collection.[77] Overnight collection therefore need not be performed.

Gastric juice volume should be collected in ten- or 15-minute intervals. The color of the gastric aspirate should be noted. If bile is aspirated during the basal collection, and if convenient, the patient should be refluoroscoped to be certain that the tube is in correct position. Sometimes the tip of the tube may pass into the duodenum and require readjustment. The tube should be adjusted so that unobstructed bile-free return is obtained. In patients who have had prior upper gastrointestinal surgery, particularly subtotal gastrectomy with Billroth II anastomosis, it may not be possible to obtain bile-free gastric juice. Despite a number of special tubes designed to occlude the gastroenterostomy, secretory testing in these subjects is frequently inaccurate.

The presence of blood in the gastric aspirate should be noted. Although there may be a small amount of blood after passage of a nasogastric tube, this should become clear with water lavage of the stomach. If there is a moderate amount of blood in the basal aspirate, the study should be postponed and appropriate studies performed to determine the bleeding site.

MEASUREMENT OF GASTRIC ACID

There are three methods to measure gastric acid: the indicator-titration method, the pH meter-titration method, and the pH method.

Of the indicators used to measure gastric acid, there are two main categories. There are indicators which change color at or near pH 3.5 (e.g., Topfer's reagent) and those which change color at approximately pH 7 to 8 (e.g., neutral red or phenol red). Those which change color at pH 3.5 were previously referred to as measuring "free" acid. Those which change color at about pH 7 measure titratable acid ("free"+ "combined" acid = titratable acid). Since there are substances (e.g., protein) in the gastric juice which are capable of combining with the hydrogen ion of the secreted HCl and thereby alter its activity coefficient, there is no rationale for separating "free" from "combined" acid.[78] It is preferable to measure total titratable acid.

Since indicators depend upon the accuracy and precision of the observer and are not usually as accurate as a good pH meter, the pH method is better. If, however, a good pH meter is not available, the indicator method (phenol red) is satisfactory for clinical testing.

The pH meter–titration method requires an accurate pH meter. A known aliquot of gastric juice is titrated to pH 7.0 with dilute NaOH (0.1 or 0.2 N). In our laboratory we use 0.2 ml samples of gastric juice diluted with 4 ml of distilled water. These are titrated with 0.2 N NaOH. The volume of titrant in milliliters (times 1000) required to reach pH 7 equals the hydrogen ion concentration in milliequivalents per liter. Gastric secretory volume multiplied by hydrogen ion concentration equals acid output per unit time. In order to maintain accuracy, the pH meter should be calibrated daily before use with two standard buffers (e.g., pH 2.0 and 7.0). In addition, control titrations should be done with a known concentration of HCl (e.g., titration of 0.2 ml of 0.1 N HCl). Accuracy should be within 3 per cent.

Since pH is a reflection of hydrogen ion activity, Moore and Scarlata have proposed using carefully measured pH and converting this into hydrogen ion concentration using a conversion table.[79] This method requires precision buffers for standardization and a moderate amount of time for measurement of each sample. Since the pH-titration method is rapid, accurate, and precise, it is our opinion that it is the method of choice for most clinical laboratories.

EXPRESSION OF RESULTS

Basal gastric acid secretion refers to interdigestive or fasting gastric secretion. Conventionally, basal secretion is referred to as "basal acid output" or "BAO," and usually refers to the sum of four 15-minute basal collections. It is expressed as milliequivalents per hour.

There has been considerable confusion regarding the expression "maximal acid output" (MAO). Makhlouf et al. reserve this phrase for calculated maximal response as calculated from dose response data of graded doses of any gastric secretagogue.[80] Others have defined MAO as the acid output obtained 15 to 45 minutes after histamine acid phosphate (40 μg per kilogram subcutaneously).[10] Baron refers to MAO as the total acid output which occurs during the first postinjection hour (i.e., 0 to 60 minutes).[81] MAO is distinguished from "peak acid output" (PAO), which represents the sum of the two highest successive 15-minute acid responses.[81] The PAO after a maximal dose of stimulant represents the most reproducible measurement of stimulated gastric acid secretion, and is a good index of the calculated maximal response of the stomach to secrete acid.

It is important that secretory terminology become standardized. For the present, the following terminology seems appropriate:

1. *Peak acid output (PAO)* equals the highest observed rate of secretion during the course of an individual test. Conventionally it is usually the sum of the two highest ten- (peak 20) or 15- (peak 30) minute periods. These can be converted into milliequivalents per hour by multiplying by 3 or 2 respectively.

2. *Maximal acid output (MAO)* equals the sum of the four highest 15-minute, or six highest ten-minute periods produced by a dose of stimulant above which (i.e., greater doses of the same stimulant) acid secretion is no greater.

3. *Calculated maximal acid output (CMAO)* equals the calculated maximal response of the stomach attainable at an infinite dose of a single stimulant. CMAO is calculated by measuring the responses to multiple doses of a gastric stimulant.[80] CMAO is not commonly measured in routine secretory testing.

4. *Calculated maximal secretory capacity (CMSC)* equals the calculated maximal secretory capacity of the stomach to single or multiple agents above which no other agent or combination of agents gives a

greater secretory response. This measurement also requires multiple dose-response studies, and has not been used in clinical studies.

ELECTROLYTES

In addition to secreting hydrochloric acid, the stomach secretes sodium, potassium, calcium, and magnesium.[82] In routine clinical gastric secretory testing, gastric electrolytes are not usually measured. In certain diseases in which the gastric mucosal barrier is damaged (see pp. 563 and 570), such as gastritis, gastric ulcer, and possibly Menetrier's disease, gastric hydrogen ion concentration may not increase to the usual value of at least 100 mEq per liter during maximal acid secretion[83] (see pp. 642 to 654 and 692 to 710). Since hydrogen ion and sodium ion in the gastric juice vary reciprocally and since gastric juice is usually isotonic with plasma, when stimulated peak hydrogen ion secretion is lower than normal (i.e., less than 100 mEq per liter) it is advisable to measure gastric sodium ion concentration. Increased sodium concentration during maximally stimulated gastric acid secretion suggests damage to the gastric mucosal barrier.[84]

PEPSINOGEN AND PEPSIN

In man, the gastric chief, mucous neck, and pyloric gland cells secrete pepsinogens in response to any of the previously mentioned stimulants for gastric acid secretion.[85] In addition, secretin is a potent stimulus of pepsinogen secretion in man.[86] There are two main groups of pepsinogens (groups I and II). In addition to having different sites of origin, these groups differ in electrophoretic motility and substrate specificity (see pp. 189 to 193).[87]

There are a number of methods for pepsin measurement. Each method is dependent upon the enzymatic action of pepsin on a substrate which results in a measurable end product. These include hemoglobin,[88] an insoluble substrate which is covalently bound with Remazobrillant Blue,[89] radioiodinated serum albumin,[90] and many others.[85] At present, pepsin measurements fail from lack of accuracy and precision

because of other acid proteases which interact in the pepsin measurement, inactivation of pepsin during collection, and the highly time-consuming methodology required to perform pepsin determinations. For these reasons most clinical secretory laboratories do not measure pepsin on patients during secretory testing. In addition, there is no known clinical situation in which pepsin measurement will establish or refute a diagnosis.

INTRINSIC FACTOR

In man, the parietal cells secrete intrinsic factor both at rest and in response to any of the agents which increase gastric acid secretion.[91] The usual semiquantitative method for measuring intrinsic factor is the Schilling test. There are other more specific and quantitative methods for measuring intrinsic factor.[92]

Intrinsic factor secretion is not usually measured during routine secretory testing. In certain gastrointestinal diseases (e.g., pernicious anemia, gastric atrophy, and gastritis) there is or may be a decrease in intrinsic factor secretion (see p. 566).[92] In patients with vitamin B_{12} deficiency, ability to secrete intrinsic factor should be determined (Schilling test).

GASTRIC MUCUS

Gastric mucus, mucoproteins, glycoproteins, and blood group secretion have been reviewed,[93] and are discussed on pages 144 to 160. These sources should be reviewed for further information on mucus secretion.

INTERPRETATION OF GASTRIC SECRETORY TESTING

IN HEALTH

Gastric acid secretion has been studied in healthy subjects.[94-96] Average basal secretion is greater in male subjects than in females, and average gastric acid secretory capacity decreases with increasing age.[96] Basal acid output (BAO) has been measured in a number of laboratories. Al-

TABLE 42–2. BASAL AND MAXIMAL STIMULATED GASTRIC ACID SECRETION IN NORMAL SUBJECTS AND PATIENTS WITH DUODENAL ULCER*

| | | | ACID OUTPUT (mEq/hr) | | | | |
| | | | Normal | | Duodenal Ulcer | | |
	SEX	N	Mean	ULN	Mean	LV-DU	REFERENCE
Basal	M	615	2.4	?6.6	5.3	0.1	95
	F	634	1.3	?4.1	2.9	0.1	95
Histamine	M	25	23.1	42.0	45.9	>0	10
	M	20	21.6	49.2	42.0	15	102
	F	20	12.3	30.2	32.0	18.8	102
Betazole	M	75	34.4	59.8	42.4	6.2	94
	M	30	21.8	45.8	35.0	14.4	126
	F	45	16.8	40.0	30.8	13.4	126
Pentagastrin	M	18	25.0	45.0	43.0	15.0	127

*N = Number. ULN = Upper limit of normal (mean + 2 SD). LV-DU = Lowest value duodenal ulcer. (Modified from Baron, J. H.: Scand. J. Gastroent. Suppl. 6:9, 1970.)

though the absolute values vary somewhat, average normal basal acid output is approximately 2 mEq per hour, and the upper limit of normal BAO is approximately 5 mEq per hour (Table 42–2).[96] It is advisable for each secretory laboratory to establish its normal values in a group of subjects whose age and sex correspond to those of its study population.

Normal peak acid output (PAO) or maximal acid output (MAO) depends on the age, sex, and health of the population studied. The average MAO in most series of reported subjects is approximately 20 mEq per hour, with an upper limit of normal of approximately 40 mEq per hour (Table 42–2).[96]

DUODENAL ULCER DISEASE

In patients with duodenal ulcer disease, average basal and peak stimulated gastric acid output is greater than in control, nonduodenal subjects. There is, however, a marked overlap between normal and duodenal ulcer patient responses, particularly during the basal hour.[96] It is uncommon to find a patient with basal achlorhydria and duodenal ulcer, but this combination occasionally occurs. It is also uncommon to find a patient with duodenal ulcer who secretes less than 12 mEq per hour in response to a dose of secretagogue capable of producing maximal acid secretion (Table 42–2).[96]

Approximately one-third to one-half of patients with duodenal ulcer are hypersecretors of gastric acid when compared with normal subjects.[96] Because of the marked overlap in acid secretion between normal and duodenal ulcer patients, the discriminatory value of secretory testing in the diagnosis of duodenal ulcer is limited.

Recent studies have shown that patients with duodenal ulcer are more sensitive to pentagastrin than nonduodenal ulcer control subjects.[97] The dose of pentagastrin required for one-half maximal response (D_{50}), and calculated maximal acid output (CMAO) was calculated. The D_{50} was significantly lower and CMR significantly greater in the duodenal ulcer subjects when compared to nonduodenal ulcer control subjects (Fig. 42–3). The explanation for the shift in the dose-response curve to the left in patients with duodenal ulcer disease is unknown. Fasting serum gastrin is usually less than or similar to normal in patients with duodenal ulcer disease.[98] It is possible that patients with duodenal ulcer might have increased "vagal tone" (see p. 182) which produces the shift in the pentagastrin dose-response curve. Another explanation might be decreased circulation or decreased release of inhibitors of gastric acid secretion. Aubrey and Forest recently reported that the results of a sin-

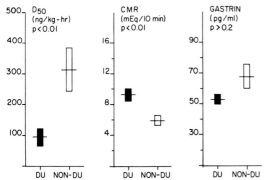

Figure 42–3. Mean D_{50} (dose of pentagastrin required for one-half maximal response) was significantly less in 20 duodenal ulcer patients when compared to 20 nonduodenal ulcer subjects. The line indicates the mean and the rectangle indicates two standard errors of the means. Mean calculated maximal response to pentagastrin (CMR) was significantly greater in the duodenal ulcer patients when compared to nonduodenal ulcer patients. Average fasting serum gastrin was not significantly different between the two groups.

gle day dose-response test with intravenous histamine acid phosphate were comparable to multiple single-day single-dose tests.[99] This study suggests that it may be possible to collect dose-response data on an individual patient on a single day study. It is possible with these data to calculate the dose required for one-half maximal response (D_{50}) and calculated maximal acid output (CMAO) (pp. 174 to 186).

There is evidence to suggest that those duodenal ulcer patients with very high rates of stimulated gastric acid secretion may have a greater incidence of complications of duodenal ulcer disease, and often may require elective surgery for duodenal ulcer disease. In addition, this group may have a greater incidence of incomplete vagotomies when compared to duodenal ulcer subjects with lower rates of acid secretion.[100]

At present, there is no evidence that secretory data give any significant information as to the type of surgery (vagotomy and drainage procedure versus vagotomy and antrectomy) which should be performed in patients requiring surgical intervention for peptic ulcer disease[101] (pp. 772 to 787).

As with acid secretion, pepsin secretion is also increased in patients with duodenal ulcer disease when compared with control subjects. There is less discriminatory in-

formation in separating duodenal ulcer from nonduodenal ulcer patients with pepsin secretion than with acid secretion.

GASTRIC ULCER

As a group, patients with gastric ulcer tend to secrete acid at lower basal and stimulated secretory rates than do normal subjects.[102] Those patients with gastric ulcer located within the body of the stomach tend to have lower secretory rates than those with gastric ulcers located in the prepyloric area.[102] Secretion in this latter group is usually normal, and in some instances may approach the hypersecretion as seen in patients with duodenal ulcer. Those patients with both gastric and duodenal ulcer tend to be hypersecretors similar to patients with duodenal ulcer alone (Table 42–2).[102]

The pathophysiological explanation for the decreased acid secretion in patients with gastric ulcers of the body of the stomach is not known (see p. 697). There is some evidence to suggest that these patients may have increased back-diffusion of gastric acid across the damaged gastric mucosa, producing spurious lowering of the measured secretory rate.[103] Also, some patients with gastric ulcer have increased bile reflux into the stomach, and bile salts are capable of damaging the gastric mucosa.

GASTRIC CARCINOMA

In patients with gastric cancer, both basal and maximal stimulated gastric acid secretion is usually subnormal, but only approximately 20 per cent of patients with gastric cancer have achlorhydria.[104] Gastric secretory rates may be normal in patients with gastric cancer. In those patients with gastric cancer who are capable of secreting acid, gastric secretory testing offers little information. In those patients with radiographic evidence of gastric ulceration and achlorhydria after a maximal stimulating dose of histamine or pentagastrin, the probability of the gastric lesion being a neoplasm approaches 100 per cent. There may be increases in protein secretion and β-glucuronidase secretion in patients with gastric cancer.[105] These measurements are not usually performed in routine clinical secretory testing, and their clinical value must be studied further (see p. 587).

AFTER GASTRIC SURGERY

VAGOTOMY

At present, vagotomy with a gastric drainage procedure (e.g., pyloroplasty or gastroenterostomy) and vagotomy with antrectomy are the most commonly performed surgical procedures for duodenal ulcer disease. Until recently, cutting the anterior and posterior vagal trunks just above the diaphragmatic hiatus was the usual method of performing a vagotomy. Recently, two variations of performing vagotomy have been introduced: (1) Selective gastric vagotomy.[106] This involves isolating the hepatic and celiac branches of the intra-abdominal vagal trunks. These branches are left intact, and the anterior and posterior gastric branches are cut. Usually a gastric drainage procedure is also performed. (2) Highly selective gastric vagotomy, i.e., parietal cell (oxyntic gland) vagotomy, which involves isolation and ligation of the vagal branches to the oxyntic gland area of the stomach.[107] The antral, hepatic, and celiac vagal branches are left intact (see pp. 772 to 787). A drainage procedure need not be performed with a highly selective vagotomy, provided the gastric outlet is not narrowed and distorted.

In normal subjects, graded doses of insulin produce graded responses. Insulin, 0.2 unit per kilogram, as a rapid intravenous injection, produces the greatest peak 15-minute acid output. In normal subjects, the peak response after 0.2 unit per kilogram occurs from 45 to 90 minutes after injection, and is approximately 85 per cent of the maximal betazole-induced peak 15-minute acid output.[60] In unoperated patients with duodenal ulcer, the peak insulin–peak histamine acid response is approximately 80 per cent.[108]

There has been considerable confusion regarding the interpretation of the post-vagotomy insulin test. Certain conclusions, however, can be made regarding the effect of vagotomy on gastric acid secretion. Complete truncal vagotomy decreases maximal stimulated gastric acid output produced by the usual maximal doses of betazole or histamine to approximately 30 per cent of the preoperative secretory rate, a decrease of about 70 per cent.[109, 110] Incomplete vagotomy also decreases histamine-stimulated maximal acid output, but usually not to the degree that follows complete vagotomy. After incomplete vagotomy, there may be a decrease ranging from 10 to 60 per cent in MAO.[110, 111]

Selective vagotomy, as performed by surgeons skilled at this procedure, may produce a greater incidence of complete vagotomies when compared to truncal vagotomy.[112] Selective vagotomy may also have a lesser incidence of postvagotomy diarrhea.[112]

There is no significant difference in the decrease in maximal response to histamine, Histalog, or pentagastrin in selective versus truncal vagotomy.[106, 108] Highly selective (oxyntic gland) vagotomy also decreases maximal acid secretion by comparable levels as produced by truncal vagotomy.[107] The two-week postvagotomy insulin response may change over a period of time. Some patients who were "late" positive responders soon after surgery (see below) may become "early" positives. Some patients who were "negative" may become "late" positives (see below). The clinical significance of this change in type of response to insulin suggests that insulin testing should be performed at least three to six months after surgery. The acid-reducing effect of vagotomy, either complete or incomplete, on maximal histamine-stimulated acid secretion remains stable over years.[113]

The method of performing the insulin test has been discussed (see above). A number of criteria for the interpretation of the secretory data have evolved in an attempt to separate patients with incomplete vagotomy from those with a complete vagotomy.[114] Criteria suggestive of an incomplete vagotomy include the following: (1) Increase in volume of gastric secretion after insulin. (2) BAO equal to or greater than 2 mEq per hour. (3) Gastric acid concentration increased by 20 mEq per liter, or increased greater than 10 mEq per liter if basal gastric juice was achlorhydric within the two postinsulin hours. (4) The same as criterion 3, except that the increase in concentration occurs in the first postinsulin hour. (5) Total acid output in excess of 2 mEq per hour in any postinsulin hour.

Grossman (personal communication) has recently suggested that, instead of arbitrarily declaring an insulin test positive, negative, or indeterminate, the data be reported as follows: (1) Average basal acid concentration. (2) Peak postinsulin acid concentration. (3) Increase in acid concentration (number 2 minus number 1). (4) Basal acid output. (5) Peak 30-minute postinsulin acid output. (6) Increase in acid output (number 5 minus number 4). Expressing insulin data in this or a similar[115] way will permit greater uniformity in the reporting, and might permit better prognostic interpretation of the data.

Ross and Kay suggested that there are three types of postvagotomy responses to insulin: (1) "early" response (i.e., an increase in acid concentration of at least 20 mEq per liter), occurring within the first 45 minutes after insulin; (2) "late" response, occurring later than 45 minutes after insulin;[116] or (3) negative response, or no increase in acid concentration after insulin injection. There is evidence to suggest that patients with the "early" type of postvagotomy insulin response may have a greater incidence of recurrent ulcer disease than do those with negative or late responses.[117]

Payne and Kay examined the effect of graded doses of histamine acid phosphate on acid secretion in postvagotomy subjects to determine whether the dose-response curve had shifted to the right after vagotomy.[118] They studied histamine acid phosphate doses of 40, 80, and 120 μg per kilogram subcutaneously. There was no evidence that the 80 or 120 μg per kilogram doses produced greater maximal acid outputs than the standard 40 μg per kilogram dose. They also tested the effect of histamine acid phosphate (40 μg per kilogram subcutaneously) plus a continuous intravenous infusion of the cholinergic agent methacholine (0.2 mg per minute). In those subjects without marked bile reflux, maximal acid secretion approached the preoperative histamine response. These data suggest that it is possible to reintroduce "vagal tone" in the postvago-

tomy patient and to restore maximal acid secretion to prevagotomy values.

As mentioned previously, peak pentagastrin-stimulated gastric acid secretion is normally achieved with a dose of 6 μg per kilogram given intramuscularly or subcutaneously. After vagotomy, the dose of pentagastrin required to produce maximal acid secretion may increase to 12 μg per kilogram.[119]

ANTRECTOMY AND VAGOTOMY

After antrectomy without vagotomy, the postoperative maximal acid secretory response to a maximal dose of histamine is decreased by approximately 50 to 80 per cent when compared with preoperative values. Adding vagotomy to this procedure decreases acid secretory response to histamine by about 85 per cent when compared with preoperative values.[121, 122]

SUBTOTAL GASTRECTOMY

Subtotal gastrectomy (approximately 75 per cent resection) without vagotomy removes the gastric antrum plus a significant portion of the parietal cell mass. After subtotal gastrectomy maximal histamine-stimulated gastric acid secretion is decreased by approximately 90 per cent. However, it is frequently difficult to obtain bile-free gastric juice in patients with subtotal gastrectomy and Billroth II anastomoses. Although a balloon has been used to occlude the stoma during secretory tests, this technique is difficult and not commonly used.[122] Retrieval of an unabsorbed marker has been studied in patients with Billroth II anastomoses, and frequently less than 60 per cent of the instilled marker is aspirated (see pp. 829 to 839).

In summary, gastric secretory testing in patients who have had gastric surgery is technically more difficult than performing secretory tests in the nonoperated patients. The discriminatory value of secretory data in the diagnosis of recurrent ulceration is marginal at best. In those patients with a BAO greater than 5 mEq per hour and/or an MAO in response to histamine greater than 15, the incidence of recurrent ulceration is high.[96] Other diagnostic procedures, such as endoscopy and radiography, are superior to secretory studies in the diagnosis of recurrent ulceration in the postoperative patient.

ZOLLINGER-ELLISON SYNDROME

Most patients with Zollinger-Ellison syndrome, i.e., gastrin-producing tumor of the pancreas (or gastrin-producing microadenomatosis of the pancreas) and peptic ulcer disease are associated with marked hypersecretion of gastric acid (see p. 743).[12] The basal gastric acid output in this condition is usually greater than 10 to 15 mEq per hour in the unoperated patient, and is usually greater than 5 mEq per hour in the postoperative patient.[12] In addition, basal acid concentration (BAC) is usually well above normal BAC (i.e., approximately 40 mEq per liter) and is in the range of 80 to 140 mEq per liter.[12] BAO divided by MAO is frequently greater than 60 per cent, as is BAC divided by MAC.[12] Each of these criteria, however, may be present in patients with duodenal ulcer disease without Zollinger-Ellison syndrome and may be absent in patients with Zollinger-Ellison syndrome.[13] Previously, overnight secretion was collected in patients suspected of having this syndrome. Not uncommonly, overnight secretion reveals greater than 100 mEq. In patients with Zollinger-Ellison syndrome the collection of gastric juice for prolonged periods of time may produce hypovolemia, hypotension, and hypochloremic alkalosis. Prolonged collection of gastric juice in hypersecretors is therefore not advised.

In summary, gastric secretory testing may give results which are suggestive of Zollinger-Ellison syndrome. However, there are both false-positive and false-negative secretory responses. If any of the aforementioned criteria are present on gastric secretory testing, Zollinger-Ellison syndrome should be suspected, and serum gastrin level measured (see pp. 555 to 558). In certain instances, a calcium infusion test with gastric acid and serum gastrin measurements may be helpful in discriminating Zollinger-Ellison syndrome patients from other hypersecretors.

PERNICIOUS ANEMIA AND GASTRIC ATROPHY

In patients with pernicious anemia and gastric atrophy, basal and stimulated gastric acid and pepsin secretion are markedly decreased. In most subjects with pernicious anemia, histamine-fast achlorhydria is noted. In some subjects with pernicious anemia and achlorhydria, there may be circulating and intragastric antibodies directed against the parietal cell, intrinsic factor (i.e., blocking antibodies), and intrinsic factor–vitamin B_{12} complex (i.e., binding antibodies) (see pp. 567 to 568).[92]

In patients with pernicious anemia and gastric atrophy, there may be increased protein secretion by the stomach. At present, these determinations are not specific, and do not establish specific diagnosis. Gastric biopsy is the method of choice for determining the histological alteration of the gastric mucosa.

MENETRIER'S DISEASE — HYPERTROPHIC HYPERSECRETORY GASTROPATHY

Classically, Menetrier's disease represents the presence of large gastric folds, hypoproteinemia, edema, and achlorhydria.[123] In these subjects gastric acid secretion is usually negligible. Gastric protein secretion is increased and is the cause of the hypoproteinemia (see pp. 35 to 48).

There have been recent reports of patients with a combination of Menetrier's disease and hypertrophic hypersecretory gastropathy.[124] The latter condition represents large gastric folds and hypersecretion of gastric acid.[125] These patients do not have elevated serum gastrin levels. In those patients with the combined syndrome there is increased secretion of gastric acid both basally and in response to histamine. Hydrogen ion concentration in response to histamine does not increase normally to at least 105 mEq per liter. The lack of normal increase in acid concentration probably represents damage to the gastric mucosal barrier. In addition, such patients have marked gastric protein loss.

Gastric secretory testing in this group can give meaningful clinical information, particularly when gastric protein loss is measured. Diagnosis is established by gastric biopsy, either by peroral technique or at surgery (see p. 570).

CONCLUSIONS

Under what circumstances does gastric secretory testing aid the clinician in the diagnosis and/or management of patients with upper gastrointestinal disease? It can be concluded that secretory testing, when properly performed, may assist in the diagnosis and management of patients with peptic ulcer disease, Zollinger-Ellison syndrome, gastritis, gastric cancer, hypertrophic hypersecretory gastropathy, and Menetrier's disease; it is also useful after acid-reducing peptic ulcer surgery.

REFERENCES

1. Beaumont, W. Experiments and Observations on the Gastric Juice and the Physiology of Digestion. New York, Dover Publications, Inc., 1959.
2. Ewald, C. A., and Boas, J. Beitrage zur Physigogie und der Verdauung. Archiv. Path. Anat. Physiol. (Virchow) *101*:325, 1885.
3. Ehrenreich, M. Ueber die kontinuierliche Untersuchung des verdauungsablaufs Mittels der Magenverrveilsonde. Z. Klin. Med. 75:231, 1912.
4. Rehfuss, M. E. Diseases of the Stomach. Philadelphia, W. B. Saunders Co., 1927.
5. Hollander, F., and Penner, A. History and development of gastric analysis procedure. Amer. J. Dig. Dis. 5:739, 786, 1939; 6:22, 1939.
6. Henning, N., and Norjsoth, L. Die Magensekretion wahrend des Sehlates. Deutsche Arch. Klin Med. *172*:558, 1932.
7. Dragstedt, L. R. Pathogenesis of gastroduodenal ulcer. Arch. Surg. 44:438, 1942.
8. Ihre, B. J. E. Human gastric secretion. Acta Med. Scand. (Suppl.) 95:1, 1938.
9. Polland, W. S., and Bloomfield, A. L. Normal standards of gastric function. J. Clin. Invest. 9:651, 1931.
10. Kay, A. W. Effect of large doses of histamine on gastric secretion of HCl. An augmented histamine test. Brit. Med. J. 2:77, 1953.
11. Card, W. I., and Marks, I. N. The relationship between the acid output of the stomach following "maximal" histamine stimulation and parietal cell mass. Clin. Sci. *19*:147, 1960.
12. Ptak, T., and Kirsner, J. B. The Zollinger-Ellison syndrome, polyendocrine adenomatosis and other endocrine associations with

peptic ulcer. Advan. Intern. Med. *16*:213, 1970.
13. Winship, D. H. Problems in the diagnosis of Zollinger-Ellison syndrome by analysis of gastric secretion. *In* Non-insulin-Producing Tumors of the Pancreas, L. Demling and R. Ottenjann, (eds.). Stuttgart, Thieme Verlag, 1969.
14. Isenberg, J. I., Spector, H., Hootkin, L. A., et al. An apparent exception to Schwarz's dictum, "no acid–no ulcer." New Eng. J. Med. *285*:629, 1971.
15. Charles, R. M., Moss, M. J., Kunz, W., et al. Gastric secretory derangement in Menetrier's disease. Amer. J. Dig. Dis. 8:191, 1963.
16. Christiansen, P. M., and Johansen, A. Single gastric biopsy in subjects with low acid secretion after maximal histamine stimulation. Scand. J. Gastroent. *1*:86, 1966.
17. MacDonald, W. C., and Rubin, C. E. Gastric biopsy—a critical evaluation. Gastroenterology 53:143, 1967.
18. Koelle, G. B. Parasympathomimetic agents. *In* The Pharmacological Basis of Therapeutics, L. S. Goodman and A. Gilman, (eds.). New York, Macmillan, 1965, p. 464.
19. Dotevall, G., Schoder, G., and Walan, A. The effect of poldine, glycopyrrolate, and l-hyoscyamine on gastric secretion of acid in man. Acta Med. Scand. *177*:169, 1965.
20. Birnbaum, D., Karmeli, F., and Tefera, M. The effect of diazepam on human gastric secretion. Gut *12*:616, 1971.
21. Linder, A. E., Cohen, N., Berkowitz, J., et al. A note on the oral dose of acetazolamide required to inhibit acid secretion. Gastroenterology 46:273, 1964.
22. Castell, D. O., Johnson, R. B., and Sparks, H. A. Abbreviated Histalog gastric analysis: Comparison with peak acid output. Amer. J. Dig. Dis. *12*:713, 1967.
23. Lawrie, J. H., and Forest, A. P. M. The measurement of gastric acid. Postgrad. Med. J. *41*:408, 1965.
24. Williams, J. A., and Benn, A. A gastric sampling tube. Lancet *1*:1309, 1965.
25. Callender, S. T., Retief, F. P., and Witts, L. J. The augmented histamine test with special reference to achlorhydria. Gut *1*:326, 1960.
26. Baron, J. H. Studies of basal and peak acid output with an augmented histamine test. Gut 4:136, 1963.
27. Hassan, M. A., and Hobsley, M. Position of subject and of nasogastric tube during a gastric secretion study. Brit. Med. J. *1*:458, 1970.
28. Hector, R. M. Improved technique of gastric aspiration. Lancet *1*:15, 1968.
29. Hobsley, M., and Silen, W. Use of an inert marker (phenol red) to improve accuracy in gastric secretion studies. Gut *10*:787, 1969.
30. Venables, C. W. The effect of measuring uncollected secretion upon the gastric pepsin-acid response to histamine and pentagastrin. Brit. J. Surg. 56:386, 1969.
31. Kunz, H. J., Norby, T. E., and Rogers, C. H. A

pH measuring radio capsule for the alimentary canal. Amer. J. Dig. Dis. 16:739, 1971.

32. Stack, B. H. R. Use of the Heidelberg pH capsule in the routine assessment of gastric acid secretion. Gut 10:245, 1969.

33. Marks, I. N., and Shay, H. Augmented histamine test, Ewald test and Diagnex test. Amer. J. Dig. Dis. 5:1, 1960.

34. Christiansen, P. M. The Azur-A method as a screening test of gastric acid secretion. Scand. J. Gastroent. 1:9, 1966.

35. Pastore, J. O., Kato, H., and Belsky, J. L. Serum pepsin and tubeless gastric analysis as a predictor of stomach cancer. New Eng. J. Med. 286:279, 1972.

36. Irvine, W. J., Stewart, A. G., McLoughlin, G. P., et al. Appraisal of the application of ^{99m} Tc in the assessment of gastric function. Lancet 2:648, 1967.

37. Roth, J. L. A. Clinical evaluation of the caffeine gastric analysis in duodenal ulcer patients. Gastroenterology 19:199, 1951.

38. Beazell, J. M., and Ivy, A. C. The influence of alcohol on the digestive tract. Quart. J. Study Alcohol 1:45, 1940.

39. Fordtran, J. S., and Collyns, J. A. H. Antacid pharmacology in duodenal ulcer. Effect of antacids on postcibal gastric acidity and peptic activity. New Eng. J. Med. 274:921, 1966.

40. Barreras, R. F., and Donaldson, R. M., Jr. Effects of induced hypercalcemia on human gastric secretion. Gastroenterology 52:670, 1967.

41. Blum, N. I., Mayoral, N. G., and Kalser, M. M. Augmented gastric analysis. A word of caution. J.A.M.A. 191:339, 1965.

42. Goldenberg, J., Cummins, A. J., and Gompertz, M. J. A clinical evaluation of the maximal Histalog test. Amer. J. Dig. Dis. 12:468, 1967.

43. Rosiere, G. E., and Grossman, M. I. An analog of histamine that stimulates gastric acid secretion without other actions of histamine. Science 113:651, 1951.

44. Carneiro de Moura, M., and Lucao, J. G. Bronchial asthma and the augmented histamine test. Gastroenterology 48:152, 1965.

45. Desai, H. G., Antia, F. P., Gupte, U. V., et al. Dose of histamine for maximal stimulation of gastric acid secretion. Gastroenterology 57:636, 1969.

46. Grossman, M. I. Histamine dosage. Gastroenterology 15:378, 1950.

47. Zaterka, S., and Neves, D. P. Maximal gastric secretion in human subjects after Histalog. Comparison with augmented histamine test. Gastroenterology 47:251, 1964.

48. Laudano, O. M., and Roncoroni, E. L. Determination of the dose of Histalog that provokes maximal gastric secretory response. Gastroenterology 49:372, 1965.

49. Ward, S., Gillespie, I. E., Passaro, E. P., and Grossman, M. I. Comparison of Histalog and histamine as stimulants for maximal gastric secretion in human subjects and in dogs. Gastroenterology 44:620, 1963.

50. Isenberg, J. I., Brooks, A. M., and Grossman, M. I. Pentagastrin versus betazole as stimulant of gastric secretion: Comparative study in man. J.A.M.A. 206:2897, 1968.

51. Gregory, R. A., and Tracy, H. J. The constitution and properties of two gastrins extracted from hog antral mucosa. Gut 5:103, 1964.

52. Makhlouf, G. M., McManus, J. P. A., and Card, W. I. Dose-response curves for the effect of gastrin II on gastric acid secretion in man. Gut 5:379, 1964.

53. Konturek, S. J., and Krol, W. The influence of gastrin-related peptides on HCl secretion in man and in cats with gastric fistulas and Heidenhain pouches. Gastroenterologia 106:281, 1966.

54. Köster, K. H., Rödbro, P., and Petersen, H. J. Comparative effects of tetragastrin and histamine on acid and intrinsic factor secretion in man. Scand. J. Gastroent. 3:23, 1967.

55. Multicentre Pilot Study. Pentagastrin as a stimulant of maximal gastric acid response in man. Lancet 1:291, 1967.

56. Wormsley, K. G. Pentagastrin snuff: A new means of stimulating gastric secretion. Lancet 1:57, 1968.

57. Jepson, K., Duthie, H. L., Fawcett, A. N., et al. Acid and pepsin response to gastrin I, pentagastrin, tetragastrin, histamine, and pentagastrin snuff. Lancet 2:139, 1968.

58. Isenberg, J. I., Csendes, A., and Walsh, J. H. Resting and pentagastrin-stimulated gastroesophageal sphincter pressure in patients with Zollinger-Ellison syndrome. Gastroenterology 61:655, 1971.

59. Brooks, F. P. Insulin hypoglycemia and gastric secretion. Amer. J. Dig. Dis. 10:737, 1965.

60. Isenberg, J. I., Stening, G. F., Ward, S., et al. Relation of gastric secretory response in man to dose of insulin. Gastroenterology 57:395, 1969.

61. Isenberg, J. I., Stening, G. F., Pitcher, J. L., and Brooks, A. M. The effect of graded insulin doses on incompletely vagotomized subjects. Gastroenterology 59:698, 1970.

62. Baron, J. H., Guttierrez, L. U., Spencer, J., Tinker, J., and Welbourn, R. B. The insulin test in the unoperated subject. Gut 10:1046, 1969.

63. Stempien, S. J. A note on the hazards of "maximal" insulin tests. Gastroenterology 60:345, 1971.

64. Hollander, F. Laboratory procedures in the study of vagotomy (with particular reference to the insulin test). Gastroenterology 11:419, 1948.

65. Bachrach, W. H., and Bachrach, L. B. Reevaluation of the Hollander test. Ann. N.Y. Acad. Sci. 140:915, 1967.

66. Greenwood, F. C., Lawson, J., and Stamp, T. C. B. The plasma sugar, free fatty acid, cortisol, and growth hormone response to insulin. I. In control subjects. J. Clin. Invest. 45:429, 1966.

67. Stempien, S. J., Lee, E. R., and Dagradi, A. E. Tolbutamide gastric analysis. Clinical correlations and interpretations. Amer. J. Dig. Dis. 13:643, 1968.

68. Thomas, D. G., and Duthie, H. L. Use of 2-

deoxy-D-glucose to test for completeness of surgical vagotomy. Gut 9:125, 1968.

69. Reeder, D. D., Jackson, M. B., Ban, J., Clendinner, B. G., Davidson, W. D., and Thompson, J. C. Influence of hypercalcemia on gastric secretion and serum gastric concentration in man. Ann. Surg. 172:540, 1970.

70. Passaro, E., Basso, N., Sanchez, R. E., and Gordon, H. E. Newer studies in the Zollinger-Ellison syndrome. Amer. J. Surg. 120:138, 1970.

71. Rune, S. J. Comparison of the rates of gastric acid secretion in man after ingestion of food and after maximal stimulation with histamine. Gut 7:344, 1966.

72. Hunt, J. N. Gastric emptying and secretion in man. Physiol. Rev. 39:491, 1959.

73. Brooks, A. M., and Grossman, M. I. Effect of secretin and cholecystokinin on pentagastrin-stimulated gastric secretion in man. Gastroenterology 59:114, 1970.

74. Brooks, A. M., Agosti, A., Bertaccini, G., and Grossman, M. I. Inhibition of gastric acid secretion in man by peptide analogues of cholecystokinin. New Eng. J. Med. 282:535, 1970.

75. Bennett, A., and Fleshler, B. Prostaglandins and the gastrointestinal tract. Gastroenterology 59:790, 1970.

76. Dreiling, D. A., and Janowitz, H. D. The effect of glucagon on gastric secretion in man. Gastroenterology 36:580, 1959.

77. Levin, E., Kirsner, J. B., and Palmer, W. L. A simple measure of gastric secretion in man. Comparison of one-hour basal secretory histamine secretion and twelve-hour nocturnal gastric secretion. Gastroenterology 19:88, 1951.

78. Moore, E. W. Terminology and measurement of gastric acidity. Ann. N.Y. Acad. Sci. 140:866, 1967.

79. Moore, E. W., and Scarlata, R. W. The determination of gastric acidity by the glass electrode. Gastroenterology 49:178, 1965.

80. Makhlouf, G. M., McManus, J. P. A., and Card, W. I. The action of the pentapeptide (ICI 50, 123) on gastric secretion in man. Gastroenterology 51:455, 1966.

81. Baron, J. H. Measurement and nomenclature of gastric acid. Gastroenterology 45:118, 1963.

82. Hunt, J. N., and Wan, B. Electrolytes in mammalian gastric juice. In Handbook of Physiology, Sec. 6, Vol. 2, C. F. Code (ed.). Washington, D.C., American Physiological Society, 1968, p. 781.

83. Hirschowitz, B. I. Electrolytes in human gastric secretion. Amer. J. Dig. Dis. 6:199, 1961.

84. Davenport, H. W. Why the stomach does not digest itself. Sci. Amer. 226:86, 1972.

85. Samloff, I. M. Pepsinogens, pepsins, and pepsin inhibitors. Gastroenterology 60:586, 1971.

86. Brooks, A. M., Isenberg, J. I., and Grossman, M. I. The effect of secretin, glucagon, and duodenal acidifications on pepsin secretion in man. Gastroenterology 57:159, 1969.

87. Samloff, I. M., and Townes, P. L. Electrophoretic heterogeneity and relationships of pepsinogens in human urine, serum, and gastric mucosa. Gastroenterology 57:659, 1970.

88. Berstad, A. A modified hemoglobin substrate method for the estimation of pepsin in gastric juice. Scand. J. Gastroent. 5:343, 1970.

89. Rinderknecht, H., Geokas, M. C., Silverman, P., et al. A new ultrasensitive method for determination of proteolytic activity. Clin. Chim. Acta 21:197, 1968.

90. Grossman, M. I., and Marks, I. N. Secretion of pepsinogen by the pyloric glands of the dog, with some observations on the Histalog of the gastric mucosa. Gastroenterology 38:343, 1960.

91. Twoney, J. J., Laughter, A. H., and Jordan, P. H. Studies into human IF secretion. Amer. J. Dig. Dis. 16:1075, 1971.

92. Jeffries, G. H. Gastric secretion of intrinsic factor. In Handbook of Physiology, Sect. 6, Vol. II, C. F. Code (ed.), Washington, D.C., American Physiological Society, 1967, p. 919.

93. Glass, G. B. J., Mori, H., and Pamer, T. Measurement of sulfated and nonsulfated glycoprotein in human gastric juice under fasting conditions and following stimulation with histamine, pentagastrin and insulin. Digestion 2:124, 1969.

94. Wormsley, K. G., and Grossman, M. I. Maximal Histalog test in control subjects and patients with peptic ulcer. Gut 6:427, 1965.

95. Grossman, M. I., Kirsner, J. B., and Gillespie, I. E. Basal and Histalog-stimulated gastric secretion in control subjects and in patients with peptic ulcer or gastric ulcer. Gastroenterology 45:14, 1963.

96. Baron, J. H. The clinical use of gastric function tests. Scand. J. Gastroent. Suppl. 6:9, 1970.

97. Isenberg, J. I., Best, W., and Grossman, M. I. The effect of graded doses of pentagastrin in gastric acid secretion in duodenal ulcer and non-duodenal ulcer subjects. Clin. Res. 20:222, 1972.

98. Hansky, J., Korman, M. G., Cowley, D. J., and Baron, J. H. Serum gastrin in duodenal ulcer. Gut 12:959, 1971.

99. Aubrey, D. A., and Forest, A. P. M. Comparison of the gastric secretory responses following the administration of histamine acid phosphate and pentagastrin by separate continuous intravenous infusions or by a step-test method. Scand. J. Gastroent. 5:449, 1970.

100. Harrison, A. M., Wechsler, R. L., and Elliott, D. W. Gastric analysis in the absence of demonstrable gastric pathology. Amer. J. Surg. 123:132, 1972.

101. Duthie, H. L. Pre-operative acid tests. In After Vagotomy, J. A. Williams and A. G. Cox, (eds.). London, Butterworth, 1969, p. 225.

102. Baron, J. H. An assessment of the augmented histamine test in the diagnosis of peptic ulcer. Correlations between gastric secretion, age and sex of patients, and site and nature of the ulcer. Gut 4:243, 1963.

103. Chapman, M. A., Werther, J. L., and Janowitz, H. D. Response of the normal and pathological human gastric mucosa to an instilled acid load. Gastroenterology 55:345, 1968.
104. Fischermann, K., and Koster, H. H. The augmented histamine test in the differential diagnosis between ulcer and cancer of the stomach. Gut 3:211, 1962.
105. Kim, Y. S., and Plaut, A. G. β-Glucouronidase studies on gastric secretions from patients with gastric cancer. Gastroenterology 49:50, 1965.
106. Kronborg, O., Malmstion, J., and Christiansen, P. M. A comparison between the results of truncal and selective vagotomy in patients with duodenal ulcer. Scand. J. Gastroent. 5:519, 1970.
107. Johnson, D., Humphrey, C. S., Smith, R. B., et al. Should the gastric antrum be vagally denervated if it is well drained and in the acid stream.? Brit. J. Surg. 58:725, 1971.
108. Kronborg, O. Results of prolonged insulin tests in patients with duodenal ulcer. Comparison between insulin and histamine activated gastric secretion. Scand. J. Gastroent. 5:695, 1970.
109. Bank, S., Marks, I. W., and Louw, J. H. Histamine and insulin stimulated gastric acid secretion after selective and truncal vagotomy. Gut 8:36, 1967.
110. Kronborg, O. Pre- and post-operative insulin tests in patients with duodenal ulcer. Scand. J. Gastroent. 5:687, 1970.
111. Bell, P. R. F., Checketts, R. G., Johnson, D., and Duthie, H. L. Augmented histamine response after incomplete vagotomy. Lancet 2:978, 1965.
112. Kennedy, T., and Connell, A. M. Selective or truncal vagotomy? A double-blind randomized control trial. Lancet 1:899, 1969.
113. Bell, P. R. F. The long-term effect of vagotomy on the maximal acid response to histamine in man. Gastroenterology 46:387, 1964.
114. Gillespie, G., Gillespie, I. E., and Kay, A. W. An analysis of the insulin test after vagotomy using simple and multiple criteria. Gut 9:470, 1968.
115. Kronborg, O. Methods and results of repeated insulin tests. Scand. J. Gastroent. 5:577, 1970.
116. Ross, B., and Kay, A. W. The insulin test after vagotomy. Gastroenterology 46:379, 1964.
117. Johnson, D., Thomas, D. G., Checketts, R. G., and Duthie, H. L. An assessment of postoperative testing for completeness of vagotomy. Brit. J. Surg. 54:831, 1967.
118. Payne, R. A., and Kay, A. W. The effect of vagotomy on maximal acid secretory response to histamine in man. Clin. Sci. 22:373, 1962.
119. Aubrey, D. A., and Forest, A. P. M. The effect of vagotomy on human gastric secretion. Brit. J. Surg. 57:332, 1970.
120. Gillespie, I. E., Clark, D. H., Kay, A. W., and Tankel, H. I. Effect of antrectomy, vagotomy with gastrojejunostomy, and antrectomy with vagotomy on spontaneous and maximal gastric acid output in man. Gastroenterology 38:361, 1960.
121. Broome, A., Bergstrom, H., and Olbe, L. Maximal acid response to histamine in duodenal ulcer patients subjected to resection of the antrum and duodenal bulb followed by vagotomy. Gastroenterology 52:952, 1967.
122. Marks, I. N. The significance of gastric secretion after partial gastrectomy and gastroenterostomy. Amer. J. Gastroent. 27:566, 1957.
123. Frank, B. F., and Kern, F. Menetrier's disease. Gastroenterology 53:953, 1967.
124. Brooks, A. M., Isenberg, J. I., and Goldstein, H. Giant thickening of the gastric mucosa with acid hypersecretion and protein-losing gastropathy. Gastroenterology 58:73, 1970.
125. Stempien, S. J., Ringold, I. M., Heiskell, C. L., et al. Hypertrophic hypersecretory gastropathy. Amer. J. Dig. Dis. 9:471, 1964.
126. Breuer, R. I., and Kirsner, J. B. Present status of Histalog gastric analysis. Ann. N.Y. Acad. Sci. 140:882, 1967.
127. Johnson, D., and Jepson, K. Use of pentagastrin in a test of gastric acid secretion. Lancet 2:585, 1967.

Chapter 43

Interpretation of Serum Gastrin Values

John H. Walsh

The technique of radioimmunoassay has been applied successfully to the measurement of physiological concentrations of gastrin in human serum or plasma.[1-4] By use of this technique some of the factors responsible for stimulation and inhibition of gastrin release in normal and pathological conditions have been defined. As the technique becomes more widely available, more studies will be performed and may provide further insight into the pathogenesis of peptic ulcer disease. Gastrin radioimmunoassay has been especially useful in establishing the diagnosis of gastrinoma (gastrin-secreting pancreatic islet cell tumor of the Zollinger-Ellison variety).[5] Measurement of circulating gastrin concentration offers the most specific method for distinguishing patients with gastrinoma from other patients with acid hypersecretion and peptic ulcer disease.

As more patients with ulcer disease are studied, it is likely that many patients with less overt clinical manifestations of the Zollinger-Ellison syndrome will be recognized. Already several gastrinoma patients have been found with only moderate basal acid hypersecretion, stimulated acid output greater than two times the basal output, and only moderately elevated serum gastrin values. Such patients will provide a diagnostic challenge, because their basal gastrin concentrations may overlap basal

and certainly postprandial values obtained in some patients with duodenal ulcer disease, especially those with prior vagotomy. Preliminary evidence suggests that the differences between gastrinoma and other ulcers can be magnified by certain stimulation tests which will be discussed in this chapter.

FASTING GASTRIN CONCENTRATIONS

Normal gastrin concentrations vary among various laboratories using different assay methods and different standards. The most sensitive and specific assays have utilized antibodies prepared against the whole gastrin molecule rather than against a C-terminal fragment. Among the several assays now being reported, normal mean values for basal gastrin concentration have been between 30 and 120 pg per milliliter (pg is the abbreviation for picogram, 10^{-12}g), with a few apparently normal subjects having values in the range of 200 to 300 pg per milliliter.[2-4, 6-9] Most patients with Zollinger-Ellison syndrome have had values well above the upper limits of normal, frequently greater than 1000 pg per milliliter and usually greater than 500 pg per milliliters.[5-10] Decreases in serum gastrin have been found in some gastrinoma patients following total gastrectomy[8, 11] and following successful parathyroidectomy for hyperparathyroidism.[12] In these circumstances serum gastrin values may fall into the normal or high normal range. In a few documented and several suspected cases of gastrinoma, fasting gastrin concentrations have ranged between 200 and 500 per milliliter prior to gastric or parathyroid surgery.

Gastrin values are usually also elevated in patients with achlorhydria or hypochlorhydria.[7, 13-15] Thus both extremes of acid secretion may be associated with elevated gastrin values; on the one hand, depressed acid secretion leads to loss of normal inhibition of gastrin release by acid and possibly to secondary hyperplasia of the gastrin-producing cells; on the other hand, autonomous release of gastrin from an extragastric tumor may produce excessive secretion of acid and hyperplasia of acid-secreting glands. Gastrin values in patients with achlorhydria tend to average between 500 and 1000 pg per milliliter and thus overlap the values found in those with the Zollinger-Ellison syndrome. In achlorhydrics there is a positive association between high gastrin values and the presence of parietal cell antibodies in the serum, which in turn usually reflects antral sparing by atrophic gastritis.[7, 15]

In the intermediate range of acid secretion there seems to be poor correlation between fasting gastrin and acid secretory rate, either basal or stimulated.[16] In the various series reported to date, there have been no large differences in fasting gastrin concentrations between normal subjects and those with duodenal ulcer, with mean values between groups usually varying by less than 20 pg per milliliter either higher or lower.[3, 4, 6, 8, 9, 16, 17] It has not been established whether normal gastrin concentrations in patients with duodenal ulcer and acid hypersecretion indicate autonomy of the gastrin cells in the sense that the usual suppression of gastrin release by acid may be inadequate or absent.[18] When patients with hypochlorhydria or with parietal cell antibodies are excluded, there seems to be no relationship between serum gastrin and age in the adult population.[7] Gastrin values average approximately twice normal in patients with gastric ulcer,[4, 9, 16] and this is correlated with the tendency for reduced acid secretion in this disease.[16]

Of the two major types of surgical procedures performed for duodenal ulcer, antrectomy or more extensive gastrectomy, with or without vagotomy, results in significant lowering of basal gastrin concentrations,[6, 15, 19] whereas vagotomy without resection results in moderate increases in basal gastrin.[6, 19, 20] The increased gastrin values found after vagotomy may reflect loss of acid inhibition of gastrin release.

Although serum gastrin concentrations are usually diminished after partial gastrectomy, increased gastrin concentrations would be anticipated in patients with the syndrome of retained antrum. This condition occurs in patients with incomplete antral resection and gastrojejunal anastomosis. A pouch of antral tissue remains attached to the duodenal stump, where it is no longer exposed to gastric acid but is subject to distention by antral mucus and potentially exposed to bile refluxed from the duodenum. In such patients gastric acid hypersecretion and recurrent ulceration persist until the remaining tissue is resected. Good examples of this syndrome have been difficult to find in recent years, because this type of resection has been avoided. Only one example of hypergastrinemia caused by retained antrum has been published.[20a]

Two other surgical procedures, portacaval shunt and massive small bowel resection, are often followed by gastric acid hypersecretion. The liver plays no apparent role in the inactivation of gastrin, and there is no evidence that gastric hypersecretion results from decreased catabolism of gastrin after portacaval shunting. Instead, there is evidence that some other humoral factor, normally inactivated by the liver, is responsible. The small intestine is a possible site for gastrin inactivation. In two patients who had intestinal resection with acid hypersecretion, however, serum gastrin concentrations were normal or low (Walsh, unpublished observations).

During a 24-hour period the serum gastrin tends to be increased after meals and falls to its lowest levels in the early morning before breakfast.[21] Nocturnal gastrin concentrations may be higher in patients with duodenal ulcer than in normal subjects.[21] In patients with gastrinoma there is little fluctuation in serum gastrin during the day, although there may be moderate fluctuations from day to day. Pyloric obstruction results in moderate increases in serum gastrin which can be decreased by nasogastric drainage.[21]

STIMULATION OF GASTRIN RELEASE

In response to a protein meal most normal subjects will have an increase in serum gastrin of 50 to 200 pg per milliliter, with a peak between 20 and 40 minutes after eating.[4, 6, 9, 22-25] Responses in normal and duodenal ulcer subjects are similar, with ulcer subjects showing a tendency toward higher responses. Patients with gastrinoma usually have no gastrin response to feeding. Hypochlorhydric patients with elevated fasting gastrin levels usually have exaggerated increases in gastrin after eating.[6] A few patients with acid hypersecretion, some of them with duodenal ulcer, and moderately elevated fasting gastrin concentrations have shown exaggerated gastrin responses to feeding. Following vagotomy the increase in serum gastrin after feeding is usually greater than in nonoperated duodenal ulcer patients.[20, 26] Resection of the gastric antrum abolishes the postprandial gastrin response in patients with gastrojejunal anastomosis,[6, 26] but patients with gastroduodenal anastomosis may have nearly normal gastrin responses, probably reflecting release of gastrin from the duodenum.[26] Carbohydrate and fat given alone are poor stimulants of gastrin release.[4, 9]

Acetylcholine in the dog is a potent gastrin releasing agent, but its effect has not been studied in man. Of the individual amino acids, only glycine has been studied and shown to be a stimulant of gastrin release in man.[22] Distention probably releases gastrin in man, as evidenced by the increased values found in patients with pyloric obstruction, but there is no standard method for demonstrating gastrin release by distention in normal subjects. It has not been established with certainty whether antral neutralization alone will release gastrin in the absence of another stimulant such as distention or a chemical releaser. Alcohol is not a potent gastrin-releasing agent in man.[6]

In response to insulin hypoglycemia definite increases in serum gastrin can be demonstrated if the pH of the stomach is maintained at neutrality, and moderate responses can be obtained during continuous aspiration of gastric contents.[3, 8, 24, 27] In a surprising preliminary report, Stadil and coworkers found that truncal vagotomy did not abolish the serum gastrin response to insulin.[28]

Two agents, calcium and secretin, may selectively increase serum gastrin concentrations in patients with gastrinoma. In normal subjects and patients with duodenal ulcer, calcium is a moderate stimulant of acid secretion (see p. 542), whereas in patients who have Zollinger-Ellison syndrome the stimulation by calcium may be pronounced. Calcium infusion may increase serum gastrin values in normal and ulcer subjects, but the increases are only approximately two times basal levels after a three-hour infusion of 4 mg per kilogram per hour.[29] In response to an infusion of 5 mg per kilogram per hour, patients with gastrinoma have shown marked increases in serum gastrin, usually to stimulated values greater than 1000 pg per milliliter.[10] The greatest increases have been found in patients with intermediate fasting gastrin concentrations of 200 to 800 pg per milliliter. Similar observations were made by Trudeau and McGuigan in a patient with normal gastrin values vollowing parathyroidectomy.[12] The change in serum gastrin after a three-hour infusion of calcium may provide a useful test for distinguishing those patients with Zollinger-Ellison syndrome who have equivocal basal levels. It has not yet been determined whether a significant number of patients with ordinary ulcer disease will have false-positive responses.

There is preliminary evidence that secretin may release gastrin in some patients with gastrinoma,[30] unlike the usual decrease in gastrin found in normal and achlorhydric patients.[14, 31] The proportion of gastrinoma patients who will show this response has not been determined. Secretin testing may have an advantage over other stimulation tests if a significant proportion of gastrinoma patients show a positive response, because it ordinarily does not increase serum gastrin.

SUPPRESSION OF GASTRIN RELEASE

In achlorhydric patients with increased serum gastrin concentrations, gastric acidification causes a prompt decline in gastrin of about 50 to 70 per cent.[2, 7, 14] The rate of decline in gastrin values has led to estimates that the half-life of circulating gastrin is in the order of 5 to 15 minutes.[2, 7] In patients with Zollinger-Ellison syndrome, gastric acidity does not suppress gastrin values. The effects of gastric acidification have not been studied extensively in other patients, but moderate decreases were noted in one study.[4] The inhibitory effect of acid on insulin stimulation of gastrin release has been noted. Little is known about the pH requirements in man for the release of gastrin by protein.

Since gastrin release is felt to be mediated by cholinergic reflexes in the gastric wall (pp. 144 to 160), it seems reasonable that anticholinergic drugs might decrease gastrin levels. Increased gastrin values found after vagotomy indicate that vagal cholinergic stimulation is not required for basal and chemical release of gastrin. Doses of atropine between 0.6 and 1 mg have generally not depressed fasting gastrin concentrations and have led to increased gastrin responses to feeding.[6, 9, 25] In the doses used, the predominant effect of atropine was probably suppression of acid secretion which led to decreased feedback inhibition of gastrin release. In several patients with gastrinoma, we have observed no change in serum gastrin following administration of atropine or propantheline bromide.

In normal subjects and patients with duodenal ulcer or pernicious anemia, parenteral administration of secretin resulted in 30 to 40 per cent decreases in basal gastrin concentrations.[14, 31] As mentioned previously, some patients with gastrinoma may show an anomalous response with stimulation of acid secretion and increase in serum gastrin.

Little is known about pharmacological agents which might decrease serum gastrin concentrations in patients with gastrinoma, although an effective nontoxic agent would have obvious clinical importance. We have preliminary evidence that parenteral administration of ethylenediaminetetraacetic acid (EDTA) in doses sufficient to produce hypocalcemia will depress serum gastrin and gastric acid secretion in some patients with gastrinoma (Passaro and Walsh, unpublished observations). This inhibition is not likely to have much clinical application, but perhaps other less toxic suppressive agents will be identified.

SUMMARY

As a diagnostic tool, gastrin radioimmunoassay is useful primarily in establishing the diagnosis of gastrinoma (Zollinger-Ellison syndrome). When antibodies are prepared against the entire human or hog gastrin molecule and suitably purified gastrin standards are used in the assay, fasting serum gastrin concentrations in normal subjects and patients with duodenal ulcer usually range between 10 and 150 pg per milliliter. Higher values found in achlorhydric patients offer no problems in the differential diagnosis from gastrinoma because of clinical dissimilarities between the two groups of patients. Patients with Zollinger-Ellison syndrome usually have fasting gastrin concentrations greater than 500 pg per milliliter and often greater than 1000 pg per milliliter. Some patients with gastrinoma, especially after correction of hyperparathyroidism, may have gastrin values in an intermediate range between normal and usual gastrinoma values. Marked stimulation of serum gastrin following infusion of calcium and lack of normal postprandial increases in gastrin after a protein meal may aid in the diagnosis. An increase in serum gastrin and in acid secretion in response to secretin may also prove to be helpful in the diagnosis of these patients. Serum gastrin measurement is a useful method for distinguishing gastrinoma patients from patients with ordinary duodenal ulcer disease, but does not distinguish ulcer patients from normals. Postoperative measurement of serum gastrin may be helpful in excluding the syndrome of retained antrum in patients with subtotal gastric resection and recurrent ulcers.

REFERENCES

1. McGuigan, J. E. Immunochemical studies with synthetic human gastrin. Gastroenterology 54:1005, 1968.
2. Yalow, R. S., and Berson, S. A. Radioimmunoassay of gastrin. Gastroenterology 58:1, 1970.
3. Hansky, J., and Cain, M. D. Radioimmunoassay of gastrin in human serum. Lancet 2:1388, 1969.
4. Ganguli, P. C., and Hunter, W. M. Radio-immunoassay of gastrin in human plasma. J. Physiol. 220:499, 1972.
5. McGuigan, J. E., and Trudeau, W. L. Immunochemical measurement of elevated levels of gastrin in the serum of patients with pancreatic tumors of the Zollinger-Ellison variety. New Eng. J. Med. 278:1308, 1968.
6. Berson, S. A., Walsh, J. H., and Yalow, R. S. Radioimmunoassay of gastrin in human plasma and regulation of gastrin secretion. Nobel Symposium XVI: Frontiers in Gastrointestinal Hormone Research, Stockholm, July 20-21, 1970. In press.
7. Ganguli, P. C., Cullen, D. R., and Irvine, W. J. Radioimmunoassay of plasma-gastrin in pernicious anaemia, achlorhydria without pernicious anaemia, hypochlorhydria, and in controls. Lancet 1:155, 1971.
8. Stadil, F., Rehfeld, J. F., and Thaysen, E. H. Variations in the concentrations of serum gastrin in the Zollinger-Ellison syndrome. In Gastrointestinal Hormones and Other Subjects, 5th Scandinavian Conference on Gastroenterology, August 25-28, 1971, E. H. Thaysen, (ed.). Copenhagen, Munksgaard, 1971, p. 125.
9. Korman, M. G., Soveny, C., and Hansky, J. Serum gastrin in duodenal ulcer. Gut 12:899, 1971.
10. Passaro, E., Jr., Basso, N., and Walsh, J. H. Calcium challenge in the Zollinger-Ellison syndrome. Surgery 72:60, 1972.
11. Friesen, S. R., Bolinger, R. E., Pearse, A. G. E., and McGuigan, J. E. Serum gastrin levels in malignant Zollinger-Ellison syndrome after total gastrectomy and hypophysectomy. Ann. Surg. 172:504, 1970.
12. Trudeau, W. L., and McGuigan, J. E. Effects of calcium on serum gastrin levels in the Zollinger-Ellison syndrome. New Eng. J. Med. 281:862, 1969.
13. McGuigan, J. E., and Trudeau, W. L. Serum gastrin concentrations in pernicious anemia. New Eng. J. Med. 282:358, 1970.
14. Hansky, J., Korman, M. G., Soveny, C., and St. John, D. J. B. Radioimmunoassay of gastrin: Studies in pernicious anemia. Gut 12:97, 1971.
15. Strickland, R. G., Bhathal, P. S., Korman, M. G., and Hansky, J. Serum gastrin and the antral mucosa in atrophic gastritis. Brit. Med. J. 4:451, 1971.
16. Trudeau, W. L., and McGuigan, J. E. Relations between serum gastrin levels and rates of gastric hydrochloric acid secretion. New Eng. J. Med. 284:408, 1971.
17. Reeder, D. D., Jackson, B. M., Ban, J. L., Davidson, W. D., and Thompson, J. C. Effect of food on serum gastrin concentrations in duodenal ulcer and control patients. Surg. Forum 21:290, 1970.
18. Berson, S. A., and Yalow, R. S. Gastrin in duodenal ulcer. New Eng. J. Med. 284:445, 1971.
19. McGuigan, J. E., and Trudeau, W. L. Serum gastrin levels before and after vagotomy and pyloroplasty or vagotomy and antrectomy. New Eng. J. Med. 286:184, 1972.
20. Korman, M. G., Hansky, J., and Scott, P. R. Serum gastrin in duodenal ulcer. III. Influence of vagotomy and pylorectomy. Gut 13:39, 1972.
20a. Korman, K. G., Scott, D. F., Hansky, J., and Wilson, H. Hypergastrinemia due to excluded gastric antrum: A proposed method for differentiation from the Zollinger-Ellison syndrome. Austral. New Zeal. J. Med. 3:266, 1972.
21. Feurle, G., Ketterer, H., Becker, H. D., and Creutzfeldt, W. Circadian serum gastrin concentrations in control persons and in patients with ulcer disease. Scand. J. Gastroent. 7:177, 1972.
22. McGuigan, J. E., and Trudeau, W. L. Studies with antibodies to gastrin. Gastroenterology 58:139, 1970.
23. Forrester, J. M., and Ganguli, P. C. The effect of meat extract (Oxo) on plasma gastrin concentration in human subjects. J. Physiol. 211:33, 1970.
24. Stagg, B. H., Lewin, M. R., Boulos, P. B., and Clark, C. G. The release of gastrin in response to insulin, food, and meat extract (Oxo). Brit. J. Surg. 58:863, 1971.
25. Walsh, J. H., Yalow, R. S., and Berson, S. A. The effect of atropine on plasma gastrin response to feeding. Gastroenterology 60:16, 1971.
26. Stern, D. H., and Walsh, J. H. Release of gastrin in postoperative duodenal ulcer patients. Gastroenterology. In press.
27. Hansky, J., Korman, M. G., Cowley, D. J., and Baron, J. H. Plasma-gastrin levels in patients with duodenal ulcer after insulin hypoglycemia. Brit. J. Surg. 58:863, 1971.
28. Stadil, F., Rehfeld, J. F., and Christiansen, P. M. Effect of vagotomy on gastrin release by insulin. In Gastrointestinal Hormones and Other Subjects, 5th Scandinavian Conference on Gastroenterology, August 25-28, 1971, E. H. Thaysen (ed.) Copenhagen, Munksgaard, 1971, p. 45.
29. Reeder, D. D., Jackson, B. M., Ban, J., Clendinnen, B. G., Davidson, W. D., and Thompson, J. C. Influence of hypercalcemia on gastric secretion and serum gastrin concentrations in man. Ann. Surg. 172:540, 1970.
30. Isenberg, J. I., Walsh, J. H., Passaro, E., Jr., Moore, E. W., and Grossman, M. I. Unusual effect of secretion on serum gastrin, serum calcium, and gastric acid secretion in a patient with suspected Zollinger-Ellison syndrome. Gastroenterology 62:626, 1972.
31. Hansky, J., Soveny, C., and Korman, M. G. Effect of secretin on serum gastrin as measured by immunoassay. Gastroenterology 61:62, 1971.

Chapter 44

Gastritis

Graham H. Jeffries

INTRODUCTION

Current knowledge of gastritis is based mainly upon studies of gastric mucosal structure and function. Although many gastrointestinal symptoms have been attributed to gastritis, it is now evident that diffuse gastric mucosal lesions are commonly asymptomatic; thus clinicians must rely on secretory, radiographic, endoscopic, and mucosal biopsy studies to characterize mucosal lesions.

Gastric secretory studies may provide quantitative information reflecting the number of parietal cells in the gastric mucosa; with maximal secretory stimulation, acid secretion is proportional to the parietal cell mass. A decrease in the number of gastric parietal cells (as in atrophic gastritis) will be reflected by a decrease in acid secretion. The composition of gastric juice also reflects the permeability characteristics of the gastric mucosa; normally, the surface epithelium is relatively impermeable to hydrogen ions, but when acute mucosal injury disrupts this barrier to ion diffusion, acid will diffuse back from the gastric lumen, and sodium and potassium ions from interstitial fluid and mucosal cells will appear in higher concentrations in the gastric juice, together with varying amounts of plasma protein and blood cells.

Radiographic studies provide limited data in patients with gastritis. Thickening of mucosal folds may be appreciated in pa-

tients with hypertrophic gastritis, and a relative decrease in the mucosal folds may reflect mucosal atrophy, but these radiographic changes must be interpreted with caution and confirmed by other studies.

Gastroscopic inspection of the gastric mucosa has been facilitated by the development of flexible fiberoptic instruments which permit not only inspection of the entire gastric mucosa but also gastrophotography and biopsy. Diffuse lesions that are not demonstrable radiographically can be seen (see pp. 521 to 535). Mucosal biopsies obtained either gastroscopically or by peroral biopsy instruments permit microscopic assessment of the complete thickness of the gastric mucosa. The histological abnormalities can be correlated with secretory, radiographic, and endoscopic findings, and a pathological diagnosis can be established. Mucosal biopsy is safe and simple, but it has the disadvantage of blind sampling of the mucosa; gastritis, however, is usually a diffuse lesion, so that blind peroral biopsies usually document the lesion.

CLASSIFICATION[1, 2]

Gastritis is best classified according to the microscopic changes observed in gastric biopsy specimens. Although the term gastritis suggests inflammation in the mucosa, it should be appreciated that the ter-

560

minology is descriptive and does not necessarily reflect basic disease mechanisms. The pathogenesis of many gastric lesions is still poorly understood.

Acute Gastritis. Lesions of varying severity may be caused by a wide variety of agents or conditions (vide infra). The terms *acute gastritis, acute erosive gastritis, acute hemorrhagic gastritis,* and *acute stress erosion* refer to varying manifestations of the acute mucosal reaction.

Chronic Gastritis. This term includes a variety of lesions (probably of varying etiology) which persist over long periods. In *chronic superficial gastritis* the lamina propria adjacent to the mucosal surface and between gastric pits is infiltrated with mononuclear cells; the glands remain normal. In *atrophic gastritis* the infiltration with mononuclear cells is more diffuse and accompanies a variable loss of gland cells; the lesion may be graded according to the degree of gland atrophy. *Gastric atrophy* is characterized by a complete loss of gastric glands, with thinning of the mucosa and minimal infiltration; gastric glands may be variably or completely replaced by intestinal epithelium (*intestinal metaplasia*). *Granulomatous gastritis* has been described in patients with tuberculosis, sarcoidosis, or regional enteritis. *Eosinophilic gastritis* may be a localized granulomatous lesion, or may be a diffuse infiltration of the entire thickness of the stomach from mucosa to serosa; this infiltration usually involves the pylorus and proximal small bowel. *Hypertrophic gastritis* refers to an increase in mucosal thickness resulting from hyperplasia of the surface epithelial cells. The lesion may be localized or diffuse.

THE NORMAL STRUCTURE AND FUNCTION OF THE GASTRIC MUCOSA

Knowledge of normal mucosal structure and function provides a basis for understanding the pathophysiology and clinical manifestations of gastric mucosal disease.

The Surface Epithelium. Columnar mucus-secreting cells line the gastric pits and extend over the luminal surface. These cells differentiate from a population of rapidly proliferating cells at the base of the gastric pits; they migrate to the surface and continuously replace surface cells which are shed into the gastric lumen. The mean life span of these cells is approximately three days.[3]

An important function of the surface epithelium of the stomach is its relative impermeability to ions, particularly H^+.[4] This relative impermeability ("mucosal barrier") retains the high concentration of hydrogen ions secreted by parietal cells within the gastric lumen and normally protects the mucosa from acid-peptic digestion. The small amounts of H^+ which may normally diffuse across the epithelium in spite of the barrier are effectively neutralized in interstitial fluid. It was once thought that surface mucus formed a protective layer on the mucosa, but in vitro studies suggest that this is not the case; it is more likely that the mucosal barrier to ion diffusion is a metabolic function of the surface epithelial cells.

It is of particular interest that the antral mucosal epithelium has a greater permeability to ions than the mucosa of the body and fundus of the stomach. This difference has been demonstrated experimentally in isolated pouches of fundic or antral mucosa.[5] Antral mucosal permeability to H^+ may permit gastrin cells located deep in the pyloric glands to monitor changes in the composition of luminal content (particularly with respect to H^+, amino acid, and peptide concentration) and to regulate the secretion of gastrin in response to these changes.

Glands of the Body and Fundus. These glands consist of tubular acini extending from the base of gastric pits to the muscularis mucosae and lined by specialized secretory cells — parietal cells secreting hydrochloric acid and intrinsic factor, chief cells secreting pepsinogens, and mucous neck cells secreting both mucoproteins and pepsinogen.[6]

The population of cells in the gastric glands is a relatively stable one with a long life, in contrast to the short life of surface epithelial cells. Both cell populations, however, may be derived from primitive cells at the base of the gastric pits.[6, 7] The hormonal and vagal control of secretion from the gastric glands is relatively well defined. Much less is known about the factors which regulate the proliferation of cells in the gastric mucosa. Recent experimental studies suggest that gastrin may not only have a secretory function, but may also exert a trophic effect on gastric parietal cells;[8] this would explain the increase in parietal cell population in patients with gastrin-secreting tumors of the pancreatic islets (Zollinger-Ellison syndrome).

Gastric secretory function can be measured in a reproducible manner when large doses of histamine phosphate (0.04 mg per kilogram of body weight) with an antihistaminic agent, the histamine analogue Histalog (100 mg subcutaneously), or synthetic gastrin peptide, Pentagastrin (6 μg per kilogram), are used as secretory stimulants. Acid secretion, expressed as the maximal acid output (MAO in milliequivalents per hour), is a direct reflection of the number of gastric parietal cells (see pp. 536 to 550). The same secretory stimuli cause the secretion of intrinsic factor which appears to be released from mucosal storage.[9]

Secretory studies which do not utilize maximal stimulation of the gastric glands are of limited clinical value, because acid secretion does not parallel the parietal cell population; maximal stimulation is necessary to establish achlorhydria (i.e., the absence of gastric parietal cells) and to estimate gastric hypersecretion.

Glands of the Antral (Pyloric) Mucosa. Pyloric glands are more convoluted than those of the fundus, and are lined by cuboidal or columnar cells which secrete an alkaline mucus containing pepsinogens. The antrum has an important function in regulating gastric secretion and emptying. Gastrin released from gastrin cells in the pyloric glands in response to food and distention at pH values >3.5 mediates the gastric phase of acid secretion and stimulates contractions of the stomach.

ACUTE GASTRITIS

Pathologically, the lesions of acute hemorrhagic or erosive gastritis (Fig. 44–1) may be localized or diffuse. Necrosis of surface cells with extravasation of blood and plasma from damaged vessels in the lamina propria produces superficial erosions; deeper erosions may involve the underlying gastric glands. Surface mucous cells between erosions may exhibit degenerative changes, or there may be evidence of mucosal regeneration with basophilic flattened or cuboidal surface epithelial cells containing little mucus.[10] More severe lesions which extend to the submucosa and muscularis (i.e., acute ulcers) may develop from superficial erosions.

Clinical and Laboratory Manifestations. Acute gastrointestinal bleeding is the major clinical manifestation of acute gastritis. Early gastroscopic examination in patients admitted to hospital with acute hematemesis has revealed that erosive gastritis is a common cause of massive bleeding; this lesion may account for up to 30 per cent of bleeding episodes, and can only be diagnosed by gastroscopy.[11, 12] Beaumont first observed in his classic gastric fistula studies that erosive gastritis was often unaccompanied by symptoms; endoscopic studies following aspirin ingestion have confirmed this. Patients with gastritis associated with acute infection (e.g., salmonella or staphylococcal food poisoning) may suffer epigastric discomfort, anorexia, nausea, and vomiting; these symptoms may be due to stimulation of visceral afferent nerves which is independent of gastric mucosal changes.

Transient hypochlorhydria or achlorhydria may be observed during episodes of acute gastritis; this may be explained in part by the back-diffusion of H^+ through the damaged mucosa.

On gastroscopic examination, the mucosa may appear to be edematous and hyperemic with surface erosions and mucosal hemorrhages.[11] It is important to distinguish the lesions of acute gastritis from small erosions that may result from aspiration of the mucosa into the sampling orifices of a nasogastric tube. Serial gastroscopic observations or mucosal biopsies usually show complete recovery within several days of the onset of acute bleeding; this recovery is consistent with the rapid proliferation and replacement of surface epithelial cells.

Pathogenesis. Acute gastritis has been well documented following ingestion of aspirin and alcohol, during treatment with antitumor agents, following gastric irradiation or gastric freezing, as a terminal event in uremia, in association with infection, in staphylococcal food poisoning, and as a complication of several stress situations—particularly severe trauma, operations, or infection accompanied by shock.

Two experimental approaches have provided information that may relate to the pathogenesis of acute gastric mucosal injury in man. Studies on the *gastric mucosal barrier to* H^+ have shown that a variety of exogenous agents alter mucosal permeability. At an acid pH, acetylsalicylic acid is un-ionized and relatively lipid soluble; this solubility permits aspirin to diffuse through the lipid membrane of surface epithelial cells and to damage the epithelium. Epithelial cell injury causes a reversible loss of the mucosal barrier and permits back-diffusion of H^+ into the mucosa. This acid back-diffusion extends mucosal injury and leads to acid-peptic digestion with erosions and hemorrhage.[13] Similar changes in the gastric mucosal barrier have been demonstrated in experimental animals subjected to hemorrhagic shock and in critically ill patients;[14] a decrease in gastric mucosal blood flow may be an important cause for mucosal injury in ill patients with a variety of disorders. Studies of *cell proliferation in the gastric mucosa* of animals exposed to conditions that may experimentally mimic human stress have documented changes in mucosal cell regeneration accompanying mucosal injury.[15] Mucosal erosions in animals subjected to restraint stress are preceded by a decrease in mucosal blood flow, a decrease in the activity of cellular enzymes which synthesize DNA, and an inhibition of cell division in the proliferation compartment at the base of gastric pits.

Endoscopic observations and studies of gastric mucosal permeability in man suggest that erosive gastritis is caused by exogenous and endogenous influences which increase mucosal permeability and directly injure surface cells and/or impair the regenerative capacity of the mucosal epithelium. When the noxious influence is transient, varying degrees of acute injury (from superficial erosions to acute penetrating ulcers) are followed by rapid recovery unless serious complications (massive bleeding with shock, or perforation) modify the clinical course. When the mucosa is subjected recurrently or chronically to a noxious influence—e.g., with chronic aspirin ingestion or reflux of bile following gastrojejunostomy—recurrent erosion and repair of the mucosa may lead to gland atrophy, or acute lesions may be replaced by chronic ulcers.

Management of Acute Hemorrhagic Gastritis. Many patients with hemorrhagic gastritis stop bleeding spontaneously when they enter hospital. Continued bleeding from documented gastritis may be controlled by ice water lavage of the stomach and by correction of bleeding or clotting defects. When acute bleeding has stopped, vigorous antacid therapy to neutralize all secreted acid has been recommended because of the impaired ability of the mucosa to withstand acid injury.[16] When massive uncontrolled bleeding demands operative intervention, a vagotomy with gastric drainage may provide better control of hemorrhage than gastric resection. The mortality of patients with bleeding from acute gastritis is related to liver failure complicating cirrhosis, or to cardiovascular disease.

Following recovery from an episode of hemorrhagic gastritis, the patient should avoid aspirin, phenylbutazone, and other agents which may cause acute gastric mucosal injury.

CORROSIVE GASTRITIS

Corrosive gastritis results from accidental or suicidal ingestion of strong acids, bichloride of mercury, carbolic acid, or Lysol. Although ingestion of strong alkali may cause gastritis, esophagitis is usually a greater clinical problem. Tissue necrosis may lead to perforation of the stomach, chronic scarring, or obstruction. Treatment includes the administration of an appropriate antidote, gastric lavage, and general supportive therapy—maintenance of an adequate airway and of circulating blood require corrective surgery (see pp. 605 to 607).

GASTRITIS DUE TO PHYSICAL AGENTS: IRRADIATION AND FREEZING

Acute gastritis has been observed during the course of gastric irradiation. Acute injury may be followed by a reduction in the parietal cell population and hypochlorhy-

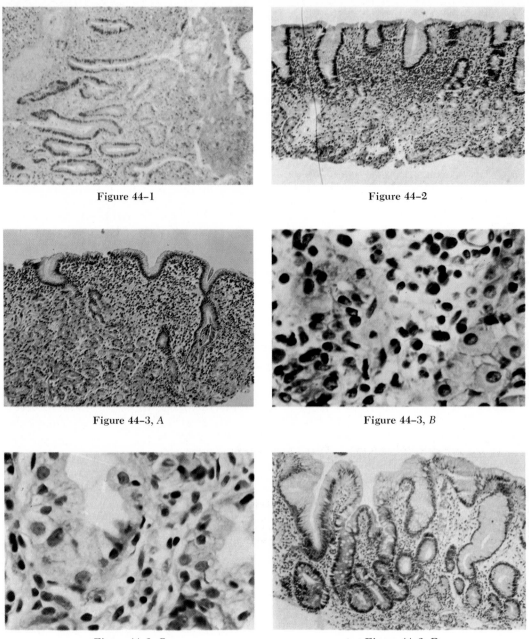

Figure 44–1

Figure 44–2

Figure 44–3, *A*

Figure 44–3, *B*

Figure 44–3, *C*

Figure 44–3, *D*

Figure 44–1. Acute hemorrhagic gastritis. Peroral gastric mucosal biopsy from a 32-year-old male who presented with massive hematemesis following ingestion of alcohol and aspirin. Gastroscopic examination revealed diffuse hemorrhagic erosions of the gastric body and fundus. There is necrosis of the surface epithelium and gastric glands with early regeneration of mucous cells. Hematoxylin and eosin stain.

Figure 44–2. Chronic superficial gastritis. The lamina propria between the gastric pits is infiltrated with mononuclear cells; this infiltrate does not extend to the deeper glandular compartment. The surface mucous cells are relatively flattened, compared with the columnar cells of the gastric pits. Gastric secretion of acid was in the normal range.

Figure 44–3. Chronic atrophic gastritis. *A*, Gastric mucosal biopsy from a 40-year-old asymptomatic sister of a patient with pernicious anemia. Gastric acid secretion was in the low normal range, vitamin B_{12} absorption was normal, and serum contained parietal cell antibody. There is infiltration of the lamina propria between gastric pits and extending between gland acini; the glandular compartment is reduced. *B*, High power view of *A* demonstrates infiltration of lymphocytes, plasma cells, and eosinophils between acini of parietal cells. *C*, Residual gastric gland acinus from a mucosal biopsy exhibiting partial atrophic gastritis; several gland cells show evidence of degeneration. *Figure 44–3 continued on opposite page.*

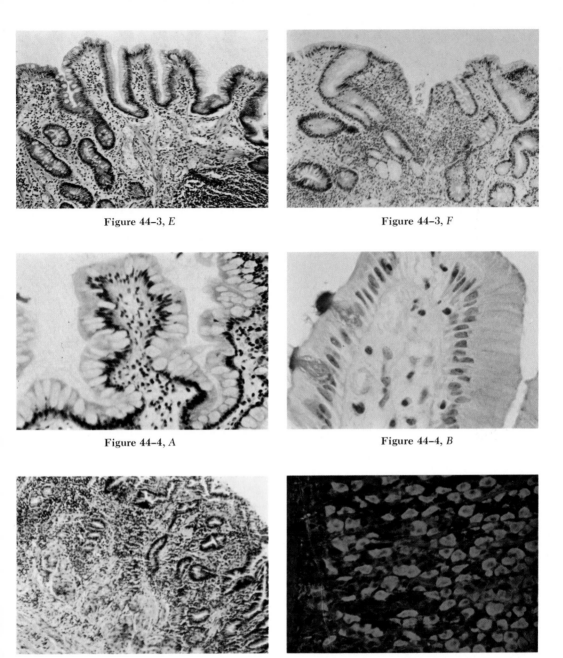

Figure 44–3, E

Figure 44–3, F

Figure 44–4, A

Figure 44–4, B

Figure 44–5

Figure 44–6

Figure 44–3 *Continued.* *D*, *E*, and *F*, Biopsies of fundic mucosa from patients with pernicious anemia. *E*, Gastric atrophy with absent gastric glands (right) and partial intestinal metaplasia (left); there is a lymphoid follicle in the lamina propria. In *D* and *F* the mucous cells of the gastric pits and surface are retained, but residual gastric glands are devoid of chief and parietal cells and consist of undifferentiated and pyloric-type mucous gland cells. There is patchy intestinal metaplasia. There is a superficial erosion in *F* which may represent a source of occult bleeding which is not uncommon in patients with pernicious anemia.

Figure 44–4. Intestinal metaplasia. *A*, Mucosa that is totally replaced by intestinal villi and crypts. *B*, Intestinal goblet cells (left) and gastric mucous cells (right) stained with alcian blue. Both mucosal biopsies were from a patient with pernicious anemia.

Figure 44–5. Chronic gastritis associated with gastric ulcer disease. This mucosal biopsy was from the antrum of a patient with a lesser curve gastric ulcer. There is severe superficial gastritis with inflammatory cells extending into the deeper zone of pyloric glands.

Figure 44–6. Gastric parietal cell antibodies. Serum from a patient with pernicious anemia was incubated with a frozen section of rat gastric mucosa, and the section was subsequently stained with fluorescein-labeled antiserum to human gamma globulin. Parietal cell cytoplasmic antigen which has combined with antibody in the serum shows fluorescent staining under ultraviolet illumination.

dria or achlorhydria of several months' duration. Reduction in acid secretion induced by irradiation may be of benefit to patients with intractable duodenal ulcer disease when operation is contraindicated by other disease.[17] Gastric freezing, recently in vogue for the treatment of duodenal ulcer, causes hemorrhagic necrosis of the gastric mucosa; this is followed by rapid restoration of normal structure and function. Controlled therapeutic trials have not established the value of this procedure.[18, 19]

It has been suggested that ingestion of hot foods and particularly hot tea may cause thermal injury to the gastric mucosa. In one study it was observed that subjects who drank tea at temperatures between 130° and 135° F exhibited gastritis more often than subjects who drank their tea at lower temperatures.

CHRONIC SUPERFICIAL GASTRITIS

Pathologically, chronic superficial gastritis (Fig. 44–2) is characterized by excessive lymphocytic and plasma cell infiltration of the lamina propria adjacent to the surface and gastric pits. There may also be a polymorphonuclear infiltrate penetrating the superficial epithelium. The surface mucous cells may be irregular in shape or flattened, with a decrease in mucus in their apical cytoplasm. The gastric glands remain normal, and the cellular infiltrate does not extend between gland acini. The pathogenesis of this lesion, particularly its relationship to acute gastritis, has not been defined.

The clinical significance of chronic superficial gastritis remains uncertain. It is not known whether this abnormal mucosa is more susceptible to acute injury with erosion and hemorrhage. In a 20-year follow-up of 93 patients with superficial gastritis, Siurala and Salmi found that the lesion commonly progressed to atrophic gastritis; they observed only one patient who developed gastric carcinoma during the period of follow-up.[20]

CHRONIC ATROPHIC GASTRITIS AND GASTRIC ATROPHY

Atrophic gastritis (Fig. 44–3) is a diffuse lesion of the gastric mucosa that particularly involves the body and fundus. There is a partial or complete loss of gastric gland cells, with variable thinning of the mucosa and infiltration with lymphocytes, plasma cells, and occasional eosinophils. In severe atrophic gastritis, the residual glands may contain undifferentiated or pyloric-type cells. The gastric pits are decreased in number, but may retain normal gastric mucus cells. There may be a patchy or diffuse replacement of surface gastric epithelium by intestinal type mucosa (intestinal metaplasia), with all the cellular elements of the normal intestinal epithelium (Fig. 44–4).

Clinical and Laboratory Manifestations. There are no specific symptoms associated with atrophic gastritis. The majority of patients remain asymptomatic, but some complain of ill-defined dyspepsia. The clinical manifestations of vitamin B_{12} deficiency are often the only overt evidence of underlying atrophic gastritis. There may be bleeding from the atrophic mucosa; this is usually occult and should raise the suspicion of gastric malignancy. Occasionally, bleeding may be massive and recurrent.

There is evidence that the frequency of atrophic gastritis increases with age, and that the lesion is more common in women. Atrophic gastritis has a higher frequency in the relatives of patients with pernicious anemia[21] and in patients with diabetes mellitus, thyroid disease (thyrotoxicosis, myxedema, and Hashimoto's thyroiditis), idiopathic Addison's disease, and iron deficiency anemia.[22, 23]

Atrophy of the gastric glands in the fundic mucosa leads to gastric hyposecretion. The reduction in acid secretion with maximal stimulation parallels the decrease in parietal cells; in patients with advanced atrophic gastritis or gastric atrophy, histamine-fast achlorhydria is usual. Loss of parietal cells depresses the secretion of gastric intrinsic factor. Normally, intrinsic factor is secreted in considerable excess of the amount necessary for optimal vitamin B_{12} absorption;[9] thus many patients with atrophic gastritis and achlorhydria may secrete sufficient intrinsic factor to permit normal vitamin B_{12} absorption. Vitamin B_{12} malabsorption is seen in patients with gastric atrophy with total lack of intrinsic factor. Vitamin B_{12} deficiency is a late manifestation of vitamin malabsorption, because it takes several years for the hepatic vitamin B_{12} store to be depleted. The loss of chief cells in atrophic gastritis decreases the secretion of pepsinogens, but does not have nutritional consequences; protein digestion by pancreatic enzymes and intestinal peptidases permits normal amino acid and peptide absorption. A depression of urinary pepsinogen excretion reflects the decrease in gastric enzyme.

Idiopathic atrophic gastritis is usually confined to the acid-secreting mucosa of the gastric body and fundus.[24] This localization explains a recent observation that serum gastrin levels are greatly elevated in patients with pernicious anemia. In these patients, the pyloric mucosa may appear histologically normal with an excessive number of gastrin cells in the glands. Hypergastrinemia results from loss of the normal acid inhibition of gastrin release; perfusion of the gastric antrum with acid restores normal serum gastrin levels in these patients.[25, 26]

On endoscopic examination, severe atrophic gastritis and gastric atrophy may be recognized by visualization of submucosal vessels through the thinned mucosa. Endoscopic diagnosis of lesser degrees of atrophic gastritis is unreliable. Radiographically, air contrast studies may reveal a paucity of mucosal folds in the distended gastric body and fundus. Only biopsy of the fundic mucosa can establish accurately the diagnosis of atrophic gastritis. Multiple biopsies provide a better assessment of the lesion when atrophy or intestinal metaplasia is patchy and variable.

The demonstration of circulating antibodies reactive with gastric mucosal antigens (parietal cell, or intrinsic factor) may suggest the diagnosis of atrophic gastritis (vide infra).

Pathogenesis. Although it has been suggested that a variety of extrinsic influences may cause atrophic gastritis, particularly with repeated exposure, there is currently no evidence that the agents which commonly cause acute gastritis—aspirin and alcohol—are also etiological factors in chronic atrophic gastritis.

There is growing evidence, both clinical and experimental, that bile salts may cause acute and chronic injury to the gastric mucosa. This may follow reflux of bile through the pylorus, or may complicate gastric resection with gastrojejunal anas-

tomosis. In acute experiments, bile salts disrupt the gastric mucosal barrier to ion diffusion;[27] although it has not been established experimentally, chronic exposure may lead to degeneration of the deeper glandular layer. Patients with gastric ulcer disease usually exhibit chronic gastritis in the antrum (Fig. 44–5); this extends proximally to replace part of the mucosa of the body of the stomach, and may precede the development of gastric ulceration. Reflux of bile into the stomach occurs with significant frequency in patients with gastric ulcer disease.[28] Gastric resection with gastrojejunal anastomosis is often followed by progressive atrophy of the gastric mucosal remnant. This atrophy may be due in part to removal of trophic influences by vagectomy and antrectomy, but the frequent demonstration of gastritis proximal to the anastomosis, often with superficial erosions and gland atrophy, suggests alternate mechanisms—possibly bile salt damage.

Chronic infection, particularly syphilis, has been implicated as a rare cause for chronic gastritis.

The demonstration of specific immunological phenomena in patients with idiopathic chronic atrophic gastritis (and pernicious anemia) has led to the hypothesis that immune mechanisms may be of importance in the pathogenesis of this mucosal lesion. Antibodies reactive with parietal cell cytoplasmic antigen (parietal cell antibody) and with intrinsic factor have been detected in the serum of patients with pernicious anemia or atrophic gastritis. Parietal cell antibody (Fig. 44–6), detected by complement fixation tests using gastric mucosal homogenate, or by indirect immunofluorescence on sections of gastric mucosa, is present in serum of approximately 60 per cent of patients with idiopathic atrophic gastritis and in 80 to 90 per cent of patients with pernicious anemia.[22, 29] Intrinsic factor antibodies combine with intrinsic factor at two sites. Type I antibody combines with intrinsic factor and prevents vitamin B_{12} binding, i.e., the antibody reacts at or near the vitamin B_{12} binding site or modifies this site. Type II antibody combines with intrinsic factor without impairing vitamin B_{12} binding.[30] With the rare exception of patients with diabetes mellitus or thyrotoxicosis, intrinsic factor antibodies have been detected only in patients with pernicious anemia (60 to 70 per cent). The association between thyroid disease, Addison's disease, diabetes mellitus, and atrophic gastritis or pernicious anemia may be related to immunological mechanisms; these patients have in common a high incidence of specific antibodies reactive against tissue antigens. Approximately 25 per cent of patients with Hashimoto's thyroiditis exhibited circulating parietal cell antibodies;[22] those with antibody have atrophic gastritis.[23] Conversely, patients with pernicious anemia or atrophic gastritis exhibit a high incidence of specific thyroid antibodies and a high frequency of thyroid disease.[22]

It has not been established that circulating parietal cell or intrinsic factor antibodies cause atrophic gastritis. A significant number of patients with atrophic gastritis do not exhibit gastric antibodies, and patients with hypogammaglobulinemia, deficient in circulating antibody, may develop atrophic gastritis.[31] Studies in experimental animals have failed to show gastric mucosal changes following injection of parietal cell antibody. With repeated injections, however, a decreased number of gastric parietal cells and a parallel decrease in gastric secretion were observed in rats.[32] The striking difference in the frequency of intrinsic factor antibodies in patients with atrophic gastritis (none) and pernicious anemia (60 to 70 per cent) suggests that this antibody may modify vitamin B_{12} absorption. Intrinsic factor antibodies have been detected in the gastric juice of patients with pernicious anemia; there the antibody may inactivate small amounts of intrinsic factor which would otherwise be adequate to maintain normal vitamin B_{12} absorption.[3]

Cell-mediated, delayed hypersensitivity is an alternative mechanism for immunological damage to the gastric glands in atrophic gastritis. The atrophic mucosa is heavily infiltrated by lymphocytes and plasma cells which contain immunoglobulins reactive with gastric antigens. Blast cell transformation of peripheral lymphocytes and the production of migration inhibition factor by blood leukocytes in response to gastric antigens provide evidence of delayed hypersensitivity in pernicious anemia (Fig. 44–7).[34, 35]

Although present evidence is consistent with the hypothesis that immunological mechanisms are of etiological importance in atrophic gastritis, this remains unproved. The alternative possibility that the immunological phenomena are secondary to mucosal injury is not supported by clinical and experimental evidence. Damage to the mucosa by chemical or physical agents does not stimulate the appearance of immunological phenomena, and does not cause lesions that are confined to the acid-secreting mucosa. Further development of animal experimental models of atrophic gastritis may clarify the cause of human disease and the role of immunological processes. In both the dog and primates, atrophic gastritis can be produced by immunization with gastric antigens.[36, 37] These animals develop circulating antibodies to parietal cells and intrinsic factor. The animal model presents the opportunity to relate the kinetics of mucosal cell turnover to immunological phenomena, and to determine whether parietal cells are thus destroyed.

Course and Prognosis. There is little evidence to support the concept that the varying degrees of mucosal atrophy represent progressive stages in the evolution of atrophy in individual patients.[38] It is more likely that the residual gland cell population represents a varying balance between cell renewal and destruction in the mucosa; this may not change over many years or, alternatively, may change abruptly. The ability of corticosteroids to stimulate regeneration of gastric parietal cells in some patients with pernicious anemia documents the fact that this atrophic mucosa has not lost its potential to form gastric glands.[39] One difficulty in evaluating the course of atrophic gastritis lies in the fact that severe atrophy with gastric secretory failure precedes the development of vitamin B_{12} deficiency by several years. A prospective study of the families of patients with pernicious anemia may yield important information on the course of atrophic gastritis; these subjects are at high risk for the development of mucosal disease.[21]

Vitamin B_{12} therapy restores normal cell proliferation and maturation in patients with pernicious anemia and arrests the development of neurological disease. The gastric mucosal lesion remains, and its

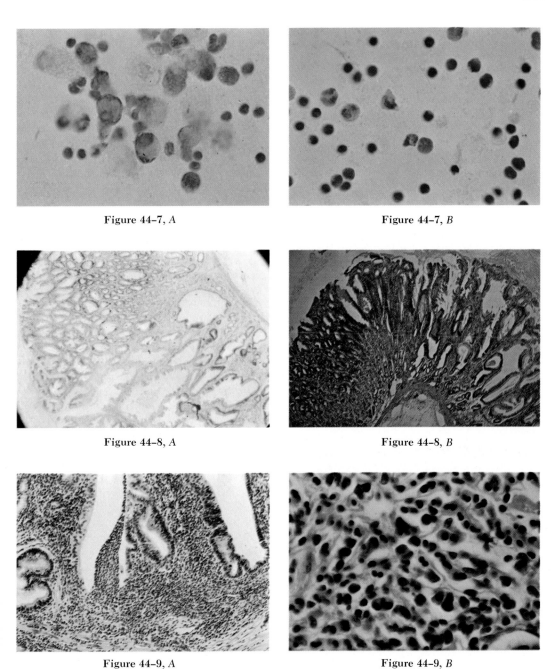

Figure 44–7, *A*

Figure 44–7, *B*

Figure 44–8, *A*

Figure 44–8, *B*

Figure 44–9, *A*

Figure 44–9, *B*

Figure 44–7. Peripheral lymphocyte response to gastric mucosal antigens in pernicious anemia. Peripheral lymphocytes in suspension culture with gastric parietal cell antigen; lymphocytes from a patient with pernicious anemia (*A*) exhibit clumping and blast-cell transformation (15 per cent of cells transformed), whereas cells from a control subject (*B*) remain unstimulated.

Figure 44–8. Giant hypertrophic gastritis. Sections of gastric mucosa from a surgical specimen. *A*, The normal mucosa is replaced by hyperplastic surface epithelial cells which form convoluted or cystic acini extending to the muscularis mucosae and replacing the normal gastric glands. *B*, A transition zone between normal mucosa on the left and abnormal mucosa on the right.

Figure 44–9. Eosinophilic infiltration. An 18-year-old male presenting with iron deficiency anemia from occult bleeding, and hypoproteinemia. An upper gastrointestinal series showed thickening of the mucosal folds in antrum and proximal duodenum. At operation there was diffuse thickening of the distal stomach. Sections revealed focal mucosal erosions (*A*) and diffuse infiltration with eosinophils (*B*).

malignant potential is a persisting threat to the patient with treated pernicious anemia (or atrophic gastritis). In a follow-up of 116 patients with atrophic gastritis over a ten- to 15-year period, nine developed gastric carcinoma and two developed benign polyps.[38] It has been estimated that atrophic gastritis increases the risk of carcinoma of the stomach 20-fold over age-matched controls.[40]

Management. Patients who develop evidence of vitamin B_{12} deficiency (either low serum vitamin B_{12} levels or overt pernicious anemia) should receive a monthly injection of vitamin B_{12} (100 μg intramuscularly). All patients with atrophic gastritis should be screened prospectively to establish the early diagnosis of gastric carcinoma. Unfortunately, elderly patients may have a poor tolerance for repeated cytologic, endoscopic, or radiographic examinations of the stomach which would optimally define gastric neoplasms. Repeated examinations of the stool for occult blood are mandatory in these high-risk patients.

HYPERTROPHIC GASTRITIS

Giant hypertrophic gastritis (Menetrier's disease) is an uncommon pathological condition in which there is massive enlargement of the gastric mucosal folds by hyperplastic surface mucus cells. Macroscopically and radiographically the mucosal folds (either generalized or localized) are particularly prominent, with a tortuous nodular or polypoid distribution, and with surface edema, congestion, hemorrhage, or erosion. Microscopically, there is a benign hyperplasia of surface epithelial cells which line elongated, tortuous, branched, or dilated gastric pits that may extend to or through the muscularis mucosae. The normal gastric glands are often replaced by the hypertrophic surface epithelium; in uninvolved mucosa, the gastric glands are normal. There is a variable infiltration of the lamina propria by inflammatory cells which may be secondary to mucosal ulceration and infection.

Clinical Features. Patients with hypertrophic gastritis may seek medical attention because of epigastric pain, vomiting,

fluid retention secondary to hypoproteinemia, or gastrointestinal bleeding. Enlarged mucosal folds may be demonstrated radiographically and endoscopically, but these studies do not establish the diagnosis. Peroral gastric biopsy is of limited value because of the thickness of the mucosa. Only a full-thickness surgical biopsy provides a reliable diagnosis (Fig. 44–8).[41] Gastric acid secretion may be within the normal range, or may be depressed by replacement of normal gastric glands and/or altered mucosal permeability. Achlorhydric gastric juice or secretions neutralized by intragastric instillation of alkali contain excessive amounts of plasma proteins. It has been well established that excessive intraluminal losses of plasma protein may lead to hypoproteinemia with edema in these patients; indeed, the first demonstration of protein-losing gastroenteropathy was in a patient with Menetrier's disease.[42]

Differential Diagnosis. Enlargement of gastric mucosal folds observed by the radiologist or endoscopist may be due to mucosal hyperemia and edema or to mucosal infiltration by granuloma or neoplasm; or it may represent hypertrophy of normal cellular elements. In many of these patients, mucosal biopsies reveal normal histology. In some there may be hyperplasia of gastric parietal cells with acid hypersecretion; this should raise the suspicion of hypergastrinemia (Zollinger-Ellison syndrome) or of hypertrophic hypersecretory gastropathy, a condition of unknown cause which may also be associated with excessive leakage of plasma protein[43] (see p. 527). A diagnosis of gastric carcinoma or lymphoma can usually be established by endoscopic examination, with multiple mucosal biopsies and direct brushings for gastric exfoliative cytology.

Treatment. When hypertrophic gastritis is localized, a partial gastric resection may relieve dyspeptic symptoms and control enteric loss of protein. More radical surgery to excise diffuse disease may not be justified by the patient's disability. Medical management with antacids and a high protein diet with frequent small meals may give symptomatic relief, but these do not modify the gastric loss of plasma protein. Rarely, there may be spontaneous remission.

EOSINOPHILIC GASTRITIS

Eosinophilic gastroenteritis is a disorder of unknown cause in which there is a diffuse infiltration of the distal stomach and/or proximal small bowel with eosinophils without evidence of granuloma or vasculitis.[44] In the stomach, infiltration may be confined to the mucosa or muscle layers, or may extend from mucosa to serosa. Mucosal involvement causes enlargement of antral folds, which may simulate other infiltrative processes; ulceration may lead to bleeding or plasma protein leakage (Fig. 44–9). Symptoms and signs of pyloric obstruction result from thickening of the muscularis by infiltrating cells. Patients with serosal infiltration may present with signs of peritonitis and may develop ascites. Peripheral eosinophilia is present before therapy in the majority of patients. The management of these patients should be directed toward excluding neoplasm or granulomatous disease of the stomach. Treatment with corticosteroids is usually effective in maintaining these patients in remission (see p. 576).

GRANULOMATOUS DISEASE OF THE STOMACH

The gastric mucosa may be involved in regional enteritis. This is uncommon, and is usually associated with extensive small bowel involvement. Mucosal ulceration is complicated by bleeding. Symptoms suggestive of peptic ulcer disease may result from pyloric and duodenal involvement. Tuberculosis of the stomach has usually been associated with open pulmonary disease; this is an autopsy finding in patients with advanced tuberculosis. Sarcoidosis involves the lymphoid tissue of the antral mucosa and submucosa with typical granulomas. Eosinophilic granuloma is usually localized as a sessile or polypoid lesion in the distal stomach (see pp. 573 to 577).

REFERENCES

1. Wood, I. J., and Taft, L. I. Diffuse Lesions of the Stomach. London, Edward Arnold, Ltd., 1958.
2. MacDonald, W. C., and Rubin, C. E. Gastric biopsy—a critical evaluation. Gastroenterology 53:143, 1967.
3. Lipkin, M., Sherlock, P., and Bell, B. Cell proliferation kinetics in the gastrointestinal tract of man. II. Cell renewal in stomach, ileum, colon, and rectum. Gastroenterology 45:721, 1963.
4. Davenport, H. W. Physiology of the Digestive Tract. 3rd ed. Chicago, Year Book Medical Publishers, 1971, pp. 113–114.
5. Dyck, W. P., Werther, J. L., Rudick, J., et al. Electrolyte movement across canine antral and fundic gastric mucosa. Gastroenterology 56:488, 1969.
6. Rubin, W., Ross, L. L., Sleisenger, M. H., and Jeffries, G. H. The normal human gastric epithelia. A fine structural study. Lab. Invest. 19:598, 1968.
7. Ragins, H., Wincze, F. M., Liu, S. M., and Dittbrenner, M. The origin and survival of gastric parietal cells in the mouse. Anat. Rec. 162:99, 1968.
8. Willems, G., Vansteenkiste, Y., and Limbosch, J. M. Stimulatory effect of gastrin on cell proliferation kinetics in canine fundic mucosa. Gastroenterology 62:583, 1972.
9. Jeffries, G. H. Gastric secretion of intrinsic factor. In Handbook of Physiology, Sect. 6, Vol. II, C. F. Code (ed.). Washington, D.C., American Physiological Society, 1967, pp. 919–924.
10. Lev, R., Siegel, H. I., and Glass, G. B. J. Effects of salicylates on the canine stomach: A morphological and histochemical study. Gastroenterology 62:970, 1972.
11. Katz, D., Douvres, P., Weisberg, H., McKinnon, W., and Glass, G. B. J. Early endoscopic diagnosis of acute upper gastrointestinal hemorrhage. Demonstration of relatively high incidence of erosions as a source of bleeding. J.A.M.A. 188:405, 1964.
12. Palmer, E. D. The vigorous diagnostic approach to upper gastrointestinal tract hemorrhage. J.A.M.A. 207:1477, 1969.
13. Davenport, H. W. Salicylate damage to the gastric mucosal barrier. New Eng. J. Med. 276:1307, 1970.
14. Skillman, J. K., Gould, S. A., Chung, R. S. K., and Silen, W. The gastric mucosal barrier: Clinical and experimental studies in critically ill and normal man, and in the rabbit. Ann. Surg. 172:564, 1970.
15. Kim, Y. S., Kerr, R., and Lipkin, M. Cell proliferation during the development of stress erosions in mouse stomach. Nature 215:1180, 1967.
16. Ivey, K. J. Acute haemorrhagic gastritis: Modern concepts based on pathogenesis. Gut 12:750, 1971.
17. Levin, E., Clayman, C. B., Palmer, W. L., and Kirsner, J. B. Observations on the value of gastric irradiation in the treatment of duodenal ulcer. Gastroenterology 32:42, 1957.
18. McIlrath, D. C., and Hallenbeck, G. A. Review of gastric freezing. J.A.M.A. 190:715, 1964.
19. Perry, G. T., Dunphy, J. V., Fruin, R. C., and Littman, A. Gastric freezing for duodenal ulcer. A double blind study. Gastroenterology 47:6, 1964.
20. Siurala, M., and Salmi, H. J. Long-term follow-up of subjects with superficial gastritis or a

normal gastric mucosa. Scand. J. Gastroent. 6:459, 1971.

21. teVelde, K., Abels, J., Anders, G. J. P. A., Arends, A., Hoedemaeker, P. J., and Nieweg, H. O. A family study of pernicious anemia by an immunologic method. J. Lab. Clin. Med. 64:177, 1964.

22. Doniach, D., Roitt, I. M., and Taylor, K. B. Autoimmune phenomena in pernicious anaemia. Serologic overlap with thyroiditis, thyrotoxicosis, and systemic lupus erythematosus. Brit. Med. J. 1:1374, 1963.

23. Irvine, W. J., Davies, S. H., Teitelbaum, S., Delamore, I. W., and Williams, A. W. The clinical and pathologic significance of gastric parietal cell antibody. Ann. N.Y. Acad. Sci. 124:657, 1965.

24. Magnus, H. A., and Ungley, C. C. The gastric lesion in pernicious anaemia. Lancet 1:420, 1938.

25. McGuigan, J. E., and Trudeau, W. L. Serum gastrin concentrations in pernicious anemia. New Eng. J. Med. 282:358, 1970.

26. Yalow, R. S., and Berson, S. A. Radioimmunoassay of gastrin. Gastroenterology 58:1, 1970.

27. Ivey, K. J., Den Besten, L., and Clifton, J. A. Effect of bile salts on ionic movement across the human gastric mucosa. Gastroenterology 59:683, 1970.

28. Rhodes, J., Barnado, D. E., Phillips, S. F., et al. Increased reflux of bile into the stomach in patients with gastric ulcer. Gastroenterology 57:241, 1969.

29. Jeffries, G. H., and Sleisenger, M. H. Studies of parietal cell antibody in pernicious anemia. J. Clin. Invest. 44:2021, 1965.

30. Samloff, I. M., Kleinman, M. S., Turner, M. D., Sobel, M. V., and Jeffries, G. H. Blocking and binding antibody to intrinsic factor and parietal cell antibody in pernicious anemia. Gastroenterology 55:575, 1968.

31. Twomey, J. J., Jordan, P. H., Jarrold, T., et al. The syndrome of immunoglobulin deficiency and pernicious anemia. Amer. J. Med. 47:340, 1969.

32. Tanaka, N., and Glass, G. B. J. Effect of prolonged administration of parietal cell antibodies from patients with atrophic gastritis and pernicious anemia on the parietal cell

mass and hydrochloric acid output in rats. Gastroenterology 58:482, 1970.

33. Schade, S. C., Feick, P., Muckerheide, M., and Schilling, R. F. Occurrence in gastric juice of antibody to a complex of intrinsic factor and vitamin B_{12}. New Eng. J. Med. 275:528, 1966.

34. McGuigan, J. E. In vitro behavior of lymphocytes from patients with pernicious anemia. J. Clin. Invest. 46:1094, 1967.

35. Rose, M. S., Chanarin, I., Doniach, D., Brostoff, J., and Ardeman, S. Intrinsic factor antibodies in absence of pernicious anaemia. Three- to seven-year follow-up. Lancet 2:9, 1970.

36. Hennes, A. R., Sevelios, J., Lewellyn, T., Joel, W., Woods, A. H., and Wolf, S. Atrophic gastritis in dogs. Arch. Path. 73:281, 1962.

37. Krohn, K. Experimental gastritis in the dog. 1. Production of atrophic gastritis and antibodies to parietal cells. Ann. Med. Exp. Fenn. 46:249, 1968.

38. Siurala, M., Varis, K., and Wiljasalo, M. Studies of patients with atrophic gastritis: a 10- to 15-year follow-up. Scand. J. Gastroent. 1:40, 1966.

39. Jeffries, G. H., Todd, J. E., and Sleisenger, M. H. The effect of prednisolone on gastric mucosal histology, gastric secretion and vitamin B_{12} absorption in patients with pernicious anemia. J. Clin. Invest. 45:803, 1966.

40. Hitchcock, C. R., MacLean, L. D., and Sullivan, W. A. The secretory and clinical aspects of achlorhydria and gastric atrophy as precursors of gastric cancer. J. Nat. Cancer Inst. 18:795, 1957.

41. Schindler, R. On hypertrophic glandular gastritis, hypertrophic gastropathy, and parietal cell mass. Gastroenterology 45:77, 1963.

42. Citrin, Y., Sterling, K., and Halsted, J. The mechanism of hypoproteinemia associated with giant hypertrophy of the gastric mucosa. New. Eng. J. Med. 257:906, 1957.

43. Overholt, B. F., and Jeffries, G. H. Hypertrophic, hypersecretory protein-losing gastropathy. Gastroenterology 58:80, 1970.

44. Klein, N. C., Hargrove, R. L., Sleisenger, M. H., and Jeffries, G. H. Eosinophilic gastroenteritis. Medicine 49:299, 1970.

Chapter 45

Granulomatous and Infectious Disease of the Stomach

Steven Raffin

GRANULOMATOUS DISEASE OF THE STOMACH

The reticuloendothelial system responds in a stereotyped manner to a variety of infectious agents, foreign materials, and as yet uncharacterized stimuli with a nodular, proliferative reaction. This "basic lesion, a granuloma ... , contains at the periphery concentric reticular fibers, while at the center [it] is occupied by epithelioid cells, with or without giant cells."[1] When physicians found such a histological picture in stomachs 30 years ago, syphilis and tuberculosis were the obvious diagnostic considerations. Today, these two infections rarely involve the stomach but have been replaced by less understood processes, including Crohn's disease, disseminated sarcoidosis, isolated granulomatous gastritis, and eosinophilic granuloma of the stomach.

There is little that is specific in the mode of clinical presentation or roentgenological appearance of these uncommon lesions. In fact, differentiation from one another or from peptic ulceration or gastric malignancy may be exceptionally difficult. However, the physician must be aware of the possibility that his patient's gastric ulcer may heal not with antacids but with penicillin therapy, or that his patient's intragastric mass may require only limited resection or antituberculous drugs rather than radical cancer surgery.

CLASSIFICATION

Gastric granulomas associated with chronic beryllium poisoning,[2] sutures, or talc[3] are not included in this discussion.

I. Infectious granulomas of the stomach
   A. Tuberculosis[4-6]
   B. Tertiary syphilis[7-9]
   C. Histoplasmosis[10, 11]
   D. Eosinophilic granuloma associated with larval nematodes[12]
II. Granulomas of unknown etiology
   A. Systemic sarcoidosis with gastric involvement[13]
   B. Crohn's disease of small or large bowel with gastric involvement[14-16]
   C. Circumscribed eosinophilic granuloma of the stomach[17-19]
   D. Isolated granulomatous gastritis; i.e., none of the above[3, 20]

573

From the diverse nature of the lesions outlined, one may notice that specific clinical and diagnostic features do exist but that their striking similarities allow a general discussion of the group as a whole.

CLINICAL PICTURE

Apart from the extragastric signs and symptoms associated with either the disseminated infection or the granulomatous process, the clinical features of granulomatous gastritis are nonspecific and may include postprandial epigastric pain, vomiting, weight loss and weakness, hematemesis, and gastric outlet obstruction.[3, 9, 14, 19-22] Diarrhea is an infrequent sign, most commonly associated with concurrent extragastric Crohn's disease.[14, 20] Either hypo- or achlorhydria is a frequent finding.[3, 9, 14, 19-23] The degree of anemia seen parallels the course of extragastric involvement or subsequent hemorrhage.

A remarkably similar spectrum of roentgenological appearances of the stomach has been described for each of the granulomatous processes; these are enumerated as follows: (1) gastric ulceration;[3, 6, 11, 15, 19-24] (2) "tumor";[5, 6, 10, 13, 19, 21, 22, 24] (3) pyloroantral stenosis;[3, 5, 6, 9, 13-15, 19-24] (4) a constricting lesion in body of stomach (hourglass lesion);[3, 9-11] (5) concurrent duodenal involvement;[3, 15, 19-21] and (6) a picture resembling linitis plastica.[3, 6, 9, 13, 22-24]

Confusion may arise when reviewing gastric cytology in a patient with unsuspected granulomatous gastric ulceration. Multinucleated giant cells have been misdiagnosed as being malignant in cases of gastric syphilis and sarcoidosis. These bizarre cells must not be confused with swallowed respiratory giant cells, which usually contain dust particles. When found, they are evidence of benign granuloma formation and give no clue to the specific diagnosis.[1, 25, 26]

Definitive diagnosis relies upon either isolation of the offending infectious agent or documentation of a concurrent extragastric granulomatous process, either by appropriate serological testing or by biopsy. The details of specific diagnosis and treatment will be delineated subsequently.

INFECTIOUS GRANULOMAS OF THE STOMACH

Tuberculosis. A tabulation of the medical literature prior to 1950 revealed 159 cases of gastric tuberculosis in 96,251 autopsies (0.16 per cent) and 117 cases among 20,585 autopsies on patients whose primary disease was tuberculosis (0.57 per cent).[27] Several factors have been postulated to explain the extreme rarity of gastric involvement in patients with pulmonary or intestinal tuberculosis: (1) the sparsity of lymphoid follicles in the gastric wall, (2) the acidity of the stomach, and (3) rapid passage of the ingested organisms through the stomach.[5, 21] Today this entity is even less common, especially in Western Europe and the United States.

Semispecific roentgenologic features include the presence of fistulas and simultaneous ulceration of both the antrum and duodenum,[4, 6, 21] although these same findings may be found in Crohn's disease (Fig. 45–1). The most frequent site of gastric involvement is the antrum.[6] Angiographic demonstration of marked hypervascularity

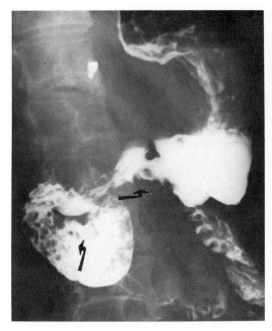

Figure 45–1. Gastroduodenal tuberculosis. Ulceronodular inflammation (arrows) has resulted in marked antral and duodenal deformity. (From Goldberg, H., and Reeder, M.: In Alimentary Tract Roentgenology, 2nd ed., A. R. Margulis and H. J. Burhenne [eds.]. St. Louis, C. V. Mosby Co., 1973.)

as well as thickening of the stomach wall and omentum without tumor blush also suggests tuberculosis,[6] although tumor-like capillary blushes have been noted.[28]

Diagnosis must depend upon the demonstration of either acid-fast bacilli or caseating granulomata in the stomach by endoscopic or surgical biopsy. Demonstration of bacilli in tissue occurs in only one-third of the cases,[4] and they are rarely cultured from gastric washings.[29]

Medical treatment is effective. Surgery should be reserved to remove irreversibly destroyed tissue.[6, 29] Standard "triple therapy," i.e., isonicotinic hydrazide (INH), streptomycin, and para-aminosalicylic acid (PAS), should be employed for primary treatment. There are no statistics documenting the use of the newer antituberculous drugs such as ethambutol or rifampin, although there is no reason to doubt their effectiveness in gastric tuberculosis. Gastric tuberculosis has been reported as the seat of carcinoma in more than 20 cases.[30]

Tertiary Syphilis. Secondary syphilis frequently involves the stomach transiently without granuloma formation. Twelve men with healed penile lesions, maculopapular eruptions, positive serologies, and no gastrointestinal symptoms were endoscoped. Eleven had gastritis, consisting of edematous, erythematous mucosa with scattered hemorrhage and erosions. Concurrent sigmoidoscopic examinations in all revealed hyperemic, friable, edematous bowel. After 2.4 million units of penicillin therapy, almost all experienced healing of the rectal and gastric mucosal inflammation.[31] Others report a similar experience in early syphilis[32] and go as far as saying that the stomach is always involved during the spirochetemia of primary and secondary lues.[33]

Significant gastric disease is limited to cases of tertiary lues, with an incidence of about 0.1 per cent.[8] Rigid proof that *T. pallidum* is responsible for the rather nonspecific, pleomorphic picture of granulomatous gastritis is possible. Macerated material from the lesion in question may be injected into rabbit testes with subsequent recovery of spirochetes;[34] however, most cases are not diagnosed by finding the organism. The accepted criteria for diagnosis are as follows: (1) untreated tertiary

lues, (2) a roentgen defect in the stomach, (3) presence of "gastric" symptoms, (4) inability to alleviate these symptoms or effect any improvement in the anatomical defect by orthodox management without luetic therapy, (5) symptomatic relief with disappearance of the roentgen defect after intensive penicillin treatment, and (6) tissue removed at biopsy showing histological changes compatible with lues, namely a fibrosing, obliterative panvasculitis.[7, 8, 35] The most diagnostic roentgen findings include the so-called hourglass stomach and large, shallow ulcerations.[8, 9] Differentiation from linitis plastica may be exceptionally difficult (Fig. 45–2). The syphilitic ulcer has a different endoscopic appearance from peptic ulcer. A violaceous, purple hue may be seen on the irregular mucosal borders of a large, shallow, yellow crater.[7, 35]

Treatment of this lesion is based on anecdotal reports. Most physicians feel that if the diagnostic criteria outlined are fulfilled, an intensive course of penicillin that produces signs of healing is sufficient evidence to forestall cancer surgery. Complicating this regimen is the well known

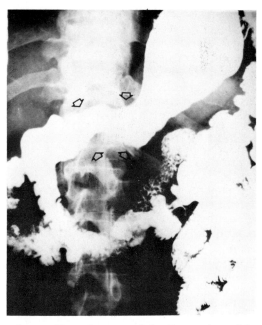

Figure 45–2. Gastric syphilis. Tertiary lues of the stomach has produced marked rigidity and narrowing of the distal stomach (arrows) and is indistinguishable from linitis plastica.

variability in the rate of healing of these lesions, some showing only slight changes after six months of therapy.[8, 9]

Histoplasmosis. Sparse reports describe gastric involvement in disseminated histoplasmosis.[10, 11] Histoplasmin skin test during initial dissemination of the organism may be negative, whereas cultures of blood, lymph nodes, bone marrow, sputum, and liver are positive. After the initial infection is suppressed with amphotericin B, the patient may be well until presenting later with dysphagia or an annular, malignant-appearing lesion of the fundus and cardia of the stomach. Open biopsy of such lesions may reveal non-caseating granulomas, and a silver stain will demonstrate the organism. Although such lesions may be treated with amphotericin B with relief of the dysphagia, the constricting lesion may be refractory and surgery necessary. One must be aware of this mode of presentation, especially in the endemic areas bordering the Mississippi River.

Eosinophilic Granuloma Secondary to Larval Nematodes. Eating raw cod or herring in Japan allows the larvae of *Anisakis sp.*, a nematode, to penetrate human gastric mucosa and establish a symptomatic, ulcerating eosinophilic granulomatous reaction. Meticulous serial sectioning of the lesions often allows morphologic identification of the genus of the immature worms. If the lesion is indolent, treatment is local resection. This unusual form of visceral larval migrans "may become recognized as a public health problem in Japan."[12]

GRANULOMAS OF UNKNOWN ETIOLOGY

Systemic Sarcoidosis with Gastric Involvement. "Sarcoidosis is a chronic systemic disease of undetermined etiology or etiologies.... Diagnosis is dependent upon clinical as well as histological evidence of disseminated disease and the exclusion of other etiologic agents."[13] With this partial definition in mind, one can discard the vast majority of reports of "isolated sarcoid of the stomach."[13, 24] One cannot make the diagnosis without some evidence of dissemination; i.e., enlarged

hilar nodes, fibronodular pulmonary parenchymal disease, decreased pulmonary compliance, lytic lesions in the phalanges, hyperglobulinemia, hypercalciuria or hypercalcemia, cutaneous anergy, or positive Kveim test.[3, 13]

Asymptomatic scattered granulomata of the stomach as documented by mucosal biopsy have been reported in as many as 10 per cent of sarcoid patients,[36] but the true incidence of significant gastric sarcoid is not known. The gastric component is rarely clinically important, having been discovered in only two of 257 patients with sarcoidosis.[37] When pain and vomiting result from gastric involvement, one must be sure that hypercalcemia is considered, because the symptoms may abate following medical lowering of the elevated serum calcium.[38] Verified sarcoid of the stomach is indistinguishable from other granulomatous processes; if the question of malignancy arises or massive hemorrhage supervenes, surgery is indicated.[23]

Crohn's Disease of Small or Large Bowel with Gastric Involvement. As with sarcoid of the stomach, granulomatous gastritis due to Crohn's disease can be diagnosed *only* if coexisting extragastric disease is present; i.e., in the small or large bowel.[14-16, 39] Gastric Crohn's disease is twice as frequent in males as in females, and most patients are younger than 30 years of age. To date, there are approximately 30 case reports in the medical literature.[14-16, 40]

Symptoms are the same as for other granulomatous infiltrations of the stomach, but may be overshadowed by concurrent intestinal disease. Gastric outlet obstruction has been reported in as many as two-thirds of patients.[16] The antrum is involved most frequently, with narrowing and ulceration seen on upper gastrointestinal series, and a cobblestone mucosa may be seen on endoscopy. The contiguous duodenum is often also diseased (Fig. 45–3).

Reports of treatment emphasize the favorable results of posterior gastrojejunostomy, bypassing the diseased antrum and relieving any obstructive component.[14, 16, 40] No conclusions can be drawn concerning the efficacy of steroid therapy.[16]

Eosinophilic Granuloma of the Stomach. A careful distinction must be made be-

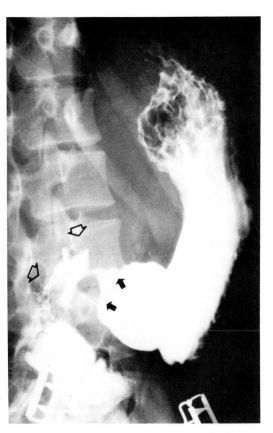

Figure 45–3. Gastroduodenal Crohn's disease. Marked inflammation and narrowing of the stomach (solid arrows) and duodenum (hollow arrows) has resulted in severe deformity mimicking peptic disease or tuberculosis (see Fig. 45–1).

tween circumscribed eosinophilic granuloma of the stomach and diffuse (allergic?) eosinophilic gastroenteritis. The former lesion is rarely associated with peripheral eosinophilia, is usually polypoid or nodular and confined to the gastric antrum, becomes symptomatic from local ulceration or outlet obstruction, and responds poorly to corticosteroids and well to local resection. The latter lesion is often accompanied by striking peripheral eosinophilia, and 50 per cent of the patients suffer from allergy or asthma. Many present with fever, cramping abdominal pain, diarrhea, and serositis (ascites or hydrothorax) and respond well to corticosteroids, although the course is usually characterized by exacerbations and remissions (see pp. 1066 to 1081).[17, 18, 41, 42] The medical literature often

fails to make this distinction, rendering incidence statistics misleading.[41]

Microscopically, the basic cell types in these granulomata are the fibroblast and eosinophil, in contrast to the unrelated eosinophilic granuloma of bone in which reticulum cells and histiocytes predomnate.[41] Perhaps a better name for the gastric lesion might be "eosinophil-infiltrated granuloma of the stomach."[19] It seems likely that this localized histopathology represents no more than a response to varied topical antigens, although this hypothesis is pure speculation arising from extrapolation from animal models.[18]

Isolated Granulomatous Gastritis. This lesion is diagnosed by exclusion. It closely resembles sarcoid and Crohn's disease of the stomach without the systemic or intestinal components.[3, 20] There is some merit to considering it as a distinct entity at present, although the symptomatology and pathology are the same as that described for the other types of granulomatous gastritis. In contrast to patients with gastric sarcoid or Crohn's disease in whom the peak age of onset is under 40 years, patients with isolated granulomatous gastritis are most often older.[20] No case of isolated granulomatous gastritis has been described which has evolved into Crohn's disease or sarcoidosis.[3] Thoughts regarding pathogenesis parallel the "local antigen" hypothesis proposed to explain the genesis of circumscribed, eosinophil-infiltrated gastric granulomatosis. There is no experience with corticosteroids in treating this lesion, and local surgical resection is curative.

SUPPURATIVE GASTRITIS

This exceedingly rare condition is usually referred to as phlegmonous gastritis, the term "phlegmonous" being derived from a Greek word referring to one of the "humors" of the body. It is often used instead of the term "suppurative" in this disease process to add historical authenticity. The earliest descriptions date to Galen in 160 A.D., who "described symptoms that point to an abscess or a phlegmonous or erysipelatous tumor of the stomach."[43] During the past 150 years, 390 cases have been reported, for an estimated world incidence of 2.5 cases per year.[44]

PATHOGENESIS AND PATHOLOGY

Predisposing factors, culled from the literature, include chronic gastritis, trauma, alcoholism, hypoacidity, "hard work," infections elsewhere in the body, increased age, low socioeconomic environment, and chronic malnutrition.[44]

The pathological findings (usually at autopsy) include a dilated viscus with thickened walls (1.0 to 1.5 cm) and discolored mucosa (deep red to purple). The submucosa is usually edematous and may ooze pus. Thrombosed vessels are also commonly found, although vasculitis is uniformly absent. The bacteria can usually be seen enmeshed in a fibrinopurulent exudate on sections of the stomach wall. There is usually a sparing of the duodenum and esophagus.[45] In over 70 per cent of patients, alpha hemolytic streptococci have been isolated from the lesions cultured,[44] although pneumococci (associated with pneumonia and endocarditis),[46] staphylococci, E. coli, and rarely Proteus vulgaris and Clostridium welchii have been isolated.[46, 47]

CLINICAL PICTURE

The patient usually presents with an acute abdominal catastrophe, with abrupt onset of mid-epigastric pain, nausea, and vomiting. Purulent emesis, a rare occurrence, is specific for this entity. Diarrhea is usually not present, but fever, chills, and severe prostration are frequent ominous signs of bacteremia.[45, 46] Peritoneal irritation with muscle guarding and rebound tenderness on palpation are found in 80 per cent of patients.[45] Disappearance of abdominal pain upon assuming a sitting position (Dienenger's sign) is touted as being specific for diffuse phlegmonous gastritis.[46, 47] Roentgenographic findings are nonspecific. A picture resembling infiltrating carcinoma or linitis plastica has been reported.[44, 45] There is no experience with fiberoptic, flexible endoscopy in this disease.

Death usually ensues from massive circulatory collapse. Owing to the limited number of cases treated at one time, a rational basis for therapy has not been established.[45] Survival has increased from 16 per cent in 1938 to 67 per cent in 1970.[44] An increased awareness of this rare entity, adequate antimicrobial therapy, and more aggressive surgery have accounted for the improvement in statistics. Of 14 survivors in the last ten years, nine underwent some form of gastric resection. Of the seven patients who died during this period, only one expired after surgery.[44] Surgery must be accompanied by vigorous antimicrobial therapy. Ampicillin or Keflin will usually be appropriate in light of the high incidence of Streptococcus viridans and occasional coliform infections.

Emphysematous Gastritis. This disease is a less common, but more lethal, suppurative process, with 15 cases and only six survivors reported in the world literature to date.[48] The lesion arises from phlegmonous gastritis caused by gas-forming organisms (the coliforms or C. welchii) rather than from invasion by the pyogenic cocci.[49] The roentgenological appearance is striking, consisting of bubbles of varying sizes in the thickened stomach wall. The rugal folds are often edematous. There may be submucosal blebs of gas which impart a cobblestone texture to the mucosa. Intramucosal penetration of the contrast medium and sinus tracts may also be seen. This roentgenographic picture in a patient who is not prostrate may be encountered in association with pneumatosis cystoides intestinalis and traumatic emphysema of the stomach secondary to endoscopic perforation or rupture of a pulmonary bullus into the esophageal wall.[49, 50] A frequent pathognomonic event in a large percentage of patients is the recovery of a necrotic cast of the stomach wall after emesis.[49]

Usually a pre-existing disease of the stomach such as malignancy,[50] damage from corrosive agents,[48] viral or alcoholic gastroenteritis, or recent gastroduodenal surgery may be implicated in the pathogenesis. With only 15 cases to review and a mortality of 60 per cent, one cannot propose definitive therapy; the program for the nonemphysematous variety of suppurative gastritis applies also to this variant. One late complication in survivors may be cicatricial constriction of the

stomach which eventually requires subtotal gastrectomy.[49]

REFERENCES

1. Goldgraber, M., Kirsner, J., and Raskin, H. Nonspecific granulomatous disease of the stomach. Arch. Intern. Med. 102:10, 1958.
2. Negus, D. Giant-cell granuloma of the stomach. Brit. J. Surg. 53:475, 1966.
3. Present, D., Lindner, A., and Janowitz, H. Granulomatous diseases of the gastrointestinal tract. Ann. Rev. Med. 17:243, 1966.
4. Chazan, B., and Aitchison, J. Gastric tuberculosis. Brit. Med. J. 2:1288, 1960.
5. Tuchel, V., Macarie, R., Lauch, E., Fesiuc, P., and Zaharia, M. Gastric tuberculosis simulating a complicated tumor-like form. Digestion 2:237, 1969.
6. Pinto, R., Zausner, J., and Beranbaum, E. Gastric tuberculosis — report of a case with discussion of angiographic findings. Amer. J. Roent. 110:808, 1970.
7. Knight, W., and Falk, A. Tertiary gastric syphilis. Gastroenterology 9:17, 1947.
8. Cooley, R., and Childers, J. Acquired syphilis of the stomach. Gastroenterology 39:201, 1960.
9. Madding, G., Baer, L., and Kennedy, P. Gastric syphilis — a case report. Ann. Surg. 159:271, 1964.
10. Nudelman, H., and Rakatansky, H. Gastric histoplasmosis — a case report. J.A.M.A. 195:44, 1966.
11. Perez, C., Sturim, H., Kouchoukos, N., and Kamberg, S. Some clinical and radiographic features of gastrointestinal histoplasmosis. Radiology 86:482, 1966.
12. Asami, K., Watanuki, T., Sakai, H., Imano, H., and Okamoto, R. Two cases of stomach granuloma caused by Anisakis-like larval nematodes in Japan. Amer. J. Trop. Med. Hyg. 14:119, 1965.
13. Kremer, R., and Williams, J. Gastric sarcoidosis — a difficult diagnosis. Amer. Surgeon 36:686, 1970.
14. Johnson, O., Hoskins, W., Todd, J., and Thorbjarnarson, B. Crohn's disease of the stomach. Gastroenterology 50:571, 1966.
15. Cohen, W. Gastric involvement in Crohn's disease. Amer. J. Roent. 101:425, 1967.
16. Fielding, J., Toye, D., Beton, D., and Cooke, W. Crohn's disease of the stomach and duodenum. Gut 11:1001, 1970.
17. Ureles, A., Alschibaja, T., Lodico, D., and Stabins, S. Idiopathic eosinophilic infiltration of the gastrointestinal tract, diffuse and circumscribed. Amer. J. Med. 30:899, 1961.
18. O'Neill, T. Eosinophilic granuloma of the gastrointestinal tract. Brit. J. Surg. 57:704, 1970.
19. Schwinger, A. Eosinophilic granuloma of the upper GI tract. Amer. J. Dig. Dis. 10:58, 1965.
20. Fahimi, H., Deren, J., Gottlieb, L., and Zamcheck, N. Isolated granulomatous gastritis:
Its relationship to disseminated sarcoidosis and regional enteritis. Gastroenterology 45:161, 1963.
21. Balikian, J., Yenikomshian, S., and Jidejian, Y. Tuberculosis of the pyloro-duodenal area. Amer. J. Roent. 101:414, 1967.
22. Kune, G., and Fullerton, J. Crohn's disease of the stomach. Postgrad. Med. J. 41:100, 1965.
23. Ramirez, J., Ponka, J., and Haubrich, W. Massive hemorrhage from sarcoid ulcers in the stomach. Henry Ford Hosp. Med. Bull. 12:15, 1964.
24. Wadina, G., and Melamed, A. Gastric granuloma (sarcoidosis?). Amer. J. Gastroent. 45:11, 1966.
25. Prolla, J., Kobayashi, S., Yoshii, Y., Yamaoka, Y., and Kasugai, T. Diagnostic cytology of the stomach in gastric syphilis — report of two cases. Acta Cytol. 14:333, 1970.
26. Bennington, J., Porus, R., Ferguson, B., and Hannon, G. Cytology of gastric sarcoid — report of a case. Acta Cytol. 12:30, 1968.
27. Palmer, E. Tuberculosis of stomach and stomach in tuberculosis: Review with particular reference to gross pathology and gastroscopic diagnosis. Amer. Rev. Tuberc. 61:116, 1950.
28. Kinkhabwala, M., and Dziadiw, R. Arteriographic manifestations of tuberculosis of the splenic flexure and the stomach. Brit. J. Radiol. 44:384, 1971.
29. Stirk, D. Primary tuberculosis of the stomach, caecum, and appendix treated with antituberculous drugs. Brit. J. Surg. 55:230, 1968.
30. Aird, I. Companion in Surgical Studies. Edinburgh, Livingstone, 1958, p. 745.
31. Schwartz, I. Gastroscopic observations in secondary syphilis. Gastroenterology 10:227, 1948.
32. Mitchell, R., and Bralow, S. Acute erosive gastritis due to early syphilis. Ann. Intern. Med. 61:933, 1964.
33. Palmer, E. Clinical Gastroenterology, 2nd ed. New York, Harper and Row, 1963, pp. 154–156.
34. Harris, S., and Morgan, H. The isolation of Spirochaeta pallida from the lesion of gastric syphilis. J.A.M.A. 99:1405, 1932.
35. Patterson, C., and Rouse, M. Description of gastroscopic appearance of luetic gastric lesions in late acquired syphilis. Gastroenterology 10:474, 1948.
36. Palmer, E. Note on silent sarcoidosis of gastric mucosa. J. Lab. Clin. Med. 52:231, 1958.
37. Mayock, R., Bertrand, P., Morrison, C., and Scott, J. Manifestations of sarcoidosis: Analysis of 145 patients with a review of nine series selected from the literature. Amer. J. Med. 35:67, 1963.
38. Lebacq, E., and Gossart, J. Sarcoidose gastrique avec hypercalcemie. Efficacité du traitment corticoide. Bull. Soc. Méd. Hôp. 76:706, 1960.
39. Law, D. Regional enteritis. Gastroenterology 56:1086, 1969.
40. Burgess, J., Legge, D., and Judd, E. Surgical treatment of regional enteritis of the stomach

and duodenum. Surg. Gynec. Obstet. *132*:628, 1971.

41. Higgins, G., Lamm, E., and Yutzy, C. Eosinophilic gastroenteritis. Arch. Surg. *92*:476, 1965.

42. Hardy, T., and Elesha, W. Eosinophilic granuloma of the stomach. Amer. Surgeon *34*:296, 1968.

43. Konjetzny, G. *In* Handbuch der speziellen Pathologischen: Anatomie und Histologie, Vol. 4, Ch. 3, F. Henke and O. Lubarsch (eds.). Berlin, Springer-Verlag, 1928, pp. 768–1116.

44. Stephenson, S., Yasrebi, H., Rhatigan, R., and Woodward, E. Acute phlegmasia of the stomach. Amer. Surgeon *36*:225, 1970.

45. Gonzalez-Crussi, F., and Hackett, L. Phlegmonous gastritis. Arch. Surg. *93*:990, 1966.

46. LaForce, F. Diffuse phlegmonous gastritis—a rare complication of pneumococcal endocarditis. Arch. Intern. Med. *120*:230, 1967.

47. Nevin, N., Eakins, D., Clarke, S., and Carson, D. Acute phlegmonous gastritis. Brit. J. Surg. *56*:268, 1969.

48. Meyers, H., and Parker, J. Emphysematous gastritis. Radiology *89*:426, 1967.

49. Gonzalez, L., Schowengerdt, C., Skinner, H., and Lynch, P. Emphysematous gastritis. Surg. Gynec. Obstet. *116*:79, 1963.

50. Smith, T. Emphysematous gastritis associated with adenocarcinoma of the stomach. Amer. J. Dig. Dis. *11*:341, 1966.

Chapter 46

Polyps, Tumors, and Cancer of the Stomach

Lloyd L. Brandborg

INTRODUCTION

Polyps and Benign Tumors. Polyps may be defined as nodules of tissue which protrude above the normal level of the mucosa in which they occur. They may be pedunculated, i.e., attached to a stalk, or sessile. They may be benign or malignant neoplasms, inflammatory, degenerative, infectious, proliferations of normal tissue (hamartomas), or ectopic tissue, e.g., pancreatic rests. Almost all benign tumors have a polypoid configuration.

The most common benign tumor found in the stomach at autopsy is a leiomyoma.[1] Most of these lesions are found incidentally; they are ordinarily 1 cm or less in diameter. Occasionally they may attain diameters of up to 5 cm.

The next most common benign tumor is the polypoid adenoma.[1, 2] It is found most often in patients with chronic "gastritis" or intestinal metaplasia such as that which occurs in the stomach of patients with pernicious anemia. They range in size from 1 mm to several centimeters.

Other benign tumors occurring in the stomach are rare and include lipoma, tumors of neural origin, angiomas, hemangioperiocytoma or glomus tumors, granular cell myoblastoma, and carcinoid tumors.[1, 2]

Malignant Tumors. Ninety to 95 per cent of tumors occurring in the stomach are malignant.[1] Of these, approximately 95 per cent are carcinomas and 5 per cent are sarcomas. There has been a marked decrease in death rates from gastric carcinoma over the past four decades in the United States. In 1930 the death rate from carcinoma of the stomach was approximately 33 per 100,000 population, whereas in 1972 projections are for a death rate of less than 10 per 100,000 population.[3] This striking change is due to a decrease in incidence of carcinoma of the stomach and not to earlier diagnosis or better surgical or other therapy.

ETIOLOGY AND PATHOGENESIS

The etiology of all gastric tumors is obscure. There is a particularly high incidence of adenomatous polyps in individuals with pernicious anemia in comparison with patients having a normal stomach. An incidence of approximately 8 to 10 per cent of associated benign gastric polyp is found in stomachs with gastric carcinoma. In contrast to patients with gastric carcinoma, who are able to secrete acid in approximately 70 to 75 per cent of cases, 95 per cent of gastric polyps occur in patients with achlorhydria and achylia. Patients with multiple gastric polyposis almost invariably have achlorhydria and achylia. Although gastric polyps and gastric carcinoma may occur in the same stomach, the relationship between these two lesions is obscure.[4] If a malignant polyp is found, it may be impossible to determine whether or not it developed from an adenomatous polyp or whether it was malignant at the onset. Furthermore, most of the malignant polyps which have been described have occurred in stomachs with invasive carcinoma elsewhere.[4] Although carcinoma in situ may be observed in adenomatous polyps removed surgically or studied at autopsy, no patient has been observed who had metastases at the time of operation.[4] On occasion, however, microinvasion of these carcinomata in situ may be observed. Some of the interpretations of carcinoma in situ are due to small zones of focal "atypicality" and are found in proximity to areas of acute inflammation and granulation tissue. Some patients with adenomatous polyps, including multiple gastric polyps, have been followed for several years with no change in the size of the polyps, increase in numbers, or development of carcinoma.[4] Furthermore, after resection of these polyps or partial gastrectomy, the remaining stomach does not seem to be more prone to develop new polyps or carcinoma.

Because of the frequent finding of chronic gastritis and chronic atrophic gastritis in stomachs that contain gastric carcinoma, it is tempting to assign an etiological role to gastritis. Such a role, however, has not been proved.[2] A spectrum of pathological appearances occurs in the uninvolved stomachs of patients with gastric carcinoma, ranging from a mild superficial "gastritis" to severe atrophy and intestinalization. In the presence of severe atrophy there may be few inflammatory cells in the lamina propria. Approximately 80 per cent of stomachs harboring gastric carcinoma contain some histological "gastritis." Chronic gastritis is also found with systemic illnesses such as chronic infections, gastric sarcomas and benign tumors, iron deficiency anemia, secondary vitamin B_{12} deficiency, and folate deficiency. Furthermore, histological gastritis is such a common finding on biopsy studies of otherwise healthy individuals[5] that it is difficult to assign an etiological role in the development of carcinoma of the stomach. It is found with increasing frequency with advancing age and corresponds to the reduced secretory capacity of the stomach associated with aging and may be merely a feature of senescence. Despite the lack of proof of an etiological role of gastritis, intestinalization, metaplasia, and adenomatous polyps in the etiology of gastric carcinoma, it is reasonable to assume that this is the soil in which carcinoma grows.

Chronic gastric ulcer has been regarded in the past as a precursor of gastric carcinoma. No data are available to establish this relationship. The problem is most likely insolvable, because in order to absolutely prove that a pre-existing benign ulcer became malignant, histological examination of the entire index ulcer would have to have been carried out. The finding of carcinoma cells in gastric ulcer is not even suggestive that the ulcer was benign and underwent malignant transformation. These ulcers probably result from peptic digestion of a superficial carcinoma. Although it is possible that chronic peptic ulcer within the stomach may undergo malignant degeneration, this event must be extremely rare.

Hypertrophic "gastropathy" is a rare lesion of the stomach characterized by widespread hypertrophy of the gastric mucosa.[6] There may or may not be an inflammatory component. The lesion is characterized by hyperplastic gastric glands containing large cystic spaces. These individuals are frequently achlorhydric, and histologically most specimens do not contain chief and parietal cells. The pathology probably represents a metaplastic lesion and not a hypertrophic gastritis. A few of these patients have been observed to develop successively adenomatous polyps and finally adenocarcinoma of the stomach.[6] The estimated incidence of carcinoma is approximately 8 per cent. Fewer than 200 of these patients have been reported since Menetrier's description in 1888[7] (see p. 570).

Another situation which may be associated with the development of carcinoma of the stomach is previous partial gastrectomy or gastroenterostomy for benign gastric or duodenal ulcer disease.[8-10] The incidence of carcinoma of the gastric remnant following the surgical procedure is approximately the same in gastric and duodenal ulcer. The interval between the surgical therapy of ulcer and the diagnosis of carcinoma varies between six and 37 or more years. This extremely long interval virtually excludes carcinoma as the initial lesion. Various hypotheses have been advanced to explain the development of gastric carcinoma in the postoperative stomach. Although data are not available, an important factor may be the reflux of bile and intestinal and pancreatic juices into the stomach through the gastroenterostomy. It appears that the incidence of carcinoma of the stomach in patients treated surgically for duodenal ulcer is increased to the level occurring in the general population.[11] The chance for subsequent development of carcinoma in the operated patient with gastric ulcer may conceivably be somewhat reduced as compared with the unoperated patient.

ADENOMATOUS POLYPS

CLINICAL FEATURES

History. The most common symptom of benign adenomatous polyp is nondescript upper abdominal pain. The pain is usually not related to food; it is a dull ache, occasionally a gnawing sensation, and is not relieved by antacids. Rarely, nausea and vomiting may be present. In very rare instances, large distal gastric polyps may prolapse into the duodenum and produce gastric obstruction. Overt hemorrhage is uncommon, but occult bleeding occurs frequently. Occasionally, polyps may infarct, slough, and be vomited. Weight loss and anorexia are uncommon. The only complaints may be easy fatigability and weakness caused by iron deficiency anemia or pernicious anemia. However, many patients are asymptomatic or have other symptoms for which an incidental upper gastrointestinal X-ray is obtained.

Physical Examination. The physical examination is usually noncontributory. In the presence of iron deficiency anemia there may be pallor, spooning of the nails, and other signs of iron deficiency. In patients with overt hemorrhage, the signs of hypovolemia may be present, manifested by hypotension, tachycardia, and, rarely, shock. Patients with untreated pernicious anemia characteristically have a lemon-yellow pallor of the skin. The hair is frequently white or gray, the ear lobes long, and the tongue smooth. There may be the findings of combined system disease. These patients may also have a low-grade fever of 100° to 101°F. A mass or tenderness on palpation caused by gastric polyp is almost never present.

Laboratory Data. The hematocrit, red blood cell count, and hemoglobin are usually normal. With occult bleeding, iron deficiency anemia may be present, in which case the bone marrow will not contain iron. With untreated pernicious anemia, the peripheral blood smear is macrocytic and hyperchromic with hypersegmented polymorphonuclear leukocytes, and the bone marrow is megaloblastic. Gastric analysis will demonstrate histamine- or Histalog-fast achlorhydria in 95 per cent of patients. None of the routine laboratory findings are specific for polyps.

Roentgenological Diagnosis. Radiology is a fairly sensitive technique for detecting gastric polyps. Caution must be used by the radiologist to procure good mucosal detail, because small polyps, particularly those 1 cm or less in diameter, may be obscured if the stomach is full of barium. They are seen as round, translucent filling defects within the stomach (Fig. 46–1). The presence of a stalk and a small size support a diagnosis of benignancy. Polyps larger than 2 cm in size, particularly sessile ones, are more likely to be malignant, although many are benign.[4]

Gastroscopy. Gastroscopy (see pp. 521 to 531) is more sensitive than radiology in detecting small polypoid lesions. It also assists in differentiating the nature of the polyp. In patients with adenomatous polyps of the stomach it is common to detect one by roentgenological methods and to find several endoscopically. Adenomatous polyps are usually somewhat more hyperemic than the surrounding mucosa and often have small focal hemorrhages. Many of the newer fiberoptic endoscopes have the capability for procuring directed biopsy and directed exfoliative cytology. Disadvantages are that in some instances it is technically not possible to direct the biopsy forceps or the cytological sampling device to the lesion. The biopsies are tiny fragments, and obtaining even multiple benign specimens does not exclude the

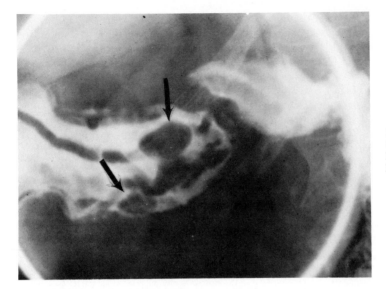

Figure 46–1. Two antral polyps (arrows). One is on a long stalk, the other is sessile. This patient had more than a dozen polyps seen at gastroscopy.

possible presence of malignancy at another site within the polyp. These instruments are also adaptable to both still and motion picture color photography, providing a permanent record of the appearance of the lesion and a basis for comparison in follow-up studies.

Exfoliative Cytology. Exfoliative cytology, if properly done and expertly interpreted, is the most sensitive technique for establishing a diagnosis of malignancy or excluding it if suspected by other methods (see p. 589). Patients with untreated pernicious anemia invariably have large benign epithelial cells with a varying morphology.[12-14] Large "active" benign gastric cells may be regularly recovered from their stomachs (Figs. 46–2 and 46–3). The persistence of large, "active" benign gastric cells after adequate vitamin B_{12} replacement is almost invariably associated with adenomatous polyp. Patients with adenomatous polyps may also exfoliate small tissue particles resembling fronds,[13] supporting a diagnosis of benign polyp. Intramucosal malignancies which radiologically may resemble benign polyps[13] and which do not penetrate into the lumen

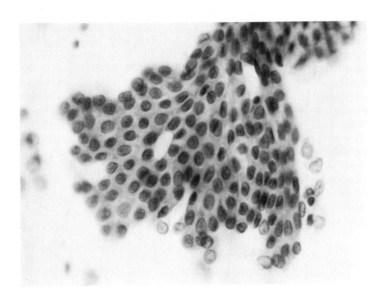

Figure 46–2. Benign gastric surface cells. × 400.

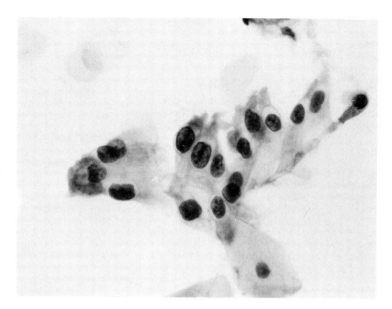

Figure 46–3. Large "active" gastric cells from a patient with untreated pernicious anemia and gastric polyps. × 400.

of the stomach cannot be diagnosed by exfoliative cytology. Except for the presence of fronds, the exfoliative cytological appearance is nonspecific. Large gastric cells may be seen in other situations, such as healing benign gastric ulcer, folate deficiency, and "gastritis," and in some elderly patients without obvious disease or nutritional deficiency.[13, 14]

TREATMENT

Although controlled data are not available, the consensus is that gastric polyps should be surgically excised.[2] The indication for excision in the past has been the malignant potential of these lesions.[4] In view of the low potential for malignant transformation,[4] this indication in itself is probably not valid. If there are sufficient reasons to believe that the patient's symptoms are due to gastric polyps or if complications result from them, surgical excision is warranted. The surgery of choice is local excision, including the stalk if one is present. Even when several polyps are present, extensive gastrectomy is not warranted. In multiple gastric polyposis, a subtotal gastrectomy may be the therapy of choice.

In patients whose symptoms are clearly not or probably not due to gastric polyps, nonsurgical observation is warranted if the polyps are smaller than 2 cm in diameter. Many of these polyps, even in patients followed for several years, do not grow or increase in number and do not appear to have a very high potential for malignant degeneration.[4] In patients in whom observation is elected, periodic X-ray, endoscopy, and exfoliative cytology should be done. Polyps larger than 2 cm in diameter, particularly sessile lesions, have a higher potential for containing malignancy; if surgical contraindications are not present, these lesions should be locally excised.

PROGNOSIS

Prognosis in patients with adenomatous polyps is excellent. If individuals who have associated invasive carcinoma are excluded, virtually none with adenomatous polyp, including multiple gastric polyposis, die from gastric carcinoma,[4] whether they receive surgical therapy or are simply followed. Although the groups of patients treated surgically as compared with those who are observed may not be comparable, the fact that these polyps undergo little change in size and rarely if ever become malignant supports a period of observation if other surgical indications are not present.

CARCINOMA OF THE STOMACH

Advanced carcinoma of the stomach is a dismal disease with a low cure rate. During the past three to four decades five-year survival in the United States increased from 7 per cent to only 9 per cent of all patients.[2] Most patients do not seek medical care until they are symptomatic, by which time they already have advanced disease. The diagnosis of carcinoma of the stomach confined to the mucosa is rare in most countries.

If gastric carcinoma can be detected while it is still confined to the mucosa, as it is in Japan through the mass surveys, cure rates are higher than 90 per cent.[15] Despite the increasing numbers of patients with gastric carcinoma confined to the mucosa that are being diagnosed in Japan,[16] the majority still have advanced gastric carcinoma at the time of diagnosis. In these patients the prognosis is equally as dismal as it is elsewhere throughout the world.

EPIDEMIOLOGY

Striking differences occur in death rates and incidence of gastric cancer throughout the world.[2, 17] The highest occurrence is in Chile, followed closely by Japan. Other countries with high incidences include Iceland, China, Austria, Finland, and Hungary. On the other hand, death rates from carcinoma of the stomach are extremely low in Egypt and Malaysia.[1, 17] In almost every country for which data are available, male incidences are higher than female. In the United States, nonwhites have approximately twice the incidence seen in whites in both males and females. Unexplained regional differences occur within countries, even in those with a homogeneous population. Low incidences in some countries may be explained, in part, by low life expectancy.

The reasons for these striking differences are not known. Various statistical correlations have been made with the incidence of gastric cancer. Among some of the factors which have been related to its occurrence have been low socioeconomic levels, urban dwelling, diet, background irradiation, presence of trace metals in soil, types of soil, occupation, and genetic factors. However, the decreased incidence in people migrating to the United States from countries of high occurrence, particularly in the second and third generations, suggests some environmental factor in most victims.

GENETIC FACTORS

Several families have been described with an unusually high occurrence of carcinoma of the stomach.[18, 19] A genetic factor of obscure significance is an approximately 10 per cent increase of gastric cancer in blood group A compared with suitable controls.[2] In patients with pernicious anemia, a genetic disease, who are estimated to have a 10 per cent chance of developing gastric cancer,[20] blood group A is also increased. Another genetic marker, which may be related, is the finding of Lewis group-specific substance, either Le[a] or Le[b] or both, in saliva in all patients with gastric carcinoma examined, whereas in the normal population approximately 7 per cent of subjects are Lewis negative.[21]

CLINICAL FEATURES

History. The most common symptom of gastric carcinoma is weight loss, which occurs in up to 96 per cent of patients.[2] Pain occurs in approximately 70 per cent. In some it is mild and a vague discomfort. In approximately 25 per cent it is similar to the pain of peptic ulcer. It may or may not be relieved by food or antacids and in some patients is of long duration, up to four or more years. The symptoms are thus completely nonspecific. Approximately 50 per cent of patients have vomiting. Other symptoms relating to the gastrointestinal tract are changes in bowel habits, such as constipation or diarrhea, which may direct investigation to the wrong level of the gut. Anorexia occurs in about 25 per cent of patients; this must be differentiated from early satiety, easy filling with eating, which occurs in only about 10 per cent. Dysphagia is a common symptom of carcinoma of the fundus and cardia of the stomach. Gross hematemesis is unusual and occurs in less than 10 per cent. Although overt hemorrhage is rare, occult bleeding is extremely common. A number of other systemic symptoms may occur, including weakness, easy fatigability, a sensation of abdominal fullness, fever, abdominal tenderness, ascites with peritoneal metastases, and angina pectoris which may be related to the degree of anemia.

Physical Examination. Forty-five to 50 per cent of patients with advanced gastric carcinoma will have a palpable mass on physical examination.[2] The liver may be palpable even though it does not contain metastases, and this should not be a contraindication to surgical therapy. Approximately 20 per cent of patients will be cachectic or emaciated. Abdominal tenderness, however, is present in only approximately 20 per cent. Five per cent of patients have palpable peripheral lymph nodes. Metastases may also be detected in hard nodular livers and on rectal examination because of metastases to the pelvic organs. Ascites may be present in a few patients with peritoneal and/or hepatic metastases. If ascites or jaundice is present owing to gastric carcinoma, the patient is almost invariably inoperable.

Laboratory Findings. The gastric analysis is of substantial clinical usefulness. In the presence of an ulcerating lesion of the stomach, achlorhydria demonstrated with adequate stimulation is virtually pathognomonic of a malignant lesion. On the other hand, the finding of acid is of no significance whatsoever in excluding a diagnosis of carcinoma of the stomach, nor can benign ulcer be differentiated from malignant ulcer on the basis of acid concentration or the amount secreted.[22] Anemia occurring in gastric carcinoma may be of several types. The most common is iron deficiency anemia caused by chronic occult blood loss. Macrocytic anemia may be seen in patients with gastric carcinoma and untreated pernicious anemia or folate deficiency. Patients with pernicious anemia or folate deficiency and combined iron deficiency will have a mixed type of anemia. A normochromic normocytic anemia may be seen even though bone marrow metastases are not present. Occult blood is often present in the stool. The routine laboratory data provide few clues to the diagnosis of gastric carcinoma, although many patients are hypoproteinemic. In the pres-

ence of hepatic metastases there may be bilirubin and alkaline phosphatase may be elevated but metastases may be present with entirely normal liver function tests. An isolated, elevated alkaline phosphatase may betoken bone metastases and not necessarily indicate liver involvement.

A number of substances have been measured in the gastric contents. It has been shown that β-glucuronidase activity,[23] lactic dehydrogenase, and other nonproteolytic enzymes are elevated in gastric cancer. Also increased is lactic acid.[24] There are changes in gastric mucosubstances as well.[2] These determinations are not clinically available. The overlap between noncancer and cancer patients also limits their usefulness and specificity.

Carcinoembryonic antigen, which is found in the sera in most patients with carcinoma of the colon and pancreas, is also found in approximately 50 per cent of patients with gastric carcinoma.[25] As the assay has become more sensitive, the specificity has decreased. The antigen may also be present in those with alcoholic liver disease, inflammatory bowel disease, and collagen-vascular disease. Other tumor-specific antigens are under study but not available for clinical application.

Roentgenological Diagnosis. X-ray is one of the more sensitive techniques for detecting lesions within the stomach. The radiologist must be cautious to procure good mucosal detail,[22] because smaller lesions may not be apparent in the stomach that is filled with barium. One of the more common causes for incorrect diagnosis is the technically inadequate examination.[22] With technically adequate examinations, the detection rate for lesions is in the order of 95 per cent. However, in the case of ulcers it may frequently be impossible on the basis of roentgenological features to distinguish between benign and malignant lesions. Some features which may aid in differentiating these lesions from benign ulcers are effacement or abnormal mucosal folds on films with adequate mucosal detail,[22] "niche encastrée" (niche in a notch), "niche enplateau," an ulcer with a flat, slightly wavy base, and "grosse niche triangulaire," a triangular, widebased ulcer.[26] Carman's sign (Figs. 46–4 and 46–5) indicates a mass with an ulceration within it. Benign ulcers with a large

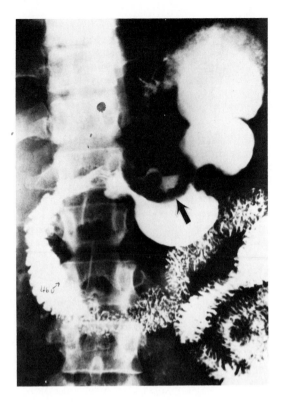

Figure 46–4. An ulcerated carcinoma in a 46-year-old man, demonstrating both crescentic crater within the contour of the lesser curvature (arrow) and the area of radiolucency between the gastric wall and lumen (Carman's sign). (Courtesy of Dr. M. H. Sleisenger.)

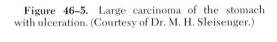

Figure 46–5. Large carcinoma of the stomach with ulceration. (Courtesy of Dr. M. H. Sleisenger.)

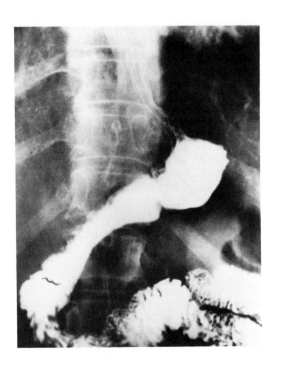

Figure 46–6. Diffusely infiltrative carcinoma of the stomach, linitis plastica. (Courtesy of Dr. M. H. Sleisenger.)

amount of surrounding edema may be indistinguishable. The diffuse infiltrating carcinomas, linitis plastica (Fig. 46–6), are usually diagnosable by failure of the stomach to distend when filled with barium and the absence or marked reduction of motor activity. Polypoid carcinomas (Fig. 46–7) may occasionally be confused with intramural, extramucosal tumors. Many carcinomatous ulcers are apparently benign by roentgenological criteria.[22] A large group of ulcers have an indeterminate appearance, with features of both benignancy and malignancy. Most of these lesions prove ultimately to be benign.[22] It is crucial in any medically treated ulcerating lesion to procure suitable follow-up examinations to assess progress toward healing (see pp. 692 to 710).

Gastroscopy. Gastroscopy is an important procedure which aids in the differential diagnosis of gastric lesions.[16] Linitis plastica may be recognized by failure of the stomach to distend with air and the frequent absence of mucosal folds. The gross appearance is less sensitive in ulcerating lesions in which many small carcinomas may be indistin-

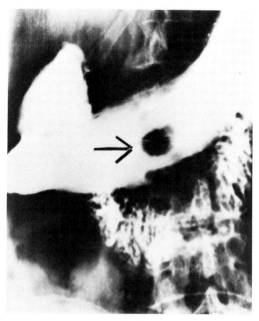

Figure 46–7. Gastric polyp (arrow) discovered in 1955 at yearly X-ray examination in 69-year old patient with pernicious anemia for 19 years. Later, cytological examination revealed malignant cells. (Courtesy of Dr. M. H. Sleisenger.)

guishable from benign ulcer.[27] Large benign ulcers with substantial surrounding inflammatory reaction and edema may have the appearance of malignant ulcers. The newer fiberoptic instruments frequently have biopsy and directed cytology attachments. This adds another dimension to the differential diagnosis of benign versus malignant lesions. The new instruments also have movable tips which increase the amount of the stomach that can be visualized.[16] The accuracy of gastroscopic biopsy with the fiberoptic instrument ranges from 80 per cent to more than 90 per cent in malignancy.[16] If exfoliative cytology obtained by direct sampling is added, this accuracy may be increased to the range of 96 to 98 per cent. Positive biopsy samples may be obtained in approximately 86 per cent of those with advanced cancers and 89 to 90 per cent of those with early carcinomas of the stomach.[16] It may be impossible, using the end-viewing instruments, to biopsy the proximal edge of an ulcerating lesion. Care should be taken to avoid hemorrhagic- and necrotic-appearing areas, because these may not yield the diagnosis. Because of the small size of the biopsy, six to ten should be procured from each lesion if possible, although on occasion this may be technically difficult. The disadvantages of the directed biopsy and cytology are that, on occasion, lesions cannot be visualized for technical reasons. In some lesions that are visualized, it may be impossible to place the biopsy forceps and cytological sampling device on the lesion. It is impossible with directed biopsy and cytology to sample the entire stomach wherein malignancy may exist and be unrecognized (see pp. 521 to 531).

An important place exists for lavage cytology in the detection and exclusion of gastric malignancy. Overconfidence, to the exclusion of other techniques, should not be placed in any diagnostic method, including fiberoptic endoscopy with directed biopsy and cytology, exfoliative cytology, or radiology.

Exfoliative Cytology. If its limitations are recognized, exfoliative cytology is an extremely useful diagnostic method for detection and exclusion of malignancy if other procedures suggest its presence. Cytology is of no use in diagnosing submucosal malignancies which do not penetrate into the lumen of the stomach. Malignancies such as leiomyosarcomas, even when ulcerated, do not exfoliate diagnostic cells. Some tumors may have necrotic or fibrin membranes overlying them, preventing exfoliation of diagnostic cells. The nature of these malignancies is usually apparent by the radiographic and gastroscopic appearance.

Lavage techniques are superior to any abrasive instrument for obtaining the specimen.[28-31] Cytological smears are optimal for diagnosis. The preparation of a "button" for histological examination is unnecessary, creates a great deal of additional work for the technologist, at best provides a pseudoarchitecture, and decreases accuracy.

The technique is simple and is performed by technologists without a physician in attendance. Several conditions must be observed. The collection of the specimen, processing, and scanning are best performed by trained cytotechnologists. Patients who are dehydrated do not exfoliate optimally; accordingly, adequate hydration is necessary. Patients with gastric obstruction require careful cleansing with a large-lumen Ewald tube and occasionally may require overnight gastric suction. Specimens must be rapidly processed, smeared, and fixed while wet to minimize digestion. Sending gastric contents to the laboratory for "cytology" is useless and should be condemned. The final diagnosis of benignancy, malignancy, or unsatisfactory must be made by an interested and skilled pathologist or clinician. Unsatisfactory examinations require a repeat study. These include specimens containing no normal gastric surface cells (Fig. 46–2) and those in which the cellular material is obscured by barium, food, and other debris. The presence of normal surface cells indicates an adequate cell collection if precautions are taken to minimize procurement of small suction biopsies by too vigorous aspiration of the gastric contents.

The highest accuracy has resulted from the utilization of chymotrypsin to procure the gastric specimen.[28, 30] How chymotrypsin works in gastric cytology is unknown. On the basis of histochemical studies, it removes substantial polysaccharide from cartilage.[32] It clearly promotes exfoliation

of both benign and malignant epithelial cells from gastric mucosal specimens in vitro.[33] The optimal concentration is in the range of 5 mg per 100 ml in a suitable buffer solution. Its action may be related to a mucolytic effect or may possibly be through a proteolytic action disrupting intercellular bonds.[33] Accuracy in the diagnosis of proved gastric malignancy is in excess of 90 per cent, and false-positive diagnosis when no malignancy is present is ordinarily less than 1 or 2 per cent (Table 46–1). Lavage with saline or Ringer's solution results in an acceptable accuracy in the range of 80 to 85 per cent in the hands of some skilled investigators.[29, 31] Saline lavage appears to be less sensitive than chymotrypsin lavage in the diagnosis of malignant ulcers (Table 46–1).[28, 31] Chymotrypsin lavage is not more difficult than saline lavage, and the increase in accurate diagnosis suggests that the technique should be more widely adopted.

The interpretation of the cellular material should include only three possible diagnoses: (1) malignant cells present (with an interpretation of cell type), (2) no malignant cells present, and (3) unsatisfactory. "Diagnoses" by such meaningless terminology as "class I, II, III, IV, V," "suspicious," "doubtful," "atypical," "highly atypical," and so forth reflect insecurity with cellular morphology and should be discouraged. This sort of diagnosis often leads to unjustified surgery. The "Class III," "suspicious," "doubtful," "atypical," and "highly atypical," cells usually occur in patients with benign dis-

TABLE 46–1. GASTRIC CYTOLOGY, VETERANS ADMINISTRATION HOSPITAL, SAN FRANCISCO, 1961–1971

| | CYTOLOGY | |
	Malignant No. (%)	Benign No. (%)
Carcinoma	90 (93)°	7 (7)†
Lymphoma	9 (90)	1 (10)
Benign disease	3 (0.5)	581 (99.5)

°Includes 43 ulcerating carcinomas.

†False-negatives include two ulcerating carcinomas, one linitis plastica, and four large necrotic carcinomas.

ease[12-14] who can be managed medically. Furthermore, in almost every instance the malignant or benign nature of the cells can be determined if the individual responsible for the diagnosis is versed in cellular morphology.[28]

Patient preparation is crucial, particularly hydration. On the night prior to the examination the patient is given a clear liquid supper followed by three to five glasses of water. On the morning of the examination, breakfast is withheld and another three to five glasses of water are given.

The chymotrypsin lavage is performed as follows:[34] On arrival at the laboratory, the patient is given a glass of water containing 30 mg of α-chymotrypsin. He is instructed to expectorate oral secretions and sputum, to minimize confusing cellular material from the lungs and nasopharynx. He remains recumbent for 30 minutes after this drink. A chilled Levin tube is then passed through the mouth without lubricants, and the residual gastric contents are aspirated and saved. The stomach is then vigorously lavaged for three minutes with 100 ml volumes of Ringer's solution, utilizing a 100-ml glass syringe while the patient rotates to the supine, right lateral decubitus, prone, and left lateral positions. This solution is aspirated and saved for processing. Next, 500 ml of acetate buffer at pH 5.6 (13.6 g of sodium acetate and 0.6 ml glacial acetic acid per liter of distilled water) containing 30 mg of α-

chymotrypsin is instilled into the stomach through the tube. The patient rotates through 360 degrees, spending two minutes each in the supine, right lateral decubitus, prone, and left lateral decubitus positions. This permits the lavage fluid to contact all the gastric mucosa. This solution is then rapidly aspirated and processed. It is not necessary to remove the last possible drop from the stomach for an adequate examination.

The lavage fluids are placed in 50-ml plastic tubes in an ice bath to retard digestion. The residual gastric contents and the Ringer's solution are centrifuged in the 50-ml plastic tubes for three minutes at 5000 rpm in an angle head centrifuge while the chymotrypsin solution is in the patient's stomach. The supernatant fluid is decanted and the sediment removed from the tubes with a small spatula. The smears are prepared by smearing the sediment between pairs of glass slides. They are immediately fixed, while wet, in alkaline alcohol (3.0 ml of 0.1N NaOH and 97 ml of 95 per cent ethanol). Usually five pairs of slides are made, one from the residual contents, one from the Ringer specimen, and three from the chymotrypsin specimen. The slides are stained by Rubin and Benditt's modification of Papanicolaou's technique.[35]

One slide from each pair, prepared in the preceding manner, is scanned by the cytotechnologist, who marks interesting, abnormal, and malignant cells. Also,

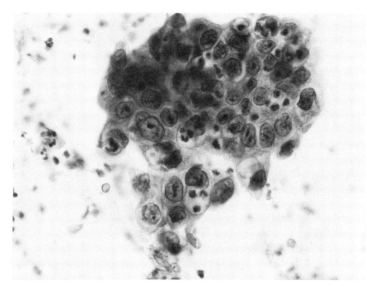

Figure 46-8. Adenocarcinoma. × 400.

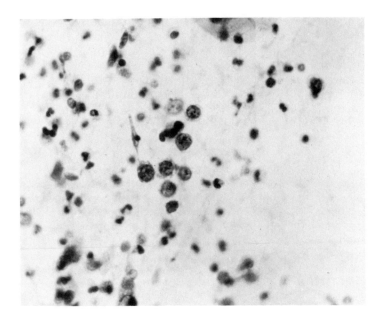

Figure 46-9. Reticulum cell sarcoma. Note finely vacuolated rim of cytoplasm. Lymphosarcoma cells are similar but slightly smaller. × 400.

benign gastric columnar cells are marked as an indication of a satisfactory test. It is unnecessary to scan both slides prepared in this way (the reason for doing it is a better distribution of cells), because it is rare to find malignant cells on one slide and not on its mate. The final diagnosis is the responsibility of the clinican or pathologist.

INTERPRETATION OF THE CYTOLOGICAL SPECIMEN. Squamous epithelium, cells of respiratory origin, histiocytes, and inflammatory cells are almost invariably present in the smears. The cytological diagnosis of malignancy is made on alterations in the nucleus. These include irregular chromatin distribution, hyperchromatism, excessive variation in the size of the nuclei, increased nuclear to cytoplasmic ratio, enlarged and multiple nucleoli, empty spaces within the nucleus, and irregular "pseudopods" protruding from the nucleus ("Idaho potato" nucleus). The cell of origin can often be determined from the cytoplasmic features. Thus cytoplasmic basophilia, vacuolization, crowded

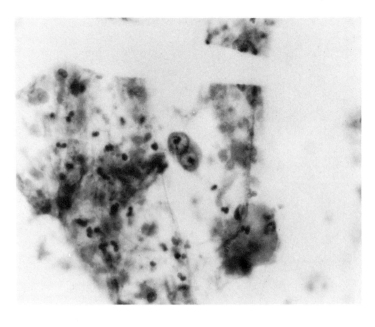

Figure 46-10. Reed-Sternberg cell from gastric Hodgkin's disease. × 400.

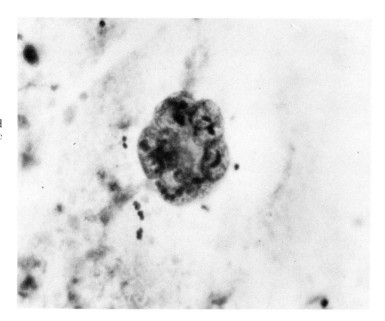

Figure 46–11. Multinucleated malignant giant cell from gastric Hodgkin's disease. × 400.

clumps, and a syncytial appearance without distinct cellular borders favor adenocarcinoma (Fig. 46–8). Orangophilic staining, malignant pearls, tadpole cells, and fiber cells indicate a squamous origin (see pp. 601 to 602). Malignant lymphoma almost invariably exfoliates single cells and not clumps of cells (Fig. 46–9). The nuclear criteria of malignancy are present. These cells are small, approximately the size of a benign gastric surface cell. It may be possible to differentiate reticulum cell sarcoma from lymphosarcoma, because it is a slightly larger cell with a more prominent, finely vacuolated rim of cytoplasm. The finding of Reed-Sternberg cells (Fig. 46–10 and 46–11) in the gastric cytology establishes a diagnosis of Hodgkin's disease.[36] The slides from patients with malignant lymphoma almost invariably contain large numbers of inflammatory cells which provide a clue to the possible diagnosis. Examination of slides containing large numbers of inflammatory cells requires frequent switching to the high dry objective (×400) so as not to overlook malignant lymphoma. In some undifferentiated tumors, it may not be possible to distinguish between malignant lymphoma and undifferentiated carcinoma by cytological appearance. Scanty numbers of malignant-appearing "lymphoid" cells may be recovered from patients with viral respiratory infections. Ideally, patients with colds should not have a gastric cytology until they have recovered.

The interpretation of the nature of the cells is made on morphological grounds. Fluorescent staining, whether induced by the previous administration of tetracycline or by staining the material with acridine orange, results in such high false-positive and false-negative rates of diagnosis that these techniques are to be discouraged. Furthermore, the nature of the fluorescent cells must be confirmed by morphology.

INDICATIONS FOR CYTOLOGY. Ideally, all gastric ulcers should be examined cytologically prior to embarking upon a course of medical therapy. If endoscopy with directed biopsy and cytology yields a diagnosis of malignancy, lavage cytology is not necessary. However, if the directed biopsy and cytology do not diagnose the presence of malignancy, lavage cytology is indicated. Although it has been shown that some "early" malignant ulcers have substantial healing,[27] the expert utilization of endoscopy with directed biopsy and cytology and lavage exfoliative cytology should correctly detect the vast majority of these lesions. The very few which are missed would likely be diagnosed on the basis of nonhealing.

Another indication is the presence of overt tumor. Cytology is the most sensitive nonhistological technique of correctly predicting the cell type of a tumor prior to surgery. This is of practical importance in the differential diagnosis between carcinoma and malignant lymphoma. If the surgeon has a firm diagnosis of malignant lymphoma, he may be encouraged to remove the bulk of the tumor, which theoretically would make postoperative irradiation therapy more effective. The test is of particular help in the differential diagnosis of the narrow antrum, i.e., antral "gastritis," enlarged rugal folds, and problems in the cardia and fundus. Patients with dysphagia should also have an esophageal cytology (see pp. 111 to 112 and 455 to 463).

Although cytological screening for occult or "early" malignancy would appear desirable, in the United States it has proved to be impractical, even in patients with a suspected high risk, because of the low incidence.[37] It would seem reasonable to periodically, e.g., annually, examine patients with a suspected high risk, such as those with pernicious anemia, gastric polyposis, and achlorhydria, even though the yield would be low.

Cytology is useful in patients who may develop carcinoma of the stomach after surgery for benign peptic ulcer disease. Even if a lesion cannot be demonstrated by radiology or endoscopy, patients who develop symptoms after several years of good health following ulcer surgery should be examined cytologically. Although recurrent gastric carcinoma may appear some months or years after primary surgical therapy, cytology is not so sensitive in these patients, because the recurrence or incompletely extirpated tumor is often extraluminal and cannot be diagnosed by this technique. Metastatic tumors to the stomach are ordinarily submucosal, and for the most part cannot be diagnosed by exfoliative cytology. An exception is an occasional ulcerated malignant melanoma.[38]

TREATMENT

The only curative therapy for gastric carcinoma is surgical excision.[2] The type of operation performed must be left to the discretion and experience of the surgeon doing the procedure. As a generality, large polypoid lesions may be treated with a limited gastrectomy, particularly if evidence of metastases is absent. Antral lesions, both polypoid and ulcerating but not infiltrating, may be treated by a partial or subtotal gastrectomy. Total gastrectomy is almost never indicated in the therapy of gastric carcinoma.

More radical surgery, which includes removal of all lymph node areas where carcinoma may be predicted to metastasize as well as resection of contiguous organs (e.g., partial colectomy, partial pancreatectomy, splenectomy), results in an operative mortality approximately twice that of the less radical procedures.[39] Radical total gastrectomy is associated with an operative death rate of approximately 50 per cent. In patients who are operated on for cure by super-radical resection, overall five-year survival decreases by approximately 25 per cent. The decrease in survival is most marked in the patients with lymph node metastases who undergo the super-radical procedure in anticipation of cure.[39]

Although many patients, at the time of laparotomy, are found to be inoperable for cure, palliative resection or gastroenterostomy may be indicated. Although the overall survival is improved but little in most, some patients with slow-growing carcinomas may receive substantial comfort, decrease in obstruction and hemorrhage, and improvement in nutrition. On the other hand, patients with esophageal obstruction caused by inoperable carcinomas of the cardia or fundus invading the esophagus may be given a "feeding" gastrostomy, but this will only prolong their agony.

Chemotherapy. Chemotherapy of metastatic gastric carcinoma is noncurative, but may provide palliation. Although several drugs have been studied, 5-fluorouracil (5-FU) has had the widest clinical application. It is the third drug of choice; the first two have not yet been discovered. An objective response, defined as a 50 per cent regression in measurable tumor mass, may be expected in 20 per cent of patients. Subjective improvement occurs in approximately 40 per cent of patients.[40] The responses are usually of short duration, a matter of a few months at most. Prolongation of life has not been proved. Although no predictive factors are available, an occasional patient will have a dramatic clinical response which may last for up to a year or more.

Outpatient treatment is practical in most instances. A recommended regimen is 5-FU given once weekly at a dosage of 15 mg per kilogram either intravenously or orally.[40] The differences in antitumor effect by either route of administration are insignificant. The weekly, rather than daily, administration of the drug has significantly decreased mortality and toxicity without any apparent decrease in antitumor effect. Patients who have an objective or a subjective response usually do so within the first six weeks of treatment.

The major toxicity associated with 5-FU includes diarrhea, stomatitis, nausea, vomiting, anorexia, leukopenia, and thrombocytopenia. The gastrointestinal toxicity is more prominent with orally administered drug, and the hematopoietic toxicity is more common with the intravenous route. Other, rarer side effects include renal, hepatic, and central nervous system toxicity and alopecia. Theoretically, oral administration should benefit patients with hepatic metastases owing to a higher concentration in the portal venous blood. However, this assumption has not been established; most tumors receive their blood supply through the hepatic artery.

Combination drug therapy has not been widely used in gastrointestinal carcinoma. Theoretically, multiple agents should be more effective than single drugs, because each is cytotoxic at a different stage of cell division or metabolism. A combination which has apparently increased objective response rates is 1,3-bis-(2-chlorethyl)-1-nitrosourea (BCNU) and 5-FU.[41] The regimen examined was BCNU, 35 mg per m², and 5-FU, 7 mg per kilogram, given daily for five days and repeated in eight weeks. On this program, four of six patients with gastric carcinoma had an objective response. The number of patients treated is too small to draw conclusions, but this approach requires further study.

A large effort is directed toward finding useful chemotherapeutic agents. However, these investigations have been largely unrewarding. Adriamycin, an antibiotic with antitumor activity, has recently been shown to have induced a response in seven of nine patients with metastatic gastrointestinal cancer (M. R. Dollinger, personal communication).

Even though the response rates are low and the failure rates high, chemotherapy should be offered to patients with incurable gastric carcinoma. Because of the serious toxicity associated with all the available drugs, they should be used only by skilled oncologists or by units specializing in chemotherapy. These physicians and centers also have investigative drugs which are not released for more general use and which may prove to be valuable. Although the current agents give little cause for other than pessimism, it is to be hoped that more effective chemotherapy will be discovered in the future.

Radiation Therapy. Systematic studies of radiation therapy of gastric carcinoma are not available. However, it should be considered in the patient with unresectable gastric carcinoma, particularly if the tumor is largely localized to the vicinity of the stomach.[2] Although it has been held in the past that adenocarcinomas are not radiosensitive, there are no predictive factors in either the gross or the histological classification. In general, the mucinous carcinomas are less responsive than the more undifferentiated varieties.[2] Although adenocarcinomas of the stomach are not radiocurable, some are radioresponsive. This cannot be determined without attempting therapy.

The usual tissue dose of irradiation is in the order of 6000 rads. This therapy may result in some local control of the disease. Irradiation therapy is of some use in selected patients in controlling hemorrhage.[2]

Immunotherapy. The demonstration of antitumor antibodies to tumor extract in patients with regressing gynecological cancers[42] has stimulated investigation of possible immunotherapy in a large number of different types of cancers. Attempts at immunization with autogenous tumor cells and Freund's adjuvant in similar patients produced no vaccine-related remissions.[43] A wide variety of antigens such as BCG and Freund's adjuvant, chemicals, such as 2,3,5-triethylene-imino-benzoquinone (TEIB), dinitrochlorobenzene (DNCB), with or without added tumor cells, homogenates, or tumor fractions have been administered to cancer patients.

Topical immunotherapy with TEIB and DNCB is as effective as topical chemotherapy in cutaneous malignancy.[44] Fewer data are available for similar procedures in gastrointestinal carcinomas. A tumor vaccine prepared by using bisdiazobenzidine to couple autologous tumor cells to rabbit gamma globulin and given with Freund's adjuvants[45] may produce objective tumor regression in up to 38 per cent of gastrointestinal carcinomas.[46] Unfortunately, in many of these patients, the role of immunotherapy is unclear, because some received radiotherapy or chemotherapy or both.[45-47] Another added procedure was plasma–white blood cell exchanges.[46]

There are almost an infinite number of substances which can be administered which induce "immunity" as estimated by circulating antibody titers or delayed hypersensitivity. Before benefit to patients with incurable carcinoma can be concluded, controlled clinical studies are mandatory. Randomized studies comparing immunotherapy alone with the various combinations of chemotherapy with and without added radiation therapy are crucial. This approach opens an entire new field which may, in the future, be of great clinical value.

PROGNOSIS

The prognosis in patients with advanced carcinoma of the stomach is poor. Sixty-five per cent of those subjected to surgery are found to be incurable at the time of operation.[2] Of all the patients seen with the disease, fewer than 10 per cent are cured by surgery. The factor which seems to determine a favorable outlook is a long history as opposed to a brief history. Patients with achlorhydria and with pernicious anemia tend to develop carcinoma in the proximal stomach. These tumors tend to be polypoid, often multicentric, and generally of a relatively low-grade malignancy.[48] Patients who secrete hydrochloric acid tend to develop ulcerating carcinomas of a high-grade malignancy in the antrum.[48]

The gross characteristics of the tumor are important prognostically. Thus the Borrmann 1, polypoid, and Borrmann 2, ulcerating but noninfiltrating, carcinomas have the best prognosis.[2] The Borrmann 3, ulcerative infiltrating, and the diffuse infiltrating varieties, including linitis plastica, Borrmann 4, have an extremely low cure rate. Superficial, spreading carcinoma and carcinoma in situ, the diagnosis which is usually made cytologically, have an excellent prognosis. So does "early" carcinoma as detected in asymptomatic individuals through the mass surveys in Japan. It is still unknown whether untreated superficial spreading carcinoma or carcinoma in situ always becomes invasive cancer. Despite the lack of this knowledge, current practice indicates surgical extirpation if a gross lesion can be detected. It is difficult to recommend total gastrectomy in patients who have a positive exfoliative cytological diagnosis of carcinoma but in whom no lesion can be detected. Positive cytologies may occur in some patients, particularly those with pernicious anemia, for several years before an overt carcinoma is diagnosable.[49]

Virtually all carcinomas of the stomach are adenocarcinomas derived from the epithelium. The histological classification is somewhat less sensitive in predicting prognosis. Generally, the less differentiated and more widely invasive tumors are associated with a shorter course and early death.

Some individuals with long survival have tumors which are advancing en bloc and have a substantial rim of lymphocytes and plasma cells adjacent to the advancing border and focal necrosis of tumor cells in the vicinity of inflammatory response.[50] These histological features suggest a favorable reaction on the part of the host to his tumor. Even in the presence of metastases, some of these individuals may survive for several years.[50] Some other long-term survivors do not have these histological features and their significance is as yet obscure.[22]

SARCOMAS OF THE STOMACH

Although gastric sarcomas are said to account for only approximately 5 per cent of all gastric malignancies,[2] their recognition is important because of their substantially higher curability. As the incidence of gastric carcinoma in the United States is decreasing, the percentage of gastric cancer patients having lymphoma is increasing.[16] Lymphoma may account for as much as 8 to 10 per cent of gastric cancer currently (see Table 46–1).[16] The higher curability is observed in those patients with sarcomas that are limited to, or have not extended far beyond, the vicinity of the stomach. Patients with disseminated lymphomas have gastric involvement in about 40 per cent of cases.[2] In these individuals, death is usually due to disseminated malignancy and not to the gastric involvement. Occasionally death may result from overt gastrointestinal hemorrhage.

For clinical purposes the sarcomatous lesions of the stomach include the lymphomas (lymphosarcoma, reticulum cell sarcoma, and Hodgkin's disease) and the leiomyosarcomas. The lymphomas occur at a ratio of approximately 4 to 1 over the leiomyosarcomas. Other tumors, such as fibrosarcomas and angiosarcomas, are extremely rare in the stomach.

MALIGNANT LYMPHOMA

History. It is not possible to differentiate carcinoma of the stomach from lymphosarcoma of the stomach on the basis of the patient's clinical history.[2, 51, 52] Lymphosarcomas have approximately the same age distribution as carcinoma of the stomach, with a somewhat increased incidence in younger individuals. The disease has occurred in childhood.

The most common symptom of gastric lymphoma is abdominal pain, which occurs in approximately 90 per cent of patients. The duration of pain is variable and ranges from a few days to several years. The pain may be vague and nondescript or indistinguishable from the pain of peptic ulcer disease.[51] Approximately 50 per cent of patients with gastric lymphoma have either had a past history of peptic ulcer disease or symptoms that are highly suggestive of it. The next most common symptom, which occurs in more than 50 per cent of the patients, is weight loss of more than 10 pounds; in some patients weight loss is massive. Vomiting occurs in approximately 25 to 30 per cent of patients and nausea in approximately 15 to 20 per cent. Other symptoms are weakness and fatigue, "indigestion," a feeling of abdominal fullness, and eructation. Hematemesis occurs in 20 per cent of patients, but it is massive in less than 5 per cent. Ten to 15 per cent of patients have melena,

but it is rarely massive. Although overt bleeding is relatively uncommon, occult bleeding is frequent.

Physical Examination. Patients with malignant lymphoma confined to the stomach usually have no significant physical findings. Occasionally, an epigastric mass may be present. Patients with disseminated lymphoma frequently have multiple abdominal masses, and localization in the stomach is difficult to determine on physical examination. There may be pallor and other signs of anemia. Peripheral lymphadenopathy, hepatomegaly, and splenomegaly are common in patients with disseminated lymphoma.

Laboratory Findings. The routine laboratory data provide no clues to the diagnosis of lymphoma confined to the stomach. When it is present, anemia is usually iron deficiency in type. The differential white blood cell count is usually normal. These patients do not have a "leukemic" peripheral blood smear. The gastric analy-

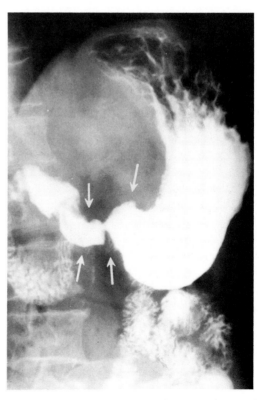

Figure 46–12. Narrow, irregular antrum (arrows) caused by reticulum cell sarcoma. Considered to be antral "gastritis" for more than one year. Correctly diagnosed by exfoliative cytology.

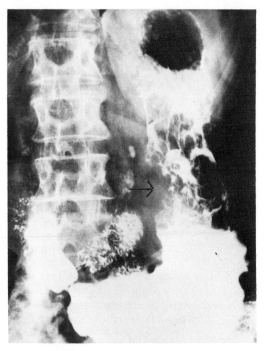

Figure 46–13. Lymphosarcoma of the stomach. Note infiltration, enlargement of folds of this tumor. (Courtesy of Dr. M. H. Sleisenger.)

sis is variable; most are capable of secreting hydrochloric acid.

Roentgenological Diagnosis. Malignant lymphoma is a great imitator of benign and malignant disease.[2, 53] Although X-ray is a sensitive method for detection of lesions, it is frequently impossible to differentiate malignant lymphoma from carcinoma of the stomach. Several different gross types of malignant lymphoma occur in the stomach. These include ulcerative lesions, polypoid lesions, diffuse infiltrating lesions (Fig. 46–12), giant hypertrophy of the gastric rugal pattern (Fig. 46–13), and various combinations. It is usually only with the marked hypertrophy of the rugal folds that the examining roentgenologist suggests the possibility of malignant lymphoma.[2, 53] These tumors are often quite large on radiographic examinations, often multicentric, and occur in all parts of the stomach but appear to have some predilection for the antrum.

Endoscopy. Most lymphomas of the stomach cannot be differentiated from carcinoma on gross appearance. The endo-

scopic appearance may be that of an erosive, hemorrhagic gastritis superimposed on large rugal folds, polypoid lesions, ulcerative lesions, and combinations of the above. Too few data are available to assess the role of directed biopsy and cytology of malignant lymphoma.[16] The preparation of imprint cytology slides from the biopsy specimens may increase accuracy.[54] The wider application of these procedures should permit a more precise differential diagnosis between malignant lymphoma and carcinoma of the stomach.

Exfoliative Cytology. Exfoliative cytology may be the most sensitive technique for differentiating carcinoma from lymphoma prior to surgery (see Table 46–1). The cytological characteristics of malignant lymphoma are well established (see Figs. 46–9, 46–10, and 46–11). In some very undifferentiated malignancies the differentiation of carcinoma and lymphoma may not be possible on cytological appearance. Giant follicular lymphoma, which is rarely found in the stomach, cannot be diagnosed by exfoliative cytology. These tumors exfoliate only benign-appearing lymphocytes, and the diagnosis can be made only on histological criteria.

Treatment. The therapy of malignant lymphoma of the stomach is surgery followed by postoperative irradiation therapy.[2, 51-53] The best survival data have been generated from institutions where this approach is applied. Postoperative irradiation is indicated even though the surgeon may think that he has removed all the cancer. This is due to the fact that, although frequently localized, these lesions are often multicentric.[51-53] Theoretically, the patient who has an unresectable lesion of the stomach would respond better to irradiation therapy if the bulk of the tumor could be excised.[2] This would provide a smaller mass of tissue for the radiotherapist to direct his attention to. The usual dosage of postoperative radiation is in the order of 3000 to 4000 rads to the tumor-bearing area. Long survival has followed postoperative irradiation therapy for patients in whom no resection was attempted.

Lymphomas are not necessarily radiosensitive. In general, the small cell lymphosarcomas appear to be more radiosensitive and probably more radiocurable than some of the reticulum cell sarcomas.

Hodgkin's disease may be radiosensitive and radiocurable when confined to the stomach.

Chemotherapy is indicated in disseminated lymphoma or in patients with such widespread abdominal disease that irradiation cannot be safely undertaken. The drugs which may be tried include the nitrogen mustards and chlorambucil, vincristine, vinblastine, methotrexate, and high-dose prednisone. These drugs should be given only by physicians skilled in their use because of their serious toxicity.

Prognosis. In general, the small cell lymphosarcomas have a better prognosis than reticulum cell sarcoma or Hodgkin's disease. This is due to their more favorable response to radiation therapy. Small tumors have a better prognosis than large lesions. Peritoneal involvement apparently does not influence cure, whereas lymph node involvement is associated with lower cure rates.[55] Thirty to more than 50 per cent of patients will survive for more than five years,[2, 51-53] with apparent cure, and 13 to 50 per cent will survive for ten years or longer.[51]

It is difficult to compare various reports, because often the basis for selecting a particular therapy is not described. Thus, whether or not surgery is followed by irradiation may depend upon whether or not the surgeon believes that the tumor was completely removed. Occasional patients who have biopsy alone followed by postoperative irradiation therapy appear to do almost as well as those who are resected and irradiated.

LEIOMYOSARCOMA OF THE STOMACH

Gastric leiomyosarcoma accounts for between 0.25 and 1.5 per cent of all gastric malignancies.[2, 56] Whether this malignancy arises from a pre-existing benign leiomyoma is a possibility that is difficult, if not impossible, to prove. The tumor occurs in approximately equal frequency in both sexes. It is seen at a somewhat younger age than carcinoma of the stomach and has been observed in childhood.

Most leiomyosarcomas are intramural, extramucosal tumors. However, they may be attached to the stomach and not present within the lumen. Rarely they are dumbbell shaped and have an intra- and exogastric component. They are frequently ulcerated or necrotic.

History. The average duration of symptoms is somewhat less than in malignant lymphoma or carcinoma of the stomach. There is a wide variation, ranging from a few days to several years.[2, 56] Pain, which occurs in about 50 per cent of patients, is highly variable in character and intensity. It is usually located in the epigastrium and varies from a vague, nondescript "indigestion" to peptic ulcer-like pain of a severe intensity. Hematemesis and melena are more common than with other gastric malignancies and tend to be repeated and copious. Anorexia and weight loss occur in approximately 20 per cent. Nausea and vomiting are infrequent, as is dysphagia. Weight loss occurs in 25 per cent of subjects. Occasionally, leiomyosarcoma may be asymptomatic and discovered either by the patient finding a palpable epigastric mass or on roentgenological examination of apparently healthy individuals.

Physical Examination. The most common physical finding is a palpable epigastric mass which occurs in up to 75 per cent of patients. It is usually spherical and firm and is often mobile. Abdominal tenderness is common, but may be absent. Anemia is frequent, and there may be pallor. Physical findings of excessive weight loss are usually not present.

Laboratory. Anemia when present is iron deficiency in type, and occurs in approximately 75 per cent of patients. Gastric analysis is of little value in the diagnosis; acid secretion varies from achlorhydria to hypersecretion.

Roentgenological Diagnosis. Most leiomyosarcomas appear as spherical, intramural, extramucosal tumors on roentgenological examination. It is not possible to differentiate malignant tumors from benign leiomyomas on the basis of the radiographic appearance. Large lesions are more probably cancerous than small lesions.[2, 58] Frequently there is a central ulceration within the mass.

Gastroscopy. The major contribution of gastroscopy is the confirmation of a tumor in the stomach. Gastroscopy will frequently reveal lesions in which a central ulceration is not identified on radiographic examination as a site of hemorrhage. No data are available on the role of directed biopsy or directed cytology in the diagnosis of leiomyosarcoma. It is unlikely that these procedures will contribute substantially to the correct differential diagnosis of extramucosal lesions. This is due to the fact that, fortunately, the biopsy forceps is too small to procure more than a superficial specimen.

Exfoliative Cytology. Exfoliative cytology is of no use whatsoever in the diagnosis of leiomyosarcoma.

Treatment. The only curative treatment of leiomyosarcoma is surgical extirpation.[2, 56] The type and extent of the operation depend upon the size and extent of the cancer. In patients with tumor confined to the stomach, a partial or subtotal gastrectomy is usually adequate. Occasionally, in tumors of the proximal stomach, a total gastrectomy or a proximal gastrectomy may be necessary. Radiation therapy has not been shown to be effective in leiomyosarcoma. No information is available on chemotherapy.

Prognosis. More than 50 per cent of patients with leiomyosarcoma will be cured by surgery. Patients with metastases in lymph nodes or liver, or with direct extension beyond the confines of the stomach, have a poor prognosis. Other factors which influence outcome are large size and anaplasia. Even if the tumors are small, anaplastic lesions are associated with a poor prognosis. However, despite the presence of metastases, palliative surgery may be indicated for control of hemorrhage; because of the unpredictability of cancer, some patients may receive substantial benefit.

LEIOMYOMAS OF THE STOMACH

Leiomyomas are the most common benign tumor of the stomach detected at autopsy.[1, 2] The incidence depends upon how carefully the prosector searches for these lesions, because they are often small. In 16 per cent of autopsies in patients not suspected of having gastric disease, leiomyomas ranging from 0.2 to 1.9 cm have been observed.[2] Clinically significant leiomyomas of the stomach, however, are rare lesions.[57] They are often found incidentally at the time of surgery for other

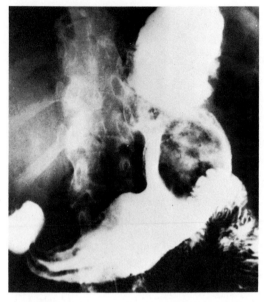

Figure 46–14. Large leiomyoma of the stomach. (Courtesy of Dr. M. H. Sleisenger.)

conditions. It is rare for a leiomyoma less than 3 cm in diameter to be responsible for symptoms.

The larger leiomyomas, on the other hand, may be clinically significant. The symptoms are indistinguishable from those associated with leiomyosarcomas. It is not possible to differentiate leiomyoma from leiomyosarcoma by any of the clinical techniques currently available short of excision and histological examination.

Symptomatic leiomyomas are usually detectable by roentgenological examination (Fig. 46–14). They have a similar or identical appearance to leiomyosarcomas except for a generally smaller size. None of the routine laboratory tests, endoscopy, or exfoliative cytology is capable of providing a firm preoperative histological diagnosis.

Treatment. Symptomatic leiomyomas responsible for pain or hemorrhage should be treated surgically.[2, 57] It is also reasonable to excise those leiomyomas which are incidentally found at the time of surgery for other conditions. The surgical excision need only be a limited local removal of the tumor. If a frozen section at the time of surgery is diagnostic of, or strongly suggestive of, a leiomyosarcoma, the margins of the resection should be at least 2 cm.[57]

ECTOPIC PANCREAS (PANCREATIC RESTS)

Pancreatic rests or ectopic pancreas are relatively rare tumors occurring in the stomach and may mimic other polypoid lesions such as adenomatous polyp or leiomyoma. Ordinarily, they are small, *intramural, extramucosal* lesions located on the distal greater curvature of the antrum. They are rarely larger than 2 cm in diameter. Approximately 25 per cent of ectopic pancreatic tissue occurs in the stomach.[2]

History. Approximately 50 per cent of pancreatic rests are symptomatic, and half of them are asymptomatic and detected at the time of surgery for other indications or found at the time of autopsy. The symptoms may include vague, nondescript abdominal pain, nausea, and occasionally vomiting. Bleeding occurs only when the overlying mucosa becomes ulcerated. Since ectopic pancreas is an embryologic anomaly, it is frequently observed in the first and second decades of life. More than 50 per cent of patients with pancreatic rests have a diagnosis made before the age of 40 years.[2]

Physical Examination. The physical examination provides no clues to the diagnosis of pancreatic rests. They are rarely if ever large enough to detect by palpation.

Laboratory Findings. The routine laboratory data are of little use in establishing a diagnosis of pancreatic rest. If the lesion has ulcerated and bled, iron deficiency anemia may be present. The gastric analysis, on the other hand, is of substantial use in differentiating these lesions from benign adenomatous polyps. The large majority of patients with ectopic gastric pancreas are capable of secreting varying levels of hydrochloric acid, whereas 95 per cent of patients having adenomatous polyps are achlorhydric. The gastric analysis is of little use in differentiating ectopic pancreas from a small leiomyoma, leiomyosarcoma, or other intramucosal, extramural tumors, because most of these patients secrete acid.

Roentgenological Diagnosis. A preoperative diagnosis may be made on radiographic criteria. Pancreatic rests usually present as distal greater curvature, intramural, extramucosal tumors, or polypoid lesions. There is often a central pit with elevation of the mucosa overlying the lesion. If a secretory duct is visualized, the preoperative diagnosis is established.

Gastroscopy. Gastroscopy will confirm the presence of an extramucosal, intramural tumor. There are no specific features, however, which conclusively establish a diagnosis of pancreatic rests. The most usual gross appearance is that of a sessile, polypoid, umbilicated, somewhat yellowish submucosal tumor. Pancreatic rests can be confused with lipoma. Further support of the gastroscopic diagnosis of pancreatic rest is the distal antral location.

Exfoliative Cytology. Exfoliative cytology is of no assistance in making a diagnosis of pancreatic rest.

Treatment. The treatment of choice for symptomatic pancreatic rest is distal gastrectomy.[2] The incidentally discovered lesions may be locally excised.

Prognosis. The prognosis in patients with surgically treated pancreatic rests is excellent. Unless the lesion has undergone malignant change, extirpation is curative.

MISCELLANEOUS TUMORS OF THE STOMACH

A number of other rare tumors occur in the stomach. Some are benign, and some have malignant potential. The correct diagnosis is frequently not made prior to the time of surgery or autopsy and is based on histological criteria. The rare malignant lesions cannot be differentiated on clinical and radiographic criteria from carcinomas or lymphomas of the stomach.

SQUAMOUS NEOPLASMS OF THE STOMACH

Squamous cell carcinomas of the stomach are extremely rare,[58] and benign squamous cell neoplasms are even rarer.[59] Fewer than 100 malignant cases have been recorded.[58] Clinically and radiographically, they do not differ from other carcinomas of the stomach. The differential diagnosis should be made by exfoliative cytology.

The prognosis of squamous neoplasms of the stomach appears to be the same as the usual gastric carcinoma. Since squamous neoplasms tend to be somewhat more radioresponsive than adenocarcinoma, it would appear to be reasonable upon confirmation of the diagnosis to treat those lesions that are not resectable with irradiation therapy. Perhaps postsurgical irradiation therapy similar to that employed in patients with lymphoma would be of use.

GASTRIC LEIOMYOBLASTOMAS

Leiomyoblastoma is a rare tumor of the stomach which has a malignant potential.[60] The clinical features are similar to those of leiomyosarcoma, and surgical excision is the therapy of choice. Too few data are available to assess the role of irradiation therapy, but in the few patients so treated, it appears to be ineffective. Approximately 40 per cent of patients with gastric leiomyoblastoma will die of their tumor because of metastatic disease.

PLASMACYTOMA OF THE STOMACH

Plasma cell neoplasms occur most often in the bone marrow. Rarely they may involve the stomach.[61] Clinically, gastric plasmacytomas resemble carcinoma of the stomach. Differentiation from carcinoma or lymphoma on radiographic or endoscopic criteria is not possible. No data are available as to whether or not exfoliative cytology can diagnose this lesion. The laboratory is of virtually no help. Only one instance of Bence Jones proteinuria has been recorded. Serum protein electrophoresis may rarely reveal a myeloma "spike."

Therapy is surgical resection followed by irradiation therapy. Chemotherapy may be of some value. This cancer apparently has a predisposition to dissemination, and these individuals may ultimately develop other visceral and osseous disease. Chemotherapy may be of some use. One apparent remission has been recorded after treatment with nitrogen mustard for a recurrent tumor in the rectum.

GLOMUS TUMORS OF THE STOMACH

Glomus tumors are considered to be benign proliferations of glomus cells, blood vessels, and occasionally nervous elements.[62] It is uncertain as to whether they are neoplasms, hamartomas, or a functional hyperplasia. The most common symptoms are peptic ulcer-like pain and hemorrhage. The radiographic findings have included interpretation of ulcer, carcinoma, polyps, and extramucosal intramural filling defects. True glomus tumors do not apparently have a potential to metastasize. They may be locally aggressive and invasive. Treatment is surgical excision; the prognosis is good.

CARCINOSARCOMA OF THE STOMACH

Carcinosarcoma of the stomach is a rare neoplasm which contains both carcinomatous and sarcomatous elements in the same tumor.[63] The clinical features do not differ from other cancers of the stomach. Many of the described lesions have been polypoid, fungating, necrotic tumors. The prognosis appears to be similar to that of carcinoma of the stomach. There is no clinical way of establishing a diagnosis with certainty prior to surgery or autopsy. Therapy is surgical excision if possible. No data are available on irradiation or chemotherapy.

METASTATIC CANCER TO THE STOMACH

In patients dying of advanced cancer, metastases to the stomach are not rare.[2] The most usual malignancies which metastasize to the stomach are mammary carcinoma and malignant melanoma. The stomach is frequently involved by direct extension with carcinoma of the pancreas. Malignancies from other primary lesions, exclusive of disseminated malignant lymphoma, rarely involve the stomach. Mammary carcinoma metastatic to the stomach resembles linitis plastica roentgenologically. It is not possible to determine on radiographic appearance whether the gastric metastases represent a possible second primary lesion. Malignant melanoma metastatic to the stomach is part of widely metastatic disease, with many other organs also involved. The gastric tumors are frequently multiple and often ulcerated;

other levels of the gastrointestinal tract are frequently involved.

The differential diagnosis in these unfortunate patients is rarely of practical importance. Their deaths are ordinarily due to widespread metastases to other vital organs and not to direct involvement of the stomach. Occasionally they may expire from an exsanguinating hemorrhage, but this is uncommon.

Other than the various forms of chemotherapy, no treatment is available. If a patient who has been successfully treated for another cancer develops a gastric lesion without any other evidence of metastatic disease, surgical intervention is indicated. These lesions may as well represent a new primary as metastatic cancer.

REFERENCES

1. Cox, A. J., Jr. Pathology. In Surgery of the Stomach and Duodenum, 2nd ed., H. N. Harkins and L. M. Nyhus (eds.). Boston, Little, Brown and Co., 1969.
2. McNeer, G., and Pack, G. T. Neoplasms of the Stomach. Philadelphia, J. B. Lippincott Co., 1967.
3. Silverberg, E., and Holleb, A. I. Cancer statistics 1972. CA 22:2, 1972.
4. Monaco, A. P., Sanford, I. R., Castleman, B., and Welch, C. E. Adenomatous polyps of the stomach. A clinical and pathological study of 153 cases. Cancer 15:456, 1962.
5. Siurala, M., Isokoski, M., Varis, K., and Kekk, M. Prevalence of gastritis in a rural population. Bioptic study of subjects selected at random. Scand. J. Gastroent. 3:211, 1968.
6. Chusid, G. L., Hirsch, R. L., and Colcher, H. Spectrum of hypertrophic gastropathy. Arch. Intern. Med. 114:621, 1964.
7. Menetrier, P. Des polyadénomes gastriques et de leurs rapports avec le cancer de l'estomac. Arch. Physiol. Norm. Path. 1:32, 226, 1888.
8. Pygott, F., and Shah, V. L. Gastric cancer associated with gastroenterostomy and partial gastrectomy. Gut 9:117, 1968.
9. Stalsberg, H., and Taksdal, S. Stomach cancer following gastric surgery for benign conditions. Lancet 2:1175, 1971.
10. Kobayashi, S., Prolla, J. C., and Kirsner, J. B. Late gastric carcinoma developing after surgery for benign conditions. Amer. J. Dig. Dis. 15:905, 1970.
11. Saegesser, F., and Jämes, D. Cancer of the gastric stump after partial gastrectomy (Billroth II principle) for ulcer. Cancer 29:1150, 1972.
12. Rubin, C. E. The diagnosis of gastric malignancy in pernicious anemia. Gastroenterology 29:563, 1955.
13. Rubin, C. E. Newer advances in the exfoliative cytology of the gastrointestinal tract. Ann. N.Y. Acad. Sci. 63:1377, 1956.
14. Brandborg, L. L., Taniguchi, L., and Rubin, C. E. Exfoliative cytology in non-malignant conditions of the upper intestinal tract. Acta Cytol. 5:187, 1961.
15. Kasugai, T. Prognosis of early gastric cancer. Gastroenterology 58:429, 1970.
16. Morrissey, J. F. Gastrointestinal endoscopy. Gastroenterology 62:1241, 1972.
17. Kurihara, M., and Segi, M. Mortality statistics on gastrointestinal cancer in some countries. Recent Advan. Gastroent. 1:58, 1967.
18. Woolf, C. M., and Isaacson, G. A. An analysis of five "stomach cancer families" in the state of Utah. Cancer 14:1005, 1961.
19. Dubarry, J. J., Faivre, J., and Pillegand, B. Digestive cancers in the same family. Cancerous predestination. Recent Advan. Gastroent. 1:130, 1967.
20. Zamcheck, N., Grable, E., Ley, A. B., and Norman, L. R. Occurrence of gastric cancer among patients with pernicious anemia at the Boston City Hospital. New Eng. J. Med. 252:1103, 1955.
21. McConnell, R. B. Genetic factors in carcinoma of the stomach. Recent Advan. Gastroent. 1:481, 1967.
22. The Veterans Administration Cooperative Study on Gastric Ulcer. Gastroenterology 61:No. 4, Part 2, 1971.
23. Kim, Y. S., and Plaut, A. β-Glucuronidase studies in gastric secretions from patients with gastric cancer. Gastroenterology 49:50, 1965.
24. Piper, D. W., Kemp, M. L., Fenton, B. H., Croydon, M. J., and Clarke, A. D. Gastric juice lactic acidosis in the presence of gastric carcinoma. Gastroenterology 58:766, 1970.
25. Moore, T. L., Zupchik, H. Z., Marcon, N., and Zamcheck, N. Carcinoembryonic antigen assay in cancer of the colon and pancreas and other digestive tract disorders. Amer. J. Dig. Dis. 16:1, 1971.
26. Gutmann, R. A., Bertrand, I., Peristiany, T. J. Le cancer de l'estomac au debut. Paris, G. Doin et Cie., 1939.
27. Sakita, T., Ogura, Y., Takasu, S., Fukutomi, T., Miwa, T., and Yoshimori, M. Observations on the healing of ulcerations in early gastric cancer. The life cycle of the malignant ulcer. Gastroenterology 60:835, 1971.
28. MacDonald, W. C., Brandborg, L. L., Taniguchi, L., and Rubin, C. E. Gastric exfoliative cytology: An accurate and practical diagnostic procedure. Lancet 2:83, 1963.
29. Raskin, H. F., Kirsner, J. B., Palmer, W. L., and Pleticka, S. The clinical value of the negative gastrointestinal exfoliative cytology examination in cancer suspects. Gastroenterology 42:266, 1962.
30. Brandborg, L. L., MacDonald, W. C., Rubin, C. E., and Gottlieb, S. Cytological diagnosis of gastric cancer by chymotrypsin lavage. Recent Advan. Gastroent. 1:300, 1967.
31. Taebel, D. W., Prolla, J. C., and Kirsner, J. B. Exfoliative cytology in the diagnosis of stomach cancer. Ann. Intern. Med. 63:1018, 1965.
32. Benditt, E. P., and French, J. E. Histochemistry of connective tissue: I. The use of enzymes as specific histochemical reagents. J. Histochem. Cytochem. 1:315, 1953.

33. Yamada, T. Basic study of the proteolytic enzyme lavage method in the gastric diagnosis, especially in the comparative analysis of exfoliative tendency of malignant and benign gastric epithelial cells. Acta Cytol. 8:19, 1964.
34. Brandborg, L. L., Tankersley, C. B., and Uyeda, F. "Low" versus "high" concentration chymotrypsin in gastric exfoliative cytology. Gastroenterology 57:500, 1969.
35. Rubin, C. E., and Benditt, E. P. Simplified technique using chymotrypsin lavage for cytological diagnosis of gastric cancer. Cancer 8:1137, 1955.
36. Rubin, C. E., and Massey, B. W. The preoperative diagnosis of gastric and duodenal malignant lymphoma by exfoliative cytology. Cancer 7:271, 1954.
37. MacDonald, W. C., Brandborg, L. L., Taniguchi, L., Beh, J. E., and Rubin, C. E. Exfoliative cytology screening for gastric cancer. Cancer 17:163, 1964.
38. Reed, P. I., Raskin, H. F., and Graff, P. W. Malignant melanoma of the stomach. J.A.M.A. 182:298, 1962.
39. Gilbertsen, V. A. Results of treatment of stomach cancer. An appraisal of efforts for more extensive surgery and a report of 1983 cases. Cancer 23:1305, 1969.
40. Bateman, J. R., Pugh, R. P., Cassidy, F. R., Marshall, G. J., and Irwin, L. E. 5-Fluorouracil given once weekly: Comparison of intravenous and oral administration. Cancer 28:907, 1971.
41. Reitemeier, R. J., Moertel, C. G., and Hahn, R. G. Combination chemotherapy in gastrointestinal cancer. Cancer Res. 30:1425, 1970.
42. Graham, J. B., and Graham, R. M. Antibodies elicited by cancer in patients. Cancer 8:409, 1955.
43. Graham, J. B., and Graham, R. M. The effect of vaccine on cancer patients. Surg. Gynec. Obstet. 109:131, 1959.
44. Williams, A. C., and Klein, E. Experiences with local chemotherapy and immunotherapy in premalignant and malignant skin lesions. Cancer 25:450, 1970.
45. Czajkowski, N. P., Rosenblatt, M., Wolf, P. L., and Vasquez, J. A new method of active immunization to autologous human tumour tissue. Lancet 2:905, 1967.
46. Humphrey, L. J., Murray, D. R., Boehm, O. R., Jewell, W. R., and Griffen, W. O., Jr. Immunotherapy of cancer in man. VII. Studies of patients with cancer of the alimentary tract. Amer. J. Surg. 121:165, 1971.
47. Cunningham, T. J., Olson, K. B., Laffin, R., Horton, J., and Sullivan, J. Treatment of advanced cancer with active immunization. Cancer 24:932, 1969.
48. Kuster, G. G. R., ReMine, W. H., and Dockerty, M. E. Gastric cancer in pernicious anemia and in patients with and without achlorhydria. Ann. Surg. 175:783, 1972.
49. Loux, H. A., and Zamcheck, N. Cytological evidence for the long "quiescent" stage of gastric cancer in two patients with pernicious anemia. Gastroenterology 57:173, 1969.
50. Steiner, P. E., Maimon, S. N., Palmer, W. L., and Kirsner, J. B. Gastric cancer: Morphologic factors in five-year survival after gastrectomy. Amer. J. Path. 24:947, 1948.
51. Joseph, J. I., and Lattes, R. Gastric lymphosarcoma: Clinicopathologic analysis of 71 cases and its relation to disseminated lymphosarcoma. Amer. J. Clin. Path. 45:653, 1966.
52. Loehr, W. J., Mujahed, Z., Zahn, F. D., Gray, G. F., and Thorbjernarson, B. Primary lymphoma of the gastrointestinal tract: A review of 100 cases. Ann. Surg. 170:232, 1969.
53. Sherrick, D. W., Hodgson, J. R., and Dockerty, M. B. The roentgenologic diagnosis of primary gastric lymphoma. Radiology 84:925, 1965.
54. Yoshii, Y., Takahashi, J., Yamaoka, Y., and Kasugi, T. Significance of imprint smear in cytologic diagnosis of malignant tumors of the stomach. Acta Cytol. 14:249, 1970.
55. Stobbe, J. A., Dockerty, M. B., and Bernatz, P. E. Primary gastric lymphoma and its grades of malignancy. Amer. J. Surg. 112:10, 1966.
56. Burgess, J. N., Dockerty, M. B., and ReMine, W. H. Sarcomatous lesions of the stomach. Ann. Surg. 173:758, 1971.
57. Kavlie, H., and White, T. T. Leiomyomas of the upper gastrointestinal tract. Surgery 71:842, 1972.
58. Boswell, J. T., and Helwig, E. B. Squamous cell carcinoma and adenocarcinoma of the stomach: Clinicopathologic study. Cancer 18:181, 1965.
59. Parks, R. E. Squamous neoplasms of the stomach. Amer. J. Roent. 101:447, 1967.
60. Lavin, P., Hajdu, S. I., and Foote, F. W., Jr. Gastric and extragastric leiomyoblastomas. Clinicopathologic study of 44 cases. Cancer 29:305, 1972.
61. Remigio, P. A., and Klaum, A. Extramedullary plasmacytoma of the stomach. Cancer 27:562, 1971.
62. Appelman, H. D., and Helwig, E. B. Glomus tumors of the stomach. Cancer 23:203, 1969.
63. Tanimura, H., and Furuta, M. Carcinosarcoma of the stomach. Amer. J. Surg. 113:702, 1967.

Chapter 47

Corrosive Damage

Steven Raffin

The gastrointestinal tract above the ligament of Treitz has more than its fair share of endogenous erosion and ulceration. This discussion will focus on the even more dire consequences of exogenous corrosive assault on the gastric mucosa. The populations at risk include the suicidal patient and the alcoholic who inadvertently drinks acid or alkaline material. Children are not well represented in the gastric corrosion literature, as the majority accidentally swallow only enough lye to develop esophageal injury.[1]

TYPES OF CORROSIVES

Corrosive substances may be classified into four major categories: "fixers, such as formaldehyde or phenolic acid; destructive substances, such as hydrochloric, glacial acetic, sulfuric, or nitric acid; softeners, such as lye; and weak substances, such as oxalic acid or arsenic."[2] Agents from all four classes have been reported to cause antral stenosis, the major subacute complication of ingestion survivors. Sulfuric acid ingestion is more likely to result in early death caused by perforation and gangrene.[3] Lye has caused severe gastric necrosis despite its more frequent association with esophageal stricture.[4] Formaldehyde is unique in causing a picture resembling linitis plastica. The corrosive gastritis can be so marked that the whole stomach is involved and eventually becomes thickened and scarred. The reported patients required total gastrec-tomy.[4-6] Household sources of these agents are unfortunately common. Lye is found in washing powders, paint removers, drainpipe and toilet bowl cleaners, detergents, and Clinitest tablets. Hydrochloric or muriatic acid is found in metal, swimming pool, and toilet bowl cleaners. Formaldehyde has occasionally been compounded in deodorizing tablets and plastic menders.[7]

PATHOLOGY

The pathology of corrosive gastritis is variable, depending upon the species, quantity, and concentration of the agent ingested and the duration of tissue contact. A partially full stomach is somewhat protected, and antral damage predominates. An empty stomach is usually half to two-thirds involved, as its surface-to-volume ratio is quite high, allowing diffuse contact of mucosa with the corrosive agent.[8] Concentrated acids produce a coagulative necrosis with a protective eschar, whereas alkalis cause a liquefying necrosis with saponification of tissue fat and a solvent action on tissue protein.[7, 8] Alkalis are more corrosive than acids and have a greater effect on esophageal squamous epithelium.[3]

PATHOGENESIS

Oversimplified schema are rampant in the literature, explaining the usual localization of lye burns to the esophagus and

605

acid burns to the stomach, but there is no way for the physician to be certain that this relationship holds true in a particular patient. The more concentrated the corrosive, the more probable that severe damage to both organs will result. Lye, being more corrosive, damages the esophagus in transit to the stomach where it is neutralized by gastric acid and rendered inert. Many exceptions to this theory exist. One study of corrosive injury containing a large number of alkali ingestions documented necrosis of esophagus, stomach, and rarely small bowel when the lye was taken in large quantities.[4] Another recent report describes esophageal sparing and antral ulceration leading to perforation from alkali ingestion in the form of Clinitest tablets.[9] Obviously, the heat and sodium hydroxide liberation did not begin until the tablets contacted water in the dependent gastric pool. Acid, on the other hand, superficially burns the mouth and oropharynx and rapidly traverses the relatively resistant esophagus. In the stomach it sears the mucosa from "magenstrasse" to antrum where it causes intense pylorospasm and entrapment of acid. This antral pooling fosters intense local corrosion and, later, stricture formation.[3, 8, 10] The spectrum of acid changes in the antrum ranges from edema and petechiae to destruction of mucosa with loss of glands, discrete ulceration, and transmural spread to serosa. With serosal involvement, diffuse peritonitis with or without associated perforation is inevitable. Immediate or delayed hemorrhage and eventually fibrosis and gastric outlet obstruction are additional complications three or four weeks after the ingestion.[3, 7, 8] Overlap exists, because 15 per cent of esophageal strictures are associated with acid ingestion,[11] and pyloric stenosis has been the outcome in approximately 20 per cent of alkali ingestions.[3, 4, 7-9] Several bizarre cases of suicide attempts using gelatin capsules or tissue paper containing crystalline lye have led to total sparing of the esophagus and extensive gastric injury.[4] The duodenum is almost always spared, because the spastic pylorus proves to be an effective barrier.[12]

CLINICAL PICTURE

Clinical features of corrosive ingestion begin with oropharyngeal discomfort.

Most striking is the sudden onset of severe epigastric pain and hematemesis almost immediately after ingestion. The gastric bleeding may regress promptly, only to reappear several months after injury, but the pain is usually persistent from the onset.[12] As antral stenosis progresses, vomiting may increase over a two- to six-week period. Obviously, the massive burn with either perforation or transmural diffuse peritonitis presents as an acute abdominal catastrophe.[1, 4, 8]

Two cases of fatal gas emboli in the portal veins have been reported. One case arose secondary to corrosive perforation and peritonitis with two gas-forming organisms, *Clostridium welchii* and *Escherichia coli*, and the other was sterile, presumably resulting from dissection of air into gastric venules draining the denuded stomach.[13]

Interesting associations with the subacute cases are protein loss through the damaged mucosa as documented by labeled albumin studies and the finding of hypo- or achlorhydria.[12] The lack of acid

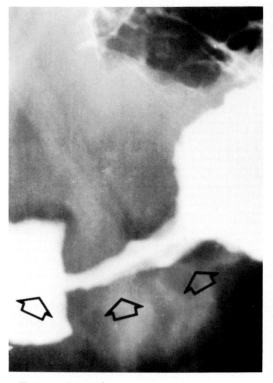

Figure 47–1. The arrows point to a stenosed antrum in a patient several months after acid ingestion. Note that the duodenal bulb appears normal.

cannot be explained by loss of parietal cell mass, because the lesions are almost always confined to the antrum. Radioimmunoassay of gastrin has not yet been studied in this clinical setting.

One may see how difficult the exclusion of carcinoma might be in a chronic case with delayed symptoms presenting without a history of ingestion. The patient will complain of weight loss and obstructive symptoms and have roentgenographic evidence of antral stenosis, and, occasionally, ulceration (Fig. 47-1), hypo- or achlorhydria, and hypoproteinemia.[3, 7, 11, 12] Surgeons have been led to the incorrect diagnosis at laparotomy when palpating just such a fibrosed, rigid antrum.

TREATMENT

The literature is divided in suggesting diagnostic and therapeutic approaches in the acute patient. All agree to the institution of supportive measures, including nasogastric suction, antacids, the maintenance of plasma chemistry and volume, blood replacement, bronchopulmonary toilet, and close observation. The earlier reports warn against the danger of perforating a necrotic gut wall with rigid endoscopes or even large-bore stomach tubes.[8, 12] They also describe a nonperforating diffuse peritonitis that ensues from severe necrosis of the gastric wall, and state that surgery is contraindicated in the immediate postingestion period.[7, 8, 12] In these earlier series, few patients survived the initial 24 hours after a large ingestion.[8] The few who did had their surgery eight to ten weeks later when the damaged portion of stomach had fully demarcated itself in the usual form of antral stenosis.

Recent reports admonish this expectant "wait and see" attitude.[1, 4] Aggressive but cautious fiberoptic endoscopy is suggested, using an end-viewing scope; if findings of necrosis are present, the scope should not be forced past this area. Emergency laparotomy may be indicated, with resection of the potentially perforating section of stomach.[1, 3, 4] Occasionally, total gastrectomy is required with bowel interposition.[4, 14] These series suggest increased survival in patients who would not have survived to be included in the older, more conservative reports.

The only specific medical antidotes outlined in various reports seem homeopathic in the face of large corrosive ingestion: "weak alkalis for acids, lemon juice for alkali, table salt for nitric acid, and alcoholic beverages for carbolic acid."[7, 8] These measures must not be substituted for the aggressive approach just outlined. More experience is needed with the four-way, fiberoptic, end-viewing scopes in corrosive ingestions; but at present, if survival is to be increased in the severe cases, prompt endoscopic visualization and appropriate surgical management are essential.

REFERENCES

1. Asbaugh, D., Jenkins, D., and Gainey, M. Gastroscopy in corrosive burn of the stomach. J.A.M.A. 216:1638, 1971.
2. Bosch del Marco, L. Contribucion al estudio de la gastritis corrosiva: Estudio clinico y experimental. An Fac. de Med. de Montevideo 34:891, 1949.
3. Poteshman, N. Corrosive gastritis due to hydrochloric acid ingestion. Amer. J. Roent. 99:182, 1967.
4. Allen, R., Thoshinsky, M., Stallone, R., and Hunt, T. Corrosive injuries of the stomach. Arch. Surg. 100:409, 1970.
5. Bartone, N., Grieco, V., and Herr, B. Corrosive gastritis due to ingestion of formaldehyde without esophageal impairment. J.A.M.A. 203:104, 1968.
6. Roy, M., Calonje, M., and Mouton, R. Corrosive gastritis after formaldehyde ingestion. New Eng. J. Med. 266:1248, 1962.
7. Citron, B., Pincus, I., Geokas, M., and Haverback, B. Chemical trauma of the esophagus and stomach. Surg. Clin. N. Amer. 48:1303, 1968.
8. Steigmann, F., and Dolehide, R. Corrosive acid gastritis. Management of early and late cases. New Eng. J. Med. 254:981, 1956.
9. Messersmith, J., Oglesby, J., Mahoney, W., and Baugh, J. Gastric erosion from alkali ingestion. Amer. J. Surg. 119:740, 1970.
10. Testa, G. Contribito radiologio e sperimentale allo studio della lesioni esofage e gastriche nelle causticazioni da alcali. Radiol. Med. Torino 25:17, 1938.
11. Holzbach, R. Corrosive gastritis resembling carcinoma due to ingestion of acid. J.A.M.A. 205:175, 1968.
12. Marks, I., Bank, S., Werbeloff, M., Farman, J., and Louw, J. The natural history of corrosive gastritis. Amer. J. Dig. Dis. 8:509, 1963.
13. Fink, D., and Boyden, F. Gas in the portal veins. Radiology 87:741, 1966.
14. Shaw, A., Garvey, J., and Miller, B. Lye burns requiring total gastrectomy and colon substitution for esophagus and stomach. Surgery 64:837, 1969.

Chapter 48

Diverticula, Rupture, and Volvulus

Steven Raffin

GASTRIC DIVERTICULA

As contrasted with the spectrum of disease emanating from colonic diverticulosis, the solitary gastric diverticulum barely warrants consideration. It is a rare roentgenological discovery, with an incidence ranging from 1 in 600 to 1 in 2400 routine upper gastrointestinal series.[1, 2] First described by Thomas Baille in 1793,[3] gastric diverticula have now been reported in over 500 patients,[4] and have an incidence of 0.0043 per cent of hospital admissions.[5] Most are discovered in persons between the fourth and sixth decades of life, with equal sexual and racial prevalence.[5]

The term diverticulum is descriptive of the gross anatomy, a bypath, in Latin. Gastric ulcers, excavating neoplasms, surgical artifacts, traction pouches, and pristine gastric diverticula unassociated with other pathological processes all fulfill the simple criterion of being a bypath to the normal contour of the barium-filled stomach. Seventy-six per cent of gastric diverticula occur high on the posterior wall of the stomach, approximately 2 cm below the esophagogastric junction and 3 cm from the lesser curvature. These pouches are almost never associated with peptic, granulomatous, or neoplastic processes.[1, 4-6] Fifteen per cent of diverticula are prepyloric and are usually the result of antecedent peptic, granulomatous, or neoplastic disease.[7] The remaining 8 to 10 per cent of pouches are located along the intervening mucosa.[2, 8]

A smoldering controversy exists in the literature as to the nomenclature of gastric diverticula. The original dichotomy states that "true," congenital or juxtacardiac diverticula contain all layers of the stomach, whereas "false," acquired or juxtapyloric diverticula contain only mucosa.[1, 5] A recent study reporting seven cases of juxtacardiac diverticula found that none had an outer muscular coat, and hence all would be labeled false despite their classic locations and lack of association with either intra- or perigastric inflammation.[4] It seems reasonable to conclude that the hoary classification of these rare pouches perpetuates misconceptions and that notation of location plus the presence or absence of associated pathological processes serves the clinician best.[1, 4]

PATHOGENESIS

The pathophysiology of the juxtapyloric or traction diverticulum is obvious. The pouch develops from the addition of abnormal stresses to the gastric wall from surgery, healing ulcer, or periantral inflammation.[7] Differentiation from ulcer or malignancy may be very difficult without

608

endoscopic visualization, cytology, and biopsy. The juxtacardiac diverticulum with or without a full complement of muscularis propria most probably arises from either a defect in a specific area high on the posterior gastric wall[1] or the presence of abnormal intraluminal pressures at this unique point.[2] Some clinicians state that the only true or primary gastric diverticula arise in the juxtacardiac region.[4] Congenital diverticula containing all layers of the gastric wall must be very uncommon indeed, because very few have been found in autopsies of newborns or infants.[1]

DIAGNOSIS

All positive defects of the barium-filled stomach must be diagnosed. The juxtapyloric pouch is more difficult to distinguish from a peptic or malignant process than is the juxtacardiac diverticulum. The criteria for diagnosis of the former are a pliable contour on multiple spot films and the presence of grossly normal mucosa on endoscopy. The latter has a characteristic roentgenological appearance of a solitary pouch, 2 to 4 cm in diameter, with a smooth, rounded, pliable contour on barium study (Fig. 48–1).[1, 5] Both X-ray and endoscopy may reveal rugal folds entering the pouch through a narrow neck.[1]

The gastroscopic view of the mouth of a juxtacardiac diverticulum is usually diagnostic; i.e., a small round stoma with sharp margins which may change size in synchrony with peristalsis. The histology of such a diverticulum obtained at surgery in symptomatic patients always shows chronic inflammatory changes.[4]

Gastric diverticula not located in the antrum or cardia are extremely unusual, and find their way into case reports.[2, 8] In fact the tenth greater curvature diverticulum was recently described as a radiological curiosity; it contained all layers of the normal stomach wall.[2] Another report emphasized the value of compression films in the upper gastrointestinal series to demonstrate a pliable wall in the case of two intramural diverticula.[8] Careful roentgenographic technique is required for both small and large pouches. A giant 10-cm diverticulum was missed totally during a barium study until the examiner positioned the patient so that the small stoma was dependent.[6]

CLINICAL PICTURE

The clinical importance of gastric diverticula has been a controversial subject for years, because more than 50 per cent of patients are asymptomatic.[1, 7] Typical ulcer-

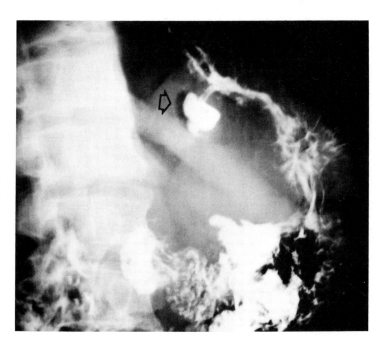

Figure 48–1. This solitary juxtacardiac gastric diverticulum (arrow) is easily seen on upper gastrointestinal series.

like pain or vomiting is rare in some reports[5] but common in others.[4] One study concluded that this lesion was a "potent source" of "entirely nonspecific" symptoms such as vague high abdominal pain usually precipitated by a meal, with postprandial relief upon lying down.[9] Other reports describe exactly the opposite picture, with pain in the fasting state and upon lying down and relief with meals.[1, 4] The larger lesions with mucosal inflammation most probably account for this spectrum of complex, nonspecific dyspepsia. Based solely upon history and physical examination, clinical differentiation of a juxtacardiac gastric diverticulum from an atypical peptic ulcer, pancreaticobiliary disease, or even functional complaints may be difficult.

Complications and associations of gastric diverticula are few in number. Unanticipated hemorrhage and perforation are the two catastrophic events that rarely occur.[1, 5] There is no obvious tendency toward carcinogenesis in these pouches, but occasionally incidental mucosal or submucosal tumors may be found inside, with aberrant pancreas heading the list. Finally, there is no correlation between gastric diverticula and other gastrointestinal diseases, including small and large bowel diverticula.[5]

TREATMENT

Treatment of a very rare lesion that is predominantly asymptomatic and that has few complications is impossible to evaluate statistically. Medical therapy encompasses such diverse maneuvers as postural drainage, bland diet, antacids, and water-induced emesis. It is usually unsuccessful in affording more than temporary relief.[1, 4] Many physicians claim total relief of dyspeptic upper abdominal pain with surgical ablation of the pouch.[4-6, 9] One must be concerned, however, about the false-positive effects of sham surgery in a patient with nonspecific gastrointestinal complaints.

GASTRIC RUPTURE

A very rare, devastating, and poorly understood catastrophe involving the upper gut is spontaneous rupture of the stomach,[10] which by definition excludes those cases associated with penetrating abdominal wounds or those resulting from involvement of the stomach by adjacent destructive processes or by ulcer or carcinoma. These obvious causes will not be discussed further; rather, spontaneous gastric perforation and rupture following blunt abdominal trauma will be examined.

ETIOLOGY

Traumatic. Up to the late 1930's, approximately 800 cases of abdominal contusion had been reported, with only 60 or so cases of rupture of the stomach.[10] A recent series of 200 nonpenetrating abdominal injuries contained only two cases of gastric rupture, but damage to liver, spleen, and bowel was frequent.[11] The explanation for this apparent sparing of the stomach lies with an understanding of its anatomical position. It is well protected, lying snugly against the spine, and is partially covered by ribs, diaphragm, lung, liver, and transverse colon.[10, 12] It is also very mobile and tolerates distortion well, requiring more than 4 liters of fluid in its lumen before rupturing.[13, 14] Finally, the cardioesophageal junction and pylorus act as escape valves for excessive gastric contents.[12, 15, 16] Further attesting to the resistance of the stomach to rupture from blunt trauma, an early investigator "directed a blow with a knobbed stick against the abdominal wall . . . but never produced rupture; . . . [and] filled the stomachs of animals and then struck them them over this area with a club . . . but [produced] no complete rupture."[17] Hence the stomach appears to be the least vulnerable of the abdominal viscera to blunt trauma.

On the other hand, the gastric lumen is one of the most accessible areas of the gut to direct visualization and subsequent internal contusion. Iatrogenic perforation during gastroscopy has been evaluated with both the standard and new fiberoptic gastroscopes by the American Society for Gastrointestinal Endoscopy.[18] There were 151,652 standard gastroscopies evaluated with 76 perforations (50 per 100,000) and five subsequent deaths (3.3 per 100,000), as compared with 32,237 fibergastroscopies with 24 perforations (74 per

100,000) and six subsequent deaths (19 per 100,000). The lack of improvement in morbidity and mortality statistics with the concomitant gain in visualization is most likely related to overconfidence in the fiberscopes' "total" flexibility and proclaimed safety, along with failure to appreciate the danger of their still rigid and traumatic business ends. Rarely, pneumoperitoneum may follow endoscopy without evidence of perforation. This event is benign, resolving spontaneously with nasogastric suction. Air dissecting along intramural vessels into the peritoneal cavity is the postulated mechanism, as no rents in the gastric wall are found at laparotomy.[19]

Nontraumatic. Nontraumatic, spontaneous gastric perforation was first described in 1845 by James Carson,[20] 16 years after Cruveilhier showed that prior reported perforations were the result of peptic disease.[12] Spontaneous perforation, exclusive of the newborn, is more common in females in the fifth decade,[12] in contrast to a peak incidence of young males sustaining rupture following blunt trauma.[10]

Several conceptual notions help to explain the pathogenesis in most of the reported cases. The "magenstrasse" is firmly bound by the gastrohepatic ligament[12, 20] and is less distensible than the greater curvature, which is composed of pliable rugal folds. Seventy-three per cent of spontaneous gastric ruptures in adults occur on the lesser curvature,[12] whereas in children the greater curvature perforates more frequently.[16, 21]

Distention of the stomach caused by overindulgence was recorded in over 60 per cent of ruptures in a recent review of 44 cases.[12] Overdistention of the stomach has been shown to acutely kink the gastroesophageal junction, which then can act only as a one-way valve. With the addition of pylorospasm, the stomach becomes a taut bladder susceptible to rupture by increases in intra-abdominal pressure.[12, 16] Attempts at retching against an occluded cardia have been proposed as the pressure-generating mechanism for spontaneous perforation in this setting.[12]

Besides gluttony, overdistention and rupture of the stomach have been described with sodium bicarbonate ingestion.[20] Cadaver studies have shown that sodium bicarbonate will release enough carbon dioxide when mixed with dilute hydrochloric acid to cause gastric rupture.[22] An interesting combination of increased distention and pressure arises in cardiac resuscitation, in which mouth-to-mouth gastric inflation combined with external cardiac massage has led to gastric rupture.[23] In fact, nasal oxygen administration alone at 4 to 6 liters per minute has led to gastric rupture in three adults.[21] Another case of oxygen rupture occurred in a patient recovering from an inguinal herniorrhaphy.[24] Cases of gastric rupture have been associated with the strain of labor[25] and the postpartum period.[26] An unfortunate patient with an inguinal hernia containing a ptotic stomach suffered fatal gastric rupture and serves well to summarize the pathophysiology of spontaneous gastric perforation.[15] The prerequisite anatomy was present in this patient, including obstruction of the distal stomach in the hernia sac and distention of the stomach with air and beer. The additional stress of periodic increases in abdominal pressure brought about by repeated attempts at vomiting completed the necessary sequence of events.

CLINICAL PICTURE

One must consider the diagnosis of spontaneous gastric rupture in a setting of abdominal distention, shock, diffuse peritoneal irritation, gastrointestinal hemorrhage, and cervical subcutaneous emphysema.[10, 12, 24, 27] High serum amylase values may be confusing, pointing toward the false diagnosis of acute pancreatitis.[16] Some physicians suggest that a trochar be passed into the abdomen to relieve the taut distention.[12, 27] Laparotomy and repair of the rent must follow swiftly if the patient is to survive. Unfortunately, this diagnosis has never been made before operation or autopsy.[16] The prognosis is very poor, with an operative mortality of 65 per cent and an overall mortality of 85 per cent. Respiratory embarassment, shock, and peritonitis are the major factors contributing to the rapid demise of most patients.[12] A rare and fatal case of embolization of gastric contents into the systemic circulation at the time of gastric rupture has been described with bean starch cells in sections of kidney, liver, and brain.[28]

GASTRIC VOLVULUS

Gastric volvulus is an uncommon, acquired twist of the stomach upon itself. Torsion of one part of the upper gut around another without vascular compromise may be asymptomatic. On the other hand, patient complaints may range from a mild dragging in the epigastrium with bloating and early satiety to intense upper abdominal pain and shock. The subtleties of the former and the urgency of the latter presentation must be kept in mind if this purely anatomical lesion is to be diagnosed and repaired.

Gastric volvulus was first recognized by Berti in 1886[29] during a postmortem examination. Since that inauspicious description, volvulus has been reported in about 250 patients and is more than a mere medical curiosity.[30, 31] Males are involved as frequently as females, and the peak incidence occurs during the fifth decade of life.[30]

TYPES OF VOLVULUS

The anatomic classification of gastric volvulus is superficially straightforward, but much confusion arises from attempts at its clinical application. Basically, three types of volvulus exist.[32] The *organoaxial* volvulus occurs when the stomach twists along its long axis, the cardiopyloric line, in a manner analogous to the ringing out of a wet rag (Fig. 48–2, *A*). The fixed cardioesophageal junction and second duodenum act as anchor points, creating a closed loop obstruction in acute cases. A minority of physicians feel that this is the most common type,[30, 33] most often seen as

the "upside down stomach" in the patient with a large paraesophageal hiatus hernia.[34] The twist in *mesenteroaxial* volvulus occurs along an imaginary line from the middle of the lesser curvature to the middle of the greater curvature (Fig. 48–2, *B*), and is at approximately right angles to the cardiopyloric axis of the organoaxial volvulus. The consensus is that this type is most common, especially in chronic torsion without vascular embarrassment.[31, 35, 36] It is possible that the third type, or *mixed* gastric volvulus, is the most frequent form and is the source for the confusion over incidence statistics. Further discussion will deal with the clinically important recognition of acute and chronic situations resulting from obstruction or ischemia and lesser degrees of torsion, respectively.

PATHOGENESIS

The pathophysiology is not obscure. The normal stomach is well restrained by the gastrosplenic, gastrocolic, and gastrohepatic ligaments.[35, 36] From cadaver studies the stomach cannot be rotated 180 degrees unless one of these fibrous attachments is severed. If displaced with intact ligaments, the stomach will glide back into its anatomical position. Hence, in vivo, ligamentous laxity is the major factor permitting volvulus to occur. Rarely, supernumerary ligaments in the form of adhesions to the peritoneum or adjacent viscera will provoke abnormal torsion of the stomach.[34] Extrinsic pressure from enlarged adjoining organs or masses, or intrinsic tumor, may distort the normal anatomy and allow the stomach to twist. Abnormally active peristalsis after a heavy meal and a low insertion of the esophagus have also been incriminated in the pathogenesis of gastric volvulus.[36]

The final major pathophysiological event incriminated in volvulus formation is the presence of abnormal celomic extensions into which the twisted stomach may be drawn, either as a paraesophageal hiatus hernia or as a hernia associated with eventration of the diaphragm.[34] For example, the presence of a paraesophageal hiatus hernia draws up the dependent greater curvature via push from organs be-

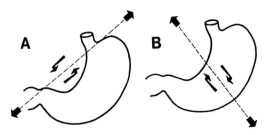

Figure 48–2. Types of gastric volvulus. The dashed line represents the axis about which the stomach twists. *A*, Organoaxial volvulus; *B*, mesenteroaxial volvulus. (Modified from Wastell, C., and Ellis, H.: Brit. J. Surg. 58:557, 1971.)

low and negative pressure in the thoracic hernia pouch. This is one of the more common presentations of chronic gastric volvulus, especially in the elderly patient with lax ligaments and ptotic viscera.

CLINICAL PICTURE

Acute volvulus with either luminal obstruction or vascular strangulation of the stomach[30] is not a subtle diagnostic dilemma, because the patient often presents in frank shock. A clinical triad was set forth in 1904,[38] describing this acute abdominal catastrophe: (1) violent retching with production of little vomitus, (2) constant, severe epigastric pain, and (3) great difficulty in advancing a nasogastric tube past the distal esophagus. The upper abdomen may be greatly distended, with the lower quadrants retaining surprisingly soft and flat contours.[36] In a patient with susceptible anatomy, acute volvulus may be precipitated by a heavy meal.[37] Reported mortality figures range from 42 to 56 per cent.[30]

In contrast, chronic volvulus or torsion may go undetected for years, the major symptoms being low-grade pain, bloating, eructation, and pyrosis.[35] Postcibal borborygmi may result from chyme passing through the entrapped gas and may be quite embarrassing at the dinner table. Patients with diaphragmatic defects may even complain of breathlessness,[34] where-as others with mild torsion may be totally asymptomatic. Without roentgenological assistance one may not be able to resolve the syndrome of chronic or intermittent torsion from chronic gallbladder disease, peptic ulcer, "gastritis," or functional complaints.[34] Mortality in chronic volvulus has been reported to vary from 10 to 13 per cent.[30]

DIAGNOSIS

Definitive diagnosis resides with the radiologist. An erect film of the abdomen may rarely show two air-fluid levels in the left upper quadrant and hence be diagnostic (Fig. 48–3).[36] The barium examination shows a tapering of the distal esophagus in acute strangulation; actual visualization of the twisted viscus in intermittent or partially obstructed cases is also diagnostic of this condition (Fig. 48–4).[35] One must be suspicious of intermittent torsion when, in a symptom-free interval, the barium examination shows only a paraesophageal hernia or eventration of the diaphragm. Fiberoptic endoscopy plays little role in the diagnosis of volvulus, because the twist precludes passage of the instrument.

TREATMENT

A conservative approach to the treatment of volvulus has been that of gastric

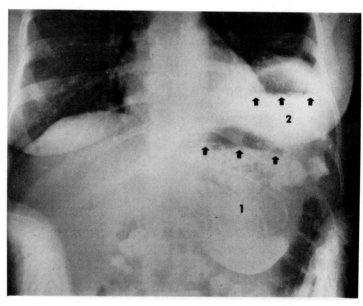

Figure 48–3. Mesenteroaxial volvulus in a patient with eventration of the diaphragm. Two air-fluid levels (arrows) are seen in this upright plain film of the abdomen. Numbers 1 and 2 indicate proximal and distal stomach, respectively.

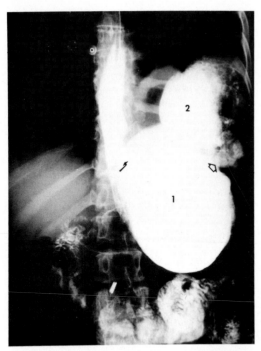

Figure 48–4. Mesenteroaxial volvulus in a patient with eventration of the diaphragm. The barium examination reveals the location of the cardioesophageal junction (solid arrow). Colon accompanies stomach above the diaphragm (hollow arrow). Numbers 1 and 2 indicate proximal and distal stomach, respectively.

decompression alone. It has been suggested that if the volvulus can be corrected by nasogastric aspiration, it will not recur. Recent evidence to the contrary exists, recommending that nasogastric decompression be considered only as a preoperative measure.[35]

The treatment of the acute strangulating twist causing vascular insufficiency is emergency laparotomy. Gastric decompression via nasogastric tube or trochar and restoration of the normal anatomy with an anterior gastropexy comprise the repair in either the acute or the recurrent case. One surgeon insists that the subphrenic space be partially and permanently occupied with transpositioned colon to ensure success of the repair.[34] If any obvious anatomic defects are present, such as a rent or bulge in the diaphragm, adhesions, or a paraesophageal hiatus hernia, they, too, should be repaired.[30, 35, 36]

The torsion involved in volvulus formation has the potential to damage other organs. A recent report described splenic rupture in a mesenteroaxial volvulus with congenital absence of the gastrocolic liga-

ment. Splenectomy accompanied by ligamentous repair and gastropexy gave a gratifying result.[33]

REFERENCES

1. Localio, S., and Stahl, W. Diverticular disease of the alimentary tract. II. The esophagus, stomach, duodenum, and small intestine. Current Prob. Surg. 21, 1968.
2. Dodd, G., and Sheft, D. Diverticulum of the greater curvature of the stomach. Amer. J. Roent. *107*:102, 1969.
3. Baille, T. The Morbid Anatomy of Some of the Most Important Parts of the Human Body. London, 1793, Chap. vii: 92.
4. Tillander, H., and Hesselsjö, R. Juxtacardial gastric diverticula and their surgery. Acta Chir. Scand. *134*:255, 1968.
5. Palmer, E. Gastric diverticula, a collective review. Int. Abstr. Surg. 92:417, 1951.
6. Seltzer, M. A huge gastric diverticulum. Amer. J. Dig. Dis. *16*:167, 1971.
7. Eras, P. The development of a false antral gastric diverticulum. Gastrointest. Endoscop. *15*:118, 1968.
8. Rabushka, S., Melamed, M., and Melamed, J. Unusual gastric diverticula. Radiology *90*:1006, 1968.
9. Palmer, E. Gastric diverticula, with special reference to subjective manifestations. Gastroenterology 35:406, 1958.
10. Wolf, N. Subcutaneous rupture of the stomach. Review of the literature and report of a case. N. Y. State J. Med. *36*:1539, 1936.
11. Fitzgerald, J., Crawford, E., and DeBakey, M. Surgical considerations of non-penetrating abdominal injuries. Amer. J. Surg. *100*:22, 1960.
12. Albo, R., de Lorimier, A., and Silen, W. Spontaneous rupture of the stomach in the adult. Surgery 53:797, 1963.
13. Revilliod, E. Rupture de l'estomac. Rev. Méd. Suisse Rom. 5:5, 1885.
14. Morris, C., Ivy, A., and Maddock, W. Mechanism of acute abdominal distention. Arch. Surg. 55:101, 1947.
15. Gue, S. Spontaneous rupture of the stomach, a rare complication of inguinal hernia. Brit. J. Surg. 57:154, 1970.
16. Mirsky, S., and Garlock, J. Spontaneous rupture of the stomach. Ann. Surg. *161*:466, 1965.
17. Ritter and Vanni: as cited by Rehn: Arch. Klin. Chir. 53:383, 1896.
18. Katz, D. Morbidity and mortality in standard and flexible gastrointestinal endoscopy. Gastrointest. Endoscop. *15*:134, 1969.
19. Brandborg, L. Upper gastrointestinal endoscopy. In Surgery of the Stomach and Duodenum, 2nd ed., H. Harkins, and L. Nyhus (eds.). Boston, Little, Brown and Co., 1969, p. 173.
20. Zer, M., Chaimoff, C., and Dintsman, M. Spontaneous rupture of the stomach following ingestion of sodium bicarbonate. Arch. Surg. *101*:532, 1970.
21. Walstad, P., and Conklin, W. Rupture of the

normal stomach after therapeutic oxygen administration. New Eng. J. Med. *264*:1201, 1961.

22. Murdfield, P. Rupture of the stomach from sodium bicarbonate. J.A.M.A. *87*:1692, 1926.

23. Demos, N., and Poticha, S. Gastric rupture occurring during external cardiac resuscitation. Surgery *55*:364, 1964.

24. Harper, F., and Roher, C. Gastric rupture complicating herniorrhaphy. South. Med. J. *62*:12, 1969.

25. Miller, J. Spontaneous rupture of the stomach during labor. New Eng. J. Med. *209*:1085, 1933.

26. Christoph, R., and Pirkham, E. Unexpected rupture of the stomach in the postpartum period, a case report. Ann. Surg. *154*:100, 1961.

27. Baglio, C., and Fattal, G. Spontaneous rupture of the stomach in the adult. Amer. J. Dig. Dis. *7*:75, 1962.

28. Graham, J., and Breitenecker, R. Embolization of gastric contents associated with rupture of the stomach. Arch. Path. *84*:659, 1967.

29. Berti, A. Sigolare attortiglamento dell'esofago col duodeno sequito da rapida morte. Gazz. Med. Ital. Prov. Ver. *9*:139, 1886.

30. Wastell, C., and Ellis, H. Volvulus of the stomach. Brit. J. Surg. *58*:557, 1971.

31. Bockus, H. Gastroenterology, Vol. I, 2nd ed. Philadelphia, W. B. Saunders Co., 1963, p. 911.

32. Buchanan, J. Volvulus of stomach. Brit. J. Surg. *18*:99, 1930.

33. Hudspeth, A., and McWhorter, J. Gastric volvulus causing rupture of the spleen. Arch. Surg. *102*:232, 1971.

34. Tanner, N. Chronic and recurrent volvulus of the stomach. Amer. J. Surg. *115*:505, 1968.

35. Gosin, S., and Gallinger, W. Recurrent volvulus of the stomach. Amer. J. Surg. *109*:642, 1965.

36. Camblos, J. Acute volvulus of the stomach. Amer. Surgeon *35*:505, 1969.

37. Dalgaard, J. Volvulus of the stomach. Acta Chir. Scand. *103*:131, 1952.

38. Borchardt, L. Pathology and therapy of volvulus of stomach. Arch. Klin. Chir. *74*:243, 1904.

Chapter 49

Bezoars

Steven Raffin

There are few areas in the study of medicine that are more steeped with a bizarre and mystical lore than the subject of bezoars. The term refers to food or foreign matter that has undergone digestive change in the gut of either man or animals. The word arose from attempts at transliteration of the Arabic "badzehr," Persian "padzahr," or Turkish "panzehir."[1] From antiquity to the eighteenth century, oriental bezoars from the stomachs of goats and gazelles and occidental bezoars from the South American vicuña were highly praised for their magical medicinal properties against such diverse ailments as old age, snakebite, plagues, and evil spirits.[2] So precious were they that a gold framed bezoar was included in the inventory of Queen Elizabeth's crown jewels in 1622.[3] Proper dosage of these animal concretions was as much a problem as was the establishment of clinical indications: "... for one bitten, poisoned, or stung, is the weight of twelve barley grains[;] the dose for weakness of the heart and loss of sexual power is one grain."[4]

More than a mere medical curiosity when found in the gut of man, bezoars present serious, current medical problems, including upper gastrointestinal ulceration with bleeding and small bowel obstruction. Bezoars have been classified into two groups: hair or trichobezoars, and plant or phytobezoars.[1, 5, 6] A third group of miscellaneous intragastric bodies includes fungal agglomerations,[7] food boli,[6, 8, 9]

chemical concretions,[1, 10] and foreign bodies.[11]

CLINICAL PICTURE

Bezoars may produce symptoms ranging from a dragging or fullness in the right upper quadrant to epigastric pain, which is the most frequent symptom (70 per cent). Periodic attacks of nausea and vomiting (64 per cent) are also common. A mass could be palpated in 57 per cent of phytobezoars as contrasted to 88 per cent of trichobezoars. Gastric outlet and intestinal obstruction are also common.[1] The incidence of associated peptic ulceration with the more abrasive phytobezoars (24 per cent) is greater than with trichobezoars (10 per cent).[5] The incidence of perforation and peritonitis is about 7 and 10 per cent, respectively — less frequent but obviously more catastrophic events.[5]

DIAGNOSIS

The laboratory is of little help in diagnosis, except that an associated hypochromic, microcytic anemia and modest leukocytosis may be present. Erect films of the abdomen may show a mass invading the gastric air bubble (Fig. 49–1). The upper gastrointestinal series usually reveals a freely movable mass in the barium field.[12, 13] There is less permeation of the

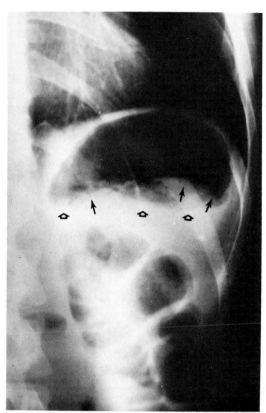

Figure 49–1. Upright plain film of the abdomen. The hollow arrows point to an air-fluid level in the stomach bubble. The solid arrows point to a bezoar floating at the air-fluid interface.

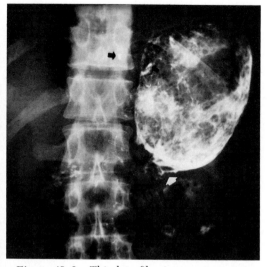

Figure 49–2. This late film in an upper gastrointestinal series of a patient following Billroth II partial gastrectomy and vagotomy demonstrates a barium-coated gastric bezoar. The white arrow points to the surgical stoma, and the solid arrows point to the vagotomy clips.

barium into the bulk of the phytobezoar than into the trichobezoar,[6] which may aid in differentiation. The postgastric emptying films should show the mass with a thin barium shell in either case (Fig. 49–2). Bezoars are black and may be tarry; endoscopic biopsy yielding hair or vegetable fibers is pathognomonic.[6] Of interest, gastric carcinoma has never been reported accompanying bezoars, although malignant and benign tumors must be considered in the radiological differential diagnosis.

TYPES

PHYTOBEZOAR

The most common bezoar in current clinical medicine is the phytobezoar. Plant bezoars may be composed of the digested fibers, leaves, roots, and skins of almost any plant matter and are usually smaller, more compact, and hence more abrasive than hair bezoars. They are most often found in males (77 per cent) over the age of 30 (70 per cent),[1] and have a prevalence in the population that now seems to parallel the number of partial gastrectomies.[10, 12-15]

Postgastrectomy Bezoar. In the late 1930's, none of the reported patients with bezoar had had prior gastric surgery.[1, 5] The literature of the last ten years contains many reports which describe phytobezoars complicating the postoperative management of patients with Billroth I and Billroth II partial gastrectomies, especially when accompanied by vagotomy.[10, 12-15] The former operation is more commonly associated with bezoars remaining in the gastric pouch, whereas in the latter situation the mass often passes through the larger surgical anastomosis into the small intestine, occasionally causing acute obstruction.[10, 14] A majority of physicians believe that a decrease in drainage through the surgical outlet, a decrease in acid-pepsin secretion, improper mastication, and diets too high in cellulose after gastric resection and vagotomy contribute to the pathogenesis of this newly recognized entity.[10, 12, 14]

Attesting to the role of vagectomy in predisposing to bezoars, a recent report described a large gastric bezoar in an autovagectomized patient, the neurolysis

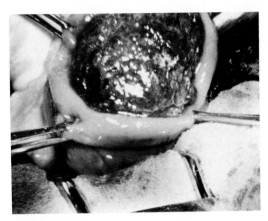

Figure 49–3. This photograph, taken during gastrotomy, demonstrates the lengthy incision needed to retrieve a large, black phytobezoar.

being secondary to encasement of the vagi by esophageal carcinoma.[16] Another recent report of phytobezoar in an unusual setting described a patient with decreased gastric motility as a result of myotonic muscular dystrophy.[17]

The standard treatment of phytobezoar includes manual attempts at external dissolution, a liquid diet, suction and lavage, or endoscopic internal fragmentation. If these methods fail, a gastrotomy must be performed (Fig. 49–3). The surgical mortality is appreciable, at about 5 per cent, but the mortality of untreated bezoar is 60 to 70 per cent.[5]

Fortunately, exciting new trials of enzymatic digestion have been described for the noninterventive treatment of phytobezoar. Papain and acetylcysteine, both proteolytic enzymes, have been tried with moderate success.[14,18] Cellulase, an enzyme specific for the damaging fibrous substrate, totally dissolved a large phytobezoar in less than two days in a man with a Billroth I gastroduodenostomy and vagotomy.[19] Further trials of cellulase preparations (Gastroenterase) are definitely warranted.

Persimmon Bezoar (Diospyrobezoar). A major subgroup of phytobezoar not related to gastric surgery is the diospyrobezoar named for a native American tree of the ebony family, *Diospyros virginiana*, the persimmon. Its fruit, a true berry, possesses little fiber but has a luxuriant pulp. In unripe and, to a lesser degree, in ripe fruit, the astringent properties are attributed to a substance called shiboul or phlobotannin which coagulates on contact with dilute acid.[20] This substance is present under the skin in ripe fruit, making the mature fruit potentially dangerous. Thus the pathophysiology is obvious. Unripe pulp or ripe skin is ingested by a patient with free acid, and a coagulum results; this sequence accounted for 73 per cent of phytobezoars in one extensive series.[1,5] Symptoms begin soon after excessive ingestion of persimmons and are potentiated by drinking copious amounts of water. The unfortunate consequence in extreme instances is severe distress which suggests an acute abdominal catastrophe to the physician.

"Cotton Bezoar." An even more bizarre phytobezoar was reported in an exheroin addict on methadone. This patient continued intravenous injections despite counseling, using cotton pledgets to filter the crushed tablet-water mixture. Afterwards, he swallowed the cotton, thus avoiding the bitter taste of methadone. A "cotton-picking stomach syndrome" resulted.[21]

TRICHOBEZOAR

Hairballs are contained within a glairy, mucoid coat and are composed of decaying foodstuff enmeshed among enormous amounts of hair. They are always black and have a fetid odor emanating mainly from undigested dietary fat and bacterial colonization. Large balls may be present for years in an asymptomatic phase, growing slowly by accretion to eventually become a J-shaped cast of the stomach. For unknown reasons hair strands are not usually passed through the pylorus, and hair is rarely found in the stool of these patients.[22] Occasionally a trichobezoar may attain a wet weight of over 6 pounds.

Trichobezoars are most often found in females (90 per cent) before the age of 30 (80 per cent). In the past they were more common than phytobezoars, but today the relative incidence has been reversed.[1,5] Hair ingestion or trichophagia, which is the cause of the disorder, is only infrequently associated with blatant neuropsychiatric disturbances, in contrast to the ingestion of inorganic foreign bodies;

however, some feel that the trait represents a personality maladjustment analogous to fingernail biting.[1]

The treatment is surgical, because there is no way to dissolve matted hair in vivo. Soilage of the peritoneum and subsequent peritonitis at laparotomy can be a grave consequence, because the stomach contains both bacteria and putrefied material enmeshed in the hairballs.[5]

FOOD BOLUS

The composition of a food bolus may vary from undigested pits, seeds, or citrus rinds to minimally digested food in a loose aggregation.[1, 6, 8, 9] This last type may closely resemble a gastric malignancy on endoscopic visualization when adherent to the mucosa and composed of fleshy-appearing fruit pulp. The literature has reports of ileal obstruction necessitating laparotomy from impacted food boli, especially in patients with partial gastrectomy.[8, 9] Early removal by gastric lavage is usually successful, and proper mastication of foodstuffs would probably eliminate this entity.[6]

CONCRETION

Concretions range from the mundane to the bizarre. Occasionally, agglomerated antacid tablets may cause small bowel obstruction in partially gastrectomized patients.[10] Youngsters ingesting rather than sniffing glue have occasionally presented with insoluble gastroliths (L. L. Brandborg, personal communication). Classically, the gastric concretion is unique to furniture finishers who drink a mixture of shellac and alcohol for the stimulating effects of the latter component. Upon subsequent ingestion of water as a chaser, the resinous contents agglutinate into a solid mass in the stomach. This lesion grows by laminar accretion, with the rate paralleling the bouts of imbibition and the gross appearance similar to growth rings on the wood furniture for which the mixture was solely concocted. These masses may exceed 4 pounds[1] and must be surgically excised.

FOREIGN BODIES

True foreign body ingestion, including such diverse items as pins, nails, razor blades, buttons, and coins, is usually seen in children or psychotic individuals. Nonspecific upper quadrant pain may be the only clue to diagnosis, although laceration of the gut wall with hemorrhage or perforation sometimes occurs. The stomach may be literally brim full of bric-a-brac, and the only therapy is gastrotomy and removal of the collection.[11]

GASTROINTESTINAL FUNGAL BALLS

Recently the presence of large, spongy yeast balls in the stomach has been described in three adult patients following Billroth I gastroduodenostomy. Only one of these patients had had a vagotomy. These patients were not taking antibiotics, steroids, or immunosuppressive agents and had no systemic diseases to account for the proliferation of Candida in their stomachs. None of the patients had free hydrochloric acid, but all had acid to histamine stimulation. Only one of the patients had narrowing at the surgical anastomosis.[7]

REFERENCES

1. DeBakey, M., and Ochsner, A. Bezoars and concretions. Surgery 4:934, 1938.
2. Dechambre, A. Dictionnaire encyclopedique des sciences medicales, Vol. 9. Paris, Victor Masson et Fils, 1868, p. 221.
3. Murdock, H. Persimmon bezoars occurring around Tulsa, Oklahoma. J. Oklahoma Med. Assn. 27:442, 1934.
4. Elgood, C. A treatise of the bezoar stone. By the late Mahmud Bin Masud the Imad-ul-din, the Physician of Ispahan. Ann. Med. Hist. 7:73, 1935.
5. DeBakey, M., and Ochsner, A. Bezoars and concretions. Surgery 5:132, 1939.
6. Sanowski, R., and DiDianco, J. Pseudotumors of the stomach. Amer. J. Dig. Dis. 11:607, 1966.
7. Borg, I., Heijkenskjold, F., Nilehn, B., and Wehlin, L. Massive growth of yeasts in resected stomach. Gut 7:244, 1966.
8. McCabe, R., and Knox, W. Phytobezoar in gastrectomized patients. Arch. Surg. 86:264, 1963.
9. Koh, I., Urca, I., and Tikva, P. Intestinal obstruction after partial gastrectomy due to orange pith. Arch. Surg. 100:79, 1970.
10. Cain, G., Moore, P., and Patterson, M. Bezoars — a complication of the postgastrectomy state. Amer. J. Dig. Dis. 13:801, 1968.

11. Cigtay, O., and Quesada, R.   Foreign bodies in the gastrointestinal tract. Amer. Family Pract. 3:104, 1971.

12. Szemes, G., and Amberg, J.   Gastric bezoars after partial gastrectomy. Radiology 90:765, 1968.

13. Rigler, R., and Grininger, D.   Phytobezoars following partial gastrectomy. Surg. Clin. N. Amer. 50:381, 1970.

14. Sparberg, M., Nielsen, A., and Andruczak, R. Bezoar following gastrectomy. Amer. J. Dig. Dis. 13:579, 1968.

15. Cohen, Y., and Heun, S. W.   Phytobezoar after gastrectomy. Brit. J. Surg. 58:236, 1971.

16. Kirks, D., and Szemes, G.   Autovagotomy and gastric bezoar. Gastroenterology 61:96, 1971.

17. Kuiper, D.   Gastric bezoar in a patient with myotonic dystrophy. Amer. J. Dig. Dis. 16:529, 1971.

18. Schlang, H.   Acetylcysteine in removal of bezoar. J.A.M.A. 214:1329, 1970.

19. Pollard, H., and Block, G.   Rapid dissolution of phytobezoar by cellulase enzyme. Amer. J. Surg. 116:933, 1968.

20. Izumi, S., Isida, K., and Iwamoto, M. Mechanism of formation of phytobezoars with special reference to persimmon ball. Jap. J. Med. Sc. Tr., II Biochem. 2:21, 1933.

21. Kaden, W. Phytobezoar in an addict: The cotton-picking stomach syndrome. J.A.M.A. 209:1367, 1969.

22. Davies, I.   Hairballs or hair casts of stomach and gastrointestinal tract. Lancet 2:791, 1921.

Chapter 50

The Pathology of Peptic Ulcer

Edwin H. Eigenbrodt

Benign peptic ulcers derive their name from the association with acid-pepsin juice in their formation. Normally the major divisions are acute and chronic peptic ulcers, although occasionally an ulcer in an intermediate stage of development is seen. Radiologists and clinicians classify ulcers on the basis of their duration, whereas pathologists utilize the morphology of the ulcers in their classification. Benign peptic ulcers occur almost exclusively in the esophagus, stomach, and duodenum. Rarely, in high gastric secretory states, ulcerations can occur farther down the gastrointestinal tract in the jejunum.[1-3] In this chapter only gastric and duodenal ulcerations are considered.

ACUTE PEPTIC ULCERATION AND EROSION

These lesions are found in a variety of clinical settings. They have been found after shock,[4] major medical illnesses,[5-7] burns (Curling's ulcers),[8-12] steroid therapy,[13, 14] and neurological disorders (Cushing's ulcers),[5, 15] and postoperatively after distant operations.[16-20] Crawford and co-workers analyzed both clinical and autopsy data on acute gastric and/or duodenal ulcers for a 12-year period from 1957 to 1969.[5] The autopsy incidence of acute ulceration was 3.6 per cent. Males predominated over females by 2 to 1. The average age of the clinical group of patients was 41 years, and the average age of the autopsy group was 51 years. Grosz and Kwang-Tzen, in a recent analysis of their data over a four-year period (1960 to 1964) on patients who had upper gastrointestinal hemorrhage, found that bleeding from acute stress ulcers was most prevalent in the 56- to 65-year age range.[6] They found an almost equal sex ratio, with a slight male predominance. Acute peptic ulcers can also be found in children and have been particularly reported after burns.[10, 21, 22]

As shown in Figure 50–1, an erosion is a circumscribed superficial necrotic defect of the gastric or duodenal mucosa which does not penetrate the muscularis mucosae. A similar acute necrotic defect which penetrates the muscularis mucosae and extends deep into the wall or perforates through it is called an acute peptic ulcer. In a majority of instances acute erosions and ulcers are shallow, multiple gastric lesions which are scattered throughout the stomach (without an antral predilection, in contrast to chronic ulcers). These ulcers elicit little inflammatory response, and no fibrosis is present.[16] The base of the lesions is usually black and hemorrhagic.

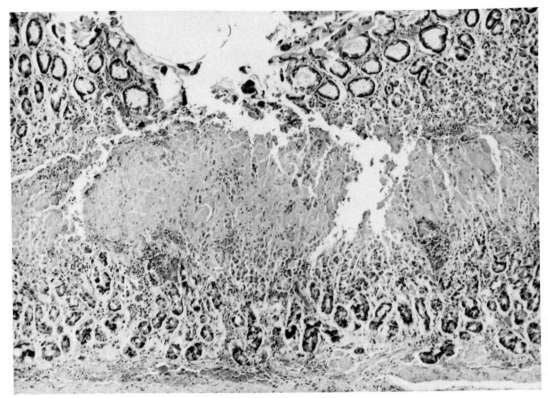

Figure 50–1. Acute gastric erosion. Note area of necrotic mucosal glands which have elicited almost no tissue inflammatory response. The necrosis does not extend to the muscularis mucosae.

The deeper, penetrating ulcers may be accompanied by some chronic inflammatory reaction.[17] Erosions heal by re-epithelialization of the mucosa with glands which are appropriate for that area, and even acute ulcers heal with little or no scarring. Consequently, it is difficult, if not impossible, to determine the site of a healed nonperforated acute ulcer or erosion. Both erosions and acute ulcers can cause hemorrhage into the gastrointestinal tract, but the most severe hemorrhages are caused by acute ulcers eroding large submucosal vessels.[8]

With fiberoptic gastroscopy it has been possible to follow the development and resolution of acute peptic ulcers and erosions.[7] Within 24 hours of sustaining severe trauma, patients were noted to have foci of pallor and hyperemia which were located almost exclusively in the proximal body of the stomach near the greater curve. By 24 hours, petechiae and 1 to 2 mm round, shallow, red-based erosions appeared in the same area of the stomach. By

48 hours the erosions were deeper, black-based, and had some marginal edema. As the disease process progressed, the erosions were seen scattered throughout the entire stomach without isolated antral involvement.

Histological progression of the lesions began with focal edema and early diapedesis of red blood cells. This was followed by mucosal hemorrhage in the lamina propria and mucosal coagulation necrosis with sloughing of the necrotic cells. Scanning electron microscopy revealed discontinuities of the limiting membranes of the altered surface epithelial cells, exposing the intracellular contents and leaving altered "empty" cells which resembled a honeycomb.

In some patients the diffuse erosions persisted for as long as three weeks. As healing progressed the lesions reversed, with diminution of the swelling and regrowth of the mucosa until it finally reverted to normal.

Lucas and colleagues concluded that

these lesions may form because of localized vascular problems but were unable to find any thrombosed vessels in the early stages.[7] Margaretten and McKay, on the other hand, found microthrombi in the base of acute lesions in 70 per cent of their patients.[23] Additionally, they present laboratory evidence that an episode of disseminated intravascular coagulation occurred in 66 per cent of their patients with acute erosions and ulcers.

CHRONIC PEPTIC ULCERS

Morphologically, the main feature which differentiates an acute peptic ulcer from a chronic peptic ulcer is the presence of fibrosis.

Grossly, a chronic peptic ulcer is usually a round or oval, sometimes elliptical crater penetrating deep into the wall of the stomach or duodenum. The ulcers may appear punched out or may have a terraced or overhanging margin. In chronic peptic ulcers of the stomach the aboral margin nearest the pylorus is often flattened and less steep than the proximal oral margin of the ulcer. The base of the ulcer may be relatively clean and granular appearing, but often is partly filled with a bloody or brown-tinged exudate. Beneath the base there is a pale, gelatinous, moderately firm material and then dense fibrous tissue.

As shown in Figure 50–2, benign peptic ulcers have four distinct layers:[24] The lumen of the crater contains an exudate (1) of predominantly polymorphonuclear leukocytes, often admixed with red blood cells or fibrin. Occasionally there is a predominance of lymphocytes and plasma cells. Beneath the exudate is a layer of eosinophilic, hyaline-appearing fibrinoid necrosis (2). This necrotic layer rests on granulation tissue (3), consisting of proliferating fibroblasts and capillaries with acute and chronic inflammatory cells. The granulation tissue gradually blends with dense fibrous tissue (4), which penetrates deeply into the muscle layers. At the

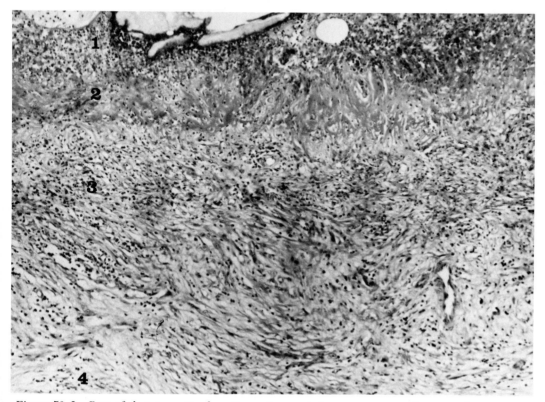

Figure 50–2. Base of chronic peptic ulcer. Four microscopic layers are present: 1, acute inflammatory exudate; 2, fibrinoid necrosis; 3, granulation tissue; and 4, scar tissue formation.

margin of the ulcer the muscularis propria often is turned up and fuses with the muscularis mucosae. The blood vessels which are seen in the scar tissue of the ulcers are thick walled and sclerotic. Immediately surrounding the margin of the ulcer there are often some edema, hemorrhage, and inflammation.

As a chronic peptic ulcer develops, the diameter may increase slightly, but the significant feature is increasing penetration in the wall.[25] If the ulcer is wholly contained within the gastric or duodenal wall, it is considered a mural ulcer. As the crater becomes deeper, fibrous adhesions develop between the ulcer and adjacent tissue. Finally, if the ulcer penetrates into an adjacent structure, it is known as a confined perforation. The pancreas is by far the most common site of confined perforation for both gastric and duodenal ulcers. Confined perforation is a major cause of intractability in chronic peptic ulcer disease.[26, 27]

As a chronic peptic ulcer heals, the lesion becomes predominantly fibrotic but the amount of fibrosis appears less than that in an active ulcer. The glandular epithelium grows over the surface, but in contrast to acute peptic ulcers, in which the mucosa appears normal, the mucosa does not regenerate normally over chronic peptic ulcers. Rather, it is simple, nonspecialized type of epithelium. With chronic gastric ulcers the retraction of the fibrous tissue often leads to a puckered area of the mucosa with radiating folds. A puckered scar can also be seen in the duodenum as the result of a healed duodenal ulcer, but in the duodenum the end result can be a small diverticulum. The serosal surface may show a thickened white scar, although often there are adhesions on the serosal surface with surrounding structures.

Almost all chronic duodenal ulcers are located in the first part of the duodenum. Portis and Jaffe reported that almost 85 per cent of duodenal ulcers were within 2 cm of the pylorus.[28] Niwayama and Terplan, including both active duodenal ulcers and duodenal scars, found that 93.4 per cent were in the first portion of the duodenum.[29] Oi and Sakurai had an even higher incidence of duodenal ulceration in the first portion of the duodenum, with 99.3 per cent of ulcers occurring in this region. Almost all the ulcers occurred in the first several centimeters of duodenum distal to the pyloric ring.[30]

Although duodenal ulcers are generally considered to be small in size, Niwayama reported only 54.5 per cent of duodenal ulcers at autopsy as being less than 2.0 cm, with an additional 11.1 per cent reported as "small".[29] In addition they had an 8.1 per cent incidence of duodenal ulcers greater than 3.0 cm. The occurrence of "giant" duodenal ulcers is relatively rare, but Mistilis and colleagues were able to collect 14 cases of giant duodenal ulcers over a three-year period, ten of which were confirmed at surgery or autopsy. The size of these ulcers varied from 3.0 to 6.0 cm, and all ten confirmed cases had confined perforation into the pancreas.[31] Lunsden et al. have reported an additional 25 cases, and many of these had also destroyed a large part of the posterior duodenal wall and penetrated to the pancreas.[32] Both groups of patients had an average age of over 60 years. Both the Mistilis and Lunsden groups were impressed with the difficulty in diagnosing these cases roentgenologically. Histological examination of the giant duodenal ulcers revealed only typical chronic peptic ulceration.

Chronic gastric ulcers are predominantly found in the antrum of the stomach. Portis and Jaffe found 59.1 per cent within 6 cm of the pyloric ring,[28] and Niwayama and Terplan showed an incidence of 64.4 per cent of gastric ulcers in the same area.[29] Oi et al. found that 96.4 per cent of all gastric ulcers occurred within 2 cm of the border zone, which they defined as the zone between the body and antrum which contains both fundic and pyloric glands. The width of this border zone was 2.0 cm or less in all their patients.[33] This group continued their investigations of the relationship of structure to ulceration and mapped out stomachs for both mucosal histology and muscle bundle structure.[34] They showed that ulcers occurred not only adjacent to the border zones of the mucosa, but also in areas where the border zone crossed large gastric muscle bundles. Schrager and coworkers also found that gastric ulcers occurred in the mucoid antral glands in the region of the body and pyloric gland junction.[35]

The most common site in the stomach for ulceration is the lesser curvature.[29] In evaluating 634 cases of gastric ulcers, Sun and Stempien found 88.3 per cent of lesions on the lesser curve and only 4.6 per cent on the greater curve of the stomach.[36] Interest had been raised as to the possible malignant potential of the greater curvature ulcers. Boudreau et al. showed that malignant gastric ulcers occurred in all areas of the stomach and that 51 per cent of gastric ulcers on the greater curvature were benign.[37] Sun and Stempien found no malignant greater curvature ulcers at all in their series.[36] Findley, in evaluating 44 cases of greater curvature ulceration, found only five malignancies.[38]

Niwayama and Terplan found that 54.5 per cent of benign gastric ulcers measured less than 2.0 cm, and 86.2 per cent of the ulcers were less than 3.0 cm.[29] Sun and Stempien record an even higher percentage of small gastric ulcers, with 78 per cent measuring less than 2.0 cm radiographically.[36] When Alvarez and McCarty published their very large series of benign and malignant gastric ulcers in 1928, it was felt that size could be a good indicator of malignancy.[39] Of 638 resected benign gastric ulcers, 92 per cent measured less than 2.4 cm and no benign ulcers exceeded 4.0 cm in diameter. Of lesions less than 2.4 cm, only one in ten was malignant. Ulcers between 2.4 and 3.7 cm were malignant twice as often as benign, and of the 682 resected malignant gastric ulcers 71 per cent were greater than 4 cm. The utilization of size to determine malignant potential has been seriously questioned in recent years. Boudreau et al. found that 10 per cent of benign gastric ulcers exceeded 4.0 cm in diameter and 38 per cent of the total mixed group of benign and malignant ulcers exceeding 4.0 cm were benign.[37] Findley also found size as a determinant of malignancy of little value, because the range of benign gastric ulcers in his series was from 0.4 to 3.0 cm and of malignant gastric ulcers, 0.7 to 3.0 cm.[38] Marshak et al. have reported seven "giant" benign gastric ulcers which measured from 3.5 to 7.0 cm.[40] In analyzing 77,000 consecutive admissions, Lulu found 400 benign gastric ulcers, of which ten were giant ulcers measuring from 3.0 to 7.0 cm. In the same series of admissions there were only seven malignant gastric ulcers of 101 gastric carcinomas, and of the seven, only four exceeded 3.0 cm in diameter.[41]

Most benign chronic gastric ulcers occur singly. Niwayama and Terplan found an incidence of 12.7 per cent of multiple benign chronic gastric ulcers,[29] whereas Portis and Jaffe report that 7.9 per cent of the chronic gastric ulcers in their series were multiple.[28] More recently, Boyle was only able to find 2.3 per cent of 634 cases of chronic gastric ulcer which were multiple.[42]

A circumstance which has generated more attention is the coexistence of benign chronic gastric and duodenal ulcers in the same patient, or the instance of an ulcer healing in the stomach or duodenum to be followed by an ulcer at the other site. In 1926, Wilkie showed a 16 per cent incidence of combined gastric and duodenal ulcers in the ulcer population he saw. He also noted that 53 per cent of patients requiring resection for a benign gastric ulcer had an associated duodenal ulcer.[43] In 1958, Mangold reported 157 cases of combined gastric and duodenal ulcer, which encompassed only 3.5 per cent of the gastric and duodenal ulcer patients if prepyloric ulcers were included.[44] Mangold reported that in most cases the duodenal ulcer preceded the gastric ulcer, but in eight patients the reverse was true. More recent series have confirmed the sequence of duodenal ulcer followed by gastric ulcer and have reported an incidence of from 6.6 to 64 per cent of this type of combined ulceration.[45-49]

One final factor deserving mention is the relationship between chronic peptic ulcer disease and chronic gastritis. A classification of chronic gastritis is given on page 561. Hebbel examined stomachs at autopsy from patients without gastrointestinal problems, with gastric, duodenal, or combined ulcers, and with carcinoma of the stomach. He noted that in the *normal* gastrointestinal group, there were many stomachs without gastritis but that the incidence and severity of gastritis increased in older patients. Almost no changes were present before age 30, and severe changes were uncommon before age 50. In *all the stomachs associated with any type of chronic peptic ulceration* there was a chronic exudative antral gastritis. Gastritis in the body of the stomach was more frequently associated with benign chronic gastric ulcers. Severe atrophic gastritis was seen in some patients with gastric carcinoma.[50]

Although chronic duodenal ulcer is associated with a chronic antral gastritis, Classen and colleagues were able to demonstrate a duodenitis in only four of the 18 patients with duodenal ulcer they examined. They found no relationship between gastritis and duodenitis.[51]

In an attempt to further explore the relationship of chronic gastritis in chronic peptic ulcer disease, two recent investigations have utilized fiberoptic gastroscopy and multiple biopsies from various areas of the stomach.[52, 53] Stadelmann et al., in addition to biopsying patients with chronic benign gastric ulcers, also studied a large, relatively comparably aged control group.[52] The control subjects showed a surprising incidence of the various types of gastritis which paralleled that of the ulcer patients although less in severity. In both control subjects and ulcer patients as age increased there was a decrease in the amount of normal mucosa and an increase in severe chronic exudative and atrophic gastritis, with the amount of chronic superficial exudative gastritis varying very little. There was a close relationship between the site of the ulcer and the extent of the gastritis. Chronic gastric ulcers, unlike acute gastric ulcers,[54] were never found in an area of normal body glands, but occurred 70 per cent of the time in antral mucoid glands just proximal to the border zone between antral and body glands. Patients with ulcers in the subcardiac region had no normal gastric mucosa remaining. The wide variation in location of chronic gastric ulcers can thus be explained in part by the shifting of the border zone. Gear and coworkers showed that the gastritis in patients with healed chronic gastric ulcers persists and even worsens following healing of the ulcer.[53]

Stadelmann and coworkers assumed that the same pathogenetic process is operative in both chronic duodenal and chronic gastric ulcers but that the occurrence differs only by local factors, of which gastritis is one. They showed that in spite of the same gastric mucosal morphology, ulcers in

younger patients occurred in the duodenum, whereas older patients would have a prepyloric localization.[52]

Other morphological features of the stomach which have been implicated in chronic gastric and duodenal ulceration include stomach size[55] and the lymphatic system in the gastroduodenal region.[56]

REFERENCES

1. Zollinger, R. M., and Ellison, E. H. Primary peptic ulcerations of the jejunum associated with islet cell tumors of the pancreas. Ann. Surg. 142:709, 1955.
2. Ross, J. R., Warren, K. W., and Rudolph, N. E. Zollinger-Ellison syndrome (report of a case with clinical appraisal of the syndrome). Med. Clin. N. Amer. 50:469, 1966.
3. Ellison, E. H., and Wilson, S. D. The Zollinger-Ellison syndrome. Ann. Surg. 160:512, 1964.
4. Editorial: Haemorrhagic ulceration of gut. Brit. Med. J. 3:132, 1971.
5. Crawford, F. A., Hammon, J. W., and Shingleton, W. W. The stress ulcer syndrome. Amer. J. Surg. 121:644, 1971.
6. Grosz, C. R., and Kwang-Tzen, W. Stress ulcers: A survey of the experience in a large general hospital. Surgery 61:853, 1967.
7. Lucas, C. E., Sugawa, C., Riddle, J., Rector, F., Rosenberg, B., and Walt, A. J. Natural history and surgical dilemma of "stress" gastric bleeding. Arch. Surg. 102:266, 1971.
8. Moncrief, J. A., Switzer, W. E., and Teplitz, C. Curling's ulcer. J. Trauma. 4:481, 1964.
9. O'Neill, J. A., Jr., Pruitt, B. A., Jr., Moncrief, J. A., and Switzer, W. E. Studies related to the pathogenesis of Curling's ulcer. J. Trauma 7:275, 1967.
10. Law, E. J., Day, S. B., and MacMillan, B. G. Autopsy findings in the upper gastrointestinal tract of 81 burn patients. Arch. Surg. 102:412, 1971.
11. Pruitt, B. A., Foley, F. D., and Moncrief, J. A. Curling's ulcer: A clinical-pathology study of 323 cases. Ann. Surg. 172:523, 1970.
12. Foley, F. D. The burn autopsy. Amer. J. Clin. Path. 52:1, 1969.
13. Brush, B. E., Block, M. A., Geoghegan, T., Ensign, D. C., and Sigler, J. W. The steroid-induced peptic ulcer. Arch. Surg. 74:675, 1957.
14. Fentress, V., Firnschild, P., and Reveno, W. S. Perforated duodenal ulcer complicating prednisone therapy. New Eng. J. Med. 254:657, 1956.
15. Dalgaard, J. B. Cerebral vascular lesions and peptic ulceration. Arch. Path. 69:359, 1960.
16. Fletcher, D. G., and Harkins, H. N. Acute peptic ulcer as a complication of major surgery, stress or trauma. Surgery 36:212, 1954.
17. Penner, A., and Bernheim, A. I. Acute postoperative esophageal, gastric and duodenal ulcerations. Arch. Path. 28:129, 1939.
18. Berkowitz, D., Wagner, B. M., and Uricchio, J. F.

Acute peptic ulceration following cardiac surgery. Ann. Intern. Med. *46*:1015, 1957.

19. McDonnell, W. V., and McCloskey, J. F. Acute peptic ulcers as a complication of surgery. Ann. Surg. *137*:67, 1953.

20. Herbut, P. A. Acute peptic ulcers following distant operations. Surg. Gynec. Obstet. *80*:410, 1945.

21. Abramson, D. J. Curling's ulcer in childhood: Review of the literature and report of five cases. Surgery *55*:321, 1964.

22. Silverberg, M., and Davidson, M. Pediatric gastroenterology: A review. Gastroenterology *58*:229, 1970.

23. Margaretten, W., and McKay, D. G. Thrombotic ulcerations of the gastrointestinal tract. Arch. Intern. Med. *127*:250, 1971.

24. Karsner, H. T. The pathology of peptic ulcer of the stomach. J.A.M.A. *85*:1376, 1925.

25. Haubrich, W. S. The clinical recognition and pathological anatomy of intractability in peptic ulcer disease. Ann. N.Y. Acad. Sci. *99*:114, 1962.

26. Powell, J. R. Intractability of ulcers of the upper gastrointestinal tract. Amer. J. Clin. Gastroent. *56*:501, 1971.

27. Ross, J. R., and Reaves, L. E. Syndrome of posterior penetrating peptic ulcer. Med. Clin. N. Amer. *50*:461, 1966.

28. Portis, S. A., and Jaffe, R. H. A study of peptic ulcer based on necropsy records. J.A.M.A. *110*:6, 1938.

29. Niwayama, G., and Terplan, K. A study of peptic ulcer based on necropsy records. Gastroenterology *36*:409, 1959.

30. Oi, M., and Sakurai, Y. The location of duodenal ulcer. Gastroenterology *36*:60, 1959.

31. Mistilis, S. P., Wiot, J. F., and Nedelman, S. H. Giant duodenal ulcer. Ann. Intern. Med. *59*:155, 1963.

32. Lunsden, K., MacLarnon, J. C., and Dawson, J. Giant duodenal ulcer. Gut *11*:592, 1970.

33. Oi, M., Oshida, K., and Sugimura, S. The location of gastric ulcer. Gastroenterology *36*:45, 1959.

34. Oi, M., Ito, Y., Kumagi, F., Yosida, K., Tanaka, Y., Yoshikawa, K., Miho, O., and Kijima, M. A possible dual mechanism in the origin of peptic ulcer. Gastroenterology *57*:280, 1969.

35. Schrager, J., Spink, R., and Mitra, S. The antrum in patients with duodenal and gastric ulcers. Gut *8*:497, 1967.

36. Sun, D. C. H., and Stempien, S. J. Site and size of the ulcer as determinants of outcome. Gastroenterology *61*:576, 1971.

37. Boudreau, R. P., Harvey, J. P., and Robbins, S. L. Anatomic study of benign and malignant gastric ulcerations. J.A.M.A. *147*:374, 1951.

38. Findley, J. W. Ulcers of the greater curvature of the stomach. Gastroenterology *40*:183, 1961.

39. Alvarez, W. C., and McCarty, W. C. Sizes of resected gastric ulcers and gastric carcinomas. J.A.M.A. *91*:226, 1928.

40. Marshak, R. H., Yarnis, H., and Friedman, A. I. Giant benign gastric ulcers. Gastroenterology *24*:339, 1953.

41. Lulu, D. J. Benign giant gastric ulcer. Amer. Surgeon *37*:357, 1971.

42. Boyle, J. D. Multiple gastric ulcers. Gastroenterology *61*:628, 1971.

43. Wilkie, D. P. D. Coincident duodenal and gastric ulcer. Brit. Med. J. *2*:469, 1926.

44. Mangold, R. Combined gastric and duodenal ulceration. Survey of 157 cases. Brit. Med. J. *2*:1193, 1958.

45. Weisberg, H., and Glass, G. B. J. Coexisting gastric and duodenal ulcers; a review. Amer. J. Dig. Dis. *8*:992, 1963.

46. Johnson, H. D. Gastric ulcer: Classification, blood group characteristics, secretion pattern and pathogenesis. Ann. Surg. *162*:996, 1965.

47. McCray, R. S., Ferris, E. J., Herskovic, T., Winawer, S. J., Shapiro, J. H., and Zamcheck, N. Clinical differences between gastric ulcers with and without duodenal deformity. Ann. Surg. *168*:821, 1968.

48. Vesely, K. T., Kubickova, Z., and Dvorakova, M. Clinical data and characteristics differentiating types of peptic ulcer. Gut. *9*:57, 1968.

49. Rumball, J. M. Coexistent duodenal ulcer. Gastroenterology *61*:622, 1971.

50. Hebbel, R. Chronic gastritis. Amer. J. Path. *19*:43, 1943.

51. Classen, M., Koch, H., and Demling, L. Duodenitis, significance and frequency. Bibl. Gastroenterol. *9*:48, 1970.

52. Stadelmann, O., Elster, K., Stolte, M., Miederer, S. E., Deyhle, P., Demling, L., and Siegenthaler, W. The peptic gastric ulcer—histotopographic and functional investigations. Scand. J. Gastroent. *6*:613, 1971.

53. Gear, M. W. L., Truelove, S. C., and Whitehead, R. Gastric ulcer and gastritis. Gut *12*:639, 1971.

54. Kawai, K., Murakami, K., and Misaki, F. Endoscopical observations of the gastric ulcer. Endoscopy *1*:97, 1969.

55. Cox, A. J., Jr. Stomach size and its relation to chronic peptic ulcer. Arch. Path. *54*:407, 1952.

56. Vojtisek, V., Jelinek, V., and Chlumska, A. Experimental gastroduodenal ulcer. Amer. J. Surg. *121*:650, 1971.

Chapter 51

The Pathogenesis of Peptic Ulcer

John S. Fordtran

The presence of gastric acid and pepsin is, by definition, a prerequisite for the development of peptic ulcer, and in general terms it may be said that the higher the rate of acid-pepsin secretion, the more likely it is that a person will develop an ulcer, and vice versa. At the two extremes, peptic ulcer develops in all but 7 per cent of patients with severe gastric hypersecretion associated with gastrin-producing islet cell tumors,[1] and never develops in patients with pernicious anemia. Very rarely what appears to be a benign peptic ulcer of the stomach occurs in a patient who secretes no acid in response to a maximal dose of histamine.[2] Whether these ulcers have a different pathogenesis from peptic ulcers, or whether acid-pepsin was secreted prior to the development of the ulcer, is not known.

Although the average secretion rate of acid-pepsin is higher in patients with duodenal ulcer than in control subjects, duodenal ulcer not uncommonly and gastric ulcer frequently develop in patients who secrete less acid-pepsin than the mean value for normal subjects. This observation proves that decreased mucosal resistance plays a role in at least some cases of ulcer. Furthermore, although a large area of sensitive mucosa is exposed to acid-pepsin, generally only a circumscribed area

becomes affected by an ulcer. This is true for massive hypersecretory states associated with gastrin-producing tumors as well as in the usual type of ulcer disease. It also holds true in experimental studies when large amounts of acid and pepsin are perfused through a loop of duodenum.[3] Therefore *locally* impaired resistance must be postulated in virtually every patient with a peptic ulcer in order to explain the fact that a focal ulcer, rather than a diffuse lesion, is produced. The anatomical location, mucosal blood flow, mucus production, cell renewal, and pre-existing inflammatory disease might all influence local tissue resistance and thus contribute to ulcer development.

It is not clear whether gastric and duodenal ulcers have a similar or a different pathogenesis. Based on their different average rates of gastric secretion, some workers consider duodenal, prepyloric, channel, and combined gastric and duodenal ulcers to be due to gastric hypersecretion, and gastric (corpus) ulcers to be due to deficient mucosal resistance.[4] Other arguments presented to justify separating the diseases with regard to etiology are that gastric and duodenal ulcer patients differ with regard to social class, genetic background, and frequency of ABO blood group and secretor status. Different personalities and anthropological differences have also been reported. On the other hand, a local defect in mucosal resistance must be postulated in both ulcers, acid-pepsin is a prerequisite for both ulcers, and there is a good deal of overlap in the level of acid secretion even among patients with duodenal and gastric (corpus) ulcers. Furthermore, the excellent twin study of Eberhard (see p. 639) has shown that duodenal and gastric ulcers share a common inheritance at least to some extent, and the evidence suggests that patients with both diseases have a higher level of anxiety and greater sensitivity to stress than do control subjects.

Although it is clear that there are important differences with regard to age, sex, and prevalence in different countries, current evidence favors a basically similar pathogenesis, i.e., too much acid-pepsin for the degree of local tissue resistance. Among patients with either gastric or duodenal ulcer, the relative importance of acid-pepsin excess and mucosal resistance deficit may be quite different. Some patients get a gastric (corpus) ulcer because of acid-pepsin excess, whereas others (the majority) get it because of decreased resistance. Similarly, some patients (the majority) get a duodenal ulcer because of acid-pepsin excess, and others because of decreased resistance. Considering all the evidence, this hypothesis seems preferable to a categorical statement that gastric ulcer develops because of decreased resistance and duodenal ulcer because of gastric hypersecretion.

The separation of the roles of acid and pepsin in the production of peptic ulcer and peptic esophagitis has been difficult. Some workers have stressed the role of acid as the ulcerogen, and others have emphasized the importance of pepsin. Pepsin activity cannot, of course, be dissociated from that of acid, because pepsin is active only in the presence of acid. Goldberg et al.[5] have carefully studied this problem, using a cat esophagitis model. Acid solutions of pH 1.0 (about 127 mEq per liter) caused a severe esophagitis, even in the complete absence of pepsin. As a matter of fact, addition of pepsin to such solutions did not increase the severity of the esophagitis, which was probably due to protein denaturation. At pH 1.6 (31 mEq

per liter) and at pH 2.0 (12 mEq per liter), esophagitis was produced only when pepsin was added to the acid solution. At these pH levels it is likely that pepsin produced esophagitis by protein digestion. Therefore it appears that with this model pepsin is an important factor in causing esophagitis within the pH range of 1.6 to 2.0. At higher levels of acidity, which are often present in the stomachs of human subjects, acid alone can produce injury.

ACID-PEPSIN

Gastric secretion in patients with peptic ulcer is described in detail on pages 144 to 160 and 174 to 193. The following brief statement summarizes current knowledge as interpreted by the author.

DUODENAL ULCER

1. The degree of hypersecretion varies markedly in different series, from a negligible to a threefold increase above the secretion rate in control subjects. These different results are largely due to differences in patient and control group selection.

2. The cause of increased acid secretion is due in part to an increased number of functioning parietal cells in the stomach. This is the entire explanation for higher peak histamine or gastrin responses, and a partial explanation for higher rates of basal secretion.

3. The cause of the elevated number of functioning parietal cells, which causes the higher peak stimulated response, is not known. Genetic factors are probably involved; chronic elevation of "secretory drive" may also be important in some cases.

4. Although patients vary widely in their secretory rate, active duodenal ulcer rarely if ever develops in a patient whose peak stimulated response is less than 12.5 mEq of acid per hour. Exceptions to this rule are almost invariably due to a recent complication, such as hemorrhage or perforation, or to an error in the test.

5. Chronic stimulation of the parietal cells, such as by hypergastrinemia caused by islet cell adenoma, elevates the parietal cell mass. It is not known whether other

forms of chronic gastric stimulation in man (frequent ingestion of food, anxiety, high "vagal tone," calcium ingestion) would have a similar effect. Pyloric obstruction is said to elevate the peak histamine response, but the evidence of such an occurrence is usually not convincing. The peak histamine response is not elevated by high coffee ingestion for four months, and it is not reduced by anticholinergic therapy for twelve months.

6. The higher average basal secretion in duodenal ulcer than in control subjects is partially due to the higher parietal cell mass. However, the ratio of basal secretion to peak stimulated response is high in some or many duodenal ulcer patients (depending upon the method of patient selection), and this *cannot* be explained by the increased parietal cell mass. These patients with "idiopathic basal hypersecretion" must have a high level of secretory drive or increased sensitivity of the parietal cells to a normal level of drive. High secretory drive could be caused by high vagal tone, a high blood concentration of a secretagogue, or a low blood concentration of an inhibitor (enterogastrone). High secretory drive or increased sensitivity of the parietal cells in these patients is apparently not due to elevated serum gastrin level (with the exception of the Zollinger-Ellison syndrome), although the issue is not completely settled. Enterogastrone levels, vagal tone, and parietal sensitivity are not subject to specific measurement at present.

Control subjects occasionally have a secretory pattern suggesting increased secretory drive or increased parietal sensitivity. If these subjects also have a normal or high functional parietal cell mass, they are presumably prone to develop a duodenal ulcer.

7. The functional parietal cell mass (as estimated by the peak stimulated response), the basal secretion, and the ratio of basal to peak stimulated secretion may change dramatically (up or down) over a period of six to twelve months. The importance of this spontaneous change is obvious, although at present its mechanism is completely unknown.

8. Whether spontaneous ulcer healing and recurrence are associated with a change in gastric acid secretion has not been definitely determined. It is also not known whether the tendency to gastric hypersecretion precedes for some time the development of a duodenal ulcer, although the evidence suggests that it does.

9. In normal subjects and in patients with duodenal or gastric ulcer, the amount of pepsinogen secretion tends to correspond to the amount of acid secretion. There is no convincing evidence that any abnormal class of pepsinogens is secreted in duodenal or gastric ulcer patients, or that gastric or duodenal ulcer is ever caused by a specific increase in pepsinogen secretion (out of proportion to the rate of acid secretion). A high value of pepsinogen-acid secretion ratio may be suggestive of increased vagal tone; if so, its value in evaluating the pathogenesis of hypersecretion has been grossly neglected in the past.

GASTRIC ULCER

1. Average acid secretion rate in gastric (corpus) ulcer patients is lower than in control subjects, but there is wide scatter in both groups. Some patients with a corpus ulcer have very high rates of secretion, whereas some are nearly achlorhydric.

2. Patients with both a duodenal ulcer and a gastric ulcer have rates of acid secretion similar to those of duodenal ulcer patients. Patients with prepyloric ulcer secrete acid at about the same rate as do control subjects.

3. To a degree, low acid secretion in gastric ulcer patients may be due to gastritis, which usually surrounds an ulcer crater and may diminish the parietal cell mass. Whether the parietal cell mass, as measured by the peak stimulated secretion rate, increases after healing of a gastric ulcer has never been adequately proved.

4. Low rates of acid secretion in patients with gastric ulcer may, to some extent, be due to enhanced permeability of the mucosa to hydrogen ions (so that secreted acid is absorbed rather than collected), but the quantitative importance of this mechanism has not been established.

5. Low acid secretion in patients with gastric ulcer tends to be associated with higher than normal levels of serum gastrin.

The high gastrin levels are probably due to decreased inhibition of antral gastrin release because of higher than normal antral pH.

DECREASED MUCOSAL RESISTANCE

As already noted, a localized area of decreased mucosal resistance must be postulated in virtually every patient with a peptic ulcer. Some of the factors which may be responsible for this local defect are the mucosal and muscular anatomy of the stomach and duodenum, derangements in mucosal blood flow, defects in mucus production, abnormalities in the rate of cell renewal, and pre-existing inflammatory disease of the gastric and duodenal mucosa.

ANATOMICAL PREDISPOSITION

A number of workers have pointed out that peptic ulcer nearly always develops in junctional epithelium.[6, 7] For instance, esophageal ulcers occur just above the junction of fundic and esophageal mucosa, gastric ulcers just below the junction of fundic and antral mucosa, and duodenal ulcers just below the junction of pyloric and duodenal mucosa. In a recent study of 855 peptic ulcers, only 3 per cent occurred in areas other than at mucosal junctions.[8] Peptic ulcer almost never occurs in acid-secreting mucosa; when this does occur, the ulcer is usually located in aberrant antral mucosa rather than in parietal mucosa.[8] The reason why gastric ulcers appear at different distances from the pyloric sphincter is that the antrum extends a variable distance from the pylorus, especially along the lesser curvature. The junction between the acid-bearing and pyloric gland areas on the lesser curvature varies from 2 to 16 cm from the pyloric ring.[7]

The cause of this striking localization of peptic ulcer to the junctional epithelium is not known. Presumably, these areas are more sensitive to acid-pepsin than other parts of the upper gastrointestinal mucosa, and perhaps they are exposed to higher acid-pepsin concentrations.

Capper and coworkers reported that the alkaline area of the stomach, which presumably corresponds to the antrum, is quite small in patients with duodenal ulcer, whereas in gastric ulcer patients the alkaline area is extensive.[9] Around all gastric ulcers there was a great deal of gastritis, but it was possible to show histologically that the alkaline area was lined by true antral mucosa and not degenerated fundic mucosa. These findings suggest that gastric ulcer develops in patients who have a large antrum, whereas duodenal ulcer occurs in patients with a small antrum. The inverse relationship between the size of the antrum and that of the parietal cell mass may be of great importance.[9] This study was based on an analysis of only a small group of patients.

It has also been shown recently that peptic ulcer tends to occur in relation to certain muscular bands in the stomach, especially where these muscular bands coincide with junctional epithelium. The effective focus of the "dual mechanism" (junctional epithelium and muscle anatomy) for gastric ulcers is located at or near the angulus, which agrees with the clinical observations that gastric ulcers tend to occur in this location. Oi et al. make the provocative statement that the development of an ulcer is not always anatomically possible in the stomach (muscular bands do not cross junctional epithelium), regardless of other influences, whereas the development of an ulcer in the duodenum is always anatomically possible.[8]

MUCOSAL BLOOD FLOW AND HYPOXIA

As illustrated in Figure 51–1, the mucous membrane of the stomach has a rich blood supply, consisting of arborizing capillaries which appear to fill almost completely the glandular area, "like a vascular sponge." The arrangement of mucosal vessels is the same in all parts of the stomach. The vessels of the stomach wall anastomose freely. The mucosal arteries of the anterior and posterior wall arise from a plexus of vessels beneath the muscularis mucosae, whereas on the lesser curvature the mucosal arteries arise from the left gastric artery, outside the stomach wall. It is possible that this different vascular supply might somehow predispose to lesser curvature ulcer.

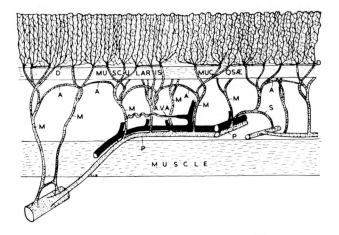

Figure 51–1. Diagram of the vascular arrangement in the stomach wall, drawn after microscopic dissections of injected stomachs. On the left is shown the lesser curve, with mucosal arteries (M) arising from the left gastric artery outside the stomach wall. On the right is the pattern as seen in the anterior and posterior wall, where the mucosal arteries arise from a plexus of vessels beneath the muscularis mucosae. In the center, an arteriovenous anastomosis (AVA) is shown. A = Anastomosis between two mucosal arteries on the under aspect of the muscularis mucosae. S = Anastomosis between ends of arteries. P = Submucous plexus. D = Anastomosing channels on the glandular aspect of the muscularis mucosae from which the capillaries of the mucosa arise. (From Barlow, T. E., Bentley, F. H., and Walder, D. N.: Surg. Gynec. Obstet. 93:657, 1951.)

Arteriovenous anastomoses are prominent beneath the muscularis mucosae, and these operate to circumvent the large mucosal capillary bed.[10-12] The effectiveness of the mucosal shunt system is striking. The arteriovenous anastomoses are responsible for the marked blanching or engorgement of the mucosa in response to various emotional and pharmacological stimuli. Observations of the capillary network in vivo show that alternative opening and closing of capillaries, and thus alternating ischemia and plethora, is a normal condition.[12] Although the majority of gastroduodenal shunts act in concert, paradoxical activity among neighboring shunts is known to occur.

Thus, whatever the physiological mechanisms of control may be, channels exist that are capable of bringing large quantities of blood to the mucosa, or transferring blood from one point to another in the stomach or duodenal mucosa. The arteriovenous (A/V) shunts provide a means of rapidly directing blood into or away from the mucous membrane, by purely local action involving relatively few vessels. Presumably, the shunts are under the control of nervous and hormonal influences. It has been shown, for instance, that anterior hypothalamic stimulation in experimental animals increases both generalized and mucosal blood flow to the stomach (acid secretion is increased simultaneously), whereas posterior hypothalamic stimulation reduces blood flow and secretion. The central nervous system can thus affect both blood flow and secretion, and an autonomic imbalance has often been proposed as an etiological factor in the development of peptic ulcer.[13]

By using the distal two-thirds of the human stomach excised at operation for duodenal ulcer, it is possible to determine the size of the A/V anastomoses in the living state and to make preliminary inquiries into the passage of circulating fluid through these channels.[10, 11] This is done by perfusing the vessels of the excised stomach with plasma; the stomach remains apparently healthy and active for at least eight hours, as judged by acid secretion. A/V shunt function is measured by the number of small glass spheres which, when injected into the arterial circulation, are recovered from the veins—the more beads recovered, the more the shunts are open, and the less the mucosa is perfused. Acetylcholine, for instance, markedly increases mucosal blood flow (i.e., reduces recovery of beads and by inference closes the shunts).

It is not known whether the shunts are normal or abnormal in peptic ulcer disease, but the system of A/V anastomoses can theoretically produce local hypoxia in two ways:[12] (1) if the shunt is open, ischemia results; (2) if the shunt is closed for prolonged periods, plethora may be produced, and this is also believed to cause hypoxia. If a focal lesion is to develop as a result of abnormal shunt activity, a prolonged abnormal function of one or two shunts must be postulated. There are several reasons to select plethoric hypoxia as the explanation for mucosal damage rather than ischemic hypoxia. First, erosion (as studied by gastroscopy or in gastrostomy patients) is said to develop as a sequel to mucosal engorgement. Second, pharmacological preparations commonly used to produce acute experimental ulcers (other than vasopressin) cause shunt closure and plethora. The same is true for vagus activity.[12]

In 1937, Necheles proposed that overproduction, and especially continuous production, of acetylcholine would produce anoxemia of tissues, and that this would be more severe in those regions in which most branches of the vagus nerve are distributed.[14] He further stated that most branches of the vagus nerve are found in the duodenal cap and lesser curvature of the stomach, thus explaining the frequency of ulcers in these areas. Unfortunately, no proof was given that vagus nerve branches are excessive in these regions, and current textbooks of neuroanatomy and anatomy do not describe any preponderance of vagal nerve endings in the duodenal bulb or on the lesser curvature of the stomach.

Although some workers believe that the local breakdown of tissue resistance has a vascular basis, this has never been proved. There simply are not any data relevant to ulcer pathogenesis. In a recent extensive symposium on gastrointestinal blood flow, the role of deranged gastric mucosal blood flow in ulcer pathogenesis was not discussed,[15] presumably indicating a lack of reliable data on the subject.

DEFECTIVE MUCUS, ABO BLOOD GROUP, AND SECRETOR STATUS

According to Menguy,[16] the "mucous barrier" is a thin layer of mucus covering the epithelial cells of the gastrointestinal mucosa. It is continuously renewed as its superficial layers are lost into the gut lumen. Mucus has extraordinary qualities of viscosity, adhesiveness, and cohesiveness which allow it to form a continuous layer separating the underlying epithelial cells from proteolytic luminal contents. Mucoprotein is relatively resistant to enzymatic hydrolysis because of the carbohydrate prosthetic groups.

The theory of the protective action of the mucous barrier is illustrated in Figure 51–2.[17] Although antral mucus, studied in vitro, does not significantly impede the diffusion rate of HCl or pepsin, it is thought to be an effective barrier by virtue of its ability to retard mixing of luminal acid-pepsin with the neutral solution that is believed to be secreted by the antral and duodenal mucosa. Thus, provided that some neutral fluid is secreted by the antral and duodenal cells, the surface of the mucosa would be in contact with neutral fluid, regardless of the amount of acid within the lumen. Pepsin would diffuse through the mucous barrier, but, on entering regions of successively higher pH, would become inactive and finally destroyed. As already noted, the organization would maintain itself by continued renewal.

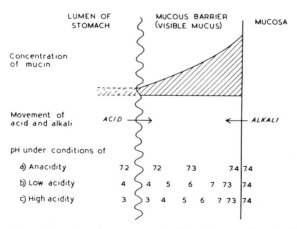

Figure 51–2.   Diagram of hypothetical concentration and pH gradients within the "visible" mucous layer on the gastric mucosa when contents of stomach are (a) anacid, (b) weakly acid, and (c) strongly acid. The directions of movement of acid and alkali are also shown. (From Heatley, N. G.: Gastroenterology 37:313, 1959.)

A qualitatively inferior mucus might not retard mixing, or on exposure to acid-pepsin it might flocculate, rather than form a protective gel. However, studies on aspirated gastric mucus (which may not accurately reflect the "mucus barrier") have failed to reveal differences which would logically suggest that ulcer patients secrete a mucus which is less protective than that secreted by control subjects.[18, 19] These studies were done on groups of control and ulcer subjects without regard to the rates of acid-pepsin secretion in the individual subjects. It would be of interest to compare gastric mucus in individuals with high acidity but no ulcer (i.e., good resistance) to the mucus from patients with ulcer and low acid secretion (low resistance groups) rather than from random groups of normal and ulcer patients.

Curt and Pringle[19, 20] reported that mucus from patients with duodenal ulcer has a higher viscosity than mucus from normals. Although this would not be expected to reduce the protective effect of mucus in the context of the hypothesis described in Figure 51-2, the authors suggested that one of the results of increased viscosity might be prevention of the pH receptors in the antrum from inhibiting the release of gastrin, and this might contribute to gastric hypersecretion.

The fact that nonsecretors of ABH blood group substance have a slight but significantly higher incidence of ulcer than those who secrete the Lewis blood group substances (all people secrete one or the other of these blood group substances, and the total amount secreted is approximately the same)[21] suggests that ABH mucoproteins might be more protective than the Lewis mucoproteins. However, a genetic association unrelated to ulcer pathogenesis is, perhaps, just as likely.

Menguy has reviewed the evidence that aspirin is injurious to the gastric mucosa (even that administered parenterally or per rectum), and that this effect is not mediated via enhanced acid and pepsin secretion.[22] Rather, he has reported that aspirin profoundly reduces the rate of mucus secretion and also alters the composition of mucus. This might represent one means by which salicylates predispose to gastric and duodenal mucosal ulceration (see p. 646).

The "defective mucus barrier" theory is alive, although it has not been proved to be of any importance in ulcer pathogenesis. In a recent symposium on gastrointestinal mucus, it was concluded that the position of mucus was still so uncertain that it might be questioned whether it protected the gut against anything.[23]

GASTRITIS

Since gastric (corpus) ulcers occur in patients whose average rate of gastric secretion is lower than normal, these lesions are, more often than duodenal ulcers, considered to occur because of decreased tissue resistance. Gastric ulcers always occur in an area surrounded by gastritis,[6, 22-25] but it is not known which comes first—the ulcer or the gastritis. If gastritis is primary, the decreased resistance theory would be reasonable, because gastritis is known to predispose to ulcer experimentally.[26] In the careful biopsy study by Gear et al.,[27] superficial or atrophic gastritis was found to persist or even worsen after healing of the ulcer, whether treatment was medical or surgical. This finding suggests that gastritis is the basic disease process and that gastric ulcer is a secondary phenomenon. On the other hand, the gastritis might be secondary to the gastric ulcer, and since the gastritis often spreads into the parietal mucosa, it might also cause gastric secretion to decrease.[6]

The gastritis in patients with gastric ulcer apparently involves what was originally the fundic as well as the antral mucosa,[6, 28] even though the ulcer is always located in the antral area. If the gastritis is primary, maximal acid secretion, which estimates the parietal cell mass, would be expected to be the same before and after the ulcer heals. On the other hand, if the gastritis is secondary to the ulcer, acid secretion might increase after healing of the ulcer. Capper suggests, from a histological study, that the parietal cell mass increases as a gastric ulcer heals,[28] and several observers have suggested that gastric secretion increases appreciably after healing of a gastric ulcer.[6, 29, 30] However, none of these reports is convincing, and the present author is not aware of a careful and systematic study of maximal acid secretion before and after healing of gastric ulcers.

Mangus has shown that chronic and even atrophic gastritis in the antrum occurs to some degree in all patients with duodenal ulcer.[31] Tanner [32] and Marks and Shay[6] believe that the onset of this gastritis reduces gastric secretion, which results in healing of the duodenal ulcer; the gastritis, however, predisposes to gastric ulcer. This would explain the facts that from 10 to 50 per cent of gastric ulcer patients have X-ray evidence of a deformed duodenal bulb, that in combined ulcer disease the duodenal almost always precedes the gastric ulcer, and that when both diseases are present concomitantly, the duodenal ulcer is inactive or healed in 90 per cent of the patients.[6, 32-34]

As discussed on page 626, duodenal ulcers may occur in an area surrounded by duodenitis, but as with the gastritis and gastric ulcer problem, it is not certain which is primary.

REFLUX OF BILE

Recently it has been shown that the pyloric sphincter, which normally is relatively competent, allows duodenal contents to reflux into the stomach of gastric ulcer patients.[35] Furthermore, the concentration of bile acids is higher in gastric contents of gastric ulcer patients than in normal subjects.[24, 26] Experimentally, exposure of the gastric mucosa to duodenal contents produces gastritis (especially in the antrum),[36] and it has been suggested that reflux of duodenal contents through the pylorus causes gastritis, which in turn predisposes to gastric ulcer.[24, 26] Two mechanisms have been suggested to explain gastric mucosal damage by bile acids—alteration of the protective mucous lining via the detergent property of bile acids, and an increased gastric permeability of hydrogen ("broken barrier"). It has never been shown, however, that the relatively small amounts of intestinal content that do reflux into the stomach of gastric ulcer patients are harmful to the gastric mucosa, and the fact that pyloroplasty does not predispose to gastric ulcer means that regurgitation cannot be the sole cause of gastric ulcer.[26]

The importance of reflux of intestinal contents into the stomach in the etiology of gastric ulcer has not been definitely settled. One major problem is that we do not know whether increased reflux precedes or follows the gastric ulcer.

THE GASTRIC MUCOSAL BARRIER

When acid secretion is negligible, acid instilled into the stomach diffuses slowly across the fundic mucosa, but when the parietal cells are secreting acid, acid back-diffusion from the stomach lumen apparently ceases.[37] These results are most consistent with the hypothesis that the surface epithelial cells of the fundic mucosa are impermeable to hydrogen but that hydrogen can diffuse slowly across some cell or cells of the gastric glands. Secretion of fluid into the lumen of the gastric glands presumably prevents acid in the lumen of the stomach from coming in contact with the permeable cells of the gastric glands. This theory would explain why the acidity of the secreting stomach contents is approximately the same when collected continuously as when left in contact with the gastric mucosa for relatively long periods.[37]

Acid disappears much more rapidly from pyloric pouches than from fundic pouches of the dog stomach.[39] This may in part be due to neutralization of the acid load by an alkaline secretion from the pyloric mucosa, but Dyck et al. believe that acid back-diffusion is also much greater across pyloric than across fundic mucosa, and postulate that this may account for the fact that almost all peptic ulcers occur in pyloric mucosa.[39]

Davenport has found that aspirin (see pp. 648 to 649) and many other substances disrupt the gastric "mucosal barrier," and allow an increased back-diffusion of hydrogen ions into the gastric mucosa. He suggested that once the barrier was broken (by aspirin, for example), hydrogen ions present in the stomach would diffuse rapidly across the gastric mucosa and cause damage and bleeding in the process.[38, 40] The pathogenesis of such injury would be as follows: aspirin → broken barrier → H^+ back-diffusion → injury.

This hypothesis has been enthusiastically accepted by a number of workers, and it is currently fashionable to speak of the broken barrier as *the mechanism* by which many drugs, bile salts, and severe stress predispose to gastric erosion, ulceration, and bleeding.[41] There is, however, no proof that this sequence is correct, and it is equally possible that the broken barrier is, like bleeding, simply an indication of injury rather than its cause. In other words, it is possible that a damaged mucosa loses its normal permeability characteristics, and that acid back-diffusion is only an index (perhaps a sensitive one) of that injury. Obviously, the fact that acid added to the gastric lumen enhances the damaging effect of drugs is equally compatible with either possibility, because there are a number of ways in which acid could potentiate the effect of other ulcerogenic agents (activation of pepsin, direct injury by acid to a susceptible mucosa).

With regard to the "broken barrier" and gastric ulcer, it should be kept in mind that animal experiments on the barrier are generally done with stomach pouches made from the fundus, whereas a gastric ulcer almost always develops in pyloric mucosa (see above).

Overholt and Pollard found that acid instilled in the stomach was somewhat more rapidly absorbed* in patients with gastric ulcer than in control subjects, suggesting increased permeability in the gastric ulcer patients.[42] On the other hand, glycine instilled in the stomach as a trap for hydrogen ions caused the same apparent increase in maximal stimulated acid secretion in normals and in gastric ulcer patients, which suggests normal permeability of the surface epithelium in gastric ulcer patients. When 30 mEq of HCl (160 mEq per liter, 200 ml) was instilled into the stomach of normal people, Chapman and coworkers found an absorption rate of 2.2 ± 0.2 mEq per 15 minutes in normal subjects. Gastric ulcer patients absorbed from 1.6 to 3.0 mEq per 15 minutes, and pernicious anemia patients absorbed 2.6 to 3.3 mEq per 15 minutes.[43] These findings suggest nearly normal gastric permeability to hydrogen ions in most patients with gastric ulcer, and slightly increased permeability in those with pernicious anemia.

---

*Absorption by H^+ diffusion has not been separated from neutralization by HCO_3^- secretion, but most estimates suggest that disappearance of H^+ is mainly due to H^+ absorption.

Much more work must be done before the significance of a broken permeability barrier to hydrogen diffusion is accepted as the initial event in the pathogenesis of gastric mucosal injury.

DEFECTS IN CELL RENEWAL

The surface epithelium of the gastrointestinal mucosa undergoes continuous renewal. It seems likely that small defects in the mucosa of the stomach and duodenum occur frequently in almost all people because of trauma, and yet rarely if ever are these defects converted into a chronic peptic ulcer. The repair of such defects must depend on the rate of renewal of surface epithelial cells. Defects in renewal could theoretically play a role in the conversion of small erosions into chronic ulcers. Although cell renewal rates have apparently not been studied in relation to the etiology of peptic ulcer, it has been suggested that ACTH and adrenal steroids reduce cell renewal rate and that this might predispose to ulcer in patients receiving these drugs (see pp. 644 to 646).[44]

SALIVARY SECRETION

Malhotra has shown, with either fluid or solid meals, that mucus in the stomach content arises almost exclusively from the salivary glands rather than from mucus secretion by the stomach.[45] Many have postulated that saliva protects against peptic ulcer because of its bicarbonate content (neutralization of HCl), because saliva under some circumstances reduces acid secretion, and because of the protective effect of its mucus. Since mastication increases salivary flow, the types of food ingested markedly influence the amount of saliva swallowed during a meal.[45]

There is, however, no direct evidence for a link between salivary flow or composition and peptic ulcer. The incidence of peptic ulcer is apparently not increased in Sjögren's syndrome.

DEFICIENT NEUTRALIZATION OF ACID

In man, in contrast to dogs, the bicarbonate output from the pancreas can match the acid output from the stomach.[46] Increased duodenal acidity theoretically could result from decreased pancreatic and biliary bicarbonate as well as from increased gastric acid secretion. This mechanism of ulcer pathogenesis was considered in the past, but interest waned when it was found that duodenal ulcer patients secreted pancreatic bicarbonate at least as rapidly as normal subjects in response to secretin.[47] Furthermore, there is no evidence that pancreatic bicarbonate secretion is important in regulating the acidity of the duodenal bulb, and patients with pancreatic insufficiency do not have an increased incidence of duodenal ulcer.

A resurrection of this hypothesis is currently under way in view of the report that nicotine and smoking reduce pancreatic and biliary bicarbonate secretion in response to endogenous and exogenous secretin.[48] These findings provide a mechanism whereby smoking might increase the incidence of duodenal ulcer. However, there is no convincing evidence that smoking and peptic ulcer are *causally* related, and the data presented so far on the effect of smoking on pancreatic bicarbonate secretion in human subjects are not particularly convincing. Several reports have indicated that smoking decreases gastric acid secretion; if gastric acid and duodenal bicarbonate were reduced equally by smoking, duodenal acidity would not be affected.

ABNORMAL MOTILITY

Abnormal motility might predispose to gastric ulcer in several ways. First, incompetence of the pyloric sphincter would allow bile to reflux into the stomach, produce gastritis, and thus predispose to ulcer. Second, antral hypomotility and stasis might favor the development of gastritis. Third, pyloric spasm (or stenosis) might result in antral distention and potentiate gastrin release. To date, there is no strong support for any of these theories, although it is possible that one or all of these mechanisms may be a contributing factor in selected cases. It is unlikely that abnormal motility is the underlying basic cause of most cases of gastric ulcer.

A good deal of work has been done on gastric emptying in patients with duodenal ulcer. Shay used a barium and water test meal and by X-ray found that patients with duodenal ulcer have rapid gastric emptying.[49] Hunt used test meals of saline, glucose, and glucose plus acid and found that gastric emptying as measured by the serial sampling technique was the same in patients with duodenal ulcer and in normal students.[50] Brömster and colleagues found no difference in ulcer and control subjects in the half-life in the stomach of a liquid test meal (Lundh) as measured by external isotope counting,[51] whereas Griffith et al., using a similar method, found that a meal of porridge, eggs, milk, and bread was emptied more rapidly in duodenal ulcer patients than in control subjects.[52] George reported that by a double sampling technique and water as a test meal, duodenal ulcer and normal subjects have similar rates of gastric emptying.[53] Finally, it was recently reported that buffer emptying after a steak meal is more rapid in patients with duodenal ulcer than in control subjects.[54] The results of these studies are thus contradictory, and it is not definitely established whether duodenal ulcer subjects have normal or increased rates of gastric emptying. It seems best to tentatively conclude that liquid test meals are emptied at a normal rate, but that solid meals are emptied more rapidly in duodenal ulcer patients.

Various mechanisms whereby rapid gastric emptying could contribute to the development of duodenal ulcer have been offered. These include increased force of the gastric juice impinging on the duodenal cap,[55] more rapid delivery of acid into the duodenum,[52] and rapid buffer emptying, reducing the effectiveness by which food buffer can reduce gastric acidity.[54] It should be noted that rapid gastric emptying and gastric hypersecretion could be caused by a single underlying abnormality, such as high vagal tone or high blood level of a substance that stimulates both motility and secretion.

SEX HORMONES

Women have a relatively low incidence of peptic ulcer, especially prior to menopause and during pregnancy.[56] Furthermore, it is rare for a premenopausal woman with a peptic ulcer to sustain a perforation.[55,57] The mechanism by which the female sex and pregnancy protect against ulcer is not clear. At least two studies have shown that estrogen treatment hastens ulcer healing,[58,59] whereas a third study failed to show a difference in treated and untreated groups.[60] Acid and pepsinogen secretion are not decreased by estrogen treatment in humans,[59,61] although it has been suggested that mucus production is increased during such therapy.[59] Acid secretion does not apparently fall significantly during pregnancy.[62] Progesterone given intramuscularly lowered acid secretion modestly in five patients with duodenal ulcer.[59] Estrus in female dogs depresses acid secretion from vagally denervated gastric pouches, suggesting that hormonal changes can influence gastric secretion by a humoral mechanism, at least in this species.[63]

THE ADRENAL GLAND

A popular theory in the 1950's was that the adrenal gland is intimately involved in the pathogenesis of chronic peptic ulcer. This was based upon the claim that corticosteroids increase gastric acid secretion, that these agents are ulcerogenic when used therapeutically, and that peptic ulcer occurs rarely, if at all, in patients with untreated adrenal insufficiency (normal acid secretion is dependent on a normal background of adrenal activity). It was suggested that emotional and other forms of stress acted upon the hypothalamus, caused ACTH release, and thereby stimulated the adrenal cortex to secrete adrenal hormones in excess amounts. These hormones then produced peptic ulcer by increasing gastric acid secretion and/or by reducing mucosal resistance. The theory, therefore, rested on two assumptions: (1) that emotional and other forms of stress are ulcerogenic, and (2) that the ulcerogenic effect of stress is mediated via adrenocortical hormones.[56]

For a number of reasons it seems safe to conclude that this theory is probably not valid. First, although stress may well be ulcerogenic, its effect could be mediated by the vagus nerve as well as hormonally.

Second, it was never established that adrenal hormones in physiological doses influence gastric secretion rate or are ulcerogenic. Indeed, it is questionable whether adrenal steroids are ulcerogenic even in pharmacological doses. Finally, blood corticosteroid concentration and urinary excretion of adrenal hormone metabolites are normal or low in patients with peptic ulcer, but never higher than normal.[56]

Thus there is no convincing evidence that adrenocortical hyperactivity is a cause of chronic gastric or duodenal ulcer. The incidence of peptic ulcer is apparently not increased in patients with Cushing's syndrome.

ENVIRONMENTAL INFLUENCES

Peptic ulcer has become much more prevalent in the past 40 to 50 years. Part of this increase is due to better methods of diagnosis and cure and control of other diseases, but a real increase in ulcer frequency also seems to have occurred. Although this has been attributed variously as being due to anything from increased use of cigarettes to methods of food preparation, the general belief is that it is due mainly to modern civilization with its tendency to dissolve the existing social structures. This would explain why the increased incidence of ulcer is mainly noted in large modern cities, whereas the ulcer rate in rural districts and among primitive races remains relatively low. Only some types of sociopsychological events seem to increase ulcer incidence. For example, ulcer incidence was not increased in frontline German troops in World War II but was high among the services behind the lines. Also, ulcer incidence decreased in concentration camps but increased after liberation from the prisons. Pflanz et al. believe that the common denominator tending to cause ulcer occurrence or recurrence is voluntary exclusion or forced expulsion from a community or group.[64]

Various occupations are said to be associated with a high ulcer incidence. In London, for example, foremen, doctors, and business executives were found to have a high frequency of duodenal ulcer, whereas agricultural workers have a low incidence.[55, 65] However, the results of studies in different cities and countries often conflict, and it is the present writer's conclusion that a generally valid association between occupation and incidence of peptic ulcer has not been demonstrated.

Social class is also thought to affect ulcer incidence. For example, duodenal ulcer is said to be evenly distributed throughout the entire population, but gastric ulcer is seen infrequently in professional groups and is found in excess in the laboring classes. Possibly these social class differences, if they are valid, may be one factor in causing geographical differences in the ratio of duodenal to gastric ulcer.[55]

It is generally believed that ulcer symptoms and complications, especially those caused by duodenal ulcer, exhibit a seasonal periodicity. This impression was confirmed in two recent studies.[66, 67] In 198 patients with duodenal ulcer, Demole and Hecker[66] found that about 73 per cent had a typical periodicity and about 27 per cent were nonperiodic. Of the 73 per cent with periodic symptoms, 36 per cent occurred in the spring, 29 per cent in the fall, 22 per cent in the winter, and only 14 per cent in the summer. These differences were statistically highly significant, tending to prove the validity of *seasonal* periodicity in the 73 per cent of the overall group who exhibited any type of periodic recurrence. Periodic variations, when observed, have been related to climatic conditions, meteorological variations, dietary habits, and emotional strain.

This brief review indicates that environmental and constitutional factors influence ulcer occurrence and recurrence. How these effects are mediated, i.e., via increased acid-pepsin or decreased mucosal resistance, is not at all clear.

HEREDITY

There is a strong familial tendency in duodenal ulcer, and there is evidence that the propensities to develop gastric and duodenal ulcer are independently inherited.[55] Although this might be due to environmental as well as genetic factors, the excellent twin study of Eberhard leaves little doubt that the genetic influence is predominant.[68] In a study of 34 pairs of monozygous and 78 pairs of dizygous twins, one of each pair having been discovered to have a duodenal ulcer, this worker assessed the importance of heredity, environment, and personality in the etiology of ulcer pathogenesis. His analysis assumes that the early environmental influence of twins is similar, whether the twins are monozygous or dizygous, and he reviews evidence to support the validity of this assumption. He found that 50 per cent of the monozygous twins showed concordance for ulcer, whereas only 14 per cent of the dizygous twins were concordant. These results strongly suggest that genetic inheritance is of great importance in the pathogenesis of ulcer. Results of previous twin studies were reviewed; they also show a higher frequency of concordance in monozygous than in dizygous twin pairs, although the ratio was about 2:1 instead of 3.6:1 as found by Eberhard.

How genetic make-up determines ulcer susceptibility is not known, but by definition its effect must be mediated by decreased tissue resistance or increased acid-pepsin secretion. As noted on page 176, there is suggestive but by no means definitive evidence that the rate of acid secretion and the parietal cell mass are under genetic control. The fact that ABO blood groups and secretor status are different in ulcer and control populations suggests the possibility that defective resistance, mediated by qualitatively inferior mucus production, might be a mechanism of genetic influence in the tendency to develop peptic ulcer.

This study suggests that gastric and duodenal ulcer may be inherited together, at least to some extent. Out of 23 dizygous propositi with gastric ulcer, only three were found to have a partner with peptic ulcer, and in all these cases the ulcer was duodenal in location. For five monozygous propositi with gastric ulcer, two partners had ulcer, one duodenal and the other gastric.[68]

PSYCHOSOMATIC FACTORS AND DRUGS

These are judged to be of such great interest and practical significance that they are reviewed in detail on pages 163 to 172 and 642 to 654.

A MODUS OPERANDI FOR CLINICAL USE

Although ulcer pathogenesis is multifactorial and usually not specifically definable in an individual patient, *on a clinical level* it is useful to classify patients into one or more of the following etiological groups. This helps focus a patient's understanding of his disease, aids in therapy, and probably has a good deal of validity.

1. Anxiety and stress-induced.
2. Drug-induced: salicylates, caffeine, alcohol, steroids, other. See pages 642 to 654.
3. Associated with chronic debilitating illness.
4. Familial.
5. Large stomach: peak stimulated secretion rate >60 mEq per hour.
6. Increased secretory drive: basal–peak acid secretion ratio >0.2 (endocrine-induced [elevated gastrin, hypercalcemia] or idiopathic).
7. Decreased resistance: lower than expected rates of acid secretion.
8. No identifiable etiology.

If one wishes to study ulcer pathogenesis in a given patient in greater detail, ABO blood group and secretor status, gastric and duodenal histology (for gastritis and duodenitis), gastric acid absorption rates (as indication of injured mucosa), buffer emptying rate, dose-response curves with histamine or gastrin and studies to evaluate pyloric competence could be employed.

REFERENCES

1. Ellison, E. H., and Wilson, S. D. The Zollinger-Ellison syndrome: Re-appraisal and evaluation of 260 registered cases. Ann. Surg. *160*:512, 1964.
2. Isenberg, J. I., Spector, H., Hootkin, L. A., and Pitcher, J. L. An apparent exception to Schwarz's dictum, "no acid – no ulcer." New Eng. J. Med. *285*:620, 1971.
3. Ivy, A. C., Grossman, M. I., and Bachrach, W. H. Peptic Ulcer. Philadelphia, The Blakiston Co., 1950.
4. Menguy, R. Pathophysiology of peptic ulcer. Amer. J. Surg. *120*:282, 1970.
5. Goldberg, H. I., Dodds, W. J., Gee, S., Montgomery, C., and Zboralske, F. F. Role of acid and pepsin in acute experimental esophagitis. Gastroenterology *56*:223, 1969.
6. Marks, I. N., and Shay, H. Observations on the pathogenesis of gastric ulcer. Lancet *1*:1107, 1959.

7. Oi, M., Oshida, K., and Sugimura, S. The location of gastric ulcer. Gastroenterology *36*:45, 1959.
8. Oi, M., Ito, Y., Kumagai, F., Yoshida, K., Tanaka, Y., Yoshikawa, K., Miho, O., and Kijima, M. A possible dual control mechanism in the origin of peptic ulcer. A study on ulcer location as affected by mucosa and musculature. Gastroenterology *57*:280, 1969.
9. Capper, W. M., Laidlaw, C. D'A., Buckler, K., and Richards, D. The *p*H fields of the gastric mucosa. Lancet *2*:1200, 1962.
10. Barclay, A. E., and Bentley, F. H. The vascularization of the human stomach. A preliminary note on the shunting effect of trauma. Brit. J. Radiol. *22*:62, 1949.
11. Barlow, T. E., Bentley, F. H., and Walder, D. N. Arteries, veins, and arteriovenous anastomoses in the human stomach. Surg. Gynec. Obstet. *93*:657, 1951.
12. Sherman, J. L., Jr., and Palmer, E. D. Hypoxia of vascular origin in the development of gastroduodenal ulcer disease. *In* Pathophysiology of Peptic Ulcer, S. C. Skoryna (ed.). Philadelphia, J. B. Lippincott Co., 1963, p. 339.
13. Leonard, A. S., Gilsdorf, R. B., Pearl, J. M., Peter, E. T., and Ritchie, W. P. Hypothalamic influence on gastric blood flow, cell counts, acid and mucus secretion – factors in ulcer provocation. *In* Gastric Secretion, T. K. Shnitka, J. A. L. Gilbert, and R. C. Harrison (eds.). New York, Pergamon Press, 1967, p. 149.
14. Necheles, H. A theory on the formation of peptic ulcer. Amer. J. Dig. Dis. Nutr. *4*:643, 1937.
15. Jacobson, E. D. (ed.). Symposium on the gastrointestinal circulation. Gastroenterology *52*:327, 1967.
16. Menguy, R. Regulation of gastric mucus secretion. *In* Gastric Secretion, T. K. Shnitka, J. A. L. Gilbert, and R. C. Harrison (eds.). New York, Pergamon Press, 1967, p. 177.
17. Heatley, N. G. Mucosubstance as a barrier to diffusion. Gastroenterology *37*:313, 1959.
18. Hoskins, L. C., and Zamcheck, N. Studies on gastric mucus in health and disease. II. Evidence for a correlation between ABO blood group specificity, ABH (O) secretor status, and the fucose content of the glycoproteins elaborated by the gastric mucosa. Gastroenterology *48*:758, 1965.
19. Curt, J. R. N., and Pringle, R. Viscosity of gastric mucus in duodenal ulceration. Gut *10*:931, 1969.
20. Pringle, R., and Curt, J. R. N. The viscosity of gastric mucus in chronic duodenal ulcer. Gut *12*:418, 1971.
21. Muschel, L. H. Blood groups, disease, and selection. Bact. Rev. *30*:427, 1966.
22. Menguy, R. Gastric mucosal injury by aspirin. Gastroenterology *51*:430, 1966.
23. Symposium on mucus. Gut *12*:417, 1971.
24. Du Plessis, D. J. Pathogenesis of gastric ulceration. Lancet *1*:974, 1965.
25. Leading article. Gastric ulcer and gastritis. Lancet *2*:481, 1966.
26. Delaney, J. P., Cheng, J. W. B., Butler, B. A., and

Ritchie, W. P., Jr. Gastric ulcer and regurgitation gastritis. Gut 11:715, 1970.

27. Gear, M. W. L., Truelove, S. C., and Whitehead, R. Gastric ulcer and gastritis. Gut 12:639, 1971.

28. Capper, W. M. Factors in the pathogenesis of gastric ulcer. Hunterian Lecture delivered at the Royal College of Surgeons of England on 18 January 1966. Ann. Roy. Coll. Surg. Eng. 40:21, 1967.

29. Hurst, A. F., and Venables, J. F. True incidence of hyperchlorhydria in gastric and duodenal ulcer. Guy's Hosp. Rep. 79:249, 1929.

30. Watkinson, G. A study of the changes in pH of gastric contents in peptic ulcer using the twenty-four hour test meal. Gastroenterology 18:377, 1951.

31. Mangus, H. A. In Modern Trends in Gastroenterology, 1st Series, F. Avery Jones (ed.). London, Hoeber, 1952, p. 346.

32. Tanner, N. C. Surgery of peptic ulceration and its complications. Postgrad. Med. J. 30:448, 1954.

33. Mangold, R. Combined gastric and duodenal ulceration: A survey of 157 cases. Brit. Med. J. 2:1193, 1958.

34. Aagaard, P., Andreassen, M., and Kurz, L. Duodenal and gastric ulcer in the same patient. Lancet 1:1111, 1959.

35. Flint, F. J., and Grech, P. Pyloric regurgitation and gastric ulcer. Gut 11:735, 1970.

36. Lawson, H. H. Effect of duodenal contents on the gastric mucosa under experimental conditions. Lancet 1:469, 1964.

37. Altamirano, M. Back-diffusion of H⁺ during gastric secretion. Amer. J. Physiol. 218:1, 1970.

38. Davenport, H. W. Damage to the gastric mucosa: Effects of salicylates and stimulation. Gastroenterology 49:189, 1965.

39. Dyck, W. P., Werther, J. L., Rudick, J., and Janowitz, H. D. Electrolyte movement across canine antral and fundic gastric mucosa. Gastroenterology 56:488, 1969.

40. Davenport, H. W. Back diffusion of acid through the gastric mucosa and its physiological consequences. In Progress in Gastroenterology, Vol. 2, G. B. J. Glass (ed.). London, Grune & Stratton, Inc., 1970, p. 42.

41. Smith, B. M., Skillman, J. J., Edwards, B. G., and Silen, W. Permeability of the human gastric mucosa. Alteration by acetylsalicylic acid and ethanol. New Eng. J. Med. 285:716, 1971.

42. Overholt, B. F., and Pollard, H. M. Acid diffusion into the human gastric mucosa. Gastroenterology 54:182, 1968.

43. Chapman, M. A., Werther, J. L., and Janowitz, H. D. Response of the normal and pathological human gastric mucosa to an instilled acid load. Gastroenterology 55:344, 1968.

44. Max, M., and Menguy, R. Influence of adrenocorticotropin, cortisone, aspirin, and phenylbutazone on the rate of exfoliation and the rate of renewal of gastric mucosal cells. Gastroenterology 58:329, 1970.

45. Malhotra, S. L. A study of the effect of saliva on the concentration of mucin in gastric juice and its possible relationship to the aetiology of peptic ulcer. Gut 8:548, 1967.

46. Wormsley, K. G. Inhibition of gastric acid secretion. Gastroenterology 62:156, 1972.

47. Comfort, M. W., and Osterberg, A. E. External pancreatic secretion in cases of duodenal ulcer. Gastroenterology 4:85, 1945.

48. Solomon, T. E., and Jacobson, E. D. Cigarette smoking and duodenal ulcer disease. New Eng. J. Med. 286:1212, 1972.

49. Shay, H. The pathologic physiology of gastric and duodenal ulcer. Bull. N.Y. Acad. Med. 20:264, 1944.

50. Hunt, J. N. Some notes on the pathogenesis of duodenal ulcer. Amer. J. Dig. Dis. 2:445, 1957.

51. Brömster, D., Carlberger, G., and Lundh, G. Measurement of gastric emptying rate. Lancet 2:224, 1966.

52. Griffith, G. H., Owen, G. M., Campbell, H., and Shields, R. Gastric emptying in health and in gastroduodenal disease. Gastroenterology 54:1, 1968.

53. George, J. D. Gastric acidity and motility. Amer. J. Dig. Dis. 13:376, 1968.

54. Fordtran, J. S., and Walsh, J. H. Gastric acid secretion rate and buffer content of the stomach after eating. J. Clin. Invest. 52, 1973, in press.

55. Jones, F. A. Clinical and social problems of peptic ulcer. Brit. Med. J. 1:719, 1957.

56. Crean, G. P. The endocrine system and the stomach. Vitam. Horm. 21:215, 1963.

57. Clark, D. H. Peptic ulcer in women. Brit. Med. J. 1:1254, 1953.

58. Truelove, S. C. Stilboesterol, phenobarbitone and diet in chronic duodenal ulcer. Brit. Med. J. 2:559, 1960.

59. Parbhoo, S. P., and Johnston, I. D. A. Effects of oestrogens and progestogens on gastric secretion in patients with duodenal ulcer. Gut 7:612, 1966.

60. Connell, A. M., Fletcher, J., Jones, J. H., Langman, M. J. S., Leonard Jones, J. E., and Pygott, F. Oestrogens and high protein and high carbohydrate diets in the treatment of duodenal ulcer (abstract). Gut 7:717, 1966.

61. Kaufmann, H. J., and Spiro, H. M. Estrogens and gastric secretion. Gastroenterology 54:913, 1968.

62. Clark, D. H., and Tankel, H. I. Gastric acid and plasma-histaminase during pregnancy. Lancet 2:886, 1954.

63. Landon, J. H., and Wild, R. A. Oestrus and gastric secretion in the dog. Gut 11:855, 1970.

64. Pflanz, M., Rosenstein, E., and von Uexküll, T. Socio-psychological aspects of peptic ulcer. J. Psychosomatic Res. 1:68, 1956.

65. Welsh, J. D., and Wolf, S. Geographical and environmental aspect of peptic ulcer. Amer. J. Med. 24:754, 1960.

66. Demole, M. J., and Hecker, G. Seasonal periodicity of duodenal ulcer. A statistical study. Gastroenterologica 105:82, 1966.

67. Gardiner, G. C., Pinsky, W., and Myerson, R. M. The seasonal incidence of peptic ulcer activity. Fact or fancy? Amer. J. Gastroent. 45:22, 1966.

68. Eberhard, G. Peptic ulcer in twins. A study in personality, heredity, and environment. Acta Psychiat. Scand. 44:Suppl. 205, 1968.

Chapter 52

Drugs and Peptic Ulceration

Allan R. Cooke

INTRODUCTION

The frequent concurrence of peptic ulcer, a common disease, and the use of various common drugs has led to the general impression that certain drugs increase the incidence of peptic ulcer in man. This impression is often the result of a general tendency to extrapolate valid experimental evidence of drugs causing gastric ulceration in animals to human subjects. This type of evidence is useful and the inference is often helpful, but the degree to which it is relevant in man is often not examined critically. The evidence for an ulcerogenic effect in man has usually rested on data of experimental production of ulcers in animals, of an effect on a mechanism suspected of participating in the pathogenesis of a peptic ulcer, and of a temporal relationship with manifestation of an ulcer or reactivation of a previous ulcer. Rarely, evidence of differences in ulcer incidence in a treated and controlled population has been provided.

All the drugs to be discussed, with the possible exception of ethanol, cause gastric lesions (erosions or ulcer) in animals and thus can be considered ulcerogenic. Reviews dealing with dosage, method of administration, and animal species for most of the drugs (corticosteroids, salicylates, phenylbutazone, reserpine, caffeine) have been published and will not be discussed further here.[1-3] Indomethacin

causes gastric ulceration in the dog,[4] and nicotine does so in the rat.[5]

The aim of this chapter is to review the evidence associating certain drugs with chronic peptic ulcer and gastric damage.

FREQUENCY OF PEPTIC ULCER IN THE GENERAL POPULATION°

To determine whether drugs cause peptic ulceration it is necessary to know the frequency of the disease in the general population. The definitive study of this type was done by Doll and colleagues[6] in a field survey of about 6000 workers living in London. The incidence of peptic ulcer between age 15 and age 64 when corrected for age and sex was 5.8 per cent for men and 1.9 per cent for women. The highest incidence was 9.6 per cent in men 45 to 54 years old, and 6.1 per cent for women 55 years old or older. Many had little disability from this ulcer. In a survey of the literature, it was stated that "from 5 per cent to 10 per cent of most populations develop an ulcer in a lifetime, [and] that the total incidence of those afflicted at any one annual survey will vary from 1 per

---

°The term frequency is used to include incidence and prevalence rates. The incidence rate is the number of new cases occurring annually, and the prevalence rate is the number of cases of the disease present at one moment in time. Both are often expressed per 100,000 population or as a percentage.

642

cent to 3 per cent of the population above 20 years of age...."[7]

Blumenthal gathered data from a variety of sources in the United States (Selective Service examinations, autopsies, and health insurance plans) and derived an average prevalence rate for peptic ulcer of 25 per 1000 adults per year.[8]

The frequency of peptic ulcer estimated by autopsy data can be misleading. Hospital populations differ from one area to another, and interest of the pathologist is another important factor. Frequently, statistical principles are ignored, and all lesions from varying age groups are expressed as a single percentage without regard for age distribution of the ulcers found or the autopsy population at risk. Watkinson[9] was fully aware of these inadequacies and reduced these defects in his study. All autopsies performed over a 20-year period (1930–1949) at the University of Leeds were analyzed retrospectively by one expert observer under whose supervision they had been performed. A second, concurrent investigation of the incidence of ulcers at eleven teaching and seven nonteaching hospitals in London, Oxford, Newcastle, Bristol, Birmingham, Manchester, Leeds, York, and Glasgow was undertaken in 1956, so that it was possible to estimate the national and regional frequency of peptic ulcer. Watkinson's conclusions were that the best estimate of ulcer frequency from the national survey was 8.3 per cent for men and 3.9 per cent for women and for the Leeds study was 14.2 per cent for men and 7.7 per cent for women. Watkinson stated that the excellent care taken by the Leeds autopsy staff "makes it likely that these figures (i.e., the Leeds) approximate more nearly the true ulcer frequency in the population as a whole." He also noted a uniform pattern of the frequency of peptic ulcer in three cities, Leeds, Rotterdam, and Stockholm.

These studies give a reasonable estimate of the frequency of peptic ulcer in the general population. The difficulty in obtaining these data is obvious. Estimates of the incidence of peptic ulceration in patients with various chronic diseases — e.g., rheumatoid arthritis, ulcerative colitis, collagen diseases — have been little better than guesses. Since these are the diseases for which salicylates, corticosteroids, in-domethacin, and other drugs are given, it is important to know the frequency of peptic ulcer in this population.

FREQUENCY OF PEPTIC ULCER IN PATIENTS WITH CHRONIC DISEASES

Estimates have varied of the frequency of peptic ulceration in patients with rheumatoid arthritis before the introduction of corticosteroids. Values of 4.5 per cent[10] and 6 to 8 per cent[11] have been suggested. Bowen et al.[12] found that 3.3 per cent of 830 patients with rheumatoid arthritis had a peptic ulcer when assessed at the Mayo Clinic in 1947. During the period from 1954 to 1957 at the same clinic, an incidence of 8.1 per cent was reported for 877 patients with rheumatoid arthritis not receiving corticosteroids. Whether this change was due to increasing frequency, better diagnosis, or use of other drugs is pure speculation. Gibberd[13] did an interesting retrospective study on the incidence of dyspepsia and peptic ulceration in 533 patients with rheumatoid arthritis. He found that 3.4 per cent of the patients complained of dyspepsia before the onset of rheumatoid arthritis, whereas 15.9 per cent had it after the onset. Independent of drug therapy, the frequency of dyspepsia was estimated to range from 6.4 to 15.9 per cent. He found that 2 per cent of 533 patients had peptic ulceration before and 3.7 per cent after the onset of rheumatoid arthritis, at which time they were receiving salicylates, corticosteroids, and phenylbutazone.

Peptic ulceration was found in 4 per cent of 600 patients with Crohn's disease attending the Mayo Clinic.[14] Recently in a series of 300 patients with Crohn's disease, the reported incidence of peptic ulceration was 8 per cent.[15] It was interesting that 4 per cent of 124 patients receiving corticosteroids developed peptic ulceration. If these figures are taken at face value, one could conclude that corticosteroids protect against the development of peptic ulceration in patients with Crohn's disease.

These types of reports may indicate approximately the frequency of peptic ulceration in special groups of patients reporting to clinics for assessment and treatment of their disease, but give no indication as to the overall frequency of either the disease or associated peptic ulceration in the general population. Furthermore, the association of two common diseases may occur by chance alone if the population sample is not representative of the general population.[16] Finally, in nearly all studies corrections for age, sex, geographical location, and social class have been ignored, and thus the sample groups are not representative of the general population.

Since good estimates are not available of the frequency of peptic ulceration in diseases in which the ulcerogenic drugs are commonly used, this author has assumed that the incidence in these various chronic diseases is at least that in the normal population. On the basis of the studies just described, the frequency of peptic ulceration will be assumed to be about 8 to 14 per cent for men and 4 to 8 per cent for women. These figures probably underestimate the incidence in the population with chronic illnesses, but they are the best estimates that can be made with the data available.

Both retrospective and prospective studies have been used to show an association between peptic ulcer and ulcerogenic drugs. Retrospective studies have been of two types: those without controls, which indicate that an association may exist but do little else; and those designed with both control and test groups. The difficulty is to find suitable controls. A prospective, controlled study is the ideal, but there have been very few of these.

The literature on ulcerogenic drugs is interspersed with case reports suggesting a cause-and-effect relationship. Although these are useful to draw attention to the problem, little weight can be given them unless they are reported as part of a population receiving the drug so that some estimate of incidence can be made. With a disease as common as peptic ulcer, an isolated case report of ingestion of an ulcerogenic drug and subsequent development of a peptic ulcer is very difficult to interpret.

With these difficulties in mind, the evidence relating peptic ulceration and ulcerogenic drugs will be considered for each drug.

EVIDENCE OF ASSOCIATION BETWEEN DRUGS AND PEPTIC ULCER

CORTICOSTEROIDS

It has been held for some time that the "steroid ulcer" was relatively painless ("silent"), developed rapidly, and often presented with complications such as perforation.[17] The "steroid ulcer" was described radiologically as being shallow, often multiple, and usually located in the pyloric antrum. It was described macroscopically as being pliable with little fibrous reaction.[17]

The basis for an entity, steroid ulcer, has been questioned. Garb and coworkers[18] examined the records of 1084 patients who underwent gastric resection for gastric ulcer and found 57 (5.6 per cent) who had received adrenal corticosteroids; in about half (23 patients) of these 57, the ulcer was thought to be directly attributable to the corticosteroids. Twenty-three patients who had undergone gastric resection for benign gastric ulcer but had not received corticosteroids were selected as control subjects and were matched as far as possible for sex, age, location, and use of salicylates.

The authors found neither specific radiological differences between the two groups nor correlation with duration or dosage of corticosteroids. Multiple ulcers occurred equally in both groups, and differences in size were not found. Finally, the steroid ulcers were similar histologically to those controls. It appears that the steroid ulcer in man is identical to the nonsteroid ulcer.

Studies of the relationship between corticosteroids and peptic ulceration can be considered as follows:

RETROSPECTIVE STUDIES

Patients with Diseases Other Than Rheumatoid Arthritis. In a literature survey in 1954, Sandweiss[19] found 980 patients with various diseases who were receiving corticosteroids for long or short periods. He found 34 new or reactivated peptic ulcers, a prevalence of 3.5 per cent.

In a comprehensive, critical survey of the literature in 1967, Cooke[20] found in nine studies a total of 1699 patients with asthma, ophthalmic diseases, various allergic disorders, dermatoses, malabsorption syndrome, ulcerative colitis, and various pediatric conditions who had received corticosteroids. Only six instances of peptic ulceration were recorded, a prevalence of 0.3 per cent (range zero to 1.1 per cent). In a recent study,[15] 4 per cent of 124 patients with Crohn's disease receiving corticosteroids were found to have a peptic ulcer. It was suggested by Cooke[20] that corticosteroids did not increase the incidence of peptic ulceration, a view confirmed in a recent survey.[21] However, a firm conclusion is not justified on the basis of these reports, because the studies were from selected groups of patients and no control groups of any kind were studied.

Patients with Rheumatoid Arthritis. Cooke[20] reviewed 23 separate studies (containing two previous surveys) with a total of 4278 patients, in whom 286 had a peptic ulcer attributed to corticosteroids. This is a prevalence of 6.7 per cent (range, zero to 38.4 per cent) and not greater than the figure stated above for the frequency in the general population. For the vast majority of the patients (3796 in 16 studies) the range was zero to 7.5 per cent. In all the studies with the exception of that of Kern et al.,[22] virtually no attempt was made to assess the role of other potentially ulcerogenic drugs. Very few patients had radiological studies or endoscopic examinations, and rarely was a pretreatment control X-ray done.

In the study by Kern et al.,[22] 21 of 169 patients with rheumatoid arthritis were found to have a peptic ulcer, a prevalence of 12.5 per cent (18.2 per cent for males, 8.7 per cent for females). Some patients were receiving acetylsalicylic acid or phenylbutazone as well as corticosteroids. It was estimated that 4 per cent of the patients had developed a peptic ulcer directly attributable to corticosteroids. This study suggests that patients with rheumatoid arthritis may have an increased incidence of peptic ulceration, but whether this was due to corticosteroids, to other drugs, or to unknown causes is unresolved.

PROSPECTIVE STUDIES

There have been a few prospective studies. Sherwood and coworkers, using radiological examinations every three to four months, followed for 17 to 28 months 24 patients with allergic diseases treated with triamcinolone (2 to 16 mg daily).[23] Peptic ulcer was not found in any patient. Meltzer et al. studied two groups of patients, one consisting of 55 patients (Group 1, 35 of whom had rheumatoid arthritis) taking long-term prednisone (average dose, 14 mg. per day) and the other consisting of 60 patients (Group 2, 36 of whom had rheumatoid arthritis) who were to be treated with corticosteroids.[24] All the patients in Group 2 were assessed clinically and radiologically before starting corticosteroids. In Group 1, six patients (10.9 per cent) were found to have a peptic ulcer and in two of them it became active during therapy. In Group 2, six patients (10 per cent) were found to have a peptic ulcer, but there was no evidence for the development of a new ulcer or reactivity of an old ulcer upon X-ray examination five months later. These two studies indicate that corticosteroids in moderate doses do not cause peptic ulcer.[23, 24]

In two widely quoted radiological studies in patients with rheumatoid arthritis treated with corticosteroids and other ulcerogenic drugs, the prevalence of peptic ulceration was 19 and 31 per cent, respectively.[25, 26] In both studies pretreatment baseline X-ray studies were not done; thus it is impossible to implicate corticosteroids or other ulcerogenic drugs as the cause for the high prevalence of peptic ulceration. Furthermore, many patients presented atypically, and thus the radiological findings should have been confirmed by other methods. These two studies do suggest, however, that patients with rheumatoid arthritis have a higher prevalence of peptic ulceration than the general population, thus confirming the findings of Kern et al.[22] Recently, Strickland and coworkers gave 20 mg per day of prednisone to 14 healthy subjects and compared them with a control group. No ulcers were found on X-ray examinations one month later.[27]

In the studies reviewed it was difficult to determine whether dose was a determining factor in developing a "steroid ulcer." In general, in animal studies with ulcerogenic drugs, the development of an ulcer is dose related. It was not obvious that this was so in the studies in man.

The question of whether corticosteroids

interfere with the healing of chronic peptic ulcers has not been investigated. There is adequate evidence that corticosteroids do interfere with the healing of experimental ulcers,[1] and it would seem reasonable that this may be its effect in man.

In summary, from the prospective and retrospective studies it is concluded that patients with rheumatoid arthritis probably have a higher frequency of peptic ulceration, the cause of which is unclear. Corticosteroids in moderate doses (there is little evidence for high doses) do not increase the incidence of peptic ulceration.

SALICYLATES

The salicylate in common use is aspirin, and studies relating this to peptic ulcer will be discussed. Aspirin is well documented as causing occult bleeding and acute gastric erosions, but there is little evidence to suggest that it causes peptic ulceration.[28, 29]

It was not until the study by Douglas and Johnston in Australia that there was evidence indicating a relationship between aspirin ingestion and chronic peptic ulceration.[30] During three and one-half years they observed that 55 of 77 patients admitted with chronic gastric ulcer had been chronically ingesting a proprietary compound containing aspirin, phenacetin, and caffeine (APC). A similar association, which applied particularly to women with gastric ulcer, was later reported from the same country.[31] No control subjects were studied in either instance.

In case-controlled studies, Gillies and Skyring examined various social and environmental factors in peptic ulcer. In their first study[32] of inpatients in a Sydney hospital (100 patients with gastric ulcer, 50 with duodenal ulcer, and 25 with gastric cancer, with age- and sex-matched controls) they found that patients with gastric ulcer smoked more $(P < 0.001)$, ingested more APC $(P < 0.001)$, and had more marital disharmony, more divorce, and lower educational attainment than their controls. No association was found for ethanol consumption and peptic ulceration. The consumption of other drugs (indomethacin, steroids, phenylbutazone) was not different in controls and ulcer patients. This study suggested a relationship between the development of peptic ulcer and smoking and APC consumption.

In their second study, the association of APC ingestion, smoking, and family history of ulcer was examined in a working population in the Sydney area.[33] They confirmed their previous findings. Among subjects with gastric ulcers there were more APC taken $(P < 0.001)$, more smokers $(P < 0.001)$, and more persons with a family history of ulcer $(P < 0.05)$ than expected if the ulcer and nonulcer populations were homogeneous. Family history of ulcers $(P < 0.05)$ and smoking $(P < 0.01)$ were both associated with duodenal ulcer. Using morbidity ratios (observed–expected frequency times 100), they found that smoking was more strongly associated with gastric ulcer but very weakly with duodenal ulcer. A positive family history of ulcer was associated with gastric and duodenal ulcer to the same degree.

These studies imply that smoking, family history, and APC ingestion are strongly associated with the development of a peptic ulcer, particularly gastric ulcer. This is good evidence for the ulcerogenic role of smoking and APC in a population in the Eastern states of Australia, but it is difficult to decide which factor is preeminent. It is likely that aspirin (or phenacetin and caffeine) is ulcerogenic, but the data do not allow a firm conclusion. Phenacetin and caffeine are unproved to be ulcerogenic per se in man, but may well be when combined with aspirin. Smoking appears to be an important factor.

SMOKING

One of the early studies of an association between smoking and peptic ulceration was that by Doll and coworkers.[34] They studied the smoking habits of 327 patients with gastric ulcers, 338 patients with duodenal ulcers, and 1143 control subjects with diseases unrelated to smoking and matched for age, sex, and type of place of residence. For both sexes the proportion of nonsmokers was smaller in the ulcer groups than in the corresponding control groups: gastric ulcer, men 1.3 per cent against 4.7 per cent, women 51.1 per cent against 66.8 per cent; duodenal ulcer, men 2.1 per cent against 5.8 per cent, women 53.7 per cent against 62.0 per cent. In the case of gastric ulcer the differences were statistically significant for both sexes, but with duodenal ulcer significant differences were found for men only.

These studies were extended to examine the effect of smoking on the healing of gastric ulcers in inpatients. It was found that the ulcer niche diminished in size by two-thirds in 30 of 40 patients who were advised to stop smoking as against 23 of 40 who were not so advised. The average reduction in size of the ulcer niche was 78.1 per cent (stopping smoking) and 56.6 per cent (continued smoking).[34]

This study provides strong evidence that smoking may be a factor in the production or maintenance (delayed healing) of a peptic ulcer. Other data supporting this conclusion were presented by Doll and Hill,[35] who found that death from peptic ulcer among medical practitioners in Great Britain was lowest among nonsmokers (no ulcer deaths), and increased with the amount of tobacco smoked. The total number of deaths was small (21 deaths), and not statistically significant. Results from two other studies have indicated that smoking was associated with an increase in deaths from gastric ulcer, but there was conflicting evidence for duodenal ulcer.[36,37]

Brown and colleagues studied about 1000 men aged 60 to 69 and recorded their smoking history.[38] The prevalence of peptic ulcer increased from 6.6 per cent among nonsmokers to 8.3 per cent among smokers of 1 to 9 cigarettes per day; to 9.2 per cent (10 to 19 cigarettes per day); and to 13 per cent (20 or more cigarettes per day). Smoking was considered unlikely to be a direct cause of peptic ulcer by Doll and co-workers, because the consumption of cigarettes "has increased in Britain over the past two or three decades, while the incidence of gastric ulcer is thought to have diminished. . . . Furthermore the distribution of gastric ulcer mortality throughout the world . . . is quite unlike the distribution of tobacco-smoking."[34]

Smoking probably interferes with the healing of gastric ulcer and thus maintains its chronicity, but probably is not a direct causal agent. When considered in relation to the data from Australia concerning aspirin ingestion,[32,33] smoking plus aspirin may be more ulcerogenic than either alone.

INDOMETHACIN

Indomethacin was introduced into clinical medicine about 1963. Hart and Boardman in a study of 123 patients with various rheumatic diseases found no occurrence of peptic ulcer in periods of up to one year follow-up.[39] Lövgren and Allander reported three exacerbations of peptic ulcer and two new peptic ulcers among 18 patients with rheumatoid arthritis receiving indomethacin for six months.[40] In 1968, Taylor et al. reported nine new ulcers and one exacerbation of a pre-existing ulcer in patients with rheumatoid arthritis.[41] The number of patients followed was not given, pretreatment barium meal X-rays were not done, and some patients were receiving other drugs as well.

Lockie and Norcross found 14 peptic ulcers in a series of 180 patients, a prevalence of 7.8 per cent.[42] However, only six of the 14 developed a new ulcer (3.3 per cent), the other eight having had pre-existing ulcer disease. Furthermore, 11 of the 14 patients had received salicylates or corticosteroids. Katz et al. found six ulcers (one pre-existing) in 97 patients with rheumatoid arthritis, a prevalence rate of 6 per cent.[43]

The study by Rothernich is of interest because it was prospective.[44] He followed 216 patients (mainly with rheumatoid arthritis) receiving indomethacin for periods up to 30 months. Barium meals were given to 12 patients at random, all of whom had dyspepsia. Gastrointestinal symptoms occurred in 25 per cent of the patients, but most had a prior history and about three-fourths were receiving other drugs. Ten of the 216 patients receiving indomethacin and other drugs developed a peptic ulcer (four exacerbations of a pre-existing ulcer), a prevalence rate of 4.6 per cent and an incidence rate of 2.8 per cent. Two of 74 patients receiving only indomethacin developed an ulcer, an incidence of 2.7 per cent. Thus the incidence of peptic ulcer as a result of indomethacin therapy was between 2.7 and 2.8 per cent. These figures are similar to the incidence of peptic ulcer in the general population. Furthermore, even with correction for age and sex and other factors (these were not given), it is doubtful whether indomethacin was ulcerogenic in this study.

The paucity of reports and complete lack of prospective studies of indomethacin ingestion with matched controls make it impossible to decide whether indomethacin is ulcerogenic. What evidence that is available from five studies (634 patients, 35 new or reactivated ulcers) indicates a prevalence of 5.5 per cent (a maximal figure). This figure is no greater than that given for the frequency in the general population.

PHENYLBUTAZONE

This author is not aware of any controlled prospective studies examining the relationship between phenylbutazone and peptic ulceration, and thus all data are retrospective.

Mauer, in 1955, in a survey of 23 publications containing 3934 patients, found 40 patients in whom gastric complications occurred (1 per cent); there were 22 patients with acute peptic ulcers (0.6 per cent) and 18 patients with exacerbations of pre-existing ulcers.[45] This evidence indicates that peptic ulceration is a doubtful complication of phenylbutazone. In the study by Kern and coworkers,[22] two of 40 males (5 per cent) and five of 67 females (7.5 per cent) with rheumatoid arthritis were identified as receiving phenylbutazone and developing a peptic ulcer. Kuzell et al. reported that of 200 patients with gout receiving phenylbutazone over 30 months, none were found to have a peptic ulcer, although seven complained of epigastric pain.[46] Since the review by Mauer, only a few isolated case reports have appeared in the literature. A review of the subject in 1963[1] added little to the evidence obtained by Mauer. In the most recent study,[47] in which 562 patients (about 50 per cent with rheumatoid arthritis) were treated for two to ten years (mean, 4.1 years) with daily doses of 100 to 800 mg (mostly < 200 mg daily), only three patients developed a peptic ulcer. Gastrointestinal symptoms occurred in 25 patients, ten of whom were X-rayed and found to have a normal stomach.

These studies indicate that peptic ulceration is probably not a complication of phenylbutazone.

RESERPINE

In a review in 1959, and from his own experience, Bachrach concluded that reserpine was not responsible for peptic ulceration.[48] At that time reserpine had been in general use for four years, and Bachrach found only ten patients reported in eight publications in whom peptic ulcer was attributed to reserpine. One of the series reviewed was that of Hollister, who found three instances of gastrointestinal bleeding without peptic ulcer in 600 patients receiving psychiatric doses of reserpine.[49] Drenick observed no adverse effects over 30 days when giving reserpine, 0.25 mg three times a day, to ten ulcer patients.[50] In his review, Kirsner mentioned isolated case reports, but concluded that the incidence of peptic ulcer was low.[3]

It seems very doubtful that reserpine is ulcerogenic in man.

CAFFEINE AND ETHANOL

This author is unaware of any evidence directly implicating caffeine or ethanol as a cause of peptic ulcer in man. Reviews by Roth[51] and Kirsner[3] did not implicate caffeine as a cause of peptic ulceration. No evidence is available implicating ethanol as being ulcerogenic.

EVIDENCE OF DAMAGING EFFECTS OF DRUGS ON THE STOMACH IN MAN

CHANGES IN THE GASTRIC MUCOSAL BARRIER

Davenport has indicated that the stomach has a barrier to the absorption of hydrogen ion and that this can be disrupted by various agents, so that there is a loss of hydrogen ion from and a gain of sodium into the stomach lumen.[52] In animal studies it has been found that with this disruption of the barrier, the electrical potential difference (PD) decreases.[53, 54]

Geall and coworkers instilled aspirin and ethanol into the stomachs of volunteer subjects and caused a marked fall in the PD which was used as an index of a

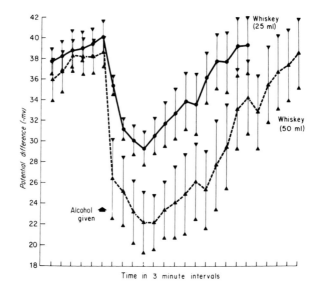

Figure 52–1. Effect of alcohol on PD of human gastric mucosa. Mucosa negative to peripheral blood (mean ± SE, n = 7). (From Geall, M. G., et al.: Gastroenterology 58:437, 1970.)

change in the barrier (Fig. 52–1).[55] As yet, the effects of other drugs have not been tested.

OCCULT BLOOD LOSS (MICROBLEEDING)

Normal subjects lose up to 1.5 ml blood daily when studied by the Cr[51]-labeled red cell technique. Most subjects (over 70 per cent) when given about 2 g of unbuffered aspirin daily for three days will increase this fecal blood loss to a mean value of about 3 to 5 ml per day.[56, 57] Within individual subjects this increased blood loss is reproducible.[58] Buffering the aspirin to maintain a neutral pH so that acetylsalicylate ion is formed and no hydrogen ions are present in the stomach results in virtually no gastric absorption of aspirin[59] and no detectable increase in normal occult bleeding.[60, 61]

Ethanol did not cause occult bleeding when given as 180 ml of whiskey (31.8 per cent weight per volume) on each of three days[62] or as 140 ml of cocktail (40 per cent weight per volume) for one day.[61] However, when combined with unbuffered aspirin, ethanol increased significantly the blood loss induced by the unbuffered aspirin.[62]

Scott and coworkers examined fecal blood loss in 83 patients with rheumatoid arthritis or miscellaneous diseases, and 13 normal volunteers after ingestion of salicy-lates, corticosteroids, and phenylbutazone.[63] The doses were 2 to 6 g per day of salicylates, 5 to 20 mg per day of prednisolone or its equivalent, and 200 to 400 mg per day of phenylbutazone. They found that salicylates caused occult bleeding in 70 per cent of their patients (mean loss was 4.9 ml per day). Two patients in 44 patient trials receiving corticosteroids increased their fecal blood loss; one had a gastric ulcer and the other may have bled from preceding aspirin. Two patients of 22 studied bled in response to phenylbutazone; one was probably due to preceding aspirin ingestion; blood loss in the other was just above normal (2.3 ml per day).

Wanka et al. compared fecal blood loss in response to unbuffered aspirin and indomethacin (200 to 250 mg per day) in 13 patients with rheumatic diseases.[64] They found that of 12 patients tested, 11 bled in response to aspirin (range, 3 to 18 ml per day, mean = 5.9 ml per day), whereas with indomethacin, eight did not bleed and five bled (range 2 to 4 ml per day, mean = 1.2 ml per day).

These studies indicate that unbuffered aspirin will reproducibly (> 70 per cent population) cause occult bleeding, whereas ethanol, corticosteroids, and phenylbutazone probably do not do so. Indomethacin causes a mild increase in occult bleeding much less than in response to unbuffered aspirin.

EROSIONS OR ACUTE GASTRITIS

Although there are isolated case reports of some ulcerogenic drugs causing acute erosions or acute gastritis, they are difficult to evaluate. It is unlikely that phenylbutazone, caffeine, or reserpine causes acute gastritis or erosions in man, but no firm conclusions are warranted. It is interesting that in a group of patients and normal subjects treated with prednisone (20 to 40 mg per day) and followed with gastric biopsies for 14 weeks, some with atrophic gastritis showed regeneration of the gastric glands, whereas no change was found in normal subjects and those with superficial gastritis. These findings were confirmed in another study.[27] The point is that corticosteroids did not cause gastritis or erosions.[27, 65]

Unbuffered aspirin is well documented by gastroscopy as a cause of acute erosions in man.[66-68] Highly buffered aspirin does not cause acute erosions.[68]

When taken in excessive quantities (to drunkenness), ethanol caused acute gastritis and gastric erosions documented by gastroscopy and biopsy.[69] The changes were reversible and the mucosa returned to normal by seven to 20 days.[69] The evidence available suggests that this type of acute gastritis does not go on to chronic gastritis.[70, 71]

HEMATEMESIS OR MELENA (MACROBLEEDING)

There has been no systematic study of an association between corticosteroids, phenylbutazone, reserpine, caffeine, or smoking and the occurrence of upper gastrointestinal bleeding. However, there have been a number of studies in which the association of overt bleeding with unbuffered aspirin ingestion was examined.

Recent reviews have been written by Salter,[72] Cooke,[70] and Langman,[73] whose review is most detailed and informative.

From the evidence above, the lesions one would expect to find in those patients said to have bled as a result of unbuffered aspirin ingestion would be acute erosions. If the erosions were situated such that a large vessel was involved, overt bleeding would be expected to occur.

On this basis therefore one would expect on epidemiological data that if aspirin were a cause of hematemesis or melena, the lesions found most commonly would be gastric erosions (if gastroscopy or a normal, i.e., negative, barium meal X-ray examination were performed).

The data appear to confirm this prediction. There is a greater association of aspirin ingestion in those with acute erosions than in those with chronic peptic ulceration.[74-77] Parry and Wood[74] found that in 637 general admissions, 542 patients did not bleed and 32 per cent of these took aspirin. Of the 95 who had hematemesis or melena, 69 per cent gave a history of having taken aspirin within seven days. Of these 95 patients, 45 were found to have a chronic peptic ulcer (22 took aspirin, 23 did not) and 35 had erosions (of these, 33 took aspirin).

It is very difficult to interpret the evidence associating aspirin with overt gastrointestinal bleeding. The ideal (and almost impossible) study would be a prospective case-controlled study of documented aspirin intake and subsequent gastrointestinal bleeding. To date, such a study has not been designed and so the evidence rests on retrospective studies.

Retrospective studies have been of two types: studies without controls which indicate that the association is worthy of further investigation, and studies with a control and test group. Although finding suitable controls would seem a simple problem, this has not proved to be the case.

The types of controls selected by eight groups of investigators have borne out these difficulties (Table 52–1).[74, 76-82] The use of a patient in the right-hand bed[76, 78] would include patients who may have a stroke or some other cause of memory loss, just as the study by Brown and Mitchell[81] may have included some control neurological patients who may have taken aspirin. Dyspeptic outpatients[79] as control subjects would include people warned against salicylates by their referring doctor. Even general medical admissions may be unsatisfactory, because Parry and Wood[74] found that 25 per cent of their control patients admitted with gastrointestinal, cardiovascular, hematological, and neurological disorders took aspirin, whereas 50 per cent of the remainder of controls gave a positive history.

TABLE 52–1. COMPARISON OF ASPIRIN INGESTION IN CONTROL AND TEST GROUP (HEMATEMESIS OR MELENA) IN EIGHT STUDIES

REFERENCE	CONTROL GROUP	No. PATIENTS	ASPIRIN	%	TEST GROUP	No. PATIENTS	ASPIRIN	%
Kelly, 1956	Myocardial infarction	100	4	4	GI bleeding	49	16	33
Muir and Cossar, 1955	Right hand bed	–	–	5	" "	166	73	44
Muir and Cossar, 1959	Right hand bed	106	17	16	" "	106	57	54
Alvarez and Summerskill, 1958	Dyspeptic outpatients	103	17	16	" "	103	55	53
Lange, 1957	General medical admissions	31	7	23	" "	96	43	45
Parry and Wood, 1967	General medical admissions	542	174	32	" "	95	65	68
Brown and Mitchell, 1956	Medical, surgical, gynecological, and neurological patients	100	40	40	" "	70	36	51
Allibone and Flint, 1958	Nonthoracic surgical or accident patients	129	59	46	" "	129	61	47

Thus there are difficulties in choosing suitable controls, and the incidence of aspirin ingestion as indicated in Table 52–1 varies from 4 to 46 per cent, an 11-fold variation. Langman[73] attempted to standardize results by comparing four studies[74, 76, 79, 81] in which data were given about aspirin ingestion 48 hours before admission. He found that the aspirin and bleeding groups had a range of 51 to 58 per cent, but by contrast the control groups still showed a twofold range (11 to 26 per cent).

Added to these difficulties are the following problems in history taking: (1) During the course of a medical or surgical catastrophe, patients may forget that they took a simple remedy such as aspirin. (2) It is difficult to determine if aspirin was taken for symptoms of bleeding, e.g., malaise, abdominal discomfort, or whether the symptoms of bleeding occurred after aspirin ingestion. (3) Most of the studies have been done in Great Britain. Banks and Baron, writing in Lancet, indicated that in 1964 there were 300 commercial preparations containing aspirin.[83] Unless patient and doctor knew this list, a positive history of aspirin ingestion may have been missed.

In recent study of hematemesis and melena, Schiller and coworkers found that in three five-year periods the incidence of admission to hospital for upper gastrointestinal bleeding was constant, whereas the ingestion of drugs (mainly aspirin) in the third quinquennium was four times that in the first.[84] If aspirin was a significant cause for admission to hospital with upper gastrointestinal bleeding, then it would be expected that the incidence would not have remained constant in the face of increased aspirin ingestion.

In summary, there is a great deal of evidence of an association between aspirin ingestion and overt upper gastrointestinal bleeding. This association is strongest for bleeding caused by gastric erosions. The lack of satisfactory control groups and difficulties in history taking do not allow a firm conclusion.

PATHOGENESIS

As indicated in the preceding discussion, there is inadequate evidence in man to indicate that corticosteroids, indomethacin, phenylbutazone, caffeine, reserpine, and ethanol are ulcerogenic. There is evidence that aspirin (given as a mixture containing phenacetin and caffeine) and smoking may be ulcerogenic. If these drugs are to be considered ulcerogenic in man, it is necessary to consider how they may induce peptic ulceration.

There are a number of theories about the mechanisms by which drugs may cause peptic ulceration. In general terms, these drugs may result in a stimulation of acid output or a change in the mucosal defense mechanisms.

STIMULATION OF ACID SECRETION

Caffeine is a moderately strong stimulant of acid secretion in man.[85, 86] Adrenal corticosteroids are mild stimulants of acid secretion.[27, 87] Phenylbutazone[3] was found to cause mild stimulation of basal secretion in about half the subjects tested. Indomethacin was not found to alter gastric secretion.[88] Reserpine in a single dose stimulates acid secretion but in repeated doses does not.[89] Aspirin and other salicylates decrease gastric secretion by causing increased back-diffusion of hydrogen ion.[52]

Ethanol may be a stimulant of acid secretion at low concentrations in man, but this was not found in a recent study.[90] At higher concentrations ethanol may decrease acid secretion by causing increased back-diffusion of hydrogen ion similar to that of unbuffered aspirin.[90]

Smoking and nicotine have variable effects on gastric secretion in man, a conclusion reached by Packard in a review of the literature.[91] More recent studies in man have not resolved the problem; pentagastrin-stimulated acid secretion was decreased[92] or unchanged.[93]

The absence of any marked effect of the ulcerogenic drugs on gastric acid secretion in man has led investigators to examine other mechanisms.

MUCOSAL RESISTANCE

This can be divided into the gastric mucous barrier and the gastric mucosal barrier.

Gastric Mucous Barrier. Menguy and coworkers have found that cortisone, ACTH, aspirin, indomethacin, and phenylbutazone reduce the secretory rate and change the composition of gastric mucus. He has summarized this work in a recent review and suggests that the protective role of mucus is decreased as a result of drug treatment and leads to ulceration.[94]

The protective role of mucus has been subject to question.[95] Mucus is a thin, unstirred layer which has weak neutralizing and buffering capacity, and acid diffuses rapidly through it.[96] Its main function is lubrication. If these are the properties of mucus, then it is difficult to understand whether alterations in its properties are of any significance except to indicate that the cells producing it may be damaged, i.e., a change in the gastric mucosa.

Gastric Mucosal Barrier. Davenport has found that salicylates, ethanol, and other agents will increase the permeability of the gastric mucosa to water-soluble compounds and other ions.[52] In the presence of acid (1 mM or 100 mM) aspirin is absorbed and the barrier is disrupted, but bleeding occurs only when the mucosa is simultaneously exposed to aspirin and strong acid (100 mM). Aspirin induces the abnormal permeability (indicated by a loss of hydrogen ion, a gain in sodium ion, and a fall in potential difference), and acid back-diffusion damages the capillaries. This damage may be the mechanism by which gastric erosions induced by unbuffered aspirin are produced. Occult bleeding, overt bleeding, and possibly peptic ulceration may ultimately result. A schematic diagram of these effects is given in Figure 52–2.

Recently, studies on the mucosal barrier of the dog similar to those by Davenport have been made, using caffeine, phenylbutazone, indomethacin, and adrenal corticosteroids.[54] Indomethacin (pH 7 or 1) disrupted the mucosal barrier and caused bleeding, but the other drugs were without effect.

The results of these studies suggest that unbuffered aspirin, ethanol (> 8 g per 100 ml) and indomethacin have similar effects on the gastric mucosal barrier and may induce gastric erosions by this mechanism. How corticosteroids, caffeine, and phenylbutazone act is unclear, but from the evidence discussed above it is likely they do not cause erosions or ulceration in man. In a recent study in dogs, nicotine was found to depress pancreatic and biliary secretion, but was without effect on gastric secretion or the gastric mucosal barrier.[97] This effect on pancreatic and biliary secretion may be a mechanism by which smoking could be ulcerogenic.

In summary, the evidence in man suggests that only unbuffered aspirin (combined with phenacetin and caffeine) and smoking lead to clinically evident ulcers or erosions. There is good experimental evidence in man and animals for the ulcerogenic effect of unbuffered aspirin; that for smoking is unresolved.

SUMMARY AND CONCLUSION

1. The ulcerogenic drugs discussed are those that are in common use in man and

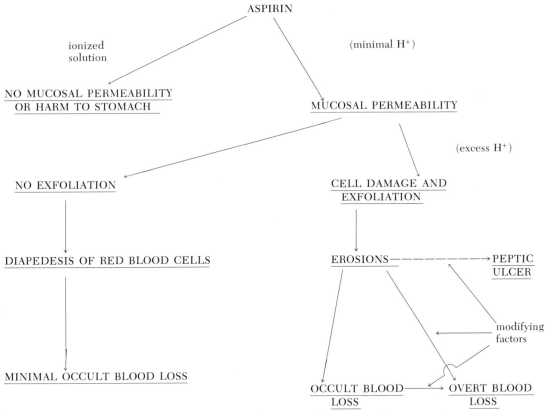

Figure 52-2. A schematic diagram to explain some of the effects of aspirin on the stomach.

cause experimental gastric ulceration or erosions (ethanol excepted) in animals. They are adrenal corticosteroids, salicylates, smoking and nicotine, indomethacin, phenylbutazone, reserpine, caffeine, and ethanol.

2. The frequency of peptic ulceration in the general community is estimated as about 8 to 14 per cent for men and 4 to 8 per cent for women.

3. The frequency of peptic ulceration in the population with chronic diseases is very difficult to obtain. Figures vary widely, biased selections have usually been made, and often it has been impossible to find a group who have not been receiving ulcerogenic drugs.

4. It seems likely that patients with rheumatoid arthritis have a greater propensity for peptic ulceration than do the normal population. Whether this is due to the disease itself or to drug therapy is unresolved.

5. Because of a variety of problems, including lack of controls and failure to match control subjects for sex and age, few prospective studies, and use of multidrug therapy, it is extremely difficult to reach firm conclusions concerning drug-induced peptic ulceration.

6. Adrenal corticosteroids probably do not cause peptic ulceration in the usual doses. The "steroid ulcer" does not exist as a pathological entity. There is little evidence to indicate that indomethacin, phenylbutazone, reserpine, caffeine, and ethanol are ulcerogenic in man. However, the data do not allow a firm conclusion.

7. Unbuffered aspirin (combined with phenacetin and caffeine) may be ulcerogenic. This conclusion rests on studies from the eastern states of Australia and needs confirmation from studies in other countries.

8. Smoking is possibly ulcerogenic but more likely maintains the chronicity of an ulcer.

9. In man: (a) Ethanol and unbuffered aspirin are capable of disrupting the gastric mucosal barrier; the other drugs have

not been tested. (b) Unbuffered (but not highly buffered) aspirin and indomethacin induce occult bleeding. Phenylbutazone, ethanol, and corticosteroids do not. (c) Unbuffered (but not highly buffered) aspirin and ethanol cause gastric erosions. Corticosteroids do not. No firm conclusions can be reached regarding phenylbutazone, caffeine, or reserpine. (d) There is little literature about hematemesis and melena with the ulcerogenic drugs except aspirin. It seems likely (but firm conclusions cannot be made) that unbuffered aspirin ingestion is associated with overt bleeding. The bleeding is possibly due to gastric erosions induced by unbuffered aspirin.

10. All the ulcerogenic drugs have little or no effect or decrease acid secretion. Only caffeine is a moderately strong stimulant of acid secretion, and it is unproved as a cause of peptic ulceration in man.

Unbuffered aspirin, ethanol, and indomethacin (tested only in the dog) but not caffeine, phenylbutazone, and adrenal corticosteroids (the last three drugs have been tested only in the dog) break the gastric mucosal barrier. However, of these drugs only unbuffered aspirin is possibly ulcerogenic in man. Smoking and nicotine have little effect on acid secretion, and, when tested in the dog, were without effect on the gastric mucosal barrier; a decrease in biliary and pancreatic secretion has been found.

A clear mechanism by which drugs induce ulceration in man is not yet evident.

REFERENCES

1. Skoryna, S. C. (ed.). Pathophysiology of Peptic Ulcer. Montreal, McGill University Press, 1963, pp. 213–322.
2. Segal, H. L. Ulcerogenic drugs and technics. Amer. J. Med. 29:780, 1960.
3. Kirsner, J. B. Drug-induced peptic ulcer. Ann. Intern. Med. 47:666, 1957.
4. Nicoloff, D. M. Indomethacin. Arch. Surg. 97:809, 1968.
5. Robert, A. The pro-ulcer effect of nicotine. An experimental study in the rat. J. Lab Clin. Med. 78:831, 1971.
6. Doll, R., Jones, F. A., and Buckatzsch, M. M. Occupational factors in the aetiology of gastric and duodenal ulcers. Med. Res. Council Spec. Report No. 276. London, His Majesty's Stationery Office, 1951, pp. 1–96.
7. Ivy, A. C., Grossman, M. I., and Bachrach, W. H. Peptic Ulcer. Philadelphia, The Blakiston Co., 1950, p. 608.
8. Blumenthal, I. S. Digestive disease as a national problem. III. Social cost of peptic ulcer. Gastroenterology 54:86, 1968.
9. Watkinson, G. The incidence of chronic peptic ulcer found at necropsy. Gut 1:14, 1960.
10. Bauer, W. In Proceedings of the Conference on the Effects of Cortisone. Rahway, N. J., Merck and Co., 1952, p. 56.
11. Ragan, C. In Proceedings of the Conference on the Effects of Cortisone. Rahway, N. J., Merck and Co., 1952, p. 55.
12. Bowen, R., Mayne, J. G., Cain, J. C., and Bartholomew, L. G. Peptic ulcer in rheumatoid arthritis and relationship to steroid treatment. Proc. Mayo Clin. 35:537, 1960.
13. Gibberd, F. B. Dyspepsia in patients with rheumatoid arthritis. Acta Rheum. Scand. 12:112, 1966.
14. Van Patter, W. N., Bargen, J. A., Dockerty, M. B., Feldman, W. H., Mayo, C. W., and Waugh, J. M. Regional enteritis. Gastroenterology 26:347, 1954.
15. Fielding, J. F., and Cooke, W. T. Peptic ulceration in Crohn's disease (regional enteritis). Gut 11:998, 1970.
16. Berkson, J. The statistical study of association between smoking and lung cancer. Proc. Mayo Clin. 30:319, 1955.
17. Spiro, H. M. Stomach damage from aspirin, steroids and antimetabolites. Amer. J. Dig. Dis. 7:733, 1962.
18. Garb, A. E., Soule, E. H., Bartholomew, L. G., and Cain, J. C. Steroid-induced gastric ulcer. Arch. Intern. Med. 116:899, 1965.
19. Sandweiss, D. J. Effects of adrenocorticotrophic hormone and of cortisone on peptic ulcer. Gastroenterology 27:604, 1954.
20. Cooke, A. R. Corticosteroids and peptic ulcer: Is there a relationship? Amer. J. Dig. Dis. 12:323, 1967.
21. Cushman, P. Glucocorticoids and the gastrointestinal tract: Current status. Gut 11:534, 1970.
22. Kern, F., Clark, G. M., and Lukens, J. G. Peptic ulceration occurring during therapy for rheumatoid arthritis. Gastroenterology 33:25, 1957.
23. Sherwood, H., Epstein, J. I., and Buckley, W. E. Peptic ulcer among allergic patients on long term triamcinolone therapy. J. Allergy 31:21, 1960.
24. Meltzer, L. E., Bockman, A. E., Kanenson, W., and Cohen, A. The incidence of peptic ulcer among patients on long-term prednisone therapy. Gastroenterology 35:351, 1958.
25. Gedda, P. O., and Moritz, U. Peptic ulcer during treatment of rheumatoid arthritis with cortisone derivatives. Acta Rheum. Scand. 4:249, 1959.
26. Kammerer, W. H., Freiberger, R. H., and Rivelis, A. L. Peptic ulcer in rheumatoid patients on corticosteroid therapy. Arthritis Rheum. 1:122, 1958.
27. Strickland, R. G., Fisher, J. M., and Taylor, K. B. Effect of prednisolone on gastric function and structure in man. Gastroenterology 56:675, 1969.
28. Bockus, H. L. (ed.). Gastroenterology, Vol. I,

2nd ed. Philadelphia, W. B. Saunders Co., 1963, p. 445.

29. Baragar, F. D., Duthie, J. J. R. Importance of aspirin as a cause of anaemia and peptic ulcer in rheumatoid arthritis. Brit. Med. J. 1:1106, 1960.

30. Douglas, R. A., and Johnston, E. D. Aspirin and chronic gastric ulcer. Med. J. Australia 2:893, 1961.

31. Duggan, J. M., and Chapman, B. L. The incidence of aspirin ingestion in patients with peptic ulcer. Med. J. Australia 1:797, 1970.

32. Gillies, M., and Skyring, A. Gastric ulcer, duodenal ulcer and gastric carcinoma: A case-control study of certain social and environmental factors. Med. J. Australia 2:1132, 1968.

33. Gillies, M., and Skyring, A. Gastric and duodenal ulcer. The association between aspirin ingestion, smoking and family history of ulcer. Med. J. Australia 2:280, 1969.

34. Doll, R., Jones, F. A., and Pygott, F. Effect of smoking on the production and maintenance of gastric and duodenal ulcers. Lancet 1:657, 1958.

35. Doll, R., and Hill, A. B. Lung cancer and other causes of death in relation to smoking. Brit. Med. J. 2:1071, 1956.

36. Hammond, E. C., and Horn, D. Smoking and death rates—report on 44 months of follow-up of 187, 783 men. J.A.M.A. 166:1294, 1958.

37. Weir, J. M., and Dunn, J. E. Smoking and mortality: A prospective study. Cancer 25:105, 1970.

38. Brown, R. G., McKeown, T., and Whitfield, A. G. W. A note on the association between smoking and disease in men in the seventh decade. Brit. J. Prev. Soc. Med. 11:162, 1957.

39. Hart, F. D., and Boardman, P. L. Indomethacin: A new non-steroid anti-inflamatory agent. Brit. Med. J. 2:965, 1963.

40. Lövgren, O., and Allander, E. Side effects of indomethacin. Brit. Med. J. 1:118, 1964.

41. Taylor, R. T., Huskisson, E. C., Whitehouse, G. H., Hart, F. D., and Trapnell, D. H. Gastric ulceration occurring during indomethacin therapy. Brit. Med. J. 4:734, 1968.

42. Lockie, L. M., and Norcross, B. M. In Arthritis and Allied Conditions, 7th Ed., J. L. Hollander (ed.). Philadelphia, Lea & Febiger, 1966, p. 345.

43. Katz, A. M., Pearson, C. M., and Kennedy, J. M. A clinical trial of indomethacin in rheumatoid arthritis. Clin. Pharm. Ther. 6:25, 1965.

44. Rothernich, N. O. An extended study of indomethacin. I. Clinical pharmacology. J.A.M.A. 195:531, 1966.

45. Mauer, E. F. The toxic effects of phenylbutazone (Butazolidin). New Eng. J. Med. 253:404, 1955.

46. Kuzell, W. C., Schaffarzick, R. W., Naugler, W. E., Gaudin, G., Mankle, E. A., and Brown, B. Phenylbutazone (Butazolidin) in gout. Amer. J. Med. 16:212, 1954.

47. Sperling, I. L. Adverse reactions with long-term use of phenylbutazone and oxyphenbutazone. Lancet 2:535, 1969.

48. Bachrach, W. H. Reserpine, gastric secretion and peptic ulcer. Amer. J. Dig. Dis. 4:117, 1959.

49. Hollister, L. E. Hematemesis and melena complicating therapy with rauwolfia alkaloids. Arch. Intern. Med. 99:218, 1957.

50. Drenick, E. J. Reserpine in peptic ulcer. Amer. J. Dig. Dis. 1:521, 1956.

51. Roth, J. L. A. Peptic ulcer disease: Iatrogenic factors. In The Stomach, C. M. Thompson, D. Berkowitz, and E. Polish (eds.). New York, Grune and Stratton, 1967, pp. 291–305.

52. Davenport, H. W. Salicylate damage to the gastric mucosal barrier. New Eng. J. Med. 276:1307, 1967.

53. Davenport, H. W., Warner, H. A., and Code, C. F. Functional significance of gastric mucosal barrier to sodium. Gastroenterology 47:142, 1964.

54. Chvasta, T. E., and Cooke, A. R. The effect of several ulcerogenic drugs on the canine gastric mucosal barrier. J. Lab. Clin. Med. 79:302, 1972.

55. Geall, M. G., Phillips, S. F., and Summerskill, W. H. J. Profile of gastric potential difference in man. Effects of aspirin, alcohol, bile and endogenous acid. Gastroenterology 58:437, 1970.

56. Holt, P. R. Measurement of gastrointestinal blood loss in subjects taking aspirin. J. Lab. Clin. Med. 56:717, 1960.

57. Grossman, M. I., Matsumoto, K. K., and Lichter, R. J. Fecal blood loss produced by oral and intravenous administration of various salicylates. Gastroenterology 40:383, 1961.

58. Croft, D. N., and Wood, P. H. N. Gastric mucosa and susceptibility to occult gastrointestinal bleeding caused by aspirin. Brit. Med. J. 1:137, 1967.

59. Cooke, A. R., and Hunt, J. N. Absorption of acetylsalicylic acid from unbuffered and buffered gastric contents. Amer. J. Dig. Dis. 15:95, 1970.

60. Leonards, J. R., and Levy, G. Reduction or prevention of aspirin-induced occult gastrointestinal blood loss in man. Clin. Pharmacol. Ther. 10:571, 1969.

61. Bouchier, I. A., and Williams, H. S. Determination of fecal blood loss following combined alcohol and sodium acetylsalicylate intake. Lancet 1:178, 1969.

62. Goulston, K., and Cooke, A. R. Alcohol, aspirin and gastrointestinal bleeding. Brit. Med. J. 4:664, 1968.

63. Scott, J. T., Porter, I. H., Lewis, S. M., and Dixon, A. St. J. Studies of gastrointestinal bleeding caused by corticosteroids, salicylates and other analgesics. Quart. J. Med. 30:167, 1961.

64. Wanka, J., Jones, L. I., Wood, P. H. N., and Dixon, A. St. J. Indomethacin in rheumatic diseases: A controlled clinical trial. Ann. Rheum. Dis. 23:218, 1964.

65. Siurala, M., Peltola, P., and Varis, K. The effect of long-term treatment with prednisone upon the state of the human gastric mucosa. Scand. J. Gastroent. 3:407, 1968.

66. Douthwaite, A. H., and Lintott, G. A. M. Gastroscopic observation of the effect of aspirin and certain other substances on the stomach. Lancet 2:1222, 1938.

67. Weiss, A., Pitman, E. P., and Graham, E. C. Aspirin and gastric bleeding. Amer. J. Med. 31:266, 1961.

68. Thorsen, W. B., Western, D., Tanaka, Y., and Morrissey, J. F. Aspirin injury to the gastric mucosa. Arch. Intern. Med. 121:499, 1968.

69. Palmer, E. D. Gastritis: A revaluation. Medicine 33:199, 1954.

70. Cooke, A. R. Aspirin, ethanol and the stomach. Aust. Ann. Med. 19:269, 1970.

71. Wolff, G. Does alcohol cause chronic gastritis? Scand. J. Gastroent. 5:289, 1970.

72. Salter, R. H. Aspirin and gastrointestinal bleeding. Amer. J. Dig. Dis. 13:38, 1968.

73. Langman, M. J. S. Epidemiological evidence for the association of aspirin and acute gastrointestinal bleeding. Gut 11:627, 1970.

74. Parry, D. J., and Wood, P. H. N. Relationship between aspirin taking and gastroduodenal haemorrhage. Gut 8:301, 1967.

75. Valman, H. B., Parry, D. J., and Coghill, N. F. Lesions associated with gastroduodenal haemorrhage in relation to aspirin intake. Brit. Med. J. 4:661, 1959.

76. Muir, A., and Cossar, I. A. Aspirin and gastric hemorrhage. Lancet 1:539, 1959.

77. Allibone, A., and Flint, F. J. Bronchitis, aspirin, smoking and other factors in the aetiology of peptic ulcer. Lancet 2:179, 1958.

78. Muir, A., and Cossar, I. A. Aspirin and ulcer. Brit. Med. J. 2:7, 1955.

79. Alvarez, A. S., and Summerskill, W. H. J. Gastrointestinal haemorrhage and salicylates. Lancet 2:920, 1958.

80. Kelly, J. J. Salicylate ingestion: A frequent cause of gastric hemorrhage. Amer. J. Med. Sci. 232:119, 1956.

81. Brown, R. K., and Mitchell, N. The influence of some of the salicyl-compounds (and alcoholic beverages) on the natural history of peptic ulcer. Gastroenterology 31:198, 1956.

82. Lange, H. F. Salicylates and gastric haemorrhage. I. Occult bleeding II. Manifest bleeding. Gastroenterology 33:778, 1957.

83. Banks, C. N., and Baron, J. H. Drugs containing aspirin (letter). Lancet 1:1165, 1964.

84. Schiller, K. F. R., Truelove, S. C., and Williams, D. G. Haematemesis and melaena with special reference to factors influencing the outcome. Brit. Med. J. 2:7, 1970.

85. Roth, J. A., and Ivy, A. C. The effect of caffeine upon gastric secretion in the dog, cat and man. Amer. J. Physiol. 141:454, 1944.

86. Chvasta, T. E., and Cooke, A. R. Emptying and absorption of caffeine from the human stomach. Gastroenterology 61:838, 1971.

87. Cooke, A. R. The role of adrenocortical steroids in the regulation of gastric secretion. Gastroenterology 52:272, 1967.

88. Winship, D. H., and Bernhard, G. C. Basal and histamine-stimulated human gastric acid secretion. Lack of effect of indomethacin in therapeutic doses. Gastroenterology 58:762, 1970.

89. Emas, S. Mechanisms of action of reserpine on gastric secretion of acid. Amer. J. Dig. Dis. 13:572, 1968.

90. Cooke, A. R. Ethanol and gastric function. Gastroenterology 62:501, 1972.

91. Packard, R. S. Smoking and the alimentary tract: A review. Gut 1:171, 1960.

92. Wilkinson, A. R., and Johnston, D. Inhibitory effect of cigarette smoking on gastric secretion stimulated by pentagastrin in man. Lancet 2:628, 1971.

93. Debas, H. T., Cohen, M. M., Holubitsky, I. B., and Harrison, R. C. Effect of cigarette smoking on human gastric secretory responses. Gut 12:93, 1971.

94. Menguy, R. Gastric mucus and the gastric mucous barrier. Amer. J. Surg. 117:806, 1969.

95. Cooke, A. R. Mucosal resistance and corticosteroids. Gastroenterology 53:506, 1967.

96. Heatley, N. G. Muco-substance as a barrier to diffusion. Gastroenterology 37:313, 1959.

97. Konturek, S. J., Solomon, T. E., McCreight, W. G., Johnson, L. R., and Jacobson, E. D. Effects of nicotine on gastrointestinal secretions. Gastroenterology 60:1098, 1971.

Chapter 53

Acute Gastroduodenal Stress Ulceration

Robert N. McClelland

Acute gastroduodenal ulceration caused by stress is encountered with increasing frequency. According to Robbins and associates, the incidence in various series varies from zero to 35 per cent, depending upon the nature of the stress and the types of patients studied.[1] The increasing incidence of stress ulceration is probably related to the fact that more patients sustaining severe stress, caused by sepsis, shock, head injuries, or burns, now survive long enough to develop acute gastroduodenal stress ulceration, whereas in the past they succumbed before this complication could occur.

ETIOLOGY

The cause of stress ulceration is still unknown; however, there are sufficient data to provide some basis for reasonable theories concerning the etiology. It is probable that stress ulceration may be caused by one or both of two basic mechanisms. The first mechanism relates to the hypersecretion that occurs in human beings during stress, resulting in acid-peptic mucosal autodigestion, and thus acute gastroduodenal stress ulceration.[1-4] The levels of gastric acid secretion noted by various investigators may depend upon when gastric acid secretion is measured after the onset of stress and also upon the

nature of the stress. One major type of stress ulceration, however, is probably directly caused by marked hypersecretion of gastric acid. This is so-called Cushing's ulcer, which occurs after severe brain injuries or intracranial neurosurgical procedures. The incidence of Cushing's ulcer is reflected by a recent report of 960 severe brain injuries by Heiskanen and Torma, who noted that 1.1 per cent of these patients developed gross upper gastrointestinal hemorrhage from such ulcers.[5] Watts and Clark demonstrated that gastric acid secretion in patients who bled from Cushing's ulcers after severe brain trauma often reached levels occurring in patients with the Zollinger-Ellison syndrome. They found that parenteral anticholinergics invariably reduced such very high levels of gastric acid secretion to normal and apparently prevented Cushing's ulcers in such neurosurgical patients.[6, 7] This work was recently confirmed by Norton and his associates.[8] None of the head injury patients in either of these studies had received or were receiving adrenal steroids or other ulcerogenic agents at the time their gastric acidity increased and bleeding occurred. Idjadi and associates also found high levels of gastric acid and pepsin secretion and deficient production of gastric mucus in seven patients with severe brain injuries, two of whom bled from Cushing's ulcers.[9] The blocking of such gastric hypersecretion with anticholinergics in patients with severe brain trauma and recent experiments by Berman and Ducker[10] and by Norton and associates[11] indicate that the cause of this type of gastric acid hypersecretion may be direct stimulation of the vagal nuclei by increased intracranial pressure. This peculiar type of early, excessive parasympathetic activity associated with serious central nervous system injury probably does not originate in the same manner as do the excessive parasympathetic stimuli arising later after other types of stress. This second type of excessive parasympathetic stimulus caused by non-neurological stress is discussed in the following paragraphs.

The second possible cause of acute gastroduodenal stress ulceration relates to the development of ischemic areas in the gastroduodenal mucosa. Leonard and associates,[12, 13] Nicoloff and associates,[14] and Goodman and Osborne[15] have postulated that any severe stress may cause prolonged ischemia of the gastroduodenal mucosa. They note that the strong sympathetic stimulus and high circulating catecholamine levels caused by severe and prolonged stress may open arteriovenous shunts in the gastroduodenal submucosa (see Fig. 51–1, p. 632). Because of this phenomenon, blood which normally flows through the capillary bed of the gastroduodenal mucosa then flows instead through the submucosal arteriovenous shunts and is thus diverted from the gastroduodenal mucosa. The mucosa therefore may remain ischemic for several hours or days during periods of severe stress and ultimately is severely injured by such ischemia. Stress ulceration then develops when the areas of mucosal ischemia undergo necrosis. The necrosis and ulceration of the gastroduodenal mucosa may develop because of ischemia alone, or may be hastened by the autodigestion activity of normal or elevated levels of gastric acid and pepsin which digest ischemic gastroduodenal mucosa much more readily than normal mucosa.

In experimental animals, Leonard and associates have also shown that after the cessation of the initial stress-induced excessive sympathetic nervous stimulus (which causes mucosal ischemia) there is a rebound, or pendular, excessive parasympathetic stimulus, which closes submucosal gastroduodenal arteriovenous shunts and diverts excessive amounts of blood through the previously ischemic gastroduodenal mucosa.[12, 13] Such an abnormally high mucosal blood flow might be detrimental in that the ischemic gastroduodenal mucosa would become engorged with blood and this could cause further mucosal injury and necrosis, resulting in ulceration and subsequent bleeding or perforation of the stress ulcers. Ischemic mucosal damage might then be further compounded by increased gastric acid and pepsin secretion caused by excessive parasympathetic stimuli acting on undamaged parietal cells to cause gastric acid hypersecretion after the excessive sympathetic stimuli of stress have abated. Such pendular or markedly variable autonomic nervous activity might explain why some workers have found decreased gastric acidity and others increased gastric acidity during stress. If so, it is possible that the timing of the collection of gastric secretions in relation to the state of autonomic nervous stimuli could markedly affect the results obtained upon measuring gastric acidity.

Another possible cause of ischemic injury to the gastric mucosa which may lead to acute stress ulceration is the occurrence of acute thrombosis within the gastric mucosal blood vessels caused by disseminated intravascular coagulation. The syndrome of disseminated intravascular clotting is being recognized with increasing frequency as a complication of many serious illnesses. Interestingly, disseminated intravascular coagulation occurs most often as a complication of severe sepsis and burns; it is tempting to speculate that this could account for the high incidence of stress ulceration seen in patients with sepsis or burns. Disseminated intravascular coagulation should be strongly suspected if patients with gastric hemorrhage are found to have low platelets, prolonged prothrombin times, and serum fibrinogen levels below 160 mg per 100 ml, with severe illnesses, such as sepsis, which are known to cause consumptive coagulopathy. If this diagnosis is made promptly, treatment with sufficient intravenous heparin may stop the gastric hemorrhage. However, until more experience accumulates with the diagnosis and treatment of disseminated intravascular coagulation, great caution should be taken in managing stress ulcer bleeding on this basis, because obviously the bleeding might increase with heparinization if these diagnostic and therapeutic concepts are wrong. Margaretten and McKay[16] and Colman and associates[17] have recently written interesting reviews on the possible association of bleeding stress ulcers and disseminated intravascular clotting.

Recent work by Silen (personal communication) and others[18-20] indicates that there is "back-diffusion" of gastric acid through the gastroduodenal mucosa in patients who develop stress ulceration. Such back-diffusion may occur because of prior ischemic injury of the mucosa, but it seems probable that this is not the basic cause of stress ulceration. The initial ischemic mucosal injury may increase mucosal permeability and permit acid back-diffusion to occur. The acid back-diffusion may then further damage the mucosal cells previously injured by ischemia and thus increase the likelihood of stress ulceration. Incidentally, the amount of gastric acid which back-diffuses may also be another factor which accounts for the variable quantities of gastric acid secretion reported during stress by various investigators.

Menguy and others[21, 22] postulate that loss of the normal gastric mucus barrier may be the primary cause of stress ulceration. There is, however, conflicting evidence as to whether gastric mucus secretion is altered by stress in human beings. Two recent studies show that gastric mucus secretion is not depressed or altered in composition and may even be increased during stress.[3, 4] Another recent study, however, shows quantitative depression and qualitative alteration of gastric mucus in human beings under prolonged, severe stress.[1] Here too, however, these conflicting data regarding gastric mucus secretion in relation to stress may (as with gastric acid and pepsin measurements) relate to the time the gastric mucus secretion is measured after the onset of stress, the type of stress, methodological differences in measurement of gastric

mucus, and other as yet unappreciated variables. In summary, the accumulated evidence indicates that the basic event in the development of all gastroduodenal stress ulcerations (with the possible exception of Cushing's or central nervous system stress ulcerations) is gastric mucosal ischemia probably induced by an excessive sympathetic discharge, or, in some instances, disseminated intravascular coagulation occurring because of many kinds of stress. These essential vascular events may explain all the variable changes seen in gastric acid, mucus, and pepsin secretions as well as gastric mucosal back-diffusion.

The ischemic origin of gastroduodenal stress ulceration has recently been further corroborated by Lucas and associates, who have made gastrocamera photographs of the gastric mucosa of human beings undergoing severe stress.[3] These photographs of the gastric mucosa showed areas of marked mucosal ischemia which, in some instances, were beginning to undergo necrosis and ulceration. Attempts are currently being made to develop methods of directly measuring gastric mucosal blood flow in human beings. Such direct measurements of gastroduodenal mucosal blood flow in persons undergoing stress may also aid in determining whether the ischemic theory of gastroduodenal stress ulceration is valid.

Probably the most frequent type of stress causing stress ulceration is bacterial sepsis. Billroth first observed this fact in 1867, and many others have noted that at least 70 per cent of those developing stress ulcers have some form of significant sepsis.[23-27] The mechanism whereby sepsis induces stress ulceration is unknown, but more than likely sepsis is simply one, albeit the most common, of many types of stress which may induce excessive autonomic splanchnic nervous stimuli which ultimately cause ischemic necrosis of the gastroduodenal mucosa and stress ulceration. Other factors which may also be involved in the development of stress ulceration resulting from sepsis are the possible increases of gastric acid[28] and pepsin secretion and the decreased effectiveness of the gastric mucus barrier against mucosal autodigestion which may be directly affected by severe sepsis.

PREVENTION OF STRESS ULCERATION

As suggested by Watts and Clark,[6, 7] it is important that all patients suffering severe intracranial injury or having major neurosurgical procedures have measurements of their gastric acid secretions. Any elevation of gastric acid secretion in these patients should be treated by immediate and frequent administration of parenteral anticholinergics and antacids which block acid secretion and apparently prevent development of Cushing's ulcers in most instances.

Recently, Silen has found that other types of stress ulcers can often be prevented by the frequent instillation of antacids into the stomachs of severely ill patients who are likely to develop stress ulcers (personal communication). Sufficient antacid is given to maintain a constant intragastric pH greater than 6. Although nonneurosurgical stress ulcers are probably not primarily caused by acid hypersecretion, even low levels of gastric acid may contribute to stress ulcer formation. If all gastric acid is kept constantly neutralized, such additional mucosal injury and ulceration may not occur.

Another critical factor to consider in the prevention of stress ulcers is sepsis. In many cases sepsis cannot be quickly controlled; but when it can be (such as by drainage of abscesses and appropriate antibiotic therapy), bleeding from stress ulcers often promptly ceases and gastric surgery may thus be avoided.

It has been suggested that the incidence of stress ulceration may be significantly less in severely ill patients who are maintained on central intravenous hyperalimentation until stress relents.[29] More recently, additional data indicating the importance of nutritional and metabolic requirements in the prevention of stress ulcer have been reported by Chernov and associates.[30] They suggest that large doses of intramuscular vitamin A may aid in preventing stress ulceration. Vitamin A increases the regeneration of gastric mucous cells and the production of protective gastric mucus.

This observation concerning the importance of vitamin A in the prevention of stress ulceration is also interesting in relation to independent work done by Ehrlich and Hunt showing that vitamin A also has a specific role in preventing the adverse effects of adrenal corticosteroids on the healing of laparotomy wounds.[31] Patients under stress have high levels of circulating adrenal corticosteroids. Although it seems less likely now than previously that adrenal steroids cause stress ulcers by increasing gastric acid secretion, such steroids may have at least two other adverse effects. (1) They may increase initial gastric mucosal ischemia by potentiating the effect of high levels of circulating catecholamines in severely ill patients. In other words, adrenal corticosteroids may increase the tendency of excessive splanchnic sympathetic stimuli to open splanchnic submucosal arteriovenous shunts, thus increasing gastroduodenal mucosal ischemia. (2) High levels of adrenal corticosteroids might interfere with the ability of the gastroduodenal mucosa to heal when it is injured in any manner.

The importance of good nutrition in preventing stress ulceration is further emphasized by the recent work of Bounous and associates, who have shown in dogs that necrosis and ulceration of the mucosa of a loop of small bowel to which the arterial blood supply has been interrupted may be prevented by instilling hypertonic glucose solutions into the loop of bowel prior to arterial ligation.[32] They have shown that this probably restores and maintains levels of high energy phosphate molecules within the intestinal mucosal cells and thus makes the cells more resistant to ischemic injury and permits more rapid regeneration of mucosal cells to replace those which do undergo necrosis despite a superabundance of intracellular metabolic substrate.

TREATMENT OF ACUTE GASTRODUODENAL STRESS ULCERATION

Bleeding is the chief manifestation of acute gastroduodenal stress ulceration. About half of all stress ulcer patients who bleed massively require surgery, because stress ulcers are less likely to stop bleeding spontaneously than are ordinary gastroduodenal ulcers. If surgery for bleeding stress ulcers is excessively delayed, the mortality will exceed 80 per cent, whereas, with timely and appropriately selected surgery, mortality may still be high but may fall to 35 to 40 per cent.[33]

If, despite all methods of prevention, the patient bleeds massively from acute gastroduodenal stress ulceration, treatment should initially consist of accurate blood replacement, iced saline gastric lavage with added antacid solution, and parenterally administered anticholinergic drugs. Anticholinergic drugs should be used because they may shunt blood away from the bleeding gastric mucosa by blocking excessive splanchnic parasympathetic activity and thus opening gastric submucosal arteriovenous shunts. In addition, anticholinergic drugs may further lower even normal or subnormal levels of gastric acid and pepsin which may compound the is-

chemic injury to the gastric mucosa. LeVeen and associates have also recently described a limited but interesting experience with gastric lavage and intraperitoneal injection of Levophed solutions in stopping various types of gastrointestinal hemorrhage.[34, 35]

Patients with persistent bleeding should be checked for coagulation defects, and specific clotting defects should be corrected. Blood should be replaced with the freshest blood possible, and fresh frozen plasma may be helpful if fresh blood is not available.

Atik recently demonstrated that intravenous infusions of fresh platelet packs may cause cessation of bleeding from stress ulcers (unpublished data). He indicated that even though patients with bleeding stress ulcers may have normal

TABLE 53–1. SURGICAL TREATMENT OF STRESS ULCER

AUTHOR	No. CASES	TYPE TREATMENT			SURVIVAL			REBLED		
		Local	V. & P.	Resect.	Local	V. & P.	Resect.	Local	V. & P.	Resect.
Kirtley (Vanderbilt)	41	20% (8)°	63% (26)	17% (7)	50% (4)	70% (18)	43% (4)	25% (2)	15% (4)	14% (1)
Fogelman and Garvey (Baylor)	9	11% (1)	33% (3)	56% (5)	0% (0)	33% (1)	80% (4)	100% (1)	67% (2)	20% (1)
O'Neill et al. (Brooke)	22	5% (1)	14% (3)	81% (18)	0% (0)	0% (0)	67% (12)	100% (1)	33% (1)	? ?
David et al. (Mayo Clinic)	33	9% (3)	58% (19)	33% (11)	100% (3)	80% (15)	90% (10)	0% (3)	40% (8)	27% (3)
	18†	16% (3)	22% (4)	62% (11)	100% (3)	0% (0)	90% (10)	0% (3)	100% (4)	27% (3)
Kunzman (Viet Nam)	43	12% (5)	68% (29)	20% (9)	80% (4)	80% (23)	45% (4)	80% (4)	52% (15)	44% (4)
Goodman (U. of Michigan)	13	15% (2)	70% (9)	15% (2)	0% (0)	67% (6)	0% (0)	100% (2)	44% (4)	50% (1)
Hoerr (Cleveland Clinic)	16	6% (1)	50% (8)	44% (7)	Not specified—75% overall and none died from rebleed			0% (0)	13% (1)	0% (0)
Bryant (U. of Kentucky)	5	0% (0)	100% (5)	0% (0)	0% (0)	20% (1)	0% (0)	0% (0)	100% (5)	0% (0)
Beil (Cornell)	15	0% (0)	0% (0)	100% (15)	0% (0)	0% (0)	40% (6)	0% (0)	0% (0)	7% (1)
Total cases and means of nine series	197	11% (21)	52% (102)	37% (74)	57% (12)	70% (70)	60% (44)	62% (13)	40% (40)	23% (17)

°Actual numbers of cases in parentheses.
†Number of cases which were gastric or gastroduodenal ulcers rather than single duodenal ulcers in Mayo series.

TABLE 53–2.   CRITERIA FOR SELECTION OF OPERATION FOR STRESS ULCER

Vagotomy and Gastrectomy	Vagotomy-Pyloroplasty and Suture of Bleeding Points
1. Large solitary ulcer greater than 2.5 cm in diameter, unless in very poor risk, elderly patient	1. Solitary ulcer less than 2.5 cm in diameter
2. Many bleeding ulcers scattered throughout the stomach and duodenum which cannot be securely sutured	2. Solitary ulcer greater or less than 2.5 cm in diameter in very poor risk patients
3. Diffusely bleeding "stress hemorrhagic gastritis"	3. Relatively few, closely grouped, small ulcers which can be readily sutured to stop bleeding

numbers of platelets, the adhesiveness of the platelets may be greatly diminished; therefore they cannot form adequate clots in the bases of their ulcers, and bleeding continues.

Several investigators have recommended that intra-arterial infusions of splanchnic vasoconstrictive agents such as epinephrine or Pitressin should be carried out through catheters selectively placed in various visceral arteries.[36-38] Experience with this technique is limited, but it seems to have been very effective in a number of cases. The only concern one might have regarding such vasoconstrictive treatment would be that mucosal ischemia might be aggravated and additional stress ulcers might form and bleed after cessation of such vasoconstrictive therapy, if indeed mucosal ischemia does induce stress ulceration. However, the relatively brief period of splanchnic vasoconstriction would probably permit clot formation without inducing significant mucosal damage.

If the patient loses more than 3 units of blood within less than 24 hours and significant bleeding is continuing, operation should not be delayed; otherwise the mortality rate will increase rapidly.[33]

Unfortunately, no experience with stress ulceration is yet extensive enough to make definite statements about the proper surgical management of this disease. There are, however, sufficient clinical data in several recent reports to allow reasonable recommendations for the surgical treatment of stress ulcers. As with other types of gastroduodenal ulcers, it seems that no single operation is best for all cases of bleeding stress ulcers. Table 53–1 summarizes the results of various methods of surgical treatment of bleeding stress ulcers attained in nine recently reported series.[24, 33, 39-45] It will be noted that the overall surgical mortality from bleeding stress ulcers is about 35 to 40 per cent regardless of whether vagotomy-gastrectomy or vagotomy-drainage with suture of bleeding ulcers is selected as treatment. An additional 35 to 40 per cent of these patients, however, will die later of causes unrelated to stress ulcer bleeding. The rebleeding rate from stress ulcers is higher if vagotomy-drainage with suture of the bleeding ulcers is done; however, the mortality rate may be slightly lower.

In view of these clinical data, and until well controlled, larger prospective and randomized studies comparing results of various operations for bleeding stress ulcers become available, we generally treat stress ulcers in the following manner. In younger, relatively better risk patients, vagotomy-gastrectomy (usually 70 to 75 per cent gastric resection) with removal of the bleeding ulcers is done. Bleeding ulcers remaining in the gastric fundus are oversewn. In poorer risk, older patients, however, vagotomy-pyloroplasty with suture of the bleeding ulcers is done, unless very extensive multiple, shallow bleeding ulcers cannot be controlled by suture, in which case vagotomy-gastrectomy is performed with removal of as many of the bleeding ulcers as possible and suture of the remaining bleeding points. These criteria for selection of the type of operation to be done for bleeding stress ulcers are summarized in Table 53–2. Perforation of stress ulcer occurs less frequently than does hemorrhage, and it is best treated by simple closure unless there is associated hemorrhage.

REFERENCES

1. Robbins, R., Idjadi, F., Stahl, W. M., and Essiet, G.   Studies of gastric secretion in stressed patients. Ann. Surg. 175:555, 1972.
2. Lucas, C. E., Sugawa, C., Riddley, J., Rector, F., Rosenberg, B., and Walt, A. J.   Natural history and surgical dilemma of "stress" gastric bleeding. Arch. Surg. 102:266, 1971.
3. Lucas, C. E., Sugawa, C., Friend, W., and Walt, A. J.   Therapeutic implications of disturbed gastric physiology in patients with stress ulcerations. Amer. J. Surg. 123:25, 1972.
4. McClelland, R. N., Shires, G. T., and Prager, M.   Gastric secretory and splanchnic blood flow studies in man after severe trauma and hemorrhagic shock. Amer. J. Surg. 121:143, 1971.
5. Heiskanen, O., and Torma, T.   Gastrointestinal ulceration and hemorrhage associated with severe brain injury. Acta Chir. Scand. 143:562, 1968.
6. Watts, C. C., and Clark, K.   Gastric acidity in the comatose patient. J. Neurosurg. 30:107, 1969.
7. Watts, C., and Clark, K.   Effects of an anticholinergic drug on gastric acid secretion in the comatose patient. Surg. Gynec. Obstet. 130:61, 1970.
8. Norton, L., Greer, J., and Eiseman, B.   Gastric secretory response to head injury. Arch. Surg. 101:200, 1970.
9. Idjadi, F., Robbins, R., Stahl, W. M., and Essiet, G.   Prospective study of gastric secretion in stressed patients with intracranial injury. J. Trauma 11:681, 1971.
10. Berman, I. R., and Ducker, R. B.   Pulmonary, somatic, and splanchnic circulatory responses to increased intracranial presssure. Ann. Surg. 169:210, 1969.
11. Norton, L., Fuchs, E., and Eiseman, B.   Gastric secretory response to pressure on vagal nuclei. Amer. J. Surg. 123:13, 1972.
12. Leonard, A. S., Engle, J. C., Peter, E. T., Long, D., and Wangensteen, O. H.   Gastric blood flow and inhibition of histamine-stimulated gastric secretion. J.A.M.A. 187:121, 1964.
13. Leonard, A. S., Long, D., French, L. A., Peter, E. T., and Wangensteen, O. H.   Pendular pattern in gastric secretion and blood flow following hypothalamic stimulation—origin of stress ulcer? Surgery 56:109, 1964.
14. Nicoloff, D. M., Peter, E. T., Leonard, A. S., and Wangensteen, O. H.   Catecholamines in ulcer provocation. J.A.M.A. 191:111, 1965.
15. Goodman, A. A., and Osborne, M. P.   An experimental model and clinical definition of stress ulceration. Surg. Gynec. Obstet. 134:563, 1972.
16. Margaretten, W., and McKay, D. G.   Thrombotic ulcerations of the gastrointestinal tract. Arch. Intern. Med. 127:250, 1971.
17. Colman, R. W., Robboy, S. J., and Minna, J. D.   Disseminated intravascular coagulation (DIC): An approach. Amer. J. Med. 52:679, 1972.
18. Skillman, J. J.   Acute gastroduodenal "stress" ulceration. Barrier to disruption of varied pathogenesis? Rev. Surg. 59:478, 1970.
19. Skillman, J. J., Gould, S. A., Chung, R. S. K., and Silen, W.   The gastric mucosal barrier: Clinical and experimental studies in critically ill and normal man, and in the rabbit. Ann. Surg. 172:564, 1970.
20. Smith, B. M., Skillman, J. J., Edwards, B. G., and Silen, W.   Permeability of the human gastric mucosa. Alteration by acetylsalicylic acid and ethanol. New Eng. J. Med. 285:716, 1971.
21. Menguy, R., and Desbaillets, L.   The gastric mucous barrier: Influence of protein-bound carbohydrate in mucus on the rate of proteolysis of gastric mucus. Ann. Surg. 168:475, 1968.
22. Menguy, R.   Gastric mucus and the gastric mucous barrier. Amer. J. Surg. 117:806, 1969.
23. Billroth, T.   Über duodenalgeschwüre bei Septicämie. Wien Med. Wochenschrift 17:705, 1867.
24. David, E., and Kelly, A.   Acute postoperative peptic ulceration. Surg. Clin. N. Amer. 49:1111, 1969.
25. Douglass, H. O., Jr., and LeVeen, H. H.   Stress ulcers. Arch. Surg. 100:178, 1970.
26. Douglass, H. O., Jr., Falk, G. A., and LeVeen, H. H.   Infection: A cause of acute peptic ulceration in hypersecreting animals. Surgery 68:827, 1970.
27. Rosoff, C. B., and Goldman, H.   Effect of the intestinal bacterial flora on acute gastric stress ulceration. Gastroenterology 55:212, 1968.
28. Howe, C. W., Wigglesworth, W. C., and Porell, W. J.   Gastric secretory responses to surgical stress and infection. Surg. Forum 2:34, 1952.
29. Gurd, F. N., and McClelland, R. N.   Trauma workshop report: The gastrointestinal tract in trauma. J. Trauma 11:1089, 1970.
30. Chernov, M. S., Hale, H. W., Jr., and Wood, M.   Prevention of stress ulcers. Amer. J. Surg. 122:674, 1971.
31. Ehrlich, H. P., and Hunt, T. K.   The effects of cortisone and anabolic steroids on the tensile strength of healing wounds. Ann. Surg. 170:203, 1969.
32. Bounous, G., Sutherland, N. G., McArdle, A. H., et al.   The prophylactic use of an "elemental" diet in experimental hemorrhagic shock and intestinal ischemia. Ann. Surg. 166:312, 1967.
33. Beil, A. R., Jr., Mannix, H., Jr., and Beal, J. M.   Massive upper gastrointestinal hemorrhage after operation. Amer. J. Surg. 108:324, 1964.
34. LeVeen, H. H., Diaz, C., Piccone, V. A., Langsam, A. A., and Pedowitz, W. J.   Control of gastrointestinal bleeding. Amer. J. Surg. 123:154, 1972.
35. LeVeen, H. H., Diaz, C., Falk, G., Piccone, V. A., Yarnoz, M., Wynkoop, B. J., Nelson, J., Pedowitz, W., Belfasky, R. B., and Borek, B.   A proposed method to interrupt gastrointestinal bleeding: preliminary report. Ann. Surg. 175:459, 1972.
36. Morello, D. C., Klein, N. E., Wolferth, C. C., Jr., and Matsumoto, T.   Management of diffuse hemorrhage from gastric mucosa. Amer. J. Surg. 123:160, 1972.
37. Nusbaum, M., Baum, S., Blakemore, W. S., and

Tumen, H. Clinical experience with selective intra-arterial infusion of vasopressin in the control of gastrointestinal bleeding from arterial sources. Amer. J. Surg. 123:165, 1972.

38. Rosch, J., Dotter, C. T., and Rose, R. W. Selective arterial infusions of vasoconstrictors in acute gastrointestinal bleeding. Radiology 99:27, 1971.

39. Bryant, L. R., and Griffen, W. O., Jr. Vagotomy and pyloroplasty. Arch. Surg. 93:161, 1966.

40. Fogelman, M. J., and Garvey, J. M. Acute gastroduodenal ulceration incident to surgery and disease. Amer. J. Surg. 112:651, 1966.

41. Flowers, R. S., Kyle, K., and Hoerr, S. O. Post-operative hemorrhage from stress ulceration of the stomach and duodenum. Amer. J. Surg. 119:632, 1970.

42. Goodman, A. A., and Frey, C. F. Massive upper gastrointestinal hemorrhage following surgical operations. Ann. Surg. 167:180, 1968.

43. Kirtley, J. A., Scott, H. W., Jr., Sawyers, J. L., Graves, H. A., Jr., and Lawler, M. R. The surgical management of stress ulcers. Ann. Surg. 169:801, 1969.

44. Kunzman, J. Management of bleeding stress ulcers. Amer. J. Surg. 119:637, 1970.

45. O'Neill, J. A., Jr., Pruitt, B. A., Jr., and Moncrief, J. A. Surgical treatment of Curling's ulcer. Surg. Gynec. Obstet. 126:40, 1968.

Chapter 54

Chronic Duodenal Ulcer

Charles O. Walker

The understanding of duodenal ulcer remains uneven. The clinical description of the disease continues to be improved, and diagnostic tools multiply beyond our ability to evaluate them. Great strides have been made in elucidating the hormonal and nervous control of gastric secretion; yet the pathophysiology of duodenal ulcer remains elusive, and medical treatment has not been proved to significantly alter the clinical course.

INCIDENCE AND PREVALENCE

How frequently ulceration of the stomach or duodenum is found depends upon the technique used to detect the disease and how vigorously the search is pressed. If the investigator makes a careful search for evidence of ulcer, whether by symptoms, endoscopy, X-ray, or autopsy, he will doubtless find more ulcers than in a routine examination not done with peptic ulcer disease specifically in mind.

Incidence. Incidence is defined as the number of individuals within a population group who have active duodenal ulcer within a given year. Depending on the study, activity may be based on symptoms, X-ray evidence of an active ulcer, surgery, autopsy, or some combination of these techniques. An estimated incidence of duodenal ulcer in males and females is shown in Figure 54–1. These are average results based on two large autopsy studies,[1] symptomatic patients seen in a private practice,[2] a United States National Health Survey based on a well balanced sample of 235,000 persons,[3] and a survey of Massachusetts physicians.[4] The autopsy series exclude those patients who died of duodenal ulcer disease. In spite of the different methods of data collection, the various studies closely agree; they show that duodenal ulcers first appear in significant numbers at about age 20 and by age 30 are seen in 2 per cent of males and 0.5 per cent of females. From 40 to 45 years of age on, 3 per cent of males and 1 per cent of females will have an active duodenal ulcer during each year. None of these stud-

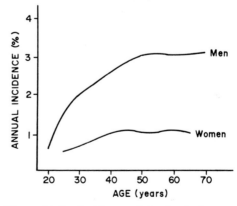

Figure 54–1. Incidence of duodenal ulcer: percentage of the general population who have an active ulcer crater at some time during a given year. The incidence figures shown are an overall estimate, based on both clinical and autopsy studies.[1-4]

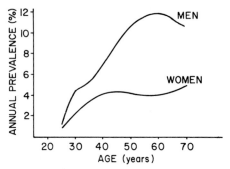

Figure 54-2. Prevalence of duodenal ulcer: percentage of the general population with evidence of active or inactive duodenal ulcer at some time during a given year. The prevalence figures shown are overall estimates, based on both clinical and autopsy studies.[1, 4]

ies is broken down to yield racial propensities, but it is apparent that in the United States, Caucasians, Negroes, and Latin Americans are frequently affected.

Prevalence. Prevalence is the percentage of the population that has duodenal ulcer, whether active or inactive, within a given year. The estimated prevalence of duodenal ulcer in males and females is shown in Figure 54-2. The prevalence increases rapidly in males and females during their late twenties and thirties. A peak prevalence of 4 per cent is achieved in females by age 40 with little subsequent increase, whereas male prevalence is 4 per cent at 30, is 7 per cent at 40, and slightly exceeds 10 per cent at 50. After age 50, males have no further significant increase.[1, 4]

Ulcer Mortality. There were 6.5 deaths per 100,000 population caused by gastric

and duodenal ulcer in males in the United States in 1963.[3] As shown in Figure 54-3, deaths per 100,000 population are infrequent under age 30, become much more frequent after age 60, and achieve a rate of 80 per 100,000 by age 80. The age-specific male death rate, shown in Figure 54-3, applies to both gastric and duodenal ulcer. In another study, it was shown that of all deaths caused by peptic ulcer, 75 per cent were due to duodenal ulcers and only 25 per cent due to gastric ulcers.[1] About three times more men than women die of gastric and duodenal ulcer.

CLINICAL COURSE

Although sporadic cases appear in individuals under age 20, duodenal ulcer first appears in significant numbers in patients in their early twenties and then the disease steadily increases in frequency and reaches a peak incidence and prevalence in the 40- to 50-year age group.[1-6] In most cases, symptoms precede actual objective evidence of ulceration by five to ten years.[2, 7] Few ulcers have their symptomatic onset after 60 years of age.

Duodenal ulcer is a chronic and recurrent disease, and there is an old saying, "once an ulcer, always an ulcer." Although this adage is useful in teaching, its validity is not clearly established.

In typical chronic duodenal ulcer disease, the first episode is seldom the patient's last. In 371 duodenal ulcer patients followed for 25 years, 40 per cent had a first recurrence during the first year, and 70 per cent had at least one recurrence by the fifth year.[5] During each subsequent year, 5 per cent of the remaining ulcer-free patients had a relapse. Not until 20 years elapsed did this annual relapse rate drop below 2 per cent. During the 25 years Krause followed these 371 duodenal ulcer patients, *all initially seen in the hospital,* only 11 per cent of the males and 18 per cent of the females had no recurrences.[5] Seventy per cent of the males and two-thirds of the females were either operated upon, died of their ulcer disease, or had severe symptoms at some time during their course. This study indicates that only about 15 per cent of a hospitalized population will escape a first recurrence,

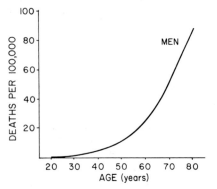

Figure 54-3. Age specific death rates in men due to peptic ulcer in the United States.[3]

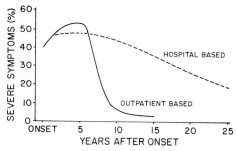

Figure 54–4. Persistence of severe ulcer symptoms in two duodenal ulcer populations in any given year. The hospital-based patients[5] have a much greater tendency to have persistent severe ulcer symptoms than the patients initially seen as outpatients.[2]

and that the physician should shy away from proclaiming a patient cured until at least 20 years have elapsed without a recurrence.

However, not all studies portray such a high recurrence rate and such chronicity. Thus, in Fry's study of ulcer patients seen in a *private practice* (most of whom were not hospitalized), peak symptoms occurred 7.5 years after onset, and attacks then became less frequent and less severe. After ten years, 90 per cent of these patients were either free of disease or minimally symptomatic.[2] In addition, several other studies reveal a decrease in recurrence rate in male duodenal ulcer disease in the fifth and sixth decades.[3, 6-9]

The difference between Krause's hospitalized patients and Fry's outpatients is diagrammed in Figure 54–4. For the first five to eight years almost 50 per cent of the patients in each group had moderately severe to incapacitating disease. By ten years severe symptoms were unusual in Fry's patients, whereas many of the hospital-based patients continued to have severe symptoms up to 25 years following onset.

In summary, duodenal ulcer is clearly a chronic disease with a strong predisposition to relapse. Only 10 to 15 per cent of patients will not suffer a relapse, and most of those relapsing will be severely affected for at least five to ten years. It appears that the disease wanes with the passage of time, especially in patients seen only as outpatients, but more data are clearly needed to determine the natural history of duodenal ulcer.

ASSOCIATED DISEASES

Certain chronic diseases are considered to be more frequently associated with duodenal ulcer and gastric ulcer than would be expected by chance alone (Table 54–1). Many studies have suggested that peptic ulcer is more frequent in patients with pulmonary disease and tuberculosis than in the general population.[2, 10, 11] Likewise, rheumatoid arthritis, even excluding the influence of aspirin and steroids, may be associated with a higher frequency of peptic ulcer (see pp. 643 to 644).[10-12] Cirrhosis of the liver, particularly in its advanced stages, with or without a surgically created portacaval shunt, has a high incidence of peptic ulcer.[13]

These various correlations, if true, are still clinical, and pathogenesis is speculative. Most of these patients have muscle wasting and negative nitrogen metabolism; possibly some aspect of protein malnutrition is involved. In many of the studies reporting these associations the controls are poor, the selection great, and the conclusions tenuous, but the best guess would be that individuals with chronic pulmonary disease, pulmonary tuberculosis, rheumatoid arthritis, cirrhosis

TABLE 54–1. DISEASES ASSOCIATED WITH DUODENAL ULCER AND GASTRIC ULCER

Positive Correlates
1. Chronic obstructive lung disease
2. Pulmonary tuberculosis
3. Rheumatoid arthritis
4. Cirrhosis of liver
5. Gastrin-secreting tumor

Possibly Positive Correlates
1. Coronary heart disease
2. Crohn's disease (small bowel)
3. Aortic aneurysm
4. Myasthenia gravis
5. Polycythemia vera
6. Hyperparathyroidism

Negative Correlates
1. Carcinoma
2. Diabetes mellitus
3. Obesity
4. Hypertension
5. Myocardial infarction
6. Gallbladder disease
7. Addison's disease

of the liver, and, of course, gastrin-secreting tumors, have an increased incidence of peptic ulcer.

A number of diseases have enough evidence suggesting an increased incidence of peptic ulcer that further study is warranted.[2, 10, 14-17] These include coronary heart disease, Crohn's disease, aortic aneurysm, myasthenia gravis, polycythemia vera, and hyperparathyroidism. Table 54–1 also gives a list of diseases that have either no increase or even a lower incidence of duodenal and gastric ulcer than in the general population.[2, 10, 11, 18] Considering the many theories that have linked stress, the adrenal glands, and peptic ulcer, it is noteworthy that patients with Cushing's disease are not reported to have an increased incidence of peptic ulcer. Individuals with Addison's disease are almost always achlorhydric or hyposecretors. With replacement therapy, acid secretion rises; a few patients will develop a duodenal or gastric ulcer, but even in those treated for Addison's disease the incidence of ulcer is low.[19-21]

SYMPTOMS OF PEPTIC ULCER

PEPTIC ULCER PAIN

Visceral vs. Somatic. Uncomplicated peptic ulcer pain is an example of visceral pain (see p. 330). As such, it is poorly localized and midline in location. Referred pain is rarely associated with the visceral pain of uncomplicated chronic peptic ulcer. With penetration to the serosa or into other organs, somatic pathways are stimulated; intense, circumscribed, steady somatic pain is produced, and referred pain becomes common. The somatic pain is appreciated in an area closely approximating the region being stimulated. The referred pain is sharp and also well circumscribed, but is localized in a site distant to the stimulus. The somatic component of the pain may occur in conjunction with the original visceral pain, in which instance the usual ulcer pattern remains with superimposed somatic symptoms; or the somatic pain may mask the visceral pain entirely, in which case the diagnosis may become difficult unless the patient is asked about preceding visceral pain.[22, 23] At times, the patient may present with a somatic pain pattern without preceding visceral pain.

Character, Location and Radiation of Pain. No matter how a patient characterizes his pain, i.e., burning, boring, aching, hunger-like, or gnawing, or if he only describes it as a vague discomfort, careful questioning will reveal it to be a fluctuating (but not colicky) pain, often poorly localized, and perceived to be deep to the abdominal wall.[20-23] The specific words or phrases the patient uses to describe his pain are not so important as other properties of this pain, such as the response to food and alkali and a history of recurrences and remissions. A flutter or nervousness of the stomach relieved by milk is more suggestive than burning epigastric pain present continuously for ten years. The pain of duodenal ulcer is usually epigastric in location (often just above the umbilicus). The pain is almost always in the middle of the epigastrium or just to the right of the midline. Gastric ulcers also produce visceral pain in the epigastrium, but it is located higher in the epigastrium and is sometimes to the left of the midline. These differences are only apparent when large numbers of patients are surveyed and are of little help in differential diagnosis in the individual patient.[23] Only rarely do uncomplicated peptic ulcers cause pain outside the epigastrium.

With large or penetrating ulcers, steady and severe pain may be present. This somatic pain is well localized, and referred pain is common. Upon penetration, duodenal ulcers tend to produce pain that radiates to the right upper quadrant and back, whereas somatic gastric ulcer pain lateralizes to the left upper quadrant, thorax, and back (see p. 761).

Rhythm of Pain. The classic pattern for peptic ulcer pain, duodenal or gastric, is for the pain to begin one to three hours postprandially and for relief to be obtained by eating food (especially milk or other protein-rich foods), taking antacids, or vomiting. Pain is not present upon awakening in the morning or after an eight- to ten-hour fast, but it does occur late in the evening, and it may wake the patient after two to three hours of sleep.

This pain pattern is easy to remember and understand if correlated with gastric acidity. An idealized acid pattern is shown in Figure 54–5. When a meal is eaten, in-

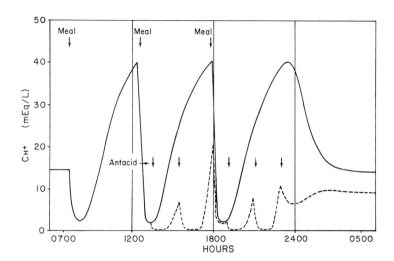

Figure 54–5. Gastric acidity (milliequivalents per liter) over a 24-hour period in a hypothetical duodenal ulcer patient. These curves are estimates based on the combined results presented in references 29, 104, and 106. The solid curve portrays acid concentration occurring in a duodenal ulcer patient who eats three meals a day, eats no snacks, and takes no antacids. The dashed curve indicates the effect of an antacid taken one and three hours after the noon and evening meals, and at bedtime.

tragastric acid concentration falls precipitously as the food, especially the protein component, buffers gastric acid. This buffering is the mechanism by which food relieves ulcer pain. In spite of acid production in response to the meal, the buffer capacity of the food maintains a relatively low intragastric acid concentration for one to two hours postprandially. Pain is absent during this period. As the meal buffer is emptied, acid concentration rises owing to a continued high rate of acid secretion, and pain occurs. If the patient eats the evening meal at 6:00 P.M., his acid secretion rates will be back to near-basal levels by 11:00 P.M. However, if he eats a bedtime snack at 11:00 P.M., high rates of acid secretion will continue until about 3:00 A.M. Such patients tend to wake up with pain around 1:00 to 2:00 A.M.

A classic pattern is not seen in every patient. Pain patterns vary, depending upon the sensitivity of the ulcer to acid-pepsin, on the rate of acid secretion by the patient, and on the specific timing of his meals.

Certain empiric characteristics and differences, present in the pain patterns of duodenal and gastric ulcers and in other dyspepsia, will now be considered.

NIGHT PAIN. Night pain occurs in almost 50 per cent of peptic ulcer patients and is justifiably used as a strong clue for the presence of organic disease. Its value in the diagnosis of peptic ulcer is enhanced if it is relieved by food, antacids, or vomiting. It must be emphasized, however, that 20 per cent of patients with epigas-

tric distress of nonpeptic origin, i.e., gastritis or functional dyspepsia, also have night pain.[24]

POSTPRANDIAL PAIN. Onset of pain one to two hours after a meal is common in patients with both duodenal and gastric ulcers. Pain within the first 30 minutes of eating occurs in about 20 per cent of gastric ulcer patients, but in only a few patients with duodenal ulcer. This is because acid produced in the body of the stomach bathes an ulcer in the stomach earlier than one in the duodenum and, in addition, some work suggests that gastric ulcers may be more sensitive to acid than duodenal ulcers, with pain occurring at a lower acid concentration.[25, 26]

PAIN PRECEDING A MEAL. Highly suggestive of ulcer disease is pain beginning three or more hours after a meal or preceding the next meal.[24] Such a pattern is particularly helpful because functional pain rarely occurs with such timing.[24, 27, 28]

DURATION OF PAIN. In the careful study of Edwards and Coghill, duodenal ulcer pain came on later and lasted longer than gastric ulcer pain, with 33 per cent of duodenal ulcer distress and 16 per cent of gastric ulcer distress continuing until the next meal.[24]

MORNING PAIN. Pain typically does not precede breakfast, because the stomach's acid output, which has not been stimulated by food for the past eight to 12 hours, is at its lowest ebb at this time.[29] Duodenal ulcers causing gastric outlet obstruction may be associated with morning pain, and ulcers in children are reported to cause morning pain.[30]

RELIEF OF PAIN WITH FOOD AND AL-KALI.   Relief of pain by alkali is typical of both gastric and duodenal ulcers, although gastric ulcer pain is slightly less responsive. The major difficulty with the use of this finding in differential diagnosis is that many patients with functional gastrointestinal complaints get partial or complete relief with alkali.[24, 27, 28] Relief of ulcer pain by food may not be as frequent as with alkali, but appears to be more specific, because pain relief by food is not as common in functional dyspepsia as is relief with alkali.

PAIN EXACERBATED BY FOOD.   Exacerbation or precipitation of pain by food is rare in duodenal ulcer, common in functional disease (45 per cent), and of intermediate frequency in gastric ulcer (24 per cent).[24] It is not unusual for a patient with a gastric ulcer to have both aggravation and subsequent relief of pain by food. In fact, such a pattern coupled with periodicity of symptoms was found to be the most predictive clinical syndrome for the diagnosis of gastric ulcer in a computer analysis of ulcer symptoms.[27]

Clusters (Remissions and Relapses). Duodenal ulcer is a chronic and recurrent disease with a tendency to heal and recur spontaneously. Pain has usually been present for several years when the diagnosis is first made. Depending upon the selection of patients, the mean duration of symptoms prior to diagnosis will be from five to ten years. The range is obviously wide, from the individual without pain at first diagnosis to the patient with a 25-year history of pain. This ulcer pain, which remits only to be followed by another bout of pain, has been said to exhibit "periodicity"; more recently, these episodes of pain have been descriptively designated as pain "clusters"[27] The chronicity of ulcer and the tendency of pain to occur in clusters in a typical group of ulcer patients are shown in Figure 54–6.[31] Retrospective histories will reveal similar clusters of pain occurring over many years in most duodenal ulcer patients.[32]

In Edwards and Coghill's survey of duodenal and gastric ulcer, the pain attacks (relapse) varied from slightly less than a week to eight weeks in duration. A small

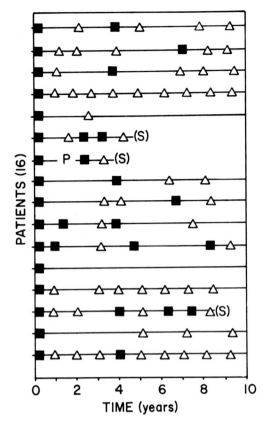

- ■ Course of ulcer treatment
- △ Ulcer distress - no formal treatment
- S Surgery
- P Perforation

Figure 54–6. Chronicity and periodicity of duodenal ulcer in 16 patients with duodenal ulcer. (Redrawn from Malmros, H., and Hiertonn, T.: Acta Med. Scand. 133:229, 1949.)

percentage of patients (less than 10 per cent) had relapses for three months or longer; in most instances these were gastric ulcer patients. However, variations among groups are so great that the duration of attacks does not allow one to distinguish between gastric and duodenal ulcer.

When remissions occur, they are usually longer than the episodes of pain. In duodenal ulcer, the remissions tend to be short (one to three months), with each one of similar length, whereas gastric ulcer patients have remissions of variable lengths. However, once again, similarities are greater than differences, and the length of remissions in a given patient would be of limited value in differential diagnosis.

Although gastric and duodenal ulcers have more similarities than differences in

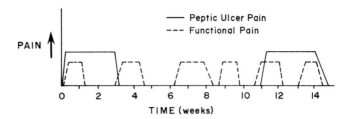

Figure 54–7. Pain clusters in peptic ulcer and functional dyspepsia. Pain relapses and remissions are longer and more regular in patients with peptic ulcer than in those with functional gastrointestinal disorders.

their pain periodicity, the pattern of dyspepsia found in functional gastrointestinal disease is different from that in peptic ulcer disease, and these differences are valuable in differential diagnosis. Typical cluster patterns of peptic ulcer and functional gastrointestinal disease are illustrated in Figure 54–7. In sharp contrast to duodenal and gastric ulcer patients, both relapses and remissions of pain in functional gastrointestinal disease are of short duration.

The occurrences of pain in clusters, followed by one- to three-month periods without pain, have long been recognized to be of particular value in diagnosis, and are said to be present in 70 to 90 per cent of ulcer patients when first diagnosed.[33-35] As patients are followed, this percentage rises as those ulcer patients who initially presented without pain or with ill-defined dyspepsia develop the more typical cluster pain of peptic disease. However, a note of caution is needed; a few individuals with peptic ulcer may have constant pain without periodicity and have a pain pattern indistinguishable from that of nonulcer (functional) dyspepsia.[34] This constant pain is apparently not due to persistence of an active ulcer crater, and such patients probably have pain that is not related to the ulcer itself. These patients tend to maintain this pain pattern and it may be difficult to tell when an ulcer crater is present, because the crater is not heralded by new symptoms.

PATHOGENESIS OF PEPTIC ULCER PAIN

Most observers believe that the visceral pain of peptic ulcer is due to stimulation of nerves within the gastric wall by acid and/or altered gastric motility.

Acid-Induced Pain. Palmer was a leading advocate of the acid-peptic etiology of ulcer pain. He felt that the concentration

of acid, its duration of action, and the sensitivity of the lesion (i.e., depth of penetration, amount of inflammation) determined the presence or absence of pain.[36]

The concept that gastric acid is somehow important in the genesis of ulcer pain is readily accepted by most physicians. That acid is important is eminently reasonable, because the production and relief of symptoms appear to be closely correlated with those events which either increase or decrease gastric acid. For example, pain commonly appears one and one-half to three hours postprandially at a time when gastric acidity is the highest, and ingestion of food or alkali reduces gastric acidity and relieves ulcer pain. (The absence of such a response casts doubt on the diagnosis of peptic ulcer.) Likewise, vomiting, which empties the stomach of acid, will frequently relieve the pain of peptic ulcer, so much so that some patients learn to induce vomiting for the relief which it brings. Furthermore, aspiration of gastric acid will yield prompt relief of pain,[25, 26, 28, 36, 37] and reintroduction of the gastric contents will cause pain to reappear, but not if the gastric juice is neutralized prior to reintroduction.[26]

Bönninger, in 1908, and Palmer, in 1926, devised protocols for acid infusion tests. If an individual was having spontaneous pain, although pain need not be present at the onset of the test, a dilute solution of hydrochloric acid (200 ml of 0.1 N HCl) was introduced into his stomach. In the hands of many investigators, the introduction of the acid was followed, after a lag period of up to 20 minutes, by the intensification or appearance of typical ulcer pain in most patients. The great majority of duodenal and gastric ulcer patients had a positive test. Friedman, while studying servicemen with dyspepsia, was careful to control the test so that the expectations of the physician or patient did not influence the results.[28] He found an extremely good correlation between the presence of peptic ulcer and the acid test.

As further proof that acid induces pain, Dragstedt demonstrated under local anesthesia that a duodenal ulcer was sensitive to acid and that pain so induced could be relieved with alkali.[38]

Finally, Bonney and Pickering found that in a given patient there was a general pH range at which pain appeared and disappeared.[26] Pain occurred if hydrogen ion concentration exceeded a certain level for a long time, and disappeared if the acidity fell much below this level. The pH threshold for pain was 1.5 to 2.5 for duodenal ulcer and 2.2 to 3.0 for gastric and anastomotic ulcers.

The Contribution of Motility. Although it is generally accepted that acid stimulation of nerve endings in the ulcer crater is the major cause of visceral ulcer pain, there is suggestive evidence that abnormalities in motility may, at least in some instances, also be important.[39, 40] Even Palmer, the champion of acid-induced pain, states "that in an occasional instance of intermittent and also remittent pain, the waves of pain, or the exacerbations in it, corresponded exactly with the peristaltic contractions of the stomach."[36]

For years, observers have noted that ulcer pain was frequently associated with hyperperistalsis as measured by kymography or X-ray.[36, 40, 41] The type of gastroduodenal peristalsis most frequently associated with ulcer pain has been the type II antral waves. These are spiking contractions of the stomach that produce pressure of up to 30 cm of water and last about 20 seconds. In normal subjects they are associated with hunger, and they may be increased in frequency and last longer in some patients with peptic ulcer.[34, 42] Anticholinergics inhibit antral type II waves as they relieve ulcer pain. Other abnormalities of motility, such as increased intragastric tension and alterations of gastric emptying, have never been established as a cause of pain. The relief of pain by anticholinergic drugs may be mediated by reduced acid secretions as well as by decreased motility.[25, 26, 41, 43]

In the study of Patterson and Sandweiss, patients did not develop spontaneous pain unless gastric or duodenal peristalsis, measured by kymography, was present and active.[44] However, with the addition of alkali, the pain could be abolished while duodenal activity continued. The various issues raised by these studies are not entirely resolved, and the interested reader can pursue the issue further.[41, 45]

In conclusion, when the pH at an ulcer site is greater than 2 to 3 in duodenal ulcer patients and greater than 3 in gastric ulcer patients, pain will usually be absent. Acid directly stimulating nerve endings must for now be considered the major cause of visceral ulcer pain. Changes in peristalsis are likely a secondary response to the ulcer but may at times aggravate or cause pain.

VOMITING

In some older studies, vomiting was prominently mentioned and was said to be present in 50 per cent or more of patients.[35, 46] However, vomiting to relieve pain made up a significant proportion (40 per cent) of those who vomited. Vomiting also represented outlet obstruction in some, and in many others it was a minor part of the disease sequence.[32] In more recent studies in which uncomplicated ulcer patients were carefully followed, vomiting was found to be infrequent.[28, 33, 34] Gastric ulcer patients have a slightly higher incidence of vomiting than patients with duodenal ulcer. A patient who obtains complete pain relief only when he vomits is more likely to have a gastric ulcer than a duodenal ulcer. Interestingly, patients with gastritis (a frequent concomitant of gastric ulcer) also have a high incidence of vomiting, which is said to relieve epigastric pain.[24]

WEIGHT LOSS

Weight loss is present in many patients with peptic ulcer.[34, 47] Its frequency appears to be higher in gastric (60 per cent) than in duodenal (48 per cent) ulcer, and significant weight loss (greater than 10 pounds) is also more frequent in those with gastric ulcers (37 per cent versus 24 per cent). In a study which compared weight loss in persons with benign and malignant gastric ulcers, weight loss greater than 10 pounds was present in 42 per cent of each group.[47] Thirty-five per cent of each group had no weight loss. When weight loss in persons with peptic ulcer was compared with weight loss in individuals with nonulcer dyspepsia, the percentages for each category were similar.[24]

EPIGASTRIC TENDERNESS

Epigastric tenderness is common in patients with ulcer. In uncomplicated disease, the tenderness is modest, without rigidity or rebound. It is doubtful that the presence of tenderness should be given much weight in differential diagnosis, because patients with nonulcer dyspepsia also exhibit epigastric tenderness; its absence should cast some doubt on a diagnosis of active ulceration.

OTHER SIGNS AND SYMPTOMS

In patients with uncomplicated peptic ulcer, a number of nonspecific symptoms such as constipation, epigastric fullness, belching, pyrosis, anorexia, weakness, nausea, and diarrhea are noted.[35, 48] The frequency of these symptoms is not high, few are mentioned in most reviews, and such complaints are frequent enough in the normal population that they do not help diagnostically. Obviously, constipation or diarrhea may be induced by medication, epigastric fullness may be seen if the ulcer is complicated by obstruction, and diarrhea may occur if the ulcer is induced by a Zollinger-Ellison tumor, but their occurrence confounds rather than aids the diagnosis.

PSYCHIC MANIFESTATIONS

Individuals with duodenal ulcer do not have a characteristic personality (see p. 164). However, anxiety and depression are often associated with peptic ulcer, and patients with severe anxiety and/or depression obtain a poor response from treatment, either medical or surgical.[49-51] Since both anxiety and depression are common in nonpeptic (functional) dyspepsia, their recognition is not as important diagnostically as it is therapeutically.[52]

CLINICAL SPECTRUM OF DUODENAL ULCER

The preceding section has described the symptoms of duodenal ulcer. Not every duodenal ulcer patient has a classic ulcer history, because symptoms depend on the pathology, physiology, and psyche of the particular patient. The duodenal ulcer variants, recognized because of distinctive diagnostic, therapeutic, or pathological features, are listed in Table 54–2. As shown in the table, ulcer patients can be divided into two major categories, dyspeptic or asymptomatic. If dyspeptic, they may have either typical or atypical ulcer symptoms. Those with typical symptoms may be further subdivided into groups with or without concomitant somatic symptoms and a group with typical symptoms in whom an ulcer cannot be demonstrated (the pseudoulcer-duodenitis complex). Atypical symptoms are found in two situations: first, when the somatic pain of a complication is the only pain appreciated; and second, when a duodenal ulcer occurs in an individual with functional pain.

CLASSIC DUODENAL ULCER

The following symptoms, listed more or less in order of importance, are the pri-

TABLE 54–2. CLINICAL SPECTRUM OF PEPTIC ULCER DISEASE

I. Dyspepsia
  A. Typical or suggestive of peptic ulcer disease
    1. Peptic ulcer disease with visceral pain (classic syndrome)
    2. Peptic ulcer disease with visceral and somatic pain
      a. Obstruction
      b. Penetration
      c. Perforation
    3. Pseudoulcer-duodenitis syndrome
  B. Atypical symptoms
    1. Somatic pain
    2. Functional-like symptoms
  C. Ulcers with special features
    1. Postbulbar duodenal ulcer
    2. Pyloric channel ulcer
    3. Combined gastric and duodenal ulcer
    4. Ulcer symptoms in children and elderly
II. Asymptomatic
  A. Radiological diagnosis
  B. Presentation as a complication
    1. Hemorrhage
    2. Perforation

mary components of the classic duodenal ulcer history:

1. Chronic nonradiating epigastric pain with clusters of pain.
2. Rhythmic pain which coincides with the acid cycle:
   a. Onset of pain preceding a meal.
   b. Onset of pain one to three hours postprandially.
   c. Pain occurring one to two hours after retiring.
   d. Relief of pain by food.
3. Pain not present on awakening in the morning.
4. Relief of pain by alkali.

Patients with all four of the aforementioned components most likely have a peptic ulcer. Most patients with duodenal ulcer will, after thoughtful questioning, give a close approximation of this history. The cataloguing of duodenal ulcer pain as epigastric and nonradiating is helpful, but the quality of the pain is not too important.

ASYMPTOMATIC PEPTIC ULCER

There are patients with chronic ulcer who have no pain. They are diagnosed by an upper gastrointestinal series done for another reason, or they present with a complication of peptic ulcer without a history of prior ulcer symptoms.[53, 54]

In surveys of apparently healthy, asymptomatic individuals, the prevalence of duodenal deformity and ulcer is reported to be from 8 to 50 per cent.[55] In the study of Dunn and Etter, 650 male executives aged 35 to 65 underwent an upper gastrointestinal barium examination as part of a routine annual health examination. They found that the incidence of duodenal deformity or ulcer crater was 30 per cent in subjects whose history did not suggest peptic disease.[53] Each X-ray considered positive was read as positive independently by three radiologists, but the criteria for deformity and the number of patients who actually had a crater were not given. If ulcer disease is present in these asymptomatic individuals, it may be more benign than in symptomatic individuals, but this cannot be answered until the clinical course is established. These individuals appeared to have fewer complaints in general, and the investigators suggest that

they may have a higher threshold to pain or are less aware of symptoms.[53] Whether this lack of awareness is physiological or psychological is speculative.

However, it seems unlikely that 30 per cent of asymptomatic persons have duodenal ulcers, for the following reasons: (1) To justify the diagnosis of an asymptomatic state, careful inquiry must be made about symptoms compatible with peptic ulcer disease for the previous five years.[5] (2) Although extreme "cloverleaf" deformity is closely correlated with chronic duodenal ulcer, less severely distorted bulbs may have multiple causes.[56] (3) Long-term follow-up of these individuals should reveal a higher proportion developing symptoms of peptic ulcer than controls without "deformity," and this has not been demonstrated. (4) In very detailed autopsy studies, the highest prevalence of ulcer (acute plus scar) is only 16 per cent during the years of highest prevalence.[1]

The second way in which the incidence of asymptomatic ulcers may be discovered is to determine how frequently patients with complications of ulcer disease admit to previous ulcer symptoms. Between 3 and 14 per cent of individuals who present with a perforated ulcer deny previous pain.[33, 57, 58] Histology of many perforated asymptomatic ulcers reveals a chronic ulcer, and a large percentage of these individuals subsequently develop symptoms.[59]

Upper gastrointestinal bleeding, apparently from painless peptic ulcer, is more frequent than previously painless perforation. However, histological proof of chronic peptic ulcer is usually not obtained in the bleeding patient.[33, 54]

In summary, it is still not clear how frequently chronic peptic ulcers are asymptomatic. Considering the frequency of ulcer at autopsy plus clinical studies (with their invariable selection of patients), it is reasonable to conclude that about 10 per cent of chronic peptic ulcers are asymptomatic, at least during their initial stage.

DUODENAL ULCER WITH FUNCTIONAL-LIKE PAIN

A few patients with duodenal ulcer have symptoms that are identical with functional dyspepsia (see p. 683).[34] Their pain is chronic and often in the epigastrium, but lacks the usual ulcer periodicity, is not in rhythm with the acid cycle, and is poorly relieved by food. The pain is often aggravated by stress, and some relief may be obtained from antacids. Neurotic personalities are present in most such patients.[28, 60]

An upper gastrointestinal X-ray series, often ordered in a perfunctory manner, is the usual route of discovery for this ulcer. Hemorrhage and perforation are also seen during the course of the disease, and at times the ulcer is first diagnosed after an ulcer complication reveals its presence.

Long-term follow-up is not available, but at least for several years most patients will continue to have functional rather than ulcer-type pain. Ulcers tend to come and go without a change of symptoms.[34]

Pathophysiology is not clear, but could represent asymptomatic ulcers occurring in subjects with fortuitous functional pain or the presence of the ulcer diathesis in an individual so neurotic that his pain is distorted by his psyche.

Treatment of such patients by the usual ulcer regimen is not very helpful, and antianxiety drugs or sedative drugs are only slightly better.[28]

ULCERS WITH SOMATIC PAIN

The complications of duodenal ulcer, i.e., penetration, perforation, and obstruction, produce severe somatic pain. Visceral ulcer pain may be obliterated, as all the patient's attention is focused on the arresting pain of the complication (see pp. 758 to 764). The typical visceral pain of duodenal ulcer has usually preceded the somatic pain, but sometimes, especially with perforation, the history of previous pain may not be elicited. Later, after resolution of the complication, the typical visceral pain may reappear or occur for the first time.

PSEUDOULCER-DUODENITIS

The preceding presentations are acknowledged manifestations of duodenal ulcer; although further effort is needed to more fully delineate their scope, there is no real argument as to their place in the disease spectrum. However, duodenitis and/or pseudoulcer are seldom considered

as diagnostic possibilities, and, when they are, it is usually in a condescending manner. Although they have been under- and overdiagnosed in the past, there is adequate evidence that these are valid entities, with a pathogenesis similar to that of duodenal ulcer, representing one of the variants of duodenal ulcer.

Beck and coworkers selected patients with peptic ulcer symptoms and normal X-rays and contrasted the histology of their duodenal bulb by biopsy to those of three control groups: individuals with negative history and normal X-rays, individuals with normal X-rays and atypical upper gastrointestinal symptoms in no way suggestive of peptic ulcer, and patients with peptic ulcer disease established by X-ray and history.[61] The biopsy specimens were read blind on two separate occasions. The results indicate that normal control subjects and those with gastrointestinal complaints atypical for ulcer had only a modest cellular infiltrate. By contrast, the ulcer patients and those with ulcer symptoms but normal X-rays had biopsy specimens that were heavily infiltrated with chronic inflammatory cells.

This well controlled study strongly suggests, along with other less well controlled studies, that duodenitis is a clinical entity. Patients are characterized by the following features:

1. Symptoms highly suggestive of peptic ulcer appear; although obstruction and perforation are not seen, bleeding does occur.[62, 63]

2. Radiology reveals a bulb without an ulcer niche or gross deformity; coarse folds are common in the bulb and postbulbar area, although the folds may also be entirely normal.[64, 65] Some patients will have a normal X-ray, which has been preceded by or will be followed by X-rays showing coarse duodenal folds.[66]

3. Histologically, a heavy cellular infiltrate (largely mononuclear) and microscopic ulceration are seen. The mucosa may take on the appearance of gastric epithelium, and in severe cases there will be flattening of the villi.

4. Acid secretory studies may be normal or high.

Coarse duodenal folds are more frequent when hyperchlorhydria is present; most authors who have found hypersecretion in their "duodenitis" patients have established the presence of coarse duodenal folds as a major criterion for placing patients in this category.[62, 67, 68]

Duodenoscopy is the technique for future research evaluation and for current diagnosis. Initial work by fiberduodenoscopy suggests that duodenitis may be present independent of or accompanying duodenal ulcer (see pp. 531 to 534).[64]

The natural history of duodenitis may be exemplified by the study of Krag.[65] He reviewed 174 patients who had characteristic ulcer symptoms but no X-ray evidence of peptic ulcer, the bulb being completely normal in 64 per cent, and coarse folds without deformity or ulcer being found in the rest. This syndrome, which he called pseudoulcer, was most frequently diagnosed in younger patients, the peak incidence preceding that of duodenal ulcer by about a decade. Acid secretion rates by Ewald test meal were higher than normal, and thus similar to the values of duodenal ulcer patients. Ninety-two per cent of the patients were successfully followed over the next ten to 20 years. During follow-up, 40 per cent developed a definite ulcer by X-ray or surgery. Older patients and those with coarse folds had a higher incidence of ulcer on follow-up than did younger patients or patients with normal duodenal folds.

In summary, it seems apparent that duodenitis may precede frank duodenal ulceration by months to years when follow-up is sufficiently long and complete. It is still conjectural whether duodenitis is one form of peptic ulcer disease, its constant companion, or a separate disease.

POSTBULBAR DUODENAL ULCER

The bulb forms about two-thirds of the first part of the duodenum. Its mucosa is fine and granular, and the mucosal folds run parallel to its long axis. Beyond the bulb, the mucosal folds become transverse, and any ulcer found at or beyond the transition to transverse folds is postbulbar.[69-71] Most occur in the first part of the duodenum or in the second part of the duodenum proximal to the ampulla of Vater.[71, 72]

The reported incidence of postbulbar ulceration has a wide range (1 to 30 per cent of all peptic ulcers). The true incidence is probably less than 5 per cent; one surgeon who routinely opened the duodenum found that less than 3 per cent of duodenal ulcers were postbulbar.[69, 73]

Although in many instances the symptoms are similar to those of other duodenal ulcers, most investigators stress two major concepts in the clinical description of postbulbar ulcer: first, that pain is often atypical, and second, that complications, particularly hemorrhage, are frequent.[69-71, 73, 74]

Approximately 90 per cent of patients with postbulbar ulcer present with pain.[69, 71] In the largest clinical series (99 patients), 80 per cent of those presenting with pain were said to have had ulcer pain with periodicity, rhythmicity, and treatment response fairly typical of duodenal ulcer.[71] However, in several other series, most of the patients had atypical pain patterns.[69, 70, 73] The most common site of pain is the epigastrium, but concomitant pain in the right upper quadrant is frequent (15 per cent), and at times pain may be found only in the right upper quadrant (8 per cent). Radiation of pain to the back, especially at night, is two to three times more frequent than in bulbar ulcers.[69-71] Although only about 50 per cent of ulcers in the duodenal bulb produce night pain, 90 per cent of patients with postbulbar ulcer have night pain. Thus almost all individuals with painful postbulbar ulcers will have night pain which frequently radiates through to the back; at times, nocturnal back pain may be the only pain appreciated.

When the pain is atypical in location (right upper quadrant or back), the usual ulcer periodicity is often lacking and response to treatment is usually poor.[69, 70, 73] Although not carefully correlated in most studies, penetration of these ulcers is not unusual, and many patients with severe and bizarre symptoms probably have penetrated ulcers.[69]

Hemorrhage is by far the most common of the complications of postbulbar ulcers. It appears to be two to four times more frequent than would be expected in bulbar ulcers, and ranges from 40 to 66 per cent.[69-71, 73] In the series with the least surgical selection, the rate was 40 per cent.[71] The bleeds are often massive, with emergency surgery needed to prevent exsanguination.

Duodenal obstruction, with a slowly progressive intermittent course, will supervene in 15 per cent of the patients. The obstructive episodes consist of severe pain of sudden onset, with continuous vomiting lasting for up to several days, followed by gradual abatement to an asymptomatic interlude.[69] Edema and scarring can on rare occasions induce obstruction of the biliary outflow tract. Free perforation is rare.

Individuals with a postbulbar ulcer often have symptoms that fail to respond to prescribed medical treatment. This ineffectual treatment is the product of missed diagnosis (because of a vague history or incomplete radiological examination) and also because frequently the ulcer has penetrated.

The specific diagnosis of postbulbar ulcer is almost never made from the initial history, although the physician usually suspects that peptic disease is present. The radiologist must take particular care to fill the area just distal to the bulb if the diagnosis is to be made. If the upper gastrointestinal series is equivocal, hypotonic duodenography or gastroduodenoscopy may resolve the issue.

In the differential diagnosis, duodenal diverticula, pancreatic tumors, pancreatitis, and tumors of the duodenum will cause confusion.[69] Normal mucosa will be seen in diverticula, and there will be no stenosis or spasm of the opposite wall, which is typical of postbulbar ulcer. Tumors and pancreatitis usually do not cause ulceration in this region; but if the issue remains unclear, hypotonic duodenography and gastroduodenoscopy will clarify the diagnosis. Typical X-rays are shown in Figures 40–25 to 40–28, pages 511 to 512.

PYLORIC CHANNEL ULCERS

The pyloric channel is that segment of the gastrointestinal tract, approximately 2 cm long, that forms the oscillating junction between the duodenal bulb and gastric antrum.[75] Its distal margin is the histological gastroduodenal junction, and it extends proximally 2 cm.[76] Ulcers in this location have a propensity to cause obstruction, to penetrate, and to run an accelerated clinical course; they are thereby difficult to treat medically.[75, 77-79] However, an ulcer of the pyloric channel which did not penetrate, obstruct, or prove intractable would be very unlikely to be included in a surgical review of channel ulcers. Since most series are composed predominantly of ulcers proved at surgery, there is a bias for inclusion of the more virulent cases.

Typical peptic ulcer pain is rather infrequent in patients with pyloric ulcer; when typical pain is present, it is common to find an active duodenal ulcer in addition to the channel ulcer.[75, 77-79] Typical ulcer periodicity and rhythmicity are frequently absent. Pain coming on either immediately or very soon after eating is frequent (35 per cent). Relief of pain by food and alkali is still found in the majority of patients (65 per cent), but this is less effective than in comparable patients with duodenal ulcers. Attempts to correlate the atypical pain with posterior penetration are inconclusive.[75, 77]

Vomiting, which is very frequent and at times the major method used by the patient to obtain relief, correlates very well with the presence of outlet obstruction.[78] However, when the ulcers causing outlet obstruction are excluded, vomiting is no more common than in routine gastric or duodenal ulcers.[75]

These ulcers run an accelerated clinical course.[77, 78] More specifically, the duration of symptoms from onset until surgery is shorter than in duodenal ulcers (7.7 vs. 14.5 years), but longer than for gastric ulcers (7.7 vs. 3.5 years), and in 70 per cent of individuals developing obstruction the total duration of symptoms is less than one year. This, coupled with a somewhat poorer response to medical treatment, has led to the concept that a channel ulcer should be treated surgically (see pp. 772 to 787).[77] The tendency to treat these ulcers surgically reflects more than just virulence. If the ulcer is considered a gastric ulcer rather than duodenal or channel, the specter of cancer is raised and more rapid referral is likely. However, gastric cancer rarely occurs in the pyloric channel and therefore almost never presents as an apparent benign pyloric channel ulcer.[75, 77-79] If those patients with outlet obstruction are treated for their obstruction as outlined on pages 767 and 768, thereby eliminating most of the obstructing ulcers from further consideration, a group of patients remain with unobstructing ulcer in the channel;

these patients should be treated medically with the expectation that many will respond favorably to medical treatment. Typical X-rays are shown in Figures 40–16 and 40–17, pages 505 and 506.

COMBINED GASTRIC AND DUODENAL ULCERS

When peptic ulcers occur simultaneously in the stomach and duodenal bulb, the frequency of certain complications and the response to treatment are sufficiently characteristic to justify separate consideration of these patients. The age range in which this association is found is the same as that for gastric ulcer, with a peak incidence between 40 and 70 years.[80]

Approximately 7 per cent of all peptic ulcers will be gastric-duodenal combinations.[80, 81] About one in 20 to 30 duodenal ulcer patients will have an associated gastric ulcer, and one in five gastric ulcer patients will have an associated duodenal ulcer.[80, 81] In radiological surveys, supplemented by surgical results, the duodenal ulcer is active in about 45 per cent of the patients and the gastric ulcer is active in 98 per cent. Thus when both ulcers are present, it is statistically more likely that the gastric ulcer is the cause of symptoms or bleeding than the duodenal ulcer. In 38 per cent of combined ulcers found in autopsy series, both ulcers were healed.[80]

The most frequent clinical sequence is for a patient to have a duodenal ulcer which progresses to chronicity or healing and then becomes complicated by a gastric ulcer. Thus 80 per cent are either patients in whom both ulcers are active or in whom a duodenal ulcer has progressed to complete healing, leaving an active gastric ulcer.[80] A less common but well documented sequence is for a gastric ulcer to be complicated by a duodenal ulcer (6.5 per cent).[80-82]

Although symptoms may change in some patients coincident with the appearance of the new ulcer, there is nothing characteristic about the change which would allow a prospective diagnosis. A patient whose duodenal ulcer has been in remission may have his symptoms return, not because of duodenal ulcer activity, but because he now has a gastric ulcer.[80, 81]

Three complications of peptic ulcer—

pyloric stenosis, hemorrhage, and intractability—appear to be more frequent in those with combined disease than in those with either gastric or duodenal ulcer as a single entity. Gastric retention has been said to occur in as many as 64 per cent of these concomitant ulcers, but documentation of true outlet obstruction is usually lacking.[83] A composite of many series suggests that 12 per cent may actually have gastric outlet obstruction.[80-83] Presumably, the outlet obstruction is largely due to the duodenal disease, with the gastric lesion only a contributing factor.

The incidence of hemorrhage is quite high (30 to 50 per cent) in patients with the combined lesion.[80-82] In most instances, bleeding is from the gastric ulcer. The incidence of bleeding is much greater, i.e. 47 per cent versus 8 per cent, than in gastric ulcers occurring alone.[80]

Finally, this combination ulceration frequently appears to be intractable to medical therapy, and this, coupled with the high incidence of hemorrhage and pyloric stenosis, results in surgery often being utilized.[80-84] However, clinical data reveal that at least 30 per cent of patients will have a good response to medical therapy, and this impression is confirmed by autopsy series which show that combined gastric and duodenal ulcers are frequently both healed.[80-82]

ULCER SYMPTOMS IN CHILDREN AND ELDERLY

The symptoms of ulcer disease in children are qualitatively different from those seen in adults. In addition, there are significant differences between the various age groups in children. In infants, most ulcers are associated with stress and present as bleeding or perforation.[85] In older children (aged two to 16 years) complications remain frequent, being greater than 50 per cent in several series, with bleeding being most common.[30, 86, 87] Pain is almost always present, but it may be quite atypical, especially in children less than nine years old. Epigastric, periumbilical, or generalized abdominal pain may be seen. Relief by food is not consistent, early morning pain may occur, and nausea and vomiting are common. Night pain, relief of pain by vomiting, and a good response to antacids are similar to findings in adults. In younger children, diarrhea, anorexia, and headaches may be manifestations of peptic ulcer.

Several features of peptic ulcer disease as seen in the elderly (over 60 years old) should be emphasized. First, many concomitant diseases are seen.[48] Forty per cent of these patients have some manifestation of cardiovascular disease, and the majority have some other serious disease. Second, relatively few ulcers develop for the first time after the age of 60, and those that do often manifest themselves by hemorrhage or perforation, with either no prior symptoms or previous symptoms of only short duration.[48] In the elderly, as in younger adults, there does not appear to be much difference between the symptoms or complications of gastric and duodenal ulcers.

DIAGNOSIS OF DUODENAL ULCER

HISTORY

Many individuals with duodenal ulcers may only complain of mild epigastric distress or dyspepsia. They may consistently deny pain. Thus the first and most important phase of diagnosis is to decide if any discomfort compatible with peptic ulcer pain is actually present. A patient may complain of heartburn, indigestion, gas, aches, discomfort, hunger pains, or only a flutter, but these may implicate peptic disease as surely as burning, gnawing, or boring pain if used in the proper context. If it is a chronic, epigastric sensation that occurs in clusters, has its onset one to two hours after meals, and is relieved by food or antacids, it is probably due to peptic disease regardless of how it is described by the patient. The patient should be asked not only whether he takes antacids but also whether he uses Tums, Rolaids, baking soda, Alka Seltzer, or other proprietary drugs.

If the pain pattern suggests that a peptic ulcer is present, the illness must be further characterized by gathering details about the patient's personality, eating and drinking habits, drug usage, family history, concomitant diseases, and symptoms compatible with ulcer complications or unusual ulcer presentations.

Anxiety and Depression. Although any personality type may acquire a duodenal ulcer, anxiety and depression are two symptoms which should be carefully quantified. These symptoms are important, because when they are prominent the patient is likely to have a poor response to medical or surgical therapy.[49-52] In addition, such individuals are frequently habitual users of alcohol, tobacco, and caffeine products. The physician must explore the content of the patient's life. For example, he should ask about interpersonal relationships with wife, family, friends, and associates, about financial problems and employment, and about current or recurrent events that precipitate relapses. The patient must be given time to digress, ramble, and ventilate. The time required to obtain this information is well spent for several reasons. First, the doctor will determine whether anxiety and depression are present; second, he will discover the structure of the ulcer patient's life; and, third, he will establish a rapport with the patient which is treatment in and of itself.

Eating Habits. The patient should be asked if any particular food aggravates his symptoms (often none will) and how many meals and snacks he eats and at what time. Particular attention should be given to late evening snacks, because these increase the likelihood of night pain and prevent attainment of the nocturnal basal secretory state (see pp. 628 to 640, 668 to 672, and 685 to 688).

Caffeine and Alcohol. The physician should ascertain how many cups of coffee and/or tea are drunk. Some individuals drink large amounts of cola-type and other soft drinks which contain caffeine. How much alcohol is used and whether the patient is addicted to alcohol must be known for both prognosis and treatment.

Drugs. Aspirin use must be diligently sought and quantified, because aspirin may initiate and perpetuate gastric mucosal damage and may induce gastrointestinal bleeding. Since the patient will often not be aware that many drugs contain aspirin, the physician must explore this subject in depth. Other drugs such as reserpine, phenylbutazone, indomethacin, and corticosteroids may or may not generate, perpetuate, or induce ulcers or bleeding of ulcers, but the physician must be aware of their use so that he may decide, in each case, whether to continue or modify their use (pp. 642 to 654). The number of cigarettes smoked per day and the number of years they have been used must be noted.

Family History. Certain families have a high incidence of duodenal ulcer, and the history of ulcers in other family members will strengthen clinical suspicion in the current patient and perhaps give some insight into why the patient developed an ulcer. The polyendocrine syndrome should be ruled out in any patient with a strong family history of ulcer, but in fact most patients with a strong family history have no specific endocrine abnormality (p. 639).

Concurrent Diseases. Chronic obstructive lung disease, pulmonary tuberculosis, rheumatoid arthritis, and cirrhosis of the liver appear to be associated with a higher incidence of peptic ulcer. In addition, these diseases plus other chronic illnesses, such as atherosclerotic heart disease, diabetes, and hypertension, will increase the morbidity and mortality of any ulcer complications.

Symptoms of Ulcer Complications. Hematemesis, melena, previous transfusions, vomiting (ask about the presence of old food in the vomitus), abdominal distention, recent changes in ulcer pain pattern, and back pain must be specifically asked about, because the patient may not volunteer this information (see pp. 757 to 770).

Symptoms of Unusual Ulcer Presentations. When the Zollinger-Ellison syndrome is present, symptoms are the same as in other peptic ulcers, only more virulent and often refractory to therapy. Prominent diarrhea and stearrhea may occur and even precede the ulcer symptoms. Channel ulcers frequently obstruct, and postbulbar ulcers produce frequent night pain, back pain, and bleeding.

PHYSICAL EXAMINATION

Except for epigastric tenderness, the physical examination is unrewarding in patients with uncomplicated duodenal ulcer. Epigastric tenderness is common, but not invariable, and many of the diseases from which duodenal ulcer must be differentiated (pancreatitis, cholecystitis, gastric ulcer and cancer, and even functional dyspepsia) may have epigastric tenderness. These diseases may produce abdominal masses, organomegaly, or severe tenderness in other parts of the abdomen, and may be reflected systemically in jaundice, weight loss, and lymphadenopathy. In addition, the complications of ulcer may produce masses, acute abdomen, distention, and a succussion splash.

LABORATORY STUDIES

Routine laboratory studies should include a hemoglobin, stool test for occult blood, and serum calcium.

Gastric Secretory Tests (Basal and Peak Stimulated Response). Although history and radiology are clearly much more important, secretory tests can be quite helpful if the following guidelines are adopted (pp. 174 to 186 and 536 to 550).

1. Gastric secretory studies should be done by trained personnel who fluoroscopically place sump tubes in the midantrum and accurately collect and analyze the specimens.

2. Studies are done after an overnight fast, and both basal and maximally stimulated secretory rates are determined.

3. All patients with a complicated clinical course, in whom surgery is planned, or in whom the diagnosis is in doubt are studied.

If these guidelines are followed, the following diagnostic and management clues will be obtained.

1. The individual with the Zollinger-Ellison syndrome will be discovered early rather than tragically late. This diagnosis is strongly suspected when high basal output is found (greater than 15 mEq per hour) or when the basal output is 60 per cent or more of the peak acid output (see pp. 746 to 747). Even basal secretory rates of greater than 10 mEq per hour and basal-peak ratios greater than 0.3 are suggestive of the Zollinger-Ellison syndrome, and patients with results that fall in this range should be further evaluated by measuring serum gastrin levels.

2. Hypersecretors (those whose maximally stimulated acid output is clearly above the upper limits of normal, i.e., greater than 50 mEq per hour in men and greater than 40 mEq per hour in women) will be identified. These patients are prime candidates for current or future duodenal ulcer and/or duodenitis.[65, 88] In addition, ulcer disease in hypersecretors often pursues a more virulent course with earlier surgery than in duodenal ulcer patients with acid outputs in the normal range (see pp. 536 to 550).

3. Hyposecretors (those whose maximally stimulated acid output is less than 14 mEq per hour in men and 12 mEq per hour in women) will also be identified. Such individuals are extremely unlikely to currently have a duodenal ulcer.

4. Comparison of pre- and postoperative acid values is an effective way to gauge the success of surgery. Successful vagotomy lowers the maximally stimulated acid output 70 per cent, the addition of antrectomy decreases output by 85 per cent, and a subtotal gastrectomy lowers maximally stimulated output by 90 per cent. If the basal acid output is greater than 5 mEq per hour or if the maximal acid output is greater than 15 mEq per hour postoperatively, the frequency of marginal ulceration is high and Zollinger-Ellison syndrome or retained antrum should be suspected. Because of difficulty in carrying out acid studies after gastric surgery, low values should not be given too much emphasis, especially on the basis of a single test (see pp. 536 to 550).

Serum Gastrin. Serum gastrin level tests are not yet freely available in the medical community, and until they are their use will be limited. Even so, serum gastrin should be determined on any patient with virulent ulcer disease, basal hypersecretion (see preceding section), stomal ulcer, and elevated blood calcium concentration, as well as when the Zollinger-Ellison syndrome is suspected for any reason (see pp. 555 to 558).

RADIOLOGY (see pp. 496 to 519)

If the diagnosis of duodenal ulcer disease has not previously been documented, if the symptoms have undergone recent change, suggesting a complication or secondary diagnosis, or if the patient has recently bled, an upper gastrointestinal barium study should be done. If the diagnosis has been previously confirmed, the course is not virulent, and surgery is not contemplated, then additional radiological evaluation is not needed.

An ulcer niche in the bulb confirms the diagnosis of an active duodenal ulcer. A classically deformed bulb (not just spastic or poorly filled) is practically pathognomonic of previous duodenal ulcer disease, but does not necessarily indicate that an active ulcer is present. Coarse duodenal folds without duodenal deformity are compatible with the diagnosis of duodenitis.

The radiologist and gastroenterologist must be constantly on guard against the following errors:

1. Inadequate filling of the postbulbar area and lack of care in scrutinizing it.

2. Over- or underdiagnosis of an active crater when the duodenal bulb is grossly deformed.[56, 64]

3. Poor-filling duodenal bulbs that are assumed to be deformed.

4. Interpreting a bulb in which mucosal detail is not secured.

Duodenal Ulcers with Normal Radiographs. There are a number of reasons why the radiologist may not identify an ulcer when other methods establish the presence of such a lesion.

1. Large or edematous folds may prevent barium from entering an ulcer, or a spastic bulb may prevent filling of the bulb or ulcer by barium.

2. Blood clots, mucus, or detritus may lodge in folds and cover the ulcer.

3. The crater may be shallow and not retain enough barium for visualization, or a long linear ulcer may not be appreciated because of its unusual shape.

4. The ulcer may have healed prior to examination or may appear afterward and be detected by another technique.

5. The X-ray technique may have been hasty and proper views and compression not done.[56, 89]

In spite of the many possible reasons why an ulcer might be overlooked, it turns out that in a nondeformed bulb, ulcer niches are seldom missed. Less than 5 per cent of all ulcers subsequently shown to be present at duodenoscopy will have been missed by the radiologist. In addition, fewer than 5 per cent of nondeformed bulbs will have an ulcer diagnosed by X-ray which cannot be later confirmed.[64]

It is thus apparent that if good films are obtained with adequate mucosal detail, a normal bulb is good evidence against a duodenal ulcer. In many instances the radiologist will alert the physician to the possibly of duodenitis by describing coarse duodenal folds.

DUODENOSCOPY

The new duodenoscopes enable the endoscopist to enter the bulb in almost every instance in which the scope is successfully passed into the stomach (see pp. 531 to 534). The endoscopist has no difficulty identifying the normal bulb, the grossly deformed bulb, the active duodenal ulcer, and bleeding points. Visual inspection plus biopsy may also enable him to diagnose duodenitis. It has not been established that this technique will allow diagnosis of inactive early duodenal ulcer when deformity is slight.

It is not yet clear whether the improved diagnosis and management resulting from duodenoscopy are worth the discomfort and slight risk associated with the procedure. However, as shown in the following breakdown of diagnostic problems, most patients can be successfully handled without duodenoscopy.

1. A probable ulcer niche in an individual with ulcer symptoms — duodenoscopy is usually not indicated.

2. A probable ulcer niche in an asymptomatic patient — duodenoscopy is usually indicated.

3. A grossly deformed bulb in either an asymptomatic patient or a patient with typical ulcer symptoms — duodenoscopy is usually not indicated.

4. Typical ulcer symptoms with the bulb either normal or exhibiting only coarse folds — duodenoscopy is indicated.

5. Diagnostic problems in which a duodenal ulcer could possibly explain the symptoms but no ulcer niche appears on X-ray — duodenoscopy is indicated.

This approach to duodenoscopy is adopted in the hope that the following goals can be achieved:

1. Prevention of labeling patients as having duodenal ulcer when one is not present.

2. Establishment of duodenal ulcer or duodenitis as present and producing symptoms previously felt to have some other explanation, i.e., cholelithiasis, functional dyspepsia, or pancreatitis.

3. Prevention of duodenoscopy being performed when there is little chance that the findings will alter the diagnosis or therapy.

OTHER DIAGNOSTIC PROCEDURES

The placement of a nasogastric tube on the first hospital day will often be the most rewarding procedure conducted. The gastric residual volume should be less than 200 cc after an overnight fast or less than 300 cc four hours postprandially. If larger volumes are returned, gastric retention is present. The presence of blood is of obvious importance. The pH of the gastric contents can be helpful, because if the patient is having pain and the gastric pH is greater than 3, doubt is cast on the diagnosis of uncomplicated duodenal ulcer.

If perforation is suspected, a three-way abdominal series (supine, cross-table lateral, and upright pain abdominal film) is obtained. Free air will be seen in 75 to 85 per cent of patients with perforations. The serum amylase is elevated in 20 per cent of the posterior penetrating ulcers and is modestly elevated in a similar percentage of perforated ulcers (see p. 761).

DIFFERENTIAL DIAGNOSIS

GASTRIC ULCER AND GASTRIC CARCINOMA

The symptoms of a duodenal ulcer are so similar to those of a gastric ulcer that it is futile, except in a statistical sense, to predict which will be present in a given individual. This is evident from Table 54–3, which depicts the frequency of various symptoms and clinical manifestations in these two diseases. The major manifestations of gastric carcinoma are also shown in the table, and it is evident that gastric carcinoma sufficiently differs from duodenal ulcer that distinction is often possible. However, the definitive diagnosis will be made by X-ray, endoscopy, and histology (see pp. 586 to 596).

TABLE 54–3. DIFFERENTIAL DIAGNOSIS

	DUODENAL ULCER	GASTRIC ULCER	GASTRIC CARCINOMA
Pain			
Present	++++	+++	+++
Location	Epigastric	Epigastric	Epigastric
Duration	Years	Years	Months
Clusters	++++	+++	+
Constant	+	++	++++
Acid rhythm	++++	+++	++
Food relief	++++	+++	+
Food-induced	±	+	++
Easy satiety	±	+	++
Vomiting	±	+	+
Weight loss	+	++	+++

FUNCTIONAL DYSPEPSIA

At first glance, it would appear that the overlap in symptoms between peptic ulcer and functional dyspepsia is extensive enough to make the diagnosis difficult. However, as shown in Table 54–4, in most patients the separation of duodenal and gastric ulcers on the one hand and functional dyspepsia on the other is quickly appreciated by history alone.[24, 27, 28, 34]

Pain in functional dyspepsia is usually less severe but definitely as chronic as that found in peptic disease. It is a strong clinical impression that females and individuals under age 40 are more frequently affected than males and those over age 40, but specific age and sex incidence figures are lacking. Remissions are of short duration, and clusters of pain are not distinct. The history may be inconsistent and rambling. The correlation of symptoms with acid production peaks is usually poor, and relief of pain by food is infrequent. However, partial relief of symptoms by alkali is seen and may cause confusion. Stress frequently causes an increase in symptoms in peptic ulcer and in functional dyspepsia. In contrast to peptic ulcer, vomiting is relatively common. Weight loss is of the same magnitude as that seen in peptic ulcer.[24] Nonspecific complaints, such as belching, nausea, constipation, food intolerances, and nongastrointestinal complaints (specifically headaches and arthralgias) are common. Relief with an ulcer regimen is difficult to achieve and, if a response is seen, it is short lived. Treatment with sedative or tranquilizing drugs is more effective, but symptoms soon recur in many instances.

TABLE 54–4. DIFFERENTIAL DIAGNOSIS

	DUODENAL ULCER	GASTRIC ULCER	FUNCTIONAL DYSPEPSIA
Pain			
Present	++++	+++	+++
Location	Epigastric	Epigastric	Variable, often epigastric
Duration	Years	Years	Years
Clusters	++++	+++	++
Constant	+	++	++
Acid rhythm	++++	+++	+
Food relief	++++	+++	++
Food induced	±	+	++
Easy satiety	±	+	+
Vomiting	±	+	+++
Weight loss	±	+	±
Nausea, belching, flatulence	+	+	+++
Neurotic traits	±	±	++

Usually barium meal studies will be obtained and are useful in convincing patient and doctor that an ulcer or cancer is not present. If doubt persists, gastroscopy and duodenoscopy may be helpful.

Functional dyspepsia is a chronic disease of many years' duration. In contrast to many peptic ulcer patients, these individuals are seldom incapacitated and function well in their occupations.[34] Follow-up of three to five years reveals the disease to persist basically unchanged, but long-term studies are lacking. It is a clinical impression that the disease often remits spontaneously after five to ten years.

ESOPHAGITIS

Peptic inflammation of the esophagus may be manifested by pain clusters, rhythmicity of the pain related to the acid cycle, pain relief from food and antacids, and night pain. The pain of esophagitis (pyrosis) can usually be distinguished from that of peptic ulcer. Pyrosis is a retrosternal burning which starts at the xiphoid and moves up toward the sternal notch. Patients usually describe it with hand motion; i.e., they put their hand at the xiphoid and then sweep upward in the midline to the sternal notch. Postural aggravation of pyrosis is typical. Symptoms of esophagitis are considered in detail on pages 433 to 435.

PANCREATITIS

Episodes of pancreatitis may simulate peptic ulcer. It is not the severe, acute episodes which cause diagnostic difficulties, but rather the recurrent episodes or relapses associated with chronic pancreatitis. The relapses may suggest periodicity, and the epigastric pain is often aggravated by meals. In addition, abdominal findings are not always striking, fever is uncommon in such relapses, and the serum amylase is often normal.

Directing the physician away from ulcer and toward a diagnosis of pancreatitis would be back pain, elevated serum amylase (especially if greater than twice normal), postural relief of pain (sitting up and leaning forward), subcostal pain, poor relief with antacids, abdominal mass, and evidence of weight loss. Vomiting is often present; yet it affords no relief as it usually does in peptic ulcer. A history of alcoholism and the presence of steatorrhea, diabetes, and/or pancreatic calcifications suggest that pancreatitis is responsible for the pain. Upper gastrointestinal X-rays may not solve the dilemma, because pancreatitis may cause edema of the duodenum and simulate duodenitis and/or peptic ulcer disease.[56] Of course, penetrating ulcer may cause pancreatitis, and at times both may be present independently. If it is not clear which is present, nasogastric suction, which is beneficial in both, should be begun.[90]

BILIARY PAIN

Severe attacks of biliary pain, frequently weeks to years apart, may have to be differentiated from a perforated ulcer but should not be confused with chronic duodenal ulcer pain.[91] It is the mild biliary tract pain (sometimes called minor colic) that may cause confusion.[92] This is often referred to by the patient as an ache or discomfort rather than as pain; it is steady, usually occurs in the right upper quadrant or epigastrium, and lasts for one to four hours. At times it may occur daily, but it is typically spaced at intervals of weeks to months. This pain often occurs at night and is associated with vomiting.

Points which separate these episodes of biliary pain from chronic duodenal ulcer pain are the following:

1. Biliary pain is often in the right upper quadrant and may radiate to just below the right scapula and to the tip of the right shoulder, whereas uncomplicated duodenal ulcer is almost never found in the right upper quadrant or with scapular or shoulder radiation.

2. Biliary pain is not relieved by food or antacids and does not possess the rhythmicity of the acid cycle.

3. Biliary tract pain does not usually occur as clusters of pain separated by pain-free intervals.

4. Vomiting is common in biliary tract disease, but does not relieve pain. Vomiting is unusual in uncomplicated duodenal ulcer disease, but when it occurs pain is usually relieved.

5. Fever, leukocytosis, and right upper

quadrant abdominal signs would be uncommon in duodenal ulcer but occur in biliary tract disease.[92, 93]

SMALL BOWEL AND VASCULAR DISEASE

Small bowel pain is typically a periumbilical cramping pain which can usually be readily distinguished from peptic disease. Terminal ileal pain may begin several hours postprandially and, in this way at least, suggest a duodenal ulcer. In abdominal angina, pain begins after eating; it is quite severe, and the larger the meal, the worse the pain. Relief cannot be obtained with antacids or additional food. The patient voluntarily decreases his consumption of food to prevent the pain, and weight loss is usually marked.

VARIOUS DUODENAL LESIONS

Polyps, webs, tumors, and inflammations may bleed, obstruct, or produce ulcer-like symptoms. X-ray and/or duodenoscopy will usually clarify these problems.

ETIOLOGIC CLASSIFICATION

At the completion of the clinical evaluation, the physician has determined the diagnosis and, in addition, has obtained data from the patient relevant to the cause of his duodenal ulcer. Since treatment will be predicated not only on standard empirical grounds but also on the specific causes of the ulcer in each patient, it behooves the doctor to classify each patient into one or more "etiological" groups, as described on page 640.

1. Anxiety and stress-induced.
2. Drug-induced.
3. Associated with chronic debilitating illness.
4. Familial.
5. Hypersecretion (large stomach)—high maximal stimulated acid output.
6. Increased secretory drive: basal-peak acid secretion ratio greater than 0.2.
    a. Endocrine-induced (autonomous gastrin secretion, hypercalcemia).
    b. Idiopathic.

7. Decreased resistance: anatomical location, duodenitis, lower than expected rates of acid secretion.
8. Idiopathic.

This type of systematic classification will individualize treatment, add clarity to discussion, and help the patient understand his disease.

TREATMENT

The physician must not lose sight of what he can expect to accomplish with treatment of duodenal ulcer. Peptic ulcer of the duodenum is a chronic disease with many remissions and relapses. Although its intensity may wane with time, permanent remissions occur in only 10 to 25 per cent of patients who are ill enough at the outset to require hospitalization. The cures that do occur are spontaneous and probably not in response to medical treatment. Surgical treatment can with relatively low mortality and morbidity effect a cure in about 80 to 90 per cent of patients, depending upon the type of surgery, but this cure is produced at the expense of significant side effects in a troublesome minority and a postoperative recurrence rate of 5 to 15 per cent.

Medical therapy is directed at relieving symptoms, hastening healing, and decreasing the frequency of relapse. It clearly relieves symptoms and probably hastens healing, but it is not known whether medical therapy decreases relapses.

Since duodenal ulcer is a very chronic disease, therapy must be efficient, effective, and tolerable.

AVOIDANCE OF NOXIOUS AGENTS

Any drug or food which damages the gastroduodenal mucosae should not ordinarily be given to a duodenal ulcer patient. Aspirin (acetylsalicylic acid) clearly damages the mucosae and should not be used. Darvon or Tylenol should be prescribed as substitutes, and the patient should be repeatedly cautioned that many proprietary drugs contain aspirin. Heavy ethanol consumption causes a gastritis which predisposes the mucosae to injury from aspirin and possibly other agents.[94] The exact role of alcohol itself in producing or maintaining ulceration is not clear; but it and caffeine can induce acid production and possess no acid-neutralizing capability, so both should be avoided if possible. Sanka and Postum can be offered as substitutes for coffee and tea. Many cola drinks contain caffeine and should be used in moderation by duodenal ulcer patients.

Reserpine and phenylbutazone (Butazolidin) have not been shown statistically in man to cause or perpetuate peptic ulceration or bleeding, but each has been implicated as causing indigestion in man and ulceration in animals, and they should be used cautiously in ulcer patients.[95-98]

Glucocorticoids, such as prednisone (in low to moderate doses), have not been proved ulcerogenic.[14, 99-102] However, there is still sufficient uncertainty about a causal relationship between steroid therapy and peptic ulcer that the presence or history of duodenal ulcer is a relative contraindication to steroid therapy.[103] If the need for the glucocorticoids is great, ulcer therapy should be started or maintained concomitantly in such patients.

There are no data as to the influence of large doses of steroids, i.e., greater than 40 mg of prednisone per day, but there is a widespread clinical impression that large doses may induce ulcers. This impression must be viewed critically, however, as patients sick enough to receive high-dose steroid therapy are quite likely to form ulcers without steroid therapy. Regardless of whether they actually induce ulceration, large-dose steroid therapy may mask the symptoms of ulceration, and even penetration and perforation may not be associated with abdominal pain.

Smoking, which is associated with many diseases, may also be an important cause of duodenal ulcer disease, although the relationship may be indirect rather than one of cause and effect. Smoking should be stopped, but it may be practical to plan its discontinuation so that the patient does not alter his entire life style at once.

DIET

The only foods which should be restricted in the usual duodenal ulcer pa-

tients are caffeine, alcohol, and those foods which the patient feels induce pain. The administration of milk induces acid production, and although the milk has some neutralizing capacity, the acid secretion it stimulates will continue after the milk has emptied from the stomach. Evidence suggests that hourly ingestion of milk or protein is associated with higher gastric acidity than when three regular meals are ingested.[104, 105] The duodenal ulcer patient should eat three meals a day, and snacks should be discouraged. The patient should be especially advised not to eat a bedtime snack, because this delays the appearance of the basal secretory state for several hours and is associated with high nocturnal acidity (Fig. 54–5).

Most patients will accept a noncaffeine coffee, but many will balk at a total restriction of ethanol. Alcohol with a meal or immediately preceding the meal is an acceptable compromise when the ulcer is not active, but alcohol should be avoided completely for six weeks after treatment for active ulcer has begun.

ANTACIDS

Adequate neutralization of gastric contents can be achieved with hourly antacids, but the inconvenience and expense of such therapy guarantees that it will be of short duration. The most effective manner of using antacids is to give them at a time of maximal acid production and when they will be retained the longest in the stomach. One hour after a meal, gastric hydrogen ion secretion is near its maximal rate but gastric contents still have a relatively high pH owing to the buffer of the meal.[106] After one hour, the buffer of the stomach becomes progressively less in amount, acid secretion continues at a high rate, and the pH of the stomach contents drops progressively. Antacids administered one hour after eating will be retained with the remainder of the meal in the stomach for several hours and reduce gastric acidity for at least two hours (see Fig. 54–5). A second dose, approximately three hours after the meal, will not reduce acidity as long as the first dose (because of more rapid gastric emptying three hours after a meal than one hour after eating), but will lower acidity almost up to the next meal. The larger the dose, the longer the period of reduced acidity.[106] A large bedtime dose is important to reduce acidity for as long as possible during the night. A complete discussion of antacid therapy, including dose, frequency, complications, and choice of antacid agents, is contained on pages 721 to 728.

ANTICHOLINERGICS

Since nocturnal secretion is effectively suppressed by anticholinergics and since side effects are not appreciated by the patient when he is asleep, it is logical to use anticholinergics at bedtime. Anticholinergic drugs (in an effective dose) taken before or after a meal will reduce gastric acidity better than when antacids alone are given. Provided there are no contraindications, anticholinergic drugs may therefore be prescribed during the day, as well as at bedtime, although there is no proof that such treatment will hasten healing or reduce recurrences. See page 734 for a detailed discussion of the action, indications, dosages, and contraindictions of antichloinergic drugs in peptic ulcer patients.

RADIATION THERAPY

Duodenal ulcer patients with severe pain who do not respond to maximal medical therapy, including hospitalization, are intractable. In the elderly or debilitated patient, surgery is often unacceptable because of the expected high morbidity and mortality. In such circumstances, the parietal cells of the stomach can be irradiated in an attempt to induce a gastritis with subsequent loss of secretory capacity.[107] Sixteen hundred fifty rads is directed at the fundus through anterior and posterior ports over two weeks.[108] In one large series, 23 per cent of individuals developed histamine-fast achlorhydria, and 34 per cent had a 50 per cent or greater reduction in acid secretion. These reductions are not permanent; much of the secretory capacity returns within one to two years.[109] Those individuals with a significant depression of acid output appear to have fewer recurrences compared with those in whom irradiation failed to reduce acid production.[109] Those with pyloric ob-

struction should not receive radiation therapy. In the past, treatment was repeated once, but radiation skin burns have occurred after a second course, and in most instances a second course should be avoided.[110] In one report radiation nephritis developed after a latent period of 9.3 years (11 months to 19 years) in 40 per cent of 67 patients who received 2000 rads to the parietal areas as an adjunct to surgical therapy.[111] Nine patients died of chronic renal disease. Cause and effect were shown by the severe involvement of the left kidney as compared with the right kidney. The incidence of cancer does not appear to be increased.

In summary, radiation therapy should be used when (1) standard medical therapy cannot control the disease, (2) surgical therapy is contraindicated because of severe concomitant disease states, and (3) life expectancy is less than ten years. Patients who fit this definition will usually have advanced atherosclerotic heart disease, chronic lung disease, or severe liver disease. Radiation should not be given as an adjunct to standard surgical therapy.

PSYCHIC STRESS

Anxiety and depression, especially if coupled with alcoholism, are associated with a poor symptomatic response to therapy, either medical or surgical. Since they impair the effectiveness of other forms of therapy, it would seem logical to treat the anxiety and/or depression with the hope that ulcer symptoms and ulcer prognosis could be improved, but there is no evidence that antianxiety or antidepression drug therapy decreases ulcer symptoms or alters the natural history of the disease. These drugs should be used with discretion, because they are expensive and potentially harmful. On the other hand, a concerned physician who relates to his patient can, without any special effort at delving into the patient's subconscious problems, be a calming and strengthening influence. An attempt should be made to eliminate excesses, as many patients are obviously driving themselves either mentally or physically. Suggestions by the physician are often quite effective in allowing a patient to gracefully slow down his hectic pace. Some patients benefit from the addition of physical activity, whereas others need to find work to occupy themselves.

MAINTENANCE THERAPY

Major therapeutic endeavors are difficult when the patient is in remission, for the following reasons:

1. Patients take medication sporadically or not at all when asymptomatic.[28, 34]
2. The patient who has been told to take prophylactic medications may lose confidence in them when he relapses unless the natural course of his disease has been explained.
3. Since duodenal ulcer is a chronic disease, the continuous administration of medicine to an asymptomatic individual could continue for years.

Many physicians doubt the wisdom of continuous therapy during asymptomatic interludes, because proof that treatment prevents relapse is lacking. However, prophylactic therapy should seldom be harmful, may be helpful, and will be adhered to fairly well in some patients if the physician thoughtfully presents the program. It appears reasonable until evidence to the contrary is forthcoming to utilize as much therapy during the remissions as will be reasonably tolerated.

During maintenance treatment, the diet remains the same except that some modest ethanol intake, if used with meals, is acceptable. Harmful drugs, especially aspirin, are still rigorously avoided. Smoking should be discouraged. The patient should continue to take anticholinergics and antacids at bedtime. This maintenance program should be easy to adhere to; with proper physician guidance, all but the most obstinate patients will comply. For the patient who has had several recurrences, maintenance therapy should include anticholinergics before or after each meal and antacids taken one hour after each meal, in addition to the bedtime dosages.

SUMMARY OF THERAPY

When the patient has an *acute* relapse, the following measures should be instituted:

1. Bedrest for several days, usually at home, should be used unless the relapse is quite mild.
2. Three normal meals a day, excluding caffeine, alcohol, and foods that aggravate an individual patient's symptoms, should be encouraged. Snacks between meals and at bedtime should be specifically discouraged.
3. Hourly antacids are taken during the day, and a large dose is taken at bedtime.
4. An anticholinergic should be taken just before or just after each meal and at bedtime, and the dose should be large enough to induce mild side effects. Anticholinergic complications should be watched for carefully. These drugs should not be used in elderly patients, or in patients with partial outlet obstruction or prostatism.
5. If possible, all potentially harmful drugs should be restricted or discontinued, especially salicylates. Tylenol or Darvon should be given to the patient for use instead of aspirin.
6. Smoking should be discouraged (although there is no proof of a causal association).

When the patient has been pain free for about seven days, *subacute* therapy can be started. This differs from the above in that antacids are taken one and three hours after each meal and at bedtime. This treatment is continued for six weeks.

Once an episode has been controlled, the patient enters on *maintenance* therapy, which should include the following:

1. Avoidance of excesses.
2. Diet: ethanol or caffeine only with meals, and no snacks.
3. Antacids at bedtime only, except when the disease is virulent with frequent relapses; then antacids are prescribed one hour after each meal and at bedtime.
4. Anticholinergics at bedtime only, except when the disease is virulent with frequent relapses; then anticholinergics are prescribed before each meal and at bedtime.
5. Avoidance of aspirin; Tylenol or Darvon is kept on hand for headache.

When a recurrence of dyspepsia occurs, the patient should be taught to immediately increase his medication to at least the level of the subacute regimen. If this does not induce a remission within 48 hours, the acute regimen should be started.

REFERENCES

1. Watkinson, G. The incidence of chronic peptic ulcer found at necropsy. Gut 1:14, 1960.
2. Fry, J. Peptic ulcer: A profile. Brit. Med. J. 2:809, 1964.
3. Blumenthal, I. S. Digestive disease as a a national problem. III. Social cost of peptic ulcer. Gastroenterology 54:86, 1968.
4. Monson, R. R., and MacMahon, B. Peptic ulcer in Massachusetts physicians. New Eng. J. Med. 281:11, 1969.
5. Krause, V. Long-term results of medical and surgical treatment of peptic ulcer. Acta Chir. Scand. Suppl. 310, 1963.
6. Norbye, E. Ulcer statistics from Drammen Hospital, 1936–1945. Acta Med. Scand. 143:50, 1952.
7. Weir, R. D., and Backett, E. M. Studies of the epidemiology of peptic ulcer in a rural community: Prevalence and natural history of dyspepsia and peptic ulcer. Gut 9:75, 1968.
8. Knutsen, B., and Selvaag, O.: The incidence of peptic ulcer. Acta Med. Scand. Suppl. 196:341, 1947.
9. Hunt, J. N., and Wales, R. C. Progress in patients with peptic ulceration treated for more than five years with Poldine, including a double-blind study. Brit. Med. J. 2:13, 1966.
10. Monson, R. R. Duodenal ulcer as a second disease, Gastroenterology 59:712, 1970.
11. Cobb, S., and Hall, W. Newly identified clusters of diseases: Rheumatoid arthritis, peptic ulcer and tuberculosis. J.A.M.A. 193:1077, 1965.
12. Gibberd, F. B. Dyspepsia in patients with rheumatoid arthritis. Acta Rheum. Scand. 12:112, 1966.
13. Phillips, M. M., and Conn, H. O. Portacaval anastomosis and peptic ulcer: A coincidental relationship. Gastroenterology 62:876, 1972.
14. Fielding, J. E., and Cooke, W. T. Peptic ulceration in Crohn's disease. Gut 11:998, 1970.
15. Barbaras, A. P., Bouhoutsos, J., and Martin, P. Aortic aneurysm and peptic ulcer. Brit. Med. J. 1:768, 1971.
16. Jones, A. W., Kirk, R. S., and Blour, K. The association between aneurysm of the abdominal aorta and peptic ulceration. Gut 2:679, 1970.
17. Sanders, D. B., and Johns, T. R. Peptic ulcer in myasthenia gravis. J.A.M.A. 207:1857, 1969.
18. Ross, R. J., and Pudvan, W. R. Peptic ulcers and gallbladder disease. Radiology 96:119, 1970.
19. Stempien, S. J., and Dagradi, A. The histamine response of the gastric mucosa in a patient with adrenal insufficiency: Effect of cortisone administration. Gastroenterology 27:358, 1954.
20. Engel, F. L. Addison's disease and peptic ulcer. J. Clin. Endocrinol. Metabol. 15:1300, 1955.
21. Gray, S. J., Ramsey, L. G., and Thorn, G. Adrenal influences on the stomach: Peptic ulcer in Addison's disease during adrenal steroid therapy. Ann. Intern. Med. 45:73, 1956.
22. Smith, L. A. The pattern of pain in the diagnosis of upper abdominal disorders. J.A.M.A. 156:1566, 1954.
23. Rivers, A. B. Pain in benign ulcers of the esophagus, stomach and small intestine. J.A.M.A. 104:169, 1935.
24. Edwards, F. C., and Coghill, N. F. Clinical manifestations in patients with chronic atrophic gastritis, gastric ulcer, and duodenal ulcer. Quart. J. Med. 37:337, 1968.
25. Woodward, E. R., and Schapiro, H. Relationship of ulcer pain to pH and motility of stomach and duodenum. Proc. Soc. Exp. Biol. Med. 85:504, 1954.
26. Bonney, G. L. W., and Pickering, G. W. Observations on the mechanism of pain in ulcer of the stomach and duodenum. Clin. Sci. 6:63, 1948.
27. Rinaldo, J. A., Scheinok, P., and Rupe, C. E. Symptom diagnosis. A mathematical analysis of epigastric pain. Ann. Intern. Med. 59:145, 1963.
28. Friedman, M. Peptic ulcer and functional dyspepsia in the Armed Forces. Gastroenterology 10:586, 1948.
29. Moore, J. G., and Englert, E. Circadian rhythm of gastric acid secretion in man. Nature 226:1261, 1970.
30. Muggia, A., and Spiro, H. Childhood peptic ulcer. Gastroenterology 37:715, 1959.
31. Malmros, H., and Hiertonn, T. A post-investigation of 687 medically treated cases of peptic ulcer. Acta Med. Scand. 133:229, 1949.
32. Edwards, H., and Copeman, W. S. C. Dyspepsia: An investigation. Brit. Med. J. 2:640, 1943.
33. Radloff, E. Observations on five hundred and forty-three cases of peptic ulcer. Gastroenterology 8:343, 1947.
34. Rae, J. W., and Allison, R. S. The effect of diet and regular living conditions on the natural history of peptic ulcer. Quart. J. Med. 22:439, 1953.
35. Emery, E. S., and Monroe, R. T. Peptic ulcer: A study of five hundred and fifty-six cases. Arch. Intern. Med. 43:846, 1929.
36. Palmer, W. L. The mechanisms of pain in gastric and in duodenal ulcer. Arch. Intern. Med. 39:109, 1927.
37. Palmer, W. L., and Heinz, T. E. Mechanisms of pain in gastric and in duodenal ulcer. Arch. Intern. Med. 53:269, 1934.
38. Dragstedt, L. R., and Palmer, W. L. Direct observations on the mechanism of pain in duodenal ulcer. Proc. Soc. Exp. Biol. Med. 29:753, 1932.
39. Cannon, W. B., and Washburn, A. L. An explanation of hunger. Amer. J. Physiol. 29:441, 1912.
40. Bolton, C. Interpretation of gastric symptoms. Lancet 1:1159, 1928.
41. Ruffin, J. M., Baylin, G., Legerton, C. W., and Texter, E. C. Mechanism of pain in peptic ulcer. Gastroenterology 23:252, 1953.
42. Shirokova, K. I. Periodic activity of the stomach in normals and peptic ulcer disease. Trudx I Mosk. Med. Inst. 8:133, 1960.

43. Hightower, N. C., and Gambill, E. F. The effects of Banthine on pain and antral gastric motility in patients with duodenal ulcer. Gastroenterology 23:224, 1953.

44. Patterson, T. L., and Sandweiss, D. J. The relationship between gastro-duodenal motility phases and symptoms associated with duodenal ulcer in the human. Amer. J. Dig. Dis. 9:375, 1942.

45. Kasich, A. M., Fein, H. D., and Boleman, A. P. Pain in peptic ulcer. Amer. J. Med. Sci. 241:483, 1961.

46. Kirk, R. C. Differential diagnosis in 207 cases of peptic ulcer of the duodenum. Gastroenterology 7:168, 1946.

47. Smith, F. H., Boles, R. S., and Jordan, S. M. Problem of gastric ulcer reviewed. J.A.M.A. 153:1505, 1953.

48. Cutler, C. W. Clinical picture of peptic ulcer after sixty. Surg. Gynec. Obstet. 107:23, 1958.

49. Hojer-Pedersen, W. On the significance of psychic factors in the development of peptic ulcer. Acta. Psychiat. Neurol. Scand. Suppl. 119, 33, 1958.

50. Weiner, H., Thaler, M., Reiser, M. F., and Mirsky, T. A. Etiology of duodenal ulcer. 1. Relation of specific psychological characteristics to the rate of gastric secretion (serum pepsinogen). Psychosomat. Med. 19:1, 1957.

51. Jorgensen, T. G., Christensen, J. K., Fischer, P. A., and Stvandbygaard, N. Preoperative prediction of results following surgery for chronic duodenal ulcer. Gastroenterology 60:680, 1971.

52. Hamilton, M. The personality of dyspeptics with special reference to gastric and duodenal ulcer. Brit. J. Med. Psychol. 23:182, 1950.

53. Dunn, J. P., and Etter, L. E. Inadequacy of the medical history in the diagnosis of duodenal ulcer. New Eng. J. Med. 266:68, 1962.

54. Chinn, A. B., and Werkesser, E. C. Acute hemorrhage from peptic ulceration: An analysis of 322 cases. Ann. Intern. Med. 34:334, 1951.

55. Daily, M. E., and Miller, E. R. A search for symptomless gastric cancer in 500 apparently healthy men of 45 and over. Gastroenterology 5:1, 1948.

56. Templeton, F. E. Peptic ulcer. X-ray examination of the stomach. Chicago, University of Chicago Press, 1964, pp. 386–397.

57. Turner, F. P. Acute perforations of stomach, duodenum and jejunum. Surg. Gynec. Obstet. 92:281, 1951.

58. DeBakey, M. Acute perforated gastroduodenal ulceration. Surgery 8:825, 1028, 1940.

59. Tolley, J. P. Definitive surgical therapy for perforated peptic ulcer. Amer. J. Surg. 113:327, 1967.

60. Martin, L., and Lewis, N. Peptic ulcer cases reviewed after ten years. Lancet 2:1115, 1949.

61. Beck, I. T., Kahn, D. S., Lacerte, M., Solgmar, J., Callegavini, U., and Geolres, M. C. Chronic duodenitis: A clinical pathological entity. Gut 6:376, 1965.

62. Ostrow, J. D., and Resnick, R. H. Hyperchlorhydria, duodenitis and duodenal ulcer: A clinical study of their interrelationships. Ann. Intern. Med. 51:1303, 1959.

63. Rivers, A. B. A clinical study of duodenitis, gastritis and gastrojejunitis. Ann. Intern. Med. 4:1265, 1931.

64. Belber, J. P. Endoscopic examination of the duodenal bulb: A comparison with X-ray. Gastroenterology 61:55, 1971.

65. Krag, E. Pseudoulcer and true peptic ulcer. Acta Med. Scand. 178:713, 1965.

66. Schulman, A. The cobblestone appearance of the duodenal cap, duodenitis and hyperplasia of Brunner's glands. Brit. J. Radiol. 43:787, 1970.

67. Fraser, M., Pittman, R. G., Lowrie, H., Smith, G., Forrest, A., and Rhodes, J. Significance of the radiological finding of coarse mucosal folds in the duodenum. Lancet 2:979, 1964.

68. Rhodes, J., Evans, K. T., Lawril, J. H., and Forrest, A. P. M. Coarse mucosal folds in the duodenum. Quart. J. Med. 37:151, 1968.

69. Cooke, L., and Hutton, C. F. Postbulbar duodenal ulceration. Lancet 1:754, 1958.

70. Pattison, A. C., and Stellar, C. A. Surgical management of postbulbar duodenal ulcers. Amer. J. Surg. 111:313, 1966.

71. Ramsdell, J. A., Bartholomew, L. G., Cain, C. R., and Davis, G. S. Postbulbar duodenal ulcer. Ann. Intern. Med. 47:700, 1957.

72. Kaufman, S. A., and Levene, G. Postbulbar duodenal ulcer. Radiology 69:848, 1957.

73. Harkins, H. N. Duodenal ulcer. In Surgery of the Stomach and Duodenum, 2nd ed., H. N. Harkins and L. M. Nyhus (eds.). Boston, Little, Brown, & Co. 1969, pp. 227–248.

74. Swarts, J. M., and Rice, M. L. Postbulbar ulcer with particular reference to its hemorrhagic tendency. Gastroenterology 26:251, 1954.

75. Foulk, W. T., Comfort, M. W., Butt, H. R., Dockerty, M. B., and Weber, H. M. Peptic ulcer near the pylorus. Gastroenterology 32:395, 1957.

76. Minoru, O., and Sakurai, Y. The location of duodenal ulcer. Gastroenterology 36:60, 1959.

77. Murray, G. F., Ballinger, W. F., and Stafford, E. S. Ulcers of the pyloric channel. Amer. J. Surg. 113:119, 1967.

78. Texter, E. C., Smith, H. W., Bundisen, W. E., and Barborka, C. J. The syndrome pylorique. Gastroenterology 36:573, 1959.

79. Texter, E. C., Baylin, G. J., Ruffin, J. M., and Legerton, C. W. Pyloric channel ulcer. Gastroenterology 24:319, 1953.

80. Weisberg, H., and Glass, G. B. J. Coexisting gastric and duodenal ulcer; a review. Amer. J. Dig. Dis. 8:992, 1963.

81. Mangold, R. Combined gastric and duodenal ulceration. Brit. Med. J. 2:1193, 1958.

82. Welsh, J. S., Floyd, E. C., McKeon, S. A., Moore, K., and Cohn, I. Combined gastric and duodenal ulcer, comparison of medical and surgical treatment. Amer. Surgeon 31:590, 1965.

83. Johnson, D. Associated gastric and duodenal ulcers. Surg. Gynec. Obstet. 102:287, 1956.

84. McCray, R. S., Ferris, E. J., Herskovic, J., Winawer, S. J., Shapiro, J. H., and Zamcheck, N. Clinical differences between gastric ulcers with and without duodenal deformity. Ann. Surg. 168:821, 1968.

85. Lukash, W. M., Candela, H. J., Ryan, R. R., and Nielsen, O. F. Gastric ulceration in infancy. Amer. J. Dig. Dis. 12:318, 1967.

86. Milliken, J. C. Duodenal ulceration in children. Gut 6:25, 1965.

87. Wells, R. F. Peptic ulcer in adolescent and young adults. Military Med. 132:680, 1967.

88. Harrison, A. M., Wechsler, R. L., and Elliott, D. W. Gastric analysis in the absence of demonstrable gastric pathology. Amer. J. Surg. 123:132, 1972.

89. Prevot, R. Roentgenology of the duodenum. In Alimentary Tract Roentgenology, A. R. Margulis and H. J. Burhenne (eds.). St. Louis, C. V. Mosby Co., 1967, pp. 528–532.

90. Cogbill, C. L., and Song, K. T. Acute pancreatitis. Arch. Surg. 100:673, 1970.

91. French, E. B., and Robb, W. A. T. Biliary and renal colic. Brit. Med. J. 2:135, 1963.

92. Littler, T. R., and Ellis, G. R. Gallstones: A clinical survey. Brit. Med. J. 1:842, 1952.

93. Price, W. H. Gallbladder dyspepsia. Brit. Med. J. 2:138, 1963.

94. Needham, C. D., Kyle, J., Jones, P. F., Johnston, S. J., and Kerridge, D. F. Aspirin and alcohol in gastrointestinal hemorrhage. Gut 12:819, 1971.

95. Marser, E. F. The toxic effects of phenylbutazone (Butazolidin). New Eng. J. Med. 253:404, 1955.

96. Sperling, I. L. Adverse reactions with long-term use of phenylbutazone and oxyphenbutazone. Lancet 2:535, 1969.

97. Bachrach, W. H. Reserpine, gastric secretion and peptic ulcer. Amer. J. Dig. Dis. 4:117, 1959.

98. Drenick, E. J. Reserpine in peptic ulcer. Amer. J. Dig. Dis. 1:521, 1956.

99. Cooke, A. R. Corticosteroid and peptic ulcer: Is there a relationship? Amer. J. Dig. Dis. 12:323, 1967.

100. Kern, F., Clark, G. M., and Lukens, J. G. Peptic ulceration occurring during therapy for rheumatoid arthritis. Gastroenterology 33:25, 1957.

101. Sherwood, H., Epstein, J. I., and Buckley, W. E. Peptic ulcer among allergic patients on long-term triamcinolone therapy. J. Allergy 31:21, 1960.

102. Meltzer, L. E., Bockman, A. E., Kanenson, W., and Cohen, A. The incidence of peptic ulcer among patients on long-term prednisone therapy. Gastroenterology 35:351, 1958.

103. Max, M., and Menguy, R. Influence of adrenocorticotropin, cortisone, aspirin, and phenylbutazone on the rate of exfoliation and the rate of renewal of gastric mucosal cells. Gastroenterology 58:329, 1970.

104. Kirsner, J. B., and Palmer, W. L. The effects of various antacids on the hydrogen ion concentration of the gastric contents. Amer. J. Dig. Dis. 7:85, 1940.

105. Bingle, J. P., and Lennard-Jones, J. E. Some factors in assessment of gastric antisecretory drugs by sampling technique. Gut 1:337, 1960.

106. Fordtran, J. S., and Collyns, J. A. H. Antacid pharmacology in duodenal ulcer. New Eng. J. Med. 274:921, 1966.

107. Goldgraber, M. C., Rubin, C. E., Palmer, W. L., Dobson, R. L., and Massey, B. W. The early gastric response to irradiation. A serial biopsy study. Gastroenterology 27:1, 1954.

108. Hodges, P. H. In The physiology and treatment of peptic ulcer, J. G. Allan (eds.). Chicago, University of Chicago Press, 1959, pp. 89–139.

109. Levin, E., Chapman, C. B., Palmer, W. L., and Kirsner, J. B. Observations on the value of gastric irradiation in the treatment of duodenal ulcer. Gastroenterology 32:42, 1957.

110. Clayman, C. B., Palmer, W. L., and Kirsner, J. B. Gastric irradiation in the treatment of peptic ulcer. Gastroenterology 55:403, 1968.

111. Thompson, P. L., MacKay, I. R., Robson, G. S., and Wall, A. J. Late radiation nephritis after gastric X-irradiation for peptic ulcer. Quart. J. Med. 40:145, 1971.

Chapter 55

Chronic Gastric Ulcer

Charles T. Richardson

INCIDENCE

The incidence of gastric ulceration varies with the type of population examined, the age of the population, and the type of study conducted (antemortem vs. postmortem). The incidence of gastric ulcer in Norway was 1 per 1000 (0.1 per cent) in 1942.[1] Fourteen of 13,885 (0.1 per cent) employees of the Metropolitan Life Insurance Company were found to have a gastric ulcer during a ten-year period of observation.[2] It has been estimated that 3,500,000 persons in the United States were affected annually by peptic ulcer disease during the period 1963 to 1965.[3] This figure included persons with both duodenal and gastric ulcerations. If the usual ratio for duodenal ulcer to gastric ulcer of 4:1 is correct,[4] then approximately 700,000 persons per year in the United States, or 0.4 per cent of the total population, would have had a gastric ulcer.

Autopsy studies demonstrate a somewhat higher incidence of gastric ulceration. In a well planned prospective study by Watkinson,[5] the incidence of active gastric ulcer as well as ulcer scars seen at autopsy was reported. Benign gastric ulcers were determined as the cause of death in 1.7 per cent of males and in 1.1 per cent of females in the population autopsied. After eliminating the ulcer deaths, approximately one in 34 men (2.9 per cent) and one in 59 women (1.7 per cent) demonstrated evidence of either an active gastric ulcer or an ulcer scar at the time of death.

It has been noted that the incidence of gastric ulcer was two-thirds less than expected in professional and business executives and two-thirds more than expected in unskilled and heavy manual laborers.[6] In another study, gastric ulcer was two to five times more common in men in the less prosperous classes than in the upper social classes.[7]

Most series report a male-to-female ratio of from 3:1 to 4:1 for benign gastric ulcers.[8-12] The age distribution for both men and women is almost identical,[8] with the highest incidence occurring in the sixth decade of life. In a review by Gill,[13] it was stated that gastric ulcers become more common as age advances; a definite increased incidence was noted in women after the menopause.

CLINICAL FEATURES

Pain. The patient with a benign gastric ulcer will present most frequently with abdominal pain or discomfort,[14-16] which is typically epigastric in location. Numerous terms are used by patients to describe their pain or discomfort, but the words most often used are "aching," "nagging," "cramplike," or "dull." Less frequently mentioned adjectives are "hot," "burning," "sore," or "fiery." Two-thirds of the patients experience radiation of their pain, and the most frequent site of radiation is through to the back. Less frequently encountered sites of radiation are to the ster-

692

num, to the epigastrium in patients whose pain did not originate in the epigastrium, to the hypochondria, and around one or both sides to the back.[16]

Pain may occur within 30 minutes of the completion of a meal, or it may be delayed to as long as three hours after eating. Most patients will describe immediate relief of pain following the ingestion of food, although in one study[16] food aggravated or precipitated the pain in 25 per cent of the patients. A number of patients (43 per cent in one series)[16] will describe nocturnal pain or discomfort which usually occurs one to two hours after going to bed. This probably occurs more frequently in patients who eat a bedtime snack.

The pain in most patients (two-thirds or more) with a gastric ulcer will be decreased or relieved by antacids. In the small group that do not receive relief from antacids, the pain may stop spontaneously, or it may continue until the ingestion of the next meal.

Although the pain of patients with gastric ulcer is often characterized by remissions and exacerbations, this is more commonly seen in patients with a duodenal ulcer (see p. 670). In one review,[17] there was no correlation between exacerbation and remissions of pain (pain clusters) and the symptomatic diagnosis of benign gastric ulcer.

Abdominal Tenderness. Tenderness may be present in a number of gastric ulcer patients; when present, it is usually epigastric in location. The tenderness will often be relieved by flexing the muscles of the anterior abdominal wall.

Anorexia. Although often equated with malignancy, anorexia has been reported in as many as 46.4 per cent of patients with a presumably benign ulcer.[16] It is possible that some patients who describe anorexia do so because food precipitates or increases their pain, and they are therefore hesitant to eat.

Weight Loss. A modest loss of weight is not an uncommon finding in patients with benign gastric ulcer. This weight loss is almost certainly secondary to the decreased appetite of these individuals, and a weight gain should be anticipated as the ulcer heals.

Nausea and Vomiting. Nausea with or without vomiting may be an important symptom of patients with a gastric ulcer. Nausea occurred in 53.6 per cent of patients studied by Edwards and Coghill,[16] whereas vomiting occurred in 38.1 per cent. Vomiting may decrease or relieve pain in some patients. Six per cent of the patients in the aforementioned review reported that pain always persisted until relieved by vomiting.

Hematemesis and Melena. Patients with a gastric ulcer may present with hematemesis, melena, or occult gastrointestinal bleeding. Bleeding occurs in approximately 25 per cent of gastric ulcer patients at some time during the course of their disease.

Water Brash. Salivation may occur as a reflex phenomenon secondary to irritation of the esophageal, gastric, or duodenal mucosa. When this reflex secretion is excessive, the saliva may, without the individual's knowledge, pass down the esophagus and collect above the cardiac sphincter. This collection of saliva may suddenly be brought into the mouth without any vomiting effort. This condition is known as water brash.[18] It is reported by one-third of the patients with a gastric ulcer.[16]

DIFFERENTIAL DIAGNOSIS

Unnecessary delays often occur in evaluating patients with signs or symptoms suggesting peptic ulcer disease. In one review,[15] the average duration of symptoms from the time of onset of the illness until a correct diagnosis was made was 14.2 months. The patient waited an average of 7.8 months before consulting a physician, whereas the physician was responsible for 6.4 months of delay. The vagueness of the early symptoms of ulcer disease, especially gastric carcinoma, should be given greater emphasis in an effort to avoid diagnostic delays.[4]

BENIGN VS. MALIGNANT GASTRIC ULCER

A gastric malignancy cannot be differentiated from a benign ulcer on the basis of symptomatology.[19] Epigastric pain, anorexia, vomiting, and bleeding are of about equal frequency in the two diseases,[14, 15] whereas weight loss is more frequent and more marked in cancer than in benign gastric ulcer.[14] This, however, is of little help in the individual patient. The physical examination may be helpful if an abdominal mass is palpated or if there is evidence of metastatic disease such as the presence of an enlarged supraclavicular lymph node. Although the history and physical examination may be helpful, the differentiation between a benign and a malignant gastric ulcer is usually made by X-ray, endoscopy, cytology, secretory studies, and response to medical therapy. These specific diagnostic tools are discussed in the next section.

DUODENAL ULCER

It is almost impossible to differentiate a patient with a gastric ulcer from a patient with a duodenal ulcer on the basis of signs or symptoms. There are, however, a few differences in the natural history of gastric and duodenal ulcers that deserve mentioning. In one series,[16] the mean age of patients with a gastric ulcer was nine years higher than that of those with a duodenal ulcer; duodenal ulcers tend to occur in the third and fourth decades, whereas gastric ulcers reach their highest incidence in the sixth and seventh decades. In addition, there is apparently no significant trend toward a seasonal incidence in patients with a gastric ulcer as has been reported in patients with a duodenal ulcer.[20]

OTHER DISEASES

The differential diagnosis of gastric and duodenal ulcer from esophagitis, pancreatitis, small bowel disease, biliary tract disease, and functional dyspepsia is covered in detail on pages 682 to 685.

DIAGNOSTIC TECHNIQUES

X-RAY

The barium X-ray examination remains the single most widely used diagnostic tool in gastric ulcer. The value of this method, however, is in direct proportion to the skill, experience, interest, and facilities of the examiner; the cooperation of the patient; the index of suspicion of the clinician; and the opportunity for repetition of the examination during therapy.[21] As soon as possible after the patient is first seen, the barium X-ray should be performed. Although this method is accurate in detecting over 90 per cent of all gastric ulcers, its accuracy in distinguishing benign from malignant gastric ulcers is not that good. In a review of 550 patients with a preoperative radiological diagnosis of benign ulcerating lesions of the stomach, Lampert et al. found that 13 per cent had malignant lesions at the time of surgery.[14] Walters stated that an X-ray diagnosis of benign gastric ulcer was made in 10 per cent of patients who at the time of surgery were found to have carcinoma.[22] Dodd and Nelson studied 100 patients with a gastric ulcer; they found that the ulcer was detected by X-ray in 91 per cent of the cases, and of the detected ulcers 91.2 per cent were correctly interpreted as being either benign or malignant.[23] The overall accuracy of X-ray detection and interpretation was 83 per cent. These data are summarized in Table 55–1 and are compared with endoscopic results. In a review by Browne et al.,[24] the correct diagnosis of benign or malignant gastric ulcer was made in 87.9 per cent of 228 patients examined.

Criteria Suggesting Benignancy. When present, probably the most reliable sign of benign gastric ulceration is Hampton's sign (see Fig. 40–1, p. 497).[23] This is characterized by a radiolucent line, usually not more than 1 mm in width, which may partially or completely traverse the orifice of an ulcer. Shumacher and Hampton conclusively demonstrated that the radiolucency is due to the thin, undermined marginal mucosa of the crater.[25] Although an incomplete Hampton line was demonstrated by the Veterans Administration study in one patient with gastric carcinoma, Kirsh considers that a true Hampton line is indicative of a benign ulcer.[26] The line cannot be demonstrated in many patients with benign gastric ulcer, and its absence is not of diagnostic significance.

The ulcer collar is another radiological finding that is suggestive of a benign gastric ulcer (see Fig. 40–2, p. 498).[23] This term refers to the translucent band which may intervene between the ulcer crater

TABLE 55-1. ACCURACY OF DIAGNOSTIC METHODS FOR DETECTION OF GASTRIC ULCER*

	ROENTGENOLOGIC EXAMINATION	GASTROSCOPIC EXAMINATION
Percentage of all lesions detected	91%	86%
Percentage of detected lesions correctly interpreted	91.2%	94.2%
Overall accuracy of detected and interpreted lesions	83%	81%
Overall accuracy of combined methods of examination	95%	

*Data derived from Dodd, G. D., and Nelson, R. S.: Radiology 77:177, 1961.

and the lumen of the stomach. This most likely represents edema and inflammatory exudate which may surround the ulcer crater. It is imperative that the ulcer collar be distinguished from a mass with central ulceration, especially when the collar is of sufficient size that the term ulcer mound is used to describe it. Wolf and Marshak state that the surface of the benign ulcer mound is sharply demarcated and smooth, and it is covered by intact folds.[27] In most instances the margins join the adjacent stomach in a smooth manner and without sharp discontinuity.

The presence of folds that radiate to the very edge of the crater is a third sign that may be useful in diagnosing a benign gastric ulcer.[28] If the folds radiate in the vicinity of the crater but are interrupted near the crater, a malignant lesion should be considered. The aforementioned criteria are only valid in the absence of a mass.[23]

There are other criteria that have been mentioned as indicative of a benign gastric ulcer. An incisura has been considered as a sign of benignancy, and when present it does suggest a benign process. However, it is seen very infrequently. In the review by Kirsh, it was demonstrated in only 10 per cent of 118 benign lesions and was demonstrated in none of the 22 malignant lesions.[28]

The penetration of an ulcer beyond the gastric lumen on X-ray has been reported as a sign of benignancy, but in the study by Kirsh,[28] penetration beyond the gastric lumen was demonstrated in 93 per cent of the 118 benign gastric ulcers and in 82 per cent of the 22 malignant ulcers. It therefore should not be considered a highly reliable radiological sign of benignancy; on the other hand, if the ulcer does not penetrate beyond the gastric lumen, malignancy should be suspected.

Criteria Suggesting Malignancy. The most valuable signs of malignancy are a negative filling defect either in the crater itself or at its upper or lower margins, and abnormal or effaced mucosal folds.[26, 28] In 19 of the 22 malignant ulcers reviewed by Kirsh, a filling defect was demonstrated, and in the same number of patients abnormal folds were present near the base of the crater. These signs were also present in a small percentage (14 per cent and 13 per cent, respectively) of the 118 patients with a benign ulcer. Although these signs imply a malignant ulcer, they cannot therefore be considered an absolute criterion for malignancy. According to Dodd and Nelson, the only valid X-ray sign of malignant ulceration is the demonstration of a tumor in the vicinity of the crater.[23] This may vary from an unmistakable ulcer within a mass to interruption or distortion of the mucosal folds on a limited segment of the periphery of the crater. A nodular or irregular base cannot be assumed to indicate malignancy, because blood clots, granulation tissue, and food particles may be indistinguishable from tumor nodules.[21, 29] See pages 497 to 502 for a detailed description of the X-ray findings in malignant gastric ulcer.

Location and Size. The location, size, configuration, and depth of an ulcer crater as determined by X-ray should not be utilized as absolute criteria in differentiating a benign from a malignant gastric ulcer.[30, 31] As recently as 1950, it was thought that almost all ulcers on the greater curvature were malignant. In 1961, Findley reviewed 44 cases in which an ulcer was located on the greater curvature, and of the 44 only five were malignant.[32] In the recent Veterans Administration cooperative study,[33] none of the 25 gastric carcinomas discovered in the 638 patients admitted to the study were located on the greater curvature. In this same study, Sun and Stempien reported a total of 29 benign ulcers that were located on the greater curvature.[34] The aforementioned data would suggest that patients with a benign-appearing greater curvature ulcer can be managed therapeutically in the same manner as patients with a benign-appearing ulcer in other parts of the stomach.

Historically, the location of an ulcer in relation to the pylorus has also been used as a differentiating point between benign and malignant ulcers. Allen stated that 65 per cent of all ulcers in the 2-cm area proximal to the pylorus were malignant.[35] Ivy and coworkers also indicated an increased incidence of malignancy in the prepyloric region, although they did cite contradictory reports.[36] In a large series of gastric ulcers, Singleton reported 15 that were located in the inch proximal to the pylorus.[37] Seven were benign histologically, and the other eight healed completely with medical therapy, strongly suggesting that all 15 of the ulcers were benign. In the Veterans Administration cooperative study,[33] out of 216 ulcers located in the 3 cm proximal to the pylorus, only five were malignant. Stated in another way, only 20 per cent of the gastric carcinomas occurred in the 3 cm proximal to the pylorus, whereas 35.5 per cent of all ulcers occurred within the proximal 3 cm. This certainly supports the concept that there is no higher incidence of malignancy in prepyloric ulcers. Elliott et al., in their review, determined that there was no statistical evidence to lend credence to the dogma of "malignant until proved otherwise" when an ulcer was located in the prepyloric area.[30]

There is evidence in the literature that ulcer size as determined by X-ray may aid in differentiating a benign from a malignant lesion. For many years clinicians have been taught that ulcers measuring greater than 4.0 cm in diameter were malignant until proved otherwise. In 1929, Alvarez and McCarty reviewed 638 gastric ulcers and 682 gastric carcinomas and stated that if a gastric ulcer was larger than a quarter (2.4 cm) but smaller than a silver dollar (3.7 cm), the chances were two to one that it was malignant.[38] If the ulcer was larger than a dollar, it was almost certainly malignant. Robbins contradicted the 4.0 cm rule as being absolute.[31] Fifty-three patients were reported with ulcers measuring 4.1 cm or larger; of this group 20 ulcers were benign and 33 were malignant. Marshak and his colleagues described seven patients with benign gastric ulcer in whom the crater exceeded 3.5 cm in diameter.[39] Comfort et al., however, observed that the larger the ulcer, the more frequently the radiologists found features sufficiently suggestive of malignancy to equivocate.[8] In the recent Veterans Administration study, 10.4 per cent of ulcers larger than 2.0 cm were malignant.[33] Thus it may be concluded that although there is insufficient evidence to equate a large ulcer with malignancy, there is a higher incidence of malignancy in large gastric ulcers when compared with small gastric ulcers.

Kirsh has emphasized two significant weaknesses in X-ray technique which might lead to a wrong diagnosis and which, when possible, should be avoided.[26] The omission of mucosal relief films or the inability to obtain adequate mucosal relief films is one of the principal defects in technique. A second fault is the use of too dense barium or the use of an insufficiently penetrating radiographic technique which may lead to nonvisualization of a filling defect. A high kilovolt technique should be used in order to adequately visualize a filling defect in the stomach.

GASTROSCOPY

With the introduction of fiberoptics, the addition of photography, and the development of biopsy capabilities, gastroscopy has become an important tool in the diagnosis of gastric ulcers and in the differentiation of benign from malignant ulcers (see pp. 521 to 531). When gastroscopy, performed by a competent endoscopist, is combined with good barium X-rays of the stomach, the diagnostic accuracy of differentiating a benign from a malignant gastric ulcer increases to 95 per cent.[23] When gastroscopy alone is utilized, the overall diagnostic accuracy ranges from 73 per cent in one series[40] to 81 per cent in another.[23] As is demonstrated in the review by Dodd and Nelson (Table 55–1), a slightly greater number of ulcers were detected by roentgenology than by endoscopy, but of those that were detected the diagnostic accuracy of endoscopy was greater than that of roentgenology.[23]

The addition of gastroscopic photography as a diagnostic aid obviously provides an opportunity to follow an ulcer to healing by means of serial photographs. The stages of healing or nonhealing in response to therapy may be recorded during serial examinations. With the further addition of biopsy capabilities and in some cases cytological brush smears, the diagnostic usefulness of gastroscopy is increased. In a series by Williams et al., 46 patients were subjected to gastroscopy combined with histological examination either by biopsy or by cytological smear.[41] There was agreement between the gastroscopic and histological diagnosis in 89 per cent of the cases. Usually the biopsy specimen or cytological smear served to confirm the gastroscopic diagnosis, but in some of the cases in which disagreement occurred, the histological or cytological appearance served to correct an incorrect gastroscopic diagnosis.

Although gastroscopy is an important diagnostic tool and is associated with relatively little discomfort or risk to the patient, the procedure should be considered as a valuable adjunct and not as an alternative to the barium X-ray examination.[40-42]

ACID SECRETION STUDIES

Numerous studies have demonstrated that patients with a gastric ulcer have on the average a lower basal acid output, peak acid output, and maximal acid output than do normal individuals.[43-45] The overlap, however, between the two groups is tremendous, and the values for the BAO, PAO, and MAO are of no diagnostic value in most instances. Whether the decrease in measured acid in patients with a gastric ulcer is secondary to decreased acid production or to increased back-diffusion of acid through an abnormal mucosa[46] has not been clearly established.

The prime reason for performing secretory studies in patients with a gastric ulcer is to determine whether or not they are achlorhydric when stimulated with his-

tamine, Histalog, or pentagastrin, and thus to aid in differentiating a benign from a malignant gastric ulcer. It has been stated[44, 47] that patients with gastric carcinoma have a 20 to 25 per cent incidence of histamine and Histalog-fast achlorhydria, whereas achlorhydria is almost never seen in patients with a benign gastric ulcer.

Benign gastric ulcers have on very rare occasions been described in patients who have histamine-fast achlorhydria.[48-50] These observations would serve to challenge the dictum of "no acid, no ulcer."[51, 52] The phenomenon, however, which might explain the occurrence of a benign gastric ulcer in the presence of apparent achlorhydria, would be that the measured absence of acid was actually secondary to the back-diffusion of hydrogen ions through an altered gastric mucosa and not to true histamine-fast achlorhydria.

It is the opinion of this author and others[50] that a patient with a gastric ulcer and apparent histamine-fast achlorhydria whose condition is documented by a repeat study should be considered as having gastric carcinoma.

CYTOLOGY

The role of exfoliative cytology in the early diagnosis of gastric carcinoma and in the differentiation between benign and malignant lesions in the stomach has been reviewed numerous times during the past 20 years and is discussed in detail on pages 589 to 594. The technique was advocated by Beale over 100 years ago, when he examined vomitus by a paraffin block technique.[53] It was, however, the development of a staining technique by Papanicolaou[54] in the 1940's that stimulated interest in gastric exfoliative cytology. The fundamental concepts have remained unchanged, and only the manner of obtaining material—by balloons, abrasive brushes, mucosal sponging devices, and the use of enzymes—has varied.[55]

The most important limiting factor in the use of cytology is the lack of skilled and interested cytologists and cytotechnologists. Exfoliated gastric cells are under continuous enzymatic digestion prior to their removal from the stomach, and this must be overcome by proper aspirating techniques. The aspiration of only fasting gastric contents or the delay in processing of carefully obtained lavage specimens is to be deplored.[56]

Because of the inaccuracy of some of them, the potential danger of others, and the discomfort to the patient, abrasive techniques are considered to be inferior to properly executed lavage techniques.[56-58] Rosenthal and Traut first introduced the use of mucolytic or proteolytic enzymes to liquefy the mucous barrier and aid in obtaining fresh cells by gastric lavage.[59] They introduced buffered papain for gastric lavage, but papain did not always yield well preserved cells.

Rubin and Benditt found that fresh cells could be obtained by using chymotrypsin lavage.[57] The original chymotrypsin lavage technique was later modified and shortened and was described by Brandborg et al.[56] and MacDonald et al.[58] This modified technique is more applicable for widespread use than the longer procedure, and it was reported that more than 80 per cent of gastric carcinomas could be diagnosed in good routine laboratories using this method. In laboratories interested specifically in gastric cytology, the accuracy is much higher. In the aforementioned authors' own laboratories,[58] they report a diagnostic accuracy of 93 per cent with malignant lesions of the stomach and an accuracy of 99.7 per cent with benign lesions.

Gastric cytology was thought at one time to be a useful screening test for the early diagnosis of asymptomatic gastric carcinoma. This was evaluated by MacDonald and coworkers[60] in two groups of patients thought to be more likely to have or to develop gastric carcinoma than the general population. One group was composed of patients with pernicious anemia, and the other group contained elderly patients who were either hypochlorhydric or achlorhydric. Five hundred patients were evaluated by exfoliative cytology, and three gastric carcinomas were discovered. In two of the three patients, the lesion was diagnosed as a carcinoma on the X-ray examination of the stomach. In this study cytological screening of a highly selected population diagnosed only one gastric carcinoma that was not detected by the radiol-

ogist. It can be concluded that cytological screening should not be employed in the general population but that cytology should be used as an adjunct to radiography and endoscopy in differentiating a benign from a malignant gastric lesion.

GASTRIN

As reported by Trudeau and McGuigan, serum gastrin concentrations are higher in patients with presumably benign gastric ulcers than in the control population and in the population with duodenal ulcer.[61]

In a recent study, serum gastrin determinations were obtained in patients with gastric carcinoma localized to the antrum, the antral body junction, and the body of the stomach.[62] In the patients with antral carcinoma, the fasting mean serum gastrin level (80 ± 18 pg per milliliter SEM) was essentially the same as the control population (92 ± 8 pg per milliliter). In the other groups, however, the gastrin levels were significantly higher than the control population. In those with a carcinoma in the antral body junction region, the average gastrin level was 257 ± 32 pg per milliliter, whereas the value in the patients with a malignant ulcer in the body was 1028 ± 389 pg per milliliter. As might be anticipated, there was an inverse relationship between the serum gastrin levels and the rates of gastric acid secretion. Four of the five patients with carcinoma in the body of the stomach were achlorhydric.

At present, the finding of elevated serum gastrin concentrations in certain patients with malignant gastric ulcers is extremely interesting, but for clinical purposes it does not seem practical to recommend the routine acquisition of serum gastrin levels for diagnostic purposes in patients with either a benign or a malignant gastric ulcer. Interpretation of serum gastrin concentrations is discussed in detail on pages 555 to 558.

IMMUNOLOGICAL STUDIES

Several investigators have evaluated the possibility of developing an immunological test for gastric carcinoma. Hakkinen et al. in Scandinavia,[63, 64] and Stoebner and colleagues in this country,[65] have been developing an antibody to react with an antigen in the gastric juice of patients with carcinoma. Patterson reports that unfortunately 10 to 15 per cent of patients with apparent benign gastric ulcers also react with the antibody (personal communication). False-negative tests in patients with gastric carcinoma, on the other hand, are rare. At present, this test is not sufficiently specific to be of diagnostic value in differentiating gastric carcinoma from benign gastric ulcer.

There have been several recent reports in which alpha$_1$-fetoglobulin has been found in the serum of patients with adenocarcinoma of the stomach with hepatic metastasis.[66-68] In another report, alpha$_1$-fetoglobulin was found in the tumor of a patient with a gastric carcinoma with liver and lymph node metastasis.[69] This is of no practical diagnostic value at present, but it indicates that further investigation may lead to a diagnostically significant serological test for gastric carcinoma.

MANAGEMENT

IMMEDIATE

If the ulcer is diagnosed as malignant by X-ray, gastroscopy, cytology, or biopsy, the mode of therapy has already been determined. A quick but thorough evaluation for metastatic disease should be performed; if there is no evidence of metastases, patients with gastric carcinoma should be submitted to immediate surgery. If, however, the ulcer by all diagnostic criteria is either clearly benign or indeterminate, should the patient be submitted to a trial of medical therapy? This question has been debated for many years, and an answer based on well controlled studies is still not available. There are those who would recommend immediate surgical intervention in all patients with a gastric ulcer whether the ulcer is apparently benign or malignant. In other areas of the human body, when the diagnosis is uncertain, the physician readily recommends a surgical procedure which will yield a definitive diagnosis. Palumbo and Sharpe[70] and others[14, 71-73] have stated that the current rationale of watchful waiting in patients with a gastric ulcer which may be malignant is more hazardous than

that of performing a surgical procedure. These investigators also state that delays encountered by medical observation often lead to great socioeconomic loss, disruption of the patient's normal daily life, and development of complications secondary to the lesion. The possibility also exists that the chance of cure may be lost if the lesion is malignant. Other investigators have advocated early surgery because of a high recurrence rate in patients with initially healed gastric ulcers.[74, 75]

There is, however, an equally impressive argument against early surgery.[24, 76, 77] First, most gastric ulcers are benign; second, essentially all malignancies can be detected by a lack of complete symptomatic, radiological or gastroscopic response to medical therapy; third a significant number of patients will not have a recurrence, and this group will be spared a surgical procedure; fourth, there is an admittedly low but definite mortality rate associated with surgery; and finally, a certain number of patients will experience morbidity in the form of a postgastrectomy syndrome.

It is this author's opinion that the most reasonable synthesis of the aforementioned information indicates that a trial of medical therapy is justified in those gastric ulcers that are, according to good diagnostic criteria, probably benign. A number of different regimens have been included in trials of medical therapy, but only three factors—hospitalization, carbenoxolone, and the discontinuation of smoking—have been demonstrated by controlled clinical trials to increase the rate of healing of gastric ulcers.

Hospitalization. Hospitalization has been associated in at least one randomized study with an increased rate of healing of benign gastric ulcers.[78] When comparing the group that was hospitalized for four weeks with the control group that was treated for the same period as outpatients, the rate of healing was statistically different. Forty-one per cent of the ulcers in the hospitalized group were healed by two-thirds or more of their original size by the end of one month, compared with 13 per cent of the ulcers in the control group.

Because of the economic impact that three or four weeks of hospitalization can have on the patient and his family, it seems reasonable not to hospitalize every patient with a gastric ulcer. There are some patients who will require hospitalization, at least initially, to expedite their evaluation and to properly introduce them to a good medical regimen for treatment of their ulcer. There is a second group who for psychological reasons must be hospitalized in an effort to isolate them from a stressful home or employment environment. In these patients the hospital can be a very important and necessary adjunct to their therapy. The third group who obviously must be hospitalized are those with complications such as bleeding, perforation, or obstruction.

Smoking. In a controlled study by Doll and coworkers, inpatients with gastric ulcers who at the time of admission were regular smokers were divided at random into groups.[79] In one group the patients were advised to stop smoking, whereas in the other group nothing was said in reference to smoking. All the patients were treated in bed for four weeks, and all other therapy was equal in both groups. In the 40 patients advised to stop smoking, the ulcer healed by two-thirds or more in 75 per cent; whereas in the group not advised to quit smoking, the ulcer healed by two-thirds or more in 58 per cent (p value not given). The average reduction in size of the ulcer was 78.1 per cent in the first group and 56.6 per cent in the second group ($p = 0.03$). The average gain in weight and the severity of symptoms were not significantly different in the two groups. Although these statistics are not overly impressive, they at least suggest that the rate of healing of gastric ulcers is greater in patients who stop smoking.

It is not likely that smoking is a direct cause of gastric ulceration. In Great Britain, the smoking of cigarettes has actually increased during the past 30 years, whereas the incidence of gastric ulcer has decreased. Although cigarette smoking may not be an etiological factor, it may interfere with the healing of an ulcer and may aid in the maintenance of its chronicity. Patients with a gastric ulcer should therefore be advised to stop smoking.

Carbenoxolone Sodium. For a number of years extracts of licorice have been used in Europe in the treatment of peptic ulcer. The active portion of the extract is be-lieved to be the glycoside glycyrrhizinic acid. When this acid is hydrolyzed, a pentacyclic triterpenoid is formed, and it is the disodium salt of a derivative of this compound that is referred to as carbenoxolone sodium (Biogastrone).[80] Animal studies have demonstrated that carbenoxolone sodium and similar preparations have anti-inflammatory properties but also that they may cause salt and water retention.

The first double-blind controlled clinical trial of carbenoxolone sodium was reported by Doll et al. in 1962.[80] All patients in this study were advised to continue working unless they had severe pain, to eat a normal diet except for fried foods, to stop smoking, and to limit alcohol intake. Thirty patients were given the active drug, and 20 patients received a placebo. In the group receiving the active drug, the ulcer disappeared radiographically within five weeks in 11 (37 per cent), and the ulcer niche, on the average, was reduced in size by 72 per cent. In the placebo-treated group, the ulcer disappeared completely within five weeks in only one patient (5 per cent), and the ulcer niche, on the average, was reduced in size by 34 per cent.

At least two additional studies have confirmed that reduction of ulcer size and increased rate of healing are associated with carbenoxolone therapy.[81, 82] Unfortunately, in each of these studies salt and water retention was a significant complication. Peripheral edema was the most common manifestation, but dyspnea and congestive heart failure also occurred. In an effort to circumvent this complication, Horwich and Galloway introduced a five- or six-day regimen in which carbenoxolone was omitted on one or both days of the weekend in individuals likely to develop edema.[82] With this regimen side effects were less marked and less frequent. There was no mention, however, of whether the ulcer healing rate was affected.

In a further attempt to reduce the side effects of carbenoxolone, Doll et al. treated one group of patients with carbenoxolone in combination with spironolactone and another group with carbenoxolone and a thiazide diuretic.[83] There was a decreased incidence of edema in the group receiving spironolactone, but there was also a decrease in the rate of ulcer healing. It was thought that the aldosterone antagonist might interfere with ulcer healing by altering electrolyte transport across the gastric mucosa. In the group treated with carbenoxolone and, if necessary, a thiazide diuretic, ulcer healing was not retarded by the thiazide, and the previously reported increased healing with carbenoxolone was demonstrated. Carbenoxolone is not available in the United States.

Estrogens. Doll et al. studied the effect of estrogens on the rate of gastric ulcer healing in men and in women 60 years of age or older.[81] Even though Truelove demonstrated a beneficial effect from estrogen therapy in the treatment of duodenal ulcer,[84] the present study demonstrated no statistically significant difference between the rate of healing of gastric ulcers in the estrogen-treated group and the placebo-treated group.

Cholestyramine. Since it has been suggested that reflux of bile into the stomach may be an etiological factor in the development of gastric ulceration,[85-88] a double-blind controlled trial was performed, using cholestyramine, an exchange resin that binds bile acids,[89] in the treatment of gastric ulcers. The patients treated with cholestyramine had a greater reduction in the size of the ulcer, had less pain, and used fewer antacid tablets than did the patients in the placebo group, but the differences were not statistically significant.

Diet. The long-established medical regimens for the treatment of gastric ulcers have invariably included dietary restrictions. Almost every practicing clinician has been taught during the course of his training that patients with either gastric or duodenal ulcer should be provided a bland diet with frequent feedings, including the liberal use of milk and cream. The purpose of the dietary management is an attempt to eliminate all irritating foods and to provide adequate and continuous neutralization of acid. Although there is no evidence that dietary restrictions have a deleterious effect on the patient, the experimental evidence supporting the use of such diets is extremely poor.

Until the beginning of the twentieth century Leube's starvation regimen was the accepted treatment for gastric ulcer.[90] In 1901 Lenhartz introduced the concept of frequent small feedings, and in 1904 he published data supporting this therapy.[91] The barium X-ray had not been introduced at the time of Lenhartz's studies, and the diagnosis of ulcer was primarily based on the presence of hematemesis or melena. Many of the patients treated in the early 1900's with the Lenhartz diet were actually pain-free at the time of their dietary treatment. It is very likely that many of the patients did not have an ulcer and that the etiology of the hemorrhage was not peptic ulcer as assumed.

After the introduction of the bismuth or barium X-ray study, the diagnosis of peptic ulcer could be made in the absence of hemorrhage, and the Lenhartz dietary regimen was then utilized in the treatment of almost all patients with peptic ulcer. Through the years the dietary regimen was modified by various individuals, and milk and cream were added to it. It was not until 1939 that a serious attempt was made to adequately evaluate the true effectiveness of dietary restrictions. In 1939, Nicol found that the mean acidity of gastric contents aspirated at hourly intervals through a nasogastric tube was only slightly different in patients receiving milk, cream, and vegetable purée from what it was in those who ate a diet composed of four main meals daily and 150 ml of milk at night.[92] Other studies have confirmed the premise that a bland diet and/or the frequent drinking of milk will not decrease gastric acidity and may indeed cause an increase in gastric acid secretion.[93, 94] Of even greater significance than the fact that a bland diet and milk regimens do not reduce gastric acidity is the fact that two controlled clinical trials have supported the view that dietary restrictions will not enhance the healing rate of a gastric ulcer.[95, 96] There is also no evidence to suggest that, once remission has occurred, dietary restrictions will protect against or delay a relapse.[97]

Although it seems reasonable to allow patients with a gastric ulcer free access to food, there are several restrictions that should be imposed, and these are discussed below:

COFFEE AND TEA. Coffee and tea contain caffeine, and tea also contains theophylline. Caffeine and theophylline are methylated xanthines,[98] and as such they inhibit phosphodiesterase.[99, 100] As a result of this inhibition, 3'5'-cyclic AMP is not converted to 5'AMP, and thus excessive amounts of cyclic AMP are present. This is thought to be the mechanism by which the xanthine derivatives cause an increase in acid secretion. Although there are no studies demonstrating that coffee and tea are ulcerogenic, it would seem appropriate to eliminate substances from the diet which clearly stimulate acid and which in themselves have no neutralizing capacity.

ALCOHOL. There are no studies demonstrating that ethanol is ulcerogenic, but there is evidence that ethanol damages the gastric mucosal barrier.[101-103] Once this barrier is broken, hydrogen ion back-diffusion occurs,[102, 104-106] and pepsin secretion may be stimulated.[107] There is some evidence that ethanol in low concentrations also stimulates gastric acid secretion.[108] It seems reasonable to eliminate any substance from the diet such as ethanol which damages the mucosal barrier, allows hydrogen back-diffusion, and stimulates (but does not neutralize) gastric acid secretion.

SALICYLATES. Salicylic acid and acetylsalicylic acid damage the gastric mucosal barrier,[101, 102, 104-106] predispose to hemorrhage from an ulcer crater, and may produce mucosal erosions and bleeding at any site in the stomach or duodenum. For these reasons patients with a gastric ulcer should be strongly advised not to take any compound containing aspirin, and they should be provided with a list of all medicines, both proprietary and prescription, that contain salicylates. A complete list of drugs containing salicylates was published in Lancet in 1963.[109] Patients should also be provided with a nonsalicylate-containing medication such as acetaminophen for pain or fever.

BEDTIME FEEDING. Patients with ulcer should be asked not to eat a bedtime snack and not to eat or drink anything except water and medication within the three-hour period prior to retiring. Almost all foods will stimulate hydrochloric acid secretion; after the initial neutralizing effect of the ingested food, the hydrochloric acid content in the stomach is often higher than basal values. Since the patient is not awake to take antacids one to two hours after retiring, his ulcer crater will be exposed to higher concentrations of acid during the night if he eats a bedtime snack than if he does not; thus eating of a bedtime snack probably increases the likelihood of awakening at night with pain and may delay healing.

Antacids. Antacids are administered to patients with a presumably benign gastric ulcer because they relieve pain, and it is hoped that they hasten healing and prevent recurrences. That they relieve pain is generally accepted, but whether or not antacids hasten healing or prevent recurrences has not been established.

It is the present policy of this author to prescribe antacids every hour while the patient is awake until there is complete radiographic or gastroscopic healing of the ulcer. The reader is referred to pages 732 to 734 for detailed information on the type and dosage of antacids recommended.

Whether antacids should be continued after the ulcer has healed is not known. It is the policy of this author to prescribe antacids one hour after meals and at bedtime for an indefinite period in the hope of preventing a recurrence.

Anticholinergics. If one accepts the premise that the hydrogen ion concentration of the stomach in gastric ulcer should be maintained at a minimum, every effort should be made to attain this goal. This would include the use of anticholinergic drugs. If a patient is taking antacids every hour while awake, it is reasonable to give anticholinergic therapy only at bedtime to help maintain a low overnight secretion of acid. Anticholinergics should be given in a dose sufficient to produce mild symptoms (i.e., a slightly dry mouth).

There are certain contraindications and objections to the use of anticholinergics. Anticholinergics must be used very cautiously in men who have even a slightly enlarged prostate gland, because urinary retention may ensue. If, however, anticholinergics are given only at bedtime, this is usually not a major problem. Since anticholinergics delay gastric emptying, the hypothesis that gastric retention is important in the etiology of a benign gastric ulcer has been mentioned as an objection to their use. This theory has not been established, and there is no convincing evidence that it is correct. At present, therefore, the advantage of a bedtime anticholinergic in decreasing nocturnal acid secretion seems to outweigh this objection to its use. A recently published controlled study indicates that anticholinergics increase the healing rate of gastric ulcer and also decrease the recurrence rate. This is discussed in more complete detail on pages 739 to 740.

Reduction of Anxiety. The exact role of anxiety in the development of a gastric ulcer is not known. Emotional stress, however, is apparent in a number of patients with a gastric ulcer, and may or may not have etiological significance.

If emotional conflicts are recognized by the physician, every effort should be made to resolve these conflicts. Many times a frank discussion of the problems will sufficiently allay anxiety. As stated above, one of the indications for hospitalizing patients with a gastric ulcer is the need for removing them from a stressful environment. In some individuals mild sedatives may also be helpful in relieving anxiety.

FOLLOW-UP

If the ulcer is visible by X-ray, this technique is used in the follow-up examinations, either exclusively or in combination with endoscopy. On the other hand, if the ulcer is not visible by X-ray and the initial diagnosis was made by endoscopy, then follow-up to complete healing by endoscopy is mandatory.

The first follow-up examination should be performed three weeks after the initial diagnosis is made. This is only to determine whether healing is occurring and whether the ulcer is decreasing in size. The absolute rate of healing is not of major importance at this time. If the ulcer has remained the same size as on the initial examination, if it has increased in size, or if it has begun to demonstrate any of the radiographic or gastroscopic signs of malignancy, the patient should be considered an immediate surgical candidate. A few ulcers may be healed completely at this time; for those that have completely healed, a repeat X-ray should be obtained in two or three months to make certain that the ulcer has not recurred.

The second follow-up examination for those patients who have not healed completely at the time of the first follow-up should be performed six weeks after the initial diagnosis. At this time a high percentage of ulcers should be healed completely. Of those that are not healed completely, the ulcer should be reduced by 90 per cent of its original size. If these two criteria are not satisfied, the patient should be considered for surgery. In the Veterans Administration study, 70.4 per cent of the 638 patients had complete healing at the end of six weeks, and satisfactory progress (90 per cent reduction in size) had been made in an additional 7.7 per cent.[110]

Twelve weeks from the time of the initial diagnosis, the third follow-up examination should be performed on those patients who have made satisfactory progress but have not healed completely at the time of the six-week examination. It is generally accepted that all patients having an incompletely healed ulcer at the end of 12 weeks should be referred for surgery. The patient with a large gastric ulcer (over 2.5 cm in width) is the possible exception to this rule. The rate of healing in both large and small gastric ulcers is approximately 3 mm per week.[111] It is obvious therefore that the percentage rate of healing at a given time after beginning therapy will be lower for large than for small ulcers. Large ulcers may require 15 weeks or possibly longer to heal completely rather than the 12 weeks allowed for small and medium-sized ulcers. This fact was demonstrated by the Veterans Administration study.[34] The percentage of each ulcer size (expressed as width) healed at three, six, and 12 weeks is shown in Figure 55-1. For large ulcers only 15 per cent were healed at three weeks, 36 per cent at six weeks, and 52 per cent at 12 weeks. Since the percentage of patients with large ulcers that are healed at a given time forms a straight line, it might be assumed that an increasingly larger number of patients might have completely healed if treatment had been prolonged beyond 12 weeks. It is also apparent, however, from Figure 55-1 that it might require as long as 21 weeks for the complete healing of some large ulcers. To observe an ulcer for 21 weeks seems unreasonable and dangerous.

It is the opinion of this author that the 12-week rule should be followed in all ulcers less than 2.5 cm in width and that all

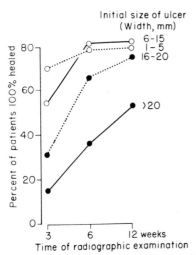

Figure 55–1. Percentage of patients with complete healing at three, six, and 12 weeks in relation to initial size of ulcer.

ulcers regardless of size should be submitted to surgery if not completely healed at the end of 15 weeks. This, of course, is only valid if there is no endoscopic or radiographic evidence of malignancy and if the ulcer demonstrates evidence of progressive healing with each follow-up examination.

OTHER FACTORS AFFECTING RATE OF HEALING

Age. In the study by Steigmann and Shulman, healing appeared to progress more rapidly in the younger patients (less than 45 years of age) than in the older patients.[111] The Veterans Administration study, however, revealed no difference in the healing rates between the various age groups.[110]

Anemia. There is no evidence to suggest that anemia adversely affects the rate of healing. Patients admitted with hematemesis and melena and a decreased hematocrit heal just as rapidly as those patients who have never had a decreased hematocrit.

Sex, Duration of Symptoms, and Weight Loss. These factors could not be correlated with the rate of healing in the Veterans Administration study.[110]

AFTER HEALING, ARE FOLLOW-UP EXAMINATIONS INDICATED?

Banks and Zetzel state that a presumably benign gastric ulcer should be followed by uninterruped medical supervision for at least five years and that this follow-up should include periodic X-ray examinations even in the absence of clinical symptoms.[71] There is no evidence based on controlled studies that there is a need for additional follow-up once an ulcer has healed as clearly documented by X-ray or endoscopy. Considering the frequency with which gastric ulcers recur, however, it seems advisable to repeat the X-ray or endoscopic procedure three months after documented healing to make certain that the ulcer has remained healed.

If symptoms recur, the recurrent symptoms should be evaluated in the same manner as the initial ulcer. It is unwise to assume that because the initial gastric ulcer was benign, the recurrent ulcer is also benign. A recurrent ulcer must be evaluated and treated with the same diligence as was the initial ulcer.

CAN MALIGNANT ULCERS DEMONSTRATE HEALING?

Since one of the most important signs of benignancy is the complete healing of a gastric ulcer on medical therapy, it becomes extremely important to know whether or not ulcerations within a gastric carcinoma can heal or at least demonstrate a progressive healing trend over the initial weeks of therapy. Bachrach reported in 1962 a search of the world literature from 1950 to 1960 along with the combined experience of 76 radiologists in an effort to determine the incidence of complete X-ray disappearance of malignant ulcerations of the stomach.[112] In his search, only ten cases were found which might meet the criteria of complete healing. If, however, complete healing is defined as complete normalization of the stomach, including the return of the pliability of the wall of the stomach both under the fluoroscope and with multiple views of the stomach, it is questionable whether complete healing of a neoplastic ulcer ever occurs. Although it is not well documented, there are individual reports of at least partial healing of malignant gastric ulcers.

It was the conclusion of Bachrach that the documented instances of complete radiographic disappearance of malignant gastric ulcers are much too infrequent to endanger the validity of the therapeutic trial as an important test for benign ulcer.[112] His review of the ten "possible" cases of complete healing of neoplastic ulcerations should not place the therapeutic trial in jeopardy, but instead should emphasize the importance of improved barium X-ray examinations, including air contrast studies, improved interpretation of the examinations, and improved endoscopic and biopsy techniques.

DIAGNOSIS, MANAGEMENT, AND FOLLOW-UP SUMMARIZED

X-Ray. If the ulcer is visualized by X-ray and is apparently benign, a follow-up examination should be performed at three, six, and 12 weeks. A large ulcer may be followed to 15 weeks. All studies must demonstrate a progressive healing trend. An additional study should be performed three months after documented healing.

Gastroscopy. If this technique is available, every gastric ulcer should be visualized by endoscopy and several biopsies should be obtained from the ulcer margin. If the ulcer is not visualized by X-ray, it should be followed to complete healing by endoscopy.

Secretory Studies. If achlorhydria is demonstrated on two occasions after histamine or pentagastrin stimulation, carcinoma should be assumed.

Cytology. This procedure should be performed on all patients with a gastric ulcer in hospitals and clinics where the technique is available.

Serum Gastrin and Immunological Techniques. These studies offer only minor diagnostic assistance at present.

Medical Therapy. In patients in whom the initial clinical studies suggest that the gastric ulcer is benign, a very vigorous therapeutic approach is justified, because healing with medical therapy is utilized as further proof that the ulcer is benign. Failure of the ulcer to heal, on the other hand, suggests that the ulcer is likely to be malignant.

HOSPITALIZATION. Hospitalization should be utilized in most patients for initial evaluation and introduction to medical regimen, in patients who for emotional reasons require isolation from family and employment, and in patients with complications of gastric ulcer disease.

SMOKING. Patients should be advised to stop smoking.

DIET. Patients are allowed free access to food with the exception of foods that specifically cause pain, coffee, tea, and alcohol. Patients should have nothing to eat or drink except medications and water within three hours of bedtime. No salicylates should be taken. Patients should be advised specifically which drugs contain salicylates and should be provided with a substitute medication for pain or fever.

ANTACIDS. Antacids should be given hourly while the patient is awake.

ANTICHOLINERGICS. Anticholinergics should be given at bedtime in a dose sufficient to cause mild dryness of the mouth, unless there is a specific medical contraindication to their use.

REDUCTION OF ANXIETY. Patients should be made aware that emotional factors may play a role in the development or prolongation of their disease. Sedatives and tranquilizers may be advisable in some.

PROGNOSIS AND NATURAL HISTORY

Natvig and coworkers reviewed the histories of 152 gastric ulcer patients three years after the initial diagnosis and found that only 44 per cent had remained well, whereas 56 per cent had developed a recurrent ulcer.[74] Smith and Jordan reviewed patients with a presumably benign gastric ulcer and found recurrences in 20.1 per cent of 104 patients who had been followed for less than two years, 31.4 per cent recurrence in 76 patients followed for two to five years, and 46.8 per cent recurrence rate in 111 patients followed for five years or longer.[75] In their review of 101 patients followed for an average of 5.6 years, Flood and Hennig reported one or more recurrent ulcers in all but two patients.[20] In the Veterans Administration study, there were 377 patients whose initial ulcer healed completely and who were followed for two years.[113] Of this group, 41.9 per cent had one or more recurrent ulcers. There were 114 patients or 30.2 per cent who had one documented recurrence during the follow-up period, whereas there were 44 patients, or 11.6 per cent, who had two episodes of recurrent ulceration.

FACTORS ASSOCIATED WITH RECURRENCE

Age and Sex. Flood and Hennig followed 101 patients for an average of 5.6 years.[20] Eighteen of the patients were less than 40 years of age when first admitted to the study. The patients in the younger age group were symptomatic during a greater percentage of the follow-up period than were the patients in the older age group. Hanscom and Buchman in the Veterans Administration study, on the other hand, reported that age had no effect on recurrence.[113] In the report by Flood and Hennig, a comparison of the incidence of recurrent ulceration in males and females of all ages revealed no significant difference between the sexes.[20] Krag, on the other hand, stated that men have a poorer prognosis than women and that the difference between the two sexes is significant (P < 0.05).[114]

Duration of Symptoms. Thirty-six of the patients followed by Flood and Hennig had symptoms of ulcer disease for less than one year when first admitted to the study.[20] The incidence of recurrence was slightly lower in this group than in those patients with a history of symptoms for more than a year. The difference, however, was not significant, and therefore duration of symptoms was not thought to be related to incidence of recurrence.

Length of Time Required for Healing. If it could be ascertained that the length of time required for initial healing had prognostic significance in regard to the likelihood of recurrent ulceration, it might be reasonable to recommend early surgery for those patients whose initial ulcer healed more slowly than the average ulcer. It was suggested by Flood and Hennig that a slower rate of healing meant a slightly poorer than average clinical course.[20] Hanscom and Buchman, however, considered that the question of whether the time required for initial healing affected recurrence rate was still unsettled.[113]

Location and Size of Initial Ulcer. As demonstrated by the Veterans Administration study, the location or size of the initial ulcer did not affect the likelihood of recurrent ulceration.[34]

Hemorrhage. In the study reported by Flood and Hennig, hemorrhage occurred at some time during the course of the ulcer in 37 per cent of patients.[20] The recurrence rate however, was essentially the same in this group as it was in the patients with no history of bleeding.

Gastric Acid Secretion. There was no definite correlation between gastric acidity and prognosis in one study.[115] In another study, however, patients with a high gastric acid secretion as measured by an Ewald test meal had a poorer prognosis than those with a lower secretory capacity (P < 0.01).[114]

LOCATION AND SIZE OF RECURRENT ULCERS

In the Veterans Administration study, the recurrent ulcer often occurred at a different site from the original ulcer. This is illustrated in Figure 55–2.[116]

On the other hand, the percentage of ulcers in the various anatomic segments and curvatures of the stomach is almost the same for the original and recurrent ulcers. For example, 88 per cent of initial ulcers and 94 per cent of the recurrent ulcers were on the lesser curvature. Three recur-

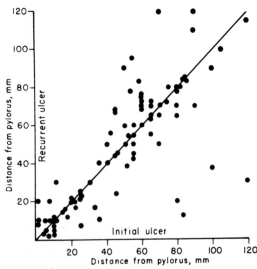

Figure 55–2. Location of recurrent ulcer compared with location of the initial ulcer in the same patient. Each point represents one patient.

rent ulcers were located on the greater curvature, and in each case the original ulcer was located on the greater curvature.[116] In regard to distance from the pylorus, the recurrent ulcer group on the average closely resembled the initial ulcer group, with the exception that there were no recurrent ulcers located more than 12 cm from the pylorus, whereas there were 26 initial ulcers located in that area.

Many of the recurrent ulcers were small in comparison with the original ulcer. The median product size for the initial ulcer was 97 sq mm; for the first recurrence, 35 sq mm; and for the second recurrence, 20 sq mm. The difference between the size of the initial ulcer and the first recurrence was statistically significant, whereas the difference in size between the first and second recurrences was not significant. The most likely explanation for the difference in the size of the initial ulcer and the recurrences was that the recurrences were detected at an earlier stage of development than was the initial ulcer.[116]

CLINICAL COURSE OF RECURRENT ULCERS

There is evidence to suggest that a benign recurrent ulceration heals as readily as does an initial ulcer. Seventy-three of the 84 patients (86.9 per cent) with recurrent ulceration in the Veterans Administration study healed within the allotted 12-week period.[116] This figure certainly compares favorably with and actually surpasses the 75.9 per cent healing rate of initial ulcers that healed within the protocol time period. It must be remembered, however, that any recurrent ulcer group may be a select group in that the patients with a tendency for slow healing have already been labeled as "refractory" on the basis of their initial ulcer and channeled to surgery.

IS SURGERY INDICATED FOR RECURRENT ULCER?

Surgery for recurrent ulceration has been advocated by numerous investigators. One of the important reasons for this attitude is the supposedly increased incidence of malignancy in recurrent ulcer-

ation. Smith and Jordan stated that in their opinion a recurrent ulcer harbored potential malignancy, and any recurrence was an adequate indication for surgery.[75] This expected increased incidence of malignancy in recurrent ulceration did not prove to be true in the Veterans Administration study, and therefore Littman and Hanscom could not recommend surgery for recurrent ulceration on this basis.[116]

Surgery has also been advised in patients with recurrent ulceration because of the possibility of more frequent complications; i.e., bleeding and perforation in these patients as compared with patients experiencing their first gastric ulcer. The complication rate was low, however, in the Veterans Administration study in the patients with recurrent ulceration.[116] Therefore it does not seem reasonable to recommend surgery for recurrent ulceration because of the possibility of complications.

As stated earlier, recurrent ulcers heal as frequently as do initial ulcers. This observation, made in the Veterans Administration study,[116] is supported by Steigmann and Shulman[111] and Pollard et al.[117] It does not, therefore, seem reasonable to recommend surgery on the basis of potentially poor healing of the recurrent ulcer.

The most frequently mentioned indication for surgery has been the development of two recurrences. This indication is based on the theory that those patients who have had two recurrences over a specified period are more likely to have further recurrences. Although the rate for second recurrences was approximately equal to the rate for first recurrences in the Veterans Administration study,[116] the data were not adequate to either defend or disprove the assumption that a higher incidence of recurrences is to be expected in those persons having had two recurrences.

Even though the necessity for surgery has not been established by prospective studies in patients with two recurrences, it has been the policy of our group to recommend surgery for patients having had a second recurrence. The reader is referred to pages 838 to 839 for details on the surgical approach to recurrent gastric ulcer.

It is interesting to note that it is uncommon to see patients with more than two or three recurrences of a gastric ulcer. This is in contrast to patients with duodenal ulcer disease in whom numerous recurrences may be noted over a period of several years. There are two possible explanations for this. It is possible that after two or three recurrences all patients with a benign gastric ulcer are treated surgically; or it may be that gastric ulcer is a self-limited disease, and eventually the tendency to develop an ulcer spontaneously disappears. In order to settle this question, long-term prospective studies are needed.

GASTRIC ULCER WITH COEXISTENT DUODENAL ULCER

One of the first investigators to report the relatively frequent association of gastric and duodenal ulcers was Wilkie in 1926.[118] He reported that 53 per cent of 79 patients with a gastric ulcer also had a concomitant duodenal ulcer. In 1929, Hurst and Stewart reported figures which contradicted the results of Wilkie.[119] Based upon 4000 autopsy studies, they reported coexistent gastric and duodenal ulceration in 5.5 per cent of the cases. Johnson stated that of the patients admitted to the hospital for evaluation of ulcer disease, approximately 7 per cent have both duodenal and gastric lesions.[120] A report by McCray et al. in 1968 supported the original report by Wilkie in that the incidence of concomitant ulceration was 48 per cent at Boston City Hospital and 64 per cent at University Hospital.[121] In the Veterans Administration study, Rumball reports an overall incidence of 41.6 per cent of patients with a gastric ulcer having coexistent deformity of the duodenal bulb, a duodenal ulcer, or both.[122]

RELATION TO THE SITE AND SIZE OF THE GASTRIC ULCER

Data reported both by the Veterans Administration study[122] and by Vesely and coworkers[123] demonstrate a higher incidence of duodenal ulceration when the gastric ulcer is located below the angulus (approximately 50 per cent) than when the gastric ulcer is located above the angulus (approximately 35 per cent). In the Veter-

ans Administration study, the size of the gastric ulcer was not related to the incidence of concomitant duodenal ulcers.[122]

RELATION TO RATE OF HEALING OF GASTRIC ULCER

In a study by McCray et al. it was reported that gastric ulcers when associated with duodenal ulcers were more frequently chronic or recurrent and typically produced symptoms for more than one year.[121] Pollard and colleagues, on the other hand, found that associated duodenal ulcer or duodenal bulb deformity had no effect on the healing rate of gastric ulcers.[117] This finding was substantiated by the Veterans Administration study.[122]

RELATION TO RECURRENCE OF GASTRIC ULCER

In the study by McCray et al., there was a definitely increased incidence of recurrent gastric ulceration when an associated duodenal ulcer or deformity of the bulb was present. Krause likewise reported an increased incidence of recurrent ulceration in the presence of concomitant duodenal ulcer.[124] Dworken et al.[125] and Flood and Hennig,[20] on the other hand, observed that an associated duodenal ulcer had no effect on the recurrence rate. The data reported in the Veterans Administration study demonstrated the effect of coexistent duodenal ulcer disease on the recurrence rate of gastric ulcer to be somewhere between the two extremes.[122] There was a slight but definite increased frequency of recurrent gastric ulcer among the Caucasian patients with coexistent duodenal ulcer. The recurrence rate in the Negro patients, however, was higher than the Caucasian rate, regardless of whether or not a coexistent duodenal ulcer was present.

RELATION TO GASTRIC CARCINOMA

It has been accepted by many individuals that the chances of an apparently benign gastric ulcer actually being malignant were decreased if a coexistent duodenal ulcer or duodenal bulb deformity was demonstrated. This premise, however, was not supported by the study of Smith et al., who reported coexistent duodenal deformities in 19.7 per cent of 879 patients with benign gastric ulcer and in 20.2 per cent of 84 patients with a malignant ulcer.[76] In the Veterans Administration study there were only three patients (1.2 per cent) with gastric carcinoma in the 259 gastric ulcer patients demonstrating evidence of duodenal ulcer disease.[122] On the other hand, there were 22 gastric carcinomas (6.0 per cent) in the 359 patients who did not demonstrate evidence for coexistent duodenal ulceration. Three (12 per cent) of the 25 patients with malignant ulcers had evidence for coexistent duodenal ulcer, whereas 256 (42.7 per cent) of the 599 patients with a benign ulcer had evidence indicating a diseased duodenum. These data would certainly lend credence to the theory that a benign-appearing gastric ulcer is more likely to be benign if associated duodenal ulcer disease is present, but in an individual patient a deformed duodenal bulb does not rule out a gastric malignancy.

SIGNIFICANCE OF MULTIPLE GASTRIC ULCERS

Instances of simultaneous, multiple, chronic ulcerations of the stomach constitute only a small percentage of the large numbers of recorded cases of chronic peptic ulcer.[126] The term "multiple chronic gastric ulcer" is reserved for use in patients who have two or more chronic ulcers as visualized by X-ray. This is in contrast to the multiple acute gastric ulcerations or erosions that are often seen with acute gastritis or after salicylate ingestion and demonstrated by endoscopy but not by X-ray. Judd and Proctor in 1925 reported that in 1475 cases of gastric ulcer, 87 patients (6 per cent) had two or more gastric ulcerations.[127] Welch and Allen reported an 8 per cent incidence of multiple gastric ulceration in 512 cases of gastric ulcer at the Massachusetts General Hospital.[9] Katz and Bierenbaum reported the case history of a patient with four simultaneous chronic gastric ulcerations.[126]

A total of 22 patients with two or more gastric ulcerations were reported in the Veterans Administration study, but of these 22, only 15 were usable cases and included in the study.[128] These 15 patients comprised 2.3 per cent of the 653 ulcer cases included in the study. Thirteen of the 15 patients had two ulcers, one had three ulcers, and one had four ulcers.

CLINICAL FEATURES

In the Veterans Administration study, the patients with multiple chronic gastric ulceration did not differ from the patients with a single ulcer as far as age or sex was concerned.[128] There were a total of 33 ulcers in the 15 patients with two or more ulcerations. Sixteen (48.5 per cent) were located in the antrum, nine (27 per cent) were located in the body, and one (3 per cent) was located in the fundus. It was Judd and Proctor's experience that most of the multiple gastric ulcers in their study were located in the antrum.[127] The clinical features of patients with multiple gastric ulcers were no different from those of patients with single ulcers.[127, 128]

INITIAL RESPONSE TO TREATMENT AND RECURRENCE

Based on the data obtained in the Veterans Administration study, patients with multiple gastric ulcers have a slightly decreased rate of healing when compared with persons with a solitary ulcer.[128] This decrease was, however, not statistically significant. Because of the small number of patients with multiple ulcers, the recurrence rate could not be reliably estimated. It was noted, however, that patients who initially have two or more gastric ulcers and who have recurrent disease have no greater propensity to develop multiple ulcers during the recurrent episode than do persons with an initially solitary lesion.

The same indications for surgical intervention should be applied to patients with multiple gastric ulcers as to patients with single ulcers. Multiple gastric ulcerations in themselves are not an indication for surgery.

CARCINOMA AND MULTIPLE GASTRIC ULCERS

It has been stated that the presence of more than one chronic gastric ulcer in an individual patient was evidence that the ulcers were benign.[9] This fact is certainly not well documented in the literature, and lymphosarcoma has been implicated as the cause of some cases of multiple gastric ulcerations.[129]

It should not be assumed that because one ulcer in a patient with multiple chronic gastric ulcers is benign, all ulcers are benign. Each ulcer must be evaluated independently.

CAN MALIGNANT DEGENERATION OCCUR IN A BENIGN GASTRIC ULCER?

Although many individuals have supported the premise that malignant degeneration of a benign gastric ulcer can occur, this is very difficult to prove histologically. In 1924, Finsterer stated that malignant degeneration of a benign ulcer was so frequent an occurrence that resection of a gastric ulcer might be regarded as an early operation for cancer of the stomach.[130] Swynnerton and Truelove reviewed 375 cases of proved carcinomas and stated that in 26 patients there was some evidence that the carcinoma may have originated in a chronic gastric ulcer.[131] Ekström provided strong evidence that in 138 patients undergoing gastric resection carcinoma may have arisen from a chronic gastric ulcer in 16 of the patients.[132]

Mallory, in 1940, expressed an opinion quite different from the aforementioned authors.[133] He concluded that chronic gastric ulcers rarely, if ever, degenerate to form carcinomas. Ewing stated that malignant degeneration of a benign gastric ulcer probably accounted for not more than 2 to 3 per cent of gastric carcinomas.[134] In a review of 411 patients with gastric ulcers, Marshall stated that there was insufficient histologic evidence to warrant a conclusion that gastric ulcers present a high potential origin for malignancy.[135]

REFERENCES

1. Knutsen, B., and Selvaag, O. The incidence of peptic ulcer. Acta Med. Scand. (Suppl.) 196:341, 1947.
2. Jennison, J. Observations made on a group of employees with duodenal ulcer. Amer. J. Med. Sci. 196:654, 1938.
3. Blumenthal, I. S. Digestive disease as a national problem. Gastroenterology 54:86, 1968.
4. Kukral, J. C. Gastric ulcer: An appraisal. Surgery 63:1024, 1968.
5. Watkinson, G. The incidence of chronic peptic ulcer found at necropsy. Gut 1:14, 1960.
6. Doll, R., Jones, A. F., and Buckatzsch, M. M. Occupational factors in the aetiology of gastric and duodenal ulcers with an estimate of their incidence in the general population. Spec. Rep. Ser. Med. Res. Council 276:1 1951.
7. Doll, R. Epidemiology of peptic ulcer. In Modern Trends in Gastroenterology, Jones, F. A.(ed.). New York, Paul B. Hoeber, Inc., 1952.
8. Comfort, M. W., Priestley, J. T., Dockerty, M. B., Weber, H. M., Gage, R. P., Solis, J., and Epperson, D. P. The small benign and malignant gastric lesion. Surg. Gynec. Obstet. 105:435, 1957.
9. Welch, C. E., and Allen, A. W. Gastric ulcer study of Massachusetts General Hospital cases during the ten year period 1938–1947. New Eng. J. Med. 240:277, 1949.
10. Cain, J. C., Jordan, G. L., Comfort, M. W., and Gray, H. K. Medically treated small gastric ulcer. J.A.M.A. 150:781, 1952.
11. Larson, N. E., Cain, J. C., and Bartholomew, L. G. Prognosis of the medically treated small gastric ulcer. New Eng. J. Med. 264:119, 1961.
12. Swynnerton, B. F., and Tanner, N. C. Chronic gastric ulcer. Brit. Med. J. 2:841, 1953.
13. Gill, A. M. Gastric ulcer. Brit. Med. J. 3:415, 1968.
14. Lampert, E. G., Waugh, J. M., and Dockerty, M. B. The incidence of malignancy in gastric ulcer believed preoperatively to be benign. Surg. Gynec. Obstet. 91:673, 1950.
15. Gray, D. B., and Ward, G. E. Delay in diagnosis of carcinoma of the stomach. Amer. J. Surg. 83:524, 1952.
16. Edwards, F. C., and Coghill, N. F. Clinical manifestations in patients with chronic atrophic gastritis, gastric ulcer, and duodenal ulcer. Quart. J. Med. 37:337, 1968.
17. Rinaldo, J. A., Scheinok, P., and Rupe, C. E.: Symptom diagnosis. A mathematical analysis of epigastric pain. Ann. Intern. Med. 59:145, 1963.
18. Best, C. H., and Taylor, N. B. The Physiological Basis of Medical Practice. Baltimore, Williams and Wilkins Co., 1961, p. 597.
19. Grimes, O. F., and Bell, H. G. Clinical and pathological studies of benign and malignant gastric ulcers. Surg. Gynec. Obstet. 90:359, 1950.
20. Flood, C. A., and Hennig, G. C. Recurrence in gastric ulcer under medical management. Gastroenterology 16:57, 1950.
21. Kirsner, J. B., Clayman, C. B., and Palmer, W. L. The problem of gastric ulcer. Arch. Intern. Med. 104:995, 1959.
22. Walters, W. Gastric ulcer, carcinomatous ulcer or ulcerating carcinoma? Ann. Surg. 115:521, 1942.
23. Dodd, G. D., and Nelson, R. S. The combined

radiologic and gastroscopic evaluation of gastric ulceration. Radiology 77:177, 1961.

24. Browne, D. C., Welch, G. E., Moss, J. B., and McHardy, G. Gastric ulcer—Better criteria for benignancy and malignancy. Amer. J. Gastroent. 23:211, 1955.

25. Shumacher, F. V., and Hampton, A. O. Radiographic differentiation of benign and malignant gastric ulcers. Ciba Clinical Symposia 8:161, 1956.

26. Kirsh, I. E. Radiological aspects of cancer after apparent healing. Gastroenterology 61:606, 1971.

27. Wolf, B. S., and Marshak, R. H. Profile features of benign gastric niches on roentgen examination. J. Mt. Sinai Hosp., New York 24:604, 1957.

28. Kirsh, I. E. Benign and malignant gastric ulcers. Roentgen differentiation. Radiology 64:357, 1955.

29. Sussman, M. L., and Lipsay, J. J. Roentgen differentiation of benign and malignant ulcers. Surg. Clin. N. Amer. 27:273, 1947.

30. Elliott, G. V., Wald, S. M., and Benz, R. I. A roentgenologic study of ulcerating lesions of the stomach. Amer. J. Roent. 77:612, 1957.

31. Robbins, S. L. Contributions of the pathologist to the present-day concepts of gastric ulcer. J.A.M.A. 171:2053, 1959.

32. Findley, J. W., Jr. Ulcers of the greater curvature of the stomach. Gastroenterology 40:183, 1961.

33. Wenger, J., Brandborg, L. L., and Spellman, F. A. Clinical aspects. Veterans Administration Cooperative Study on Gastric Ulcer. Gastroenterology 61:598, 1971.

34. Sun, D. C. H., and Stempien, S. J. Site and size as determinants of outcome.. Gastroenterology 61:576, 1971.

35. Allen, A. W. Gastric ulcer and cancer. Surgery 17:750, 1945.

36. Ivy, A. C., Grossman, M. I., and Bachrach, W. H. Peptic Ulcer. Philadelphia, Blakiston Division, McGraw-Hill Book Co., 1950.

37. Singleton, A. C. Benign prepyloric ulcer. Radiology 26:198, 1936.

38. Alvarez, W. C., and McCarty, W. C. Sizes of resected gastric ulcers and gastric carcinomas. J.A.M.A. 91:226, 1928.

39. Marshak, R. H., Yarnis, H., and Friedman, A. I. Giant benign gastric ulcers. Gastroenterology 24:339, 1953.

40. Baker, L., Gorvett, E. A., and Spellberg, M. A. Diagnostic accuracy of gastroscopy in neoplasms of the stomach. Cancer 5:1116, 1952.

41. Williams, D. G., Truelove, S. C., Gear, M. W. L., Massarella, G. R., and Fitzgerald, N. W. Gastroscopy with biopsy and cytological sampling under direct vision. Brit. Med. J. 1:534, 1968.

42. Gibbs, D. D., and Parry, D. J. Gastroscopy combined with intragastric photography. Postgrad. Med. J. 45:577, 1969.

43. Sircus, W. The aetiology of peptic ulcer. In Peptic Ulcer: A symposium for Surgeons, C. Wells and J. Kyle (eds.). Edinburgh, Livingstone, 1960, p. 11.

44. Grossman, M. I., Kirsner, J. B., and Gillespie, I.

45. Wormsley, K. G., and Grossman, M. I. Maximal Histalog test in control subjects and patients with peptic ulcer. Gut 6:427, 1965.

46. Davenport, H. W. Is the apparent hyposecretion of acid by patients with gastric ulcer a consequence of a broken barrier to diffusion of hydrogen ions into the gastric mucosa? Gut 6:513, 1965.

47. Shearman, D. J. C., Finlayson, N. D. C., and Wilson, R. Gastric function in patients with gastric carcinoma. Lancet 1:343, 1967.

48. Levin, E., Kirsner, J. B., and Palmer, W. L. Benign gastric ulcer with apparent achlorhydria. Gastroenterology 17:414, 1951.

49. Cocking, J. B., and MacCaig, J. N. Effect of low dosage carbenoxolone sodium on gastric ulcer healing and acid secretion. Gut 10:219, 1969.

50. Isenberg, J. I., Spector, H., Hootkin, L. A., and Pitcher, J. L. An apparent exception to Schwartz's dictum, "no acid—no ulcer." New Eng. J. Med. 285:620, 1971.

51. Schwarz, K. Ueber Penetrierende Magen und Jejunalgeschwüre. Beitr. Klin. Chir. 67:96, 1910.

52. Bralow, S. P. Current concepts of peptic ulceration. Amer. J. Dig. Dis. 14:655, 1969.

53. Beale, L. S. The Microscope in Medicine. 2nd Ed. London, J. & A. Churchill, Ltd., 1858.

54. Papanicolaou, G. N. New procedures for staining vaginal smears. Science 95:438, 1942.

55. Taebel, D. W., Prolla, J. C., and Kirsner, J. B. Exfoliative cytology in the diagnosis of stomach cancer. Ann. Intern. Med. 63:1018, 1965.

56. Brandborg, L. L., Taniguchi, L., and Rubin, C. E. Is exfoliative cytology practical for more general use in the diagnosis of gastric cancer? A simplified chymotrypsin technique. Cancer 14:1074, 1961.

57. Rubin, C. E., and Benditt, E. P. A simplified technique using chymotrypsin lavage for the cytological diagnosis of gastric cancer. Cancer 8:1137, 1955.

58. MacDonald, W. C., Brandborg, L. L., Taniguchi, L., and Rubin, C. E. Gastric exfoliative cytology: an accurate and practical diagnostic procedure. Lancet 2:83, 1963.

59. Rosenthal, M., and Traut, H. F. The mucolytic action of papain for cell concentration in the diagnosis of gastric cancer. Cancer 4:147, 1951.

60. MacDonald, W. C., Brandborg, L. L., Taniguchi, L., Beh, J. E., and Rubin, C. E. Exfoliative cytological screening for gastric cancer. Cancer 17:163, 1964.

61. Trudeau, W. L., and McGuigan, J. E. Relations between serum gastrin levels and rates of gastric hydrochloric acid secretion. New Eng. J. Med. 284:408, 1971.

62. Trudeau, W. L., and McGuigan, J. E. Serum and tissue measurements in patients with carcinoma of the stomach. Gastroenterology 62:822, 1972.

63. Hakkinen, I. P. T. An immunochemical

method for detecting carcinomatous secretion from human gastric juice. Scand. J. Gastroent. 1:28, 1966.

64. Hakkinen, I. P. T., Jarvi, O., and Gronroos, J. Sulphoglycoprotein antigens in human alimentary canal and gastric cancer. An immunohistological study. Internat. J. Cancer 3:572, 1968.

65. Stoebner, R. C., Cain, G. D., and Patterson, M. A rapid screening test for detection of gastric carcinoma. Clin. Res. 18:39, 1970.

66. Geffroy, Y., Metayer, P., Denis, P., et al. Alpha foeto-proteine et cancer secondaire du foie, Presse Méd. 78:1896, 1970.

67. Mehlman, D. J., Bulkley, B. H., and Wiernik, P. H. Serum alpha₁fetoglobulin with gastric and prostatic carcinomas. New Eng. J. Med. 285:1060, 1971.

68. O'Conor, G. T., Tatarinov, Y. S., Abelev, G. I., et al. A collaborative study for the evaluation of a serologic test for primary lever cancer. Cancer 25:1091, 1970.

69. Geffroy, Y., Boureille, J., Denis, P., Colin, R., and Metayer, P. Sem. Hôp. Paris 47:1281, 1971.

70. Palumbo, L. T., and Sharpe, W. S. Gastric ulcer: Is it benign or malignant? Arch. Surg. 85:705, 1962.

71. Banks, P. M., and Zetzel, L. The prognosis in peptic ulcer treated conservatively. New Eng. J. Med. 248:1008, 1953.

72. Hayes, M. A. The gastric ulcer problem. Gastroenterology 29:609, 1955.

73. Johnson, S., Lindholm, H., and Stenstrom, T. Should gastric ulcer as a rule be treated surgically? Acta Med. Scand., Suppl. 246:80, 1950.

74. Natvig, P., Römcke, O., and Swaar-Seljesaeter, O. Results of medical treatment of gastric and duodenal ulcer. Acta Med. Scand. 113:444, 1943.

75. Smith, F. H., and Jordan, S. M. Gastric ulcer: A study of 600 cases. Gastroenterology 11:575, 1948.

76. Smith, F. H., Boles, R. S., Jr., and Jordan, S. M. Problem of the gastric ulcer reviewed. J.A.M.A. 153:1505, 1953.

77. Gott, J. R., Jr., Shapiro, D., and Kelty, K. C. Gastric ulcer: A study of 138 patients. New Eng. J. Med. 250:499, 1954.

78. Doll, R., and Pygott, F. Factors influencing the rate of healing of gastric ulcers. Lancet 1:171, 1952.

79. Doll, R., Jones, F. A., and Pygott, F. Effect of smoking on the production and maintenance of gastric and duodenal ulcers. Lancet 1:657, 1958.

80. Doll, R., Hill, I. D., Hutton, C., and Underwood, D. J. II. Clinical trial of a triterpenoid liquorice compound in gastric and duodenal ulcer. Lancet 2:793, 1962.

81. Doll, R., Hill, I. D., and Hutton, C. F. Treatment of gastric ulcer with carbenoxolone sodium and estrogens. Gut 6:19, 1965.

82. Horwich, L., and Galloway, R. Treatment of gastric ulceration with carbenoxolone sodium: Clinical and radiological evaluation. Brit. Med. J. 2:1274, 1965.

83. Doll, R., Langman, M. J. S., and Shawdon, H. H. Treatment of gastric ulcer with carbenoxolone: Antagonist effect of spironolactone. Gut 9:42, 1968.

84. Truelove, S. C. Stilboestrol, phenobarbitone, and diet in chronic duodenal ulcer. Brit. Med. J. 2:559, 1960.

85. DuPlessis, D. J. Pathogenesis of gastric ulceration. Lancet 1:974, 1965.

86. Rhodes, J., Barnado, D. E., and Phillips, S. F. Increased reflux of bile into the stomach in patients with gastric ulcer. Gastroenterology 57:241, 1969.

87. Davenport, H. W. Destruction of the gastric mucosal barrier by detergents and urea. Gastroenterology 54:175, 1968.

88. Ivey, K. J., DenBesten, L., and Clifton, J. A. Effect of bile salts on ionic movement across the human gastric mucosa. Gastroenterology 59:683, 1970.

89. Black, R. B., Rhodes, J., Davies, G. T., Gravelle, H., and Sweetnam, P. A controlled clinical trial of cholestyramine in the treatment of gastric ulcer. Gastroenterology 61:821, 1971.

90. Lawrence, J. S. Dietetic and other methods in the treatment of peptic ulcer. Lancet 1:482, 1952.

91. Lenhartz, H. A. D. Eine neue Behandlung des Ulcus Ventriculi. Dtsch. Med. Wchr. 30:412, 1904.

92. Nicol, B. M. Control of gastric acidity in gastric ulcer. Lancet 2:881, 1939.

93. Bingle, J. P., and Lennard-Jones, J. E. Some factors in the assessment of gastric antisecretory drugs by a sampling technique. Gut 1:377, 1960.

94. Lennard-Jones, J. E., and Babouris, N. Effect of different foods on the acidity of the gastric contents in patients with duodenal ulcer. Gut 6:113, 1965.

95. Evans, P. R. C. Value of strict dieting, drugs and Robaden in peptic ulcerations. Brit. Med. J. 1:612, 1954.

96. Doll, R., Friedlander, H., and Pygott, F. Dietetic treatment of peptic ulcer. Lancet 2:5, 1956.

97. Langman, M. J. S. The medical treatment of gastric and duodenal ulcer. Postgrad. Med. J. 44:603, 1968.

98. Goodman, L. S., and Gilman, A. The Pharmacological Basis of Therapeutics. London, Macmillan, 1970.

99. Butcher, R. W. Role of cyclic AMP in hormone action. New Eng. J. Med. 279:1378, 1968.

100. Harris, J. B., Nigon, K., and Alonso, A. Adenosine-3',5'-monophosphate: Intracellular mediator for methyl xanthine stimulation of gastric secretion. Gastroenterology 57:377, 1969.

101. Geall, M. G., Phillips, S. F., and Summerskill, D. M. Profile of gastric potential difference in man. Effects of aspirin, alcohol, bile, and endogenous acid. Gastroenterology 58:437, 1970.

102. Smith, B. M., Skillman, J. J., Edwards, B. G., and Silen, W. Permeability of the human gastric mucosa: Alteration by acetylsalicylic

acid and ethanol. New Eng. J. Med. 285:716, 1971.

103. Ivey, K. J. Gastric mucosal barrier. Gastroenterology 61:247, 1971.

104. Davenport, H. W. Gastric mucosal injury by fatty and acetylsalicylic acids. Gastroenterology 46:245, 1964.

105. Davenport, H. W. Damage to the gastric mucosa. Effects of salicylates and stimulation. Gastroenterology 49:189, 1965.

106. Davenport, H. W. Potassium fluxes across the resting and stimulated gastric mucosa. Injury by salicylic and acetic acids. Gastroenterology 49:238, 1965.

107. Johnson, L. R. Pepsin stimulated by topical hydrochloric and acetic acids. Gastroenterology 62:33, 1972.

108. Davenport, H. W. Ethanol damage to canine oxyntic glandular mucosa. Proc. Soc. Exp. Biol. Med. 126:657, 1967.

109. Banks, C. N., and Baron, J. H. Drugs containing aspirin. Lancet 1:1165, 1964.

110. Roth, H. P. Healing of initial ulcers in relation to age and race. Gastroenterology 61:570, 1971.

111. Steigmann, F., and Shulman, B. The time of healing of gastric ulcers. Implications as to therapy. Gastroenterology 20:20, 1952.

112. Bachrach, W. H. Observations upon the complete healing of neoplastic ulcerations of the stomach. Surg. Gynec. Obstet. 114:69, 1962.

113. Hanscom, D. H., and Buchman, E. The follow-up period. Gastroenterology 61:585, 1971.

114. Krag, E. Long-term prognosis in medically treated peptic ulcer. Acta Med. Scand. 180:6,657, 1966.

115. Barsby, B. Prognosis of healed gastric ulcers. Lancet 2:59, 1951.

116. Littman, A., and Hanscom, D. H. The course of recurrent ulcer. Gastroenterology 61:592, 1971.

117. Pollard, H. M., Bachrach, W. H., and Block, M. The rate of healing of gastric ulcers. Gastroenterology 8:435, 1947.

118. Wilkie, D. P. D. Coincident duodenal and gastric ulcer. Brit. Med. J. 2:469, 1926.

119. Hurst, A. F., and Stewart, M. J. Gastric and Duodenal Ulcer. New York, Oxford University Press, 1929.

120. Johnson, H. D. The special significance of concomitant gastric and duodenal ulcers. Lancet 1:266, 1955.

121. McCray, B. S., Ferris, E. J., Herskovic, T., Winawer, S. J., Shapiro, J. H., and Zamcheck, N. Clinical differences between gastric ulcers with and without duodenal deformity. Ann. Surg. 168:821, 1968.

122. Rumball, J. M. Coexistent duodenal ulcer. Gastroenterology 61:622, 1971.

123. Vesely, K. T., Kubrickova, Z., and Dvorakova, M. Clinical data and characteristics differentiating types of peptic ulcer. Gut 9:57, 1968.

124. Krause, V. Long-term results of medical and surgical treatment of peptic ulcer. Acta Chir. Scand. Suppl. 310, 1963.

125. Dworken, H. J., Roth, H. P., and Duben, H. C. Observations on the course of benign gastric ulcer and factors affecting its prognosis. Gastroenterology 33:880, 1957.

126. Katz, I., and Bierenbaum, M. L. Multiple chronic gastric ulcers. Amer. J. Roent. 77:623, 1957.

127. Judd, E. S., and Proctor, O. Multiple gastric ulcers. Med. J. Rec. (Suppl.) 121:93, 1925.

128. Boyle, J. D. Multiple gastric ulcers. Gastroenterology 61:628, 1971.

129. Snoddy, W. T. Primary lymphosarcoma of the stomach. Gastroenterology 20:537, 1952.

130. Finsterer, H. Ulcer-cancer of stomach. Arch. Klin. Chir. 131:71, 1924.

131. Swynnerton, B. F., and Truelove, S. C. Simple gastric ulcer and carcinoma. Brit. Med. J. 2:1243, 1951.

132. Ekström, T. On the development of cancer in gastric ulcer and ulcer symptoms in gastric cancer. Acta Chir. Scand. 102:387, 1952.

133. Mallory, T. B. Carcinoma in situ of stomach and its bearing on histogenesis of malignant ulcers. Arch. Path. 30:348, 1940.

134. Ewing, J. Neoplastic Disease. 3rd Ed. Philadelphia, W. B. Saunders Co., 1928, p. 674.

135. Marshall, S. F. The relation of gastric ulcer to carcinoma of the stomach. Ann. Surg. 137:891, 1953.

Chapter 56

Peptic Ulcer in Childhood

Mervin Silverberg

Although peptic ulcer is common in adults, too often it is loosely diagnosed as the cause for unexplained, ubiquitous abdominal pain of children. Thus its incidence varies between institutions. Despite some unusually large series of cases,[1, 2] random reports of the incidence appear to be quite stable in 29 major pediatric centers, averaging about two new cases per year.[3] A Registry for peptic ulcer cases has been available for about a decade, but it suffers from the lack of criteria for objective and uniform reporting. Up to the end of 1971, the Registry had received reports on 772 cases throughout the United States.[4]

SYMPTOMATOLOGY AND CLINICAL FEATURES

Four distinct types of ulcer can be described.

Acute Infantile. This form is usually found in newborns and infants under two years of age and presents with bleeding, perforation, or obstruction. The full-term infant may be particularly vulnerable, with a relatively high gastric acidity and large parietal cell mass during the early newborn period.[5] In many instances the manifestations can be managed conservatively without surgical intervention. In the age group between two weeks and two years peptic ulcer disease is relatively uncommon.

Acute and Secondary. These ulcers are related to serious systemic disorders such as sepsis, central nervous system disease,[6] and the administration of corticosteroids. They appear randomly in all age groups, but are more likely to occur in those patients either with previously proved ulcer disease or with diseases which are more likely to be complicated by ulcer. Pediatric disorders which are associated with an incidence of ulcer disease greater than expected are cirrhosis, chronic pulmonary disease, hypoglycemia, congenital pyloric stenosis,[7] and short bowel syndrome.[8] They occur with equal frequency in the stomach and duodenum and show no sex predilection. It should be mentioned that peptic ulcer may occur at a third site; namely, in Meckel's diverticulum.[9] It is often associated with lower bowel bleeding, intestinal obstruction, or recurrent abdominal pain, particularly in a male child.

Adult or Chronic. This type is found predominantly in children from school age upward, and increasingly resembles the adult disease as the child grows older. Chronic peptic ulcer has been noted in infants of one and one-half years;[10] however, most occur in children between five and 16 years of age. In comparison with ulcer manifestations in adults, pain, particularly in the younger child, tends to be diffuse and periumbilical, is unrelated to meals, and is frequently associated with vomiting. The typical pain-food-relief pattern tends to emerge in the adolescent patient, and the gnawing hunger pains are usually localized to the epigastrium. Night pain is often noted and emphasized;[11] however, its significance must be considered in the light of its moderate frequency in functional abdominal pain. Although infrequently studied, a significantly increased incidence of blood group O patients has been noted with duodenal ulcer, as compared with a control group.[12] After initial recovery, more than 50 per cent of ulcer patients have recurrent distress when followed for more than one year, despite energetic treatment.[11, 12] It is believed furthermore that there is a 50 per cent chance that a duodenal ulcer noted in childhood will cause symptoms when the patient is an adolescent or adult.[13] In general, males outnumber females in a ratio of 3:2, and one gastric ulcer is noted for every eight duodenal lesions.

Ulcers Associated with Adenomata of Endocrine Glands. Such ulcers have been reported in older children, particularly with non-beta cell adenoma of the pancreas (Zollinger-Ellison syndrome).[14] In this condition, unlike ordinary peptic ulcer, high blood gastrin levels are found; also, these lesions are usually more resistant to traditional therapy, tend to recur, and more often are multiple and involve the postbulbar area. The excessive gastrin produced by the tumors induces maximal gastric hypersecretion, resulting in diarrhea and malabsorption.[15] Such patients occasionally also have adenomas of the parathyroid, adrenal, and pituitary glands, some of which (usually parathyroid) may be active. These tumors occur singly or in combination. For more detailed discussion of the Zollinger-Ellison syndrome, see pages 743 to 754.

DIAGNOSIS

Demonstration of an ulcer crater or persistent deformity of the duodenal bulb endoscopically or radiographically affords the most incontrovertible basis for diagnosis. Duodenal irritability and pylorospasm are usually unreliable signs of the diagnosis in children who are particularly anxious and frightened during the studies. Gastric acid studies, including histamine or Histalog stimulation, have not been of diagnostic value in children. An unusually broad range of results is reported in normal children, not significantly different from the results of many ulcer patients who are studied.[16] Unlike that of older children, the acid secretion during the first months of age appears to be a function of age rather than weight. Achlorhydria may be noted immediately after birth, but high acid concentrations are often found by the end of the first day of life. The high acid values persist from two to 15 days, although total gastric juice volumes are always well below adult values.[17, 18] Pepsin secretion generally follows a similar pattern to acid output. After three months of age, both acid and pepsin excretion in normal infants remain below adult values.[17] Unfortunately, adequate control studies and gastric analysis performed during comparable periods of ulcer activity are not available.

A family history of peptic ulcer is a valuable aid because it is reported to occur in one-quarter of pediatric patients with proved ulcers. Melena is relatively uncommon, although insidious, virtually painless bleeding may occur with occult blood in the stools. In long-standing undiagnosed cases, iron deficiency anemia develops; it is the presenting problem in 20 per cent of ulcer patients. Significant emotional disorders are said to occur in 25 per cent of the patients, with school phobias most frequently noted.

TREATMENT

Therapeutic measures vary according to the type of ulcer. Acute infantile and secondary ulcers require immediate attention for bleeding or perforation. These patients are often critically ill, and the ulcer usually presents at the time the primary disease is poorly controlled. Antacids and anticholinergic agents are often used prophylactically in patients with severe burns (see p. 660). Children receiving corticosteroids rarely develop ulcerative disease except when the underlying disorder predisposes them. In patients given long courses of steroids, the traditional prophylactic regimen is instituted whenever they present with ulcer complaints.

In the acute stage of the adult type of chronic ulcer, treatment is directed to frequent neutralization of gastric acidity by nonabsorbable antacid or food. Initially, an hourly regimen of 1 to 2 ounces of antacid or antacid alternating with 1 to 3 ounces of milk-cream mixture is administered. Longer intervals of time are used with improvement, and a liberal regular diet with frequent feedings is introduced as soon as the child is asymptomatic. Rigid dietary and activity restrictions in children are usually both unnecessary and frustrating. Reliance on antacids is relatively unnecessary, because snacks appear empirically to be just as effective and easily form part of a child's routine. Postcibal anticholinergic agents such as propantheline (1.5 mg per kilogram per 24 hours) or methantheline bromide (6.0 mg per kilogram per 24 hours), are prescribed three times a day and before bedtime. The dosage may be raised to a maximal level which can be used without producing intolerable side effects. In the very anxious patient a tranquilizer such as hydroxyzine in the prepuberal child and diazepam in the adolescent may be a useful adjunct. As a rule, this kind of antiulcer regimen, with minor modifications, is maintained for about one year, or longer if the child is still symptomatic.

SPECIAL PROBLEMS

Mild or chronic blood loss is treated with oral or parenteral iron to keep the hematocrit above 30 per cent. Transfusion, usually with packed erythrocytes, is necessary only with more severe blood losses. If large infusions are required, 5 to 10 ml of 10 per cent calcium gluconate should be given intravenously at regular intervals to obviate depletion of calcium.

Intractable persistence of pain is usually due to inadequate therapy or to penetration of the ulcer through the wall of the viscus. Hospitalization and appropriate studies should delineate both the problem and the associated underlying pathology which may interfere with recovery.

Obstruction may occur in those with chronic ulcer disease, associated with edema or fibrous deformity. Pylorospasm or transitory edema may be differentiated by decompressing the stomach with nasogastric aspiration for two to three days, and then introducing 100 to 500 cc of saline and aspirating for residual contents one hour later.

Intractable pain or bleeding, fibrous obstruction, and perforation frequently require surgical intervention. Elective surgery in chronic cases varies from one center to another, although vagotomy with pyloroplasty and antrectomy seem to be most popular and are associated with the least morbidity.[19] Sufficient data regarding the relationship of procedure and recurrence are not yet available. In patients with the Zollinger-Ellison syndrome total gastrectomy with removal of accessible adenomas or their metastases is the procedure of choice.[20] Contrary to previous opinion, children of any age are able to thrive after successful total gastric resection.[14]

REFERENCES

1. Girdany, B. R. Peptic ulcer in children. Pediatrics 12:56, 1953.
2. Tudor, R. B. Peptic ulceration in childhood. Pediat. Clin. N. Amer. 14:109, 1967.
3. Singleton, E. B., and Faykus, M. H. Incidence of peptic ulcer as determined by radiologic examinations in the pediatric age group. J. Pediat. 65:858, 1964.
4. Tudor, R. B. Gastric and duodenal ulcers in children. Gastroenterology 62:823, 1972.
5. Polacek, M. A., and Ellison, E. H. Gastric acid secretion and parietal cell mass in the stomach of a newborn infant. Amer. J. Surg. 111:777, 1966.
6. Rosenlund, M. L., and Koop, C. E. Duodenal ulcer in childhood. Pediatrics 45:283, 1970.
7. Kelsey, D., Stayman, J. W., McLaughlin, E. D., and Mebane, W. Massive bleeding in a newborn infant from a gastric ulcer associated with hypertrophic pyloric stenosis. Surgery 64:979, 1968.
8. Avery, G. B., Randolph, J. G., and Weaver, T. Gastric response to specific disease in infants. Pediatrics 38:874, 1966.
9. Rutherford, R. B., and Akers, D. R. Meckel's diverticulum: A review of 148 pediatric patients with special reference to the pattern of bleeding and to mesodiverticular vascular bands. Surgery 59:618, 1966.
10. Ravitch, M. M., and Duremdes, G. D. Operative treatment of chronic duodenal ulcer in childhood. Ann. Surg. 171:641, 1970.
11. Milliken, J. C. Duodenal ulceration in children. Gut 6:25, 1965.
12. Habbick, B. F., Melrose, A. G., and Grant, J. C. Duodenal ulcer in childhood: Study of predisposing factors. Arch. Dis. Child. 43:23, 1968.
13. Michener, W. M., Kennedy, R. L. J., and DuShane, J. W. Duodenal ulcer in childhood. Amer. J. Dis. Child. 100:814, 1960.

14. Rosenlund, M. L. The Zollinger-Ellison syndrome in children: A review. Amer. J. Med. Sci. *254*:884, 1967.
15. Rosenlund, M. L., Crean, G. P., Johnson, D. G., Holtzapple, P. G., and Brooks, F. P. The Zollinger-Ellison syndrome in a 10-year-old boy. J. Pediat. *75*:443, 1969.
16. Ghai, P. M. S., Walia, B. N. S., and Gadekar, N. G. An assessment of gastric acid secretory response with "maximal" augmented histamine stimulation in children with peptic ulcer. Arch. Dis. Child. *40*:77, 1965.
17. Agunod, M., Yamaguchi, N., Lopez, R., Huhby, A. L., and Glass, G. B. J. Correlative study of hydrochloric acid, pepsin, and intrinsic factor secretion in newborns and infants. Amer. J. Dig. Dis. *14*:400, 1969.
18. Avery, G. B., Randolph, J. G., and Weaver, T. Gastric acidity in the first day of life. Pediatrics *37*:1005, 1966.
19. Johnston, P. W., and Snyder, W. H., Jr. Vagotomy and pyloroplasty in infancy and childhood. J. Pediat. Surg. *3*:238, 1968.
20. Wilson, S. D., and Ellison, E. H. Total gastric resection in children with the Zollinger-Ellison syndrome. Arch. Surg. *91*:165, 1965.

Chapter 57

Reduction of Acidity by Diet, Antacids, and Anticholinergic Agents

John S. Fordtran

THE RATIONALE

It is reasonable to assume that gastro-duodenal and esophageal mucosa becomes ulcerated whenever acid-pepsin concentrations are too high for too long a period for the natural resistance of a local area of mucosa (see p. 628), and that reduction in acidity will aid in healing even though acid is not completely eliminated or even decreased to the degree necessary to reduce "peptic activity."* These assertions are supported by the following facts:

First, peptic ulcer does not develop in the absence of gastric acid. Second, there is a threshold level of peak stimulated acid output (about 14 mEq per hour) below which patients do not develop or maintain an active duodenal ulcer. Third, in experimentally induced peptic esophagitis, reduction of acid concentration from about

---

*The popular idea that gastric acidity must be reduced to pH 3 or 4 (the pH at which peptic activity is zero with artificial substrates) in order to be effective in ulcer therapy was never based on any kind of experimental evidence. In fact, the degree to which acidity must be reduced to hasten healing and prevent recurrences depends upon the sensitivity of the local area of mucosa in question and probably differs in different people.

60 to about 10 mEq per liter eliminates esophagitis, even though pepsin concentrations and "peptic activity" with hemoglobin as the substrate were equal at both concentrations of acid.[1] Finally, antacid therapy reduces the frequency of Mann-Williamson ulcers in dogs even though gastric acid is not completely neutralized.[2]

On the basis of these considerations, it is reasonable and logical to attempt to reduce gastric acidity in the various peptic diseases. The medical methods currently used to achieve this are diet and antacid and anticholinergic drugs. Their emphasis in this chapter is not intended to deny the importance of newer forms of possible ulcer therapy — prostaglandins to reduce gastric secretion, secretin to stimulate pancreatic bicarbonate secretion and inhibit gastric acid secretion, antipepsin agents, gastrin inhibitors, and so forth. All these are potentially important, but at present none has been adequately evaluated on a clinical level to warrant a detailed discussion. Since each of these newer agents is designed to reduce acid-pepsin, it is evident that no conceptual breakthrough is on the visible horizon. The value of such new therapies will presumably depend strictly upon their ability to reduce acid-pepsin in relation to the severity of undesirable side effects. Carbenoxolone treatment for gastric ulcer is discussed on page 700.

SECRETORY RESPONSE TO A MEAL

The acid secretory pattern before and after a steak and toast meal in six normal subjects and in seven patients with duodenal ulcer is shown in Figure 57–1. The peak secretory response to the meal was 16 per cent higher than the peak histamine response in the ulcer patients and 14 per cent lower than the peak histamine response in the normal subjects. Additional studies in these same patients revealed that the meal buffer was emptied more rapidly in the duodenal ulcer patients than in the normal subjects.[3] The combined effects of increased secretion of acid (owing to higher parietal cell mass and to hyperresponsiveness to the meal) and rapid buffer emptying resulted in higher acid concentration of the gastric contents in the duodenal ulcer patients than in the normal subjects. A major aim of diet, antacid, and anticholinergic therapy is effective and safe reduction of acid secretion and the acidity of gastric contents stimulated by the ingestion of food.

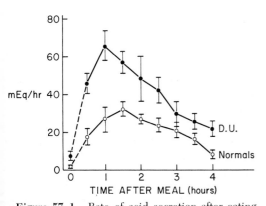

Figure 57–1. Rate of acid secretion after eating a meal of steak, toast, butter, and water in six normal subjects and in seven patients with duodenal ulcer. Mean ± SE. The rate of basal secretion, measured by standard methods, is shown for comparison at zero time. (From Fordtran, J. S., and Walsh, J. H.: J. Clin. Invest., 1973, Vol. 52, in press.)

DIET THERAPY

It has been conclusively proved, in my opinion, that hourly milk therapy and bland diets do not reduce gastric acidity. Evidence in support of this statement is reproduced in Figure 57–2.[4-6] In fact, hourly milk and cream ingestion stabilizes acid concentration at a *high* level.[4, 5] Furthermore, four controlled studies have shown no benefit of a bland diet on the clinical course of peptic ulcer.[7-10]

Other aspects of ulcer diets have been considered, but have been less extensively tested in the laboratory. Fruit juices contain weak organic acids which dissociate appreciably at and below pH 4. The pH of fruit juices ranges from 2.2 for lemon juice to 4.2 for tomato juice.[11] (The pH of a large number of other liquids was also recently reported.)[12] Fruit juices contain a significant amount of buffer, and therefore tend to maintain a pH near their own level in spite of the addition of alkali or acid. Thus in vitro addition of fruit juice to gastric juice, or the ingestion of fruit juices on an empty stomach, will raise the pH of gastric juice if it is below that of the fruit juice and lower it if it is above.[13] The effect of citrus juices on gastric acidity also depends upon the effect of the juice on acid secretion. In dogs, 100 calories of orange juice caused 25 per cent as much acid secretion as 100 calories of beef.[14] This seems high, but in fact was one of the lowest rates of acid secretion in response to any of a large number of foods. Similar data in humans are not available, and measurements of gastric acidity after a meal, with and without citrus juice, have rarely been reported. Haggard and Greenberg fed eight normal subjects a mixed protein meal and found that pineapple, grape, orange, and grapefruit juices increased average gastric acidity at one hour compared with water as a control. Tomato juice had the opposite effect. By 90 minutes after the meal, all the juices except grapefruit were associated with *less* acidity than with water.[11] Dimmler et al. fed two normal subjects a normal type breakfast with and without orange juice and noted no difference in postprandial pH.[13] Claytor and colleagues compared the effects of 250 cc of orange juice, 250 cc of milk and cream, and an

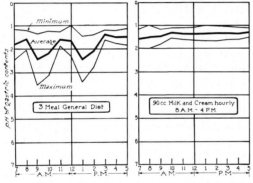

The effect of a general diet (17 experiments) and of milk and cream (20 experiments) on the pH of the gastric contents.

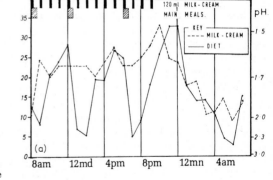

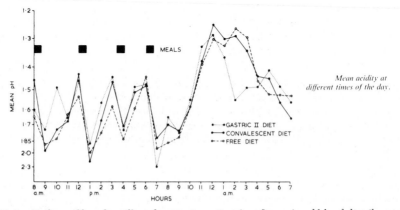

Mean acidity at different times of the day.

Figure 57–2. Failure of hourly milk and cream ingestion (top figures) and bland diet (lower figure) to reduce gastric acidity when compared with three regular meals. (From Kirsner, J. B., and Palmer, W. L.: Amer. J. Dig. Dis. 7:85, 1940; Bingle, J. P., and Lennard-Jones, J. E.: Gut *1*:337, 1960; and Lennard-Jones, J. E., and Barbouris, N.: Gut 6:113, 1965.)

Ewald meal (toast and tea) on gastric acidity. They found much higher "free acidity" from 45 to 75 minutes after the orange juice meal than after the other foods. Since there are only slight traces of free acid in orange juice, they concluded that these results were due to increased secretion of acid induced by orange juice, rather than to its own acidity.[15]

Some physicians have advocated the elimination of acid-containing beverages from the diet of peptic ulcer patients,[12] whereas others allow free use of citrus juices because of the fact that they are less acid than even normal gastric juice.[13] It is my opinion that the data at hand are insufficient to allow a judgment either way. If citrus juices cause increased acidity, it is probably due to stimulation of acid secretion or reduction of the effective buffer of a mixed meal, rather than because they have a relatively low *p*H to begin with.

Urgently needed is a detailed study of many foods in human subjects, which should include an analysis of their effect on gastric secretion and postprandial gastric acidity in comparison with other foods in equicaloric amounts. It is likely that there are foods which cause increased secretion and increased acidity out of proportion to their caloric value. At present, however, no specific food (with the possible exception of caffeine, which is considered a drug) has been shown to have this effect.

The discomfort noted by some patients and some normal subjects after the ingestion of orange and other citrus juices is probably due at times to factors other than the acidity of these fluids or their effect on acid secretion. They are very hypertonic, and some studies have suggested that the discomfort they produce is due to a specific volatile organic molecule in the juice.[16]

Spices are also often restricted in the diet prescribed to ulcer patients. There is no evidence that a wide variety of spices in small or large amounts stimulate acid secretion when placed in the stomach or when held in the mouth.[17] The administration of huge amounts of spices to dogs in conjunction with histamine in beeswax injection increased the incidence of histamine-provoked gastric and duodenal ulceration.[17] These results are meaningless in terms of normal pathophysiology, because the dose of spice was so large and the stomach was irrigated with spice without food or other buffering agent. In a clinical study, Schneider and coworkers showed that large amounts of most spices can be ingested without altering the rate of ulcer healing.[18] No untoward symptoms were noted if these spices were ingested with food. Black pepper and cloves were considered as gastric irritants, because they tended to produce epigastric distress in patients with inactive duodenal ulcer. Pepper, mustard seed, and thyme irrigated into the stomach in the absence of food produced hyperemia, edema, and/or erythema. No evidence was presented that the use of spices in normal amounts with food was ulcerogenic or that spices delayed the healing of peptic ulcers.

Ulcer patients are often advised to eat a "soft" rather than a "rough" diet. The rationale of such therapy is based upon "clinical experience," the only experimental evidence being a study of excisional gastric ulcer in rabbits. In 1930 Fauley and Ivy reported that excision ulcers in the rabbit heal irrespective of diet, but that if a silk suture is placed in the ulcer base, it heals on a soft diet but becomes chronic on a rough diet. The rough diet consisted of hay, oats, and raw carrots.[19] As far as I am concerned, this is insufficient evidence to warrant placing peptic ulcer patients on a "soft diet."

In summary, the available experimental evidence does not suggest that deletion of any specific foods from the diet (caffeine and alcohol excluded) will hasten ulcer healing, prevent ulcer recurrence, or decrease ulcer symptoms in patients with uncomplicated peptic ulcer. Nor is there convincing evidence that any specific diet will be associated with less gastric acidity than a normal diet of a patient's own choosing. It is logical therefore to allow patients with peptic ulcer to eat a normal diet of their own choosing. To prescribe a bland diet, frequent feedings, or frequent milk ingestion is illogical, based on current evidence. To continue such therapy because "if you told a patient that he need follow no dietary restriction, he might well conclude that you were ill informed, if not a quack" is to be condemned. This is a poor reason to perpetuate illogical and unpleasant therapy that serves to divert attention from methods of treatment that are more likely to be of benefit.

Although it is my opinion that patients with peptic ulcer should be allowed to eat a completely normal diet, it seems best to avoid any food after the dinner meal so as to reduce nocturnal acid secretion. It is evident from Figure 57–1 that food induces a dramatic and prolonged stimulation of acid secretion, especially in patients with duodenal ulcer. To eat a meal or snack at 10:00 P.M. assures high rates of acid secretion until at least 2:00 A.M. Although it has not been proved, bedtime feedings may enhance the frequency of waking at night with pain, and would be expected to reduce the effectiveness of anticholinergic agents in reducing nocturnal acidity. By the same token, frequent feedings, as opposed to three meals a day, are illogical. Patients with duodenal ulcer have an exaggerated secretory response to eating,[3] repeated stimulation may cause parietal cell hyperplasia (this has not been proved), and frequent meals (of milk at least) do not reduce gastric acidity.

ANTACID THERAPY

Theoretically antacids are useful in treating peptic ulcer because they reduce both acidity and peptic activity. Peptic activity is reduced by virtue of the fact that pepsin is maximally active between pH 1.5 and 2.0, and is inactive above pH 2.3 to 4.0, depending on the substrate (see pp. 189 to 193 and reference 1 of this chapter). Some antacids are said to bind pepsin directly and to coat an ulcer crater, but neither of these actions is well substantiated.

CHEMICAL BASIS OF ANTACID ACTION

Most antacids in current use are combinations of aluminum, magnesium and calcium salts. Although single salts are not often used (with the exception of calcium carbonate), the major ones are described individually in order to provide a basis for understanding antacid action.

SODIUM BICARBONATE

$$NaHCO_3 + HCl \rightarrow NaCl + H_2O + CO_2$$

Sodium bicarbonate is highly soluble and reacts almost instantaneously and irreversibly with hydrochloric acid (see Fig. 57–3). For every equivalent of acid neutralized, the body receives an equivalent of bicarbonate, because acid secretion into the stomach is balanced exactly by bicarbonate addition to the extracellular fluid (ECF). Sodium bicarbonate is usually ingested in excess of the amount of acid present in the stomach; being highly soluble, the excess is emptied rapidly into the small bowel, where it is absorbed. The net effect of giving sodium bicarbonate, whether it reacts with gastric acid or is delivered to the small intestine, is the delivery to the extracellular fluid of an amount of sodium bicarbonate equal to that ingested. The kidneys excrete the excess bicarbonate and sodium, provided there is no renal insufficiency.

Sodium bicarbonate is not recommended for long-term use because of its tendency to produce alkalosis and because its high degree of solubility causes it to be emptied relatively rapidly from the stomach; as the result of rapid emptying, its duration of antacid effect is short, at least when it is ingested by fasting patients. This drug is commonly used by the lay public for relief of "acid indigestion" or "upset stomach," either in the form of baking soda or in effervescent tablets combined with aspirin.

CALCIUM CARBONATE

$$CaCO_3 + 2HCl \rightarrow CaCl_2 + H_2O + CO_2$$

This reaction is not so rapid as the reaction of HCl and $NaHCO_3$ (Fig. 57–3). The calcium chloride formed in this reaction is highly soluble. However, in the small bowel about 90 per cent of the calcium chloride is reconverted to insoluble calcium salts (mainly calcium carbonate and to a lesser extent calcium phosphate) and to insoluble calcium soaps. Because of this, relatively little of the calcium re-

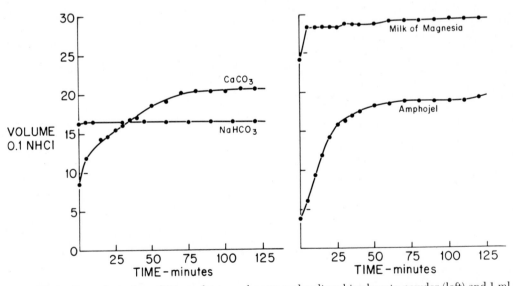

Figure 57–3. Rate of reaction of 0.1 g calcium carbonate and sodium bicarbonate powder (left) and 1 ml of magnesium hydroxide (milk of magnesia) and aluminum hydroxide (Amphojel) with 0.1 N HCl. These in vitro titrations were carried out by adding HCl at intervals to the antacid (dissolved in or suspended in water) in amounts required to keep the pH at 3.0 The stirring rate was 60 rpm; the temperature, 37°C.

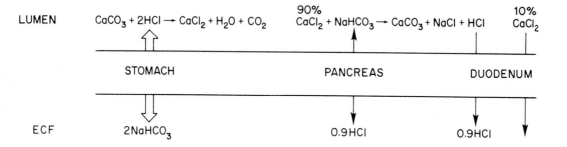

$$\text{For every 2 mEq of HCl neutralized, 0.2 mEq of } HCO_3^- \text{ added to ECF}$$

Figure 57–4. Mechanism by which neutralization of gastric acid with calcium carbonate results in a modest net addition of sodium bicarbonate to the extracellular fluid (ECF).

mains in a soluble form, and thus calcium absorption is limited.[20-22]

The neutralization of gastric HCl, the formation of soluble calcium chloride, and its reconversion to calcium carbonate are illustrated in Figure 57–4. Note that about 90 per cent of the calcium chloride reacts with sodium bicarbonate to reform calcium carbonate (based on the data of Clarkson and coworkers[22]). This reaction releases HCl, which can be absorbed as such or react with additional sodium bicarbonate of pancreatic or intestinal origin. To the extent that calcium chloride is reconverted to calcium carbonate (or to calcium phosphate), acid-base balance is not disturbed. The reason for this is shown in Figure 57–4. However, to the extent that calcium chloride does not react with sodium bicarbonate in the intestinal lumen (estimated at 10 per cent), the extracellular fluid receives a bicarbonate load. This will tend to raise the serum bicarbonate concentration and reduce urinary hydrogen excretion. If kidney function is normal, the excess sodium and bicarbonate load is readily handled, and a significant alkalosis does not develop. For this reason, calcium carbonate is often referred to (somewhat inaccurately) as a nonsystemic antacid.

The effects of calcium absorption on serum and urinary calcium and phosphorus concentration and on renal function are discussed on page 729.

The advantages of calcium carbonate are that it is a potent antacid and that it is inexpensive. Because it is insoluble, it is emptied from the stomach at a slower rate

than sodium bicarbonate, which prolongs its antacid action. The disadvantages of calcium carbonate are the chalky taste, the tendency to constipation (caused by the formation of insoluble calcium salts), the production of hypercalcemia and the milk alkali syndrome, and acid rebound.

ALUMINUM HYDROXIDE

$$Al(OH)_3 + 3HCl \rightarrow AlCl_3 + 3H_2O$$

Both aluminum hydroxide and aluminum oxide react with HCl in the stomach to form aluminum chloride. Depending upon the manufacturer's process, there are great differences in the solubility of different preparations in acid solution, and, consequently, wide variations in the rate of acid neutralization.[20, 21, 23] The rate of reaction of one preparation with acid at pH 3.0 is shown in Figure 57–3.

In the small intestine aluminum chloride reacts to form insoluble basic aluminum salts; thus there are very little aluminum chloride absorption and little effect on acid-base balance. The reason why acid-base balance is not significantly affected is the same as that described for calcium carbonate.

The advantages of aluminum hydroxide are its relative palatability and the lack of any clinical evidence of toxicity. It has been suggested that aluminum salts bind and inactivate pepsin, but there is no evidence that this occurs under conditions in which these drugs are actually used in patients. The disadvantages of this antacid are that it tends to constipate (because of insoluble salts), it is expensive, and it has a relatively low neutralizing capacity.

Aluminum phosphate is one of the insoluble aluminum salts precipitated in the small bowel, and phosphate absorption is reduced by aluminum hydroxide therapy. This action provides a basis for lowering serum phosphate levels in patients with chronic renal disease, but it is a potential hazard in causing phosphorus depletion (see complications of antacid therapy). Aluminum compounds also reduce the absorption of tetracycline and possibly of atropine and iron.[20, 21]

MAGNESIUM HYDROXIDE (MILK OF MAGNESIA)

$$Mg(OH)_2 + 2HCl \rightarrow MgCl_2 + 2H_2O$$

Magnesium hydroxide is highly insoluble in water but readily soluble in dilute acid. It reacts promptly with gastric acid (Fig. 57–3), and is a relatively potent antacid. Magnesium hydroxide remaining in the stomach (after acid is neutralized) is insoluble, and is thus emptied at a slower rate than are soluble antacids such as sodium bicarbonate. This prolongs its antacid action, to some degree at least.

After ingestion of magnesium hydroxide, a combination of magnesium chloride (equal to the amount that reacted with HCl in the stomach) and magnesium hydroxide is delivered to the small bowel. The magnesium hydroxide is presumably changed in the small bowel to soluble but poorly absorbable magnesium salts, and their osmotic effect produces a tendency to diarrhea. Because of reactions in the small bowel similar to those described with calcium carbonate therapy, there is little effect on acid-base balance. About 15 per cent of the ingested magnesium is absorbed, and this is readily excreted in the urine if kidney function is normal. In patients with renal disease, magnesium retention may result from the chronic use of magnesium salts.

CLINICAL ANTACID PHARMACOLOGY

The effect of antacids on postcibal gastric acidity, correlated with the rate of meal-stimulated acid secretion, is shown in Figure 57–5. Acid secretion, measured by in vivo titration to pH 5.0,[3] is recorded in the top panel of the figure for seven patients with duodenal ulcer. On two other test days these same patients were fed the meal, and either water as a control or 156 mEq of antacid was ingested one hour after eating. When water was taken after the meal, gastric acidity remained at relatively low levels for the first hour and a half, in spite of the fact that acid was secreted at near maximal rates during this period.[3, 24] The change from a slow to a rapid rate of increase in gastric acidity occurred at the time when gastric acidity was about 8 mEq per liter and the pH about 2.2. The meal used in these studies buffered hydrochloric acid in vitro down to but not below a pH of 2.2. These results suggest therefore that in spite of high rates of acid secretion, gastric acidity rises slowly until the meal's buffer (the part that is not emptied from the stomach) is fully titrated to pH 2.2.[24] This required about one and one-half hours in the seven subjects reported in Figure 57–5. After this time acid secretion continues at a rapid rate; since no unacidified protein (buffer) remains in the stomach, acidity rises rapidly, to a maximum of about 65 mEq per liter in these seven patients.

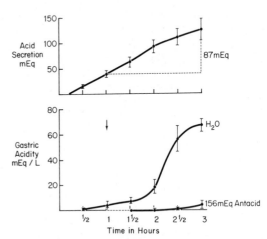

Figure 57–5. Correlation of acid secretion rate in response to a steak, toast, butter, and water meal (upper panel) with gastric acidity in the presence and absence (H_2O given as control) of 156 mEq of antacid ingested one hour after eating (lower panel). These studies were conducted on the same seven patients on three different test days. (From Fordtran, J. S., et al.: New Eng. J. Med., 1973, in press.)

The striking effect on gastric acidity of ingesting 156 mEq of antacid is also shown in Figure 57–5. Acidity was near zero for two hours after the antacid was ingested, rising to only about 3 mEq per liter by the end of the experiment. The pH of the gastric contents 30 minutes after the antacid was about 5.8, compared to 2.2 at this time interval when no antacid was ingested. It should be noted that it required 156 mEq of antacid to effectively buffer the 87 mEq of acid secreted from one to three hours after the meal. This inefficiency is caused by gastric emptying of antacid before it reacts with acid.

Antacids ingested in the fasting state have a much shorter duration of action (20 to 40 minutes) than antacids ingested after a meal.[25] This is presumably due to the fact that gastric emptying of excess antacid is more rapid in the fasting state than after a meal.

RELATIVE POTENCY OF DIFFERENT ANTACIDS

Although it is well recognized that components of various commercial preparations have markedly different buffering capacities in vitro, it is not possible to accurately predict the relative antacid potency of commercial antacids from product labels. This is because the amounts of different components are often not specified, and because of varying degrees of solubility ("reactivity") of aluminum and magnesium salts, depending on the specific method employed in their manufacture. Furthermore, in vitro tests can be carried out in many different ways, and the relative effectiveness of antacids may change dramatically from one in vitro assay to another.

Recently it has been shown that the amount of 0.1 N HCl that can be added over a two-hour period to 1 ml of liquid antacids without reducing the pH below 3.0, with a stirring rate of 60 rpm, correlates very well with relative antacid potency in vivo in patients with gastric and duodenal ulcer.[24] (It is stressed that the choice of pH 3.0 as an endpoint in the in vitro test does not imply that this is the pH level that should be aimed for in treating patients; this is simply the in vitro endpoint that correlated best with in vivo results.) Some liquid antacids, in decreasing order of in vitro antacid potency, are listed in Table 57–1. Note that the neutralizing capacity of 15 ml of liquid antacid might vary from 6 to 105 mEq. These results and their companion in vivo studies reported in reference 24 contradict the popular view among physicians that there is little difference in the effectiveness of the various liquid antacids.

DOSE-RESPONSE RELATIONSHIPS

The dose of antacid drugs has been little studied, partly because experiments carried out in fasting patients have revealed such short duration of action that dose seemed much less important than frequency of ingestion. With the realization that antacids have substantially longer action when given after meals, a consideration of dose-response relationships becomes of clinical importance. The average hydrogen ion concentration of the gastric contents two hours after various doses of liquid aluminum-magnesium hydroxide (Maalox) is shown in Figure 57–6. The antacid was ingested one hour after a standard steak meal.[24] In patients whose peak histamine response was greater than 25 mEq per hour (designated "hypersecretors"), the hydrogen ion concentration with no antacid was about 50 mEq per liter, and increasing doses of antacid resulted in a progressive fall in gastric acidity. A dose of 78 mEq of antacid (30 ml) was required to reduce acidity by half. In contrast, in patients whose peak histamine response was less than 17 mEq per hour (designated "hyposecretors") gastric acidity with no antacid was only 14 mEq per liter, and a dose of only about 20 mEq (9 ml) of antacid would reduce acidity by half.[24]

The results just presented are average results in high and low secretors. Results in different patients vary widely, and cannot be accurately predicted from the peak histamine response or from other clinical studies.[24] A five-fold reduction in gastric acidity for two hours in high secretor groups is usually achieved only by a dose of about 156 mEq of antacid. Of course, if

TABLE 57–1. TITRATION TO pH 3.0 OF 1 ML OF ANTACID WITH 0.1 N HCl, 60 RPM, 37°C

ANTACID	CONTENTS	0 TIME		10 MIN		30 MIN		60 MIN		120 MIN°
		ml	%†	ml	%†	ml	%†	ml	%†	ml
Ducon	Al and Mg hydroxides, Ca carbonate	20.2	29	29.9	43	45.7	65	58.3	83	70.4
Mylanta II	Mg and Al hydroxides, simethicone	4.3	10	8.2	20	17.3	42	27.9	67	41.4
Titralac	Glycine, Ca carbonate	32.9	85	36.0	93	37.4	97	37.9	98	38.7
Camalox	Al and Mg hydroxides, Ca carbonate	12.7	49	20.6	80	32.5	91	35.6	99	35.9
Aludrox	Al hydroxide gel, Mg hydroxide	6.4	23	12.3	44	24.8	88	27.9	99	28.1
Maalox	Mg and Al hydroxide gel	5.5	21	10.8	42	19.9	77	24.5	95	25.8
Creamalin	Hexitol stabilized Al hydroxide gel, magnesium hydroxide	11.1	43	17.8	69	25.6	99	25.7	100	25.7
Di-Gel	Al and Mg hydroxides, simethicone	5.6	23	12.4	50	22.8	93	24.1	98	24.5
Mylanta	Mg and Al hydroxides, simethicone	4.1	17	7.2	30	15.8	66	21.4	90	23.8
Silain-Gel	Mg and Al hydroxides, simethicone	3.3	14	6.6	29	14.0	61	20.1	87	23.1
Marblen	Mg and Ca carbonates, Al hydroxide, Mg phosphate, Mg trisilicate	17.2	75	19.5	86	20.6	91	21.7	95	22.8
WinGel	Al and Mg hydroxides, hexitol stabilized	8.4	37	13.1	58	19.6	87	20.5	91	22.5
Gelusil M	Mg trisilicate, Al hydroxide, Mg hydroxide	11.1	49	17.9	80	20.0	89	20.9	94	22.3
Riopan	Mg and Al hydroxides	3.5	16	6.2	28	12.6	57	18.0	81	22.1
Amphojel	Al hydroxide gel	3.9	20	9.3	48	16.4	85	18.5	96	19.3
A-M-T	Mg trisilicate, Al hydroxide gel	6.5	36	10.4	58	13.3	74	15.2	85	17.9
Kolantyl Gel	Bentyl, Al hydroxide, Mg hydroxide, methylcellulose	5.7	34	9.7	57	14.6	86	15.3	90	16.9
Trisogel	Mg trisilicate, Al hydroxide gel	7.2	43	10.9	66	13.7	83	16.0	97	16.5
Malcogel	Mg trisilicate, Al hydroxide gel	3.9	25	8.0	50	10.7	67	12.8	81	15.9
Gelusil	Mg trisilicate, Al hydroxide	4.1	31	7.2	54	10.5	79	11.0	83	13.3
Robalate	Dihydroxyaluminum aminoacetate	3.4	30	7.7	68	10.4	92	10.8	95	11.3
Phosphaljel	Al phosphate gel	2.5	59	2.9	68	3.8	90	3.9	93	4.2

°The value in this column, divided by 10, is a measure of buffer capacity of the antacid in milliequivalents per milliliter after 120 minutes. This applies to the special circumstances of this in vitro test.

†Percentage of final volume added at 120 minutes. These data are reproduced from reference 24, slightly modified.

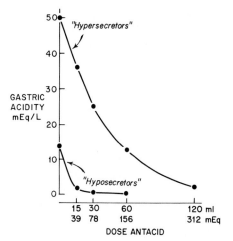

Figure 57–6. Average antacid dose response (Maalox) in a group of patients whose peak histamine response was greater than 25 mEq per hour ("hypersecretors") and in a group of patients whose peak histamine response was less than 17 mEq per hour ("hyposecretors"). Patients were fed a meal of steak, toast, butter, and water; one hour later from zero to 120 ml of antacid was ingested, and gastric acidity was measured two hours later (i.e., three hours after the meal). (From Fordtran, J. S., et al.: New Eng. J. Med., 1973, in press.)

gastric sampling is carried out at shorter intervals after the antacid, gastric acidity is reduced to a greater extent for each dose of antacid.

Dose-response curves carried out in individual patients have emphasized that the degree to which a given patient responds to antacids depends not only on his parietal cell mass, but also on the rate at which he empties the antacid from the stomach, and on his gastric secretory response to eating.[24] Which of these factors varies in different patients, and thus accounts for the different results with antacids even in patients with a similar parietal cell mass, is not known. How well an antacid will reduce acidity in a given patient must be determined by direct testing.

LIQUIDS VS. TABLETS AND POWDERS

There is no a priori reason to prefer antacid in liquid over tablet or powder form. However, in vivo–in vitro comparisons of various tablet preparations have not been made, and in vitro studies show that it takes several tablets to equal even a small dose of the same liquid antacid.

Some tablet antacids must be chewed thoroughly or they will not disintegrate and react with acid in the stomach. Powders have to be suspended in liquid before they can be swallowed. It is generally easier to ingest large amounts of antacid in liquid form.

RATE OF REACTION WITH ACID

As shown in Figure 57–3 antacid constituents vary with respect to their rate of reaction with acid. Even the same chemical may vary in its reaction rate, depending upon the method of its preparation. Commercial antacid combinations also vary in the rapidity with which they react with acid,[24] and "rapid action" is stressed in some advertisements as an advantage. Ironically, slow reactivity was at one time stressed as an advantage, on the false assumption that it could be equated with a long duration of action.[26]

Whether reaction rate is important is unknown. Since antacids are usually ingested in amounts in excess of the acid content of the stomach, complete reaction in a short period of time may not be necessary. Slow development of reactivity of the antacid that remains in the stomach could even be construed as an advantage, because it might prevent development of unnecessarily high pH levels. Also, slow reaction generally means that the unreacted antacid is insoluble, and hence might be emptied from the stomach at a slower rate than more readily soluble antacids. On the other hand, the amount of initially reactive antacid in the stomach should be large enough to raise the pH of the stomach contents to near 5.5 in order to fully reconstitute acidified protein as a buffer. The amount of antacid required will vary from patient to patient, depending upon the volume, hydrogen ion concentration, and amount of protein in the stomach when the antacid is ingested. Very slow reacting antacids might be emptied from the stomach before accomplishing this objective.

As indicated, no data are available to decide whether the rate of reaction with acid, within the range of differences that occur with commercial antacids, is clinically significant. I suspect that it is not important.

COMPLICATIONS OF ANTACID THERAPY

The constipating effect of calcium carbonate and aluminum hydroxide and the cathartic effect of magnesium salts have already been described. These are usually of little consequence and are handled by the combined use of a constipating and a cathartic antacid. Renal disease caused by potassium depletion with diarrhea-producing antacids and concretions in the gut with constipating antacids are very rare but serious related complications. Magnesium retention in patients with renal disease is a potential but rare problem. Many commercial antacids contain a relatively large amount of sodium, which may accentuate fluid retention in patients with congestive heart failure, hypoproteinemia, or ascites.[27, 28] Aluminum hydroxide reduces the absorption of tetracycline and possibly of iron and atropine.[20, 21]

Acid rebound, hypercalcemia and the milk alkali syndrome, phosphorus depletion and aluminum toxicity will be discussed in greater detail.

ACID REBOUND

Since acid in the antrum and duodenum is postulated to inhibit further acid secretion by the feedback loops shown in Figure 14–4 (p. 181), neutralization of gastric acid should cause an enhanced rate of acid secretion. The data to support or refute the existence of this type of acid rebound were extensively reviewed in 1959; no convincing evidence for such a phenomenon in either man or laboratory animals was found.[29] Recently it has been shown that human subjects develop acid rebound following the ingestion of calcium carbonate.[30, 31] Since other antacids failed to show this effect, even when given frequently in large amounts, it seems likely that hypersecretion after calcium carbonate ingestion is related to calcium and not to reduction of gastric acidity. It is likely that species variation accounts for the fact that calcium-induced hypersecretion has not been consistently produced in animals. For instance, hypercalcemia stimulates acid secretion in humans but depresses acid secretion in the dog and rat.[32, 33]

Several features of the acid rebound induced by calcium carbonate should be noted. First, experiments to demonstrate rebound in humans involve measuring acid secretion at a time when all the antacid has been removed from the stomach. The hypersecretion that has been demonstrated after oral calcium carbonate therapy is therefore prolonged (lasting for several hours after the drug), and it occurs at a time when the antrum has been reacidified. Thus alkalinization of the antrum is not present at the time the hypersecretion has been demonstrated. Second, such experiments do not test whether hypersecretion is produced during the time that the gastric pH is high as a result of antacid ingestion. The negative results with sodium bicarbonate and magnesium–aluminum hydroxide do not necessarily mean that these agents do not stimulate acid secretion during the time these drugs are in the stomach and are reducing gastric acidity. Third, all studies that have shown acid rebound with calcium carbonate have been acute rather than long-term studies. It is not known for sure that calcium carbonate ingested for weeks or months would continue to cause rebound hypersecretion. Fourth, acid hypersecretion after oral calcium carbonate has to date been demonstrated mainly in patients with duodenal ulcer. There is, however, no reason to doubt its occurrence in other patients and in normal subjects, provided they secrete enough HCl to convert insoluble calcium carbonate into soluble calcium chloride (see below). Finally, it is theoretically possible that magnesium might inhibit calcium-induced hypersecretion, because these ions have opposite effects on many transport systems. However, preliminary results in my laboratory suggest that magnesium hydroxide does not prevent acid rebound caused by calcium carbonate.

The mechanism of acid rebound after oral calcium carbonate is not clear. It is known that other calcium salts also induce secretion, so the effect is not specific for the carbonate salt; in fact, it is likely that soluble calcium chloride, resulting from reaction of insoluble calcium salts with gastric HCl, is the active principle. (Whether or not high calcium foods, such as milk, will produce acid rebound has not been tested.) The phenomenon can be demonstrated in both fasting[31] and fed subjects, but a meal seems to potentiate the effect.[30] Since hypercalcemia stimulates acid secretion (probably by gastrin release), hypercalcemia is one possible mechanism for acid rebound. However, the response in different subjects correlates poorly with the degree of rise in ionized or total serum calcium concentration.[30] In one patient, calcium carbonate infused into the small intestine was shown to stimulate acid secretion, demonstrating that contact of calcium with the antrum was not a requirement.[30] It is my guess that most of the hypersecretion noted after oral calcium carbonate therapy is due to a local effect of calcium acting within the stomach and proximal small bowel, and that this is mediated by antral and duodenal gastrin release. Inhibition of enterogastrone secretion is another possible mechanism. In individual subjects, hypercalcemia may also be involved, but it is clear that oral calcium therapy can induce acid secretion in some patients without a significant rise in serum calcium concentration.

Regardless of the mechanisms, therapeutic amounts of calcium carbonate stimulate gastric secretion. The clinical significance of this finding deserves careful consideration, because calcium carbonate is considered by many authorities to be the antacid of choice in the treatment of peptic ulcer. The degree of hypersecretion induced by a single dose after meals is not marked in most patients, but some are quite sensitive and secretion rate may increase greatly, even approaching the peak histamine response.[30] When calcium carbonate is given repeatedly to fasting duodenal ulcer patients, the average rate of acid secretion is doubled.[31] Under normal conditions (that is, when gastric contents are not disturbed as part of an experimental procedure), the effect of hypersecretion on gastric acidity is mitigated by the buffering capacity of antacid that remains in the stomach, or by a second meal or a second dose of antacid. The major exception would be that calcium carbonate would probably cause higher nocturnal gastric acidity than if no antacid or a noncalcium-containing antacid had been ingested. (This has not actually been demonstrated.)

It seems likely therefore that calcium therapy will result in sustained but, for the most part, buffered gastric hypersecretion. Whether this has a deleterious effect on the long-term course of peptic ulcer is not known, but chronic gastric secretion stimulated by other means leads to parietal cell hyperplasia.

HYPERCALCEMIA AND THE MILK ALKALI SYNDROME

The three types of the milk alkali syndrome are depicted in Table 57–2. The main features of the syndrome in all its stages are hypercalcemia, elevated blood urea nitrogen and creatinine, and frequently the presence of alkalosis as manifested by high serum CO_2 content. Many patients have a high phosphorus level because of the large amount of this substance in milk and because of decreased excretion of phosphate in the urine. The acute stage is readily reversible when alkali and calcium are withdrawn. In the subacute stage there is marked improvement in renal function (but not necessarily to normal) when calcium and alkali intake are withheld, but this may take several weeks. In contrast, improvement in the chronic stage is usually incomplete, and the patient is left with significantly reduced renal function.

The symptoms are those of hypercalcemia, renal insufficiency, and acid-base disturbance; these are listed in Table 57–2. Abnormal calcification is present in the chronic stage.

This disease can develop any time there is a high calcium intake combined with any factor tending to produce alkalosis. Thus it may develop in patients who ingest large amounts of milk plus an absorbable alkali such as sodium bicarbonate, in patients who ingest milk and vomit (alkalosis caused by loss of gastric acid), or in patients who take only large amounts of calcium carbonate. This is more likely to happen in patients with marked gastric acid hypersecretion because a higher fraction of ingested calcium carbonate would be converted to soluble calcium chloride, which in turn increases the fraction of calcium absorbed and in-

TABLE 57–2. TYPES OF MILK ALKALI SYNDROME*

	ACUTE	SUBACUTE	CHRONIC
Blood chemistry	Elevated Ca, BUN, and creatinine. Normal or elevated PO_4 and CO_2	Same as acute	Same as acute
Symptoms	Frequent nausea, vomiting, anorexia, weakness, lethargy, mental changes (psychosis or encephalitis-like), headache, dizziness	Same as acute, plus asthenia, muscle aching, polydipsia and polyuria, occasional conjunctivitis	Infrequent nausea, vomiting; anorexia, occasional mental changes, asthenia, muscle aching, pruritus, polydipsia and polyuria
Other findings		Occasional band keratopathy. Soft tissue calcifications absent	Band keratopathy and other abnormal calcifications, including nephrocalcinosis (histological, but not necessarily radiological)
Response to withdrawal of milk and alkali	Rapid relief of symptoms, return of renal function to normal	Rapid relief of some symptoms; others clear gradually. Gradual but marked improvement in renal function. Serum calcium level returns to normal, but not as rapidly as in acute stage	Muscle aching and pruritus clear slowly. Little or no improvement in renal function. Serum calcium gradually returns to normal. Some reduction in abnormal calcification
Circumstance in which the type is seen	Complication of treatment with milk and alkali, usually after about one week of such treatment	Usually seen during therapy with milk and alkali used intermittently for years	Occurs after long history of high milk or alkali intake or both

*Modified from McMillan, D. E., and Freeman, R. B.: Medicine 44:487, 1965.

creases the tendency to alkalosis (see Fig. 57–4). A preceding renal disease probably facilitates development of the syndrome, but is definitely not a prerequisite.

The pathogenesis of this disorder is probably as follows:[34]

1. The level of serum calcium rises mildly in most patients treated with large amounts of calcium (milk or calcium antacids).

2. This suppresses parathyroid function.

3. This leads to phosphorus retention via reduced renal phosphorus excretion.

4. If homeostatic mechanisms are not adequate, hypercalcemia develops.

5. Hypercalcemia plus hyperphosphatemia produces a high calcium-phosphorus product, which is critical in producing renal damage.

6. Reduced glomerular filtration impairs calcium and phosphorus excretion and may lead to higher blood calcium and phosphorus levels with further damage to the kidneys.

7. Alkalosis, if present, is due to absorbable alkali or to vomiting. The vomiting may be related to the peptic ulcer or to the hypercalcemia.

Although the syndrome has rarely been recognized by gastroenterologists, even when phenomenal amounts of milk and calcium carbonate have been prescribed for relatively long periods, the results of the study by McMillan and Freeman are alarming.[34] These workers gave a group of ulcer patients six ounces of milk every other hour and on alternate hours either 15 ml of aluminum hydroxide or one teaspoon of calcium carbonate powder (about 3.6 g). There were 20 patients in each group, and allocation to the calcium and noncalcium antacid was random. The average rise in serum calcium, phosphorus creatinine, and CO_2 content observed in the calcium-treated group is shown in Figure 57–7. These are average figures; the deleterious effect on some patients was even more striking.

Hyperparathyroidism and vitamin D intoxication are the main diseases to be considered in the differential diagnosis. Both may be associated with peptic ulcer. The single most useful method of separating hyperparathyroidism and milk alkali syndrome is the fall in serum calcium levels once calcium intake is withdrawn. Other distinguishing features are the alkalosis and elevated serum phosphate levels in many patients with milk alkali syndrome; these are almost never seen in those with hyperparathyroidism. The

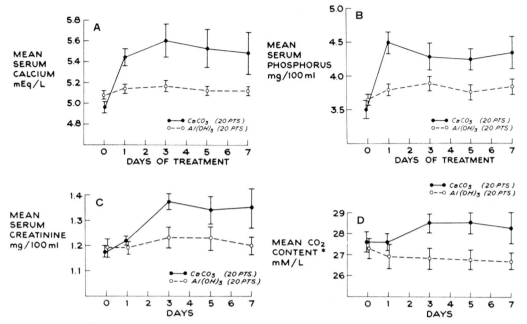

Figure 57–7. Effect of calcium carbonate and aluminum hydroxide, ingested every two hours, on serum calcium, phosphorus, creatinine, and bicarbonate concentrations. On alternate hours both groups of ulcer patients received milk. (From McMillan, D. E., and Freeman R. B.: Medicine 44:485, 1965.)

hypercalcemia of milk alkali syndrome is said to respond to adrenal steroid therapy,[35] but the number of times such a response has been documented must be quite small; the hypercalcemia of hyperparathyroidism rarely responds to steroid therapy. Urinary calcium excretion is elevated in hyperparathyroidism prior to the development of renal failure; it is elevated in acute but not chronic milk alkali syndrome.

In vitamin D intoxication the history will usually be diagnostic if the disease is considered. These patients often have renal failure, increased urinary calcium, and elevated serum phosphate levels; therefore their condition may closely simulate the milk alkali syndrome. The hypercalcemia of vitamin D intoxication responds dramatically to steroids.[36]

Other diseases to consider in the differential diagnosis are malignant tumors, sarcoidosis, hyperthyroidism, acute bone atrophy, and adrenal insufficiency.

PHOSPHORUS DEPLETION

Aluminum salts bind phosphorus in the diet and in intestinal secretions and thus reduce the rate of phosphorus absorption.

This effect is put to advantage in patients with renal failure in order to lower serum phosphorus concentration toward normal. However, if renal function is normal and dietary intake of phosphorus is low, it is possible to produce phosphorus depletion by aluminum hydroxide therapy.[2, 37] Malabsorption syndromes also reduce phosphorus absorption and would be expected to predispose to phosphorus depletion. Similarly, relative hypersecretors of gastric acid will change a higher fraction of the ingested aluminum hydroxide into aluminum chloride, and there will be a greater tendency to react with soluble phosphate to form insoluble aluminum phosphate. The absence of alkaline pancreatic juice from the upper small bowel might also favor the formation of aluminum phosphate, because the aluminum would exist longer in the form of chloride rather than undergo rapid conversion to the less reactive, insoluble aluminum hydroxide.[2]

Phosphorus depletion is characterized by marked decrease in urinary phosphorus, hypercalciuria, and hypophosphatemia. The hypercalciuria is due in part to increased calcium absorption from the gut, but is due also to skeletal resorption.[37] The symptoms of phosphorus depletion are anorexia, weakness, and malaise. The development of these symptoms in patients taking aluminum hydroxide antacids should suggest the diagnosis. If severe and prolonged, phosphorus depletion may lead to osteomalacia, osteoporosis, and fracture, especially if it occurs in patients with some other cause of bone disease, such as steroid therapy. In such patients (postrenal transplant patients, for instance) it is especially important to guard against phosphorus depletion.

Prevention is usually simple: Make sure the phosphorus content of the diet is adequate. If urinary phosphorus excretion is greater than 300 mg per day, phosphorus depletion is unlikely.[37]

In patients predisposed to phosphorus depletion or in those with other factors tending to produce osteoporosis or osteomalacia, aluminum hydroxide antacids should be used with special caution. Theoretically, aluminum phosphate would be an ideal antacid in such circumstances. Practically, it has very little antacid activity. Probably the best solution would be to give phosphate supplements (in the form of sodium and potassium phosphate, Neutro-Phos) if aluminum hydroxide antacids are to be used in such patients.

ALUMINUM TOXICITY

Aluminum salts are poorly absorbed as a result of the formation of insoluble aluminum salts in the gastrointestinal tract. What little is absorbed (presumably as aluminum chloride) is readily excreted in the urine if renal function is normal. However, aluminum toxicity develops if uremic rats are fed a *soluble* aluminum preparation (or if aluminum is injected systemically). Toxicity is manifested by lethargy, periorbital bleeding, anorexia, and finally death.[38] The studies by Thurston and coworkers show that small amounts of aluminum are retained when aluminum hydroxide is administered in experimental renal failure, but there is no evidence that such amounts are toxic per se.[39] (Phosphorus depletion may develop, but this has nothing to do with aluminum toxicity.)

Some controversy exists about the safety of aluminum hydroxide in uremic patients. At present, the evidence that aluminum-containing antacids are toxic in uremic patients is not convincing.

CLINICAL INTERPRETATION

Because antacids have not been proved by clinical trial to favorably influence the healing of peptic ulcer or to aid in preventing recurrences, some experienced clinicians and investigators downgrade the importance of antacids and recommend using them only for pain relief. I cannot agree with this position, because there are no good studies suggesting that antacids are not helpful, and because, when properly used, these drugs will reduce gastric acidity rather markedly. What can be accomplished with one or two doses of antacid taken at appropriate intervals after eating is shown in Figure 57–8. Note that acidity can be markedly reduced by antacids during the time when postcibal acid secretion is maximal (compare with Fig. 57–1). Therefore, although admitting on an intellectual level the tenuous basis on which all ulcer therapy rests, I believe that based on current knowledge of ulcer pathogenesis and clinical pharmacology antacids are important in treating active ulcer and that they should be used in an attempt to prevent relapses. Having made this judgment, it is important that

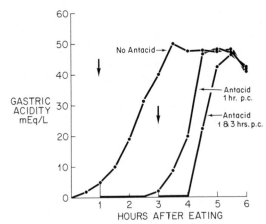

Figure 57–8. Average gastric acidity in a group of patients with duodenal ulcer after a steak meal, and the effect of 80 mEq antacid given one hour after the meal or one and three hours after the meal. (This figure is a composite of data reported in Fordtran, J. S., and Collyns, J. A. H.: New Eng. J. Med. 274:921, 1966, and previously unpublished data from the author's laboratory.)

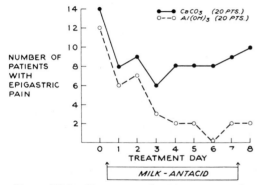

NUMBER OF PATIENTS WITH EPIGASTRIC PAIN

MILK - ANTACID

Figure 57-9. Frequency of pain in peptic ulcer patients treated with calcium carbonate or aluminum hydroxide every other hour. (From McMillan, D. E., and Freeman, R. B.: Medicine 44:485, 1965.)

antacids be used in such a manner that they have as large an effect on gastric acidity as possible. The following guidelines are suggested, with full recognition of their arbitrary nature.

For reasons already discussed, it is my opinion that calcium carbonate should not constitute the mainstay of antacid therapy. This decision is strengthened by the fact that two controlled studies have suggested that intensive calcium carbonate therapy delays pain relief and delays healing of peptic ulcer.[34, 40] The result of one of these studies is shown in Figure 57-9. Assuming that observer bias is not involved, it seems likely that these poor results are related to calcium-induced gastric hypersecretion. Whether smaller amounts of calcium carbonate added to magnesium and aluminum hydroxide have a beneficial effect because of enhanced potency or a detrimental effect because of rebound hypersecretion is unknown. It is my present practice not to use calcium-containing antacids but to use larger volumes of noncalcium preparations to achieve the desired antacid dose.

Patients are therefore given a choice of two or three of the more potent aluminum-magnesium hydroxide antacids; they can select one according to cost or their taste preference, or can use them alternately to avoid "taste fatigue." Preparations containing anticholinergic drugs are avoided, because antacid and anticholinergic dosage must be individualized. If the patient has diarrhea, or if antacids containing

magnesium hydroxide have produced diarrhea in the past, the most potent antacids containing only aluminum hydroxide (Amphojel, for example) are used (Table 57-1). It may be necessary to alternate between a diarrhea-producing and a constipating antacid. If the patient has salt retention, an antacid with low sodium content is advisable; Riopan has less sodium than many other antacids. If the patient is taking adrenal steroids or has osteoporosis, phosphate supplements are prescribed. If the patient has renal disease, magnesium blood levels must be monitored if magnesium-containing antacids are used. Some nephrologists prescribe calcium to patients with chronic renal disease (hoping to prevent bone disease), and if these patients have peptic ulcer, calcium carbonate is a logical antacid. Serum calcium and phosphorus should be measured at intervals to detect hypercalcemia or a high $CaPO_4$ product. Aluminum hydroxide antacids may be used to lower serum phosphorus in these patients, so this also may be a logical antacid for peptic ulcer in this group.

The recommended dose of antacid depends upon the condition being treated and upon the stage of the disease (active ulcer vs. preventive therapy). In general, the dose should be as large as is reasonably tolerable. Large doses taken less frequently are better tolerated than small doses taken hourly. If for any reason the less potent antacids are prescribed, the volume of each dose is adjusted upward by a factor easily calculated from the data in Table 57-1.

Antacid therapy should be explained to the patient with the aid of hand-drawn charts, such as those shown in Figures 57-1, 57-5, and 57-8. This is essential, because when the patient does not understand the rationale, he will very soon give up on antacids, or may become confused on timing in relation to meals. Even with thorough explanation, patients often believe that they can make up for missed doses by doubling the next dose, or get "one hour before meals" (a ridiculous time to take antacids except for pain relief) confused with "one hour after meals."

Suggested programs in specific clinical situations are as follows:

Gastric Ulcer. Hourly, while the patient is awake, because response to therapy is a major criterion of whether or not the ulcer is benign. If the ulcer fails to heal in the preallotted time (see pp. 703 to 704), there should be no question about the adequacy of antacid administration, which only causes procrastination. A dose of about 40 mEq antacid is reasonable in most patients, but if the patient has a relatively high peak secretory capacity (> 20 mEq per hour), it would be advisable to double the dose. After healing is complete, approximately 80 mEq of antacid one hour after meals and at bedtime is strongly advised indefinitely, in the hope of preventing a recurrence (which occurs in about 50 to 60 per cent of patients on unspecified and presumably very little maintenance therapy).

Duodenal Ulcer. Hourly antacid while awake in about an 80-mEq dose until the patient is pain free for seven to ten days. Then about 80 mEq one and three hours after each meal and at bedtime for six weeks. Then, if the patient has demonstrated a tendency to have frequent relapses, from 80 to 160 mEq one hour after meals and at bedtime indefinitely, in the hope of preventing a recurrence. Most patients will not stay on this therapy for long periods, but some will, especially if the preventive program is presented with enthusiasm.

Inadequate Relief of Pain, Inadequate Healing, or Frequent Relapses. Determine the effectiveness of antacid therapy and adjust the antacid dose accordingly.* Rule out the Zollinger-Ellison syndrome, and consider the possibility that the patient's symptoms are caused by something other than peptic ulcer.

Zollinger-Ellison Syndrome During Diagnostic Studies. Antacids in a dose of about 75 mEq should be given every 30 minutes or by continuous intragastric drip.[41-43] (Anticholinergic therapy also is advisable.) This is essential, because many patients perforate or bleed massively while the physician is preoccupied with diagnostic studies.

---

*This can easily be done by having the patient eat the same breakfast or lunch on four separate days, and measuring acidity of the gastric contents three hours after the meal when different doses (zero to 150 mEq) of antacid are ingested one hour after the meal.

ANTICHOLINERGIC DRUGS

MECHANISM OF ACTION

These drugs competitively inhibit the action of acetylcholine on structures innervated by postganglionic cholinergic nerves and on smooth muscles that respond to acetylcholine. Thus, they antagonize the muscarinic action of acetylcholine.[44] Although the synthetic and semisynthetic quaternary ammonium agents also have ganglionic blocking potential, in the dosages that can be employed clinically these drugs are also considered as purely antimuscarinic agents.[45] Some anticholinergic drugs have an effect on the central nervous system—stimulation in small doses, depression in high doses.

The results of anticholinergic action on exocrine glands and smooth and cardiac muscle may be summarized as follows: Salivary, bronchial, and sweat secretion are depressed. The pupils dilate and eye accommodation is diminished or abolished. The heart rate may be transiently depressed, but the major effect is inhibition of vagal input, so that heart rate is increased. The tone and contractile force of the urinary bladder, biliary tract, and gastrointestinal tract are reduced, and gastric and pancreatic secretion are inhibited.

Some workers have concluded that gastric secretion is relatively resistant to depression by anticholinergic agents. For instance, Innes and Nickerson claim that small doses inhibit salivary, bronchial, and sweat secretion, that larger doses dilate the pupils, inhibit accommodation, increase heart rate, and reduce bladder and gastrointestinal motility, whereas still larger doses are required to inhibit gastric secretion.[44] The results of Juniper would appear to contradict this thesis, at least as a generalization applicable to all such drugs, because he found that one anticholinergic agent had a significantly greater effect on basal gastric than on sweat or salivary gland secretion.[46] These results are shown in Figure 57–10.

CLINICAL PHARMACOLOGY

The belladonna alkaloids are readily absorbed from the gastrointestinal tract,

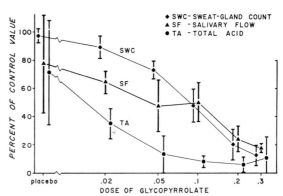

Figure 57–10. Effect of graded doses of intramuscular glycopyrrolate on sweat, salivary flow, and basal gastric acid secretion in five subjects. The value representative of drug effect is plotted as a percentage of control value. Mean results ± 1 SD. (From Juniper, K.: Amer. J. Dig. Dis. *12*:439, 1967.)

whereas the quaternary ammonium agents are absorbed relatively poorly.[44] The latter drugs have relatively little effect on the central nervous system, presumably because they do not pass the blood-brain barrier.

The clinical usefulness of anticholinergic drugs is limited by the production of generalized blockade of parasympathetic function. Whether any particular anticholinergic drug has a selective action in inhibiting a particular parasympathetic activity is controversial. Bachrach reviewed an extensive literature in 1958 and concluded that there was no evidence that any anticholinergic drug selectively alters a particular parasympathetic function.[47] Innes and Nickerson agreed, saying that there is no evidence of a greater margin between desired effects and undesirable side effects for synthetic agents than for the natural belladonna alkaloids.[44] According to this thesis, all anticholinergic drugs are equally efficacious in inhibiting acid secretion provided the dose is titrated to the limits of tolerance (dry mouth, photophobia, blurring of vision). On the other hand, Sun concluded in 1964 that certain drugs do have a special affinity for inhibiting certain effector organs.[45] For instance, he reported that for a number of anticholinergic drugs, the occurrence of dryness of the mouth and blurring of vision does not assure an antisecretory effect in the stomach, whereas for other drugs rather pronounced antisecretory activity can be demonstrated at a dose just below that which produces dryness of the mouth or visual changes.

Unfortunately, this important controversy has not been settled. The results of Mitchell and colleagues would favor some degree of selectivity of anticholinergic action, because these workers found

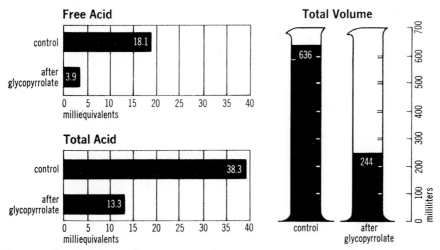

Figure 57–11. Effect of glycopyrrolate on nocturnal gastric secretion in peptic ulcer patients. (From Barman, M. L., and Larson, R. K.: Amer. J. Med. Sci. *246*:325, 1963.)

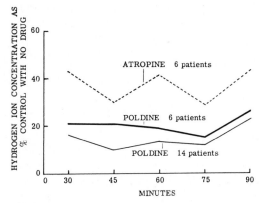

Figure 57–12. Geometric mean hydrogen ion concentration of gastric contents after atropine or poldine as percentage of control. The meal used in these studies was apple juice, milk, toast, butter, and eggs. (From Mitchell, R. D., et al.: Gastroenterology 43:400, 1962.)

that poldine, a quaternary ammonium agent, inhibited acid secretion much better than atropine, even though both were

given in amounts slightly below the dose which produced troublesome side effects.[48] The data of Dreiling and Janowitz on the effect of anticholinergic drugs on pancreatic secretion also favor selectivity.[49] However, neither of these studies is conclusive insofar as the present argument is concerned.

When given orally in an amount just below the dose which produces side effects, anticholinergic drugs reduce basal acid secretion by about 50 per cent and maximal histamine (or gastrin) secretion by about 40 per cent of the control rate of acid secretion.[50] The reduction in peak histamine- or gastrin-stimulated secretory response by anticholinergic drugs is probably due to a diminished sensitivity of the parietal cells to histamine and gastrin.[50] An example of the effect of anticholinergic drugs on nocturnal acid output is shown in Figure 57–11. Excellent reduction was noted even though the dose was fixed at a low level in these experiments.[51]

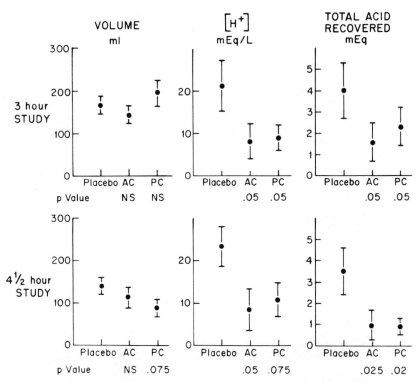

Figure 57–13. Effect of an "optimal effective dose" of poldine (Nacton) on postcibal gastric volume, hydrogen ion concentration, and total recoverable gastric acid. Four g of calcium carbonate was ingested one hour after the meal. Gastric contents were removed at either three hours after the meal (ten patients, top panel) or 4½ hours after the meal (eight patients, lower panel). Each patient was studied on three test days; on one day he received Nacton 30 minutes before the meal (AC), on another he received Nacton 60 minutes after the meal (PC), and on a third day he received a placebo. (Data of D. E. Polter and J. S. Fordtran, previously unpublished.)

Some studies have shown no inhibition by anticholinergic drugs of gastric acidity following ingestion of normal food, but other experiments have clearly demonstrated that at least some anticholinergic drugs reduce postcibal gastric acidity.[48, 52] (The results of one of these studies are shown in Fig. 57–12.) This effect could be mediated by decreased emptying of the meal buffer, by reduced acid secretion rate, or both. It seems likely that the major effect is on reduction of gastric acid secretion, because postcibal gastric volume is not increased by an optimal effective oral dose of anticholinergic drugs (Figs. 57–13 and 57–14).[6]

Some investigators have the impression that anticholinergic drugs given for weeks to months exert an antisecretory effect not present after short-term therapy. Furthermore, the antisecretory effect is thought to persist for several days to several months after the drugs are discontinued. However, no evidence in favor of this hypothesis was found in the studies by Norgaard et al.,[53] Kaye et al.,[54] or Walan.[55] For instance, poldine and glycopyrrolate reduced histamine-stimulated acid secretion to the same degree in patients who had been on anticholinergic therapy only long enough to titrate them to an effective dose (three to five days) as in patients who had been on these drugs continuously for one year.[53] Moreover, secretion had returned to control level within 48 hours after discontinuing long-term anticholinergic therapy.[53]

At times a patient may develop an increased tolerance to anticholinergic drugs. For instance, two tablets may produce mild side effects initially, but some months later three tablets may produce negligible side effects. Whether this tolerance to side effects signifies a diminished effect on gastric secretion has not been definitely determined, but studies which have correlated salivary and gastric secretory data while on a fixed dose of atropine, and gastric secretory studies over a two- to four-year period while on a fixed dose of l-hyoscyamine,[55] suggest that inhibition of gastric secretion by anticholinergics may decrease with time owing to acquired tolerance. Thus it would seem wise to periodically retitrate patients to the optimal effective dose, rather than to remain indefinitely with the initially determined dose.

The duration of action of various anticholinergic drugs has not been carefully and systematically studied. The synthetic drugs are said to have a longer action than atropine. Mitchell and co-workers claim that an oral dose of poldine has anticholinergic action for eight hours,[48] whereas atropine action is considerably shorter. Dotevall et al. claim that when l-hyoscyamine, the most active part of atropine, is administered in tablets with sustained release, its effect is prolonged for at least eight to nine hours.[50]

All investigators agree that the dose of an anticholinergic drug should be titrated to that level which is at or just below the dose which produces mild side effects. This "optimal effective dose"[45] will be markedly different in different patients, but those who require only a small dose (to produce mild side effects) will have as much inhibition of gastric secretion as

Figure 57–14. Effect of an "optimal effective dose" of poldine (Nacton) on acid secretion rate four to five hours and five and one-half to six and one-half hours after a standard steak meal. See Figure 57–13 legend for experimental details. Acid secretion rate was measured by continuous gastric suction, starting one hour after all gastric contents were removed by a Levin tube. The four- to five-hour secretion rates were measured in the ten patients referred to in Figure 57–13 (tube inserted three hours after the meal), and the five and one-half- to six and one-half-hour secretion rates were measured in the eight patients referred to in Figure 57–13 (tube inserted four and one-half hours after the meal). (Data of D. E. Polter and J. S. Fordtran, previously unpublished.)

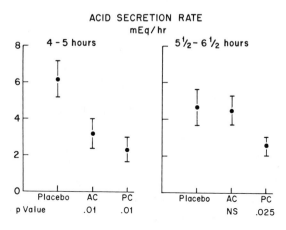

those patients who have a larger tolerance and thus receive a larger dose.[55] Since the evidence favors some selectivity of anticholinergic action, it would seem best for physicians to use only anticholinergic drugs which have been demonstrated to substantially reduce meal-stimulated acidity and basal and nocturnal acid secretion when given in a dose just below the amount which produces side effects.

When used to reduce postcibal gastric acidity, these drugs are usually given about 15 to 30 minutes before meals. However, it has been argued on theoretical grounds[56] that it would be preferable to give the drugs after meals, in order to get a sustained effect owing to slower emptying of the drug from the stomach. With this regimen the peak effect would theoretically be one to two hours after eating, when patients often have the onset of ulcer pain. By contrast, when given 30 minutes before meals the drug will be emptied sooner from the stomach and have a shorter duration of action, with a peak effect soon after eating (while the food is still buffering gastric acid and the anticholinergic effect is not needed). This question has been recently investigated in our laboratory, and the results are shown in Figures 57–13 and 57–14. Patients with duodenal ulcer were fed a standard steak meal and one hour later were given an antacid. Poldine (Nacton) was given 30 minutes before the meal on one test day, and one hour after eating on another. On a third test day the patients were given a placebo. With each therapeutic regimen, gastric acidity and total acid in the stomach were reduced when gastric contents were sampled three hours (ten patients) and 4½ hours (eight patients) after eating. Acid secretion rate was reduced for about five hours with both schedules. On the basis of these results and the pattern of acid secretion rate and gastric acidity after eating (Figs. 57–1 and 57–5), we give anticholinergic drugs 30 minutes before eating rather than after a meal. The peak action probably occurs when acid secretion is maximal, and the antisecretory effect lasts for at least five hours (four and one-half hours after the meal). By that time the patient is ready to redo the cycle with another

dose of anticholinergic and then another meal.

These studies demonstrate that anticholinergic drugs reduce gastric acidity even in patients who have taken an antacid one hour after eating. This effect of the anticholinergic drug is probably due mainly to reduced acid secretion, although delayed emptying of antacid and protein buffer may also play a role. If emptying was delayed, it was not enough to cause gastric volume to increase. These results show that anticholinergic drugs taken before or after meals have an additive effect with antacids taken one hour after meals in reducing gastric acidity. However, when antacids were ingested hourly, Soergel and Hogan found no additional reduction of gastric acidity by anticholinergic drugs.[57]

Some workers have postulated that chronic anticholinergic therapy reduces the functional parietal cell mass. Prolonged stomach rest might cause parietal hypoplasia much as prolonged work stimulated by hypergastrinemia causes hyperplasia of the parietal cells. However, there is at present no evidence for such an occurrence in patients treated for 12 to 18 months with various anticholinergic drugs.[53–55]

EFFECT ON PANCREATIC BICARBONATE SECRETION

Theoretically the benefits of reduced acid secretion in duodenal ulcer might be mitigated if there were a corresponding reduction of bicarbonate secretion into the proximal duodenum, resulting in decreased neutralization of acid. The degree to which anticholinergic drugs inhibit pancreatic and biliary bicarbonate secretion after a meal is not known. Innes and Nickerson claim that atropine has little effect on the secretion of pancreatic juice or bile.[44] On the other hand, Dreiling and Janowitz found a marked reduction (about 80 per cent) in basal and secretin-stimulated pancreatic output of bicarbonate in response to anticholinergic therapy.[49] The significance of this study to the question at hand is reduced by the fact that the anticholinergic drugs were given intravenously; however, the authors did use an optimal therapeutic dose, determined by prior titration in each subject.

These results aside, the importance of pancreatic bicarbonate in protecting against duodenal ulcer in man has not been established. Complete or near complete diversion of pancreatic juice from the duodenum predisposes to duodenal ulceration in experimental animals,[41] but patients with exocrine pancreatic insufficiency have not been shown to have an increased incidence of duodenal ulcer. This does not settle the question, however, because such patients may also have reduced acid secretion (this has apparently not been carefully studied). We are not aware of any careful study of duodenal bulb pH with and without anticholinergic therapy.

RESULTS OF CLINICAL TRIALS

The effect of anticholinergic drugs can be assessed by means of controlled clinical trials, but it is doubtful if these can be "double-blind," because side effects often identify which patients are on placebo and which are on active drugs. Furthermore, specific identification of a recurrence of duodenal ulcer is difficult, and unless observer bias is completely eliminated (which is extremely difficult with the drugs in question), the effect of anticholinergics on "ulcer recurrence" is of doubtful significance. The frequency of complications is probably the most objective criterion that can be assessed, but the relatively low complication rate in most groups requires large numbers of patients followed for long periods of time, and observer bias can also influence the interpretation of the frequency of complications.

Considering these problems, it is not surprising that controlled trials have given conflicting results on the value of anticholinergic drugs in duodenal ulcer. Data prior to 1958 were reviewed by Bachrach,[47] who concluded that there was no convincing evidence that these drugs improve the results of treatment in uncomplicated duodenal ulcer or that they prevented recurrences. Sun,[45] Walan,[55] Kaye et al.,[58] and Trevino et al.[59] have reviewed most

of the recent studies, which are about evenly divided between those which claim that anticholinergic drugs prevent recurrence and complications to a statistically significant degree, and those which reveal completely negative results. The opinion of the experts is sharply divided,[60, 61] with some considering these drugs to be of proved benefit, and others strongly of the opinion that they are merely "logical placebos."[62]

The possible reasons for the discrepancy among different studies has been discussed,[60, 61] but no generally accepted explanation is available. Bias of the investigator, variable criteria of a "recurrence" or "complication," variable definition of what constitutes a beneficial effect, inadequate observation periods, low incidence of recurrence and complications in the placebo group, variations in concomitant therapy, and different "ulcer populations" are probably important in some instances.

Owing to the divergent results of controlled clinical trials, it is not possible to say whether or not anticholinergic therapy is beneficial in the long-term management of duodenal ulcer. This is, in our opinion, not evidence that these drugs are probably ineffective. Rather, the dramatically different results indicate the difficulty in doing controlled studies in duodenal ulcer with drugs that preclude a double-blind approach. When prejudice cannot be eliminated, results are suspect, and it is obvious from reading the literature that investigators are as often prejudiced against as for anticholinergic drugs. Few studies in gastric ulcer have been reported. Recently, Baume et al. reported that glycopyrronium bromide (Robinul) accelerated initial healing and reduced recurrence rate in patients with gastric ulcer.[63]

CLINICAL INTERPRETATION AND APPLICATION

It is obvious that a scientifically valid judgment cannot be made as to whether anticholinergic drugs are helpful, are harmful, or make no difference in the treatment of patients with peptic ulcer. Nevertheless, physicians have to make a decision about whether or not to use anticholinergic drugs in the treatment of their patients. Everything considered, it is my decision to use anticholinergic drugs in patients with both gastric and duodenal ulcer, provided there are no relative or absolute contraindications (see below). Having made this decision, patients are carefully titrated to the optimal effective dose, and the drugs are described to the patient with enthusiasm. The optimal effective dose is redetermined at intervals of six to twelve months because of the likelihood that some patients will develop acquired tolerance. Only those drugs which have been demonstrated to reduce postcibal acidity and nocturnal acid secretion in a dose below the toxic level are used. The drugs are prescribed at bedtime. It seems likely that they will be more effective in reducing nocturnal acidity and acid secretion if the patient does not eat a bedtime meal; for this reason, patients are advised not to eat after supper. If patients are taking antacids only once or twice after each meal, anticholinergics are prescribed 30 minutes prior to eating. If antacids are used hourly, anticholinergics are not prescribed prior to eating, but are still used at bedtime.

Mild dryness of the mouth, blurred vision, and photophobia are useful signs of anticholinergic action and are not considered as complications. Their occurrence is an indication for a slight reduction in dosage. Constipation may be bothersome to some patients; if it occurs without other evidence of toxicity, it may be treated with small amounts of laxative antacids, without a reduction in anticholinergic dose. Such patients should be watched for evidence of intestinal atony. Mild and questionable urinary hesitancy is an indication for a reduction in anticholinergic dosage. A definitely weakening urinary stream and definite urinary hesitancy are indications for a temporary suspension of anticholinergic therapy; when restarted, the drugs should only be used at bedtime in order to guard against possible development of urinary retention.

Central nervous system symptoms may develop, especially in elderly patients. These occur in about 10 per cent of patients titrated to an optimal effective dose,

and include nervousness, dizziness, insomnia, headache, loss of taste, nausea, and vomiting.[47] Usually these symptoms will develop soon after the start of anticholinergic therapy if they are going to occur; occasionally such symptoms may be delayed, suggesting a cumulative intolerance. The secondary effects of these drugs may in some instances not be identified in terms of a specific objective sensation. In these cases the patient can only state that he feels better without than with the drug, and he may not realize how much better until a period of time without the drug.[47]

Occasionally gastric retention may be precipitated in patients with a narrowed gastric outlet. This should be watched for by physical examination (succussion splash) as well as by history and laboratory tests.

Acute glaucoma, impotence, and pulmonary complications caused by dry bronchial secretions are rare but serious complications of anticholinergic therapy. Anhidrosis caused by anticholinergic agents would be dangerous under conditions that might lead to heat stroke.

Anticholinergic drugs should not be prescribed to any patient with gastric retention, partial gastric outlet obstruction, prostatism, glaucoma, or achalasia. These drugs reduce lower esophageal sphincter tone, but whether they are helpful or harmful in reflux peptic esophagitis has not been determined. Anticholinergic agents should not be used (or should be used with extreme caution) in elderly and debilitated patients; their use in such patients often leads to central nervous system derangements, intestinal atony, and urinary retention.

REFERENCES

1. Goldberg, H. I., Dodds, W. J., Gee, S., Montgomery, C., and Zboralske, F. F. Role of acid and pepsin in acute experimental esophagitis. Gastroenterology 56:223, 1969.
2. Fauley, G. B., Freeman, S., Ivy, A. C., Atkinson, A. J., and Wigodsky, H. S. Aluminum phosphate in the therapy of peptic ulcer. Arch. Intern. Med. 67:563, 1941.
3. Fordtran, J. S., and Walsh, J. H. Gastric acid secretion and buffer content of the stomach after eating: Results in normal subjects and in patients with duodenal ulcer. J. Clin. Invest. Vol. 52, 1973 (in press).

4. Kirsner, J. B., and Palmer, W. L. The effect of various antacids on the hydrogen-ion concentration of the gastric contents. Amer. J. Dig. Dis. 7:85, 1940.

5. Bingle, J. P., and Lennard-Jones, J. E. Some factors in the assessment of gastric antisecretory drugs by a sampling technique. Gut 1:337, 1960.

6. Lennard-Jones, J. E., and Barbouris, N. Effect of different foods on the acidity of the gastric contents in patients with duodenal ulcer: A comparison between two "therapeutic" diets and freely chosen meals. Gut 6:113, 1965.

7. Lawrence, J. S. Dietetic and other methods in the treatment of peptic ulcer. Lancet 1:482, 1952.

8. Doll, R., Friedlander, P., and Pygott, F. Dietetic treatment of peptic ulcer. Lancet 1:5, 1956.

9. Truelove, S. C. Stilboestrol, phenobarbitone, and diet in chronic duodenal ulcer. Brit. Med. J. 2:559, 1960.

10. Buchman, E., Kaung, D. T., Dolan, K., and Knepp, R. N. Unrestricted diet in the treatment of duodenal ulcer. Gastroenterology 56:1016, 1969.

11. Haggard, H. W., and Greenberg, L. A. The influence of certain fruit juices on gastric function. Amer. J. Dig. Dis. 8:163, 1941.

12. Flick, A. L. Acid content of common beverages. Amer. J. Dig. Dis. 15:317, 1970.

13. Dimmler, C., Power, M. H., and Alvarez, W. C. The effect of orange juice on gastric acidity. Amer. J. Dig. Dis. 5:86, 1938.

14. Saint-Hilaire, S., Lavers, M. K., Kennedy, J., and Code, C. F. Gastric acid secretory value of different foods. Gastroenterology 39:1, 1960.

15. Claytor, F. W., Smith, W. L., and Turner, E. L. The effect of orange juice on gastric acidity. Amer. J. Dig. Dis. 8:43, 1941.

16. Alvey, C., and Cahn, A. Orange juice and digestive dysfunction. Med. J. Austral. 2:11, 1956.

17. Sanchez-Palomera, E. The action of spices on the acid gastric secretion, on the appetite, and on the caloric intake. Gastroenterology 18:254, 1951.

18. Schneider, M. A., DeLuca, V., and Gray, S. J. Amer. J. Gastroent. 26:722, 1956.

19. Fauley, G. B., and Ivy, A. C. Experimental gastric ulcer: The effect of the consistency of the diet on healing. Arch. Intern. Med. 46:524, 1930.

20. Harvey, S. C. Gastric antacids and digestants. In The Pharmacological Basis of Therapeutics, L. S. Goodman and A. Gilman (eds.), 3rd ed. New York, Macmillan, 1965, p. 990.

21. Brody, M., and Bachrach, W. H. Antacids. I. Comparative biochemical and economic considerations. Amer. J. Dig. Dis. 4:435, 1959.

22. Clarkson, E. M., McDonald, S. J., and DeWardner, H. W. The effect of a high intake of calcium carbonate in normal subjects and patients with chronic renal failure. Clin. Sci. 30:425, 1966.

23. Littman, A. Reactive and nonreactive alumi-

num hydroxide gels: Dose-response relationships in vivo. Gastroenterology 52:948, 1967.

24. Fordtran, J. S., Morawski, S. G., and Richardson, C. T. In vivo and in vitro evaluation of liquid antacids. New Eng. J. Med., 1973, in press.

25. Fordtran, J. S., and Collyns, J. A. H. Antacid pharmacology in duodenal ulcer. New Eng. J. Med. 274:921, 1966.

26. Grossman, M. I. Duration of action of antacids. Amer. J. Dig. Dis. 1:453, 1956.

27. Bleifer, K. H., Belsky, J. L., and Bleifer, D. J. Sodium content of four antacids. New Eng. J. Med. 261:604, 1959.

28. Rimer, D. G., and Frankland, M. Sodium content of antacids. J.A.M.A. 173:995, 1960.

29. Pereira-Lima, J., and Hollander, F. Gastric acid rebound: A review. Gastroenterology 37:145, 1959.

30. Fordtran, J. S. Acid rebound. New Eng. J. Med. 279:900, 1968.

31. Barreras, R. F. Acid secretion after calcium carbonate in patients with duodenal ulcer. New Eng. J. Med. 282:1402, 1970.

32. Ward, J. T., Adesola, A. O., and Welbourn, R. B. The parathyroids, calcium and gastric secretion in man and the dog. Gut 5:173, 1964.

33. Barreras, R. F., Greenlee, H. B., and McConnell, C. Species and individual variations in gastric response to hypercalcemia. Clin. Res. 17:524, 1969.

34. McMillan, D. E., and Freeman, R. B. The milk alkali syndrome. A study of the acute disorder with comments on the development of the chronic condition. Medicine 44:485, 1965.

35. Goldsmith, R. S. Differential diagnosis of hypercalcemia. New Eng. J. Med. 274:674, 1966.

36. Dent, C. E. Cortisone test for hyperparathyroidism. Brit. Med. J. 1:230, 1956.

37. Lotz, M., Zisman, E., and Bartter, F. C. Evidence for a phosphorus-depletion syndrome in man. New Eng. J. Med. 278:409, 1968.

38. Berlyne, G. M., Yagil, R., Benari, J., Weinberger, G., Knopf, E., and Danovitch, G. M. Aluminum toxicity in rats. Lancet 1:564, 1972.

39. Thurston, H., Gilmore, G. R., and Swales, J. D. Aluminum retention and toxicity in chronic renal failure. Lancet 1:881, 1972.

40. Baume, P. E., and Hunt, J. H. Failure of potent antacid therapy to hasten healing in chronic gastric ulcers. Austral. Ann. Med. 18:113, 1969.

41. Woldman, E. E., and Rowland, V. C. Continuous acid adsorption by aluminum hydroxide drip in the treatment of peptic ulcer. Rev. Gastroent. 3:27, 1936.

42. Cornell, A., and Hollander, F. The efficacy of the drip method in the reduction of gastric acidity. Amer. J. Dig. Dis. 9:332, 1942.

43. Lennard-Jones, J. E., Hart, J. C. D., and Wilcox, P. B. Acidity of gastric contents during nocturnal intragastric drip therapy in patients with duodenal ulcer. Gut 6:274, 1965.

44. Innes, I. R., and Nickerson, M. Drugs inhibiting the action of acetylcholine on structures innervated by postganglionic parasympa-

thetic nerves. Antimuscarinic or atropinic drugs. *In* The Pharmacological Basis of Therapeutics, L. S. Goodman and A. Gilman (eds.), 3rd ed. New York, Macmillan, 1965, p. 521.

45. Sun, D. C. H. Long-term anticholinergic therapy for prevention of recurrence in duodenal ulcer. Amer. J. Dig. Dis. *9*:706, 1964.

46. Juniper, K. The relative effective dose of an anticholinergic drug, glycopyrrolate, on basal gastric secretion and sweat- and salivary-gland activity. Amer. J. Dig. Dis. *12*:439, 1967.

47. Bachrach, W. H. Anticholinergic drugs. Survey of the literature and some experimental observations. Amer. J. Dig. Dis. *3*:743, 1958.

48. Mitchell, R. D., Hunt, J. W., and Grossman, M. I. Inhibition of basal and postprandial gastric secretion by poldine and atropine in patients with peptic ulcer. Gastroenterology *43*:400, 1962.

49. Dreiling, D. A., and Janowitz, H. D. Inhibitory effect of new anticholinergics on the basal and secretin-stimulated pancreatic secretion in patients with and without pancreatic disease. Amer. J. Dig. Dis. *5*:639, 1960.

50. Dotevall, G., Schroder, G., and Walan, A. Effect of poldine, glycopyrrolate and *l*-hyoscyamine on gastric secretion of acid in man. Acta Med. Scand. *177*:169, 1965.

51. Barman, M. L., and Larson, R. K. The effect of glycopyrrolate on nocturnal gastric secretion in peptic ulcer patients. Amer. J. Med. Sci. *246*:325, 1963.

52. Collyns, A. H., and Fordtran, J. S. Controlled analysis of antacids and anticholinergics in modifying gastric acidity and peptic activity after steak in patients with duodenal ulcer. Gastroenterology *48*:812, 1965.

53. Norgaard, R. P., Polter, D. E., Wheeler, J. W., and Fordtran, J. S. Effect of long term anticholinergic therapy on gastric acid secretion, with observations on the serial measurement of peak Histalog response. Gastroenterology *58*:750, 1970.

54. Kaye, M. D., Beck, P., Rhodes, J., and Sweetnam, P. M. Gastric acid secretion in patients with duodenal ulcer treated for one year with anticholinergic drugs. Gut *10*:774, 1969.

55. Walan, A. Studies on peptic ulcer disease with special reference to the effect of *l*-hyoscyamine. Acta Med. Scand. (Suppl.) 516, 1970.

56. Ingelfinger, F. J. Anticholinergic therapy of gastrointestinal disorders. New Eng. J. Med. *268*:1454, 1963.

57. Soergel, K. H., and Hogan, W. J. Rationale for the use of anticholinergic agents in management of duodenal ulcer. Amer. J. Dig. Dis. *9*:657, 1964.

58. Kaye, M. D., Rhodes, J., Beck, P., Sweetnam, P. M., Davies, G. T., and Evans, K. T. A controlled trial of glycopyrronium and *l*-hyoscyamine in the long term treatment of duodenal ulcer. Gut *11*:559, 1970.

59. Trevino, H., Anderson, J., Davey, P. G., and Henley, K. S. The effect of glycopyrrolate on the course of symptomatic duodenal ulcer. Amer. J. Dig. Dis. *12*:983, 1967.

60. Dotevall, G. Comment. Selected summaries. Gastroenterology *60*:1142, 1971.

61. Kaye, M. D. Anticholinergic drugs in duodenal ulcer. Gastroenterology *62*:502, 1972.

62. Leading article. Anticholinergics and duodenal ulcer. Lancet *2*:1173, 1970.

63. Baume, P. E., Hunt, J. H., and Piper, D. W. Glycopyrronium bromide in the treatment of chronic gastric ulcer. Gastroenterology *63*:399, 1972.

Chapter 58

The Zollinger-Ellison Syndrome and Related Diseases

James E. McGuigan

THE ZOLLINGER-ELLISON SYNDROME

In 1955, Zollinger and Ellison described a syndrome[1] characterized by extremely elevated rates of gastric acid secretion, severe and recalcitrant upper gastrointestinal ulcerative disease, and non-beta islet cell tumors of the pancreas. Although others[2, 3] had previously recognized the association of noninsulin secreting islet cell tumors of the pancreas and severe ulcerative disease of the upper gastrointestinal tract, Zollinger and Ellison[1] first suggested that the disease was due to a humoral material secreted by the tumor which might stimulate gastric acid secretion enormously. Time has confirmed this hypothesis. The two original patients described by Zollinger and Ellison had relentlessly progressive and extraordinarily severe ulcer disease, requiring, for each, numerous surgical procedures with eventual total gastrectomy and the identification of non-beta islet cell tumors of the pancreas.

The Zollinger-Ellison syndrome, although distinctly uncommon, is not extremely rare; approximately 700 cases have been recorded in the literature to date. Sixty per cent of patients with the Zollinger-Ellison syndrome are males.[4] The disease has been recognized from early childhood to patients in the tenth decade, but is most common in patients from 20 to 50 years of age.[4, 5] It is a potentially, and often, lethal disease; mortality is usually not due to malignancy, but rather usually results from the extreme effects of hypergastrinism in stimulating enormous amounts of gastric hydrochloric acid, resulting in virulent ulcerative disease of the upper gastrointestinal tract.

Etiology and Pathogenesis. Approximately five years after the suggestion by Zollinger and Ellison of a gastric secretagogue liberated by these tumors, it was demonstrated in tumor extracts.[6, 7] Its biological behavior, virtually from the outset, strongly suggested the hormone gastrin, a known potent stimulant of gastric acid secretion. Subsequent studies, including chemical isolation of a polypeptide with the amino acid composition and peptide mapping pattern identical with that of human gastrin, and demonstration by radioimmunoassay of large amounts of gastrin in the Zollinger-Ellison tumors as well as in sera from patients with the Zollinger-Ellison syndrome have established that gastrin is the agent responsible for the Zollinger-Ellison syndrome.[8-10]

The non-beta islet cell tumors of the pancreas (Figs. 58–1 to 58–3) may be either single or multiple within the substance of the pancreas. In addition, they have been found in the hilus of the spleen, in the

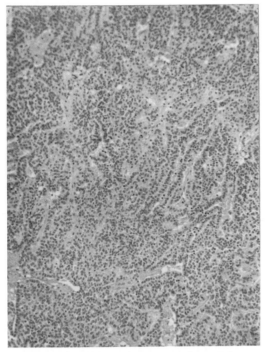

Figure 58–1. Non-beta islet cell, ulcerogenic tumor of the pancreas (Zollinger-Ellison syndrome). Hematoxylin and eosin stain. × 125. (Courtesy of Dr. Marie Greider.)

is more likely a metastatic lesion than an independent focal tumor. The tumors vary enormously in size, ranging from approximately 2 mm up to 20 cm or more in diameter. In approximately 50 per cent of patients with the Zollinger-Ellison syndrome a single tumor is found within the pancreas; further, they are most commonly found in the head and tail of the pancreas, and least commonly in the body. Approximately two-thirds of Zollinger-Ellison tumors are malignant in respect to their biological behavior, histological appearance, or both. Metastases may involve regional lymph nodes, liver, spleen, bone, mediastinum, skin, or peritoneal surfaces.[4, 11]

The original description of the syndrome recognized that these tumors did not contain insulin, giving rise to the term "non-beta islet cell tumor." Insulin-containing and -secreting beta cells may be readily identified by specific staining techniques used with light microscopy and by the morphological characteristics of their granules on electron microscopy. The early suspicion that the tumors might arise from alpha cells of the islets which secrete glucagon has subsequently not been borne out. There is at least one additional class of cells (and perhaps more) in the pancreatic islets: these are the delta cells (also designated as D cells or A_1 cells of Hellmann and Hellerstrom).[12, 13] Approximately 5 to 10 per cent of cells in the islets are delta cells. Recently, fluorescent antibody techniques have demonstrated gastrin to be

walls of the stomach and duodenum, and in regional lymph nodes. Often there is a marked disparity between the biological behavior and the histological appearance of these non-beta islet cell tumors; therefore a nonmalignant appearing adenoma in a lymph node in a patient with the disease

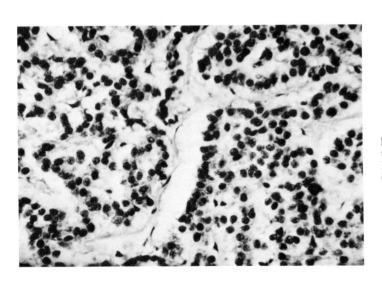

Figure 58–2. Same tumor as in Figure 58–1, at higher magnification (× 400). Cells are malignant. Hematoxylin and eosin stain. (Courtesy of Dr. Marie Greider.)

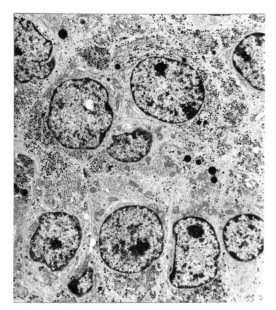

Figure 58–3. Electron photomicrograph of an ulcerogenic tumor of the pancreas (Zollinger-Ellison syndrome). The well differentiated cells contain small secretory granules. The large black granules are lipid bodies. × 4000. (Courtesy of Dr. Marie Greider.)

contained in or on abundant granules which pack the cytoplasm of delta cells in normal human pancreatic tissue.[14, 15] Thus it appears likely that gastrin-containing pancreatic tumors of the Zollinger-Ellison variety originate from delta cells of the pancreatic islets of Langerhans. In many respects they are similar to cells located along the course of the pyloric glands in the antrum of the stomach, which have been shown also by immunofluorescence to contain gastrin (see p. 482).[16, 17]

The parietal cell mass is often greatly enlarged[18] in patients with the Zollinger-Ellison syndrome, and volume may be from three to six times normal. Since studies in experimental animals have demonstrated that the parietal cell mass may be expanded by secretagogues, including pentagastrin,[19] it is likely that the increased numbers of parietal cells in this disease result from their continuous maximal, or near maximal, stimulation by gastrin.

In addition to the presence of the often multiple ulcerations in the upper gastrointestinal tract, there may be other functional and morphological changes in the upper small intestine. The duodenal and proximal jejunal mucosa is often abnormal,[20, 21] with areas of denuded villi, infiltration of the lamina propria by eosinophils and polymorphonuclear leukocytes, edema, hemorrhage, and multiple superficial mucosal erosions. Remaining villi in the regions of abnormal small intestinal mucosa are often stunted and wider than normal. Brunner's glands, which are usually restricted to the proximal duodenum, may also be found in the region of the ligament of Treitz.

Clinical Features and Diagnosis. Patients with the Zollinger-Ellison syndrome usually present to the physician with symptoms referable to ulcer disease of the upper gastrointestinal tract.[11] Often these symptoms are the same as in the common varieties of peptic ulcer disease; however, they are usually much more persistent and more progressive. The distribution of the ulcers, on the other hand, is similar to ordinary peptic ulcer; i.e., the most common site is the first part of the duodenum, and the stomach is second in frequency.[11] Indeed, 75 per cent of ulcers in this disease are located in these positions and are usually not multiple. However, ulceration distal in the second, third, or fourth portions of the duodenum raises the suspicion of the Zollinger-Ellison syndrome, because these sites are unusual for peptic ulcer disease.[4, 11, 22] Further, as in the two patients originally described by Zollinger and Ellison, the jejunum may contain an ulcer. This phenomenon is consistent with an upper jejunal pH of 1.0 to 2.0 in patients with the Zollinger-Ellison syndrome. In a large series,[4] 25 per cent of ulcers were located in sites in which ulcer disease is not usually present, 14 per cent being in the distal duodenum and 11 per cent in the jejunum. Patients with Zollinger-Ellison tumors have two or more ulcerations at adjacent sites or widely separated; thus they have been noted simultaneously in the stomach, duodenum, and jejunum in some patients.

Ulcers are often large, frequently exceeding 2 cm in diameter; they also may be moderate or small in size. Although giant ulcer is by no means pathognomonic of the Zollinger-Ellison syndrome, it should alert the physician to the possibility of the Zollinger-Ellison syndrome.

Another feature which characterizes the Zollinger-Ellison syndrome is the frequent failure of patients to respond satisfactorily to conventional methods of treatment for peptic ulcer disease. It should be emphasized, however, that some patients will respond in some degree to medical management of their peptic ulcer disease.[23-25] In addition, conventional surgical procedures directed to the correction of usual peptic ulcer disease may relieve signs and symptoms caused by ulcerogenic tumor of the pancreas; however, this is usually transient, with symptoms returning shortly after surgery. Ulceration at the anastomosis and at sites distal to the surgical procedure is common when surgery for peptic ulcer is performed and the ulcerogenic tumor of the pancreas is unrecognized. Following partial gastric resection or vagotomy and pyloroplasty, the ulcerations are usually multiple and often penetrate or perforate.[5] To summarize, the Zollinger-Ellison syndrome is suspect under the following circumstances: in multiple ulcers of the upper gastrointestinal tract; in ulcers distal to the duodenal bulb; when medical treatment of peptic ulcer disease is ineffective; with rapid recurrence of peptic ulcer following surgery for ulcer disease; and when giant ulceration is noted.

Some characteristic radiographic abnormalities may assist in the diagnosis of the Zollinger-Ellison syndrome (Fig. 58–4). Often the gastric rugal folds will be extremely prominent, and in the absence of demonstrable obstruction the stomach may contain large amounts of fluid.[26] The prominence of the gastric folds may also suggest Menetrier's disease or gastric lymphoma; such prominent gastric mucosal folds, particularly along the greater curvature, may also occasionally be found in apparently normal individuals. Prominence of the mucosal folds may also be found throughout the duodenum and, in some instances, in the jejunum. The normally fine mucosal folds may be thickened, widened and abnormally separated from each other (Fig. 58–5). Large amounts of fluid may be contained in the lumen of the upper gastrointestinal tract.

The diagnosis of the Zollinger-Ellison syndrome is strongly suspected in patients with a compatible clinical history, particularly those in whom rates of gastric acid secretion are generously increased. Slightly more than half of patients with the Zollinger-Ellison syndrome have basal gastric acid secretory rates which exceed 15 mEq per hour, and approximately two-thirds of patients with the Zollinger-Ellison syndrome have acid secretory rates which exceed 10 mEq per hour. This excessive acid secretion, as indicated previously, is the result of liberation of gastrin from the tumor. Additional information may be gained, in some patients, by measuring gastric acid secretory rates following maximal stimulation with histamine or Histalog (betazole). Such stimulation of patients with the Zollinger-Ellison syndrome does not increase the rate of gastric acid secretion nearly so much as in normal individuals or those with common peptic ulcer disease. In the latter group basal gastric acid per hour is usually less than 60 per cent of the amount secreted after a maximal dose of histamine or Histalog,[27, 28] whereas it is greater than 60 per cent in many patients with the Zollinger-Ellison

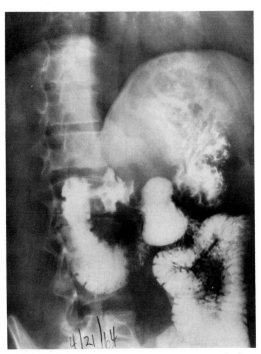

Figure 58–4. Large greater curvature and duodenal ulcers associated with the Zollinger-Ellison syndrome. Note also the edematous gastric and small bowel folds. (Courtesy of Dr. M. H. Sleisenger.)

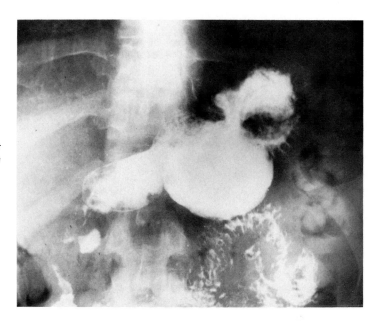

Figure 58–5. Postbulbar ulcer and enlarged jejunal folds in the Zollinger-Ellison syndrome.

syndrome. Comparison of the *concentration* of acid before and after stimulation may be more helpful than the measurement of acid output per unit time, in distinguishing usual peptic ulcer disease from this syndrome.[29] Gastric acid secretory studies assist in the diagnosis, but do not make it certain. There is substantial overlap in rates of basal gastric acid secretion among normal individuals, those with duodenal ulcer, and those with the Zollinger-Ellison syndrome.[28] It is not always possible to distinguish between patients with the Zollinger-Ellison syndrome and those with common peptic ulcer disease by comparison of their basal and stimulated rates of gastric acid secretion.[28] Arteriography is only occasionally helpful in identifying tumors of the Zollinger-Ellison variety.[30, 31]

Bioassay, i.e., the capacity of serum or urine to stimulate gastric acid secretion in the experimental animal, has been used as a method for identifying patients with the Zollinger-Ellison syndrome.[32-34] This method is less sensitive and specific than radioimmunoassay for gastrin.

At present, the most reliable method for establishing the diagnosis of the Zollinger-Ellison syndrome is the measurement of increased serum or plasma concentrations of gastrin by radioimmunoassay.[9, 35] Patients with Zollinger-Ellison syndrome usually have gastrin levels which are greater than 300 pg per milliliter, whereas most normal individuals, and persons with other varieties of peptic ulcer disease, usually have serum gastrin concentrations of less than 200 pg per milliliter (averaging approximately 80 pg per milliliter).[36, 37] Thus a markedly elevated fasting serum or plasma gastrin concentration in a patient with compatible clinical features establishes the diagnosis. (See pp. 555 to 558.)

It is worth pointing out, however, that marked hypergastrinemia is not specific for the Zollinger-Ellison syndrome. Markedly elevated serum or plasma gastrin levels are found in many patients with pernicious anemia,[35, 38] which in terms of gastric acid secretion represents the antithesis of the Zollinger-Ellison syndrome. In the latter the marked elevations in serum gastrin concentrations are due to gastrin liberation from the islet cell tumors. The mechanism by which hypergastrinemia occurs in pernicious anemia appears to be entirely different. In normal man and in other mammals the most effective mechanism for inhibition of gastrin release is that of acidification of the antral contents; antral acidification effectively inhibits gastrin release because of a variety of stimuli, including feeding, antral distention, vagal stimulation, and other varieties of cholinergic stimulation. When the pH of the antral contents is reduced to 3 or lower, gastrin release is inhibited; when the pH is reduced to 1.5, gastrin release is completely eliminated.[39] Pernicious anemia is characterized by gastric achlorhydria, and the pH of the gastric contents in this disease is 6 or higher even following maximal histamine stimulation. Since inhibition is not present in pernicious anemia, the hypergastrinemia represents a defect in the normal mechanism for feedback control of gastrin release. That this hypothesis is correct is supported by observations that marked reductions in serum gastrin follow instillation of 0.1 N hydrochloric acid in the stomach in these patients.[35]

Patients with Zollinger-Ellison tumors may have other symptoms in addition to those associated with ulcers of the upper gastrointestinal tract. Diarrhea is frequent, and it may precede symptoms of ulcer by as much as eight years; 7 per cent of patients have diarrhea without ulcer disease.[4] Diarrhea is due principally to the effects of large amounts of hydrochloric acid poured into the upper gastrointestinal tract. It may be reduced or eliminated by aspiration of gastric juice from the stomach. In addition to excessive hydrochloric acid secretion, hypergastrinemia also stimulates pepsin release by gastric chief cells. Since pH values as low as 1 and 3.6 have been recorded in the proximal and distal jejunum, respectively, pepsin is activated, contributing to ulcerations and other inflammatory changes at these loci. Large amounts of circulating gastrin may contribute to the problems by increasing intestinal secretion of potassium and reducing jejunal absorption of water and sodium, an effect unrelated to the pH of the intestines because it has been noted in the absence of gastric acid hypersecretion.[40] These patients do not have watery diarrhea, although they have measurable decreases in sodium and water absorption. It is possible that gastrin may inhibit small bowel absorption, but gastric hypersecretion is necessary for clinical symptomatology, including diarrhea. In addition, patients with Zollinger-Ellison tumors may have malabsorption of a variety of other substances, including fat. The often associated steatorrhea results from inactivation of pancreatic lipase at low pH in the upper small intestine.[20] Pancreatic lipase is exquisitely susceptible to acidification, becoming irreversibly denatured and therefore ineffective. The result is that triglycerides are not split into fatty acids, monoglycerides, and diglycerides. Bile salts may be also precipitated in the small intestine in the acid milieu, further contributing to steatorrhea, because micelles, necessary for the facilitation of fatty acid and monoglyceride absorption, are not formed (see pp. 250 to 277). Patients with the Zollinger-Ellison syndrome may also develop vitamin B_{12} malabsorption which is not correctable by the addition of intrinsic factor.[20] Although secretion of intrinsic factor appears to be normal, the low pH in some way interferes with its role in facilitation of absorption of vitamin B_{12}. The precise mechanism by which the low pH reduces the activity of intrinsic factor is not known; however, when the pH is adjusted to 7, inhibition disappears.

A relationship exists between serum gastrin levels and calcium administration in patients with the Zollinger-Ellison syndrome.[41] During and after intravenous infusion of calcium, serum gastrin concentration increases markedly.[41] Perhaps calcium infusion stimulates gastrin release,[41] because it also increases the rate of gastric acid secretion to 75 per cent (or greater) of those achieved with maximal Histalog stimulation in patients with the Zollinger-Ellison syndrome.[42, 43] In contrast, the acid response to calcium infusion in duodenal ulcer patients is only approximately a third as great as the response to Histalog.

Patients with the Zollinger-Ellison syndrome may also have tumors, benign or malignant, of other endocrine organs, the most common of which are parathyroid tumors (vide infra).

Treatment. Long-term medical treatment is uniformly unsatisfactory for patients with the Zollinger-Ellison syndrome; it may, however, benefit some patients transiently. For this reason a favorable temporary response to medical treatment does not eliminate the diagnosis of the Zollinger-Ellison syndrome. Intensive medical therapy, including the use of frequent and effective antacids, has an important role in the preparation of patients for surgery and for treatment prior to surgical intervention (see p. 734). Patients have responded symptomatically to intensive treatment with anticholinergic agents associated usually with transient reduction in rates of gastric acid secretion.

The treatment of patients with ulcerogenic tumors of the pancreas is surgical. In considering the indicated mode of surgical treatment, one must remember that the major clinical threat is the physiological effect of continuous excessive gastrin release, not the biological effects of the tumors. Despite their frequent metastases and their malignant histological appearance, these tumors usually do not cause death. Major morbidity and death usually result from complications of ulcer: perforation, fistula formation, hemorrhage, and all the ravages of a physiologically malignant and relentless ulcerative disease of the upper gastrointestinal tract.

Subtotal resection is often followed by ulcer of the jejunum (Fig. 58–6). The results of surgery for the Zollinger-Ellison syndrome indicate that total gastrectomy is the treatment of choice for this disease. This conclusion is based on observations that mortality is lowest in patients with the Zollinger-Ellison syndrome in

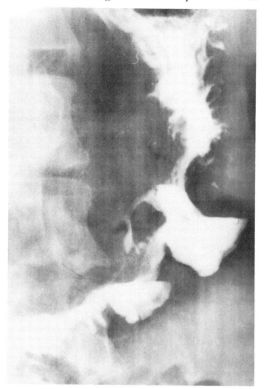

Figure 58–6. Huge jejunal ulcer in Zollinger-Ellison syndrome after subtotal gastrectomy. (Courtesy of Dr. M. H. Sleisenger.)

whom total gastrectomy is performed as the initial surgical procedure.[44] A review of the literature up to 1966 reveals that of patients with the Zollinger-Ellison syndrome receiving total gastrectomy as the first operation, 87 per cent were alive. With multiple surgical procedures, 73 per cent were alive. Among 400 patients who did not undergo surgery, only 27 per cent survived. Thus whether the patient has multiple tumors or even metastatic tumor, total gastrectomy is the surgical procedure of choice. What decision should be made for the patient who, after careful examination, appears to have a solitary, circumscribed, and apparently readily resectable ulcerogenic islet cell tumor? Is resection of the tumor alone satisfactory treatment? It must be considered, in view of the frequent complications of total gastrectomy and the potentially long life span of these patients after diagnosis and treatment. The application of gastrin radioimmunoassay in this clinical situation may permit tumor resection alone in such individuals. Reduction in gastrin levels to normal following tumor resection, accompanied by clinical improvement, would provide strong evidence for complete removal of tumor. The patient should then be followed by serum gastrin measurements to help detect early tumor recurrence.

Gastric irradiation has been used in isolated instances to reduce gastric acid secretion in patients with Zollinger-Ellison tumors. However, this therapy has not generally been satisfactory, and is not recommended.

Prognosis. After total gastrectomy, patients with the Zollinger-Ellison tumor, even without resection of the tumor, usually improve markedly and ulcers disappear. Although these patients are subject to the same complications as other patients following total gastrectomy, they live longer than patients on whom total gastrectomy is performed for carcinoma of the stomach, and therefore they have need for exogenous vitamin B_{12} administration, because vitamin B_{12} stores in the liver will be depleted within two to four years after gastrectomy. In addition, since hepatic storage of vitamin B_{12} may be reduced preoperatively, it is wise to treat such patients with 50 μg of parenteral vitamin B_{12}

monthly indefinitely after total gastric resection.

In some instances pancreatic tumor, both primary and metastatic, of the Zollinger-Ellison syndrome has been observed to regress and even—in the case of metastatic tumor—to disappear after total gastric resection.[45] The explanation for this phenomenon is not clear, although a trophic influence exerted by the stomach on the tumor has been suggested. It must be stressed that the tumor does not regress in most of these patients after total gastric resection. After total gastric resection fasting serum gastrin concentrations may remain relatively stable, may fall toward normal (in those individuals in whom tumor has apparently regressed), or may progressively increase.[46] In our experience a progressive and continuing increase in serum gastrin concentrations has been associated with unusually rapid progression of the tumor and a poor prognosis.

The presence of extensive metastases at the time of recognition does not contraindicate total gastrectomy, because many of these patients markedly improve following resection and live for many years. In approximately 10 per cent of patients with Zollinger-Ellison tumors, there is also diffuse islet cell hyperplasia. The islet cell hyperplasia may be an isolated finding, or it may accompany a demonstrated islet cell tumor.

DIARRHEA AND HYPOKALEMIA WITH NON-BETA ISLET TUMORS OF THE PANCREAS (THE PANCREATIC CHOLERA SYNDROME)

There are some patients with non-beta islet tumors of the pancreas who have voluminous diarrhea and massive losses of fluid and electrolytes, often with the development of profound hypokalemia and metabolic acidosis; the rates of gastric acid secretion are not increased in these patients.[47-49] Because of the extreme losses of fluid and electrolytes in this disorder, it has been referred to by some as "pancreatic cholera." This entity is discussed in detail on pages 365 to 370, and is reviewed here only briefly.

Etiology and Pathogenesis. In these patients, just as in patients with the Zollinger-Ellison syndrome, the cause of the disease is non-beta islet cell tumors of the pancreas; however, in contrast to the Zollinger-Ellison syndrome these tumors neither contain nor secrete gastrin. It is suspected that they liberate a humoral agent which results in the massive losses of fluid and electrolytes. The precise nature of this postulated physiologically active agent has not been defined, but some investigators suspect that it may be secretin;[50] others have suspected prostaglandins. Convincing evidence for either hypothesis is not available. The gastric inhibitor peptide (GIP) has also been proposed as a potential cause for this syndrome.

Clinical Features and Diagnosis. In this syndrome the stool volume may be enormous—often as much as 5 to 8 liters per day. The watery diarrhea is associated with losses of potassium which may be as great as 100 to 200 mEq per day. Profound hypokalemia and metabolic acidosis may develop; indeed, all the serious signs and symptoms of hypokalemia, including nephropathy, are commonly found in these patients. Gastric acid secretion is normal or, more frequently, reduced or absent. After resection of the islet cell tumors in some patients, markedly reduced or absent gastric acid secretion has returned to normal.[49, 51] This finding suggests that, in addition to promoting intestinal losses of fluids and electrolytes, the humoral agent released by these tumors inhibits gastric acid secretion. Unlike patients with the Zollinger-Ellison syndrome, aspiration of the gastric contents does not relieve or diminish the watery diarrhea. In order to prevent hypovolemia, shock, and death, large volumes of fluid containing electrolytes must be administered. Hypercalcemia, caused by the circulation of a parathormone-like material, which also may be liberated from these tumors, is also evident during the course of some patients with this syndrome. The exact cell type of the pancreatic islet from which these tumors arise is not known.

Treatment. The treatment of this hypokalemic diarrheal syndrome is resection of the islet cell tumor. After complete resection of the tumor the symptoms dramatically disappear. As indicated, reduced or absent gastric acid secretion may return to normal. Corticosteroid administration has been successful in the temporary treatment of this syndrome;[49] however, in view of the severity of symptoms and the effectiveness of resection, corticosteroid therapy cannot be substituted for surgery.

Prognosis. Complete excision of the tumor is usually followed by dramatic cessation of symptoms and return to health.

MULTIPLE ENDOCRINE ADENOMAS

In some patients multiple endocrine tumors, adenomas or carcinomas, may arise simultaneously or at different times from several endocrine organs; this disorder has been referred to as Wermer's syndrome.[52-54] An instance of two or more tumors arising in different endocrine glands was described in 1903.[52] Its recognition is of historical interest, because it shortly followed the description of the first hormone, secretin, and actually preceded by two years Edkin's discovery of gastrin.[55] Ulcer disease of the gastrointestinal tract occurring with endocrine tumors was first recognized in 1939.[53] Ulceration of the upper gastrointestinal tract occurs at some time in over 50 per cent of patients with multiple endocrine adenomas. The adenomas, although demonstrable histologically in their respective endocrine glands, do not in all instances give clinical or physiological evidence of hormone secretion.

Etiology and Pathogenesis. Wermer's studies have indicated that the development of multiple endocrine tumors may be transmitted as an autosomal dominant gene with variable expressivity.[54] Clinical symptoms of hormone excess may result from endocrine cell hyperplasia, adenoma, or carcinoma. The factor or factors responsible for stimulation of the development of changes leading to the hyperendocrine activity in the various organs have not been defined.

Clinical Features and Diagnosis. In an extensive evaluation of patients with this syndrome, pancreatic islet cell involvement was found in 69 of 85 patients.[56] Islet cell involvement included disorders of both beta cells and other cell types. Hypoglycemia, the cause of death in five patients, was found in approximately 36 per cent of these patients. Although islet cell carcinoma was histologically demonstrable in 21 patients, only one patient at the time of review was known to have died of carcinoma.

Ulcer disease of the upper gastrointestinal tract is present in more than 50 per cent of patients with multiple endocrine adenomas. The ulcerations are found in atypical locations and are multiple in approximately half these patients.[56, 57] They are almost invariably found in patients with adenomas or adenocarcinomas of the pancreatic islets. In this syndrome gastrin-containing tumors arising in the islets of the pancreas may be present in association with other endocrine adenomas. Within our present framework of knowledge it appears that the Zollinger-Ellison syndrome fits within the broad spectrum of the multiple endocrine adenoma syndrome. This view is further supported by the frequent finding of additional endocrine tumors in patients with the Zollinger-Ellison syndrome and the frequency of the latter in families with multiple endocrine adenomatosis. In patients with the Zollinger-Ellison syndrome, 21 per cent were found to have additional endocrine disease; pituitary tumors were found in 17 of these 56 patients.[4] The most common endocrine abnormality found in association with the Zollinger-Ellison syndrome is that of adenomas of the parathyroid glands. Hypoglycemia, caused by insulin-secreting beta cell adenomas or carcinomas, may also be associated with the Zollinger-Ellison tumors.

Treatment. The treatment of endocrine adenomas is surgical. Required treatment is dictated by the recognition of endocrine abnormalities resulting from excessive hormone release. It is now evident that many tumors found at postmortem examination in patients with multiple endocrine adenomas or the Zollinger-Ellison syndrome go unrecognized during life because of the absence of overt clinical manifestations.

Prognosis. Just as the gravity of the Zollinger-Ellison syndrome lies in hypergastrinemia, the life of the patient with the multiple endocrine adenoma syndrome is threatened by the physiological effects of the hormones of the hyperfunctioning endocrine glandular elements. Death may result from the malignant behavior of these tumors; it is much less likely than that caused by the action of excessive hormone release. Symptoms of excessive endocrine activity are relieved when the offending tumor or hyperplastic gland is removed.

ISLET CELL TUMORS OF THE PANCREAS WITH MULTIPLE ENDOCRINE EXPRESSIONS

Isolated cases have been reported of pancreatic islet tumors which secrete multiple hormones with their respective, diverse physiological effects.

Etiology and Pathogenesis. Tumors arising at various sites in the body, including from islets of the pancreas, may contain and release multiple hormones. For example, an islet cell carcinoma of the pancreas has been described which contained and released large amounts of ACTH, melanocyte-stimulating hormone, gastrin, and glucagon.[58] In addition, this particular tumor may have contained excessive amounts of parathormone and antidiuretic hormone. The mechanisms responsible for development of tumors liberating multiple hormonal substances have not been elucidated. It is evident that ACTH release is particularly common in such tumors. The tumors releasing more than one hormone have included islet cell carcinoma, carcinoid, pheochromocytoma, and oat cell carcinoma.[58, 59] Ulcerations of the upper gastrointestinal tract, with or without the demonstration of hypergastrinemia, are common among such patients.

Clinical Features and Diagnosis. The patient is often brought to the attention of the physician by the endocrine manifestations of the tumor. Tumors releasing multiple substances may arise in the pancreas, the adrenal cortex, the mediastinum, and the lung. Carcinomas of the ileum have also been described as releasing multiple endocrine substances, including ACTH and serotonin.

Treatment. Although the numbers of reported cases of multiple endocrine

agents being released from single tumors is small, the available literature suggests a high incidence of malignancy in such tumors.[58, 59] The treatment of the tumor is resection, which, when complete, results in the relief of symptoms caused by release of multiple physiologically active agents.

Prognosis. Total removal of the tumor is associated with clinical improvement. The numbers of patients with such abnormalities are too small to be certain of long-term prognosis, particularly in view of their relatively recent recognition and their apparent tendency to be malignant.

ISLET CELL HYPERPLASIA (NESIDIOBLASTOSIS)

In some patients with the clinical features of the Zollinger-Ellison syndrome, marked hyperplasia of the islets of Langerhans may be found in the pancreas.

Etiology and Pathogenesis. Islet cell hyperplasia is characterized by the increased numbers and size of islet cells in the pancreas; frequently they are also more densely cellular. The difficulty in characterizing these multiple or frequently densely cellular islets has given rise, in some instances, to the use of the term *microadenomatosis*. The term *nesidioblastosis* has also been applied to describe diffuse proliferation of islet cells of the pancreas.

Islet cell hyperplasia, in patients with the clinical symptom complex of the Zollinger-Ellison syndrome, has been observed both in the presence and in the absence of simultaneously recognizable Zollinger-Ellison tumors.[60] The relationship between the islet cell hyperplasia and the Zollinger-Ellison tumors has not been defined. It is not certain that islet hyperplasia of this variety is present without tumor; or perhaps in some instances the ulcerogenic islet cell tumor may escape recognition. It has been speculated that these hyperplastic islet cells contain and release a humoral agent, i.e., gastrin, which participates in the pathogenesis of the Zollinger-Ellison syndrome. This suggestion has not been proved.

Clinical Features and Diagnosis. The symptoms and complications in these patients with hyperplasia of the islet cells are not distinguishable from those of patients with the Zollinger-Ellison syndrome with adenomas or carcinomas of the islets. Islet cell hyperplasia may be recognized surgically, early in its course; later, tumors of the pancreas, which have escaped prior recognition, may be found.

Treatment. The treatment of patients with symptoms and complications characteristic of the Zollinger-Ellison syndrome caused by islet cell hyperplasia is surgical. In many instances these patients have been treated successfully by total gastrectomy. Some patients have improved substantially after resection of a substantial portion of the pancreas containing islet cell hyperplasia.

Prognosis. In general, patients with hyperplasia of the islets of Langerhans with symptoms characteristic of the Zollinger-Ellison syndrome have the same potential complications as those with tumors.

HYPERPARATHYROIDISM AND PEPTIC ULCER DISEASE

An assortment of questions remain to be answered concerning possible relationships between hyperparathyroidism and peptic ulcer disease. Some authors have suggested that there is an increased incidence of peptic ulcer disease in patients with hyperparathyroidism; however, at present such an increased association of peptic ulcer disease with hyperparathyroidism has not been proved. The incidence of peptic ulcer disease in the general population in the United States has been estimated as approximately 15 per cent;[61] however, the varying expressions of peptic ulcer disease make it difficult to establish this incidence with satisfactory confidence. Some retrospective studies of patients with hyperparathyroidism have suggested incidences of peptic ulcer disease ranging from 20 to 30 per cent.[62, 63] Conversely, there have been reports of the incidence of ulcer disease and hyperparathyroidism at as low as 9.1 per cent, failing to affirm a clear-cut statistical association between hyperparathyroidism and peptic ulcer disease.[64]

Clinical Features and Diagnosis.

When peptic ulcer disease occurs in association with hyperparathyroidism and is not due to a simultaneously occurring islet cell tumor of the pancreas, the clinical features are those of common peptic ulcer disease. The ulcer disease is more prevalent in males; 80 per cent of the ulcers are in the duodenum, and, just as with usual peptic ulcer disease, almost always in its first portion. Unlike the Zollinger-Ellison syndrome the patients do not have marked gastric hypersecretion. Following parathyroidectomy there have been instances in which the rate of gastric acid secretion has decreased substantially; however, usually no significant changes in acid secretory rates are observed,[65-68] and the procedure may be followed by no significant change in the status of the ulcer disease. In some patients the peptic ulcer disease responds to conventional therapy without parathyroidectomy. In other instances symptoms improve remarkably after parathyroidectomy.

Because of potential relationships between peptic ulcer disease and hyperparathyroidism, a variety of studies have been conducted in attempts to define the relationships between the serum calcium levels and gastric acid secretion. Patients with hypoparathyroidism, whose serum calcium levels are usually less than 7.0 mg per 100 ml, are usually achlorhydric. Following treatment with calcium, vitamin D, or parathormone with subsequent elevation of plasma calcium to eucalcemic levels, gastric acid secretory rates in such patients usually return to normal.[69] Calcium infusion with consequent increased plasma calcium concentrations in man results in increases in gastric acid secretion.[70] It has been suggested that calcium may exert its effect on acid secretion by promoting gastrin release.[41] Studies in normal individuals and those with the Zollinger-Ellison syndrome[41] show increases in serum and plasma gastrin concentrations after intravenous infusion with calcium. In dogs calcium infusion does not raise serum gastrin levels or stimulate gastric acid secretion. These related, and perhaps relevant, observations do not, however, substantiate the relationship between hyperparathyroidism and peptic ulcer disease, nor do they prove that peptic ulcer disease, if resulting from hyperparathyroidism, necessarily results from excessive gastrin release.

Treatment. The treatment of peptic ulcer disease in association with hyperparathyroidism would appear, at present, to be that indicated for the treatment of the two individual diseases. Approach to the hyperparathyroidism would usually be surgical, and the treatment of the peptic ulcer would be that indicated by the clinical features in the individual patient. Certainly the occurrence of peptic ulcer disease in association with hyperparathyroidism should make the physician alert to the possibility that the patient may have multiple endocrine adenoma syndrome, with excessive gastrin release, perhaps from an islet cell tumor of the pancreas. It is probable that some of the observed association between ulcer disease of the upper gastrointestinal tract and hypercalcemic hyperparathyroidism may be that caused by the presence of gastrin-releasing tumors of the pancreas, which may or may not be recognized.

Prognosis. The bulk of currently available information would indicate that the prognosis of peptic ulcer disease in association with hyperparathyroidism is similar to the usual, more common variety of peptic ulcer disease. When the ulcer disease represents an associated Zollinger-Ellison syndrome, conventional medical and surgical modes for common peptic ulcer disease, as already noted above, will not be successful.

REFERENCES

1. Zollinger, R. M., and Ellison, E. H.   Primary peptic ulcerations of the jejunum associated with islet cell tumors of the pancreas. Ann. Surg. 142:709, 1955.
2. Seiler, S., and Zinninger, M. M.   Massive islet cell tumor of pancreas without hypoglycemia. Surg. Gynec. Obstet. 82:301, 1946.
3. Forty, R., and Barrett, G. M.   Peptic ulceration of third part of duodenum, associated with islet cell tumors. Brit. J. Surg. 40:60, 1952.
4. Ellison, E. H., and Wilson, S. D.   The Zollinger-Ellison syndrome: Reappraisal and evaluation of 260 registered cases. Ann. Surg. 160:512, 1964.
5. Wilson, S. D., and Ellison, E. H.   Total gastric resection in children with the Zollinger-Ellison syndrome. Arch. Surg. 91:165, 1965.
6. Gregory, R. A., Tracy, H. J., French, J. M., and Sircus, W.   Extraction of gastrin-like substance from pancreatic tumour in case of Zollinger-Ellison syndrome. Lancet 1:1045, 1960.
7. Rawson, A. B., England, M. T., Gillam, G. G., French, J. M., and Stammers, F. A. R.   Zollinger-Ellison syndrome with diarrhoea and malabsorption: Observations on patient before and after pancreatic islet-cell tumour removal without resort to gastric surgery. Lancet 2:131, 1960.
8. Gregory, R. A., Grossman, M. I., Tracy, H. J., and Bentley, P. H.   Nature of gastric secretagogue in Zollinger-Ellison tumours. Lancet 2:543, 1967.
9. McGuigan, J. E., and Trudeau, W. L.   Immunochemical measurement of elevated levels of gastrin in the serum of patients with pancreatic tumors of the Zollinger-Ellison variety. New Eng. J. Med. 278:1308, 1968.
10. Gregory, R. A., Tracy, H. J., and Agarwal, K. L.   Amino acid constitution of two gastrins isolated from Zollinger-Ellison tumour tissue. Gut 10:603, 1969.
11. Way, L., Goldman, L., and Dunphy, J. E.   Zollinger-Ellison syndrome: An analysis of twenty five cases. Amer. J. Surg. 116:293, 1968.
12. Bloom, N.   New type of granular cell in islets of Langerhans of man. Anat. Rec. 49:363, 1931.
13. Hellerstrom, C., and Hellman, B.   Some aspects of silver impregnation of the islets of Langerhans in rat. Acta Endocr. 35:518, 1960.
14. Lomsky, R., Langr., F., and Vortel, V.   Immunohistochemical demonstration of gastrin in mammalian islets of Langerhans. Nature 223:618, 1969.
15. Greider, M. H., and McGuigan, J. E.   Cellular localization of gastrin in the human pancreas. Diabetes 20:389, 1971.
16. McGuigan, J. E.   Gastric mucosal intracellular localization of gastrin by immunofluorescence. Gastroenterology 55:315, 1968.
17. McGuigan, J. E., and Greider, M. H.   Correlative immunochemical and light microscopic studies of the gastrin cell of the antral mucosa. Gastroenterology 60:223, 1971.
18. Zollinger, R. M., and Moore, F. T.   Zollinger-Ellison syndrome comes of age. J.A.M.A. 204:361, 1968.
19. Crean, G. P., Marshall, M. W., and Rumsey, R. D.   Parietal cell hyperplasia induced by the administration of pentagastrin (ICI 50,123) in rats. Gastroenterology 57:147, 1969.
20. Shimoda, S. S., Saunders, D. R., and Rubin, C. E.   The Zollinger-Ellison syndrome with steatorrhea. Mechanisms of fat and vitamin B_{12} malabsorption. Gastroenterology 55:705, 1968.
21. Mansbach, C. M., Wilkins, R. M., Dobbins, W. O., and Taylor, M. P.   Intestinal mucosal function and structure in the steatorrhea of Zollinger-Ellison syndrome. Arch. Intern. Med. 121:487, 1968.
22. Guida, P. M., Todd, J. E., Moore, S. W., and Beal, J. M.   Zollinger-Ellison syndrome with interesting variations. Amer. J. Surg. 112:807, 1966.
23. Shimoda, S. S., and Rubin, C. E.   The Zollinger-Ellison syndrome with steatorrhea. Anticholinergic treatment followed by total gas-

trectomy and colonic interposition. Gastroenterology 55:695, 1968.

24. Cook, B. H., and Lennard-Jones, J. E. Effect of antisecretory drugs on gastric hypersecretion in endocrine adenoma syndromes. Lancet 2:247, 1966.

25. Shuster, F., and Alexander, H. C. Antacid relief of diarrhea in Zollinger-Ellison syndrome. J.A.M.A. 208:2162, 1969.

26. Melnyk, C. S., Krippaehne, W. W., Benson, J. A., Jr., and Dunphy, J. E. Spontaneous remission of Zollinger-Ellison syndrome. Arch. Intern. Med. 115:42, 1965.

27. Marks, I. N., Selzer, G., Louw, J. H., and Bank, S. Zollinger-Ellison syndrome in Bantu woman, with isolation of gastrin-like substance from primary and secondary tumors. I. Case report. Gastroenterology 41:77, 1961.

28. Ayogi, T., and Summerskill, W. H. J. Gastric secretion with ulcerogenic islet cell tumor: Importance of basal acid output. Arch. Intern. Med. 117:667, 1966.

29. Ruppert, R. D., Greenberger, N. J., Beman, F. M., and McCullugh, F. M. Gastric secretion in ulcerogenic tumors of the pancreas. Ann. Intern. Med. 67:808, 1967.

30. Alfidi, R. J., Skillern, P. F., and Crile, G. Arteriographic manifestations of the Zollinger-Ellison syndrome. Cleveland Clin. Quart. 36:41, 1969.

31. Thomas, R. L., Robinson, A. E., Johnsrude, I. S., Goodrich, J. K., and Lester, R. G. The demonstration of an insulin and gastrin producing tumor by angiography and pancreatic scannings. Amer. J. Roent. 104:646, 1968.

32. Bader, J. P., Bonfils, S., Laudat, P., Dubrasquet, M., and Lambling, A. Le pouvoir gastro-secretagogue des urines dans le syndrome de Zollinger-Ellison. Rev. Internat. Hepat. 16:723, 1966.

33. Lai, S. K. Studies on gastrin. Gut 5:327, 1964.

34. Moore, F. T., Murat, J. E., Endahl, G. L., Baker, J. I., and Zollinger, R. M. Diagnosis of ulcerogenic tumor of the pancreas by bioassay. Ann. J. Surg. 113:735, 1967.

35. Yalow, R. S., and Berson, S. A. Radioimmunoassay of gastrin. Gastroenterology 58:1, 1970.

36. Trudeau, W. L., and McGuigan, J. E. Serum gastrin levels in patients with peptic ulcer disease. Gastroenterology 59:6, 1970.

37. Trudeau, W. L., and McGuigan, J. E. Relations between serum gastrin levels and rates of gastric hydrochloric acid secretion. New Eng. J. Med. 284:408, 1971.

38. McGuigan, J. E., and Trudeau, W. L. Serum gastrin concentrations in pernicious anemia. New Eng. J. Med. 282:358, 1970.

39. Uvnäs, B. Discussion of Schofield, B.: Inhibition by acid of gastrin release. Gastrin (UCLA Forum in Medical Sciences No. 5), M. I. Grossman (ed.). Berkeley, University of California Press, 1966, p. 186.

40. Wright, H. K., Hersh, T., Floch, M. H., and Weinstein, L. D. Impaired intestinal absorption in the Zollinger-Ellison syndrome independent of gastric hypersecretion. Amer. J. Surg. 119:250, 1970.

41. Trudeau, W. L., and McGuigan, J. E. Effects of calcium on serum gastrin in the Zollinger-Ellison syndrome. New Eng. J. Med. 281:862, 1969.

42. Basso, N., and Passaro, E., Jr. Calcium-stimulated gastric secretion in the Zollinger-Ellison syndrome. Arch. Surg. 101:399, 1970.

43. Passaro, E., Jr., Basso, N., Sanchez, R. E., and Gordon, H. E. Newer studies in the Zollinger-Ellison syndrome. Amer. J. Surg. 120:138, 1970.

44. Wilson, S. E., and Ellison, E. H. Survival in patients with the Zollinger-Ellison syndrome, treated by total gastrectomy. Ann. Surg. 111:787, 1966.

45. Friesen, S. R. A gastric factor in the pathogenesis of the Zollinger-Ellison syndrome. Amer. J. Surg. 168:483, 1968.

46. Friesen, S. R., Bolinger, R. E., Pearse, A. G. E., and McGuigan, J. E. Serum gastrin levels in malignant Zollinger-Ellison syndrome after gastrectomy and hypophysectomy. Ann. Surg. 172:504, 1970.

47. Verner, J. E., and Morrison, A. B. Islet cell tumor and a syndrome of refractory watery diarrhea and hypokalemia. Amer. J. Med. 25:374, 1958.

48. Edmeads, J. G., Matthews, N. T., McPhedran, N. T., and Ezrin, C. Diarrhea caused by pancreatic islet cell tumors. Canad. Med. Assn. J. 86:847, 1962.

49. Marks, I. N., Bank, S., and Louw, J. H. Islet cell tumor of the pancreas with reversible watery diarrhea and achlorhydria. Gastroenterology 52:695, 1967.

50. Tompkins, R. K., Kraft, A. R., and Zollinger, R. M. Secretin-like choleresis produced by a diarrheogenic non-beta islet cell tumor of the pancreas. Surgery 66:131, 1969.

51. Murray, J. S., Paton, R. R., and Pope, C. E., II. Pancreatic tumor associated with flushing and diarrhea: Report of case. New Eng. J. Med. 264:436, 1961.

52. Erdheim, J. Zur normalen und pathologischen Histologie der Glandula thyreoides, parathyreoides und hypophysis. Beitr. Path. Anat. 33:158, 1903.

53. Rossier, P. H., and Dressler, M. Familiäre Erkrankung innersekretorischer Drüsen, kombinieret mit Ulcuskrankheit. Schweiz. Med. Wchnschr. 69:985, 1939.

54. Wermer, P. Genetic aspects of adenomatosis of endocrine glands. Amer. J. Med. 16:363, 1954.

55. Edkins, J. S. On the chemical mechanism of gastric secretion. Proc. Roy. Soc. London B76:376, 1905.

56. Ballard, H. S., Frame, B., and Hartwik, R. J. Familial multiple endocrine adenoma–peptic ulcer complex. Medicine 43:481, 1964.

57. Huizenga, K. A., Goodrick, W. I. M., and Summerskill, W. H. J. Peptic ulcer with islet cell tumor. Amer. J. Med. 37:564, 1964.

58. O'Neal, L. W., Kipnis, D. M., Luse, S. A., Lacy, P. E., and Jarett, L. Secretion of various endocrine substances by ACTH-secreting tumors — gastrin, melanotropin, norepinephrine, serotonin, parathormone, vasopressin, glucagon. Cancer 21:1219, 1968.

59. Liddle, G. W., Givens, J. P., Nicholson, W. E.,

and Island, D. P. The ectopic ACTH syndrome. Cancer Res. 25:1057, 1965.

60. Bloodworth, J. M. B., Jr., and Elliott, D. W. The histochemistry of pancreatic islet cell lesions. J.A.M.A. 183:1011, 1968.

61. Kirsner, J. B. The parathyroids and peptic ulcer. Gastroenterology 34:145, 1958.

62. Black, B. H. Hyperparathyroidism. Springfield, Ill., Charles C Thomas, Publisher, 1953.

63. Ellis, C., and Nicoloff, D. M. Hyperparathyroidism and peptic ulcer disease. Arch. Surg. 96:114, 1968.

64. Ostrow, J. D., Blandshard, G., and Gray, S. J. Peptic ulcer in primary hyperparathyroidism. Amer. J. Med. 29:769, 1960.

65. Ward, J. T., Adesola, A. O., and Welbourne, R. B. The parathyroids, calcium and gastric secretion in man and the dog. Gut 5:173, 1964.

66. Barrearas, R. F., and Donaldson, R. M. Role of calcium in gastric hypersecretion parathyroid adenoma and peptic ulcer. New Eng. J. Med. 276:1122, 1967.

67. Barrearas, R. F., and Donaldson, R. M. Effects of induced hypercalcemia on human gastric secretion. Gastroenterology 52:670, 1967.

68. Patterson, M., Wolma, F., Drake, A., and Ong, H. Gastric secretion and chronic hyperparathyroidism. Arch. Surg. 99:9, 1969.

69. Donegan, W. L., and Spiro, H. M. Parathyroids and gastric secretion. Gastroenterology 38:750, 1960.

70. Smallwood, R. A. Effect of intravenous calcium administration on gastric secretion of acid and pepsin in man. Gut 8:592, 1967.

Chapter 59

Complications of Peptic Ulcer Disease

Charles O. Walker

HEMORRHAGE

INCIDENCE

The exact incidence of bleeding from peptic ulcer is not known. Surveys based on hospital admissions overestimate bleeding frequency, and some patients with ulcer who bleed are not bleeding from their ulcer. Based on four extensive studies, it seems reasonable to conclude that 15 to 20 per cent of patients with peptic ulcer will have at least one hemorrhage during a 15- to 25-year period of follow-up.[1-4] Duodenal ulcer patients bleed somewhat more frequently (17 per cent) than do patients with gastric ulcers (12 per cent). Some studies show a higher frequency of bleeding in elderly (greater than 60 years) duodenal ulcer patients,[3] whereas other surveys have revealed no particular tendency for older patients to bleed.[5]

ASYMPTOMATIC HEMORRHAGE

Although hemorrhage may be the first manifestation of chronic peptic ulcer, it is difficult to estimate the incidence of this presentation for three reasons.[1-9]

1. The presence of a duodenal ulcer and/or duodenal deformity in a bleeding patient does not prove that the ulcer is the bleeding site.

2. Bleeding may be from an acute ulcer (induced by either stress or drugs), and yet be lumped with chronic duodenal ulcers.

3. An admission history taken from a frightened or obtunded patient may be incomplete, yielding the erroneous impression that the bleed was not preceded by peptic ulcer symptoms.

RECURRENT HEMORRHAGE

In five series, the incidence of rebleeding in duodenal ulcer patients varied from 30 to 51 per cent.[2, 5, 7, 10, 11] This is approximately twice the estimated incidence of bleeding in the general duodenal ulcer population, indicating that one bleeding episode increases the chance of a second bleed. The incidence of rebleeding after a first, second, or third bleed remains constant at about 40 to 50 per cent.

In gastric ulcer patients, from 6 to 40 per cent rebleed for a second time. After a first, second, or third bleed, the rebleeding incidence is constant at about 25 to 30 per cent.[2, 5, 12]

It is not possible to predict the risk of a second bleed from age, type of ulcer, or severity of the index hemorrhage.[5] The severity of subsequent hemorrhages cannot be predicted from the severity of the current bleed.[11] If no ulcer or deformity can be detected by radiology (suggesting that the bleeding is from a superficial site and not a chronic peptic ulcer), the recurrence rate is significantly reduced, i.e., 14 per cent vs. 50 per cent.[5]

POSTOPERATIVE HEMORRHAGE

When gastric resection is performed for perforation, obstruction, or intractability, the incidence of bleeding over the next five years is very low. When the resection is done for hemorrhage, bleeding is distressingly frequent during the next five years. For instance, when 164 patients were followed for five years after an index bleed, 38 per cent had a subsequent bleed. When gastric resection was performed after an index bleed, bleeding, often of a serious degree, recurred in 32 per cent over the next five years.[7] In another study, 21 per cent bleed after gastric resection, whereas 43 per cent rebleed without surgical treatment.[11] Although some of the rebleeding events after surgery were serious, others were mild. Some of the rebleeding is from marginal ulcer, and some is from stomatitis or gastritis. Finally, these studies indicate what can be expected following gastric resection. It has been suggested that the addition of vagotomy will significantly reduce the incidence of bleeding after gastric surgery performed for bleeding (see pp. 774 to 777).

CLINICAL MANIFESTATIONS

Upper gastrointestinal hemorrhage from peptic ulcer may become dramatically apparent via hematemesis or melena, or it may be insidious and first suspected when a hypochromic microcytic anemia is detected. In the latter instance, occult blood may be found only intermittently in the stool. On admission to a hospital, a bleeding duodenal ulcer is twice as likely to exhibit melena as hematemesis, whereas gastric ulcers present with hematemesis and melena with equal frequency.[3]

Many varied and complicated physiological responses, such as hypotension, tachycardia, and syncope, will be seen in patients with sudden acute blood loss; these are covered in detail under diagnosis and management of gastrointestinal bleeding (see pp. 195 to 214). All these manifestations of bleeding are the result of underperfusion of various organs and segments of organs secondary to decreased perfusion pressure (shock), decreased oxygen-carrying capacity of the blood (anemia), and localized vascular disease (arteriosclerosis). Strokes, transient ischemia attacks, changes in personality, blindness, angina, myocardial infarction, congestive heart failure, and intestinal ischemia may be precipitated by a gastrointestinal hemorrhage, and the patient may present with symptoms of these complications rather than a history of gastrointestinal bleeding.

PRECIPITATING FACTORS

Attempts to discover events that might precipitate bleeding from chronic peptic ulcers have, except for aspirin, not been particularly convincing or very helpful clinically. Drugs such as ethanol, reserpine, butazolidine, and corticosteroids, infections, and anxiety may at times predispose to bleeding, but their role is more likely permissive than the cause of most hemorrhages (see pp. 195 to 214). Certainly aspirin is quite an important cause of upper gastrointestinal bleeding, but how often it induces a chronic peptic ulcer to bleed is speculative.

PHYSICAL EXAMINATION

If the hemorrhage is from a chronic peptic ulcer without concomitant obstruction or perforation, the physical findings except for manifestations of the vascular complications considered above will be normal. On the other hand, the physical examination may quickly alert the physician to the possibility of another source for the upper intestinal bleeding.[13] Various physical findings and some of the syndromes to consider are listed in Table 59–1. The list of considerations is not exhaustive, but it clearly demonstrates the value of a careful examination of each bleeding patient.

PERFORATIONS

Peptic ulcers that extend through the serosa may open into the free abdominal

TABLE 59–1. PHYSICAL FINDINGS IN HEMORRHAGE

EXAMINATION SITE	FINDINGS	CONSIDER
Eyes	Jaundice	Ampullary carcinoma, hematobilia, alcoholic liver disease with varices
	Angioid streaks retina	Pseudoxanthoma elasticum
Face	Ruddy complexion	Polycythemia
	Perioral pigmentation	Peutz-Jeghers syndrome
	Perioral telangiectasia	Hereditary hemorrhagic telangiectasia
Buccal cavity	Varicosities under tongue	Phlebectasia of jejunum
Vasculature	Nodular arteritis	Periarteritis nodosa
	Collaterals-periumbilical	Portal hypertension
	Periumbilical + flank	Vena caval obstruction
Liver	Hepatomegaly	Portal hypertension, carcinoma, hereditary hemorrhagic telangiectasia
Spleen	Splenomegaly	Portal hypertension, lymphoma, leukemia
Abdomen	Mass	Aneurysm, gastric and renal carcinoma, carcinoma of head of pancreas
Extremities	Hyperextension of joints	Ehlers-Danlos syndrome
Scrotum	Varicosities (Fordyce lesions)	Phlebectasia of jejunum
Skin	Bruising, petechia	Hemorrhagic diathesis
	Coarse, yellow, thick skin of axillae, neck, and periumbilical regions	Pseudoxanthoma elasticum
	Telangiectasia	Hereditary hemorrhagic telangiectasia
	Spider angiomata	Liver disease
	Rash (lower extremities)	Henoch-Schönlein disease

cavity with dramatic suddenness; burrow into the pancreas, liver, or greater omentum, causing chronic intractable symptoms; or exit into the biliary tract, filling it with air. Although penetration and perforation both begin with extension of the ulcerative process beyond the serosa of the stomach or duodenum, the site of exit (either free or into a contiguous organ) results in clinically and prognostically distinct syndromes.[14]

INCIDENCE

Eight per cent of 2607 peptic ulcer patients reviewed in 1940 by DeBakey from Charity Hospital in New Orleans had been admitted for acute perforation.[15] More recently, Tolley tabulated the incidence of perforation from several large series.[16] He found that the incidence of perforation ranged from 5 to 11 per cent. In Fry's careful, prospective, long-term evaluation of peptic ulcer disease in his private practice (comprised largely of outpatients), 6 per cent of the patients perforated.[2] Among

430 patients more than 60 years of age, the incidence of free perforation was 10 per cent.[17] In reviews in which both hemorrhage and perforation are evaluated, bleeding occurs two to three times more frequently than perforation. Perforation is much more frequent in males than in females.

SITE OF PERFORATION

The site of perforation for duodenal ulcers is usually the anterior wall of the first part of the duodenum.[18] A small percentage (less than 10 per cent) may perforate posteriorly. Sixty per cent of perforated gastric ulcers are on the lesser curvature, with the rest occurring on the anterior, posterior, or prepyloric areas of the stomach with about equal frequency.

PERFORATION IN PREVIOUSLY ASYMPTOMATIC PATIENTS

An average of 7.5 per cent of perforations occur in individuals who deny previous symptoms of peptic ulcer.[15, 18, 19] Postperforation, a number of these patients will develop typical ulcer symptoms.

ACUTE VS. CHRONIC ULCERS

Attempts are frequently made to classify perforations as to whether the ulcer which perforated was acute or chronic. Presumably, if the ulcer is acute, there would be a good possibility that further symptoms would not occur and that minimal therapy is adequate. Perforations which were not preceded by pain and which were classified as acute at surgery were shown by Gilmour to have a more benign course than ulcers which appeared chronic.[20] Seventy-seven per cent of his patients with "acute" perforations did well, whereas none of those with "chronic" perforations did well. Subsequent studies have not shown such a sharp distinction between the subsequent course of acute and chronic perforations.[16, 18, 19, 21] These studies strongly suggest that the occurrence of any perforation places the individual in a virulent class of peptic ulcer disease, although they also show that if peptic symptoms preceded the perforation, the prognosis is worse.

MULTIPLE COMPLICATIONS

Perforation complicated by concomitant hemorrhage or gastric outlet obstruction represents a serious event.[22] Approximately 8 per cent of perforations are complicated by hemorrhage. If the hemorrhage is massive, mortality approaches 50 per cent. Clinical and autopsy figures reveal that most bleeding perforated ulcers are chronic and that they frequently occur in patients with severe unrelated disease, especially malignancy.

GASTROJEJUNAL ULCERS

Gastrojejunal ulcers frequently penetrate, but because of the proximity of the lesion to adjacent structures free perforation seldom occurs.[23]

MANIFESTATIONS

As an inordinate amount of time is spent discussing perforations without preceding symptoms, physicians may forget that most perforations are preceded by ulcer symptoms which not infrequently have intensified in the days and weeks before the perforation.[24]

In most patients who suffer a free perforation, it is clear that a catastrophic event has taken place. When viewed by skilled observers, diagnostic accuracy approaches 100 per cent.[25] The pain of perforation begins suddenly, often following a meal, and quickly attains maximal intensity. It is severe pain, variously described as excruciating, knife-like, or agonizing, and it is constant and unrelenting.[15, 24, 26] The pain is initially appreciated in the epigastrium or right upper quadrant, but soon spreads throughout the abdomen. Shoulder top pain may occur, back pain is uncommon (perforations are anterior), and nausea and vomiting are not prominent.

The patient is obviously in great distress and lies immobile in bed with grunting, shallow respirations. The blood pressure and pulse are normal (the patient is normovolemic at the onset), but the patient may be cold and clammy. The abdominal muscles are in spasm, and, if the patient has adequate abdominal musculature, his abdominal wall will exhibit board-like rigidity. Tenderness, especially in the epigastrium, is marked, bowel sounds are absent, and there may be a loss of hepatic dullness.

The classic lull (intermediate or second stage) may sometimes be seen. The patient feels better and appears improved, but examination will reveal that abdominal tenderness and rigidity are still prominent and bowel sounds are still absent. As peritonitis progresses, pneumoperitoneum increases, bowel distention appears, and the abdomen becomes distended (third stage). Parietal peritoneal irritation decreases, and tenderness and rigidity are less marked. Hypovolemia with hypotension and tachycardia commonly supervenes.

Leukocytosis usually appears quickly, and pneumoperitoneum is found in 75 per cent of those with perforation. The amylase was modestly elevated in 16 per cent of 1000 cases.[27] The amylase level seldom exceeds twice normal, but when it does, large perforations and a high mortality are predictable.

Diagnosis becomes difficult in perforation when one of several variant syndromes is present. The ulcer may seal soon after perforation; the resulting pain and abdominal findings are less intense than those seen with large soilage, and soon clear. A pneumoperitoneum must usually be present before this forme fruste perforation can be diagnosed. In similar fashion, spillage from an early sealing or slowly leaking perforation may be diverted by the falciform ligament down the right gutter to the cecal fossa. This will produce right lower quadrant pain, tenderness, and rigidity, and thus simulate appendicitis. Finally, an ulcer may perforate posteriorly into the lesser sac. In this instance, symptoms are less severe and pain is felt in the back.

PENETRATION

INCIDENCE

The frequency of penetration in patients with uncomplicated peptic ulcer disease has not been carefully documented. Two surgical series have carefully reviewed the frequency of penetration in ulcer patients coming to surgery.[28, 29] In approximately 20 per cent of 672 patients, confined perforations were found. Duodenal ulcers had penetrated in 26 per cent of those operated on, whereas confined perforations were present in 17 per cent of those with gastric ulcers coming to operation.

SITES OF PENETRATION

Many peptic ulcers which extend beyond the serosa do not perforate freely into the abdominal cavity but are limited by fibrous adhesions or penetration into an adjacent structure. These adjacent structures, in order of frequency, are pancreas, gastrohepatic omentum, biliary tract, liver, greater omentum, mesocolon, colon, and abdominal wall. The pancreas, biliary tract, and colon are more frequently involved by duodenal ulcers, whereas the gastrohepatic ligament and mesocolon are usually invaded by gastric ulcers.[30, 31]

MANIFESTATIONS

Symptoms have usually been present for many years, and asymptomatic penetration is rare.[28, 32] The penetrating ulcer exemplifies substitution of somatic pain for visceral pain.[33] If the patient does not volunteer and the physician fails to ask about previous abdominal symptoms, a straightforward diagnosis is made obscure. The previous visceral peptic symptoms may be altered, abruptly or insidiously, or they may be replaced completely by somatic pain.

The following manifestations of penetration are the most helpful in diagnosis:

1. Back pain is referred pain that is appreciated in the lower thoracic or upper lumbar area. It may occur in the absence of anterior abdominal pain. Back pain is present in 50 per cent of ulcer patients who are found to have penetration at the time of surgery; only 20 per cent of patients without penetration have back pain.

2. The pain clusters become less distinct and may even merge, producing constant pain.

3. In 20 per cent of those with penetrating ulcers, the usual clear relationship of the pain to the acid cycle (rhythmicity) is lost.

4. The pain often becomes intractable to medical management.

5. The superimposed somatic pain results in unusual patterns of anterior abdominal pain in one-fifth of penetrating ulcers. Pain may radiate to the chest, right upper quadrant (especially duodenal ulcer), left upper quadrant (especially gastric ulcer), and back.

A number of other symptoms are common but are less specific for penetration. Thus vomiting is much more frequent than in the uncomplicated ulcer patient.[29] Night pain is statistically more frequent than in noncomplicated ulcer, but it is only when this night pain is refractory to treatment or recurs many times each night that it suggests penetration.[28]

Common complications related to the penetration are hemorrhage (33 per cent), chemical pancreatitis (16 to 20 per cent), and anemia and weight loss. Rare complications are jaundice from biliary tract involvement, abscess, and clinically significant pancreatitis.

DIAGNOSIS

The diagnosis of posterior penetration is made by taking a careful history. In a small percentage, hyperamylasemia or radiological evidence of penetration will be helpful (see p. 509). If back pain, night pain, distortion of epigastric pain, or intractability to treatment are not present, less than 15 per cent of such patients will have anatomical evidence of penetration. A nondeformed duodenal bulb weighs against the presence of a posteriorly penetrating duodenal ulcer.[28]

GIANT DUODENAL ULCER

Because of its particular virulence, one subgroup of penetrating ulcer, giant duodenal ulcer, is worth considering in more detail. These large ulcers (3 to 6 cm) may be mistaken on X-ray for a normal, somewhat rounded, duodenal bulb (see Fig. 40–22, p. 508.[34-36] The alterations of symptoms, refractoriness to therapy, and complications seen in varying proportions in many penetrating ulcers culminate in the giant duodenal ulcer. The ulcer base is invariably located in the pancreas, and additional adhesions to the liver, gallbladder, and bile ducts are common. These patients are often acutely ill, with diffuse epigastric pain without rhythmicity or periodicity, and with radiation of pain to the back or right upper quadrant. Many years of typical peptic ulcer pain have preceded their current illness.

In addition to severe intractable pain, bleeding or pyloroduodenal obstruction with vomiting and weight loss occurs in most patients with giant duodenal ulcers. Even though the ulcer lies within the pancreas, it is rare for the serum amylase level to be elevated.

Treatment consists of resuscitation of the patient and early operation.

GASTRIC OUTLET OBSTRUCTION (PYLORIC STENOSIS)

A generally accepted definition of gastric outlet obstruction does not exist. Total obstruction is no diagnostic problem, but

TABLE 59–2.   CRITERIA FOR GASTRIC RETENTION

History
  1. Vomiting of stale food (food ingested over four hours previously)
  2. Repetitive vomiting, often projectile or nocturnal
Physical examination
  1. Visible gastric peristalsis
  2. Succussion splash more than four hours after eating
Gastric aspirate
  1. Gastric residue greater than 300 cc four hours after eating
  2. Overnight fasting gastric residue greater than 200 cc
  3. Twelve-hour gastric secretion greater than 750 cc
Radiology
  1. Retention of barium, 50 per cent at four hours
  2. Large atonic stomach
Special studies
  1. Saline load: Positive for obstruction when more than 400 cc of 750 cc of normal saline is retained after 30 minutes
  2. Barium-burger: Barium residue after six hours in intact stomach and three hours in resected stomach

partial outlet obstruction will be missed by some and overdiagnosed by others. Some of the more reasonable proposed criteria are listed in Table 59–2.[37-42] Although no systematic attempt has been made to compare these various criteria, the postprandial and nocturnal gastric residue and the saline load test appear to be the most objective and reproducible methods defining the presence of partial obstruction.

INCIDENCE

Gastric outlet obstruction is less common in peptic ulcer than hemorrhage or perforation. Ten and one-half per cent of 8451 patients seen at Cook County Hospital with gastroduodenal ulcer had gastric outlet obstruction, but in a series without surgical selection, the incidence was less than 5 per cent.[43] In two series, which reviewed consecutive cases of outlet obstruction, duodenal ulcers were responsible for the obstruction in 82 per cent of the cases, whereas gastric ulcers were responsible in 6.5 per cent of those obstructed.[39, 42] When one considers that duodenal ulcers are two to three times more frequent than gastric ulcers, outlet obstruc-

TABLE 59–3. CAUSES OF OUTLET OBSTRUCTION

1. Peptic ulcer disease
   A. Duodenal ulcer
   B. Antral ulcers
   C. Channel ulcers
2. Tumors
   A. Benign
      (1) Adenomatous polyp
      (2) Ectopic pancreas
   B. Malignant
      (1) Antral carcinoma
      (2) Carcinoma of the pancreatic head
      (3) Lymphomas
3. Inflammatory
   A. Cholecystitis
   B. Acute pancreatitis
   C. Regional enteritis
4. Miscellaneous
   A. Adult hypertrophic pyloric stenosis
   B. Postsurgical stenosis
   C. Pyloric diaphragm
   D. Duodenal diaphragm
   E. Caustic stricture
   F. Annular pancreas

tion is decidedly more frequent in duodenal than in gastric ulcers.

The causes of gastric outlet obstruction are listed in Table 59–3. Most of them are infrequent except for peptic ulcer disease and carcinoma of the stomach.

MANIFESTATIONS

PRECEDING PEPTIC ULCER SYMPTOMS

A long history of peptic ulcer disease is present in nearly all patients who present with gastric outlet obstruction caused by peptic diseases.[37-39, 41, 42] In one study, the average duration of symptoms was 12 years and only 6 per cent had symptoms less than one year.[41] Clusters of abdominal pain, usually typical for ulcer, have occurred in the vast majority of patients. Those with duodenal ulcer are more likely than those with gastric ulcer to have had typical pain.[37-39, 42]

DURATION OF OBSTRUCTIVE SYMPTOMS

The symptoms of obstruction which bring the patient to the physician are usually measured in months rather than in years. Obstructive symptoms have been present for less than one month in 50 per cent and for less than three months in approximately 80 per cent.[38, 41, 42] Symptoms have been present for longer than one year in 10 per cent. Obviously the latter patients are not severely affected throughout the year, but their year-long disability represents a little-appreciated fact; i.e., that outlet obstruction may produce chronic symptoms lasting a year or longer.[38, 42]

SYMPTOMS OF OBSTRUCTION

Vomiting. Pain is replaced by vomiting as the most frequent clinical manifestation when obstruction supervenes in peptic ulcer. Vomiting is found in the large majority (77 to 97 per cent) of obstructed individuals.[37, 42] Although pain was still more common than vomiting in some series, including the large review of Kozoll, the frequency of vomiting is still the most striking feature of retarded gastric emptying.

Balint and Spence carefully analyzed the vomiting of pyloric stenosis. They found that emesis was the presenting symptom in 90 per cent of their patients. It was copious in about 50 per cent, occurred daily in 26 per cent, and occurred more than once a day in 30 per cent of their cases. In 18 per cent it was nonspecific, being erratic in timing and frequency. Nocturnal vomiting was seen in 19 per cent, and stale food was produced in 15 per cent.[42] Other authors report variations on these percentages, but the agreement is surprisingly close, and a consensus of various reports is presented in Table 59–4. Nausea is usually associated with the vomiting, and vomiting is more frequent late in the day.

Pain. The pattern of pain is frequently altered with the onset of obstruction.[37, 42] The pain tends to become more constant, i.e., without remission, but it may maintain its daily rhythmicity and continue to respond to treatment.[38] In fact, 70 per cent of patients still respond to treatment, but vomiting is frequently the major means of relief. Thirty per cent of patients cannot obtain relief by alkali, food, or vomiting, and many patients feel that eating aggravates their pain.[38, 39] Pain continues to occur after meals in 62 per cent of duodenal and in 83 per cent of gastric ulcer pa-

TABLE 59–4. CLINICAL FEATURES OF GASTRIC OUTLET OBSTRUCTION

Vomiting:
    Absent   10%
    Nonspecific 18%
    Obstructive 72% (copious—one or more times
                           per day)
        Nocturnal 16%
        Stale food 29%
Pain:
    Absent—rare, less than 5%
    Epigastric—83%
    Description—fullness 28%, cramping 23%,
        burning 24%
    Periodicity—daily pain is typical
    Rhythmicity—postprandial 70%, noctural 37%
    Relief with treatment
        Alkali   46%
        Vomiting   40%
        Food   25% (may aggravate pain)
        None   33%
    Anorexia (35–65%)
    Weight loss (pounds)
        None   30%
        Greater than 10, 21%; greater than 15, 22%;
           greater than 20, 14%
    Constipation (33%)
    Diarrhea (10%)

tients.[38] One clear difference is that the epigastric pain is frequently described as a fullness with obstruction and is rarely so classified when obstruction is absent.

Other Symptoms. Anorexia may be present instead of vomiting, particularly if the patient has curtailed his food consumption. With or without vomiting, anorexia is seen in 35 to 65 per cent of those with outlet stenosis.[38, 42]

In patients with uncomplicated peptic disease, weight loss greater than 10 pounds is seen in approximately 37 per cent of gastric and 24 per cent of duodenal ulcers, whereas 58 per cent of patients with outlet obstruction caused by peptic ulcer have lost more than 10 pounds. Fourteen per cent lose greater than 20 pounds, and 30 per cent report no weight loss at all.[37, 39–42, 44]

Constipation, occasionally severe, is present in at least one-third, and diarrhea may be present in 10 per cent of patients with outlet obstruction.[38, 39, 42]

PHYSICAL EXAMINATION

The physical examination may reveal evidence of weight loss or malnutrition.[38]

Abdominal tenderness is common but nonspecific. The incidence of a succussion splash ranges from 2 to 66 per cent and of visible peristalsis from 1 to 25 per cent, depending upon the method of patient selection.

LABORATORY CHANGES

Anemia and a low serum albumin are seen in 20 per cent of patients with obstructing gastroduodenal ulcer.[39, 41, 42] Bleeding and nutritional deficiencies are responsible for the anemia. Alcoholism, poor dietary habits, and the pyloric obstruction are the factors responsible for the nutritional deficiencies.

Prerenal azotemia, hypokalemia, hypochloremia, and alkalosis are found in up to one-fifth of patients presenting with pyloric obstruction.[39, 41, 42] The incidence of these electrolyte changes will vary with the severity of obstruction; if the diagnosis is made early, metabolic complications will rarely be seen.

If severe, decreased dietary intake and vomiting result in metabolic alkalosis. The gastric mucosa secretes hydrochloric acid into the stomach lumen and adds bicarbonate to the venous system. With vomiting, hydrogen and chloride are lost and bicarbonate thus achieves an excess in the body. At this point, it could be anticipated that the kidneys would excrete the excess bicarbonate as sodium bicarbonate. However, the situation is complicated by a sodium and water deficit produced by decreased intake and loss of Cl^-, Na^+, K^+ and H_2O in the vomitus. In addition, the body continues to produce organic acids whose anions ($SO_4^=$, $PO_4^=$, etc.) are nonreabsorbable in the nephron.[45]

Thus we have an individual with a contracted extracellular fluid volume (ECF), excess bicarbonate anions, hypochloremia, and organic acid anions which will be excreted short of renal failure. What happens is that (1) in the face of ECF depletion, most of the sodium is conserved by the kidney for volume protection in spite of HCO_3^- excess; (2) since chloride, which would normally be reabsorbed with the sodium to maintain electrochemical neutrality, has been depleted, bicarbonate is reabsorbed instead, perpetuating the alkalosis;

and (3) the organic acids which must be excreted are done so with hydrogen and potassium which have been exchanged for sodium.[45-48]

These renal events result in protection of the ECF; retention of HCO_3^- and perpetuation of the alkalosis; loss of potassium in the urine, which, coupled with modest losses in the vomitus and decreased intake, may produce a large potassium deficit; and hydrogen losses into the urine, yielding an acid urine (paradoxical aciduria).

Treatment directed at replacement of the chloride loss will produce a bicarbonate diuresis because Cl^- will then be reabsorbed instead of HCO_3^-. If NaCl is used, ECF contraction is lessened and a brisk sodium bicarbonate diuresis will ensue.[45]

An intracellular acidosis is common when a hypokalemic metabolic alkalosis eventuates.[45, 49] In these circumstances, potassium moves out of the cell and hydrogen fluxes inward. With correction of the alkalosis, potassium moves back into the cell and a modest hypokalemia may become profound. Thus even though the alkalosis could be corrected with sodium chloride alone, potassium supplementation, as a KCl solution, should be begun early in treatment. Another reason for using KCl is that, if there is a large potassium deficit (greater than 400 mEq), the alkalosis may be refractory to correction with saline alone.[45, 50]

Clinically, the severity of the metabolic alkalosis is best correlated with measurement of the standard bicarbonate or calculated base excess. When the bicarbonate is from 5 to 25 mEq per liter greater than normal or the base excess is from +7 to +20 mEq per liter, clinical symptoms of irritability, lethargy, confusion, and weakness are usually present.[48] With values greater than these, tetany may appear. These patients need careful but vigorous treatment, and surgery is contraindicated until correction is achieved, which may take several days.

PROGNOSIS

Mortality. Most of the factors associated with an increased mortality could be reasonably predicted; they include increasing age (especially over 60), other complicating medical illnesses, and the need for preoperative transfusion. With obstruction secondary to gastric ulcers, overall mortality increases from approximately 8 per cent in the sixth decade to greater than 20 per cent in patients over 70 years.[51] When the obstruction is caused by duodenal disease, mortality is 7 per cent in the sixth decade, but rises to 12 per cent and 26 per cent in the seventh and eighth decades, respectively.[51] Concomitant cardiac disease, if severe enough to require cardiac drugs, was associated with a 50 per cent mortality.[51]

The combination of massive hemorrhage and obstruction is not uncommon in patients with peptic ulcer disease.[22] Mortality rates appear to double in such circumstances. Minor bleeds frequently accompany obstruction, and this type of bleeding does not change the prognosis but may initially confuse the physician. Obstruction plus perforation is uncommon but increases mortality six- or seven-fold.

A number of related factors representing a high degree of obstruction are associated with a poor prognosis. Weight loss, alkalosis, prolonged preoperative suction, and inability to resume a diet preoperatively are such factors. When suction is needed beyond four days, mortality doubles.[51] If nightly aspiration alone can be utilized instead of continuous suction, mortality does not increase with time. However, it cannot be concluded that nightly aspiration is better treatment than continuous suction, because patients who can be managed by night suction undoubtedly have less severe obstruction.

Reversibility. When gastric retention is a product of outlet obstruction, the nature of this obstruction plus the integrity of the gastric musculature determines whether the obstruction will respond to medical therapy and, more important, whether the obstruction will recur. Although it is often assumed that outlet obstruction is synonymous with stenosis from scar tissue, this is not the case when the stomachs are carefully examined pathologically.[40, 52] What is found is that stenosis, often accompanied by a penetrating ulcer, is present in 50 per cent of patients with peptic outlet obstructions. In those without stenosis, an inflammatory mass or penetrating ulcer is usually present. However, 19 per cent of all patients have neither stenosis nor a penetrating ulcer. Except for a few of the patients with fibrotic stenosis, active ulcers are usually present. Symptoms in these various groups are very similar. The retention caused by nonstenotic, nonpenetrating ulcers responds more frequently to preoperative medical treatment, and it is in this group of patients that medical therapy should be most successful. It must be stressed that these patients, who are potentially curable by medical means, represent a minority of those who develop outlet obstruction.

The duration and type of clinical symptoms do not clearly separate medically reversible and nonreversible gastric outlet obstruction. Even the signs and symptoms of severe obstruction, such as the vomiting of stale food, succussion splash, and alkalosis, may at times be associated with a reversible lesion. It has not been determined whether the clinical criteria of outlet obstruction, listed in Table 59–2, will predict which patients will respond to medical therapy. One procedure, the saline load test, has been evaluated and seems to be of distinct value.[53] To perform the saline load test, the tip of a nasogastric tube is placed fluoroscopically so that it lies in the middle of the gastric antrum. Sodium chloride, 750 cc of 0.9 per cent solution, is rapidly infused. Thirty minutes later, with the patient rotated to ensure good emptying, the contents are aspirated. The volume of saline removed 30 minutes later is recorded. "At the end of the first 24 hours of suction, a saline load test result of 200 ml or less is an extremely favorable sign. Such patients tolerate progressive feedings normally at the end of a 72-hour period of suction and have done well subsequently, except for one who returned 18 months later with recurrent retention. Patients with a saline load test result of 300 ml or more, at the end of 24 hours, have almost always required surgery, either at the end of the 72-hour period of suction or soon thereafter."[53]

DIAGNOSIS

If a patient presents with vomiting and worsening of peptic symptoms or if he complains of anorexia and weight loss, consideration must be given to the possibility that he has gastric retention. The clinician must first decide if gastric retention is present, and then, after treatment has been started, he decides if an organic gastric outlet obstruction is present.

The first step is *not* to order an upper gastrointestinal barium study but to make the diagnosis of gastric retention by direct means. A nasogastric tube, preferably a 32 F Ewald tube or a 34 F Edlich gastric lavage tube, is inserted into the stomach under fluoroscopic control, after an overnight or eight-hour fast or four hours postprandially. If after an overnight fast there is more than 200 cc of fluid, or if four hours postprandially more than 300 cc is present, it is quite likely that gastric retention is present. These aspirations should be performed with the patient sitting rather than lying. Then the patient should be moved from side to side to ensure complete recovery.

If retention is diagnosed, the large bore tube is left in place and the stomach is meticulously washed. This lavage is important if the subsequent diagnostic (saline load test) and therapeutic endeavors (continuous suction) are to be effective.

Once the stomach is clean, and this may take several hours, the large bore tube is removed and a 16 F sump-type nasogastric tube is inserted. This is a convenient time to perform a saline load test. It will help confirm the presence of obstruction, and the results can be compared with later saline loads to document response to treatment.

The diagnosis of gastric retention has now been made and quantified, the stomach is clean, and a well positioned nasogastric tube is in place. Continuous nasogastric suction and treatment of metabolic abnormalities are undertaken, and the search for the cause of the gastric retention is begun.

Other causes of gastric retention, such as atropine-like drugs, diabetes, and electrolyte abnormalities, can inhibit gastric emptying. If they are present, the physician should suspect that either outlet obstruction is not present or that it may be mild enough to respond to medical therapy. The most common causes of nonobstructive gastric retention are listed in Table

TABLE 59–5. CAUSES OF GASTRIC RETENTION WITHOUT OUTLET OBSTRUCTION

1. Atropine-like drugs
2. Diabetic neuropathy
3. Immobilization
4. Severe pain or trauma, especially involving the peritoneum
5. Contiguous inflammation
    Gastric ulcer
    Pancreatitis
6. Infection
    Septicemia, viral or bacterial
    Pneumonia
7. Central nervous system disease
8. Electrolyte and acid-base disorders
    Hyper- and hypocalcemia
    Hypokalemia
    Uremia
    Acidosis
9. Emotional stress

59–5.[54] Any of these factors could cause retention, and final disposition must be temporized until they are discounted or treated.

If it becomes apparent that some nonobstructive cause of retention is present and if it can be alleviated, further therapy and diagnostic maneuvers may not be needed. Most of the causes of nonobstructive retention will be apparent on careful evaluation. Medications should always be scrutinized carefully for drugs with anticholinergic effects. Peripheral diabetic neuropathy will be present in diabetics with gastric stasis.

The major problem in the differential diagnosis of organic outlet obstruction is between peptic ulcer disease and carcinoma of the stomach. The physical signs and laboratory findings are identical, and most of the symptoms, such as vomiting, weight loss, constipation, diarrhea, and gastrointestinal bleeding, are likewise similar.[39, 42] However, the absence of pain or a history of previous dyspeptic-like pain of less than one year's duration is a solid clue to the possible presence of malignancy.

The search for the cause continues during the initial period of treatment, which should be continuous nasogastric suction. If the nonstimulated output of acid from the stomach is absent or very low, cancer should be suspected; if acid output is greater than 5 mEq per hour, peptic ulcer is likely; if acid is greater than 10 to 15 mEq per hour, Zollinger-Ellison syndrome is likely. To further evaluate these possibilities, maximal acid output can be stimulated by histamine, Histalog, or gastrin. Gastric cytology can likewise be done during the initial period of nasogastric suction. Finally, after the stomach has been well decompressed for 72 hours, upper gastrointestinal series and/or endoscopy are performed. Because of fibrosis, edema, and spasm, these studies may not reveal an active ulcer even if one is present. On the other hand, if these studies fail to reveal evidence of carcinoma, such a diagnostic possibility is extremely unlikely. These studies will also detect polyps, ectopic pancreas, carcinoma of the pancreas, pancreatitis, and adult hypertrophic pyloric stenosis; if completely normal, a nonobstructive cause of gastric retention is implicated.

Peptic ulcer patients with outlet obstruction are frequently hospitalized for long periods before a definitive diagnosis or treatment is rendered.[52] There are four reasons for this delay:

1. The diagnosis is not suspected from the history, and a succussion splash is not checked for on the physical examination.

2. The concomitant presence of mild bleeding may delay attention to obstructive symptoms.

3. The diagnosis is suspected, but the proper studies (the three-hour postprandial gastric aspiration or saline load study) are not performed.

4. Retention of barium may not be noted on the upper gastrointestinal series.[52, 55] Contrary to popular opinion, this does not exclude a partial outlet obstruction.

TREATMENT

It is apparent that treatment and diagnosis proceed together. The initial step in treatment and diagnosis, after a history and physical examination, is gastric aspiration and lavage with a large bore tube. This allows further diagnostic maneuvers and, by removing detritus, enables nasogastric suction to better decompress the stomach.

In those with prominent and long-standing obstruction, an extracellular fluid deficit may exist; if the deficit is severe, prerenal azotemia may complicate the picture. The loss of HCl, K^+, and water in the vomitus and K^+ and H^+ in the urine produces a hypochloremic, hypokalemic, metabolic alkalosis. The best way to treat these problems is with isotonic NaCl. Once an adequate urine output is apparent, KCl should be added to the infusion solution at 10 mEq per hour until potassium balance becomes positive. Once this happens, 40 to 80 mEq per day may be adequate during the decompression phase of therapy. Adequate calories (at least 1200 per day) as D10W must be given to inhibit gluconeogenesis. If dehydration is extreme, large volumes of saline may be needed. A central venous catheter is helpful in avoiding overhydration, but left heart failure may develop in patients with impairment of left ventricular function, whereas right-sided pressure remains within normal limits.[56]

Continuous nasogastric suction is maintained for at least 72 hours. This period is adequate to decompress most atonic stomachs, but is not so long as to greatly extend negative nitrogen balance if adequate calories are given; unless extreme medical contraindications exist, retention after 72 hours means that the patient is probably a surgical candidate.

If the patient has high grade obstruction at 72 hours, as manifested by large 24-hour aspirations and high saline load values (greater than 400), particularly if there are other indications for surgery, such as previous perforation, obstruction, or massive hemorrhage, the problem becomes *when* rather than *whether* to perform surgery. If nutritional and fluid and electrolyte status are good and diagnostic tests are complete, there is probably little to gain by delaying definite treatment (see pp. 778 to 779).

If, as sometimes happens, it is not clear whether partial outlet obstruction is present, there are two paths open. First, nasogastric suction can be continued for several days while diagnostic tests are repeated, or, second, clear liquids as high in nitrogen as possible may be started, and the gastric residual aspirated at bedtime, with continuous suction during the night to maintain gastric tone. If the degree of obstruction is not extreme, sufficient nutri-

tion can be given in this way to put the patient in positive nitrogen balance while diagnostic procedures are repeated. Patients can be treated in this way for weeks and have a low operative mortality when finally operated upon.[51]

In those who present with extreme malnutrition and high grade obstruction, intravenous hyperalimentation will probably improve their chances for successful surgical repair. In such patients, hyperalimentation is begun as soon as their potassium deficit is replaced (p. 33).

If the patient responds quickly to nasogastric suction, as exemplified by a normal saline load test at 24 hours and falling gastric aspirates, he is likely to respond to medical treatment alone, but the aspiration should still be continued for 72 hours. Then he is started on clear liquids and hourly antacids, followed by graduation to a regular diet several days later.

INTRACTABILITY

Intractability is the most common reason for surgical treatment of peptic ulcer disease.[24, 52] The decision to call a patient's peptic symptoms intractable is a subjective one. Therefore great care must be taken in evaluating the patient. The temporal pattern of the patient's pain and a detailed history of measures giving relief of any anorexia, weight loss or vomiting must be obtained. Failure to obtain this information will deny surgery to some who need it and subject others to it too hastily.

Pain which is continuous, unresponsive to good care given in a hospital, and associated with vomiting and weight loss is clearly refractory. However, pain need not be continuous and totally refractory to treatment to qualify as intractable. When periods of remission get shorter and relapses become longer, and when during each relapse the pain becomes progressively more severe and of longer duration, the patient's ulcer is probably best classified as refractory. This is particularly so if relief from food and alkali is becoming less effective. Likewise, pain relieved by hospitalization which recurs promptly upon return home or any pain that recurs under all but the most stringent of medical regimens is refractory.[29, 52]

TABLE 59-6. FACTORS RESPONSIBLE FOR INTRACTABILITY

Intrinsic
  Penetration of ulcer
  Pyloric obstruction
  Postbulbar ulceration
  Channel ulcer
  Hypersecretory drive states
  Other chronic diseases (see p. 667)

Extrinsic
  Drugs
    Acetylsalicylic acid
    Corticosteroids (?)
  Smoking (?)
  Caffeine (?)

Neuropsychiatric
  Psychic stress
  Inadequate personality

ETIOLOGY

Some of the factors responsible for intractability are listed in Table 59-6. *Penetration* of peptic ulcers appears to be the most important cause.[30, 31] It is probably at least part of the reason for intractability in 50 per cent of patients coming to operation.[30] The symptoms of penetration are in many respects identical with those of intractability catalogued above.

Pyloric obstruction by chronic peptic ulcer disease represents a form of intractability, whether or not pain is prominent. In one-third of patients, the pain, even if not severe, is more or less unrelenting and unrelieved even by vomiting. In many others, symptoms of posterior penetration, which is a frequent concomitant, are superimposed.

Postbulbar ulcers frequently become intractable to medical therapy.[57] This, coupled with atypical symptoms and frequent delays in diagnosis, may condemn the patient to years of disability before diagnosis and effective treatment are achieved.

Channel ulcers exhibit a high incidence of pain that is incompletely relieved by treatment.[58, 59] Commonly present in channel ulcers and undoubtedly often responsible for their intractability are partial outlet obstruction and penetration.

The various *hypersecretory drive states* are frequently associated with severe unrelenting symptoms (see pp. 743 to 756). If they are considered and the appropriate studies (gastric secretion and serum gas-

trin) performed, these diseases are usually easily diagnosed.

Chronic bronchopulmonary disease, rheumatoid arthritis, pulmonary tuberculosis, and *advanced cirrhosis* have a high incidence of peptic ulcer disease. Ulcers, particularly gastric ulcers, tend to heal slowly in patients with these diseases, and such slow healing may be a factor in intractability.

Aspirin and *smoking* (see pp. 646 to 647) appear to increase the incidence of peptic ulcer disease and to retard healing. Thus they could contribute to the persistence of ulceration. Many other drugs have been implicated as factors in ulcer formation, but none have been proved either to increase the incidence or to retard the healing of peptic ulcer.

Anxiety and *depression* are tremendously important in precipitating, prolonging, and intensifying peptic disease (see pp. 687 to 689). The relief of some of this stress by hospitalization, by appropriate drug therapy, and by establishment of a good doctor-patient relationship can frequently decrease the patient's symptoms.

How a patient appreciates and verbalizes his symptoms will obviously influence the physician's interpretation of the patient's pain. The patient, depending on his personality and self-image, may be a stoic or a complainer, and the physician must decide in each patient what his complaints denote.

An even more difficult problem is the patient with ulcer disease who obtains secondary gain from his illness. In these patients, relief by any means may be impossible.

DIAGNOSIS

In the diagnosis of intractability, the history will emphasize the progression of symptoms and their temporary response to treatment. Once the physician feels that he is dealing with intractable disease, he should proceed more or less by a checklist through the various possible factors that may be responsible (Table 59-6). Most of the intrinsic factors, such as pyloric obstruction and secretory drive states, should be diagnosed if the proper studies are ordered. One exception is penetration, because the radiologist infrequently makes the diagnosis and the serum amylase level is usually normal. Thus one of the major causes of an unresponsive ulcer can seldom be verified by ancillary techniques, and the history remains the only way to diagnose both penetration and intractability.

The extrinsic insults to the stomach, aspirin, caffeine, corticosteroids, smoking, and possibly other drugs, can be discontinued and the patient observed to see if this has a salutary effect.

The effect of stress and emotions, family structure, and secondary gain must be evaluated as to their role in the intractability.

TREATMENT

The diagnosis of intractability usually implies that medical therapy has failed. If it is not clear that medical therapy has failed, it can be attempted once again, preferably in the hospital. However, care must be taken not to treat "one more time" as a form of procrastination.

Current data suggest that about 75 per cent of those treated surgically will obtain good to excellent results (see pp. 772 to 774). Many of the remainder will be unhappy because of early dumping, diarrhea, and vague dyspeptic symptoms. One recent study was able to predict both those who would be satisfied and those who would be dissatisfied with their surgical results.[60] Alcohol abuse, character disorders, and neurosis were very significantly correlated with symptoms after surgical procedures. None of the following were of help in predicting the results of surgery at one year: sex, age, socioeconomic status, duration of symptoms, time lost from work, a history of bleeding or perforation, the preoperative augmented histamine test result, or a positive postoperative insulin test. This study would suggest that certain persons often offered surgery, i.e., the alcoholic or dependent individual with an inadequate personality, are the ones who will continue to have disabling symptoms postoperatively; whereas patients who do not exhibit character deviation, character neurosis, or alcohol abuse will obtain good symptomatic response.

Some individuals may have frequent, severe recurrence of their ulcer symptoms, yet, because of concomitant medical disease, be very poor operative candidates. In these patients, irradiation of the gastric parietal cell mass could prove to be of great benefit.

REFERENCES

1. Chinn, A. B., and Weckesser, E. C. Acute hemorrhage from peptic ulceration; an analysis of 322 cases. Ann. Intern. Med. 34:339, 1951.
2. Fry, J. Peptic ulcer: A profile. Brit. Med. J. 2:809, 1964.
3. Norbye, E. Ulcer statistics from Drammen Hospital, 1936–1945. Acta Med. Scand. 143:50, 1952.
4. Krag, E. Pseudo-ulcer and true peptic ulcer. Acta Med. Scand. 178:713, 1965.
5. Wenckert, A., Borg, I., and Lindtlom, P. Review of medically treated bleeding gastric and duodenal ulcers. Acta Chir. Scand. 120:66, 1960.
6. Radloff, F. F. Observations on five hundred and forty-three cases of peptic ulcer. Gastroenterology 8:343, 1947.
7. Serebro, H. A., and Mendeloff, A. I. Late results of medical and surgical treatment of bleeding peptic ulcer. Lancet 2:505, 1966.
8. Heraldson, S. Prognosis in conservative treatment of bleeding peptic ulcer. Nord. Med. 38:778, 1948.
9. Welch, C. E. Treatment of acute massive gastroduodenal hemorrhage. J.A.M.A. 141:1113, 1949.
10. Boles, R. S., Cassidy, W. J., and Jordan, S. M. Medical versus surgical management for complication of hemorrhage in duodenal ulcer. Gastroenterology 32:52, 1957.
11. Donaldson, R. M., Handy, J., and Papper, S. Five-year follow-up study of patients with bleeding duodenal ulcer with and without surgery. New Eng. J. Med. 259:201, 1958.
12. Arias, I. M., Zamcheck, N., and Thrower, W. B. Recurrence of hemorrhage from medically treated gastric ulcers. Arch. Intern. Med. 101:369, 1958.
13. Jones, F. A. Problems of alimentary bleeding. Brit. Med. J. 2:267, 1969.
14. Haubrich, W. S., Roth, J. L., and Bockus, H. L. The clinical significance of penetration and confined perforation in peptic ulcer disease. Gastroenterology 25:173, 1953.
15. DeBakey, M. Acute perforated gastroduodenal ulceration. Surgery 8:852, 1028, 1940.
16. Tolley, J. A. Definitive surgical therapy for perforated peptic ulcer. Amer. J. Surg. 113:327, 1967.
17. Cutler, C. W. Clinical patterns of peptic ulcer after sixty. Surg. Gynec. Obstet. 107:23, 1958.
18. Balasegaram, M. Immediate definitive surgery for perforated peptic ulcers. Amer. J. Surg. 115:642, 1968.
19. Turner, F. P. Acute perforations of stomach,

duodenum and jejunum. Surg. Gynec. Obstet. 92:281, 1951.

20. Gilmour, J. Prognosis and treatment in acute perforated peptic ulcer. Lancet 1:870, 1953.
21. Hofkin, G. A. Course of patients with perforated duodenal ulcer. Amer. J. Surg. 111:193, 1966.
22. Moore, S. W., and Fuller, F. W. Multiple simultaneous complications of peptic ulcer. Amer. J. Surg. 97:184, 1959.
23. Wychulis, A. R., Priestley, J. T., and Foulk, W. T. A study of 360 patients with gastrojejunal ulceration. Surg. Gynec. Obstet. 122:89, 1966.
24. Berne, C. J., and Mikkelsen, W. P. Management of perforated peptic ulcer. Surgery 44:591, 1958.
25. Seeley, S. F., and Campbell, M. D. Nonoperative treatment of perforated peptic ulcer. Surg. Gynec. Obstet. 102:435, 1956.
26. Botsford, T. W., and Wilson, R. E. The Acute Abdomen. Philadelphia, W. B. Saunders Co., 1969.
27. Rogers, F. A. Elevated serum amylase. Ann. Surg. 153:228, 1961.
28. Norris, J. R., and Haubrich, W. S. The incidence and clinical features of penetration in peptic ulceration. J.A.M.A. 178:386, 1961.
29. Caruolo, J. E., Hallenbeck, G. A., and Dockerty, M. B. A clinicopathologic study of posterior penetrating gastric ulcers. Surg. Gynec. Obstet. 101:759, 1955.
30. Haubrich, W. S. The clinical recognition and pathological anatomy of intractability in peptic ulcer disease. Ann. N.Y. Acad. Sci. 99:114, 1962.
31. Ross, J. R., and Reaves, L. E. Syndrome of posterior penetrating peptic ulcer. Med. Clin. N. Amer. 50:461, 1966.
32. Cassel, C., Ruffin, J. M., and Bone, F. C. The clinical features of walled-off perforated peptic ulcer. South. Med. J. 44:1021, 1951.
33. Rivers, A. B. Syndrome of peptic ulcer perforating into pancreas. Proc. Mayo Clin. 22:290, 1947.
34. Mistilis, S. P., Wiot, J. F., and Nedelman, S. H. Giant duodenal ulcer. Ann. Intern. Med. 59:155, 1963.
35. Berkowitz, D., and Glassman, S. Giant duodenal ulcer. Gastroenterology 42:743, 1962.
36. Bullock, W. K., and Snyder, E. N. Benign giant duodenal ulcer. Gastroenterology 20:330, 1952.
37. Goldstein, H., Jamin, M., Schapiro, M., and Boyle, J. D. Gastric retention associated with gastroduodenal disease. Amer. J. Dig. Dis. 11:887, 1966.
38. Kozoll, D. D., and Meyer, K. A. Obstructing gastroduodenal ulcer, symptoms and signs. Arch. Surg. 89:491, 1964.
39. Kreel, L., and Ellis, H. Pyloric stenosis in adults: A clinical and radiological study of 100 consecutive patients. Gut 6:253, 1965.
40. Dworken, H. J., and Roth, H. P. Pyloric obstruction associated with peptic ulcer. J.A.M.A. 180:1007, 1962.
41. Moody, F. G., Cornell, G. N., and Beal, J. M.

Pyloric obstruction complicating peptic ulcer. Arch. Surg. 84:462, 1962.
42. Balint, J. A., and Spence, M. P. Pyloric stenosis. Brit. Med. J. 1:890, 1959.
43. Kozoll, D. D., and Meyer, K. A. Obstructing gastroduodenal ulcers, general factors influencing incidence and mortality. Arch. Surg. 88:793, 1964.
44. Kozoll, D. D., and Meyer, K. A. Computer analysis of 2639 painful gastroduodenal ulcers. Arch. Surg. 91:983, 1965.
45. Schwartz, W. B., Van Ypersele de Strihou, C., and Kassirer, J. P. Role of anions in metabolic alkalosis and potassium deficiency. New Eng. J. Med. 279:630, 1968.
46. Aber, G. M., Sampson, P. A., Whitehead, T. P., and Brooke, B. N. The role of chloride in the correction of alkalosis associated with potassium depletion. Lancet 2:1028, 1962.
47. Kassirer, J. P., and Schwartz, W. B. The response of normal man to selective depletion of hydrochloric acid and correction of metabolic alkalosis in man without repair of potassium deficiency. Amer. J. Med. 40:10, 1966.
48. Clark, R. G., and Norman, J. N. Metabolic alkalosis in pyloric stenosis. Lancet 1:1244, 1964.
49. Saunders, S. J., Irvine, R. O. H., Crawford, M. A., and Milne, M. D. Intracellular pH of potassium deficient voluntary muscle. Lancet 1:468, 1960.
50. Walker, G. W., and Jost, L. J. Relative roles of potassium and chloride in correction of hypokalemic hypochloremic alkalosis. Johns Hopkins Med. J. 120:148, 1967.
51. Kozoll, D. D., Mittelpunkt, A. I., and Meyer, K. A. Obstructing duodenal ulcers; effects of treatment on morbidity and mortality. Arch. Surg. 91:431, 1965.
52. Thomson, F. B., McDougall, E. P., and McIntyre, D. I. Follow-up study of 500 patients with chronic duodenal ulcer admitted to a veterans hospital. Surg. Gynec. Obstet. 110:51, 1960.
53. Boyle, J. D., and Goldstein, H. Management of pyloric obstruction. Med. Clin. N. Amer. 52:1329, 1968.
54. Rimer, D. G. Gastric retention without mechanical obstruction. Arch. Intern. Med. 117:287, 1966.
55. Raskin, H. F. Barium-Burger roentgen study for unrecognized, clinically significant gastric retention. South. Med. J. 64:1227, 1971.
56. Rapaport, E., and Scheinman, M. Rationale and limitations of hemodynamic measurements in patients with acute myocardial infarction. Mod. Concepts Card. Dis. 38:55, 1969.
57. Cooke, L., and Hutton, C. F. Postbulbar duodenal ulceration. Lancet 1:754, 1958.
58. Folk, W. T., et al. Peptic ulcer near the pylorus. Gastroenterology 32:395, 1957.
59. Murray, G. F., Ballinger, W. F., and Stafford, E. S. Ulcers of the pyloric channel. Amer. J. Surg. 113:199, 1967.
60. Jorgensen, T. G., et al. Preoperative prediction of results following surgery for chronic duodenal ulcer. Gastroenterology 60:680, 1971.

Chapter 60

Indications for Surgery and Selection of Operation in Peptic Ulcer Disease

Robert N. McClelland

INDICATIONS FOR SURGERY IN PEPTIC ULCER DISEASE

In general, about 85 per cent of duodenal ulcers and 50 per cent of gastric ulcers may be managed by nonsurgical means. The classic indications for surgical treatment of peptic ulcer are intractability, hemorrhage, perforation, and obstruction. The ensuing discussion delineates the judgments and decisions made in the clinical applications of these surgical indications.

INTRACTABILITY

Duodenal Ulcer. Intractability is the principal surgical indication in about 40 to 50 per cent of peptic ulcer patients undergoing surgery. It is, however, the most difficult indication to apply, because its evaluation is entirely subjective. Nevertheless, there are good guidelines for the proper definition of intractability. First, there must be an accurate diagnosis of the ulcer. There should be a history of chronic ulcer symptoms which have responded poorly to medical treatment for many months and preferably for several years.

An intensive attempt to treat the ulcer medically must be made. Generally, outpatient treatment is instituted under close guidance of the physician. The details of medical therapy are dealt with elsewhere and will not be repeated here. If outpatient medical treatment is unsuccessful, the patient is hospitalized and treated intensively. Inpatient treatment should continue for at least three to four weeks for an adequate trial of medical therapy. If possible, the patient may be treated at home on a semi-ambulatory basis during the latter part of the therapy. After this, if the patient continues having disabling ulcer symptoms, or has prompt symptomatic recurrence despite continuing adequate medical treatment, surgery should be considered. In some instances, even though the patient responds completely for several months to medical treatment, it is good judgment to operate if the patient has a long chronic history (over two years), has been incapacitated frequently in the past despite good medical treatment, and is a good operative risk. In such severe ulcer diatheses it is probably good judgment to operate electively before major ulcer complications or severe complicating medical diseases develop which

772

would considerably increase surgical mortality.

Certain types of duodenal ulcers are more likely to require surgery on the basis of intractability. These are chronic posterior penetrating ulcers (especially when associated with pancreatitis),[1] postbulbar ulcers,[2] pyloric channel ulcers,[3] ulcers which have previously caused a major complication, ulcers developing before age 20 or after age 65 (especially in males),[4] and chronic ulcers in alcoholics and psychologically unstable patients who are unlikely to maintain a suitable medical regimen.

Gastric Ulcer. The treatment of choice for chronic or recurrent gastric ulcer is surgical, because mortality and morbidity are somewhat less than with medical therapy, the cure rate is much higher, and the possibility of missing a potentially curable gastric carcinoma is avoided. Chronic gastric ulcer may be defined as one which fails to heal completely after good medical treatment or promptly recurs in spite of suitable continuing medical treatment. If an ulcer recurs several months or years after medical treatment and there is no evidence of malignancy, it may still be considered an acute gastric ulcer and medically treated intensively once more. However, if it does not promptly heal or recurs for a second time, it should be defined as a chronic gastric ulcer and treated surgically.

When a gastric ulcer is detected, intensive study to determine whether it is malignant is undertaken. Surgery should be performed immediately if any of the following pertain: radiological or gastroscopic suggestion of malignancy,[5-7] histamine-fast achlorhydria,[8] positive cytology[9] or biopsy (preferably obtained through the fiberoptic gastroscope), or chronic ulcer. If none of these criteria pertain, Paustian et al. suggest intensive in-hospital medical treatment for a period of three weeks.[10] In this time, a benign ulcer will usually diminish in size by at least 50 per cent. Paustian and colleagues found a final diagnostic error of only 2.7 per cent when using this criterion. If the ulcer diminishes more than 50 per cent after three weeks, treatment is continued for a total of six to eight weeks. If 50 per cent healing has not occurred after three weeks, or complete healing after six to eight weeks, surgery is performed in good risk patients, because the possibility of malignancy or chronicity (with associated complications of bleeding or perforation) increases after that time. After successful medical treatment, the patient should be X-rayed again four to six weeks after complete healing has been demonstrated and while continuing medical treatment. If recurrence is noted then, the ulcer should be removed immediately, because the chronicity of the ulcer is then apparent and the danger of persistent medical treatment is thus increased.

Approximately 30 to 70 per cent of benign gastric ulcers recur even with adequate medical therapy.[11, 12] The incidence of serious complications developing because of ill-advised persistent medical treatment of chronic or recurrent gastric ulcers is quite high. The mortality for medical treatment (mostly resulting from hemorrhage or perforation) in a large review (3208 cases) of gastric ulcer patients was 5.4 per cent and for surgical therapy was 3.4 per cent.[12] Much of the surgical mortality arose from emergency operations for hemorrhage, perforation, and obstruction. The surgical mortality fell to 1.8 per cent, however, if only elective surgical mortality was considered. Moreover, many deaths from emergency gastric ulcer surgery might have been prevented if elective surgery had been performed as soon as it was apparent that medical treatment of gastric ulcers had failed. The morbidity of medical treatment in this series of patients was 11.5 per cent, and was mostly related to development of life-endangering hemorrhage or perforation, whereas the morbidity of surgical treatment was 7.1 per cent and was mostly related to postoperative complications and postgastrectomy symptoms which, although undesirable, were not life threatening in most instances. Also significant was the difference in clinical cure rate without recurrence during the average seven-year follow-up. The cure rate for medical treatment was only 48 per cent vs. 90 per cent for surgical treatment. Theoretically, by selecting some gastric ulcer patients for medical treatment and others for surgical treatment, according to the criteria discussed above, better overall therapeutic results, in terms of morbidity and mortality, should be attained than if medical treatment only or surgical treatment only is recommended.

Many clinicians have the erroneous conception that gastric cancer and duodenal ulcer rarely occur simultaneously. Other misconceptions are that gastric cancers are almost invariably associated with achlorhydria and with short clinical histories. However, several large studies show that more than 20 per cent of patients with malignant gastric ulcers also have or have had duodenal ulcers,[13, 14] that acid is secreted in about 75 per cent of malignant gastric ulcers,[15] and that up to 28 per cent of malignant gastric ulcer patients have gastric ulcer histories of more than five years.[16] Therefore none of these criteria should lull the clinician into a false sense of security. If any improvement in treatment of gastric carcinoma occurs, it will be by removing malignant gastric ulcers quickly. The overall five-year survival for malignant gastric ulcers is 41 per cent, whereas it is 15 per cent or less for all other forms of gastric cancer.[12] This presupposes that the malignant ulcer was not thought likely to be malignant prior to its removal (see pp. 705 to 710).

HEMORRHAGE

As an Indication for Peptic Ulcer Surgery. Approximately 20 per cent of peptic ulcers will bleed at some time, and nearly one-third of the patients who undergo operation do so because of hemorrhage. About half of all deaths from peptic ulcer are due to hemorrhage.[17, 18] The possibility of hemorrhage sufficiently severe to require surgery is more likely in patients with gastric ulcer, posterior penetrating duodenal ulcer, and postbulbar ulcer. Ulcers in these sites not only are more likely to bleed, but are more likely to bleed massively and to continue bleeding once they have begun. Approximately 75 per cent of peptic ulcers will cease bleeding with medical treatment, but the remainder will require emergency surgery. About one-third of patients undergoing surgery for hemorrhage bleed severely enough to require emergency operation.

Peptic ulcer hemorrhage must usually be massive to serve as an indication for surgery. Massive peptic ulcer hemorrhage is defined as follows: acute blood loss sufficient to reduce serum hemoglobin to less than 8 g per 100 ml and serum hematocrit to less than 24, to produce signs of clinical shock, and to require more than 1500 cc of whole blood to replace blood loss and restore vital signs. The presence of any of these criteria is sufficient to define massive hemorrhage[19, 20] (see pp. 195 to 214).

Surgery might be done in some cases for repeated nonmassive hemorrhages, especially if these occur in patients more than 60 years old, in patients who have another major ulcer complication such as perforation or obstruction, in patients who cannot be maintained on a good ulcer regimen, or in those who suffer some degree of intractable pain.

Clinical data indicate that a single massive hemorrhage after the age of 60, more than one massive hemorrhage, or one massive hemorrhage plus another previous major ulcer complication under the age of 60 is generally an indication for peptic ulcer surgery.[17, 18, 21-24] The rationale for allowing only one massive hemorrhage in the older patient is based upon average mortality figures of 15 per cent for massive hemorrhage and 4 per cent for lesser hemorrhage in patients over 60 and less than 5 per cent for massive hemorrhage and approximately 1 per cent for lesser hemorrhage in patients under 60. In other words, although mortality does not rise with repeated hemorrhages in either age group and although it is doubtful that the elderly are more likely to rebleed than younger patients, the fact that any single hemorrhage is at least three times more likely to be fatal in patients over 60 is sufficient reason to perform elective surgery on such patients unless other serious associated diseases contraindicate surgery.

In those under 60 suffering more than one massive hemorrhage or one massive hemorrhage plus another major ulcer complication, current data support the conclusion that such virulent ulcers (arbitrarily defined as any ulcer associated with two or more major complications) are extremely likely to develop additional life-threatening complications which may require emergency surgery.[4] At this point, it becomes more likely that the patient will die of repeated ulcer complications than that he will die following elective surgery to correct the ulcer diathesis.

Some clinicians state that surgery may not really protect against repeated duodenal ulcer hemorrhage,[21, 25-27] citing a mean incidence of 18 per cent rebleeding after duodenal ulcer surgery (when the surgery was done initially for bleeding); however, the gravity of the rebleeding after surgery must be considered. In less than one-third of patients is the rebleeding sufficient to require several transfusions and thus endanger life significantly. Moreover, most of these series are based on rebleeding after subtotal gastrectomy. More recently, however, Hallenbeck, in a review of several series of gastric surgery for duodenal ulcer, noted a mean incidence of postoperative rebleeding of only 6 per cent when vagotomy and antrectomy was done for bleeding.[24] This is probably because the more physiologically sound vagotomy and antrectomy controls the more severe ulcer diathesis associated with bleeding better than subtotal gastrectomy, which does not incorporate the additional protection of vagotomy. Thus life-threatening hemorrhage is expected after vagotomy and antrectomy in less than 2 per cent of all cases. In contrast, if gastric surgery is not performed for bleeding duodenal ulcer, Donaldson and coworkers report a rebleeding rate of 40 per cent,[26] and Gardner and Baronofsky, 51 per cent.[28] If an ulcer crater was seen on upper gastrointestinal series, the rebleeding rate within five years rose to 70 per cent, according to Gardner and Baronofsky. Consequently, at least 15 per cent of duodenal ulcer patients not operated upon after massive hemorrhage would have at least one episode of potentially fatal bleeding within five years of the initial hemorrhage. This is more than seven times the expected rate of significant rebleeding after vagotomy and antrectomy for hemorrhage.

Borland et al.[21] and Grace and Mitty[27] contend that surgery is not indicated in the management of bleeding peptic ulcer except for emergency surgery for unrelenting hemorrhage. Significantly, they make no distinction between minor and massive hemorrhages or between younger or older patients in their series. It is generally agreed that surgery is not required for minor hemorrhage (with the exceptions previously noted), especially in younger patients. Also, it is agreed that emergency surgery is required for exsanguinating peptic ulcer hemorrhage. The chief point of contention therefore is whether to perform elective surgery for one massive hemorrhage over age 60 or for two or more massive hemorrhages under age 60. Only large, prospective controlled studies will settle the issue with certainty, but the bulk of current opinion favors elective surgery in such cases.[22-24, 29]

Leape and Welch further point out that patients must be followed for at least five years to determine the true incidence of morbidity and mortality from recurrent bleeding.[29] In Borland's medical series, only a third of the patients were followed more than five years (only 5 per cent of these were patients over 60 who suffered massive hemorrhage) and another third were followed for less than a year.[21]

Table 60-1, based upon generally accepted figures from the medical and surgical literature, shows a comparison of the expected mortality and rebleeding rates from medical and elective surgical treatment of patients over 60 suffering a massive peptic ulcer hemorrhage. There is a more than twofold difference in mortality in favor of surgical therapy. In addition to reduced mortality from recurrent hemorrhage, surgical therapy also greatly reduces the morbidity of often-repeated hemorrhages in medically treated patients. Furthermore, better protection is provided by surgical treatment against intractable pain, perforation, and obstruction, complications which are also quite likely to cause mortality in patients with peptic ulcers which have demonstrated their virulence by massive bleeding. Certainly the morbidity of gastric surgery must also be considered, but with better surgical procedures it should be minimal and should only infrequently endanger life, in contrast to recurrent hemorrhage.

As an Indication for Emergency Peptic Ulcer Surgery. In order to appraise accurately and quickly the rate and amount of bleeding from a peptic ulcer, a large-bore nasogastric tube should be inserted immediately. In no other way can a dangerously increased rate of bleeding be recognized quickly enough to take adequate and rapid surgical measures against

TABLE 60–1. MORTALITY IN MASSIVE BLEEDERS OVER 60 (WITHIN FIVE YEARS OF INITIAL HEMORRHAGE) (BASED ON 40 PER CENT REBLEED RATE)

MEDICAL TREATMENT		SURGICAL TREATMENT	
Survived first hemorrhage	1000		1000
		Elective surgery	1000 (15)
	Minor hemorrhage Major hemorrhage		Minor hemorrhage Major hemorrhage
Second hemorrhage	265 135		40 20
	(10) (20)		(2) (3)
	370		55
Third hemorrhage	100 50		15 7
	(4) (8)		(1) (1)
	138		20
Fourth hemorrhage	38 18		6 3
	(1) (3)		(0) (0)
TOTAL DEAD	46		22

Number dead in parentheses.
Twenty-four more dead of recurrent hemorrhage with medical treatment.

the hemorrhage. In addition, the nasogastric tube also provides a good means of stopping the bleeding. Many times merely evacuating blood clots from the stomach and allowing its contraction to an empty, quiescent state help bleeding cease rapidly. This is probably due to contraction of gastric submucosal blood vessels and generally decreased gastric blood flow induced by decompression of the dilated stomach. Also, cold saline lavage through the nasogastric tube is often conducive in several ways to stopping the hemorrhage. The cold lavage dilutes and removes acid and pepsin, and local hypothermia induces blood vessel contraction and clot formation and reduces autodigestive enzyme activity. Lavage is continued until the return is essentially clear of blood or until it is apparent that bleeding is persistent and surgery is required. When hemorrhage stops and the Levin tube is clear of blood for several hours, the tube is removed and the regular medical ulcer regimen is begun. It is a common experience to see a patient with a massively bleeding ulcer being treated without nasogastric suction and with hourly milk and antacids who continues to bleed despite such treatment. Such patients often promptly stop bleeding as soon as the dilated stomach is

evacuated with a nasogastric tube and cold saline lavage is begun. Nasogastric tubes are now available which function on a sump principle and are much more efficient for emptying and lavaging the stomach (Salem sump tube; Anderson tube[30]).

There is probably no place for control of bleeding by hypothermia machines. The technique is difficult, associated with significant morbidity and mortality, and probably no more effective than simple iced saline lavage.[31, 32]

As mentioned, approximately 75 per cent of bleeding peptic ulcers stop bleeding without requiring emergency surgery. Emergency surgery to stop bleeding is avoided if possible, because the mortality for emergency surgery for bleeding is at least five times the mortality for elective peptic ulcer surgery, especially in poor risk patients. This statement must not be interpreted to mean that emergency surgery is avoided until the patient is in serious condition from continuing hemorrhage. Continuing massive bleeding is unlikely to stop and the mortality and the morbidity increase greatly unless operation is promptly performed. This is particularly true for elderly, poor risk patients for whom the physician might be unwisely inclined to delay surgery even longer.

Hoerr and colleagues,[33] Foster et al.,[17] and many others have documented the marked reduction in mortality rate from persistently bleeding peptic ulcers which is achieved if certain guidelines are followed to decide when to operate. Surgery should be immediately performed for exsanguinating hemorrhage which is evidenced by massive hematemesis or steady and rapid flow of blood from a nasogastric tube, with development of shock which persists after rapid administration of 1000 cc of whole blood. Surgery should also be done when more than 1500 cc of whole blood is given in less than 24 hours and significant bleeding continues, or when more than 2500 cc of blood is given during three consecutive days and significant bleeding persists, or when significant recurrent bleeding occurs during the same hospitalization for an episode of massive ulcer bleeding. If there is a shortage of an unusual blood type or crossmatching problems exist, even earlier operation may be wise.

PERFORATION

As an Indication for Peptic Ulcer Surgery. Approximately 5 per cent of peptic ulcers perforate at some time. The likelihood that a gastric ulcer will perforate is less. The ratio of duodenal ulcer to gastric ulcer perforation is 15:1, whereas the ratio of duodenal to gastric ulcer incidence is 4 or 5:1. Most perforations are free perforations into the peritoneal cavity, but may also be confined. In fact, in all peptic ulcer patients coming to surgery, about 20 per cent present with confined perforations. Most confined perforations occur in ulcers on the posterior duodenal or gastric wall and erode into the pancreas. The confined perforation is often associated with intractable pain or bleeding.[1] Only rarely does a primary peptic ulcer penetrate into surrounding viscera such as the colon, common duct, or kidney.

Treatment of Free Perforation. Immediate surgery is the treatment of choice for free perforation, with two possible exceptions.[34] The first exception is the so-called forme fruste ulcer.[35] A forme fruste ulcer leaks into the free peritoneal cavity and causes a moderate localized peritonitis and usually pneumoperi-

toneum, but the ulcer is promptly sealed off by omentum or surrounding viscera and further leakage of gastroduodenal content stops. The typical patient has a history of dramatic onset of abdominal signs and symptoms which may diminish rapidly in intensity and may almost disappear. In other cases, there is a slower atypical onset of abdominal signs and symptoms which fail to advance or diminish over several hours. Perforation may not be suspected until free air is detected in the abdominal cavity by suitable X-ray studies (i.e., upright chest or left lateral decubitus films of the abdomen). Adequate therapy of the spontaneously sealed ulcer consists of nasogastric intubation with a large-bore tube and constant suction drainage of the stomach to prevent recurrent leakage of the sealed ulcer. Nasogastric suction is continued for two or three days or until associated ileus and all clinical findings completely resolve. Intravenous fluid and broad-spectrum parenteral antibiotic therapy are also given (see pp. 338 to 351). The patient is evaluated very frequently during such therapy; if any suggestion of increasing peritonitis or clinical deterioration develops, surgery is immediately performed.

The second possible exception to operative treatment of a free ulcer perforation may be made in the management of patients with other grave illnesses which significantly increase surgical mortality. Usually this would include patients with recent transmural myocardial infarctions or other grave cardiopulmonary disease. Intensive medical treatment with continuous nasogastric suction, intravenous fluids, and broad-spectrum antibiotics would be instituted even though the ulcer had not sealed off when the patient was first seen. Even in such high risk patients, surgery must be performed after a reasonable trial of medical therapy indicates that peritonitis is not resolving or is advancing. The advancing peritonitis from continued ulcer leakage is more dangerous to the patient than judiciously performed surgery.

Despite some reports that medical treatment is suitable for many free perforations, the general conclusion is that surgery is preferable, because it more quickly and surely stops gastroduodenal leakage and permits thorough cleansing of the peritoneal cavity. For these reasons mortality and morbidity should be lower with surgical than with medical treatment.

Treatment of "Contained Perforations" of Peptic Ulcers. The indications for treatment of this condition are less well defined than for free perforations. Surgery is often performed on the basis of indications related to intractable pain or hemorrhage with which contained perforations are likely to be associated. In more unusual cases persistent or recurrent pancreatitis may be caused by a contained perforation into the pancreas, and surgery to correct the ulcer is indicated on this basis if medical therapy is not successful in relieving the pancreatitis. Surgery is also indicated to correct the very rare perforation of peptic ulcer into other viscera such as the common duct or colon as soon as such a condition is recognized.

OBSTRUCTION

As an Indication for Peptic Ulcer Surgery. Approximately 10 per cent of operations for peptic ulcer are performed primarily for obstruction.[36] Most patients with peptic ulcer obstruction are managed by medical therapy alone unless they are immediately prepyloric or pyloric channel ulcers, in which case surgery is more likely to be required.[3] Pyloric obstruction caused by peptic ulcer has an inflammatory and fibrotic component. Usually three days or less of continuous nasogastric suction suffices to resolve inflammatory edema at the pylorus and relieve the obstruction. If obstruction does not relent, however, after five to seven days of nasogastric suction, it is unlikely that medical management will be effective and surgery must be performed. It will be apparent that obstruction has relented when the amount of 12-hour gastric secretion drops below 750 cc and the brilliant green color (caused by biliverdin) of the gastric aspirate changes to a darker green or amber color. This is confirmed by the saline load test (less than 400 cc of 750 cc of normal saline injected into the stomach retained after 30 minutes)[37, 38] or by upper gastrointestinal barium series. The saline load test, if found positive on admission, indicates that surgery will most probably be required, but a period of preoperative nasogastric suction and preparation of at least five to seven days is usually necessary (see pp. 757 to 770).

In patients with marked weight loss caused by chronic pyloric obstruction, it is wise to begin intravenous hypertonic feedings of protein hydrolysate and dextrose through a central venous catheter, as described by Dudrick and colleagues.[39] Before beginning central intravenous hyperalimentation, however, particular care should be taken to correct hypokalemic, hypochloremic alkalosis often present in patients with chronic pyloric obstruction.[40] Hyperalimentation causes considerable potassium loss and might compound the difficulty of potassium replacement in patients already severely depleted. These patients may have total body deficits of potassium of up to 800 to 1000 mEq. Mortality and morbidity from surgery may be reduced from over 20 per cent to less than 5 per cent by reversal of negative nitrogen balance in severely depleted patients.[41] Until central intravenous hyperalimentation was developed, it was sometimes necessary in severely depleted patients to feed them per jejunostomy for several days before definitive gastric surgery. Now this is seldom necessary.

In some instances, even though nasogastric suction relieves an initially complete or very high grade pyloric obstruction, elective surgery should be performed during that hospital admission after the patient is suitably prepared. This should be done in patients previously having at least one other major ulcer complication such as perforation, hemorrhage, or a previous obstructive episode, or in patients who had intractable pain in spite of adequate medical therapy prior to the obstruction. Patients should also have surgery, even though the obstruction does relent with nasogastric suction, when they are demonstrated by upper gastrointestinal series to have pronounced fixed pyloric narrowing caused by marked scarring of the duodenal bulb, a pyloric channel ulcer, or an immediately prepyloric ulcer, or by a definitely positive saline load test, because of the great likelihood that recurrent obstruction will develop in these circumstances.

The general recurrence rate of complete or virtually complete pyloric obstruction caused by ulcer after medical treatment of an episode of such obstruction is 20 to 25 per cent,[38] and, in the instances just mentioned, would very probably be significantly higher. In view of the evidence that operative mortality for patients with obstructing ulcers is four to five times less in the better-nourished patient,[41] it seems wise perhaps to operate electively on patients with a first episode of severe pyloric obstruction, even though they respond to medical therapy. It seems likely that they will soon reobstruct and perhaps then require surgery under less than optimal conditions. The post-treatment saline load test,[37] in addition to an upper gastrointestinal series, may help greatly in deciding which of these patients are likely to reobstruct soon and therefore to be candidates for elective surgery after an initial bout of pyloric obstruction. If the patient is reliable and can be followed adequately, medical treatment may be tried; but if this is unsatisfactory, surgery should be performed promptly before debilitation occurs.

SELECTION OF OPERATION FOR PEPTIC ULCER

For many years the search has continued for the "ideal" peptic ulcer operation. Surgeons and gastroenterologists still have a penchant for recommending one operation for peptic ulcer to the general exclusion of others, often on the basis of somewhat questionable clinical impressions that a certain operation gives "better results." Out of this cloud of dissension and mass of data a more rational concept for selecting the proper operation for peptic ulcer is emerging. This more rational concept proposes no single ideal operation but, instead, several. It therefore becomes the clinician's task to learn how to select the most suitable operation for a particular patient. This concept is so recent that the criteria for selection currently used in many centers are not so well defined by large randomized prospective clinical studies. There are, however, sufficient restrospective clinical data from many centers to be able to outline certain criteria to use in the selection of a reasonable operative procedure for a specific patient. In the following discussion an attempt will be made to outline the method

of selection we use, which is similar to that used by several other centers.[42–46]

SELECTION OF ELECTIVE OPERATION FOR DUODENAL ULCER

There are currently three basic operations in general use for the treatment of duodenal ulcer. These operations are vagotomy and antrectomy,[42, 47-49] vagotomy and drainage,[50-52] and subtotal gastrectomy.[42, 53]

Vagotomy and Antrectomy. This operation is the most rational physiologically, because it controls most certainly both the chief phases of gastric acid secretion. The cephalic secretory phase is controlled by vagotomy and the gastric secretory phase by antrectomy. This is borne out by several very large clinical series which have accumulated since the mid 1940's, showing an ulcer recurrence rate of less than 1 per cent after vagotomy and antrectomy. An additional advantage of this operation is a smaller incidence of unacceptable weight loss and inability to eat normal amounts of food (small stomach syndrome) than with subtotal gastrectomy. This is due to the smaller amount of stomach resected (less than 50 per cent) with antrectomy and vagotomy than with subtotal gastrectomy (65 to 75 per cent). Indeed, Palumbo and associates maintain that only a distal antrectomy (25 per cent resection or less) is required and support this statement by reporting a recurrence rate of 0.4 per cent in 510 patients followed up to 16 years.[47] There has not, however, been a lesser incidence of dumping syndrome than with subtotal gastrectomy, although this has not been a frequent problem with either operation when a small gastrointestinal stoma is constructed. The great majority of patients report excellent long-term satisfaction with vagotomy and antrectomy.

The principal disadvantage of vagotomy and antrectomy is a mortality rate which is somewhat higher than after vagotomy and drainage. The average mortality for an elective vagotomy and antrectomy is 1.5 to 2.0 per cent; the average mortality of elective vagotomy and drainage is 0.5 to 1.0 per cent. The average mortality, however, in poor-risk patients for emergency vagotomy and antrectomy (for bleeding or perforation) is approximately 20 per cent; it is about 10 per cent for emergency vagotomy and drainage. The emergency operative mortality, however, should be less than 3 per cent for both operations in younger, better risk patients.

On the basis of the foregoing figures, vagotomy and antrectomy is the operation of choice for duodenal ulcer patients with the following characteristics: male sex, history of major complications (especially hemorrhage), high basal and histamine-stimulated gastric acid secretion,[43, 46, 54] relative youth, no complicating medical diseases, and good nutritional state. In short, when possible recurrence is judged a more significant problem than operative risk, vagotomy and antrectomy should be done. It is not critical whether a Billroth I or Billroth II gastrointestinal reconstruction is performed when vagotomy is done, although the Billroth II is probably technically safer when the duodenum is significantly scarred because of the decreased chance of gastroduodenal leak.

Vagotomy and Drainage. The chief advantage of this procedure is low operative mortality. Another major advantage is that it has the lowest incidence of nutritional problems and dumping syndrome.

The principal disadvantage of vagotomy and drainage, which is a relative one, however, is its higher recurrence rate. In most large series which have been followed for up to ten years, the recurrence rate for vagotomy and pyloroplasty is about 6 to 10 per cent, being perhaps somewhat higher for vagotomy and gastroenterostomy. The recurrence rate may be less than 3 per cent in some series in which the main indication for surgery was intractability or the average follow-up period was short. However, in series in which many of the patients underwent surgery for major duodenal ulcer complications rather than intractability and in which there was a preponderance of young males, i.e., series of more virulent ulcers, the recurrence rate is probably much higher after vagotomy and drainage.[42] Nobles reports a recurrence rate after vagotomy and drainage of 23.5 per cent after 15 years.[55]

One technical factor which may cause higher recurrence rates after vagotomy and pyloroplasty is failure to construct a pyloroplasty which adequately drains the

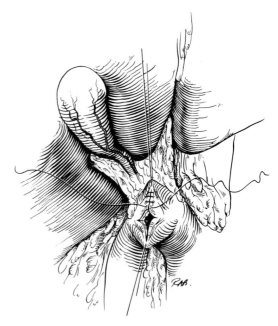

Figure 60–1. Heineke-Mikulicz pyloroplasty.

gastric antrum. The classic Heineke-Mikulicz pyloroplasty (Fig. 60–1) most commonly used may be more likely to cause antral stasis than other pyloroplasties. The Finney and Jaboulay pyloroplasties (Figs. 60–2 and 60–3, respectively) are now performed more often to afford more adequate antral drainage and probably lower recurrence rates. Bryant and as-

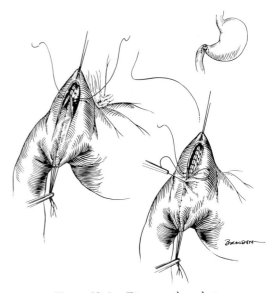

Figure 60–2. Finney pyloroplasty.

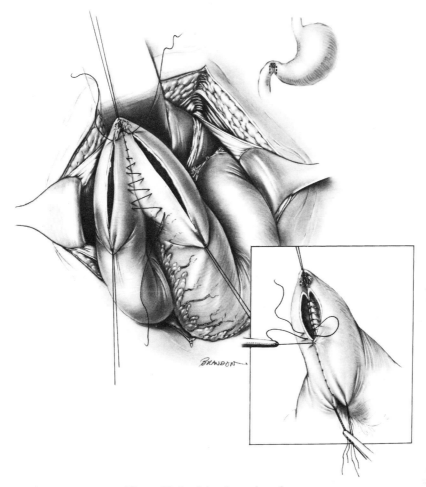

Figure 60–3. Jaboulay pyloroplasty.

sociates noted a recurrence rate of 22 per cent after Heineke-Mikulicz pyloroplasties vs. 10 per cent with Finney pyloroplasties.[56] Hayden and Read noted antral retention in 58 per cent of patients with Heineke-Mikulicz pyloroplasties and in less than 10 per cent of patients with Finney pyloroplasties.[57] The more patulous opening provided by the Finney and Jaboulay pyloroplasties probably accounts for their better antral drainage. In most instances, the Finney pyloroplasty is used, the Jaboulay pyloroplasty being reserved for very severe duodenal bulb scarring and inflammation. The Finney and Jaboulay pyloroplasties are safer in that a two-layer anastomosis is performed without fear of obstruction; only one layer of sutures should be used in constructing the Heineke-Mikulicz pyloroplasty in order to

avoid obstructing the gastric outlet. Leakage of pyloroplasties of which we are aware all occurred in one-layer Heineke-Mikulicz pyloroplasties.

On the basis of its associated advantages and disadvantages, vagotomy and drainage (preferably vagotomy and Finney pyloroplasty), should be the elective procedure of choice in duodenal ulcer patients with the following characteristics: advanced age, female sex, significant complicating medical disease increasing operative risk, poor nutritional state, not markedly elevated basal and histamine-stimulated gastric acid secretion, intractability as the sole reason for surgery, no previous major ulcer complications (especially hemorrhage), or severe scarring around the duodenum (making gastric resection excessively dangerous). In short, in poor risk patients or patients without too severe ulcer diathesis but with indications for surgery, vagotomy and drainage is the procedure of choice.

Subtotal Gastric Resection. Although this operation, consisting of removal of 65 to 75 per cent of the distal stomach, was the standard operation for duodenal ulcer for many years, it currently has little to recommend it in comparison to the two procedures previously discussed, although it may be performed in otherwise good risk patients who have excessive gastric dilatation and edema caused by chronic pyloric obstruction, in which case vagotomy may cause prolonged gastric atony and retention.

Subtotal gastrectomy gives less protection against recurrent ulcer than vagotomy and antrectomy. The average ulcer recurrence rate in more recent series is 5 per cent after Billroth II subtotal gastric resection and 13.8 per cent after Billroth I subtotal gastric resection.[58] The recurrence rate is higher after Billroth I gastrectomy, probably because insufficient stomach is often resected in order to approximate the stomach and duodenum without suture line tension. When the vagus nerve is resected, either Billroth I or II reconstructions are acceptable, because high gastric resection is not necessary with a vagotomy. Another disadvantage of subtotal gastric resection is an elective mortality of 1.5 to 2.0 per cent and an emergency mortality rate of 20 per cent or more in poor risk patients.[17] The mortality is the same as for vagotomy and antrectomy, but without the advantage of the low recurrence rate of vagotomy and antrectomy. The mortality of subtotal gastrectomy is significantly higher than that of vagotomy and drainage, with questionably fewer recurrences.[53]

Truncal vs. Selective Vagotomy. The only possible advantage of subtotal gastrectomy is the lack of vagotomy complications. Generally, the incidence of troublesome postvagotomy diarrhea is only 5 per cent, and even then the diarrhea can usually be controlled by dietary and medical treatment, with the exception of about 0.5 to 1 per cent who respond poorly, if at all, to treatment (see p. 814). The only other noteworthy late complication of vagotomy is the possibility that the incidence of gallstones may increase after truncal vagotomy.[59] Many reports comparing selective vagotomy and truncal vagotomy have appeared recently.[60-62] Selective vagotomy is performed by cutting only the vagal fibers to the stomach while leaving the hepatic and celiac branches of the anterior and posterior vagal trunks intact (Fig. 60–4).[63] It was postulated that selective vagotomy would be associated with fewer instances of postvagotomy diarrhea, but might cause a greater incidence of incomplete vagotomy. The opposite has proved to be true, however, in that there has been no difference in the incidence of postvagotomy diarrhea, but surprisingly a complete gastric vagotomy has been more frequently achieved than with truncal vagotomy.[61] No data are available now, but selective vagotomy may be associated with a smaller incidence of gallstone formation than is truncal vagotomy (perhaps because of preservation of the hepatic branch of the vagus nerve and of gallbladder innervation). Selective vagotomy is technically more difficult to perform, but not excessively so, and if its advantages are confirmed by additional experience, it may replace truncal vagotomy.

Recently, Amdrup and Jensen have reported results in patients with duodenal ulcer undergoing an even more selective, or "super-selective," vagotomy.[64] In this operation, not only are the celiac and hepatic vagal branches left intact, the vagal

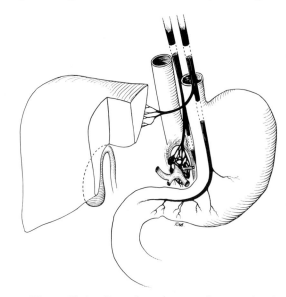

Figure 60–4. Sites of vagal section for truncal and selective vagotomies.

branches to the gastric antrum are also preserved. The intact antral innervation permits normal gastric emptying and obviates the need for a gastric drainage procedure, so the pylorus is left undisturbed. The intact pylorus is said to eliminate dumping. It will be interesting to see what continued experience with "super-selective" vagotomy reveals, but present experience with it is much too limited to make any meaningful judgments concerning it.

SELECTION OF EMERGENCY OPERATION FOR BLEEDING DUODENAL ULCER

The mortality from duodenal ulcer hemorrhage can be decreased even in poor risk patients by prompt operation when it is apparent that hemorrhage is not responding to medical treatment and by selection of the proper operation to stop the hemorrhage. All patients with bleeding ulcers should ideally be managed from admission by a "hematemesis team," consisting of an internist and a surgeon, both of whom have a large experience in managing gastrointestinal bleeding. In this way the most appropriate therapy for a particular patient is likely to be chosen (see pp. 195 to 214). The timing of surgical therapy has already been discussed. Foster and associates,[17] Weinberg,[65] Farris and Smith,[66] and many others have shown that the mortality from emergency surgery for bleeding duodenal ulcer can be decreased from 20 per cent or more when gastric resection is performed to about 10 per cent or less in elderly poor risk patients when the lesser procedure of vagotomy and pyloroplasty with suture of the bleeding vessel is performed.

The exception to the rule of performing emergency vagotomy and pyloroplasty with suture for bleeding duodenal ulcer would be a duodenal ulcer in younger, better risk patients, especially if the ulcer is a "giant" posterior penetrating one.[67, 68] A giant ulcer is arbitrarily defined as one larger than 2.5 cm in diameter. At least 20 per cent of giant posterior penetrating ulcers will rebleed in the immediate postoperative period if vagotomy and pyloroplasty with suture is done (some surgeons report up to 35 per cent) and will require immediate reoperation with an additional

mortality rate of up to 40 per cent for the reoperation.[68-70] If, however, the giant ulcer is instead oversewn and removed from the "alimentary stream" by a Billroth II gastric resection, the rebleeding rate is about 6 per cent in the immediate postoperative period, with a consequent reduction in emergency reoperation and mortality rate. In poor risk patients one must nevertheless accept the 20 per cent rebleeding incidence and perform vagotomy and pyloroplasty with suture of the giant ulcer, because the total mortality would still be less than if all very poor risk patients with giant posterior penetrating ulcers underwent initial gastric resections. In younger, better risk patients with giant ulcers it is wiser to perform initial emergency Billroth II gastric resection with exclusion of the bleeding ulcer from the "alimentary stream," because they would thus have less mortality than they would from rebleeding if vagotomy and pyloroplasty were performed initially.[67] It is also sound judgment to perform emergency vagotomy and antrectomy in good risk patients bleeding from a small ulcer, because the mortality is essentially the same as in emergency vagotomy and pyloroplasty among such patients. It is preferable, because, as discussed earlier, the late rebleeding rate is much less when vagotomy and antrectomy is done,[24] especially as an emergency procedure for hemorrhage, than when vagotomy and pyloroplasty is done. Any question, however, of a patient's ability to withstand a resection dictates that the surgeon perform vagotomy and pyloroplasty with ulcer suture.

In summary, older, poor risk patients undergoing emergency operation for bleeding duodenal ulcer should have vagotomy and pyloroplasty with suture regardless of ulcer size. The younger, good risk patients should have vagotomy and antrectomy, *especially* in the presence of a bleeding giant, posterior, penetrating duodenal ulcer.

SELECTION OF EMERGENCY OPERATION FOR PERFORATED DUODENAL ULCER

The standard operation for management of acute free perforation of a duodenal ulcer is immediate laparotomy and closure of the perforation. Several recent reports, however, suggest that it may be good judgment to perform more definitive surgery during the emergency operation.[71-75] After perforation, as many as two-thirds of the patients will require additional ulcer surgery within the next five years. About half of these will require surgery for recurrent major ulcer complications such as hemorrhage, obstruction, or reperforation and the other half for intractable ulcer pain. These figures are somewhat lower when perforation is the initial ulcer manifestation and somewhat higher when there is a chronic history of duodenal ulcer. Many clinicians maintain that most perforations occur in those with chronic rather than acute ulcers, although the prevailing opinion has been that about 50 per cent of perforations occur in patients with acute duodenal ulcers.

Therefore in younger patients without complicating medical diseases, who have perforated only a few hours before surgery, are in good general condition, and have minimal peritonitis, either a vagotomy and pyloroplasty or vagotomy and antrectomy may be safely performed. In most instances, vagotomy and pyloroplasty is adequate, but when systemic and local conditions seem suitable and there is a history of previous major ulcer complications, especially hemorrhage, a vagotomy and antrectomy is indicated for better control of the more virulent ulcer diathesis. If conservative judgment is used in selecting patients for definitive operation as against simple closure of the perforation, the mortality and morbidity for definitive emergency operation in good risk patients is no higher than if a simple closure is done; i.e., about 1 to 2 per cent. The great gain will be that when definitive operation is performed, less than 6 to 10 per cent will require reoperation instead of a minimum of 35 per cent who will require reoperation within five years if a simple closure only is done, not to speak of another 30 to 35 per cent who may not require ulcer surgery but who will continue to have troublesome symptoms. If there is any doubt of the safety of performing definitive emergency operation, however, simple closure of the perforation should be performed.

SELECTION OF OPERATION FOR OBSTRUCTING PEPTIC ULCER

The management of obstructing duodenal, pyloric channel, and immediately prepyloric gastric ulcer is essentially the same, because similar pathophysiology pertains to all. In general, the same criteria should be used in selecting the operation for obstruction as have already been discussed; i.e., in young, good risk patients without excessive duodenal scarring and inflammation, and without excessive gastric dilatation and edema, vagotomy and antrectomy should be performed; in older, poor risk patients or those with excessive duodenal scarring and inflammation, vagotomy and drainage (usually Jaboulay pyloroplasty or gastroenterostomy) should be performed.

It is, however, unsafe to perform vagotomy, especially vagotomy and drainage, if the stomach has not returned to normal size and muscle tone after an adequate period of nasogastric decompression before surgery for obstruction.[41, 76-79] Otherwise, the incidence of prolonged gastric atony and failure of gastric emptying will be prohibitively high (see p. 795). For this reason, it is suggested by some surgeons that gastroenterostomy alone or subtotal gastric resection without vagotomy be performed by choice for chronic pyloric obstruction. Certainly this suggestion should be followed if it is found upon exploration that the stomach is still significantly dilated and thick walled as a result of the obstruction. In that case, gastroenterostomy alone, with a Stamm tube gastrostomy for postoperative suction,[80] should be performed on poor risk patients or those with excessive reaction about the duodenum; subtotal gastrectomy alone should be performed on better risk patients without excessive reaction about the duodenum.

The foregoing should be the exception rather than the rule, however. In most instances, after five to seven days of preoperative nasogastric decompression, the stomach will be well compensated and vagotomy can safely be performed with either antrectomy or drainage as indicated, although antrectomy is preferred, because gastric atony is probably less likely after vagotomy and antrectomy. Gastric suction should also be maintained for four or five days postoperatively before beginning feedings as a further safeguard against postoperative atony. When possible, such postoperative gastric suction should be performed through a Stamm gastrostomy tube placed during surgery. This will avoid the discomfort and complications of prolonged nasogastric intubation. Placement of a gastrostomy tube is simple when vagotomy and drainage is done and the entire stomach remains; however, this may be more difficult or impossible because of the physical configuration of some patients after a vagotomy and antrectomy, in which case the nasogastric tube must be accepted. Such prolonged periods with no oral feedings are tolerated much better now than previously because of the development of central intravenous hyperalimentation,[39] which has almost entirely obviated the need for feeding jejunostomies, often required by these patients in the past.

When feedings are begun, it is wise to begin immediately with low residue solids with little or no intake of liquids orally for a day or so until one is sure the stomach is emptying adequately. Aspiration of stomach contents at bedtime two to three hours after the last meal allows documentation of gastric emptying. Although perhaps somewhat paradoxical, the stomach in these cases is more likely to regain normal tonus and peristalsis and to empty with solid food than with liquid.[81] The required fluids are, of course, given parenterally for a day or so after gastric suction is discontinued and solid feedings are started. When solids have been taken well, liquids can then be given in gradually increasing quantities, although they should still be withheld during meals and for 30 minutes before and after meals (see p. 794).

SELECTION OF ELECTIVE OPERATION FOR GASTRIC ULCER

The elective operation of choice for benign gastric ulcer is antrectomy with removal of the ulcer and Billroth I or II gastrointestinal reconstruction. In those with gastric ulcer without associated duodenal ulcer, the recurrence rate should be only 2 per cent and the mortality rate less than 1 to 2 per cent.

Some surgeons have recently reported good results by treating gastric ulcer with vagotomy and pyloroplasty with or without wedge excision of the ulcer.[82-85] This may be suitable for elderly, poor risk patients, but otherwise, as will be discussed further below, the recurrence rate as reported by some is excessively high.

Postgastrectomy symptoms are much less after antrectomy for gastric ulcer than after subtotal gastrectomy for duodenal ulcer because of the significantly smaller amount of stomach removed when antrectomy only is performed.

If gastric ulcer is associated with duodenal ulcer, as it is in about 20 per cent of gastric ulcer cases,[86] or if there is a high level of basal or histamine stimulated gastric acidity, a vagotomy should be added to the antrectomy for gastric ulcer. Antrectomy without vagotomy in these instances is likely to be associated with an inordinate recurrence rate.

Ulcers in the proximal stomach are a more controversial problem, especially those near the esophagogastric junction; they lend themselves poorly to treatment by resection or vagotomy because of their much less accessible locations—high in the stomach near the esophagus surrounded by severely inflamed and edematous tissue. Such conditions make it likely that resections will be associated with a high incidence of suture line leakage and that it will be difficult to locate the vagi and perform a safe and complete vagotomy. The several methods proposed for dealing with such proximal gastric ulcers are proximal gastrectomy, the Schoemaker gastrectomy, vagotomy and pyloroplasty with or without wedge excision of the ulcer, and the Kelling-Madlener operation. Proximal gastrectomy gives poor results because of a mortality rate approaching 10 per cent in some series (a result mostly of leakage of the esophagogastric anastomosis). The Schoemaker operation is antrectomy plus excision of a tongue of proximal lesser curvature, including the proximal ulcer.[87] It is suitable for some high gastric ulcers which are not too large, not surrounded by too much inflammatory reaction, and not too near the esophagogastric junction. If these limitations of the Schoemaker gastrectomy are not considered, however, the gastric suture line will be placed insecurely in inflamed, edematous tissue precariously near the esophagogastric junction and will be very prone to leak. Vagotomy and pyloroplasty are recommended in several recent papers as adequate treatment for benign proximal gastric ulcer.[82-84] Many recommend that wedge excision of the ulcer also be performed, but others assert that the ulcer will usually heal if left in situ after vagotomy and pyloroplasty is performed. In older, poor risk patients with high proximal gastric ulcers, vagotomy and pyloroplasty without ulcer excision may be safe and effective treatment; if the proximal ulcer is excised, however, the mortality from leakage at the site of ulcer excision may be inordinately high. Another problem possibly associated with treatment of proximal gastric ulcers by vagotomy and pyloroplasty is the difficulty of exposing the vagi when there is extensive periesophageal inflammatory reaction in association with the high gastric ulcer. There might be a high incidence of esophageal injury and incomplete vagotomy in such cases. A major

objection to vagotomy and pyloroplasty, not only as treatment for proximal gastric ulcers, but also for distal gastric ulcers, is the inordinately high recurrence rate reported by some after vagotomy and pyloroplasty. Zahn and associates report a recurrence rate of 38 per cent, with a follow-up period averaging over seven years and extending up to 15 years.[88] Other reports of lower recurrence rates with this procedure have significantly shorter follow-up periods than that of Zahn and associates. Admittedly, in elderly, poor risk patients ulcer recurrence is not so critical as a low mortality rate which is gained by vagotomy and pyloroplasty. Also, recurrence may not develop before older patients' deaths from other causes. The Kelling-Madlener operation, however, is simpler and more advantageous than all the foregoing procedures for proximal gastric ulcers, insofar as both mortality and recurrence rates are concerned. This operation, described by Kelling in 1918[89] and Madlener in 1923,[90] is often neglected in discussions

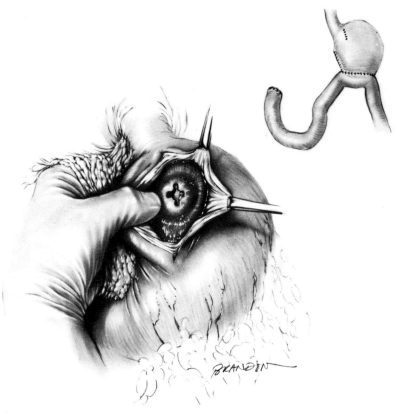

Figure 60–5. Kelling-Madlener operation. Treatment of high, proximal gastric ulcer by distal antrectomy, leaving the ulcer in situ to heal after four-quadrant frozen section biopsy proves it to be benign.

of proximal gastric ulcer surgery. It consists of an antrectomy with either Billroth I or II reconstruction; the ulcer is left in situ after first proving its benign nature by four-quadrant biopsy by frozen section during surgery. When the gastric antrum is removed, the proximal ulcer virtually always heals very quickly. In fact, it is probably not necessary to remove all the antrum — the pylorectomy is probably the critical part of the operation. The Kelling-Madlener operation has the great advantage of avoiding a suture line in inflamed, edematous tissue near the esophagus, thus avoiding suture line leakage while achieving excellent healing of the ulcer. A more recent series reported by Maurer confirms the efficacy of this operation in 55 patients with proximal gastric ulcers.[91] The Kelling-Madlener operation is our operation of choice for benign high proximal gastric ulcer (see Fig. 60–5).

In summary, antrectomy is the operation of choice for all benign gastric ulcers, with removal of distal ulcers and biopsy only of proximal ulcers.

At times the question arises of whether to reoperate and perform a radical subtotal gastrectomy when simple antrectomy has been done for a supposed benign gastric ulcer which proves to be malignant upon examining permanent tissue sections. The consensus is that reoperation should not be done, because the risk of immediate reoperation does not justify the questionable benefit of more extensive radical subtotal gastric resection, unless resectable tumor was left at the line of resection in a good risk patient.

SELECTION OF EMERGENCY OPERATION FOR BLEEDING GASTRIC ULCER

In general, antrectomy with removal of the bleeding gastric ulcer and Billroth I or II reconstruction is the emergency treatment of choice unless the patient is too poor a risk to tolerate resection or the ulcer is in a position in which resection is difficult and likely to be associated with a high incidence of suture line leakage near the esophagogastric junction. In these cases, the better treatment is to leave the ulcer in situ, oversew the bleeder in its base with nonabsorbable suture material,

and perform vagotomy and pyloroplasty.[92] If the gastric ulcer is distal, it may be preferable to wedge excise the ulcer rather than oversew it. Biopsy of the ulcer during surgery should always be performed by frozen section; if it is found to be malignant, resection is done.

GASTRIC ULCER PERFORATION

Essentially the same criteria are used to select the operation of choice for perforated gastric ulcer as for perforated duodenal ulcer. If the patient is a good risk and peritonitis is minimal, a definitive operation may be safely performed. This would consist of an antrectomy and removal of a distal ulcer or an antrectomy and closure of a proximal ulcer with an omental patch. Even if the ulcer proves to be malignant on frozen section, radical subtotal gastrectomy should not be performed, because the patient would not be likely to tolerate it under emergency conditions; moreover, operation could only be considered palliative in any event, because tumor cells have been spilled from the perforation into the peritoneal cavity.

In poor risk patients or those with excessive peritonitis, biopsy and closure of a perforated gastric ulcer are all that should be done. After closure, intensive medical treatment is instituted; if complete healing of the ulcer has not occurred at six to eight weeks or if there is a history of chronic gastric ulcer, a reoperation for definitive treatment of the ulcer should be undertaken. If the ulcer proves to be malignant on biopsy at surgery for perforation, but is not suitable for resection then, reoperation for possible palliative resection can be done within three to four weeks, if the patient is judged a suitable risk for reoperation at that time.

REFERENCES

1. Ross, J. R., and Reaves, L. E., III. Syndrome of posterior penetrating peptic ulcer. Med. Clin. N. Amer. 50:461, 1966.
2. Pattison, A. C., and Stellar, C. A. Surgical management of postbulbar duodenal ulcers. Amer. J. Surg. 111:313, 1966.
3. Murray, G. F., Ballinger, W. F., II, and Stafford, E. S. Ulcer of the pyloric channel. Amer. J. Surg. 113:199, 1967.
4. Moore, F. D., Peete, W. P. J., Richardson, J. E.,

Erskine, J. M., Brooks, J. R., and Rogers, H. The effect of definitive surgery on duodenal ulcer disease: A comparative study of surgical and non-surgical management in 997 cases. Ann. Surg. 132:652, 1950.

5. Carandang. N., Schuman, B. M., and Priest, R. J. The gastrocamera in the diagnosis of stomach disease. J.A.M.A. 204:171, 1968.

6. Dodd, G. D., and Nelson, R. S. The combined radiologic and gastroscopic evaluation of gastric ulceration. Radiology 77:177, 1961.

7. Hara, Y., Tobita, Y., Tsunoda, H., Sugiyama, K., Arakawa, M., Ansfield, F. J., and Hoon, J. R. Intragastric photography: Gastrocamera with fiberscope. Arch. Surg. 94:337, 1967.

8. Welch, C. E., and Allen, A. W. Gastric ulcer. New Eng. J. Med. 240:277, 1949.

9. Brandborg, L. L., MacDonald, W. C., Rubin, C. E., and Gottlieb, S. Cytological diagnosis of gastric cancer by chymotrypsin lavage. Proceedings of the Third World Congress of Gastroenterology 1:300, 1967.

10. Paustian, F. F., Stein, G. N., Young, J. F., Rogh, J. L. A., and Bockus, H. L. The importance of the brief trial or of rigid medical management in the diagnosis of benign vs. malignant gastric ulcer. Gastroenterology 38:155, 1960.

11. Angel, R. T., Giacobine, J. W., and Jordan, G. L. A current evaluation of the problem of gastric ulcers. Amer. J. Surg. 114:730, 1967.

12. Kukkral, J. C. Gastric ulcer: An appraisal. Surgery 63:1024, 1968.

13. Kirsner, J. B., Clayman, C. B., and Palmer, W. L. The problem of gastric ulcer. Arch. Intern. Med. 104:995, 1959.

14. Lampert, E. G., Waugh, J. M., and Dockerty, M. B. The incidence of malignancy in gastric ulcers believed preoperatively to be benign. Surg. Gynec. Obstet. 91:673, 1950.

15. Comfort, M. W., Priestley, J. T., Dockerty, M. B., Weber, H. M., Gage, R. P., Solis, J., and Epperson, D. P. The small benign and malignant gastric lesion. Surg. Gynec. Obstet. 105:435, 1957.

16. Gray, D. B., and Ward, G. E. Delay in diagnosis of carcinoma of the stomach: An analysis of 104 cases. Amer. J. Surg. 83:524, 1952.

17. Foster, J. H., Hall, A. D., and Dunphy, J. E. Surgical management of bleeding ulcers. Surg. Clin. N. Amer. 46:387, 1966.

18. Kozoll, D. D., and Meyer, K. A. Massively bleeding gastroduodenal ulcers. Effects of treatment on morbidity and mortality. Arch. Surg. 89:250, 1964.

19. Stewart, J. D., Sanderson, G. M., and Wiles, C. E., Jr. Blood replacement and gastric resection for massively bleeding peptic ulcer. Ann. Surg. 136:742, 1952.

20. Stewart, J. D., Schaer, S. M., Potter, W. H., and Massover, A. J. Management of massively bleeding peptic ulcer. Ann. Surg. 128:791, 1948.

21. Borland, J. L., Sr., Hancock, W. R., and Borland, J. L., Jr. Recurrent upper gastrointestinal hemorrhage in peptic ulcer. Gastroenterology 52:631, 1967.

22. Brooks, J. R., and Eraklis, A. J. Factors affecting the mortality from peptic ulcer. New Eng. J. Med. 271:803, 1964.

23. Editorial: Recurrent gastrointestinal bleeding. Lancet 1:220, 1971.

24. Hallenbeck, G. A. Elective surgery for treatment of hemorrhage from duodenal ulcer. Gastroenterology 59:784, 1970.

25. Coe, J. D., McLaughlin, C. W., Jr., and Walker, E. Recurrent gastrointestinal bleeding after definitive gastric surgery. Arch. Surg. 88:888, 1964.

26. Donaldson, R. M., Jr., Handy, J., and Papper, S. Five-year follow-up study of patients with bleeding duodenal ulcer with and without surgery. New Eng. J. Med. 259:201, 1958.

27. Grace, W. J., and Mitty, W. F. Does subtotal gastrectomy in bleeding peptic ulcer prevent recurrence of bleeding? Amer. J. Dig. Dis. 7:69, 1962.

28. Gardner, B., and Baronofsky, I. D. The massively bleeding duodenal ulcer with especial reference to crater. Surgery 45:389, 1959.

29. Leape, L. L., and Welch, C. E. Late prognosis of patients with upper gastrointestinal hemorrhage. Amer. J. Surg. 107:297, 1964.

30. Hughes, R. K., and Wootton, D. G. Gastric sump drainage with a water seal monitor. Surgery 61:192, 1967.

31. McFarland, J. B. Gastric hypothermia. Rev. Surg. 55:552, 1968.

32. Rodgers, J. B., Older, T. M., and Stabler, E. V. Gastric hypothermia: A critical evaluation of its use in massive upper gastrointestinal bleeding. Ann. Surg. 163:367, 1966.

33. Hoerr, S. O., Dunphy, J. E., and Gray, S. L. The place of surgery in the emergency treatment of acute massive upper gastrointestinal hemorrhage. Surg. Gynec. Obstet. 87:338, 1948.

34. Seeley, S. F. Nonoperative treatment of perforated duodenal ulcer. Postgrad. Med. 10:359, 1951.

35. Singer, H. A., and Vaughan, R. T. The "forme fruste" type of perforation peptic ulcer. Surg. Gynec. Obstet. 50:10, 1930.

36. Kozoll, D. D., and Meyer, K. A. Obstructing gastroduodenal ulcers. Arch. Surg. 88:793, 1964.

37. Boyle, J. D., and Goldstein, H. Management of pyloric obstruction. Med. Clin. N. Amer. 52:1329, 1968.

38. Goldstein, H., Janin, M., Schapiro, M., and Boyle, J. D. Gastric retention associated with gastroduodenal disease: A study of 217 cases. Amer. J. Dig. Dis. 11:887, 1966.

39. Dudrick, S. J., Wilmore, D. W., Vars, H. M., and Rhoads, J. E. Can intravenous feeding as the sole means of nutrition support growth in the child and restore weight loss in an adult? Ann. Surg. 169:974, 1969.

40. Black, D. A. K., and Jepson, R. P. Electrolyte depletion in pyloric stenosis. Quart. J. Med. 23:367, 1954.

41. Judd, D. R., Simmons, R. D., Kelley, W., and Newton, W. T. Gastric outlet obstruction due to peptic ulcer. Arch. Surg. 100:90, 1970.

42. Farmer, D. A., Harrower, H. W., and Smithwick, R. H. The choice of surgery in peptic ulcer disease. Amer. J. Surg. 120:295, 1970.

43. Frankel, A., Finkelstein, J., and Kark, A. E.   The selection of operation for peptic ulcer. The use of the gastric secretory response to the augmented histamine test as a guide. Amer. J. Gastroent. 46:206, 1966.

44. Harrington, J. L., Jr.   A possible solution to the vagotomy-antrectomy and vagotomy-pyloroplasty controversy. Amer. J. Surg. 121:215, 1971.

45. Rosemond, G. P., and Reichle, F. A.   The operation of choice for peptic ulcer disease. Amer. J. Gastroent. 48:392, 1967.

46. Silberman, V. A., and Winkley, J. H.   Surgical treatment of peptic ulcer. Arch. Surg. 97:84, 1968.

47. Palumbo, L. T., Sharpe, W. S., Lulu, D. J., Bloom, M. H., and Dragstedt, L. R.   Distal antrectomy with vagectomy for duodenal ulcer. Arch. Surg. 100:182, 1970.

48. Scott, H. W., Jr., Sawyers, J. L., Gobbel, W. G., Jr., Herrington, J. L., Jr., Edwards, W. H., and Edwards, L. W.   Vagotomy and antrectomy in surgical treatment of duodenal ulcer disease. Surg. Clin. N. Amer. 46:349, 1966.

49. Thoroughman, J. C., Walker, L. G., Jr., and Raft, D.   A review of 504 patients treated by hemigastrectomy and vagotomy. Surg. Gynec. Obstet. 119:257, 1964.

50. Eisenberg, M. M., Woodward, E. R., Carson, T. J., and Dragstedt, L. R.   Vagotomy and drainage procedure for duodenal ulcer. Ann. Surg. 170:317, 1969.

51. Weinberg, J. A., Stempien, S. J., Movius, H. J., and Dagradi, A. E.   Vagotomy and pyloroplasty in the treatment of duodenal ulcer. Amer. J. Surg. 92:202, 1956.

52. Whittaker, L. D., Jr., Judd, E. S., and Stauffer, M. H.   Analysis of use of vagotomy with drainage procedure in surgical management of duodenal ulcer. Surg. Gynec. Obstet. 125:1018, 1967.

53. Rhea, W. G., Jr., Killen, D. A., and Scott, H. W., Jr.   Long term results of partial gastric resection without vagotomy in duodenal ulcer disease. Surg. Gynec. Obstet. 120:970, 1965.

54. Landor, J. H.   Gastric secretory tests and their relevance to surgeons. Surgery 65:523, 1969.

55. Nobles, E. R., Jr.   Vagotomy and gastroenterostomy; 15-year follow-up of 175 patients. Ann. Surg. 32:182, 1966.

56. Bryant, W. M., Klein, D., and Griffin, W. O., Jr.   The role of vagotomy in duodenal ulcer surgery. Surgery 61:864, 1967.

57. Hayden, W. F., and Read, R. C.   A comparative study of the Heineke-Mikulicz and Finney pyloroplasty. Amer. J. Surg. 116:755, 1968.

58. Harkins, H. N., and Nyhus, L. M.   Surgery of the Stomach and Duodenum, 2nd ed. Boston, Little, Brown and Company, 1969, p. 491.

59. Clave, R. A., and Gaspar, M. R.   Incidence of gallbladder disease after vagotomy. Amer. J. Surg. 118:169, 1969.

60. Kraft, R. O., Fry, W. J., Wilhelm, K. G., and Ransom, H. K.   Selective gastric vagotomy, Arch. Surg. 95:625, 1967.

61. Sawyers, J. L., Scott, H. W., Jr., Edwards, W. H., Shull, H. J., and Law, D. H., IV.   Comparative studies of the clinical effects of truncal and selective gastric vagotomy. Amer. J. Surg. 115:165, 1968.

62. Smith, G. K., and Farris, J. M.   Reappraisal of the long-term effects of selective vagotomy. Amer. J. Surg. 117:222, 1969.

63. Griffith, C. A., and Harkins, H. N.   Selective gastric vagotomy: Physiologic basis and technique. Surg. Clin. N. Amer. 42:1431, 1962.

64. Amdrup, E., and Jensen, H. E.   Selective vagotomy of the parietal cell mass preserving innervation of the undrained antrum. Gastroenterology 59:522, 1970.

65. Weinberg, J. A.   Treatment of the massively bleeding duodenal ulcer by ligation, pyloroplasty and vagotomy. Amer. J. Surg. 102:158, 1961.

66. Farris, J. M., and Smith, G. K.   Appraisal of the long-term results of vagotomy and pyloroplasty in 100 patients with bleeding duodenal ulcer. Ann. Surg. 166:630, 1967.

67. Silen, W., and Moore, F. D.   Editorial: Surgical treatment of bleeding duodenal ulcer: A plea for caution. Ann. Surg. 160:778, 1964.

68. Snyder, E. N., Jr., and Stellar, C. A.   Results from emergency surgery for massively bleeding duodenal ulcer. Amer. J. Surg. 116:170, 1968.

69. Cogbill, C. L., and Kinkade, P. T.   Emergency operation for massive hemorrhage from peptic ulcer. Amer. Surgeon 32:283, 1966.

70. Kelley, H. G., Grant, G. N., and Elliott, D. W.   Massive gastroduodenal hemorrhage. Arch. Surg. 87:6, 1963.

71. Donaldson, G. A., and Jarrett, F.   Perforated gastroduodenal ulcer disease at the Massachusetts General Hospital from 1952 to 1970. Amer. J. Surg. 120:306, 1970.

72. Hamilton, J. E., and Harbrecht, P. J.   Growing indications for vagotomy in perforated peptic ulcer. Surg. Gynec. Obstet. 124:61, 1967.

73. Hinshaw, D. M., Pierandozzi, J. S., Thompson, R. J., Jr., and Carter, R.   Vagotomy and pyloroplasty for perforated duodenal ulcer. Amer. J. Surg. 115:173, 1968.

74. Jordan, G. L., Jr., Angel, R. T., and DeBakey, M. E.   Acute gastroduodenal perforation. Arch. Surg. 92:449, 1966.

75. Smith, L., and Beehan, P. J.   Definitive operations for perforated duodenal ulcers. Surg. Gynec. Obstet. 129:465, 1969.

76. Bergin, W. F., and Jordan, P. H.   Gastric atonia and delayed gastric emptying after vagotomy for obstructing ulcer. Amer. J. Surg. 98:612, 1959.

77. Harper, F. B.   Gastric dysfunction after vagectomy. Amer. J. Surg. 112:94, 1966.

78. Hermann, G., and Johnson, V.   Management of prolonged gastric retention after vagotomy and drainage. Surg. Gynec. Obstet. 130:1044, 1970.

79. Kraft, R. O., Fry, W. J., and DeWeese, M. S.   Postvagotomy gastric atony. Arch. Surg. 88:865, 1964.

80. Cox, W. D., and Gillesby, W. J.   Gastrostomy in postoperative decompression. Amer. J. Surg. 113:298, 1967.

81. Dunphy, J. E.   Discussion in: Postoperative ileus. Amer. J. Surg. 116:369, 1968.

82. Farris, J. M., and Smith, G. K. Treatment of gastric ulcer (in situ) by vagotomy and pyloroplasty: A clinical study. Ann. Surg. *158*:461, 1963.

83. Farris, J. M., and Smith, G. K. Some other operations for gastric ulcer. Surg. Clin. N. Amer. *46*:329, 1966.

84. Kraft, R. O., Fry, W. J., and Ransom, H. K. Surgery for gastric ulcer. Rev. Surg. *51*:730, 1966.

85. McNeill, A. D., McAdam, W. A. F., and Hutchison, J. S. F. Vagotomy and drainage in the treatment of gastric ulcer. Surg. Gynec. Obstet. *128*:91, 1969.

86. Athanassiades, S., and Charalambopoulou, J. Coexistent gastric and duodenal ulcer. Amer. J. Surg. *120*:381, 1970.

87. Schoemaker, J. Zur Technik der Magenresektion nach Billroth I. Arch. Klin. Chir. *121*:268, 1922.

88. Zahn, R. L., Stemmer, E. A., Hom, L. W., and Connolly, J. E. Delayed recurrence of gastric ulcer following vagotomy and drainage procedures. Amer. Surgeon *34*:757, 1968.

89. Kelling, G. Über die operative Behandlung des chronischen Ulcus ventriculi. Arch. Klin. Chir. *109*:775, 1911.

90. Madlener, M. Über Pylorektomie bei pylorusfernem Magengeschwur. Zentr. Chir. *50*:1313, 1923.

91. Mauer, H. Die Operation nach Madlener und ihre Ergebnisse. Bruns. Beitr. Klin. Chir. *182*:266, 1951.

92. Dorton, H. E. Vagotomy, pyloroplasty, and suture for bleeding gastric ulcer. Surg. Gynec. Obstet. *122*:1015, 1966.

Chapter 61

Peptic Ulcer Surgery: Postoperative Care and Immediate Complications

Robert N. McClelland

The postoperative management of patients undergoing peptic ulcer surgery requires the close attention of the clinician to all aspects of the patient's physiology. Thus there are many phases of care, such as those dealing with the cardiopulmonary and urinary systems; these are the same as those of all surgical patients, and they are well covered in textbooks of general surgery. The following discussion will emphasize the details of postoperative care and immediate complications which relate more specifically to gastric surgery.

MANAGEMENT OF NASOGASTRIC AND GASTROSTOMY TUBES

In most gastric operations a nasogastric tube of adequate size (at least No. 18 French) is inserted by the anesthesiologist into the patient's stomach, usually after the abdomen is opened. This permits the surgeon to direct the proper positioning of the tube within the stomach and spares the patient the needless discomfort of preoperative nasogastric tube insertion. The nasogastric tube is inserted before surgery, however, in emergency situations involv-ing active hemorrhage or acute perforation or in patients who require preoperative nasogastric intubation for pyloric obstruction. The most effective nasogastric tube to maintain constant gastric decompression and allow easy irrigation is a "sump" tube.[1] Two sump nasogastric tubes are available commercially—the Salem and the Anderson nasogastric sump tubes. Both tubes are made of clear, soft plastic and incorporate a small external air vent connected to a small air channel which runs the length of the tube beside the main suction lumen. The decompressive vent prevents blockage of the suction lumen by gastric mucosa, as often happens with the nonsump nasogastric tube when suction is applied. The nasogastric tube is usually maintained on suction until normal peristalsis returns and it is apparent that there is no gastric hemorrhage, that bile is in the nasogastric aspirate, and that the volume of aspirate is small enough to indicate no obstruction of the gastrointestinal stoma or efferent jejunal loop. Occasionally the sump nasogastric tube removes swallowed air and fluid so completely that the audibility of peristalsis is diminished even though ileus has relented and the passage of flatus may be delayed because the gut is kept so empty by the sump tube. This is not a disadvantage, however, but a testimony to the effectiveness of the tube. In such cases of apparently delayed resumption of peristalsis and passage of flatus, the sump tube is removed on the third postoperative day if the patient's abdomen is flat and soft, his temperature and white blood count are normal, and the quantity and nature of the nasogastric aspirate are considered normal. Agents to stimulate peristalsis are avoided because of the danger of causing excessive pressure on a fresh suture line and inducing anastomotic leakage. Use of such peristaltic agents later in some instances of prolonged gastric atony will be discussed subsequently.

Gastrostomy tube suction is preferable in patients who tolerate nasogastric suction poorly or who require prolonged decompression. These include very elderly patients, patients with significant chronic pulmonary disease, and patients with chronic pyloric obstruction and severe gastric dilatation and edema.[2] Gastrostomy is most often required and performed with vagotomy and drainage operations. Gastrostomy is technically easier in these in-stances than after gastric resections, because mobilization of the stomach to the abdominal wall for suture is easier with an intact stomach than after subtotal gastrectomy. Fortuitously, vagotomy and drainage is more likely to be done in elderly patients and patients with chronic pulmonary disease—those who benefit most from gastrostomy as opposed to nasogastric suction. As Herrington and colleagues state, gastrostomy is associated with some complications and even fatalities and should not be used routinely after gastric surgery.[3] It should be used only when prolonged gastric ileus is expected in elderly, poor risk patients; otherwise, nasogastric suction should be employed.

In our experience, the gastrostomy tube functions more safely and effectively if inserted into the stomach, as shown in Figure 61–1. A No. 22 French red rubber catheter, with additional holes cut into its distal third, is inserted through a stab wound at the midpoint of the anterior gastric wall and secured with two concentric purse string sutures placed in the gastric wall surrounding the tube. The tube is inserted into the gastric lumen far enough to lie along the posterior gastric

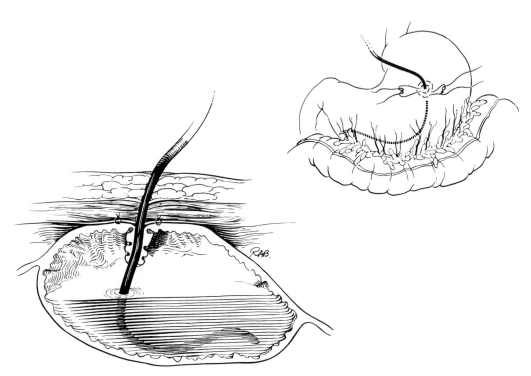

Figure 61–1. Method of inserting a gastrostomy tube.

wall. This tube, so positioned, more completely empties both fluid and air from the stomach than does a Foley catheter. The gastrostomy tube is kept on suction for about five days postoperatively, after which it is clamped and oral feedings are given. If oral intake is tolerated, the tube is removed about the seventh postoperative day.[2] The serosal-lined tract of the Stamm gastrostomy promptly closes. If oral intake is not accepted, feeding is stopped and the gastrostomy tube is placed on suction again until it seems safe to attempt oral feeding again.

Several surgeons suggest that gastric decompression is unnecessary in most patients undergoing gastric surgery.[4, 5] Herrington usually maintains gastric decompression throughout the operation and removes the nasogastric tube about eight hours postoperatively if the patient is doing well and is fully recovered from anesthesia.[3, 6] Rachlin and MacDonald and Byrd not only stop gastric decompression so quickly, but also feed solid food on the first or second postoperative day.[7, 8] Although these surgeons' data suggest that routine postoperative gastric decompression may *not* be necessary, abandonment of postoperative decompression and early feeding cannot be recommended now on the basis of their limited experience. The chief advantage cited for early discontinuance of postoperative gastric decompression relates mostly to patient comfort rather than to safety, whereas the potential disadvantages of even the occasional case of gastric dilatation, vomiting and aspiration, or suture line disruption from gastric distention, when postoperative gastric decompression is not used, relate to patient safety and to potential serious morbidity and even mortality.

FLUID AND ELECTROLYTE THERAPY

The Na^+, K^+, and Cl^- concentrations of gastric juice secreted by the normal, unobstructed stomach are similar to that in the extracellular fluid of the body.[9] It is therefore more appropriate to replace nasogastric aspirate with equivalent amounts of intravenous Ringer's lactate (Hartmann's) solution with added potassium chloride

than with 0.9 per cent NaCl solution. Normal saline solution contains excessive amounts of both sodium and chloride ions in comparison with gastric juice and may therefore induce hypernatremia, hyperchloremia, and metabolic acidosis if given in excessive quantities.[10] Potassium losses, amounting to 5 to 15 mEq per liter of gastric juice from the unobstructed stomach, are adequately replaced by adding 15 to 20 mEq of KCl to each liter of Ringer's lactate or other intravenous solution, providing that renal function, serum levels of potassium, and acid-base balance are normal.[10, 11]

Fluid replacement must be modified in patients with chronic pyloric obstruction and/or prolonged periods of associated vomiting and water drinking. In these instances, excessive loss of chloride and potassium ions from the stomach and kidney relative to loss of hydrogen, sodium, and bicarbonate ions causes hypochloremic, hypokalemic metabolic alkalosis.[11, 12] The typical serum chemistry findings in such cases are low K^+, high CO_2 combining power, low Cl^-, and low Na^+. The serum pH will usually be 7.4 or higher, depending upon the severity of electrolyte losses and degree of compensation. In the early stages of vomiting caused by chronic pyloric obstruction, serum potassium may not fall to reflect the amount of loss of intracellular potassium, but almost invariably the serum bicarbonate level is elevated and the serum chloride level is depressed. If the patient vomits and drinks no water, a more severe extracellular fluid volume deficit develops in addition to the serum compositional defects. The extracellular fluid volume deficit is manifested by loss of tissue turgor and inadequate filling of the vascular tree; i.e., by rapid pulse, hypotension, drowsiness (but not disorientation), oliguria, weakness, and loss of tissue elasticity and volume. The serum sodium level is usually normal, but may be slightly depressed or elevated.

If the patient continues to drink large volumes of water and to vomit, essentially the same serum electrolyte compositional defects and acid-base balance defects are present, although they may be somewhat altered by the dilutional effect of ingested water. With much water drinking and vomiting and only partial pyloric obstruction, signs of extracellular fluid volume deficit may be less, but evidence of relative or absolute water excess may be noted instead. The signs of water excess are low serum sodium, mental confusion and disorientation, ultimate severe central nervous system irritability and convulsions, oliguria, and, rarely, when free water overload is severe, excessive tearing, salivation, edema, and hypertension.[10]

Replacement of fluid and electrolyte losses associated with chronic pyloric obstruction and vomiting differs significantly from that of replacement of fluid and electrolytes lost from the unobstructed stomach. Attempts should be made to correct compositional and volume defects simultaneously.[10, 12] In general, with normal renal function, replacement begins with judicious intravenous infusions of 0.9 per cent NaCl solution containing 40 mEq of KCl per liter. *As a rule, intravenous potassium chloride should be infused no faster than 20 mEq per hour to prevent problems with cardiac rhythm.* This solution provides sufficient potassium and chloride ions to correct the metabolic alkalosis and sufficient volume to correct the extracellular fluid volume deficit. Unless the potassium deficit is corrected, it is very difficult, or perhaps impossible, to elevate serum chloride levels, reduce the elevated serum bicarbonate, and correct metabolic alkalosis. This is because adequate hydrogen ion to correct metabolic alkalosis is not available until intracellular potassium losses are replaced. Severe electrolyte disturbances may require replacement of up to 800 mEq of potassium.[11] Correction of these deficiencies must proceed cautiously, with appraisal of serum electrolyte concentrations, serum pH, urine output (hourly), central venous pressure, and vital signs at appropriate, frequent intervals. If extracellular fluid deficiency persists after correction of serum electrolyte composition and metabolic alkalosis, additional intravenous fluids are given as Ringer's lactate solution containing smaller amounts of KCl to avoid excessive quantities of potassium and chloride ions.

A 70-kg adult must lose at least 6 per cent of his body weight as extracellular fluid to show obvious signs of extracellular fluid volume depletion;[10] therefore severely depleted patients may require as much as 6 liters of intravenous fluids per day for two or three days when first hospitalized for chronic pyloric obstruction and protracted vomiting.

These special requirements for fluid and electrolytes related to gastric surgery for peptic ulcer are modified by other losses from nasogastric suction, fistulous drainage, sweating, and insensible water loss caused by fever, diarrhea, and urine. Very careful intake and output records must be maintained.[10]

POSTOPERATIVE FEEDING, GASTRIC ATONY, AND RETENTION

The stomach more readily empties itself of small amounts of dry, low residue food than of liquids after various gastric surgical procedures (reference 13 and unpublished data). This is probably because liquid, particularly in significant amounts and in combination with solid food, causes excessive gastric distention postoperatively and exaggerated stretching of gastric smooth muscle fibers. According to Starling's law governing the contraction of smooth muscle fibers, gastric peristalsis then becomes inadequate for gastric emptying, resulting in postoperative gastric atony, retention, and vomiting. This is more likely if gastric smooth muscle fibers which were previously badly stretched by gastric distention resulting from chronic pyloric obstruction are then denervated by vagotomy.[2, 14-18] After gastric surgery for peptic ulcer, it is therefore advisable to use one of two basic feeding regimens, depending upon whether chronic pyloric obstruction and gastric decompensation were present preoperatively. If there was no preoperative chronic pyloric obstruction and gastric resection instead of a gastric drainage procedure was performed, oral liquids should not be given just before, during, or for one hour after a meal. This helps prevent dumping and uncomfortable gastric distention. All food should have high protein, moderate fat, and low carbohydrate content to reduce the incidence of dumping. Milk and carbonated beverages are avoided in the early postoperative period, because these liquids often cause uncomfortable flatulence and fullness in gastric surgery patients. High residue fibrous foods should also be avoided, especially citrus pulps which can cause bolus obstruction of the gastric stoma or of the small bowel.[19-21]

All these dietary recommendations in the early postoperative period apply equally to postgastric surgery patients having preoperative chronic pyloric obstruction and gastric decompensation, but in addition it is important to avoid all oral liquids for 24 to 48 hours after the patient begins taking solid food orally.[13] This is especially true if preoperative gastric dilatation was severe or if vagotomy and drainage is performed. Fluid requirements are supplied intravenously until it is certain that the patient is taking small frequent dry feedings without gastric retention. Oral fluids are given in small quantities usually 24 to 48 hours after solid food is begun, again with care taken that no liquid is ingested just before, during, or for one hour after a meal of solid, low residue dry food.

The mean incidence of troublesome postoperative gastric atony is at least 4 per cent after various types of gastric surgical procedures for peptic ulcer, and about half these patients require reoperation. Because of the relatively low incidence of significant gastric retention with vomiting and because of the great variability of gastric surgical technique and postoperative management, it is virtually impossible to determine with certainty from current data whether gastric atony is more common after vagotomy and after chronic pyloric obstruction and gastric distention.[2, 4, 5, 14-18, 22] Practically speaking, it is best to assume that it is and to take measures to prevent this possible complication.

It is important therefore, when surgery for chronic pyloric obstruction is done, that gastric decompression be maintained for four or five days preoperatively and four or five days postoperatively by nasogastric or gastrostomy tube suction, especially if vagotomy is done. Subsequent gastric distention may be prevented by frequent, small postoperative *dry* feedings initially (see p. 767 for management of obstructing peptic ulcer).[2, 13, 17] If gastric dilatation and edema are still notable during surgery for obstructing peptic ulcer, either subtotal gastrectomy without vagotomy or gastroenterostomy without vagotomy (the latter procedure being preferred in poorer risk patients) should be done to decrease the possibility of prolonged postoperative gastric atony and retention which is increased significantly (from 5 to 20 per cent) when vagotomy is done for such severe, chronic pyloric obstruction.[2, 14-17]

If postoperative atony and persistent vomiting develop despite the precautions discussed above, they must be treated promptly before massive gastric dilatation and decompensation and fluid and electrolyte depletion occur; otherwise treatment is much more difficult and protracted (L. Dragstedt, personal communication, and reference 18). All oral intake should be quickly stopped and gastric suction and intravenous feeding reinstituted. An upper gastrointestinal contrast X-ray study is obtained, using thin barium, to rule out obvious mechanical obstruction.[23] If no mechanical obstruction is detected, gastric suction is maintained for four or five days. It is wise to maintain central intravenous feedings with Dudrick and coworkers' regimen of hyperalimentation with concentrated glucose and protein hydrolysates.[24] Since it is never possible to determine exactly how long these patients will be unable to take oral feedings, central intravenous hyperalimentation should be given at the onset of gastric atony before inanition develops. In some instances, a small nasogastric polyethylene tube may be passed through the gastroenteric stoma into the upper jejunum as described by Bachrach and Tecimer, and the patient can be given jejunostomy feedings through this tube.[25] The nasogastric tube is removed after four or five days (the nasogastric tube should not be left in and clamped, because this may cause air swallowing and dangerous acute gastric dilatation). The patient is given nothing orally for another 24 to 48 hours. If no vomiting occurs, small dry feedings are given six times daily in gradually increasing amounts and central intravenous hyperalimentation is continued until it is certain that oral intake is tolerated. If dry food is tolerated for 48 hours, liquids in small, gradually increasing amounts are given between meals only. The patient should eat sitting up, avoid reclining, and, while in bed, lie on his right side as much as possible. These maneuvers promote gastric emptying by gravity. A nasogastric tube should be passed each evening before bedtime and at least two hours after the last oral intake. The stomach is evacuated with this tube; if more than 200 to 300 cc of gastric content remains, gastric suction is maintained overnight and the nasogastric tube is removed and oral feeding resumed the following morning. Such nocturnal intubation may be required for several days before it is apparent that gastric emptying is adequate.

If significant gastric fullness and vomiting recur during a second attempt at feeding, oral intake is again stopped and constant gastric suction reinstituted. When the stomach is completely empty (about 24 hours after starting gastric suction again) a repeat upper gastrointestinal X-ray series is obtained. If no contrast material passes through the gastroenteric stoma, it is likely that mechanical obstruction is present, and reoperation is probably necessary. If some contrast material passes the stoma, as it will in 93 per cent of functional gastric atony cases according to Hermann and Johnson,[23] a trial of bethanechol (Urecholine) therapy, as suggested by Vasconez and associates (personal communication and reference 26) and Roth and associates[18] may be tried, if at least 21 days have elapsed since the initial gastric surgery.

The technique of Vasconez and associates is quoted as follows:

Initial roentgenographic studies of the stomach should be obtained with dilute contrast material to establish the diagnosis of gastric retention. The stomach is then emptied and any pre-existing fluid and electrolyte deficits are corrected (hypokalemia may greatly aggravate gastric atony). A plain roentgenogram of the abdomen is obtained to serve as a baseline, and the patient is skin tested with bethanechol to exclude an idiosyncratic sensitivity to the drug. The patient is then given a regular meal (without liquids except for contrast media) which he must usually be encouraged to eat because of reluctance based on previous unsuccessful attempts to retain food. Two hundred and fifty ml of barium sulfate is given with the meal to provide radiographic contrast while following the bolus of food under fluoroscopy. A second upright film of the abdomen is then obtained which will usually again show a distended stomach. By turning and positioning the patient under fluoroscopy, an attempt is made to locate the anastomosis and situate the patient so that the gastric contents will be in the most dependent position for drainage. The patient is then given 2.5 mg of bethanechol chloride subcutaneously at 15-minute intervals for six to eight doses while the gastric contents are followed fluoroscopically. Within 30 minutes after the first bethanechol is given, vigorous intestinal contractions will usually be apparent. Shortly thereafter, gastric peristalsis will follow, with weak fibrillating movements which progress to a stronger coordinated contraction. The other parasympathomimetic actions of bethanechol will be manifest within one hour. These include sweating, flushing, nausea, and the urge to urinate and defecate. Unless the side effects are particularly severe, it is not necessary to discontinue the treatment. With vomiting of a small amount, the procedure should still be continued, but if most of the gastric contents are vomited, a rest period is given and the entire process is repeated, including reingestion of food and barium. After administration of approximately six to eight doses of bethanechol and in the absence of mechanical outlet obstruction, it will be observed that a large portion of the food and contrast material will have passed from the stomach into the intestine, and in one and one-half to two hours the stomach will be virtually empty. When this has been accomplished, the patient is ready to begin a regular fixed schedule of feedings and bethanechol chloride medication. Three feedings a day of a regular diet (but with no liquids during meals) are given, with nothing between meals except water. Fifteen mg of bethanechol chloride is given orally 30 minutes before each meal, and 5 mg is given subcutaneously at hourly intervals between 7 A.M. and midnight. If the patient tolerates this regimen for 24 hours, parenteral bethanechol is decreased to 5 mg every two hours from 7 A.M. to midnight and he continues also to receive 15 mg of bethanechol chloride orally 30 minutes before each meal. This regimen continues for another 48 hours. After that, parenteral bethanechol chloride is stopped, but oral bethanechol chloride is continued in a dosage of 15 mg 30 minutes before meals three times daily. One week after beginning therapy, the patient should be ready to continue treatment at home. A repeat upper gastrointestinal X-ray series is not essential. Oral administration of bethanechol chloride is continued at home 30 minutes before meals in a lesser dosage of 10 mg three times a day for about two more weeks. The last week of therapy the patient is given 5 mg of bethanechol chloride orally 30 minutes before meals three times daily. In one month bethanechol chloride therapy is usually stopped completely.*

---

*From Vasconez, L. D., et al.: Arch. Surg. *100*:693, 1970. Copyright 1970, American Medical Association.

With this therapy, Vasconez and his associates successfully treated five of six patients suffering from prolonged gastric atony following vagotomy and antrectomy. One successfully treated patient's gastric atony had persisted for 46 days after surgery. Three patients had had unsuccessful reoperations for failure of gastric emptying, but responded subsequently to bethanechol chloride treatment. The one failure proved to be a mechanical obstruction caused by a constricted gastroduodenostomy found at reoperation; this was successfully treated by revision of the anastomosis (personal communication and reference 26).

Roth et al. also suggested that bethanechol chloride is useful in managing postoperative gastric atony. In one patient they found it necessary to continue oral bethanechol chloride for six months after surgery.[18]

If bethanechol chloride and all other conservative methods fail, if there is sufficient gastric retention to prevent adequate oral nutrition, and if at least three weeks have passed since the initial gastric surgery, reoperation should be performed. Three weeks are sufficient for the disappearance of stomal edema or hematoma or local peritonitis and for correction of fluid and electrolyte disturbances (especially hypokalemia) which may have caused or contributed to gastric atony and retention. In about half the patients with gastric retention, no obvious mechanical obstruction of the gastric stoma is discovered upon re-exploration. Whether obvious mechanical obstruction is present or not, reconstruction of the gastroenteric anastomosis is done. If vagotomy and drainage was done originally, an antrectomy with a Billroth II retrocolic reconstruction should be performed. If a Billroth I gastrectomy was done originally, this is also changed to a Billroth II retrocolic gastrectomy; whereas if a Billroth II gastrectomy was done initially, a small reresection of the gastrojejunostomy stoma is performed and a careful complete reconstruction of the stoma is performed. A feeding jejunostomy is also constructed, and a tube gastrostomy is inserted into the gastric remnant if possible.[27] If a gastrostomy tube cannot be in-

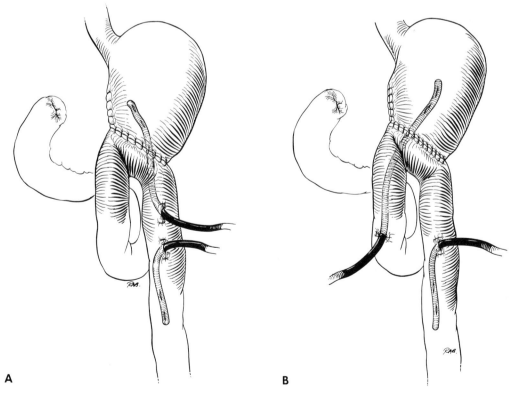

A   **B**

Figure 61–2. Method of inserting jejunostomy tubes. *A*, Efferent loop insertion. *B*, Afferent and efferent loop insertion.

serted easily through the anterior gastric wall, as is usually the case, a retrograde jejunostomy tube is passed from the small bowel back through the gastroenteric stoma into the stomach for gastric suction.[28] This permits postoperative gastric suction without the discomfort of a nasogastric tube. This is particularly desirable in those patients who may have already suffered a nasogastric tube for many days and may require gastric suction for an additional prolonged period before gastric emptying resumes (Fig. 61–2).

After reoperations for delayed gastric emptying, especially when no mechanical cause is found, oral feeding is begun in the same manner as discussed earlier.

It must again be emphasized that reoperations for prolonged gastric atony are much better tolerated if normal nutrition is maintained with central intravenous hyperalimentation from the onset of gastric retention.[24]

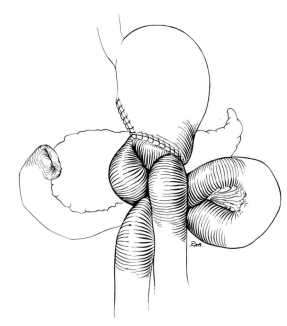

Figure 61–3. Retroanastomotic hernia.

MECHANICAL CAUSES OF POSTOPERATIVE GASTRIC RETENTION AND VOMITING

POSTGASTRECTOMY HERNIA

Obstruction of the gastric outlet after a Billroth II gastrectomy or gastrojejunostomy may occur in the early or late postoperative periods when either the efferent or afferent jejunal limb herniates through the retroanastomotic space, as shown in Figure 61–3. According to Sebesta and Robson,[29] there have been 171 cases of such postgastrectomy hernias since the original description by Petersen in 1900.[30] Half of these hernias occur within one month of the original gastric operation, another 25 per cent within one year, and the remaining 25 per cent more than one year after operation. Probably because of failure to recognize these hernias and the rapid development of strangulation of the small bowel, the mortality has been 30 per cent in the operated patients and 100 per cent in those not operated upon. These hernias may develop after any type of gastrojejunostomy construction, but more commonly occur after retrocolic isoperistaltic anastomosis. More commonly the efferent limb herniates, although the afferent limb may herniate if it is too long. Markowitz suggests that the hernias may be prevented by closure of the retroanastomotic hiatus.[31] This may be done by suturing the efferent limb, the afferent limb, or the mesentery of the loop to the posterior parietal peritoneum when retrocolic anastomosis is done. If there is an antecolic anastomosis, the loop can be sutured to the transverse colon and mesocolon. The afferent limb should not be excessively long.

The symptoms of postgastrectomy hernia are often not dramatic, and may be attributed to gastric atony or stomal edema, with the unfortunate result that the correct diagnosis is often delayed until intestinal strangulation develops. If the hernia involves the efferent loop, a clinical picture of intestinal obstruction will likely develop. Such patients will have abdominal distention and generalized colicky pain and will vomit bile-stained material. Upper gastrointestinal contrast X-rays are helpful in showing that the site of obstruction is below the gastric stoma. On the other hand, if the hernia involves the afferent limb, the patient most often develops sudden onset of constant pain in the upper abdomen, vomiting is in-

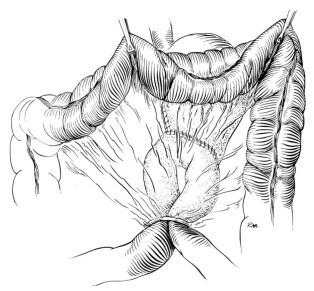

Figure 61–4. Hernia through the meso-colon.

frequent, and vomitus does not contain bile. Contrast X-rays reveal no obstruction of the gastric outlet or in the efferent loop. The serum amylase level may be elevated, perhaps caused by retrograde pressure within the afferent loop transmitted to and partially obstructing the pancreatic duct.[32]

Treatment of retroanastomotic postgastrectomy hernia is surgical, with reduction of the hernia and resection of any bowel that is thought to be nonviable. The gastroenteric anastomosis is then reconstructed and care is taken to close the retroanastomotic space, as mentioned earlier.[31]

Another type of internal hernia which may also cause mechanical obstruction of the gastric outlet is herniation of the gastrojejunostomy limbs through the opening in the transverse mesocolon (Fig. 61–4). This hernia occurs after a retrocolic Billroth II gastrectomy because of failure to suture the edges of the opening in the mesocolon to the anterior and posterior gastric wall superior to the gastrojejunostomy, or because of the later disruption of such sutures.[33] The symptoms are similar to those of the retroanastomotic hernia of the efferent loop. An upper gastrointestinal contrast study may be quite helpful, because such a study often indicates a characteristic constriction of the gastrojejunostomy limbs a short distance below the gastroenteric anastomosis. The

treatment is prompt reoperation, reduction of the hernia, and careful suturing of the edges of the mesocolon circumferentially around the stomach above the gastrojejunostomy.

OBSTRUCTION DUE TO ADHESIONS AFTER GASTRIC SURGERY

Postoperative adhesions may cause kinking, constriction, or volvulus of the small bowel and result in partial or complete obstruction of the efferent or afferent limbs of the gastrojejunostomy after a Billroth II gastrectomy. The symptoms are persistent vomiting and varying amounts of abdominal pain. The more characteristic findings, often present when the afferent jejunal limb of the gastroenterostomy is obstructed, are discussed in the section on afferent loop obstruction. An upper gastrointestinal contrast X-ray study may be helpful in indicating mechanical obstruction and the need for early surgery, but is unlikely to indicate that the obstruction is due to adhesions. In the early postoperative period if it is felt likely that mechanical obstruction secondary to kinking or adhesions is present, an attempt may be made to pass a long intestinal tube (i.e., a Cantor or Miller-Abbott tube) into the upper small bowel if there is no evidence of intestinal strangulation or peritonitis. If this is done with fluoroscopic guidance and without vigorous manipulations so as to avoid possible suture line disruption, the obstruction may be relieved by the passage of the long intestinal tube. When the tube passes into the upper jejunum it should be left in place for several days to act as a splint to prevent recurrent obstruction, and jejunostomy feedings may be given through it. If more than two or three weeks have elapsed since surgery, the adhesions are apt to be so dense that they are unlikely to yield to the passage of the long tube, and immediate surgery is usually indicated. In any case, attempts to pass a long intestinal tube should be continued for only a short time; if the tube does not pass quickly, attempts to use it should be abandoned, and surgery to correct the obstruction should be promptly performed before bowel necrosis occurs.

Postoperative adhesions may also cause obstruction of pyloroplasties in the early or late postoperative periods. Occasionally the pyloroplasty suture line adheres to the inferior surface of the liver, with resultant kinking and obstruction of the pyloroplasty. This complication can probably be prevented by interposing the greater omentum between the pyloroplasty and liver, after construction of the pyloroplasty. Several fine silk sutures are necessary to secure the omentum over the pyloroplasty. Herrington states that since employing this maneuver he has encountered no more pyloroplasty obstructions from adhesions.[34]

AFFERENT LOOP SYNDROME AFTER SURGERY FOR PEPTIC ULCER

This problem is uncommon and occurs after either Billroth II gastrectomy or gastrojejunostomy. Either operation creates a short segment of bowel, consisting of the duodenum and proximal jejunum, in which varying degrees of stasis may develop if there is partial obstruction by kinking, twisting, adhesions, internal hernia, intussusception, or stomal stenosis, as illustrated in Figure 61–5. If such obstruction develops soon after surgery, it may be one of the chief causes of duodenal stump dehiscence. If duodenal stump dehiscence does not occur, the more classic chronic or acute "afferent loop syndrome" may de-

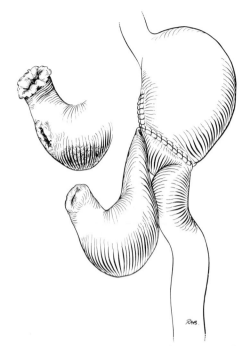

Figure 61–5. Afferent loop obstruction. Inset shows blowout of duodenal stump.

velop in the early postoperative period or years later.[32, 33, 35-37]

The classic "chronic afferent loop syndrome" consists of postprandial epigastric fullness associated with variable nausea and upper abdominal pain which are relieved suddenly by copious vomiting of bile containing little or no food. In thin patients, the distended afferent loop may be palpated as an epigastric mass especially prominent shortly after meals. X-ray studies are usually unrevealing, but occasionally show marked dilatation of the afferent jejunal loop.

The classic afferent loop syndrome is caused by an accumulation of biliary-pancreatic secretions in the afferent loop during a meal. The stomach usually empties itself of food before vomiting occurs. Distention of the afferent loop with biliary-pancreatic secretions which accumulate within the loop proximal to a partial obstruction finally causes nausea and vomiting. Since the food has already left the stomach, only the biliary-pancreatic secretions, which are suddenly ejected from the afferent loop into the stomach, appear in the vomitus. Other causes of bilious vomiting after gastric surgery are discussed on pages 137 and 138.

If afferent loop obstruction is complete, pain and nausea are more severe and unrelenting, rather than mild and episodic. No bile is present in the vomitus. The serum amylase level may be elevated owing to mild pancreatitis caused by partial pancreatic duct obstruction; the obstruction occurs because of high intraluminal pressure within the obstructed afferent loop. This is an acute rather than chronic condition, and complete obstruction of the afferent loop may mimic other acute intraabdominal conditions such as acute pancreatitis, intestinal obstruction, or perforated ulcer. Prompt surgical correction must be made before perforation of the loop occurs.[32, 35]

The best treatment for the afferent loop syndrome is prevention. In order to lessen the chances for obstruction when constructing the gastrojejunostomy, the afferent limb should be neither too long nor too short. The gastrojejunostomy should be performed 5 to 15 cm distal to the ligament of Treitz and preferably should be retrocolic. The gastroenterostomy stoma should be placed so that it is horizontal when the patient stands erect, and the gastroenterostomy limbs should be placed as they naturally lie in relation to the stomach without kinking or distortion. The afferent limb should be attached to the greater curve of the stomach (isoperistaltic). Mitty and coworkers note that 91 of the 105 cases of afferent loop obstructions reported occurred in antiperistaltic loops.[37] Finally, the development of internal hernia, which may produce afferent loop obstruction, is prevented by careful suturing of the mesocolon around the stomach above the gastroenterostomy and closure of the retroanastomotic space.

There are many corrective operations for the afferent loop syndrome. Most operations eliminate the afferent loop or reconstruct it so that it is no longer obstructed,

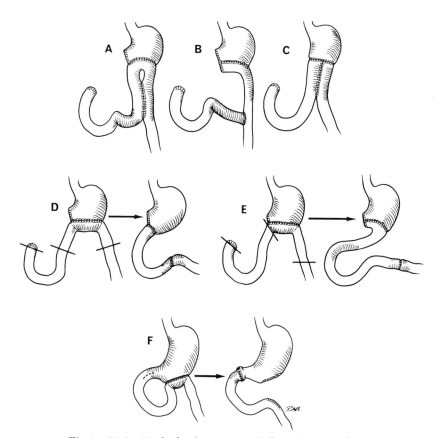

Figure 61–6. Methods of treatment of afferent loop syndrome.

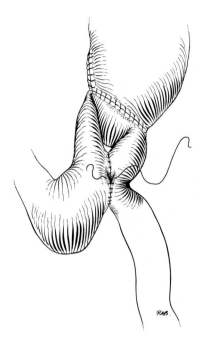

Figure 61-7. Emergency method for correcting acute afferent loop syndrome in critically ill patients.

as illustrated in Figure 61-6. If the afferent loop is hugely distended and the clinical situation is desperate, a simple enteroenterostomy between the two limbs of the gastrojejunostomy may be performed despite the somewhat increased possibility of subsequent recurrent ulceration, as illustrated in Figure 61-7.[33] The likelihood of such recurrent ulceration, however, is greatly diminished by vagotomy after such enteroenterostomy or other corrective operations in which a jejunal loop is interposed between the gastric remnant and the distal bowel. In general, attempts to "free up adhesions" and "straighten out kinks" should be avoided in favor of complete reconstruction of the gastrojejunostomy, or elimination of the afferent loop by conversion of a Billroth II to a Billroth I reconstruction with or without an interposed jejunal segment.

JEJUNOGASTRIC INTUSSUSCEPTION

This form of gastric outlet obstruction occurring after gastric surgery was first described in 1914 by Bozzi; since then, more than 150 cases have been reported.[38-43] Jejunogastric intussusception occurs

most frequently after antecolic Billroth II Polya gastric resections, although it has been described after all types of gastric operations. It has been reported to occur from five days to 35 years postoperatively, but 50 per cent of all cases occur between one and ten years after surgery. Only 8 per cent of reported cases have occurred within one month of surgery. It is impossible to state the incidence of this complication, but Caudell and Lee propose that the chronic recurring or intermittent form may account for many of the symptoms of the postgastrectomy syndrome.[38] The types of jejunogastric intussusception are efferent loop intussuscepting into the stomach, 75 to 80 per cent; afferent loop intussuscepting into the stomach, 10 to 15 per cent; and both loops intussuscepting into the stomach, 5 to 10 per cent (see Fig. 61-8). Shackman felt that the first two types were more likely to occur late and that the last type was more apt to occur soon after surgery.[42] The chronic form is more common, and the patient typically complains of recurring epigastric distress and occasional severe vomiting. As Dolan and Hockman state, diagnosis may be difficult in the chronic recurring form, because an upper gastrointestinal contrast X-ray study is diagnostic only at the time of actual intussusception.[40] The barium sulfate ingested during fluoro-

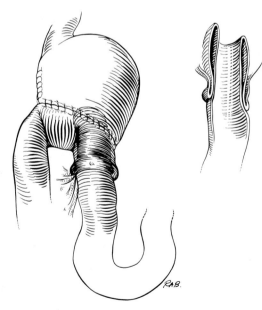

Figure 61-8. Jejunogastric intussusception.

scopic examination may reduce the intussusception before it is recognized by the radiologist.

The acute form of jejunogastric intussusception presents with a sudden onset of abdominal pain, nausea and vomiting, and a mass in the left upper abdomen (palpable in less than 50 per cent). Hematemesis, first of coffee ground-like material, and ultimately of bright red blood, frequently occurs. The classic X-ray appearance is shown in Figure 61–9.[43] The barium produces a "coiled spring" sign within the gastric pouch. This is caused by barium coating of the jejunal valves of Kerckring, which are intussuscepted into the stomach. Often this classic X-ray finding may not be seen in the more frequent chronic form of jejunogastric intussusception. In some of the chronic recurring or intermittent cases intussusception is seen only on gastroscopy (however, many minimal intussusceptions seen occurring intermittently during gastroscopy are asymptomatic). It is always important to perform the upper gastrointestinal contrast study with the patient in the extreme Trendelenburg position, both prone and supine, especially in chronic cases, to avoid missing a significant jejunogastric intussusception which may slide in and out and quite possibly not be seen in the erect or semierect position.

Devor and Passaro recommend nonoperative care of acute cases if there is no shock, hematemesis, prolonged obstruction, or evidence of peritonitis.[39] Probably about two-thirds of the acute cases may be treated conservatively, with reduction occurring spontaneously or after an upper gastrointestinal contrast series and nasogastric suction. About one-third, however, require operation. Bowel must be resected in about two-thirds of those operated upon, because the intussusception cannot be reduced. When incarceration occurs, mortality rises, with delay in operation, to 10 per cent within 48 hours and more than 50 per cent beyond 48 hours. Early postoperative intussusception

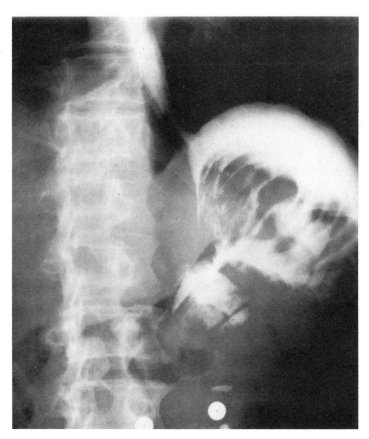

Figure 61–9. Appearance of jejunogastric intussusception on barium contrast study.

does not require surgical treatment, because there are no reports of incarceration associated with early postoperative intussusception, according to Devor and Passaro.[39] These authors also recommend that emergency operation for incarcerated acute jejunogastric intussusception be confined to reduction of the intussusception, resection of nonviable bowel, and stabilization of the loop by suturing it to the transverse mesocolon. Correction of chronic intussusception is attained by conversion of a gastrojejunostomy to a gastroduodenostomy; alternatively, Devor and Passaro suggest a new retrocolic Hofmeister anastomosis with suture of the efferent loop to the transverse mesocolon.

POSTGASTRECTOMY SMALL BOWEL OBSTRUCTION BY BOLUS

The first case of small intestinal obstruction after partial gastrectomy caused by a bolus of food (red cabbage) was reported by Seifert in 1930.[21] Since that time, various other kinds of phytobezoars have been reported to cause this condition after gastric surgery.[44] In most cases, the obstruction is caused by orange pulp (85 cases).[20] The condition is caused by inadequate mastication of fibrous, high residue food, and by inadequate fragmentation and digestion of the fibrous pulp within the partially excised stomach, with resultant passage of a large bolus of tenacious material into the small bowel where it impacts and produces intraluminal obstruction. In most cases, poor dentition leads to inadequate mastication of food. The condition is readily prevented if postgastric surgery patients have their dentition repaired, chew all food well, and avoid eating fibrous foods, particularly citrus fruit, after their operations. The condition should be suspected in any patient who develops a clinical picture of small bowel obstruction after gastric surgery, particularly when a history is given of inadequate dentition or mastication and ingestion of fibrous, pulpy foods. The treatment in such conditions is prompt operation and location of the bolus of food within the lumen of the small bowel. Usually enterotomy can be avoided by manual milking of the obstructing bolus into the cecum. Obviously, this problem may occur any time after gastric surgery.

A phytobezoar may also remain in the stomach; instead of producing small bowel obstruction, it may cause acute or chronic gastroenterostomy obstruction, with intermittent or intractable abdominal pain, nausea, and vomiting.[44]

IMMEDIATE POSTOPERATIVE HEMORRHAGE

Hemorrhage immediately after gastric surgery may occur in the peritoneal cavity or within the lumen of the gastrointestinal tract. Intraperitoneal bleeding should be suspected in any patient who develops "idiopathic" shock soon after gastric surgery. Most often, intraperitoneal hemorrhage comes from the mesentery or omentum when a ligature slips off a vessel or from an unrecognized intraoperative splenic injury. If this is suspected, transfusions are begun and the patient is promptly reoperated.[33, 45] Intraperitoneal bleeding may occur more slowly and present not as shock, but as an unexplained fall in hemoglobin. Intraperitoneal needle paracentesis, splenic scan, or visceral arteriography may be helpful in detecting cases of suspected slow intraperitoneal bleeding, thus permitting earlier reoperation for control of the bleeding.

Intraluminal bleeding soon after gastric surgery occurs in about 5 per cent of all postgastric surgery patients when all possible causes for bleeding are considered. About one-third of these cases bleed severely enough to require reoperation to control the bleeding. Hardy notes that about one-third of early postoperative bleeds are due to continuation of hemorrhage for which the operation was performed and that nearly half these patients die of this complication. Another third bleed from an anastomotic suture line shortly after surgery. The final third bleed several days following operation, and it usually cannot be determined whether the bleeding arises from the suture line or from peptic ulceration.[33]

The best means of preventing continuation of hemorrhage for which the operation was performed is to be certain of the cause of the hemorrhage and take adequate measures to control it during the initial surgery. Before operation for upper gastrointestinal hemorrhage, careful preoperative workup should ideally consist of history, physical examination, and appropriate laboratory and X-ray studies, including liver function and coagulation tests (minimal coagulation tests include prothrombin time, partial thromboplastin time, platelet count, clotting time, and bleeding time; the last test may be the only one which will detect von Willebrand's disease), upper gastrointestinal series, and esophagogastroscopy. Esophagogastroscopy is highly desirable if bleeding is not too massive, because Palmer has shown that the supposed site of bleeding is not the actual source in about 40 per cent of all cases of upper gastrointestinal bleeding.[46]

If there is no time to perform these studies because of the severity of the bleeding, the bleeding site may still be detected in most patients during surgery. Through a longitudinal gastroduodenostomy a careful inspection is made for lesions in the duodenum or distal stomach after blood clots are removed. The gastroduodenostomy incision is usually made initially only in the distal stomach and slightly across the pylorus. This exploratory incision readily permits detection and oversewing of the usual bleeding bulbar duodenal or prepyloric gastric ulcer; yet it still leaves the option of performing vagotomy and pyloroplasty or vagotomy and antrectomy. If the initial longitudinal duodenal incision is made too long, it is difficult to close the duodenum securely if gastrectomy is done. If, on the other hand, a pyloroplasty is done, the longitudinal incision can be extended farther down the duodenum, allowing closure of the gastroduodenostomy as a Finney pyloroplasty. If the bleeding site is not in the duodenum or distal half of the stomach, a separate high transverse gastrotomy is made on the anterior gastric wall about 7 cm long and about 5 cm below the cardioesophageal junction. Through this high gastrotomy, bleeding sites in the proximal stomach and at the cardioesophageal junction can be readily visualized and oversewn. A sterile, lighted proctoscope should be available for visualizing bleeders higher in the esophagus, if it is not possible to perform esophagoscopy before or during surgery. The sterile proctoscope is readily introduced into the lower esophagus through the high gastrotomy. Additional information about the source of questionable bleeding should be obtained by measuring portal venous pressure in an omental vein during laparotomy with a water manometer.

Bleeding from an anastomotic suture line, causing about one-third of early postgastric surgery bleeding, results from failure to place properly all hemostatic sutures, loosening of suture knots, or breaking of sutures. Such bleeding usually occurs immediately or shortly after surgery, but another group may have secondary hemorrhage about eight to ten days after surgery.

Early postgastric surgery bleeding is not usually due to recurrent ulceration, but this can occur and can cause suspicion of the Zollinger-Ellison syndrome. Way and colleagues describe several patients with ulcerogenic tumors who bled from recurrent ulcers even before their Levin tubes were removed after initial surgery for peptic ulcer; unfortunately, the surgery consisted of less than a total gastrectomy.[47]

When bleeding occurs in the early postoperative period, initial treatment should consist of gastric lavage with cold saline solution and blood replacement. Clotting parameters should be rechecked and any clotting defects treated specifically. Regardless of the cause of postoperative bleeding, it stops with conservative treatment in about two-thirds of patients, unless the bleeding appears to be very brisk, in which case immediate reoperation is required. The usual criteria for reoperating are essentially the same as those indicating surgery for peptic ulcer bleeding before the initial ulcer surgery; i.e., when 1500 cc of blood is given within less than 24 hours and bleeding is unabated, reoperation should be done; or if slower bleeding, requiring 1 or 2 pints of blood daily, persists for more than 72 hours, the patient should be re-explored to search for the point of bleeding.[48]

At re-exploration for early rebleeding, the gastric pouch is reopened by a transverse gastrotomy at a convenient point above the previous gastroenterostomy. Bleeding points from anastomotic suture lines are oversewn, and other bleeding sites within the stomach, esophagus, and jejunum can be seen and managed through this gastrotomy. If a duodenal ulcer has been oversewn and left in situ within the closed duodenal stump after a Billroth II gastrectomy, it may be necessary to reopen the duodenal stump to inspect the ulcer and resuture the bleeding vessel in the ulcer if no bleeding site is found within the stomach. When the duodenal stump is reopened, it should be very carefully reclosed and decompressed, with a small duodenostomy tube and Penrose drains placed near it, as described on page 809.[49] If the gastric remnant is too small to perform gastrotomy safely above the gastroenterostomy, the anterior portion of the gastroenterostomy is opened for inspection of the interior of the stomach. If a pyloroplasty was done originally, it is simply reopened to look for bleeding and then carefully reclosed; a gastrostomy tube should be placed in the stomach for decompression postoperatively.

DUODENAL STUMP DEHISCENCE AFTER BILLROTH II GASTRECTOMY

The incidence of duodenal stump dehiscence after Billroth II gastrectomy ranges from 1 to 6 per cent in various reports, and the mean incidence is about 3 per cent.[49] This serious complication causes half the deaths from Billroth II gastrectomy, and the average mortality rate for the "duodenal stump blowout" is about 50 per cent.[50] The peak incidence of duodenal stump dehiscence occurs on the fourth or fifth postoperative day; however, it may occur as late as the twelfth postoperative day.[50]

The principal causes of duodenal stump dehiscence are (1) duodenal distention from afferent limb obstruction; (2) duodenal ischemia from excessive dissection and mobilization of the duodenal stump; (3) insecure closure of the duodenal stump caused by technical errors; (4) insecure duodenal closure caused by edema, scarring, and rigidity of the duodenum; (5) periduodenal infection and abscess; and (6) pancreatic injury and fistula, with digestion of the duodenal suture line.[33, 51, 52]

Prevention of Duodenal Stump Dehiscence. Obviously the best means of preventing duodenal stump dehiscence is avoidance of a duodenal stump. This is achieved by performing a vagotomy and gastroenterostomy or a vagotomy and Jaboulay pyloroplasty if there is excessive duodenal scarring and the surgeon feels that duodenal closure will be too difficult if a gastrectomy is done. In some cases, however, it is not apparent that duodenal dissection will be inordinately difficult and closure insecure until the surgeon is committed, for various technical reasons, to a gastrectomy.[51-53] Also, in some instances, the surgeon may feel that antrectomy and vagotomy is strongly indicated in a young, good risk male patient with a virulent ulcer diathesis and high gastric acid secretion even though the duodenal dissection may be somewhat difficult. Even in these patients, however, if it seems that duodenal dissection and closure will be inordinately difficult, resection should not be done.

When performing gastric resection, excessive mobilization and dissection with resulting devascularization of the scarred duodenum are avoided. Lahey suggested placing a T-tube in the common bile duct during gastrectomy if one is unsure of the duct's relationship to the duodenum to avoid damaging the common duct.[54] However, if there is such excessive scarring and contraction superior to the duodenum near the common duct, it is better to avoid gastrectomy and perform a vagotomy and drainage procedure.[54]

In patients with posterior penetrating duodenal ulcer, when the ulcer cannot be safely removed to allow mobilization of the posterior duodenal wall for secure duodenal closure, the Nissen maneuver is utilized to obtain satisfactory duodenal closure (Fig. 61–10).[51, 55] When the Nissen maneuver is done, or the duodenal closure is the least bit tenuous, a decompressive duodenostomy tube should be inserted into the duodenal stump. Protective, decompressive duodenostomy to avoid duodenal stump leakage was first described by Friedemann in 1936.[56] Since then, other authors have described the decompressive tube duodenostomy.[49, 52, 53] Most of these techniques involve insertion of a large-bore catheter into the duodenal stump,

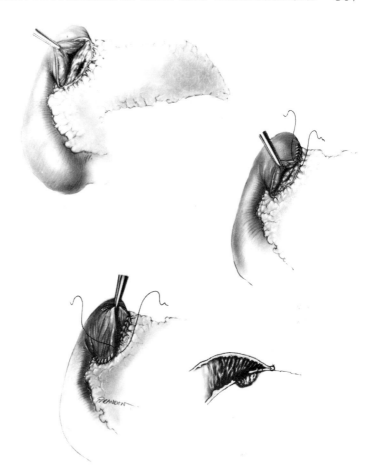

Figure 61–10. Modified Nissen procedure for closure of difficult duodenal stump following Billroth II gastrectomy.

with establishment of a purposeful, controlled duodenal fistula in order to prevent a later, more dangerous, uncontrolled fistula.

The technique we have used since 1958 in about 120 cases differs from the previously described techniques of tube duodenostomy in that a smaller catheter (No. 10 Foley) is inserted into the duodenum and very effective duodenal decompression is obtained with it, sufficient to prevent high postoperative intraduodenal stump pressures that may ultimately cause leakage through an insecure duodenal stump suture line. The smaller tube, however, does not cause a fistula when it is removed as do the larger duodenostomy tubes.[49]

The insertion and management of the small duodenostomy tube we use is simple. A No. 10 Foley catheter is inserted into the duodenum either through the line of closure or preferably into the anterior duodenal wall, as shown in Figure 61–11.

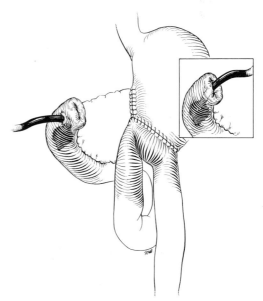

Figure 61–11. Method of inserting a No. 10 Foley duodenostomy tube to decompress duodenal stump after Billroth II gastrectomy and to prevent duodenal stump dehiscence.

The duodenostomy tube is brought out through a small stab wound in the right upper quadrant of the abdomen and fixed to the skin with a suture. The tube is connected to low intermittent suction from a Gomco suction machine. The duodenal secretions are sufficiently thin to flow very easily through the small tube. The duodenostomy tube is kept on suction until postoperative ileus abates and the nasogastric tube is removed. Duodenostomy tube suction is then discontinued, and the tube is connected to gravity drainage. The duodenal drainage usually decreases markedly by the ninth postoperative day; the small balloon on the No. 10 French duodenostomy tube is then deflated, and the tube is slightly withdrawn from the duodenal stump so that its tip lies just outside the tiny opening in the duodenal wall. Suction is again applied to the duodenostomy tube with a Gomco suction machine and is continued overnight. The following day, if the overnight duodenostomy tube drainage is less than 100 cc, the duodenal catheter is removed. Rarely is there any persistent drainage after the tube is removed, because the small duodenal opening rapidly seals. The patient is usually ambulatory (being able to carry the dependent drainage bottle to which the duodenostomy tube is attached) after the third postoperative day, and no restriction of normal convalescent activity is necessary.

Our experience with the small No. 10 French Foley catheter duodenal stump decompression was reported in 1967; in a group of more than 68 difficult duodenal stump closures protected by the duodenostomy in a series of 420 Billroth II gastrectomies, only two patients developed duodenal stump dehiscences. These leaks occurred in debilitated patients who had emergency operations for bleeding duodenal ulcers and had insecure duodenal stump closures. Only one of the 352 other Billroth II gastrectomy patients during the period of that review in whom it was deemed unnecessary to perform tube duodenostomy had a duodenal stump dehiscence, and this was also a debilitated patient undergoing emergency surgery for bleeding. All three of these duodenal stump dehiscences could have been avoided by suturing the bleeding ulcer and performing vagotomy and pyloro-

plasty instead of emergency gastrectomy. This, nevertheless, represents an overall incidence of duodenal stump dehiscence of only 0.7 per cent in a series of 420 Billroth II gastrectomies. This is a fourfold reduction below the average 3 per cent incidence of duodenal stump dehiscence occurring in a recently collected series of over 3000 gastrectomies, and is considerably below the 6 per cent rate of duodenal stump dehiscence reported in one series in which duodenostomy was never used.[49]

There has been no significant morbidity after this type of duodenostomy other than occasional transient drainage around the duodenostomy catheter when the catheter temporarily became occluded. This ceased when the duodenostomy catheter was flushed with a few cubic centimeters of saline solution. The catheters should be routinely flushed by the surgeon twice daily with 3 to 4 cc of normal saline solution. Two minor subcutaneous infections about the tubes cleared promptly with adequate drainage.

Our experience with approximately 50 additional cases of small tube duodenostomy since our initial report remains essentially the same.

Although not routinely recommended, if any duodenal stump closure causes much concern, it should be drained with Penrose drains (the drains should be placed near but not on the duodenal closure; otherwise the drains may contribute to the likelihood of leakage). These drains are used in conjunction with the tube duodenostomy, but should be brought out through a separate opening in the abdominal wall. The Penrose drains may be gradually removed after a week if the patient is doing well and no evidence of duodenal leakage has appeared.[51, 55]

If an ulcer has been excluded from the duodenal closure and left on the surface of the pancreas (since it is very dangerous and unnecessary to attempt to remove such posterior penetrating ulcers), it should also be drained with Penrose drains. Such ulcer beds may contain inapparent pancreatic ducts and thus require external drainage to prevent catastrophic leakage of pancreatic secretions into the abdomen postoperatively.[57-60]

Management of Duodenal Stump Dehiscence and End Duodenal Fistula. If duodenal stump dehiscence occurs, peritonitis and sepsis develop rapidly (unless the stump is adequately drained). If a Penrose drain is present, duodenal dehiscence is recognized much earlier by the appearance of duodenal content in the drain tract, and there is usually only local, rather than generalized, peritonitis. Thus a more rapid institution of treatment and significant reduction in mortality are possible.[50, 51, 55] If the duodenal fistula is controlled by the previously placed drains and there is no spreading peritonitis or sepsis, nonoperative management is the treatment of choice.[50, 61-63] If possible, a sump drain should be inserted into the fistulous tract beside the Penrose drains and constant suction applied to it. Sump suction removes fluids and reduces skin digestion by pancreatic juice, makes the spread of fistulous drainage within the peritoneal cavity less likely, and induces more rapid closure of the fistula. Skin digestion about the external opening of the duodenal fistula is further reduced by keeping the skin near the fistula covered with gum karaya powder, which is much more satisfactory for this purpose than is aluminum paste. Oral intake is stopped, nasogastric suction is reinstituted (preferably with the more efficient Salem sump suction nasogastric tube), and central intravenous hyperalimentation is begun.

Recent reports and our own experience suggest that hyperalimentation tends to markedly decrease gastrointestinal secretion. Intravenous hyperalimentation therefore may contribute directly to the closure of gastrointestinal fistulas and control of excessive fluid and electrolyte losses from fistulas by significantly reducing the volume and digestive enzyme content of fistulous discharge; this effect is over and above the important role of intravenous hyperalimentation in maintaining good nutrition in such debilitating conditions.[62, 64, 65]

In some instances, parenterally administered anticholinergic drugs may also diminish fistulous drainage, and these agents may be tried unless they are felt to be contraindicated. They may, however, compound problems with ileus, inspissation of pulmonary secretions, and thirst.

After an initial period of nasogastric suction, when ileus has abated, the duodenal fistula seems controlled by adequate drainage, no peritonitis or sepsis is evident, and the patient is otherwise clinically stable, the nasogastric tube is removed. The next day, small, frequent oral feedings are started cautiously if removal of the nasogastric tube is tolerated. If oral feedings do not excessively increase duodenal fistulous drainage, the amount of feeding is slowly increased, with central intravenous hyperalimentation maintained. If oral feeding is not tolerated or increases duodenal fistulous drainage excessively, one of the elemental, nonresidue diets now available, such as Vivonex (Eaton Laboratories), may be suitable when given in frequent, small quantities. Such an elemental diet consists of a mixture of glucose, amino acids, electrolytes, and vitamins.

If neither of these methods of oral feeding is possible, a small plastic feeding tube may be inserted through the nose into the gastric remnant and passed through the gastroenterostomy well into the upper jejunum and used for infusing jejunostomy feedings.

The method of inserting such a nasojejunal feeding tube is described by Bachrach and Tecimer.[25] Their method is as follows: Through a small polyethylene 190 tube long enough to reach the upper jejunum from the nose, a long wire is inserted. A No. 1 silk thread is attached to the wire, and the wire is withdrawn from the polyethylene tube, thus pulling the silk thread into the polyethylene tube throughout the length of the tube. A rubber finger cot containing about 2 cc of mercury is securely tied on the silk thread to serve as a weight at the end of the tube (much like a small Cantor tube), and the silk thread is fixed in place at the nasal end of the polyethylene tube. This assemblage is passed through the nose into the gastric remnant. With fluoroscopic aid this tube is passed through the gastroenterostomy into the upper jejunum. Its position should be checked by injecting water-soluble contrast medium into the polyethylene tube while making an X-ray film of the abdomen. When the tube is positioned properly in the proximal jejunum, the silk thread is released from the proximal (nasal) end of the tube and the small mercury-weighted finger cot and its attached silk thread are carried out of the polyethylene tube (which has been fixed in place at the nose) by intestinal peristalsis. Both the silk thread and the mercury-weighted finger cot then pass readily through the gut and are passed per rectum. The indwelling nasojejunal tube may then be left in place for long periods and used for continuous or intermittent jejunostomy feedings or for feedings of one of the newer elemental diet preparations. A Barron pump is very useful in allowing slow, continuous 24-hour infusion of diet through this tube. The tube should be flushed with water several times daily to prevent plugging. In very debilitated patients such tube feedings may be given in conjunction with central intravenous hyperalimentation. Ultimately, however, if sufficient feeding is tolerated through the nasojejunal tube, or orally, intravenous hyperalimentation may be discontinued.

The nasojejunal feeding tube may also be used to return duodenal fistulous fluid to the jejunum. When the quantity of duodenal fistulous drainage is large, intravenous replacement of the fluid and electrolytes which are lost may be very difficult. If the fluid is collected and refed, however, the problem of fluid and electrolyte replacement is less. When the duodenal fistulous drainage is refed to the patient, the bottle in which it is collected must be kept in a container of ice and the accumulated duodenal drainage should be removed and refed slowly through the nasojejunal feeding tube in small increments every two to four hours throughout the day and night, or, preferably, it should be refed slowly and constantly with a Barron pump. Cooling of the fistulous fluid and prompt return of it to the gut prevent bacterial overgrowth in the fluid which may cause severe enteritis and diarrhea. If there is gross purulent material or heavy bacterial contamination in the fistulous fluid, it should not be refed. Refeeding of duodenal fistulous drainage is probably unnecessary when the volume of drainage is less than 1500 to 2000 cc per 24-hour period. The fluid and electrolyte losses must still be carefully measured, however, and replaced by suitable intravenous or oral fluids and electrolytes. As much as 4 or 5 liters of fluid per day may be lost from some duodenal fistulas, and at least a significant portion of this drainage must be refed to the patient.

If it is impossible to insert the nasojejunal feeding tube, it may be necessary to perform a feeding jejunostomy for supplemental feeding.[27] Since the advent of parenteral hyperalimentation and the small nasojejunal feeding tube, however, the usual feeding jejunostomy has not been required nearly so often as in the past.[24, 25]

With such conservative treatment of duodenal fistulas, Edmunds and associates noted that less than 5 per cent of duodenal stump fistulas require definitive surgery for closure. They also reported in their series of 55 duodenal and gastric fistulas that all 17 of the fistulas which closed spontaneously did so in less than two months (the remainder died before operative attempts at closure were made or as a result of operations to close the fistulas).[50] In our experience, if operation becomes necessary to close the fistula, the most effective surgical technique is to dissect out the fistulous tract to its origin at the duodenal stump and suture the open end of a defunctionalized Roux-en-Y limb of proximal jejunum directly over the fistulous opening in the duodenal stump, thus draining the fistula internally into the defunctionalized limb. If this is done in conjunction with a vagotomy, it is unlikely to cause recurrent ulcer resulting from diversion of duodenal content from the gastrojejunostomy. In contrast, direct attempts to suture the fistulous opening are likely to be difficult, dangerous, and ineffective, and a jejunal onlay patch to close the fistula is probably more likely to be associated with persistent leakage or infection. Penrose drains are left near the site of these repairs.

If a duodenal stump dehiscence occurs and prior Penrose drainage to the duodenal stump was not established, or if drainage is inadequate and spreading peritonitis or sepsis develops, adequate drainage with Penrose and sump suction drains to the area of the duodenal leak must be immediately established. Usually this is done through a right upper quadrant abdominal incision. Attempts, at this time, to directly close the duodenal dehiscence are usually ill advised, unless the dehiscence occurs and is detected very early before the patient's general condition deteriorates and the inflammatory reaction about the duodenal stump becomes severe.[50] In such unusual instances, if it appears technically feasible, the duodenum may be reclosed, a small decompressive duodenostomy tube inserted as described above, and good drainage established to the area of stump closure. In most cases, however, prompt, adequate Penrose and sump suction drainage alone is the surgical treatment of choice for duodenal stump dehiscence.

The overall mortality of duodenal stump dehiscence varies from 15 to 70 per cent, but at present probably averages about 30 per cent.[50, 63]

GASTROJEJUNAL, GASTRODUODENAL, AND GASTRIC FISTULAS

The incidence of these fistulas after gastric surgery ranges from 0.5 to 1 per cent. They most commonly arise at the anterior or posterior suture lines of the gastroenteric anastomosis or in the Hofmeister suture line of the gastric remnant.[33, 50, 63] The Hofmeister suture line leak is especially likely to occur at the so-called angle of sorrow where the anterior and posterior gastrojejunal or gastroduodenal suture lines meet each other at the Hofmeister suture line of the stomach. Much more rarely, they may occur in the fundus or body of the stomach away from the anastomotic suture lines.[66]

The principal causes of these fistulas are technical errors and partial devascularization of the gastric remnant after a gastric resection. Partial gastric remnant devascularization causing suture line leakage probably occurs more often than is recognized.[33, 67, 68] Such devascularization is most likely to occur after high gastric resections. The gastric pouch generally receives adequate blood supply even though all four major arteries supplying the stomach are ligated, if collateral supply to the gastric remnant through the inferior phrenic arteries and/or vasa brevia of the splenic artery is preserved. Excessively high ligation of the left gastric artery at the celiac trifurcation may, however, interrupt collateral gastric arterial flow through the inferior phrenic arteries. The left gastric artery therefore should not be ligated at its origin, but should be ligated distally at its entry into the lesser curvature of the stomach. Avoidance of high ligation of the left gastric artery may also prevent inadvertent interruption of the blood supply to the left hepatic lobe, because in about 25 per cent of all individuals part or all of the blood supply of the left hepatic lobe arises from an accessory or replaced left hepatic artery arising from the left gastric artery near its celiac origin.[67, 68] Another cause of partial devascularization of the gastric remnant and gastric fistulization is concomitant splenectomy, which may be required by splenic injury or purposeful removal of the spleen as part of radical subtotal gastrectomy for gastric cancer.[66, 69] Usually loss of the short gastric arteries arising from the splenic artery to supply the gastric fundus will not cause gastric devascularization unless blood flow through the inferior phrenic arteries is also compromised. Occasionally fistulas have been reported high in the gastric fundus along the greater curvature of the stomach after splenectomy even though the stomach has not been removed. These fistulas are caused by inclusion of the gastric wall in clamps placed on the short gastric arteries during splenectomy, thus causing necrosis of the gastric wall and gastric fistula formation. This is prevented by careful placement of clamps in this area to avoid including the gastric fundus when removing the spleen. The gastric fundus should be imbricated on itself with a single row of interrupted sutures if it is feared that the wall of the gastric fundus was possibly damaged during splenectomy and that gastric fistulization at the fundus may result. Penrose drains should also be placed in the splenic bed after splenectomy so any such gastric fistulization will be controlled, generalized peritonitis prevented, and gastric fistulas promptly recognized. Gastroenteric or gastric fistulas should always be considered in the differential diagnosis of peritonitis or subphrenic abscess which occurs after gastric or splenic surgery.

Gastroenteric, duodenal, and gastric fistulas may also initially appear to be wound infections or dehiscences until bowel content appears in the abdominal wound. The site of the fistula may usually be located by an upper gastrointestinal contrast X-ray study, using a water-soluble radiopaque medium. When external fistulous drainage occurs, visual confirmation of the gastroenteric leak may be made by feeding the patient grape juice, methylene blue dye, or charcoal by mouth and watching for the appearance of these substances in the external fistulous drainage. If the fistula cannot be confirmed by these means but is strongly suspected because of sepsis and peritonitis, immediate surgery to establish drainage is required as described for duodenal stump dehiscence.[63]

Pettersson and Wallensten comment that the choice of drainage, suture closure, or re-resection of gastroenteric fistulas is much the same, and that the type of surgical therapy depends upon the extent of the suture line disruption, the condition of the patient at the time of the operation to correct the fistula, and whether the fistula is walled off. The mortality is about 40 per cent for each method of treatment. The mortality of nonsurgical treatment, however, without drainage is 80 per cent. Pettersson and Wallensten base these mortality statistics on 45 cases of gastroenteric fistulas occurring after Billroth I or Billroth II gastrectomy. One-third of the fistula patients in their series were managed "conservatively," i.e., without surgery, and the remaining two-thirds were treated surgically, as follows: 43 per cent had drainage only, 27 per cent were resutured, and 30 per cent had re-resections. In eight of nine patients on whom re-resection was done, the earlier Billroth I gastrectomy was changed to a Billroth II gastrectomy.[63]

In some cases, the fistula, if it is not too large, may be closed about a small catheter which is placed on constant suction postoperatively for better control of the fistula. This may be done if it seems technically possible to do more than simply drain the fistula externally with Penrose and sump drains, but inadvisable to resuture or resect the fistula.[61] The area about the fistula should, however, be drained with Penrose and sump suction drains in addition to inserting the catheter directly into the fistula.

After corrective surgery for gastroenteric fistulas, supportive care, including central intravenous hyperalimentation, is very important. Nasogastric decompression is perhaps more important in cases of gastroen-

teric fistulas to reduce the volume of fistulous drainage than in most cases of end duodenal fistula. The small Bachrach-Tecimer nasojejunal feeding tube may also be used to great advantage in the care of these patients.[25] Intrajejunal feeding through this tube beyond the fistula and central intravenous hyperalimentation will probably greatly reduce the need for feeding jejunostomy in these patients, and the intravenous hyperalimentation will encourage spontaneous closure of these fistulas not only by marked improvement of nutrition, but also by significantly reducing the volume and enzyme content of the fistulous drainage.[24, 62, 64, 65]

INFECTIOUS COMPLICATIONS AFTER GASTRIC SURGERY

The incidence of wound and intra-abdominal abscesses is significantly increased after gastric surgery for chronic pyloric obstruction and emergency surgery for hemorrhage and perforation of peptic ulcers. Chronic pyloric obstruction may allow bacterial growth caused by gastric stasis, increasing the incidence of wound infections and other septic complications. This may probably be reduced in incidence by giving oral nonabsorbable antibiotics 24 hours preoperatively to those with chronic pyloric obstruction. Snyder and Stellar report a wound infection rate of 10 per cent in a large series of patients with duodenal ulcers in whom emergency surgery was performed for massive bleeding,[48] whereas Gardner et al. report an overall wound infection rate of only 3.3 per cent in a large series of patients undergoing elective gastric surgery.[15] Rapid overgrowth of bacteria in the gastric blood clots and hemorrhagic shock probably account for the increased rate of sepsis seen in patients undergoing emergency surgery for gastroduodenal hemorrhage. Because of the increased rate of wound infections after emergency gastric surgery for hemorrhage or perforation or after surgery for chronic pyloric obstruction, it is wise to close only the deeper layers of the abdominal incision. The fascia of the potentially infected abdominal wound should be closed with wire or similarly nonreactive monofilament synthetic suture. The skin and subcutaneous tissue are left open, and gauze dressings are changed twice daily. After three or four days, if the abdominal wound appears clean, the skin and subcutaneous tissue are closed with sterile tape strips. This management does not delay wound healing, and indeed may hasten it by preventing infection.

Glotzer and associates have recently reported that wound infections in contaminated abdominal incisions may be prevented by lavaging the wound with an antibiotic solution before primary closure.[70] This method may prove to be an acceptable alternative to leaving the contaminated wound open; however, we have been well satisfied with open treatment of such wounds. In either case, the patient should receive broad-spectrum parenteral antibiotic therapy before and for several days after emergency gastric surgery for hemorrhage, perforation, or chronic pyloric obstruction. Antibiotics are most effective if they are started before surgery; otherwise, an effective antibiotic blood level is not present at the time of greatest tissue contamination, i.e., during the operation.

Reduction of septic complications after elective surgery for gastric ulcer or cancer in achlorhydric or hypochlorhydric stomachs may also be achieved by placing the patient on clear liquids, a mechanical bowel cleansing routine (i.e., enemas and mild cathartics), and oral Neothalidine suspension and tetracycline for 24 hours before elective gastric surgery. This is done for two reasons. First, in achlorhydric or hypochlorhydric stomachs there is often a heavy growth of pathogenic organisms which may be eliminated by broad-spectrum oral antibiotics given shortly before surgery. Thus the chance of contamination of the peritoneal cavity and abdominal wound from the open stomach during surgery is greatly reduced. Second, if resection of a portion of transverse colon is required by invasion or adherence of a benign or malignant gastric ulcer to the colon or mesocolon, the colon has been adequately prepared to permit safe resection and primary anastomosis of the involved colon during the gastric surgery.

SUBPHRENIC AND INTRA-ABDOMINAL ABSCESS AFTER GASTRIC SURGERY

Sherman and associates reported that subphrenic abscess followed 1.4 per cent of a series of 3000 gastric operations at Ohio State University Hospital.[71] This figure is consistent with other series.[72] They also noted that 34 per cent of a series of 130 patients with subphrenic abscess developed the abscess after gastroduodenal surgery. Probably most such abscesses occurred because of leakage of suture lines. Parenteral antibiotics do not seem to have significantly reduced the incidence of postoperative subphrenic abscess, although they may often alter the clinical findings of subphrenic or intra-abdominal abscesses and make diagnosis more difficult. The more liberal use of preoperative oral antibiotics, as discussed above, or lavage of the peritoneal cavity with broad-spectrum antibiotics during surgery may, however, reduce the incidence of postoperative peritonitis and intra-abdominal abscess more than have parenteral antibiotics. Several recent reports cite the efficacy of peritoneal antibiotic lavage in the prevention and treatment of peritonitis and intra-abdominal abscesses.[73-75] Antibiotic lavage should not be done routinely after gastric surgery, but in patients with a higher potential of septic postoperative complications, i.e., after emergency and reoperative gastric surgery of all types, it may be advisable. A solution of 2 g of kanamycin in 800 cc of normal saline (0.25 per cent solution) plus 50,000 units of bacitracin may be used for such intra-abdominal lavage. After surgery and careful mechanical cleansing of the peritoneal cavity with copious saline lavage, the abdominal cavity is washed with 800 cc of this antibiotic solution. It remains in the peritoneal cavity for 15 to 20 minutes during abdominal closure; just before the last sutures are tied, about half the antibiotic solution is aspirated from the abdominal cavity. We have used this antibiotic lavage solution frequently for the last several years, and have had no problems with respiratory depression or eighth nerve or renal toxicity, in contrast to earlier experiences with 1 per cent solutions of kanamycin or neomycin which often caused respiratory depression or arrest.

Intra-abdominal abscesses suspected after gastric surgery because of unexplained fever can usually be diagnosed and localized by physical examination and X-ray studies. A thorough discussion of the diagnosis and management of subphrenic and intra-abdominal abscess is beyond the scope of this review; however, the principal point to emphasize is that one must suspect, diagnose, and treat them early if the still significant mortality (about 30 per cent) is to be reduced. Barnard's aphorism must be kept in mind: "Pus somewhere, pus nowhere, pus under the diaphragm!"[71, 72]

VAGOTOMY COMPLICATIONS

DIARRHEA

The incidence of slight or transient postvagotomy diarrhea may approach 60 per cent. Persistently troublesome postvagotomy diarrhea, however, occurs in less than 5 to 6 per cent of all patients.[33] Even in more severe instances, the diarrhea can usually be controlled medically. Postvagotomy diarrhea requiring surgical treatment for possible correction probably occurs after less than 0.3 per cent of all vagotomies.[76, 77]

The exact cause of postvagotomy diarrhea is unknown. Dragstedt postulates that some postvagotomy diarrhea may be caused by enteritis produced by overgrowth of pathogenic bacteria (personal communication). The bacteria may flourish because of small bowel stasis caused by vagotomy. Another potential source for such pathogenic bacteria is the gastric pouch. Reduction of gastric acid levels and gastric stasis caused by vagotomy and gastric resection or drainage may permit bacterial overgrowth in the stomach which may cause enteritis and diarrhea.

Treatment. In most instances, postvagotomy diarrhea is transient and mild and requires minimal or no treatment. Several means are available for treating more troublesome cases. An adjustment of diet with deletion of foods which cause increased diarrhea is most effective at times. As in the dumping syndrome, small frequent feedings of a low residue, high protein, moderate fat, low carbohydrate diet with no fluid intake during meals are preferable. Often milk or other foods containing high quantities of lactose may aggravate the condition.

If alterations in diet do not control postvagotomy diarrhea, medications such as anticholinergics and diphenoxylate (Lomotil) may be helpful. Although at times quite effective, these agents, by reducing bowel motility, might increase intestinal bacterial overgrowth and enteritis caused by intestinal stasis and possibly aggravate rather than alleviate diarrhea, but this is probably unlikely.

Although seemingly paradoxical, postvagotomy diarrhea may respond to oral bethanechol chloride (Urecholine), 10 to 20 mg 30 minutes before each meal and at bedtime. Urecholine may diminish intestinal stasis caused by vagotomy and thus theoretically eliminate the potential for intestinal bacterial overgrowth and enteritis, or it may correct altered small bowel motility induced by vagotomy and relieve the diarrhea whether bacterial overgrowth is involved or not.

In cases of more severe postvagotomy diarrhea it may be necessary, Dragstedt states, to intermittently induce gastrointestinal "rest" by stopping all oral intake and placing the patient on nasogastric suction and intravenous fluids for a few days. The severe diarrhea usually subsides within a day or so of beginning this regime; when this occurs and fluid and electrolyte balance are corrected, the nasogastric tube is removed and the patient begins frequent small, low residue feedings, taking oral liquids only between meals. A course of oral tetracycline, 250 mg every six hours for five to seven days, is also given after the nasogastric tube is removed. Tetracycline theoretically decreases pathogenic intestinal organisms possibly caused by postvagotomy intestinal stasis and stops diarrhea caused by such organisms (personal communication).

For rare cases of postvagotomy diarrhea in which vigorous medical treatment fails and progressive debility is occurring, Sawyers and Herrington describe a surgical procedure which has been quite effective

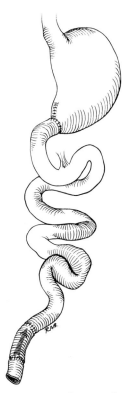

Figure 61–12. Reversed jejunal segment for treatment of a rare form of intractable postvagotomy diarrhea.

in the small number of cases in which it has been tried. A 10-cm segment of upper jejunum is reversed to form an antiperistaltic portion of bowel 90 to 100 cm distal to the ligament of Treitz (Fig. 61–12). They stress that the reversed segment must be located in this area, as otherwise it is unlikely to arrest the diarrhea. This operation corrected diarrhea and weight loss in all of nine patients thus far treated in this manner.[77] It must be stressed, however, that this operation might be required in no more than about 0.3 per cent of all patients having vagotomies, i.e., those with truly intractable, debilitating diarrhea. A similar operation has been described by Craft and Venables.[76] The possible placebo effect of this procedure must be recognized, although previous attempts to correct postvagotomy diarrhea surgically by placing the reversed bowel segment more distally have been unsatisfactory. Fortuitous, coincidental cessation of the diarrhea also seems unlikely, because prolonged unsuccessful medical treatment of the diarrhea,

which often had been present for months, was carried out in Herrington's patients before performing the surgery which apparently promptly and persistently corrected or greatly improved the diarrhea in the small number of cases reported. Admittedly, this is an operation which, by purposely inducing intestinal stasis, would seem illogical if Dragstedt's theory that intestinal bacterial overgrowth resulting from stasis causes postvagotomy diarrhea is correct. This dilemma merely emphasizes the lack of understanding of the cause of postvagotomy diarrhea. Until a better etiological understanding is obtained, treatment of postvagotomy diarrhea must necessarily be empiric.

TECHNICAL COMPLICATIONS AFTER VAGOTOMY

The chief technical problems arising from vagotomy are splenic rupture, esophageal perforation, and periesophageal or mediastinal hemorrhage.

The incidence of splenic rupture during vagotomy varies considerably, but in a recent collected series of more than 5000 vagotomies, the average incidence of splenic rupture was 3 per cent.[78] Splenic rupture is usually caused by traction on the splenic capsule during esophageal mobilization preparatory to performing truncal vagotomy. To lessen the incidence of splenic rupture during vagotomy, caudad traction to make the vagi taut for easier identification should be placed on the lesser curvature of the stomach rather than on the greater curvature, as suggested by Wangensteen and Kelly.[79] If traction is exerted on the greater curvature of the stomach, more direct pull is placed on the spleen with greater likelihood of capsular tearing. Splenic rupture is also less likely if the esophagus is mobilized primarily from the medial rather than the lateral aspect; thus the surgeon's finger, in bluntly dissecting around the esophagus, is directed toward rather than away from the spleen, and excessive traction on the splenic capsule and short gastric arteries is avoided. After completion of esophageal mobilization and just before abdominal closure, the spleen is carefully inspected; if there is any splenic capsular tear, the spleen must be removed. Attempts to "patch" even small capsular tears are ill advised and may lead to catastrophic postoperative splenic hemorrhage.

Esophageal perforation occurs during esophageal mobilization to perform vagotomy in about 1 per cent of all cases. If such mobilization is done cautiously, however, with good exposure and lighting, and with a large-bore Levin tube in the esophagus to serve as a guide for the esophageal mobilization, the incidence of perforation should be lower than 1 per cent. Esophageal perforation is recognized either by direct visualization or by the appearance of a few bubbles of gastric fluid through an otherwise unrecognized esophageal tear. Also, if the esophageal perforation is posterior, it may be noted only by feeling the Levin tube directly through the esophageal tear. Esophageal perforation is a potentially fatal injury and is the chief cause of death resulting from technical error after vagotomy. Most reviews of vagotomies, however, report a very low mortality rate from this complication. Most esophageal perforations are detected immediately, and usually only the unrecognized ones cause death. Perforations should be closed with two inverting layers of interrupted nonabsorbable sutures, and should be drained externally with several Penrose drains. With adequate repair, the mortality of esophageal perforation is less than 10 per cent. Since the incidence of esophageal perforation is less than 1 per cent, the overall mortality from iatrogenic esophageal perforation should be less than 0.1 per cent after truncal vagotomy.[78, 80-82]

Periesophageal and/or mediastinal hemorrhage may occur when small vessels on the esophageal surface are torn during vagotomy. If such bleeding vessels are not ligated, postoperative intra-abdominal hemorrhage or, less frequently, intramediastinal hemorrhage may occur.[78, 82, 83]

Complications may also develop when the left lobe of the liver is mobilized to expose more adequately the periesophageal area during vagotomy. Some surgeons prefer to retract the left hepatic lobe superiorly with a Weinberg vagotomy retractor to avoid potential complications of left hepatic lobar mobilization, but this may not afford good exposure for vagotomy if the left hepatic lobe is large. If division of the left triangular ligament of the liver (the Grey Turner maneuver) is carried too far medially toward the vena cava, the left hepatic vein or vena cava may be injured; however, with good visualization this should not happen. Another complication of the Grey Turner maneuver relates to failure to replace the left lobe of the liver into its normal anatomic position after it has been folded and retracted to the right to expose the vagi. Left hepatic lobe infarction can occur when the lobe has remained or has fallen back into this "folded" position after abdominal closure. To avoid this problem, some surgeons recommend reattachment of the left hepatic lobe to the left triangular ligament when the lobe has been mobilized.[78]

POSTVAGOTOMY DYSPHAGIA OR TRANSIENT ACHALASIA

After vagotomy, some patients complain of mild dysphagia, usually only with solid food, for a few days. It is usually transient and requires no treatment except reassurance of the patient. Mild dysphagia is probably due to periesophageal edema and possibly partial denervation of the lower esophageal sphincter by avulsion of its vagal nerve supply. Mild dysphagia is usually *not* painful, but is described as a painless "sticking" of food in the esophagus. If dysphagia persists for more than a few days, however, esophagrams and esophagoscopy should be done. Dilatation of the distal esophagus may be done, if necessary, at the time of esophagoscopy. Usually, esophageal dilatation relieves mild postvagotomy "achalasia" readily and permanently. Patients with this problem should be cautioned to chew very thoroughly and swallow only small boluses of food until the dysphagia disappears.

Infrequently, postvagotomy dysphagia is considerably more severe and persistent and is associated with pain upon swallowing. In such cases, periesophageal inflammation and fibrosis are more likely the cause of severe, persistent dysphagia than is mild periesophageal edema or esophageal vagal denervation. Severe, painful dysphagia is less likely to relent spontaneously, and such cases may require more careful and repeated dilatations. More severe dysphagia tends to appear later after vagotomy than the milder, more transient cases of dysphagia. Severe, persistent postvagotomy dysphagia, fortunately, is quite unusual.[19, 84, 85]

POSTVAGOTOMY HIATUS HERNIA

Hiatus hernia developing after abdominal vagotomy occurs in about 10 to 15 per cent of all patients undergoing vagotomy. The frequency with which it is described, however, depends upon the vigor of the diagnostic approach. In patients with postvagotomy hiatus hernia, esophageal reflux may occur very frequently, but it is unusual for such reflux to be symptomatic or to cause esophagitis. Thus it is probably not essential to perform hiatus herniorrhaphy routinely after abdominal vagotomy, although some surgeons recommend it. It may be wise, however, if there was preoperative evidence of peptic esophagitis or symptomatic hiatus hernia, to perform a Hill hiatus herniorrhaphy at the time of abdominal vagotomy. The simplicity and effectiveness of the Hill hiatus herniorrhaphy, especially during vagotomy, recommends it as the procedure of choice.[82, 86]

POSTVAGOTOMY GALLBLADDER DISEASE

There is some suggestion that the incidence of gallstones following vagotomy is significantly increased. This incidence may rise to 20 per cent or more of all patients having truncal vagotomies who are followed for five to 15 years. This may be related to gallbladder stasis induced by truncal vagotomy. Therefore one of the possible advantages of selective gastric vagotomy, which leaves the gallbladder vagal innervation intact, is that the incidence of gallstones may not be increased by that operation. However, there is currently a paucity of data on this long-term complication of vagotomy, so opinions regarding it should be reserved for the present.[87]

ACUTE PANCREATITIS FOLLOWING GASTRIC SURGERY

The incidence of acute pancreatitis occurring early postoperatively after gastric surgery is less than 1 to 2 per cent. This low incidence is fortunate, for the mortality of postoperative acute pancreatitis ranges from 30 to 50 per cent in various reports.[88, 89]

Acute pancreatitis after gastric surgery may be caused by several factors, such as direct trauma to the pancreas (usually from dissecting in the area of an ulcer penetrating into the pancreas with or without injury to pancreatic ducts), vascular impairment of the pancreas, or pancreatitis secondary to postoperative biliary tract disease, sepsis, or hyperparathyroidism.[57-59]

The diagnosis of acute postoperative pancreatitis is difficult in the first few postoperative days, because abdominal pain from surgery and narcotics may mask the usual signs and symptoms. Several other postoperative complications of gastric surgery, such as duodenal stump dehiscence, anastomotic leak, intestinal obstruction and infarction, or acute afferent loop syndrome, may mimic acute postoperative pancreatitis. Acute pancreatitis must be considered in any postgastric surgery patient who appears unusually ill postoperatively. At times, the only manifestations of acute postoperative pancreatitis are unexplained hypotension and tachycardia. Unfortunately, serum amylase levels are normal in about one-third of such patients, and other conditions such as duodenal stump dehiscences and anastomotic leaks may, on the other hand, cause elevated serum and urine amylase levels not associated with acute postoperative pancreatitis.[88, 89]

If the clinical condition of a patient with possible acute postoperative pancreatitis is deteriorating, i.e., if unexplained shock and/or sepsis develop postoperatively, the patient's abdomen should be re-explored at once. The chief purpose of re-exploration is not to treat pancreatitis, but to rule out with certainty other intra-abdominal catastrophes such as hemorrhage, anastomotic and duodenal stump leaks, common duct and pancreatic duct injuries, intestinal obstruction and infarction, acute afferent loop syndrome, and acute postoperative cholecystitis, which may exactly mimic acute postoperative pancreatitis and which must be treated surgically. Several recent reports state that judicious abdominal exploration does not increase mortality from acute pancreatitis and often leads to discovery of remedial surgical conditions resembling acute pancreatitis which would have caused death had they not been surgically corrected.[90, 91] If no serious intra-abdominal conditions other than acute pancreatitis are found on re-exploration, however, the pancreas is not disturbed, but Penrose and sump suction drains are placed into the lesser peritoneal sac about the pancreas. Whether or not a cholecystostomy should be done in such cases is debatable. From the technical standpoint, it may be readily done in most cases with no significant trauma to the patients. In those instances in which a "common channel" between the biliary and pancreatic ducts contributes to a "reflux" pancreatitis, or in which pancreatic edema obstructs the distal common bile duct, biliary decompression may be helpful. Since there is no way of being certain whether a common channel is present or not, we would usually advise cholecystostomy in these cases. After this, the patient is treated medically for acute pancreatitis by a continuation of nasogastric suction, intravenous fluids (perhaps central intravenous hyperalimentation to reduce pancreatic secretory activity), broad-spectrum antibiotics, anticholinergic agents, and other appropriate means. Parenthetically, it is not necessary to perform later cholecystectomy routinely when a cholecystostomy has been done for acute pancreatitis, unless gallbladder disease was present.

UNUSUAL OR RARE COMPLICATIONS OF GASTRIC SURGERY

A number of complications such as inadvertent gastroileostomy, infarction of the gastric remnant, infarction of the omentum, and unusual types of jaundice may occur rarely after gastric surgery.

Inadvertent gastroileostomy should be suspected if a patient develops diarrhea and malnutrition soon after gastric resection or gastroenterostomy. This can usually be confirmed by upper gastrointestinal X-ray contrast studies, but such studies may fail to establish the diagnosis in approximately 25 to 30 per cent of patients. The lesion may be detected by barium enema in 35 to 40 per cent of all patients. Recognition may be delayed because of the varied symptoms and findings associated with it and because of its rarity. Bachulis and Thomford recorded only 88 cases reported up to 1969. It should obviously be repaired as soon as it is detected.[92]

Infarctions of the gastric remnant and the greater omentum rarely occur after gastric surgery. They are caused by virtually total destruction of the gastric collateral blood supply, arising mainly from the inferior phrenic and short gastric arteries in cases of infarction of the gastric remnant and from the right and left gastroepiploic arteries in cases of greater omental infarction. The chief clinical findings in both instances are unexplained persistent postoperative fever and evidence of peritonitis. Gastric remnant infarction may also cause upper gastrointestinal bleeding resulting from necrosis of the gastric mucosa. The treatment is prompt total gastrectomy or total omentectomy. As mentioned earlier, lesser degrees of ischemia occur more frequently and may often be the cause of gastroenterostomy leaks, fistulas, and associated intra-abdominal abscesses.

The many causes of jaundice occurring after gastric surgery are too numerous to discuss fully in a brief review, but the reader is referred to a good summary article by Lester on causes of postoperative jaundice.[93] Other than jaundice caused by injury to the bile ducts, pancreas, or hepatic artery, none of the causes of jaundice after gastric surgery are peculiar to gastric surgery alone.[57-59]

It must be recalled that all or part of the arterial blood supply to the left hepatic lobe arises from the left gastric artery near the celiac axis in about 15 to 25 per cent of all individuals. In a similar percentage of patients, all or part of the arterial blood supply to the right hepatic lobe arises from the superior mesenteric artery. Because of these arterial anomalies, the left gastric artery should not be ligated proximally near its origin during gastrectomy; its branches should be ligated instead where they enter the lesser gastric curvature. Similar care should be taken to avoid injuring an anomalous right hepatic artery while dissecting the duodenum during gastric resection. This artery may pass immediately posterior to the duodenum and be mistaken for the right gastric or gastroduodenal artery. Inadvertent ligation of these anomalous hepatic arteries does not usually cause fatal hepatic necrosis, but may cause temporary jaundice and fever postoperatively. Undoubtedly, because of the rich collateral arterial blood supply to the liver, in more instances than one would think likely, these anomalous hepatic arteries are accidentally ligated during gastric surgery with no untoward sequelae.[67, 68]

REFERENCES

1. Hughes, R. K., and Wootton, D. G. Gastric sump drainage with a water seal monitor. Surgery 61:192, 1967.
2. Kraft, R. O., Fry, W. J., and DeWeese, M. S. Postvagotomy gastric atony. Arch. Surg. 88:865, 1964.
3. Herrington, J. L., Jr., Edwards, W. H., and Sawyers, J. L. Elimination of routine use of gastric decompression following operation for gastroduodenal ulcer. Ann. Surg. 159:807, 1964.
4. Argyropoulos, G. D., and White, M. E. E. Gastrointestinal function following vagotomy and pyloroplasty. Arch. Surg. 93:578, 1966.
5. Collins, C. D., Difford, F., Homer, C. B., and Duthie, H. L. Indications for gastrostomy after vagotomy. Arch. Surg. 93:451, 1966.
6. Herrington, J. L., Jr. Methods of postoperative gastric decompression, including an experience with the omission of its routine use. Amer. J. Surg. 110:424, 1965.
7. MacDonald, R. F., and Byrd, C. W. Early postoperative oral feeding. Surg. Gynec. Obstet. 110:510, 1960.
8. Rachlin, L. A rationale for postgastric surgery care. Amer. J. Surg. 111:496, 1966.
9. Menguy, R. Stomach. In Principles of Surgery, S. I. Schwartz (ed.). New York, McGraw-Hill Book Co., 1969.
10. Shires, G. T., and Canizaro, P. Fluid and electrolyte therapy. In Surgery Annual 1971, P. Cooper and L. M. Nyhus (eds.). New York, Appleton-Century-Crofts, 1971.
11. Whitten, T. A., and Bickel, J. G. Potassium in gastric juice. Gastroenterology 59:330, 1970.
12. Black, D. A. K., and Jepson, R. P. Electrolyte depletion in pyloric stenosis. Quart. J. Med. 23:367, 1954.
13. Dunphy, J. E. Discussion in Harrower, H. W.: Postoperative ileus. Amer. J. Surg. 116:369, 1968.
14. Bergin, W. F., and Jordan, P. H., Jr. Gastric atonia and delayed gastric emptying after vagotomy for obstructing ulcer. Amer. J. Surg. 98:612, 1959.
15. Gardner, B., Butler, E. D., and Goldman, L. Early complications of gastrectomy. Arch. Surg. 89:475, 1964.
16. Harper, F. B. Gastric dysfunction after vagectomy. Amer. J. Surg. 112:94, 1966.
17. Latchis, K. Delayed gastric emptying in the immediate postoperative period. Rev. Surg. 26:217, 1969.
18. Roth, J. L. A., Vilardell, F., and Affolter, H. Postvagotomy gastric stasis. Ann. N. Y. Acad. Sci. 99:203, 1962.
19. Pierandozzi, J. S., and Ritter, J. H. Transient achalasia, a complication of vagotomy. Amer. J. Surg. 111:356, 1966.
20. Schlang, H. A., and McHenry, L. E. Obstruction of the small bowel by orange in the postgastrectomy patient. Ann. Surg. 159:611, 1964.
21. Seifert, E. Über Krautileus. Deutsche Zeitschr. Chir. 222:96, 1930.
22. Fisher, R. D., Ebert, P. A., and Zuidema, G. D. Obstructing peptic ulcers. Arch. Surg. 94:724, 1967.
23. Hermann, G., and Johnson, V. Management of prolonged gastric retention after vagotomy and drainage. Surg. Gynec. Obstet. 130:1044, 1970.
24. Dudrick, S. J., Wilmore, D. W., Vars, H. M., and Rhoads, J. E. Can intravenous feeding as the sole means of nutrition support growth in the child and restore weight loss in an adult? Ann. Surg. 169:974, 1969.
25. Bachrach, W. H., and Tecimer, L. B. Use of a feeding tube in the management of gastric retention following gastro-enteric anastomosis. Amer. Surgeon 30:476, 1964.
26. Vasconez, L. O., Adams, J. T., and Woodward, E. R. Treatment of reluctant postvagotomy stoma with bethanechol. Arch. Surg. 100:693, 1970.
27. Rogers, J. C. T. Jejunostomy in the high risk gastrectomy patient. Surg. Gynec. Obstet. 125:333, 1967.
28. Madding, G. F. Malignant stomal obstruction following subtotal gastric resection. Amer. J. Surg. 97:326, 1959.
29. Sebesta, D. G., and Robson, M. C. Petersen's retroanastomotic hernia. Amer. J. Surg. 116:450, 1968.
30. Petersen, W. Concerning twisting of the intestines following a gastroenterostomy. Arch. Klin. Chir. 62:94, 1900.
31. Markowitz, A. M. Internal hernia after gastrojejunostomy. Surg. 49:185, 1961.
32. Sisler, G. E., Haims, B. W., and Spencer, F. C. Postgastrectomy afferent loop volvulus and gangrene; a late complication simulating pancreatitis. Amer. J. Surg. 114:932, 1967.
33. Hardy, J. D. Problems associated with gastric surgery: A review of 604 consecutive patients with annotation. Amer. J. Surg. 108:699, 1964.

34. Herrington, J. L., Jr. Delayed gastric outlet obstruction occurring after pyloroplasty or gastroduodenostomy: A simple surgical maneuver for its prevention. Surgery 56:1035, 1964.

35. Buckberg, G. D. Acute obstruction of the afferent loop after gastrectomy. Amer. J. Surg. 113:682, 1967.

36. Herrington, J. L., Jr. The afferent loop syndrome: Additional experience with its surgical management. Amer. Surgeon 34:321, 1968.

37. Mitty, W. F., Jr., Grossi, G., and Nealon, T. F., Jr. Chronic afferent loop syndrome. Ann. Surg. 172:996, 1970.

38. Caudell, W. S., and Lee, M. L., Jr. Acute and chronic jejunogastric intussusception. New Eng. J. Med. 253:635, 1955.

39. Devor, D., and Passaro, E., Jr. Jejunogastric intussusception: Review of 4 cases, diagnosis and management. Ann. Surg. 163:93, 1966.

40. Dolan, K. D., and Hockman, R. E. Jejunogastric intussusception ten years after gastric surgery. J.A.M.A. 205:128, 1968.

41. Reyelt, W. P., Jr., and Anderson, A. A. Retrograde jejunogastric intussusception. Surg. Gynec. Obstet. 119:1305, 1964.

42. Schackman, R. Jejunogastric intussusception. Brit. J. Surg. 27:475, 1940.

43. Tuschka, O. Jejunogastric intussusception. J.A.M.A. 186:126, 1963.

44. Moseley, R. V. Pyloric obstruction by a phytobezoar following pyloroplasty and vagotomy. Arch. Surg. 94:290, 1967.

45. Harvey, H. D. Complications in hospital following partial gastrectomy for peptic ulcer, 1936 to 1959. Surg. Gynec. Obstet. 117:211, 1963.

46. Palmer, E. D. The vigorous diagnostic approach to upper gastrointestinal tract hemorrhage. J.A.M.A. 207:1477, 1969.

47. Way, L., Goldman, L., and Dunphy, J. E. Zollinger-Ellison syndrome; an analysis of twenty-five cases. Amer. J. Surg. 116:293, 1968.

48. Snyder, E. N., Jr., and Stellar, C. A. Results from emergency surgery for massively bleeding duodenal ulcer. Amer. J. Surg. 116:170, 1968.

49. Jones, R. C., McClelland, R. N., Zedlitz, W. H., and Shires, G. T. Difficult closures of the duodenal stump. Arch. Surg. 94:696, 1967.

50. Edmunds, L. H., Jr., Williams, G. M., and Welch, C. E. External fistulas arising from the gastro-intestinal tract. Ann. Surg. 152:445, 1960.

51. Harrower, H. W. Closure of the duodenal stump after gastrectomy for posterior ulcer. Amer. J. Surg. 111:488, 1966.

52. Rodkey, G. V., and Welch, C. E. Duodenal decompression in gastrectomy; further experience with duodenostomy. New Eng. J. Med. 262:498, 1960.

53. Austen, W. G., and Baue, A. E. Catheter duodenostomy for the difficult duodenum. Ann. Surg. 160:781, 1964.

54. Lahey, F. H. The use of an identifying "T" tube in the common bile duct in gastric resection for duodenal ulcer adherent to the bile ducts. Surg. Gynec. Obstet. 80:197, 1945.

55. Nissen, R. Duodenal and Jejunal Peptic Ulcer. Technique of Resection. New York, Grune & Stratton, Inc., 1945.

56. Friedemann, M. Über Hilfen und Sicherungen bei gefahrvollen und technisch schwierigen Magenoperationen. Beitr. Klin. Chir. 163:293, 1936.

57. Carpenter, J. C., and Crandell, W. B. Common bile duct and major pancreatic duct injuries during operations on the stomach: A report of three cases. Ann. Surg. 148:66, 1958.

58. Ehrlich, E. W., and Howard, J. M. Ampullary disconnection during gastrectomy. Ann. Surg. 170:961, 1969.

59. Roe, C. F., Gazzangia, A., McNamara, J., and Moore, F. D. Aberrant intrapancreatic ducts leading to fatality after gastrectomy. Amer. J. Surg. 105:685, 1963.

60. White, T. T., Sanderson, E. R., and Morgan, A. Injury to the sphincter of Oddi in the course of gastric and duodenal surgery. Amer. J. Surg. 114:247, 1967.

61. Carter, B. N. II, and Bruck, W. E. The repair of leaks in the line of anastomosis after the Billroth I gastric resection. Ann. Surg. 146:816, 1957.

62. Dudrick, S. J., Wilmore, D. W., Steiger, E., Mackie, J. A., and Fitts, W. T., Jr. Spontaneous closure of traumatic pancreatoduodenal fistulas with total intravenous nutrition. J. Trauma 10:542, 1970.

63. Pettersson, S., and Wallensten, S.: Leakage at suture lines after partial gastrectomy for peptic ulcer. Acta Chir. Scand. 135:229, 1969.

64. Hamilton, R. F., Davis, W. C., Stephenson, D. V., and Magee, D. F. Effects of parenteral hyperalimentation on upper gastrointestinal tract secretions. Arch. Surg. 102:348, 1971.

65. Wilmore, D. W., Daly, J. M., Dudrick, S. J., and Vars, H. M. Gastric secretion after parenteral fluid administration. Arch. Surg. 102:509, 1971.

66. Graves, H. A., Jr., Nelson, A., and Byrd, B. F., Jr. Gastrocutaneous fistula as a postoperative complication. Ann. Surg. 171:656, 1970.

67. Rodgers, J. B. Infarction of the gastric remnant following subtotal gastrectomy. Arch. Surg. 92:917, 1966.

68. Thompson, N. W. Ischemic necrosis of proximal gastric remnant following subtotal gastrectomy. Surgery 54:434, 1963.

69. Bryk, D., and Petigrow, N. Postsplenectomy gastric perforation. Surgery 61:239, 1967.

70. Glotzer, D. J., Goodman, W. S., and Geronimus, L. H. Topical antibiotic prophylaxis in contaminated wounds. Arch. Surg. 100:589, 1970.

71. Sherman, N. J., Davis, J. R., and Jesseph, J. E. Subphrenic abscess. Amer. J. Surg. 117:117, 1969.

72. Ariel, I. M., and Kazarian, K. K. Classification, diagnosis and treatment of subphrenic abscesses. Rev. Surg. 28:1, 1971.

73. Crook, J. N., Cotlar, A. M., Bornside, G. H., and Cohn, I., Jr. Intraperitoneal cephalothin in the treatment of experimental appendiceal peritonitis. Amer. Surgeon 34:736, 1968.

74. DiVincenti, F. C., and Cohn, I., Jr. Intraperitoneal kanamycin in advanced peritonitis: A

preliminary report. Amer. J. Surg. *111*:147, 1966.

75. McKenna, J. P., Currie, D. J., MacDonald, J. A., Mahoney, L. J., Finlayson, D. C., and Lanskail, J. C. The use of continuous postoperative peritoneal lavage in the management of diffuse peritonitis. Surg. Gynec. Obstet. *130*:354, 1970.

76. Craft, I. L., and Venables, C. W. Antiperistaltic segment of jejunum for persistent diarrhea following vagotomy. Ann. Surg. *167*:282, 1968.

77. Sawyers, J. L., and Herrington, J. L., Jr. Antiperistaltic jejunal segments for control of the dumping syndrome and postvagotomy diarrhea. Surgery *69*:263, 1971.

78. Simmons, R. L., Back, V. R., Harvey, H. D., and Herter, F. P. Technical complications of transabdominal vagotomy. Arch. Surg. *92*:922, 1966.

79. Wangensteen, S. L., and Kelly, J. M. Gastric mobilization prior to vagotomy to lessen splenic trauma. Surg. Gynec. Obstet. *127*:603, 1968.

80. Hauser, J. B., and Lucas, R. J. Esophageal perforation during vagotomy. Arch. Surg. *101*:466, 1970.

81. McBurney, R. P. Perforation of the esophagus: A complication of vagotomy or hiatal hernia repair. Ann. Surg. *169*:851, 1969.

82. Postlethwait, R. W., Kim, W. K., and Dillon, M. L. Esophageal complications of vagotomy. Surg. Gynec. Obstet. *128*:481, 1969.

83. Marty, A. T., and Watson, C. G. Hemopneumothorax following transabdominal vagotomy. Amer. Surgeon *36*:674, 1970.

84. Guillory, J. R., Jr., and Clagett, O. T. Post-vagotomy dysphagia. Surg. Clin. N. Amer. *47*:833, 1967.

85. Harris, J., and Miller, C. M. Cardiospasm following vagotomy. Surgery *47*:568, 1960.

86. Tolstedt, G. E., and Bell, J. W. Hiatus hernia; an unusual complication of transabdominal vagotomy. Amer. J. Surg. *107*:895, 1964.

87. Clave, R. A., and Gaspar, M. R. Incidence of gallbladder disease after vagotomy. Amer. J. Surg. *118*:169, 1969.

88. Saidi, F., and Donaldson, G. A. Acute pancreatitis following distal gastrectomy for benign ulcer. Amer. J. Surg. *105*:87, 1963.

89. White, T. T., Morgan, A., and Hopton, D. Postoperative pancreatitis: A study of seventy cases. Amer. J. Surg. *120*:132, 1970.

90. Diaco, J. F., Miller, L. D., and Copeland, E. M. The role of early diagnostic laparotomy in acute pancreatitis. Surg. Gynec. Obstet. *129*:263, 1969.

91. Trapnell, J. E., and Anderson, M. C. Role of early laparotomy in acute pancreatitis. Ann. Surg. *165*:49, 1967.

92. Bachulis, B. L., and Thomford, N. R. Gastroileostomy. Arch. Surg. *98*:786, 1969.

93. Lester, R. Causes of postoperative jaundice. Amer. J. Surg. *116*:342, 1968.

Chapter 62

Late and Persistent Postgastrectomy Problems

Frederic W. Smith, Graham H. Jeffries

Afferent loop obstruction, gastroileostomy, gastric outlet and intestinal obstruction, and postvagotomy complications are discussed in detail on pages 791 to 819. Recurrent ulcer is described on pages 829 to 837, and bilious vomiting on pages 800 to 802. This chapter is concerned with systemic infections, gastric carcinoma, the dumping syndrome, and diarrhea and malabsorption after gastric surgery.

INFECTION AFTER GASTRIC RESECTION

There is an increased frequency of active pulmonary tuberculosis in patients who have had subtotal gastrectomy. This is probably related to postgastrectomy malnutrition with activation of pre-existing disease, in addition to the higher frequency of both tuberculosis and ulcer disease in the chronic alcoholic patient.[1] When gastric surgery is necessary in patients with pulmonary tuberculosis, a conservative procedure less likely to be complicated by postoperative weight loss is indicated. Prophylactic isoniazid, 300 mg. daily, has been recommended for the postgastrectomy patient with a positive, intermediate strength tuberculin test.[2] Salmonella enteritis has been described with increased frequency in patients with subtotal gastric resections. This increased susceptibility may be due to loss of the protective effect of gastric acidity.[3]

GASTRIC CARCINOMA

Gastric carcinoma may develop as a late complication of gastric surgery for benign disease.[4, 5] In one series of patients carcinoma was observed with a frequency that was six times greater than in the control population. The location of lesions adjacent to the anastomosis in patients who had surgery 25 or more years previously suggests a relationship of the neoplasm to atrophic gastritis.

THE DUMPING SYNDROME

The clinical manifestations of the dumping syndrome result from the rapid introduction of hyperosmolar solutions into the proximal jejunum. Although dumping is more frequent and of greater severity after Billroth II type procedures with a high gastric resection and gastrojejunostomy, it complicates all surgical procedures for duodenal ulcer, including vagotomy and pyloroplasty. As many as 20 to 40 per cent of patients suffer from dumping symptoms immediately after operation, but symptoms usually decrease with time; 5 to 10 per cent of patients may suffer persisting disability because of dumping. Occasionally symptoms of dumping will appear for the first time after a period of months or years after surgery.

The dumping syndrome may be separated into early and late phases. The onset of the early phase is typically during or shortly after a meal and appears to be related to jejunal distention and the release of vasoactive hormones into the circulation. Gastrointestinal symptoms include nausea, eructation, a sensation of epigastric fullness or distention, abdominal cramping, and occasionally vomiting and diarrhea. The "small stomach syndrome" relates specifically to symptoms of fullness, bloating, or distention caused by rapid jejunal filling. Vasomotor symptoms include palpitations, weakness or fainting, a feeling of cold or warmth, drowsiness, dyspnea, and sweating. During this early symptomatic phase, lasting 30 to 60 minutes, there is an elevation of blood glucose, an increase in the peripheral hematocrit, a decrease in circulating blood volume, and a decrease in serum potassium and phosphorus levels.

Jejunal distention results from both rapid passage of food through the anastomosis and the secretion of water and electrolytes into the proximal jejunum as the hyperosmolar content is diluted. Symptoms of nausea and fullness can be duplicated by balloon distention of the jejunum, and X-ray studies of patients with the dumping syndrome, using a hypertonic solution of sucrose with barium sulfate, have demonstrated small bowel hypersecretion associated with fluid levels and flocculation of the barium. Although a decreased blood volume is a characteristic finding during the early phase of the dumping syndrome, vasomotor symptoms do not depend on changes in plasma volume; vasomotor symptoms may be experienced during dumping when the blood volume is maintained at a normal level by infusion.

The current view is that vasomotor symptoms are related to the release of one or more vasoactive substances into the circulation; both serotonin and bradykinin have been suggested as such agents.[6] In both experimental animals and patients with the dumping syndrome, significant elevations of both serotonin and bradykinin have been measured in the peripheral blood. Bradykinin may cause flushing, sweating, peripheral vasodilatation, tachycardia, and postural hypotension, whereas serotonin may be responsible in part for the diarrhea.

Symptoms associated with bradykinin are early and transient, and are related to a brief increase in cardiac output. Bradykinin is rapidly hydrolyzed by serum carboxypeptidase. Serotonin, which has a later appearance than bradykinin, is associated with peripheral vasoconstriction and a decrease in cardiac output. The mechanism for the release of serotonin and bradykinin is not well defined. Argentaffin cells in the jejunal mucosa are rich in serotonin and other vasoactive amines; experimentally, hypertonic glucose has been shown to release secretory granules and to increase blood serotonin levels.[7]

The late phase of dumping is associated with symptoms of hypoglycemia. Early hyperglycemia together with the release of intestinal hormones leads to excessive insulin secretion with reactive hypoglycemia which reaches a peak about two hours after carbohydrate ingestion. Faintness, sweating, palpitations, tiredness, and headache are common symptoms; hypoglycemic coma is a rare complication.[8]

Medical management of patients with the dumping syndrome is usually effective. This consists of a high protein, low carbohydrate diet given in multiple small feedings (Table 62-1). Fluids are restricted at mealtimes and are provided between meals. Some patients benefit from anticholinergic drugs. Other agents, including serotonin antagonists, glucagon, insulin, and oral hypoglycemic agents, have been used without convincing evidence of efficacy.[9] Symptomatic patients may gain relief by lying flat for a short period after meals.

When patients remain disabled in spite of medical therapy, a variety of surgical procedures may be considered.[10-12] These include conversion of the gastrojejunal anastomosis to a gastroduodenal anastomosis, the creation of a jejunal pouch to increase reservoir capacity, a reduction in the size of the gastric outlet, the interposition of an isoperistaltic loop of jejunum, or the interposition of a reversed jejunal segment between stomach and duodenum or jejunum. Between 50 and 70 per cent of satisfactory results have been reported after interposition of a reversed segment.[12]

POSTGASTRECTOMY DIARRHEA

Although not always disabling, diarrhea is a common problem after gastric surgery, particularly with vagotomy. Several causes for diarrhea must be considered in the individual patient with a significant problem.

Diarrhea is one component of the dumping syndrome; increased secretion by the small bowel and increased peristaltic activity may result in several liquid stools shortly after meals. Treatment with an antidumping diet may be of benefit. After vagotomy many patients experience diarrhea which is not particularly related to meals, may be explosive in onset, and may awaken the patient at night. The precise mechanism for postvagotomy diarrhea has not been defined. Diarrhea after gastric surgery usually decreases over a period of months; intractable diarrhea may require therapy with antidiarrheal agents, and in some instances has been treated surgically with a reversed jejunal segment.[13]

Lactase deficiency should be considered as a diagnostic possibility in patients with postgastrectomy diarrhea. Patients who were previously able to tolerate an ulcer diet containing milk may observe a relationship between diarrhea and milk ingestion after operation. Lactase deficiency has been documented by enzyme assay in mucosal biopsies from symptomatic patients.[14, 15] Surgery may precipitate symptoms by causing more rapid gastric emptying, thus exposing the lactase-deficient mucosa to a higher concentration of lactose. Patients with documented lactase deficiency should be treated by dietary restriction of milk and milk products; these patients should be given adequate calcium supplements as prophylaxis against the development of bone disease.

TABLE 62–1. ANTIDUMPING DIET

GENERAL RULES	DAILY MEAL PLAN	
1. No fluids of any kind during meals.	*Breakfast:*	
	Fruit	1/2 cup
2. Avoid concentrated sweets such as sugar, jelly, cake, pie, puddings, candy, and sugar-sweetened fruit.	Cereal	1/2 cup
	Eggs	2
	Bacon	2–4 strips
	Bread	1 slice
3. The use of sugar substitutes is permissible.	Butter or margarine	2 teaspoons
	Midmorning:	
4. The diet may require modification in individual cases.	Milk	1 cup
	Skim milk powder	2 tablespoons
	Dinner:	
5. The meals should be eaten slowly.	Meat, fish or fowl	2–4 ounces
	Vegetable	1 serving
6. Plan six feedings a day, varying amounts as tolerated, and including amounts listed in daily meal plan.	Salad	1 serving
	Bread	1 slice
	Butter or margarine	2 teaspoons
	Fruit	1/2 cup
	Midafternoon:	
	Milk	1 cup
	Skim milk powder	2 tablespoons
	Supper:	
	Meat, fish, or fowl	2–4 ounces
	Vegetables	1 serving
	Bread	1 slice
	Butter or margarine	2 teaspoons
	Gelatin dessert	1/2 cup
	Bedtime feedings:	
	Milk	1 cup
	Skim milk powder	2 tablespoons
	Cheese	2 ounces

Table 62–1 *continued on opposite page.*

TABLE 62–1. ANTIDUMPING DIET (*Continued*)

FOODS ALLOWED	FOODS OMITTED
Beverages: All meals—One hour before or after. Coffee, tea, decaffeinated coffee, fruit juice sweetened with sugar substitute, milk if tolerated.	*Beverages:* All not listed under foods allowed.
Cereal, bread and crackers: All prepared without sugar.	*Cereal, bread and crackers:* All prepared with sugar.
Cheese: All, may be used in unlimited amounts.	*Dessert:* All prepared desserts except those listed under Foods allowed.
Desserts: Part of milk, egg, and fruit allowance may be used in preparing desserts; rennet, custard, or gelatin desserts sweetened with sugar substitute.	*Fruit:* All sugar-sweetened fruits, banana, fresh figs, or dried fruit.
Egg: Use three or more daily.	*Meat, fish, fowl:* All prepared with cream sauce or gravy.
Fat: All in unlimited amounts; butter, margarine, vegetable oils and fats, salad dressings, lard.	*Potato or substitute:* Sweet potato, hominy.
Fruit: Unsweetened fruit except banana, fresh figs, or dried fruit.	*Soups and sauces:* Cream sauces, gravy, or soups with meals.
Meat, fish, fowl: All except creamed.	*Sweets:* All sweets, including sugar, candy, jam, jelly, marmalade, preserves, molasses, honey, syrups.
Potato or substitute: White potato, rice, macaroni, spaghetti, noodles; one half cup may be substituted for one slice bread.	*Vegetables:* All not listed under Foods Allowed.
Soups: Broth, bouillon, consommé and soup made with allowance of milk and vegetables. Use only one hour before or after meals.	*Miscellaneous:* Sweet pickles, relishes, popcorn, meat sauces.
Sweets: See Foods omitted.	

Vegetables:

Asparagus	Kale
Broccoli	Mustard
Brussels sprouts	Spinach
Cabbage	Turnip greens
Cauliflower	Lettuce
Celery	Mushrooms
Chicory	Okra
Cucumber	Parsley
Dill pickle	Pepper, green
Endive	Radish
Escarole	Sauerkraut
Eggplant	String beans, young
Greens	Summer squash
Beet greens	Tomatoes
Chard	Tomato juice
Collard	Watercress
Dandelion	

POSTGASTRECTOMY MALABSORPTION

Mild steatorrhea is to be expected after gastric resection with gastrojejunal anastomosis.[16] This can be attributed in large part to delayed stimulation of pancreatic secretion and gallbladder emptying, and incomplete, late mixing of the food bolus with digestive secretions.[17] In this respect a gastroduodenal anastomosis is more physiological, as it permits more optimal secretion of pancreatic juice which is coordinated with gastric emptying. True pancreatic insufficiency may be a rare consequence of postoperative pancreatitis or may be the result of atrophy secondary to prolonged periods of inadequate hormonal stimulation. In patients with marked steatorrhea, bacterial overgrowth in association with afferent loop stasis or a jejunocolic fistula must be considered (see p. 927). Gastric surgery may precipitate malabsorption in patients with previously latent adult celiac disease (gluten enteropathy). These patients exhibit typical atrophy of the proximal jejunal mucosa; prior to operation normal absorption may have been maintained by more normal distal small bowel[18] (see pp. 864 to 884).

Weight loss and malnutrition after gastric surgery are usually related to a decrease in food intake; this problem is most common after extensive gastric resection with gastrojejunostomy complicated by dumping.[19-23] Malabsorption contributes to this problem. Maldigestion of dietary protein and bacterial degradation of essential amino acids may lead to a negative nitrogen balance with relative protein malnutrition and hypoproteinemia. The latter may be accentuated by an increase in the enteric loss of plasma protein.

Bone disease after partial gastric resection is associated with defects in the absorption of both calcium and vitamin D.[24, 25] Fat-soluble vitamin D is normally absorbed after solubilization in bile acid micelles; when disturbances in the metabolism or distribution of bile salts lead to steatorrhea, vitamin D malabsorption usually follows. Clinical and/or laboratory evidence of metabolic bone disease has been documented in 30 per cent or more of patients after gastric resection. Osteomalacia is the most common bone lesion, and is usually associated with an increase in the level of serum alkaline phosphatase. An elevation of the serum alkaline phosphatase, however, may also be due to liver disease or Paget's disease. Osteoporosis is encountered less frequently than osteomalacia. Treatment with vitamin D supplements and calcium may control bone pain, but will not restore deformities caused by pathological fractures and vertebral collapse.

Anemia is a common finding in the postgastrectomy patient;[26] in one series 53 per cent of 292 patients were found to be anemic.[27] Iron deficiency is the most common mechanism for anemia. Although a decrease in dietary iron intake, together with increased gastrointestinal blood loss from marginal ulceration and/or gastritis, may contribute to iron deficiency, the major defect may be the malabsorption of dietary organic iron. A reduction in gastric acidity, loss of iron binding substances from the gastric juice, bypass of the duodenum, and incomplete digestion of organic iron may each reduce iron absorption. Patients with iron deficiency alone usually respond to therapy with oral preparations of inorganic iron. In view of the high frequency of iron deficiency anemia after partial gastrectomy, there is a rational place for prevention of anemia with prophylactic ferrous sulfate.

A significant number of patients develop megaloblastic anemia caused by folic acid and/or vitamin B_{12} deficiency. Folic acid deficiency may be due in part to decreased intake, and in part to reduced absorption. Vitamin B_{12} deficiency is usually secondary to malabsorption caused by deficient secretion of intrinsic factor. Progressive atrophy of the gastric remnant may be a consequence of bile reflux, coupled with the removal of the trophic effect of vagal innervation and gastrin stimulation; this appears to be most common after surgery for gastric ulcer disease, but has also been documented after surgery for duodenal ulcer. In addition to a decrease in the secretion of intrinsic factor, overgrowth of bacteria in the proximal intestine may compete for available vitamin B_{12}. The presence of folic acid and/or vitamin B_{12} deficiency should be assessed by examination of bone marrow aspirates and by measurement of the serum levels of these vitamins. Appropriate replacement therapy should be given together with iron if the vitamin deficiency is associated with iron deficiency.

AN OVERVIEW

Although 90 per cent of patients are said to be satisfied with their gastric surgery, the frequency and the nature of postgastrectomy problems, particularly with advancing years, indicate that gastric resection should not be undertaken lightly. The surgical procedure of choice in the management of ulcer disease is the one that will cause the least disturbance of gastrointestinal function while controlling gastric acid secretion. At present, vagotomy with drainage (either pyloroplasty or gastroenterostomy) provides the closest approach to this goal.

Patients with persisting and severe postgastrectomy complaints may represent major problems in management. Several studies have attempted to correlate the frequency of complaints or disability with the presence of psychiatric disorders preor postoperatively.[28, 29] It will be found, however, that the majority of patients with postgastrectomy symptoms will have significant organic disease; endoscopic examination of the gastric remnant, stoma, and afferent loop will reveal many abnormalities that are not detected by other means. The treatment of postgastrectomy problems is facilitated by an understanding of the pathophysiology of these disorders.

REFERENCES

1. Hanngren, A., and Reizenstein, P. Studies in dumping syndrome. V. Tuberculosis in gastrectomized patients. Amer. J. Dig. Dis. 14:700, 1969.
2. Brummer, D. L. Prophylaxis of tuberculosis after gastrectomy. Amer. J. Dig. Dis. 14:753, 1969.
3. Waddell, W. R., and Kunz, L. J. Association of salmonella enteritis with operations on the stomach. New Eng. J. Med. 255:555, 1956.
4. Stalsberg, H., and Sigbjörn, T. Stomach cancer following gastric surgery for benign conditions. Lancet 2:1175, 1971.
5. Kobayashi, S., Prolla, J. C., and Kirsner, J. B. Late gastric carcinoma developing after surgery for benign conditions. Amer. J. Dig. Dis. 15:905, 1970.
6. Macdonald, J. M. Serotonin and bradykinin in the dumping syndrome. Amer. J. Surg. 117:204, 1969.
7. Tobe, T., Kimura, C., and Fujiwara, M. Role of 5-hydroxytryptamine in the dumping syndrome after gastrectomy: Histochemical study. Ann. Surg. 165:382, 1967.
8. Bacon, P. A., and Myles, A. B. Hypoglycaemic coma after partial gastrectomy. Postgrad. Med. J. 47:134, 1971.
9. Sullivan, M. B., Jr., and Patton, T. B. Insulin, tolbutamide, serotonin and the dumping reaction. Ann. Surg. 159:742, 1964.
10. Herrington, J. L. Remedial operations for severe postgastrectomy symptoms (dumping): Emphasis on an antiperistaltic (reverse) jejunal segment interpolated between gastric remnant and duodenum and role of vagotomy. Ann. Surg. 162:789, 1965.
11. Jordan G. L., Jr. Surgical management of postgastrectomy problems. Arch. Surg. 102:251, 1971.
12. Sawyer, J. L., and Herrington J. L., Jr. Antiperistaltic jejunal segments for control of the dumping syndrome and postvagotomy diarrhea. Surgery 69:263, 1971.
13. Herrington, J. L., Jr., Edwards, W. H., Carter, J. H., and Sawyers, J. L. Treatment of severe postvagotomy diarrhea by reversed jejunal segment. Ann. Surg. 168:522, 1968.
14. Gryboski, J. D., Thayer, W. R., Jr., Gryboski, W. A., Gabrielson, I. W., and Spiro, H. M. A defect in disaccharide metabolism after gastrojejunostomy. New Eng. J. Med. 268:78, 1963.
15. Welsh, J. D., Shaw, P. W., and Walker, A. Isolated lactase deficiency producing postgastrectomy milk intolerance. Ann. Intern. Med. 64:1252, 1966.
16. Lawrence, W., Jr., Vanamee, P., Peterson, A. S., McNeer, G., Levin, S., and Randall, H. T. Alterations in fat and nitrogen metabolism after total and subtotal gastrectomy. Surg. Gynec. Obstet. 110:601, 1960.
17. Lundh, G. The mechanism of postgastrectomy malabsorption. Gastroenterology 42:637, 1962.
18. Hedberg, C. A., Melnyk, C. S., and Johnson, C. F. Gluten enteropathy appearing after gastric surgery. Gastroenterology 50:796, 1966.
19. Goldstein, F. Mechanisms of malabsorption and malnutrition in the blind loop syndrome. Gastroenterology 61:780, 1971.
20. Wall, A. J., Ungar, B., Baird, C. W., Langfold, I. M., and Mackay, I. R. Malnutrition after partial gastrectomy. Influence of site of ulcer and type of anastomosis and role of gastritis. Amer. J. Dig. Dis. 12:1077, 1967.
21. Pryor, J. P., O'Shea, M. J., Brooks, P. L., and Datar, K. M. The long-term metabolic consequences of partial gastrectomy. Amer. J. Med. 51:5, 1971.
22. Editorial. Postgastrectomy malnutrition. Brit. Med. J. 1:396, 1969.
23. Hillman, H. S. Postgastrectomy malnutrition. Gut. 9:576, 1968.
24. Eddy, R. L. Metabolic bone disease after gastrectomy. Amer. J. Med. 50:442, 1971.

25. Bordier, P., Matrajt, H., Hioco, D., Hepner, G. W., Thompson, G. R., and Booth, C. C. Subclinical vitamin D deficiency following gastric surgery. Histologic evidence in bone. Lancet 1:437, 1968.

26. Johnson, H. D., Kahn, T. H., Srivatsa, R., Doyle, F. A., and Welbourn, R. B. The late nutritional and haematological effects of vagal section. Brit. J. Surg. 56:4, 1969.

27. Hines, J. D., Hoffbrand, A. V., and Mollin, D. L. The hematologic complications follow-ing partial gastrectomy. A study of 292 patients. Amer. J. Med. 43:555, 1967.

28. Mason, M. C., and Clark, L. G. Psychiatric disorders after surgery for duodenal ulcer. Gut 11:258, 1970.

29. Johnstone, F. R. C., Holubitsky, I. B., and Debas, H. T. Postgastrectomy problems in patients with personality defects: The "albatross" syndrome. Canad. Med. Assn. J. 96:1559, 1967.

Chapter 63

Stomal and Recurrent Gastric Ulcer

Robert N. McClelland

RECURRENT PEPTIC ULCER

The classic causes of recurrent ulcer after gastric surgery are incomplete vagotomy, inadequate gastric resection, retained gastric antrum in the excluded duodenal stump, ulcerogenic tumor syndromes, and ulcerogenic drugs.[1-8] An excessively long afferent loop is also usually listed as a cause of ulcer recurrence, but this is probably unusual, especially if a vagotomy is performed.

Recurrent ulcer caused by inadequate vagotomy may decrease as technical improvements in performing this operation are developed.[9, 10] Selective gastric vagotomy may achieve more complete vagotomy than does truncal vagotomy. Incomplete vagotomy after truncal vagotomy (according to the Hollander test) approaches 25 to 30 per cent, but this has now been reduced to less than 5 to 6 per cent in some series after selective vagotomy.[11-13] It remains to be seen whether the incidence of more complete vagal nerve section achieved by selective vagotomy will significantly decrease duodenal ulcer recurrence. Some have recently questioned the accuracy of the Hollander test in determining the *clinical* significance of a vagotomy said to be "incomplete" by the Hollander test, and in predicting the incidence of re-

current ulcer caused by so-called "failed" vagotomy.[14, 15] Attempts have been made by Burge and associates to determine by electrical vagus nerve stimulation during surgery whether a complete vagotomy has been achieved. A recent report of their work with 600 vagotomized patients is very encouraging. The simple instrument they use is now available commercially; hopefully the method will soon be validated by other workers.[9]

Inadequate gastric resection is now less important as a cause of recurrent duodenal ulcer, because vagotomies and antrectomies are being performed more often than subtotal gastric resections without vagotomies. Obviously, in view of the low recurrence rates seen after vagotomy and antrectomy (less than 1 per cent), the importance of a high gastric resection is less than when subtotal gastric resection was the standard duodenal ulcer operation.

Retention of gastric antrum within the duodenal stump after Billroth II gastric resection has, in the past, been a significant cause of recurrent ulcer. If a small gastric antral fragment is left in the alkaline environment of the duodenal stump postoperatively, large amounts of gastrin are produced continuously by the excluded gastric antral mucosa, stimulating gastric acid secretion and predisposing to recurrent ulcer. Serum gastrin levels in patients with this condition have not been reported, but presumably would be elevated. In 1960, workers at the Lahey Clinic reported that 40 per cent of their recurrent ulcer patients with initial Billroth II gastric resections were found to have retained gastric antrum within the duodenal stump at reoperation.[3] The importance of removing all gastric antral tissue from the duodenum before closing the duodenal stump is now recognized, and ulcer recurrences caused by this have dropped precipitously. We have seen only one duodenal ulcer recurrence probably caused by retained gastric antrum within the duodenal stump within the last ten years. The decreased incidence of retained gastric antrum is attributed to obtaining a frozen section of the circumference of the duodenal stump during surgery for microscopic examination for gastric antral tissue before closing the duodenum. If retained gastric antrum is found on biopsy during surgery, a more distal duodenal resection is done and the resected tissue is examined microscopically until all gastric antral tissue is removed from the duodenal stump. It is impossible to determine by gross inspection, particularly of a scarred duodenum, whether all gastric antral tissue has been resected. Gastric antral tissue sometimes extends in small, irregular projections across the pylorus into the duodenum, and this is not detectable except by microscopic examination.

The fourth of the classic causes of recurrent duodenal ulcer is the Zollinger-Ellison syndrome. This unusual condition increases in incidence as means of diagnosing it improve. Currently, the Zollinger-Ellison syndrome is usually suspected by determination of preoperative basal and histamine- or Histalog-stimulated gastric acid secretory levels.[16] Also, routine serum gastrin assays must become even more vital as a part of the preoperative studies performed on peptic ulcer patients (see pp. 743 to 754 for a complete discussion of the Zollinger-Ellison syndrome).[17, 18] Several studies at different times may be needed if normal serum gastrin levels are found on an initial study in patients in whom the Zollinger-Ellison syndrome is strongly suspected, because serum gastrin levels may fluctuate in patients with ulcerogenic tumors. Careful preoperative work-up for ulcerogenic tumors of the pancreas will permit initial appropriate treatment by total gastrectomy and greatly reduce the morbidity and mortality of rapidly recurrent and virulent ulcers caused by gastrin-producing tumors.[19]

DIAGNOSIS OF RECURRENT DUODENAL ULCER

Recurrent duodenal ulcer symptoms may differ from preoperative ulcer symptoms. After a Billroth II gastric resection, the recurrent ulcer is in the left upper quadrant of the abdomen and the patient may have pain in that area and in the epigastrium if there is much inflammatory reaction about the ulcer. The pain may be quite variable in intensity, periodicity, and location, and at least 20 to 30 per cent of recurrent ulcer patients have little or no pain, presenting only with gastrointestinal bleeding.[4] In some cases, pain after peptic ulcer surgery may be due to alkaline reflux gastritis[20] or gastritis caused by various gastric irritants such as alcohol, coffee, tea, cola beverages, aspirin, phenylbutazone, indomethacin, or reserpine. Of course, these ulcerogenic agents may actually induce recurrent ulcer as well as gastritis.

At least 50 to 60 per cent of recurrent ulcer patients have overt hematemesis or melena. Melena is more likely to occur than hematemesis. Occult gastrointestinal bleeding can be detected intermittently in nearly all recurrent ulcer patients. There is a greater bleeding tendency for recurrent ulcers than for the previously unoperated duodenal ulcers. This is probably because virulent duodenal ulcers are more likely to bleed, to require surgery, and to recur than less virulent ulcers. Patients who have initial duodenal ulcer surgery for bleeding are about three times more likely to rebleed later and require reoperation for bleeding than is the patient originally operated for indications other than hemorrhage. Certainly not all patients who have gastrointestinal bleeding after duodenal ulcer surgery are bleeding from a recurrent ulcer. The rebleeding is probably due to gastritis or other causes in about half the cases, especially if the bleeding is of minor to moderate degree and requires no transfusions.[4]

Determination of basal and histamine-stimulated gastric acid secretory levels may provide suggestive information regarding the likelihood of recurrent ulceration. Unfortunately, the accuracy of postoperative gastric acid determinations may be seriously impaired by reflux of alkaline gastrointestinal secretions into the gastric pouch during postoperative gastric acid determinations. Such alkaline reflux may partially or completely neutralize any gastric acid present, giving a falsely low level of gastric acid secretion. This should not imply that postoperative gastric acid secretory studies are not valuable, for they may be very helpful in suggesting (but not confirming) the presence of a recurrent ulcer if high levels of gastric acid secretion are demonstrated. Indeed, if postoperative basal gastric acid secretion is greater than 5 mEq per hour, the Zollinger-Ellison syndrome should be strongly suspected and may be confirmed now by simultaneous determination of serum gastrin levels.[16-18] In any patient suspected of recurrent ulcer, serum gastrin levels should be obtained routinely, if possible, even though high gastric acid levels are not found. Even the high levels of gastric acid secretion occurring in the Zollinger-Ellison syndrome may be almost completely neutralized by reflux of alkaline gastrointestinal secretions into the stomach during postoperative gastric acid secretory studies; in such instances serum gastrin determinations are critical in diagnosing and treating properly, by total gastrectomy, recurrent ulcers caused by the Zollinger-Ellison syndrome.

An increasing number of patients developing recurrent duodenal ulcer have had a vagotomy during their initial ulcer surgery; thus it is desirable to determine whether the recurrent ulcer is due to a failed vagotomy. The average incidence of failed truncal vagotomy is 25 to 30 per cent, according to the original criteria of the Hollander test, whereas the incidence after selective vagotomy employing similar criteria may be as low as 5 per cent.[11-13, 22] The methods of performing the insulin and 2-deoxy-D-glucose tests[23] are described on pages 181 and 542.

The Hollander test is potentially hazardous. Dangerous hypoglycemic reactions may occur; aside from the central nervous symptoms caused by such reactions, severe cardiac arrhythmias may develop suddenly and insidiously when the blood sugar falls rapidly. Such arrhythmias are especially prone to occur in patients with arteriosclerotic heart disease, those taking digitalis, and those with hypokalemia. For these reasons, Read recommends that the Hollander test not be performed on patients in any of those categories. He also recommends that all patients undergoing the Hollander test receive an intravenous infusion containing 40 to 80 mEq KC1 per liter during the test to offset cardiac arrhythmias caused by hypokalemia, because the insulin injection and hypoglycemia may suddenly induce hypokalemia in marginally normokalemic patients. It is also wise to maintain patients on a cardiac monitor throughout the Hollander test; if arrhythmias occur, the test should be promptly terminated by an intravenous injection of 50 cc of 50 per cent glucose solution. This should always be immediately available in a syringe kept at the patient's bedside during the test.[21] Undoubtedly, many Hollander test protocols recommend giving excessively high doses of insulin (i.e., over 20 units).

Because of the potential danger and perhaps questionable significance of the Hollander test, a case may be made for not performing the test in any patient suspected of recurrent ulceration after a vagotomy. If the test is negative, thus indicating a "complete" vagotomy, the result may be falsely negative because of neutralization of gastric acid by reflux of alkaline gastrointestinal juices into the stomach. Therefore, whether the Hollander test is positive or negative, we re-explore the periesophageal area for missed vagal fibers during laparotomy for recurrent ulcer in *any* patient, except those with the Zollinger-Ellison syndrome. We no longer perform the Hollander test. The 2-deoxy-glucose test is also dangerous.[24]

Recent studies indicate that postoperative maximal histamine (or Histalog) acid secretory studies may indicate adequacy of vagotomy when compared with similar, preoperative studies. It is stated that vagotomy should decrease the postoperative response to maximal histamine or Histalog stimulation to below 50 to 70 per cent of the preoperative acid secretory response.[25, 26] There are insufficient data at present to determine the accuracy of this statement. Certainly, the maximal histamine or Histalog response would be an appealing substitute for the more dangerous Hollander test.

Unfortunately, the accuracy of an upper gastrointestinal barium contrast study in detecting recurrent ulcer ranges only from 25 to 70 per cent. Small recurrent ulcers are especially likely to be missed by a standard barium contrast study. The Japanese have significantly increased the diagnostic accuracy of upper gastrointestinal barium contrast studies by performing barium–air contrast X-ray studies of the stomach or gastric remnant. Air is injected into the stomach after evacuating most of the barium from the stomach, or air is injected into the stomach after spraying the gastric wall with a thin layer of barium from a special spray tube inserted into the stomach. These contrast techniques may demonstrate even a small, shallow, primary, or recurrent ulcer by causing it to stand out in relief against a background of intragastric air when the ulcer is covered with a thin barium layer.

About four weeks after peptic ulcer surgery, it is helpful to obtain a baseline upper gastrointestinal barium contrast X-ray study to determine what variations of the upper gastrointestinal outline were caused by the surgical procedure. If symptoms develop later and a repeat upper gastrointestinal X-ray series is done, the earlier baseline barium study is examined and it may thus be determined whether a defect in the later X-ray study was present in the earlier one, in which case a suspicious lesion may be assumed with more certainty to be a surgical artifact, rather than a recurrent ulcer or a gastric tumor.

Without doubt, the most helpful modality for diagnosing recurrent ulcer is the flexible fiberoptic gastroscope. With this device, endoscopy is readily done with little discomfort or danger to the patient, and a complete survey of the entire gastric remnant, gastroenteric anastomosis, and efferent and afferent jejunal limbs is possible. By direct visualization and photography virtually certain diagnosis of most recurrent peptic ulcers may be made[27] (see pp. 528 to 529).

SURGICAL TREATMENT OF RECURRENT PEPTIC ULCERS

Generally, the accepted treatment for recurrent peptic ulcer is surgical. Patients who are poor operative risks because of advanced age or associated disease may be treated medically under close supervision. This is not the treatment of choice, however, because recurrent ulcers are usually more resistant to medical treatment than primary peptic ulcers and are more likely to be accompanied by serious complications.[2] The mortality for medical treatment of recurrent peptic ulcer is approximately 10 per cent. This may partially reflect the fact that poor risk patients were treated medically instead of surgically in some cases; however, the deaths are chiefly due to ulcer complications rather than to concomitant diseases. Mortality for surgical treatment of recurrent duodenal ulcers may also approach 10 per cent, but the mortality mostly arises from emergency surgery for bleeding and perforation. The mortality for elective surgery for recurrent ulcer is about 2 per cent.

Clayman and associates report a large experience with radiation treatment of duodenal ulcers, indicating ulcer recurrence in about 20 per cent of patients so treated.[28] When standard medical treatment is ineffective and surgery is considered too dangerous, gastric irradiation might be considered in poor risk patients with recurrent peptic ulcer, as an alternative to surgical treatment. Irradiation of the gastric remnant has also been reported to be effective in the management of patients with the Zollinger-Ellison syndrome by reducing gastrin production from the ulcerogenic tumor and reducing gastric acid secondary to a radiation-induced gastritis. Certainly, this would not be the treatment of choice for patients with recurrent ulcers caused by the Zollinger-Ellison syndrome.

SURGICAL MANAGEMENT OF RECURRENT DUODENAL ULCER AFTER VAGOTOMY AND ANTRECTOMY

The mean incidence of recurrent duodenal ulcer after vagotomy and antrectomy is less than 1 per cent, which is lower than that after any other surgical procedure for duodenal ulcer (see p. 779). Recurrences after vagotomy and antrectomy are usually caused by inadequate vagotomy, ulcerogenic tumor, or retained gastric antral tissue in the duodenal stump. If repeated serum gastrin and gastric acid secretory levels are not elevated, the recurrent ulcer is almost certainly due to an incomplete vagotomy. At laparotomy, the periesophageal area is re-explored for vagal fibers. Persistent posterior vagal fibers are most likely to be found, according to Demos.[10] These posterior vagal fibers are most often located away from the esophagus directly overlying the right crus of the diaphragmatic esophageal hiatus. All retained vagal fibers are removed and their identity confirmed by frozen section biopsy during surgery. After all retained vagal fibers are removed and if no ulcerogenic tumor is noted, a gastric re-resection is performed so the patient has a 66 to 75 per cent gastric resection instead of the previous antrectomy. It may be argued that completion of the vagotomy alone would theoretically permit healing of the ulcer without gastric re-resection, but the uncertainty of obtaining a complete vagotomy in these circumstances makes it desirable to obtain additional protection against ulcer recurrence by performing a moderate gastric re-resection, especially if only a few small intact vagal fibers are found. If, on the other hand, a *large* intact vagal trunk is found, probably representing the entire posterior or anterior vagus which was missed during the initial operation, it may be elected not to perform gastric re-resection unless the recurrent ulcer is large or the stoma is stenotic.

If no retained vagal fibers are found, a search for a gastrin-producing tumor should be made to further confirm the preoperative evidence against the Zollinger-Ellison syndrome. If incomplete vagotomy and ulcerogenic tumor are eliminated as causes of recurrence and if a Billroth II operation was performed initially, the duodenal stump should be opened and examined for retained gastric antral tissue; any retained antrum should be removed. Examination of the duodenal stump for retained antral tissue is only necessary, however, if adequate frozen

section examination of the circumference of the duodenal stump for gastric antral tissue was not done during the original Billroth II gastrectomy.

As more experience is gained with serum gastrin determinations, it may be found that the presence of retained gastric antrum in the duodenal stump may be ruled out by finding normal serum gastrin levels preoperatively, thus obviating the need for opening the duodenal stump. There are currently no data indicating what levels of serum gastrin may be produced by retained gastric antral fragments within the duodenal stump, but it is probable that there would be a significant increase, possibly even within the range of levels found in patients with the Zollinger-Ellison syndrome.

If inadequate vagotomy, ulcerogenic tumor, and retained gastric antrum are not found, it must be assumed that there is an unusually virulent duodenal ulcer diathesis which requires a higher gastric resection with vagotomy instead of antrectomy and vagotomy for its control. Therefore a gastric re-resection is performed, leaving the patient with 20 to 25 per cent of his stomach instead of the 50 to 60 per cent which remained after the original antrectomy. The surgeon should decreasingly be confronted with this situation, however, because of spreading adoption of secretory tests and of measurement of serum gastrin along with improving surgical technique for antrectomy and vagotomy.

If preoperative serum gastrin levels are markedly elevated, or if basal gastric acid secretory levels are greater than 5 mEq per hour, the Zollinger-Ellison syndrome is probably the cause of the recurrent ulcer. It is possible, however, that retained gastric antral tissue in the duodenal stump of a patient who has had a Billroth II gastrectomy might also have caused the recurrent ulcer and the high basal levels of gastric acid secretion and high serum gastrin levels. Thus the duodenal stump must be opened and searched for retained gastric antral tissue if no evidence of Zollinger-Ellison tumor is found on exploration. If obvious retained antral tissue is found within the duodenal stump and no Zollinger-Ellison tumor is detected on exploration, the retained antral tissue is removed completely, the duodenum is

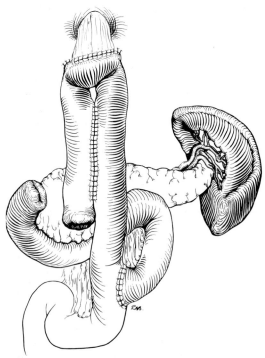

Figure 63–1. Method of construction of a Lawrence pouch after total gastrectomy.

closed, and no further gastric resection is performed, because removal of the gastric antral tissue from the duodenal stump should remove the source of gastrin which induced the high gastric acid levels and the recurrent ulcer. Additional serum gastrin levels should be determined in the early postoperative period to confirm this etiology.

If retained gastric antral tissue is not found in the duodenal stump when repeated high serum gastrin levels are found after an initial vagotomy and antrectomy, it must be assumed that the recurrent ulcer is due to the Zollinger-Ellison syndrome even though no ulcerogenic tumor is found. (The Zollinger-Ellison syndrome may be due to pancreatic islet cell hyperplasia rather than to tumor; it is dangerous, however, to attempt to confirm this by pancreatic biopsy because of the well recognized morbidity of pancreatic biopsy.[29]) When confronted with this situation, a total gastrectomy should be performed along with the creation of a Lawrence jejunal pouch to replace the stomach (Fig. 63–1). Several reports confirm that the technical and postgastrectomy problems

associated with this simply constructed pouch are significantly less than those encountered with other gastric replacement pouches after total gastrectomy.[30, 31] There are far fewer nutritional problems after total gastrectomy for the Zollinger-Ellison syndrome than for gastric malignancies, although the reasons for this empiric observation are not understood.[19]

RECURRENT DUODENAL ULCER AFTER VAGOTOMY-DRAINAGE PROCEDURES

Recurrence after vagotomy-drainage procedures develops in about 6 to 10 per cent of cases after a ten-year follow-up period. If basal acid secretory and serum gastrin levels do not cause suspicion of the Zollinger-Ellison syndrome, laparotomy is performed and the periesophageal area reexplored to remove any intact vagal trunks. If the patient is elderly, underweight, or otherwise a poor risk and preoperative basal and histamine-stimulated acid levels are relatively low, the surgeon may elect only to remove the intact vagus nerve with good prognosis for ulcer healing. Thus the poor risk patient is spared a longer procedure and loss of gastric reservoir. This is not the procedure of choice, however, because many of these patients may have had ulcer recurrences because of poorly functioning drainage stomas which only gastric resection will correct. One cannot determine at surgery whether drainage is adequate.

In a younger, better risk, better nourished patient, especially one having higher acid secretory levels, an antrectomy is therefore performed in addition to removal of obviously intact vagal nerves for better prevention of further ulcer recurrence. In such patients only minimal postoperative problems should be encountered.

If no intact vagal fibers are found in patients having ulcer recurrences after vagotomy and drainage procedures, an antrectomy is indicated.

Obviously, if gastric acid secretory levels and serum gastrin levels indicate the presence of the Zollinger-Ellison syndrome, a total gastrectomy is the only safe means of controlling this virulent ulcer diathesis.[19]

RECURRENT DUODENAL ULCER AFTER SUBTOTAL GASTRECTOMY WITHOUT VAGOTOMY

The mean incidence of recurrent duodenal ulcer after 65 to 75 per cent subtotal gastrectomy without vagotomy is approximately 5 to 6 per cent; most recurrences are within two years. Duodenal ulcer recurrences after this procedure should become a less frequent problem, because fewer subtotal gastrectomies are now being performed.

The Zollinger-Ellison syndrome and retained gastric antral tissue in the duodenal stump must be ruled out in patients with ulcer recurrences after subtotal gastrectomy by appropriate gastric acid secretory and serum gastrin studies and by re-exploration of the duodenal stump for retained gastric antrum (in those who have had Billroth II resections).

If the Zollinger-Ellison syndrome is present, a total gastrectomy and Lawrence pouch reconstruction are performed (see p. 834). If no Zollinger-Ellison tumor is found, but retained gastric antrum is in the duodenal stump, the retained antral tissue is removed and the duodenum is reclosed. Removal of retained antral tissue in the duodenal stump would probably permit ulcer healing, but a vagotomy should also be done for additional assurance of ulcer healing. Gastric re-resection should be performed only if the recurrent ulcer is large and it is feared that obstruction of the gastroenteric stoma by scarring may occur as the ulcer heals or that the ulcer may bleed or perforate before it heals. These same considerations apply in the case of recurrence following vagotomy and antrectomy. If gastric re-resection is done for such reasons, it should be limited to the amount required to remove the ulcer safely; otherwise postsurgical nutritional problems are likely to occur because of the small gastric pouch which remains.

If Zollinger-Ellison tumor and retained gastric antrum in the duodenal stump are eliminated as causes of ulcer recurrence after subtotal gastrectomy, vagotomy is performed. Again, re-resection of the stomach is done only for the "local" or "mechanical" reasons given in the previous paragraph. An "inadequate" subtotal gastric resection becomes an "adequate" one when vagotomy is added to it. Although some surgeons recommend vagotomy and gastric re-resection in all cases of ulcer recurrence after subtotal gastrectomy, there is no physiological basis for gastric re-resection and practical experience reveals no better recurrent ulcer prevention by vagotomy and gastric re-resection than by vagotomy alone when ulcer recurrence follows subtotal gastrectomy.[1, 8]

DUODENAL ULCER RECURRENCE AFTER GASTROENTEROSTOMY WITHOUT VAGOTOMY

Although gastroenterostomy without vagotomy was the operation of choice for duodenal ulcer more than a generation ago, it is now usually performed only as a compromise procedure in poor risk patients requiring relief of chronic pyloric obstruction in the presence of severe edema and dilatation of the stomach. The mean ulcer recurrence rate following gastroenterostomy is 35 to 40 per cent, but the mean time of recurrence is 10 to 11 years, much longer (for unknown reasons) than the mean recurrence time following other ulcer operations.[6]

In poor risk, underweight patients, after ruling out the Zollinger-Ellison syndrome, the surgeon should probably perform vagotomy alone to treat recurrent ulcer after simple gastroenterostomy.

In better risk patients with no nutritional problems, however, it is preferable to perform vagotomy and antrectomy for better control of the ulcer diathesis after simple gastroenterostomy. This is especially true if gastric acid secretory levels are high, if ulcer recurrence was relatively soon after the original gastroenterostomy, or if the recurrent ulcer is so large that it may obstruct the gastroenterostomy by scarring or may bleed or perforate before it heals. These factors, obstruction, bleeding, or perforation, may indicate resection of the gastroenterostomy and recurrent ulcer with reconstruction of a new gastroenterostomy or with substitution of a pyloroplasty for the gastroenterostomy even in some of the poorer risk patients.

EMERGENCY MANAGEMENT OF BLEEDING OR PERFORATION OF A RECURRENT STOMAL ULCER

In many instances, unfortunately, there will be no opportunity to obtain preoperative gastric acid and serum gastrin levels before emergency surgery for a bleeding recurrent ulcer. After controlling hemorrhage and shock by transfusion and direct suture of the bleeding point, the surgeon should make a careful search for an ulcerogenic tumor of the pancreas. If this is found, a total gastrectomy is performed. In such emergency situations, it is probably best to attempt no construction of any type of complicated gastric replacement pouch. Instead, a simple Roux-en-Y end-to-side esophagojejunostomy should be constructed after the emergency total gastrectomy. If necessary, a jejunal replacement pouch of a more complicated type can be made later, after the patient's full recovery.

Although this may seem to be radical surgery under emergency conditions, it is safer to remove all the stomach to prevent early rebleeding in the immediate postoperative period. Way and associates report several cases among 25 Zollinger-Ellison syndrome patients who bled and required emergency reoperation even before their nasogastric tubes were removed when anything less than a total gastrectomy was done initially![19] This has also been our experience. If, in the surgeon's judgment, total gastrectomy cannot be performed initially because of the patient's extremely precarious condition, the bleeding recurrent ulcer may be resected in a limited fashion or, more probably, securely oversewn with nonabsorbable suture and the operation terminated when the bleeding has been adequately controlled. After this, the patient should be treated with continuous infusion of antacid into the stomach through a nasogastric tube to make rebleeding somewhat less likely. Anticholinergic drugs should also be used. Intensive efforts are then made to improve the patient's general condition so that, within a few hours or days when he has suitably improved and before he rebleeds, a total gastrectomy may be more safely done.

If there is no evidence of a Zollinger-Ellison tumor during emergency surgery for recurrent stomal ulcer bleeding, the management may vary according to the original ulcer operation and the patient's condition. If antrectomy and vagotomy was the original operation, the bleeding is immediately controlled by direct ligation of the bleeding vessel with nonabsorbable suture. Periesophageal exploration for retained vagal fibers is done, and any retained vagal fibers are removed. If the patient's condition is suitable, a limited resection of the ulcer and gastroenterostomy is done to reduce the chance of early rebleeding from the ulcer before it heals, especially if the ulcer is large (>2.5 cm). If, however, the patient is not in good enough condition for emergency resection, the surgeon may simply depend upon the suture of the ulcer to prevent rebleeding until the completed vagotomy allows ulcer healing.

If no Zollinger-Ellison tumor or retained vagal fibers are found, the surgeon must consider the possibility of retained gastric antral tissue within the duodenal stump as a possible cause of the massively bleeding recurrent ulcer if a Billroth II gastrectomy was done originally and there was not histological confirmation of complete removal of gastric antral tissue from the duodenal stump during the original operation. The duodenal stump is opened and examined circumferentially by frozen section biopsy for retained gastric antral tissue, which is completely removed if found. The duodenum is closed, and a limited resection of the gastroenterostomy and bleeding ulcer is done.

If no Zollinger-Ellison tumor, incomplete vagotomy, or retained gastric antral tissue is discovered, a higher gastric resection is done, leaving a gastric remnant of 25 to 35 per cent.

If the original duodenal ulcer operation was a vagotomy-drainage procedure and emergency surgery is done for bleeding recurrent ulcer, the ulcer is first visualized and oversewn with nonabsorbable suture to stop the bleeding. The periesophageal area is then re-explored, and any intact vagal fibers are removed. If the patient is a poor risk and intact vagal fibers are found and removed, no more is done. If the patient is a good risk, however, in addition to completing the vagotomy, the surgeon should perform antrectomy and ulcer removal for more certain control of the ulcer diathesis. If no intact vagal fibers are found and the vagotomy thus seems complete, antrectomy should be performed, unless the patient is a very poor risk, in which case only suture of the bleeding ulcer is done and more definitive surgery is performed later when the patient's condition has improved; meanwhile the patient should receive intensive antacid and anticholinergic therapy.

If the original ulcer operation was a subtotal gastrectomy, a vagotomy is done after first stopping hemorrhage by suturing the bleeding ulcer. If the patient is in poor condition, or the ulcer is small and bleeding is readily controlled by suture, no gastric re-resection or ulcer removal is done. If the recurrent ulcer is large (greater than 2.5 cm) and therefore apt to be difficult to control by suture and to rebleed, or is likely to cause obstruction of a small gastroenteric stoma by scarring as it heals, a small gastric re-resection should be done, with removal of the ulcer and reconstruction of the gastroenteric stoma. Wedge removal of recurrent ulcers should generally be avoided, because this may distort the gastroenteric stoma and cause obstruction, or the suture line in the edematous tissue about the ulcer may be prone to leak.

In all these instances of emergency surgery for recurrent ulcer bleeding, gastric acid secretory levels and serum gastrin levels should be obtained immediately after surgery. If these studies indicate an ulcerogenic tumor or retained gastric antrum, intensive antacid and anticholinergic treatment is begun to control hypersecretion and to prevent rebleeding until total gastrectomy or removal of retained gastric antrum can be done when the patient recovers sufficiently from the emergency operation.

EMERGENCY MANAGEMENT OF PERFORATED STOMAL ULCER

In most cases of perforated recurrent stomal ulcer, it is probably safest to close the perforation by patching it with an omental tag and to allow the patient to recover, meanwhile maintaining intensive antacid and anticholinergic therapy. Gastric acid and serum gastrin levels are ob-

tained immediately postoperatively. After this, appropriate definitive surgery is performed, using the previously described guidelines.[32]

If the patient is a good risk and does not have excessive peritonitis, in addition to patching the perforation the periesophageal area is explored and a vagotomy is done if one was not done previously, or retained vagal fibers are removed if vagotomy done during initial ulcer surgery was inadequate; this may permit the ulcer to heal and obviate additional surgery later.

If a complete vagotomy was done previously, or after it is completed, antrectomy is performed in good risk patients. It offers the most complete protection against ulcer recurrence, and is especially desirable if it is feared that a large ulcer may bleed or obstruct the stoma.

If a vagotomy and antrectomy was performed previously in a patient who has suffered perforation of a recurrent ulcer and the vagotomy is found apparently to be complete at re-exploration, it is probable that the patient has an ulcerogenic tumor even though no obvious pancreatic tumor is found, or has retained gastric antrum in the duodenal stump. It is probably inadvisable, however, to do total gastrectomy or to open the duodenal stump during emergency surgery for perforation of a recurrent ulcer, and a less than total gastrectomy would most likely be ineffective in preventing prompt ulcer recurrence. Accordingly, under these circumstances, the perforated ulcer should only be closed. When the patient recovers and diagnostic studies, including gastric acid secretory levels and serum gastrin levels, are obtained, appropriate definitive surgery may be performed.

In some cases, it may be impossible to close a large perforation of a recurrent ulcer securely or without obstructing the gastroenteric stoma. In such instances, resection of the ulcer and gastric re-resection or resection may be the only safe means of mangagement.

GASTROJEJUNOCOLIC FISTULA SECONDARY TO RECURRENT PEPTIC ULCER

Gastrojejunocolic fistula is much less frequent now than when simple gastroenterostomy was performed for most duodenal ulcers; however, it is still encountered and must be considered in any patient with a gastrojejunostomy or a Billroth II gastrectomy who develops persistent severe diarrhea, steatorrhea, and weight loss.[33, 34] The profuse diarrhea and inanition are caused by a proliferation of bacteria in the small bowel produced by passage of feces into the proximal small bowel through the fistula (pp. 927 to 936). There may or may not be pain, bleeding, and other clinical signs of recurrent ulcer. Barium enema is the principal means of diagnosis of the fistula. It is more likely than an upper gastrointestinal contrast study to reveal all visceral components of a gastrojejunocolic fistula.

Before adequate means of correcting fluid, electrolyte, and nutritional deficits and sterilizing the bowel were available, a staged operation to correct the fistula was done. The first stage of the operation consisted of a completely diverting right transverse colostomy. The diverting colostomy prevented further fecal spill into the small bowel through the fistula, thus alleviating the diarrhea and allowing correction of fluid and electrolyte deficits and weight loss. After the patient's condition improved, the second stage operation consisted of resection of the fistula and performance of a more effective ulcer operation. After this, the colostomy was closed at the third stage operation about a month later.[34]

Alternatively, the first stage operation may be an end-to-side ileosigmoidostomy, which defunctionalizes the fistula as does the colostomy, but it may be more stressful to a markedly debilitated patient than the transverse colostomy which can be done more quickly and less traumatically.

The staged procedure is still recommended in seriously ill patients, but in better risk patients the treatment of choice is a one-stage resection of the fistula and corrective ulcer surgery after suitable preoperative correction of metabolic deficits and bowel sterilization.[33]

RECURRENT GASTRIC ULCER

The incidence of gastric ulcer recurrence following antrectomy without vagotomy is about 2 per cent. After vagotomy and drainage procedures, however, the recurrence rate may rise to 30 to 40 per cent.[35] If recurrence does develop, however, the usual preoperative work-up for the Zollinger-Ellison syndrome or retained gastric antrum within the duodenal stump is done; if these are detected, they are managed by total gastrectomy or removal of retained antral tissue, as discussed previously in the management of recurrent ulcer after surgery for duodenal ulcer.

If the Zollinger-Ellison syndrome and retained antral tissue are ruled out and gastric ulcer recurs after antrectomy, a vagotomy and moderate re-resection are performed. If recurrence follows a vagotomy-drainage operation, this is converted to an antrectomy. Recurrences of gastric ulcers after antrectomy and vagotomy not caused by the Zollinger-Ellison syndrome or retained antrum within the duodenal stump are unusual, but should be managed by periesophageal re-exploration to complete a possibly incomplete vagotomy and performance of a moderate gastric re-resection.

As discussed on page 786, the recurrence rate following vagotomy-drainage procedures performed for gastric ulcers ultimately approaches 40 per cent.[35] Thus it seems that vagotomy-drainage is not the operation of choice for most gastric ulcers. If such an operation has been performed and the gastric ulcer recurs, the obvious conclusion is that the patient must now be subjected to an antrectomy; in most instances this will adequately control the gastric ulcer diathesis and prevent further recurrence.

Some gastric ulcers recur after a simple antrectomy because they are actually a part of a duodenal ulcer diathesis. This is true of approximately 20 per cent of all gastric ulcers.[36] In that instance, if there were a high gastric acid secretory level in the range of a duodenal ulcer diathesis, an antrectomy would not have been an adequate operation for such gastric ulcers. This would be suspected in patients with a recurrent gastric ulcer who had elevated postoperative gastric acid levels on either basal or histamine-stimulated studies. In those cases, the corrective procedure of choice would be to perform a vagotomy and perhaps moderate re-resection of the stomach. Such recurrences may be prevented by performing antrectomy *and* vagotomy as an initial procedure on all gastric ulcer patients with associated duodenal ulcers and/or high preoperative basal or histamine-stimulated gastric acid levels.

The consensus of recent studies is that satisfactory results will ultimately be obtained in approximately 80 to 90 per cent of recurrent peptic ulcer patients if the treatment regimens outlined herein are followed in a logical and rational fashion.[1-8]

REFERENCES

1. Andros, G., Donaldson, G. A., Hedberg, S. E., and Welch, C. E. Anastomotic ulcers. Ann. Surg. 165:955, 1967.
2. Beal, J. M. The surgical treatment of marginal ulcer. Amer. Surgeon 25:1, 1959.
3. Boles, R. S., Jr., Marshall, S. F., and Bersoux, R. V. Follow-up study of 127 patients with stomal ulcer. Gastroenterology 38:763, 1960.
4. Jaffe, B. M., Newton, W. T., Judd, D. R., and Ballinger, W. F., II. Surgical management of recurrent peptic ulcers. Amer. J. Surg. 117:214, 1969.
5. Meyer, K. A., and Stein, I. F., Jr. Management of recurrent peptic ulcer. Surg. Clin. N. Amer. 32:35, 1952.
6. Priestley, J. T., and Gibson, R. H. Gastrojejunal ulcer: Clinical features and late results. Arch. Surg. 56:625, 1948.
7. Wychulis, A. R., Priestley, J. T., and Foulk, W. T. A study of 360 patients with gastrojejunal ulceration. Surg. Gynec. Obstet. 122:89, 1966.
8. Young, G. A., and Movius, H. J. Surgical treatment of gastrojejunal stomal ulcer. Amer. J. Surg. 104:231, 1962.
9. Burge, H., Roberts, T. B. L., Stedeford, R. D., and Lancaster, M. J. Present position of the electrical stimulation test. Gut 10:155, 1969.
10. Demos, N. J. The elusive posterior vagus: Its identification by palpation. Amer. Surgeon 32:317, 1966.
11. Kraft, R. O., Fry, W. J., Wilhelm, K. G., and Ransom, H. K. Selective gastric vagotomy. Arch. Surg. 95:625, 1967.
12. Sawyers, J. L., Scott, H. W., Jr., Edwards, W. H., Shull, H. J., and Law, D. H., IV. Comparative studies of the clinical effects of truncal and selective gastric vagotomy. Amer. J. Surg. 115:165, 1968.
13. Smith, G. K., and Farris, J. M. Reappraisal of the long-term effects of selective vagotomy. Amer. J. Surg. 117:222, 1969.
14. Gillespie, G., Gillespie, I. E., and Kay, A. W. Response to insulin of the intact stomach in patients with duodenal ulcer. Gut 10:744, 1969.
15. Thompson, B. W., and Read, R. C. Clinical significance of the positive response to the Hollander test. Amer. J. Surg. 120:660, 1970.
16. Aoyagi, T., and Summerskill, W. H. J. Gastric secretion with ulcerogenic islet cell tumor. Arch. Intern. Med. 117:667, 1966.
17. McGuigan, J. E., and Trudeau, W. L. Immunochemical measurement of elevated

levels of gastrin in the serum of patients with pancreatic tumors of the Zollinger-Ellison variety. New Eng. J. Med. 278:1308, 1968.
18. Yalow, R. S., and Berson, S. A. Radioimmunoassay of gastrin. Gastroenterology 58:1, 1970.
19. Way, L. Goldman, L., and Dunphy, J. E. Zollinger-Ellison syndrome. An analysis of twenty-five cases. Amer. J. Surg. 116:293, 1968.
20. vanHeerden, J. A., Priestley, J. T., Farrow, G. M., and Phillips, S. F. Postoperative alkaline reflux gastritis. Amer. J. Surg. 118:427, 1969.
21. Read, R. C., and Doherty, J. E. Cardiovascular effects of induced insulin hypoglycemia in man during the Hollander test. Amer. J. Surg. 119:155, 1970.
22. Hollander, F. The insulin test for the presence of intact nerve fibers after vagal operations for peptic ulcer. Gastroenterology 7:607, 1946.
23. Thomas, D. G., and Duthie, H. L. Vagal test with 2-deoxyglucose to test for the completeness of surgical vagotomy. Gut 9:125, 1968.
24. Himsworth, R. L., and Colin-Jones, D. G. Factors which determine the gastric secretory response to 2-deoxy-D-glucose. Gut 10:1015, 1969.
25. Bell, P. R. F. The long term effect of vagotomy on the maximal acid response to histamine in man. Gastroenterology 46:387, 1964.
26. Konturek, S. J., Wysocki, A., and Oleksy, J. Effect of medical and surgical vagotomy on gastric response to graded doses of pentagastrin and histamine. Gastroenterology 54:392, 1968.
27. Benfield, J. R., Tanaka, Y., and Morrissey, J. The role of the gastrocamera in the diagnosis of marginal ulcer. Arch. Surg. 95:609, 1967.
28. Clayman, C. B., Palmer, W. L., and Kirsner, J. B. Gastric irradiation in the treatment of peptic ulcer. Gastroenterology 38:763, 1960.
29. Potet, F., Martin, E., Thierry, J. P., Bader, J. P., Bonfils, S., and Lambling, A. A histological study of the pancreas in the Zollinger-Ellsion syndrome. Rev. Internat. Hepat. 16:737, 1966.
30. Lawrence, W., Jr. Reservoir construction after total gastrectomy; an instructive case. Ann. Surg. 155:191, 1962.
31. Scott, H. W., Jr., Law, D. H., IV, Gobbel, W. G., Jr., and Sawyers, J. L. Clinical and metabolic studies after total gastrectomy with a Hunt-Lawrence jejunal food pouch. Amer. J. Surg. 115:148, 1968.
32. Thoroughman, J. C., Walker, L. G., Jr., Taylor, B. G., and Dunn, T. Free perforation of anastomotic ulcers. Ann. Surg. 169:790, 1969.
33. Amlicke, J. A., and Ponka, J. L. Gastrocolic and gastrojejunocolic fistulas. Amer. J. Surg. 107:744, 1964.
34. Marshall, S. F., and Knud-Hansen, J. Gastrojejunocolic and gastrocolic fistulas. Ann. Surg. 145:770, 1957.
35. Zahn, R. L., Stemmer, E. A., Hom, L. W., and Connolly, J. E. Delayed recurrence of gastric ulcer following vagotomy and drainage procedures. Amer. Surgeon 34:757, 1968.
36. Athanassiades, S., and Charalambopoulou, J. Coexistent gastric and duodenal ulcer. Amer. J. Surg. 120:381, 1970.

Section 11

The Small Intestine

Chapter 64

Anatomy

Jerry S. Trier

Remarkable structural specializations greatly facilitate the digestive and absorptive functions of the small bowel.[1, 2] The clinician should be familiar with these morphological features, because their alteration in disease results in defective intestinal function as well as significant and often predictable clinical symptoms.[3]

GROSS MORPHOLOGY

A detailed description of the anatomy of the small intestine is not within the scope of this book, and the interested reader is referred to standard reference texts of gross anatomy.[4, 5] The few points which follow merit emphasis because of their potential clinical importance.

The small intestine is efficiently designed. Its many redundant loops allow it to occupy limited space within the abdominal cavity. The adult human small intestine is an elongated tube 12 to 22 feet long, its length depending on both the tone of the muscular wall and the way in which it is measured. The small intestine lies free in the peritoneal cavity and is mobile except for its proximal 10 inches, the duodenum, which is retroperitoneal

and, hence, immobile. The anatomical relationship of the duodenum to other viscera is important because disease of the duodenum may extend into these adjacent organs and vice versa (Fig. 64–1). The duodenum is molded around the head of the pancreas in a horseshoe fashion. Coincident with this intimate contact between the pancreas and all portions of the duodenum, disease of the pancreas may distort or invade adjacent duodenal tissue. On the other hand, duodenal disease, especially peptic ulceration, may penetrate into and involve pancreatic tissue. Disease of the duodenum in the region of the ampulla of Vater may obstruct the distal portion of the common bile duct and the main pancreatic duct, thus interfering with normal delivery of bile and pancreatic secretions into the duodenum.

Both the liver and the gallbladder are in immediate contact with the anterosuperior aspect of the proximal or first portion of the duodenum (Fig. 64–1). Disease of these organs may involve each other and result in complications such as cholecystoduodenal fistulas or penetration of peptic duodenal ulcerations into either the quadrate or right lobe of the liver. Less often, the common bile duct, which passes

840

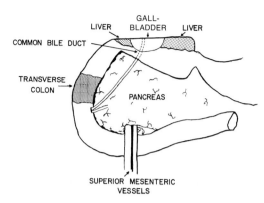

Figure 64-1. Diagram showing relationship of the duodenum to adjacent viscera.

behind the proximal duodenum en route to its entry into the descending duodenum, may be jointly involved with the proximal duodenum by disease. Carcinoma of the transverse colon may extend into and involve the descending or second portion of the duodenum, because the transverse colon crosses it anteriorly (Fig. 64-1). The superior mesenteric artery and vein cross the transverse or third portion of the duodenum near the midline as they emerge from the root of the mesentery of the small intestine. It is alleged that these vessels may produce functional obstruction of the third portion of the duodenum by compressing it as it crosses the spine, especially in thin individuals. The descending aorta passes directly behind to the duodenum, and aneurysms of this major vessel may rupture into the lumen of the duodenum, causing catastrophic gastrointestinal bleeding.

Unlike the fixed retroperitoneal duodenum, the jejunum and the ileum are suspended by an extensive mesentery, and have considerable mobility within the abdominal cavity. Usually, the jejunal loops lie over the duodenum, pancreas, and left kidney in the upper abdomen and thus may be affected by disease of those organs. For example, the radiolucent "sentinel" loop seen by X-ray in patients with acute pancreatitis results from ileus localized to a loop of jejunum overlying the pancreas (see p. 1174). The ileum generally occupies the lower abdomen and a portion of the pelvis. The distal few inches of ileum are the least mobile, be-

cause the cecum is usually affixed to the posterior abdominal wall.

There is no specific anatomical structure which marks the end of the jejunum and the beginning of the ileum; instead, the proximal two-fifths of mobile small intestine are arbitrarily considered jejunum and the distal three-fifths are designated ileum. However, significant differences in the structure of the proximal jejunum and the distal ileum facilitate their identification by the radiologist and surgeon.

The diameter of the proximal jejunum is almost twice that of the distal ileum, and its wall is considerably thicker. The spiral or circular folds, the *plicae circulares*, which consist of a fold of submucosa covered by a full thickness of mucosa, are most abundant and well developed (up to 1 cm in height) in the distal duodenum and proximal jejunum. These folds gradually become sparser and less elaborate, and often disappear entirely in the distal third of the ileum. Elliptical aggregates of lymphoid tissue (Peyer's patches) up to 1 inch or more in length are present along the antimesenteric border in the distal half of the ileum, but are not normally found in the jejunum. Peyer's patches are most prominent in young individuals; they atrophy toward middle age and may be difficult to identify in old age. The amount of fat in the mesentery adjacent to the jejunum is very small; hence the mesentery appears translucent. In contrast, the mesentery adjacent to the ileum contains much fat and appears opaque, another difference which helps the surgeon identify the level of a specific segment of small intestine.

The anatomy of the blood supply to the small intestine is discussed in detail on pages 378 to 381.

HISTOLOGY

The wall of the small intestine consists of four layers, the serosa, the muscularis, the submucosa, and the mucosa (Fig. 64-2).

The *serosa* or outermost layer is an extension of the peritoneum. It encircles the jejunum and ileum but covers only a part of the anterior portion of the retroperitoneal duodenum. Like the peritoneum, the serosa consists of a single layer of flat-

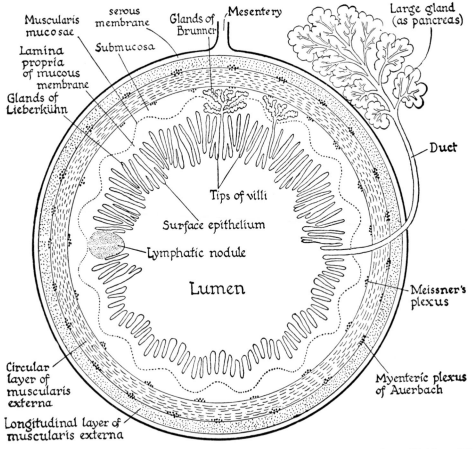

Figure 64–2. Schematic diagram of a cross section of the intestinal tract. (From Bloom, W. N., and Fawcett, D. W.: A Textbook of Histology. Philadelphia, W. B. Saunders Co., 1968.)

tened mesothelial cells overlying some loose connective tissue.

The *muscularis* consists of two layers of smooth muscles, an outer or longitudinal layer in which the long axis of the individual smooth muscle cells parallels the long axis of the intestine, and a thicker inner or circular layer in which the individual muscle cells tend to encircle the bowel (Fig. 64–2). This arrangement of muscle cells facilitates efficient propulsion of the intraluminal contents of the gut. Ganglion cells and nerve fibers of the myenteric plexus are interposed between these two layers of muscle.

The *submucosa* consists largely of dense connective tissue sparsely infiltrated by cells including lymphocytes, macrophages, eosinophils, mast cells, and plasma cells. The submucosa also contains elaborate lymphatic and venous plexuses which drain the lymphatic and venous capillaries of the lamina propria of the mucosa. It also contains an extensive network of arterioles and the ganglion cells and nerve fibers which form the autonomic submucous plexus.

Elaborately branched acinar glands, Brunner's glands, which contain both mucous and serous secretory cells, fill much of the submucosal space of the duodenal cap and the proximal half of the descending duodenum. Small islands of Brunner's glands are regularly present in the submucosa of the distal duodenum, and isolated islets may extend well into the jejunum. There is evidence that the secretion elaborated by Brunner's glands, which is rich in both mucus and bicarbonate, protects the proximal duodenum from acid-peptic digestion. Moreover, these glands are of additional clinical im-

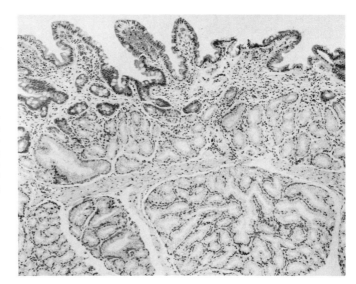

Figure 64–3. Normal human duodenal mucosa. Brunner's glands are infiltrating the submucosa and the lamina propria. As a result, the villous architecture appears distorted. Hematoxylin and eosin stain. Approximately × 70. (From Brandborg, L. L., et al.: Gastroenterology 37:1, 1959.)

portance in that they regularly penetrate and extend into the lamina propria of the mucosa of the proximal duodenum (Fig. 64–3). This often results in marked distortion of the so-called normal villous pattern in this segment of small intestine. Failure to appreciate this normal variant in *proximal* duodenal tissue has often resulted in serious misinterpretation of peroral biopsies obtained from this region, including incorrect diagnoses of primary mucosal disease in individuals whose biopsy specimens from the *distal* duodenum or proximal jejunum would have revealed mucosa with perfectly normal villous architecture.[6]

The numerous villi which greatly amplify the absorptive and digestive surface which is in contact with the intraluminal intestinal contents are a striking structural feature of the innermost layer of the small intestine, the *mucosa*. Although the villi are often described as finger-like structures 0.5 to 1 mm in height, their appearance in man may vary with their location in the small intestine and from individual to individual. The villi are normally broad and ridge shaped in the proximal duodenum where the lamina is infiltrated with Brunner's glands and, especially in young individuals, with lymphoid follicles. Sectioned biopsies from this area often fail to show discrete villi and may resemble superficially the flattened mucosa found in the more distal bowel in patients with celiac sprue.[6] In the more distal duodenum and proximal jejunum, the villi are often leaf shaped, but may be finger shaped. In the distal jejunum and ileum, finger-shaped villi are the rule. The villi are tallest in the distal duodenum and proximal jejunum and progressively appear shorter toward the ileocecal valve.

The villous architecture of the small intestine varies significantly among normal inhabitants of different parts of the world. There are convincing data that the intestinal mucosa of residents of India,[7] Southeast Asia,[8] and the Caribbean Islands[9] is commonly characterized by shorter villi, deeper crypts, and increased cellularity in the lamina propria than is the mucosa of residents of Europe and North America. The factors responsible for this morphological variation have not been defined. The suggestion that the milieu of the intestinal lumen differs in various parts of the world owing to diverse dietary habits and distinctive intraluminal intestinal microbial ecology is attractive but unproved. Nevertheless, awareness of this sometimes striking geographic variability of "normal" villous architecture is imperative for proper interpretation of intestinal mucosal biopsies.

The intestinal mucosa itself can be conveniently divided into three distinct layers (Figs. 64–4 and 64–5). The deepest of these is the *muscularis mucosae*, a thin sheet of smooth muscle, three to ten cells

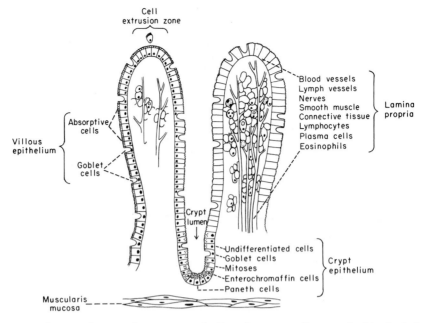

Figure 64–4. Schematic diagram of two sectioned villi and a crypt to illustrate the histological organization of the small intestinal mucosa.

thick, which separates the mucosa from the submucosa.

The middle layer, the *lamina propria*, is a continuous connective tissue space bounded below by the muscularis mucosae and above by the intestinal epithelium. The lamina forms the connective tissue core of the numerous villi and

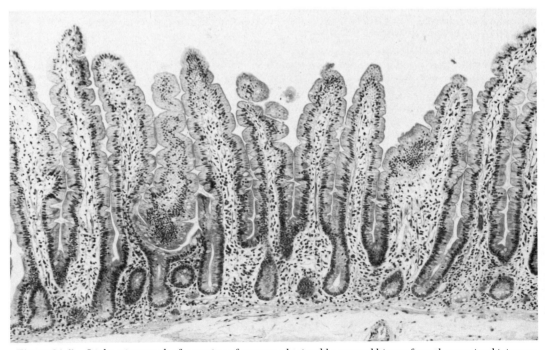

Figure 64–5. Light micrograph of a section of mucosa obtained by peroral biopsy from the proximal jejunum of a normal man. Hematoxylin and eosin stain. Approximately × 93.

surrounds the pit-like crypts which encircle villi around their base. The lamina propria normally contains many types of cells, including plasma cells, lymphocytes, mast cells, eosinophils, macrophages, smooth muscle cells, fibroblasts, and noncellular connective tissue elements (collagen, reticular, and elastin fibers).

There is increasing evidence that the lamina propria may serve important protective functions by combating microorganisms and other foreign substances that may penetrate the overlying epithelial barrier. The lamina contains cells capable of phagocytosis and, with its many plasma cells, is an active site of immunoglobulin synthesis.[10] Indeed, significant intestinal dysfunction is often seen in patients in whom the plasma cell population and immunoglobulin synthesis of the lamina propria are deficient (see pp. 55 to 58).

The lamina propria also provides important structural support, not only for its overlying epithelium but also for the many small vascular channels that nourish the mucosa and that carry away absorbed materials to the systemic circulation. These blood and lymphatic capillaries differ structurally from one another. The blood capillaries have thin endothelial walls with many tiny (0.05 to 0.1 μ) diaphragm-covered pores (Fig. 64–6). These pores have greater permeability to large molecules and particulate material than does the pore-free portion of the capillary wall.[11] In contrast, the walls of the lymphatic capillaries are continuous and contain no such discrete pores. The lamina propria also contains small unmyelinated nerve fibers. These may help regulate mucosal blood flow and, perhaps, mucosal secretory activity.

The inner layer of the mucosa consists of a continuous sheet of a single layer of columnar epithelial cells which lines both the crypts and the villi. The base of each

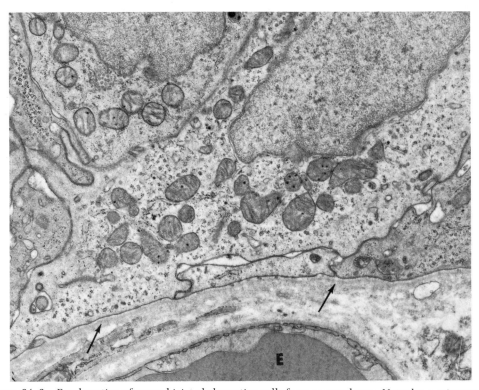

Figure 64–6. Basal portion of several jejunal absorptive cells from a normal man. Note the continuous basal lamina (arrows) which is closely applied to the basal cell membrane of absorptive cells. Part of a capillary containing an erythrocyte (E) within its lumen is seen in the underlying lamina propria. Approximately × 12,000. (From Trier, J. S.: Handbook of Physiology: Alimentary Canal, C. Code, Ed. Washington, D.C., American Physiological Society, 1968.)

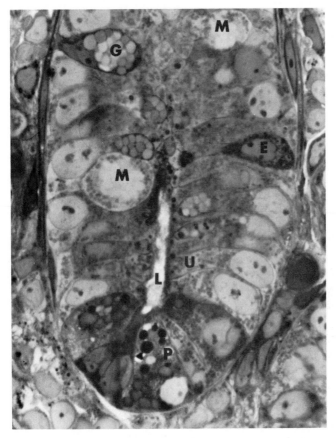

Figure 64–7. High magnification light micrograph of a jejunal crypt from a biopsy from a normal volunteer. Paneth cells (P) help form the base of the crypt. Undifferentiated cells (U), goblet cells (G), and an endocrine cell (E) are seen along the lateral wall of the crypt. Two of the undifferentiated cells are undergoing mitosis (M). The crypt lumen (L) is sectioned tangentially. Toluidine blue stain of resin-embedded section. Approximately × 1400. (From Trier, J. S.: Handbook of Physiology: Alimentary Canal, C. Code, Ed. Washington, D.C., American Physiological Society, 1968.)

epithelial cell rests on a thin, continuous basement membrane which separates the epithelium from the underlying lamina propria. The main known functions of the crypt epithelium are cell renewal and secretion; the main function of the villous epithelium is absorption. The crypt epithelium is composed of at least four distinct cell types: the Paneth, goblet, undifferentiated, and endocrine cells (Figs. 64–4 and 64–7).

Morphologically, Paneth cells strongly resemble zymogenic cells such as the pancreatic and salivary gland acinar cells which are known to secrete large amounts of protein-rich materials. The Paneth cells are readily identified by their location in the base of the crypts, by their strongly basophilic cytoplasm, and by their large eosinophilic secretory granules.

The goblet cells of the crypts are located on the lateral walls of the crypts, and their morphology resembles goblet cells elsewhere in the gastrointestinal tract. They are shaped like a brandy goblet, and the

bulk of their cytoplasm between the basally located nucleus and the apical brush border is packed with many mucous granules.

The most abundant cells in the crypts are the undifferentiated or principal cells which form the lateral walls of the crypts and which are also found in the crypt base between the Paneth cells. Their cytoplasm contains many secretory granules. These granules are quite small and not obvious in routine histological preparations, but they are easily seen in the apical cytoplasm near the crypt lumen when sections are stained for glycoprotein with the periodic acid–Schiff (PAS) technique.

The endocrine cells (also often called enterochromaffin, argentaffin, or basal granular cells) are characterized by their "inverted" appearance compared with the other crypt cells in that their small secretory granules are distributed in the basal cytoplasm between the nucleus and the cell apex (Figs. 64–4 and 64–7). This basal location suggests that the endocrine cells liberate their granules into the lamina propria. This is in contrast to the other crypt epithelial cells, which are exocrine cells in that they secrete their granules into the gastrointestinal lumen via the crypt lumen. The endocrine cell granules do not stain with hematoxylin or eosin and, hence, cannot be identified in routinely stained tissue sections. Rather, special staining methods (ammoniacal silver, potassium dichromate, etc.) which utilize the strong reducing potential of the endocrine cell granules must be employed. There are several distinct populations of small intestinal endocrine cells which can be distinguished from one another only histochemically or by subtle morphological criteria at the electron microscopic level. The heterogeneity of endocrine cell structure is not surprising, since these cells have been implicated in diverse physiological processes as described briefly below.

Although it is established that the four epithelial cell types which form the crypts are active secretory cells, remarkably little is known about the contribution of crypt secretions to normal digestive and absorptive processes. The goblet cells constantly secrete mucus into the intestinal lumen. Although this mucus is said to protect and lubricate the intestinal mucosa, firm experimental data on its role are hard to find. The endocrine cells produce significant quantities of serotonin which may stimulate intestinal smooth muscle contraction; hence these cells have been implicated in the regulation of gastrointestinal motility.[12] The endocrine cells may also produce a kallikrein-like enzyme which, when secreted, enhances formation of vasoactive polypeptides from kinin precursors in the blood.[13] The potential clinical significance of excessive secretion of substances by endocrine cell tumors in patients with carcinoid syndromes is discussed on pages 1031 to 1041. Recently there has been renewed interest in a suggestion made over 35 years ago by Parat that intestinal endocrine cells produce and secrete gastrointestinal hormones such as secretin, pancreozymin, and gastrin.[14]

Even less is known about the function of Paneth and undifferentiated cell secretions.[15] One might expect that these actively secreting cells would contribute important digestive enzymes such as proteases and lipases to the intraluminal contents. However, available data indicate that such enzymes are not produced in the crypts. Indeed, the only major digestive enzymes found in cell-free filtrates of intestinal juice are amylase and enterokinase. Thus, the significance of Paneth and undifferentiated cell secretion simply is not known.

Like other alimentary epithelia, the epithelium of the small intestine is a rapidly proliferating tissue. Although little is known about the secretory function of the crypt epithelium, its major role in the constant renewal of the intestinal epithelium has been firmly established.[16-18]

Cell proliferation in the gut is confined to the intestinal crypts; mitoses are not normally seen on the villi. Within the crypts, the undifferentiated cells divide most actively, although goblet cells are also capable of proliferating. As new cells are formed within the crypts, cells migrate up the wall of the crypts and onto the base of the villus. On the villi, the cells begin to differentiate into absorptive cells; they lose their capacity for proliferation and secretion but begin to develop the specialized features which characterize absorptive cells. Differentiation continues as the cells migrate up the villus until they reach its upper third, where their absorptive capacity reaches its peak and they are fully differentiated cells. When the absorptive cells reach the extreme villous tip, they degenerate, lose their absorptive capacity, and eventually slough off into the intestinal lumen.[16-18]

In man the entire process of cell migration and maturation from cell birth in the crypts to cell loss from the villous tips normally takes place in only five to seven days in the duodenum and jejunum and four to five days in the ileum.[17-19] Thus, the epithelium lining the absorptive surface of the small intestine is normally replaced completely every four to seven days. The rapid cell renewal of this epithelium may at times protect its integrity and, under other circumstances, increase its vulnerability to noxious substances. A continuous intestinal epithelial lining could not be maintained in patients with celiac sprue were it not for its rapid renewal rate. In this disease, absorptive cells are constantly being damaged by gluten and are rapidly sloughed into the gut lumen.[20, 21] Moreover, the rapid repair and healing seen in the small intestine of celiac sprue patients after removal of gluten from the diet is a reflection of the tremendous regenerative potential of the intestinal epithelium. On the other hand, *because* of its great proliferative activity, the intestinal epithelium is particularly susceptible to damage by mitotic inhibitors which interfere with normal cell proliferation. Thus, significant damage to the intestinal epithelium may be seen in patients receiving abdominal irradiation or cancer chemotherapeutic agents which inhibit cell renewal.[22]

In any case, the dynamic nature of this epithelium with its constant and rapid renewal rate must always be considered when one interprets its morphology in normal or pathological conditions.

The epithelium which covers intestinal villi is composed of absorptive cells, goblet cells, and a few endocrine cells. The morphology of the villous goblet and endocrine cells closely resembles that of crypt goblet and endocrine cells. Since major known functions of the villi are

digestion and absorption and the absorptive cells play a major role in these processes, their highly specialized structure will now be considered in some detail.

The absorptive cells are tall, columnar cells with basally located nuclei (Figs. 64–8 and 64–9). The surface they present to the intraluminal intestinal contents is amplified about 30-fold by the numerous finger-like microvilli which form the brush border of their luminal surface. The plasma membrane covering the microvilli is in direct contact with the contents of the bowel lumen and is both morphologically and biochemically distinctive. It is appreciably wider and contains more cholesterol than most apical plasma membranes. Although physiological studies of absorption indicate that the membrane may contain very small pore-like areas of increased permeability, it appears continuous, and pores, if present, cannot be visualized using current morphological methods.

A continuous filamentous-appearing glycoprotein coat is applied directly to the outer surface of the microvillous membrane (Figs. 64–10 and 64–11). This sur-

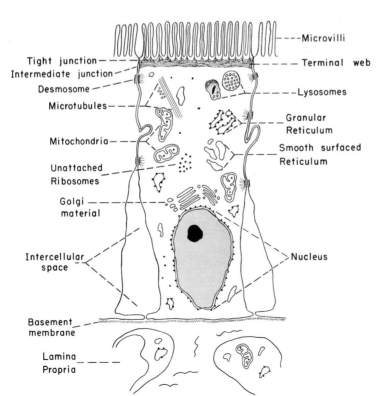

Figure 64–8. Schematic diagram of an intestinal absorptive cell. (Redrawn from Trier, J. S., and Rubin, C. E.: Gastroenterology 49:574, 1965.)

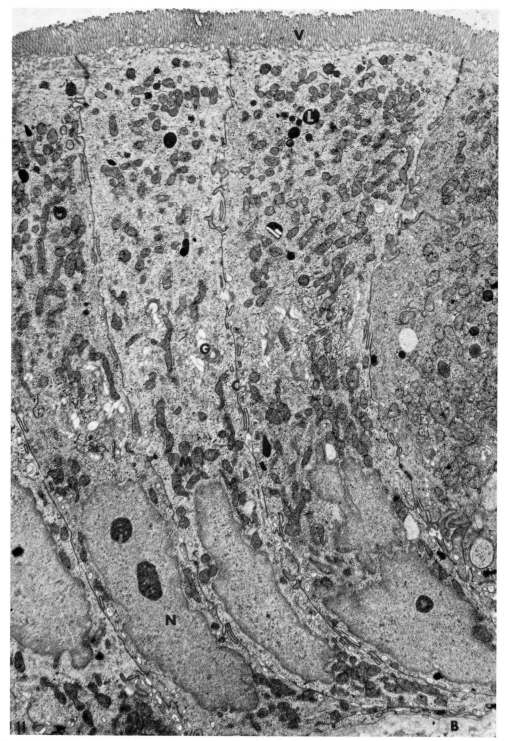

Figure 64–9. Low magnification electron micrograph of intestinal absorptive cells from the middle third of a jejunal villus from a normal man. Basal lamina (B) is seen in the lower right corner. (V) microvilli; (N) nucleus; (G) Golgi material; (L) lysosomes; (M) mitochondria; (C) lateral cell membrane. Approximately × 450. (From Trier, J. S.: Handbook of Physiology: Alimentary Canal, C. Code, Ed. Washington, D.C., American Physiological Society, 1968.)

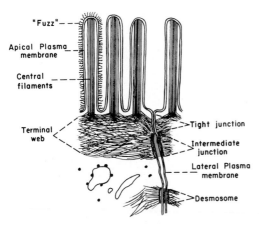

"Fuzz"

Apical Plasma membrane

Central filaments

Terminal web

Tight junction

Intermediate junction

Lateral Plasma membrane

Desmosome

Figure 64–10. Schematic illustration of the specializations of the apical cytoplasm of the plasma membrane of intestinal absorptive cells. (Redrawn from Trier, J. S., and Rubin, C. E.: Gastroenterology 49:574, 1965.)

face coat is well developed in humans and for years was thought to be goblet cell mucus which had been adsorbed onto the microvillous membrane. However, recent work has shown conclusively that this surface coat differs chemically from goblet cell mucus, that it is produced and secreted by the absorptive cells on which it is found, and that it is so firmly attached to the membrane that it cannot be removed even with potent proteolytic and mucolytic agents so long as the absorptive cells remain intact.[23] Hence this glycoprotein fuzzy coat must be considered an integral part of the microvillous membrane of the cells.

The microvillous membrane, together with its surface coat, does more than simply provide an immense surface area which facilitates absorption of nutrients previously digested within the gut lumen. The microvilli participate *actively* in absorptive and digestive phenomena in several ways. First, intraluminal digestive enzymes such as pancreatic amylase and proteases may be adsorbed onto the surface coat, and at least some digestive processes previously thought to occur exclu-

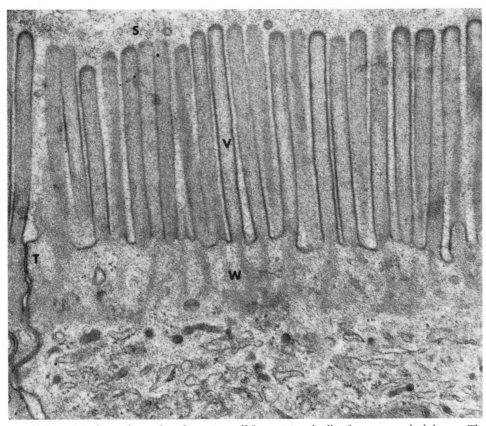

Figure 64–11. Apical cytoplasm of an absorptive cell from a jejunal villus from a normal adult man. The well developed filamentous surface coat (S) lining the microvilli (V) is apparent. A tight junction (T) between adjacent cells is seen to the left at the level of the terminal web (W). Approximately × 27,200.

sively in the lumen, such as the breakdown of large proteins into smaller peptides, actually may take place in part on the microvillous surface. Second, disaccharidases and certain peptidases have been localized to the microvillous membrane–surface coat portion of intestinal absorptive cells, and pure preparations of isolated microvillous membranes covered with their surface coat effectively hydrolyze disaccharides and polypeptides to their constituent monosaccharides and amino acids.[24, 25] Thus, the terminal digestion of carbohydrates and proteins occurs at the level of the microvillous membrane–surface coat complex prior to monosaccharide and amino acid absorption by the cells.[26] Third, there is evidence that specific receptors are located on the microvillous membrane–surface coat complex. These receptors selectively bind substances prior to their absorption and may explain the selective absorption of certain nutrients at specific sites along the small intestine. For example, ileal absorptive cells contain a specific receptor for intrinsic factor–bound vitamin B_{12} on their microvillous surface. In contrast, jejunal absorptive cells do not contain such a receptor, which may explain why normal absorption of physiological quantities of vitamin B_{12} is confined to the ileum.[27] Receptors may also play a role in the absorption of conjugated bile salts, food iron, and calcium, all of which are preferentially absorbed at specific levels of the small intestine, although specific receptors for these substances have not yet been identified.

An important morphological specialization is seen at the upper part of the lateral plasma membrane. Here, the outer leaflets of adjacent plasma membranes fuse to form a "tight junction", which completely obliterates the extracellular space for a short distance (Figs. 64–10 and 64–11).[28] This tight junction has important implications in regard to transport phenomena. It completely encircles the upper part of the lateral aspect of the cell, and it is impermeable to morphologically detectable tracer substances such as protein solutions and suspensions of small particulate material. Similarly, available physiological studies indicate that small ions and molecules which cannot be visualized, such as Na^+, Cl^-, and water, are not actively transported through the tight junction to an appreciable degree, although some passive diffusion may occur at this site. Thus, in general the contents of the gut lumen must cross at least the microvillous membrane, the apical cytoplasm, and the lateral plasma membrane of the absorptive cells to gain access to the intercellular space during absorption (Fig. 64–10).

The intercellular space between adjacent absorptive cells may vary considerably in width from a small fraction of a micron between absorptive cells at the base of the villi to a micron or more between absorptive cells near the tip of the villus. This intercellular space is considerably wider during active absorption; hence its greater width near the tip of the villi is not surprising.[29] A few lymphocytes, macrophages, and eosinophils are normally seen in the spaces between absorptive cells of a given villus. In villi from patients with mucosal disease, the number of such intrusive cells may be markedly increased.

The rim of cytoplasm immediately beneath the microvilli consists of aggregations of amorphous material and is known as the terminal web region (Figs. 64–8 and 64–9). The filaments which form the cores of the microvilli are embedded in the web (Fig. 64–11). The exact function of the web is not known, but it seems likely that it provides important structural support for the microvillous absorptive surface.

Various organelles are distributed in the cytoplasm beneath the terminal web. These include many mitochondria, a variable number of lysosomes, granular and smooth-surfaced endoplasmic reticulum, a well defined supernuclear Golgi complex, microtubules, and a moderate number of unattached ribosomes. Although all the specific functions of each of these organelles in absorptive processes have not been defined precisely, some information is available.

The mitochondria, as in other cells, participate in oxidative reactions which provide energy needed for metabolic processes. The lysosomes probably segregate waste products and cytotoxic substances until they can be either degraded by lytic lysosomal enzymes into useful substances or extruded from the cells.

The endoplasmic reticulum plays an important role in intracellular synthetic and perhaps intracellular transport processes. For example, during fat absorption, the endoplasmic reticulum resynthesizes triglyceride from absorbed monoglyceride and fatty acid (see p. 252). It has also been suggested that the thin liproprotein coat that surrounds chylomicrons is synthesized by the endoplasmic reticulum and applied to the triglyceride droplets as they travel through channels of the endoplasmic reticulum. The endoplasmic reticulum is probably also the major site for synthesis of the digestive enzymes found in absorptive cells such as peptidases and disaccharidases.

The Golgi material, regularly located in the cytoplasm above the nucleus (Figs. 64–8 and 64–9) is connected to the endoplasmic reticulum and is often considered as a specialized component of this membranous system. Available data indicate that the Golgi material segregates, stores, and chemically modifies material absorbed and synthesized by cells.

The basal plasma membrane of normal villous absorptive cells is close to the continuous thin basement membrane which bridges the gap between adjacent lateral plasma membranes (Figs. 64–6 and 64–8). The capillaries and lymphatics in the lamina propria may lie very close to the basal surface of absorptive cells (Fig. 64–6), but absorbed material must always cross the epithelial basement membrane to gain access to these vascular channels.

Thus, in the process of absorption, material first may bind with the glycoprotein surface coat of the microvilli, where some digestion of the adsorbed nutrients may occur. Products of digestion then penetrate the microvillous membrane and traverse the terminal web region and a variable amount of cytoplasmic matrix. The absorbed material may then either enter the intercellular space between absorptive cells by crossing the lateral plasma membrane, or the material may enter the intracellular channels of the endoplasmic reticulum. In the reticulum, the material may be biochemically modified and travel to the Golgi material where it may be further modified or stored. Eventually the material leaves the cell by crossing either the lateral or the basal plasma membrane. Finally, the absorbed material penetrates the epithelial cell basement membrane to enter the lamina propria in which it traverses the lymphatic or capillary endothelial cells to gain access to the lymph or the blood.

REFERENCES

1. Bloom, W., and Fawcett, D. W. The intestines. *In* A Textbook of Histology, Philadelphia, W. B. Saunders Co., 1968, pp. 560–581.
2. Trier, J. S. Morphology of the epithelium of the small intestine. *In* Handbook of Physiology—Alimentary Canal, vol. 3, pp. 1125–1176. Washington, D.C., American Physiological Society, 1968.
3. Trier, J. S. Structure of the mucosa of the small intestine as it relates to intestinal function. Fed. Proc. 26:1391, 1967.
4. Goss, C. M. The digestive system. *In* Gray's Anatomy of the Human Body, C. M. Goss (ed.). pp. 1161–1263: Philadelphia, Lea and Febiger, 1966.
5. Grant, J. C. B., and Basmiajian, J. U. The abdominopelvic cavity. *In* Method of Anatomy. pp. 200–224. Baltimore, Williams and Wilkins Co., 1965.
6. Rubin, C. E., and Dobbins, W. O., III. Peroral biopsy of the small intestine. Gastroenterology 49:676, 1965.
7. Baker, S. J., Ignatius, M., Mathan, V. I., Vaish, S. K., and Chacko, C. C. Intestinal biopsy in tropical sprue. *In* Intestinal Biopsy, G. E. W. Wolstenholme and M. P. Cameron (eds.) Boston, Little, Brown, and Co., 1962, pp. 84–101.
8. Sprinz, H., Sribhibhadh, R., Gangarosa, E. J., Benyajati, C., Kundel, D., and Halstead, S. Biopsy of the small bowel of Thai people. Amer. J. Clin. Path. 38:43, 1962.
9. Brunser, O., Eidelman, S., and Klipstein, F. A. Intestinal morphology of rural Haitians. A comparison between overt tropical sprue and asymptomatic subjects. Gastroenterology 58:655, 1970.
10. Crabbé, P. A., Carbonara, A. O., and Heremans, J. F. The normal human intestinal mucosa as a major source of plasma cells containing γ-A-immunoglobulin. Lab. Invest. 14:235, 1965.
11. Clementi, F., and Palade, G. E. Intestinal capillaries. I. Permeability to peroxidase and ferritin. J. Cell Biol. 41:33, 1969.
12. Erspamer, V., and Asero, B. Identification of enteramine, the specific hormone of the enterochromaffin cell system, as 5-hydroxytryptamine. Nature 169:800, 1952.
13. Oates, J. A., Pettinger, W. A., and Doctor, R. B. Evidence for the release of bradykinin in carcinoid syndrome. J. Clin. Invest. 45:173, 1966.
14. Parat, M. Contribution à l'histo-physiologie des organes digestifs de l'embyron. L'apparation corrélative de la cellule de Kultschitzki et de la sécrétine chez l'embryon. Compt. Rend. Soc. Biol. 90:1023, 1924.
15. Trier, J. S. The Paneth cells: An enigma. Gastroenterology, 51:560, 1966.

16. Leblond, C. P., and Messier, P. Renewal of chief cells and goblet cells in the small intestine as shown by radioautography after injection of thymidine-H[3] into mice. Anat. Rec. *132*:247, 1958.

17. Lipkin, M., Sherlock, P., and Bell, B. Cell proliferation kinetics in the gastrointestinal tract of man. II. Cell renewal in stomach, ileum, colon, and rectum. Gastroenterology *45*:721, 1963.

18. MacDonald, W. C., Trier, J. S., and Everett, N. B. Cell proliferation and migration in the stomach, duodenum, and rectum of man: Radioautographic studies. Gastroenterology *46*:405, 1964.

19. Shorter, R. G., Moertel, C. G., Titus, J. L., and Reitemeier, R. J. Cell kinetics in the jejunum and rectum of man. Amer. J. Dig. Dis. *9*:760, 1964.

20. Padykula, H. A., Strauss, E. W., Ladman, A. J., and Gardner, F. H. A morphologic and histochemical analysis of the human jejunal epithelium in non-tropical sprue. Gastroenterology *40*:735, 1961.

21. Trier, J. S., and Browning, T. H. Epithelial-cell renewal in cultured duodenal biopsies in celiac sprue. New Eng. J. Med. *283*:1245, 1970.

22. Trier, J. S., and Browning, T. H. Morphologic response of the mucosa of human small intestine to X-ray exposure. J. Clin. Invest. *45*:194, 1966.

23. Ito, S. The enteric surface coat on cat intestinal microvilli. J. Cell Biol. *27*:475, 1965.

24. Eichholz, A. Structural and functional organization of the brush border of intestinal epithelial cells. III. Enzymic activities and chemical composition of various fractions of tris-disrupted brush borders. Biochim. Biophys. Acta *135*:475, 1967.

25. Rhodes, J. B., Eichholz, A. and Crane, R. K. Structural and functional organization of the brush border of intestinal epithelial cells. IV. Aminopeptidase activity in microvillus membranes of hamster intestinal brush borders. Biochim. Biophys. Acta *135*:959, 1967.

26. Crane, R. K. Enzymes and malabsorption: A concept of brush border membrane disease. Gastroenterology *50*:254, 1966.

27. Mackenzie, I. L., Donaldson, R. M., Kopp, W. L., and Trier, J. S. Antibodies to intestinal microvillous membranes. II. Inhibition of intrinsic factor–mediated attachment of vitamin B_{12} to hamster brush borders. J. Exp. Med. *128*:375, 1968.

28. Farquhar, M. G., and Palade, G. E. Junctional complexes in various epithelia. J. Cell Biol. *17*:375, 1963.

29. Tomasini, J. T., and Dobbins, W. O. III. Intestinal mucosal morphology during water and electrolyte absorption: A light and electron microscopic study. Amer. J. Dig. Dis. *15*:226, 1970.

Chapter 65

Embryology and Congenital Abnormalities

Charles Krone

EMBRYOLOGY

The intestinal tract in man can be recognized at four weeks of embryonic development as a simple tube stretching from the stomach to the cloaca, joined ventrally to the yolk stalk, and evenly divided into cephalic and caudal limbs supported by a dorsal mesentery. Beginning in the fifth week, the tube elongates, forming a hairpin-shaped primary intestinal loop, extending ventrally into the belly stalk and joined at its apex to the yolk sac by the vitelline or omphalomesenteric duct. The cephalic limb develops into the distal duodenum to proximal ileum; the caudal limb becomes the distal ileum to proximal two-thirds of the transverse colon. The embryonic junction of the cephalic and caudal limbs in the adult can only be recognized if a portion of the vitelline duct persists as a Meckel diverticulum. Further elongation of the primary loop results in temporary umbilical herniation and counterclockwise rotation of the intestine around an axis formed by the superior mesenteric artery, which is located in the dorsal mesentery between the two limbs of the loop. Although a continuous process, it is convenient to divide rotation into three stages. The first, from the fifth to the tenth week of embryonic life, includes umbilical herniation, 90 degree counterclockwise rotation, and return of the in-testine to the abdominal cavity. The proximal jejunum is the first to re-enter the abdomen, and it comes to lie on the left side. Subsequent returning loops settle more and more to the right. The cecal swelling is the last part of the gut to re-enter the abdominal cavity, temporarily located in the right upper quadrant, directly below the right lobe of the liver. During the second stage, between ten and twelve weeks, the cephalic and caudal loops rotate an additional 180 degrees, completing a full 270 degrees with respect to the starting point. The third stage, from the twelfth week to the fifth month, includes further descent of the cecum to its normal position at the level of the iliac crest and fixation to the posterior abdominal wall of the cecum, the ascending and descending colon, and the entire mesentery of the small intestine from the ligament of Treitz to the ileocecal junction.

Histogenesis. The human digestive tract is formed from an entodermal tube, producing the epithelial cells and glands, and an encasing layer of mesoderm, yielding connecting tissue, muscle, and peritoneum. Circular muscle appears by the seventh week, longitudinal by the twelfth. Simple columnar epithelium first lines the entire gastrointestinal tract. Between the sixth and seventh weeks, the epithelial lining of the duodenum proliferates and may result in complete luminal occlusion. Formation of coalescing vacuoles eventually restores the patency of the lumen. This process may be shared to a lesser extent by the entire small and large intestine. Villi develop at the eighth week from rounded elevations in the epithelium. At the base of villi, during the third month, ingrowths of tubular epithelium form the intestinal glands of Lieberkühn. In the duodenum, Brunner's glands shortly follow. This dynamic developmental process continues, with glands and villi increasing in number through childhood. Sucrase activity has been found in the human fetus as early as eight weeks,[1] when it is present equally throughout the proximal and distal intestine and colon. Between the eighth and twenty-sixth weeks of development, a definite increase in sucrase activity of several times magnitude occurs in the proximal small intestine with a loss of activity in the colon. At approximately 20 to 32 weeks, sucrase, maltase, and isomaltase reach the lower range of normal activity found in the adult.[2] Lactase activity is low at 28 weeks of embryonic development, but increases by two- or threefold just before term.[3] Premature infants, therefore, are often lactose intolerant for a number of days until normal lactase activity is achieved. For an extensive review of the histological and biochemical development of the small intestine, the reader is referred to the monograph by Koldovsky.[4]

Spontaneous rhythmic activity of the small intestine is seen at six to seven weeks when nervous elements in Auerbach's plexus are first found. Peristaltic movements of the small intestine develop at approximately the fourth month, and the fetus begins to swallow amniotic fluid at this time. Beginning with the fourth month, an increasing amount of material accumulates in the intestine. This material, *meconium*, consists of a mixture of epithelial cells, lanugo hairs, and sebaceous secretion. The intestinal contents are sterile until postpartum oral feeding begins, at which time a bacterial flora first forms.

CONGENITAL ABNORMALITIES

Classification of the major developmental anomalies of the gastrointestinal tract includes (1) atresia and stenosis, (2) duplication, (3) persistence of vestigial structures and heterotopia, (4) errors of rotation and defective fixation, and (5) defective innervation. Symptomatic disorders resulting from congenital anomalies of the intestine most frequently appear during infancy and childhood, although the presence of a congenital defect may be discovered for the first time in the adult; frequently these are asymptomatic.

CONGENITAL ATRESIA AND STENOSIS

In the classic atresia, the proximal segment of bowel ends blindly with either complete separation of the two segments accompanied by a wedge-shaped defect of the mesentery or the two segments united by a slender, solid, fibrous cord. Stenosis implies an incomplete stricture of the intestine, without loss of continuity of the segments, proximal and distal, to the involved area. The stenotic area may be

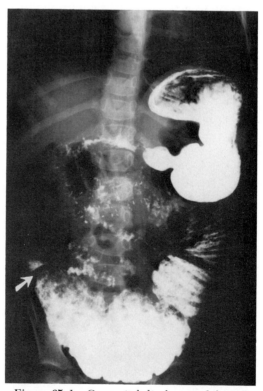

Figure 65–1. Congenital diaphragm of the proximal small intestine producing intestinal obstruction. (Courtesy of Dr. M. Pitt.)

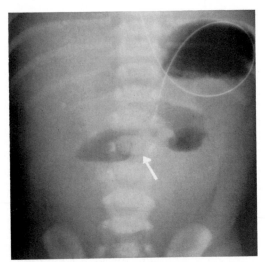

Figure 65–2. Jejunal atresia in a mongoloid. Note that the jejunum ends blindly (arrow). The infant was obstructed. (Courtesy of Dr. C. A. Gooding.)

barely perceptible with either little or no functional disturbance, or markedly strictured with high-grade obstruction (Figs. 65–1, 65–2, and 65–3). Stenosis may also take the form of an intraluminal diaphragm. Intestinal atresia is rare, with an estimated frequency of one in every 20,000 live births. Two mechanisms of pathogenesis have been proposed: a primary developmental defect caused by persistence or failure of resolution of the epithelial proliferative phase during the fifth through eighth weeks of develop-ment, or a later acquired defect caused by vascular insufficiency.[5, 6] Arrest in growth at the solid stage may result in atresia of the duodenum, but there is considerable evidence that this is not the cause of atresia in the jejunum and ileum. Observations at surgery and autopsy reveal evidence of vascular insufficiency at the segment of bowel showing atresia or stenosis. Experimentally, in utero ligation of mesenteric vessels in unborn puppies and lambs leads to intestinal atresia, and incomplete vascular occlusion leads to stenosis.[7] Observation that the bowel distal to the site of atresia frequently contains bile which is not secreted until the eleventh week, squamous cells which are not shed by the fetal skin and swallowed until the third month, and lanugo which is not present until the sixth month suggests that the jejunoileal atresia must occur relatively later in the course of fetal development.

Twenty-five per cent of the cases of intestinal atresia may be due to meconium ileus, and the frequency of mucoviscidosis in atresia is about 9 per cent. The atresia may result from reaction to inspissated meconium or volvulus of the heavy meconium-filled bowel. Intrauterine volvulus, strangulation of internal hernia, and rarely intussusception are considered the most common causes for acquired injury to the small bowel, resulting in small intestinal atresia and stenosis.[8] A report of twin premature females with jejunal atresia and

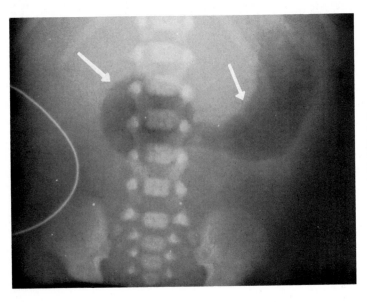

Figure 65–3. Flat film of an infant with acute, complete gastric obstruction due to duodenal atresia, showing the "double bubble" sign. There is air in the duodenum and stomach (arrows). (Courtesy of Dr. C. A. Gooding.)

evidence of congenital rubella suggests that the proliferative vascular lesions found in infants with rubella may also involve the intestine.[9] Several reports of familial intestinal atresia raise the possibility of genetic etiology in some cases, and family history of consanguinity suggests that the genetic disorder may be autosomal recessive.[10, 11]

Clinical Presentation. Intestinal atresia is the most common cause of intestinal obstruction in the first two weeks of life. Infants present with persistent vomiting of bile which may begin within minutes of birth and always within the first 24 hours (Fig. 65–4). Less severe stenosis may not manifest symptoms for weeks or months. Normally the infant evacuates meconium during the first day of life. With intestinal atresia there is usually no stool, but small amounts of grayish-green mucoid material may be passed. Hydramnios has been emphasized as a clue to the early recognition of proximal alimentary tract obstruction. Of principal diagnostic value is the plain film of the abdomen, demonstrating air-filled loops of bowel down to the site of obstruction, with no air distally. This is generally sufficient to assess the nature of the problem, and an upper gastrointestinal

series with barium is unnecessary. A contrast enema has been recommended when doubt exists concerning the location of a distal ileal or colonic obstruction. Recently the hazard of barium enema studies in infants with small bowel atresia has been emphasized, because the distal segment may open freely into the peritoneal cavity.[12] As a barium enema would be deleterious in such instances, it is recommended that water-soluble contrast material be administered routinely.

Jejunoileal atresias may be single or multiple.[13] In patients with atresia, the proximal jejunum is involved in about 30 per cent, distal jejunum 20 per cent, proximal ileum about 15 per cent, and distal ileum 35 per cent. Between 5 and 10 per cent of patients have atresia in more than one location.[14] Atresia, stenosis, and diaphragms in multiple sites having the appearance of a "string of sausages" may involve the entire small bowel, but more commonly are found confined to the middle one-third or one-half of the small intestine.[15] In jejunoileal atresias dissolution of necrotic tissue may result in disruption of the continuity of the bowel and mesentery, and the intestine may be very short, as though most were infarcted and resorbed. The mesentery may show evidence that local early damage resulted in absence of its entire midportion. The blood supply of the distal small bowel then runs through a narrow band of mesentery arising from the ileocecal region with no fixation to the posterior abdominal wall. Subsequent growth of the ileum allows for a "corkscrew" volvulus to wind around this narrow strip of mesentery.[15, 16]

Treatment. Surgical intervention is mandatory in the infant and should promptly follow decompression of the proximal gastrointestinal tract and adequate correction of fluid and electrolyte balance. The dilated, often atonic small intestine proximal to the atresia may fail to function following primary anastomosis. Postoperative obstruction results when adequate proximal resection is not achieved. End-to-end small bowel anastomosis is preferred. Side-to-side anastomoses have been discarded because of the frequent complication of blind loop syndrome[17] (Fig. 65–5). In jejunal atresia adequate resection of the proximal dilated bowel may not be possible or may result in a

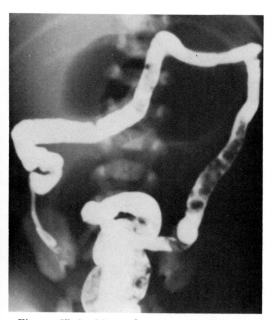

Figure 65–4. Microcolon in a newborn with atretic small bowel and complete small bowel obstruction. (Courtesy of Dr. C. A. Gooding.)

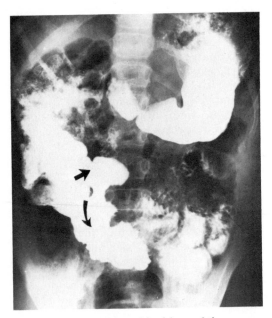

Figure 65–5. A 10-cm blind loop of ileum causing bacterial overgrowth and malabsorption syndrome in a ten-year-old girl. Extensive ileal atresia was discovered two days post partum and an ileal resection with side-to-side ileocecal anastomosis performed (straight arrow). Bacterial overgrowth and malabsorption were corrected by transection of the blind sac (curved arrow). (Courtesy of Dr. E. Weser.)

marked loss of absorptive surface. A technique for a tapering jejunoplasty with end-to-end jejunojejunostomy has recently been described which allows for conservation of bowel while promoting effective peristalsis in such situations.[18]

In 1950, Evans noted a mortality rate of 91 per cent on collected review of 1498 cases of intestinal atresia. From 1957 to 1967, survival in jejunal atresia was almost 60 per cent and in ileal atresia was about 65 per cent.[5, 14] Infant survival is significantly improving and is now principally determined by the concomitant presence of other developmental anomalies less frequently found with jejunoileal than with duodenal atresias. Congenital atresia and stenosis of the small intestine is predominantly a problem of infancy; however, recurrent attacks of abdominal pain and vomiting may be encountered as late as the fifth decade in patients with multiple congenital stenotic segments of the ileum.[19]

DUPLICATIONS

A duplication is a spherical or tubular cyst intimately attached to a portion of the gastrointestinal tract. Intestinal duplications are invariably on the mesenteric side of the gut, usually between the leaves of the mesentery. The pathogenesis remains unknown, although two theories have been popular, including the persistence of budding diverticula normally seen in early development of the gut and persistence of isolated vacuoles which are normally present within the occluded lumen during the solid stage of intestinal development. For classification as a true duplication, there must be intimate adherence of the cystic structure to the gut, a smooth muscle wall, and a gastrointestinal type mucosal lining. The duplication may or may not communicate with the gastrointestinal tract. Those with communication are most frequently lined with gastric mucosa. Most duplications are seen in the ileum, although they may occasionally be found in the jejunum.[20, 21]

There are three basic types of duplications: large single, long tubular, and smaller intramural cysts. The large single cyst may cause symptoms owing to obstruction of the attached bowel from pressure caused by distention of the cyst, or may present as a visible or palpable mass on examination. Although the large spherical cysts generally do not communicate with the bowel, the long tubular duplications commonly do (Fig. 65–6). Frequently they are lined by gastric mucosa which may cause peptic ulceration of the adjacent bowel with complications of gastrointestinal bleeding and/or perforation. The smaller intramural cysts are most common at or near the ileocecal valve and may cause intestinal obstruction by compression of the ileum at the entrance to the cecum or, more commonly, by causing intussusception (see p. 345).

Symptoms resulting from intestinal duplication may present in early life or may first be noted in adulthood. Not infrequently, asymptomatic duplications are found incidentally at laparotomy in the course of surgery for an unrelated problem. The preoperative diagnosis is often difficult and is not usually made until the time of laparotomy. Large enterogenous

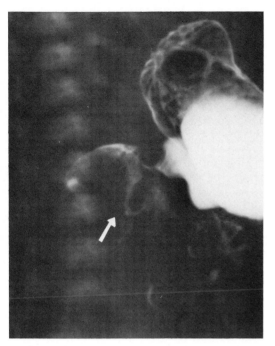

Figure 65-6. Duodenal duplication causing acute gastric obstruction by compromising the lumen. Arrow indicates the duplication, containing contrast substance. (Courtesy of Dr. C. A. Gooding.)

cysts may be readily removed at surgery, but the long duplications may require resection of both duplication and segment of the main channel because frequently blood supply and muscle layers are intimately shared.

MECKEL'S DIVERTICULUM

Meckel's diverticulum is the most frequent congenital anomaly of the intestinal tract, having an incidence of 0.3 to 3.0 per cent in autopsy reports; it most commonly remains asymptomatic throughout life.[22] Of the patients presenting with complications, 60 per cent are under two years of age and more than one-third are less than one year. At birth the vitelline duct normally is completely obliterated, the closure proceeding from the umbilicus inward. With incomplete obliteration the intestinal end of the duct persists as a sac. Occasionally the blind end is joined to the umbilicus by a fibrous band, and rarely the vitelline duct persists intact, maintaining a patent communication between ileum and the umbilicus from which intestinal con-

tents may escape. The diverticulum arises from the antimesenteric border of the ileum, usually within 100 cm of the ileocecal valve (the average being between 80 and 85 cm), is usually approximately 2 inches in length, and ends blindly.[23] It contains all the layers of the intestinal tract. The mouth of the sac is wide, often being equal to the width of the intestinal lumen itself. About 45 per cent of resected diverticula contain normal ileal mucosa. Gastric, duodenal, colonic, and pancreatic ectopic mucosa has been described, of which 80 to 85 per cent is gastric, and is most often found close to the mouth of the diverticulum. Blood is supplied through a terminal branch of the superior mesenteric artery which is carried to the diverticulum by a separate mesentery.

Complications of Meckel's diverticulum include hemorrhage, intestinal obstruction, diverticulitis, umbilical discharge, and perforation with peritonitis. Rarely the diverticulum becomes incarcerated in an indirect inguinal hernia (Littre's). Prolapse of a short segment of ileum through a patent vitelline duct may produce a complicated form of intussusception. Rarely foreign bodies may become impacted in Meckel's diverticulum and a neoplasm may develop within the wall of the diverticulum.

Bleeding is the most common complication, resulting from ulceration of ileal mucosa adjacent to contained ectopic gastric mucosa; it is most frequently painless, and is usually encountered in children less than two years of age. Meckel's diverticulum accounts for nearly half of all lower gastrointestinal bleeding in children.[24] Only infrequently can a diagnosis be made by X-ray study. Gas filling the pouch, or a large opaque stone, may occasionally be recognized on plain film of the abdomen. Less commonly, barium may fill the diverticulum (Fig. 65-7). The diagnosis is usually made in the operating room. In adults, mesenteric angiography may be helpful in identifying the site of bleeding.

The principal mechanisms causing intestinal obstruction are intussusception with the diverticulum as lead point and herniation through, or volvulus around, a persistent fibrous cord remnant of the vitelline duct which may extend to the ab-

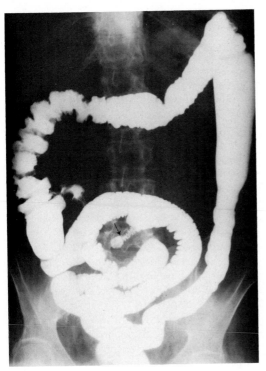

Figure 65–7. Barium-filled Meckel's diverticulum.

dominal wall, base of mesentery, or an adjacent segment of bowel. Early surgical intervention is mandatory for survival (see pp. 344 to 346).

Diverticulitis may produce a clinical picture indistinguishable from acute appendicitis. Failure to find an inflamed appendix necessitates making a search for a Meckel diverticulum. Perforation may occur, associated with thrombosis of the blood supply to the diverticulum.

Peptic ulceration may cause postprandial abdominal pain. Rarely it may result in obstruction comparable to pyloric stenosis.

Local excision should be performed whenever a Meckel diverticulum is discovered at surgery, even when found incidentally, because of the potential complications. Following local excision, the intestine is repaired in the transverse axis so that narrowing does not follow. Ligation and invagination by purse-string suture is not performed, as it frequently leads to intussusception. Occasionally, a resection of intestine containing the diverticulum is necessary and end-to-end anastomosis is performed.

ANOMALIES OF ROTATION AND FIXATION

Aberrations of intestinal rotation result in anomalous position of the small intestine and colon and abnormal fixations and bands predisposing to internal herniation and volvulus. These anomalies may be classified according to the stage of rotation in which they occur.

Malrotation in the first stage results in failure of reduction of herniated midgut back into the celomic cavity. All the midgut and often other viscera, such as liver, stomach, spleen, or colon, remain in the umbilical sac as an *omphalocele*. Coils of intestine are found protruding through the large umbilical ring covered by a protective jelly-like matrix of umbilical tissue. Immediate surgical attention is required.

Four types of anomalies may occur from faulty rotation during the second stage: nonrotation, malrotation, reversed rotation, and paraduodenal hernia. The midgut, upon returning to the abdominal cavity, may fail to rotate. In this anomaly, referred to as *nonrotation*, the duodenum descends in a straight line downward to the right of the superior mesenteric artery in direct continuity with the small bowel, and is located in the right half of the abdominal cavity with the transverse colon, looping around itself in a U-shaped fashion. The colon lies entirely on the left, and the terminal ileum enters the cecum by crossing the midline from the right. *Malrotation* is the most common of anomalies of the second stage, and is essentially a form of incomplete rotation. The midgut may fail to complete the process of rotation through the entire arc of 180 degrees. Instead, it may become arrested at any point along the way, and the cecum may be found at the splenic level, in front of the superior mesenteric vessels, or, as most frequently found, in the subhepatic position. Invariably, unusual attachments and adhesions are associated with malrotation. *Reversed rotation* is a very rare anomaly. The midgut, instead of performing a counterclockwise movement of 180 degrees, rotates in a reversed, or clockwise, direction to an arc of 90 degrees. The cecum and the transverse colon pass through the root of the mesentery behind the superior mesenteric artery with the duodenum in front.

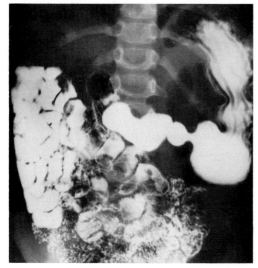

Figure 65–8. Malrotation of the small intestine in an infant with a mass felt in the right upper quadrant. Note the absence of the jejunum in the left upper quadrant. (Courtesy of Dr. C. A. Gooding.)

The opening in the mesentery through which they pass is often very small, and the risk of obstruction at this point is great. The ascending colon and cecum are not fixed posteriorly. A rare condition, *paraduodenal hernia,* may occur to the right or the left of the duodenum, resulting from incomplete rotation of either the cephalic or the caudal segment of the midgut.

Anomalous conditions arising from the third stage of rotation are generally due to deficient peritoneal fixation or incomplete fusion of the mesentery of the midgut. These commonly involve the cecum and the ascending colon also. The small bowel may have a mesentery with a long and narrow pedicle with deficient fixation (Fig. 65–8). The second or third portion of the duodenum may also be free and mobile.

Complications of anomalies in rotation include volvulus and incarceration of bowel in an internal hernia. Volvulus results from abnormal fixation of the intestine, the midgut often twisting about its long narrow pedicle during the first few days of life. In addition, obstruction may result from abnormal bands and defective fixations, causing internal hernia commonly involving the descending duodenum. Adults found to have anomalous rotation are most frequently asymptomatic, and gastrointestinal symptoms may erroneously be attributed to such abnormalities. Symptoms can be reliably attributed to malrotation only when evidence of intestinal obstruction is present. Among infants and children the major pathological

Figure 65–9. Acute gastric and duodenal obstruction in an infant with malrotation of the duodenum. Arrow indicates characteristic cone-shaped terminus. (Courtesy of Dr. C. A. Gooding.)

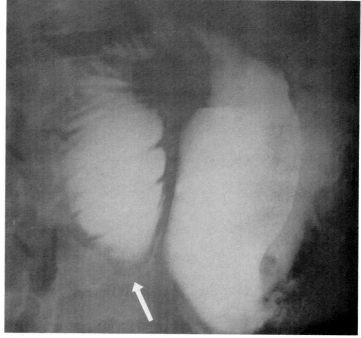

problems are obstruction of the descending duodenum and volvulus of the midgut (Fig. 65–9). In about half of such cases the two lesions occur together.[25] About half of adult cases will present with acute intestinal obstruction, principally caused by volvulus of the cecum and ascending colon; the other causes of acute obstruction are volvulus of the sigmoid flexure or of the small bowel. About one-third of patients will present with chronic intestinal obstruction; the majority of them will have chronic cecal torsion, and the remainder pyloric obstruction.[26]

Although roentgenographic examination is helpful, exploratory laparotomy systematically conducted is necessary to make an accurate anatomical diagnosis. Often the anatomical relationship of the midgut is greatly distorted, and identification and localization of various parts of the bowel are difficult. The surgical principles for orderly correction of malrotation promulgated by Ladd in 1936 still apply: (1) reduction, or resection, of midgut volvulus, if present; (2) release of peritoneal bands which hold the colon in its abnormal position; and (3) thorough exploration of the duodenum and relief of any obstruction. Other congenital abnormalities may accompany anomalies of intestinal rotation, particularly duodenal stenosis or atresia, and these must be searched for at the time of surgery.[25] Congenital short intestine has been described in association with malrotation.[27, 28]

The results of surgery are excellent and usually permanent.[29] Normal alimentary function generally follows several days after surgery. Failure to obtain a satisfactory postoperative result should suggest additional congenital anomalies not recognized at the time of surgery.

MISCELLANEOUS ABNORMALITIES

A number of rather rare congenital abnormalities of the small intestine have been described. Isolated heterotopic gastric mucosa has been found in the small intestine, appearing as tumorous, polypoid, nodular, or rugose masses of up to 3 to 12 cm in size. Lesions have resulted in intussusception or bleeding, or have been recognized as a polyp on X-ray in the absence of associated symptoms.[30] Only 16 cases have been reported in the literature,

and those most commonly in the proximal jejunum.

A very rare disorder of segmental absence of intestinal musculature may be encountered in a neonate with intestinal obstruction caused by intussusception in which segments of ileum entirely lack muscle layers and contain only mucosa and serosa.[31]

Hirschsprung's disease involving the entire colon and distal small intestine has been described.[32] Rarely, small intestinal aganglionosis may extend up to the jejunum. High mortality has been associated with failure to recognize the nature of the abnormality preoperatively. Plain film of the abdomen reveals small intestinal obstruction of a distal type, as in ileal atresia. However, gas may be seen in the rectum, and barium enema may reveal a small, but yet "used," colon (see pp. 1463 to 1471).

REFERENCES

1. Jirsova, V. Development of invertase activity in the intestines of human fetuses, appearance of jejunoileal differences. Biol. Neonat. 13:143, 1968.
2. Dahlquist, A., and Lindberg, T. Development of the intestinal disaccharidase and alkaline phosphatase activities in the human fetus. Clin. Sci. 30:517, 1966.
3. Bayless, T. M., and Christopher, N. L. Disaccharidase deficiency. Amer. J. Clin. Nutr. 22:181, 1969.
4. Koldovsky, O. Development of the Functions of the Small Intestine in Mammals and Man. New York, S. Karger, 1969, pp. 139–178.
5. White, J. J., Tecklenberg, P. L., Esterly, J. R., and Haller, J. A. Changing concepts in the management of intestinal atresia. Surg. Clin. N. Amer. 50:863, 1970.
6. Nixon, H. H., and Tawes, R. Etiology and treatment of small intestinal atresia: Analysis of a series of 127 jejunoileal atresias. Surgery 69:41, 1971.
7. Abrams, J. S. Experimental intestinal atresia. Surgery 64:185, 1968.
8. Grosfeld, J. L., and Clatworthy, H. W., Jr. The nature of ileal atresia due to intrauterine intussusception. Arch. Surg. 100:714, 1970.
9. Esterly, J. R., and Talbert, J. L. Jejunal atresia in twins with presumed congenital rubella. Lancet 1:1028, 1969.
10. Mishalany, H. G., and Najjar, F. B. Familial jejunal atresia: Three cases in one family. J. Pediat. 73:753, 1968.
11. Mishalany, H. G., and Derkaloustian, V. M. Familial multiple-level intestinal atresias: Report of two siblings. J. Pediat. 79:124, 1971.
12. Wolfson, J. J., and Williams, H. A hazard of barium enema studies in infants with small bowel atresia. Radiology 95:341, 1970.

13. Shafie, M. E., and Richham, P. P. Multiple intestinal atresia. J. Pediat. Surg. 5:655, 1970.
14. Delorimier, A. A., Fonkalsrud, E. W., and Hays, D. M. Congenital atresia and stenosis of the jejunum and ileum. Surgery 65:817, 1969.
15. Spencer, R. The various patterns of intestinal atresia. Surgery 64:661, 1968.
16. Weitzman, J. J., and Vanderhoof, R. S. Jejunal atresia with agenesis of the dorsal mesentery. With "Christmas tree" deformity of the small intestine. Amer. J. Surg. 111:443, 1966.
17. Santulli, T. V., Chen, C. C., and Schullinger, J. N. Management of congenital atresia of the intestine. Amer. J. Surg. 119:542, 1970.
18. Thomas, C. G., Jr. Jejunoplasty for the correction of jejunal atresia. Surg. Gynec. Obstet. 129:545, 1969.
19. Naunton, M. M. Multiple congenital stenoses of the ileum in an adult. Gut 6:92, 1965.
20. Anderson, M. C., Silberman, W. W., and Shields, T. V. Duplication of the alimentary tract in the adult. Arch. Surg. 85:94, 1962.
21. Chavez, C. M., and Timmis, H. H. Duplication cysts of the gastrointestinal tract. Amer. J. Surg. 110:960, 1965.
22. Johns, T. N. P., Wheeler, J. R., and Johns, F. S. Meckel's diverticulum disease: A study of 154 cases. Ann. Surg. 150:241, 1959.
23. Berne, A. S. Meckel's diverticulum. New Eng. J. Med. 260:690, 1959.
24. Rutherford, R. B., and Akers, D. R. Meckel's diverticulum: A review of 148 pediatric pa-

tients, with special reference to the pattern of bleeding and to mesodiverticula vascular bands. Surgery 59:618, 1966.
25. Gross, R. E. The Surgery of Infancy and Childhood. Philadelphia, W. B. Saunders Co., 1953, pp. 192-203.
26. Wang, C., and Welch, C. E. Anomalies of intestinal rotation in adolescents and adults. Surgery 54:839, 1963.
27. Hamilton, J. R., Reilly, B. J., and Morecki, R. Short small intestine associated with malrotation: A newly described congenital cause of intestinal malabsorption. Gastroenterology 56:124, 1969.
28. Konvolinka, C. W. Congenital short small intestine: A rare occurrence. J. Pediat. Surg. 5:574, 1970.
29. Rees, J. R., and Redo, S. F. Anomalies of intestinal rotation and fixation. Amer. J. Surg. 116:834,1968.
30. Weismann, R. R. Tumorous heterotopic gastric mucosa in the small intestine. Arch. Surg. 100:619, 1970.
31. Steiner, D. H., Maxwell, J. G., Rasmussen, B. L., and Jones, R. Segmental absence of intestinal musculature. An unusual cause of intestinal obstruction in the neonate. Amer. J. Surg. 118:964, 1969.
32. Coran, A. G., Bjordal, R., Eek, S., and Knutrud, O. The surgical management of total colonic and partial small intestinal aganglionosis. J. Pediat. Surg. 4:531, 1969.

Chapter 66

Celiac Sprue Disease

Jerry S. Trier

DEFINITION

A precise definition of celiac sprue seems essential; without one, classification of intestinal malabsorptive disease becomes hopelessly confused. The many other names used to identify patients with this disease (celiac disease, idiopathic steatorrhea, nontropical sprue, adult celiac disease, gluten-induced enteropathy, etc.) provide testimony for the confusion of the past. Since this disease has the same clinical features, etiology, pathology, and response to treatment in children and in adults, the term celiac sprue[1] seems the most suitable and will be used in this chapter.

Celiac sprue is a disease in which there is (1) actual or potential intestinal malabsorption of virtually all nutrients, (2) a characteristic if not specific lesion of the small intestinal mucosa, and (3) prompt clinical improvement following withdrawal of certain gluten-containing cereal grains from the diet. The prevalence of the disease, which has been estimated at 0.03 per cent of the general population,[2] is not really known, because the typical intestinal celiac sprue lesion and the potential for eventually developing overt disease may be present in apparently asymptomatic individuals.[3] Although for years it was thought that celiac sprue occurred only in countries with temperate climates, the disease must now be considered worldwide in its distribution, because there

have recently been convincing descriptions of celiac sprue occurring in natives of tropical countries.[4, 5]

HISTORY

Although the literature pertaining to celiac sprue is quite voluminous, a few reports have provided particularly important conceptual contributions to our understanding of this disease. Thaysen, in 1932, provided a clinical description of the disease in adults, although he was totally unaware of the pathology of the intestinal lesion.[6] In 1950, Dicke suggested, in a landmark study, that certain dietary cereal grains were harmful to children with celiac sprue.[7] He astutely noted that the incidence of celiac sprue in children in Holland during World War II was markedly reduced and that previously diagnosed celiac patients seemed to improve during the war years. During this period, grain products such as wheat and rye flour were in short supply in Holland, and dietary carbohydrate was obtained from vegetable sources. In other European countries where, during the same period, cereal grains were more available, the incidence of celiac sprue did not appear reduced. Moreover, when cereal grains again became plentiful in Holland after the war, the incidence of celiac sprue returned rapidly to prewar levels. Subsequently, van de Kamer, Weijers, and Dicke[8] showed that the water-insoluble protein or gluten moiety of wheat was the substance which damaged the small intestine of patients with celiac sprue.

In 1954, Paulley, studying surgical biopsy material, provided the first accurate description of the characteristic intestinal lesion in patients with celiac sprue.[9] With the development of effective peroral suction biopsy instruments in the late 1950's, Rubin and coworkers[10] demonstrated convincingly that celiac disease in children and idiopathic or nontropical sprue in adults were identical diseases with the same clinical and pathological features.

PATHOLOGY

Celiac sprue affects primarily the mucosa of the small intestine; the submucosa, muscularis, and serosa are usually not involved, and their histology is normal. The mucosal lesion of the small intestine in patients with celiac sprue may vary considerably in both severity and extent.[10] This spectrum of pathological involvement helps explain the striking variability of the clinical manifestations of this disease.

Examination of the mucosal surface of biopsies from untreated celiac sprue patients with severe lesions with a hand lens or a dissecting microscope reveals a flat mucosal surface with complete absence of normal intestinal villi. Histological examination of tissue sections confirms this loss of normal villous structure (Fig. 66-1, A).

The mucosal surface is flat, villi are absent, and the intestinal crypts are markedly elongated and open onto a flat, absorptive surface. The total thickness of the mucosa is normal or only slightly reduced in most cases, because hypertrophy of the crypts compensates for the absence or shortening of the villi.[11] As shown by Rubin and coworkers,[10] these architectural changes decrease the amount of epithelial surface available for digestion and absorption in the involved bowel. Striking cytological abnormalities characterize the relatively few absorptive cells that line the luminal surface. These cells, which appear columnar in normal biopsy specimens, are cuboidal or almost squamous in celiac sprue biopsies. Their cytoplasm is more basophilic, the basal po-

larity of the nuclei is lost, and the brush or striated border is markedly attenuated (Fig. 66-1, B). When viewed with the electron microscope, the microvilli of the absorptive cells appear significantly shortened and often fused (Fig. 66-2). The number of free ribosomes is increased and accounts for the increase in cytoplasmic basophilia evident in histological preparations. Moreover, degenerative changes, including cytoplasmic and mitochondrial vacuolization and the presence of many large lysosomes, are obvious in many of the absorptive cells (Fig. 66-2).[12]

Many of the enzymes which contribute to digestive-absorptive processes are decreased in these damaged absorptive cells. These include disaccharidases, peptidases, alkaline phosphatase, adenosine triphosphatase, and esterases.[13, 14] Thus, not only are absorptive cells reduced in number in celiac sprue patients, but those that are present are functionally compromised.

Unlike the absorptive cells, the undifferentiated crypt cells are markedly increased in number in severe untreated celiac sprue and this accounts for the marked lengthening of crypts. Moreover, the number of mitoses in crypts is strikingly increased.[13, 15] The cytology and histochemistry of the crypt cells are normal both by light and electron microscopy.[12] Thus there are normal numbers of normal-appearing Paneth, goblet, and enterochromaffin cells and greater than normal numbers of normal-appearing undifferentiated cells in the crypts of patients with severe lesions.

The cellularity of the lamina propria is regularly increased in the involved small intestine. The cellular infiltrate consists largely of immunoglobulin-producing plasma cells and lymphocytes. In normal bowel, IgA-producing cells are most abundant, but in many sprue patients, IgM-producing cells predominate.[16, 17] Polymorphonuclear leukocytes may contribute substantially to the increased cellularity of the lamina propria.

The length of small intestine which shows the celiac sprue lesion in untreated patients varies from patient to patient and correlates with the severity of clinical symptoms.[18] Thus the patient with a severe lesion which involves the length of the small bowel will be much sicker and

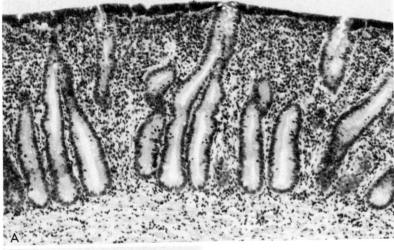

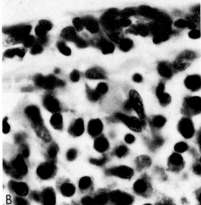

Figure 66–1. Mucosal pathology in celiac sprue. *A,* Mucosa from the duodenojejunal junction of a man with untreated celiac sprue. The mucosal surface is flat, villi are absent, and the crypts are markedly hypertrophied. There is increased cellularity of the lamina propria. × 80.

B, Higher magnification of surface absorptive cells shown in *A*. The cells are cuboidal, without a well defined apical striated border. There is marked loss of nuclear polarity. × 650.

Figure 66–1 continued on opposite page.

have far greater malabsorption than the patient with a severe duodenal lesion, a milder jejunal lesion, and a normal ileum. When the intestinal lesion does not involve the entire length of the small gut, the proximal bowel is the most severely involved and the lesion decreases in severity toward the distal small intestine. Sparing of the proximal intestine and involvement of the distal small intestine do not occur in celiac sprue.

In some untreated patients with relatively mild celiac sprue, not even the proximal intestine shows the typical severe flat lesion. Rather, some residual villous structure remains (Fig. 66–3) and the absorptive surface, although less than normal, is greater than that seen in severely diseased mucosa.[1] However, some shortening of the villi, hypertrophy of the crypts, cytologically abnormal sur-

face cells, and increased cellularity of the lamina propria must be seen in biopsies from patients with untreated disease in order to establish the diagnosis.

Appropriate treatment with a gluten-free diet results in significant improvement in intestinal structure in celiac sprue patients (Fig. 66–1, *C*). The cytology of the surface absorptive cells improves first, often within a few days.[15] Tall, columnar absorptive cells with basal nuclei and well developed brush borders replace the abnormal cuboidal surface cells which were exposed to gluten (Fig. 66–1, *D*). Subsequently, villous architecture reverts toward normal with lengthening of the villi, shortening of the crypts, and a decrease in the cellularity of the lamina propria. The mucosa of the distal small intestine improves more rapidly than that of the severely involved proximal bowel.[18] Months or even years of

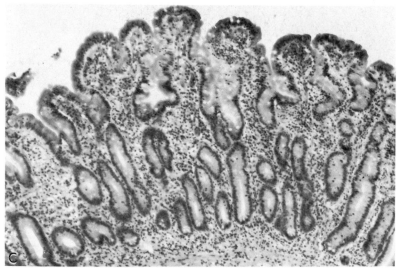

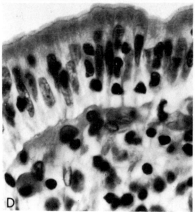

Figure 66–1 Continued. C, Mucosa from the duodenojejunal junction from the same patient shown in A after four weeks of gluten withdrawal. The mucosal architecture is definitely improved. Villi can be recognized, but mucosal architecture is still abnormal because villi are short and crypt hypertrophy and increased cellularity of the lamina propria persist. × 80.

D, Higher magnification of the surface absorptive cells from the biopsy specimen shown in C. The absorptive cells are columnar, with basally located nuclei and a well defined striated border after four weeks of gluten withdrawal. × 650.

gluten withdrawal may be required in some patients before mucosal structure reverts maximally toward normal; indeed, complete reversion to normal is relatively uncommon, and some residual abnormality, which may be striking or subtle, persists in the proximal bowel of most patients.

Patients have been described who allegedly have celiac sprue but who fail to respond to gluten withdrawal, but such reports require cautious interpretation. For example, Pink and Creamer[19] recently reported a group of patients with a flat intestinal mucosa, who they thought had celiac sprue. Not only did these patients not improve on a gluten-free diet, but their disease often progressed. Not only was their clinical response to gluten with-

drawal atypical for celiac sprue, but the histology of their mucosal lesion differed in that Paneth cells were diminished or absent and mitoses were decreased in the crypts. These patients appear to have a mucosal disease which *resembles* celiac sprue but which has distinctive histological features, a different response to treatment, and a grave prognosis. They should not be confused with celiac sprue patients.

Another rare condition which may cause confusion is collagenous sprue. Patients with this recently defined condition may present initially with symptoms and biopsy findings consistent with celiac sprue. However, they fail to respond to dietary gluten withdrawal and, with time, develop extensive deposition of collagen in the lamina propria just beneath the ab-

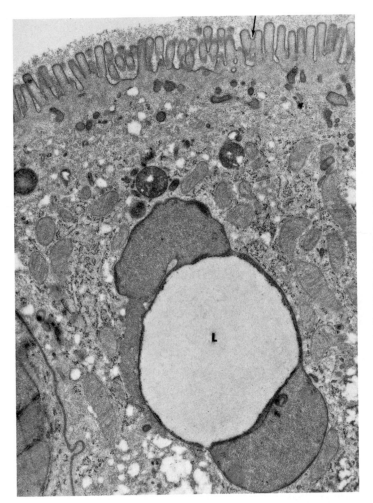

Figure 66–2. Electron micrograph of apical cytoplasm of a surface absorptive cell from a man with untreated celiac sprue. The microvilli are markedly shortened and some are fused (arrow), although the surface coat is well developed. A huge lysosome-like body (L) is prominent in the cytoplasm. There are more free ribosomes and fewer elements of membranous endoplasmic reticulum than in normal absorptive cells. × 10,000.

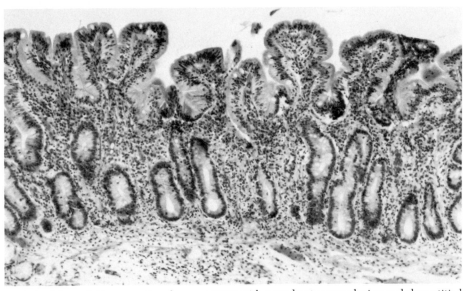

Figure 66–3. Mucosal biopsy section from a patient with a moderate sprue lesion and dermatitis herpetiformis. Villi are present but they are significantly shorter than normal and the crypts are hypertrophied. The cellularity of the lamina is increased, and the absorptive epithelium is infiltrated by mononuclear cells. × 80.

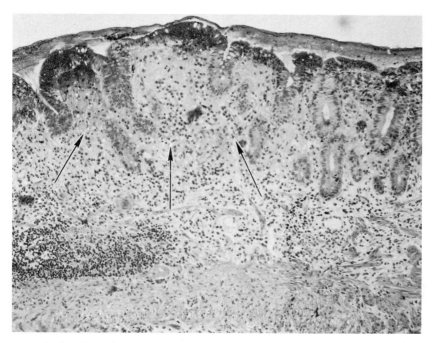

Figure 66–4. The histological appearance of jejunal mucosa from a patient with collagenous sprue. Note the deposition of collagen in the lamina propria, particularly beneath the absorptive epithelium (arrows). Crypts are decreased in number. Masson trichrome stain. × 80. (Courtesy of Dr. L. L. Brandborg.)

TABLE 66–1. EXTRAINTESTINAL MANIFESTATIONS OF CELIAC SPRUE DISEASE

ORGAN SYSTEM	MANIFESTATION	PROBABLE CAUSE(S)
Hematopoietic	Anemia	Iron, folate, vitamin B_{12}, or pyridoxine deficiency
	Hemorrhage	Hypoprothrombinemia and, rarely, thrombocytopenia due to folate deficiency
Skeletal	Osteomalacia	Malabsorption of calcium and vitamin D
	Osteoporosis	Malabsorption of amino acids causing negative nitrogen balance
	Pathological fractures	Osteomalacia and osteoporosis
	Osteoarthropathy	Unknown
Muscular	Atrophy	Malnutrition due to panmalabsorption
	Tetany	Calcium, vitamin D and/or magnesium malabsorption
	Weakness	Generalized muscle atrophy hypokalemia
Nervous	Peripheral neuropathy	Vitamin deficiencies such as thiamine and vitamin B_{12}
	Demyelinating central nervous system lesions	Unknown
Endocrine	Secondary hyperparathyroidism	Calcium and vitamin D malabsorption causing hypocalcemia
	Secondary hypopituitarism	Malnutrition due to panmalabsorption
Integument	Follicular hyperkeratosis and dermatitis	Vitamin A malabsorption, ? vitamin B complex malabsorption
	Petechiae and ecchymoses	Hypoprothrombinemia and, rarely, thrombocytopenia
	Edema	Hypoproteinemia
	Dermatitis herpetiformis	Unknown

sorptive epithelium (Fig. 66–4).[20] Unlike celiac sprue, the prognosis in collagenous sprue is grim; all reported patients have died from the disease.

In addition to the typical lesion of the small intestine, mild, nonspecific histological changes are seen in the rectal mucosa of some but not all celiac sprue patients.[21] These mimic the changes of mild proctitis and may include branching and disorganization of the rectal glands and an increase in the cellularity of the lamina propria. Also, the incidence of histologically evident gastritis is reported to be greater in celiac sprue patients than in normal individuals.

In the severely depleted patient with severe untreated celiac sprue, pathological changes may be present in many other organ systems besides the digestive tract. Detailed description and discussion of these diverse pathological changes are not within the scope of this book, but some of the more commonly encountered extraintestinal manifestations are listed in Table 66–1 (see pp. 259 to 277).

ETIOLOGY AND PATHOGENESIS

The interaction of the water-insoluble protein moiety (gluten) of certain cereal grains with the mucosa of the small intestine is crucial in the pathogenesis of celiac sprue. Instillation of wheat, barley, or rye flour into a histologically normal-appearing segment of small intestine of an asymptomatic patient with treated celiac sprue produces bloating, malaise, abdominal cramps, and diarrhea within a few hours.[8, 22, 23] The fecal fat excretion increases acutely, and the intestinal segment exposed to the gluten develops the typical mucosal lesion of celiac sprue within eight to 12 hours.[22] In contrast, instillation of rice or corn flour into a normal-appearing segment produces neither clinical symptoms nor histological changes. Instillation of oat flour seems toxic to some but not all celiac sprue patients, although the symptoms and histological changes are always less pronounced than those produced by wheat, barley, or rye flour.

Gliadin, a complex mixture of proteins obtained by alcohol extraction of wheat gluten, will also produce symptoms and histological lesions when instilled into the small intestine of asymptomatic celiac sprue patients. Similarly, certain peptic-tryptic digests of wheat gluten produce steatorrhea when fed to celiac sprue patients. The toxic substances in these digests appear to be relatively low molecular weight acidic polypeptides rich in glutamine.[24] The peptide structure seems essential for toxicity, because gliadin which has been hydrolyzed to its constituent amino acids is nontoxic and produces neither symptoms nor an intestinal lesion when fed to asymptomatic celiac sprue patients (Table 66–2).[25]

How toxic gluten damages the intestinal mucosa is not known. Two possible mechanisms which have been suggested are (1) that celiac sprue is caused by an immunological reaction to dietary gluten and (2) that celiac sprue is a metabolic disease in which gluten is incompletely digested, resulting in the accumulation of toxic substances which damage the mucosa.

Three major types of evidence are cited to support the immunological cause theory. First, circulating antibodies to gluten fractions are present in the serum of a significant percentage of celiac sprue patients.[26] However, some celiac sprue patients do not have detectable circulating antibodies to gluten, and there is no correlation between the presence of the antibodies and the severity of the disease. Moreover, some celiac sprue patients have

TABLE 66–2. TOXICITY OF GRAINS AND WHEAT FRACTIONS TO PATIENTS WITH CELIAC SPRUE DISEASE

GRAINS	TOXICITY
Wheat	+
Barley	+
Rye	+
Oats	±
Rice	−
Corn	−

WHEAT FRACTIONS	
Aqueous extract of wheat	−
Alcohol extract of wheat (gliadin)	+
Deaminated gliadin	−
Amino acids obtained by complete acid hydrolysis of gliadin	−
Glutamine-rich small polypeptides obtained by peptic-tryptic digestion of gliadin	+

circulating antibodies to nongluten dietary proteins such as milk protein, and such antibodies may simply reflect a nonspecific response to the passage of incompletely digested dietary protein across an abnormally permeable, diseased intestinal epithelium.

Second, some acutely ill celiac sprue patients improve clinically and histologically following corticosteroid administration. However, the response of celiac sprue patients to corticosteroid treatment is unpredictable and inconstant and may reflect the response of secondary adrenal insufficiency which may accompany severe celiac sprue as well as nonspecific suppression of the inflammation which accompanies the mucosal lesion.

Third, it has been pointed out that increased numbers of immunocytes are present in the lamina propria of the small intestine of untreated celiac sprue patients.[27] Though it is interesting that in many but not all celiac sprue patients the majority of immunocytes in the lamina propria produce IgM whereas in normals most of the immunocytes produce IgA, the significance of this finding is not known.[17] The increased numbers of immunocytes in the lamina propria, like the development of circulating antibodies to dietary protein, may be a secondary response to increased mucosal permeability and may have little to do with the pathogenesis of celiac sprue.

Thus, the significance of the immunological features of celiac sprue is far from clear, and much additional evidence will be needed before immunological mechanisms can be implicated in the pathogenesis of this disease.

Evidence that celiac sprue results from an inborn error of metabolism which results in accumulation of toxic material in the intestinal lumen or mucosa owing to incomplete gluten digestion is largely circumstantial. Such evidence is derived largely from experiments in which administration of gluten fractions reproduced the symptoms and typical histological lesion in celiac sprue patients in remission. It has also been shown that levels of peptidases, important in the digestion of gliadin, are reduced in the mucosa of untreated celiac sprue patients. However, following successful treatment, peptidase levels revert to normal in the histologically normal-appearing mucosa even though reingestion of gluten promptly induces clinical symptoms and recurrence of the celiac sprue lesion.[14] If deficiency of a specific peptidase were causative, deficiency of the enzyme would be apparent in the *treated* as well as in the untreated patients. Thus, the peptidase deficiencies documented thus far are nonspecific and reflect the mucosal damage. The inborn metabolic error in celiac sprue, if indeed there is one, remains to be characterized.

Although the mechanism by which gluten produces its toxic effect on the mucosa is not known, certain aspects of the interaction of the mucosa with gluten merit comment, because they help clarify the histogenesis of the mucosal lesion. There seems little doubt that certain gluten fractions are toxic to mature absorptive cells and damage them directly. These damaged and dying absorptive cells are sloughed from the mucosal surface into the gut lumen at a more rapid than normal rate. To compensate for this excessive loss of mature cells, the number of proliferative cells increases and the crypts hypertrophy. Thus, in the fully developed celiac sprue lesion, the absorptive cells are damaged and diminished in number, the villi are blunted or absent, the number of proliferating undifferentiated crypt cells is markedly increased, the crypts are markedly elongated, and cell renewal and migration are more rapid than normal.[28]

There is no doubt that genetic factors may play a role in the etiology of celiac sprue. The incidence of the disease in relatives of celiac sprue patients is significantly greater than in control populations. MacDonald and co-workers[3] found as many as four biopsy-proved cases of celiac sprue in a single family and noted a total of 11 affected relatives among 96 studied from 17 families. Symptoms were often either absent or so mild that some affected relatives were unaware of any abnormality. The detection of these "asymptomatic" celiac sprue patients casts doubt upon the accuracy of available incidence and prevalence figures and suggests that "mild" or latent celiac sprue may be more common than is currently appreciated.

Although several relatives were affected

in some kindreds, only a single case could be found in other carefully studied large families. To confuse the matter further, both concordance and discordance for celiac sprue have been documented in identical twin pairs.[29] Thus, although genetic factors are significant in the pathogenesis of at least some cases of celiac sprue, the mode of inheritance of this disease is not at all clear.

The unusual interrelationship of dermatitis herpetiformis and celiac sprue should also be mentioned in a discussion dealing with the etiology of celiac sprue. If sufficient small intestine is sampled, almost all patients with dermatitis herpetiformis have at least a mild mucosal lesion consistent with celiac sprue[30, 31] even though many patients with mild intestinal lesions have no intestinal symptoms (Fig. 66–3). The majority of patients with celiac sprue do not develop skin lesions of dermatitis herpetiformis. Moreover, the therapeutic responses of the skin and intestinal lesions are independent of each other. The skin lesion improves with sulfone administration, whereas the intestinal lesion does not. In contrast, the intestinal lesion responds to gluten withdrawal,[32] whereas the skin lesion does not. Thus dermatitis herpetiformis and celiac sprue appear to be distinct diseases, with the curious relationship that all or almost all patients with the skin disease also have celiac sprue, whereas only a few patients with celiac sprue have dermatitis herpetiformis. However, if there are clues regarding the cause of either of these diseases in this interrelationship, they still remain well hidden.

CLINICAL FEATURES AND DIAGNOSIS

The clinical manifestations of celiac sprue vary tremendously from patient to patient. Moreover, since most of the symptoms result from intestinal malabsorption, they are not specific for celiac sprue, but resemble those seen in other diseases with intestinal malabsorption (see p. 260).

The patient with a severe lesion involving the entire small intestine from proximal duodenum to distal ileum will present with devastating and life-threatening panmalabsorption. Such a patient may develop secondary involvement of many organ systems as a consequence of the extensive absorptive defects. In striking contrast, the patient with a limited lesion involving only the duodenum and proximal jejunum may have no gastrointestinal symptoms and may present only with iron deficiency anemia which is refractory to oral iron therapy[33] or with evidence of osteomalacia. Clearly, the severity of the celiac sprue lesion and its extent govern, at least in part, the severity of the clinical manifestations of the disease. However, other as yet undefined factors may be important, for the natural history of *untreated* celiac sprue is one of intermittent exacerbations and remissions.

The disease may first become apparent in infants when gluten ingestion, usually in the form of cereals, begins (pp. 286 to 287). Symptoms may persist throughout childhood if treatment is not begun, but they often diminish or disappear completely by adolescence. Symptoms generally reappear in early adult life (third and fourth decade).

In other patients, symptoms are not noted and the diagnosis is not established until middle or even old age. Whether these patients had asymptomatic or undetected celiac sprue with gluten intolerance as children (a constitutional defect) or whether they first developed gluten intolerance and the intestinal lesion as adults (an acquired defect) is not known. The finding of the typical lesion in asymptomatic relatives of celiac sprue patients[3] and the unmasking of a symptomatic disease by surgery which induces rapid gastric emptying (gastric resection, pyloroplasty)[34] suggests that adults may have clinically inapparent celiac sprue for some time.

Gastrointestinal Symptoms. The most common symptoms in patients with extensive disease include diarrhea, weight loss, and weakness. The frequency and nature of the stools vary considerably from patient to patient. Those with extensive intestinal involvement may have in excess of ten stools per day. Severe dehydration, electrolyte depletion, and even acidosis may develop, especially in infants and young children (pp. 280 to 289). The stools may be watery or semi-formed, light tan or gray, oily and frothy, and have a characteristic foul, rancid odor. Not all patients have diarrhea; some even complain of constipation. But when they do have a bowel movement they excrete immense quantities of putty-like stool that is difficult to flush down the toilet. Because of their high fat and gas content, the stools of celiac sprue patients often float on water.

The mechanisms of diarrhea in celiac sprue are not fully understood, but several factors probably contribute. First, the stool volume delivered to the colon is increased by the malabsorption of fat, carbohydrate, protein, water, electrolytes, and, indeed, all nutrients. In addition, the delivery of excessive dietary fat into the large bowel probably results in the production by bacteria of hydroxy fatty acids. These hydroxy fatty acids are potent, irritating cathartics; indeed, ricinoleic acid, a hydroxy fatty acid, is responsible for the cathartic action of castor oil. Also, Fordtran et al.[35] have shown that water and electrolytes are actually *secreted* into, rather than absorbed from, the lumen of the upper small intestine in celiac sprue patients. This secretion further increases stool volume in an intestine with already compromised absorptive capacity. Finally, if the disease extends to and involves the ileum, impaired absorption of conjugated bile salts may further aggravate the diarrhea by the direct cathartic action of the bile salts on the colon.

The amount of weight loss in a celiac sprue patient depends upon the severity and extent of the intestinal lesion which governs the degree of malabsorption and upon the ability of the patient to compensate for the malabsorption by increasing dietary intake. Many celiac sprue patients with significant malabsorption have enormous appetites and lose little or no weight. A careful dietary history from such patients often reveals tremendous hyperphagia with daily caloric intakes well in excess of normal. In severe disease, anorexia may develop with associated rapid and severe weight loss. In such debilitated patients, some of the weight loss may be masked by fluid retention caused by hypoproteinemia. In infants and young children with untreated celiac sprue, failure of weight gain and growth retardation may be the counterpart of weight loss in the adult.

In most celiac sprue patients, the weakness, lassitude, and fatigue commonly observed are not specific and are related to the general poor nutrition. In some patients, severe anemia or adrenocortical insufficiency (see below) may contribute to the weakness. In occasional patients, severe hypokalemia resulting from loss of potassium in the stool may cause severe muscle weakness.

Severe abdominal pain is rarely seen in patients with uncomplicated celiac sprue. Rather, many patients have no abdominal pain whatever. However, abdominal distention with excessive amounts of malodorous flatus is a common complaint and occurs in over half of patients with clinically apparent disease. Nausea and vomiting are uncommon in uncomplicated celiac sprue.

Extraintestinal Symptoms. The metabolic defects that may develop because of defective absorption of nutrients from the gut may involve virtually all organ systems (Table 66–1). Thus, although the gastrointestinal symptoms are often prominent, the symptoms most distressing to the patient may involve other organ systems. Many celiac sprue patients present initially with complaints not referable directly to the gastrointestinal tract. The alert physician may establish a diagnosis of celiac sprue in patients with such diverse findings as fatigue associated with refractory iron deficiency anemia or severe back pain owing to a collapsed lumbar vertebra (see pp. 259 to 277).

Anemia commonly occurs in adults with severe celiac sprue. Usually it is caused by impaired iron and perhaps folate absorption from the proximal intestine; in severe disease with ileal involvement, vitamin B_{12} absorption is also impaired. The symptoms caused by the anemia are nonspecific and may consist of weakness and fatigue, although profound anemia, which is not rare, may precipitate syncope or symptoms of congestive failure or angina pectoris in patients with occult cardiac disease. Purpura and gastrointestinal, vaginal, nasal, or renal bleeding may occur in patients with extensive disease. Such bleeding may further aggravate pre-existing anemia and is most often caused by impaired blood coagulability resulting from prothrombin deficiency secondary to impaired intestinal absorption of fat-soluble vitamin K.

Osteomalacia and osteoporosis may develop in patients with celiac sprue. Calcium absorption is impaired by (1) defective calcium transport by the diseased small intestine, (2) vitamin D deficiency caused by impaired absorption of this fat-soluble vitamin, and (3) binding of intraluminal calcium to unabsorbed dietary fatty acids, forming insoluble calcium soaps which are then excreted in the feces. In patients with severe disease, protein deficiency caused by impaired amino acid absorption may retard bone matrix formation. Bone pain, especially of the low back, rib cage, and pelvis, may develop. Pathological fractures which occur without trauma are uncommon but have been described.

Calcium depletion and/or coexistent magnesium depletion may cause paresthesias, muscle cramps, and even frank tetany. Indeed, tetany has been reported to occur in 40 to 50 per cent of patients in some series, but this figure is much too high when patients with mild celiac sprue are also considered.

Neurological symptoms caused by lesions of the central or peripheral nervous system are not common in celiac sprue patients, but occur occasionally in severely diseased individuals. Muscle weakness, paresthesias with sensory loss, and ataxia are the most common symptoms encountered. Pathological evidence of peripheral neuropathy and, very rarely, patchy demyelinization of the spinal cord, cerebellar atrophy, and capillary proliferation suggestive of Wernicke's encephalopathy have been described (Table 66–1). The cause of these phenomena is not at all clear. In most patients with neurological findings, serum vitamin B_{12} levels have been normal, although vitamin B_{12} absorption might be defective. Causative roles for thiamine, riboflavin, and pyridoxine deficiencies, although suggested, have not been established. Night blindness caused by vitamin A deficiency may occur.

Secondary hyperparathyroidism may develop in patients with severely impaired calcium absorption, a common finding in celiac sprue. The hyperparathyroidism results in mobilization of calcium from the bones in response to the low serum calcium level, and may contribute to the osteomalacia seen in such patients. The symptoms caused by secondary hyperparathyroidism reflect the osteomalacia and include bone pain and pathological fractures.

Adrenocortical insufficiency may accompany severe celiac sprue. In addition to weakness, lassitude, and dizziness related to sodium depletion and hypotension, such patients may develop increased skin and mucous membrane pigmentation reminiscent of classic Addison's disease. Adrenocortical insufficiency may be primary, or it may result from panhypopituitarism. That panhypopituitarism may accompany celiac sprue is suggested by the appearance of hypomenorrhea or amenorrhea, decreased libido and, rarely, symptoms of hypometabolism. Such endocrine insufficiencies reflect the marked malnutrition associated with severe malabsorption.

Physical Findings.   Physical findings, like symptoms, may vary considerably

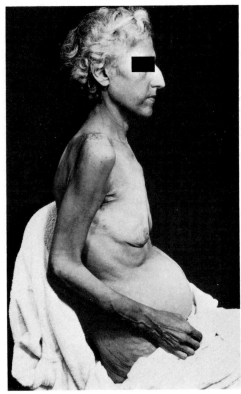

Figure 66–5. A patient with adult celiac sprue disease, before treatment. Note muscle wasting, emaciation, and abdominal distention. (Courtesy of Dr. T. P. Almy.)

among patients with celiac sprue. In the patient whose lesion is limited to the proximal small intestine, physical findings may be entirely absent or limited to pallor caused by anemia. On the other hand, the patient who has an extensive lesion involving most or all of the small intestine may have many of the findings described below.

Emaciation with evidence of recent weight loss, including loose skin folds and muscle wasting, may be prominent in patients with severe celiac sprue (Fig. 66–5). Hypotension may be related to fluid and electrolyte depletion and/or secondary adrenocortical insufficiency.

Careful examination of the integument of celiac sprue patients is important, because it is often the site of significant physical signs. Clubbing of the nails is seen in severe disease and reflects the chronic disease process. The skin may be dry with poor turgor if there is dehydration caused by excessive stool water and electrolyte loss. There may be edema, especially of the lower extremities if there is hypoproteinemia caused by deficient albumin synthesis or enteric loss of serum proteins. Increased skin pigmentation such as that seen in Addison's disease may be obvious in severely ill patients with compromised adrenocortical function. Other findings may include spontaneous ecchymoses or easy bruisability related to hypoprothrombinemia, hyperkeratosis follicularis caused by vitamin A deficiency, and pallor caused by anemia. The coexistence of celiac sprue and dermatitis herpetiformis has been discussed (see p. 872). All patients with dermatitis herpetiformis should be evaluated for celiac sprue.

Examination of the mouth may show cheilosis and glossitis with decreased papillation of the tongue.

The abdomen is often protuberant and tympanic, and has a characteristic doughy consistency when palpated owing to distention of intestinal loops with fluid and gas. Hepatosplenomegaly is uncommon, but ascites may occasionally be detected in patients with significant hypoproteinemia. Abdominal tenderness is uncommon.

The extremities may reveal loss of various sensory modalities, including light touch, vibration, and position, usually caused by peripheral neuropathy and, very rarely, demyelinating spinal cord lesions. If the neuropathy is severe, deep tendon reflexes are diminished or even absent. Hyperpathia may be present, and an ataxic gait in severely ill patients is not uncommon.

A positive Chvostek or Trousseau sign may be elicited in patients with severe calcium and/or magnesium depletion. In such individuals, bone tenderness related to osteomalacia may be prominent, especially if collapsed vertebrae or other fractures are present.

It must be emphasized that these physical findings are not specific for celiac sprue, because they may be elicited in certain patients with malabsorption caused by other diseases.

LABORATORY FINDINGS

The laboratory findings in celiac sprue, like the symptoms and signs, vary with the extent and severity of the intestinal lesion. Moreover, like other clinical findings in this disease, similar laboratory abnormalities may often be seen in patients with other diseases producing intestinal malabsorption (see Table 20–2).

Stool Examination. If malabsorption is sufficient to produce significant steatorrhea, the appearance and the odor of the stools may be typical. A watery or bulky, semi-formed, light tan or grayish, greasy-appearing stool with a rancid odor is characteristic. Microscopic evaluation of the fat content of a stool suspension stained with Sudan III or IV after hydrolysis with acetic acid and heat is a helpful bedside screening test but cannot be used to establish or exclude steatorrhea definitively. False-positive results are common, especially in hospitals in which patients receive oil-containing cathartics and suppositories in preparation for diagnostic studies.

To document steatorrhea unequivocally, the amount of fat in stool must be determined *quantitatively*, using a reliable method such as the van de Kamer chemical method. The patient should be placed on a diet of known fat content (usually 80 to 100 g per day) for a three- or four-day equilibrium period. Stools should then be collected for 72 to 96 hours, pooled, and their fat content determined quantitatively. Normal individuals excrete 2 to 7 g of fat per 24-hour period while ingesting 100 g of fat per day. Thus, if the coefficient of fat absorption

$$\frac{(\text{grams of fat ingested} - \text{grams excreted in stool} \times 100)}{\text{grams of fat ingested}}$$

is less than 93 per cent steatorrhea is present. Steatorrhea can be documented in most patients with celiac sprue and its severity correlated reasonably well with the severity and the extent of the intestinal lesion. Steatorrhea is absent, however, in some patients with disease limited to the proximal small intestine.

Hematological Tests. The anemia of celiac sprue may be secondary to iron, folate, or, rarely, vitamin B_{12} deficiency; hence red cell morphology may range from microcytic to macrocytic. A low serum iron level is very common, because the duodenal lesion invariably impairs iron absorption in the untreated patient. Leukopenia and thrombocytopenia are uncommon but may occur if severe folate or vitamin B_{12} deficiency is present. Under such circumstances, serum folate and/or serum vitamin B_{12} levels are low. The radioactive vitamin B_{12} absorption test is valuable in determining whether or not the sprue lesions involve the distal ileum. If severe ileal disease is present, vitamin B_{12} absorption is abnormally low both with and without added intrinsic factor.

The prothrombin time may be prolonged in celiac sprue owing to malabsorption of vitamin K. It is essential that the prothrombin time be evaluated prior to peroral intestinal biopsy in patients with possible celiac sprue, because serious intestinal bleeding may occur from the biopsy site if blood coagulation is abnormal. Parenteral administration of vitamin K or one of its analogues should rapidly correct the prothrombin time if the patient has no liver disease.

Oral Tolerance Tests. Certain oral tolerance tests are helpful in the evaluation of absorptive function in patients with suspected intestinal malabsorption. These tests are performed by administering an oral dose of test substance and then measuring either urinary or fecal excretion or blood levels of the substance as an index of

its transport across the intestinal mucosa. Such tolerance tests are helpful screening procedures but must be interpreted cautiously, because metabolism of the test substance may affect the test results. Moreover, oral tolerance tests are dependent upon normal gastric emptying and, if urinary excretion of the test substance is measured, normal renal function. Administration of the test substance through a tube placed in the duodenum eliminates the variable of gastric emptying.

The most useful tests are the xylose, glucose, and lactose tolerance tests. Xylose is absorbed preferentially by the proximal small intestine; hence, xylose excretion in the urine is usually markedly depressed in patients with severe, untreated celiac sprue, because the proximal intestine is most severely affected. The xylose tolerance test is therefore the most sensitive and useful oral tolerance test for evaluating patients with suspected celiac sprue. Glucose transport in celiac sprue is also diminished, because absorptive cells are both damaged and decreased in number. Hence, a flat absorption curve may be seen after oral glucose ingestion in some patients with a celiac sprue lesion. Similarly, the absorptive cell lesion also results in secondary lactase deficiency in patients with a celiac sprue lesion; thus blood glucose may fail to rise normally after lactose ingestion.

Although popular a number of years ago, the I^{131}-triolein absorption test is of relatively little clinical value. The triolein absorption test does not always establish or exclude impaired fat absorption, because false-positive and false-negative test results are commonly encountered. Moreover, differential determination of I^{131}-triolein and I^{131}-oleic acid absorption fails to distinguish defective absorption caused by impaired intraluminal digestion from defective absorption caused by mucosal disease, because commercially obtainable I^{131} triolein is unstable and heavily contaminated with I^{131} oleic acid.[36] Similarly, the vitamin A tolerance test is of little value, because it, too, is not very sensitive. Fat absorption is best evaluated by quantitative measurement of stool fat excretion, not by oral tolerance tests.

Blood Chemistries. Since many organ systems may be involved in celiac sprue, it

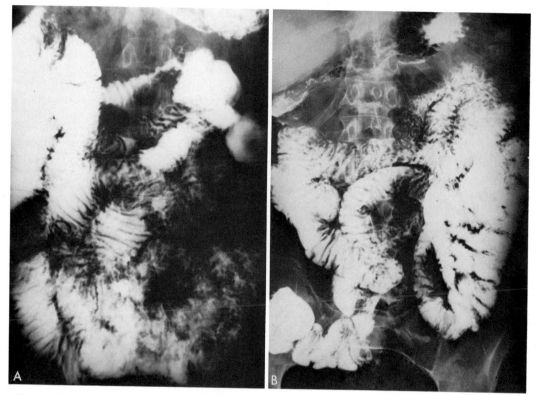

Figure 66–6. Barium contrast studies from a patient with celiac sprue. Before treatment (A), there is significant dilatation of some of the loops of small bowel, as well as marked distortion and coarsening of the mucosal pattern. After six weeks of maintenance on a gluten-free diet (B), there is a significant reduction in the dilatation and improvement in the mucosal pattern, although it has not yet returned to normal.

is not surprising that many blood chemical determinations may be abnormal in these patients.

If diarrhea is severe, marked electrolyte depletion with low serum levels of sodium, potassium, chloride, and bicarbonate can occur. In occasional patients, significant metabolic acidosis can develop in association with bicarbonate loss in the stool. Serum calcium and magnesium are often decreased in patients with diarrhea and steatorrhea. Serum phosphorus may be decreased and serum alkaline phosphatase may be increased in patients with osteomalacia. Serum albumin and, to a lesser degree, serum globulins may be diminished owing to excessive leakage of serum protein into the gut lumen. Diminished availability of amino acids for protein synthesis resulting from defective amino acid absorption might also contribute to the observed reduction in serum protein levels. In patients with sufficient intestinal involvement to produce steatorrhea, serum cholesterol and serum carotene levels are usually depressed. Indeed, the finding of a serum cholesterol level of less than 150 mg per 100 ml in an adult should alert the clinician to evaluate a patient for possible gastrointestinal malabsorption.

Miscellaneous. Abnormal tryptophan metabolism, perhaps caused by pyridoxine (vitamin B_6) deficiency, may result in elevated urinary excretion of 5-hydroxyindoleacetic acid and indican in patients with malabsorption. In patients with sufficient malnutrition to cause pituitary or adrenal insufficiency, tests of endocrine gland function such as 24-hour urinary 17-ketosteroid and 17-hydroxycorticoid excretion may be abnormal.

Roentgenographic Studies. Barium contrast roentgenograms of the gastrointestinal tract should be obtained in any patient with malabsorption. X-rays of the small intestine after a barium meal are particularly helpful in evaluating patients suspected of having untreated celiac sprue.

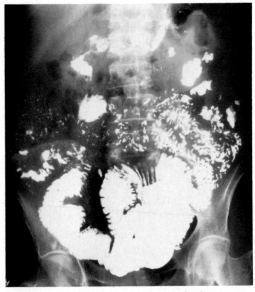

Figure 66–7. Barium contrast study from a patient with untreated celiac sprue. Note the dilated loops, coarsened mucosal folds, and "puddling" of the barium. (Courtesy of Dr. M. H. Sleisenger.)

In celiac sprue patients, abnormal findings usually include dilatation of the small intestine, replacement of the normal delicate mucosal pattern with either marked coarsening or complete obliteration of the mucosal folds, and fragmentation and flocculation of the barium meal within the gut lumen (Figs. 66–6 and 66–7). The distorted mucosal fold pattern is related to the mucosal lesion, and its distribution correlates well with the histological involvement of the mucosa. In patients with mild or moderate disease, the mucosal pattern is distorted in the proximal small intestine, whereas the ileal mucosa appears normal. In patients with severe disease, the mucosal pattern appears abnormal throughout the small intestine up to and including the ileum. The fragmentation and flocculation of intraluminal barium (usually seen best on films obtained an hour or more after ingestion of the barium meal) are not so specific and correlate less well with the severity of the disease in that dramatic

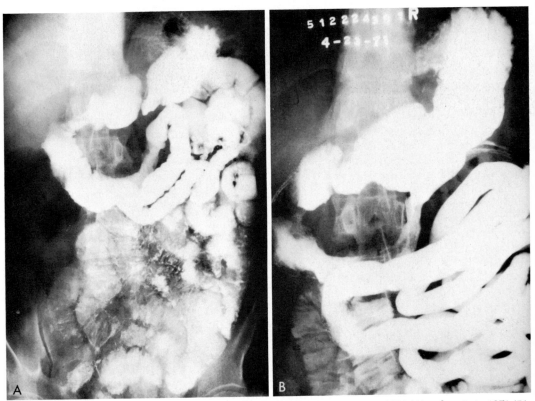

Figure 66–8. Barium contrast studies of a patient with collagenous sprue in 1964 (A) and again in 1971 (B). Note the progressive rigidity of the small bowel loops. (Courtesy of Dr. L. L. Brandborg.)

changes may be seen in patients with clinically mild disease. Excessive secretion of fluid into the proximal small intestine coupled with defective absorption of intraluminal contents probably causes dilution of the barium meal and contributes to the barium segmentation and fragmentation. A somewhat different X-ray picture will be seen in the rare disease known as collagenous sprue (Fig. 66–8).

X-rays of the bones may reveal diffuse demineralization with a generalized decrease in bone density. In addition secondary effects of osteomalacia and its associated osteoporosis, including compression fractures of vertebra and pseudofractures (Milkman's lines), are seen occasionally.

Intestinal Biopsy. Since its introduction in the mid-1950's, peroral biopsy has become an invaluable diagnostic procedure in the evaluation of patients with gastrointestinal malabsorption. Indeed, this procedure is the most valuable single diagnostic maneuver in establishing whether or not celiac sprue is the cause of malabsorption in a given patient. A variety of biopsy instruments are now available which permit relatively safe peroral biopsy of the proximal small intestine. The author uses the multipurpose biopsy tube (also called the Rubin or the Quinton tube). It has proved safe, provided there is no tendency to bleed, and it can be positioned rapidly and be easily visualized under the fluoroscope.[37] Moreover, two to four untraumatized mucosal samples are excised routinely with one passage of the tube, permitting more extensive sampling than is possible with some of the other available instruments.

To be definitive and, indeed informative, peroral biopsy must be done correctly and the tissue processed and interpreted properly. Requirements essential for biopsies to be of maximum diagnostic value include (1) precise radiological localization of the biopsy site, (2) proper orientation and prompt fixation of the biopsy samples, and (3) careful study of not one or two but of *serial sections* of the well-oriented central half or two-thirds of each biopsy. As Rubin and Dobbins have stressed,[38] the techniques of the embryologist, not the pathologist, must be used.

Biopsies for most diagnostic purposes are best obtained from the duodenojejunal junction at the ligament of Treitz. The bowel in this area is retroperitoneal and fixed; thus biopsy specimens from the same intestinal segment can be obtained serially and compared. This is of particular value in documenting histological improvement in a celiac sprue patient after treatment with a gluten-free diet. Moreover, this area is invariably involved in diffuse mucosal diseases such as celiac sprue, Whipple's disease, and a-beta-lipoproteinemia. Finally, biopsies obtained near the ligament of Treitz are usually more easily interpreted than biopsies from the more proximal duodenum where infiltration of the mucosa and submucosa with Brunner's glands and lymphoid nodules may distort villous architecture.

The biopsy findings in celiac sprue patients are described in detail on pages 865 to 866. (See Figs. 66–1, A, and 66–3.)

DIFFERENTIAL DIAGNOSIS

Although the presenting signs and symptoms are not specific and may resemble those seen with malabsorption from other causes, the diagnosis of celiac sprue can be established readily. The initial step is the suspicion of defective intestinal absorption. Malabsorption is obvious in the patient with a severe, extensive intestinal lesion and catastrophic panmalabsorption. Its recognition in the patient with a limited lesion without steatorrhea and only subtle evidence of malabsorption, such as refractory anemia, requires a high index of suspicion and an awareness that celiac sprue can present with extremely diverse clinical manifestations.

Once malabsorption has been established, the clinician must determine the nature of the underlying absorptive defect. Steatorrhea and depressed serum cholesterol, carotene, calcium, and prothrombin levels in themselves do not differentiate primary intestinal mucosal diseases such as celiac sprue from other diseases which may cause malabsorption. Indeed, these findings can all be abnormal in patients with defective intraluminal digestion caused by previous gastric or ileal resection, pancreatic insufficiency, or intraluminal bacterial overgrowth.

The presence of an abnormal xylose tolerance test is helpful in the differential diagnosis of primary mucosal disease, because xylose is usually absorbed normally by patients with defective intraluminal digestion so long as mucosal structure is normal. X-rays of the small intestine after a barium meal also help differentiate mucosal malabsorption from that of other causes; the presence of an *abnormal mucosal pattern*, not just segmentation and fragmentation of the barium meal, strongly suggests mucosal disease.

A normal biopsy sample obtained from the proximal small intestine effectively excludes the diagnosis of clinically significant untreated celiac sprue, whereas a biopsy which demonstrates the typical celiac sprue lesion strongly suggests this diagnosis. Similarly, biopsies which demonstrate the characteristic histological findings of Whipple's disease or a-beta-lipoproteinemia exclude the diagnosis of celiac sprue in patients with diffuse mucosal disease in whom the clinical picture itself is not diagnostic. Hypogammaglobulinemia may exhibit villous atrophy, that plasma cells are absent.

Since the histological appearance of the mucosa in untreated celiac sprue patients is not absolutely specific, demonstration of the mucosal histology typical of celiac sprue cannot, in itself, be considered diagnostic of this disease. A mucosal lesion identical to or closely resembling that of celiac sprue may be seen in persons with tropical sprue, although this disease occurs only in patients who have resided or traveled in areas of the world which are endemic for tropical sprue (see p. 979). But in addition, it may be difficult or impossible to distinguish the celiac sprue lesion from that seen occasionally in patients with diffuse lymphoma of the small intestine, parasitic infestation of the proximal intestine with *Giardia lamblia*, the Zollinger-Ellison syndrome with marked gastric hypersecretion, and the early lesion of collagenous sprue.

Therefore, to establish unequivocally the diagnosis of celiac sprue, a clinical response by the patient to treatment with a gluten-free diet is needed in addition to a biopsy showing the typical celiac sprue lesion. If the diet used is completely free of toxic gluten, a clinical response is usually evident within a few weeks. Indeed, some *improvement* in mucosal histology accompanies this early clinical response, although reversion of mucosal histology to normal usually requires months or even years of gluten withdrawal.

In summary, the diagnosis of celiac sprue is made by (1) demonstrating impairment of small intestinal mucosal function, (2) documenting the presence of the typical mucosal lesion, and (3) observing a prompt clinical response and, ideally, improvement in mucosal histology upon withdrawal of toxic gluten from the diet.

TREATMENT

Diet. Removal of toxic gluten from the diet is essential for the treatment of patients with celiac sprue. The need for gluten withdrawal was established by Dicke, van de Kamer, and Weijers' astute studies some 20 years ago in which the toxicity of wheat protein in children with celiac sprue was documented convincingly.[7, 8] Some ten years later, Rubin and coworkers demonstrated that instillation of wheat, barley, and rye flour into histologically normal-appearing small intestine of treated celiac sprue patients rapidly induced sprue like symptoms and that these symptoms were accompanied by the development of the typical celiac sprue lesion in the exposed mucosa.[22, 23]

Although complete dietary removal of all cereal grains known to contain toxic gluten (wheat, barley, rye, buckwheat, and probably oats) sounds simple enough, such a diet is, in reality, very difficult for most patients to achieve and maintain. Obvious sources of toxic gluten such as baked goods, wheat- or oat-containing dry cereals, noodles, spaghetti, etc., are easily avoided. But toxic glutens, especially wheat flour, are virtually ubiquitous in the normal American diet. Wheat is often used as an extender in processed foods and is present in many brands of commercially available ice cream, in salad dressing, and in many canned foods, including vegetables and soups. Indeed, wheat flour is even contained in many brands of instant coffee, catsup, mustard, and most candy bars, to give only a few examples. The rising popularity of processed foods such as frozen vegetables with wheat-containing sauces has further compounded the problem. As a result, the institution of an effective gluten-free diet requires extensive and repeated indoctrination of the patient by the physician and the dietician, as well as a motivated and basically suspicious, label-reading patient.

Aside from containing no wheat, rye, barley, or oat gluten, the diet should be well balanced and should contain normal amounts of fat, protein (at least 100 g per day), and carbohydrates.

It is not clear whether oats are toxic to all patients with celiac sprue. Some patients who are very sensitive to ingestion of small amounts of wheat flour tolerate oats without ill effects; others develop symptoms within a few hours after eating oat-containing foods. Therefore, oats are best eliminated from the diet initially, but can be carefully tried once remission has been achieved.

Rice, soybean, and corn flours are clearly nontoxic, and baked goods and cereals containing these flours can be eaten

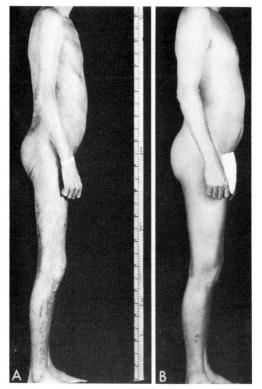

Figure 66–9. A patient with celiac sprue disease before (A) and six weeks after (B) treatment with a gluten-free diet. (Courtesy of Dr. M. H. Sleisenger.)

safely by celiac sprue patients. Helpful recipes as well as detailed instructions regarding gluten-free diets have recently been published by Marion Wood in a valuable book entitled *Gourmet Food on a Wheat-Free Diet.*[39]

Since treatment with a gluten-free diet represents a lifetime commitment for patients with celiac sprue and may carry with it significant social liability, especially in children, it should not be casually undertaken as a therapeutic trial in a patient prior to biopsy. Rather, the probable diagnosis should be established first by biopsy. Thereafter, institution of a gluten-free diet serves two functions: it initiates treatment, and, if followed by clinical improvement, confirms the histological diagnosis (Fig. 66–9).

If a patient fails to improve within a few weeks following institution of a gluten-free diet, the physician must review the patient's dietary intake meticulously. The most common cause of failure to respond to a gluten-free diet is incomplete removal of gluten from the diet. Even patients hospitalized in sophisticated university centers are often challenged inadvertently with gluten-containing foods while they are supposedly receiving gluten-free diets. It is sometimes necessary to hospitalize a patient who has not responded to gluten withdrawal on a metabolic ward under the supervision of a knowledgeable dietician to be certain that rigid gluten exclusion is in effect. By definition, celiac sprue patients respond to gluten withdrawal. Therefore if a given patient fails to improve on a gluten-free diet, either the diet is inadequate or the mucosal lesion is caused by another disease in which the intestinal histology closely resembles that of celiac sprue.

There is considerable variation among patients with celiac sprue in their ability to tolerate small amounts of toxic gluten. This difference is most apparent after patients have responded to gluten withdrawal and intestinal absorptive function has reverted to normal or near-normal. Under such circumstances, some patients can tolerate ingestion of small amounts of toxic gluten and still maintain their remission without developing symptoms. Such individuals may stray from their diets from time to time without ill effect. Other patients are exquisitely sensitive to ingestion of even minute amounts of toxic gluten and may develop massive watery diarrhea reminiscent of acute cholera within hours after ingesting as little gluten as is contained, for example, in a couple of pieces of bakery bread. The diarrhea in such patients may be so severe that it can induce clinical shock resulting from acute dehydration and be life threatening; indeed, the term gliadin shock has been applied to this condition.[40]

MacDonald and coworkers[18] have shown that during treatment with a gluten-free diet, the less severely damaged distal bowel recovers more rapidly than the maximally damaged proximal intestine. Clinical improvement correlates better with the length of histologically improved intestine than with the severity of the lesion in the proximal intestine. This helps explain the common observation that a clinical response to gluten withdrawal may precede by many months reversion of the proximal intestinal lesion to normal. Eventually, even the proximal biopsy specimens revert to normal or almost normal in about 50 per cent of patients maintained on a gluten-free diet. Most of the remaining patients show partial reversion of proximal mucosa toward normal.[18, 41] In a few patients, the proximal intestinal lesion fails to revert toward normal despite a good clinical response to prolonged gluten withdrawal. It is usually impossible to be certain that such patients are not ingesting any gluten without subjecting them to prolonged hospitalization. Moreover, if the clinical response to gluten withdrawal is equivocal in such patients, the clinician should be suspicious that the persistent flat mucosal biopsy may reflect a disease other than celiac sprue.

Some patients with untreated celiac sprue develop aggravation of their symptoms, with bloating, cramps, and diarrhea, after ingesting milk and milk products. The probable cause of this milk intolerance is secondary lactase deficiency. Lactase and other disaccharides are located in the brush border of intestinal absorptive cells, and since these cells are both reduced in number and damaged in patients with celiac sprue, the occurrence of secondary lactase deficiency is not surprising. However, milk and milk products should be omitted from the diet of celiac sprue patients only if they produce unpleasant symptoms. These foods are an excellent source of protein, calories, and calcium for the nutritionally depleted patient. Many severely ill celiac sprue patients will tolerate milk initially, and almost all develop tolerance as intestinal structure and function revert toward normal with gluten withdrawal.

Supplemental Therapy. Patients with severe disease should receive appropriate replacement therapy in addition to a gluten-free diet to help correct deficiencies caused by the absorptive defects.

Anemic patients should receive supplemental iron, folate, and/or vitamin B_{12}, depending upon the specific deficiency or deficiencies responsible for their anemia. If there is purpura or other evidence of bleeding or if there is significant prolongation of the prothrombin time, parenteral administration of vitamin K or one of its analogues is indicated.

Vigorous intravenous replacement of fluid and electrolytes may be essential in patients with dehydration and electrolyte depletion caused by severe diarrhea. Hypokalemia should be treated promptly with parenteral potassium chloride if the deficiency is severe and with oral potassium supplements if it is mild.

Intravenous calcium gluconate should be administered promptly to the rare patient who develops tetany. If there is no response to 1 or 2 g of intravenously administered calcium gluconate, the tetany may be due to hypomagnesemia. If so, 0.5 to 1 g of magnesium sulfate is given slowly intravenously in a dilute solution. All patients with hypocalcemia or with clinical or radiological evidence of osteomalacia should receive oral calcium in the form of calcium gluconate or calcium lactate, 6 to 8 g per day, as well as oral vitamin D, 50,000 units daily. In fact, it is probably desirable to administer some supplemental calcium and vitamin D to all celiac sprue patients with significant steatorrhea to help prevent mobilization of skeletal calcium. Of course, overtreatment with vitamin D and calcium may be harmful. Therefore, serum calcium must be monitored and supplementation discontinued promptly if hypercalcemia develops. Calcium and vitamin D administration should be stopped when defective fat and calcium absorption have been corrected by treatment with a gluten-free diet.

Vitamin A, thiamine, riboflavin, niacin, pyridoxine, vitamin C, and vitamin E, in the form of therapeutic formula multivitamin preparation, should probably be administered to celiac sprue patients with malabsorption, although the need for supplementation of these vitamins is not fully established (see Table 20–4).

If clinical evidence of secondary adrenal insufficiency is present, parenteral corticosteroid replacement therapy (100 to 150 mg of hydrocortisone or its equivalent daily) may be required in addition to vigorous parenteral replacement of sodium chloride. Indeed, corticosteroid administration is advocated by some authorities for all severely ill celiac sprue patients, although, in my experience, it is rarely needed unless the patient is unable to eat. Treatment with a gluten-free diet is safer and more specific, and usually results in equally rapid and more lasting improvement, even in severely ill patients. Therefore, steroids are rarely needed in the treatment of celiac sprue and then only for the acute treatment of transient adrenal insufficiency which may accompany severe malnutrition and depletion in the desperately ill patient.

Finally, it must be mentioned that drugs, like nutrients, may be absorbed capriciously by patients with severe celiac sprue. Medications considered essential for the patient's well-being should be administered parenterally until improved absorption is induced by treatment with a gluten-free diet.

PROGNOSIS AND COMPLICATIONS

If not recognized and properly treated, celiac sprue, if severe, may be fatal. Patients may develop marked malnutrition and debilitation and die of complications such as hemorrhage, intercurrent infection, or secondary adrenal insufficiency. On the other hand, death caused by celiac sprue among patients in whom the diagnosis has been established is exceedingly uncommon, because the response to gluten withdrawal is both specific and rapid.

Therefore, the prognosis for patients with correctly diagnosed and treated celiac sprue is excellent. Intestinal absorptive defects disappear promptly in infants and young children upon institution of a gluten-free diet. Growth and development usually proceed normally with continued effective treatment. The natural history of celiac sprue is such that the disease often becomes quiescent as the children approach adolescence. At this point, patients may stray from their gluten-free diet without apparent ill effects. However, their inability to tolerate gluten remains and if gluten ingestion continues into adult life, most if not all such patients eventually develop recurrent clinical evidence of celiac sprue, most often in the third or fourth decade of life. The recurrent disease may manifest itself as mild refractory iron deficiency anemia, blatant panmalabsorption, or anything in between. Therefore, patients with unequivocal evidence of celiac sprue in childhood should be encouraged to remain on a gluten-free diet indefinitely if recurrent clinical disease is to be avoided during adult life (pp. 286 to 287).

The prognosis seems equally good for patients who develop clinically apparent celiac sprue as adults. As absorptive function returns to normal on a gluten-free diet, both the primary and secondary manifestations of celiac sprue disappear. A few of the complications seen in celiac sprue such as peripheral neuropathy and pathological fractures caused by severe osteoporosis may not be totally reversible, but these are the exception, not the rule.

Two serious complications which have been associated with celiac sprue merit mention. First, there have been a number of reports which suggest that the incidence of malignant disease is greater in adults with celiac sprue than in the general population. The most worrisome study is that of Harris and coworkers,[42] who describe a series of 202 patients with a mean follow-up period of 8.2 years in whom the diagnosis of celiac sprue was documented in some and presumed in others. Malignant disease was diagnosed in 31 (15 per cent) of these patients. Thirteen patients had gastrointestinal carcinomas (esophagus, stomach, and large intestine); 14 patients had lymphomas, nine with and five without gastrointestinal involvement; and four patients had primary tumors in other sites (lung, ovary, and skin).

However, it seems doubtful that 15 per cent of *all* celiac sprue patients followed for eight or more years might be expected to develop malignant disease, as this report might suggest. Other clinicians with extensive experience have not noted such a high incidence of malignancy in patients with a documented diagnosis of celiac sprue, although sporadic cases of coexisting celiac sprue and malignancy have been observed by many. Interpretation of the data regarding the incidence of lymphoma in patients with celiac sprue is particularly difficult, because patients with primary diffuse lymphoma of the small intestine may present initially with symptoms of malabsorption and with peroral biopsy findings which are difficult or impossible to differentiate from those of patients with untreated celiac sprue. Thus, some patients initially diagnosed as having celiac sprue may, in fact, have had intestinal lymphoma simulating celiac sprue. In any case, patients with documented celiac sprue merit a careful search for a gastrointestinal malignancy if, after initially improving with gluten withdrawal, they subsequently develop symptoms such as weight loss, malabsorption, abdominal pain, or intestinal bleeding despite strict adherence to a gluten-free diet. It is not known whether treatment with a gluten-free diet reduces the incidence of malignancy in patients with celiac sprue if, indeed, it is increased.

The second serious complication associated with celiac sprue is that of ulceration and stricture of the small intestine.[43] This rare (less than 20 reported cases) complication may develop both in the untreated patient and in the patient who has responded to gluten withdrawal. The characteristic clinical findings are diarrhea, abdominal pain, intestinal bleeding, and intestinal obstruction. The ulcers occur at any level of the small intestine, and perforation with peritonitis is common. The histology of the ulceration is nonspecific and provides no clue to their pathogenesis. Seventy-five per cent of reported patients have died as a direct result of this complication, emphasizing its seriousness.[43]

Despite these two serious but uncommon complications, there are no available data which indicate that properly diagnosed and treated celiac sprue disease is associated with a shortened life expectancy.

REFERENCES

1. Rubin, C. E.   Malabsorption: Celiac sprue. Ann. Rev. Med. *12*:39, 1961.
2. Carter, C. O., Sheldon, W., and Walker, C. Coeliac disease. Ann. Hum. Gen. *23*:266, 1959.
3. MacDonald, W. C., Dobbins, W. O., and Rubin, C. E.   Studies of the familial nature of celiac sprue using biopsy of the small intestine. New Eng. J. Med. *272*:448, 1965.
4. Misra, R. C., Kasthuri, S. and Chuttani, H. K., Adult coeliac disease in tropics. Brit. Med. J. *2*:1230, 1966.
5. Walia, B. N. S., Sidhu, J. K., Tandon, B. N., Ghai, O. P., and Bhargava, S.   Coeliac disease in north Indian children. Brit. Med. J. *2*:1233, 1966.
6. Thaysen, T. E. H.   Non-tropical sprue. Copenhagen, Levin and Munksgaard, 1932.
7. Dicke, W. K.   Coeliac disease: Investigation of harmful effects of certain types of cereal on patients with coeliac disease. Doctoral thesis, University of Utrecht, Netherlands, 1950.
8. van de Kamer, J. H., Weijers, H. A., and Dicke, W. K.   Coeliac disease. IV. An investigation into the injurious constituents of wheat in connection with their action on patients with coeliac disease. Acta Paediat. *42*:223, 1953.
9. Paulley, L. W.   Observations on the aetiology of idiopathic steatorrhea. Brit. Med. J. *2*:1318, 1954.
10. Rubin, C. E., Brandborg, L. L., Phelps, P. C., and Taylor, H. C., Jr.   Studies of celiac disease. I. The apparent identical and specific nature of the duodenal and proximal jejunal lesion in celiac disease and idiopathic sprue. Gastroenterology *38*:28, 1960.
11. Mandanagopalan, N., Shiner, M., and Rowe, B. Measurements of small intestinal mucosa obtained by peroral biopsy. Amer. J. Med. *38*:42, 1965.
12. Rubin, W., Ross, L. L., Sleisenger, M. H., and Weser, E.   An electron microscopic study of adult celiac disease. Lab. Invest. *15*:1720, 1966.
13. Padykula, H. A., Strauss, E. W., Ladman, A. J., and Gardner, F. H.   A morphologic and histochemical analysis of the human jejunal epithelium in non-tropical sprue. Gastroenterology *40*:735, 1961.
14. Douglas, A. P., and Booth, C. C.   Digestion of gluten peptides by normal human jejunal mucosa and by mucosa from patients with adult coeliac disease. Clin. Sci. *38*:11, 1970.
15. Yardley, J. H., Bayless, T. M., Norton, J. H., and Hendrix, T. R.   A study of the jejunal epithelium before and after a gluten-free diet. New Eng. J. Med. *267*:1173, 1962.

16. Crabbé, P. A., and Heremans, J. F. Selective IgA deficiency with steatorrhea. Amer. J. Med. 42:319, 1967.

17. Douglas, A. P., Crabbé, P. A., and Hobbs, J. R. Immunochemical studies of the serum, intestinal secretions, and intestinal mucosa in patients with adult celiac disease and other forms of the celiac syndrome. Gastroenterology 59:414, 1971.

18. MacDonald, W. C., Brandborg, L. L., Flick, A. L., Trier, J. S., and Rubin, C. E. Studies of celiac sprue. IV. The response of the whole length of the small bowel to a gluten-free diet. Gastroenterology 47:573, 1964.

19. Pink, I. J., and Creamer, B. Response to a gluten-free diet of patients with the coeliac syndrome. Lancet 1:300, 1967.

20. Weinstein, W. M., Saunders, D. R., Tytgat, G. N., and Rubin, C. E. Collagenous sprue—an unrecognized type of malabsorption. New Eng. J. Med. 283:1297, 1970.

21. Dobbins, W. O., and Rubin, C. E. Studies of the rectal mucosa in celiac sprue. Gastroenterology 47:471, 1964.

22. Rubin, C. E., Brandborg, L. L., Flick, A. L., Mac-Donald, W. C., Parkins, R. A., Parmentier, C. M., Phelps, P., Sribhibhadh, S., and Trier, J. S. Biopsy studies on the pathogenesis of celiac sprue. In Intestinal Biopsy, Boston, Little, Brown and Co., 1962, p. 67.

23. Rubin, C. E., Brandborg, L. L., Flick, A. L., et al. Studies of coeliac sprue. III. The effect of repeated wheat instillation into the proximal ileum of patients on a gluten-free diet. Gastroenterology 43:621, 1962.

24. Bronstein, H. D., Haeffner, L. J., and Kowlessar, O. D. Enzymatic digestion of gliadin: The effect of the resultant peptides in adult celiac disease. Clin. Chem. Acta 14:141, 1966.

25. Kowlessar, O. D., and Sleisenger, M. H. The role of gliadin in the pathogenesis of adult celiac disease. Gastroenterology 44:357, 1963.

26. Taylor, K. B., Truelove, S. C., Thompson, D. L., and Wright, R. An immunological study of coeliac disease and idiopathic steatorrhea. Brit. Med. J. 2:1727, 1961.

27. Rubin, W., Fauci, A. S., Sleisenger, M. H., and Jeffries, G. H. Immunofluorescent studies in adult celiac disease. J. Clin. Invest. 44:475, 1965.

28. Trier, J. S., and Browning, T. H. Epithelial-cell renewal in cultured duodenal biopsies in celiac sprue. New Eng. J. Med. 283:1245, 1970.

29. Hoffman, H. N., Wollaeger, E. E., and Greenberg, E. Discordance for non-tropical sprue (adult celiac disease) in a monozygotic twin pair. Gastroenterology 51:36, 1966.

30. Marks, J., Shuster, S., and Watson, A. J. Small-bowel changes in dermatitis herpetiformis. Lancet 2:1280, 1962.

31. Brow, J. R., Parker, F., Weinstein, W. M., and Rubin, C. E. The small intestinal mucosa in dermatitis herpetiformis. I. Severity and distribution of the small intestinal lesion and associated malabsorption. Gastroenterology 60:355, 1971.

32. Weinstein, W. M., Brow, J. R., Parker, F., and Rubin, C. E. The small intestinal mucosa in dermatitis herpetiformis. II. Relationship of the small intestinal lesion to gluten. Gastroenterology 60:362, 1971.

33. McGuigan, J., E., and Volwiler, W. Celiac-sprue: Malabsorption of iron in the absence of steatorrhea. Gastroenterology 47:636, 1964.

34. Hegberg, C. A., Melnyk, C. S., and Johnson, C. F. Gluten enteropathy appearing after gastric surgery. Gastroenterology 50:796, 1966.

35. Fordtran, J. S., Rector, F. C., Locklear, T. W., and Ewton, M. F. Water and solute movement in the small intestine of patients with sprue. J. Clin. Invest. 46:287, 1967.

36. Tuna, N., Mangold, H. K., and Mosser, D. G. Re-evaluation of the I^{131}-triolein absorption test. J. Lab. Clin. Med. 61:620, 1963.

37. Brandborg, L. L., Rubin, C. E., and Quinton, W. E. A multipurpose instrument for suction biopsy of the esophagus, stomach, small bowel and colon. Gastroenterology 37:1, 1959.

38. Rubin, C. E., and Dobbins, W. O. Peroral biopsy of the small intestine. Gastroenterology 49:676, 1965.

39. Wood, M. N. Gourmet Food on a Wheat-Free Diet. Springfield, Ill., Charles C. Thomas, 1967.

40. Krainick, H. J., Debatin, F., Gautier, E., et al. Weitere Untersuchung über der schadlichen Voizenmehlaffekt bie der Coeliakie. I. Die akute Gliadinreaktion (gliadin shock). Helv. Pediat. Acta 13:432, 1958.

41. Benson, G. D., Kowlessar, O. D., and Sleisenger, M. H. Adult celiac disease with emphasis upon response to the gluten-free diet. Medicine 43:1, 1964.

42. Harris, O. D., Cooke, W. T., Thompson, H., and Waterhouse, J. A. H. Malignancy in adult coeliac disease and idiopathic steatorrhea. Amer. J. Med. 42:899, 1967.

43. Bayless, T. M., Kapelowitz, R. F., Shelley, W. M., Ballinger, W. F., II, and Hendrix, T. R. Intestinal ulceration—a complication of celiac disease. New Eng. J. Med. 276:996, 1967.

Chapter 67

Regional Enteritis

Robert M. Donaldson, Jr.

DEFINITION

Regional enteritis or Crohn's disease is a chronic inflammatory disease of the small bowel which is granulomatous in nature. Although the terminal ileum is most often involved, the disease may affect any part of the alimentary canal from esophagus to anus. The process is usually discontinuous, with diseased segments of bowel separated by apparently healthy segments. Inflammation extends through all layers of the gut wall and involves mesentery and regional lymph nodes. The disease is characterized by a wide variety of clinical manifestations, a prolonged, complicated, and indolent course, and unpredictable exacerbations and remissions.

HISTORY

Sporadic cases of what was almost certainly regional enteritis were described as early as 1813. Perhaps because the disease may have been confused with intestinal tuberculosis, regional enteritis was nevertheless not recognized as an entity until 1932 when Crohn, Ginzburg, and Oppenheimer first defined the clinical and pathological features of what they called "regional ileitis." More recently Crohn has summarized the events which led to present concepts about regional enteritis.[1] Crohn and his colleagues initially be-

lieved that the disorder was confined to segments of ileum, but soon recognized that any region of small bowel could be affected. Subsequently, it became apparent that the disease process could also involve duodenum, stomach, or esophagus. Within two years after Crohn's original paper, other workers began to describe patients with colonic involvement. However, it was difficult to exclude ulcerative colitis in such patients with certainty. Thus the question of whether Crohn's disease truly involved the colon remained unsettled until 1960 when Lockhart-Mummery and Morson demonstrated clinically and pathologically that Crohn's disease occurred in the colon and, in most cases, could be distinguished from ulcerative colitis.[2] Crohn's disease of the colon and its differentiation from ulcerative colitis are discussed on pages 1350 to 1352.

PATHOLOGY

Only rarely does the pathologist have the opportunity to examine tissue as early in the course of regional enteritis as during the patient's first attack of the illness. Thus there is no generally accepted concept of the earliest pathological change. In fact, most descriptions of the pathology of acute regional enteritis deal with acute inflammation superimposed on well established bowel disease. On the other hand, surgeons have become familiar with the appearance of the ileum during initial attacks of regional enteritis through laparotomies performed for suspected acute appendicitis. One or more segments of small intestine, most often the terminal ileum, appear hyperemic and somewhat boggy, but the bowel wall is thin and pliable. Although inflammation occasionally extends into the cecum, the appendix is usually normal. Uninvolved bowel adjacent to the diseased segment appears remarkably normal, and is usually, but not always, sharply demarcated from the involved segment. The extent of disease varies greatly: in many cases less than a foot of terminal ileum is inflamed; on occasion, however, most or all of the small intestine may be involved.

The mesentery is often edematous in patients with acute regional enteritis, and the peritoneal cavity may contain small amounts of serous fluid. Mesenteric lymph nodes draining involved bowel segments are usually enlarged, soft, and reddened.

Although many patients who show these early changes in the bowel and mesentery certainly develop typical regional enteritis, others, particularly those with mild ileal inflammation and minimal mesenteric involvement, recover completely from the acute attack and subsequently have no obvious bowel disease. One may justifiably ask whether this acute inflammatory process always represents a single, distinct disorder or is merely a manifestation of different disease entities, only one of which is truly regional enteritis.

Histological examination of small bowel obtained early in the course of the disease demonstrates several distinct abnormalities, but none can be considered specific for regional enteritis.[3, 4] Those findings thought to represent particularly early changes include (1) hyperplasia of perilymphatic histiocytes in all layers of the gut wall, (2) distortion and round cell infiltration of lymph nodules and Peyer's patches on the serosal surface of the bowel, (3) endothelial thickening and proliferation in mesenteric lymphatic channels, (4) sarcoid-like reactions in the lamina propria and submucosa, and (5) granulomatous inflammation of small lymphatic vessels in the lamina propria. Many reports emphasize the importance of

edema in all layers of the bowel wall. Especially marked in the submucosa, the edema is usually accompanied by hyperemia and dilatation of lymphatics. Although all these changes have been observed at one time or another early in the course of regional enteritis, none can be considered specific for the disease. Furthermore, there is little agreement as to what constitutes the primary structural change or the sequence of histological events which ultimately leads to the characteristic picture of chronic regional enteritis.

Once the disease becomes established, the small intestine appears thickened and leathery, and stenosis is common (Fig. 67–1). Although most often seen in the terminal ileum, regional enteritis may in fact involve any segment of small bowel from a few inches to several feet in length. The disease is discontinuous in the sense that involved segments are usually separated by apparently normal bowel. Intestine which lies adjacent to or between diseased segments looks perfectly normal except that healthy bowel proximal to narrowed areas may be dilated. The mesentery is markedly thickened, fatty, and edematous. Finger-like projections of thick mesentery characteristically extend over the serosal surface toward the antimesenteric border

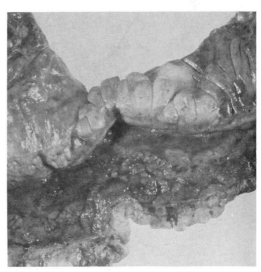

Figure 67–1. Gross specimen of ileum resected from a patient with Crohn's disease. The bowel wall is thickened as a result of involvement of all layers. Prominent mesenteric fat extends over the serosal surface. The mucosa is "cobblestoned" as a result of mucosal edema combined with linear ulceration.

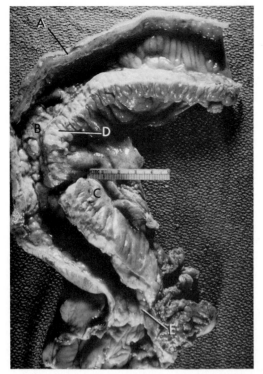

Figure 67–2. Regional enteritis. Terminal ileum is shown with thickened fibrous wall with inflammatory and proliferative changes involving all layers from the mucosa to the serosa (*A*). A "stony brook" appearance of the ulcerated mucosa is seen (*B*). The mesentery is short, thick, and retracted (*C*), sharply angulating the loop of intestine, and adipose tissue extends onto the wall of the intestine (*D*). The diameter of the ileocecal valve (*E*) is decreased. (From Mottet, K.: Histopathologic Spectrum of Regional Enteritis and Ulcerative Colitis. Philadelphia, W. B. Saunders Co., 1971.)

of the bowel. Mesenteric nodes are enlarged and firm and are often matted together to form an irregular mass.

When the diseased segment is opened, all layers of the bowel wall appear thickened, particularly the submucosa. The lumen is correspondingly narrowed. The gross appearance of the mucosal surface varies, depending upon the extent and severity of the disease. In many instances the mucosa may appear relatively normal to the naked eye except for hyperemia and edema. In advanced cases, however, normal mucosal architecture is completely destroyed by nodular swelling intermingled with deep ulcerations (Fig. 67–1). Ulcers are frequently elongated or even linear and tend to lie in the long axis of the bowel. Ulceration may occur in grossly normal mucosa or in mucosa which obviously is hyperemic, thickened, and boggy. Ulcers vary in depth but usually extend at least into the submucosa. Within the submucosal and muscular layers, two or more coalesce to form a single large intramural channel (Figs. 67–2, 67–3, 67–4, and 67–5).

Because the serosa and mesentery are regularly inflamed, a characteristic feature of this disease is the tendency for involved bowel loops, as in Figure 67–4, to be firmly matted together by fibrotic peritoneal and mesenteric bands. Mesenteric nodes

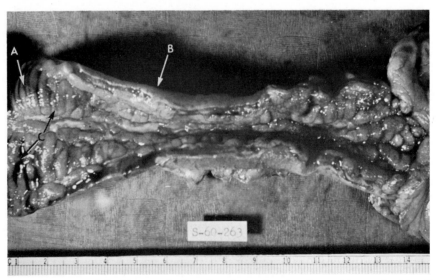

Figure 67–3. The terminal ileal lesion of relatively advanced regional enteritis, emphasizing the contrast between the flaccid uninvolved bowel (*A*) and the firm, thick, erect involved bowel (*B*). Also shown is the presence of ulcers at the bases of mucosal folds (*C*). (From Mottet, K.: Histopathologic Spectrum of Regional Enteritis and Ulcerative Colitis. Philadelphia, W. B. Saunders Co., 1971.)

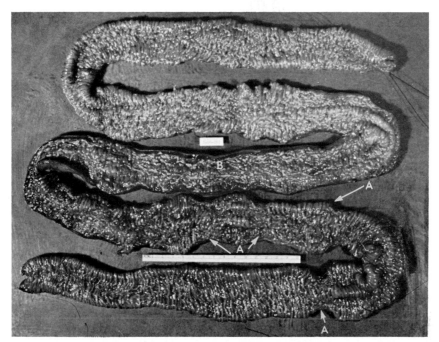

Figure 67–4. A more proximal segment of small intestine from the same patient shown in Figure 67–3, revealing the presence of multiple skip area strictures (*A*) and a less typical diffuse ulcerated lesion (*B*). (From Mottet, K.: Histopathologic Spectrum of Regional Enteritis and Ulcerative Colitis. Philadelphia, W. B. Saunders Co., 1971.)

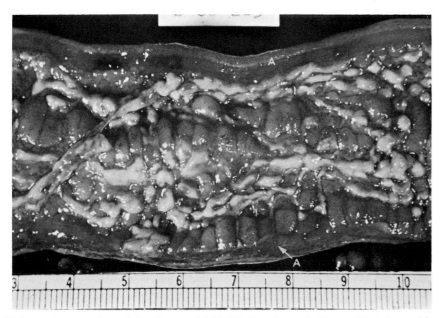

Figure 67–5. A close-up view of the elongated "skip" lesion shown in Figure 67–4. Its total length is approximately 17 cm. Shown here are the thickened bowel wall (*A*) and "stony brook" appearance of the ulcerated mucosa. (From Mottet, K.: Histopathologic Spectrum of Regional Enteritis and Ulcerative Colitis. Philadelphia, W. B. Saunders Co., 1971.)

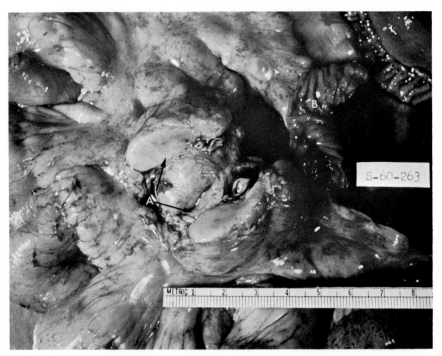

Figure 67–6. A transected enlarged mesenteric lymph node (*A*) from the patient shown in Figures 67–3 to 67–5. The node is enlarged to 2.5 cm, is firm, and the cut surface does not reveal distinctive markings. A portion of the mucosa is shown (*B*). (From Mottet, K.: Histopathologic Spectrum of Regional Enteritis and Ulcerative Colitis. Philadelphia, W. B. Saunders Co., 1971.)

are often involved also (Fig. 67–6). This adhesive process is often associated with fistula formation, another phenomenon characteristic of regional enteritis. Presumably, fistulas begin as ulcerations which gradually burrow through the serosa and into adjacent loops of bowel. Such fistulas communicate between one loop of small bowel and another or between small bowel and colon. In addition, fistulous tracts may penetrate to the skin; the umbilicus and perineum are particularly common external sites. Communicating tracts leading from bowel to bladder also occur and in fact fistulas originating in the bowel of a patient with regional enteritis are capable of involving any organ within the abdominal cavity. Most often, however, fistulas end, not in another organ, but blindly in indolent abscess cavities introperitoneally, retroperitoneally, or into the mesentery, embedded in dense, inflammatory tissue.

Examination with the light microscope shows an inflammatory response involving all layers of the bowel wall and consisting of a mononuclear infiltration in which lymphocytes and plasma cells predominate (Fig. 67–7). Characteristically, the mononuclear cells aggregate to form well defined granulomas which contain multinucleated giant cells (Fig. 67–8). Morphologically similar to sarcoid granulomas, the lesions in regional enteritis lack the acid-fast bacilli and caseation necrosis typical of tuberculosis. Endothelial thickening in small blood vessels and lymphatics, often with hyalinization, appears to be a nonspecific secondary response to inflammation. Another response to inflammation may be the gastric metaplasia occasionally observed in the mucosa of involved small bowel in which pyloric glands appear to replace normal intestinal mucosa. Rarely, chief cells and parietal cells may also be seen.

Although the presence of identifiable granulomas greatly assists in distinguishing regional enteritis from other inflammatory bowel disorders, failure to find discrete granulomas does not by itself argue against the diagnosis of regional enteritis.[5] About 25 per cent of surgical specimens from patients with well documented

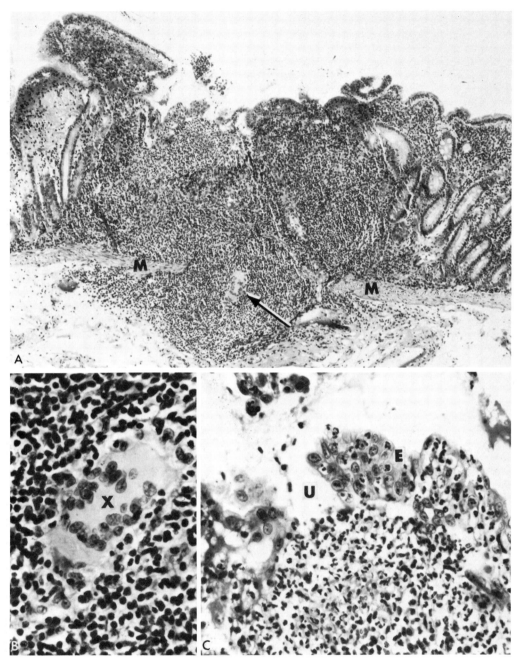

Figure 67–7. Photomicrographs of peroral small bowel biopsy specimen from a patient with duodenal involvement. Hematoxylin and eosin stain. *A*, The arrow indicates a multinucleated giant cell within a typical granuloma. The granuloma extends from submucosa to mucosa and disrupts the muscularis mucosae (M). The villous pattern is obliterated and the lamina propria heavily infiltrated with leukocytes in the region adjacent to the granuloma. × 85. *B*, Higher magnification of the giant cell (X) surrounded by mononuclear cells. × 400. *C*, In the region adjacent to the granuloma there is extensive infiltration of polymorphonuclear leukocytes among surface epithelial cells (E); a small ulceration (U) is present. × 400. (Reproduced from Hermos, J. A., et al.: Gastroenterology 59:868, 1970.)

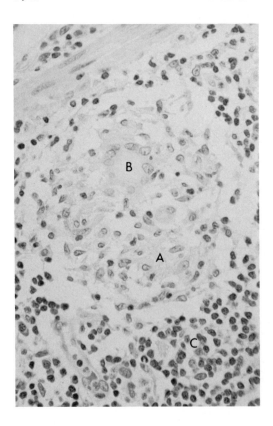

Figure 67–8. Regional enteritis. A patch of enlarged histiocytes (A) and a giant cell (B) are surrounded by a rim of lymphocytes and plasma cells (C). Necrosis is not a feature of the lesion. × 100. (From Mottet, K.: Histopathologic Spectrum of Regional Enteritis and Ulcerative Colitis. Philadelphia, W. B. Saunders Co., 1971.)

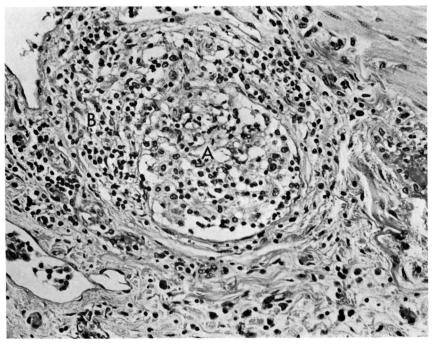

Figure 67–9. A regional enteritis granuloma located in the submucosa. A patch of histiocytes (A) is surrounded by numerous lymphocytes (B). × 64. (From Mottet, K.: Histopathologic Spectrum of Regional Enteritis and Ulcerative Colitis. Philadelphia, W. B. Saunders Co., 1971.)

regional enteritis show nonspecific transmural inflammation. A diffuse granulomatous reaction is found in another 25 per cent. Only in about one-half of the cases are "typical" focal granulomas identified. Thus, although helpful, the presence of these granulomas is not crucial to a pathological diagnosis of regional enteritis. More important is the demonstration of inflammation characterized by edema and infiltration with lymphocytes and plasma cells *in all layers* of the gut wall, particularly in the submucosal, muscular, and serosal layers.[6]

Granulomas are most often identified in the submucosa, but may be present in any layer of the bowel wall (Fig. 67–9). They may also be found in involved lymph nodes, mesentery, peritoneum, organs adjacent to diseased bowel, and liver. These granulomas consist of epithelioid cells arranged in focal aggregates which are rather vaguely limited by an outer rim of lymphocytes. One or more multinucleated giant cells may be present in the periphery. Hyalinized connective tissue occasionally occupies the central region of the granuloma, but caseation does not occur. In about 10 per cent of cases one can identify Schaumann bodies, the birefringent crystals and/or basophilic particles which tend to aggregate within foreign body giant cells.[5]

EPIDEMIOLOGY

Regional enteritis occurs throughout the world, but for the most part meaningful comparisons of incidence and prevalence rates among various populations are not possible. Reports from urban centers in England,[7] Scotland,[8] and the United States[9] indicate, however, that among industrialized Caucasians, one or two persons per 100,000 population develop the disease annually. The prevalence of regional enteritis in this setting appears to be approximately nine cases per 100,000. It is slightly more common in males than in females. Regional enteritis has been described in newborns as well as octogenarians, but symptoms most often develop when the patient is in his twenties. Those afflicted before the age of 15 are more likely to have diffuse involvement of jejunum and ileum.

The incidence of regional enteritis appears to be increasing rapidly whether one studies relatively large urban populations in Britain or selected patients referred to a medical center in the United States. Whether this rising incidence is real or merely results from increasing awareness of the disease has not been settled. Similarly, it is not clear whether regional enteritis is really more frequent in industrialized Western nations or is simply not recognized in the so-called "developing" countries.

Careful surveys indicate that in the United States, regional enteritis occurs two to three times more often among Jews than among non-Jews, but sex distribution as well as the severity and course of the illness appears to be similar in the two groups.[10] Most workers agree that whites develop the disease two to five times more often than nonwhites. The validity of this difference is difficult to determine, however, because the number of nonwhites studied has been small and diagnostic facilities have not always been comparable for the two groups. An acute, nonrecurrent form of regional enteritis appears to be unusually common among Japanese patients. In one large series reported from Japan, fewer than 10 per cent of patients had been ill for more than six months.

Many physicians have noted the presence of inflammatory bowel disease in relatives of patients with regional enteritis. Several reports indicate that 3 to 11 per cent of such patients have a family history of regional enteritis or ulcerative colitis.[11,12] Sherlock and colleagues described five patients with regional enteritis and two with ulcerative colitis in a single family, and one can find several similar, although less dramatic, examples in the medical literature.[11,12] Siblings, parents, or children constitute the relatives most likely to be affected. In their review of the literature, Sherlock et al. found four sets of monozygotic twins in which both twins had developed regional enteritis, whereas none of four patients with dizygotic twins had a similarly affected twin.[11]

ETIOLOGY AND PATHOGENESIS

The cause of regional enteritis is unknown. Indeed, we do not have enough information at present to be certain whether any single cause is responsible for all cases of what is now called regional enteritis. It remains possible, in fact, that this term merely represents a number of different diseases, each with a distinct etiology. Since this clinically dramatic disorder was only recently recognized as a clinicopathological entity, since the disease seems to occur most often in highly industrialized nations, and since the incidence apparently continues to increase in these nations, one may justifiably wonder whether regional enteritis is the product of some aspect of modern civilization. Such speculation would have a firmer basis, however, if one could be certain that data concerning prevalence and incidence did not merely reflect differences in awareness of the disease.

Because the disease is particularly common in Jews, appears to be relatively rare in nonwhites, and tends to occur in families, a constitutional predisposition seems to be important. Similar epidemiological relationships have been described for ulcerative colitis, and indeed cases of Crohn's disease and ulcerative colitis occur in the same family. Thus, similar predisposing factors may be operative in both diseases. The increased occurrence of ankylosing spondylitis, eczema, hay fever, and arthritis among relatives of patients with Crohn's disease further supports a role for an inherited constitutional predisposition.[13]

As in the case of ulcerative colitis, emotional factors have been implicated in the pathogenesis of regional enteritis,[14] but the supporting evidence is, if anything, even weaker than that for ulcerative colitis. The evidence to support this theory is derived from anecdotal, retrospective studies which report the frequent occurrence of repressed hostility and dependency among patients with regional enteritis as well as an association between psychological stress and clinical exacerbations of the disease. Such studies, however, have lacked sufficient controls to eliminate the possibility of bias. In addition in at least one prospective investigation of 19 patients with regional enteritis, no evidence was found to implicate personality or emotional factors.[15] As is true for any chronic troublesome illness, psychological and so-cial features are prominent and require rigorous attention by the physician caring for the patient with regional enteritis. At present, however, the relation between emotions and the disease remains totally undefined.

Because regional enteritis is essentially an inflammatory process, the possibility of an infectious etiology has been almost continuously considered since the disease was first described. To date, detailed examinations of diseased gut wall and of luminal contents for potentially pathogenic bacteria, fungi, or viruses have failed to identify an infectious agent. Although *Mycobacterium pseudotuberculosis* produces a subacute granulomatous inflammation of mesenteric lymph nodes in man, patients infected with this agent do not develop the small bowel pathology so characteristic of regional enteritis (see p. 1380). In fact, no known pathogen consistently produces an enteric disorder in man or experimental animals which clinically or pathologically resembles regional enteritis.[6] On the other hand, certain enteric disorders in domestic and laboratory animals have features reminiscent of regional enteritis. In cocker spaniel dogs there has been clearly described a chronic inflammatory process which affects the terminal ileum and colon with scarring, obliterative lymphangitis, thickening of the mesentery, involvement of regional lymph nodes, and skip areas. Granulomatous colitis occurs spontaneously in boxer dogs. Although this disorder is segmental, causes a symmetrical thickening of the bowel wall, and extensively involves the lymphoreticular system of the colon and its mesentery, the disease appears to be strictly limited to the colon, and deep ulceration and fistula formation do not occur. Terminal ileitis observed spontaneously in swine and hamsters bears little resemblance to the human disease. A chronic granulomatous disease of the terminal ileum and proximal colon has been described in cattle, sheep, and goats infected with *Mycobacterium johnei*, but this disorder more closely resembles intestinal tuberculosis than regional enteritis.

The chronic, inflammatory nature of the disease, the presence of granulomas, the occurrence of systemic manifestations such as arthritis and skin lesions, and the frequently observed favorable response to adrenocorticosteroid treatment all have caused speculation that altered immune mechanisms may play an important role in the pathogenesis of regional enteritis. Sarcoidosis, a disease histologically similar to Crohn's disease, is characterized by depressed delayed hypersensitivity. Diminished cellular immune responsiveness has also been implicated in regional enteritis on the basis of reports that skin tests with tuberculin and 2, 4-dinitrochlorobenzene are frequently negative.[16] It should be noted, however, that some workers have not been able to document any impairment of delayed hypersensitivity among patients with regional enteritis.[17] Similarly, Kveim tests have yielded inconsistent results. Most earlier reports indicated that the Kveim test was negative in patients with Crohn's disease. In one recent study, however, half of 74 patients were observed to have a positive Kveim test, a finding which should lead to renewed exploration of possible relationships between sarcoidosis and regional enteritis. Recently, injection of homogenates of small bowel or lymph nodes from patients with regional enteritis has produced sarcoid-like granulomas in the footpads of mice; however, the reaction may be nonspecific.[18] Finally, lymphocytes from some patients with regional enteritis exert cytotoxic effects on human colonic epithelial cells in tissue culture and show impaired blast transformation in response to phytohemagglutinin. Although these observations all point to one or more poorly delineated abnormalities of cellular immune function in regional enteritis, it is worth emphasizing that none of the observed alterations are found in all, or even most, patients with Crohn's disease. Furthermore, some of the reported abnormalities, such as impaired lymphocytic response to phytohemagglutinin, must be considered nonspecific. Because they occur in a wide variety of chronic illnesses, the meaning of such abnormalities remains unclear.

Humeral antibodies to colon cells and to *Escherichia coli* 014 are found in the sera of patients with regional enteritis with about the same frequency as is observed in that of patients with ulcerative colitis.[19] Although serum levels of immunoglobulins usually are well within normal limits, some patients with extensive or severe regional enteritis may have abnormally high levels of IgA. On the other hand, the distribution of lymphocytes which produce IgA, IgG, IgM, and IgD appears to be normal in the lamina propria of the affected bowel.

At present, firm clinical and experimental evidence is lacking to indicate whether altered immunological mechanisms play any fundamental role in the etiology of regional enteritis. Studies to date indicate that impaired cellular immunity is more likely to be important than abnormal antibody responses, but no specific immunological abnormality has yet been demonstrated consistently in patients with Crohn's disease. Furthermore, the question must always be asked whether altered immune responses represent an etiological factor or are merely the result of the disease process.

CLINICAL COURSE

Any consideration of the clinical features of Crohn's disease must continually emphasize the striking variability observed from patient to patient. The "typical" patient, such as the first case described by Crohn, is a young adult with persistent, although not usually severe, diarrhea which is not frankly bloody. The diarrhea is accompanied by fever and right lower quadrant pain. Anorexia, nausea, and vomiting may or may not be present. At this stage of illness, examination of the right lower quadrant usually elicits tenderness, often with rebound and, occasionally, a palpable, firm, irregular mass of matted loops of intestine. Since the white blood cell count may be elevated, since the illness may be relatively acute, and since diarrhea may not be prominent, the physician not infrequently makes a clinical diagnosis of appendicitis. In this situation, then, the diagnosis is first made at laparotomy.

Symptoms may persist for days to weeks but, early in the course of the disease, tend to subside spontaneously. In most cases, however, diarrhea, accompanied by fever and abdominal pain, tends to recur within several weeks or months. Diarrhea, abdominal pain, and fever are the major complaints of the patient with regional enteritis. When the disease is confined to the ileum, the diarrhea tends to be moderate in severity with usually no more than five or six bowel movements per day. Movements may be watery, but more often are soft and loose. Unless the disease involves the colon, urgency and incontinence rarely occur, and obviously bloody bowel movements are distinctly unusual. The abdominal pain tends to be steady and localized to the right lower quadrant; it usually reflects an indolent inflammatory process in the ileocecal area. Superimposed upon this steady pain is intermittent periumbilical colic usually noted just before and during bowel movements. Fever is generally moderate and, in the absence of complications, rarely exceeds 102° F. Patients may have fever without any signs or symptoms of gastrointestinal disease.

Although regional enteritis most commonly begins with intermittent attacks of diarrhea and abdominal pain, the subsequent clinical course varies greatly from patient to patient.[20, 21] In the majority of patients there is gradual deterioration over a period of years, with shorter and shorter asymptomatic intervals, progressive difficulty in maintaining body weight, and increasing fatigue and lassitude. Slow but persistent blood loss combined with poor food intake leads to anemia. The patient is particularly likely to experience intermittent episodes of partial or even complete, although temporary, small bowel obstruction with abdominal distention, colicky pain, and vomiting. Gradual progression of the disease is rather common; nevertheless, a significant number of patients remain completely asymptomatic for many years or even for the rest of their lives despite two or more attacks of regional enteritis. In approximately 20 per cent of cases the onset of the disease is sudden, the signs and symptoms strongly suggesting appendicitis; however, since the relationship of such acute ileal inflammation to regional enteritis is unclear, it is difficult to predict the subsequent course in such cases. It would appear, however, that no more than 10 to 20 per cent of patients with such acute ileitis ultimately develop chronic regional enteritis.[20, 21]

A diffuse form of the disease is seen in about 15 per cent of cases. Jejunum, ileum, and often colon are diffusely involved, and such patients tend to have particularly severe diarrhea. Fluid and electrolyte depletion, weight loss, and weakness are prominent, and the disease often seems to progress rapidly. Diffuse ileojejunitis appears to be a particularly common form of the disease in children or adolescents. As emphasized subsequently, this form of Crohn's disease must be distinguished from diffuse nongranulomatous ileojejunitis. Impaired growth represents a real threat to young patients, and surgical therapy is often required early in the course of the illness.

The variable course of Crohn's disease is dramatically emphasized by the small proportion of individuals whose otherwise unexplained fever may be the only manifestation of the disease. In other instances, the patient may be completely asymptomatic until he develops one of the "late" complications such as bowel obstruction, symptoms of serious urinary tract infection resulting from an enterovesical fistula, or ureteral obstruction or hepatic enlargement and renal failure caused by secondary amyloidosis. Anorectal or perirectal fistula or abscess often signals the presence of regional enteritis, occasionally without diarrhea and abdominal pain. When diarrhea is present, these signs strongly suggest the diagnosis. The reason for the association between regional enteritis and this complication is unknown.

Thus the course of subsequent illness is unpredictable. Although most patients have recurrent, symptomatic episodes with gradual progression, in a substantial number of patients the course of disease is rather benign. Alternatively the disorder may be rapidly progressive, sometimes even fulminant; or it may become apparent only when one of the "late" complications develops. Under such circumstances it is not surprising that meaningful evaluation of treatment for regional enteritis is, at best, extremely difficult.

COMPLICATIONS

Recurrent diarrhea associated with abdominal pain, weight loss, low-grade fever, and lassitude dominates the clinical picture of regional enteritis. Nevertheless, a wide variety of other manifestations and complications make diagnosis and management of this disease a constant challenge. *Small bowel obstruction*, a common and always serious complication, occurs in approximately 25 to 30 per cent of patients hospitalized for regional enteritis. Obstruction usually results from narrowing of a diseased segment of bowel by both scarring and acute inflammation with edema, and is therefore likely to be partial and intermittent; the occlusion usually progresses to complete obstruction, albeit slowly. Sudden, complete obstruction may also occur, however, when the small bowel becomes kinked or pinched off in an adhesive inflammatory process which involves the mesentery and peritoneum.

Fistula formation, present in at least half the patients with chronic regional enteritis, is a cardinal feature of the disease process and leads to a variety of complications. Fistulas frequently end in indolent abscess cavities which are the source of palpable masses, persistent fever, and pain. Chronic, indurated rectal fissures and fistulas with associated perirectal abscesses develop in about one-third of cases and not infrequently represent the first indication that the patient is ill. Enteroenteric fistulas between loops of small bowel may contribute to nutritional problems if such fistulas cause nutrients to bypass extensive segments of intestinal absorptive surface. In addition, enteroenteric fistulas lead to recirculation of intestinal contents, and the consequent stasis promotes bacterial overgrowth within the small bowel, which, as outlined on page 76, leads to further nutritional problems. Fistulas between bowel and the urinary bladder, although they occur in only 1 to 2 per cent of cases, invariably cause a persistent urinary tract infection and, if left unattended, will lead to irreversible renal damage. Pneumaturia with associated urinary symptoms may be the initial manifestation of regional enteritis, although this mode of presentation is rare.

Although the formation of fistulas and walled-off abscesses is very common in regional enteritis involving the small bowel, one must remember that *free perforation* of the bowel can occur; indeed the literature is replete with examples of patients with Crohn's disease of small gut who present with all the features of a perforated viscus.[22, 23]

Bleeding in regional enteritis patients, although often persistent, is usually mild. In the vast majority of patients in whom disease is limited to the small bowel, the severity of bleeding is not sufficient to change the gross appearance of the stool. Persistent slow blood loss and iron deficiency anemia are frequent, however, along with guaiac-positive feces in patients with chronic regional enteritis. Occasionally, they hemorrhage massively and require blood transfusions for repeated passages of dark red or mahogany-colored stools. Rarely, this type of bleeding is the presenting manifestation of the disease, and in those patients who are explored, the small bowel is found to be diffusely inflamed but not thickened. Hematochezia is much more obvious when Crohn's disease involves the colon, most particularly late in the course of the disease when deep ulcerations have developed.

Malignancy of the small bowel, although rare in patients with Crohn's disease, must be considered in patients who have symptoms of obstruction or who bleed continuously, or who have X-ray evidence of cancer in a small bowel segment. The risk of such malignancy is higher than in the general population; however, it does not constitute an important consideration except when clinical and X-ray findings raise the suspicion. On the other hand, in chronic inflammatory disease of the colon, the issue of malignancy becomes more significant. It is discussed on page 1330.

Systemic manifestations such as arthritis, iritis, erythema nodosum, and clubbing develop in a small proportion of patients with Crohn's disease, but are much more prominent in those with ulcerative colitis. The prevalence of arthritis, however, appears to be approximately the same in the two diseases; in most series 2 to 8 per cent of patients with regional enteritis have either a migratory polyarthritis involving large joints or ankylosing spondylitis. Usually the spondylitis is present for years before bowel symptoms appear, and there is no obvious relation between its course and the course of the regional enteritis. Although migratory monarthritis, involving large joints, afflicts patients with ulcerative colitis as well as regional enteritis, the joint and bowel symptoms tend to exacerbate or remit simultaneously in ulcerative colitis. In patients with regional enteritis, however, the arthritis is usually less severe and seems to run a course relatively independent of the state of the intestinal disease.

Clinically important *liver disease* is relatively unusual among patients with Crohn's disease, but mild abnormalities of liver function, as manifested by elevated serum alkaline phosphatase levels and abnormal sulfobromophthalein excretion, are found in approximately one-third of hospitalized patients. When the liver is involved, biopsy samples most often show a mild pericholangitis; diffuse or focal granulomatous inflammation, although it occurs, is less frequent. Fatty liver is most often seen in more severely ill and in malnourished patients. The prevalence of *cholelithiasis* has not been determined in large numbers of patients with regional enteritis, but in two studies comprising a total of 113 individuals, gallstones were found in 30 per cent (Fig. 67–10).[24, 25] The

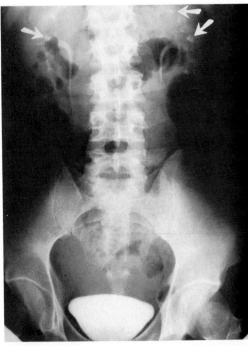

Figure 67–11. Intravenous pyelogram in a 34-year-old patient with regional enteritis and renal colic. Arrows point to radiopaque stones which were oxalate and associated with hyperoxaluria. (Courtesy of Dr. M. H. Sleisenger.)

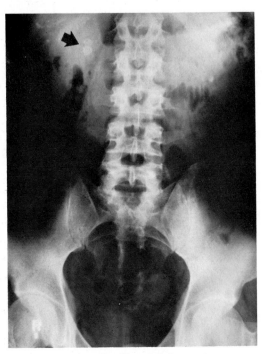

Figure 67–10. Flat film of abdomen in same patient as Figure 67–14. The patient also has cholelithiasis which caused cholecystitis and required cholecystectomy. (Courtesy of Dr. M. H. Sleisenger.)

prevalence was approximately the same in patients with and without ileal resection. Although more and better controlled observations are needed to establish whether this represents a true increase, the high incidence of gallstones in patients with ileal disease is intriguing, because such patients may well have a bile salt deficiency and thus produce bile which is conducive to cholesterol gallstone formation (see pp. 1110 to 1115).

Renal disorders are increasingly recognized as complications of regional enteritis. In addition to urinary tract infections resulting from enterovesical fistulas, patients with regional enteritis may develop ureteral obstruction and consequent hydronephrosis as a result of involvement of the ureter in the granulomatous inflammatory process. Recent reports suggest that nephrolithiasis may also be unusually frequent among patients with Crohn's disease, either with ileal dysfunction or after resection necessitated by regional enteritis. Persistent oxaluria and the formation of oxalate calculi have been observed in a small group of cases (Fig. 67–11). Glycine-conjugated bile salts, instead of being reabsorbed, are lost into the colon where colonic microorganisms convert glycine to glyoxylate which is absorbed and metabolized to oxalate.[26] Taurine is being fed to such patients in order to reduce the amount of the glycine conjugate at a few medical centers. Available data tentatively indicate that this regimen reduces oxaluria and, in some cases, is associated with disappearance of oxalate stones.[27]

A particularly serious renal complication of Crohn's disease is the development of amyloidosis with the nephrotic syndrome and/or progressive renal failure. Although this is rare, most physicians with extensive experience in caring for patients with regional enteritis have encountered at least one case in which "secondary" amyloidosis has developed. The development of hepatic and splenic enlargement and the appearance of proteinemia warrant a search for tissue evidence of this complication. The diagnosis can usually be established by rectal or liver biopsy, although renal biopsy may be necessary. Although some clinicians argue that the presence of amyloidosis constitutes a strong indication for surgical resection of diseased bowel, resection does not necessarily cure the intestinal disease permanently; further, the evidence that bowel resection arrests amyloidosis is tenuous. Thus, the decision for surgery in patients with this complication must be based upon additional indications more directly related to the diseased bowel.

Nutritional problems are extraordinarily frequent and complex. Many patients suffer from anorexia, particularly during phases of active disease; others are afraid to eat because food appears to intensify their crampy abdominal pain and distention. Still others develop rather bizarre dietary habits in the belief that only certain foods do not exacerbate symptoms. Thus, marked weight loss and manifestations of vitamin deficiencies are frequent concomitants of the disease; e.g., megaloblastic anemia caused by dietary folate deficiency is evident in a significant number of patients.

Nutritional deficiencies result not only from inadequate food intake, but also from malabsorption caused by several mechanisms operative in regional enteritis. These are as follows: (1) Diffuse granulomatous infiltration of the jejunum and ileum affects the capability of the columnar cell for absorbing multiple nutrients. (2) Intestinal lymphatics are extensively involved in regional enteritis, severely impairing fat absorption (protein and carbohydrate do not require an intact lymphatic drainage for efficient absorption). Nevertheless, patients with jejunoileitis often have abnormal xylose tolerance tests in addition to steatorrhea, and may absorb vitamins, calcium, iron, or other nutrients poorly. (3) Disaccharidase deficiency, particularly lactase deficiency, frequently results from diffuse small bowel involvement, and patients with regional enteritis may tolerate milk poorly. (4) Diseased terminal ileum may occasionally be responsible for vitamin B_{12} malabsorption, but most often the vitamin is absorbed surprisingly well even in patients with severe distal bowel disease. (5) Protein-losing enteropathy may be striking in extensive disease, particularly with ulcerations, resulting in hypoalbuminemia and edema. (6) Decreased total absorptive surface area may occur owing to widespread disease or following resection or bypass of a long segment of diseased bowel. (7) Strictures, fistulas, or enteroenterostomies or surgically produced blind pouches will cause stasis of intestinal contents and lead to proliferation of enteric bacteria in the small bowel lumen. On the basis of mechanisms outlined on page 930, vitamin B_{12} malabsorption and steatorrhea are frequent consequences of this bacterial proliferation. (8) Finally, combinations of the aforementioned mechanisms may be responsible.

Because the distal small bowel is the major site for reabsorption of conjugated bile salts, ileal resection leads to loss of these bile salts into the colon with contraction of the total bile salt pool, decreased biliary secretion of bile salts, and a diminished concentration of bile salts in the proximal gut lumen inadequate to solubilize the products of fat digestion in mixed bile salt micelles. The increased quantities of bile salts entering the colon inhibit colonic absorption of salt and water and thus contribute to the diarrhea (see pp. 231 to 233). Furthermore, resection of more than 2 feet of ileum regularly produces vitamin B_{12} malabsorption, occasionally leading to vitamin B_{12} deficiency with megaloblastic anemia and, rarely, subacute combined system disease of the spinal cord.

Whatever mechanism or combination of mechanisms may be responsible for fat malabsorption in patients with regional enteritis, diarrhea, and steatorrhea may also cause demineralization of bone, hypocalcemic tetany (vitamin D malabsorption), hypoprothrombinemia with a bleeding diathesis (vitamin K malabsorption), hyponatremia, hypokalemia and dehydration (excess water and electrolyte loss), and, finally, inanition, resulting from inadequate assimilation of dietary calories (see pp. 250 to 289).

DIAGNOSIS

Because of the complexity of regional enteritis, diagnosis can be extremely difficult, and is frequently missed unless the physician is always alert to the disease and its multiple complications. Regional enteritis must be suspected in any patient with diarrhea and abdominal pain, particularly if right lower quadrant tenderness and/or a palpable abdominal mass are also present. As noted above, the possibility of regional enteritis must also be entertained if the patient presents with unexplained fever, perirectal disease, ankylosing spondylitis, or persistent urinary tract infection. Although regional enteritis can be strongly suspected on clinical grounds, radiological demonstration of inflammatory changes in the small bowel is necessary to confirm the diagnostic impression, whereas definitive diagnosis often depends upon gross and microscopic examination of diseased bowel. Most often tissue diagnosis is based on findings in surgically resected intestine. When the duodenum or jejunum is involved, however, it is possible on occasion to establish the diagnosis by peroral suction biopsy (Fig. 67–7).

Laboratory Tests. No laboratory test or combination of tests is specific for Crohn's disease. Thus the laboratory findings assist in evaluating the patient's status, but do not in themselves support or refute the diagnosis of regional enteritis. Leukocytosis and an elevated sedimentation rate tend to suggest that the inflammatory process is active, and, as in a number of chronic or subacute disorders, thrombocytosis may be present. As a result of chronic blood loss, stools may be guaiac positive, and the patient may have a microcytic anemia with a low serum iron concentration and decreased or absent stainable iron in the bone marrow. Macrocytic, megaloblastic anemia may indicate the presence of folic acid or vitamin B_{12} deficiency. Examination of the urine may demonstrate urinary tract infection secondary to an enterovesical fistula, whereas proteinuria and the presence of Bence Jones protein in the urine may indicate the development of renal amyloidosis. The serum albumin level provides a reasonably accurate indication of the patient's overall condition; it will be low in the patient who is not eating, who has extensive malabsorption, or whose disease is causing a significant enteric loss of protein. Most often the combination of the latter two factors is responsible. Serum globulins may be elevated in some patients but are normal or low in others and thus do not provide much help. Liver function tests in most cases do not provide much useful information regarding impaired synthesis of albumin because abnormal alkaline phosphatase and sulfobromophthalein excretion are common in patients with Crohn's disease.[25] The xylose tolerance test, the Schilling test, measurement of carotene, calcium, and phosphorus, and examination of the stool for fat are all useful in determining whether or not the patient has clinically significant malabsorption. Bacterial cultures of fluid aspirated from the jejunum provide an indication of whether the disease is complicated by significant small bowel overgrowth. Since lactase deficiency may contribute to the patient's diarrhea, a lactose tolerance test is helpful in deciding whether or not the patient should avoid milk (see pp. 250 to 289).

Stool and Tissue Examinations. Since regional enteritis remains a "nonspecific" inflammatory disease of the bowel, specific, treatable causes of diarrhea must be excluded as part of the diagnostic evaluation. Fresh stool specimens and rectal contents obtained at sigmoidoscopy should be repeatedly examined for parasites, particularly for pathogenic amebae, and in acute cases the stools should be cultured for Salmonella and Shigella (see pp. 909 to 915 and 1373 to 1377). Rectal biopsy may be useful in documenting early involvement of the rectum and in ruling out schistosomiasis or amebiasis (see p. 1506). Microscopic examination of diarrheal stools may be helpful in difficult cases; the presence of large numbers of leukocytes will reassure the physician that he is not dealing with a patient who has only "functional" bowel disease.

Sigmoidoscopy. In the patient with regional enteritis limited to the small bowel, sigmoidoscopy will be normal or show only the edema and erythema seen in any patient with prolonged diarrhea. The role of sigmoidoscopy and rectal biopsy in the diagnosis of Crohn's disease of the colon is detailed on pages 1356 to 1357.

Radiology. Radiological examination of the small bowel is crucial for the diagnosis of regional enteritis. The plain film of the abdomen will demonstrate dilated small bowel loops when partial obstruction is present. Intra-abdominal masses resulting from matted, inflamed loops of bowel or from abscesses are also frequently documented on the plain film. When the diagnosis of regional enteritis is suspected clinically, a barium enema should precede radiological examination of the small bowel. The barium enema may reveal involvement of the right colon and may delineate a diseased terminal ileum (see p. 1357). Careful radiological examination of the small bowel is then performed with orally administered barium to determine the proximal extent of the disease.

The earliest changes in the small bowel pattern include thickening and distortion of the valvulae conniventes which result from submucosal infiltration and edema. When ulceration occurs, transverse and longitudinal fissures separate islands of residual swollen mucosa and, together with submucosal thickening, lead to a characteristic "cobblestone" appearance (Fig. 67–12). In more chronic and advanced cases a rather complete loss of the mucosal pattern is accentuated by the rigid thickening of the deeper layers of the bowel wall so that the involved segments of small intestine begin to assume a pipe-like appearance. As the disease progresses, the transient narrowing of involved bowel lumen

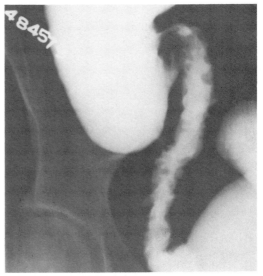

Figure 67–12. Moderate involvement of terminal ileum with typical cobblestone appearance. (Courtesy of Dr. P. Kramer.)

resulting from inflammation and spasm is replaced by a stenotic process which leads to permanent cicatricial stenosis. At this point the X-ray picture is that of a persistently narrow, rigid segment of small

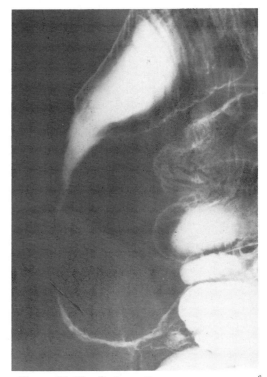

Figure 67–13. Postoperative recurrence of Crohn's disease. The small bowel at the site of anastomosis is involved and shows the typical "string" sign. (Courtesy of Dr. J. Wittenberg.)

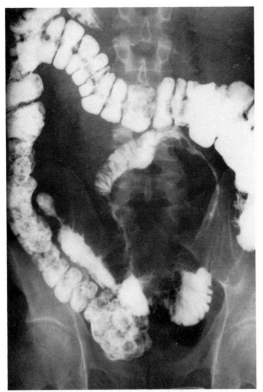

Figure 67-14. Small bowel barium study showing segments of ileum stenosed by regional enteritis. Note the cobblestones and linear ulcers. The patient had symptoms of small bowel obstruction. (Courtesy of Dr. M. H. Sleisenger.)

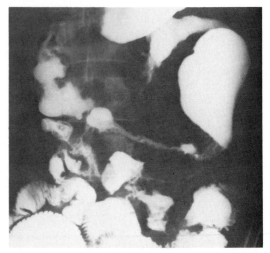

Figure 67-15. Diffuse involvement of segments of duodenum and jejunum with interspersed dilated segments of small bowel. (Courtesy of Dr. P. Kramer.)

matted lymph nodes, or from a combination of these abnormalities.

Diffuse ulceration of the mucosa combined with exudate and increased intestinal secretion often produces a hazy appearance of the barium-filled bowel. The flocculation and segmentation of barium seen in celiac sprue are not considered a radiological feature of regional enteritis, however, and the presence of unequivocal

bowel in which the mucosal pattern is lost; i.e., the well known "string sign" of regional enteritis (Figs. 67-13 and 67-14). In some cases, however, the string sign may occur in early active disease as a result of a combination of ulceration, marked spasm, and edema and thus may be completely reversible. When more than one area of bowel is diseased, involved segments of varying length are characteristically separated by radiologically normal, although sometimes dilated, segments of small intestine (Fig. 67-15). The demarcation between normal and abnormal bowel is usually quite abrupt.

In many instances loops of involved small bowel appear to be separated from one another as a result of thickening of the bowel wall. In addition, abnormal loops often appear to be closely associated with a mass lesion which results from the presence of an abscess, from thickened indurated mesentery, from enlarged and

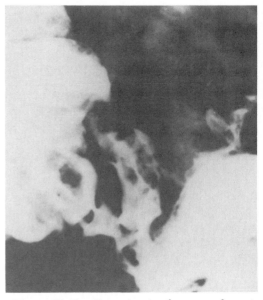

Figure 67-16. Extensive involvement of terminal ileum with burrowing ulceration, cobblestoning, and fistula formation.

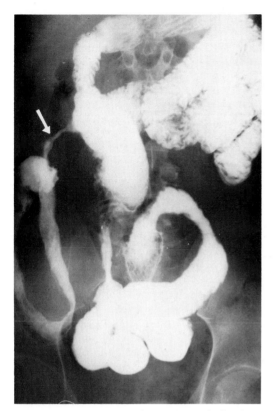

Figure 67-17. Regional enteritis of distal jejunum and proximal ileum, demonstrating narrowed, rigid loops of bowel. Arrow indicates a fistulous tract between two loops of bowel. Patient had malabsorption. Note also separation of loops and loss of normal mucosal pattern.

segmentation as well as of some proximal jejunal dilatation without obstruction should cast doubt on the diagnosis of regional enteritis in favor of celiac sprue.

Fistulas and localized perforations, although they may occur in any part of the small bowel, are most frequently seen by X-ray in the terminal ileum (Figs. 67-16 and 67-17). With terminal ileal involvement one frequently sees concomitant deformity of the cecum and ascending colon. The X-ray picture of Crohn's disease involving the colon is detailed on page 1357.

DIFFERENTIAL DIAGNOSIS

Diagnosis of regional enteritis limited to the small bowel is more difficult than the differential diagnosis, because it depends upon constant awareness of the possibility. During the early and relatively acute phase of the disease, however, regional enteritis may be confused with *appendicitis*. In general, patients with appendicitis are likely to have less diarrhea, more prominent right lower quadrant pain, more dramatic abdominal tenderness and guarding, and a more rapid course. Nevertheless, right lower quadrant pain, fever, leukocytosis, and a tender, poorly outlined right lower quadrant mass all occur frequently enough in both disorders to make differentiation between the two conditions extremely difficult. When abdominal findings rapidly worsen, however, or if doubt continues, the physician should not delay laparotomy to settle the dilemma. Less harm is done by discovering and ignoring acute ileitis at operation than by delaying necessary surgery for the patient with a gangrenous or perforated appendix (see pp. 1494 to 1499).

In patients with diffuse involvement of the small bowel, regional enteritis must be distinguished from *nongranulomatous ulcerative jejunoileitis*.[28] Abdominal pain and diarrhea are prominent features of this disorder, and the radiological appearance of the small bowel may resemble that seen in the diffuse form of regional enteritis. In nongranulomatous disease, however, weight loss, malabsorption, and hypoproteinuria tend to be much more prominent. Moreover, small bowel biopsy shows a more diffuse lesion with flattened and thickened villi, infiltration of the lamina propria, and mucosal ulcerations (see pp. 922 to 924).

Lymphoma involving the small intestine may produce a clinical picture which closely resembles regional enteritis. Diarrhea, abdominal pain, fever, weight loss, and lassitude are prominent in lymphoma, and bouts of intestinal obstruction are common. In general, however, symptoms are more constant in lymphoma and deterioration is more rapid, the average time from onset of symptoms to exploration being about six to nine months. In patients with lymphoma, palpable abdominal masses tend to be hard rather than firm, well circumscribed rather than vaguely defined, and, usually not tender. The presence of enlarged peripheral lymph nodes, pulmonary hilar adenopathy, or marked enlargement of the liver or spleen argues strongly for a diagnosis of lymphoma, but these findings are frequently absent in small bowel lymphoma. Radiologically the nodularity of thickened valvulae, the presence of distinct mass lesions within the bowel wall, and the absence of true cicatricial narrowing all serve to distinguish lymphoma from regional enteritis. Small bowel biopsy may be helpful in establishing the presence of diffuse intestinal lymphoma (pp. 950 to 958).

Chronic *fungal infections* can produce transmural inflammatory changes in the small bowel such as indolent ulcers, fistulous tracts, and abscess cavities, and thus can be confused with regional enteritis. Although patients with aspergillosis, blastomycosis, or other fungal infections often have an insidious and lengthy illness, prolonged periods of remission are rare. Furthermore, such infections are most likely to develop in patients already debilitated by an underlying disease, particularly those who are receiving adrenocorticosteroids, antibiotics, immunosuppressive agents or cancer chemotherapy. Cultures of fistulas for fungi, the finding of typical "sulfur granules," and appropriate skin tests all help to identify the presence of fungal infection (pp. 920 to 922).

Tuberculosis produces transmural inflammation of the small intestine which closely resembles the pathological process of regional enteritis. Although at one time considered a common cause of distal small bowel obstruction, enteric tuberculosis is relatively uncommon today and is now almost never seen in the absence of pulmonary tuberculosis. The disease is most commonly localized to the terminal ileum. Although fistula formation and cicatricial narrowing are frequently seen, skip areas are rare. Radiologically, however, intestinal tuberculosis is difficult to distinguish from Crohn's disease, and if acid-fast bacilli cannot be identified in the sputum, a laparotomy may be required to make the diagnosis. In many cases the cecum and right colon are also diseased (see p. 1377).

One must remember that occasionally regional enteritis can involve the duodenum. The narrowing and ulceration seen in other areas of the small bowel may be seen in the duodenum, and the X-ray appearance may mimic that of *postbulbar duodenal ulcer*. In general, however, the epigastric pain of patients with regional enteritis of the duodenum differs markedly from the typical pain pattern of peptic ulcer, being more resistant and refractory to antacids. Nevertheless, the differential diagnosis between regional enteritis involving the duodenum and postbulbar peptic ulcer may be extremely difficult clinically as well as by X-ray. Any patient with atypical gastrointestinal symptoms and X-ray findings suggestive of postbulbar ulcer should have a careful diagnostic evaluation for regional enteritis.

TREATMENT

As in all chronic diseases of unknown cause with a wide variety of clinical manifestations and complications, the management of regional enteritis is complex and individualized, depending for the most part upon the patient's condition. No single medication, surgical procedure, or therapeutic regimen can be considered appropriate for all, or even most patients with Crohn's disease; presently our knowledge permits only the outlining of some general and accepted principles.

At the onset or during an exacerbation of symptoms which suggests active disease, the patients should be placed at bedrest, sedated if necessary, and treated symptomatically. Diarrhea is often effectively reduced by codeine, Lomotil, or paregoric. In many cases these same agents simultaneously relieve the abdominal cramps with the diarrhea. On occasion, however, more potent analgesics may be required. However, in such instances perforation or obstruction should be suspected. In patients with evidence of small bowel obstruction, continuous nasogastric suction, or, rarely, small intestinal intubation and intravenous fluids will allow the acute phase of the disease with edema and spasm of the small bowel to subside. If the patient's symptoms and findings improve with such supportive therapy, including adequate replacement of electrolytes, particularly K^+, over a period of seven to ten days, there is usually no need either for more potent anti-inflammatory agents or for surgery.

In some instances, however, symptoms and signs of obstruction or of active disease persist or worsen despite symptomatic therapy. In milder cases, one can justifiably institute a trial with Azulfidine for a period of one or two weeks, although the value of this agent in regional enteritis is not established. Many experienced gastroenterologists are convinced that Azulfidine is of no benefit to patients with regional enteritis, but there are others who steadfastly believe that occasionally patients may show marked improvement in response to the drug. Objective evaluations of the efficacy of Azulfidine in regional enteritis are lacking, however, and the drug should probably not be used for longer than a week or two if the patient does not improve.

Patients whose active disease process continues in spite of bedrest and symptomatic measures are usually treated with adrenocorticosteroids. Initially at least, subjective improvement occurs in the vast majority of patients so treated. Although its effect is less clear cut and its benefit is difficult to sustain, steroid therapy is clearly indicated for patients with signs of persistent, active disease, particularly when it is extensive or associated with systemic manifestations such as arthritis, uveitis, or fever unexplained by abscess. When the disease has become well established and is complicated by fistulas, walled-off perforations with or without abscess, and strictures, steroid treatment is, on the whole, unsatisfactory compared with its effect when given to patients early in the course of their disease. Further, since there is no evidence that steroids alter the long-term course of regional enteritis, they should be given to suppress the active phase of inflammation, not to maintain the asymptomatic patient who has no evidence of continuing inflammation. In the patient who continues to have active disease, however, the presence of fistulas need not be considered a contraindication to steroid therapy for diarrhea, discomfort, or other active inflammation, provided the physician is reasonably sure intra-abdominal sepsis is not present.

In general, steroid therapy is best begun with a large dose. Patients who are severely ill appear to benefit more from seven to ten days of adrenocorticotropic hormone (40 to 60 mg in an intravenous drip over 8 to 12 hours) or from the adrenocorticosteroid administered parenterally over the same period (prednisolone, 100 mg intravenously or 100 mg intramuscularly in divided doses). In less severe cases, 60 to 80 mg of prednisolone per day should be given orally for a period of seven to ten days. If the expected improvement occurs, parenteral therapy may be replaced by oral administration and the dosage gradually reduced to a level which suppresses signs of the inflammatory process. For those on oral drugs from the onset of therapy, gradual reduction is in order also. The amount necessary for maintenance varies from patient to patient, and the physician's objective is to find the minimal dose required to suppress symptoms and signs of the disease. In general, steroids can be gradually withdrawn after a few months. If signs of inflammation recur, medication should be reinstituted or the maintenance dose again increased.

Azathioprine and other so-called immunosuppressive agents have been given to a limited number of patients with rather dramatic responses in some. At the present time, however, clinical experience is still extremely limited, and the use of these drugs for patients with regional enteritis must be considered experimental until objective evaluations of their efficacy are available. No control studies of the efficacy of steroids, Azulfidine, or azathioprine have been carried out to date.

Although many patients and a few physicians pay compulsive attention to diet, there is no evidence that what the patient eats in any way affects the symptoms or course of regional enteritis, with one notable exception: those patients with narrowing of the gut lumen caused by inflammation and spasm in the acute phase or by stenosis in the chronic phase should certainly avoid all foods which contain cellulose or other substances which are not readily digested in the upper gastrointestinal tract. Beyond the elimination of "roughage" from the diet in order to reduce the chances of partial or complete intestinal obstruction, the kinds of food eaten by the patient should not be a matter of concern for the physician. Obviously if the patient's experience indicates that certain specific foods cause symptoms, such substances must not be eaten. On the other hand, many patients with regional enteritis, as well as those with other chronic disorders of the gastrointestinal tract, eventually believe that so many foods cause symptoms that proper nutrition becomes a serious problem. In such cases, the physician must carefully discuss the patient's opinions concerning diet and provide necessary reassurance.

Of particular importance in the management of patients with regional enteritis is the provision of appropriate emotional support. In general this is best accomplished by the physician directly responsible for the patient's care and is effective only when the physician gradually comes to know his patient well. Although time-consuming, efforts directed at listening sympathetically to the patient's problems and offering helpful advice are essential in management and often yield rewarding results. Intensive psychiatric probing, although perhaps indicated in specific instances, i.e., patients with serious neuroses or psychoses, may be upsetting, occasionally has an adverse effect on the course of the disease, and should be undertaken only when the regional enteritis is relatively quiescent.

Maintenance of adequate nutrition is often difficult in patients with extensive regional enteritis, particularly in those who have been subjected to extensive small bowel resection (see pp. 250 to 289 and 971 to 977). Parenteral hyperalimentation has been advocated as a means of "resting" the bowel, allowing fistulas to heal, inducing a positive nitrogen balance, and even causing weight gain. This form of therapy, however, has not been extensively used in regional enteritis, and further experience is required for meaningful evaluation of its efficacy.[29] A similar approach consists of using an "elemental diet" which contains only monosaccharides, amino acids, vitamins, and minerals. Parenteral vitamin B_{12} should be administered regularly to all patients with ileal resections.

Specific replacement of vitamin D, calcium, vitamin K, folic acid, iron, and other nutrients which may be poorly absorbed by patients with regional enteritis is indicated whenever there is clinical or laboratory evidence of deficiency of these substances. In patients with bile salt deficiency resulting from extensive disease or resection of the terminal ileum, substitution of medium-chain triglycerides (MCT) for long-chain triglycerides in the diet re-

sults in improved lipid absorption and diminished steatorrhea. Although many patients are able to use commercially available forms of medium-chain triglycerides, these preparations usually contain considerable quantities of lactose, and patients with regional enteritis and lactase deficiency resulting from diseased or resected small bowel may tolerate this lactose poorly. Some patients, on the other hand, find MCT in oil medium quite satisfactory. Since the bile salt concentration in the proximal intestine is greatest at the time of the first meal of the day, it is probably best to recommend that larger quantities of fat be taken at breakfast than at othes meals (see pp. 259 to 277).

The diarrhea associated with disease or resection of the distal small bowel probably results in part from delivery of unabsorbed bile salts into the colon. Binding of these salts with cholestyramine has in some instances improved diarrhea. To bring this about, however, a daily dose of 8 to 12 g is usually required. Some patients are unwilling to take such a quantity of this relatively unpalatable resin. In patients with large ileal resections (more than 100 cm), moreover, binding of bile salts by the resin is of little theoretical value (see p. 971) and in fact is usually not beneficial. Although in theory the feeding of conjugated bile salts should improve fat absorption, adequate quantities of pure conjugated bile salts are not available for clinical use. Watery diarrhea may increase following the administration of pure conjugated bile salts to patients with disease or resected distal small bowel. Thus, the use of bile salts to improve lipid absorption and nutrition is at present impractical.

Bedrest, intestinal intubation when indicated, symptomatic therapy, administration of adrenocorticosteroids, and careful attention to nutrition and emotional support constitute the major aspects of long-term medical management of patients with Crohn's disease.

Operative therapy should be reserved for the complications of the disease. Recurrences of Crohn's disease develop in more than 50 per cent of patients subjected to resection and nearly always occur at the site of anastomosis of small bowel to colon. In view of this high rate of recurrence, in the absence of complications there is little or no justification for resection of diseased bowel as therapy for patients with regional enteritis. Although surgery does not play a primary role in the treatment of patients with regional enteritis, approximately 70 per cent of patients with this disease ultimately require operative treatment for one reason or another. When the disorder progresses to the point that the patient is incapacitated by symptoms in spite of intensive medical management, including the use of steroids and in some instances immunosuppressive agents such as aza-thioprine, the only recourse is primary resection or bypass of the diseased bowel. If bypass is necessary, most clinicians would agree that the diseased bowel must be excluded from the stream of intestinal contents. Although objective data are lacking to indicate which procedure is preferable, reports of persistent or reactivated disease, perforation, or even carcinoma in bypassed segments of bowel tend to argue for primary resection whenever feasible.

When acute regional enteritis is discovered during laparotomy for suspected appendicitis, no resection or bypass procedure is indicated, because the course of acute enteritis is usually self-limited and the majority of these patients do not develop chronic regional enteritis. If there is no inflammatory involvement at the base of the appendix or in the cecum, the appendix may be removed at the time of laparotomy. In the event that the patient subsequently has recurrent attacks, appendectomy at the time of operative diagnosis of regional enteritis will have resolved the vexing recurrent problem of differentiating regional enteritis from appendictis. In general, fistula formation or perforation will not occur following appendectomy if the appendix and cecum are normal. Fistulas which subsequently appear nearly always emanate from the diseased small bowel rather than from the site of appendectomy.

When an inflammatory mass is present together with fistulas or sinus tract or other evidence of extramural penetration, steroids, if used at all, must be administered with caution. The physician undertaking this course of treatment must recognize the risk of an enlarging abscess, perforation, or spreading peritonitis. Whether or not surgery is required when fistulous tracts have formed is entirely an individual matter. Rarely fistulas disappear completely when the active phase of the disease subsides either spontaneously or in response to steroid therapy. Usually, however, the draining fistulous tract, particularly those draining into the rectum or vagina, persists and causes disabling symptoms. Under these circumstances surgery is necessary. Simple local removal of the fistulous tract or fissure does not provide satisfactory results and may lead to further fistula formation and progression of the disease unless the involved segment of bowel is resected or bypassed. Because of the hazards of prolonged urinary tract infection, prompt surgical attention is indicated for enterovesical fistulas. In general, fistula formation does not usually result in the spread of regional enteritis into the viscus invaded by the fistulous tract. Thus, for example, when diseased ileum is separated from the sigmoid colon or bladder it is not unusual to find a small opening into these organs. Unless the colon or bladder is grossly involved, the defect may simply be closed. Only when the colon is obviously diseased is colonic resection necessary.

Although in most instances obstruction caused by regional enteritis can be reversed by medical measures, including in-

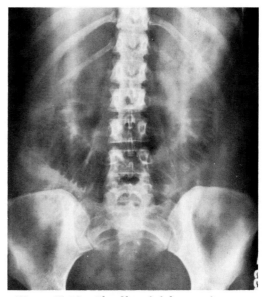

Figure 67–18. Flat film of abdomen of same patient shown in Figure 67–14 approximately one month later, when the patient had complete small bowel obstruction. Note dilated small bowel. (Courtesy of Dr. M. H. Sleisenger.)

testinal intubation, prolonged or rapidly recurrent obstruction may require a definitive surgical procedure (Fig. 67–18). Unless signs of bowel ischemia develop, it is best to operate for obstruction only after a trial of medical management and careful consideration of the need for surgery and the most suitable operative approach.

Another indication for surgery is the presence of free perforation into the abdominal cavity. Although rare, this complication can occur in either acute or chronic regional enteritis. Even though the peritoneal cavity is contaminated, the involved intestine should be resected in preference to attempting mere closure of the perforation.

When Crohn's disease involves the colon, specific surgical problems arise, and these are discussed on pages 1364 to 1365. The pathological similarities and differences between this disease and granulomatous colitis are lucidly presented in a recent monograph by Mottet.[30]

REFERENCES

1. Crohn, B. B. Granulomatous diseases of the large and small bowel. A historical survey. Gastroenterology 52:767, 1967.
2. Lockhart-Mummery, H., and Morson, B. Crohn's disease (regional enteritis) of the large intestine and its distinction from ulcerative colitis. Gut 1:87, 1960.
3. Warren, S., and Sommers, S. Pathology of regional ileitis and ulcerative colitis. J. A. M. A. 154:189, 1954.
4. Morson, B. Histopathology of Crohn's disease. Proc. Roy. Soc. Med. 61:79, 1968.
5. Williams, W. J. Histology of Crohn's disease. Gut 5:510, 1964.
6. Rappaport, H., Burgoyne, F., and Smetana, H. The pathology of regional enteritis. Military Surg. 109:463, 1951.
7. Evans, J., and Acheson, J. An epidemiological study of ulcerative colitis and regional enteritis in the Oxford area. Gut 6:311, 1965.
8. Kyle, J., and Blair, D. Epidemiology of regional enteritis in Northeast Scotland. Brit. J. Surg. 52:215, 1965.
9. Monk, M., Mendeloff, A., Siegel, C., and Lilienfeld, A. An epidemiological study of ulcerative colitis and regional enteritis among adults in Baltimore. I. Hospital incidence and prevalence, 1960 to 1963. Gastroenterology 53:198, 1967.
10. Monk, M., Mendeloff, A., Siegel, C., and Lilienfeld, A. An epidemiological study of ulcerative colitis and regional enteritis among adults in Baltimore. II. Social and demographic factors. Gastroenterology 56:847, 1969.
11. Sherlock, P., Bell, B., Steinberg, H., and Almy, T. Familial occurrence of regional enteritis and ulcerative colitis. Gastroenterology 45:413, 1963.
12. Singer, H. C., Anderson, J. G. D., Frischer, H., and Kirsner, J. B. Familial aspects of inflammatory bowel disease. Gastroenterology 61:423, 1971.
13. Hammer, B., Ashurst, P., and Naish, J. Disease associated with ulcerative colitis and Crohn's disease. Gut 9:17, 1968.
14. Ford, C., Glober, G., and Castelnuovo-Tedesco, P. A psychiatric study of patients with regional enteritis. J.A.M.A. 208:311, 1969.
15. Feldman, F., Cantor, D., Soll, S., and Bachrach, W. Psychiatric study of a consecutive series of 19 patients with regional ileitis. Brit. Med. J. 4:711, 1967.
16. Williams, W. The laboratory diagnosis of Crohn's syndrome. Proc. Roy. Soc. Med. 56:490, 1963.
17. Binder, H., Spiro, H., and Thayer, W. Delayed hypersensitivity in regional enteritis and ulcerative colitis. Amer. J. Dig. Dis. 11:572, 1966.
18. Mitchell, D. N., and Rees, R. J. W. Agent transmissible from Crohn's disease tissue. Lancet 1:168, 1970.
19. Thayer, W., Brown, M., Sangree, M., Katz, J., and Hersh, T. Escherichia coli 0:14 and colon hemagglutinating antibodies in inflammatory bowel disease. Gastroenterology 56:311, 1969.
20. Atwell, J., Duthie, H., and Goligher, J. The outcome of Crohn's disease. Brit. J. Surg. 52:966, 1965.
21. Banks, B., Zetzel, L., and Richter, H. Morbidity and mortality in regional enteritis: Report of 168 cases. Amer. J. Dig. Dis. 14:369, 1969.
22. Waye, J. D., and Lithgow, C. Small bowel perforation in regional enteritis. Gastroenterology 53:625, 1967.
23. Kyle, J., Caridis, T., Duncan, T., and Ewen, S. W. B. Free perforation in regional enteritis. Amer. J. Dig. Dis. 13:275, 1968.
24. Heaton, K. W., and Read, A. E. Gallstones in patients with disorders of the terminal ileum and disturbed bile salt metabolism. Brit. Med. J. 3:494, 1969.
25. Cohen, S., Kaplan, M., Gottlieb, L., and Patterson, J. Liver disease and gallstones in regional enteritis. Gastroenterology 60:237, 1971.
26. Dowling, R. H., Rose, G. A., and Sutor, D. J. Hyperoxaluria and renal calculi in ileal disease. Lancet 1:1103, 1971.
27. Admirand, W. H., Earnest, D. L., and Williams, H. E. Hyperoxaluria and bowel disease. Tr. Assn. Amer. Phys. 84:307, 1971.
28. Jeffries, G. H., Steinberg, H., and Sleisenger, M. H. Chronic ulcerative nongranulomatous jejunitis. Amer. J. Med. 44:47, 1968.
29. Dudrick, S. J., and Ruberg, R. L. Principles and practice of parenteral nutrition. Gastroenterology 61:901, 1971.
30. Mottet, K. M. Histopathologic Spectrum of Regional Enteritis and Ulcerative Colitis. Philadelphia, W. B. Saunders Co., 1971.

Chapter 68

Other Infectious, Inflammatory, and Miscellaneous Diseases

Lloyd L. Brandborg

BACTERIAL DIARRHEAS

Diarrheal diseases are responsible for significant worldwide morbidity and mortality.[1] They are of critical impact in countries that can least afford them. They account for the single largest cause of death in underdeveloped areas either directly or through association with malnutrition. In these countries a child has a 50 per cent chance of dying prior to the age of seven, primarily from diseases associated with diarrhea. It has been estimated that in any given 24-hour period, 200 million people on earth have gastroenteritis, most commonly diarrhea and most likely due to bacterial infections.[2] Stated another way, the amount of diarrheal water passed in any given 24 hour period equals the amount of water flowing over Victoria Falls in one minute. Even in highly developed areas, diarrhea is a major cause of childhood and infant mortality.[1] In many underdeveloped countries, "normal" bowel function is interpreted to mean two to three watery to mushy stools per day. These populations seek medical care only for symptoms of severe dehydration or severe illness. The distribution and prevalence of bacterial diarrheas are outlined in Table 68–1.

Pathogenesis of Bacterial Diarrheas. The enteropathogenic bacteria produce diarrhea by their ability to invade the mucosa, their ability to produce enterotoxins, or both. The clinical syndromes produced by these organisms depend on these factors and the level of the intestinal tract infected.[1] Shigella infection characteristically is associated with lower abdominal cramps, pus and blood in the stools, and tenesmus. On the other hand, cholera, the classic example of noninvasive enterotoxin diarrhea, results in a profuse, watery, small bowel diarrhea. The clinical correlations of enteropathogenicity of the various major pathogens are outlined in Table 68–2.

Response of the Intestine. The intestine reacts to enterotoxins by hypermotility.[3] Hypermotility also results from mucosal invasion of Shigella, Salmonella, and some strains of *Escherichia coli*. Once invasion has occurred, these bacteria release endotoxins which have potent local and systemic effects.

Vibrio cholerae, on the other hand, is the classic noninvasive diarrheagenic agent. Exposure of the intestine to the enterotoxin of this organism and that of *Shigella dysenteriae-1* (Shiga bacillus) provokes a

909

TABLE 68–1.   DISTRIBUTION AND PREVALENCE OF BACTERIAL DIARRHEAS*

CAUSATIVE ORGANISM	GENERAL DISTRIBUTION	IN NORTH AMERICA		IN DEVELOPING COUNTRIES	
		Age Group Principally Affected	Transmission Patterns	Age Group Principally Affected	Transmission Patterns
Shigella	Global	Children	Custodial institutions	0–6 yr.	Direct contact
Esch. coli	Global	Newborn	Hospital nursery	0–6 yr. ? Adults	Direct contact ? Direct contact
V. cholerae	Asia and contiguous areas	—	—	0–10 yr. All ages	Epidemic Water; ?food (epidemic)
V. parahemolyticus	Japan; ? elsewhere	Adults	Raw shellfish	?	? Raw seafood
Salmonellae	Global	All	Prepared foods; poultry; egg products	All	Food borne; direct contact
C. perfringens	? Global	Adults	Cooked meat	Children; nonimmune adults	Pork feasts ("pig bel")
Staphylococci	Industrialized nations	All	Prepared foods	—	(Rare)

*From Grady, G. F., and Keusch, G. T.: New Eng. J. Med. 285:831, 1971, with permission of the authors and publisher.

massive secretion of fluid and electrolyte into the intestine.[1]

The hypermotility and secretion of water and electrolyte into the gut are accompanied by a hyperemia of the microvasculature supplying the mucosa.[1] It is still not settled whether the increased circulation to the intestine is a primary event or secondary to the demand of the mucosa for more fluid to secrete.

Effects of Enterotoxin. Cholera toxin produces a decrease in transport of sodium from the mucosa to the serosa in rabbit and human ileal mucosa, in vitro, after a 30- to

TABLE 68–2.   CLINICAL CORRELATIONS OF ENTEROPATHOGENICITY*

ORGANISM	DIARRHEA/ DYSENTERY	ABDOMINAL PAIN	VOMITING	INCUBATION PERIOD (HR)	MUCOSAL PENETRATION	ENTERO-TOXIN	EXTRAINTESTINAL MANIFESTATIONS
Shigellae	+/+	+	±	24–72	+	+†	Seizures: meningismus
Escherichia coli	+/0 0/+	± +	0 0	24–72 24–72	0 +	+ 0(?)	Minimal Variable
Vibrio cholerae	+/0	0	±	24–72	0	+	Hypokalemic nephropathy
Salmonellae	+/±	±	±	12–36	+	0(?)	Fever: bacteremia
Clostridium perfringens	+/0 +/+§	++ ++	± +	8–15 18–48	0 ±	+‡ 0(?)	Minimal Shock
Staphylococci	+/0‡ +/+¶	± +	++ ±	4–8 Indeterminate	0 ±	+‡ +(?)	Minimal Shock

*From Grady, G. F., and Keusch, G. T.: New Eng. J. Med. 285:831, 1971, with permission of the authors and publisher.
†? only S. dysenteriae I.
‡Preformed toxin ingestion.
§Necrotizing jejunitis (enteritis necroticans) may be clinically similar to dysentery.
¶May occur when enterocolitis is produced by proliferating enterotoxin-producing organisms.

60-minute delay.[1] Chloride and bicarbonate accumulate in the mucosal perfusion solution in larger amounts than sodium. Actively transported sugars and amino acids added to the preparation enhance sodium absorption, causing a parallel isosmotic absorption of water. Clinically it has been shown that the stool volume in patients with cholera decreases substantially if they are fed glucose or amino acids.[3, 4] It has also been shown that secretion of fluid and electrolyte by jejunum and ileum can account for most of the diarrhea in patients with cholera.[5]

Intermediary Metabolites. Cholera toxin has been shown to activate adenyl cyclase and increase intestinal levels of cyclic AMP (3'-5'adenosine monophosphate).[3] Fluid hypersecretion in response to cholera toxin occurs after a minimum delay of approximately 15 minutes. Theophylline, which inhibits breakdown of cyclic AMP, produces hypersecretion almost immediately—additional evidence that cholera toxin acts through adenyl cyclase and perhaps other intermediaries. The prostaglandins can also activate adenyl cyclase, resulting in increased cyclic AMP, mimicking the action of cholera toxin. The F_{2a} subtype was effective in producing diarrhea following infusion into the mesenteric artery in dogs. The prostaglandins have also been known to play a role in stimulating contractility of smooth muscle of the intestine. Although cholera toxin is the only enterotoxin which has been shown to activate adenyl cyclase and stimulate cyclic AMP, it is probable that other toxins may also share this property (see pp. 305 to 307).

SPECIFIC BACTERIA

SHIGELLA

Shigella are capable of invading the intestinal mucosa but largely affect the colon. Whether all species have an enterotoxin similar to that recently shown in *Shigella dysenteriae*-1 (Shiga bacillus)[1] is not known. Its enterotoxin produces ileal hypersecretion to the same degree as cholera enterotoxin. Shigellae are the pathogens most often identified in field studies of diarrheal diseases. It is likely that the true incidence is underestimated because of the difficulty of culturing the organism and the failure to take mucosal swabs as specimens for culture[1] (see pp. 1373 to 1377).

ESCHERICHIA COLI

Escherichia coli are normal inhabitants of the bowel, largely the colon.[1] It had long been suspected that some strains were pathogenic, but it required the development of antigen classification and antisera to identify specific strains. Several different serotypes have been incriminated in lethal diarrhea in infants. Currently, about a dozen different enteropathogenic serotypes are known.[1]

Clinical Features. Infections with enteropathogenic *E. coli* are most important in infants and children. However, traveler's diarrhea has been reported to be due to one serotype of these organisms in British troops in Aden.[6] Typically, the diarrhea is of sudden onset, profuse and watery, and accompanied by abdominal colic. The patient is afebrile. The usual duration is short, rarely more than four to five days, and in adults no antimicrobial therapy is indicated.

Enteropathic *E. coli* are commonly responsible for epidemic diarrhea in infants and neonates. The infection can be particularly lethal in premature infants. The enteropathogenicity of strains responsible for infant diarrhea have been confirmed in adult volunteers. Epidemics of diarrhea caused by enteropathogenic *E. coli* are virtually unheard of in adults.

By virtue of their ability to penetrate the intestinal mucosa, some strains of *E. coli* produce bacillary dysentery which is clinically identical to shigellosis.[5] Some of these strains elaborate a filterable enterotoxin that is diarrheagenic in the rabbit intestinal loop.[2]

Diagnosis. Enteropathogenic *E. coli* should be suspected as a cause of epidemic diarrhea in infants and children, particularly in newborns. Specimens for culture are best obtained by rectal swabs. Specific reference antisera have been developed and incorporated into typing sets.[3] The finding of a pure culture of *E. coli* in the presence of diarrhea is strong presumptive evidence that the organism is an enteropathogen.

Treatment. Most adults with diarrhea caused by enteropathogenic *E. coli*, including traveler's diarrhea, which is probably often due to these strains, have a self-limited, afebrile course of a few days. Re-establishment of the normal gastrointestinal flora leads to rapid recovery and antimicrobial therapy is not warranted. Abdominal colic and diarrhea may be alleviated by administration of diphenoxylate with atropine (Lomotil) in dosages of 2.5 to 5 mg. every six hours.

On the other hand, the virulent enteropathogenic *E. coli* may require antimicrobial therapy.[7] In one study, seven of 13 volunteers developed a striking febrile illness with temperature to 40° C, headaches, myalgia, abdominal cramps, profuse diarrhea, or dysentery. Blood cultures of these subjects were negative. Therapy with 2 g of ampicillin daily in divided doses for three days resulted in clinical and bacteriological cure. Therapy of these virulent infections may be initiated with intramuscular ampicillin until in vitro bacterial identification and sensitivities are obtained.

One report suggests a beneficial effect of antimicrobial therapy in infants infected with an enteropathogenic *E. coli*.[8] Six of seven infants infected with *Escherichia coli* (0114) during an in-hospital epidemic were treated with gentamicin base orally, 12.5 mg per pound of body weight per 24 hours and were well within a week. The organisms had been isolated by routine daily rectal swabs and were resistant to penicillin, streptomycin, chloramphenicol, tetracycline, erythromycin, neomycin, albamycin, cloxacillin, and ampicillin, and sensitive to gentamicin. Therapy with antibiotics to which enteropathogenic *E. coli* are sensitive will abort epidemics.[8]

SALMONELLA ENTERITIDIS

Definition and Etiology. "The taxonomy of salmonellae is needlessly confusing to the nonmicrobiologist. They are easily separable into three ecological groupings according to host preference—i.e., those specifically adapted to man, those adapted to animals, and those with no specific host preference [Table 68–3]. The broad correlation of clinical

TABLE 68–3. RELATION OF SALMONELLA SPECIES AND REPRESENTATIVE SEROTYPES TO HUMAN DISEASES*

SPECIES	REPRESENTATIVE SEROTYPE†	NATURAL HOST	HUMAN DISEASE
S. choleraesuis	–	Animal (swine)	Septicemia and arteritis
S. typhi	–	Man	Enteric (typhoid fever)
S. enteritidis	Paratyphi A Schottmülleri‡	Man	Enteric fever or gastroenteritis
	Pullorum	Animal (fowl)	None
	Dublin	Animal (cattle)	Gastroenteritis
	Typhimurium		Gastroenteritis, septicemia or focal infection
	Derby Enteritidis Heidelberg and hundreds of related serotypes	Man and many animals	Gastroenteritis

*From Grady, G. F., and Keusch, G. T.: New Eng. J. Med. 285:831, 1971, with permission of the authors and publisher.
†Or serotypes.
‡Current name for Paratyphi B.

syndromes with this classification system makes it useful. The taxonomy scheme in current use recognizes three 'species' (*S. choleraesuis, S. typhi, S. enteritidis*). *S. choleraesuis and S. typhi* do not contain subtypes (serotypes), but *S. enteritidis* contains over 1500 serotypes, and all three ecological groups are represented among them. The serotypes are identified by their O and H antigens, are written in capitalized nonitalicized form (e.g., serotype Paratyphi A. of *S. enteritidis*). *S. enteritidis* serotype Typhimurium may cause septicemia and focal infection and is the most prevalent of all strains lacking a host preference and capable of producing gastroenteritis."[1]

Role of Toxins of Salmonella. The toxins of these species are endotoxins, a property held in common with all gram-negative bacteria, including the normal enteric flora. They are released on autolysis of the bacterial cell and are part of the "O" or somatic antigen. Although the exact nature of the toxin is unknown, the lipopolysaccharide which is intimately associated with the cell wall contributes to the endotoxin activity. The O antigens are toxic to man; when inoculated into the skin, they produce edema and erythema followed by necrosis. When administered intravenously in minute amounts, the subjects become ill with fever, chills, headache, malaise, and a decrease in polymorphonuclear leukocytes.[9] Since endotoxin is continuously present in the gut owing to senescence and death of bacteria, it is likely that little or none is absorbed under normal circumstances.

Clinical Features. Several forms of infection with Salmonella may be considered: gastroenteritis, enteric fever, and septicemia.

SALMONELLA GASTROENTERITIS. The enteric form of the disease is usually mild and limited to a one- to four-day period characterized by diarrhea and lower abdominal or diffuse abdominal colic. The disease has a short incubation period and results from consumption of contaminated food or water. Following infection, gastroenteritis develops after 12 to 36 hours. The onset is almost always sudden; it is accompanied by headache, chills, and abdominal distress. Nausea, vomiting, and diarrhea follow with rise in temperature and varying degrees of prostration. The course is usually between one and four days and is more severe in infants and young children. In contrast to the septicemic form of the infection, blood cultures are always negative, but organisms are frequently cultured from feces and occasionally from vomitus. *S. enteritidis* serotype Typhimurium is the most common organism, although outbreaks of other species or organisms have been reported.

The history is crucial to diagnosis. Ordinarily, Salmonella gastroenteritis is epidemic and the patient under consideration is only one of a group who has become ill as a result of the ingestion of the contaminated source. Isolated cases are occasionally seen, and in them the source of the infection cannot be accurately traced.

ENTERIC FEVER WITH SALMONELLA. This clinical form of salmonellosis is less common than gastroenteritis, but it may be seen with any of the species of Salmonella infecting man. Clinically, the illness is milder than typhoid fever, but on occasion it can be serious and rarely even fatal. The onset is usually characterized by malaise, anorexia, and diarrhea; shortly, the temperature begins to rise and will persist for one to three weeks or more if untreated. It reaches 100° F or 102° F during the first week, by which time blood cultures are

often positive. During this period stool cultures are often negative. A rash resembling the rose spots of typhoid fever may be noted in rare instances. *S. enteritidis* serotypes S. Paratyphi A and S. Schottmülleri tend to be more frequent causes of enteric fever but may also commonly cause gastroenteritis.[1]

SALMONELLA SEPTICEMIA. This is the most serious form of Salmonella infection, aside from typhoid fever. When the organism gains access to the blood stream the patient is acutely and severely ill with high fever and prostration. In most adults gastrointestinal involvement is minimal. The hallmark of this form is abscess formation in diverse areas of the body. They may be found in the pericardium, meninges, joints, lungs, endocardium, kidney, and within the peritoneal cavity. Acute cholecystitis may also occur, progressing to empyema, gangrene, and rupture of the gallbladder. Thus, local involvement must be sought in patients with high remittent fevers whose blood cultures are positive for Salmonella, because these abscesses may require surgical drainage. Any one of the species of Salmonella can cause widespread sepsis, but it is particularly noted with *S. choleraesuis*.

Diagnosis of Salmonellosis. Diagnosis may be suspected from the history, particularly during epidemics among patients ingesting common foods. Except for some nonspecific and possibly generalized abdominal tenderness, examination of the abdomen is often not remarkable. On occasion, a maculopapular pinkish eruption may be noted during the first week of illness. Splenomegaly is present only rarely but occurs in approximately 75 per cent of patients infected with *S. typhi*, usually in the second week.

Laboratory Tests. The differential white blood cell count usually shows a polymorphonuclear leukocytosis in most forms of the illness with total white blood cell counts of 15,000 to 20,000. In patients with Salmonella septicemia, leukopenia may occur. In simple gastroenteritis the white count may be normal or only slightly elevated.

Specific diagnosis depends upon the isolation and identification of Salmonella from blood, feces, or urine. The bacteriological techniques required for identification are the province of the microbiology laboratory and will not be detailed here. The most conclusive diagnosis is isolation from blood cultures, which is highly likely in individuals who have enteric fever or the septicemic type of clinical disease. Culture is most often successful early in the course of the illness during the first week. On the other hand, in Salmonella gastroenteritis, a localized form, blood culture is universally negative. Isolation of the organisms from feces is the definitive diagnostic method. They may be present in the stool for a number of weeks or months after the acute infection, so immediate identification is not critical in all cases, although early diagnosis is advisable for epidemiological purposes. In the septicemic form of salmonellosis the urine may contain the organism during the first and second week.

In Salmonella gastroenteritis or enteric fever, stool cultures should be obtained early, before overgrowth with other organisms occurs. Direct rectal swabs are probably the most productive specimens, but a fresh stool should also be submitted to the laboratory for examination.

Indirect techniques of diagnosis rely on the rise of type-specific circulating antibodies for a given organism. Thus, diagnosis may be aided by serological testing for specific agglutinins of the causative bacteria which can be demonstrated from one to two weeks after the onset of typhoid and enteric fever, septicemia, or more severe gastroenteritis. Agglutination reactions may not become positive in mild gastroenteritis until symptoms have subsided, and in some instances no rise in titer occurs. A more specific test is for the "O" agglutinin, although tests should be carried out for both O and H agglutinins. Because of the large number of Salmonella species, the antigens involved in serological testing must of necessity be limited, and only those from S. typhi, S. enteritidis serotype Schottmülleri, and S. choleraesuis are commonly used in screening for possible infection. If only a single specimen is available, an O agglutinin titer of more than 1 to 50 during the first ten days of illness is strong presumptive evidence of infection, providing the patient has not had a vaccination for salmonellosis (TAB vaccine).

Treatment for Salmonellosis. Salmonella gastroenteritis requires no specific treatment other than replacement of fluid and electrolyte losses and, rarely, administration of albumin to patients with acute protein-losing enteropathy. If the patient is not vomiting, a liquid diet may be prescribed, progressing to a soft diet with clinical improvement. The diarrhea usually responds readily to diphenoxylate with atropine (Lomotil) 5 mg every six to eight hours.

Antimicrobial therapy is indicated in patients who have enteric fever with positive blood cultures and in individuals with septicemia who may develop or who have focal infections. Abscesses may require surgical drainage. Two drugs are commonly used: chloramphenicol and ampicillin. Chloramphenicol may be given in doses of 1 to 2 g per day in four divided doses by mouth; in extremely ill individuals the initial medication may be administered intravenously. Ampicillin is preferably administered intramuscularly, in doses of 2 to 4 g per day in four divided doses. In vitro sensitivities must always be obtained because of the increasing incidence of resistant Salmonella.[1]

CARRIER STATE. It is probable that antimicrobial therapy of noninvasive salmonellosis prolongs the duration of the carrier state. One controlled study showed no clinical benefit when neomycin was compared with a placebo.[10] From the second through the eighth week a significantly larger proportion of the treated patients were still carriers.

Approximately 3 per cent of patients with typhoid fever will become permanent carriers.[9] The incidence is much less with other species of Salmonella in which the chronic carrier state tends to be of shorter duration, although some patients may harbor the organisms for years.[11] Of 3,637 known carriers in the United States in 1962, only 96 were nontyphoid salmonella carriers.[11]

Occasionally the gallbladder is the habitat for the organisms similar to S. typhi. This association is not so frequent, however. Many carriers have not had clinical infection but are found to be contacts of patients who had clinical salmonellosis. Treatment of carriers appears to be futile. Although the organism may be eradicated from the stool, its disappearance is often only temporary. Accordingly, treatment of these individuals with broad-spectrum antimicrobials is not warranted, not only because it is ineffective, but because it also may lead to resistant strains.

Some chronic carriers will spontaneously remit. All 11 chronic carriers with cholelithiasis in one study were apparently cured with cholecystectomy and antibiotic therapy.[11] Treatment consisted of 1 g of chloramphenicol and 1 g of tetracycline weekly with cholecystectomy during the third to fifth week of antibiotic therapy. In four patients who failed to cure with cholecystectomy alone, antibiotics failed in all four. Cholecystectomy alone cured four of nine patients. Although 24 of the 27 patients studied had S. typhi, two had S. typhimurium and one had S. Schottmülleri. Cholecystectomy and antibiotic therapy should be considered for the chronic carrier with cholelithiasis.

Epidemiology and Control Measures of Salmonella Infection. All Salmonella infection is derived from reservoirs in man and animals. Food, milk, and water become infected from contaminated excreta. The greatest hazards derive from the unrecognized carrier, the patient who has had subclinical disease, or animals. Except for S. typhi, salmonella infections require ingestion of a heavy inoculum in order to produce illness. The more common sources are, in addition to food and water contaminated by carriers, other contaminated drinking water, unpasteurized milk, and shellfish gathered in areas of sewage effluent. Occasionally, ingestion of insufficiently cooked meat from an infected animal will be the source of infection. Salmonellae grow between 4 and 36° C,[1] but outside this range growth ceases, although they survive. Dried foods such as powdered eggs and products containing them are particularly hard to sterilize. Occasionally salmonellosis may be acquired by ingestion of contaminated eggs from infected fowl.

The measures for control of Salmonella infection include the elimination of sources of infection and of modes and vehicles of transmission, and of measures to increase the resistance to susceptible hosts. Infected persons must be isolated to the extent that excreta are carefully disposed of. Although chronic carrier states do develop, permanent carriers analogous to those found in S. typhi infection are rare.[9] Bacteriological examinations must be carried out until Salmonella are no longer found in the feces. Individuals with positive cultures without clinical infections should not be permitted to handle food or water until several successive negative stool cultures have been obtained.

Further measures include adequate inspection of animals slaughtered for consumption. Detection of Salmonella by this manner is difficult because inactive forms of disease cannot be detected. Modern sanitation is of crucial importance, including adequate and proper sewage disposal, adequate processing of sources of drinking water, and pasteurization of milk. Rodents and flies must be excluded from premises where food is being prepared to prevent transmission by fomites. Foods prepared in large quantities must be rapidly refrigerated to less than 4° C to inhibit the growth of Salmonella. Adequate cooking of foods, particularly eggs and egg products, is also important in reducing Salmonella infection.

IMMUNIZATION. Immunization with the TAB vaccine is a measure reserved for conditions of great exposure such as in military units and is usually not used.[8] In some endemic areas, immunization may be given to new arrivals who intend to reside in these areas for varying periods of time. The TAB vaccine is made up of a heat-killed suspension of S. typhi, S. choleraesuis, and S. enteritidis serotypes S. Schottmülleri and, in some instances, S. Hirschfeldii. The vaccine is administered in three subcutaneous injections of 0.5 to 1 ml, with reinoculation with 0.5 ml every three years. The value of this immunization is difficult to assess, but the procedure is still recommended by many public health experts. It clearly reduces mortality from typhoid fever.[9] Its role in preventing other Salmonella infections is not defined.

VIBRIO CHOLERAE

Vibrios are curved, gram-negative, actively motile, flagellated rods. Most vibrios are nonpathogenic organisms. The O antigens determine the two major types (Inaba and Ogawa). The current pandemic is due to V. *cholerae*, biotype El Tor,[1] which varies from the classic strain only in a few nonimmunological characteristics. More individuals infected with El Tor vibrio are asymptomatic than those with the classic V. *cholerae*, but once symptoms develop the two conditions are indistinguishable.

The cholera vibrios are limited to man. Long-term carriers are rare, although a few individuals may have the organism in feces for a few weeks. The gallbladder has been identified as a site of infection. Endemic cholera is largely a pediatric disease. Sporadic and epidemic cholera affects all ages.

The transmission is complicated and possibly largely water borne. High rates of asymptomatic infection occur in close person-to-person contacts with patients. Food may be another means of transmission.

Clinical Features. The incubation period of cholera is not definitely known but is in the order of one to three days.[1] Usually there are no prodromal symptoms, except perhaps some malaise and simple diarrhea. The onset is abrupt and manifested by a profuse, voluminous, watery diarrhea. Originally the stools are yellowish, but they later become colorless and odorless and have the typical "rice water" appearance. There may be severe vomiting and severe prostration. There are no fevers, chills, or sweats. Severe muscle cramps, particularly of the extremities and abdominal muscles, are frequent. Colic is not a prominent feature. Oliguria and anuria are frequent. Stool volume may approach 25 liters per day. Cholera may be rapidly fulminant with death in as short a time as four hours after the onset of symptoms. The diagnosis is not difficult during epidemic cholera.

Physical Examination. The patient is severely prostrated and may be in coma or severely obtunded. There are signs of severe dehydration, including wrinkled skin with poor turgor, shrunken tongue, and soft, sunken eyeballs. Severe tachycardia is usually present as well as hypotension and often severe shock. The axillary and skin temperatures are decreased, but the rectal temperature is usually normal.

Laboratory Tests. The vibrios may be present in stool or in small intestinal contents and may be recognized in the living state in hanging drop preparations by their scintillating motion. Culture of the organism is the province of the microbiology laboratory and will not be detailed here. However, it should be recognized that the usual media used for isolating enteric pathogens, such as eosin–methylene blue, MacConkey, and Salmonella-Shigella agar, are inhibitory and the organism may not grow. The vibrios ferment lactose and can be mistaken for normal coliform bacilli.[1]

The packed cell volume, total white blood cell count, and total serum protein are increased reflecting the severe dehydration. Serum sodium, potassium, and chloride levels may be increased despite severe depletion. There is usually profound acidosis. The electrolyte content of the stool is isotonic. Average stool electrolytes are sodium, 140 mEq per liter; potassium, 10 mEq per liter; chloride, 110 mEq per liter; and bicarbonate, 140 mEq per liter. The pH of stool is alkaline.[12]

Treatment. Therapy is directed to volume-for-volume replacement of the severe fluid and electrolyte deficits and to keeping pace with fecal losses as well as insensible losses.[12] Replacement is accomplished in severe cases by intravenous administration of isotonic sodium chloride and 2 per cent sodium bicarbonate in ratios of approximately 2 to 1 by volume.[12] Ten milliequivalents per liter of potassium are added to each liter of this mixture. Since total losses in the stool may approach 25 liters per day, utilization of large vessels such as the superior or inferior vena cava and large bore catheters may be required. Tetracycline, 100 mg per liter up to 500 mg per day, added to the infusion has been shown to shorten the period of diarrhea and reduce fluid requirements.[12]

It has recently been shown in vitro that absorption of sodium by the normal human ileum is not altered in the presence of cholera toxin.[13]

Addition of glucose or actively transported amino acids causes an increased absorption of sodium. Clinical studies have shown that glucose given orally or in-traintestinal perfusion with glucose reduces the volume of choleric stools.[3, 4] This is a practical way of administering fluid and electrolytes and reducing the amount of intravenous therapy. Volume-for-volume fluid and electrolyte replacement has reduced mortality by 60 to 80 per cent in untreated persons, by 20 per cent in patients treated by previous regimens, and to zero in the uncomplicated cases.[12]

Other Vibrios. Some vibrios are not agglutinated by the O antigen which determines the two major antigenic types.[1] These are called nonagglutinable or NAG vibrios. Some have been shown to elaborate a potent enterotoxin and to produce diarrhea similar to that of classic cholera. *V. parahemolyticas*, a marine organism which is able to grow in high salt concentrations, has been responsible for important outbreaks of "food poisoning" in Japan.[1] The organism appears to have a worldwide distribution, but gastroenteritis resulting from it has not been a major problem outside the Orient.

CLOSTRIDIUM PERFRINGENS

Clostridium perfringens is the most widely distributed bacteria which is pathogenic for man and is present in human and animal feces, soils, water, air. It contaminates most commercially available food, particularly meat and poultry. Five types of the organisms are recognized, named A through E, with a number of subtypes according to the production of several toxins. In the United States in 1969, more outbreaks of food poisoning occurred from *Clostridium perfringens* than from salmonellae or staphylococci.[1] Most human diseases result from infection with the type A strains which are capable of producing spores which are heat resistant. The heat-sensitive organisms have not been associated with diarrheal disease. The illness produced by Type A *C. perfringens* is a self-limited, nonfatal diarrhea. The diagnosis is usually not made until the patient has recovered.

NECROTIZING ENTERITIS

A severe hemorrhagic necrotizing jejunitis caused by Type C *C. perfringens* has been reported from Germany[1] and from the New Guinea highlands.[14] The disease results from ingestion of contaminated food which is usually inadequately cooked. The organism produces markedly heat-resistant spores. The disease in New Guinea is directly related to pig feasting (pig bel), a sign of wealth.[14]

Clinical Features. The illness is characterized by anorexia, severe abdominal pain, bloody diarrhea, vomiting, prostration, and collapse. If untreated, it is highly lethal. It has a spectrum of presentations from the severe fulminant form to a mild gastroenteritis or dysentery.

Pathologically, the disease is characterized by a patchy, gangrenous enteritis, largely involving the jejunum. There is submucosal, subserosal, mesenteric, and lymph node gas. It occurs primarily in children.[14]

Treatment. Therapy includes blood transfusions, bowel decompression, penicillin and tetracycline, and specific *Clostridium perfringens* type C antiserum. The antiserum is administered in doses of 42,000 to 85,000 units intravenously. After these preliminary measures, the therapy of choice is resection of the involved areas of intestine. This approach has reduced the mortality from over 50 per cent to 18 per cent.

STAPHYLOCOCCI

STAPHYLOCOCCAL GASTROENTERITIS

Staphylococcal gastroenteritis is due to an enterotoxin that is heat stable, odorless, and tasteless.[1] The vast majority of organisms producing it are hemolytic *Staphylococcus aureus* and are coagulase positive, although *Staph. albus* has been incriminated in isolated instances. Virtually all staphylococcal gastroenteritis results from ingestion of food which has been contaminated with staphylococci, inadequately heated or cooked, and inadequately refrigerated. Foods containing a large proportion of protein such as salads with mayonnaise or cream pies have been most frequently incriminated.

Clinical Picture. The onset of staphylococcal gastroenteritis occurs four to eight hours after the ingestion of contaminated food. It is characterized by nausea, vomiting, a fairly profuse watery diarrhea, some abdominal colic, and, rarely, prostration. It can result in severe dehydration in infants and small children. The gastroenteritis is of usually short duration, rarely more than 24 hours, and the only therapy warranted is fluid replacement in the face of severe dehydration or clear liquids by mouth if the patient is not vomiting profusely.

Prevention. The toxogenic staphylococci are ubiquitous, and virtually all food may be contaminated with viable organisms. They survive or multiply between 4 and 36° C.[1] If contamination is not massive, heating to 50° C for one hour will sterilize food and 65° C for 12 minutes will kill 10 million staphylococci per gram of food. Following heating, the food should be rapidly chilled to less than 4° C and refrigerated until it is served.

STAPHYLOCOCCAL ENTEROCOLITIS

A fatal diarrheal disease in some patients has been described as being due to staphylococcal enterocolitis. They usually have had recent abdominal surgery and have been treated with broad-spectrum antibiotics. A few have had no surgery or have had other than abdominal surgery and have not been treated with antibiotics. Some of these individuals do not have Staphylococcus overgrowth in their intestine. "Pseudomembranous" enterocolitis should be called staphylococcal enterocolitis only when staphylococci are the predominant organism. They can usually be identified in large number by gram stain of a stool specimen (see p. 1372).

Treatment. Vancomycin hydrochloride, 500 mg every six to eight hours, is an effective antibiotic in staphylococcal enteritis. For oral administration, one ampule of the parenteral solution containing 500 mg of vancomycin hydrochloride may be diluted in 1 oz of water and given to the patient orally or administered via gastric tube.

TUBERCULOUS ENTERITIS

Prior to the development of effective chemotherapy for tuberculosis, intestinal tuberculosis was the most common complication of active pulmonary disease. The incidence was in the order of 30 per cent in autopsy studies of children with pulmonary tuberculosis and 80 per cent in autopsy studies of adults with pulmonary tuberculosis.[15] Currently, gastrointestinal involvement is an infrequent complication and is seen almost entirely in tuberculosis sanatoria. It is rarely seen in general clinical or hospital practice.[16] It is most often seen in patients with open cavitary tuberculosis with positive sputums. Rigid control of dairy herds and pasteurization of milk have virtually eliminated bovine tuberculosis in the United States (see pp. 1377 to 1381).

Pathogenesis. Intestinal tuberculosis results from swallowed human tubercle bacilli. Once swallowed, the organisms invade the intestinal mucosa and set up foci of infection in lymphatic tissue. The small intestine is the site of predilection for tuberculous infection, particularly the ileum and the region of the ileocecal valve. This area of the intestine also has the largest conglomerates of lymphatic tissue, and its presence appears to be necessary for the infection to occur.

Pathology. Three types of tuberculous intestinal lesions have ordinarily been recognized: the ulcerative type, the sclerotic or fibrous type, and hypertrophic or hyperplastic tuberculosis. The ulcerative type is by far the most common. All the stages in the evolution of tuberculosis are seen in intestinal involvement: tubercle formation, caseation, ulceration, and fibrosis.

Diagnosis. SYMPTOMS. Symptoms are of little value in making a diagnosis of tuberculous enterocolitis. Although up to 10 per cent of patients have no symptoms, most have nonspecific systemic symptoms of fever, easy fatigability, night sweats, weight loss, flu-like illnesses, and the like. Gastrointestinal symptoms are seen in less than 50 per cent of patients and include nausea and vomiting, "dyspepsia," abdominal cramps, constipation, or diarrhea, or occasionally both. Intestinal tuberculosis should be suspected when there are "(1) lung cavitation with positive sputum; (2) vague abdominal complaints; (3) temperature irregularities not related to the course of the pulmonary lesion; (4) reversal of a previously satisfactory clinical course of pulmonary tuberculosis, which is inadequately explained by the pulmonary lesion; and (5) continued unsatisfactory progress when management is adequate."[16]

PHYSICAL EXAMINATION. Other than evidence of weight loss and poor nutrition, there may be no positive physical findings. No abnormalities may be present in the abdomen. In the event of stricture or perforation, physical findings associated with these complications are evident. Occasionally there may be some tenderness over the area of intestinal involvement, usually the right lower quadrant, and if peritoneal tuberculosis is present there may be some guarding, but rigidity or rebound are usually absent. There may be a doughy feeling or sensation over the lower abdomen on palpation.

X-RAY STUDIES. Barium studies of the colon, stomach, and small bowel offer the best methods for diagnosing tuberculosis. The radiographic findings are not pathognomonic. One feature described in 1911[17] is that of altered motility. The involved bowel is difficult to fill because of irritability, and it rapidly empties itself of barium. Often the terminal ileum and cecum fail to retain barium, particularly in ulcerative disease. The differential diagnosis includes regional enteritis, amebiasis, neoplasms such as malignant lymphoma, hyperplastic lymphatics, and so forth. The differential diagnosis becomes particularly difficult with hyperplastic tuberculosis.

LABORATORY. The laboratory is of little use. Alterations in blood and urine are nonspecific. There may be occult blood in the stool. Even the finding of *Mycobacterium tuberculosis* in the stool is of little diagnostic value, because the majority of patients with pulmonary tuberculosis have tubercle bacilli in their feces.

MISCELLANEOUS. The tuberculin test is of little value except perhaps in young children. Patients with disseminated tuberculosis (miliary) are often anergic, and the tuberculin test is not positive. However, they also fail to react to other antigens such as mumps and to fungi.

Patients who have complications such as perforation or obstruction may require surgical therapy. The diagnosis may be made at the time of surgery by examination of appropriately stained sections, demonstrating the organisms in microscopic sections. Suspected tuberculosis should also be cultured and guinea pig inoculation studies performed. Grossly, the differential diagnosis from regional enteritis can be very difficult.

Treatment. Except for emergencies such as perforation or obstruction, surgery is not indicated. The discovery of effective chemotherapeutic agents has markedly altered the therapy of intestinal tuberculosis. Most patients recover without sequelae if given a regimen including rest, nutritious diet, and chemotherapy. The drugs most often used are isoniazid, para-aminosalicylic acid (PAS) and streptomycin, usually in combinations of two. The usual dosages are isoniazid, 5 to 8 mg per kilogram per day in a single dose; PAS, 200 mg per kilogram, and pyridoxine hydrochloride, 25 to 50 mg per kilogram per day. If streptomycin is used, the dosage is 20 mg per kilogram per day given intramuscularly. Its use should be restricted to in-hospital treatment because of its toxicity. Ethambutol may be used in place of PAS. Therapy should be continued for a full two years.

VIRAL GASTROENTERITIS

A number of viral infections may be associated with gastrointestinal symptoms, particularly diarrhea. These include poliomyelitis, measles, infectious hepatitis, mumps, and influenza. Upon development of the cardinal symptoms of the disease the diagnosis becomes clear. Viral "dysentery" has been considered to be more common than bacterial or protozoal diarrhea.[18] Attack rates during epidemics may reach 80 per cent of persons exposed.

The enteroviruses are normal inhabitants of the human gastrointestinal tract and include the polio viruses, Coxsackie A and B, and the echoviruses.[19] Surprisingly, they are rarely responsible for diarrheal disease except for occasional epidemics in infants. Those incriminated include echoviruses 11, 14, 17 and 18 and, questionably, the Coxsackie viruses.[19] Few data exist incriminating these agents as major causes of diarrheal diseases in individuals past infancy. Acute viral hepatitis frequently has an associated mild diarrhea and in rare individuals even steatorrhea. Mild to moderate nonspecific changes have been observed in the mucosa as studied by peroral biopsy.[20, 21] The reo- and adenoviruses have also been associated with diarrheal illness. In most instances of apparent viral gastroenteritis, a specific virus cannot be identified.

Pathogenesis. The pathogenesis of viral gastroenteritis is unclear. In infectious hepatitis, the mucosal pathology could account for the symptomatology. In the other viral infections of the gut leading to symptoms, the data are either inconclusive or not available. Symptoms of diarrhea have been produced by infecting volunteers by inhalation of nebulized bacteria-free filtrates of feces and nasopharyngeal secretions.[18] These infections may act not by a direct effect on the gut, but through infection of the central nervous system.[18]

Clinical Features. Most of the viral infections associated with diarrhea are due to organisms other than the enteroviruses and have systemic symptoms. Respiratory symptoms are prominent, particularly with reoviruses and adenoviruses. Diarrhea is usually accompanied or preceded by headache, fever, sweating, anorexia, and malaise. There may be lightheadedness, chilliness, visual disturbances, paresthesias, and vomiting. Many patients are afebrile. The stools tend to be soft to watery and rarely contain pus, blood, or mucus. Abdominal colic is usually not severe. Rarely, steatorrhea may occur.

Physical examination is noncontributory except for fever and occasionally mild abdominal tenderness. Despite the headache, there are no focal neurological findings, although occasionally meningismus may occur.

The clinical course is usually of one to four or five days, and most patients remain ambulatory.

An association between adenovirus infection and intussusception in children has been described.[22] Adenoviruses were isolated from 15 of 57 (26.3 per cent) of children with intussusception as opposed to 3 of 85 (3.5 per cent) of matched control subjects. It was suggested that hypertrophy of the lymphoid tissue infected with virus was the leading point of the intussusception.

Laboratory. Most often, the laboratory findings are normal. Occasionally, other enteric pathogens may be cultured. Viral culture requires special laboratory techniques using tissue culture and is not generally available. Serological testing will demonstrate a rise in specific antibodies but is not widely performed.

TREATMENT

Treatment is supportive. Small children and infants may require parenteral fluid replacement. Diphenoxylate with atropine (Lomotil) in dosages of 2.5 to 5 mg every four to six hours will frequently relieve the diarrhea. In the event of high fever or severe headaches, salicylates or acetaminophen frequently provide good relief. Antimicrobial therapy is contraindicated. Patients with nausea and vomiting frequently tolerate clear liquids and carbonated beverages.

FUNGAL INFECTIONS

Fungi are normal inhabitants of the human small intestine.[23] Although 19 different fungi were found in the jejunum and ileum from specimens procured from 27 entirely healthy adults, *Candida albicans* was the organism identified most frequently. Gastrointestinal disease caused by Candida in otherwise entirely healthy individuals is extremely rare. Systemic disease or gastrointestinal disease caused by Candida is usually associated with long-term chronic debilitating illness, prolonged treatment with broad-spectrum antibiotics, corticosteroids,[24] and immunosuppressive therapy and cancer chemotherapy. Occasionally, mucocutaneous candidiasis in children may disseminate to the gastrointestinal tract and end fatally.[24]

The other fungi which infect the gastrointestinal tract and produce disease are *Histoplasma capsulatum* and *Blastomyces brasiliensis*.

CANDIDIASIS

Candida albicans is a budding, yeast-like fungus which produces budding blastospores and pseudomycelia in tissue exudates and culture, both at room temperature and 37° C.

Pathogenesis. Intestinal candidiasis develops when the normal intestinal flora is suppressed or changed by broad-spectrum antibiotic therapy or when the patient's resistance is altered by therapy with corticosteroids, immunosuppressive drugs, or cancer chemotherapeutic agents.

Clinical Features. Candida infections usually involve mucous membranes of the mouth or vagina and the intertriginous areas of the skin and nails. Rarely, the fungus may spread to the gastrointestinal tract and even result in a generalized fatal candidiasis. The major symptom of intestinal candidiasis is diarrhea. It is usually watery, and at times may be quite voluminous. Abdominal cramps are sometimes present.

Physical examination is usually unrevealing, except for the findings of the various primary, debilitating diseases. There may or may not be low-grade fever. In disseminated candidiasis, even with multiple internal abscesses, many patients are afebrile.

Diagnosis. The diagnosis of intestinal candidiasis may be suspected in patients receiving long-term broad-spectrum antibiotic therapy or other drugs which alter their resistance. The fungus grows readily on all common laboratory media and is easily identifiable. Other laboratory data, such as hemoglobin, white count, differentials, and blood chemistries, provide no direct evidence of candidiasis.

Treatment. Often, discontinuing the medication with which the patient is being treated, if not contraindicated, will result in re-establishment of a normal bacterial flora and suppression of Candida. Nystatin in dosages of 500,000 to 1,000,000 units, three times daily by mouth, is effective in the treatment of intestinal candidiasis. Therapy should be continued for two days after clinical cure. If concomitant antibiotics are being administered, the therapy should continue at least as long as the antibiotic therapy. Evidence that combination therapy, e.g., tetracycline–amphotericin B when given orally, is effective in preventing the development of candidiasis is either unavailable or inconclusive. Intravenous amphotericin B should be reserved only for patients with progressive and potentially fatal fungal infections. Treatment is usually begun at 0.25 mg per kilogram of body weight and gradually increased to 1 mg per kilogram. The drug is administered intravenously over approximately six hours. Rarely, dosages of 1.5 mg per kilogram are required but except in rare refractory cases the daily dose should not exceed this amount.[24]

BLASTOMYCES BRASILIENSIS

Blastomyces brasiliensis is a large, yeast-like fungus which is thick walled, single, and multiple budding and occurs in exudates, tissues, and culture at 37° C. The fungus is confined to the South American continent. Indigenous infection does not occur in the United States.

Pathogenesis. The buccal mucosa appears to be the portal of entry. Ulcerating granulomatous disease develops in the mucous membranes of the mouth and adjacent skin. It frequently involves the lymph nodes and viscera. In intestinal involvement, infection of lymphoid tissue within the gut occurs and progresses to involve the lymphatics of the mesentery, the spleen, and the liver. It may mimic tuberculous peritonitis, abdominal lymphoma, or carcinoma. (North American blastomycosis rarely if ever has intestinal tract involvement.)

Clinical Features. The intestinal tract is rarely if ever the only site of infection in persons with South American blastomycosis. Occasionally the anogenital area appears to be the portal of entry of the fungus. The most usual area of intestinal disease is the distal ileum and the colon. The reticuloendothelial system, the liver, and other organs within the abdomen are also infected, and multiple abscesses are present.

Physical examination will reveal ulcerating, granulomatous lesions of the skin, particularly around the mouth, but sometimes generalized. Lymphadenopathy may mimic malignancy. With abdominal spread, the liver and spleen are enlarged. Other masses caused by enlarged lymph nodes and thickened bowel wall may be palpable. Tenderness is usually mild, and peritoneal signs are absent.

Diagnosis. Biopsy of ulcerating lesions for identification of the fungus is required for diagnosis.[24, 25] Abscess formation and tuberculoid and other forms of granulomas are common. There may be necrotic, caseous centers surrounded by macrophages, lymphocytes, giant cells, and fibroblasts. The fungi are large, round, 10- to 60-μ cells with multiple peripheral budding. Specimens should be submitted to the microbiology laboratory for culture. Other laboratory examinations are of little value in establishing a specific diagnosis of blastomycosis.

Treatment. Prior to the introduction of

the sulfonamide drugs, South American blastomycocis was invariably fatal in a few months to years. Prolonged therapy with sulfonamides in doses of 2 to 4 g daily will often result in substantial improvement. However, relapses are common and therapy frequently must be reinitiated. Amphotericin B in dosages up to 1.5 to 2 mg per kilogram of body weight per day, to a total dose of 8500 mg, has also been reported to be effective.[24, 25]

HISTOPLASMOSIS

Histoplasmosis is due to infection with *Histoplasma capsulatum*, a small, yeast-like, oval intracellular fungus, when found in tissues. In culture it is a yeast-like organism when grown at 37° C and at room temperature produces a mold-like filamentous fungus. Histoplasmosis is primarily a benign, self-limited, pulmonary disease. Rarely it results in chronic, malignant, and progressive disseminated infection. Occasionally the infection appears to be confined to the intestinal tract. It is most common in the north central United States but has a worldwide distribution.

Pathogenesis. The vast majority of patients with histoplasmosis have no history of any severe pulmonary disease and are detected only by positive skin test to histoplasmin.[24] Some patients acquire the infection through direct inoculation of wounds in the skin or mucous membranes. In patients with more severe pulmonary disease, the infection may be disseminated either hematogenously or through the lymphatics. The organism has a striking predilection for the reticuloendothelial system in all parts of the body. Histoplasmosis acquired through nonpulmonary routes appears to be more virulent than other forms of the disease.[24]

Clinical Features. Patients with disseminated and intestinal histoplamosis usually have symptoms of nausea, vomiting, diarrhea, abdominal colic, anorexia, and weight loss.[24, 26-29] The disease is usually marked by chronic wasting, irregular fever, and lymphadenopathy. The spleen and liver also tend to be enlarged. "Ulcerative colitis" caused by *Histoplasma capsulatum*[26, 30] has been described. One patient is recorded with small bowel histoplasmosis manifest by "giant" intestinal villi and protein-losing enteropathy.[27]

The physical examination may reveal fever, evidence of weight loss, and chronic wasting. There may be generalized lymphadenopathy mimicking malignancy. The liver and spleen are often enlarged. Tenderness or pain to palpation may be insignificant.

Laboratory Findings. Blood counts usually demonstrate an iron deficiency or normochromic normocytic anemia. Leukopenia is frequent, and rarely thrombocytopenia is present. With diffuse intestinal involvement, small bowel mucosal biopsy may demonstrate a mucosa with the lamina propria packed with macrophages filled with *H. capsulatum*.[27] A similar finding in macrophages in the rectal mucosa may be seen with colonic involvement.[30] They are particularly numerous in polypoid lesions. It may be difficult to culture or isolate *H. capsulatum* from tissues even when they are present in high numbers. They may be isolated by injection into any of a number of suitable laboratory animals; mice are usually chosen.

Radiographic Features. The radiographic signs of histoplasmosis of the intestine are not specific.[30-32] They include finely nodular infiltrated appearance of the small intestine with accentuated valvulae conniventes, "pseudopolypoid" lesions, and annular and stenosing lesions. Radiographically, they closely resemble neoplastic disease. In the small bowel, the differential diagnosis on radiographic appearance includes malignant lymphoma, regional enteritis, Whipple's disease, and carcinoma, and is very difficult. The entire intestine may be involved, or there may be focal lesions.

Treatment. The treatment of choice for histoplasmosis is intravenous amphotericin B. The same regimen is used as that for systemic candidiasis (see p. 921). If serious toxicity to amphotericin B occurs, prolonged therapy with sulfonamides (usually sulfadiazine) in very large doses has been useful in some patients.

CHRONIC ULCERATIVE (NONGRANULOMATOUS) JEJUNOILEITIS

Chronic ulcerative (nongranulomatous) jejunoileitis is characterized by chronic diarrhea, steatorrhea, weight loss, protein-losing enteropathy, abdominal pain, and fever.[33-36] The most usual lesion found on examination of peroral mucosal biopsies is a flat mucosa which may be indistinguishable from celiac sprue (see p. 879). The most characteristic pathology found at surgery or postmortem examination is multiple mucosal ulcerations between which are interspersed areas of flat mucosa and normal mucosa.

Etiology and Pathogenesis. The disease is of unknown etiology and pathogenesis. Rare individuals with celiac sprue enjoying clinical remission with a gluten-free diet have developed this complication and were no longer responsive to gluten exclusion.[37]

Clinical Features. The most prominent symptom is diarrhea which is often severe. The history of watery diarrhea may go back to childhood. Early in the course of the illness, remissions are common with occasional periods of days to months of asymptomatic good health. Ultimately, diarrhea becomes chronic, continuous, and intractable. Steatorrhea may be an initial symptom or develop later in the course of the illness. Overt intestinal hemorrhage is common. Abdominal colic is common, fever is frequent, and there is often peripheral edema because of the hypoproteinemia. Occasionally, these patients are first seen for the complications of intestinal obstruction, perforation, and massive hemorrhage. Weight loss is prominent and often marked. The diagnosis may be made only at surgery or autopsy.

Physical Examination. On physical examination, there are the findings of profound weight loss with cachexia, loss of muscle mass, marked decrease or absence of subcutaneous fat, and peripheral edema. The abdomen is usually distended. The bowel sounds are hyperactive, with visible loops of bowel through the abdominal wall. Tenderness may be mild or, in the event of penetration or perforation of the ulcers, rebound tenderness may be elicited.

Laboratory Diagnosis. Anemia is frequent and usually due to iron deficiency. The white blood cell count is variable, and ranges between 3600 and 20,000, most often with a normal differential. Total serum protein levels are decreased, with reductions in both albumin and globulin.

The albumin ranges between 1.8 and 3.5 g per 100 ml. The serum calcium level is low, reflecting the hypoalbuminemia. Steatorrhea is present on chemical analysis with up to 50 g of fecal fat per 24 hours. The five-hour urinary D-xylose test is abnormal in virtually all patients, with five-hour urinary excretions ranging between 0.3 and 4.5 g. Vitamin B_{12} absorption is variable. The stool, in the absence of overt bleeding, almost always contains occult blood. The serum sodium, potassium, chloride, and bicarbonate levels and the pH are usually normal.

Radiographic Features. All the patients reported have had abnormal small intestinal radiographs. The ulcers may not be detected on X-ray examination. In the event of stricture formation, the stenotic level may be diagnosed. The changes otherwise are nonspecific and include segmentation of barium, dilated loops of bowel which may be segmented, and irregular and coarse mucosal folds.

Intestinal Morphology. Peroral mucosal biopsy is of little use in making a diagnosis of chronic, ulcerative (nongranulomatous) jejunoileitis. The mucosa may be within normal limits[36] or it may be flat,[35] resembling celiac sprue. Many patients have been subjected to surgery for diagnosis, obstruction, or perforation. The larger surgical specimens have disclosed multiple ulcerations which contain an infiltrate of lymphocytes, plasma cells, and polymorphonuclear leukocytes.[35] Eosinophils may or may not be present in increased numbers. A patchy thickening of the bowel wall is present. No granulomas are found. Inflammation and ulceration may extend through the entire thickness of the bowel. In surgical specimens, areas of normal-appearing mucosa as well as areas of flat mucosa have been described.

Treatment. Exclusion of gluten from the diet has not resulted in any benefit. Two patients with celiac sprue had surgical resection of their ulcers followed by a favorable response to gluten exclusion.[37] Corticosteroids, e.g., prednisone or prednisolone in initial doses of 40 to 80 mg per day with reduction to maintenance doses of between 10 mg and 20 mg have produced apparent subjective and objective improvement in some of these patients. The effect of corticosteroids is, however,

924 THE SMALL INTESTINE

unpredictable. Antibiotic therapy has been of no use.

Prognosis. Patients with chronic ulcerative jejunoileitis have a poor prognosis.[35] Most expire within one to five years of the onset of their chronic diarrhea and steatorrhea. The causes of death are perforation and peritonitis, sepsis with multiple abscesses, uncontrolled gastrointestinal hemorrhage, and inanition.

PRIMARY NONSPECIFIC ULCERATION OF THE SMALL INTESTINE

Primary nonspecific ulceration of the small intestine is rare. Until 1963, only approximately 170 patients had been recorded in the world medical literature.[38] In the early 1960's, scattered case reports appeared which appeared to incriminate enteric-coated potassium salts and diuretics as etiological in some of these lesions.[39] The retrospective survey of 484 patients with primary nonspecific ulceration revealed that 275 (57 per cent) had received enteric-coated potassium chloride, a diuretic, or both.[39] The ulcer is usually single and occurs approximately twice as frequently in the ileum as in the jejunum. The differential diagnosis includes syphilis, typhoid fever, tuberculosis, embolization without infarction, vasculitis, arsenic poisoning, and incarcerated internal hernia.[40]

Etiology and Pathogenesis. The etiology of primary nonspecific ulceration of the small intestine is unknown. Vascular disease, central nervous system disease, infection, trauma, malnutrition, and hormonal causes have been proposed.[40] Enteric-coated potassium chloride tablets administered in dosages of 500 to 1000 mg readily produced ulcerative lesions of the small intestine in monkeys but rarely in dogs.[35] Enteric-coated diuretics (hydrochlorothiazide, cyclothiazide, and bendroflumethiazide) failed to produce lesions. Enteric-coated sodium chloride in dosages of 1000 mg twice daily in these experiments also failed to produce any lesions.

Clinical Features. Most patients with primary nonspecific small bowel ulceration present with symptoms of small bowel obstruction.[38] Occasionally the ulcer perforates and rarely it is responsible for gastrointestinal hemorrhage. Some patients with primary nonspecific small bowel ulceration have histories of some years' duration. Periumbilical abdominal colic, nausea, and vomiting are the most common symptoms. An occasional patient may have diarrhea, and on occasion it is massive. In the event of perforation, there is the sudden onset of severe abdominal pain which has been preceded by variable intervals with abdominal colic.

Physical Examination. Physical examination does not differentiate from other causes of small bowel obstruction. The patient may be in moderate to severe pain. Often there is diaphoresis; hypotension is not usual unless there has been hemorrhage or severe diarrhea. There is usually a tachycardia present without postural hypotension. The abdomen is distended, and if the patient's history has been of sufficient duration and associated with weight loss, visible loops of bowel may be seen through the abdominal wall. Bowel sounds are usually hyperactive and suggest obstruction. If perforation has not occurred, there may be little or no tenderness. With perforation, tenderness to light percussion and rebound tenderness are present. With perforation and peritonitis, ileus is usually present and the abdomen is silent.

Laboratory Diagnosis. The laboratory is of no specific aid in establishing a diagnosis in nonspecific small bowel ulceration. In patients who are not bleeding, the hematocrit, white blood cell count, and differential are normal. Except in patients with severe diarrhea or vomiting, the serum electrolytes and pH are normal. With perforation there is usually leukocytosis with an increase in immature polymorphonuclear leukocytes.

Radiographic Features. Plain films of the abdomen demonstrate dilated loops of small bowel with air fluid levels. Although barium studies by mouth frequently do not demonstrate the ulcerations, they may on occasion be detected by the insinuation of a long intestinal tube into the area of obstruction. Distal ileal obstruction may be detected by barium enema.

Treatment. Therapy is surgical. The entire intestine should be examined very carefully, because these ulcers may be multiple, although more often they are solitary.

Because of the apparent increase in non-specific ulceration of the intestine, enteric-coated potassium chloride with or without combinations of various diuretics is no longer manufactured. However, some pharmacies may not have returned these drugs to the manufacturer, and occasionally they are still available. If potassium supplementation is required in patients receiving diuretics, it should be administered in the form of a solution.

REFERENCES

1. Grady, G. F., and Keusch, G. T.   Pathogenesis of bacterial diarrheas. New Eng. J. Med. 285:831, 1971.
2. Gorbach, S. L.   Acute diarrhea—a "toxin" disease? New Eng. J. Med. 283:44, 1970.
3. Grady, G. F., and Keusch, G. T.   Pathogenesis of bacterial diarrheas. New Eng. J. Med. 285:891, 1971.
4. Pierce, N. F., Banwell, J. G., Mitra, R. C., Caranasos, G. J., Keimowitz, R. I., Mondal, A., and Marji, P. M.   Effect of intragastric glucose-electrolyte infusion upon water and electrolyte balance in Asiatic cholera. Gastroenterology 55:333, 1968.
5. Banwell, J. G., Pierce, N. F., Mitra, R. C., Brigham, K. L., Caranasos, G. J., Keimowitz, R. I., Fedson, D. S., Thomas, J., Gorbach, S. L., Sack, R. B., and Mondal, A.   Intestinal fluid and electrolyte transport in human cholera. J. Clin. Invest. 49:183, 1970.
6. Rowe, B., Taylor, J., and Bettelheim, K. A.   An investigation of traveller's diarrhea. Lancet 1:1, 1970.
7. DuPont, H. L., Formal, S. B., Hornick, R. B., Snyder, M. J., Libonah, J. P., Sheahan, D. G., LaBrec, E. H., and Kalas, J. P.   Pathogenesis of Escherichia coli diarrhea. New Eng. J. Med. 285:1, 1971.
8. Valman, H. B., and Wilmers, M. J.   Use of antibiotics in acute gastroenteritis among infants in hospital. Lancet 1:1122, 1969.
9. Morgan, H. R.   The enteric bacteria. In Bacterial and mycotic infections of man, R. J. Dubos and J. G. Hirsch, (Eds.). Philadelphia, J. B. Lippincott Co., 1965.
10. Effect of neomycin in non-invasive salmonella infections of the gastrointestinal tract. Lancet 2:1159, 1970.
11. Tynes, B. S., and Utz, J. P.   Factors influencing the cure of salmonella carriers. Ann. Intern. Med. 57:871, 1962.
12. Phillips, R. A.   Cholera in the perspective of 1966. Ann. Intern. Med. 65:922, 1966.
13. Grady, G. F., Madoff, M. A., Dunhamel, R. C., Moore, E. W., and Chalmers, T. C.   Sodium transport by human ileum in vitro and its response to cholera enterotoxin. Gastroenterology 53:737, 1967.
14. Murrell, T. G. C., Roth, L., Egerton, J., Samels, J., and Walker, P. D.   Pig-bel: Enteritis necro-

ticans. A study in diagnosis and management. Lancet 1:217, 1966.
15. Goldberg, B.   Tuberculous enterocolitis. In Clinical Tuberculosis, B. Goldberg, (ed.). Philadelphia, F. A. Davis Co., 1942.
16. Sauer, W. G.   Extrapulmonary tuberculosis: Diagnosis and treatment. Gastrointestinal tuberculosis. In Clinical Tuberculosis. K. H. Pfuetze and D. B. Radner, (eds.). Springfield, Ill., Charles C Thomas, 1966.
17. Stierlin, E.   Die Radiographic in der Diagnostic der Ileocöcaltuberkulose und anderer Krankheiten des Dickdarms. Muenchen. Med. Wchnschr. 1:1231, 1911.
18. Reiman, H. A.   Viral dysentery. Amer. J. Med. Sci. 246:404, 1963.
19. Horstmann, D. M.   Enterovirus infections. Etiologic, epidemiologic and clinical aspects. Calif. Med. 103:1, 1965.
20. Conrad, M. E., Schwartz, F. D., and Young, A. A.   Infectious hepatitis—a generalized disease. A study of renal, gastrointestinal and hematologic abnormalities. Amer. J. Med. 37:789, 1964.
21. Sheehy, T. W., Artenstein, M. S., and Green, R. W.   Small intestinal mucosa in certain viral diseases. J.A.M.A. 190:1023, 1964.
22. Clarke, G. J., Jr., Phillips, I. A., and Alexander, E. R.   Adenovirus infection in intussusception in children in Taiwan. J.A.M.A. 208:1671, 1969.
23. Cohen, R., Roth, F. J., Delgado, E., Ahearn, D. G., and Kalser, M. H.   Fungal flora of the normal human small and large intestine. New Eng. J. Med. 280:638, 1969.
24. Conant, N. F.   Medical mycology. In Bacterial and Mycotic Infections of Man, R. J. Dubos and J. G. Hirsch (eds.). Philadelphia, J. B. Lippincott Co., 1965.
25. Wilson, J. W., and Plunkett, O. A.   South American blastomycosis (paracoccidiodomycosis). In The Fungus Diseases of Man. Berkeley, University of California Press, 1965.
26. Shull, H. J.   Human histoplasmosis. Disease with protean manifestations; often with digestive system involvement. Gastroenterology 25:582, 1953.
27. Bank, S., Trey, C., Gans, I., Marks, I. N., and Groll, A.   Histoplasmosis of the small bowel with "giant" intestinal villi and secondary protein-losing enteropathy. Amer. J. Med. 38:492, 1965.
28. Sturim, H. S., Kouchoukos, N. T., and Ahlvin, R. C.   Gastrointestinal manifestations of disseminated histoplasmosis. Amer. J. Surg. 110:435, 1965.
29. Boone, W. T., and Allison, F., Jr.   Histoplasmosis. Amer. J. Med. 46:818, 1969.
30. Kirk, M. E., Lough, J., and Warner, H. A.   Histoplasma colitis: An electron microscopic study. Gastroenterology 61:46, 1971.
31. Perez, C. A., Sturim, H. S., Kouchoukos, N. T., and Kamberg, S.   Some clinical and radiographic features of gastrointestinal histoplasmosis. Radiology 86:482, 1966.
32. Dietz, M. W.   Ileocecal histoplasmosis. Radiology 91:285, 1968.
33. Himes, H. W., Gabriel, J. R., and Adlersberg, D.

Previously undescribed clinical and post-mortem observations in non-tropical sprue: Possible role of prolonged corticosteroid therapy. Gastroenterology 32:60, 1957.

34. Smitskamp, H., and Kuipers, F. C. Stea-torrheoea and ulcerative jejuno-ileitis. Acta Med. Scand. 177: fasc. 1, 37, 1965.

35. Jeffries, G. H., Steinberg, H., and Sleisenger, M. H. Chronic ulcerative (non-granulomatous) jejunitis. Amer. J. Med. 44:47, 1968.

36. Karz, S., Guth, P. H., and Polonsky, L. Chronic ulcerative jejuno-ileitis. Amer. J. Gastroent. 56:61, 1971.

37. Bayless, T. M., Kapelowitz, R. F., Shelley, W. M., Ballinger, W. F., and Hendrix, T. R. Intestinal ulceration—a complication of celiac disease. New Eng. J. Med. 276:996, 1967.

38. Watson, M. R. Primary nonspecific ulceration of the small bowel. Arch. Surg. 87:600, 1963.

39. Lawrason, F. D., Alpert, G., Mohr, F. L., and McMahon, F. G. Obstructive-ulcerative lesions of the small intestine. J.A.M.A. 191:641, 1965.

40. Kiser, J. L. Focal lesions of the small intestine. Amer. J. Surg. 112:48, 1966.

Chapter 69

The Blind Loop Syndrome

Robert M. Donaldson, Jr.

The development of steatorrhea and/or vitamin B_{12} deficiency in patients with any small bowel abnormality conducive to stasis of intestinal contents and small bowel bacterial overgrowth is known as the blind loop or stagnant loop syndrome.

HISTORY

In 1890, White first suspected a relation between small bowel strictures and an anemia resembling pernicious anemia, but it was not until 1924 that Seyderhelm and his colleagues demonstrated clearly that removal of an intestinal stricture cured the associated anemia. It soon became apparent that this anemia and its attendant neurological defects responded to liver therapy, that other small bowel abnormalities such as diverticula, blind pouches and enteroenterostomies could cause anemia, and that various small bowel lesions were often associated not only with anemia but also with steatorrhea. By 1939, Barker and Hummel[1] were able to document in their classic review all the salient clinical features of the blind loop syndrome. Subsequently, many workers have demonstrated that malabsorption of vitamin B_{12} and steatorrhea in patients with small bowel bacterial overgrowth can be corrected by administration of antibiotics or by appropriate surgical therapy. A detailed description of the historical development

of the blind loop syndrome may be found in a recent review.[2]

ETIOLOGY AND PATHOGENESIS

As described on page 71, the small bowel lumen normally harbors sparse numbers of gram-positive aerobes or facultative anaerobes. Any small bowel abnormality that results in local stasis or "recirculation" of intestinal contents is likely to be accompanied by marked proliferation of intraluminal microorganisms. In this situation there develops a complex small bowel flora which is predominantly anaerobic and which closely resembles the colonic flora.

A large number of disorders have been associated with proliferation of enteric microorganisms in the small bowel.[3, 4] It is important to recognize, however, that only in certain of these disorders does there develop a small bowel flora which is clinically and metabolically significant. Moreover, many patients who have intestinal abnormalities definitely conducive to bacterial overgrowth do not in fact develop steatorrhea or vitamin B_{12} deficiency.

Those small bowel disorders which have been clearly related to bacterially induced malabsorption are listed in Table 69–1.

Blind pouches of the small intestine, formed surgically by creation of an end-to-

TABLE 69-1. SMALL BOWEL ABNORMALITIES CONDUCIVE TO BACTERIAL OVERGROWTH AND CONSEQUENT MALABSORPTION

A. Following abdominal surgery
  1. "Self-filling" or "blind" pouch
  2. Enteroenterostomy
  3. Afferent loop dysfunction following gastrojejunostomy
  4. Gastrojejunocolic fistula
  5. Partial obstruction due to adhesions
B. Structural abnormalities
  1. Regional enteritis or tuberculosis
    a. Strictures with partial obstruction
    b. Enteroenteric fistulas
  2. Diverticula
C. Motor abnormalities
  1. Scleroderma
  2. Pseudo-obstruction

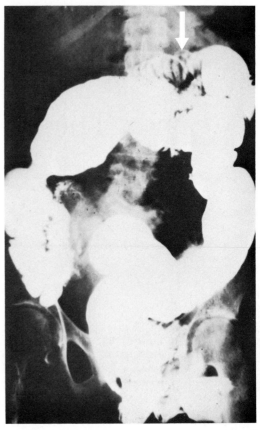

Figure 69–2. Barium enema in a 26-year-old woman with granulomatous colitis and malabsorption syndrome. Note the jejunocolic fistula and loop of jejunum (arrow). (Courtesy of Dr. M. H. Sleisenger.)

side enteroenteric anastomosis, frequently produce small bowel bacterial overgrowth (Fig. 69–1).[5] Similarly, stagnant loops of intestine resulting from fistulas or surgical enterostomies allow for continuous recirculation of small bowel contents and consequent bacterial overgrowth (Figs. 69–2 and 69–3). Following partial gastrectomy and Billroth II anastomosis, dysfunction and stasis in the afferent loop may result in

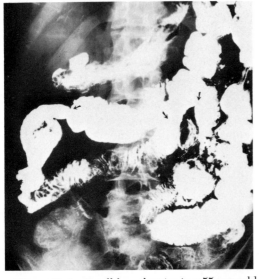

Figure 69–1. Small bowel series in a 55-year-old man with recurrent regional enteritis obstructing a prior enterocolic anastomosis (left arrow) in whom a proximal enterocolic bypass was performed (right arrows) creating a blind loop. (Courtesy of Dr. M. H. Sleisenger.)

marked intraluminal proliferation of bacteria and consequent seeding of the remainder of the small intestine.[6] In elderly people, small bowel diverticula serve as a source for bacterial overgrowth and constitute an increasingly frequent cause of the blind loop syndrome (Fig. 69–4). Partial small bowel obstruction caused by regional enteritis, adhesions, or tuberculosis frequently leads to increased numbers of microorganisms within the small bowel lumen.[8] Patients with gastric ulcers, ulcerating carcinomas of the stomach or transverse colon, or stomal ulcers following subtotal gastrectomy may develop gastrocolic or gastrojejunocolic fistulas. In this situation, food and intestinal contents are not diverted from the stomach directly into the colon, but rather colonic contents pass into the stomach and small intestine. Thus there results a massive bacterial seeding of

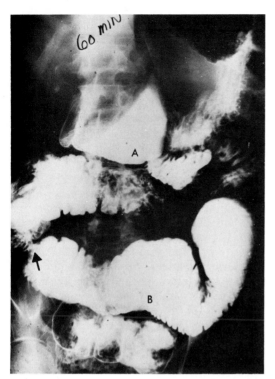

Figure 69-3. Upper gastrointestinal series in a 54-year-old man with recurrent regional enteritis after a massive resection of small intestine. Malabsorption due to dilated, partly obstructed duodenum (A), and dilated surgically reversed loop of jejunum (B) proximal to anastomosis with the colon (arrow). (From Krone, C. L., et al.: Medicine, *47*:89, 1968. © 1968, The Williams and Wilkins Co., Baltimore.)

been studied extensively, and are discussed in detail on pages 259 to 289. In brief, it appears that bacterial hydrolysis of conjugated bile salts leads to a deficiency of bile salts which is largely responsible for steatorrhea in patients with the blind loop syndrome. Vitamin B_{12} malabsorption, on the other hand, appears to result from direct bacterial uptake of the vitamin which is thus no longer available for absorption by the ileum.

CLINICAL FEATURES

Clinical manifestations of the blind loop syndrome vary greatly and depend, at least in part, upon the nature of the small bowel abnormality causing bacterial overgrowth. Patients with *jejunal diverticula* are relatively asymptomatic until small bowel bacterial populations are sufficiently established to cause steatorrhea with

the small bowel which emanates from the colon (Fig. 69-5).[9]

In addition to structural abnormalities conducive to localized intestinal stasis, more generalized alterations in small bowel peristalsis may favor bacterial proliferation and consequent metabolic abnormalities. Thus malabsorption resulting from small bowel bacterial overgrowth has been documented in patients with intestinal scleroderma and marked hypomotility.[10] "Pseudo-obstruction," a poorly understood entity characterized by hypertrophy of small intestinal smooth muscle and markedly delayed intestinal transit, can also result in significant bacterial overgrowth and associated malabsorption.[11]

The mechanisms whereby bacteria proliferating within the small bowel result in fat and vitamin B_{12} malabsorption have

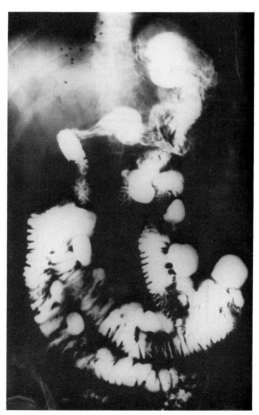

Figure 69-4. Small bowel series in an elderly male patient with blind loop syndrome due to multiple large jejunal diverticula. (Courtesy of Dr. M. H. Sleisenger.)

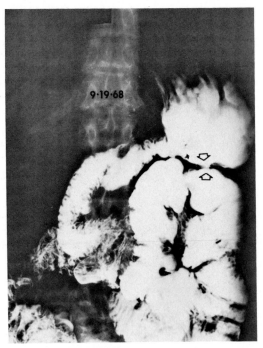

Figure 69–5. Upper gastrointestinal series in a 46-year-old man with a gastrocolic fistula (arrows) due to peptic ulcer disease causing malabsorption. (Courtesy of Dr. M. H. Sleisenger.)

increased numbers of bowel movements, weight loss, and anemia. Since most patients with steatorrhea and anemia associated with jejunal diverticula are elderly, it has been assumed that there occurs an interval of many years between the development of the diverticula and the appearance of metabolic abnormalities. Although most symptomatic patients have multiple diverticula, development of the complications of bacterial overgrowth has been reported in a few patients with a single large duodenal diverticulum. Chronic bleeding caused by ulcerations in one or more diverticula has been described, but frank hemorrhage is a rare manifestation of small bowel diverticulosis. The blood supply to very large diverticula may become compromised, leading to infarction and perforation, but such complications are also extremely uncommon. Occasionally an ingested splinter, nail, or other foreign body may lodge in a diverticulum and ultimately result in a perforation.

Patients with *strictures* or surgically formed *blind pouches* of small intestine

may note abdominal discomfort, bloating, and crampy periumbilical pain before diarrhea, steatorrhea, and the symptoms of anemia develop. In general, an interval of months to years may elapse between the time a blind pouch is formed and the onset of symptoms attributable to small bowel bacterial overgrowth. When patients have strictures or fistulas caused by *regional enteritis* or have hypomotility caused by *scleroderma*, the clinical features of the primary disease may completely overshadow any manifestations of intraluminal microbial proliferation. Furthermore, it may be difficult to determine in patients with regional enteritis or scleroderma the extent to which malabsorption is due to primary intestinal disease as compared with secondary bacterial overgrowth.

Whatever the cause of the abnormal proliferation of microorganisms within the small bowel lumen, the consequences for the patient are the same. Weight loss associated with clinically apparent steatorrhea has been observed in about one-third of patients with small bowel bacterial overgrowth severe enough to cause vitamin B_{12} deficiency.[4] Osteomalacia, vitamin K deficiency, and even hypocalcemic tetany have been known to develop as a consequence of lipid malabsorption in patients with this disorder. Furthermore, production of small bowel bacterial overgrowth in dogs and rats consistently results in increased fecal losses of lipids. The relation of bacterial overgrowth to steatorrhea has been repeatedly documented clinically as well as experimentally. Appropriate antibiotic therapy or surgical correction of the small bowel lesion conducive to stasis promptly reduces fecal fat excretion to normal or near normal levels.

Ample evidence indicates that the anemia that develops in patients with blind loop syndrome is due to vitamin B_{12} deficiency.[12] The anemia is megaloblastic and macrocytic, and serum vitamin B_{12} levels are low. Furthermore, neurological changes indistinguishable from those of pernicious anemia may develop, and the anemia can be corrected by physiological doses of the vitamin. In some patients with small bowel stasis, however, loss of blood from ulcerated areas within stagnant loops of bowel may lead to iron deficiency.

Under these circumstances, the patient may have guaiac-positive stools together with a microcytic and hypochromic or, in some instances, a "mixed" type of anemia. On the other hand, folate deficiency probably does not occur in the blind loop syndrome. Unlike the situation with vitamin B_{12}, folate synthesized by microorganisms in the small bowel appears to be available for the host, and in patients with small bowel bacterial overgrowth serum folate levels tend to be high rather than low.[13]

Hypoproteinemia is a frequent manifestation of the blind loop syndrome and is occasionally severe enough to cause edema.[14] Protein metabolism in the blind loop syndrome has not been extensively studied, however, and the. mechanism or mechanisms responsible for hypoproteinemia are poorly understood. In patients as well as in experimental animals with small bowel bacterial overgrowth, fecal losses of nitrogen tend to be increased, but there is no direct evidence that protein digestion or absorption is significantly impaired. Excessive protein losses from the gut have been implicated in one limited investigation, but this observation has not been confirmed.[15] In one carefully studied case,[16] isotopic measurements suggested that bacterial deamination of amino acids in the gut led to increased urea and ammonia formation at the expense of amino acid incorporation into protein. This would ultimately lead to a contracted amino acid pool with a rapid turnover and ultimately to hypoproteinemia. Further investigation is required to determine whether this mechanism is operative in a meaningful number of patients with small bowel bacterial overgrowth.

Little is known about the effect of intraluminal bacterial proliferation or the metabolism and absorption of carbohydrates. Abnormal xylose tolerance tests have been observed in some, but not all, patients with the blind loop syndrome, and xylose absorption is consistently impaired in rats with intestinal pouches.[17] Enteric microorganisms metabolize xylose, and it is possible that intraluminal destruction of xylose accounts for the abnormal xylose tolerance tests.[18] Intestinal bacteria also convert unabsorbed carbohydrate to organic acids and hydrogen, but the extent to which this occurs in the clinical and experimental blind loop syndrome has not been delineated.

In addition to steatorrhea, patients with the blind loop syndrome frequently complain of watery diarrhea. The mechanisms responsible for diarrhea in intestinal stasis remain to be clarified. Bacterial hydroxylation of fatty acid to form hydroxy-fatty acids has been demonstrated in dogs with experimentally produced blind pouches of jejunum.[19] Because hydroxy-fatty acids impair net sodium and water absorption by the ileum and colon and because one hydroxy-fatty acid, ricinoleic acid, is a constituent of castor oil, the formation of hydroxy-fatty acids has been implicated in the diarrhea observed in patients with small bowel bacterial overgrowth as well as in other absorptive disorders. It should be pointed out, however, that bacterial fermentation of unabsorbed sugars also occurs with the formation of lactate, butyrate, and other organic acids. These substances increase the osmotic load within the gut lumen, and it is possible that they may adversely affect salt and water transport by the gut. A possible role for the bacterial production of amines with consequent effects on bowel motility and transport also requires further investigation.

DIAGNOSIS

A small bowel abnormality associated with intraluminal bacterial proliferation should be considered in the differential diagnosis of any patient who presents with diarrhea, steatorrhea, weight loss, or macrocytic anemia, particularly if the patient is elderly and has had previous abdominal surgery. The development of diarrhea, weight loss, and macrocytic anemia months to years after gastric surgery suggests that the patient may have afferent loop dysfunction or a gastrojejunocolic fistula. A history of previous surgery for small bowel obstruction should raise the question of whether the obstruction was bypassed by an end-to-side anastomosis, leaving a blind pouch, or a side-to-side anastomosis, resulting in recirculation of small bowel contents (Fig. 69–6). On the other hand, a past history of recurrent

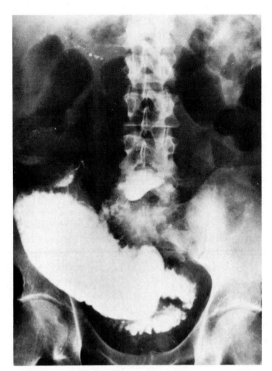

Figure 69–6. Small bowel series in a 46-year-old man with recurrent regional enteritis and malabsorption syndrome, showing a dilated loop of ileum proximal to a stenotic segment. An end-to-side ileocolostomy had previously been performed. (Courtesy of Dr. M. H. Sleisenger.)

bouts of intestinal obstruction may indicate stasis caused by a small bowel stricture or adhesions (Fig. 69–7). The presence of dysphagia and/or Raynaud's phenomenon should suggest a diagnosis of scleroderma (Fig. 69–8). In any event, a complete small bowel series should be obtained in all patients with diarrhea, steatorrhea, and/or macrocytic anemia to exclude the possibility of enteric stasis and consequent bacterial overgrowth.

When the history and small bowel X-rays suggest that proliferation of microorganisms in the small bowel lumen may cause or contribute to malabsorption, further evaluation is necessary for optimal management. The extent of steatorrhea should be determined by a fat balance study, and a test of vitamin B_{12} absorption should be carried out. If the patient has clinically significant bacterial overgrowth, vitamin B_{12} absorption is almost always impaired even though the patient may not yet have become vitamin B_{12} deficient. Intrinsic factor will not improve vitamin B_{12}

absorption in these patients. The xylose tolerance test may be normal or abnormal, because some but by no means all patients with the blind loop syndrome have diminished xylose absorption.

A small bowel biopsy is of value in excluding primary mucosal disease as the cause of disease. Although striking histological abnormalities of jejunal mucosa are not seen in patients with intraluminal bacterial proliferation, the biopsy may not be entirely normal. A patchy lesion of variable severity may be observed. This includes increased infiltration of the lamina propria with lymphocytes, plasma cells, and occasional polymorphonuclear leukocytes, together with slight thickening and blunting of villi. Penetration of the epithelial cell layer by leukocytes is also seen. Nevertheless, one does not find the distinct alterations of the surface absorptive cells regularly present in celiac sprue, and if the patient has not been in an area where

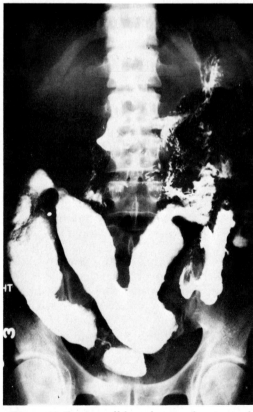

Figure 69–7. A small bowel series showing multiple strictures and blind loops in a 26-year-old man with regional enteritis and malabsorption syndrome. (Courtesy of Dr. M. H. Sleisenger.)

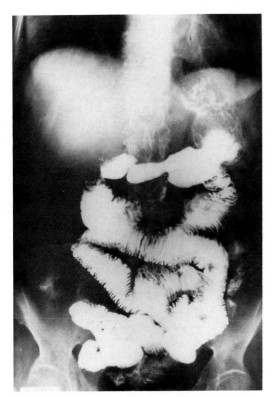

Figure 69-8. A small bowel series at one hour in a 46-year-old woman with scleroderma of the small intestine and blind loop syndrome. Note dilated loops of jejunum, delay in transit, and mucosal spiculation. (Courtesy of Dr. M. H. Sleisenger.)

tropical sprue occurs, the patchy inflammatory changes associated with intraluminal bacterial proliferation should not cause the physician to believe that any intestinal mucosal disease is responsible for malabsorption.

Once it has been established that the patient has malabsorption of fat and vitamin B_{12} as well as a small bowel abnormality possibly conducive to bacterial overgrowth, it then becomes important to demonstrate that the patient does in fact harbor increased numbers of microorganisms in the small bowel lumen and that these microorganisms are responsible for the observed malabsorption.[20] Such documentation is necessary, because it is only under these conditions that surgical or antibiotic therapy undertaken to eliminate bacterial overgrowth will actually benefit the patient.

Intubation of the small bowel allows collection of intestinal contents for bacteriological studies. The specimen should be obtained under anaerobic conditions, serially diluted, and cultured on several selective media.[21] In patients with significant bacterial overgrowth a number of different species are found, and the total concentration of bacteria generally exceeds 10^7 microorganisms per milliliter. Bacteroides, anaerobic lactobacilli, coliforms, and enterococci are all likely to be present in varying numbers. Although in most patients the intraluminal microbial proliferation can be documented in the proximal jejunum, it is important to recognize that in many instances the intestinal abnormality may result in bacterial overgrowth only in more distal portions of the small intestine.

To be certain that the observed bacterial overgrowth is responsible for the malabsorption, the patient should receive a short course of antibiotics as a therapeutic trial. After treatment with tetracycline or lincomycin for five to seven days there should be a distinct improvement in measured fecal fat excretion and vitamin B_{12} absorption if intraluminal bacteria are playing an important role in the patient.[3, 4] If one can demonstrate that antibiotic therapy reduces the number of microorganisms and at the same time corrects the absorptive defects (see Fig. 69-9), then long-term treatment directed at bacterial overgrowth can be reasonably expected to yield good results.

A number of other laboratory tests have been proposed as approaches to the diagnosis of the blind loop syndrome. Although potentially advantageous in that they might eliminate the need for small bowel intubation and for difficult and time-consuming microbiological analyses, these tests are not currently available in most routine clinical laboratories. In addition to such practical considerations, these tests also have theoretical limitations. For example, urinary indican excretion is elevated in patients with the blind loop syndrome as a result of the presence of indole-producing microorganisms in the small bowel.[4] It should be remembered, however, that indicanuria also occurs in any absorptive disorder which causes increased delivery of tryptophan to the colon, because colonic bacteria will convert unabsorbed tryptophan to indole which then can be absorbed by the colon.[22] Similarly,

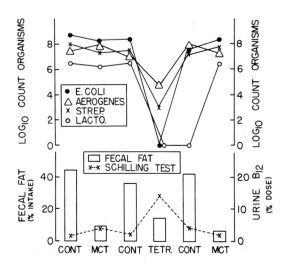

Figure 69–9. Metabolic and microbiological studies in a patient with the blind loop syndrome. The patient had afferent loop dysfunction following subtotal gastrectomy with Billroth II anastomosis. The patient was studied after two weeks of no therapy (CONT), after two weeks of treatment with medium-chain triglycerides (MCT) or after two weeks of treatment with tetracycline, 1 g daily. Only those bacterial species consistently present in large numbers are shown. Substitution of medium-chain for long-chain fatty acids in the diet corrected steatorrhea, but did not influence bacterial counts or vitamin B_{12} absorption. Tetracycline reduced bacterial counts and corrected the malabsorption of fat and vitamin B_{12}.

hydrogen production and consequent breath hydrogen excretion after an oral load of glucose measure intraluminal bacterial fermentation.[23] Although increased hydrogen production in response to glucose feeding may thus be an indication of bacterial activity in the small bowel lumen, unabsorbed glucose reaching the colon as a result of any absorptive disorder would also increase hydrogen production. Since bacteria deconjugate glycine-conjugated bile salts, a test has been proposed[24] which measures the breath excretion of radioactive carbon dioxide after administration of ^{14}C-labeled glycine conjugated to a bile salt. Again, however, bile salt hydrolysis within the colon would also result in increased excretion of radioactive carbon dioxide.

Bacterial deconjugation of bile salts can also be directly determined by subjecting jejunal aspirates to thin-layer chromatography. In health, no more than trace quantities of *free* bile salts are found in the jejunal aspirates. In patients with significant bacterial overgrowth, the concentrations of *conjugated* bile salts are reduced, particularly the concentrations of taurine conjugates; however, the concentrations of *free* bile acids are distinctly increased. *Total* bile salt concentrations are often, but not always, reduced in patients with bacterially induced steatorrhea.[4, 25, 26] When the methodology becomes practical for routine clinical use, these alterations in intraluminal bile salts may provide a use-

ful approach to the laboratory diagnosis of the blind loop syndrome.

Although currently available methods are not practical for routine use, measurement of serum bile acids constitutes another potentially useful means of identifying the blind loop syndrome. Increased serum bile acid levels have been noted in several patients with the blind loop syndrome.[27] Serum levels of conjugated bile salts are normal or only slightly elevated, and the increase is due almost entirely to increases in the concentrations of free bile acids. Following antibiotic therapy, the concentrations of free bile acids fall precipitously. Although the mechanism for this increase is not at all clear, it seems likely that bile salts deconjugated within the bowel lumen are rapidly reabsorbed by passive nonionic diffusion and, unlike conjugated bile salts, are readily bound by serum proteins. This binding might result in diminished hepatic removal from portal blood and consequent accumulation of free bile acids in the systemic circulation.

TREATMENT

The aim of therapy is reduction or elimination of the bacterial overgrowth and consists of the administration of antibiotics or, when feasible, correction of the small bowel abnormality conducive to stasis and microbial proliferation. As emphasized above, such therapy can be successful only when the patient's malabsorption directly results from intraluminal proliferation of microorganisms.[28] Surgical correction of the abnormality causing small bowel stasis is clearly the most definitive approach to management, and the feasibility of corrective surgery should be considered in all patients with the blind loop syndrome. Unfortunately, however, an operative approach is often impractical, either because extensive resection of bowel will be required or because the patient's age and debilitated condition often strongly contraindicate major surgery. In a patient with multiple jejunal diverticula involving many loops of small bowel, for example, it makes little sense to resect the diverticula which serve as a bacterial reservoir if the necessary resection is so extensive that one merely substitutes the absorptive problems caused by short bowel for the malabsorption caused by bacterial overgrowth. On the other hand, it would seem advisable to resect one or more diverticula known to be causing bacterial overgrowth and consequent malabsorption if the amount of involved bowel is slight. Correction of partial obstruction caused by stricture or adhesions is also likely to be attended by excellent long-term results, providing that such correction will not necessitate extensive resection or bypass of small intestine. In patients who have regional enteritis, a surgical approach to stricture or fistulas associated with bacterial overgrowth should be undertaken with caution because of the recurrent nature of the disease and because it may be difficult to know the extent to which malabsorption results from bacterial overgrowth rather than from the primary bowel disease.

Whether or not a surgical approach is feasible, appropriate administration of nutrients and vitamins is a crucial factor in management until the patient's malabsorption has been optimally corrected. Patients deficient in vitamin B_{12} should be treated with monthly injections of at least 100 μg of the vitamin. Whenever indicated by clinical or laboratory manifestations supplementary calcium as well as parenteral administration of vitamin D should be given. Similarly, vitamin K should be injected whenever the prothrombin time is prolonged. Steatorrhea and diarrhea can be reduced by the use of medium-chain triglycerides in place of the long-chain triglycerides which constitute the bulk of the lipids present in the conventional diet (see Fig. 69–9). Although theoretically useful in the blind loop syndrome, the administration of conjugated bile salts to correct bile salt deficiency is not a practical means of improving fat absorption because of the high cost of pure conjugated bile salts and because of the diarrhea regularly induced when bile salts are fed.

In the majority of cases, surgical correction of the small bowel abnormality is not feasible, and antibiotic therapy is required

TABLE 69–2. EFFECT OF BROAD-SPECTRUM ANTIMICROBIAL DRUGS ON MALABSORPTION IN FOUR PATIENTS WITH SCLERODERMA AND MALABSORPTION SYNDROME*

		PATIENT 1		PATIENT 2		PATIENT 3		PATIENT 4	
	Normal	Pre	Post- (48 hr)	Pre	Post	Pre	Post	Pre	Post
D-Xylose (g/5 hr)	4–8	3.78	3.5	0.3	4.2	2.7	3.9	3.7	3.8
Fecal fat (g/24 hr)	< 6	32	13	18	9.5	10	5.5	11	23
Coefficient of fat absorption (%)	> 94	68	87	80	91	85	93	84	72
Schilling (48 hr urinary excretion) (%)	> 10	24	30	1.98	7.26	15	13	9.9	23
Urinary indican (mg/24 hr)	< 100	302	112	–	170	162	76	104	136
Duodenal culture		Aerobacter > 10^6	No growth	Aerobacter > 10^6	–	–	–	Mixed flora	Mixed flora

*From Kahn, I. J., Jeffries, G. H., and Sleisenger, M. H.: New Eng. J. Med. 274:1139, 1966.

to suppress intraluminal bacterial proliferation. The agents most commonly used are tetracycline or chlortetracycline,[3, 4] the usual dosage being 250 mg four times a day. If the antibiotic is to be considered effective, diarrhea should subside and the absorption of fat and vitamin B_{12} should be distinctly improved within a week of beginning therapy (Table 69–2). Most clinicians agree that neomycin is ineffective, probably because this agent does not suppress the growth of the strict anaerobes present in large numbers in the small bowel of most, if not all, patients with the blind loop syndrome. Lincomycin, on the other hand, specifically attacks anaerobes and has been effective in improving absorption in the blind loop syndrome.[4, 29] Selection of an antibiotic on the basis of the sensitivity of the microorganisms present in the small bowel lumen is attractive in theory, but this approach is often difficult because there are usually present many different bacterial species, often with very different sensitivities. Under such circumstances it may be extremely difficult to select what could be considered the most appropriate antibiotic on the basis of microbial sensitivity. In general, once an effective agent has been found, treatment can often be maintained for months or even years with no obvious side effects and without recurrence of significant bacterial overgrowth. In many instances an excellent response can be sustained with intermittent therapy; i.e., administration of the antibiotic for two weeks out of each month. One patient has remained completely well with tetracycline administered in this fashion for 12 years.

REFERENCES

1. Barker, W. H.,and Hummel, L. E. Macrocytic anemia in association with intestinal strictures and anastomoses. Bull. Johns Hopkins Hosp. 46:215, 1939.
2. Ellis, H., and Smith, S. D. M. The blind loop syndrome. Monogr. Surg. Sci. 4:193, 1967.
3. Donaldson, R. M., Jr. Small bowel bacterial overgrowth. Advan. Intern. Med. 16:191, 1970.
4. Tabaqchali, S. The pathophysiological role of the small intestinal bacterial flora. Scand. J. Gastroenterol. 5 (suppl. 6): 139, 1970.
5. Lyall, I. G., and Parsons, P. J. Some aspects of the blind loop syndrome. Med. J. Australia 48:904, 1962.
6. Wirts, C. W., and Goldstein, F. Studies of the mechanism of postgastrectomy steatorrhea. Ann. Intern. Med. 58:25, 1963.
7. Doig, A., and Girdwood, R. G. The absorption of folic acid and labeled cyanocobalamine in intestinal malabsorption with observations on the fecal excretion of fat and nitrogen and the absorption of glucose and xylose. Quart. J. Med. 29:333, 1960.
8. Bishop, R. F., and Anderson, C. M. Bacterial flora of stomach and small intestine in children with intestinal obstruction. Arch. Dis. Child. 35:487, 1960.
9. Atwater, J. S., Butt, H. R., and Priestley, J. T. Gastrojejunocolic fistulae with special reference to associated nutritional deficiencies and certain surgical aspects. Ann. Surg. 117:414, 1943.
10. Kahn, I. J., Jeffries, G. H., and Sleisenger, M. H. Malabsorption in intestinal scleroderma. Correction by antibiotics. New Eng. J. Med. 274:1339, 1966.
11. Pearson, A. J., et al. Intestinal pseudo-obstruction with bacterial overgrowth in the small intestine. Amer. J. Dig. Dis. 14:200, 1969.
12. Badenoch, J. (ed.) The Blind Loop Syndrome. In Modern Trends in Gastroenterology. New York, Paul B. Hoeber, 1958.
13. Hoffbrand, A. V., Tabaqchali, S., and Mollin, D. L. High serum-folate levels in intestinal blind-loop syndrome. Lancet 1:1339, 1966.
14. Badenoch, J., Bedford, P. D., and Evans, J. R. Massive diverticulosis of the small intestine with steatorrhea and megaloblastic anemia. Quart. J. Med. 24:321, 1955.
15. Jeejeebhoy, K. N., and Coghill, N. F. The measurement of gastrointestinal protein loss by a new method. Gut 2:123, 1961.
16. Jones, E. A., Craigie, A., Tavill, A. S., Franglen, G., and Rosenoer, V. M. Protein metabolism in the intestinal stagnant-loop syndrome. Gut 9:466, 1968.
17. Donaldson, R. M., Jr. Role of enteric microorganisms in malabsorption. Fed. Proc. 26:1426, 1967.
18. Goldstein, F. Mechanisms of malabsorption and malnutrition in the blind loop syndrome. Gastroenterology 61:780, 1971.
19. Kim, Y. S., and Spritz, N. Metabolism of hydroxy fatty acids in dogs with steatorrhea secondary to experimentally produced intestinal blind loops. J. Lipid Res. 9:487, 1968.
20. Donaldson, R. M., Jr. Malabsorption in the blind loop syndrome. Gastroenterology 48:388, 1965.
21. Gorbach, S. L., et al. Studies of intestinal microflora. II. Microorganisms of the small intestine and their relation to oral and fecal flora. Gastroenterology 53:856, 1967.
22. Fordtran, J. S., Scroggie, W. B., and Polter, D. E. Colonic absorption of tryptophan metabolites in man. J. Lab. Clin. Med. 64:125, 1964.
23. Levitt, M. D., and Donaldson, R. M., Jr. Use of

respiratory hydrogen (H_2) excretion to detect carbohydrate malabsorption. J. Lab. Clin. Med. 75:937, 1970.

24. Sherr, H. P., Newman, A., Sasaki, Y., Banwell, J. G., and Hendrix, T. R. Detection of bacterial deconjugation of bile salts by a convenient breath analysis technique. Gastroenterology 60:81, 1971.

25. Rosenberg, I. H., Hardison, W. G. H., and Bull, D. M. Jejunal bile salt abnormalities in malabsorption with bacterial stasis (abstr.). Clin. Res. 14:304, 1966.

26. Tabaqchali, S., and Booth, C. C. Jejunal bacteriology and bile salt metabolism in patients with intestinal malabsorption. Lancet 2:12, 1965.

27. Tabaqchali, S., Hatzionnou, J., and Booth, C. C. Bile salt deconjugation and steatorrhea in patients with the stagnant-loop syndrome. Lancet 2:12, 1968.

28. Krone, C. L., Theodor, E., Sleisenger, M. H., and Jeffries, G. H. Studies on the pathogenesis of malabsorption. Medicine 47:89, 1966.

29. Polter, D. E., Boyle, J. D., Miller, L. G., and Finegold, S. M. Anaerobic bacteria as cause of the blind loop syndrome. Gastroenterology 54:1148, 1968.

Chapter 70

Whipple's Disease

Jerry S. Trier

DEFINITION

Whipple's disease is an uncommon systemic disease which invariably involves the small intestine but which may affect virtually any organ system of the body. Clinical findings may include intestinal malabsorption, fever, increased skin pigmentation, anemia, lymphadenopathy, arthralgia and arthritis, pleuritis, valvular endocarditis, and central nervous system symptoms. Patients with this disease may present with one or many of the aforementioned manifestations. The infiltration of involved tissues with large glycoprotein-containing macrophages and with small rod-shaped bacilli is specific and diagnostic for this disorder.

Until recent years, the clinical course of Whipple's disease generally progressed relentlessly to a fatal outcome. In contrast, death caused by Whipple's disease is now rare, if it occurs at all, because the institution of appropriate antibiotic therapy induces prompt, dramatic, and perhaps permanent remission.

HISTORY

The first case of Whipple's disease was described over 60 years ago by George Hoyt Whipple in a classic paper which included a remarkably thorough account of the patient's clinical illness as well as an accurate, well illustrated description of the pathological findings in the small intestine and mesenteric lymph nodes.[1] Whipple described extensive infiltration of the lamina propria with large, frothy cells (macrophages) which distorted villous architecture. He also noted the presence of large lipid deposits in the lamina propria and in the enlarged mesenteric lymph nodes. In addition he identified, in one gland stained by silver impregnation, the presence of "great numbers of a peculiar rod-shaped organism" 2 μ in length or less. Although he clearly stated that the etiology of the disease was obscure, he named the disease "intestinal lipodystrophy" and he suggested that the disease might represent a disorder of fat metabolism, because, as he put it, "this seems to offer less objections and to have more points in favor than any one word or combination of words which have been considered."

Over 40 years later, Hendrix and co-workers described involvement of the endocardium in Whipple's disease.[2] Upton subsequently demonstrated the typical foamy macrophages in peripheral lymph nodes, liver, adrenal, and valves of the heart in a patient with Whipple's disease.[3] Sieracki and Fine then documented the presence of typical macrophages in many nonintestinal tissues in four patients, clearly establishing the systemic nature of this disorder.[4]

For 45 years after its initial description,

938

the disease was considered to be a uniformly fatal and untreatable primary disorder of fat metabolism. However, in 1952, Paulley described a patient with histologically documented Whipple's disease in whom the disease remitted for a prolonged period following administration of the antibiotic chloramphenicol.[5] Despite his report, antibiotic therapy for this disease was not widely used over the next decade and many patients in whom the diagnosis had been established received only supportive treatment and, in some instances, ACTH or corticosteroids with only limited success.[6, 7]

In the early 1960's, identical rod-shaped bacilli were found within the intestinal mucosa of patients with untreated Whipple's disease in independent studies from several laboratories.[8-11] At about the same time, dramatic remission of clinical symptoms followed treatment of acutely ill Whipple's disease patients with a variety of antibiotic regimens in a number of medical centers.[11-13] More recently, the presence of bacilli identical to those seen in the intestine have been observed in nonintestinal tissues in patients with untreated Whipple's disease.[14-16] Moreover, many additional reports have clearly established that severely ill patients respond predictably and dramatically to treatment with appropriate antibiotics. Thus, if properly diagnosed, this previously fatal disease can now be treated effectively with ease.

PATHOLOGY

The pathology of Whipple's disease is distinctive; therefore histological examination of biopsies from involved tissues is usually diagnostic.

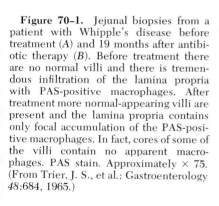

Figure 70–1. Jejunal biopsies from a patient with Whipple's disease before treatment (A) and 19 months after antibiotic therapy (B). Before treatment there are no normal villi and there is tremendous infiltration of the lamina propria with PAS-positive macrophages. After treatment more normal-appearing villi are present and the lamina propria contains only focal accumulation of the PAS-positive macrophages. In fact, cores of some of the villi contain no apparent macrophages. PAS stain. Approximately × 75. (From Trier, J. S., et al.: Gastroenterology 48:684, 1965.)

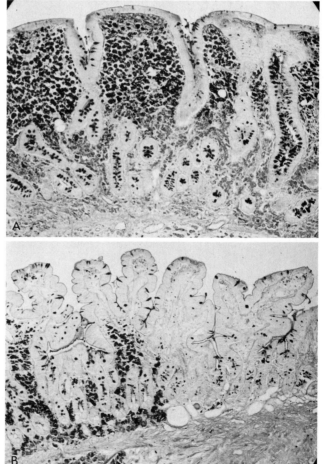

Small Intestine. The small intestine has been involved in all reported cases. Grossly, the bowel wall appears thickened and edematous. When examined with a hand lens or a dissecting microscope, the mucosa may resemble that seen in celiac sprue, in that the surface may appear flat or convoluted without apparent villi. More often, the villi are visible but markedly widened.

The abnormality in mucosal structure is readily apparent in histological sections in which extensive infiltration of the lamina propria with large macrophages markedly distorts villous architecture (Fig. 70–1, A). The cytoplasm of these macrophages is filled with many large glycoprotein granules which stain with the periodic acid–Schiff (PAS) technique.[17] The lamina propria may also contain accumulations of polymorphonuclear leukocytes. On the other hand, the cellular elements normally

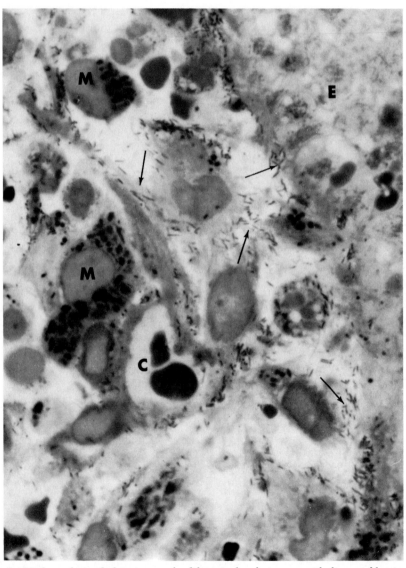

Figure 70–2. High resolution light micrograph of the interface between epithelium and lamina propria from a patient with untreated Whipple's disease. The epithelium (E) is to the right. Numerous bacilli (arrows) are seen beneath the epithelium and between the cellular elements of the lamina propria. Several typical macrophages (M) can be seen. C, capillary. Osmium-fixed, epoxy embedded tissue, toluidine blue stain. Approximately × 1500. (From Trier, J. S., et al.: Gastroenterology 48:684, 1965.)

seen in the lamina such as plasma cells, lymphocytes and eosinophils are markedly decreased, because they have been all but replaced by the large number of macrophages. The replacement of the normal cellular elements of the lamina with PAS-positive macrophages in the small intestine is of diagnostic significance, because it is specific for Whipple's disease.

Mucosal and submucosal lymphatic vessels are dilated and, in sections not exposed to lipid solvents, are filled with fat. There are fat droplets in the extracellular spaces of the lamina as well.

Although villous architecture is often markedly distorted, the absorptive epithelium shows only patchy, nonspecific abnormalities. These may include some attenuation of the brush border, some decrease in cell height, and accumulation of a moderate amount of lipid within the cytoplasm. Severe cytoplasmic abnormalities of absorptive cells such as are seen in patients with celiac sprue are not a regular feature of the intestinal lesion of Whipple's disease.

With the higher magnification of the electron microscope, many bacilli are seen in the lamina propria of the small intestine of patients with untreated Whipple's disease (Figs. 70–2 to 70–4). These tiny bacilli (0.25 μ wide and 1 to 2.5 μ long) may be located anywhere in the lamina but are usually most abundant just beneath the absorptive epithelium and around vascular channels in the upper half of the mucosa. Their fine structure, which has been identical in all patients studied to date, conclusively establishes their bacterial nature (Fig. 70–3). They have a characteristic bacterial cell wall, a pale central nucleoid and, in favorable sections, may be seen undergoing binary fission. Moreover, these bacilli are seen within the PAS-positive macrophages by which they have been phagocytosed and in which they undergo degeneration and disintegration (Fig. 70–4). It seems likely that at least some of

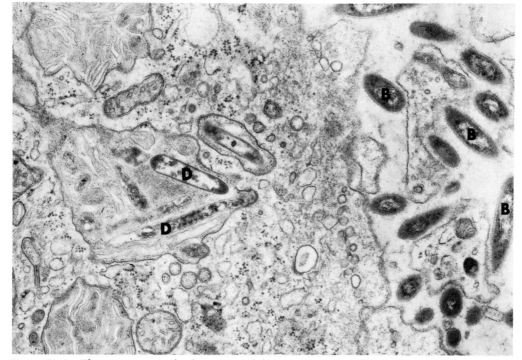

Figure 70–3. Electron micrograph of a portion of the cytoplasm of a PAS-positive macrophage and its extracellular space from a pretreatment biopsy. Many bacilli (B) are seen outside the macrophage. Within its cytoplasm, several disintegrating bacilli (D) are undergoing degeneration and contributing membranous material to a PAS-positive granule. Portions of two other typical PAS-positive granules with their closely packed membranous material are visible above and below the granule which contains the degenerating organisms. Approximately × 23,000. (From Trier, J. S., et al.: Gastroenterology 48:684, 1965.)

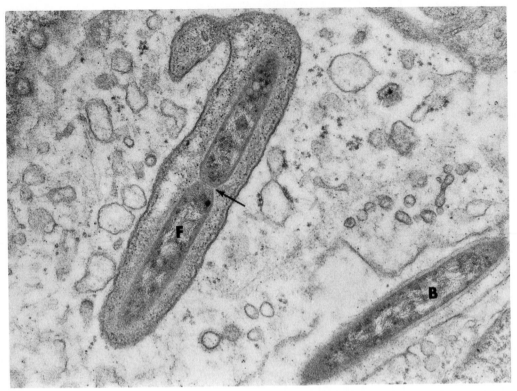

Figure 70–4. A portion of a PAS-positive macrophage from a patient with untreated Whipple's disease. A bacillus (B) is seen in the extracellular space. Within the cytoplasm of the macrophage, an organism (F) is undergoing binary fission (arrow). The dense cytoplasm immediately surrounding this organism and separated from the rest of the macrophage cytoplasm by a distinct membrane may represent an early stage in the formation of the PAS-positive granule. Approximately × 55,000. (From Trier, J. S., et al.: Gastroenterology 48:684, 1965.)

the PAS-positive glycoprotein within the macrophage granules represents remnants of the cell wall of degenerated, phagocytosed bacilli. Occasionally, the bacilli can be seen within villous absorptive cells, usually within large lysosomes in the apical cytoplasm.[18] The bacilli cannot be identified with certainty with the light microscope in routinely processed paraffin-embedded tissues; instead, electron microscopic or special high resolution light microscopic techniques must be used for positive identification.[13]

Upon treatment with appropriate antibiotics, the mucosa of the small intestine gradually reverts toward normal (Fig. 70–1, B). Bacilli disappear from the intercellular spaces within a few days, and after four to eight weeks only degenerating organisms can be identified within the cytoplasm of the PAS macrophages. Following effective treatment, the number of PAS-positive macrophages in the lamina propria gradually decreases, and plasma cells, lymphocytes, and eosinophils reappear. Concomitantly, villous architecture and absorptive cell structure return toward normal. However, in many patients, mucosal histology may not revert completely to normal for years, if ever. Patchy accumulations of PAS-positive macrophages, dilated mucosal lymphatics, and large lipid droplets often persist in the lamina propria of biopsies obtained from asymptomatic patients several years after successful antibiotic treatment.

The colonic mucosa may or may not be involved in Whipple's disease. When involved, infiltration with PAS-positive macrophages and bacilli has been documented.[15, 19] However, the finding of PAS-positive macrophages *without* demonstration of the bacilli in the colon is neither diagnostic nor specific. Similar macrophages, containing cytoplasmic PAS-positive glycoprotein, are occasionally seen in rectal and colonic mucosa of healthy individuals and are regularly found in patients with colonic histiocytosis or melanosis coli.

Extraintestinal Pathology. Systemic involvement in Whipple's disease is thoroughly documented. PAS-positive macrophages have been identified with the light microscope in most body tissues, including heart, lung, spleen, liver, endocrine glands, central nervous system, bone, lymph nodes, and kidney.[2-4] The heart lesions are of particular interest, because endocardial infiltration of macrophages may cause grossly obvious vegetative endocarditis on the heart valves. In some of these patients, secondary subacute streptococcal bacterial endocarditis has been noted at autopsy.

The typical bacilli have been demonstrated with the electron microscope in several nonintestinal tissues, including peripheral and mesenteric lymph nodes and the central nervous system in patients with active disease.[14-16]

In Whipple's disease, as in other diseases which cause severe panmalabsorption, nonspecific pathological changes secondary to severe malabsorption of nutrients may involve many organ systems. Thus, parathyroid hyperplasia, adrenocortical atrophy, severe muscle wasting, and follicular hyperkeratosis of the skin may be seen as secondary manifestations of the disease.

ETIOLOGY AND PATHOGENESIS

Although significant advances toward our understanding of the etiology and pathogenesis of Whipple's disease have been made in the past decade, many questions remain unanswered.

It is known that the mucosa of the small intestine and other involved tissues are invaded by numerous small, gram-positive bacilli in patients with active disease. The dramatic clinical improvement which parallels disappearance of these organisms during effective antibiotic therapy indicates that these bacilli play a significant role in the etiology of the disease. However, their exact role in the pathogenesis of this most unusual infection is not fully understood.

Attempts in a number of laboratories to isolate the responsible organism have yielded conflicting and, as yet, inconclusive results. Organisms which have been isolated from involved tissues and claimed to be this specific etiologic agent include aerobic corynebacteria, a Hemophilus species, a Brucella-like organism and *l*-form streptococci.[20-22] In a number of other laboratories, despite the use of sophisticated cultural techniques, a specific organism could not be isolated consistently from multiple tissue samples known to contain many bacilli.[23] Thus one must conclude that the causative organism has not been identified, and further studies will be needed to determine whether or not one of the organisms mentioned above is, indeed, the specific microbial agent responsible for Whipple's disease.

There are other factors, in addition to the difficulties in identifying the responsible organism, which suggest that Whipple's disease is a most unusual infectious disease. It occurs sporadically and is so uncommon that it has been impossible to establish any epidemiological pattern. Unlike most infectious diseases, there are no established cases of direct transmission of the illness from one patient to another, although, on two occasions, the disease has been reported in brothers. It seems likely that host susceptibility factors must play an important role in the pathogenesis of Whipple's disease in those few individuals who develop this disorder. Indeed in preliminary studies, delayed hypersensitivity as judged by phytohemagglutinin stimulation of lymphocytes and cutaneous responses to bacterial and fungal skin test antigens were depressed in patients with Whipple's disease.[24]

The nature and derivation of the peculiar macrophage which infiltrates affected tissues in Whipple's disease are also not clear. Do these cells derive from primitive reticulum cells or from the macrophages normally present in the lamina propria?

However, the extensive infiltration of affected tissues with these large macrophages contributes significantly to the clinical symptoms observed in patients. For example, infiltration of the lamina propria probably interferes with intestinal absorption. Following absorption by the relatively normal-appearing epithelial cells, nutrients are not transported properly through the diseased lamina into the mucosal vascular and lymphatic channels. Transport is further impaired by the extensively infiltrated and enlarged mesenteric lymph nodes which compromise the lymphatic drainage of the small intestine and prevent normal egress of absorbed material.

CLINICAL FEATURES AND DIAGNOSIS

The clinical presentation of patients with Whipple's disease may vary a great deal, depending upon which organ systems are involved and whether the disease is early or advanced. For example, astute clinicians have, at times, established the diagnosis in patients with fever and joint symptoms but without significant gastrointestinal complaints.[25] More commonly, the diagnosis is not suspected until patients present with prominent gastrointestinal symptoms. The disease may occur at any age[26] but is most common in the fourth and fifth decades of life. Males are affected more often than females. Most reported cases have occurred in Caucasians, but the disease has been diagnosed in Negroes and American Indians.

Symptoms. The gastrointestinal symptoms of Whipple's disease are not specific and resemble, in general, those seen in patients with other diseases in which generalized malabsorption is a feature. Diarrhea is usually a prominent complaint, and the passage of five to ten large, watery or semiformed, malodorous steatorrheal stools per day is common. Grossly bloody diarrhea has been reported, but is uncommon. When present, it may be related to impaired coagulation in patients with hypoprothrombinemia caused by defective absorption of vitamin K. As in celiac sprue, patients occasionally may complain of constipation rather than diarrhea. Abdominal bloating and poorly localized, ill-defined abdominal cramps are often present. Anorexia is more common than in patients with celiac sprue and, together with malabsorption, may produce precipitous weight loss leading to profound cachexia. Fatigue, lassitude, and weakness are particularly severe in patients with severe anorexia and diarrhea. If the malabsorption continues unchecked, specific deficiencies usually develop and these may cause extraintestinal symptoms as in other causes of malabsorption. Thus, paresthesias and hyperpathia related to peripheral neuropathy, tetany caused by hypocalcemia or hypomagnesemia, and purpura caused by impaired coagulation may be present. Loss of substantial quantities of albumin into the intestinal lumen regularly accompanies severe diarrhea in Whipple's disease;[27] hence, peripheral edema from the resultant hypoproteinemia may be a prominent complaint.

Extraintestinal symptoms may precede gastrointestinal complaints by many years in Whipple's disease. Of these, arthritis and fever are most common. About two-thirds of patients have joint symptoms, and in one large series over 30 per cent had these symptoms for over five years before the diagnosis of Whipple's disease was established.[28] The severity of the arthropathy varies from patient to patient. An intermittent migratory arthritis which may affect both large and small joints is most common. Usually, a synovial reaction which waxes and wanes is evident with tenderness, redness, swelling, and increased heat of the affected joint. Unlike rheumatoid arthritis, permanent joint deformity is rare in Whipple's disease. Many patients have arthralgia only, without objective joint findings. Severe back pains suggest the presence of spondylitis which has been documented in occasional patients.

Significant fever and chills are noted in over half of the cases of Whipple's disease. The fever is usually low grade and intermittent, although it may be high, either spiking or sustained in advanced disease. A chronic, nonproductive cough has been described in some patients and was a severe symptom in the patient reported originally by Whipple.

The central nervous system may be affected, and symptoms may include disorientation, loss of memory, and abnormal behavior associated with various cranial nerve signs such as ophthalmoplegia, nystagmus, and facial numbness.[29-31] Although these symptoms are not specific and may be related to associated nutritional deficiencies, direct involvement of the central nervous system by the Whipple's bacillus and typical PAS-positive macrophages has been documented.[16]

Physical Findings. Many of the physical findings in Whipple's disease are related to severe intestinal panmalabsorption and are identical to those discussed on pages 864 to 884. These may include profound emaciation with fat and muscle wasting, clubbing of the finger nails, hypotension caused by fluid and electrolyte loss and/or secondary adrenocortical insufficiency, increased skin pigmentation, peripheral edema related to enteric protein loss, purpura, cheilosis and glossitis, increased muscular irritability or even frank tetany caused by hypocalcemia, and loss of sensory modalities in the extremities related to peripheral neuropathy.

Palpable, moderately enlarged peripheral lymph nodes are common; these are usually firm, nontender, and freely movable. Peripheral joints may be swollen, warm, reddened, and tender if arthritis is present. Heart murmurs, when present, may be caused by vegetations on the valve surfaces, but functional systolic murmurs caused by anemia are more common. The presence of secondary acute or subacute bacterial endocarditis must be considered in febrile patients with Whipple's disease who have diastolic murmurs or changing systolic murmurs.

The abdomen is usually distended and, in about half of reported cases, is slightly to moderately tender. Periumbilical fullness or an ill-defined mass may be palpated and may be due to enlargement of the mesenteric lymph nodes. Ascites is uncommon and, when present, is usually associated with severe hypoalbuminemia. Hepatosplenomegaly is uncommon.

Neurological signs, other than those caused by peripheral neuropathy, are uncommon, but confusion, amnesia, ophthalmoplegia, and other cranial nerve signs have been noted and ascribed to primary central nervous system involvement.

Laboratory Findings. Most of the laboratory abnormalities found in Whipple's disease patients are causally related to severe intestinal malabsorption (see pp. 259 to 277). Thus, steatorrhea, defective xylose absorption, and low serum carotene and cholesterol levels are common. In patients with severe diarrhea and malabsorption, hypokalemia, hypocalcemia, hypomagnesemia, and significant hypoalbuminemia are common. Reduced 24-hour excretion of 17-hydroxycorticosteroids and 17-ketosteroids has been found in debilitated patients.

Anemia is common and is usually associated with iron deficiency. Microcytic, hypochromic red cells and a low serum iron accompany the anemia. In some patients there is macrocytosis caused by folate deficiency. In others serum iron, folate, and vitamin B_{12} are normal, and anemia may be of the type seen in chronic infection. Mild to moderate leukocytosis may be present, especially in febrile patients.

X-rays of the small intestine following a barium meal are almost invariably abnormal.[32] The most characteristic finding is marked thickening of the mucosal folds (plica circulares), especially in the duodenum and proximal jejunum (Fig. 70-5, A). In most patients there is a gradient of decreasing involvement as the distal jejunum is approached, and the ileum may appear normal. In severe disease the ileum may also appear abnormal. Dilatation of the small intestine is not usually as prominent as in other primary intestinal malabsorptive disease such as celiac sprue, and segmentation and flocculation of intraluminal barium may or may not be present. Following successful treatment with antibiotics, the thickening of the mucosal folds becomes less marked (Fig. 70-5, B); in fact, the radiological appearance of the small intestine often reverts to normal.

Biopsy Studies. Although Whipple's disease may often be suspected on the basis of symptoms, physical signs, and laboratory findings, its diagnosis can be established only by histological examination of the involved tissues.

Prior to the development of peroral intestinal biopsy methods, the diagnosis was usually established by biopsy of small intestine and/or involved mesenteric lymph nodes at laparotomy. Occasionally, biopsies of enlarged peripheral lymph nodes established the diagnosis. Now, the biopsy procedure of choice for establishing or excluding the diagnosis of Whipple's disease is peroral biopsy of the small intestine in the region of the duodenojejunal junction. This portion of the small bowel is

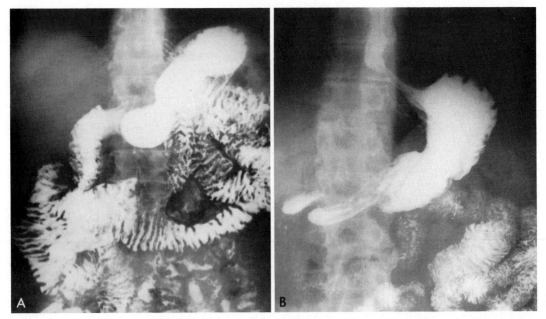

Figure 70–5. Barium contrast studies of the small intestine from a patient with Whipple's disease before (A) and after (B) treatment with antibiotics. Before treatment there are marked thickening of the plicae circulares and a loss of the normal delicate mucosal relief pattern. There is less dilatation of the small intestine than is usually seen in films of patients with severe untreated celiac sprue. After treatment the mucosal pattern appears much more normal, with a reduction in the thickness of the plicae circulares and partial return of the normal mucosal pattern. (Courtesy of Dr. Elihu Schimmel.)

involved in all symptomatic patients, even early in the disease when steatorrhea may be mild or absent.[25] Moreover, the infiltration of the lamina propria of the small intestine by PAS-positive macrophages accompanied by lymphatic dilatation is specific and diagnostic for Whipple's disease. The biopsy procedure itself is safe and can be carried out with little or no morbidity provided that blood coagulation deficiencies, if present, are corrected prior to the procedure.

In contrast, rectal biopsy may be misleading and is no substitute for peroral small intestinal biopsy. PAS-positive macrophages resembling closely those seen in Whipple's disease may be found in the rectal lamina propria in benign conditions such as melanosis coli as well as in normal patients.

DIFFERENTIAL DIAGNOSIS

It must be emphasized that joint symptoms often precede by months or years the onset of intestinal symptoms in patients with Whipple's disease.[28] Such patients may initially seek medical care in arthritis clinics. Clearly, the diagnosis of Whipple's disease must be considered in any patient with arthralgia or arthritis who develops diarrhea, malabsorption, or unexplained weight loss, especially if the arthritis cannot be precisely categorized. Tests for rheumatoid factor, including latex fixation and bentonite agglutination, are negative in patients with arthritis caused by Whipple's disease, and the serum uric acid level is usually normal.[28]

The fever of Whipple's disease may occasionally precede gastrointestinal symptoms by months. Thus, Whipple's disease must be included among the ever growing list of entities which may present with fever of unknown origin.

The lack of specificity of the gastrointestinal symptoms in Whipple's disease precludes definitive diagnosis without histological confirmation. However, the coexistence of malabsorption, arthritis, adenopathy, fever, and the rather characteristic radiological appearance of the small intestine should alert the clinician to the possible diagnosis. The diagnosis is then established by peroral intestinal biopsy which readily permits differentiation of Whipple's disease from other diffuse mucosal diseases such as celiac sprue.

TREATMENT AND PROGNOSIS

The administration of appropriate antibiotics in patients with Whipple's disease is lifesaving and results in prompt and dramatic clinical improvement. The fever and joint symptoms disappear within a few days, and the diarrhea and malabsorption disappear within two to four weeks or even sooner. A number of antibiotics, including penicillin and streptomycin in combination and broad-spectrum agents such as tetracycline, have been used with good results.[5, 12, 13, 33] However, the optimal regimen for antibiotic treatment has not yet been established. Clearly, relapses may occur following even prolonged administration of broad-spectrum bacteriostatic agents such as tetracycline, and re-

sistance to tetracycline has been documented.[13]

The author has treated five patients with penicillin alone, and all have responded dramatically with prompt relief of symptoms which correlated with the rapid disappearance of organisms from intestinal biopsies. The regimen used in these patients consisted of intramuscular administration of 600,000 units of procaine penicillin twice a day until improvement was unequivocal (usually five to ten days) followed by oral administration of penicillin G in a dose of 500 mg (800,000 units) twice daily. Penicillin therapy was discontinued when the number of macrophages in the lamina propria of the intestine had decreased significantly and villous architecture of the mucosa had returned toward normal (usually two to four months). Although empiric in terms of dosage and duration of drug administration, this regimen is effective, inexpensive, relatively safe, and well tolerated by the patient (Fig. 70–

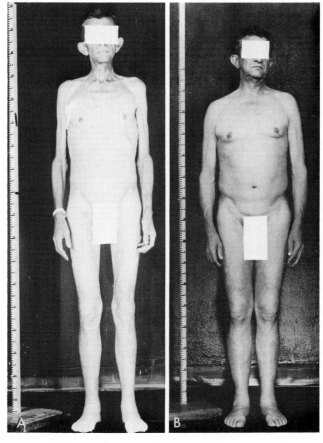

Figure 70–6. A patient with Whipple's disease, before (A) and after (B) three months of treatment with antibiotics. (Courtesy of Dr. M. H. Sleisenger.)

6). To date we have observed no relapses in patients so treated.

An appreciable number of responses to treatment with ACTH and corticosteroids were reported before the efficacy of antibiotic treatment was established. However, many patients treated with these agents failed to improve. Moreover, the widespread administration of antibiotics (often unreported) for unrelated infections in responsive patients makes it difficult to interpret the effect of corticosteroids on the basic process in Whipple's disease. There is no doubt now that antibiotics are the treatment of choice in all patients and that use of corticosteroids should be limited to the treatment of secondary adrenocortical insufficiency if it is present.

As in other diseases with severe intestinal malabsorption, appropriate replacement therapy designed to correct specific deficiencies is indicated in Whipple's disease. Since absorptive function improves rapidly after initiation of antibiotic treatment, such supplementation, discussed in detail on pages 864 to 884, usually need not be protracted. Fluid and electrolyte replacement should be administered when needed, anemic patients should receive iron or folate as indicated, vitamin D and calcium should be given at least until steatorrhea disappears, and parenteral calcium and/or magnesium are indicated in patients who develop tetany. Since most patients in whom the diagnosis is established are malnourished, the diet should be high in calories and protein and should be supplemented with a therapeutic formula vitamin preparation until absorptive function has returned to normal (Table 20–4).

The prognosis for patients with this previously fatal disease is now excellent, and most patients are completely asymptomatic within one to three months after the start of antibiotic treatment. After antibiotics are discontinued, patients must be carefully observed for symptoms of relapse, because it is not yet known whether treatment with penicillin, as outlined, effects cure of the disease in all patients. Indeed, in our experience, residual lymphatic dilatation and persistence of a few PAS-positive macrophages are seen consistently in jejunal biopsies obtained up to four years after penicillin treatment.

When relapse does occur, it is preceded by the reappearance of the typical bacilli in the mucosa of the small intestine. In fact, the bacilli have been noted to reappear several months before the recurrence of overt clinical symptoms of relapse and, when recognized, permit prediction of an impending relapse in an asymptomatic patient.[13]

REFERENCES

1. Whipple, G. H. A hitherto undescribed disease characterized anatomically by deposits of fat and fatty acids in the intestinal and mesenteric lymphatic tissues. Bull. Johns Hopkins Hosp. 18:382, 1907.
2. Hendrix, J. P., Black-Schaffer, B., Withers, R. W., and Handler, P. Whipple's intestinal lipodystrophy. Arch. Intern. Med. 85:91, 1950.
3. Upton, A. C. Histochemical investigation of the mesenchymal lesions in Whipple's disease. Amer. J. Clin. Path., 22:755, 1952.
4. Sieracki, J. C., and Fine, G. Whipple's disease—observations on systemic involvement. II. Gross and histologic observations. Arch. Path. 67:81, 1959.
5. Paulley, J. W. A case of Whipple's disease (intestinal lipodystrophy). Gastroenterology 22:128, 1952.
6. Gross, J. B., Wollaeger, E. E., Sauer, W. G., et al. Whipple's disease. Gastroenterology 36:65, 1959.
7. Puite, R. H., and Tesluk, H. Whipple's disease. Amer. J. Med. 19:383, 1955.
8. Cohen, A. S., Schimmel, E. M., Holt, P. R. and Isselbacher, K. J. Ultrastructural abnormalities in Whipple's disease. Proc. Soc. Exp. Biol. Med. 105:411, 1960.
9. Chears, W. C., and Ashworth, C. T. Electron microscopic study of the intestinal mucosa in Whipple's disease. Gastroenterology 41:129, 1961.
10. Yardley, J. H., and Hendrix, T. R. Combined electron and light microscopy in Whipple's disease. Bull. Johns Hopkins Hosp. 109:80, 1961.
11. Kurtz, S. M., Davis, T. D., Jr., and Ruffin, J. M. Light and electron microscopic studies of Whipple's disease. Lab. Invest. 11:653, 1962.
12. Davis, T. D., Jr., McBee, J. W., Borland, J. L., et al. The effect of antibiotics and steroid therapy in Whipple's disease. Gastroenterology 44:112, 1963.
13. Trier, J. S., Phelps, P. C., Eidelman, S., and Rubin, C. E. Whipple's disease: Light and electron microscope correlation of jejunal mucosal histology with antibiotic treatment and clinical status. Gastroenterology 48:684, 1965.
14. Kojecky, Z., Malinsky, J., Kodousek, R., and Marsalek, E. Frequence of occurrence of microbes in the intestinal mucosa and in the lymph nodes during long-term observations of a patient suffering from Whipple's disease. Gastroenterologica 101:163, 1964.

15. Gonzales-Licea, A., and Yardley, J. H. Whipple's disease in the rectum. Amer. J. Path. 52:1191, 1968.

16. de Groodt-Lasseel, M., and Martin, J. J. Electron microscope study of C.N.S. lesions in Whipple's disease. Path. Biol. 17:121, 1969.

17. Black-Schaffer, B. The tinctoral demonstration of a glycoprotein in Whipple's disease. Proc. Soc. Exp. Biol. Med. 72:225, 1949.

18. Dobbins, W. O., III, and Ruffin, J. M., A light- and electron-microscopic study of bacterial invasion in Whipple's disease. Amer. J. Path. 51:225, 1967.

19. Fleming, W. H., Yardley, J. H. and Hendrix, T. R. Diagnosis of Whipple's disease by rectal biopsy. New Eng. J. Med. 267:33, 1962.

20. Caroli, J., Julien, C., Eteve, J., et al. Trois cas de maladie de Whipple: Remarques cliniques, biologiques, histologiques et thérapeutiques, étude au microscope électronique de la muqueuse jejunale. Demonstration de l'origine bactérienne de l'affection. Isolement et identification du germe en cause. Sem. Hôp. Paris 39:1457, 1963.

21. Kok, N., Dybkaer, R., and Rostgaard, J. Bacteria in Whipple's disease. I. Results of cultivation from repeated jejunal biopsies prior to, during and after effective antibiotic treatment. Acta Path. Microbiol. Scand. 60:431, 1964.

22. Carache, P., Bayless, T. M., Shelley, W. M. and Hendrix, T. R. Atypical bacteria in Whipple's disease. Tr. Assn. Amer. Phys. 79:399, 1966.

23. Sherris, J. C., Roberts, C. E., and Porus, R. L. Microbiological studies of intestinal biopsies taken during active Whipple's disease. Gastroenterology 48:708, 1965.

24. Martin, F. F., Vilseck, J. R., Jr., Dobbins, W. O., and Tyor, M. P. Immunologic defect in treated Whipple's disease. Gastroenterology 60:694, 1971.

25. Hargrove, M. D., Jr., Verner, J. V., Jr., Patrick, R. L., and Ruffin, J. M. Intestinal lipodystrophy without diarrhea. J.A.M.A. 173:1125, 1960.

26. Aust, C. H., and Smith, E. B. Whipple's disease in a 3-month old infant. Amer. J. Clin Path. 37:66, 1962.

27. Laster, L., Waldmann, T. A., Fenster, L. F., and Singleton, J. W. Albumin metabolism in patients with Whipple's disease. J. Clin. Invest. 45:637, 1966.

28. Kelly, J. J., III, and Weisiger, B. W. The arthritis of Whipple's disease. Arth. Rheum. 6:615, 1963.

29. Sieracki, J. C., Fine, G., Hain, J. C., Jr., and Babin, J. Central nervous system involvement in Whipple's disease. J. Neuropath. Exp. Neurol. 19:70, 1960.

30. Badenoch, J., Richards, W. C. D., and Oppenheimer, D. R. Encephalopathy in a case of Whipple's disease. J. Neurol. Neurosurg. Psychiat. 26:203, 1963.

31. Smith, W. T., French, J. M., Gattsman, M., et al. Cerebral complications of Whipple's disease. Brain 88:137, 1965.

32. Rice, R. P., Roufail, W. M., and Reeves, R. J. The roentgen diagnosis of Whipple's disease (intestinal lipodystrophy). Radiology 88:295, 1965.

33. Maizel, H., Ruffin, J. M., and Dobbins, W. O., III. Whipple's disease: A review of 19 patients from one hospital and a review of the literature since 1950. Medicine (Balt.) 49:175, 1970.

Chapter 71

Lymphoma

Jerry S. Trier

DEFINITION

Lymphoid cells are dispersed throughout the lamina propria at all levels of the small intestine and are also present in follicular aggregates in the mucosa and submucosa which are especially prominent in the distal ileum (Peyer's patches). With its abundance of lymphoid tissue, it is not surprising that the small intestine is frequently involved in malignant disease of the lymphoid system.

Lymphoma may originate in the small intestine. Such *primary* intestinal lymphoma may be localized to a single short intestinal segment with or without involvement of its adjacent mesentery and lymph nodes, it may be multifocal and affect several intestinal segments, or it may involve diffusely the major portion of the small intestine.

On the other hand, involvement of the small intestine with lymphoma may be a *secondary* manifestation of a disseminated lymphomatous process which may affect many organs. In such patients, the tumor may be localized to one intestinal segment or it may be multifocal and invade many sites along the length of the gut.

The clinical manifestations of intestinal lymphoma vary and depend, to some degree, upon whether intestinal involvement is primary or secondary and localized or diffuse.

950

PATHOLOGY

The pathological findings in intestinal lymphoma vary both with the degree of intestinal involvement and with the histological variety of the tumor.

Primary lymphoma of the small intestine is localized most often to one segment of the small bowel, although multiple lesions are seen in 20 to 25 per cent of patients.[1] By definition, the liver, spleen, marrow, and mediastinum should be free of obvious tumor initially if the lymphoma is primary to the gut rather than an extension of disseminated disease. The ileum and jejunum are most frequently affected, whereas duodenal involvement is less common.[2-5] As in secondary lymphoma, primary intestinal lymphosarcoma and reticulum cell sarcoma are more common than primary intestinal Hodgkin's disease.[3]

In primary intestinal lymphoma, the neoplasm may arise in the lamina propria or in the lymph follicles; it may partially destroy the epithelium, causing ulceration. Large polypoid tumor masses may develop and, uncommonly, these may obstruct the intestinal lumen. Alternatively the entire circumference of the bowel wall may become infiltrated with involvement of all layers of the bowel wall, and an aneurysmal dilatation or, less commonly, a constricting, napkin ring-like lesion may

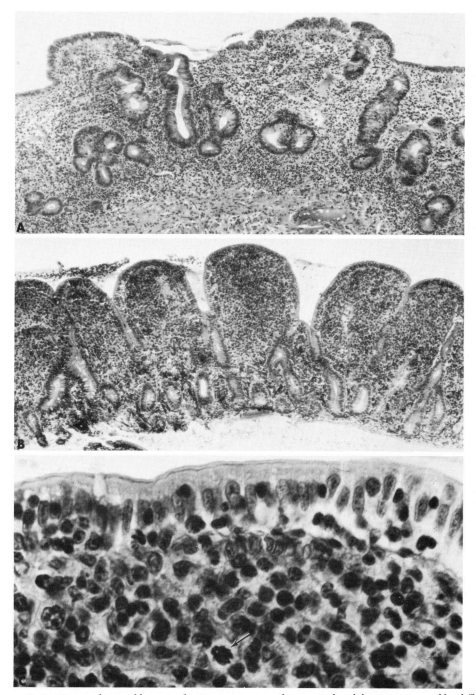

Figure 71–1. Proximal jejunal biopsies from two patients with intestinal malabsorption caused by diffuse involvement of the small intestine with lymphoma.

A, In this patient, the absorptive surface is flat and villi are absent. However, in contrast to celiac sprue, the crypts of Lieberkühn are reduced in number and their architecture is disorganized. Occasional cells in the lamina propria showed cytological evidence of lymphosarcoma at high magnification. × 100.

B, Jejunal biopsy from another patient with malabsorption caused by diffuse reticulum cell sarcoma of the small intestine. Although villi are present in this biopsy, they are markedly distorted by an expanded, tremendously cellular lamina propria. × 90.

C, Higher magnification of a portion of the biopsy shown in *B*. The pleomorphic appearance of the cells in the lamina propria is evident, and they are clearly malignant in their morphological features. The arrow indicates a mitotic figure. Unlike untreated celiac sprue, the villous epithelial cells are not markedly altered except that they are infiltrated by malignant cells. Their striated border is well preserved, and there is little vacuolization of their cytoplasm. × 624.

be formed. Involvement of the adjacent mesentery and its lymph nodes is common. In addition to ulceration, perforation and intussusception in the region of the tumor may complicate the course.[1, 2]

In a syndrome which has distinctive clinical features, including malabsorption, long segments of small intestine are diffusely invaded by the lymphomatous process.[6, 7] Mucosal involvement is extensive, and mesenteric nodes may be enlarged and contain tumor, but gross involvement of other intra-abdominal organs such as liver and spleen is not apparent, although microscopic foci of tumor may be seen in any organ at autopsy. The mucosa of the involved intestine is usually flat, the crypts are elongated, and normal villous architecture is lost (Fig. 71–1). Although the architectural appearance of the mucosa may superficially resemble that seen in celiac sprue, there are usually distinguishing features.[7] In diffuse lymphoma, unlike celiac sprue, the crypts of Lieberkühn are usually reduced in number. The lamina propria may be infiltrated by massive numbers of round cells, some of which appear malignant by cytological criteria (Fig. 71–1). The architecture of the lymphoid follicles is usually destroyed, and well defined germinal centers are absent. The presence of reticulum and blast cells lying free in the lamina propria is particularly helpful, because these cellular elements are normally confined to germinal centers of lymphoid follicles.[7] However, the malignant nature of the disease is not always revealed in peroral biopsies. In some patients with diffuse primary lymphoma, peroral biopsies may initially show only mild, nonspecific abnormalities, especially when an uninvolved segment of bowel is sampled. In others, biopsies reveal a mucosal lesion that is indistinguishable from that seen in patients with celiac sprue.[7]

Secondary involvement of the small intestine is common in patients with disseminated reticulum cell sarcoma and lymphosarcoma and is seen in about 25 per cent of these patients at autopsy.[5] Multifocal intestinal lesions are seen in over 50 per cent with intestinal involvement. On the other hand, secondary involvement in Hodgkin's disease is recognized in only about 5 per cent of patients at autopsy. Un-like primary intestinal lymphoma, the intestinal involvement in patients with disseminated lymphoma is often incidental, and specific intestinal symptoms are often absent during life. In many patients with secondary lymphoma of the small bowel, other intra-abdominal viscera, including stomach, colon, liver, and pancreas, are also invaded by the tumor.

ETIOLOGY

There is no doubt that lymphoma of the small intestine is a true neoplasm, and its cause, like that of other human neoplasms, remains unknown.

It is of great interest that a high incidence of lymphoma (both intestinal and extraintestinal) has been described in patients with celiac sprue[8] and that young adult Arabs and native Middle Eastern Jews have a high incidence of primary diffuse lymphoma of the small intestine.[7, 9] The possible frequent occurrence of this neoplasm in association with a specific disease entity and within a geographically and ethnically defined population may provide clues that may eventually help define its etiology and pathogenesis.

CLINICAL FEATURES

Primary Lymphoma with Focal Intestinal Involvement. Primary lymphoma of the small intestine may develop at any age. In general, the patient population afflicted is younger than that seen with other types of gastrointestinal malignancies. Indeed, about one-third of children with malignant lymphoma present initially with symptoms suggesting abdominal involvement.[10]

Most often, signs and symptoms of primary lymphoma of the small intestine can be attributed to a specific tumor mass. Abdominal pain is common. It is usually crampy in nature, it may be associated with nausea and vomiting, and it may reflect partial obstruction of the gut lumen by the tumor mass. Although complete obstruction may occur, it is less common than in patients with other forms of intestinal malignancy such as carcinoma. Periodic symptoms of obstruction may reflect intermittent intussusception induced by the tumor mass. The abrupt onset of continuous, severe abdominal pain may signal perforation of the friable, tumor-filled intestinal wall, which is a frequent complication. Massive intestinal hemorrhage from an ulcerated tumor mass may occasionally be the presenting symptom, but the insidious onset of anemia caused by occult intestinal bleeding is much more common. Nonspecific constitutional symptoms such as anorexia, malaise, and weight loss may precede localizing symptoms. Fever, when sustained and prominent, suggests either extensive lymphomatous involvement or the presence of a complication such as perforation or infection.

The most common physical findings are abdominal tenderness and a palpable abdominal mass. Hepatosplenomegaly and prominent peripheral lymphadenopathy suggest advanced disseminated disease. Often these organs are not palpable in primary lymphoma of the small bowel. Ascites, when present, suggests extensive mesenteric and/or retroperitoneal tumor invasion. Complications are reflected by expected physical findings such as abdominal distention and high-pitched bowel sounds in intestinal obstruction and ileus, with striking abdominal tenderness, rigidity, and rebound in patients with free intestinal perforation.

Routine hematological and chemical laboratory studies are by and large nonspecific and reflect complications. Severe anemia and guaiac-positive stools indicate intestinal bleeding; leukocytosis may reflect complicating infection; and electrolyte imbalance with hypokalemia and hypochloremia may be due to pernicious vomiting caused by intestinal obstruction.

Barium contrast study of the small intestine is helpful in raising the suspicion and defining the site and extent of primary intestinal lymphoma.[11] Contrast studies may show infiltration of the bowel wall with thickening or obliteration of mucosal folds (Fig. 71–2) or, less commonly, constriction of the involved segment of gut (Fig. 71–3). Large masses within the gut wall may necrose and cavitate, and their central core may slough into the bowel lumen. As a result, aneurysmal dilatation of the bowel may develop. On the other hand, the tumor may appear as a sizable polypoid mass projecting into the lumen. Such polypoid lesions may be associated with intussusception, especially in children. Large pressure defects which cause little or no disruption of the mucosal pattern may reflect extraintestinal tumor masses and suggest widespread involvement of the mesenteric and retroperitoneal lymph nodes with neoplasm. Lymphangiography

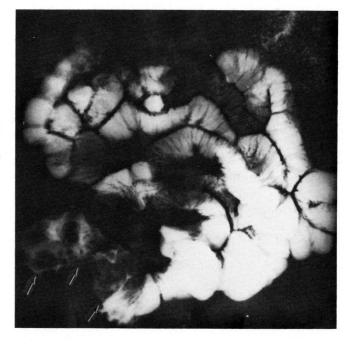

Figure 71–2. Barium contrast study of the small bowel from a patient with primary lymphosarcoma of the distal ileum and cecum. There are dilatation of the distal ileum and marked thickening and distortion of the mucosal folds in the involved area (arrows). (Courtesy of Dr. Ernest Ferris.)

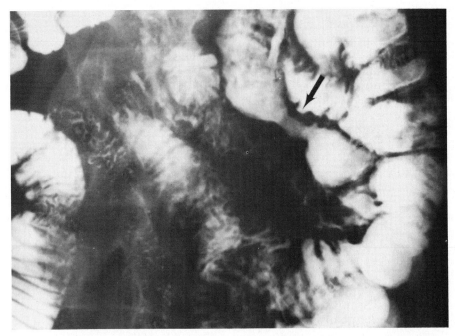

Figure 71–3. Barium contrast study of the small bowel from a patient with primary Hodgkin's disease of the proximal jejunum. There is constriction of the lumen of the involved segment of gut (arrow). (Courtesy of Dr. Ernest Ferris.)

may be helpful in determining the extent of involvement of intra-abdominal lymph nodes and retroperitoneal tissues.

Primary Lymphoma with Prominent Malabsorption. In this distinctive form of primary lymphoma, there is diffuse involvement of a large segment or of the entire small intestine.[6,7] Diffuse intestinal lymphoma has a relatively high incidence in those populations native to Middle Eastern countries. Adolescents and young adults (15 to 40 years old) are most often affected. Although this form of lymphoma occurs in the Western world, it is much less common and usually affects an older age group than in the Middle East.

Symptoms and signs of intestinal malabsorption are a prominent feature. The clinical picture may resemble celiac sprue so closely that the diagnosis of celiac sprue is considered at one time or another in many patients with primary diffuse intestinal lymphoma.[6,7] Weight loss, diarrhea, steatorrhea, malaise, and weakness are common findings. Edema, often related to loss of plasma protein into the gut, and anemia are often present. Indeed, most of the diverse signs and symptoms which characterize malabsorption caused by diffuse in-

testinal mucosal lesions have, at one time or another, been noted in patients with primary diffuse lymphoma of the small intestine (see pp. 250 to 289). On the other hand, significant and often severe abdominal pain and anorexia are usually prominent features of diffuse lymphoma, whereas they are not so common in other mucosal diseases of the small intestine, including celiac sprue, which cause malabsorption.[7]

The abdomen may be distended and tender, but a palpable abdominal mass, common in the focal form of the disease, is unusual in primary diffuse intestinal lymphoma. Clubbing of the fingernails has been noted frequently. Peripheral edema is common; ascites is less common but may be severe. Lymphadenopathy and hepatosplenomegaly are not features of primary diffuse intestinal lymphoma, whereas lymphadenopathy and hepatosplenomegaly are often seen in disseminated intestinal lymphoma.

Steatorrhea is usually a prominent feature by the time the disease is clinically apparent. Excess fat is apparent in Sudan stains of the stool, and quantitation of fecal fat excretion documents the presence of malabsorption. As would be expected, serum carotene and cholesterol levels are often depressed and the prothrombin time may be prolonged. Indeed, the laboratory findings, like the clinical symptoms, closely resemble those seen in other diseases of the small intestine with diffuse mucosal lesions and are no different from those described in detail on page 875. Thus, anemia, hypoproteinemia, hypocalcemia, hypokalemia,[12] and flat oral xylose and glucose tolerance tests are common (see also pp. 250 to 289) Recently, the presence of an abnormal serum IgA devoid of light chains has been found in some patients with diffuse intestinal lymphoma.[9]

X-ray examination of the small intestine following a barium meal is helpful in evaluating patients with diffuse primary lymphoma of the small intestine. In some patients, obliteration of mucosal folds, dilatation of the lumen, and flocculation and segmentation of barium may resemble closely the radiological picture of celiac sprue. In others, extremely coarse mucosal folds are seen and the bowel wall may be strikingly thickened (Fig. 71–4). This latter pattern may resemble that seen in Whipple's disease or amyloidosis. In Whipple's disease, however, the lesion is usually more severe in the proximal small intestine, whereas in lymphoma the distal bowel may be the most severely affected (Fig. 71–4).

Peroral biopsy of the small intestine may provide a definitive diagnosis if the intestinal segment biopsied is involved by the neoplasm. Eidelman et al.[7] emphasized that the yield of diagnostic biopsies is increased when specimens are obtained from several levels of the small intestine, thus increasing the chances of sampling involved mucosa. It must be emphasized that peroral biopsies from the proximal small intestine with mild, nonspecific changes or with histological features of celiac sprue do not preclude the diagnosis of intestinal lymphoma, because such biopsies have been obtained from patients who later were shown to have lymphoma.[7] Thus, although a biopsy which documents intestinal lymphoma is diagnostic, a biopsy which fails to show the lesion is inconclusive.

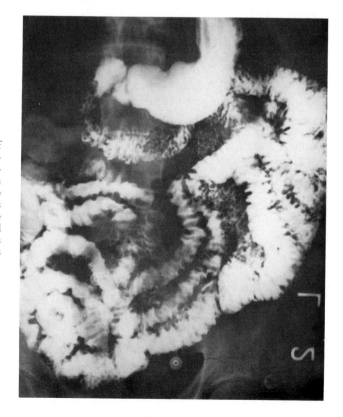

Figure 71–4. Barium contrast study of the small intestine from a patient with diffuse primary lymphoma of the small intestine. The small intestinal mucosal pattern is markedly abnormal. The mucosal folds are extremely coarse and the bowel wall is thickened. The lesion is more severe in the distal bowel than in the duodenum and proximal jejunum. This same patient's peroral biopsy of the proximal jejunum is shown in Figure 71–1, B and C.

TABLE 71–1. CLINICAL FEATURES OF LYMPHOMA OF THE SMALL INTESTINE

CLINICAL FEATURE	LOCALIZED PRIMARY LYMPHOMA	DIFFUSE PRIMARY LYMPHOMA	SECONDARY LYMPHOMA
Abdominal pain	Frequent	Frequent	Frequent
Intestinal obstruction	Frequent	Unusual	Occasional
Intestinal bleeding	Frequent	Occasional	Frequent
Intestinal malabsorption	Unusual	Frequent	Unusual
Perforation	Occasional	Occasional	Occasional
Fever	Occasional	Frequent	Frequent
Abdominal mass	Frequent	Unusual	Occasional
Hepatosplenomegaly	Occasional	Unusual	Frequent
Peripheral lymphadenopathy	Unusual	Unusual	Frequent
Positive peroral biopsy	Unusual	Frequent	Unusual

Secondary Lymphoma of the Small Intestine. Tumor invasion of the small intestine in patients with disseminated lymphoma may cause intestinal obstruction, fistulization, perforation, and/or bleeding. Indeed, the clinician is usually not aware of intestinal involvement until the patient develops signs and symptoms associated with these complications.

It must be stressed that the intestinal symptoms in patients with generalized lymphoma do not always reflect lymphomatous involvement in the gut. For example, in one series of 46 patients with widespread lymphoma and gastrointestinal bleeding, the source of the bleeding was due to gastrointestinal lesions other than neoplasm in 28 patients and was due to lymphoma in only 18 patients.[5]

Usually by the time secondary involvement of the small intestine becomes clinically apparent in patients with a disseminated lymphomatous process, the nature of the underlying disease has been established on the basis of the extraintestinal manifestations.

The clinical features of lymphoma are summarized in Table 71–1.

DIFFERENTIAL DIAGNOSIS

Primary intestinal lymphomas must be distinguished from other neoplasms, benign or malignant, which form mass lesions in a discrete segment of the small intestine. Primary intestinal carcinoma, sarcoma, fibroma, leiomyoma, and carcinoid tumors may infiltrate the bowel wall and, like lymphomas, may ulcerate and bleed. These same neoplasms may also present as intraluminal tumors, as do lipomas and adenomas, and all may intussuscept and produce symptoms of intestinal obstruction (see p. 965). Although the appearance of a mass lesion in barium contrast studies may suggest a specific type of intestinal neoplasm, definitive diagnosis requires laparotomy and histological examination of the tumor.

In many cases, it is not difficult to distinguish between lymphoma and non-neoplastic infiltrative lesions of the small bowel such as regional enteritis and tuberculous or fungal enteritis. The extraintestinal manifestations of nonmalignant diseases may help differentiate them from lymphoma (see p. 897). By and large, involvement of both small and large bowel is more common, and the total length of intestine affected is usually longer in regional enteritis than in lymphoma. In regional enteritis, stenotic lesions of the bowel are common, whereas stenosis is unusual in lymphoma; rather, the bowel is usually of normal caliber or somewhat dilated. However, occasionally the radiological appearance of non-neoplastic infiltrative lesions may resemble lymphoma so closely that surgical exploration is needed to solve the diagnostic dilemma.

The clinical and radiological picture of patients with malabsorption caused by infiltration of a long segment of the gut with lymphoma may closely mimic other intestinal mucosal diseases with malabsorption such as celiac sprue, Whipple's disease, and amyloidosis. In fact, some patients with well documented celiac sprue develop diffuse intestinal lymphoma years after the onset of their celiac sprue. However, the frequency of this relationship is not fully defined, because diffuse intestinal lymphoma in its early stages may mimic celiac sprue so closely that it is not always possible to establish whether a given patient has had lymphoma all along or whether he initially had celiac sprue and then developed lymphoma.

In patients with diffuse intestinal lymphoma with malabsorption, fever is common and treatment with a gluten-free diet fails to produce significant improvement. In marked contrast, in celiac sprue patients fever is uncommon, and withdrawal of dietary gluten, if complete, produces rapid and striking clinical improvement. Severe abdominal pain, if present, suggests lymphoma. Peroral intestinal biopsies will often, but not always, distinguish between diffuse intestinal lymphoma and celiac sprue.[7] Lymphoma can be distinguished from Whipple's disease by peroral biopsy; PAS-positive macrophages are not seen in lymphoma and are always present in Whipple's disease. Biopsy may also be helpful in distinguishing between intestinal amyloidosis and lymphoma.

The development of intestinal symptoms in patients with previously diagnosed disseminated lymphoma merits thorough diagnostic evaluation, including appropriate radiological studies, so that the nature of the lesion can be defined precisely. Although secondary intestinal involvement is common in patients with disseminated lymphoma, the incidence of such neoplastic lesions which give rise to intestinal symptoms is not high.[5]

TREATMENT AND PROGNOSIS

The therapeutic approach and the prognosis in patients with intestinal lymphoma depend upon the extent of the intestinal involvement and the presence or absence of extraintestinal neoplastic invasion.

Lymphoma confined to a single small segment of small intestine without node involvement has, by far, the best prognosis. Surgical resection is the treatment of choice for this type of lesion. Available data indicate that the expected five-year cure rate under these circumstances is on the order of 50 to 75 per cent. If adjacent tissues such as the mesentery, its lymph nodes, and adjacent organs such as the pancreas are involved, attempts at surgical resection should be followed by postoperative radiotherapy. Placing radiopaque clips at the sites of possible residual tumor at the time of surgery facilitates accurate localization of radiotherapy. With extension of the disease to extraintestinal sites, the prognosis drops precipitously and the expected five-year survival is on the order of 10 to 30 per cent. Some radiotherapists advocate postoperative radiation in all patients, including those in whom the lymphoma was thought confined to a single intestinal focus, because early involvement of adjacent tissue may be difficult to detect. Intestinal obstruction, perforation, or hemorrhage caused by primary lymphoma confined to a single site is treated surgically, and an attempt is usually made to resect the entire tumor.

Treatment of patients with malabsorption caused by primary diffuse lymphoma which involves a long segment of small intestine has been particularly disappointing. Definitive surgery is out of the question because of the length of the involved intestinal segment. Radiotherapy, employing strip or spray techniques, has been advocated, but its effectiveness in prolonging survival has not been proved. Chemotherapy with a variety of agents, including corticosteroids, vinca alkaloids, and alkylating agents such as nitrogen mustard and cyclophosphamide, either alone or in combination, has been used, but convincing data documenting effective palliation are not available. Indeed, it has been suggested that treatment with radiation or with cytotoxic drugs may predispose to intestinal perforation by causing necrosis of the neoplasm which is infiltrating the bowel wall. The incidence of sepsis and fungal infection also seems particularly high in patients treated aggressively with radiation or cytotoxic agents. The coexistence of malabsorption with severe anorexia in these patients complicates efforts to maintain adequate nutrition. Medium-chain triglyceride supplements and generous use of vitamin and mineral supplements may be helpful.

The prognosis in diffuse primary intestinal lymphoma is dismal. Cures have not been reported. In one series of nine patients, three died within a year after onset of symptoms and none survived four years.[7]

In disseminated lymphoma with secondary intestinal involvement, treatment is palliative. If a specific symptomatic lesion is confined to a localized segment of gut, radiation therapy may be used; more often, chemotherapy is employed. The five-year survival is less than 10 per cent. Palliative surgery may be needed to manage complications such as intestinal obstruction, perforation, or intractable bleeding.

REFERENCES

1. Sherlock, P., Winawer, S. J., Goldstein, M. J., and Bragg, D. G. Malignant lymphoma of the gastrointestinal tract. In Progress in Gastroenterology, G. B. J. Glass (ed.). Vol. II, pp. 369–391. New York, Grune and Stratton, 1970.
2. Rosenberg, S. A., Diamond, H. D., Joslowitz, B., and Craver, L. F. Lymphosarcoma: A review of 1269 cases. Medicine 40:31, 1961.
3. Naqvi, M. S., Burrows, L., and Kark, A. E. Lymphoma of the gastrointestinal tract: Prognostic guides based on 162 cases. Ann. Surg. 170:221, 1969.
4. Loehr, W. J., Mujahed, Z., Zahn, F. D., Gray, G. F., and Thorbjarnarson, B. Primary lymphoma of the gastrointestinal tract: A review of 100 cases. Ann. Surg. 170:232, 1970.
5. Ehrlich, A. N., Stadler, G., Geller, W., and Sherlock, P. Gastrointestinal manifestations of malignant lymphoma. Gastroenterology 54:1115, 1968.
6. Sleisenger, M. H., Almy, T. P., and Barr, D. P. The sprue syndrome secondary to lymphoma of the small bowel. Amer. J. Med. 15:666, 1953.
7. Eidelman, S., Parkins, R. A., and Rubin, C. E. Abdominal lymphoma presenting as malabsorption: A clinico-pathologic study of nine cases in Israel and a review of the literature. Medicine 45:111, 1966.
8. Harris, O. D., Cooke, W. T., Thompson, H., and Waterhouse, J. A. H. Malignancy in adult coeliac disease and idiopathic steatorrhea. Amer. J. Med. 42:899, 1967.
9. Seligman, M., and Rambaud, J. C., IgA abnormalities in abdominal lymphoma (α-chain disease). Israel J. Med. Sci. 5:151, 1969.
10. Jenkin, R. D. T., Sanby, M. J., Stephens, C. A., Darte, J. M. M., and Peters, M. V. Primary gastrointestinal tract lymphoma in childhood. Radiology 92:763, 1969.
11. Marshak, R. H., and Linder, A. E. Lymphosarcoma, Hodgkin's disease and melanosarcoma. In Radiology of the Small Intestine. Philadelphia, pp. 355-389. W. B. Saunders Co., 1970,
12. Seijffers, M. J., Levy, M., and Hermann, G. Intractable watery diarrhea, hypokalemia and malabsorption in a patient with Mediterranean type of abdominal lymphoma. Gastroenterology 55:118, 1968.

Chapter 72

Primary Tumors and Vascular Malformations

Thomas F. O'Brien, Jr.

GENERAL CONSIDERATIONS

Considering its length, total cellular volume, and diversity of structural elements, the small intestine is relatively resistant to the development of neoplasms. Yet benign and malignant growths develop in all histological components, including epithelial cells, muscular bundles, nerves, blood vessels, lymphatics, and lymphoid tissue. Both heterotopic and hamartomatous tissue may give rise to small bowel tumors (see Table 72–1).

Neoplasms of the small bowel comprise 1 to 5 per cent of all gastrointestinal tumors.[1-3] The higher figure is usually obtained from reports which include autopsy material; many small bowel neoplasms are asymptomatic and undiscovered during life. Since most of these quiescent tumors are benign, 60 to 75 per cent of all symptomatic tumors prove to be malignant. The majority of small bowel tumors are discovered during the fifth, sixth, and seventh decades of life. Usually the period from onset of symptoms to diagnosis is longer than that in neoplasms at other levels of the gastrointestinal tract, averaging six to 12 months. Delay in diagnosis is due to the rarity of such lesions (which leads to a low index of suspicion), the vague nature of early symptoms (in the absence of gross

TABLE 72–1. PRIMARY TUMORS OF THE SMALL INTESTINE

TUMOR	REFERENCES
Benign	
Adenoma	
1. Polypoid/Papillary	2, 13
2. Brunner's gland	35, 36
3. "Islet cell"	
Leiomyoma	22
Lipoma	7
Angioma	8
1. Hemangioma	
2. Telangiectasia	
3. Lymphangioma	
Fibroma	
Teratoma	13
Osteoma, osteochondroma,	
osteofibroma	13
Malignant	
Adenocarcinoma	1, 2, 3
Lymphoma	
1. Reticulum cell sarcoma	
2. Lymphosarcoma	
3. Hodgkin's disease and sarcoma	
4. Follicular lymphoma	
Leiomyosarcoma	22
Neurofibrosarcoma	30
Angiosarcoma	
1. Malignant hemangiopericytoma	8
2. Kaposi's sarcoma	37
Rhabdomyosarcoma	31
Melanosarcoma	32
Plasmocytoma	33
Intermediate	
Carcinoid	34

959

hemorrhage), the paucity of physical findings, and the inaccessibility of many of the lesions to routine diagnostic techniques. Asymptomatic intervals, often lasting weeks, are frequently described by patients with tumors in the distal half of the small bowel.

BENIGN SMALL BOWEL TUMORS

Adenomas, leiomyomas, and lipomas are the three most frequently discovered primary tumors of the small intestine. Fibromas and angiomas occur much less often, and the other benign tumors listed in Table 72–1 are rare. Benign tumors often remain asymptomatic and are found incidentally at surgery or postmortem examination. When symptomatic, the clinical picture is determined primarily by its gross structural characteristics and its distance from the pylorus, and only secondarily by its histological type. For instance, benign tumors arising in the relatively fixed duodenum often produce nausea, vomiting, and early postprandial distress. Polypoid tumors arising beyond the ligament of Treitz are more likely to produce intussusception and symptoms of intermittent bowel obstruction. As a general rule, benign tumors are least common in the duodenum, and increase in frequency toward the ileum.

ETIOLOGY

The etiology of isolated, benign small bowel tumors is unknown. No dietary, chemical, or other toxic processes have been implicated in their pathogenesis. There is no substantial evidence for malignant degeneration in these tumors. In a recent autopsy series of interest, 69 per cent of patients with benign small bowel tumors were reported to have had associated benign and malignant tumors not involving the small intestine. Twenty-three per cent of these patients had a malignant, nonintestinal neoplasm.

PATHOLOGY

ADENOMA

Three types of adenomas are found in the small intestine: islet cell adenomas, Brunner's gland adenomas, and papillary-polypoid adenomas. Only the last named result from a true neoplastic process. The so-called Brunner's gland adenomas, which most probably represent localized hyperplasia, and islet cell adenomas, which represent a heterotopic development, will not be discussed further.

Adenomas represent about 25 per cent of all benign small bowel tumors. Usually asymptomatic, they are generally discovered incidentally during surgery or at autopsy. They occur most frequently toward the ileum. Their gross and microscopic appearance is similar to that of adenomas occurring in the large intestine (see p. 1433). Although most small bowel adenomas are single, well circumscribed polyps, the rarer papillary villous adenoma has been reported.[5] Most symptomatic lesions are found in patients between 30 and 60 years of age. The symptomatic adenoma, although uncommon, often calls attention to itself by bleeding or intermittent obstruction, the latter usually because of intussusception.

LEIOMYOMA

Clinically the leiomyoma is probably the most important primary benign small bowel tumor. Although it occurs less frequently than adenomas in general, it is the most common of the symptomatic nonmalignant tumors. Leiomyomas are found at all levels of the small intestine, but occur most often in the jejunum. Grossly they may appear as submucosal or subserosal growths with either a major intraluminal or extraluminal component; dumbbell-shaped lesions with both components also occur. Central necrosis and ulceration of the overlying mucosal surface give rise to bleeding in the majority of symptomatic patients (see Fig. 72–4, C and D). Gross luminal obstruction and intussusception are uncommon; however, lesions with a large exophytic component may produce a volvulus. There is no sex predilection for the leiomyoma, and most are discovered in the later decades of life. The radiographic finding of a smooth, ovoid, intraluminal filling defect with intact overlying mucosa is highly suggestive of a leiomyoma (Fig. 72–1).

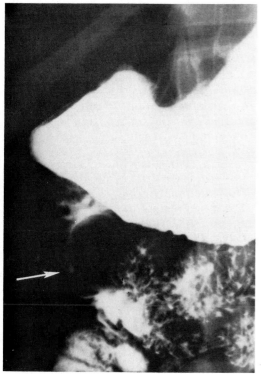

Figure 72–1. Leiomyoma of the duodenum. Note the ovoid, smooth-walled, filling defect in the descending duodenum. The arrow points to a central collection of barium within a shallow ulcer.

LIPOMA

Lipomas rank third in frequency of the benign tumors under consideration. Less than one-third of those discovered at surgery or autopsy are symptomatic.[6] Although they may occur in the duodenum, jejunum, or ileum, they are most often found in the distal ileum and ileocecal valve area (Fig. 72–2). Lipomas are rarely large, and remain submucosal and intramural in location. The principal clinical manifestations are bleeding secondary to necrosis and superficial ulceration of overlying epithelial layers. It is not uncommon for lipomas of the ileocecal valve to be discovered by barium enema during a radiographic search for occult gastrointestinal blood loss.

CLINICAL PICTURE

Benign small tumors occur approximately equally often among men and women. Symptomatic tumors are discovered most commonly in persons between 50 and 80 years old, although they have been found in persons ranging in age from nine to 90. Symptomatic tumors present obstructive features foremost, giving rise to intermittent colicky abdominal pain or, less commonly, sudden complete bowel

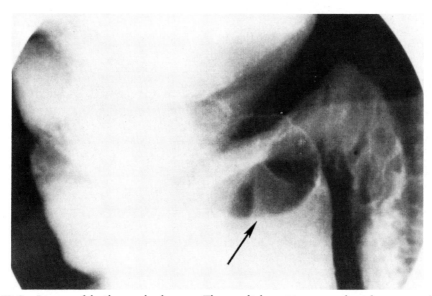

Figure 72–2. Lipoma of the ileocecal valve area. These radiolucent tumors are best demonstrated by barium enema.

obstruction. Constitutional symptoms of malignancy such as anorexia, malaise, and weight loss are distinctly uncommon. Gross or occult blood loss occurs in most patients; the degree of blood loss depends to a large extent on the histological type. A benign tumor is rarely palpable on physical examination.

DIAGNOSIS

A variety of roentgenologic techniques may be applied in the diagnosis of benign small bowel tumors, and the choice of technique should depend upon the suspected level of the lesion and probable histological type. Unfortunately, routine barium small bowel series often fail to demonstrate benign small bowel tumors, but occasionally demonstrate a localized intussusception (Fig. 72–3). The latter finding is usually indicative of a benign lesion. For tumors close to the ligament of Treitz, hypotonic duodenography often differentiates between infiltrative and inflammatory lesions of the duodenum.

Visceral angiography, via selective catheterization of the celiac and mesenteric arteries, is often useful in identifying vascular lesions such as angiomas or leiomyomas (Fig. 72–4). This technique will also establish the general locus of a lesion during an active hemorrhage. Benign tumors are invariably fed by a branch of the gastroduodenal or superior mesenteric artery. When a so-called parasitic blood supply from renal or lumbar arteries is present, a malignant lesion is most probable.[7]

A retrograde small bowel series, when the ileocecal valve is incompetent, may be useful in demonstrating some ileal tumors.

The development of more sophisticated fiberoptic instruments of greater length and biopsy capability will surely improve the preoperative diagnosis of more proximal lesions.

Exploratory laparotomy remains an important diagnostic as well as therapeutic maneuver.

TREATMENT

Surgical excision is the treatment of choice for virtually all symptomatic primary, benign small bowel tumors.

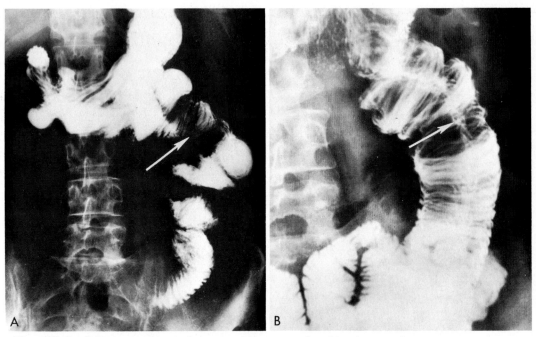

Figure 72–3. A, Intussusception in the proximal jejunum produced by a benign adenoma. B, Intussusception, close-up view. Note the typical coiled-spring appearance produced by the intussusceptum (arrow) within the intussuscipiens.

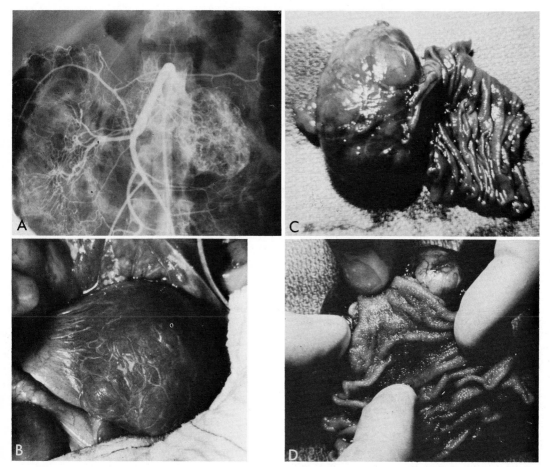

Figure 72–4. Asymptomatic leiomyoma of the small intestine which bled massively on three occasions in one year. *A*, Mesenteric arteriogram, demonstrating a large vascular mass on the left. *B*, Specimen at operation. *C*, Gross specimen, showing large extraluminal component. *D*, Ulceration of small intraluminal component.

HEMANGIOMAS AND RELATED VASCULAR MALFORMATIONS IN THE GUT

Several varieties of benign vascular lesions occur in the small bowel. They may be subclassified as either hemangiomas or telangiectasias. Hemangiomas are true tumors and represent the outgrowth of ectopic endothelium-lined blood-containing spaces, whereas telangiectasia is generally considered to be the dilatation of existing vascular structures.[8]

HEMANGIOMA

Hemangiomas of the small intestine occur with much less frequency than previously discussed tumors. They are thought to arise from the submucosal vascular plexus. They become clinically important because of their propensity for bleeding. In fact, 70 per cent of patients with small intestinal hemangiomas eventually have manifest gastrointestinal bleeding. Characteristically, there is no pain.

Although they are often small and relatively sessile lesions, they can, on occasion, become polypoid and produce obstructive symptoms. A rare variety of diffuse cavernous hemangiomatosis has been described.[9] The latter type may encircle the circumference of the small intestine and cause obstructive symptoms. Retroperitoneal hemorrhage can occur with diffuse hemangiomatosis. The presence of multiple small calcifications, resembling pelvic phleboliths, scattered throughout the abdomen is an important radiographic clue to diagnosis.

The majority of simple hemangiomas are found in the jejunum; they are less common in the ileum and uncommon in the duodenum.

Microscopically, the lesions may be capillary, cavernous, or mixed capillary-cavernous. Visceral angiography is probably the single most useful diagnostic procedure.

TELANGIECTASIA

Telangiectasias of the small bowel may be of either the hereditary or the non-hereditary type. Most clinical interest has centered around the hereditary variety known as Rendu-Osler-Weber disease. The classic features of this entity include repeated hemorrhages from the naso-pharynx and gastrointestinal tract; multiple telangiectatic lesions involving the nasopharyngeal, buccal, and gastrointestinal mucosae; and a familial history of the disorder. Telangiectatic lesions may also be seen on the skin, characteristically the palmar surfaces of the hands and within the nail beds.

Intestinal telangiectasia has been associated with Turner's syndrome, being noted in four of 55 patients in one series.[10]

Benign vascular malformations have also been the cause of repeated gastrointestinal hemorrhage with pseudoxanthoma elasticum.[11]

MISCELLANEOUS BENIGN SMALL BOWEL TUMORS

Other lesions listed in Table 72–1 are of sufficient rarity to preclude discussion here. For details of the clinical and pathological features, the reader is referred to the monographs of Wood[12] and River et al.[13]

MALIGNANT SMALL BOWEL TUMORS

Adenocarcinomas, lymphomas, and leiomyosarcomas are the three most commonly found primary malignant lesions of the small bowel, occurring in the listed order of frequency. Primary small bowel tumors (excluding carcinoids, which are discussed separately) represent 1 to 2 per cent of all malignant gastrointestinal neoplasms. Like their benign counterparts, the symptomatic tumors are usually discovered in persons beyond 50 years of age. The mean age of patients with primary small bowel lymphoma, however, averages about ten years younger than patients with adenocarcinoma or leiomyosarcoma. Other primary malignancies listed in Table 72–1 are rare. The observation of Jefferson in 1916, that "inch for inch the duodenum is more liable to cancer than the rest of the small intestine,"[14] remains valid today. Although a given type of primary malignancy may be found anywhere within the small bowel, carcinomas tend to cluster about the ligament of Treitz and sarcomas occur most frequently in the ileum.

GENERAL CONSIDERATIONS

ETIOLOGY

The etiology of small bowel malignancy remains unknown. With respect to carcinomas, there appear to be no geographic or population clusters, suggesting the absence of genetic or environmental factors in pathogenesis. Recent reports, however, make it increasingly clear that underlying chronic small bowel diseases such as celiac sprue,[15] perhaps dermatitis herpetiformis,[16] and chronic regional enteritis[17] are associated with a disproportionate number of primary bowel malignancies. It is also probable that primary small bowel lymphoma occurs with unusual frequency in the Middle East, particularly in Israel[18] and southern Iran.[19]

A single case report of two brothers differing in age by six years who both developed adenocarcinoma of the jejunum[20] is of interest, but similar cases have not been reported by others.

Carcinoma associated with chronic regional enteritis deserves special comment. An increased incidence of carcinoma as a complication of chronic inflammatory lower bowel disease (ulcerative colitis) is well recognized and accepted (see pp. 1330 to 1332). Until recent years it was generally believed that patients with Crohn's disease did not incur a similar risk. Nevertheless, over 20 cases have been compiled by several authors within the past ten years, suggesting a definite relationship between the diseases. Cancers arising in patients with chronic regional enteritis tend to develop in the ileal segments involved with the chronic inflammatory process. This is in contrast to the typical proximal location of carcinoma arising de novo. Furthermore, the mean age of patients with coexisting carcinoma and regional enteritis is a decade or more younger than that of patients with other primary carcinomas.

CLINICAL PICTURE

The sex distribution of small bowel malignancies is variably reported, occurring with equal frequency in some series and favoring males in a ratio of 2 to 1 in others. In contrast to benign tumors, malignant lesions usually become symptomatic and are discovered during life. Abdominal pain, malaise, anorexia, weight loss, and bleeding are common presenting symptoms. Sudden, complete small bowel obstruction may be the first manifestation of a small bowel malignancy. An abdominal mass or diarrhea occurs in only 25 to 30 per cent of patients; however, when a palpable abdominal mass is present, the lesion is most likely malignant. Perforation is almost invariably associated with sarcoma.

DIAGNOSIS

Since most small intestinal carcinomas arise within the 25 cm of the ligament of Treitz (in either direction) and lymphomas and sarcomas usually attain considerable size, barium contrast small bowel series identifies a considerable portion of these malignancies. When a tumor arises in more distal regions of the small intestine and considerable obstruction is present, a localized barium contrast study obtained through a decompressing Cantor tube will often demonstrate the nature of the obstructing lesion.

Certain radiographic features are helpful in predicting the histology of the lesion. Short, annular lesions are typically found with an adenocarcinoma (Fig. 72–5). Longer, ulcerating lesions producing so-called aneurysmal dilatation of the lumen favor a lymphomatous etiology (Fig. 72–6). Diffuse involvement of long segments, superficially resembling a malabsorption pattern, is uncommon but

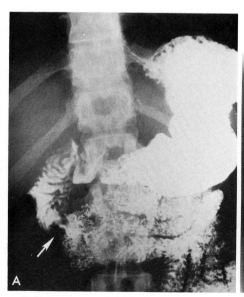
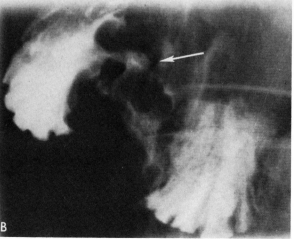

Figure 72–5. *A,* Adenocarcinoma of the duodenum. *B,* Adenocarcinoma of the duodenum, close-up view. The characteristic features of a small bowel adenocarcinoma are demonstrated here. Note the "shelving" edges at the proximal portion of the tumor. The central lumen shows destruction of the normal mucosal pattern with ulceration (arrow).

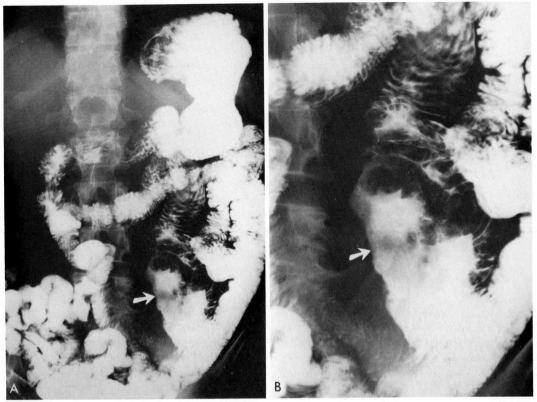

Figure 72–6. *A*, Lymphosarcoma of the small intestine. *B*, Lymphosarcoma of the small intestine, close-up view. The abnormally wide loop of intestine with tumor infiltrating the wall has been referred to as "aneursymal dilatation."

suggestive of lymphoma. Leiomyosarcomas are generally bulky tumors with displacement of adjacent, uninvolved, barium-filled bowel loops (Fig. 72–7). Intussusception is not usually seen with malignant tumors. On rare occasions lymphoma may closely resemble Crohn's disease of the terminal ileum radiographically.

The application of visceral angiography has been steadily increasing with rewarding results. As noted, the demonstration of a "parasitic" blood supply is highly suggestive of a malignant tumor.

Peroral small bowel biopsy devices may occasionally be successful in recovering diagnostic material from more proximal lesions.

Fiberoptic endoscopy has not been widely applied to the diagnosis of small bowel tumors, although the more proximal lesions are certainly within the reach of such instrumentation.

To date, tumor-specific antigens have not been identified in the sera of patients with primary small bowel malignancy.

TREATMENT

The majority of patients with primary small bowel malignancy will require surgery for definitive diagnosis, alleviation of pain, relief of obstruction, or stoppage of excessive blood loss. A wide excision with primary end-to-end anastomosis is usually attempted in lesions beyond the ligament of Treitz. Lesions proximal to the ligament of Treitz usually require a Whipple resection because of the absence of a mesentery in the duodenum. Roughly two-thirds of patients may be expected to have metastases to regional lymph nodes or beyond at the time of diagnosis.

Radiation therapy may prove helpful in the treatment of some lymphomas of the small bowel; the adenocarcinomas and

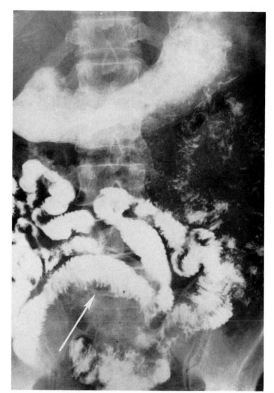

Figure 72-7. Leiomyosarcoma of the small intestine. Displacement of an uninvolved loop of ileum by a large leiomyosarcoma of the ileum.

leiomyosarcomas are characteristically resistant to such therapy, however.

Chemotherapy, like radiotherapy, has shown most effectiveness in the treatment of lymphoma. 5-Fluorouracil and its derivatives have not proved as effective in adenocarcinoma of the small intestine as they have in similar lesions arising in the large intestine.

SPECIFIC CHARACTERISTICS

ADENOCARCINOMA

Excluding carcinoids and malignancies of the ampulla of Vater, adenocarcinoma occurs with the greatest frequency among primary small bowel malignancies. Over 90 per cent are located in the duodenum or jejunum and usually within 20 cm either side of the ligament of Treitz. According to most reports, carcinoma develops more frequently in men than women, with at least a 2 to 1 preponderance. The majority

are found in patients in their sixth and seventh decades. Symptoms of intermittent obstruction are most common. Weight loss and anemia secondary to blood loss occur in most patients. Less than one-third have a palpable mass on physical examination. In younger patients, symptoms and early radiographic findings may suggest atypical peptic ulceration of the postbulbar duodenum. In this instance, cineradiography and hypotonic duodenography are quite useful in distinguishing spasm and edema from malignant invasion of the duodenal wall.

Grossly, most nonampullary duodenal carcinomas are annular in configuration (see Fig. 72–5). Microscopically, a moderate degree of differentiation is apparent in most tumors, and glandular structures may be recognized. Variable degrees of mucus may be produced. More than half the patients will have metastases to at least regional lymph nodes at the time of diagnosis. Although the prognosis for life is generally poor, some recent series have reported five-year survival rates as high as 20 per cent.[3] The prognosis for carcinomas arising in the mesenteric small bowel is slightly better than for those associated with duodenal lesions.

LYMPHOSARCOMA

Lymphomas occur next in frequency among primary small bowel malignancies, usually in the distal jejunum and ileum; the duodenum rarely gives rise to primary lymphoma. Most physicians report a definite male sex preponderance, ranging from 2 to 1 to 5 to 1. The mean age of discovery of primary lymphoma tends to be about ten years younger than that for adenocarcinoma. As these tumors arise primarily in the mesenteric small bowel, intermittent, colicky, periumbilical abdominal pain is the predominant symptom. Characteristically, lymphadenopathy, hepatosplenomegaly, and fever are absent, in contrast to lymphoma arising in other areas. Clubbing of the fingers has been mentioned as an important diagnostic clue.[19] All varieties of lymphoma, including reticulum cell sarcoma, lymphosarcoma, Hodgkin's disease. Hodgkin's sarcoma, and follicular lymphoma, can be found primarily in the small intestine. Reticulum cell sarcoma is by far the most common.

Treatment of primary abdominal lymphoma usually includes abdominal radiation therapy and alkylating agents such as cyclophosphamide (Cytoxan) and nitrogen mustard. Corticosteroids may be used for control of fever, if present, and for subjective improvement. The overall prognosis does not appear to be related to histological type, and has appeared favorable recently. Five-year survival rates of 60 per cent are commonly reported.

Lymphoma in the Middle East. A number of reports citing an unusually high incidence of primary lymphoma in Israel and southern Iran have appeared.[18, 19] These reports suggest that geographic or ethnic factors may be etiologically important. Certain distinctive clinical features are noteworthy: women are affected more commonly in both areas; the tumors tend to arise in more proximal areas of the small intestine; and the patients tend to be of rather youthful age.

Lymphoma and Malabsorption Syndromes. At least two distinctive clinical syndromes link primary lymphoma of the small intestine and steatorrhea.[21] Primary lymphoma involving principally the wall of the jejunum and/or abdominal lymphatics gives rise to a malabsorption syndrome with weight loss and steatorrhea. The clinical picture may resemble celiac sprue, and a small intestinal mucosal biopsy sample may show villous atrophy. The persistence of abdominal pain, the appearance of fever or a skin rash, and the lack of response to a gluten-free diet are signs of an underlying lymphoma (see pp. 950 to 958).

Lymphoma may also appear as a late manifestation in patients with well established gluten-sensitive celiac sprue. The association of these two diseases appears to be greater than that accounted for by chance alone. It has been speculated that neoplastic development may be the result of the rapid epithelial cell turnover or the chronic inflammatory process in the mucosa of patients with celiac sprue[15] (see pp. 864 to 884).

LEIOMYOSARCOMA

Leiomyosarcomas rank third in order of occurrence among primary small bowel malignancies. They may be found in the duodenum, jejunum, or ileum, but most occur in the latter two segments of the small intestine. In a review of 300 cases from the world's literature, Starr and Dockerty were unable to show a significant sex difference.[22] However, in their personal series of 41 patients with malignant leiomyosarcomas, males predominated in a ratio of 3 to 1. The majority of malignancies were discovered in the fifth, sixth, and seventh decades. Abdominal pain and bleeding were the most frequently observed symptoms. A mass was palpable in over half the patients. Of all the small bowel tumors, the leiomyosarcoma is most likely to be palpable on physical examination. Like lymphosarcomas, leiomyosarcomas may present clinically as bowel perforation but with much reduced frequency.

Leiomyosarcoma is the most common malignant neoplasm arising in a Meckel diverticulum.[23]

Grossly the leiomyosarcoma is most often a large lesion, usually exceeding 5 cm in diameter. Malignant smooth muscle tumors tend to be less firm and less encapsulated when compared with their benign counterparts. An abundant blood supply usually develops in association with the tumor, and together with a tendency for central necrosis and ulceration massive hemorrhage is the result.

Microscopically malignant smooth muscle neoplasms are often difficult to clearly categorize as benign or malignant. Although the usual criteria such as cellular pleomorphism and abundance of mitotic figures can be helpful, occasionally a rather benign histological appearance will be associated with spread to other areas of the body. The phrase "benign metastasizing leiomyoma" has been coined for this variety.[24] Spread of the leiomyosarcoma via the lymphatics is distinctly rare, and metastases are formed by direct extension or are blood borne.

A surgical approach is required for both treatment and palliation, because these tumors are notoriously resistant to radiation and chemotherapy. An aggressive surgical approach is recommended when distant metastases are not identified. Extensive lymph node dissection is not necessary. Following operations which the surgeon deems probable for cure, five-year survival rates approaching 50 per cent are reported.

CARCINOID TUMORS OF THE SMALL INTESTINE (EXCLUDING CARCINOID SYNDROME)

In the absence of the carcinoid syndrome (see pp. 1031 to 1041), carcinoid tumors of the intestine are difficult to classify as either unequivocally benign or unequivocally malignant. For these and other tumors with similar behavorial characteristics, the term "intermediate tumor" has been proposed.[24] Gastrointestinal carcinoids originate from the chromaffin cells of Kulchitsky which lie deep in the crypts of Lieberkühn. Carcinoids may develop anywhere in the intestinal tract from the gastric cardia to the anorectal junction. They arise most frequently, however, in the areas derived from the embryologic midgut; that is, mid-duodenum to mid-transverse colon.[25] The appendix is by far the commonest location for a gastrointestinal carcinoid.

Clinically, small intestinal carcinoids occur in men and women with equal frequency. This contrasts to the larger portion of appendiceal carcinoids which are found in women. The tumors have been reported in patients whose ages range from ten days to 89 years, with an average age of 45 years.

In the absence of metastases and the carcinoid syndrome, the majority of small intestinal carcinoids remain clinically silent. The lesions are usually found incidentally during surgery or at autopsy. An asymptomatic lesion discovered at surgery should be excised completely, and the liver examined for evidence of metastases. Postoperatively, the patient should have a quantitative determination of 5-hydroxy-indoleacetic acid at periodic intervals.

In a large review,[26] patients with carcinoids accounted for approximately 8 per cent of surgically resected small bowel neoplasms. In another series of 2500 patients with carcinoid tumors of the gastrointestinal tract, approximately one-third were found in the small intestine.[27] The ileum was the primary site eight times more frequently than the jejunum, with a predilection for the region of the ileocecal valve. Although argentaffin cells are numerous in the duodenum, primary duodenal carcinoids are rare. Most duodenal carcinoids arise in the first portion of the duodenum and in the periampullary area.

In general, the size of the primary lesion correlates well with the probability of metastases. Of 209 patients reported from the Mayo Clinic,[28] 50 per cent of the lesions were greater than 1 cm and 80 per cent of those greater than 2 cm were associated with metastases.

A carcinoid tumor may arise in a Meckel diverticulum,[29] and in this instance it will probably behave as an intestinal rather than an appendiceal variety.

The pathology and pharmacology of carcinoids and the carcinoid syndrome are further discussed on pages 1031 to 1035.

OTHER PRIMARY MALIGNANCIES OF THE SMALL BOWEL

Small intestinal malignancies which are associated with genetically determined diseases are discussed on pages 1051 to 1059. Other malignancies listed in Table 72–1 are too rare for inclusion in this text, and the reader is referred to original, referenced articles.

REFERENCES

1. Darling, R. C., and Welch, C. E. Tumors of the small intestine. New Eng. J. Med. 260:397, 1959.
2. Good, C. A. Tumors of the small intestine. Caldwell Lecture, 1962. Amer. J. Roentgenol. Rad. Therapy Nuc. Med. 89:685, 1963.
3. Hancock, R. J. An 11-year review of primary tumours of the small bowel including the duodenum. Canad. Med. Assoc. J. 103:1177, 1970.
4. Alexander, J. W., and Altemeier, W. A. Association of primary neoplasms of the small intestine with other neoplastic growths. Ann. Surg. 167:958, 1968.
5. James, A. E., Jr., and Melvin, J. Villous adenoma of the jejunum. Dig. Dis. 10:265, 1965.
6. Mayo, C. W., Pagtalunan, R. J. G., and Brown, D. J. Lipoma of the alimentary tract. Surgery 53:598, 1963.
7. Ramer, M., Mitty, H. A., and Baron, M. G. Angiography in leiomyomatous neoplasms of the small bowel. Amer. J. Roentgenol. Rad. Therapy Nuc. Med. 113:263, 1971.

8. Gentry, R., Dockerty, M. B., and Clagett, O. T. Vascular malformations and vascular tumors of the gastrointestinal tract. Int. Abstr. Surg. 88:281, 1949.

9. Nys, A., and Buyssens, N. Diffuse cavernous hemangiomatosis of the small intestine. Gastroenterology 45:663, 1963.

10. Haddad, H. M., and Wilkins, L. Congenital anomalies associated with gonadal aplasia. Review of 55 cases. Pediatrics 23:885, 1959.

11. Goodman, R. M., Smith, E. W., Paton, D., Bergman, R. A., Siegel, C. L., Ottsen, O. E., Shelley, W. M., Pusch, A. L., and McKusick, V. A. Pseudoxanthoma elasticum: A clinical and histopathological study. Medicine (Balt.) 42:297, 1963.

12. Wood, P. A. Tumors of the Intestines. A.F.I.P. Atlas of Tumor Pathology. Section VI—Fascicle 22, 1967.

13. River, L., Silverstein, J., and Tope, J. W. Benign neoplasms of the small intestine. Int. Abstr. Surg. 102:1, 1956.

14. Jefferson, G. Carcinoma of the suprapapillary duodenum causally associated with a pre-existing simple ulcer. Brit. J. Surg. 4:209, 1916.

15. Harris, O. D., Cooke, W. T., Thompson, H., and Waterhouse, J. A. H. Malignancy in adult coeliac disease and idiopathic steatorrhea. Amer. J. Med. 42:899, 1967.

16. Gjone, E., and Nordoy, A. Dermatitis herpetiformis, steatorrhea and malignancy. Brit. Med. J. 1:610, 1970.

17. Goldman, L. I., Bralow, S. P., Cox, W., and Peale, A. R. Adenocarcinoma of the small bowel complicating Crohn's disease. Cancer 26:1119, 1970.

18. Eidelman, S., Parkins, R. A., and Rubin, C. E. Abdominal lymphoma presenting as malabsorption. Medicine (Balt.) 45:111, 1966.

19. Nasr, K., Haghighi, P., Bakhshandeh, K., and Haghshenas, M. Primary lymphoma of the upper small intestine. Gut 11:673, 1970.

20. Pridgen, J. E., Mayo, C. W., and Dockerty, M. B. Carcinoma of the jejunum and ileum exclusive of carcinoid tumors. Surg. Gynec. Obstet. 90:513, 1950.

21. Dutz, W., Asvadi, S., Sadri, S., and Kohout, E. Intestinal lymphoma and sprue: A systematic approach. Gut 12:804, 1971.

22. Starr, G. F., and Dockerty, M. B. Leiomyomas and leiomyosarcomas of the small intestine. Cancer 8:101, 1955.

23. Haugen, P. A., Pegg, C. S., and Kyle, J. Leiomyosarcoma of Meckel's diverticulum. Cancer 26:929, 1970.

24. Morehead, R. E. Human pathology. New York, The Blakiston Division, McGraw-Hill Book Co., Inc., 1965.

25. Williams, E. D., and Sandler, M. The classification of carcinoid tumors. Lancet 1:238, 1963.

26. Ariel, I. M. Argentaffin (carcinoid) tumors of the small intestine: Report of 11 cases and review of the literature. Arch. Path. 27:25, 1939.

27. Sanders, R. R., and Axtell, H. K. Carcinoids of the gastrointestinal tract. Surg. Gynec. Obstet. 119:369, 1964.

28. Moertel, C. G., Sauer, W. G., Dockerty, M. B., and Baggenstoss, A. H. Life history of the carcinoid tumor of the small intestine. Cancer 14:901, 1961.

29. Roselli, A., and Paulino, F. Carcinoid tumor of Meckel's diverticulum. Amer. J. Dig. Dis. 9:509, 1964.

30. Clapp, W. A., and Haas, R. Neurofibrosarcoma of the duodenum. J. Maine Med. Assn. 62:55, 1971.

31. Moses, I., and Coodley, E. L. Rhabdomyosarcoma of duodenum. Amer. J. Gastroenterol. 51:48, 1969.

32. Beirne, M. F. Malignant melanoma of the small intestine. Radiology 65:749, 1955.

33. Douglass, H. O., Sika, J. V., and LeVeen, H. H. Plasmacytoma: A not so rare tumor of the small intestine. Cancer 28:456, 1971.

34. Simpson, A. J. The carcinoid tumor, syndrome and spectrum: A review of the literature. N. Carolina Med. J. 30:399, 452, 1969.

35. Deren, M. D., and Henry, P. D. Adenoma of Brunner's glands. Ann. Intern. Med. 44:180, 1956.

36. Lempke, R. E. Intussusception of the duodenum: Report of a case due to Brunner's gland hyperplasia. Ann. Surg. 150:160, 1959.

37. Birch, N. H. A case of Kaposi's sarcoma of the small intestine: Case report. E. African Med. J. 44:343, 1967.

Chapter 73

The Short Bowel Syndrome

Jerry S. Trier

The absorptive and digestive surface provided by the small intestinal mucosa in healthy adults is more than is needed to maintain adequate nutrition. Thus, resection of small amounts of small intestine usually causes no clinical symptoms. The severity of symptoms following resection of large segments of the small bowel is related to (1) the extent of the resection, i.e., the amount of functional absorptive and digestive surface remaining; and (2) the specific level of the resected small bowel. The latter is important, because effective absorption of certain physiologically important substances is limited to either the proximal portion (iron, calcium) or the distal portion (bile salts, vitamin B_{12}) of the small intestine. Thus, resection of up to 40 per cent of the total length of the small bowel is usually well tolerated, provided that the duodenum, the distal half of the ileum, and the ileocecal sphincter are spared. In contrast, resection of the distal two-thirds of the ileum and ileocecal sphincter alone may induce severe diarrhea and significant malabsorption even though less than 25 per cent of the total small intestine has been resected. Resection of 50 per cent or more of the small intestine usually results in significant malabsorption, and resection of 70 per cent or more of the small intestine often produces such catastrophic malabsorption that survival of the patient is threatened.

ETIOLOGY

The most common clinical conditions which require resection of massive amounts of the small intestine to preserve the life of the patient are those which compromise the blood supply of the small intestine. These include thrombosis or embolus of the superior mesenteric artery, thrombosis of the superior mesenteric vein, volvulus of the small intestine, and strangulated internal or external hernias. Less common causes for massive bowel resection include regional enteritis, neoplasm, and trauma. Rarely, surgical error such as inadvertent gastroileal anastomosis in the course of surgery for peptic ulcer may result in bypass of a major portion of the small intestine and produce a clinical picture indistinguishable from that seen following massive intestinal resection. Recent efforts to treat intractable obesity and hypercholesterolemia by jejunocolic anastomosis with bypass of the ileum and part of the jejunum have also produced, in some patients, catastrophic malabsorption of the types seen following massive resection.[1]

PATHOPHYSIOLOGY AND CLINICAL FEATURES

The minimal amount of small intestinal absorptive surface required to sustain life

971

seems to vary from patient to patient. Prolonged survival has been recorded in a number of patients with an intact duodenum and as little as 6 to 18 inches of residual jejunum.[2] However, patient survival is the exception rather than the rule if, in addition to the entire duodenum, less than 2 feet of jejunum or ileum remain. Preservation of the ileocecal sphincter seems important and appears to enhance the functional capacity of the remaining small intestine.

Virtually all nutrients, including water, electrolytes, fat, protein, carbohydrate, and all vitamins, are absorbed subnormally following massive resection of the small intestine. Fluid loss is usually greatest during the first few days after resection, and fecal effluent frequently ranges between 5 and 10 liters.[3] If vigorous fluid and electrolyte replacement is not instituted promptly, life-threatening dehydration and electrolyte imbalance may develop. As time progresses, the consequences of impaired absorption of other nutrients become evident and may affect virtually all body systems. The resulting symptoms and physical findings may resemble closely those encountered in other intestinal diseases with severe panmalabsorption such as celiac sprue or Whipple's disease, and these manifestations have been described in detail on pages 864 to 884 and 938 to 948. Briefly, severe weight loss, fatigue, lassitude, and weakness may result from caloric deprivation caused by impaired fat, protein, and carbohydrate absorption. Impaired absorption of divalent cations (Ca^{++}, Mg^{++}) may aggravate the weakness, and frank tetany may develop. As the duration of calcium and protein malabsorption lengthens, osteomalacia and osteoporosis with bone pain and even spontaneous fractures may develop. Purpura and generalized bleeding may reflect impaired coagulation caused by malabsorption of vitamin K. In time, peripheral neuropathy may develop. Excessive loss of plasma proteins into the gut does not usually occur; hence severe hypoalbuminemia with ascites and peripheral edema is much less common than in diffuse mucosal diseases of the small intestine such as celiac sprue or Whipple's disease. Mild or moderate hypoalbuminemia does occur and may reflect diminished synthesis related to impaired availability of amino acids.

There is evidence that adaptive changes occur which facilitate efficient absorption and digestion by the remaining small intestine if the patient survives the first few weeks after massive resection.[4] This adaptation to resection has been studied to a limited degree in experimental animals and in man. In rodents, small intestinal resection induces accelerated epithelial cell renewal of the small intestine and prominent hypertrophy of the villi. The mechanism for this response is not known, but it has been postulated that resection results in release of a humoral factor, perhaps somewhat analogous to erythropoietin, which stimulates enhanced production of epithelial cells in the proliferative compartment of the intestinal crypts.[5] The resulting villous hypertrophy appears

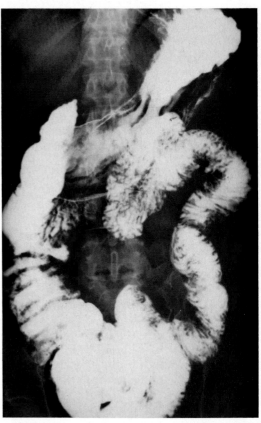

Figure 73–1. Barium contrast study of the small intestine from a patient who had undergone resection of the ileum and over half of the jejunum six months earlier. There is an increase in the caliber of the remaining small intestine, but the mucosal pattern appears normal.

to be associated with some enhancement of absorptive capacity, although this has not been studied extensively. In man, an increase in the caliber of the remaining segment of small intestine is usually seen in barium contrast X-rays several weeks to months after massive resection (Fig. 73–1). This dilatation of the bowel may reflect an increase in the total absorptive surface of the remaining small intestine. However, an increase in the length of the villi has not been found in man, although the total number of absorptive cells per unit length of villi appears increased. Thus, there appears to be hyperplasia of intestinal absorptive cells in man without true villous hypertrophy.[6] There is some clinical evidence that absorptive function improves with time after massive resection in man. For example, stool, water, and electrolyte losses appear to decrease during the first several weeks after massive resection. However, direct documentation of a compensatory increase in absorptive capacity is limited to demonstration by intraluminal perfusion of a modest increase in glucose absorption in patients who have survived massive resection.[7]

Gastric hypersecretion follows massive resection of the small intestine in approximately 50 per cent of patients and may cause serious complicating peptic ulcer disease.[2, 8] Hypersecretion has been produced experimentally in dogs and rats by massive intestinal resection, and it has been suggested but not proved that loss of an intestinal inhibitor of gastric secretion may be responsible.[9] Recently, convincing evidence has been presented that such gastric hypersecretion in man is a transient phenomenon and that gastric secretion decreases to normal levels in patients who survive the acute effects of massive resection.[8]

In striking contrast to massive resections, resections of small portions of the midintestine are usually well tolerated, because the residual bowel has sufficient reserve absorptive and digestive capacity. Indeed, clinical evidence of malabsorption may be absent in patients in whom up to 6 feet of midsmall bowel is resected. However, when much smaller segments of either the proximal or the distal small intestine are removed, significant clinical signs and symptoms usually develop.

If the entire duodenum is resected or surgically bypassed, anemia caused by malabsorption of iron frequently develops much as in a large percentage of patients who have undergone gastrojejunal anastomosis for treatment of their peptic ulcer disease. Such patients may eventually develop osteomalacia, because calcium is absorbed most efficiently by the proximal small intestine.

Resection of a limited segment of distal small intestine may cause serious diarrhea and steatorrhea. Conjugated bile salts, essential for normal fat absorption, are absorbed most effectively by an active transport mechanism present only in the ileum (see p. 252). Absence of these active absorptive sites in patients who have undergone ileal resection disrupts the enterohepatic circulation of bile salts and depletes the bile acid pool. This leads to impaired micelle formation in the intestinal lumen and compromised fat absorption by the remaining small intestine. Moreover, though the total bile salt pool is reduced in patients after ileal resection, excessive amounts pass into the colon, because their almost quantitative reabsorption by the active ileal transport mechanism no longer occurs. The cathartic properties of bile acids have been recognized for years and dihydroxy bile acids have been shown recently not only to impair absorption but also to induce secretion of water and electrolytes when placed in the colon.[10] Thus, both the fat malabsorption and severe watery diarrhea often experienced by patients with limited ileal resections can be explained by impaired ileal bile salt absorption. Indeed, this pathophysiological principle is the rationale behind employing the occasionally effective but often catastrophic maneuver of ileal bypass surgery in patients with severe obesity and hypercholesterolemia[11] (see p. 26).

Resection of the distal ileum induces predictable vitamin B_{12} malabsorption, because the specific transport mechanism for intrinsic factor mediated vitamin B_{12} absorption is localized to the ileal absorptive cells. Thus patients with total ileal resection will, in due course, develop vitamin B_{12} deficiency unless this vitamin is replaced parenterally.

Intraluminal overgrowth of bacteria may

develop in the remaining small intestine and aggravate the already severe malabsorption of fat and vitamin B_{12} (see p. 927). Loss of the ileocecal valve by resection predisposes to the development of abnormal intraluminal bacterial proliferation in the remaining small intestine.

Physical examination, as in other situations with panmalabsorption, varies with the severity and duration of the malabsorption. Initially, physical findings may be limited to poor skin turgor caused by dehydration and/or signs of hypocalcemia and hypomagnesemia, including a positive Chvostek or Trousseau sign or even frank tetany. Later, profound cachexia with purpura, increased skin pigmentation, evidence of multiple vitamin deficiency, anemia, osteomalacia, and peripheral neuropathy may be present.

The laboratory findings in patients with massive intestinal resection are predictable but not specific. Marked fluid and electrolyte derangements caused by massive initial fecal fluid loss are reflected in plasma volume determinations and serum electrolyte levels. Hypokalemia is common, as are sodium and water depletion. As mentioned above, excessive gastric secretion may occur and may aggravate the already immense fluid and electrolyte losses during the first few weeks after resection. Fecal calcium and magnesium losses may result in low serum levels of these divalent cations. If the patient survives the initial few weeks following massive resection, the laboratory abnormalities found in other clinical entities associated with severe panmalabsorption may develop. Xylose absorption is usually diminished, and low serum prothrombin, carotene, and cholesterol levels are common. As the patient is fed, marked steatorrhea develops. Hypoalbuminemia appears if prolonged negative nitrogen balance persists. Eventually, anemia caused by folate, vitamin B_{12}, or iron deficiency develops if these substances are not adequately replaced. Quantitation of vitamin B_{12} absorption with added intrinsic factor is particularly helpful in assessing the extent of ileal resection, although impaired vitamin B_{12} absorption both with and without added intrinsic factor may reflect bacterial overgrowth within the lumen of the small intestine. Careful culture of intestinal fluid on selective media is needed to establish or exclude intraluminal bacterial overgrowth in patients with ileal resections.

Barium contrast studies of the small bowel may show some adaptive dilatation of the bowel and are also helpful prognostically by providing a means of assessing the length of remaining bowel.

TREATMENT

Vigorous parenteral replacement therapy is essential and life saving during the first few weeks after massive intestinal resection. Fluid and electrolyte replacement should be guided by careful quantitation of all fluid losses in the nasogastric aspirate, fecal effluent, and urine. Serial determinations of serum electrolytes, calcium, magnesium, and body weight serve as further guides to the massive fluid and electrolyte replacement necessary in these patients.

Early initiation of total parenteral alimentation has been advocated in the treatment of patients with massive intestinal resection to prevent development of cachexia and severe nutritional deficiencies.[12] Preparation of a nutritionally balanced solution is now feasible (see Table 73–1), utilizing commercially available fibrin hydrolysate solutions. More recently, solutions of crystalline L-amino acids have become available, and these can be substituted for the fibrin hydrolysate. As little as 2 liters of fluid can provide adequate nutrition to maintain reasonable caloric intake and nitrogen balance in the adult patient (Table 73–1). Such solutions are hypertonic and must be administered into a large vein, such as the subclavian. In patients with massive intestinal resection, the solutions can and should be diluted to reduce their hypertonicity, because fecal fluid losses alone commonly exceed 2 liters per day.

While total parenteral alimentation may be life saving in patients with massive resection, it is not without danger, and numerous complications may occur.[12] These include the many complications which may be associated with prolonged subclavian catheterization (e.g., pneumothorax, hemothorax, subclavian artery injury). In addition, sepsis from contamin-

TABLE 73–1. PREPARATION OF HYPERALIMENTATION SOLUTIONS FOR ADULTS*

UNIT COMPOSITION OF BASE SOLUTION

	Bulk Method (Pharmacy)	*Single Unit Method (Ward or Pharmacy)*
Composition	165 g of anhydrous glucose (U.S.P.) + 860 ml 5% glucose in 5% fibrin hydrolysate	350 ml of 50% glucose + 750 ml of 5% glucose in 5% fibrin hydrolysate
Preparation	Sterilization through 0.22 μ membrane filter under laminar flow, filtered air hood	Aseptic mixing technique under laminar flow, filtered air hood
Volume (ml)	1000	1100
Calories (kcal)	1000	1000
Glucose (g)	208	212
Hydrolysates (g)	43	37
Nitrogen (g)	6.0	5.25
Sodium (mEq)	8	7
Potassium (mEq)	14	13

ADDITIONS TO EACH UNIT OF BASE SOLUTION†

Routine	
Sodium (2/3 chloride, 1/3 bicarbonate)	40–50 mEq
Potassium (chloride)	30–40 mEq
Magnesium (sulfate)	4–10 mEq
Optional	
Calcium (gluconate)	4–5 mEq
Phosphate (potassium acid salt)	4–5 mEq

ADDITIONS TO ONLY ONE UNIT DAILY (AVERAGE ADULT)†

Routine	
Multiple vitamin infusion	10 ml
Optional	
Vitamin K	5–10 mg
Vitamin B_{12}	10–30 μg
Folic acid	0.5–1.5 mg
Iron (dextriferron)	2.0–3.0 mg

*From Dudrick, S. J., and Ruberg, R. L.: Gastroenterology *61*:901, 1971.

†Micronutrients such as zinc, copper, manganese, cobalt, and iodine are present as contaminants in hydrolysate solutions, but may be given in plasma transfusion once or twice weekly if desired.

ated solutions or from the catheter entrance site and hyperosmolar hyperglycemic dehydration may occur. More recently, severe hypophosphatemia associated with seizures and coma has been noted.[13] Thus, conscientious attention to sterile technique and careful monitoring of the metabolic status of the patient undergoing total parenteral nutrition are essential.

Antidiarrheal agents such as Lomotil, opiates, anticholinergics, and kaolin preparations usually have little beneficial effect, although they may be tried.

Oral feedings should be initiated as soon as possible. Initial feedings should be small but frequent and consist of foodstuffs that require minimal digestion for effective absorption. Thus, initial feedings should consist primarily of simple sugars, amino acid preparations, and readily absorbable lipids such as medium-chain triglycerides. Commercial preparations of such elemental diets are useful. However, such formulations are hypertonic and should be diluted initially to avoid aggravation of the patient's diarrhea owing to administration of an excessive osmolar load. If the patient is able to tolerate these simple foodstuffs, additional, more complex foods should be added gradually until optimal nutrition is achieved. Milk must be added cautiously to the diet, because the total amount of lactase-bearing epithelium is markedly reduced following massive resection, and large amounts of milk may aggravate diarrhea. A dietary regimen in which 50 to 75 per cent of long-chain fat has been replaced by medium-chain triglyceride has been beneficial in some patients in whom a reduction in fecal water and electrolyte loss and improved overall nutrition have been noted.[3] Since some steatorrhea will always persist in patients with massive resections, total caloric intake will ultimately have to exceed that of normal individuals if the resected patient is to maintain a reasonable weight. Ideally these patients will eat at least five to six meals per day rather than the customary three.

The administration of vitamin supplements, especially fat-soluble vitamins, is essential. Calcium and, in many patients, magnesium supplements may be needed as in other patients with severe malabsorption (see Table 20–4).

If there is clinical and laboratory evidence of intraluminal bacterial overgrowth in the small intestinal remnant, intermittent courses of appropriate broad-spectrum antibiotics such as tetracycline or ampcillin should be administered.

If gastric hypersecretion has been documented in the immediate postresection period, hourly antacid therapy should be instituted. Care must be taken to avoid those antacid preparations which contain large quantities of magnesium hydroxide, because their laxative effect may aggravate the already severe diarrhea.

Under no circumstances should prophylactic ulcer surgery such as vagotomy and pyloroplasty or vagotomy and antrectomy be carried out at the time of the initial resection. As has been indicated, many patients never develop gastric hypersecretion, and in most and perhaps all of those who do, the phenomenon is transient.[8] Ulcer surgery may have disastrous consequences, because it may further impair the already compromised absorptive capacity of the resected patient.

In patients with limited resection of the small intestine, therapy is less complex. Patients with duodenal bypass or resection may require iron and calcium supplements.

In patients who have undergone ileal resections of 3 feet or less, cholestyramine in doses of 8 to 12 g per day is often effective in controlling diarrhea caused by bile acid malabsorption.[15] In patients with more extensive ileal resections, cholestyramine is usually ineffective; in fact, it may aggravate already severe steatorrhea by further depleting the patient's bile acid pool. Patients who have undergone sufficiently extensive ileal resection to have impaired vitamin B_{12} absorption should receive monthly injections of vitamin B_{12} (see Table 20–4).

SURGICAL APPROACH

Some physicians have advocated surgical intervention in patients who fail to maintain adequate nutrition and who have persistent and life-threatening malabsorption and continued weight loss after several months of intensive medical treatment, as outlined above. Reversal of a short segment of bowel at the distal margin of the remaining small intestine has been tried. Optimally, this procedure induces partial intestinal obstruction and facilitates absorption by increasing transit time. Alternatively, construction of a recirculating loop with some of the remaining small intestine has been attempted in the hope that such loops would permit nutrients to pass several times along the same segment of bowel, thus facilitating absorption. In isolated instances, such surgical intervention has appeared helpful,[14] but more often it has been of no benefit and may even have been deleterious. Such operations predispose to stasis and may induce severe bacterial overgrowth in the remaining segment of small intestine, compromising absorption even further. Moreover, there is always the risk that manipulation of the remaining intestinal segment may impair its blood supply, necessitate additional resection, and further reduce the available absorptive surface. At present, surgical treatment of massive intestinal resection must be considered experimental and should be attempted only in desperate situations.

PROGNOSIS AND COMPLICATIONS

The prognosis in patients with massive resection varies directly with the length of the remaining intestinal segment and its freedom from disease. Patients who, after resection, still have 25 per cent or more of morphologically and functionally normal small intestine have a good prognosis, whereas patients with less than 25 per cent of their small intestine have a much poorer prognosis. Patients in the latter group usually are nutritional cripples with poor general resistance to disease. In addition to the diverse complications they may develop related to their nutritional deficiencies (see above), chronic infections such as tuberculosis may complicate their already stormy course.[2]

Recently, a high incidence of oxalate stones has been reported in patients with ileal dysfunction or following resection of the ileum. This complication is discussed on page 898.

REFERENCES

1. Bondar, G. F., and Pisesky, W. Complications of small intestinal short-circuiting for obesity. Arch. Surg. 94:707, 1967.
2. Winawer, S. J., and Zamcheck, N. Pathophysiology of small intestinal resection in man. In Progress in Gastroenterology, Vol. I, G. B. J. Glass (ed.). New York, Grune and Stratton, 1968, pp. 339–356.
3. Bochenek, W., Rodgers, J. B., and Balint, J. A. Effects of changes in dietary lipids on intestinal fluid loss in the short-bowel syndrome. Ann. Intern. Med. 72:205, 1970.
4. Weser, E. Intestinal adaptation to small bowel resection. Amer. J. Clin. Nutr. 24:133, 1971.
5. Loran, M. R., and Carbone, J. V. The humoral effect of intestinal resection on cellular proliferation and maturation in parabiotic rats. In Gastrointestinal Radiation Injury, M. F. Sullivan (ed.). Amsterdam, Excerpta Medica Foundation, 1968, pp. 127–139.
6. Porus, R. L. Epithelial hyperplasia following massive small bowel resection in man. Gastroenterology 48:753, 1965.
7. Dowling, R. H., and Booth, C. C. Functional compensation after small bowel resection in man. Lancet 2:146, 1966.
8. Windsor, C. W. O., Fejfar, J., and Woodward, D. A. K. Gastric secretion after massive small bowel resection. Gut 10:779, 1969.
9. Frederick, P. L., Sizer, J. S., and Osborne, M. P. Relation of massive bowel resection to gastric secretion. New Eng. J. Med. 272:509, 1965.
10. Mekhjian, H. S., Phillips, S. F., and Hofmann, A. F. Colonic secretion of water and electrolytes induced by bile acids: Perfusion studies in man. J. Clin. Invest. 50:1569, 1971.
11. Buchwald, H. The development of the subtotal ileal bypass operation as a therapeutic approach to hypercholesterolemia and atherosclerosis: A review. Dis. Chest 51:459, 1967.
12. Dudrick, S. J., and Ruberg, R. L. Principles and practice of parenteral nutrition. Gastroenterology 61:901, 1971.
13. Silvas, S. E., and Paragas, P. D., Jr. Paresthesias, weakness, seizures and hypophosphatemia in patients receiving hyperalimentation. Gastroenterology 62:513, 1972.
14. Simons, B. E., and Jordan, G. L. Massive bowel resection. Amer. J. Surg. 118:953, 1969.
15. Hofmann, A. F., and Poley, J. R. Cholestyramine treatment of diarrhea associated with ileal resection. New Eng. J. Med. 281:397, 1969.

Chapter 74

Tropical Sprue

V. I. Mathan

DEFINITION

Tropical sprue is a syndrome of unknown cause. It should not be considered as a single disease entity.[1] All residents of or visitors to tropical regions who have malabsorption of at least two unrelated substances, such as xylose and vitamin B_{12}, and in whom no specific cause can be found for the malabsorption are considered to have tropical sprue. Histological examination reveals jejunal mucosal abnormalities in the majority of such patients, but the absence of such abnormalities does not preclude the diagnosis.[2] It must be emphasized that the many other diseases which give rise to malabsorption in temperate zones may also be found in the tropics, and it is essential to exclude these by careful evaluation before the diagnosis of tropical sprue is accepted in the individual patient.

HISTORY

A wasting disease associated with chronic diarrhea was known to the physicians of India from at least 600 B.C. In Charaka Samhita, a textbook of medicine written between 1300 and 600 B.C., it was suggested that this disease was due to "a weakness of the digestive fire" leading to "impaired assimilation of ingested food." This is remarkably similar to current concepts regarding tropical sprue.

Hillary, writing about his experiences in Barbados in 1759, was probably the first to document this disease in the English medical literature.[3] Dutch and British physicians described the clinical syndrome in great detail during the eighteenth and nineteenth centuries.[4] The multiple nutritional deficiency states (caused by malabsorption) occupied the attention of these physicians, and in the early decades of this century, tropical sprue, especially in the Caribbean, was considered a hematological disease because of the associated anemia. Only in the past 15 years, with the development of intestinal mucosal biopsy techniques and reliable methods of evaluating intestinal absorption, has the syndrome been established to be primarily of gastrointestinal origin.[5, 6]

EPIDEMIOLOGY

Tropical sprue has a peculiar geographic distribution. It supposedly does not occur in Africa south of the Sahara. Although widely prevalent in the Caribbean, it has not been reported in Jamaica. These geographic differences are as yet unexplained. Much of the early literature implied that the disease was confined to Caucasians visiting the tropics. It is now recognized that the disease is prevalent in indigenous populations, and malabsorption and asso-

978

ciated malnutrition are major public health problems in developing countries.[4] As a result of the speed and availability of modern travel and large populations of emigrants in temperate zones, some patients with tropical sprue are being seen by physicians in nontropical areas.[7]

Epidemic and endemic forms of the disease are recognized. This differentiation is only epidemiological, because the clinical manifestations are identical. All age groups are affected, although the attack rate appears significantly higher in adults. Both sexes are equally affected. Accurate figures are not available regarding the prevalence of endemic tropical sprue in indigenous populations. A high prevalence of xylose malabsorption and of minor morphological changes in the jejunal mucosa has been documented in asymptomatic subjects studied in several tropical areas.[5] This pattern of abnormalities has been termed "tropical enteropathy," but the relationship of this to tropical sprue, if any, is not clear. Nearly two-thirds of a small number of asymptomatic subjects selected from a hospital population in Haiti were found to have malabsorption of xylose and vitamin B_{12}. It is not certain that this reflects the prevalence of tropical sprue in this community. It has been estimated by studies carried out on a random sample from a rural population in southern India that three out of every 100 adults may have subclinical tropical sprue. The available data are incomplete, and the exact prevalence of tropical sprue is not known.

Several large epidemics of tropical sprue have been reported from southern India.[4] In one large epidemic during 1960 to 1962, it was estimated that 100,000 people were affected and at least 30,000 of them died.[9] Such epidemics occur without any seasonal pattern, and in any one affected village new cases continue to appear over a period of several months. The overall attack rate may be as high as 40 per 100. Diet, type and source of drinking water, and environmental factors such as housing and sanitation did not appear to influence the occurrence of these epidemics. The isolation rate of enteropathogenic bacteria from those affected in the epidemics was the same as that in control populations, and no etiological role could be ascribed to bacteria. Virological studies using limited techniques have also been unsuccessful in isolating an etiological agent. However, several epidemiological factors suggest that these epidemics are due to an infectious agent. The strongest evidence for this hypothesis is that in any given epidemic adults are symptomatically affected earlier than young children. When a village that has been affected in an epidemic is kept under surveillance, the age distribution of new cases changes, with younger age groups being most affected as the epidemic progresses.[4]

Epidemic tropical sprue was also a major problem in the Burma theater during the Second World War. It apparently accounted for at least as many repatriations to Britain as the casualties of war! Detailed etiological studies were not carried out in any of these epidemics.

PATHOLOGY

Intestinal mucosal pathology was first illustrated in autopsy material over 50 years ago.[10] These findings were later confirmed in material obtained at laparotomy. The wide availability of peroral biopsy instruments in the last 15 years has made it possible to undertake a systematic study of the intestinal mucosal morphology.

Interpretation of the mucosal pathology in patients is complicated by the presence of changes, in jejunal mucosal biopsies obtained from asymptomatic residents of the tropics, that would be considered abnormal when compared with "normal" biopsies in temperate zones. These changes consist of broadening and thickening of villi, an increase in the height of the crypts, and increased infiltration of the lamina propria and the epithelium with mononuclear cells (Fig. 74–1). Up to 40 per cent of such normal control subjects have minimal malabsorption, especially of xylose. On the other hand, only shortening of villi in a patient with unequivocal malabsorption caused by tropical sprue is shown in Figure 74–2. However, the morphological changes do not correlate well with the severity of the absorptive abnormalities and may be present in subjects without evidence of malabsorption.

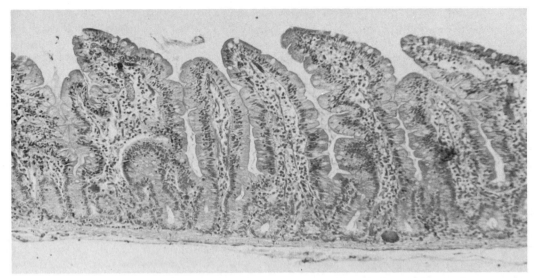

Figure 74–1. Jejunal mucosal biopsy from an asymptomatic Southern Indian adult. The thickness of the crypt layer is increased, and the number of lymphocytes in the lamina propria and the epithelium is increased. The subject had normal fat and vitamin B_{12} absorption but a slightly decreased absorption of D-xylose. × 100.

These morphological changes in asymptomatic subjects have been designated tropical jejunitis, but their pathogenesis or functional significance is not known. These geographic differences in what should be considered "normal" are important when evaluating biopsies from individual patients.

In patients with established tropical sprue, the overall thickness of the mucosa is usually within normal limits, but the villi are shortened and the crypt height is increased (Fig. 74–3). The surface epithelial cells may show severe abnormalities, cells vary in size and shape from low columnar to cuboidal, and pseudostrati-

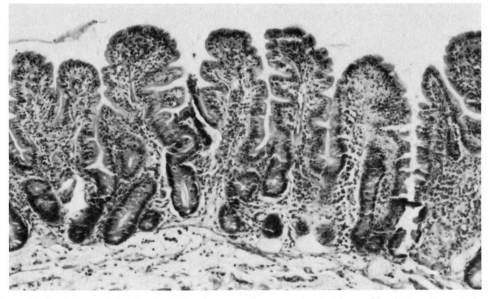

Figure 74–2. Biopsy of the duodenojejunal mucosa from a patient with a milder lesion of tropical sprue. Villous structure is preserved, but the villi are shorter than normal. The cellularity of the lamina propria is increased, and the epithelium is infiltrated with mononuclear cells. × 95.

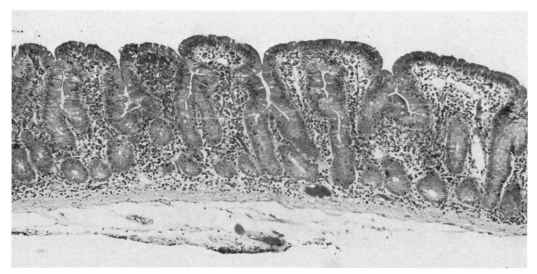

Figure 74–3. Jejunal mucosal biopsy from a patient with tropical sprue. The villi are reduced in length, with increase in the thickness of the crypts. Some of the surface epithelial cells are flattened. There is a marked increase in the number of lymphocytes in the lamina propria and epithelium. × 100.

fication may be present (Fig. 74–4). In general, surface cell alterations are much less severe than those seen in patients with untreated celiac sprue. The basement membrane is usually thickened, and fine droplets of fat may be present in both the basement membrane and surface epithelial cells even after 12 to 18 hours of fasting. The most consistent abnormality is a marked increase in the mononuclear infiltration between surface epithelial cells and in the lamina propria. These changes, although present in the majority of patients, are not specific for tropical sprue and resemble changes seen in a wide variety of pathological states, including

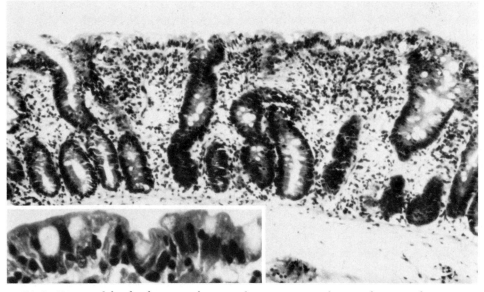

Figure 74–4. Biopsy of the duodenojejunal mucosa from a patient with tropical sprue and a severe mucosal lesion. The biopsy closely resembles the lesion seen in celiac sprue; however, the surface absorptive cells (insert) are less distorted than in most severe celiac sprue lesions. × 95; insert, × 400.

mild celiac sprue and certain parasitic infestations. Occasional patients with clinical evidence of tropical sprue have a normal or near-normal appearing jejunal mucosa on biopsy.[2]

The gastric mucosa is often characterized by atrophy and inflammation. Moreover, hypochlorhydria and diminished secretion of intrinsic factor are present in many patients.

ETIOLOGY AND PATHOGENESIS

Epidemiological and clinical evidence suggests that the syndrome of tropical sprue is the result of damage to the intestinal mucosa. The cause of this damage to the mucosa is not known, but the following have been suggested: (1) that it results from a nutritional deficiency, (2) that it is due to a dietary toxin, or (3) that it is due to a transmissible infectious organism.

The high prevalence of severe deficiency states in patients with chronic tropical sprue has led to the suggestion that it is primarily a deficiency disease. At present there is no evidence to support this claim. Tropical sprue afflicts people with no evident nutritional deficiency. The correction of deficiency states in patients with chronic sprue, although accompanied by improved general status, is not paralleled by an improvement of the intestinal absorptive capacity. Severe protein deficiency can damage the intestinal mucosa in experimental animals, but there is as yet no evidence that a similar situation occurs in adult humans. It is, however, possible that antecedent deficiency states may increase susceptibility to the damaging agent.

Occasional cases of celiac sprue have been reported from the tropics. However, tropical sprue is not improved by the institution of a gluten-free diet. Epidemiological studies so far have not revealed any evidence in favor of a dietary toxin as an etiological agent.

An infectious cause for topical sprue was suggested as early as 1905, but no causal agent, bacterial, viral, or parasitic, has so far been identified. The evidence in favor of an infectious hypothesis is primarily epidemiological. That patients develop their initial symptoms within a week of arriving in endemic areas suggests a brief incubation period. The apparent first appearance of the disease in individuals many years after leaving endemic areas suggests that factors similar to those noted in herpetic infection may play a part. The geographic differences could be explained on the basis of the prevalence of the agent or its dependence on environmental factors.

Predisposing factors may enhance susceptibility of the mucosa to the damage of the agent, which other factors may perpetuate, producing chronic malabsorption. Nutritional deficiency, especially lack of folic acid and vitamin B_{12}, may retard healing of the lesion. Bacterial colonization of the small bowel has been demonstrated in some patients with tropical sprue. These bacteria may perpetuate malabsorption by the production of toxins that interfere with fluid and electrolyte fluxes across the mucosa[11] and may also produce vitamin B_{12} malabsorption. However, several patients have been shown to have normal bacterial flora, and even when abnormal colonization is present no consistent pattern of microbial flora has been observed. Therefore, it appears at present that bacterial colonization of the small bowel, when it occurs, is probably a secondary phenomenon, although it may play a part in the perpetuation of malabsorption.

CLINICAL FEATURES

HISTORY

The majority of patients complain of diarrhea, anorexia, and abdominal distention. In addition, the symptoms associated with nutritional deficiency, especially pallor, weakness, sore tongue and mouth, edema of the legs, and night blindness, are also present. A few patients may present with only isolated sequelae of malabsorption, such as anemia, without any antecedent history of significant diarrhea.

Patients affected in epidemics and even some of the endemic patients can often name the day and sometimes the hour of onset of their symptoms. A day or two of fever, malaise, and anorexia precede the onset of diarrhea in about a quarter of such individuals. The further course of the illness can be divided into two stages. In the first stage the symptoms are predominantly gastrointestinal. The severity of the initial diarrhea differs among patients. In more than half, the stools are watery at the onset and become less fluid with the passage of time. Flecks of blood and some mucus are noted in the stools of a few patients. Nausea and vomiting, although common during the early course of the disease, tend to disappear, whereas anorexia and abdominal distention persist. In the early stage of the illness some loss of weight is common, but abdominal pain is usually not present. The second stage is characterized by the development of nutritional sequelae of persistent malabsorption in addition to continued diarrhea. The diarrhea may persist throughout the course of the illness in some patients, but, more characteristically, the course is marked with repeated remissions and relapses. Abdominal pain, usually mild, is noted by over half the patients at some point during the course of the illness. Very rarely, however, the patient has severe colicky pain which can suggest intestinal obstruction when associated with vomiting and hyperactive bowel sounds. Anorexia, abdominal distention and marked weight loss usually persist. The classic picture of tropical sprue in earlier textbooks described multiple nutritional deficiencies in the patient at this stage. The time required for such deficiencies to develop and their severity are dependent on the antecedent nutrition of the patient. Night blindness, glossitis, stomatitis, cheilosis, cutaneous and mucosal hyperpigmentation, pallor, and edema are the major symptoms of the deficiencies. Hypocalcemic tetany is rare.

PHYSICAL FINDINGS

In about half the patients there may be some abdominal distention, and when the abdominal wall is thin, peristalsis is visible. The bowel sounds are usually loud and very irregular. When the diarrhea is severe, patients may present with dehydration, acidosis, and shock.

In the chronically ill patient, the findings on abdominal examination are still minimal. Minimal hepatomegaly is pres-

ent in less than 10 per cent of patients. However, at this time the signs of nutritional deficiency dominate the picture. Pallor and mild icterus are found in patients with severe megaloblastic anemia. Over half the patients have glossitis and/or stomatitis. Cutaneous hyperpigmentation associated with vitamin B_{12} or folate deficiency is noted in one-third of the patients.[4] The characteristic distribution of this hyperpigmentation is on the dorsum of the hands, especially over the metacarpophalangeal and the interphalangeal joints, the terminal phalanges, and sometimes the nail beds. The pigmentation may be present in other parts of the skin or in the mucous membrane. Appropriate correction of the nutritional deficiencies leads to the rapid clearing of the hyperpigmentation. Edema of the dependent portions of the body is present in about one-third of patients and is associated with hypoproteinemia. Exfoliation of the skin and thin dispigmented hair associated with protein deficiency are found in only a very small number of patients.

On proctosigmoidoscopic examination the rectal mucosa appears normal in over half the patients, but in others some mucosal erythema and edema may be present. Internal hemorrhoids are present in a significant number of patients with chronic diarrhea and may produce bloody streaking of the stool.

LABORATORY FINDINGS

In each patient suspected of having tropical sprue the absorptive capacity of intestine should be evaluated, and the consequences of the observed malabsorption should be assessed.

Stool Examination. The stools are usually liquid or semi-formed, and the 24-hour stool volume is increased. The prevalence of intestinal parasites such as *E. histolytica*, *G. lamblia*, and *S. stercoralis* in patients with tropical sprue is the same as in the general population. Surveys in tropical regions have shown that pathogenic bacteria such as Salmonella, Shigella and enteropathogenic *E. coli* can be isolated from the stool in about 10 per cent of the adult population. The isolation rates of similar bacteria from patients with tropical sprue is no higher. *Capillaria philippinensis* is an important pathogen associated with malabsorption in the Pacific region.

Tests of Intestinal Absorption. The absorption of water, fat, protein, carbohydrates, vitamin B_{12}, folic acid, polyglutamates, vitamin A, and several other substances as measured by perfusion, balance studies, and tolerance tests have been found to be reduced in clinically ill patients. However, in the clinical situation, the testing of fat, xylose, and vitamin B_{12} absorption is adequate. Malabsorption of at least two of these substances should be present for the diagnosis of tropical sprue to be considered.

Steatorrhea is reflected by the presence of excessive numbers of fat droplets on a stool smear stained with Sudan III, a useful test for screening patients. Chemical determinations have shown that over 90 per cent of patients have steatorrhea, but the amount of fat in the stool is seldom as high as in clinically obvious exocrine pancreatic insufficiency. Since at least 40 per cent of the asymptomatic adults in the tropics have xylose malabsorption, its presence does not establish the diagnosis of tropical sprue, even though xylose malabsorption is present in 99 per cent of patients. In the rare patient xylose absorption may be normal. The prevalence of vitamin B_{12} malabsorption shows some geographic differences. In Caucasians with tropical sprue and in native populations in the Caribbean area, over 90 per cent of patients have vitamin B_{12} malabsorption, whereas in southern India only about 60 per cent appear to have this defect. In the majority of patients the absorption of vitamin B_{12} is not improved when additional intrinsic factor is given. In a small number of patients vitamin B_{12} malabsorption improves or becomes normal when intrinsic factor is added to the test dose.

Assessment of Nutritional Status. Dehydration associated with hypokalemia, hyponatremia, and acidosis is a frequent complication of diarrhea. Although severe dehydration is associated with hemoconcentration, hypernatremia is seldom found in these patients.

The hematological sequelae of malabsorption are frequent and led to the disease being considered of primary hematological origin for many years. Anemia may be the result of different degrees of iron, folic acid, and vitamin B_{12} deficiency. The relative importance of vitamin B_{12} and/or folate deficiency in the pathogenesis of megaloblastic erythropoiesis, present in over 60 per cent of the patients, differs according to the nutritional background and the pattern of malabsorption.

Nutritional iron deficiency is widespread in the tropics, and it is difficult to assess the additional role malabsorption in tropical sprue plays in the production of iron deficiency anemia. In temperate zones iron deficiency anemia is less common than megaloblastic anemia, unlike the situation in celiac sprue.

A prolonged prothrombin time correctable by parenteral vitamin K is found in a large number of patients. The prevalence of hypoproteinemia correlates well with the duration of illness. In addition to malabsorption, protein-losing enteropathy has been shown to play a role in the pathogenesis of this deficiency (see pp. 35 to 48).

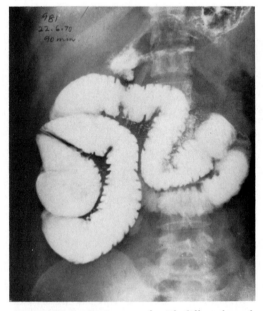

Figure 74–5. Barium meal with follow-through. The upper loops of jejunum are dilated. Edema of primary mucosal folds produces a coarse mucosal pattern. Ninety minutes after the meal, the head of the barium has progressed very little, indicating slow peristalsis.

RADIOLOGY

Dilatation of loops of small intestine, a coarse mucosal pattern with "transverse barring" or a "cog wheel" appearance, slow peristalsis with disordered forward propulsion, and flocculation of stabilized barium preparations are the major features that have been described (Fig. 74–5). When large series of patients are studied, a correlation between the degree of abnormality found radiologically and the degree of malabsorption is noted. However, these abnormalities are nonspecific in nature, and in the individual patient the importance of the radiological examination is to exclude anatomic abnormalities which can lead to secondary malabsorption.

INTESTINAL BIOPSY

The morphological changes have been described in the section on pathology. These changes are nonspecific and are not by themselves diagnostic of tropical sprue. An exact correlation between the severity of the changes noted in biopsy specimens and the degree of malabsorption has not been found. The chief reason for examining jejunal biopsy specimens is in helping to exclude diseases with specific biopsy findings such as giardiasis, Whipple's disease, and lymphoma.

DIAGNOSIS AND DIFFERENTIAL DIAGNOSIS

In the tropics the diagnosis of tropical sprue should be suspected in all patients with chronic diarrhea, malnutrition, or megaloblastic anemia. A history of having visited endemic areas is necessary before this diagnosis is entertained in temperate zones. The confirmation of the diagnosis requires establishing the presence of malabsorption and excluding the many other diseases which can give rise to intestinal malabsorption.

Acute bacillary dysentery or nonspecific diarrheal illnesses should be considered as important in the differential diagnosis in early cases in epidemic situations. The early detection of epidemics of tropical sprue is important because of the high mortality when treatment is not instituted. The diagnosis can be suspected on epidemiological and clinical grounds such as the higher attack rate in adults early in the course of the epidemic and the absence of the recognizable patterns of common diarrheal epidemics. Bacteriological and parasitological surveys should be done to exclude these causes of diarrhea. Although patients affected with epidemic tropical sprue have malabsorption even in the first week of illness, the lack of suitable tests of absorption for use in field situations makes it necessary to admit to hospital some of those affected for detailed study before the diagnosis can be confirmed.

In a patient presenting with chronic diarrhea the diagnostic problems are different. Parasitic diseases such as amebiasis can be diagnosed easily by the detection of the amebae or by the presence of appropriate serum antibodies. Parasitic diseases that are of particular importance because they are associated with malabsorption are giardiasis, strongyloidiasis, and capillariasis. These parasites are present in the upper small bowel, and examination of aspirates of jejunal juice or of jejunal biopsy specimens may be necessary to exclude them. Rapid improvement following treatment of parasitic infestations helps exclude the diagnosis of tropical sprue (see pp. 989 to 1013).

Tuberculosis of the intestines with stricture formation is still probably a most important differential diagnosis in many areas of the tropics. Careful radiological examination of the small bowel is essential in excluding this and other causes of the stagnant bowel syndrome with bacterial overgrowth (see pp. 927 to 937).

With the introduction of wheat to many traditionally rice-eating populations of the tropics, celiac sprue has become an important differential diagnosis. When a history of eating wheat is obtained, failure of response to a gluten-free diet is essential before celiac sprue can be excluded. Intestinal biopsy is of particular importance in excluding conditions such as diffuse infiltrative lymphoma and Whipple's disease.

Primary disaccharidase deficiency can be differentiated from tropical sprue by low mucosal disaccharide levels in the face of a morphologically normal mucosa.

TABLE 74–1. COMPARISON OF TROPICAL SPRUE AND CELIAC SPRUE*

	TROPICAL SPRUE	CELIAC SPRUE
Epidemiology	Tropical climate, especially Caribbean, Indian subcontinent and S.E. Asia; epidemics	Temperate zone; increased incidence in families and in blood group O Rh positive.
Etiology	? Deficiency state; ? infection	Sensitivity to gliadin fraction of gluten
Pathology	Usually partial villous atrophy; surface epithelial cells less affected; correlation with degree of malabsorption often poor	Usually total villous atrophy; surface epithelial cells more affected; correlation with degree of malabsorption often good
Extent of disease	Uniform small bowel involvement	Proximal small bowel most involved; distal small bowel less involved or normal
Clinical and laboratory findings		
Steatorrhea	Common	Common
Macrocytic anemia	Common	Uncommon
B_{12} deficiency	Common	Uncommon
Folic acid deficiency	Common	Common
Iron deficiency anemia	Common	Common
Signs and symptoms of anemia	Prominent	May or may not be prominent (variable)
Vitamin B complex deficiency	Common	Usually present (variable)
Severe hypocalcemia	Uncommon	Common
Vitamin D deficiency	Uncommon	Common
Osteomalacia	Uncommon	Common
Vitamin K deficiency	Common	Common
Urinary 5HIAA	? Normal	Uusually slightly elevated
Treatment	Vitamin B_{12}, folic acid, antibiotics	Gluten-free diet; corticosteroids in refractory cases
Response to therapy	Generally good, but may relapse if drugs not taken long enough	Usually excellent if diet remains free of gluten

*Compiled by Dr. Stephen Herr.

TREATMENT

The treatment of tropical sprue consists of controlling diarrhea, correcting nutritional deficiencies, and using measures aimed at curing the intestinal lesion.

Control of Diarrhea. This can usually be achieved by simple measures, using Lomotil (2.5 to 5.0 mg. three or four times a day) or mixtures containing belladonna and opium, paregoric, and bismuth salicylate. The exact medication and dosage must be adjusted to the individual patient. Controlling diarrhea may reduce the occurrence of fluid and electrolyte abnormalities, but it is unlikely that these measures have any effect on shortening the duration or the course of the disease.

Correction of Deficiency States. Dehydration, acidosis, hypokalemia, and hyponatremia associated with severe diarrhea can often lead to death, especially in the tropics. Severe fluid and electrolyte deficiencies must be corrected by parenteral supplementation. In the majority of cases if the diarrhea can be controlled and an adequate intake of a simple solution containing the essential electrolytes is maintained, major problems do not arise. By using these measures in epidemic situations, the mortality has been reduced to less than one per 100 (see p. 916).

Specific deficiency states such as megaloblastic anemia and iron deficiency should be appropriately treated. In the individual patient the determination of the hematological parameters should determine therapy. Orally administered iron and folic acid appear to be adequately absorbed. Vitamin B_{12} should be given parenterally, because malabsorption of this substance is frequent.

The appropriate diet for these patients has been the subject of debate for many years. Many ingeniously devised diets have had their proponents in the past. None of them have been shown to be of particular value. A diet ensuring at least

3000 calories and about 1 g of protein per kilogram body weight is adequate. In the individual patient any specific item of diet that seems to worsen his symptoms should be avoided. The ideal diet, of course, is one on which the patient gains weight. The majority of patients gain weight even when malabsorption is persistent.

Attempts at Specific Therapy. Since the agent that damages the mucosa is not known, no rational method of therapy is available. Vitamin B_{12}, folic acid, and antibiotics have all been credited with altering the course of the disease. It must be emphasized, however, that spontaneous remissions characterize the course of the disease, and the results of therapy should be evaluated only by comparison with appropriate groups of control subjects.

Administration of vitamin B_{12} and folic acid rapidly corrects deficiencies of these substances. In addition they also seem to give the patient a marked sense of well being. The effect of these agents on the absorptive abnormality is variable. In Caucasians with illness of short duration the administration of folic acid seems to result in normalization of intestinal absorption. However, in indigenous populations treated with either folic acid or vitamin B_{12} the improvement in intestinal absorption was no better than in control groups.[4] In an occasional patient there is a rapid normalization of intestinal absorption, and it is likely that the deficiency was acting as a limiting factor in the healing of the mucosal lesion.

A short course (two weeks) of sulfonamides or of broad-spectrum antibiotics such as tetracyclines has been tried, with early reports indicating that this may be curative in the majority of patients. In southern India, in a group of 57 patients not given vitamin B_{12}, folic acid, or antibiotics, the stool fat excretion became normal in 58 per cent, whereas in a comparable group of 48 treated with antibiotics a similar response was found in only 48 per cent. Vitamin B_{12} absorption became normal in 45 per cent of the controls and 50 per cent of the treated group.[4] A few patients show rapid improvement with antibiotics, similar to that seen in patients with the blind loop syndrome, and it is likely that in these patients bacterial overgrowth in the small bowel is an important contributory factor. The results of long-term antibiotic therapy (six months of tetracycline) appear more promising.[12] Fourteen of 15 patients with chronic tropical sprue treated with this regimen in Puerto Rico showed striking improvement. This form of therapy must be evaluated further.

The response to therapy appears to differ in different population groups. In the Caribbean population and in Caucasians antibiotics appear to produce better results than in Indians, and they should be used routinely in those populations. Whether these differences are the result of differences in the cause or are due to other factors is not clear at present.

PROGNOSIS

It used to be considered that repatriation to temperate zones was necessary for those affected in the tropics. More recently, the study of epidemics in India has shown that a large majority of those affected appear to recover spontaneously even in endemic zones, but sufficient data are not available to fully characterize the natural history of the disease. Longer periods of follow-up of patients treated with various regimens are necessary before prognosis can be accurately determined. It is, however, clear that if the diarrhea is controlled and nutrition is ensured, patients can lead a normal life.

REFERENCES

1. Klipstein, F. A., and Baker, S. J. Regarding the definition of tropical sprue. Gastroenterology 58:717, 1970.
2. Brunser, O., Eidelman, S., and Klipstein, F. A. Intestinal morphology of rural Haitians. A comparison between overt tropical sprue and asymptomatic subjects. Gastroenterology 58:655, 1970.
3. Hillary, W. Observations on the Changes on the Air and Concomitant Epidemical Diseases in the Island of Barbados. London, Hitch and Hawes, 1759, pp. 277–297.
4. Tropical Sprue and Megaloblastic Anaemia. A Wellcome Trust Collaborative Study. London, Churchill-Livingstone, 1971.
5. Klipstein, F. A. Progress in gastroenterology: Tropical sprue. Gastroenterology 54:275, 1969.
6. Baker, S. J., and Mathan, V. I. Tropical sprue. *In* Modern Trends in Gastroenterology,

W. I. Card and B. Creamer (eds.). London, Butterworth, 1970.

7. Klipstein, F. A., and Falaiye, J. M. Tropical sprue in expatriates from the tropics living in the continental United States. Medicine (Balt.) 48:475, 1969.

8. Klipstein, F. A., Samloff, I. M., Smarth, G., and Schenck, E. A. Malabsorption and nutrition in rural Haiti. Amer. J. Clin. Nutr. 21: 1042, 1968.

9. Mathan, V. I., and Baker, S. J. An epidemic of tropical sprue in Southern India. I. Clinical features. Ann. Trop. Med. Parasitol. 64:439, 1970.

10. Bahr, P. H. A Report on Researches on Sprue in Ceylon, 1912–1914, Cambridge, University Press, 1915.

11. Gorbach, S. L., Banwell, J. G., Jacobs, B., et al. Tropical sprue and malnutrition in West Bengal. I. Intestinal microflora and absorption. Amer. J. Clin. Nutr. 23:1545, 1970.

12. Guerra, R., Wheby, M. S., and Bayless, T. M. Long term antibiotic therapy in tropical sprue. Ann. Intern. Med. 63:619, 1965.

Chapter 75

Parasitic Diseases

Lloyd L. Brandborg

Parasitic infections of the intestine in man are an important medical problem. Frequently, they are not considered in the differential diagnosis of intestinal disease, because it is commonly held that they are largely confined to underdeveloped areas and areas of inadequate sanitation. The prevalence of these infections is probably increasing because of increasing mobility and foreign travel. Military personnel serving in the field in tropical areas are particularly susceptible to parasitic infections and constitute an important reservoir. It is possible that these persons may introduce new diseases into the United States.

The parasites infecting the small intestine may be divided into three broad groups. These include the protozoa, the roundworms, and the flatworms. The flatworms may be further divided into trematodes or flukes and cestodes or tapeworms.

PROTOZOA

GIARDIA LAMBLIA

Giardia lamblia was the first protozoan parasite to be described. It was observed by van Leeuwenhoek of Delft, who had intermittent chronic diarrhea, in his own stool and described in a letter to the Royal Society of Medicine in 1681.[1] He also made the important clinical observation that when he had liquid stools he could identify the "animalcules" but they were not identifiable in normal formed stool. *Giardia lamblia* is a cosmopolitan parasite with worldwide distribution. Incidences vary between 2 and 25 to 30 per cent.[2] In many surveys the incidences are underestimates, because they depended upon examination of a single stool specimen.

Most patients harboring this parasite are asymptomatic. However, there is general agreement that it is a pathogen and not simply a commensal. Malabsorption which is clinically identical to celiac sprue and cured by eradication of the parasite[3, 4] may occur in children. Steatorrhea is a less common finding in otherwise healthy adults.[5, 6] *Giardia lamblia* has been incriminated in epidemic diarrhea[7] and as a cause of traveler's diarrhea.[8]

PATHOGENSIS

Giardia lamblia exists in two forms, the encysted form and the trophozoite. No intermediate hosts are required. Several animal species harbor organisms of the Giardia genus; however, there appears to be a relatively high host specificity. Infection is acquired by ingestion of cysts which excyst and multiply in the duodenum and proximal small intestine.

The pathogenesis of diarrhea and steatorrhea in giardiasis is unknown. Possible factors include mechanical occlusion of

989

the mucosa[9] by massive numbers of the organism preventing passage of nutrients, competition of the parasite and host for nutrients,[5] epithelial damage, altered motility, and excessive mucous secretion.[10] Mucosal invasion has been proved,[11] and the organism has been found within epithelial cells by electron microscopy.[6] The significance of invasion is not known, because no reaction occurs within the mucosa and there is no apparent damage to the cellular organelles. The intraluminal events such as bile salt excretion and micelle formation have not been investigated.

A striking association occurs between giardiasis and the dysgammaglobulinemias (gastrointestinal immunodeficiency syndromes).[12,13] In most patients with these entities there are deficiencies of both IgA and IgM with variable levels of IgG. These immunoglobulin abnormalities occur with or without nodular lymphoid hyperplasia of the intestine. Symptomatic patients with isolated IgA deficiency may also have giardiasis. A reversible disaccharidase deficiency occurs in some patients with the immunodeficiency syndromes[13] as well as in patients who have normal immunoglobulin levels.[5] In the immunodeficiency syndromes, bacterial overgrowth has not seemed to be important, because therapy with broad-spectrum antibiotics produces no apparent benefit until the parasite is eradicated.[13]

DIAGNOSIS

History. The most common complaint of patients with symptomatic giardiasis is diarrhea.[14] It may be acute or chronic, continuous or intermittent, and may alternate with constipation. The stools are loose or watery and contain mucus but rarely blood. In a few patients, the stool may have the characteristic appearance of steatorrhea. Other symptoms include abdominal colic, nausea and vomiting, anorexia, flatulence, fatigue, weight loss, and nonspecific "nervous" symptoms. Children may have growth retardation.

Physical Examination Physical examination does not contribute to the diagnosis of giardiasis. There may be some evidence of weight loss. Sigmoidoscopy may demonstrate a nonfriable, somewhat hyperemic mucosa with a mucoid secretion in the bowel.

Laboratory Findings. The routine laboratory tests, e.g., blood counts and electrolytes, are normal in most patients. Eosinophilia is not found. Steatorrhea may be present on chemical examination for fecal fat. Serum carotene in the presence of steatorrhea may be depressed. Serum folate is low in some patients,[12] as is vitamin B_{12} urinary excretion;[12] these are reversible in most instances after eradication of the giardiae (these patients are not anemic). Protein-losing enteropathy is a rare finding and is reversible after therapy.[12] Disaccharidase deficiency is diagnosed by a lactose tolerance test after feeding 100 g of lactose or assay of a biopsy for enzyme activity.[5,12] If the true blood glucose rises more than 20 mg per 100 ml, the test is considered to be normal. Serum electrophoresis in patients with immunoglobulin deficiency diseases will reveal very low to absent gamma globulin. Immunoelectrophoresis will demonstrate the marked reduction or absence of IgA, IgM, and, in some instances, IgG.

Radiology. A nonspecific, radiographic abnormality of the small intestine is seen in some patients with giardiasis.[15] The changes consist of thickening and distortion of the mucosal folds of the duodenum and jejunum, hypersecretion, and hypermotility. These changes are reversible after therapy. On the other hand, randomized, coded films of 16 patients with invasive giardiasis compared with 16 normal control subjects revealed no abnormalities (personal observations).

Mucosal Biopsy. DUODENAL ASPIRATION. Patients without immunodeficiency diseases most often have a structurally normal small bowel mucosa (Fig. 75–1).[11] A focal acute inflammatory reaction may be present, particularly in the crypts and remote from the organisms.[16] However, these changes are seen in only a few subjects. Patients with isolated IgA deficiency may have a normal villous structure, or the mucosa may have varying degrees of abnormality and occasionally may even be flat. By light microscopy some of these individuals have absent to markedly reduced plasma cells. If normal numbers of plasma cells are present, they are producing IgM by anti-IgM fluorescent antibody

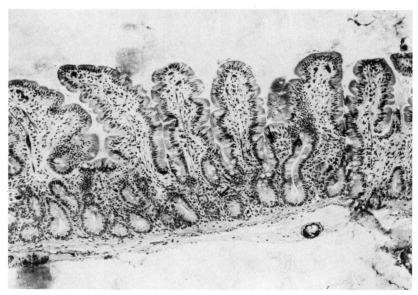

Figure 75–1. Normal proximal intestinal mucosa from a patient with invasive giardiasis. Modified Masson's stain. × 100. (From Brandborg, L. L., et al.: Gastroenterology 52:143, 1967.)

staining. Patients with giardiasis and the immunodeficiency diseases have a patchy intestinal lesion of variable severity, ranging from a normal villous structure to a severely abnormal flat mucosa similar to that seen in patients with celiac sprue.[13] The major difference from celiac sprue is the absence of plasma cells in the lamina propria.

With conventional formalin fixation and hematoxylin and eosin staining, Giardia may be very difficult to recognize, even in the luminal aspects of the biopsy.[11] They tend to stain very similar or identical to the

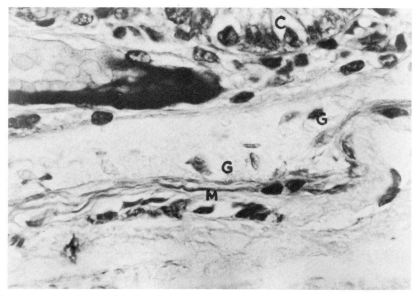

Figure 75–2. Two organisms (G) below the bases of the crypts (C) and above the muscularis mucosae (M). These organisms reside in spaces in loose connective tissue. Typically, only part of the organism is seen. One is sectioned coronally and one longitudinally. Modified Masson's stain. × 1000. (From Brandborg, L. L., et al.: Gastroenterology 52:143, 1967.)

host's tissue and, on occasion, resemble droplets of mucus between the villi and overlying the surface. Occasionally, their identity can be resolved by examination of the specimens under the oil immersion lens.

By utilizing small bowel mucosal biopsies which are fixed in Bouin's solution, serially sectioned in their entirety, and stained with a modification of Masson's trichrome stain, giardiae are easily recognizable in the luminal aspects of the biopsy.[11] By *careful* searching, small numbers of invasive giardiae may be seen in all levels of the specimen from the epithelium to below the muscularis mucosae (Figs. 75–2 and 75–3).[11] In lightly infected individuals, identification of the parasite may require exhaustive search through multiple serial sections.

Diagnosis is more easily accomplished by examining the duodenal contents[13, 14] and by gently wiping the luminal aspect of the biopsy on glass slides, which are then air dried for one hour, fixed in methanol for 30 minutes, washed in tap water, and stained with Giemsa stain. The giardiae found in this preparation are a violet-purple in color and are easily recognized.

Stool Examination.　If *Giardia lamblia* cysts or trophozoites are present on examination of feces, the diagnosis of giardiasis is established. However, as many as 50 per cent of stool specimens in patients proved to have giardiasis by duodenal intubation do not contain the parasite.[13, 14] In some patients the organism is never found in the stool. In addition to direct fecal smears in physiological saline, a stool concentration technique and permanent slides such as trichrome stains of Schaudinn-fixed material should be used.

TREATMENT

Although the majority of patients harboring giardiasis are asymptomatic, treatment is indicated, particularly if conditions are unhygienic or if there is close contact through which other individuals might become infected. The treatment of choice in both asymptomatic and symptomatic patients is quinacrine (Atabrine), 100 mg given by mouth three times daily for seven days. An initial course will cure between 90 and 95 per cent of the infections. An excellent alternative drug is metronidazole

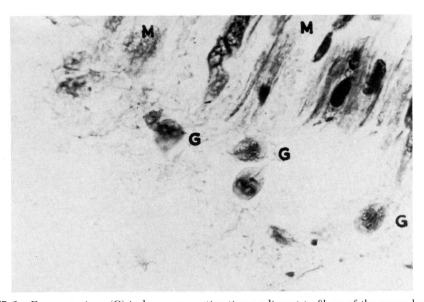

Figure 75–3.　Four organisms (G) in loose connective tissue adjacent to fibers of the muscularis mucosae (M). One is out of focus. This section is from a specimen sectioned parallel to the surface of the mucosa and is approximately 200 μ above the cut surface. This fortuitous observation of several of the parasites *en face* suggests that they may usually lie parallel to the muscularis mucosae when residing in tissue in the submucosa. Identification between epithelial cells is not simpler than with conventional sectioning. (From Brandborg, L. L., et al.: Gastroenterology 52:143, 1967.)

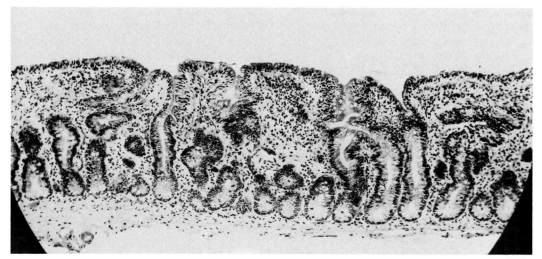

Figure 75-4. Severely abnormal intestinal lesion from a patient with a gastrointestinal immunodeficiency syndrome and giardiasis. × 120. (From Ament, M. E., and Rubin, C. E.: Gastroenterology 62:216, 1972.)

(Flagyl), administered in dosages of 250 mg three times daily for a week.

Therapy with metronidazole at this dosage for six to eight weeks in patients with giardiasis and gastrointestinal immunodeficiency syndromes results in reversal of the mucosal pathology to or toward normal in all cases (Figs. 75-4 and 75-5).[13] Patients with hypogammaglobulinemic sprue without *Giardia lamblia* infection have no improvement of the mucosal pathology on this same regimen. Some caution must be used in ascribing mucosal pathology to *Giardia lamblia*, because metro-

nidazole is an effective antibacterial agent against strict anaerobic species.[17]

COCCIDIOSIS

Two subclasses of the subphylum Sporozoa infect man. Only the coccidia which cause coccidiosis will be considered here. The *Isospora* species, *belli*, *hominis*, and *natalensis*, are found in man.[18] *I. belli* and *I. hominis* may be the same organism, and differences in oocyst

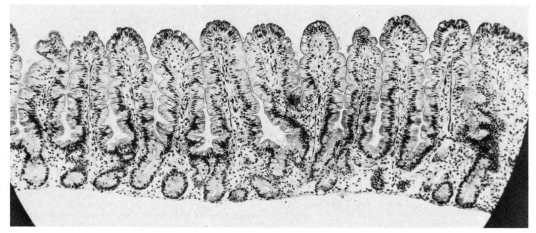

Figure 75-5. Reversal to a normal villous architecture in the same patient after eradication of Giardia. × 120. (From Ament, M. E., and Rubin, C. E.: Gastroenterology 62:216, 1972.)

appearance may simply be due to differences in maturation.[19]

Coccidia were first observed in the epithelium of the rabbit ileum in 1858[20] and in the epithelium of the human small intestine in 1860.[21] This order of parasites is an important cause of morbidity and mortality in domestic and wild animals.[22] Their distribution is limited only by the availability of hosts. Virtually every animal examined has been found to harbor its own highly species-specific coccidium. Some animals may be infected by several different species of coccidia. Infection is acquired by ingestion of viable oocysts. No vectors are required, and the oocysts may persist for long periods of time in soil.

Coccidiosis is infrequently recognized as the cause of disease in man in the United States. However, endemic areas exist in South America, Africa, and the Middle East; Chile,[18] Rotterdam,[23] and the Western Pacific[24] appear to have particularly high incidences. Failure to diagnose coccidiosis elsewhere may be due not so much to its rarity as to the failure to recognize these parasites as a cause of human disease.

PATHOGENESIS

Sporulated oocysts excyst in the proximal small intestine, where the sporozoites that are released invade the epithelium (Fig. 75–6). They become round trophozoites which enter the asexual stage of development, schizogony. The merozoites depart the mature schizont and invade adjacent epithelial cells. On invasion, they may either undergo further schizogony or become sexual gametocytes. On fertilization, the macrogametocyte (female) becomes a nonsporulated oocyst which is extruded into the intestinal lumen and eliminated in the feces.

In animals, the symptoms may be explained by the amount of intestinal epithelial destruction. Most coccidia are strictly intestinal parasites. Chickens and lambs infected with their own species-specific coccidia have been shown to develop "villous atrophy" when compared with suitable control animals.[25] Some species develop a necrotizing enteritis.

Human intestinal pathology in coccidiosis represents a spectrum of damage. Included are necrotizing enterocolitis,[26] a flat mucosa similar to celiac sprue,[27] tall clubbed villi with a marked excess of collagen and dilated vessels in the lamina propria,[27] "stubby" residual villi with elongated crypts,[27] eosinophilic infiltration similar to eosinophilic enteritis,[27] and mild nonspecific changes in lightly infected patients.[27] Organisms are not found in post mortem specimens,[26] possibly because of autolysis. Although it is not proved that coccidia cause intestinal pathology in man, the lesions are severe enough to account for the diarrhea and steatorrhea occurring in these infections.

DIAGNOSIS

History. Coccidiosis usually has an acute onset, with fever, headache, and asthenia. Diarrhea occurs in 98 per cent of patients, weight loss in 86 per cent, and colicky abdominal pain in 61 per cent.[18] Tetany, muscle cramps, paresthesias, and night blindness may occur.[27] The stools frequently contain undigested food, and often appear grossly steatorrheal. Steatorrhea has been proved in a small number of patients.[27, 28] The illness is usually of limited duration, rarely more than six months.

Physical Examination. Physical examination does not contribute to the diagnosis of coccidiosis. If the disease has been

SCHIZOGONY   GAMETOGONY

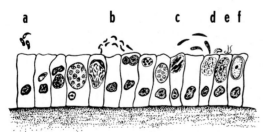

Figure 75–6. Diagrammatic representation of the life cycle of Coccidia. Sporozoites about to invade epithelium (a); first generation merozoites departing schizont and invading adjacent epithelia (b); second generation merozoites invading epithelia (c), microgametocyte (d), macrogametocyte (e), and unsporulated oocyst (f). (From Brandborg, L. L., Goldberg, S. G., and Breidenbach, W. C.: New Eng. J. Med. 283:1306, 1970.)

chronic, there may be evidence of weight loss which at times is profound. Visible loops of bowel may be seen through the abdominal wall, if the weight loss has been severe. Auscultation will often reveal hyperactive bowel sounds which are not obstructive in nature. Characteristically, there is no tenderness on palpation of the abdomen.[18]

Laboratory Findings. Depending upon the severity of the diarrhea and steatorrhea, there may be no to very severe electrolyte abnormalities. These include hyponatremia, hypocalcemia, hypokalemia, metabolic acidosis, and, rarely, uremia. Direct and indirect evidence of malabsorption would include increase in fecal fat, hypocarotenemia, and reduction in D-xylose absorption. The blood counts are usually within normal limits, except for the differential white blood cell count in which there are both a relative and an absolute eosinophilia in 54 per cent of patients.[18] (This is extremely unusual in other protozoan infections.)

The diagnosis may be made by finding oocysts in the stool.[18, 19, 28] This may prove to be extremely difficult, because they are frequently very scanty or absent even in the presence of severe diarrhea and steatorrhea. In contrast to usual techniques, the fecal specimen should be incubated for two days at room temperature to allow maturation of oocysts. Concentration techniques such as zinc sulfate floatation should be used. Staining does not aid in diagnosis.

The mature oocyst of *I. belli* is a thick-walled ovoid structure which is elongated at one end and somewhat constricted at the other.[19] The dimensions range between 11 to 16 μ and 22 to 33 μ. The mature forms contain two sporocysts which measure 7 to 9 microns by 12 to 14 microns, each containing four sporozoites and a large residual mass. *I. hominis* is supposed to have a thin cyst wall, to be sporulated on passage, and to contain one or two sporocysts.

Mucosal Biopsy. DUODENAL DRAINAGE. Peroral small bowel mucosal biopsy is probably the most sensitive way of making the diagnosis of coccidiosis.[27] The pathology is variable, ranging from a flat mucosa to mild nonspecific abnormalities (Figs. 75–7, 75–8, and 75–9). The mucosal morphology is not diagnostic. However, various forms of the parasite may be seen within epithelial cells.[27] All the various stages of the life cycle of the organism are present, but the most easily recognizable forms are the various stages of schizogony which are also the most numerous[7] (Figs. 75–10, 75–11, and 75–12).

Great care must be taken in handling, preparation, and examination of the biopsy

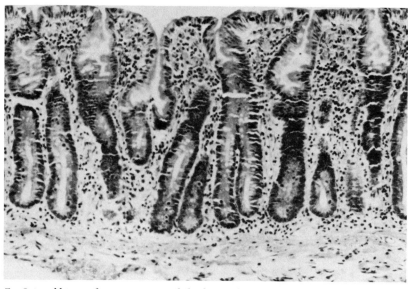

Figure 75–7. Jejunal biopsy from a patient with fatal coccidiosis. Hematoxylin and eosin stain. × 100. (From Brandborg, L. L., Goldberg, S. G., and Breidenbach, W. C.: New Eng. J. Med. 283:1306, 1970.)

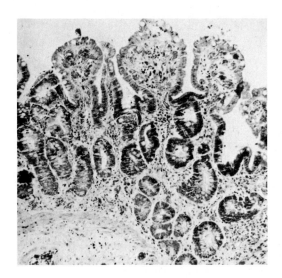

Figure 75–8. Jejunal biopsy in coccidiosis with tall, clubbed villi, dilated vascular spaces and a marked excess of collagen in the lamina propria. Giemsa stain. × 100. (From Brandborg, L. L., Goldberg, S. G., and Breidenbach, W. C.: New Eng. J. Med. 283:1306, 1970.)

Figure 75–9. Jejunal biopsy in coccidiosis with residual "stubby" villi and elongated crypts. Hematoxylin and eosin stain. × 100. (From Brandborg, L. L., Goldberg, S. G., and Breidenbach, W. C.: New Eng. J. Med. 283:1306, 1970.)

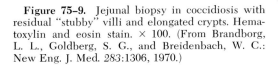

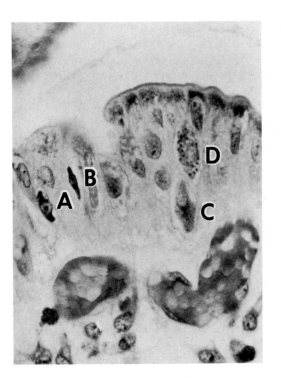

Figure 75–10. Merozoites which are developing into either schizonts or gametocytes (A and B), immature schizont (C) and macrogametocyte (D). Colophonium Giemsa stain. × 1000. (From Brandborg, L. L., Goldberg, S. G., and Breidenbach, W. C.: New Eng. J. Med. 283:1306, 1970.)

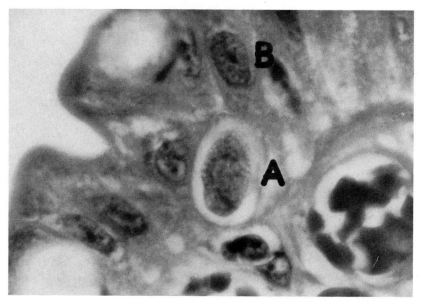

Figure 75–11. Immature schizont (A), and immature macrogametocyte (B). Overstained Giemsa. × 1000. (From Brandborg, L. L., Goldberg, S. G., and Breidenbach, W. C.: New Eng. J. Med. *283*:1306, 1970.)

specimen. Since coccidia in the epithelium in man are not nearly so numerous as in many animal species, the specimen should be processed in the following manner. Bouin's fixed specimens (two hours following which they are transferred to 70 per cent alcohol and run up in the usual techniques to paraffin embedding) are used. Each biopsy should be, serially and entirely, sectioned perpendicular to the luminal surface at 4μ. Giemsa stain or colophonium Giemsa offers the best differential stain for recognizing the various forms of schizogony.[27] *Multiple* sections must be scanned before coccidiosis is discarded as a diagnosis.

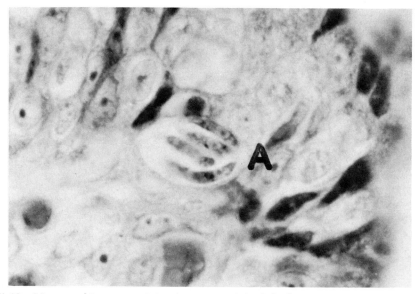

Figure 75–12. Mature schizont containing merozoites (A). Colophonium Giemsa stain. × 1000. (From Brandborg, L. L., Goldberg, S. G., and Breidenbach, W. C.: New Eng. J. Med. *283*:1306, 1970.)

Examination of the intestinal secretions may provide the diagnosis. Immature schizonts and unsporulated and sporulated oocysts are present in the intestinal secretions in some patients.[27]

Radiology. Few data are available on the radiographic appearance of the small intestine in patients with coccidiosis. In some patients, the small bowel series is normal.[18] In some there is obstruction of the duodenum.[18] There may be thickened folds in the duodenum and proximal jejunum with an infiltrated, rigid appearance, excessive secretions within the small bowel, and a rapid transit time.

TREATMENT

Most patients with coccidiosis have a benign and self-limited illness of a few days' to six months' duration. No effective therapy is known. The agents which have been administered include multivitamins, folic acid, vitamin B_{12}, tetracycline, ampicillin, prednisone, quinacrine hydrochloride, diiodohydroxyquin hydrochloride, triple sulfonamide, metronidazole, nitrofurantoin, chloroquine hydrochloride, and primaquine phosphate, all without any benefit.[27] Nitrofurantoin may conceivably shorten the course in patients who are destined for a spontaneous recovery.[27,28] Dietary therapy with a gluten-free, lactose-free, high protein diet has not proved to be of benefit.[27]

No data are available, but in patients with the benign and less chronic diseases whose diarrhea is troublesome, diphenoxylate with atropine (Lomotil) in doses of 2.5 to 5 mg every six hours may be of some benefit.

HELMINTHS — ROUNDWORMS*

ASCARIASIS

Ascaris lumbricoides is a large (about 20 cm long) roundworm with a worldwide distribution. The highest prevalence is in the hot and humid tropics. Infection is through the ingestion of embryonated eggs contaminating food or drink. The larvae

---

*For illustrations of eggs and larvae of roundworms, flatworms and flukes, the reader is referred to Figure 75–13.

emerge from the ovum in the duodenum, from which they migrate through the epithelium of the small bowel into the portal venous system and pass through the liver into the lungs. The incubation period is not precisely known, but within four to 16 days after infection a pneumonitis develops, with fever, cough, sputum production, and pulmonary infiltrates. At this time, the larvae may be found in the sputum.

After several days in the lung, the larvae break through the pulmonary capillaries into the alveoli and migrate up the bronchioles and bronchi to the pharynx, whence they are ultimately swallowed. On arrival in the small intestine, they develop into the adult males and females.

PATHOGENESIS

The pulmonary lesions are produced as the larvae rupture into the alveoli and include small hemorrhages at each site. An inflammatory reaction or a hypersensitivity reaction to various components of the larvae may also occur, which is more severe on reinfection.

The adult worms in the small intestine may produce either traumatic or toxic damage.[2, 29] Large masses of worms may produce intestinal obstruction, usually in the region of the ileocecal valve. There may be perforation of the bowel wall with peritonitis or penetration into other ectopic areas. Ascaris in the appendix may lead to appendicitis and in the common bile duct to obstructive jaundice or pancreatitis. The lungs, heart, and genitourinary systems have been invaded.[2] Sensitization and allergic symptoms may be caused by absorption of products of the living or dead worm. Massive numbers of worms, particularly in children, may lead to malnutrition caused by competition of the organism with the host.[2]

DIAGNOSIS

Clinical Features. The most common symptoms caused by Ascaris infestation are vague abdominal discomfort and abdominal colic which is usually epigastric.[2] Occasionally, diarrhea is present. Children characteristically have fever. The symptoms may suggest abdominal tumor or peptic ulcer disease.

Intestinal obstruction results when worms migrate. In this circumstance, perforation, appendicitis, and peritonitis may occur. On migration into the biliary or pancreatic ducts, jaundice, right upper quadrant pain, and colic and epigastric pain boring through to the back may occur.

Allergic reaction such as asthma, hay fever, urticaria, or conjunctivitis may also be the result of absorption of toxins derived from the worm.

Individuals harboring only a small number of worms may have few or no symptoms.

Physical Examination. Unless there are complications caused by the Ascaris infestation, there are no helpful physical findings. With bowel obstruction, the abdomen is distended with hyperactive, obstructive, high-pitched bowel sounds. Tenderness may or may not be present. If worms have perforated the intestine into the peritoneal cavity, tenderness to light percussion and rebound tenderness are found. The findings of acute appendicitis caused by Ascaris cannot be differentiated from other appendicitis. If the worm has migrated into the common bile duct or pancreatic ducts, the patient may be jaundiced. However, no specific physical findings will differentiate obstructive jaundice or pancreatitis caused by Ascaris from those of other causes.

Laboratory Findings. Routine laboratory data are of little value in diagnosing ascariasis. There may be a mild eosinophilia ranging between 5 and 10 per cent of the differential white blood cell count.[2, 29] The diagnosis is based mainly on finding eggs, adult worms, or larvae. Since each female worm excretes 200,000 eggs per day, two or three direct fecal smears are ordinarily sufficient to make the diagnosis. The eggs vary in appearance; fertilized eggs are ovoid, have a thick, double transparent mammillated wall, and are 50 to 75 μ in diameter. When first passed, the fertilized egg contains a mass of granular amorphous protoplasm. Unfertilized eggs are longer and narrower, contain a thin inner shell, and measure 40 to 90 μ. If the outer shell of the egg is lost, it can be confused with the ova of hookworm.[29] If only male worms are present, no ova will be recovered and diagnosis depends upon demonstration of the adult worm, its detection by radiographic methods, or a therapeutic trial. Occasionally, adult worms may be found in vomitus. On occasion they have been vomited, aspirated into the lungs, and caused asphyxiation, the diagnosis being made on post mortem examination. Adult worms may also be passed in the feces. Larvae may be recovered from sputum, and occasionally from vomitus.[29]

Radiographic Features. Small bowel and colon barium studies may reveal the presence of the worm as a long, translucent filling defect. If large numbers of worms are present, they may be seen as parallel filling defects in either the small bowel or the colon.[29] After the bowel is emptied of barium, the diagnosis of ascariasis may be made upon finding the intestinal tract of the worm filled with barium.

TREATMENT

Uncomplicated ascariasis is best treated by piperazine citrate, 75 mg per kilogram, with a maximum of 3.5 g daily for two days.[30] Thiabendazole is the best alternative drug and is given in a dosage of 25 mg per kilogram twice daily for two days.[30] If hookworm is present, ascariasis should be treated first because tetrachloroethylene will cause the Ascaris to migrate and they may enter ectopic sites.

Bowel obstruction may be treated by a long intestinal tube through which piperazine citrate is injected. If the drug does not cause the bolus of worms to be passed spontaneously and the obstruction is unrelieved, laparotomy is indicated. With perforation and peritonitis, hemorrhagic pancreatitis, or obstructive jaundice caused by Ascaris, laparotomy is indicated.

STRONGYLOIDIASIS

Strongyloides stercoralis exists in two forms, the free-living and parasitic forms.[2, 29] It exists in warm, moist climates in areas where there is frequent fecal contamination of the soil. In the free-living cycle, the male and female rhabditoid larvae develop into free-living adults and repeat the cycle. The rhabditoid larvae may develop into the infective form, the filariform larvae which are capable of penetrating the skin or buccal mucosa.

PATHOGENESIS

On penetration of the skin, the filariform larvae are carried in the circulation to the lungs. They rupture into the alveoli and develop into adolescent worms. Occasionally, females may invade the bronchial or tracheal mucosa and deposit eggs. Usually they are swallowed and invade the small bowel mucosa where they reside. The parasitic males are rhabditoid forms, are not tissue parasites, and soon disappear in the feces. Parasitic females invade the mucosa. Infection usually occurs in the proximal small intestine but may extend from the stomach to the anus. The female deposits thin-walled, ovoid eggs which are 50 to 60 μ long within tissue. The eggs usually develop into rhabditoid larvae which escape into the gut and are passed in the stool. The transformation to filariform larvae usually occurs in soil. If transformation to this stage occurs within the intestine, auto- or hyperinfection results. Mucosal destruction or migration of the worm to other sites is responsible for the clinical features of strongyloidiasis.

CLINICAL FEATURES

History. After cutaneous invasion by the filariform larvae, petechial hemorrhages, pruritus, papular rashes, edema, and urticaria occur.[2, 29] The pulmonary symptoms result from the pneumonitis and, depending upon the severity of the infection, include fever, cough, dyspnea, hemoptysis, chest pain, and pleural effusions. There may also be malaise and anorexia; in severe infections pulmonary edema and bronchial asthma may occur. The cutaneous and pulmonary symptoms are usually of one to two weeks' duration.

Light infections of the intestine may cause no symptoms. More severe involvement results in malaise, fever, nausea, weight loss, vomiting, and abdominal pain which is usually epigastric. Strongyloidiasis may resemble acute tropical sprue with severe diarrhea and steatorrhea.[31] Hepatomegaly, jaundice, bloody diarrhea, intestinal obstruction and death have all resulted from strongyloidiasis.

Because of the autoinfection, symptoms may be present for up to 40 or more years.[32] In chronic infection the most common complaints are nausea and abdominal pain which is usually epigastric and may be similar to peptic ulcer. Diarrhea may or may not be present.

Physical Examination. Physical examination is not specific for strongyloidiasis. In acute infections, the maculopapular rash, urticaria, and petechial hemorrhages may give a clue to the diagnosis. Once the worm is established in the small intestine, the physical findings may include epigastric tenderness to palpation.

DIAGNOSIS

Laboratory Findings. The differential white blood cell count typically shows an eosinophilia between 8 to 10 per cent and, in very severe infections, up to 50 per cent. In some patients, there may be a very marked leukocytosis. Anemia, when it occurs, is usually iron deficiency in type. Hypoalbuminemia and hypergammaglobulinemia have been observed. The stools frequently contain occult blood, mucus, and Charcot-Leyden crystals, and may contain larvae.

Mucosal Biopsy. DUODENAL DRAINAGE. Mucosal suction biopsy is an inefficient and inaccurate way of making the diagnosis, detecting the worms in only 2 per cent of patients,[33] although they may be present in the biopsy specimen.[33] The definitive diagnosis is made by examination of the duodenal secretions.[2, 29, 33] One duodenal drainage is equal to ten concentrated stool specimens as a means of diagnosing strongyloidiasis.

Radiology. The radiographic features of strongyloidiasis are nonspecific and include irritability and thickening of the mucosal folds of the duodenum and proximal jejunum. In very heavy infections, the entire intestine may be involved.

TREATMENT

The therapy of choice is thiabendazole, 25 mg per kilogram twice daily for two days.[30] There are no effective or safe alternative drugs. Strongyloidiasis should always be treated, even in asymptomatic patients when detected, because of the possibility of hyperinfectivity. Corticosteroid drugs should *never* be administered to patients with strongyloidiasis, because such therapy results in a fatal dissemination of the organism to all areas of the body.[34, 35]

CAPILLARIASIS

Intestinal capillariasis is caused by *Capillaria philippinensis* and is found only in the Philippines. The only known host is man, and the mode and source of infection are completely unknown. This roundworm produces a severe malabsorption syndrome with protein-losing enteropathy that is frequently fatal when untreated.[36]

PATHOGENESIS

The worm lies burrowed in the mucosa of the small intestine, particularly the jejunum. All stages of the parasite, including adult worms, larviparous adult females, embryonated eggs, and all stages of larval development are found within the mucosa and in the luminal contents of the gut.[36] Little inflammatory reaction is observed in the vicinity of penetrating organisms. Mucosal destruction may be apparent in the vicinity of the parasite. There are disorganization of the epithelial surface and various abnormalities of villous structure, but these findings are not specific. Comparison of mucosal biopsies procured from patients with capillariasis and suitable healthy, uninfected relatives as controls demonstrates no histological differences except for the presence of the worm.[36]

CLINICAL FEATURES

History. The symptoms of capillariasis are borborygmi, diarrhea of up to eight to ten voluminous, watery stools daily, recurrent vague abdominal pain, weight loss, malaise, anorexia, and vomiting. Diarrhea usually begins two to six weeks after the onset of abdominal pain and borborygmi.[36]

Physical Examination. Most patients have evidence of muscle wasting and weakness. The weakness is so profound that half the patients are unable to stand up. They are hypotensive with distant heart sounds, gallop rhythms, and pulsus alternans. Borborygmi are prominent, as is abdominal distention. About half the patients have abdominal tenderness. Edema and hyporeflexia are usual. Hepatosplenomegaly does not occur.

DIAGNOSIS

Laboratory. Anemia when it occurs is iron deficiency in type. Macrocytic anemia has not been described. The major electrolyte abnormalities are hypocalcemia and hypokalemia, which may be severe and associated with nephropathy, neuropathy, and cardiomyopathy. The total plasma protein levels are reduced. Fecal fat is increased to a mean of 25 g per day. (Stool volume averages 1200 g per day.) The D-xylose excretion is reduced in most patients and approximates 2.5 g in a five-hour urine specimen after a 25-g oral dose. [51]Chromium-labeled albumin studies document the protein-losing enteropathy, with stool radioactivity ranging from 6 to 43 per cent of the injected dose in five days.

The eggs of *C. philippinensis* are somewhat similar to those of *T. trichiura*. However, they are somewhat smaller, 45 by 21 μ in size. They are shaped like a peanut and are not operculated; the shell is pitted rather than smooth.

Small bowel mucosal biopsies have demonstrated the worms in approximately 50 per cent of specimens. Thus, biopsy is not a sensitive technique for making the diagnosis. Examination of the duodenal contents will reveal ova, larvae, and adult Capillaria and aid in the diagnosis.

TREATMENT

Treatment for tropical sprue, i.e., high protein diet supplemented by vitamins, tetracycline, folic acid, and diphenoxylate (Lomotil), does not lower egg counts or improve symptoms, excluding tropical sprue as a diagnosis. Thiabendazole in divided doses of 25 mg per kilogram per day has proved to be effective. Following the onset of therapy, stool egg counts decrease dramatically, the quantity of stool decreases, and the clinical condition improves. In contrast to therapy of most roundworms, therapy should be continued for 30 days. Relapses are heralded by the reappearance of ova in the stools prior to the recurrence of clinical symptoms.

ANCYLOSTOMIASIS

Intestinal hookworm disease in man is caused by *Ancylostoma duodenale* and

Necator americanus.[2, 29] The life cycles of these species are similar. Eggs in feces, when deposited in soil, hatch in one to two days to a rhabditoid larvae which develops into a filariform larvae within a week. On penetration of the skin, the larvae reach venules and are carried to the lung. When they break out of the alveolar capillaries, they pass up the respiratory tree and are swallowed. On arrival in the small intestine, they attach themselves to the mucosa and mature in approximately six weeks. Occasionally, female worms have been found to be depositing eggs in the submucosa. As with other worm infections, hookworm is common where warm, moist soil occurs and fecal contamination is common.

PATHOGENESIS

The worm, on attachment to the small intestinal mucosa, may remove as much as 0.67 ml of blood per worm per day.[2] This may be reduced with worms which have been in the intestine for months or years.[2] Mechanical blood loss from the site of attachment also contributes to the anemia. Disruption of the mucosa and heavy hookworm infestation may also contribute to the hypoproteinemia. Increased fecal loss of albumin and decreased synthesis, presumably caused by malnutrition, occurs in some patients.[37] Whether the worms produce intestinal pathology other than at the site of attachment is unknown. The intestinal pathology and malabsorption in malnourished patients are reversible with a nutritious diet even though the hookworm disease is not treated.[38] In the vicinity of the worm, there is an increase in plasma cells, lymphocytes, and eosinophils. There are associated erosions, ulcerations, and, occasionally, secondary bacterial infection.[2, 29]

Whether or not hookworm disease results in malabsorption is controversial. Malabsorption associated with hookworm disease occurs in regions of endemic tropical sprue and malnutrition. In patients with steatorrhea caused by pancreatic exocrine insufficiency, hookworm infestation does not contribute to the malabsorption.[39] The consensus is that hookworm disease does not cause malabsorption.[39, 40]

Patient resistance is important in the production of hookworm disease. Children and females are less resistant than males. Most patients suffering from severe hookworm disease are malnourished, which appears to enhance their susceptibility to infection.

CLINICAL FEATURES

History. On penetration of the skin, hookworm larvae produce local tissue reactions with pruritus which may be aggravated by secondary bacterial infections. Pneumonitis and pulmonary symptoms are not so common as those seen in strongyloidiasis and ascariasis.[2, 29] Small worm loads do not produce symptoms. Moderate or severe infestation may result in anorexia or a voracious appetite, abdominal discomfort, flatulence, and epigastric pain which is peculiarly relieved by eating bulky food or ingesting clay (geophagia). In the heavier infections, there may be abdominal distention, weight loss, nausea and vomiting, and intermittent constipation and diarrhea. With very heavy infections, edema of the face and extremities and emaciation are present.

Physical Examination. Lightly infected patients have no significant physical findings. In the presence of moderate to severe hookworm disease, the skin is dry and has a yellow pallor which is striking in light-skinned patients. Perspiration is decreased. There is edema, particularly of the face and extremities. The abdomen may be distended with prominent borborygmi. There may be tenderness to palpation which in some patients will be limited to the upper abdomen, whereas in others it may be present over the entire abdomen. Rebound tenderness is unusual. In very severe, untreated cases, there may be marked congestive heart failure and anasarca.

DIAGNOSIS

Laboratory. Anemia occurring in hookworm disease is a classic iron deficiency anemia. Folic acid-deficient megaloblastic anemia may be masked by the severe iron deficiency. The differential white blood cell count generally demonstrates an eosinophilia of 7 to 15 per cent, and it may exceed 50 per cent in severe cases. There is hypoalbuminemia, hypercholesterol-emia, and, occasionally, proteinuria.

The eggs of all the species of hookworm are very similar. They are ovoid with a thin hyaline shell and rounded ends; they measure 35 to 40 μ by 55 to 75 μ.[2, 29] Within the egg varying stages of development may be observed. There may be a morula, or they may contain differentiated larvae. In light infections, concentration techniques are required to identify the ova. In heavy infections, direct fecal smears will contain sufficient eggs to permit diagnosis. Stool specimens which are allowed to stand for several hours may contain rhabditoid larvae which have hatched from the eggs. These may be differentiated from the rhabditoid larvae of other roundworms.[29]

Adult worms, when recovered, may be identified by the anatomy of the buccal capsule. A. duodenale has a buccal capsule containing ventral teeth, and N. americanus has semilunar plates.

Mucosal Biopsy—Duodenal Drainage. Pathologic findings vary in the small bowel mucosa studied by peroral small bowel mucosal biopsy, ranging from a normal mucosa to a severely abnormal flat mucosa. Occasionally a specimen may be obtained to which an adult worm is attached. The pathological appearance is not diagnostic of hookworm disease and probably represents the severe malnutrition from which most of these patients are suffering. Occasionally, adult worms may be recovered in the duodenal contents.

Radiographic Findings. Nonspecific radiographic findings are seen in hookworm disease. These include thickening and coarsening of the mucosal folds, flocculation and segmentation of barium, and hypermotility.

TREATMENT

The therapy of choice for A. duodenale is bephenium, one 5 g packet twice a day for one day.[30] For N. americanus bephenium, one 5 g packet twice daily for three days is given. Although tetrachloroethylene (0.12 ml per kilogram for a maximum of 5 ml) is an equally effective preparation, this agent may cause Ascaris, if present, to migrate. For both these species thiabendazole, 25 mg per kg twice daily

for two days, has been shown to be effective.[30]

TAPEWORMS OR CESTODES OF MAN

A number of adult tapeworms parasitize the intestinal tract of man.[2, 29] Some depend primarily or exclusively on man as the definitive host. The more important intestinal tapeworms of man are Diphyllobothrium latum, Taenia saginata, Taenia solium, and Hymenolepis nana.[2, 29] Echinococcus disease caused by Echinococcus granulosus and Echinococcus multilocularis will not be considered, because the manifestations of these diseases are not intestinal.

Infection is acquired through the ingestion of infected flesh of the intermediate host which is raw or inadequately cooked. Infection with H. nana occurs through contact with human feces; it is the most common tapeworm found in the southern United States.[2, 29]

Adult tapeworms consist of a scolex or head which anchors the worm to the intestinal mucosa of the host. The egg-producing units, which are known as proglottides, develop from the distal end of the scolex. The proglottides include immature, mature, and gravid forms. The worm does not contain an intestinal system and absorbs its nutrients through the integument from the host's intestinal contents or the host's intestinal mucosa. The entire tapeworm is called a strobila.

DIPHYLLOBOTHRIUM LATUM

D. latum, the fish tapeworm, is 3 to 10 meters long and may contain as many as 3000 or more proglottides. The scolex is a small spatulate structure with a pair of deep sulci which provide the attachment to the intestine. As with the other tapeworms, D. latum is hermaphroditic. Each proglottid contains both the male and the female genitalia.

PATHOGENESIS

Infection in man results from ingestion of infected raw fish.[2, 29] The patient may harbor single or multiple worms. The presence of more than one worm probably represents repeated consumption of the infected source.

The host may harbor large numbers of *D. latum* for decades without symptoms or ill effects. A small proportion of patients, most of whom are reported from Finland, develop tapeworm pernicious anemia. The worm most frequently attaches to the wall of the ileum, occasionally to the jejunum, and seldom to the colon. It has been found in the gallbladder.

The worm produces vitamin B_{12} deficiency in the host by competing with him for available vitamin B_{12}. Both the host and the worm are capable of taking up vitamin B_{12} whether or not tapeworm pernicious anemia is present.

DIAGNOSIS

History. Probably most patients with *D. latum* infestation are asymptomatic. If megaloblastic anemia caused by vitamin B_{12} deficiency develops, it cannot be differentiated from other types of megaloblastic anemia on the basis of a clinical history other than ingestion of raw fish. The nonspecific symptoms of anemia such as pallor, weakness, fatigue, and, in severe cases, congestive heart failure or angina pectoris may be present.

Occasionally the presence of large numbers of worms will cause a mechanical bowel obstruction. The excretory products from the worm may on occasion result in a systemic toxemia.

Laboratory. Diagnosis is made by finding the ova or proglottides of *D. latum* in the feces. The ovum measures 40 to 50 μ by 58 to 76 μ. It has a small operculum at one end of the egg and a tiny knob at the other. The proglottides may crawl around and deposit eggs in the perianal area. They may be found by swabbing or using cellophane tape to sample this particular region of the body. The proglottides of *D. latum* are somewhat wider than they are long. The mature proglottides are packed with genital organs. There are myriads of testes and a symmetrical bilobed ovary. A convoluted uterus is present which terminates in the uterine pore. A single worm may discharge as many as 1,000,000 ova per day.

Routine laboratory data are of little use in making a specific diagnosis of *D. latum* infection. There may be a mild eosinophilia, between 5 and 10 per cent, in the differential white blood cell count. When it is present, anemia is macrocytic and the bone marrow is megaloblastic.

Radiographic Features. The worm may cause some mild irritation of the intestinal mucosa at the point of attachment. This may be manifest by some minor thickening of the mucosal folds and perhaps some motor abnormalities. In small bowel barium studies and barium enemas, the worm may be apparent as a long, thin, translucent filling defect extending over a long length of intestine.

TREATMENT

The drug of choice is niclosamide, four 500 mg tablets chewed thoroughly in a single dose after a light meal.[30] Another drug of equal efficacy is paramomycin given in four doses of 1 g 15 minutes apart, followed by a purgative in one hour. The alternative drug of choice is quinacrine hydrochloride administered in four doses of 200 mg ten minutes apart, giving 600 mg of sodium bicarbonate with each dose.[30]

On passage of the worm, cure should not be assumed unless the scolex can be found and identified. If more than 10 meters of worm is recovered, it is likely that more than one worm is parasitizing the host.

TAENIA SOLIUM (PORK TAPEWORM)

PATHOGENESIS

Man acquires pork tapeworm infection through ingestion of raw or inadequately cooked pork. The larvae are digested from the pork flesh; the heads evaginate from the cysticerci and attach to the wall of the small intestine, developing into adult worms in five to 12 weeks. Patients usually harbor only one adult worm, although more than one may be present. They may live up to 25 years or more and be resistant to multiple attempts to evacuate them. Hyperinfection in untreated patients is common and leads to cysticercosis.

Cysticercosis occurs when man or other mammals ingest the egg of *T. solium*. On contact with gastric juices and subsequently with intestinal contents, the emergent oncospheres penetrate through the intestinal wall into the mesenteric vasculature and are distributed throughout the body. They are typically filtered out between muscles, where in 60 to 70 days they become cysticerci. This larval stage of the worm has been found in every organ and tissue of the body. The symptoms produced depend upon the location and the number present. Most frequently they are found in subcutaneous tissues, followed in frequency by eye, brain, musculature, heart, liver, lungs, and abdominal cavity.[2] The larvae provoke a typical cellular reaction, including infiltration of neutrophils, eosinophils, lymphocytes, plasma cells, and occasionally giant cells. Fibrosis follows necrosis of the capsule, with caseation and calcification of the larvae as the final events.

CLINICAL FEATURES

History. The adult worm does not result in serious illness, and its presence may provoke no symptoms. Occasionally vague abdominal discomfort, hunger pains, "chronic indigestion," and diarrhea or alternating diarrhea and constipation may occur.[2, 29] It may be responsible for anorexia, hyperesthesia, and nervous disorders caused by absorption of toxic substances from the worm. Rarely, the scolex perforates the intestinal wall and peritonitis results.

The symptoms of cysticercosis depend upon the location of the parasite. The precysticercus larvae in brain may produce little functional or symptomatic abnormality. When the larvae die, tissue reactions result in a great variety of cerebral symptoms and may result in a rapidly fatal course. Convulsive disorders are the most common manifestation of cerebral cysticerci, but they may also produce behavioral disorders, paresis, obstructive hydrocephalus, dysequilibrium, meningoencephalitis and failing vision.[2] Ocular cysticercosis results in uveitis, iritis, retinitis, choroidal atrophy, palpebral conjunctivitis, or cyst formation.

Physical Examination Physical examination does not contribute to the diagnosis of *T. solium* infection. Occasionally the presence of proglottides may be found on the finger following a rectal examination, or they may be seen through the sigmoidoscope.

The physical manifestations of cysticercosis do not permit differentiation from other space-occupying lesions, whether cerebral or visceral. Ocular involvement of cysticercosis may be detected by retinoscopy.

DIAGNOSIS

Laboratory Findings. Other than a moderate eosinophilia, up to 13 per cent, the routine laboratory studies are usually within normal limits. The ova of *T. solium* are spherical or slightly ovoid in configuration and measure 31 to 43 μ in diameter. The ova have a thick-walled shell consisting of many truncated prisms and originally are provided with a thin, hyaline mother embryonic membrane. The fully developed oncosphere within the ova usually has three pairs of hooklets. The ova of *T. solium* cannot be distinguished from those of *T. saginata*. Definitive diagnosis depends upon the recovery of typical gravid proglottides. They are longer than they are wide, and the main lateral side arms of the uterus number from seven to 13 on each side. Identification of the scolex on evacuation differentiates it from that of *T. saginata*. It is about 1 mm in diameter, and has four large, deeply cupped suckers and a conspicuous rounded rostellum with a double row of large and small hooklets.

The definitive diagnosis of cysticercus disease depends on excision and microscopic examination. The invaginated scolex of the larvae has four suckers and anterior hooklets that are an exact miniature of the scolex of the adult.[2]

Radiographic Features. The worm may be detected in the intestine on barium studies. Radiographs are useful in making a diagnosis of cysticercosis after the parasite has calcified. They may be found in the musculature and in the central nervous system by high penetration X-ray films. Although calcification usually occurs in the scolex, the cyst wall may resemble an enveloping eggshell.

TREATMENT

Treatment is indicated as soon as possible after the identification of *T. solium* infection because of the serious danger of autoinfection and cysticercosis.[2,29] The therapy of choice for the adult worm is quinacrine hydrochloride in four doses of 200 mg, ten minutes apart, giving 600 mg of sodium bicarbonate with each dose.[30] An effective alternative drug is paramomycin, four doses of 1 g 15 minutes apart, followed by a purgative one hour later.

No medical therapy is available for cysticercus disease. Excision is indicated whenever possible. Ocular cysticercosis may be treated by removal of the cyst rather than enucleation of the eye. Optimal therapy is removal of the cysticercus while it is still living.[2]

T. SAGINATA (BEEF TAPEWORM)

PATHOGENESIS

Infection with *Taenia saginata* is through the ingestion of inadequately cooked or raw beef containing viable cysticercus larvae. The mature eggs are ingested by cattle; on hatching in the duodenum they penetrate the intestinal mucosa and are carried in the circulation to the striated muscle. They develop into *Cysticercus bovis* in 60 to 75 days. On digestion of the infected flesh in the intestine, the cysticercus is released and the scolex evaginates and attaches to the intestinal wall. The adult lives with its scolex embedded in the mucosa of the small bowel.

T. saginata is considerably longer than *T. solium* and may attain lengths of 25 meters or more. Ordinarily, they measure between 12 and 15 feet and have between 1000 and 2000 proglottides at any given time. Their effects on the host are due to their large size, which may result in mechanical bowel obstruction, undernutrition, and release of toxic metabolites which are absorbed.

CLINICAL PICTURE

History. The worm produces substantial disturbance in normal intestinal function. It derives its nutrition by diverting digested material from the host. Diarrhea and hunger pains frequently develop, and loss of weight may occur. Its presence may result in hyperphagia or in anorexia. Oc-

casionally it may produce acute intestinal obstruction. Proglottides lodged in the appendix have caused acute appendicitis. Absorption of toxic products of the worm may result in allergic symptoms in the form of edema of the face, abdomen, and lower limbs. The most common symptoms are the discomfort and embarrassment of proglottides crawling from the anus.

Cysticercosis caused by the larvae of *T. saginata* is not nearly so common as that occurring in the presence of *T. solium*. Beef cysticercosis, however, has the same manifestations, depending upon the site and number of cysticerci present.

Physical Examination. There may be edema of the face and extremities in patients having allergic reactions to absorbed toxins. Physical evidence of weight loss may occasionally be present. Proglottides may be observed around the anus, may be recovered on the examining finger following rectal examination, or may be seen occasionally at sigmoidoscopy.

DIAGNOSIS

Laboratory Findings. Except for a moderate eosinophilia of the differential white blood cell count, the laboratory findings are usually normal. The presence of ova in feces establishes infection with a species of Taenia, but differentiation from *T. solium* is not possible. No eggs may be present in the stool, but all patients pass gravid proglottides. The definitive diagnosis is established by examining the proglottid, which is pressed between two slides, and counting the main lateral arms of the uterus. There are usually 15 to 20 main lateral branches on each side of the main uterine stem in *T. saginata*. Overripe proglottides lose the distinctive appearance. Administration of a purgative will cause discharge of more proximal proglottides and aid in establishing the diagnosis. Identification of the scolex after therapy also aids diagnosis and ensures that the entire worm has been evacuated. The head is quadrate with a diameter of 1 to 2 mm, and has four hemispherical suckers. The apex is somewhat concave and may be pigmented. There are no hooklets. Diagnosis of cysticercosis depends upon excision and microscopic examination.

Radiographic Features. The worm may

be detected as a long, translucent filling defect on barium studies of the small intestine and colon. Cysticercus lesions may be identified by radiographic techniques similar to those used in the identification of cysticercosis caused by *T. solium*.

TREATMENT

The treatment of *T. saginata* is the same as that of *D. latum*, i.e., niclosamide, four 500 mg tablets chewed thoroughly in a single dose after a light meal, or paromomycin, four doses of 1 g 15 minutes apart followed by a purgative in one hour. Quinacrine hydrochloride in dosages of 200 mg 10 minutes apart each given with 600 mg of bicarbonate is an effective alternative drug.[30]

HYMENOLEPIS NANA (DWARF TAPEWORM)

PATHOGENESIS

H. nana is the only human tapeworm which has no intermediate host. Infection is direct from patient to patient upon ingestion of embryonated eggs. It occurs more often in children than in adults and has a higher incidence in family and institutional groups. The worms hatch in the stomach or small intestine, and the free oncospheres penetrate the villi and metamorphose into cercocysts. When the larvae migrate into the lumen of the intestine, they become attached by their scolices to the mucosa and mature into adult worms in two weeks. Continued heavy infection in man is probably due to internal autoinfection.

CLINICAL PICTURE

History. Large numbers of *H. nana* within the intestine produce considerable irritation. The more common symptoms are due to absorption of metabolic waste products of the parasite.[2] The major symptoms are headache, dizziness, anorexia, inanition, pruritus of the nose and anus, intermittent diarrhea, and abdominal distress.[2] Most patients are restless and irritable, and a few have convulsive disorders.

Physical Examination. There are no specific physical findings to indicate *H. nana* infection. Evidence of weight loss may be seen.

DIAGNOSIS

Laboratory Findings. The laboratory findings are nonspecific. An eosinophilia of 5 to 15 per cent of the differential white blood cell count may be observed.

The diagnosis is based upon finding characteristic eggs of *H. nana*. They are spherical, have a hyaline membrane, and measure 30 to 40 μ in diameter. The egg contains an oncosphere enclosed in an inner envelope with two polar thickenings each having four to eight polar filaments.[2] Within the oncosphere are three pairs of lancet-shaped hooklets. The adult worm is 25 to 30 mm in length by 1 mm in diameter. The tiny scolex is 0.2 mm in diameter, rhomboidal and has four hemispherical suckers. There is a short rostellum containing 20 to 30 spines in one ring.

Radiographic Features. Few data are available of the small intestinal appearance in *H. nana* infection. There may be nonspecific changes, including thickening and coarsening of the mucosal folds, excess secretions within the intestine, and rapid transit of barium.

TREATMENT

Niclosamide at a dosage of four 500 mg tablets chewed thoroughly in a single daily dose for five to seven days is the treatment of choice. Paromomycin is another effective drug given in a dosage of 45 mg per kilogram daily for five days. Quinacrine hydrochloride is the recommended alternative drug. It is given in four doses of 200 mg ten minutes apart, with 600 mg of sodium bicarbonate with each dose. The regimen may be repeated in one to two weeks if necessary.[30]

TREMATODES (FLATWORMS)

SCHISTOSOMIASIS (SCHISTOSOMA JAPONICUM)

The lesions produced by *Schistosoma japonicum* are the same as those seen in *S.*

mansoni and *S. haematobium*[2] (see p. 1396). Since the egg-laying female resides in the superior mesenteric venous system, the small bowel is more severely affected than with other species of Schistosoma, although *S. mansoni* involvement of the small intestine is exceeded only by that of the colon.[2]

PATHOGENESIS

The schistosome ova are the cause of overt disease. Few data support the contribution of toxins produced by worms, dead worms, or malnutrition.[41] The granulomatous reaction in the host appears to be due to a delayed hypersensitivity; in experimental animals this can be partially suppressed by immunosuppressive drugs.[2, 41]

The ova are deposited in small branches of the mesenteric venules in the submucosa. Some are extruded through the mucosa and discharged in the stools. As increasing numbers of ova become lodged in the submucosa and mucosa, infiltration of eosinophils, plasma cells, lymphocytes, and polymorphonuclear leukocytes results in pseudoabscesses.[2] The adult worms migrate to other sites and deposit ova at increasingly long levels of the intestine. Occasionally, they migrate into the vena cava and deposit eggs in the pulmonary vasculature and at other diverse areas throughout the body, including the brain. The late events in the granulomatous reaction include fibrosis, polypoid lesions, and stenosis of multiple segments of the small bowel. Intestinal obstruction is a common outcome in *S. japonicum* infection. Although few data are available, there appears to be little interference with digestion and absorption even with extensive parasitization of the intestine.[42, 43] *S. japonicum* infection should be considered in any patient with liver or bowel disease who has resided in an endemic area. Living *S. japonicum* ova have been demonstrated in such a patient in whom there was no possibility of reinfection for 47 years.[44]

CLINICAL PICTURE

History. The manifestations of schistosomiasis are protean and depend upon the number and location of the ova.[2] In acute schistosomiasis caused by *S. mansoni*, watery diarrhea occurs in all patients.[42] In some cases it is bloody. The clinical manifestations of *S. japonicum* infection include dysentery, cirrhosis of the liver, splenomegaly, appendicitis, intestinal obstruction, pulmonary hypertension, vascular occlusion, varying cerebral disorders, and varying hypersensitivity syndromes caused by products of the ova.[2] With bowel obstruction or stenosis, abdominal colic and distention may be prominent. With increasing cirrhosis and portal hypertension, the development of ascites is seen.

Physical Examination. The patient is frequently weak, pallid and cachectic. There may be marked dyspnea on slight exertion. Dilatation of the superficial veins of the abdomen and thorax is frequent. Ascites may or may not be present. The liver may or may not be palpable, but with cirrhosis and portal hypertension, splenomegaly is present. The diaphragms may be high owing to encroachment of the abdominal viscera upon the thorax. There may be both upper and lower abdominal distention caused by thickening of the mesentery and the omentum. Occasionally, the thick mesentery and omentum are palpable as masses of irregular nature within the abdomen.[2]

DIAGNOSIS

Laboratory Findings. There are ordinarily an eosinophilia and a leukocytosis which tend to decrease with chronicity. There may be hypoalbuminemia caused by either malnutrition or protein-losing enteropathy.[45] This has only been reported with schistosomal polyposis of the colon. Hypergammaglobulinemia may be present. Unless there is severe diarrhea or dysentery, more usual in acute schistosomiasis, the electrolytes are normal.

Specific diagnosis depends upon identification of the characteristic eggs in the stools or in rectal, small bowel mucosal, or liver biopsy. Although *S. japonicum* affects the small bowel largely, *S. mansoni* has also occasionally been diagnosed on the basis of small bowel mucosal biopsy.[43] Examination of feces requires the use of concentration techniques, particularly in the late chronic stages. The egg of *S. ja-*

ponicum contains a miracidium within it.[2] It has a depression at one end and a tiny lateral spinous process. It measures 70 to 100 μ by 50 to 65 μ. The ova are best found in tissue by examining a fresh crushed preparation. The biopsy specimen, rectal, small bowel, or liver, is placed in water for three to five minutes. It is compressed tightly between two microscopic slides. On separation of the slides a drop of water is added to the tissue and the slide cover-slipped.[29] Schistosome ova are easily identified with a low power objective.

Radiographic Features. No specific radiographic features establish a diagnosis of schistosomiasis. However, plain films of the abdomen may reveal air fluid-filled loops of small intestine with dilatation in the presence of stenotic or obstructing lesions of the small intestine. In the absence of obstruction, barium studies of the small intestine may demonstrate dilatation interspersed with stenoses.

TREATMENT

The treatment of choice is antimony potassium tartrate in a 0.5 per cent solution.[30] It is administered in intravenous doses of 8, 12, 16, 20, 24, and 28 ml on alternate days continuing at 28 ml on alternate days for ten doses. Stibophen, which contains 8.5 mg of antimony per milliliter, has been given in dosages of 8 to 10 ml per day, but is extremely toxic. Administration is intramuscular for ten days or longer. Another alternative drug is antimony sodium dimercaptosuccinate, administered intramuscularly at a dosage of 40 mg per kilogram in five divided doses given once or twice a week.

FASCIOLOPSIS BUSKI (GIANT INTESTINAL FLUKE)

F. buski is a common parasite in the Orient. Indigenous cases have not been described elsewhere. It is a common parasite of man and swine.[2]

PATHOGENESIS

Man is infected when he ingests the raw pods, roots, stems, and bulbs of certain water plants which grow in endemic foci containing the appropriate molluscan hosts.[2] Water in the shallow ponds or lakes containing the plant vectors is contaminated by human or swine feces which contain immature viable eggs. The eggs mature, hatch, and infect suitable snails. The cercariae escape the snails and encyst on the plants. The larvae of *F. buski* excyst in the duodenum and attach to the duodenal and jejunal mucosa. In about 90 days they develop into large, elongated, ovoidal worms measuring 20 to 75 mm in length, 8 to 20 mm in breadth, and 0.5 to 3 mm in thickness. They damage the mucosa and cause deep ulcerations at the site of attachment; large numbers may produce intestinal obstruction, and absorption of toxic products of the worm results in systemic symptoms. In very heavy infections, they may be found adherent to the pyloric mucosa and even in the large bowel. Erosions lead to hemorrhage, abscesses may develop, and large numbers of parasites result in acute ileus.[2]

CLINICAL PICTURE

History. Initial symptoms of diarrhea with hunger pains occur toward the end of the incubation period. In light infections these may be the only symptoms. In heavy infections, pain may mimic peptic ulcer and the patient may become asthenic. Edema of the face, abdominal wall, and lower extremities is common. Ascites commonly develops, accompanied by generalized abdominal pain. There may be intermittent constipation. The stool is typically greenish yellow and foul-smelling, and contains undigested food. There may be hyperphagia or anorexia with nausea and vomiting. Ultimately, there is extreme prostration, which may be followed by death in untreated patients.[2]

Physical Examination. Edema of the face and extremities may be prominent. Ascites is present frequently. There may be severe weakness or even coma.[2]

DIAGNOSIS

Laboratory Findings. Leukocytosis is often found with an absolute eosinophilia and a neutrophilic leukopenia. Occasionally there is lymphocytosis. Other laboratory abnormalities depend upon the duration and magnitude of the diarrhea.

The diagnosis rests specifically on recovery of the eggs. They are large, shaped like a hen's egg, and almost identical to the ova of *F. hepatica*. They measure 130 to 140 μ by 80 to 85 μ, and are operculated and unembryonated when passed. Each worm is capable of discharging 25,000 eggs per day. The miracidium does not develop within the egg until it is deposited in water.

TREATMENT

Hexylresorcinol crystoids in dosages of 0.4 g in patients one to seven years of age and to 1 g in patients 13 or over produce cure in 54 per cent of patients, and a 90 to 99 per cent reduction in worm load in the remainder.[2] Tetrachloroethylene as administered for *N. americanus*, i.e., a single dose of 0.12 ml per kilogram up to a maximum of 5 ml, is also effective.

MISCELLANEOUS PARASITIC INFECTIONS

A number of other parasites whose major manifestations are primarily nonintestinal may produce small bowel symptoms. Some of these organisms gain access to the body through the intestinal tract.

TRICHINELLA SPIRALIS

PATHOGENESIS

Man acquires trichinosis through the ingestion of raw or rare flesh infected with cysts of *Trichinella spiralis*.[2, 29] These cysts are digested from the meat in the stomach, and on passage into the small intestine they excyst and the larvae invade the intestinal mucosa. The larvae mature into adults in five to seven days, at which time the adult worms mate and the female begins discharging larvae in the tissues. The larvae have a predilection for striated muscle and myocardium, where they ultimately encyst. Although both adults and encysted larvae of *T. spiralis* may develop in the same host, two hosts are required to complete the life cycle. The infection is propagated in nature by the black rat and the brown rat which are cannibalistic. Although pork is the main source of infection in man, trichinosis has resulted from the ingestion of flesh from wild boars, bears, and other mammals.

DIAGNOSIS

History. The intestinal symptoms of trichinosis may begin within 24 hours of ingestion of the infective organism.[2, 29] During the five- to seven-day incubation period, irritation and inflammation of the intestine occur at the site of larval invasion. The symptoms of nausea, vomiting, diarrhea or dysentery, colic, and profuse diaphoresis may mimic acute food poisoning or bacterial infection. Bright scarlet macules or maculopapular rashes may occur on the trunk and limbs.

During the period of larval migration to the muscles, there are muscular pains, dyspnea, difficulty with mastication, pharyngeal and laryngeal dysfunction, and at times spastic paralysis. There is frequently a tender lymphadenopathy, at times salivary gland enlargement mimicking mumps, and a remittent fever of 40 to 41°C. There may be periorbital edema. Central nervous system symptoms include those of encephalitis and meningitis, ophthalmoplegia, or deafness, or the infection may resemble amyotrophic lateral sclerosis.

During the period of encystation, there may be cachexia, edema, and extreme dehydration. There may be protean neurological signs resulting from cerebral damage. In severe cases, the patient may expire from toxemia, myocarditis, pneumonitis, peritonitis, pleurisy, nephritis, or central nervous system involvement.

The great majority of patients with trichinosis do not have any symptoms, the clinical disease occurring in only approximately 5 per cent of individuals infected.[2, 29]

Physical Examination. During the incubation or diarrheal phase there may be few or no physical findings to suggest trichinosis. During the phase of larval migration, the cardinal physical finding is muscle tenderness. There may be spasticity of the limbs. Periorbital edema may be prominent. There is frequently a tender lymphadenitis. Cardiac arrhythmias may occur and congestive heart failure may be present.

Laboratory Findings. The white blood cell count typically reveals a leukocytosis with a marked hypereosinophilia ranging between 20 and 75 per cent or more. Rarely, adult worms may be recovered in the feces during the diarrheal stage of the disease. Larvae may rarely be found in the blood or spinal fluid or in the mother's milk during migration. The definitive diagnosis is made by muscle biopsy after the larvae have lodged in muscle. If they cannot be identified in small compressed samples of deltoid, biceps, pectoralis, or gastrocnemius muscle, digestion with artificial gastric juice will provide a concentrate, increasing diagnostic accuracy.[2]

TREATMENT

Trichinosis is frequently not considered during the incubation period. However, it should be considered in the differential diagnosis in any patient presenting with the aforementioned symptoms and findings. It is particularly important to procure a history of ingestion of raw meat, particularly pork. During the acute stage, piperazine citrate may be of use in ridding the intestine of adult worms.[29] Thiabendazole has been shown to be of effect in experimental animals when given 24 hours after inoculation.[2, 29] Otherwise, there is no specific therapy, but corticosteroids should be used for severe symptoms during the period of migration and encystation. Prednisone in dosages of 20 to 40 mg daily and tapered after three to five days is customarily used. Thiabendazole in dosages of 25 mg per kilogram twice daily until symptoms subside or severe toxic effects occur has been suggested as an alternative drug.[30]

AMERICAN TRYPANOSOMIASIS (CHAGAS' DISEASE)

Although symptomatic Chagas' disease has been confined to the South American continent and Central America, two indigenous cases and nine seropositive asymptomatic patients have been diagnosed in south Texas.[46, 47] In patients surviving acute infection with *T. cruzi* and developing the chronic form of illness, myocardial disease is the most common manifestation. Megaesophagus and megacolon are the most common intestinal manifestations of American trypanosomiasis. However, small intestinal dilatation and aperistalsis are also seen. At postmortem examination, even in patients with asymptomatic *T. cruzi* involvement of the intestine, the small intestine has a significant reduction in submucosal and myenteric autonomic plexuses.[47, 48]

American trypanosomiasis could prove to be a significant health problem in the United States. There is a large reservoir of *T. cruzi* infection in animals in the southern United States. Infection has been detected in Arizona, California, New Mexico, Texas, Louisiana, Georgia, Florida, and Maryland.[46] The epidemiologically important insects, the reduviid bugs of the *Triatominae* group, also have the same wide geographic distribution.[46] Infection is transmitted when the reduviid bug infected with *T. cruzi* bites the victim. On biting, the arthropod discharges feces. The parasite is introduced through the skin by the patient scratching the bite. The apparent difference between the South American reduviid bugs and those occurring in the United States is that the species in the United States do not defecate upon biting. It is possible that effective vectors may be introduced in the United States through routes such as the opening of the Pan-American highway.

PATHOGENESIS

Metacyclic trypanosomes are deposited from the feces of the bug during the time he is taking a blood meal.[2] Characteristically, deposition occurs on or near mucous membranes, particularly on the outer canthus of the eye or around the nose or lips. The invading organisms are phagocytosed by histiocytes in the corium and invade adipose and subcutaneous muscle cells. They multiply in this location as Leishmania. When the histiocytes and other parasitized cells rupture on the fourth or fifth day, the Leishmania forms are taken up by regional lymph nodes, from where at variable intervals they are discharged through the blood and lymphatic circulation and spread to diverse areas of the body.

The signs and symptoms of Chagas' disease are due to the intracellular Leishmania forms. When the host cell ruptures, large numbers escape and temporarily enter the circulation as trypanosome forms. In the intestine, escaping leishmaniae apparently result in release of a toxin which destroys the submucosal and the myenteric plexuses.[48] The end result is enteromegaly which at times may be massive.[48]

DIAGNOSIS

History. Acute Chagas' disease occurs most often in children. It is characterized by high fever and marked edema, particularly with a periorbital distribution and often involving the entire body. The acute stage lasts approximately 20 to 30 days.

Chronic Chagas' disease depends upon the major involvement within the body. Most commonly the symptoms are cardiac, primarily manifested as arrhythmias and congestive heart failure. With megaesophagus the history is indistinguishable from achalasia. With megacolon infrequent bowel movements and chronic constipation are the cardinal symptoms. With dilatation of the small intestine diarrhea or constipation may be part of the picture. Data are not available, but in the presence of stasis one could speculate that bacterial overgrowth may play an important part in the pathogenesis.

PHYSICAL EXAMINATION

In patients with acute Chagas' disease, the periorbital edema of one or both eyes is spectacular. The victim may appear to be suffering from myxedema. There is usually enlargement of the thyroid, lymph nodes, and salivary glands, and hepatosplenomegaly is present. In chronic Chagas' disease involving the intestine, there may be evidence of weight loss and abdominal distention caused by the markedly dilated bowel.

LABORATORY FINDINGS

Routine laboratory data provide no clue to the diagnosis of Chagas' disease. Diagnosis depends upon demonstration of the trypanosome forms in blood during periods when the leishmaniae rupture cells.[2] During febrile periods if the blood films are negative, guinea pig inoculation will frequently recover the organism.[2] Leishmania forms may be detected in bone marrow, spleen, or enlarged lymph nodes. The most usual immunological method for diagnosis of American trypanosomiasis is a complement fixation technique.[2] Other immunological tests are under investigation but not widely applied. Xenodiagnosis has been used but is relatively insensitive, diagnosing fewer than 50 per cent of patients infected with chronic Chagas' disease. Trypanosome-free laboratory reduviid bugs are allowed to bite suspected victims. The trypanosomes multiply rapidly in the intestinal tract of the insect, and examination of the intestine will reveal flagellated trypanosomes in ten to 30 days.

TREATMENT

There is no successful treatment available for either acute or chronic Chagas' disease. Primaquine phosphate, 10 mg daily for 21 days, has been recommended for acute Chagas' disease.[30] Patients with achalasia caused by Chagas' disease may be treated with either brusque pneumatic dilatation of the esophagus or esophagomyotomy. Occasionally, aperistaltic segments of intestine which are responsible for symptoms may be resected.

OTHER PATHOGENIC INTESTINAL PARASITES

An astonishingly large number of other parasites have been identified and incriminated in human intestinal disease.[2] Many are primary parasites of animals, or even plants, and human infection has been accidental. In others, the intestinal involvement has been coincidental with a wider systemic parasitism.

A fatal leishmanial enteritis occurs during epidemic kala-azar.[49] Sections and scrapings of the intestinal mucosa contain myriads of Donovan bodies. It is likely that many patients with visceral leishmaniasis terminating with a fatal enteritis have parasitism of the small intestine. In the past this has been dismissed as typhoid fever.

NONPATHOGENIC PARASITES

A number of parasites are frequently recovered in stool for which no evidence of pathogenicity exists.[2, 29] Even though they are most frequently found in diarrheal stools, it is probable that they are not responsible for the patient's symptoms. These are most commonly protozoa and include *Retortamonas intestinalis, Enteromonas hominis, Chylomastix mesnili, Trichomonas hominis*, and a large number of nonpathogenic amebae. If these sorts of organisms are detected and are the only ones present in feces, no treatment is indicated.

CONTROL AND PREVENTION OF INTESTINAL PARASITES

The control and prevention of intestinal parasitic diseases are the joint provinces of the practicing physician, the epidemiologist, public health experts, food inspectors, sanitary engineers, educators, and social agencies. Intestinal parasitism reflects deficiencies in standard of living, sanitation facilities, and personal hygiene. Infections acquired through the ingestion of food indicate poor control of sources of food production such as slaughterhouses as well as the personal and social behavior and eating habits of the patient. High rates of arthropod-borne diseases reflect low socioeconomic conditions, poor housing, and inadequate sanitation. In all areas of high prevalence of intestinal parasitism, lack of education and ignorance of the victims are prominent factors.

The practicing physician shares a primary role in control and prevention of parasitic diseases. It is he who is responsible for the accurate diagnosis, evaluation, and successful treatment of the patient. He is the individual upon whom the responsibility should fall to examine the family and close contacts for other infections or to refer them to appropriate public health facilities. He may be in the best position to determine the source of infection and to report it promptly. He can best advise the patient and family on means of avoiding reinfection. He should be the individual to initiate control and preventive measures through support of local health officials and educational activities.

The foundation of successful control of the protozoa and roundworms is adequate sanitation. Most important are sanitary disposal of human excreta, adequate processing of sewage, and the avoidance of promiscuous defecation. Adequate processing of water supplies will eliminate waterborne infection. The simple expedient of

wearing shoes could eliminate hookworm disease and strongyloidiasis.

Control of trichinosis, the tapeworm infections, and cysticercosis includes adequate inspection at the slaughterhouse, condemnation of infected meat, and thorough cooking or freezing of the meat prior to ingestion.

Control of schistosomiasis, which is estimated to affect 300,000,000 persons, could develop in several different directions. These would include adequate sewage treatment and sanitary disposal of human feces, the use of chemicals to eliminate the intermediate hosts and the free-living cercariae, education of populations in endemic areas to avoid infested water, and effective therapy of infected patients. Posted warnings in the vicinity of infested water could be successful if the population is literate.

A distinctive feature of parasitic infection as opposed to many viral and bacterial diseases is that no successful immunization is available. Nor does a previous infection confer any degree of immunity which might prevent reinfection. Accordingly, the most effective preventive measures are those which eliminate the possibility of exposure.

REFERENCES

1. Dobell, C. Discovery of intestinal protozoa in man. Proc. Roy. Soc. Med. *13*:1, 1920.
2. Faust, E. C., Russell, P. F., and Jung, B. C. Craig and Faust's Clinical Parasitology. 8th ed. Philadelphia, Lea and Febiger, 1970.
3. Veghelyi, P. Celiac disease imitated by giardiasis. Amer. J. Dis. Child. 57:894, 1939.
4. Cortner, J. A. Giardiasis, a cause of celiac syndrome. A.M.A. J. Dis. Child. 98:311, 1959.
5. Hoskins, L. C., Winawer, S. J., Broitman, S. A., Gottlieb, L. S., and Zamcheck, N. Clinical giardiasis and intestinal malabsorption. Gastroenterology 53:265, 1967.
6. Morecki, R., and Parker, J. G. Ultrastructural studies of the human *Giardia lamblia* and subadjacent mucosa in a subject with steatorrhea. Gastroenterology 52:151, 1967.
7. Moore, G. T., Gross, W. M., McGuire, D., Mollahan, C. S., Gleason, N. N., Healy, G. S., and Newton, L. H. Epidemic giardiasis at a ski resort. New Eng. J. Med. 281:402, 1969.
8. Babb, R. R., Peck, O. C., and Vescia, F. G. Giardiasis. A cause of traveler's diarrhea. J.A.M.A. 217:1359, 1971.
9. Veghelyi, P. V. Giardiasis. Amer. J. Dis. Child. 59:293, 1950.
10. Yardley, J. H., and Bayless, T. M. Giardiasis. Gastroenterology 52:301, 1967.
11. Brandborg, L. L., Tankersley, C. B., Gottlieb, S.,

Barancik, M., and Sartor, V. E. Histological demonstration of mucosal invasion by *Giardia lamblia* in man. Gastroenterology, 52: 143, 1967.

12. Hermans, P. G., Huizenga, K. A., Hoffman, H. N., Brown, A. L., Jr., and Markowitz, H. Dysgammaglobulinemia associated with nodular lymphoid hyperplasia of the small intestine. Amer. J. Med. 40:78, 1966.

13. Ament, M. E., and Rubin, C. E. Relation of giardiasis to abnormal intestinal structure and function in gastrointestinal immunodeficiency syndromes. Gastroenterology 62: 216, 1972.

14. Petersen, H. Giardiasis (lambliasis). Scand. J. Gastroent. 7: (Suppl. 14), 1972.

15. Block, C., and Tuckman, L. R. Diffuse small intestinal abnormality due to *Giardia lamblia* with roentgen and clinical reversibility after therapy: Case report. J. Mt. Sinai Hosp. 36:116, 1967.

16. Yardley, J. H., Takano, J., and Hendrix, T. R. Epithelial and other mucosal lesions of the jejunum in giardiasis. Jejunal biopsy studies. Bull. Johns Hopkins Hosp. 116:413, 1964.

17. Finegold, S. M., Bartlett, J. G., and Sutter, V. L. New antimicrobial drugs for anaerobic infections. Clin. Res. 20:165, 1972.

18. Jarpa Gana, A. Coccidiosis humana. Biologica (Santiago) 39:3, 1966.

19. Zaman, V. Observations on human *Isospora*. Trans. Roy. Soc. Trop. Med. Hyg. 62:556, 1968.

20. Klebs, E. Psorospermein in Innern von thierischen Zellen. Virchow's Arch. Pathol. Anat. Physiol. Klin. Med. 16:188, 1858.

21. Virchow, R. Helminthologische Notizen. 4. Zur Kenntniss der Wurmknoten. Virchow's Arch. Pathol. Anat. Physiol. Klin. Med. 18:523, 1860.

22. Davies, S. F. M., Joyner, L. P., and Kendall, B. S. Coccidiosis. Edinburgh and London, Oliver and Boyd, 1963.

23. Smitskamp, H., and Oey-Muller, E. Geographical distribution and clinical significance of human coccidiosis. Trop. Geogr. Med. 18:133, 1966.

24. Barksdale, W. L., and Routh, C. F. *Isospora hominis* infections among American personnel in the Southwest Pacific. Amer. J. Trop. Med. 28:639, 1948.

25. Pout, D. D. Villous atrophy and coccidiosis. Nature 213:306, 1967.

26. Webster, B. H. Human isosporiasis: A report of three cases with necropsy findings in one case. Amer. J. Trop. Med. Hyg. 6:86, 1957.

27. Brandborg, L. L., Goldberg, S. G., and Breidenbach, W. C. Human coccidiosis—a possible cause of malabsorption. The life cycle in small bowel mucosal biopsies as a diagnostic feature. New Eng. J. Med. 283:1306, 1970.

28. French, J. M., Whitby, J. L., and Whitfield, A. G. W. Steatorrhea in a man infected with coccidiosis (*Isospora belli*). Gastroenterology 47:642, 1964.

29. Juniper, K., Jr. Parasitic diseases of the intestinal tract. *In* Gastroenterologic Medicine, M. Paulson (ed.). Philadelphia, Lea and Febiger, 1969.

30. Handbook of Antimicrobial Therapy, 14: No. 2, Issue 340. New Rochelle, N. Y., The Medical Letter, Inc., 1972.

31. O'Brien, W., and England, M. W. S. Military tropical sprue from Southeast Asia. Brit. Med. J. 2:1157, 1966.

32. Giles, H. M. Gastrointestinal helminthiasis. Brit. Med. J. 2:475, 1968.

33. DeFigueiredo, N. J., Rubens, J., DeCarvalho, H. T., and daSilva, Jr. R. Hallazgos histopatologicos del intestino delgado en diferentes enteroparasitosis. Bol. Chileno Parasitol. 28:57, 1968.

34. Cruz, T., Reboucas, G., and Rocha, H. Fatal strongyloidiasis in patients receiving corticosteroids. New Eng. J. Med. 275:1093, 1966.

35. Civantos, F., and Robinson, M. J. Fatal strongyloidiasis following corticosteroid therapy. Amer. J. Dig. Dis. 14:643, 1969.

36. Whalen, G. G., Strickland, G. T., Cross, J. H., Rosenberg, G. B., Gutman, R. A., Walton, R. H., Vylanglo, R. H., and Dizon, J. J. Intestinal capillariasis. A new disease in man. Lancet 1:13, 1969.

37. Blackman, V., Marsden, P. D., Banwell, J., and Craggs, M. H. Albumin metabolism in hookworm disease. Trans. Roy. Soc. Trop. Med. 59:472, 1965.

38. Mayoral, L. G., Tripathy, K., Garcia, F. T., and Ghitis, J. Intestinal malabsorption and parasitic disease. The role of protein malnutrition. Gastroenterology 50:856, 1966.

39. Banwell, J. G., Marsden, P. D., Blackman, V., Leonard, P. G., and Hutt, M. S. R. Hookworm infection and intestinal absorption among Africans in Uganda. Amer. J. Trop. Med. Hyg. 16:304, 1967.

40. Tandon, B. N., Kohli, R. K., Saroya, A. K., Ramachandran, K., and Prakash, P. M. Role of parasites in the pathogenesis of intestinal malabsorption in hookworm disease. Gut 10:293, 1969.

41. Marsden, P. D., and Schultz, M. G. Intestinal parasites. Gastroenterology 57:724, 1969.

42. Domingo, E. O., and Warren, K. S. Pathology and pathophysiology of the small intestine in murine *Schistosomiasis mansoni*, including a review of the literature. Gastroenterology 50:231, 1969.

43. Halsted, C. H., Sheir, S., and Raasch, F. O. The small intestine in human schistosomiasis. Gastroenterology 57:622, 1969.

44. Lehman, J. S., Jr., Faird, Z., Bassily, S., Haxton, J., Wahab, M. F. A., and Kent, D. C. Intestinal protein loss in schistosomal polyposis of the colon. Gastroenterology 59:433, 1970.

45. Hall, S. C., and Kehoe, E. L. Prolonged survival of *Schistosoma japonicum*. Calif. Med. 113:75, 1970.

46. Woody, N. C., and Woody, H. B. American trypanosomiasis. I. Clinical and epidemiologic background of Chagas' disease in the United States. J. Pediat. 58:568, 1961.

47. Winslow, D. J., and Chaffee, E. F. Preliminary investigations on Chagas' disease. Military Med. 130:826, 1965.

48. Köberle, F. Enteromegaly and cardiomegaly in Chagas' disease. Gut 4:399, 1963.

49. Sati, M. H. Leishmanial enteritis as a cause of intractable diarrhoea and death. Sudan Med. J. 1: (NS) 216, 1962.

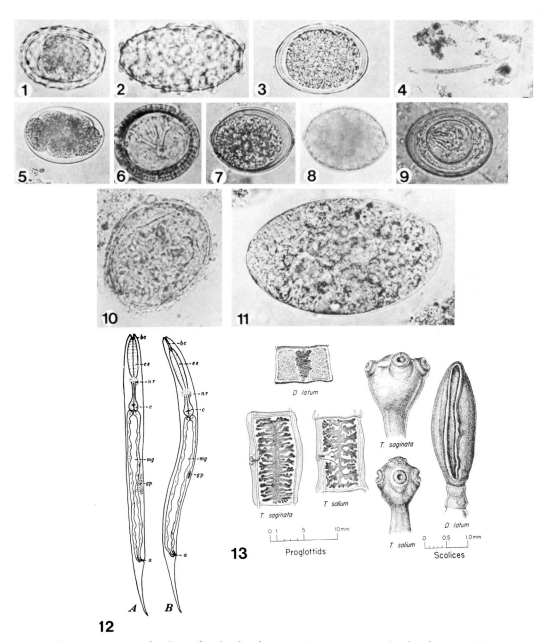

Figure 75–13. *1, Ascaris lumbricoides,* fertilized egg, × 500. *2, Ascaris,* unfertilized egg, × 500. *3, Ascaris,* decorticated egg, × 500. *4,* Rhabditiform larva of *Strongyloides stercoralis,* × 75. *5,* Hookworm egg, × 500. *6, Taenia* sp. ovum, × 750. *7, Diphyllobothrium latum* ovum, × 500. *8, D. latum* ovum, × 500. *9, Hymenolepis nana* ovum, × 750. *10, Schistosoma japonicum* ovum, × 500. *11, Fasciolopsis buski* ovum, × 500. *12,* Diagram of rhabditoid larvae of *(A) S. stercoralis,* and *(B)* hookworm, a, anus; bc, buccal chamber; c, cardiac bulb of esophagus; es, esophagus; gp, germinal primordia; mg, midgut; × 400. *13,* Scolices and gravid proglottids of some tapeworms of man. (From Hunter, G. W., III, Frye, W. W., and Swartzwelder, J. C.: A Manual of Tropical Medicine. 4th ed. Philadelphia, W. B. Saunders Co., 1966.)

Chapter 76

Carbohydrate Intolerance

Robert M. Donaldson, Jr., Joyce D. Gryboski

DISACCHARIDASE DEFICIENCY

DEFINITION

Disaccharidase deficiency refers to any congenital or acquired disorder in which the patient lacks sufficient quantities of one or more sugar-splitting enzymes required for the digestion and subsequent absorption of disaccharides. Since these enzymes are located on the surface of small bowel epithelium, disaccharidase deficiency may develop in any disease which damages small bowel mucosa. In most cases, however, intestinal epithelial structure appears normal, and disaccharide intolerance constitutes the only identifiable absorptive defect. Ingestion of the inadequately hydrolyzed and therefore poorly absorbed disaccharide may induce abdominal discomfort and diarrhea.

DEVELOPMENTAL ASPECTS

All the intestinal disaccharidases may be demonstrated in the intestinal mucosa of the three-month fetus, with lactase the least active.[1-3] The enzyme distribution is fairly uniform over the small intestine, with the least activity in duodenum and terminal ileum. Trehalase, however, remains high in the terminal ileum. Disaccharidase activity has been detected in the large intestine of the 15- to 20-week fetus,

but with differentiation of the colon it is minimal at birth. Maltase 1 activity is low and remains so even in the newborn. The other alpha-glycosidases (maltase, sucrase, isomaltase, palatinase, trehalase, dextranase, and amylase) increase in activity and reach their maximal values by the eighth fetal month. Lactase activity rises markedly during the last trimester and reaches its maximum at the end of gestation (Table 76–1).

Active hexose transport mechanisms may be detected in the ten-week fetus and increase primarily in the jejunum, leading to the development of a proximodistal difference.[2] This system can function under anaerobic as well as aerobic conditions.

The normal intestine, infant as well as adult, contains three separate lactases.[4] Enzyme I hydrolyzes lactose and cellobiose and functions at an optimal pH of 6: Enzyme II is capable of hydrolyzing lactose and a synthetic substrate, BNG (6-bromo-2-naphthyl-β-galactose), and has an optimal pH of 4.5: Enzyme III hydrolyzes only synthetic BNG and functions at a pH of 6. It is likely that Enzyme I plays the major role in lactose digestion, and that presumably Enzyme II takes over any lactase activity in patients with lactose intolerance. Enzymes I and III have been shown to be deficient in cases of lactose intolerance and lactase insufficiency.

The lactose tolerance test is normal in full-term infants after the first few days of

1015

TABLE 76–1. DISACCHARIDASE ACTIVITY IN THE FETUS AND THE ADULT

| | UNITS/G PROTEIN Fetus | | | |
	3–4 mo.	7–8 mo.	8–9 mo.	Adult
Maltase	104	235	281	300–1200
Sucrase	40	91	101	70–325
Isomaltase	36	74	85	65–270
Trehalase	11	49	42	–
Lactase	5–9	20	20	39–258
Cellobiose	0.88	4.7	4.3	9–21

life.[5-8] Early it may seem abnormal if one measures blood glucose, which may show a rise of less than 20 mg. per 100 ml, but if total reducing sugar in the blood is measured, there is also a significant amount of galactose present. Lactase activity is diminished in the premature infant because of two factors: there is less intestinal surface area and the enzyme does not develop maximally until the end of gestation. Normal lactose tolerance tests using 1.75 g per kilogram of sugar have been reported in two-week-old premature infants. No difference in the blood sugar response is noted whether lactose was present or not in the diet before testing. Others have noted, however, that although the premature infant may apparently tolerate this amount of sugar loading and may have normal elevation of blood sugar, he will develop a metabolic acidosis within 15 minutes after loading.[9] The blood pH, serum HCO_3', and serum Cl^- decrease, and the serum lactate and other organic anions increase. Undoubtedly not all the ingested disaccharide is metabolized, and the rapid formation of lactic acid in the bowel contributes to the acidosis. A lactose-free diet has not been shown to induce lactase insufficiency in man.

HISTORY

Understanding of how specific sugars might cause gastrointestinal symptoms in susceptible individuals has emerged in the past decade. Congenital lactose intolerance caused by lactose malabsorption was first identified in 1959 by Holzel and coworkers who described two infants with diarrhea relieved by elimination of milk from the diet.[10] Although lactose was poorly absorbed by these two infants, glucose and galactose absorption were normal. Thus digestion of lactose by intestinal lactase was impaired, but not the absorption of the constituent monosaccharides. Many cases of lactose intolerance have subsequently been recorded among adults as well as children. In 1960 Weijers and his colleagues studied three children with watery diarrhea caused by sucrose malabsorption.[11] Stool pH was markedly reduced in these children, and diarrhea was promptly corrected either by withdrawal of sucrose from the diet or by feeding a powerful bacterial sucrase. Subsequently it was found that most children with sucrase deficiency are also unable to digest and absorb isomaltose.

ETIOLOGY AND PATHOGENESIS

The intestinal enzymes which split the common dietary disaccharides into their monosaccharide components are listed in Table 76–2. All these disaccharidases are situated on the luminal surface of intestinal microvillous membranes. Thus disaccharides are digested at the absorptive surface of the small bowel, a site which allows for immediate absorption of the released monosaccharides. In health there appears to be a relative excess of intestinal disaccharidase activity, so that monosaccharide transport rather than disaccharide hydrolysis is the rate-limiting step in carbohydrate absorption. The mechanisms involved in carbohydrate digestion and absorption are described in detail on pages 253 to 254.

As outlined in Table 76–3, disaccharidase deficiency may be classified on the basis of whether the defect is a primary

TABLE 76-2. HUMAN INTESTINAL DISACCHARIDASES*

ENZYME	DISACCHARIDE SUBSTRATE	MONOSACCHARIDE PRODUCTS
Isomaltase (maltase Ia)	Isomaltose	Glucose
	Maltose	Glucose
Sucrase (maltase IB)	Sucrose	Glucose, fructose
	Maltose	Glucose
Maltase II	Maltose	Glucose
Maltase III	Maltose	Glucose
Lactase	Lactose	Glucose, galactose

*As classified by Dahlqvist.[14]

phenomenon with no other apparent small bowel dysfunction or whether it is secondary to disease or loss of small intestinal mucosa.[12, 13] Primary deficiencies may be further classified depending upon whether they develop at birth or are acquired in adult life. Cases of primary sucrase deficiency have been described in the past, but most workers now agree that a constitutional lack of sucrase is always associated with isomaltase deficiency.[14] It is not clear, however, whether sucrase and isomaltase are hydrolyzed by a single enzyme which contains two distinct reactive sites, or whether sucrase and isomaltase are two distinct enzymes controlled by a single genetic mechanism.[15] Of interest, but not understood, is the fact that sucrose-isomaltose intolerance present in infancy usually improves as the child grows older. Primary sucrase-isomaltase deficiency has been observed most often in infants and is extremely rare in adults.

Primary lactase deficiency, on the other hand, may occur during infancy, but more often develops in adults with no previous history of lactose intolerance.[16,17] When disaccharidase deficiency results from intestinal mucosal disease, hydrolysis of more than one disaccharide is impaired, but lactase is the disaccharidase most frequently and most severely affected.[13]

As shown in Table 76-2, maltose is hydrolyzed by at least four different enzymes. Thus it is not surprising that a primary deficiency of maltase has not been described. Furthermore, maltase activity is less likely to be severely impaired in patients with mucosal disease than is the activity of other disaccharidases.[13]

In patients with disaccharidase deficiency secondary to small bowel disease or resection, the defect simply represents a manifestation of diseased or absent small bowel mucosa. Much more difficult to understand are those primary disaccharidase deficiencies which develop in the absence of any other recognizable small bowel abnormality. Presently available evidence suggests that sucrase-isomaltase deficiency constitutes an inherited disorder transmitted as an autosomal recessive.[15]

TABLE 76-3. CLASSIFICATION OF DISACCHARIDASE DEFICIENCIES

I. Primary
　Congenital—isolated enzyme deficiency present in infancy
　　Sucrase-isomaltase deficiency
　　Sucrase deficiency (?)
　　Lactase deficiency
　Acquired—isolated enzyme deficiency which develops in adult life
　　Lactase deficiency
　　　With no other gastrointestinal disorder
　　　With other gastrointestinal disorders
　　　　Gastrectomy
　　　　Ulcerative colitis
　　　　"Irritable colon"
II. Secondary—multiple enzyme deficiencies associated with small bowel disease. Well documented in:
　　Celiac sprue
　　Tropical sprue
　　Whipple's disease
　　Small bowel resection
　　Gastroenteritis
　　Cystic fibrosis
　　Lymphoid hyperplasia
　　Giardiasis
　　Malnutrition

Constitutional lactase deficiency, on the other hand, is relatively common, and a mode of inheritance has not been identified. Although lactase deficiency can reasonably be attributed to a genetic defect when present from birth, the development of enzyme deficiency for the first time in adult life is more difficult to explain.

Since man is the only mammal that continues to drink milk in adult life, one might suppose that continued ingestion of lactose results in maintenance of lactase activity in adult humans. There is little to support this line of reasoning, however. Changes in dietary carbohydrate can alter intestinal sucrase and maltase activity, but several studies in man and experimental animals have failed to show that lactase activity is either reduced by lactose withdrawal or stimulated by prolonged feeding of lactose. Indeed, if avoidance of milk is at all responsible for the development of lactase deficiency in man, the defect must be acquired very slowly and established only over several generations. Elaboration of an acquired enzyme inhibitor has been proposed as an alternative explanation for the *de novo* appearance of lactase deficiency in adults. Since lactose malabsorption occurs transiently during bacterial, parasitic, and nonspecific diarrheas, it is of course possible that lactase deficiency might develop as a permanent sequel of otherwise transient small bowel disease. Unfortunately, evidence to support or refute these possibilities is lacking, and the mechanisms responsible for the development of acquired lactase deficiency remain poorly defined.

PATHOGENESIS OF DIARRHEA IN DISACCHARIDASE DEFICIENCY

More readily understood is the pathogenesis of symptoms in patients with disaccharidase deficiency. When lactose is ingested by lactase-deficient patients, for example, only trace amounts of the undigested disaccharide can be absorbed; most of the sugar remains in the bowel lumen. When unabsorbed disaccharide reaches the distal intestine, enteric bacteria ferment the sugar to form lactic acid, other organic acids, carbon dioxide, and hydrogen. The unabsorbed sugar in-

creases the osmotic load delivered to the distal bowel, and water enters the gut lumen. The osmotic load is further increased by the bacterial formation of two to four organic acid molecules from each disaccharide molecule. Proprionic and butyric acids are not increased. In a 24-hour stool sample there is normally no more than 35 mg of lactic acid, but in this type of diarrhea it may rise to several grams. The presence of the low molecular weight organic acids causes a change in the stool pH from a normal of 7 to 8 down to 5 or 6. The normal quantity of stool excreted by breast-fed infants is 20 to 30 g per day, by normal milk-fed infants, 40 to 50 g per day, and by those with a disaccharidase deficiency diarrhea, 100 to 300 g per day.

Although unsubstantiated, the possibility has also been raised that these organic acids may serve as "irritants" with a deleterious effect on normal fluid and electrolyte absorption by the bowel. In any event, the capacity of the distal bowel to reabsorb water is exceeded and diarrhea ensues. Transudation of fluid into the bowel lumen and bacterial formation of gases result in distention of the gut with bloating and abdominal discomfort.

DIAGNOSIS

The diagnosis of disaccharide intolerance depends upon several methods of testing: the examination of the stool for reducing sugars, the disaccharide tolerance test, and disaccharidase assay of the small bowel mucosa.

The presence of disaccharides in the urine or in the stool may be a normal finding in the premature or in the young, full-term infant.[5-9] Lactosuria has been reported in from 28 to 50 per cent of normal full-term infants and in 46 to 60 per cent of premature infants taking milk formula.[18-20] Lactose, glucose, and galactose may be present in the stools during the first week of life. The pH of the stools is often acid and may give a strongly positive reaction to Clinitest. The stools from infants taking breast milk or breast-milk simulated formulas contain more sugar than the stools from infants taking milk or an evaporated milk formula. Sucrose is not a reducing sugar and will not be detected by Clinitest. Lactulose, a synthetic sugar formed from lactose during the commercial preparation and storage of milk formula, is composed of a nonreducing galactose-fructose linkage. It is not acted upon by any of the beta-galactosidases and may be detected in the urine and the stool of infants after chromatographic or electrophoretic study.[20-22] A simple screening test for disaccharide in the stool may be performed with Clinitest tablets.[23] The results are graded from 0 to 4+, with values greater than 1+ in older children considered abnormal. In studies of neonatal stools it was noted that nearly half give greater than 1+ Clinitest results, with some up to 4+.

Measurement of lactic acid in the stool may be helpful because the technique is not difficult, and, although normally present only in negligible amounts, it increases significantly in disaccharide malabsorption. Radiologically, there is dilatation of the bowel, dilution of barium, and rapid transit after the ingestion of barium sulfate mixed with disaccharide. The histology of the intestinal mucosa is usually normal in patients with primary disaccharide malabsorption. Partial villous atrophy may rarely be noted, but the columnar epithelium is normal, the nuclei regular, and the striated border and basement membrane clear.

Experiments in which intravenously administered C^{14}-labeled disaccharides were administered indicate that maltose can be metabolized to CO_2 almost as completely as glucose, but that lactose and sucrose are poorly oxidized and are excreted in the urine.[24] The principal tests, however, remain measurement of blood glucose after an oral disaccharide load and direct enzyme assays of jejunal mucosa. (See below.)

LACTOSE INTOLERANCE

INCIDENCE AND ETIOLOGY

Although familial studies support a genetic origin in cases of lactose intolerance in infancy, the ethnic origin is the apparent determinant of who will develop lactose intolerance in later infancy or beyond. Racial patterns persist despite migration to different hemispheres and cultural habitats. Although induction of lactase has been reported in animals, the feeding of high milk intake or of no milk does not affect the lactose tolerance of humans. In adults, lactase intolerance is frequent in blacks (40 to 100 per cent),[25] Jews (nearly two-thirds),[26] Orientals (85 to 100 per cent),[27] and Indians (63 per cent).[28] The incidence in Caucasians is between 2 and 19 per cent, and is generally accepted as 10 per cent. Lactose intolerance is more common in children of affected racial and ethnic groups, but is usually not apparent until one and one-half to three years of age, although noted in Bagandan infants as early as six months of life[29] and in unweaned Thai children of one to 12 months old.[30] When the total population of breast-fed infants involved is considered, it is not a great problem. The incidence increases in a linear fashion after four to five years of age.

There are now two primary lactose intolerance disorders in infancy.

1. *Familial lactose intolerance* is that originally described and associated with vomiting, failure to thrive, dehydration, acidosis, disacchariduria, and aminoaciduria.[10, 31-33] Renal tubular disorders and central nervous system damage have been reported, as well as hemorrhagic diatheses and subdural hematoma. The vomiting may be so severe as to suggest pyloric stenosis. Siblings and distant relatives may be affected, but parental consanguinity has not been described. The parents of these children have normal lactose tolerance test results and are asymptomatic. A number of the reported infants expired, and not all those treated with a lactose-free diet responded. When lactose tolerance tests have been performed in this group, they have been within normal limits. Lactosuria and aminoaciduria followed the oral ingestion of lactose in one infant recently studied, but did not follow the intraduodenal administration of the sugar. It is postulated that some defect exists within the gut which permits or causes the abnormal transport of lactose into the circulation.

2. *Congenital lactose intolerance*, directly related to lactase insufficiency, develops shortly after the initiation of milk feedings.[14, 34] The infants exhibit abdominal distention, and pass explosive or watery, frothy, acid stools. The odor may be described as sour or even like vinegar.

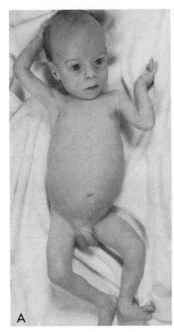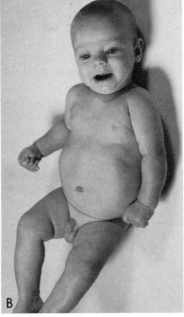

Figure 76–1. *A*, Four-month-old infant with congenital lactose intolerance. Note the abdominal distention and marked wasting of the gluteal and other musculature. *B*, The same infant at six months after two months of a lactose-free diet.

There is usually no aminoaciduria. Disacchariduria, usually considered diagnostic of the familial lactose intolerance and not found with this type, may indeed be present. The presence or absence of lactosuria is dependent upon the intraluminal concentration of the sugar and its degree of passive diffusion through the intestinal cells. Because of the rapid transit caused by the osmotic diarrhea, steatorrhea and a mild, generalized malabsorption may be present. The small bowel biopsy is normal, and there is diminished or absent lactase activity.

This disorder is more frequent in males than females. Siblings or a parent may be affected, and an autosomal dominant inheritance is suggested. The complete elimination of lactose from the diet results in a total symptomatic cure (Fig. 76–1). Many infants may tolerate low lactose diets as they grow but will develop diarrhea when challenged beyond their enzymatic capacities. The substitution of Nutramigen or soy-based formulas containing sucrose provides adequate nutritional replacement. Any infant or growing child not taking the full requirements as provided in these formulas should be given supplemental calcium.

SECONDARY LACTOSE INTOLERANCE
(Table 76–3)

Celiac Disease. In celiac disease all the disaccharidases are depressed, with lactase being the most severely affected. In cases of celiac disease, treated or untreated, sugar loading may not be followed by watery diarrhea after lactose, although lactase levels may be low.[35, 36] Some patients with celiac disease, however, develop pain and diarrhea after milk ingestion, and this has led some investigators to recommend a lactose-free, as well as a gluten-free, diet.

Small Bowel Resection or Gastrojejunostomy. Lactose intolerance has been reported in patients after extensive small bowel resection.[37, 38] This may be explained by reduction of the total lactase content of the small bowel and by increased intestinal transit, particularly if the ileocecal valve is resected. It has also been noted after gastrojejunostomy of the Billroth II type.

Gastroenteritis. Viral or bacterial gastroenteritis may be followed by a lactose intolerance which might persist for one to eight months.[39] Disacchariduria and steatorrhea may be present during the acute stages. A majority of patients with acute diarrhea, if tested during the acute stage, will also demonstrate lactose intolerance.[40,41] Some of these may even develop a generalized disaccharide or monosaccharide intolerance. The impairment is transient, and within four months there is usually a return to maximal functioning enzyme capacity. It is felt that the elimination of lactose from the diet in those proved to have lactose intolerance may prevent the subsequent development of the more serious generalized disaccharide or monosaccharide intolerance. Hypoglycemia is a significant problem in early management of these infants.

Cystic Fibrosis. Lactose intolerance has been reported in isolated patients with cystic fibrosis, but in a later study it was confirmed in 25 per cent of patients with cystic fibrosis after small intestinal enzyme assay.[42] Intolerance to lactose and sucrose has been described in several infants with this disease, and they were treated successfully with a monosaccharide-containing diet during the first year of life. Clinical tolerance to disaccharides develops by one year of age. Some consider lactose intolerance a separate genetic defect in these patients.

Lymphoid Hyperplasia of the Small Bowel. Two children with lymphoid hyperplasia of the small bowel have had lactose intolerance and secondary gluten sensitivity. Neither patient had giardiasis. One had an associated deficiency of immunoglobulin A, and the other had an elevated immunoglobulin A and hypogammaglobulinemia G.

Giardiasis. Several clinical disorders are associated with giardiasis in infancy and childhood. There may be a celiac-type picture with lactose intolerance, loose bulky stools, abdominal distention and steatorrhea. Others may have recurrent periumbilical or epigastric pain. In severe infestations there may be a bloody, mucoid diarrhea resembling that of ulcerative colitis. Lactase insufficiency may be present. Biopsies of the duodenum from patients with Giardia infestation reveal little change other than minimal inflammation of the lamina propria, edema, and slight mononuclear cell reaction.[43] Trophozoites may be found in the sections but do not penetrate the mucosa. Some abnormalities of the villous architecture have been noted, with an infiltrate of polymorphonuclear cells. There are small changes in intraluminal pH accompanying giardiasis, but these are not enough to account for the extent of carbohydrate absorption. In older individuals the lactose tolerance test may revert to normal shortly after elimination of the parasite, but in infants and young children several weeks to months may be required. The cysts may not always be detected in the stool, and a duodenal intubation with examination of duodenal fluid might be necessary to establish the diagnosis.

Malnutrition. Lactose intolerance has been noted in infants with intrauterine malnutrition syndrome who were small for term.[44] It is also frequent in infants with malnutrition and kwashiorkor. It is the last of the enzyme functions to return and follows the other disaccharidases and pancreatic enzymes.

Regional Enteritis. Lactose intolerance is associated with regional enteritis in 20 per cent of children with this disease. Since regional enteritis may appear in infancy, it must be considered before congenital lactose intolerance is accepted as the diagnosis.

CLINICAL PICTURE AND DIAGNOSIS

Lactase deficiency is by far the most common of the disaccharidase deficiencies. Although it should be suspected in any patient with unexplained diarrhea, the clinical features of this condition are in fact extremely varied. Some lactase-deficient individuals experience nausea, abdominal bloating and cramps, flatulence, and diarrhea after drinking milk. Recurrent, severe abdominal pain may be the principal symptoms in older infants and children. Others, however, find that ingestion of milk causes minimal or no symptoms. The rate of delivery of the disaccharide into the bowel is probably an important determinant of the severity of symptoms. Thus, for example, the defect often becomes clinically apparent only after gastric resection and consequent "dumping" of ingested sugar into the small bowel lumen.[12]

Because milk is the only common foodstuff which contains significant quantities of lactose, most patients with primary lactase deficiency are well aware that they develop symptoms whenever they drink milk. Most patients simply avoid milk except when needed as a laxative. Usually symptoms are brought to the physician's attention only when the patient is advised to drink milk regularly, as in the treatment of peptic ulcer or during pregnancy. Occasionally, however, the association between milk and gastrointestinal symptoms is not recognized, and lactase deficiency has been discovered in some individuals whose symptoms were previously attributed to irritable colon or functional bowel disease.[45]

The diagnosis of disaccharidase deficiency can be confirmed by determining the patient's response to an oral load of lactose. Normally, digestion and absorption will lead to the same rise in blood glucose as will the ingestion of an equivalent amount of glucose and galactose. In most patients with lactase deficiency, however, the blood glucose will not increase more than 20 mg per 100 ml following the ingestion of 100 g of lactose. Children are given 2 mg per kilogram, and capillary blood is taken at 15, 30, 60, and 120 minutes. Although a "flat" lactose tolerance curve usually represents lactase deficiency, slow gastric emptying may interfere with the diagnostic accuracy of the tolerance test.[12] In such instances in the adult, 30 g of lactose infused into the duodenum in 300 ml of water in 30 minutes will produce a normal rise in blood glucose levels. Whether the lactose is administered orally or intraduodenally, equivalent amounts of glucose and galactose must be administered in a separate control test in order to be certain that patients with apparent lactase deficiency are able to absorb the constituent monosaccharides. Since colonic bacteria convert unabsorbed sugars to hydrogen, measurement of breath hydrogen after an oral disaccharide load can provide a sensitive test of disaccharide maldigestion and malabsorption.[46] This approach has the advantage that a more physiological load of carbohydrate can be administered.

As noted, children with lactase deficiency have low pH of stools and often explosive diarrhea following an oral load of lactase. This low pH results from conversion of unabsorbed disaccharide to organic acid such as lactic and acetic acid by colon bacteria. Fecal lactic acid is generally increased in lactase-deficient patients fed lactose, but in adults the stool pH is usually not low despite a high lactate content. Presumably the increased buffering capacity of the adult colon is responsible for this difference. Steatorrhea, probably resulting from rapid transit to the small bowel, may be detected in the occasional lactase-deficient patient, but this is the exception rather than the rule.

When lactose is given together with barium to patients with lactase deficiency, X-rays taken 45 to 60 minutes later often show distention of the small bowel and dilution of contrast medium by intraluminal fluid together with rapid movement of barium into the colon.[47] Control examinations should fail to show these changes when barium is mixed with sugars other than lactose.

After an oral load of lactose, the urine of disaccharidase-deficient individuals usually contains small but measurable quantities of lactose. However, the diagnostic significance of this finding is questionable, because at most only a few hundred milligrams of disaccharide are excreted, and even in normal subjects a small amount of unhydrolyzed lactose diffuses across the intestine and appears in the urine after an oral load of 20 g or more of lactose. The small and questionably significant lactosuria observed in intestinal lactase deficiency contrasts strikingly with the severe lactosuria which occurs in "familial lactose intolerance." The latter condition is most likely unrelated to intestinal lactase deficiency and consists of severe lactosuria, diarrhea, occasional aminoaciduria, renalaciduria, and nonspecific "toxic changes in kidney, liver, and central nervous system."[48]

Although the measurements in blood, breath, stool, and urine after an oral disaccharide load offer supporting evidence for disaccharidase deficiency, definitive diagnosis requires evidence that intestinal disaccharidase activity is indeed decreased or absent. This is readily accomplished by assay of the appropriate sugar-splitting enzymes in jejunal biopsies obtained with a peroral suction biopsy tube. Dahlqvist describes in detail the optimal conditions for handling biopsies, the methods for performing disaccharidase measurements, and the criteria for normal and abnormal results.[49] Since the defect can be documented for certain only by enzyme assay of small bowel mucosa, this seems to be the logical way to demonstrate intestinal disaccharidase deficiency.

TREATMENT

Symptomatic improvement can be expected when the offending disaccharide is removed from the diet. Patients with lactase deficiency, for example, note disappearance of diarrhea and bloating when milk intake is curtailed and in fact have usually discovered this fact before seeing the doctor. If milk withdrawal does not suffice, however, all milk products should be eliminated from the diet. Diets used in the treatment of galactosemic children contain a complete list of lactose-containing foods to be avoided.[50] Similarly, infants with sucrase and isomaltase deficiency require substitution of glucose or other sugars for sucrose. Restriction of dietary sucrose in these infants regularly corrects diarrhea and restores growth rates to normal. A compilation of the carbohydrate content of various foods is helpful in planning diets for patients with symptomatic disaccharide intolerance.[51]

SUCROSE INTOLERANCE

Unlike lactase insufficiency, in which there is intolerance to only one sugar, sucrase insufficiency is also accompanied by a deficiency of isomaltase and a diminished maltase activity.[52-55]

INCIDENCE

Over 100 cases have been reported in the literature since the disease was first reported ten years ago.

INHERITANCE

The inheritance is likely of the autosomal recessive type.[15] Other affected siblings have been reported in some families, and there has been frequent consanguinity of parents. Small bowel enzyme activity has varied in the parents. In one study those from fathers were normal, but all the mothers had decreased maltase, sucrase, and isomaltase levels. In another, all parents had enzyme activity 50 per cent below normal. In a third group of four parents, one had normal, two had borderline, and the last had definitely abnormal values. It has been suggested that the homozygous individual has symptoms all his life, and the heterozygote may either be asymptomatic or affected only in childhood. γ-Amylase is reduced to 35 per cent of normal in affected individuals, perhaps the result of a single genetic mutation affecting the enzyme with maltase-sucrase activity.[56]

PATHOLOGY AND PATHOPHYSIOLOGY

Five intestinal maltase activities have been identified. Maltase I and II hydrolyze only maltose; maltase III and IV hydrolyze maltose and sucrose, but the activity of III is extremely low, and maltase V hydrolyzes maltose, isomaltose, and palatinose. Maltases IV and V are the predominant intestinal disaccharidases. Enzyme determinations reveal absent sucrase activity (maltase Ib), only trace amounts of isomaltase activity (maltase Ia), and low or absent palatinase and dextrinase activity. Total maltase activity is reduced, owing to the almost total absence of maltases III, IV, and V. Normally maltases I and II compose only 4 to 29 per cent of total maltase activity, but in these patients they total 71 to 90 per cent of total maltase function. Total functioning maltase activity is about 10 to 20 per cent of normal. The nonabsorbed sugars accumulate within the intestinal lumen and produce an osmotic and fermentative diarrhea.

SYMPTOMS

The infant is without symptoms while taking breast milk or simulated breast-milk formulas. Symptoms begin with the introduction of sucrose, dextrins, or starch into the diet. Diarrhea is explosive, watery, and acid. Its severity is proportionate to the amount of sucrose in the diet. The weight of the stools may rise to 300 to 500 g per day. There are abdominal distention and flatulence. There is usually no associated steatorrhea, but severe chronic diarrhea and the extremely rapid transit may cause a mild generalized malabsorption.

DIFFERENTIAL DIAGNOSIS

Disorders often considered in the differential diagnosis are cow's milk allergy because of its later onset than lactose intolerance, starch intolerance, or even early-onset celiac disease.

DIAGNOSIS

The diarrheas of sugar intolerance are often described as having a vinegar-like odor, owing to the excess acetic acid. The stool pH is low, invariably between 4 and 5. Stool lactic acid may measure 1 or more g per day. Since sucrose is not a reducing sugar, it will not be detected by the stool Clinitest test. Paper chromatography or electrophoretic separation of sugars will reveal its presence in the stool extract. The oral tolerance tests for palatinose and for sucrose are followed by no rise in blood sugar. The maltose tolerance test is usually normal and attributed to the functional maltase I and II enzymes. Monosaccharide and lactose tolerance tests are normal. The small intestinal histology is usually normal, although villous atrophy has been noted in the rare case, but this has reverted to normal after initiation of the diet.

TREATMENT

The treatment consists of the elimination of sucrose, dextrins and starches from the diet. Breast-milk simulated formulas or carbohydrate-free soy formulas are available commercially. The symptoms gradually improve with age, although the primary pathological disorder remains. Some may tolerate a bit of starch from rice or corn, because these contain fewer alpha 1-6 bonds than others. In patients with extreme symptoms a secondary lactose intolerance may be present and require the temporary removal of lactose from the diet.

PROGNOSIS

Although the symptoms improve with age and the diet may be somewhat broadened, enzyme levels remain unchanged. Attempts at enzyme induction by the feeding of high sucrose diets to these patients have been unsuccessful.

SECONDARY SUCROSE INTOLERANCE

Secondary sucrose intolerance is invariably associated with lactose intolerance and may therefore follow infectious diarrhea, malnutrition, kwashiorkor, intestinal resection, and giardiasis. Sucrosuria and diminished sucrase activity are noted in celiac disease, although the children are not clinically intolerant to the sugar. They have also been described in patients with cystic fibrosis, although it seems to be a problem primarily in the young infant with the disease.

Moncrieff's syndrome of hiatus hernia, sucrosuria, and mental retardation is rare. Abnormal lactose as well as sucrose tolerance tests have been noted in these patients.

TREHALOSE INTOLERANCE

Trehalose is a l-α-glucosido-l-α-glucoside. It is found in lower plants and insects but is pertinent in our diet in the form of mushrooms. In the young mushrooms its concentration is 1.4 per cent, but in older mushrooms it is converted to glucose. Its rarity is indicated by the report of only one case to 1971.[57] However, it is not unusual to encounter the individual who avoids mushrooms because of gastrointestinal symptoms after their ingestion.

ETIOLOGY AND PATHOPHYSIOLOGY

The enzyme trehalase is present in human intestinal mucosal brush border and in aging mushrooms. It hydrolyzes the glycoside into glucose. Its deficiency will produce symptoms similar to those of di- or monosaccharide malabsorption. A moderate amount of mushrooms ingested during a meal provides only a few grams of trehalose, but this appears adequate to produce symptoms.

SYMPTOMS AND DIAGNOSIS

Watery diarrhea develops within 15 minutes after the ingestion of mushrooms and continues over the following two to three hours. It is accompanied by abdominal bloating and cramping. The diagnosis is made by the trehalose tolerance test. The dosage arrived at for the adult is 50 g sugar in 400 ml of water. The test is performed and interpreted like the other sugar tolerance tests, for it measures the rise in blood glucose. In a person with trehalase deficiency the gastrointestinal symptoms are immediately reproduced after ingestion of the pure sugar. If tissue is obtained by biopsy, direct assay of the enzyme can be made.

Treatment consists of elimination of young mushrooms from the diet. It will cure the patient of all symptoms.

DIARRHEA FROM "SUGAR-FREE" CANDIES[58]

Diarrhea may rapidly follow the ingestion of dietetic products containing sorbitol, mannitol, and even cyclamates. These substances replace the sucrose or starch in cookies, candies, and soft drinks. Dietetic products have appeared in abundance on the consumer market and are being purchased by diabetics, dieters, and mothers anxious to protect their children from tooth decay.

ETIOLOGY AND PATHOLOGY

The hexitols are acted upon slowly by oral bacteria and are absorbed by passive transport mechanisms in the gastrointestinal tract. These dietary properties lead to the development of an osmotic diarrhea if a sufficient quantity of hexitol is ingested. Twenty to 30 g of sorbitol will cause diarrhea in a normal adult, and the diarrhea threshold seems to be on a dosage:weight ratio. Approximately 9 g of sorbitol is contained in a package of dietetic mints or fruit-flavored lozenges, a comparatively massive osmotic load for the toddler.

CLINICAL PICTURE AND TREATMENT

Typically, a perfectly well toddler develops explosive, watery diarrhea within two hours after ingestion of a quantity of "dietetic candy." The stool is often the color of the candy consumed. Over the next four hours there may be up to ten more watery movements. The child is well thereafter with normal bowel habits until the situation is repeated. At lower dosages, these products may simply cause flatulence and cramping. Since the symptoms are self-limited, there is no treatment. Determination of the child's threshold of tolerance should be made if the candies are to be continued.

GLUCOSE-GALACTOSE MALABSORPTION

DEFINITION

Glucose-galactose malabsorption is an inherited, congenital disorder characterized by watery diarrhea resulting from selectively impaired intestinal transport of glucose and galactose. The small bowel mucosa appears intact, and other substances are absorbed normally. Whether ingested as monosaccharides, disaccharides, or polysaccharides, glucose and galactose are poorly absorbed and regularly induce diarrhea in patients with this disorder. Fructose absorption is normal, however, and diarrhea is promptly corrected by a diet in which fructose serves as the only source of carbohydrate.

HISTORICAL ASPECTS

The disorder was apparently not recognized until 1962, when almost simultaneously Lindquist et al. in Sweden and LaPlane et al. in France described a total of six patients.[59-61] Subsequently, other well documented cases have been reported from Australia, Germany, and the United States.[62-67] Although many workers indicate that glucose-galactose malabsorption probably occurs more often than is generally recognized, no one has yet described a large series of patients, and to date the total number of reported patients does not reach 20.

INCIDENCE

The disease is extremely rare, as only 18 cases have been reported until 1971.

GENETICS AND PATHOPHYSIOLOGY

The familial nature of glucose-galactose malabsorption seems certain. Investigators in Sweden, France, and Australia have noted occurrence of the disorder in siblings, but parents of affected individuals have no symptoms suggestive of sugar malabsorption. Melin and Meeuwisse described six cases in one large family.[66] Since both males and females were affected, since five of the cases occurred in three sibships, and since none of the patients had sugar intolerance, these workers concluded that the disorder has an autosomal recessive mode of inheritance.

Studies using glucose tolerance tests have not demonstrated abnormalities in glucose absorption in parents of affected children. In one study of glucose transport by jejunal mucosa of parents of an affected child, Meeuwisse and Dahlqvist demonstrated a rather small accumulation of the sugar in the jejunal tissue of the father. Impaired glucose transport[68] has been shown in both parents and a half-sister of an affected child. The levels of glucose uptake by their jejunal mucosa were intermediate between those of the patient and of normal control subjects. It is apparent that the heterozygote may be detected by measuring the ability of the jejunal mucosa to concentrate glucose.

This genetically determined abnormality appears to be impaired intestinal transport of glucose and galactose. The defect is apparently specific in that intestinal absorptive cells appear normal by light and electron microscopy, and intestinal absorption of other substances is not impaired. Indeed, the fact that the disorder exists supports the concept that certain monosaccharides are transported by a specific active transport mechanism present in the intestine.

Active monosaccharide transport by the intestine exhibits considerable substrate specificity. Small bowel mucosa actively transports only those sugars which contain six or more carbon atoms, form a pyranose ring, and have a free hydroxyl group at C_2 and a methyl group at C_5. Glucose and galactose possess these structural requirements for active transport and in fact compete with each other for uptake by the intestinal cell. On the other hand, fructose forms a furanose ring and, unlike glucose and galactose, shows a significant blood sugar rise after it is fed. Similarly, sugar appears in the stool when glucose or galactose is fed but not when fructose is fed. Although the amounts are small, some glucose is absorbed as shown by blood sugar values and particularly by intestinal perfusion studies. The stool contains large quantities of glucose or galactose, or both, even when disaccharides or polysaccharides are fed. Thus monosaccharide absorption is impaired, whereas carbohydrate digestion is not.

Investigations on small bowel biopsies further support the concept that glucose-galactose transport is specifically impaired in this disorder.[67] Biopsies from affected individuals reveal normal disaccharidase and alkaline phosphatase activities. When incubated in vitro with radioactive labeled sugars, however, these biopsy specimens fail to accumulate glucose or galactose from the incubation medium, whereas cellular uptake of alanine proceeds normally. The "metabolic block" for glucose and galactose most likely occurs at the cell-entry step of active sugar transport. The finding of glycosuria in most patients with glucose-galactose malabsorption raises the possibility that the transport defect also occurs in the renal tubule but is not so severe.

Studies have been undertaken to evaluate this intermittent glycosuria which appears in the presence of a normal blood sugar. There is no phosphaturia or aminoaciduria, and glomerular filtration rates are normal. Maximum tubular reabsorption of glucose is normal or only slightly depressed, but a reduced minimal threshold has been demonstrated, using renal glucose titration techniques. This suggests that the kidney contains glucose transport systems which are different from those in the intestine.

As is the case in disaccharidase deficiency, diarrhea apparently results from the increased intraluminal osmotic load produced by the unabsorbed sugar molecules. Water flows into the gut lumen in response to this increased osmolarity, whereas electrolyte losses are minimal. Thus fluid depletion greatly exceeds electrolyte losses so that the patient becomes dehydrated and serum osmolarity is increased. Since unabsorbed sugars are converted by bacteria to organic acids, thus lowering stool pH, the possibility remains that a low intraluminal pH or one of the bacterial metabolites is responsible for impaired gut function and further contributes to the diarrhea. Although this question remains open, reduction of enteric bacteria by antibiotic therapy increases fecal pH but does not correct the diarrhea.

CLINICAL PICTURE AND DIAGNOSIS

Within a few days after birth, the breast-fed or formula-fed infant with glucose-galactose malabsorption develops watery diarrhea. Stools may bear such a striking resemblance to urine in this condition that a congenital communication between rectum and urinary tract is often suspected. The patient's appetite and general condition are remarkably good at the beginning, but gradually dehydration and attendant fever become prominent. If untreated, the patient may gradually deteriorate within a period of a few weeks or months. In other cases, however, the defect appears less severe, and chronic diarrhea persists for years. At the onset the patient is usually thought to have severe gastroenteritis. Diarrhea stops, however, as soon as intravenous nutrition is instituted, only to return when oral feeding is resumed. In children and young adults with this disorder, ingestion of a carbohydrate load regularly induces abdominal distress and loose stools.

Blood sugar levels tend to be low, and the blood sugar curve is essentially flat during all glucose or galactose tests, but blood sugar values increase normally after oral fructose. Increased quantities of glucose can be readily demonstrated in the feces, and a Clinistix test (specific for glucose) on the watery stools is strongly positive. Bacterial fermentation of unabsorbed

sugars results in lowering of stool pH. Glycosuria, although usually mild, is almost always present when the diet contains substantial carbohydrates other than fructose. Increased urinary excretion of β-aminoisobutyric acid has been noted in one family afflicted with this disorder.

Blood sugar rises significantly after fructose and moderately after sucrose. The normal sugar content of the stool is usually not over 0.1 per cent wet weight, but may rise to 39 per cent after monosaccharide loading. In older individuals an oral sugar load may be followed by a relatively normal rise in blood sugar, and intubation studies may be necessary for a definitive diagnosis. In such cases, glucose will always be absorbed more slowly than fructose. Normally 50 per cent of glucose and 30 per cent of fructose are absorbed in the jejunum, but in glucose-galactose malabsorption only 10 per cent of glucose is absorbed.

The histological appearance of the small bowel is normal, and intestinal mucosal disaccharidase and alkaline phosphatase activities are not diminished. Although xylose absorption may be slightly diminished, malabsorption of glucose and galactose is the only definite absorptive disorder. Mild steatorrhea is occasionally observed but is probably due to unusually rapid transit through the small bowel.

Although the symptoms are similar to those of congenital lactase deficiency, the presence of glucose in the diarrheal stools, the slight glycosuria, and the somewhat low blood sugar levels strongly suggest the diagnosis of glucose-galactose malabsorption. This diagnosis can be readily established by sugar tolerance tests together with the finding of glucose in the stool after an oral glucose load. Clinical response to a diet which contains fructose as the only carbohydrate should be favorable. Onset during the first few days of life and the normal histological appearance of the jejunal mucosal biopsy should readily distinguish glucose-galactose malabsorption from celiac sprue.

TREATMENT

During the acute phase of diarrhea, intravenous replacement of fluid and electrolyte losses is required. The reader is referred to the general discussion of diarrhea on pages 291 to 316. The best therapeutic response is obtained with a synthetic formula which contains 4 to 8 per cent fructose as the only carbohydrate ingredient. All sources of glucose and galactose, including starches and lactose, are eliminated. Since sucrose is a disaccharide composed of fructose linked to glucose and since fructose is readily absorbed in this disorder, some patients can tolerate small amounts of sucrose. Casein or soy flour provides a source for protein in the formula, and the diet must of course be supplemented by appropriate vitamins.

Although several formula adaptations have been prepared, the CHO-free diet available commercially from Borden Co., New York, N.Y., is preferred.

Absorption of the sugars does not seem to improve with age. Any tolerance in the older individual is in fact a reflection of a smaller sugar load with relation to body size and a longer intestinal transit time. These patients may still experience flatulence, cramping, and diarrhea after taking small amounts of starch, sugar, or milk.

As the infant grows older, meat, fish, and eggs are introduced, and gradually limited quantities of carbohydrates other than fructose can be added without inducing symptoms.

SECONDARY MONOSACCHARIDE MALABSORPTIONS

Infants who develop severe diarrhea during the first week of life may not tolerate any of the monosaccharides, glucose, galactose, or fructose, and a pathogenic strain of *Escherichia coli* has been implicated.[69] Although they are not clinically acidotic, these infants have hyperchloremic acidosis. Duodenal biopsy and disaccharidase levels are normal. They tolerate only a sugar-free, casein, glycerol, butterfat formula to which electrolytes, calcium, and magnesium are added; after one to six months they recover completely. A similar intolerance may develop in newborn infants operated on for high intestinal obstruction. An overgrowth of abnormal intestinal bacterial flora has been found above the area of anastomosis.

In older infants this type of intolerance may develop after infectious gastroenteritis.[40] It is usually of short duration, lasting from only a few days to several weeks, but it may be fatal if it is not diagnosed and accurately treated. A marked hypoglycemia has been noted in these infants, and intravenous glucose is necessary to supplement the carbohydrate-free feedings. After being free of diarrhea for 15 days, most infants are then able to maintain the blood sugar at 40 mg per 100 ml or above. During the acute stage of their illness they may now show an elevation in blood sugar after epinephrine or glucagon and may become hypovolemic after a small load of an amino acid mixture. Ephedrine sulfate, 5 mg every six hours, may be effective in those infants who had previously shown a response to ephedrine stimulation but who later demonstrate adrenal medullary unresponsiveness. The diagnosis and treatment of disaccharide intolerance early in acute diarrheal states may prevent the development of the severe monosaccharide intolerance.

REFERENCES

1. Auricchio, S., Rubino, A., and Murset, E. Intestinal glycosidase activities in the human embryo, fetus and newborn. Pediatrics 35:944, 1965.
2. Koldovsky, O. Development of the Functions of the Small Intestine in Mammals and Man. Basel, S. Karger, 1969. pp. 165-177.
3. Dahlqvist, A., and Lindberg, T. Development of the intestinal disaccharidase and alkaline phosphatase activities in the human foetus. Clin. Sci. 30:517, 1966.
4. Gray, G., Santiago, N., Colver, E., et al. Intestinal β-galactosidases. II. Biochemical alteration in human lactase deficiency. J. Clin. Invest. 48:729, 1969.
5. Anyon, C. P., and Clarkson, K. G. Lactose metabolism in the newborn. New Zeal. Med. J. 64:694, 1965.
6. Boellner, S. W., Beard, T. C., Panos, T. C., et al. Impairment of lactose hydrolysis in newborn infants. Pediatrics 36:542, 1965.
7. Sampayo, R. R. L., Sosa Miatello, C., Higa, J., et al. Disaccharidase activity of the intestinal mucosa in infants. Presna Med. Argent. 55:891, 1968.
8. Jarrett, E., and Holman, G. H. Lactose absorption in the premature infant. Arch. Dis. Child. 41:525, 1966.
9. Lifshitz, F., Diaz-Bensussen, S., Martinez-Garza, V., et al. Influence of disaccharides on the development of systemic acidosis in the premature infant. Pediat. Res. 5:213, 1971.

10. Holzel, A., Schwarz, V., and Sutcliffe, K. W. Defective lactose absorption causing malnutrition in infancy. Lancet 1:1126, 1959.
11. Weijers, H. A., van De Kamer, J. H., Mossel, D. R. A., and Dicke, W. K. Diarrhea caused by deficiency of sugar-splitting enzymes. Lancet 2:296, 1960.
12. Kern, F., and Struthers, J. E. Intestinal lactase deficiency and lactose intolerance in adults. J.A.M.A. 195:927, 1966.
13. Plotkin, G. R., and Isselbacher, K. J. Secondary disaccharidase deficiency in adult celiac disease (non-tropical sprue) and other malabsorption states. New Eng. J. Med. 271:1033, 1964.
14. Dahlqvist, A. Specificity of the human intestinal disaccharidases and implications for hereditary disaccharide intolerance. J. Clin. Invest. 41:463, 1962.
15. Kerry, K. R., and Townley, R. R. W. Genetic aspects of intestinal sucrase-isomaltase deficiency. Aust. Pediat. J. 1:223, 1965.
16. Haemmerli, U. P., Kistler, H., Amman, R., Marthaler, T., Semenza, G., Auricchio, S., and Prader, A. Acquired milk intolerance in the adult caused by lactose malabsorption due to a selective deficiency of intestinal lactase activity. Amer. J. Med. 38:7, 1965.
17. Gudmand-Hoyer, E., Dahlqvist, A., and Jarnum, S. Specific small intestinal lactase deficiency in adults. Scand. J. Gastroent. 4:377, 1969.
18. Davidson, A. G. F., and Mullinger, M. Reducing substances in neonatal stools detected by Clinitest. Pediatrics 46:632, 1970.
19. Ford, J. D., and Haworth, J. C. The fecal excretion of sugars in children. J. Pediat. 63:988, 1963.
20. Gryboski, J. D., Zilis, J., and Ma, O. H. A study of fecal sugars by high voltage electrophoresis. Gastroenterology 47:26, 1964.
21. Dahlqvist, A., and Gryboski, J. D. Inability of the human small intestine to hydrolyze lactulose. Biochim. Biophys. Acta 110:635, 1965.
22. Gryboski, J. D., and Boehm, J. Lactulosuria in the neonate: A preliminary report. Pediatrics 35:340, 1965.
23. Kerry, K. R., and Anderson, M. A ward test for sugar in feces. Lancet, 1:981, 1964.
24. Weser, E., and Sleisenger, M. H. Metabolism of circulating disaccharides in man and the rat. J. Clin. Invest. 46:499, 1967.
25. Bayless, T. M., and Rosensweig, N. S. A racial difference in the incidence of lactase deficiency. J.A.M.A. 197:968, 1966.
26. Gilat, T., Kuhn, R., Gelman, E., et al. Lactase deficiency in Jewish communities in Israel. Amer. J. Dig. Dis. 15:895, 1970.
27. Huang, S. S., and Bayless, T. M. Milk and lactose intolerance in healthy orientals. Science 160:83, 1968.
28. Leichter, J., and Lee, M. Lactose intolerance in Canadian West Coast Indians. Amer. J. Dig. Dis. 16:809, 1971.
29. Cook, G. C. Lactase activity in newborn and infant Baganda. Brit. Med. J. 1:527, 1967.
30. Bolin, T. E., and Davis, A. E. Asian lactose intolerance and its relationship to intake of lactose. Nature 222:382, 1969.
31. Berg, N. O., Dahlqvist, A., Lindberg, T., et al. Severe familial lactose intolerance—a gastrogen disorder? Acta Pediat. Scand. 58:525, 1969.
32. Darling, S., Morteson, O., and Sondergaard, G. Lactosuria and aminoaciduria in infancy. Acta Paediat. Scand. 49:281, 1960.
33. Holzel, A. Sugar malabsorption due to deficiency of disaccharidase activities and of monosaccharide transport. Arch. Dis. Child. 42:341, 1967.
34. Lifshitz, F. Congenital lactase deficiency. J. Pediat. 69:229, 1966.
35. Nordio, S., Lamedica, G. M., Vignolo, L., et al. Six cases of lactose intolerance. Lactose intolerance and coeliac disease. Ann. Paediat. 204:3, 1965.
36. Lubos, M. C., Gerrard, J. W., and Buchan, D. Disaccharidase activities in milk-sensitive and celiac patients. J. Pediat. 70:325, 1967.
37. Howatt, J. M., and Aaranson, I. Sugar intolerance in neonatal surgery. J. Pediat. Surg. 6:719, 1971.
38. Richards, A. J., Condon, J. R., and Mallinson, C. N. Lactose intolerance following extensive small intestinal resection. Brit. J. Surg. 58:493, 1971.
39. Sunshine, P., and Kretchmer, N. Studies of small intestine during development. III. Infantile diarrhea associated with intolerance to disaccharides. Pediatrics 34:38, 1964.
40. Lifshitz, F., Coello-Ramirez, R., and Guiterrez-Topete, G. Monosaccharide intolerance and hypoglycemia in infants with diarrhea. I. Clinical course of 23 infants. J. Pediat. 77:595, 1970.
41. Lifshitz, F., Coello-Ramirez, P., Guiterrez-Topete, G., et al. Carbohydrate intolerance in infants with diarrhea. J. Pediat. 79:760, 1971.
42. Antonowicz, I., Reddy, V., Khaw, K. T., et al. Lactase deficiency in patients with cystic fibrosis. Pediatrics 42:492, 1968.
43. Hoskins, L. C., Winawer, S. J., Broitman, S. A., et al. Clinical giardiasis and intestinal malabsorption. Gastroenterology 53:265, 1967.
44. Fekete, M., Galfi, I., Soltesz, G., et al. Lactose absorption in growth retarded newborn infants. Acta Paediat. Acad. Sci. Hung. 10:303, 1969.
45. Weser, E., Rubin, W., Ross, L., and Sleisenger, M. H. Lactase deficiency in patients with the irritable-colon syndrome. New Eng. J. Med. 273:1070, 1965.
46. Levitt, M. D., and Donaldson, R. J., Jr. Use of respiratory hydrogen (H_2) excretion to detect carbohydrate malabsorption. J. Lab. Clin. Med. 75:937, 1970.
47. Laws, J. W., and Neale, G. Radiological diagnosis of disaccharidase deficiency. Lancet 2:139, 1966.
48. Durand, P. Lattosuria idiopatica in una paziente con diarrhea cronica et acidosis. Minerva Pediat. 10:706, 1958.
49. Dahlqvist, A. Assay of intestinal disaccharidases. Enzym. Biol. Clin. 11:52, 1970.
50. Koch, R., Acosta, P., Ragsdale, N., and Donnell, G. N. Nutrition in the treatment of galactosemia. J. Amer. Diet. Assn. 43:216, 1963.

51. Hardinge, M. G., Swarner, J. B., and Crooks, H. Carbohydrates in foods. J. Amer. Diet. Assn. 46:197, 1965.
52. Auricchio, S., Rubino, A., Prader, A., et al. Intestinal glycosidase activities in congenital malabsorption of disaccharides. J. Pediat. 66:555, 1965.
53. Frezel, J. F., Rey, J., and Lamy, M. Disaccharide malabsorption. Sympos. Intest. Absorpt. and Malabsorpt. Mod. Prob. Pediat. 11:113, 1968.
54. Anderson, C. M., Messer, M., Townley, R. R. W., et al. Intestinal sucrase and isomaltase deficiency in 2 siblings. Pediatrics 31:1003, 1963.
55. Burgess, E. A., Levin, B., Mahalanabis, D., et al. Hereditary sucrose intolerance: Levels of sucrase activity in jejunal mucosa. Arch. Dis. Child. 39:431, 1964.
56. Eggermont, E. The molecular lesion of saccharose intolerance. Mod. Prob. Pediat. 11:121, 1968.
57. Bergoz, R. Trehalose malabsorption causing intolerance to mushrooms. Gastroenterology 60:909, 1971.
58. Gryboski, J. D. Diarrhea from dietetic candy. New Eng. J. Med. 275:818, 1966.
59. Laplane, R., Polonovski, C., Etienne, M., Debray, P., Lods, J. C. and Pissarro, B. L'intolerance aux sucres a transfert intestinal actif. Ses rapports avec l'intolerance au lactose et le syndrome coeliaque. Arch. Franc. Pediat. 19:895, 1962.
60. Lindquist, B., Meeuwisse, G. W., and Melin, K. Glucose-galactose malabsorption. Lancet 2:666, 1962.
61. Lindquist, B., and Meeuwisse, G. W. Chronic diarrhea caused by monosaccharide malabsorption. Acta Paediat. Scand. 51:674, 1962.
62. Lindquist, B., and Meeuwisse, G. W. Diets in disaccharidase deficiency and defective monosaccharide absorption. J. Amer. Diet. Assn. 48:307, 1966.
63. Marks, J. F., Norton, J. B., and Fordtran, J. S. Glucose-galactose malabsorption. J. Pediat. 69:225, 1966.
64. Meeuwisse, G., and Dahlqvist, A. Glucose-galactose malabsorption. Acta Paediat. Scand. 57:273, 1968.
65. Meeuwisse, G. W., and Melin, K. Glucose-galactose malabsorption. A clinical study of 6 cases. Acta Paediat. Scand. Suppl. 188:1, 1970.
66. Melin, K., and Meeuwisse, G. W. Glucose-galactose malabsorption. A genetic study. Acta Paediat. Scand. Suppl. 188:19, 1970.
67. Schneider, A. J., Kinter, W. B., and Stirling, C. E. Glucose-galactose malabsorption. Report of a case with autoradiographic studies of a mucosal biopsy. New Eng. J. Med. 274:305, 1966.
68. Elsas, L. J., Hillman, R., Patterson, J. G., et al. Renal and intestinal hexose transport in familial glucose-galactose malabsorption. J. Clin. Invest. 49:576, 1970.
69. Burke, V., and Kands, D. M. Monosaccharide malabsorption in young infants. Lancet 1:1177, 1966.

Chapter 77

Carcinoid Tumors and the Carcinoid Syndrome

O. Dhodanand Kowlessar

Carcinoid tumors are a heterogeneous group of neoplasms of either the enterochromaffin cells of the gastrointestinal tract or the enterochromaffin cell equivalents in other organs with characteristic clinical, histochemical, and biochemical features dependent upon their sites of origin. Over 90 per cent of carcinoid tumors originate in the gastrointestinal tract; they comprise 1.5 per cent of gastrointestinal neoplasms. The most frequent enteral sites are the appendix, terminal ileum, and rectum. The colon, stomach, duodenum, and Meckel's diverticulum are less frequently involved. Although rare, carcinoid tumors have been reported to develop in the biliary tract, pancreatic duct, and gonadal teratomas. Bronchial carcinoids, originating from the enterochromaffin cells in the epithelium of the bronchial tree, have been reported with increasing frequency during the past decade.

Carcinoid tumors secrete a variety of potent humoral agents in relationship to their site of origin, and there are several variants of the classic carcinoid syndrome such that the term "malignant carcinoid spectrum" appears to be a more appropriate designation.[1] The complex of symptoms and signs that encompass the carcinoid spectrum includes diarrhea, abdominal cramps, borborygmi, episodic flushing, telangiectasia, cyanosis, pellagra-like skin lesions, bronchospasm with wheezing and asthmatic-like attacks, dyspnea, and valvular lesions of the heart. These signs and symptoms in turn are due in part to increased production of a variety of substances with pharmacological and physiological actions represented by 5-hydroxytryptamine (serotonin), bradykinin, histamine, catecholamines, insulin, adrenocorticotropic hormone (ACTH), melanocyte stimulating hormone (MSH), and probably prostaglandins.

PATHOLOGY

Significant evidence has accumulated that carcinoid tumors arise from enterochromaffin cells. These cells are widely distributed in tissues derived from the primitive gut, including the gastrointestinal tract, the pancreatic ducts, the gallbladder and bile ducts, and the bronchi. Classically, it has been thought that the entire enterochromaffin cell system from which these tumors are derived arises from a single type of progenitor cell. This "unitarian concept" is based on the assumption that the enterochromaffin cell and tumors derived from it represent variations in the stage of maturity or activity of the cells which comprise the tumors. Re-

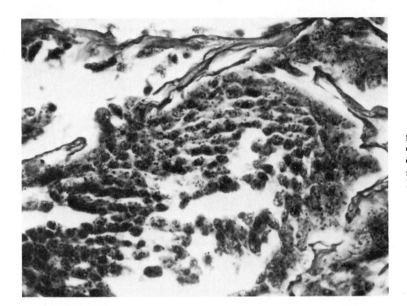

Figure 77–1. Photomicrograph of a carcinoid tumor demonstrating argentaffin cells: × 640. (From Kowlessar, O. D., et al.: Amer. J. Med. 27:673, 1959.)

cent evidence indicates that they are a variety of enterochromaffin cell types with a wide range of distribution throughout the gastrointestinal tract (Fig. 77–1). Furthermore, the carcinoids tend to correspond cytologically to the type of enterochromaffin cell which predominates in the site of origin.[2]

Utilizing a new electron-histochemical technique to study various carcinoid tumors and normal gastrointestinal mucosa, Black[2] has shown that both gastric mucosa and gastric carcinoids contained enterochromaffin cells with relatively small and uniformly rounded granules which stained with silver ultrastructurally (argyrophilic), but were argentaffin negative. Since both the stomach and the bronchi are derived from the primitive foregut, it is not surprising that Bensch et al.[3] have described similar cells in bronchial carcinoids. On the other hand, Black[2] found that the small intestinal mucosa as well as ileal and appendiceal carcinoids, of primitive midgut origin, contained argentaffin granules which were large, pleomorphic, and of uniform density. Rectal mucosa and rectal carcinoids derived from the primitive hindgut contained rounded granules larger than those of the gastric tumors, and gave neither an argyrophil nor an argentaffin reaction. Thus, it is not surprising that carcinoids of foregut (bronchus, stomach, and pancreas), midgut (jejunum, ileum,

and appendix), and hindgut (colon and rectum) origin will differ in their cytological, histochemical, biochemical, and clinical characteristics.[2,4]

PHARMACOLOGICALLY ACTIVE SUBSTANCES

In order to appreciate the various clinical manifestations of the "malignant carcinoid spectrum" it is essential to clearly understand the pharmacologically active substances derived from the tumor and/or its metastases. Among these substances are 5-hydroxytryptamine (serotonin), 5-hydroxytryptophan, histamine, catecholamines, bradykinin, and possibly prostaglandins.

SEROTONIN

Although carcinoid tumors differ widely in their ability to produce or store 5-hydroxytryptamine, the excessive production of this substance remains their most characteristic chemical abnormality. Normally 99 per cent of dietary tryptophan is available for the formation of niacin and protein. In patients with a large mass of carcinoid tumor, more than half the tryptophan intake is hydroxylated by the enzyme tryptophan hydroxylase to 5-hydroxytryptophan, which has a high affinity

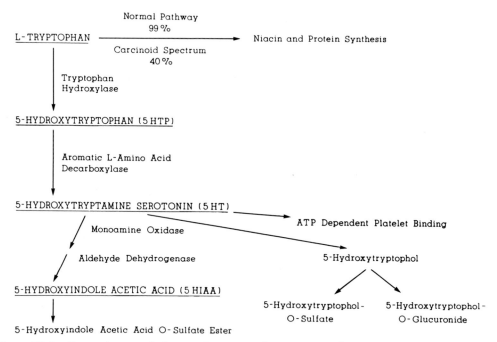

Figure 77-2. Tryptophan metabolism in the carcinoid spectrum. Underlined metabolites are those most frequently encountered.

for aromatic-L-amino acid decarboxylase which converts 5-hydroxytryptophan (5-HTP) to 5-hydroxytryptamine (5-HT) (Fig. 77–2).[5] Serotonin is the most active pharmacological indole produced by the tumor. It may be metabolized by the enzyme monoamine oxidase in the tumor (in which case it will produce little pharmacologic effect) or in the blood after release from the tumor. Serotonin is oxidized to 5-hydroxyindoleacetaldehyde which is converted to 5-hydroxyindoleacetic acid by aldehyde dehydrogenase. Small amounts of circulating serotonin are inactivated by ATP-dependent binding to platelets, or by conversion to the alcohol 5-hydroxytryptophol or its conjugates 5-hydroxytryptophol-o-sulfate and 5-hydroxytryptophol-o-glucuronide.[5] Most of the 5-hydroxyindoleacetic acid is excreted in the urine as the free acid, although small amounts may be conjugated to the o-sulfate ester before excretion. Patients with the carcinoid spectrum usually have expansion of the serotonin pool size,[6] a striking increase in blood and platelet concentration of serotonin, and elevations of 5-hydroxyindoleacetic acid in the urine.

The physiological effects of serotonin are diverse. There is good evidence that serotonin mediates the diarrhea and possibly the malabsorption, intestinal hypermotility, abdominal cramps, nausea, and vomiting observed in patients with the carcinoid syndrome.[6] Both the tone and motility of the human jejunum are increased with infusions of serotonin.[7] It has been suggested that the stimulation of peristalsis by serotonin results from a reduction of the threshold of intraluminal pressure required to elicit the peristaltic reflex, with a resultant increase in both the frequency of contraction and the volume of fluid transported.[8] Although the valvular and endocardial lesions seen in patients with the carcinoid syndrome suggest a circulating humoral substance, no direct correlation exists between the cardiac changes and the blood levels of either serotonin or other substances. Likewise, serotonin can produce bronchoconstriction in the isolated lung, but once again correlation of the release of serotonin with bronchoconstriction and wheezing is lacking at present. The edema seen in some patients has in the past been ascribed to renal factors, and may represent a direct effect of serotonin promoting sodium retention via the renal tubule, or possibly to secondary aldosteronism. Serotonin has been shown to reduce renal blood flow in the carcinoid state, and this diminution may stimulate the release of aldosterone from the adrenal cortex.[5]

HISTAMINE; CATECHOLAMINES; KININS; PROSTAGLANDINS

Other amines have been found in the urine of carcinoid patients. Those with gastric carcinoids have been shown to have frequent and consistent elevations of histamine, which is inconsistently elevated in those with ileal tumors. Increased histamine excretion is often seen in patients with gastric and bronchial carcinoids, who lack the enzyme aromatic-L-amino acid decarboxylase. Although catecholamines and their metabolites have been elevated in the urine of some patients with the carcinoid syndrome, this abnormality is unusual and to date has not been correlated with specific symptoms or origins of the tumors.[5]

In earlier studies, serotonin was thought to be primarily responsible for the carcinoid flush. Considerable evidence has been marshaled that serotonin is not the sole mediator. Intravenous injection of 5-hydroxytryptamine does not reproduce the characteristic spontaneous attacks of flushing in carcinoid patients, nor is there a correlation between the levels of free plasma 5-hydroxytryptamine and flushing episodes. Although the infusion of epinephrine or norepinephrine provokes typical flushing attacks, it is not often accompanied by increased levels of 5-hydroxytryptamine in blood obtained from either the brachial artery or the hepatic vein. Metastatic carcinoid tumors can occur without the syndrome in the presence of elevations of urinary 5-hydroxyindoleacetic acid. Recent evidence implicates a group of vasodilator peptides as the mediators of the flush in some patients with carcinoid syndrome. It is currently held that the flush in any given patient with the carcinoid syndrome is caused by a variety of biologically active substances, among which are lysyl-bradykinin and bradykinin.

These kinins (lysyl-bradykinin and bradykinin) are produced by the enzymatic action of kallikrein on an alpha-2-globulin substrate kininogen (Fig. 77-3). When synthetic bradykinin was infused rapidly into patients with the carcinoid syndrome, the flush produced was similar to the spontaneous flushes. Elevated levels of bradykinin were present in the hepatic venous blood of some patients during spontaneous and epinephrine-induced flushes. The enzyme kallikrein has been extracted from the carcinoid tumors of patients with flushing. It has also been localized in a carcinoid tumor by immunofluorescent techniques.

Epinephrine, sympathetic discharge, and alcohol ingestion, which are flush-provoking stimuli, are capable of liberating kallikrein from the tumor. Once liberated, kallikrein splits lysyl-bradykinin from kininogen. The lysyl-bradykinin is rapidly converted to bradykinin by a plasma amino peptidase, after which it is rapidly broken down to inactive smaller peptides and amino acids.[9] Besides the ability of lysyl-bradykinin and bradykinin to induce flushing, these polypeptides are capable of producing profound vasodilatation, systemic hypotension, increased salivation, lacrimation, and cardiac output, and edema and tachycardia. They may also play a contributory role in the asthmatic-like attacks and increased fibrosis seen in patients with the carcinoid syndrome.

Prostaglandins are widely distributed in human tissues, but their functions are largely unknown despite much speculation. The recent observation that prostaglandin $F_{2\alpha}$ was found in a bronchial carcinoid and an unidentified hydroxy fatty acid, most likely a prostaglandin, was also found in two ileal carcinoids[10] raises the possibility that prostaglandins must be considered in relationship to the diarrhea,

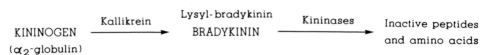

KININOGEN $\xrightarrow{\text{Kallikrein}}$ Lysyl-bradykinin / BRADYKININ $\xrightarrow{\text{Kininases}}$ Inactive peptides and amino acids
(α_2-globulin)

Figure 77-3. The formation and destruction of kinin in man. Increased production of bradykinin has been observed in some patients with the carcinoid syndrome.

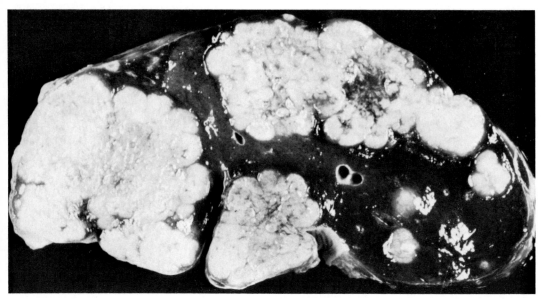

Figure 77–4. Liver with metastatic tumor. In the majority of cases with carcinoid syndrome the liver contains tumor. (From Kowlessar, O. D., et al.: Amer. J. Med. 27:673, 1959.)

flushing, and other symptoms associated with the carcinoid spectrum.

NATURAL HISTORY

The *natural history* of carcinoid tumors has traditionally been thought to vary with the location of the lesion. Metastases are infrequent in carcinoids of the appendix, but are common in extra-appendiceal carcinoids (Fig. 77–4). Intra-abdominal carcinoids spread in a progressive, stepwise pattern, initially involving the muscle coats by direct invasion, and then involving the regional lymph nodes and the liver. These tumors tend to be less aggressive than adenocarcinomas, and survival of five to ten years or longer is not uncommon, even after hepatic metastases have occurred. Bronchial carcinoids tend to be more aggressive, with earlier metastases to liver, bone, skin, and brain. The morbidity from these tumors appears to be directly related to the pharmacologically active substances secreted by the tumors. Congestive heart failure, shock, fluid and electrolyte disturbances, intestinal obstruction, and the sequelae of metastases eventually lead to death in these patients.

CLINICAL PICTURE

Carcinoid tumors may occur at any age, with an age incidence ranging from 14 to 88 years. These lesions are most common in the fifth decade of life, except for the appendiceal carcinoids which appear earlier. This is probably because the appendiceal lesions are commonly found at the time of abdominal exploration for other reasons and because the signs and symptoms of acute appendicitis necessitate appendectomy. It is possible that if appendiceal lesions were not discovered under these circumstances, they would have grown slowly and produced symptoms around the fifth decade of life.

The majority of patients with nonmetastatic carcinoids are usually free of symptoms. Symptoms caused by tumor include nonspecific crampy abdominal pain, intermittent or chronic intestinal obstruction, diarrhea, alternating bouts of constipation and diarrhea, weight loss, melena, hematemesis, rectal bleeding, and, less often, biliary obstruction. Clearly, these symptoms are not characteristic of carcinoid tumors alone, because they are observed in a wide variety of gastrointestinal lesions. On the other hand, patients may develop symptoms secondary to the pharmacological or endocrine effects of the tumor and have one or more of the characteristic features of the carcinoid syndrome.

CARCINOID SYNDROME
(Table 77–1)

The earliest manifestations of the classic carcinoid syndrome are episodic. The patients may complain of palpitations, swelling of the face, and diarrhea. Later in the course, they will experience episodes of tenseness, weakness, and nausea. Eventually, the classic vasomotor episodes appear, comprising repeated episodes of cyanotic, tricolored or bright red flushes over the face, upper extremities, and chest. They can be brought on or aggravated by anger, tension, active exercise, and the ingestion of alcohol and certain foods such as cheese. The flushes may occur repeatedly during the day, lasting for minutes, and are usually associated with perspiration, a feeling of warmth, palpitation, and tremulousness. On occasion, they are associated with conjunctival injection or increased lacrimation and salivation (bronchial carcinoid). With severe flushing, the patient may experience striking hypotension, increased respiratory rate, wheezing, borborygmi, and diarrhea. During episodes of prolonged flushing, periorbital and facial edema and oliguria may occur. On rare occasions, intense generalized pruritus and pressure-induced orange blotching of the skin have been described. In far advanced disease, chronic manifestations may develop in addition to the episodic phenomenon.

The patient is usually cachectic from severe weight loss. Funduscopic examination of the eye may reveal pigment clumping in the region of the macula, exudative punched-out lesions, pigment deposits, and colloid degeneration.[11] The skin may show bluish-red discoloration of the face, trunk, and arms with associated telangiectasia. Pellagra and scleroderma-like changes have also been described. The characteristic auscultatory finding of the heart is a precordial murmur representing valvular pulmonic stenosis. Congestive changes secondary to right-sided heart failure occur with the findings of pleural effusion, hepatic congestion, ascites, and edema of the legs. The superficial jugular veins are often distended and in association with a pulsatile liver suggest tricuspid regurgitation. If there is evidence of mitral or aortic valvular disease, one should suspect an atrial septal defect with right-to-left shunt, a bronchial carcinoid, or acquired or congenital valvular defects unrelated to the carcinoid tumor.[5] Evidence of high cardiac output at rest has been reported in patients with flushing and has been attributed to the release of a vasodilator substance (possibly bradykinin) by the tumor. The abdominal examination may reveal the signs of ascites, striking hyperactive bowel sounds, and an enlarged, firm, and nodular liver. Occasionally, an epigastric or right lower quadrant mass may be felt. Systolic bruits may be heard in the left upper quadrant secondary to involvement of the splenic artery by carcinoid tumors of the pancreas. Occasionally, a friction rub may be heard over the liver secondary to necrosis of metastatic lesions in the liver. The joints of the fingers may show changes of arthritis. Early in the disease, one may note brawny edema with resultant disabling stiffness of the legs. Peripheral edema secondary to heart failure and hypoproteinemia is a late manifestation.

The physical findings associated with acromegaly, Cushing's syndrome, and

---

TABLE 77–1. PRINCIPAL MANIFESTATIONS OF THE CARCINOID SYNDROME

1. Vasomotor disturbances—cutaneous flushes and "cyanosis"
2. Hepatomegaly—large nodular liver
3. Intestinal hypermotility—borborygmi, cramps, diarrhea, vomiting, nausea
4. Bronchoconstriction—cough, dyspnea, wheezing
5. Cardiac involvement—endocardial fibrosis with valvular deformity
6. Absence of hypertension—incidence no greater than general population
7. Prolonged clinical course—patients survive years longer than those with other tumors with metastases

pluriglandular adenomatosis have been described in association with the carcinoid spectrum on rare occasions. The signs, symptoms, and physical findings of the malabsorption syndrome can occur in some patients with the carcinoid syndrome.[12]

CARCINOID VARIANTS

Bronchial Carcinoids. These tumors produce the most striking clinical features of any of the variants of the carcinoid syndrome. Characteristically, the flushing attacks are more prolonged and severe, lasting for as long as three to four days. The flushes are frequently associated with or preceded by disorientation, tremulousness of the hands, severe anxiety, temperature elevations, periorbital and facial edema, increased salivation and lacrimation, rhinorrhea, and diaphoresis. Nausea, vomiting, explosive diarrhea, and wheezing, which are commonly encountered during the flushing episode, are usually absent between flushes. Likewise, the flushes may be associated with severe hypotension, oliguria, and, in the presence of left-sided cardiac lesions, pulmonary edema. Other unusual features of this variant include the prevalence of left-sided cardiac lesions, increased incidence of Cushing's syndrome, pluriglandular adenomatosis, acromegaly, and frequent metastasis to bone. Biochemically, the tumors appear to produce large amounts of 5-hydroxytryptophan as well as 5-hydroxytryptamine.[13] It has been recommended that patients with asymptomatic pulmonary "coin" lesions discovered during routine roentgenograms of the chest be screened with quantitative urinary excretion of 5-hydroxyindoleacetic acid.

Gastric Carcinoid Tumors. Patients with gastric carcinoids have frequently shown a characteristic clinical and biochemical syndrome. The flushes in these patients begin with a bright red patchy erythema with sharply delineated serpentine borders. The patches tend to coalesce as the blush intensifies. Certain highly spiced foods and cheeses tend to aggravate and precipitate the flushes. Increased production of large amounts of histamine may contribute to the peculiar geographic distribution of the flushes. The excessive production of histamine may in part be re-

sponsible for the increased production of hydrochloric acid and the concomitant increase of peptic ulcers seen in some of these patients.

In association with the fairly consistent histaminuria, the pattern of urinary excretion of tryptophan metabolites appears to be distinct from that of other carcinoid patients. The tumor usually lacks aromatic-L-amino acid decarboxylase and consequently releases 5-hydroxytryptophan rather than 5-hydroxytryptamine into the blood. A portion of the released 5-hydroxytryptophan is decarboxylated in the kidney with a resultant increase in urinary serotonin; 5-hydroxyindoleacetic acid may not be increased above 15 mg per 24 hours. It has been observed that these patients are less likely to have diarrhea and cardiac lesions.[9]

DIAGNOSIS

The diagnosis of carcinoid tumors is made by serendipity, by specific symptoms such as rectal bleeding, or by the patient's having developed the classic clinical syndrome. A high index of suspicion in patients with unexplained intermittent diarrhea, telangiectasia over the face, episodic flushing, wheezing, or psychosis will suggest the diagnosis of metastatic carcinoid. Isolated hepatomegaly or unilateral wheezing may give a clue to the underlying pathological process.

Routine clinical laboratory tests are rarely helpful. Leukocytosis, thrombocytosis, fever, hepatomegaly, and a friction rub over the liver suggest the intra-abdominal spread of the carcinoid tumor. Liver function tests may reveal only a modest elevation of the alkaline phosphatase with normal serum bilirubin. As the disease progresses, hypoproteinemia and hypoalbuminemia will develop. A liver scintigram after injection of radioactively labeled gold (^{198}Au) or more recently ^{99m}Tc sulfur colloid will reveal multiple filling defects in patients with hepatic metastases. A liver biopsy will reveal tumor with histology compatible with carcinoid.

Occult malabsorption, although rare, can be revealed by 72-hour quantitative stool fat, the measurement of serum carotene, prothrombin time, cholesterol level, and d-xylose excretion. This latter determination should be viewed in relationship to the age of the patient as well as the effects of serotonin on the kidney.

Roentgenographic examination of the chest will demonstrate a carcinoid lesion or metastases to the lung. Pleural biopsy may reveal the characteristic histological features of the carcinoid tumor. Upper gastrointestinal series can reveal polypoid lesions of the stomach, duodenum, and jejunum. Gastroscopy may demonstrate the lesion in the stomach and duodenum, and biopsy under direct vision will establish the diagnosis. Multiple lesions in the ileum should arouse suspicion of carcinoid. Narrowing of the intestinal lumen secondary to tumor mass and adjacent fibrous tissue reaction with associated kinking and buckling of the small intestine and mesentery in the region of the tumor have been described (Fig. 77–5). Intussusception with the polypoid

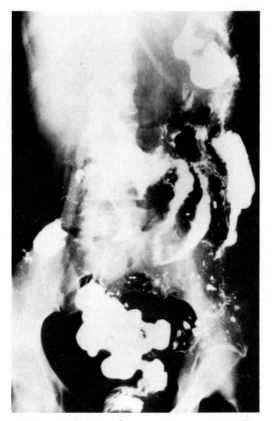

Figure 77–5. Four-hour roentgenogram of a small bowel series in a patient with a malignant ileal carcinoid, showing rigid loops of ileum and mucosal irregularities. (From Kowlessar, O. D., et al.: Amer. J. Med. 27:673, 1959.)

tumor acting as the leading point is also seen.

The majority of colonic carcinoids are small, are grossly noninvasive, and are found in the appendix incidentally or in the rectum on proctoscopic examination. However, a small number will be bulky and invasive, reminiscent radiographically of the more common adenocarcinoma or lymphomatous tumor involving the colon. A large polypoid or fungating colonic lesion with prominent extraluminal mass should suggest the possibility of a rare feature of colonic carcinoid.[14]

Selective celiac and superior mesenteric arteriography may reveal any of the following findings in ileal carcinoids — stellate arterial pattern, narrowing of the deep mesenteric branches, poor to moderate accumulation of contrast medium, and nonvisualization of veins. The metastases to the liver are highly vascular with accumulated contrast material.[15] Recently, the angiographic findings in a nonmetastatic gastric carcinoid revealed intense accumulation of contrast material in the tumor, with identification of several larger veins draining the area of the tumor. The arteries were regular, of normal caliber, and without any stellate pattern.[16]

SPECIAL STUDIES

The biochemical hallmark of the majority of metastatic carcinoids is the increased excretion of 5-hydroxyindoleacetic acid (5HIAA). The qualitative test is invariably positive and suggests a urinary excretion greater than 30 mg per 24-hour period. Since some carcinoids, e.g., gastric, do not produce enough serotonin to elevate urinary 5HIAA above 15 mg, it is essential to perform the quantitative test. Urinary excretion of 5HIAA in the range of 9 to 25 mg per 24-hour period has been described in patients with untreated celiac disease, tropical sprue, and Whipple's disease. The urinary levels of 5HIAA in patients with classic carcinoid syndrome vary widely, from 60 to 1000 mg per 24 hours. Great care should be taken to see that the patients are taking no drugs, especially medications containing glyceryl guaiacolate, acetanilid, mephenesin, and methocarbamol, all of which cause false-positive increases in 5HIAA level. Methenamine mandelate (Mandelamine) and phenothiazine derivatives with N-substituted aliphatic groups, such as promethazine hydrochloride (Phenergan), promazine hydrochloride (Sparine), prochlorperazine (Compazine), and chlorpromazine (Thorazine), result in false-negative tests for 5HIAA.[17] All foods rich in serotonin should be discontinued, especially bananas, pineapple, walnuts, and avocados. In patients with low excretion of 5HIAA, paper chromatography should be used to determine whether there are increases in 5-hydroxytryptamine and 5-hydroxytryptophan. Quantitative urinary 5-hydroxytryptamine higher than 1 to 2 mg per 24 hours in a patient with the carcinoid syndrome indicates that the tumor is a variant derived from the embryonic foregut, particularly the stomach, which releases the serotonin precursor 5-hydroxytryptophan.

Intermittent increased histamine excretion should be looked for in patients with gastric and bronchial carcinoids, especially in patients whose tumors secrete 5-hydroxytryptophan.

Determination of the 5-hydroxytryptamine content of whole blood, plasma, or platelets may help to confirm the diagnosis. Measurements of bradykinin or the tumor-kallikrein released into the peripheral circulation are possible, but the methodology is tedious and cumbersome.

In view of the known production of ectopic hormones by carcinoid tumors derived from the pancreas, bronchus, and other organs, determinations of 17-hydroxy- and ketosteroids, adrenocorticotropic hormone, melanocyte stimulating hormone, insulin, and other hormones should be performed when the clinical picture suggests overproduction of these substances. In a similar vein, it should be kept in mind that a number of pluriglandular adenomatoses have been seen in conjunction with carcinoid tumors arising from organs of the embryonic foregut. The associated tumors are diverse and have included parathyroid adenomas, pancreatic tumors producing Zollinger-Ellison syndrome, and acromegaly (see pp. 365 to 375).

In patients with carcinoid tumors complaining of intermittent flushing, an epinephrine test may be helpful. One or two minutes after the injection of 5μg of epinephrine, the patients will experience a flush similar to the spontaneous flush, with associated conjunctival suffusion, increased lacrimation and respiratory rate, and a decrease in both systolic and diastolic pressure of 40 mm Hg. However, a hypertensive response does not exclude a malignant carcinoid tumor. The test may also be positive in patients who have never experienced flushing, or who have been unaware of spontaneous flushing.[5]

DIFFERENTIAL DIAGNOSIS

The differential diagnosis of carcinoid tumors without metastases is dependent on the location of the tumor. Bronchial carcinoids must be differentiated from other solitary lung lesions, especially carcinoma. Other polypoid lesions of the stomach and small intestine will enter into the differential diagnosis. Similarly, in patients with right lower quadrant pain, other considerations will have to be taken into account, especially acute appendicitis and regional enteritis. Indeed, the X-ray may resemble Crohn's disease (Fig. 77–5). Colonic carcinoids with associated bleeding or obstruction must be differentiated from carcinomas, lymphomas, and leiomyomas in these areas.

Other clinical syndromes characterized by flushing, such as menopause, cirrhosis, and idiopathic flushing, can be differentiated by measuring urinary 5HIAA and by the epinephrine test which give uniformly negative results in these patients.[5] In some patients with systemic mastocytosis, the differentiation from the carcinoid syndrome may be difficult. Flushing, hepatomegaly, diarrhea, and occasionally steatorrhea and either osteoblastic or osteolytic bone lesions occur in both diseases. However, both urinary 5HIAA and the epinephrine provocative test are uniformly negative in systemic mastocytosis.[5]

TREATMENT

Surgical removal of the primary tumor is the best treatment. It is crucial under these circumstances that microscopic evidence of neoplastic invasion of the muscularis of the bowel wall be absent. If it is present, more extensive resection is indicated, especially in rectal carcinoids.[4] Unfortunately, in many patients with carcinoid tumor, the diagnosis is seldom made before it has metastasized. Even if metastasis has occurred, removal of a large functioning tumor will substantially reduce and eliminate symptoms or relieve intestinal obstruction. In rare instances, resection of isolated hepatic metastases may ameliorate the symptoms. The complications of surgery in patients with the carcinoid syndrome are increased. These include susceptibility to adhesion formation and the danger that anesthesia or surgical manipulation of the tumor may induce the carcinoid crisis. In view of this the patient should be pretreated with high doses of serotonin antagonists such as methysergide maleate or cyproheptadine (Periactin). Ampules of these antagonists should be available at all times during surgery. In prolonged postoperative hypotension, metaraminol bitartrate (aramine bitartrate) or angiotensin amide may restore blood pressure.[18]

The medical therapy of patients who are symptomatic from the various substances elaborated by the tumor and metastases can be divided conveniently into the following categories:

Inhibition of Serotonin Synthesis. Parachlorophenylalanine[19] can be given in a daily dosage of 3 to 4 g maximum in four equally divided doses. This medication effectively relieves nausea, vomiting, and diarrhea, and may decrease the intensity (but not the number) of flushes. The side effects are altered central nervous system function and, rarely, hypothermia.

Serotonin Antagonists. Methysergide maleate (Sansert) is given in a dose of 6 to 24 mg per day orally. One to 4 mg can be given as a single intravenous dose for an acute attack or 10 to 20 mg in 100 to 200 ml saline infusion for one to two hours or longer.[20] It irregularly controls flushes, asthmatic attacks, and diarrhea. It is more effective against the diarrhea than cyproheptadine. The side effects of this drug are hypotension, syncope, lassitude, and development of resistance. Cyproheptadine (Periactin) can be given in a dose of 6 to 30 mg per day orally. For relief of acute attacks 50 to 75 mg in 100 to 200 ml saline infused over one to two hours may be beneficial. It is as effective as methysergide, but seems to control flush better. The side effects are similar to methysergide.[20]

Other Drugs. 1. Antihistamines appear to be helpful in controlling the flush in rare patients with histamine elevation as part of the carcinoid syndrome.

2. Corticosteroid (prednisone) in doses of 15 to 40 mg per day may be dramatically beneficial in bronchial carcinoids with the carcinoid syndrome; otherwise it is usually ineffective.

3. Prochlorperazine, in doses of 10 mg three to four times daily, is occasionally helpful in controlling the flush.

4. Phenoxybenzamine, 10 to 30 mg daily, may diminish flushing by preventing kallikrein release.

Chemotherapy. A wide variety of chemotherapeutic agents have been tried. These agents have not been successful over a long period, although some remissions have been obtained with 5-fluorouracil, cyclophosphamide, and melphalan (Alkeran). Mengel[20] has observed that cyclophosphamide (Cytoxan) given in an initial dose of 40 mg per kilogram of body weight in two or three divided doses on successive days with maintenance therapy of either 10 or 15 mg per kilogram of body weight intravenously every 10 to 14 days, or 100 to 150 mg orally each day, is the most consistently effective chemotherapeutic agent. Radiotherapy (4000 to 4500 rads) may produce relief of pain from bony metastasis.

Supportive Measures. A nutritious diet, containing 70 gm of protein and high in fat and calories, with vitamin supplementation, especially niacin, is recommended. Some patients will notice that some foods may initiate episodes of flushing and diarrhea. The common offenders appear to be milk, cheeses, eggs, and citrus fruits, and these should be avoided. A high fluid intake to ensure a proper state of hydration is recommended. In the event of cardiac failure, the patient should be digitalized and given diuretics. In severe intractable diarrhea, one may have to resort to deodorized tincture of opium, 10 to 20 drops in water every four to six hours alone or in conjunction with one of the antiserotonin agents.

PROGNOSIS

Despite metastasis of the tumor, supportive and symptomatic treatment is extremely important. It should be kept in mind that patients with ileal carcinoids have lived as long as 23 years, whereas others have lived for ten or more years after the syndrome appeared. On the other hand, patients with bronchial carcinoids, oat cell carcinoma, and anaplastic pancreatic carcinoma with the carcinoid syndrome appear to have a much poorer prognosis.

REFERENCES

1. Sjoerdsma, A., and Melmon, K. L. The carcinoid spectrum. Gastroenterology 47:104, 1964.
2. Black, W. C., III. Enterochromaffin cell types and corresponding carcinoid tumors. Lab. Invest. 19:473, 1968.
3. Bensch, K. G., Gordon, G. B., and Miller, L. R. Electron microscopic and biochemical studies on the bronchial carcinoid tumor. Cancer 18:592, 1965.
4. Orloff, M. J. Carcinoid tumors of the rectum. Cancer 28:175, 1971.
5. Melmon, K. L. The endocrinologic manifestations of the carcinoid tumor. In Textbook of Endocrinology, R. H. Williams (ed.). 4th ed. Philadelphia, W. B. Saunders Co., 1968, p. 1161.
6. Sjoerdsma, A., Weissbach, H., Terry, L. L., and Udenfriend, S. Further observations on patients with malignant carcinoid. Amer. J. Med. 23:5, 1957.
7. Haverback, B. J., and Davidson, J. D. Serotonin and the gastrointestinal tract. Gastroenterology 35:570, 1958.
8. Bullbring, E., and Lin, R. C. Y. The effect of intraluminal application of 5-hydroxytryptamine and 5-hydroxytryptophan on peristalsis; the local production of 5-HT and its release in relation to intraluminal pressure and propulsive activity. J. Physiol. (London) 140:381, 1958.
9. Oates, J. A., and Butler, C. Pharmacologic and endocrine aspects of carcinoid syndrome. Advan. Pharmacol. 5:109, 1967.
10. Sandler, M., Karmin, S. M., and Williams, E. D. Prostaglandins in amine-peptide-secreting tumors. Lancet 2:1053, 1968.
11. Wong, V. G., and Melmon, K. L. Ophthalmic manifestations of the carcinoid flush. New Eng. J. Med. 277:406, 1967.
12. Kowlessar, O. D., Law, D. H., and Sleisenger, M. H. Malabsorption syndrome associated with metastatic carcinoid tumor. Amer. J. Med. 27:673, 1959.
13. Melmon, K. L., Sjoerdsma, A., and Mason, D. T. Distinctive clinical and therapeutic aspects of the syndrome associated with bronchial carcinoid tumors. Amer. J. Med. 39:568, 1965.
14. Shulman, H., and Giustra, P. Invasive carcinoids of the colon. Radiology 98:139, 1971.
15. Reuter, S. R., and Joijsen, E. Angiographic findings in two ileal carcinoid tumors. Radiology 87:836, 1966.
16. Andersen, J. B., Madsen, B., and Skjoldborg, H. Angiography in a case of carcinoid tumor in the stomach. Brit. J. Radiol. 44:218, 1971.
17. Pedersen, A. T., Batsakis, J. G., Vanselow, N. A., and McLean, J. A. False-positive tests for urinary 5-hydroxyindoleacetic acid. Error in laboratory determinations caused by glyceryl guaiacolate. J.A.M.A. 211:1184, 1970.
18. Martin, R. G. Management of carcinoid tumors. Cancer 26:547, 1970.
19. Engelman, K., Lovenberg, W., and Sjoerdsma, A. Inhibition of serotonin synthesis by parachlorophenylalanine in patients with the carcinoid syndrome. New Eng. J. Med. 277:1103, 1967.
20. Mengel, C. E. Therapy of the malignant carcinoid syndrome. Ann. Intern. Med. 62:587, 1965.

Chapter 78

Intestinal Lymphangiectasia and A-Beta-Lipoproteinemia

O. Dhodanand Kowlessar

INTESTINAL LYMPHANGIECTASIA

Intestinal lymphangiectasia is a generalized disorder of the lymphatic system characterized by the early onset of severe, frequently asymmetrical peripheral edema, hypoproteinemia, lymphocytopenia, and mild gastrointestinal symptoms. It is invariably accompanied by dilated telangiectatic lymphatic vessels of the submucosa of the small intestine.[1] The disease was originally called "idiopathic hypoalbuminemia," then termed "hypercatabolic hypoproteinemia," and later "primary protein-losing gastroenteropathy." These terms, however, do not characterize the anatomic and morphological abnormalities but only detail the secondary phenomenon of protein loss into the gastrointestinal tract.

ETIOLOGY AND PATHOGENESIS

In spite of intensive investigation, the pathogenesis of the lymphatic abnormalities remains obscure. In those patients with onset at birth and with a family history of hypoproteinemia it may well result from a congenital malformation of the lymphatic system.[1] Lymphangiography demonstrates obvious stasis and reflux in the abdominal lymphatics and consistent hypoplasia of the lymphatics of the involved extremities.[2] This observation may account for the asymmetry of the edema.

In other instances in which the onset is delayed and appears later in life, it is probably the result of an acquired defect[1] or secondary to a number of disease processes, including retroperitoneal fibrosis, retroperitoneal tumors, intestinal scleroderma, pancreatitis, constrictive pericarditis, congestive heart failure, regional enteritis, radiation enteritis, mesenteric and diffuse lymphomas, and abdominal tuberculosis.

The pathogenesis of the transudation of plasma proteins in patients with intestinal lymphangiectasia is thought to be related to increased intestinal lymphatic pressure with subsequent dilatation of the lymphatic vessels and discharge of their contents into the bowel lumen.[1] The discharge of lymph into the gastrointestinal tract has been demonstrated both by lymphangiography and by the finding of lymph in the bowel lumen by intestinal intubation (see pp. 35 to 47).

Utilizing electron microscopy, Dobbins[3] showed that the lymphatic endothelial cells of the small intestinal mucosa of a patient with intestinal lymphangiectasia contained unusually prominent intracellular filaments thought to be related to the increased hydrostatic pressure within the lymphatic lumina. The basal lamina, supporting cells, and collagen fibers surrounding the lymphatic endothelium were more prominent than in a normal subject. Numerous chylomicrons were noted in the epithelial intercellular peg areas, in the extracellular spaces of the lamina propria, and within the lymphatic lumina, suggesting that the retention of lipid within the absorptive cell is secondary to an "exit block." A further evidence of the mechanical block is the finding of large, dense lipid droplets in the lymphatic endothelium. These findings may account for the fat malabsorption seen in some of these patients.

NATURAL HISTORY

The disease primarily affects children and young adults. The mean age of onset of symptoms is around ten years, and the majority of reported patients had their initial symptoms before 28 years of age.[1] Although the disease is sporadic, there are at least four families with a number of affected members. Rarely, patients under ten years of age die after prolonged periods of severe debilitation associated with frequent infections.[4] Despite the fact that these patients have significant disorders of delayed hypersensitivity, frequent infections do not appear to be a major complication in this disease. In patients with secondary lymphatic abnormalities, the natural history is directly related to the disease process responsible for the lymphatic changes.

CLINICAL PICTURE

Significant edema, usually generalized, is regularly observed at some time during the course of the disease. The patients may be seen at birth or at a few weeks of age with markedly asymmetrical edema. Rarely, they may present with blindness secondary to macular edema. Later, there are listlessness, weakness, generalized anasarca, intermittent diarrhea, and steatorrhea in the majority of patients.[1]

A few patients develop striking gastrointestinal complaints with diarrhea, extreme steatorrhea, nausea, vomiting, abdominal pain, and abdominal distention. Generally, the gastrointestinal symptoms are mild.[1] Occasionally the disease is associated with chyluria, chylous ascites, and chylous effusions.

Physical examination reveals a well developed and usually well nourished infant, child, or adult with asymmetrical edema or generalized anasarca (Fig. 78–1). There may be evidence of pleural effusion. The abdomen may be markedly distended with prominent superficial veins, fluid wave, and shifting dullness.

DIAGNOSIS

In a patient without liver, kidney, or heart disease, with significant edema, the diagnosis of intestinal lymphangiectasia should be seriously considered. Protein and immunoelectrophoresis reveal a marked reduction of albumin, IgA, IgG,

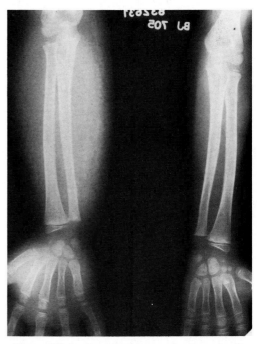

Figure 78–1. Lymphedema and enlarged radius and ulna of right arm in a ten-year-old boy with lymphangiectasia. (Courtesy of Dr. M. H. Sleisenger.)

and IgM globulins. Quantitative protein studies reveal a moderate reduction of transferrin and ceruloplasmin levels, with normal levels of fibrinogen and α_2-macroglobulin.[1] These protein abnormalities are related to severe gastrointestinal protein loss. There is at least a 25 per cent reduction of the mean survival half-time for albumin, γ-globulin, α_2-macroglobulin, and ceruloplasmin, with either a normal or a slightly increased synthetic rate for these proteins.[1] These abnormalities can be detected by iodinated polyvinyl pyrrolidone and a wide variety of labeled proteins, including iodinated serum proteins, chromium[51]-labeled proteins, copper[67]-labeled ceruloplasmin, and purified radioiodinated IgG, IgA, and IgM[1,4] (see also pp. 35 to 47).

The cholesterol may be slightly low or normal. Lymphocytopenia with a mean of 600 per mm^3 is a universal finding. Anemia is rare. Hypocalcemia low enough to cause tetany has been described in a few instances. In spite of the hypogammaglobulinemia and lymphocytopenia, these patients are capable of synthesizing antibodies to antigenic challenge in a nearly normal manner. However, they do

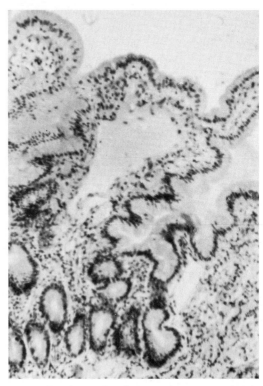

Figure 78–3. Dilated lacteal in a slightly "clubbed" villus in a biopsy specimen from a patient with lymphangiectasia. Hematoxylin and eosin stain. × 200. (Courtesy of Dr. M. H. Sleisenger.)

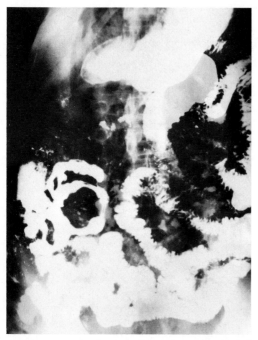

Figure 78–2. Small bowel series in a woman with lymphangiectasia, showing edematous mucosal folds and some retained secretions. (Courtesy of Dr. M. H. Sleisenger.)

have skin anergy and a striking failure to reject skin homografts.[4]

Moderate impairment of fat absorption is seen, but it is rarely massive and on occasion there is no increase in fat excretion. The fecal nitrogen excretion is normal, and tests to determine carbohydrate malabsorption, i.e., glucose and d-xylose, are usually within normal limits.

The radiographic findings in the usual case with small intestinal involvement are variable. In some cases, no abnormality is seen. In others, hypoproteinemia and secondary edema of the small intestine are obvious (Fig. 78–2). Marshak et al.[5] believe that diffuse, symmetric thickening of mucosal folds with increased secretions are the main features. They consider nodular defects unusual and segmentation and dilatation minimal or nonexistent. However, segmentation and dilatation have been observed.

Lymphangiograms will reveal stasis and reflux into the abdominal lymphatics, and significant hypoplasia of the peripheral

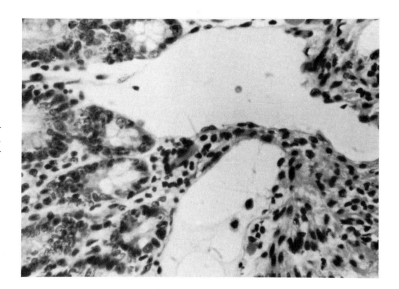

Figure 78–4. Same specimen as Figure 78–3. × 500. (Courtesy of Dr. M. H. Sleisenger.)

lymphatics with dermal back flow. Other lymphangiographic findings include partial obstruction or absence of the thoracic duct, a tortuous double thoracic duct, and the absence of periaortic lymph nodes.[2]

Peroral biopsy of the involved jejunal mucosa will show dilatation of the intramucosal lymphatics which, at times, may be so severe as to distort the villous architecture (Figs. 78–3 and 78–4). These dilated lymphatics contain large, lipid-filled macrophages in the lamina propria and submucosa.[1] It is impossible to differentiate congenital intestinal lymphangiectasia from the acquired form by biopsy alone.

In patients with ascites and/or pleural effusion, diagnostic paracentesis or thoracentesis should be performed to determine whether the patient has chylous ascites or chylous effusion, which occasionally accompany this disease. The removed fluid should be studied for proteins, lipids, acid-fast organisms, amebae, and malignant cells.

DIFFERENTIAL DIAGNOSIS

In childhood, the disease should be differentiated from celiac disease with protein weeping. The characteristic biopsy seen in untreated celiac disease and the response to a gluten-free diet should readily differentiate the two diseases. Transient hypoproteinemia, frequently associated with anemia and eosinophilia and lasting for a few weeks to a few months, has been described in a number of children and adults. Anemia is rare in patients with intestinal lymphangiectasia, and eosinophilia does not occur. Furthermore, transient hypoproteinemia is a self-limited disease. A group of young children have been described with a syndrome characterized by edema, with striking periorbital edema, iron deficiency anemia, eosinophilia, hypoalbuminemia, hypogammaglobulinemia, growth retardation, and characteristic features of allergy, including eczema, asthma, and allergic rhinitis. Unlike patients with intestinal lymphangiectasia, the jejunal biopsies in these patients are normal. The stools contain Charcot-Leyden crystals, and there is no steatorrhea. They respond clinically and biochemically to a hypoallergenic diet, specifically a milk-free diet[6] (see pp. 1075 to 1079).

Unusual causes of hypoproteinemia should be looked for in children. Among these are such entities as congenital ileal stenosis, nonspecific stenosis and inflammatory lesions of the jejunum, eosinophilic gastroenteritis, regional enteritis, lymphoma, and hookworm infestation.[7] Besides disease of the gastrointestinal tract, excessive loss of protein into the gut has been described in constrictive pericarditis, agammaglobulinemia, and the nephrotic syndrome.[1]

In the adult patient, the secondary diseases listed under etiology and pathogenesis should be considered in the differential diagnosis. Furthermore, adult celiac disease, Whipple's disease, nonspecific jejunitis, eosinophilic gastroenteritis, agammaglobulinemia, and a wide variety of diseases affecting the esophagus, stomach, and colon as well as the heart and kidney should be considered in the differential diagnosis[1] (see pp. 35 to 47).

A recent description of a patient with congenital β-lipoprotein deficiency and intestinal lymphangiectasia has been reported by Dobbins.[8] Chronic diarrhea, steatorrhea, intestinal protein loss, and dilated lacteals filled with lipid as well as club-shaped villi packed with lipid macrophages were the features of this entity. The lipophage infiltration of the abdominal lymph nodes was postulated as the mechanism of the lymphangiectasia and protein-losing enteropathy.

TREATMENT

Excessive protein loss into the gastrointestinal tract is not represented by a single disease entity. Therefore medical or surgical therapy will be dependent on the underlying process.

The medical therapy of intestinal lymphangiectasia is either a low-fat diet with less than 5 g per day or a formula diet in which long-chain fatty acids are substituted by medium-chain triglycerides (MCT) (C 6:0 to C 12:0).[9] In infants, Portagen is given as a formula which provides 20 kcal per fluid oz, whereas older children and adults are given 30 kcal per fluid oz. Each 8 fluid ounces provides 11.0 g of MCT and 0.5 g of safflower oil (the latter to provide essential fatty acids). The beverage also contains 9.6 g of protein and 24.6 g of carbohydrate (about half lactose and half sucrose) per glassful, with ample vitamins and minerals. If the patient has an associated lactase deficiency, Portagen without lactose should be used. This substitution of medium-chain triglycerides for long-chain fatty acids will result in a marked reduction of intestinal protein losses with the disappearance of the edema, ascites, pleural effusions, and gastrointestinal signs and symptoms. It would appear that the absorption of lipids containing long-chain fatty acids which are normally transported by the thoracic duct enhances intestinal protein losses in intestinal lymphangiectasia.

Surgical resection in patients with localized involvement of the small intestines with intestinal lymphangiectasia has been effective. However, in the majority of cases, the lesion is too diffuse for resection. Mistilis et al.[10] have successfully anastomosed the right saphenous vein, end-to-side, with a dilated lymphatic channel near the right external iliac vein. This lymph venous anastomosis resulted in the correction of diarrhea, steatorrhea, edema, and tetany. There was also significant reversal of the mucosal changes, but there was no significant improvement in the hypoproteinemia or in the degree of enteric protein loss. This technique is worthy of consideration in patients who do not respond to medical therapy and in those in whom the lymphangiogram shows marked abnormalities. In patients in whom chronic constrictive pericarditis is responsible for the protein-losing enteropathy and the morphological changes in the small intestine, pericardiectomy will improve the serum protein, bring about a cessation of the protein loss, and restore the microscopic appearance of the jejunal mucosa to normal.

PROGNOSIS

In the majority of cases, the response to therapy with a low-fat diet or a diet containing only medium-chain triglycerides as the source of fat is excellent. Early diagnosis, dietotherapy, and, in some instances, surgery, will correct the protein loss, edema, ascites, pleural effusion, and gastrointestinal symptoms and lead to a state of well being in patients with congenital or acquired lymphangiectasia. In secondary lymphangiectasia the prognosis will depend upon the underlying disease.

A-BETA-LIPOPROTEINEMIA

A-beta-lipoproteinemia is a rare inherited disease whose major biochemical and clinical manifestations are severe hypolipidemia, fat malabsorption, acanthocytosis of erythrocytes, cerebellar ataxia, and "atypical" retinitis pigmentosa. The disease has also been called acanthocytosis and Bassen-Kornzweig syndrome. It is genetically transmitted in an autosomal recessive fashion. Most of the reported cases have been in individuals of Jewish ancestry or Mediterranean origin.[11]

ETIOLOGY AND PATHOGENESIS

The primary underlying defect in this disorder remains unknown. The biochemical defect appears to be an inability to transport preformed triglyceride from the epithelial cells of the small intestinal mucosa and apparently also from the liver.

Characteristically, there is an absence of chylomicrons and very low density (VLDL) or pre-beta-lipoprotein, which respectively transport through plasma the glycerides derived from the dietary intake and those synthesized from endogenous precursors. Low density lipoproteins (LDL) or beta-lipoproteins which appear to be the result of the partial catabolism of VLDL and chylomicrons are also absent.[12]

The major protein constituent (apoprotein) of both VLDL and LDL, and probably also of chylomicrons, is apoLP-ser (referring to its carboxyl-terminal serine residue).[12]

Recently, Gotto et al.[12] have shown that both low density lipoprotein and its principal protein component apoLP-ser are absent from the plasma of a patient with a-beta-lipoproteinemia. On the other hand, the major protein constituents of the very low density lipoproteins other than apoLP-ser, as well as the two predominant proteins of high density lipoproteins, are present in the plasma of a-beta-lipoproteinemic patients. These authors acknowledge that their results do not conclusively establish the exact nature of the defect, because the possibility remains that undetected apoLP-ser (either in modified or in an incomplete form) is present in the plasma of these patients.[13] This finding suggests that apoLP-ser is necessary for the release of triglyceride from the small intestine and lymph into plasma. This will result in the accumulation of triglycerides in the small intestinal mucosa and the delayed appearance of chylomicrons in the circulation with resultant hypolipidemia. Since these patients are unable to form chylomicrons, it seems paradoxical that they only excrete a moderate amount of fat, rather than demonstrate a complete inability to absorb any fat.[14] It has been proposed that an alternative pathway is used to a greater extent than normal to transport long-chain fatty acids by way of the portal vein, unesterified and complexed with albumin.[12]

The decrease in serum cholesterol and triglyceride levels is probably due to the absence or deficiency of the lipoprotein involved in their transport. The cause of the acanthocytosis is unknown. It is evident that it may occur in the absence of beta-lipoprotein deficiency, because it has been described after splenectomy, in cirrhosis, and with red cell pyruvate kinase deficiency.[14] The decreased red cell linoleate levels alone will not lead to acanthocyte formation. It is possible that the changes in the lecithin-sphingomyelin composition of the red cell membrane may be responsible for the structural changes, but the reason for this change in the phospholipid composition of the red cells is not known.[11] The mechanism for the neurological findings in this disease is also unknown. It has been proposed that they might be related to the deficient transport of lipids to the central nervous system, and that beta-lipoproteins are essential for the normal structure and function of nerve cells.[14] The etiology of the retinal changes is also unclear. It may be related to the neurologic disease or to a deficiency of vitamin A or its precursors.

NATURAL HISTORY

The disease follows a fairly uniform course, beginning in childhood, usually before the age of one year. The child born of normal parents (who are often cousins) appears in good health at birth, but fails to grow and gain weight. In the first year of life, bulky stools and abdominal distention appear. In late childhood, progressive neurological dysfunction ensues. Pigmentary retinal dysfunction develops during adolescence. Progressive severe disability is the usual sequel of this disease, and many of the patients survive to adulthood, when death may be due to cardiac failure.

CLINICAL PICTURE

The earliest manifestation of this disease is failure to grow and gain weight during the first year of life. Subsequently, diarrhea and steatorrhea ensue. Associated with the fat malabsorption are abdominal distention, weight loss, and continued failure to grow. The neurological manifestations tend to occur in late childhood, after onset of the gastrointestinal symptoms. Classically, there is involvement of the central nervous system, especially the basal ganglia and cerebellum, posterolateral column, and peripheral nerves.[11] The patients demonstrate ataxia, intention tremors, nystagmus, absent deep tendon reflexes, and loss of vibratory and position sense, especially in the lower extremities. Athetoid movements and diminished pain and temperature sensation occur rarely. Muscle weakness may involve the lower extremities as the disorder progresses. In association with the progressive neuromuscular dysfunction is development of kyphosis or kyphoscoliosis, lordosis, abdominal protrusion, and pes cavus deformity.[11]

The retinal changes rarely occur before adolescence, but appear with great frequency thereafter and are invariably progressive. The retina shows the presence of pigmentary degeneration (atypical retinitis pigmentosa), and with macular involvement there is progressive blindness. Cardiomegaly, cardiac arrhythmias, and signs of congestive heart failure may develop during the course of the disease.[15]

DIAGNOSIS

In the presence of the full-blown clinical picture, with neurological deficits, steatorrhea, acanthocytosis, and hypolipoproteinemia, the diagnosis is obvious.

In most of the patients with this entity *acanthocytes* have been noted, sometimes as early as 17 months of age, and are presumably present throughout life.[11] On a wet preparation of fresh blood they are crenated spheres and cells which appear normal in size with several spiny or thorny excrescences (Fig. 78–5). Less commonly, one sees densely staining microspherocytes with long tentacle-like protuberances.[11] The acanthocytes retain their abnormal shape when incubated with normal serum. Rouleaux formation is absent, sedimentation rates are exceedingly slow, the

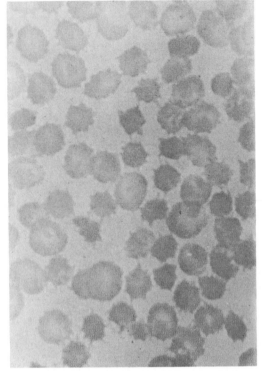

Figure 78–5. Red cells showing crenated spheres with spiny excrescences.

life span is normal or slightly decreased, and osmotic fragility is probably normal, but there is increased susceptibility to mechanical trauma. The white cells and platelets are normal. Anemia secondary to iron and folic acid malabsorption has been described.

Blood Lipids and Lipoproteins. The cholesterol content of the serum is consistently low, usually in the range of 30 to 80 mg per 100 ml, and the plasma triglycerides are usually less than 15 mg per 100 ml.[11] Characteristically, the beta-lipoprotein either is not detectable or is present in minute concentrations when analyzed by electrophoresis, by ultracentrifugation, or by specific immunological methods. In patients with A-beta-lipoproteinemia, the morphology of the upper intestinal absorptive cell is highly characteristic. The villi are normal in shape and length, but an abundance of lipid droplets is seen in the mucosal cells, especially at the tips of the villi (Fig. 78–6).[14] The submucosa and lamina propria show practically no fat droplets in the intercellular spaces or lacteals. Electron   microscopic   studies   reveal

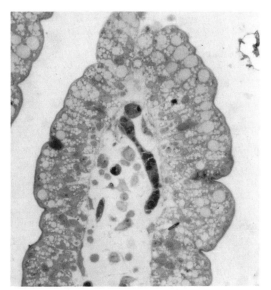

Figure 78–6. Jejunal biopsy showing a villus with striking lipid accumulation in the intestinal absorptive cells. × 400. (From Dobbins, W. O., III: Gastroenterology 50:195, 1966.)

normal-appearing microvilli, mitochondria, endoplasmic reticulum, and lipid droplets throughout the epithelial cells.[14]

Fat excretion is modest, usually less than 40 g per 24-hour period. The d-xylose and Vitamin B_{12} absorptions are usually normal. Serum vitamin A and carotene levels are low, and the prothrombin time is abnormal.

There is usually no hepatomegaly, but the liver biopsy usually shows a significant degree of fatty infiltration on light microscopy. All the fat is in the form of triglycerides, in contrast to the lipid composition of normal or alcoholic fatty liver in which a moderate amount of fatty acid is also present.[14]

DIFFERENTIAL DIAGNOSIS

In childhood, the symptoms of increased fat excretion, low carotene, and abnormal vitamin A tolerance are indistinguishable from those of celiac disease and cystic fibrosis of the pancreas, although the latter can be excluded by the finding of normal pancreatic secretions and normal concentration of sodium and chloride in the sweat. A markedly abnormal small intestinal biopsy specimen and a dramatic response to a gluten-free diet are characteristic of celiac disease. Later, when the neurological symptoms develop, the disease is readily confused with Friedreich's ataxia. There are no known abnormalities in plasma lipoproteins, red cells, or fat-laden epithelial cells in Friedreich's ataxia. In familial hypobeta-lipoproteinemia, the onset of symptoms is usually delayed into maturity and the severity of the clinical manifestations ranges from poor responsiveness to local anesthesia to a moderately progressive demyelinating disease. Retinitis pigmentosa is absent, and acanthocytosis has not been a consistent finding.[16] The chylomicrons are usually present, and serum triglyceride concentrations are normal or slightly decreased.

TREATMENT

No treatment has arrested the neurological component of this disease. A low-fat diet coupled with a daily intake of 30 to 46 g of medium-chain triglycerides has brought about a decrease in fat excretion, increased muscle strength, and weight gain. Supplementary linoleic acid, vitamin K, and vitamin A should also be given. If the patient is anemic, iron or folic acid should be prescribed.

PROGNOSIS

The prognosis is guarded. Patients may die relatively young, especially from cardiac arrhythmias and rapidly progressive congestive failure.

REFERENCES

1. Waldmann, T. A. Protein-losing enteropathy. Gastroenterology 59:422, 1966.
2. Bookstein, J. J., French, A. B. and Pollard, M. H. Protein-losing gastro-enteropathy. Concepts derived from lymphangiography. Amer. J. Dig. Dis. 10:573, 1965.
3. Dobbins, W. O., III. Electron microscope study of the intestinal mucosa in intestinal lymphangiectasia. Gastroenterology 51:1004, 1966.
4. Strober, W., Wochner, R. D., Carbone, P. P., and Waldmann, T. A. Intestinal lymphangiectasia: A protein-losing enteropathy with hypogammaglobulinemia, lymphocytopenia and impaired homograft rejection. J. Clin. Invest. 46:1643, 1967.

5. Marshak, R.D., Wolf, B. S., Cohen, N., and Janowitz, H. D.   Protein-losing disorders of the gastrointestinal tract: Roentgen features. Radiology 77:893, 1961.

6. Waldmann, T. A., Wochner, R. D., Laster, L., and Gordon, R. S.   Allergic gastroenteropathy: A cause of excessive protein loss. New Eng. J. Med. 276:761, 1967.

7. Gorske, K., Winchester, P., and Grossman, H. Unusual protein-losing enteropathies in children. Radiology 92:739, 1969.

8. Dobbins, W. O., III.   Hypo-β-lipoproteinemia and intestinal lymphangiectasia: A new syndrome of malabsorption and protein-losing enteropathy. Arch. Intern. Med. 122:31, 1968.

9. Holt, P.   Dietary treatment of protein loss in intestinal lymphangiectasia. Pediatrics 34:629, 1964.

10. Mistlis, S. P., and Skyring, A. P.   Intestinal lymphangiectasia: Therapeutic effect of lymph venous anastomosis. Amer. J. Med. 40:634, 1966.

11. Farquhar, J. W., and Ways, P.   A-beta-lipoproteinemia. In The Metabolic Basis of Inherited Disease, J. B. Stanbury, J. B.

Wyngaarden, and D. S. Fredrickson (eds.), 2nd ed. New York, McGraw-Hill Book Co., 1966, p. 509.

12. Gotto, A. M., Levy, R. I., John, K., and Fredrickson, D. S.   On the protein defect in a-beta-lipoproteinemia. New Eng. J. Med. 284:813, 1971.

13. Lees, R. S.   Immunological evidence for the presence of β protein (apoprotein of β-lipoprotein) in normal and a-beta-lipoproteinemic plasma. J. Lipid Res. 8:396, 1967.

14. Isselbacher, K. J., Scheig, R., Plotkin, G. R., and Caulfield, J. B.   Congenital β-lipoprotein deficiency: Defect in the absorption and transport of lipids. Medicine (Balt.) 43:347, 1964.

15. Dische, M. R., and Porro, R. S.   The cardiac lesions in Bassen-Kornzweig syndrome. Report of a case, with autopsy findings. Amer. J. Med. 49:568, 1970.

16. Mars, H., Lewis, L. A., Robertson, A. L., Butkus, A., and Williams, G. H., Jr.   Familial hypo-β-lipoproteinemia. A genetic disorder of lipid metabolism with nervous system involvement. Amer. J. Med. 46:886, 1969.

Chapter 79

Hereditable Multiple Polyposis Syndromes of the Gastrointestinal Tract

John Q. Stauffer

INTRODUCTION

Since the heredo-familial aspects of multiple adenomatous polyps of the colon and the subsequent development of adenocarcinoma of the colon were described by Cripps in 1881, the list of gastrointestinal polyposis syndromes with possible in-

herited causes has grown considerably (Table 79–1).[1, 2] Recognition and classification of these syndromes are important for a number of clinical and theoretical reasons. First, the cutaneous manifestations which are often disregarded as incidental findings on physical examination are unique to each syndrome and may be

TABLE 79–1. HEREDITARY POLYPOID DISEASES
OF THE GASTROINTESTINAL TRACT

DISEASE	PATHOLOGY	LOCATION	EXTRA-ABDOMINAL MANIFESTATIONS	MALIGNANT POTENTIAL
Familial polyposis	Adenomatous polyps	Colon	None	At least 95% of patients will develop colorectal carcinomas
Gardner's syndrome	Adenomatous polyps	Colon	Osteomas, epidermoid cysts, fibrous tumors dental abnormalities, and osseous abnormalities	At least 95% of patients will develop colorectal carcinomas
Peutz-Jeghers syndrome	Hamartomas of muscularis mucosa	Stomach, small intestine, colon	Buccal and cutaneous pigmentation	Carcinoma (rare); association with ovarian tumors, 5%
Generalized gastrointestinal juvenile polyposis	Juvenile polyps	Stomach, small intestine, colon	None	None
Cronkhite-Canada (? inherited)	Juvenile polyps	Stomach, small intestine, colon	Alopecia, nail dystrophy, hyperpigmentation, protein-losing enteropathy	None
Juvenile polyposis coli	Juvenile polyps	Colon	None	None
Turcot syndrome	Adenomatous polyps	Colon	Tumors of the central nervous system	Probably premalignant

the only diagnostic clues to the underlying gastrointestinal polyposis. Furthermore, these cutaneous changes often precede the onset of polyposis and alert the physician to potentially serious occult gastrointestinal disease. Secondly, in certain of these syndromes, familial polyposis and Gardner's syndrome, there is a strong potential for the colonic epithelium to undergo malignant transformation. The association of multiple polyps and adenocarcinoma circumstantially implicates the polyp as the precursor for the adenocarcinoma. However, the exact relationship between the adenomatous polyp and the development of an adenocarcinoma is no clearer than it is with isolated polyps (see p. 1433). Finally, the dominant mode of inheritance raises additional considerations: genetic counseling and tactful inquiry into the family in search of affected members.

Well documented pedigree analyses have clearly established many of these syndromes as genetic traits transmitted by a dominant gene. Furthermore, it has been reported that certain families are "cancer prone," with many members developing adenocarcinoma of the colon.[3] These observations suggest that at least one component in the pathogenesis of carcinomas of the colon involves the genetic composition of the individual. Other factors such as failure of the immune surveillance mechanisms or the presence of carcinogens in the colon must also certainly play a role in the pathogenesis of malignancy.

The following sections will discuss these syndromes: familial polyposis, Gardner's syndrome, Peutz-Jeghers syndrome, generalized juvenile polyposis, Cronkhite-Canada syndrome, juvenile polyps, and the Turcot syndrome.

FAMILIAL POLYPOSIS OF THE COLON

Familial polyposis is an inherited disease in which multiple adenomas are present throughout the large intestine.[1, 2, 4] The condition is transmitted as an autosomal dominant and may occur as often as once in 8300 births, thus having a gene frequency of at least 1:16000. McKusick[4]

has emphasized that, as in most traits inherited as autosomal dominants, the severity and age of onset are highly variable. The disease usually becomes clinically apparent in adolescence and early adulthood, although it has been reported to occur as early as four months of age and as late as 74 years. Veale[5] states that patients with polyposis but without a family history of the disease suffer the clinical symptoms and the tendency to develop carcinoma of the colon at an earlier age. Although this form has been termed the mutant variety, it may really be only the variation in gene penetrance referred to by McKusick. A mutation rate of 2 per 100,000 genes per generation has been estimated as necessary to replace genes lost through reduced reproductivity of affected individuals, so a

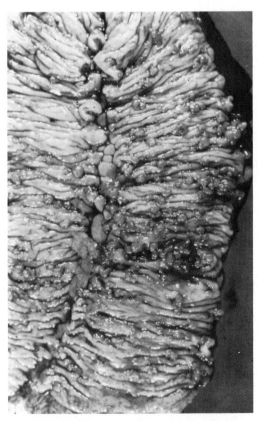

Figure 79–1. Gross specimen of a colon from a patient with familial polyposis. Note that the colon is diffusely studded with sessile and pedunculated adenomatous polyps. Although no carcinoma was seen in this specimen, nearly all patients will eventually develop a colorectal carcinoma if a total colectomy is not performed.

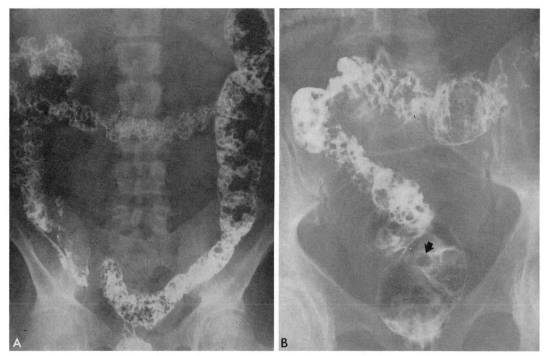

Figure 79–2. Barium enema examination of a patient with familial polyposis *(A)*. Note the marked variation in size of the polyps. Although this patient did not have osteomas or epidermoid cysts, the barium enema is similar to those seen in patients with Gardner's syndrome. Arrow indicates higher magnification of rectosigmoid shown in *B*.

mutant type of colonic polyposis would be expected.

PATHOLOGY

Sigmoidoscopic examination will reveal that the rectum and colon are diffusely studded with sessile and pedunculated polyps, ranging in size from tiny mammillations to masses several centimeters in size (Figs. 79–1 and 79–2). Histologically, the polyps do not differ from typical adenomas of either the glandular or villous type. Invariably, these patients will develop adenocarcinoma of the colon. It is not clear whether or not the adenomatous polyps themselves undergo malignant transformation any more than do single polyps (see pp. 1433 to 1436).

CLINICAL CONSIDERATIONS

The most important consideration is the high incidence of malignancy in these patients, which necessitates early diagnosis in suspected individuals. Although some

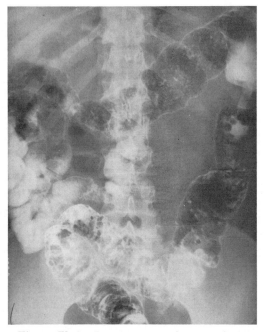

Figure 79–3. Barium enema from another patient with familial polyposis. There is an annular adenocarcinoma in the descending colon. When patients present with obstructive symptoms, often a carcinoma has already developed and metastases are present. In this case a right hemicolectomy had been performed several years ago; this obviously was inadequate therapy (see text).

patients are asymptomatic, many present with diarrhea and often with blood and mucus mixed in the stool. Abdominal cramps, weight loss, and anemia may be present. Signs and symptoms of obstruction usually indicate an already existing malignancy (Fig. 79–3). A normal sigmoidoscopic examination usually excludes a diagnosis of polyposis, as the rectum and sigmoid are the most severely affected.

TREATMENT AND PROGNOSIS

The progression of the disease must be followed by sigmoidoscopic and radiological examination with the intention of performing a total colectomy at the earliest sign of malignancy. In any event, affected individuals without a family history of the disease should undergo colectomy early (late teens or early twenties); in those patients with a family history, colectomy may be delayed until the mid-twenties. If the patient has a subtotal colectomy and ileorectal anastomosis, then periodic proctoscopy with fulguration of new polyps must be done periodically. A number of individuals will have spontaneous regression of the rectal polyps after ileorectal anastomosis.[6]

Currently, the surgical results with either ileorectal anastomosis or total colectomy and ileostomy have improved to the extent that these procedures should not be considered as a last resort. In fact, a patient with an ileorectal anastomosis may lead an almost normal existence with minimal problems with diarrhea.

Almost as important as treating the affected individual is the physician's obligation to search for other members of the family who may carry the defective gene. The physician must also counsel the patient concerning the likelihood of his transmitting the genetic defect to 50 per cent of his progeny. The polyps in familial polyposis must also be distinguished from inflammatory polyps in ulcerative colitis (Fig. 79–4). Sigmoidoscopic examination and excision of a polyp with histological study usually resolve the question.

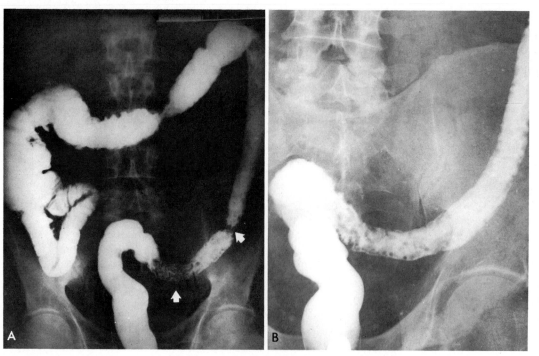

Figure 79–4.   A and B, Barium enema from a patient with ulcerative colitis. The inflammatory polyps are hard to distinguish from those in familial polyposis; the associated mucosal findings seen at sigmoidoscopy will establish the diagnosis. Inflammatory polyps are not premalignant. Arrows indicate area of higher magnification shown in B.

INTESTINAL POLYPOSIS ASSOCIATED WITH OSTEOMAS AND SOFT TISSUE TUMORS (GARDNER'S SYNDROME)

In 1953, Gardner and Richards[7] described a kindred in which multiple polypoid adenomas of the colon indistinguishable from those of familial polyposis were found in association with bone tumors and tumors confined to the cutaneous and subcutaneous tissues. Since then, many observers[2, 4, 8] have confirmed the close relationship of colonic polyposis, osteomas, and soft tissue tumors. They agree that this triad may be inherited as a single autosomal dominant, although closely linked defective dominant genes cannot be excluded. Reviews of the literature[8] and careful pedigree analysis stress that the finding of either osteomas or multiple cutaneous soft tissue tumors requires a careful search for colonic polyps.

PATHOLOGY

The adenomatous lesions of the colon are identical to those described in familial polyposis (see Figs. 79–1 through 79–4), and the colonic epithelium in these individuals has the same malignant potential. Although the bone tumors occur primarily in the mandible, sphenoid, and maxilla, they may also be found in other parts of the skeleton. The involvement of the calvarium and long bones of the extremities is more diffuse and is suggestive of osteosclerosis. The soft tissue abnormalities (Fig. 79–5) are diffuse and may be sebaceous cysts, lipomas, fibromas, fibrosarcomas, or leiomyomas. These lesions may be cutaneous, subcutaneous, mesenteric, or retroperitoneal, depending upon the cellular origin of the tumor. Often the affected individuals have an intense desmoplastic reaction around scars and incisions as the only cutaneous manifestation of the underlying colonic polyposis. Rarely, polyps have been reported in the terminal ileum in patients with Gardner's syndrome.

CLINICAL CONSIDERATIONS, TREATMENT, AND PROGNOSIS

Knowledge of this syndrome adds immense importance to "incidental" findings on physical examination. The soft tissue tumors and bone tumors often precede the onset of intestinal polyposis. The discovery of multiple polyps or the associated skin and bone tumors forces the physician to initiate an investigation of all relatives. It is also important to inform the patient of the likelihood of his transmitting the disease to 50 per cent of his offspring.

Like familial polyposis, Gardner's syndrome should be managed by total colectomy or ileorectal anastomosis followed by periodic proctoscopic examinations. Surgical intervention may be delayed to the mid or later twenties, because there is some suggestion that the malignant transformation occurs later in this syndrome than in familial polyposis.[2]

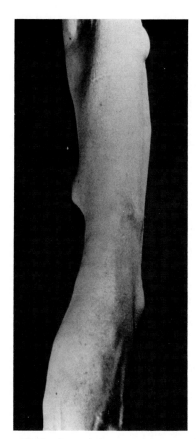

Figure 79–5. Several lipomas are seen in the forearm of this patient with Gardner's syndrome. Osteomas of the mandible and soft tissue tumors are characteristic of this syndrome.

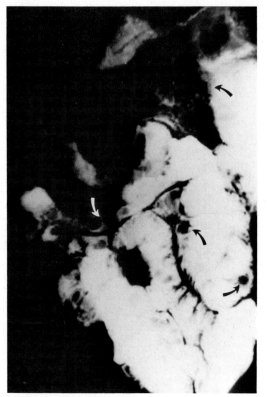

Figure 79-6. This small bowel series demonstrates the multiple hamartomas (arrows) of the gastrointestinal tract in Peutz-Jeghers syndrome. These hamartomas rarely become malignant.

POLYPOSIS OF THE SMALL INTESTINE WITH MUCOCUTANEOUS PIGMENTATION (PEUTZ-JEGHERS SYNDROME)

In 1921, Peutz described a family who manifested the association of skin pigmentation (Fig. 79–6) and polyps of the small intestine (Fig. 79–7). Later, Jeghers and coworkers reviewed several cases[9] and confirmed the association of multiple gastrointestinal polyps and mucocutaneous pigmentation. The syndrome is firmly entrenched in the medical literature as the Peutz-Jeghers syndrome and is probably inherited as a single, dominant pleiotropic gene with a high degree of penetrance.[4, 10]

PATHOLOGY

Although originally reported as restricted to the small intestine, the polyps may occur at any level in the gastrointestinal tract. Furthermore, contrary to the earlier reports, the polyps are not adenomatous but are hamartomas which rarely undergo malignant transformation. Histologically,[11, 12] these hamartomas are formed on an arborizing fibromuscular stroma which originated from a central smooth muscle mass in the muscularis mucosae of the bowel. The glandular elements are well differentiated, and Paneth, goblet, and argentaffin cells are present. These glandular elements may be deep within the muscularis mucosae and give an artifactual appearance of invasion. There are now several case reports of Peutz-Jeghers polyps undergoing malignant transformation.[13, 14] Payson reported a well documented case of Peutz-Jeghers syndrome in which a gastric polyp clearly progressed to an adenocarcinoma which subsequently metastasized into the liver. As a rule, however, malignant transformation is rare. An increased incidence of ovarian tumors of the theca cell type has been reported in Peutz-Jeghers syndrome.[15]

The cutaneous pigmentation represents areas of increased melanin deposits. These are most striking on the lips and buccal mucosa; this distribution helps distinguish them from ephelides (freckles), which are usually concentrated over the cheeks and bridge of the nose. The distribution also helps distinguish them from chloasma, xeroderma pigmentosa, or von Recklinghausen's syndrome. The lack of diffuse increase in skin pigmentation and lack of accentuation of pigmentation in body folds or about the nipples are also helpful differential points.[9]

CLINICAL CONSIDERATIONS, TREATMENT, AND PROGNOSIS

The finding of the mucocutaneous pigmentation should alert the physician to the underlying gastrointestinal polyposis. These patients are usually asymptomatic but may present with intussusception, abdominal pain, and gastrointestinal bleeding. The extensive review of patients with this syndrome by Jeghers et al.[9] in 1949 emphasizes that the pigmentation of the mucosal membranes is the sine qua non of the syndrome. They were unable to find

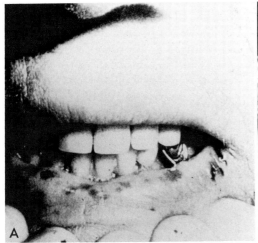

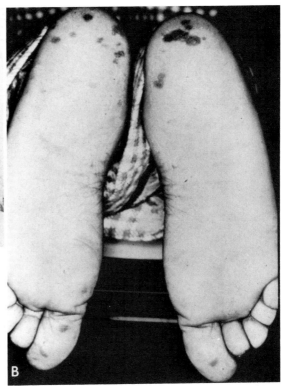

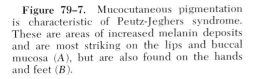

Figure 79-7. Mucocutaneous pigmentation is characteristic of Peutz-Jeghers syndrome. These are areas of increased melanin deposits and are most striking on the lips and buccal mucosa (A), but are also found on the hands and feet (B).

any patient with pigmentation who did not have intestinal polyposis.

These polyps, as a rule, do not undergo malignant transformation. Furthermore, the intestinal involvement is usually so extensive that surgical intervention, except for the specific problems of intussusception, bleeding, or obstruction, would be impossible.

GENERALIZED JUVENILE POLYPOSIS

The finding of a kindred spanning four generations with generalized juvenile gastrointestinal polyposis has led Sachatello et al.[2] to postulate that this is another hereditary syndrome of gastrointestinal polyposis distinct from Peutz-Jeghers syndrome or familial polyposis. This entity must also be distinguished from juvenile polyposis coli[5] and isolated juvenile retention polyps. Generalized juvenile polyposis is characterized by the development of numerous juvenile polyps of the stomach, small intestine, colon, and rectum.

There are no cutaneous manifestations in this entity.

HISTOLOGY

Characteristically, the juvenile polyp is smooth, although it may have a lobulated surface pattern. The cut surface of the juvenile polyp shows multiple cysts filled with mucin, a feature which distinguishes it from true adenomas (Fig. 79-8). The multiple cysts within the polyp has led to the name "retention polyp." These polyps may vary in diameter from a few millimeters to several centimeters. They may appear hemorrhagic owing to infarction from torsion of the polyp on its pedicle.

The typical juvenile polyp consists of an epithelial component surrounded by abundant connective tissue stroma which often displays a primitive mesenchymal appearance. The surface of the polyp is covered by a single layer of columnar epithelial cells often containing mucus within their cytoplasm and on their surface. The epithelial cells show no signs of

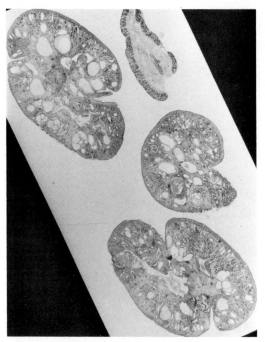

Figure 79–8. Low power magnification of a juvenile polyp. Note the multiple cysts filled with mucin and the extensive connective tissue stroma. These polyps vary in size and ulcerate and bleed easily. The epithelial cells show no signs of atypia or dedifferentiation. These polyps are benign.

increased nuclear activity such as hyperchromatism and mitosis; there may be some diminution in the number of goblet cells. The most striking feature of juvenile polyps is the increased connective tissue stroma. True bone has been reported in this stroma. No malignant transformation has been reported with these polyps.

CLINICAL CONSIDERATIONS, TREATMENT, AND PROGNOSIS

Persons affected with this syndrome present with recurrent bouts of abdominal pain secondary to repeated episodes of intussusception. They may also pass parts of the polyps per rectum and have chronic gastrointestinal blood loss. As these polyps are hamartomas and, therefore, do not undergo malignant transformation, management should be conservative. The extensive gastrointestinal involvement makes surgical intervention impossible except for treatment of intussusception and obstruction. The absence of mucocutaneous pigmentation distinguishes this entity from the Peutz-Jeghers syndrome. Histologically, they are distinct: the Peutz-Jeghers polyps have a pronounced fibromuscular stroma, and these polyps have little or no muscle tissue.

CRONKHITE-CANADA SYNDROME

In 1955, Cronkhite and Canada[16] described a syndrome which may be a variant of generalized juvenile polyposis. In this syndrome, the diffuse gastrointestinal polyposis is associated with alopecia, nail dystrophy, and hyperpigmentation. Ruymann[17] reviewed a case which occurred in an infant and was able to compare the polyps with those that occurred in adults. He concluded that these polyps were all of the juvenile type.

Although some observers feel that the nail and skin changes may be secondary to the severe malnutrition that these patients have, others state that the cutaneous changes occurred early enough in the illness to suggest a primary ectodermal defect. These polyps are benign, but they are associated with severe diarrhea which leads to water and electrolyte depletion as well as a protein-losing enteropathy. The combination of ectodermal and endodermal defects suggests a genetic defect with one or more closely linked genes involved. These polyps are benign, and management should be directed at specific complications.

JUVENILE POLYPOSIS COLI

Juvenile polyposis coli is an entity distinct from generalized juvenile polyposis. Veale and colleagues[5] have described 11 patients from four families who had multiple juvenile polyps confined to the colon. The frequent occurrence within a family suggested a genetic mechanism to them. Furthermore, all the families studied had relatives known to have died with large bowel cancer. Veale speculates that multiple juvenile polyps might be a manifestation of the polyposis gene in these children. They stress, however, that the juvenile polyps themselves are not premalignant lesions.

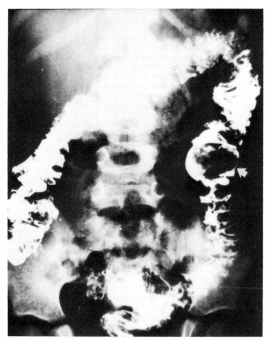

Figure 79–9. Barium enema from a patient with a single large juvenile polyp (arrow). Intestinal obstruction and intussusception are clinical complications of these polyps.

CLINICAL CONSIDERATIONS, TREATMENT, AND PROGNOSIS

The treatment is simple and direct. Polyps within reach of the sigmoidoscope should be removed, whereas those above may be watched. Removal is required if intussusception or obstruction occurs. In the case of multiple polyps, if those in the rectum are of the juvenile type, then those higher up may be considered to be the same and no surgical intervention is necessary.

THE TURCOT SYNDROME

Turcot and colleagues[18] described a brother and sister with polyposis of the colon in association with a tumor of the central nervous system. In one, a medulloblastoma of the spinal cord was found; in the other, a glioblastoma of the frontal lobe. The patients' parents were third cousins. This is probably an inherited syndrome, but experience thus far is too limited for a definite conclusion. The syndrome, if it is one, must be very rare.

Juvenile polyps may appear in children without a family history. They usually appear in the first decade, although a few may appear after the age of 20. The polyps may be solitary (Fig. 79–9) and should be differentiated from lymphoid polyps, lipomatous polyps, and adenomatous polyps. These juvenile polyps tend to occur more frequently in males.

HISTOLOGY

The polyps are identical to the juvenile polyps seen in generalized juvenile polyposis. They are composed of multiple retention cysts and microscopically have a large amount of connective tissue stroma with a few glands of varying size containing mucus and inflammatory cells. The epithelial cells lining these glands may occasionally be cuboidal, but there is no atypia or basophilic change. The surface of these polyps ulcerates and bleeds easily. Of great import is the fact that these lesions are not premalignant.

REFERENCES

1. Calabro, J. J. Hereditable multiple polyposis syndromes of the gastrointestinal tract. Amer. J. Med. 33:276, 1962.
2. Sachatello, C. R., Pickren, J. W., and Grace, J. T. Generalized juvenile gastrointestinal polyposis. Gastroenterology 58:699, 1970.
3. Lynch, H. T., and Krush, J. A. Heredity and adenocarcinoma of the colon. Gastroenterology 53:517, 1967.
4. McKusick, V. A. Genetic factors in intestinal polyposis, J.A.M.A. 182:271, 1962.
5. Veale, A. M., McColl, I., Bussey, H. J., and Morson, B. C. Juvenile polyposis coli. J. Med. Genet. 3:5, 1966.
6. Localio, S. A. Spontaneous disappearance of rectal polyps following subtotal colectomy and ileoproctostomy for polyposis of the colon. Amer. J. Surg. 103:81, 1962.
7. Gardner, E. J., and Richards, R. C. Multiple cutaneous and subcutaneous lesions occurring simultaneously with hereditary polyposis of osteomatosis. Amer. J. Human Genet. 5:139, 1953.
8. Gorlin, R. J., and Chaudhry, A. P. Multiple osteomatosis, fibromas, lipomas, and fibrosarcomas of the skin and mesentery, epidermoid inclusion cysts of the skin, leiomyomas and multiple intestinal polyposis: A hereditable disorder of connective tissue. New Eng. J. Med. 263:1151, 1960.

9. Jeghers, H., McKusick, V., and Katz, L. Generalized intestinal polyposis and melanin spots of the oral mucosa, lips and digits. New Eng. J. Med. 241:993, 1949.

10. Dormandy, T. L. Gastrointestinal polyposis with mucocutaneous pigmentation—Peutz-Jeghers syndrome. New Eng. J. Med. 256:1093, 1141, 1186, 1957.

11. Farmer, G. G., Hawk, W. A., and Turnbull, R. B. The spectrum of the Peutz-Jeghers syndrome. Amer. J. Dig. Dis. 8:953, 1963.

12. Bartholomew, L. G., Dahlin, D. C., and Waugh, J. M. Intestinal polyposis associated with mucocutaneous melanin pigmentation. Peutz-Jeghers syndrome. Review of the literature and report of six cases with special reference to pathologic findings. Gastroenterology 32:434, 1957.

13. Bernfield, M. S., and Changus, G. W. Peutz-Jeghers syndrome: Report of a case of small intestinal polyposis and carcinoma associated with melanin pigmentation of the lips and buccal mucosa. Gastroenterology 35:543, 1958.

14. Payson, B. A., and Merimgis, B. Metastasizing carcinoma of the stomach in Peutz-Jeghers syndrome. Ann. Surg. 165:145, 1967.

15. Humphries, A. L., Shepard, M. H., and Peters, J. H. J. Peutz-Jeghers syndrome with colonic adenocarcinoma and ovarian tumors. J.A.M.A. 197:296, 1966.

16. Cronkhite, L. W., and Canada, W. J. Generalized gastrointestinal polyposis, an unusual syndrome of polyposis, pigmentation, alopecia, and onychotropia. New Eng. J. Med. 252:1011, 1955.

17. Ruymann, F. G. Juvenile polyps with cachexia. Report of an infant and comparison with Cronkhite-Canada syndrome in adults. Gastroenterology 57:431, 1969.

18. Turcot, J., Despres, M. P., and St. Pierre, F. Malignant tumors of the central nervous system associated with familial polyposis of the colon. Dis. Colon Rectum 2:465, 1959.

Chapter 80

Amyloidosis and the Small Intestine

Charles Krone

INTRODUCTION

Small intestinal involvement occurs in at least 70 per cent of cases of generalized amyloidosis and may lead to widespread disruption of intestinal structure and function, producing disturbance of motility, intestinal obstruction, ischemia and infarction, ulceration, bleeding, perforation, protein-losing enteropathy, and malabsorption.[1]

Amyloid, an amorphous, eosinophilic, hyaline extracellular scleroprotein, has a unique ultrastructure of fine rigid non-branching fibrils distinct from other extracellular connective tissue elements. Current data suggest that reticuloendothelial cells produce the amyloid fibril which is then deposited into a ground substance, possibly containing abnormal mucopolysaccharides.[2, 3] Classifications have distinguished specific types of amyloidosis, such as primary, secondary, heredofamilial, and amyloidosis associated with multiple myeloma.[4, 5] Yet in all types, the ultrastructure and known chemical composition of amyloid is identical, and organ system involvement is too similar to regularly distinguish these entities pathologically.[4, 5] The location of earliest deposition of amyloid in blood vessels may be distinguished as either perireticular or pericollagen, and there is a demonstrable correlation of these patterns with specific categories of amyloidosis. Nevertheless, with our present state of knowledge, it remains most useful to consider amyloidosis in terms of clinical classification, such as presence or absence of other disease and genetic associations, and to make no conclusions about organ and tissue distribution. There does not appear to be any pattern of small intestinal involvement unique to either primary or secondary amyloidosis.

DIAGNOSIS

Diagnosis of amyloidosis is made by histological demonstration of amyloid in affected tissue. In the alimentary tract, biopsy diagnosis may be made from gingiva to the rectum. Rectal biopsy is most convenient with a 75 per cent positive yield in all patients with generalized amyloidosis (Fig. 80–1).[6] Renal biopsy has had somewhat greater reported success, 87 per cent but is more hazardous. Recently, peroral jejunal biopsy has been found to be safe and to have an equivalently positive diagnostic yield.[7, 8] The single most useful histological test is the Congo red-stained section viewed in the polarizing microscope, revealing a unique green birefringence indicating groups of parallel oriented fibrils specific for amyloid.[3]

1061

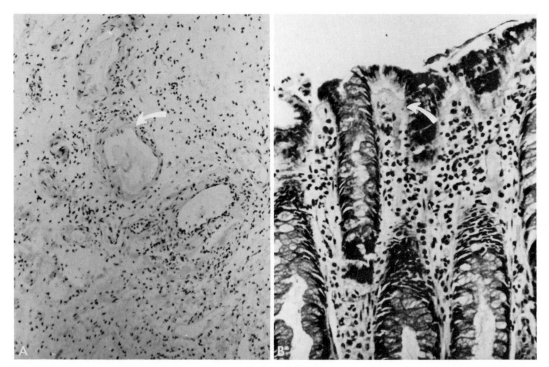

Figure 80–1.   *A*, Amyloid deposition in the wall of small blood vessels of the submucosa. From rectal biopsy stained with Congo red. ×100. *B*, Amyloid deposition in the lamina propria just below the epithelium. Rectal biopsy stained with periodic acid–Schiff stain. × 225.

PATHOLOGY

The presence of amyloid in a tissue does not evoke an inflammatory response, and damage is apparently caused by local replacement of tissue. Therefore knowledge of the anatomicohistological site of amyloid deposition helps in understanding the clinical manifestations. Earliest gastrointestinal infiltration probably occurs in and about blood vessels of the submucosa. Initial deposition may be in the intima (perireticular) or adventitia (pericollagen), according to type of amyloidosis.[4] Eventually the whole wall is thickened, the lumen becomes increasingly narrower, and complete occlusion may result, with subsequent infarction of the area it serves.[4] Involvement of the bowel musculature is relatively frequent. The muscularis mucosae and outer layers may be more involved than the inner circular layer. Amyloid is deposited between muscle fibers and may cause pressure atrophy. Ultimately, the whole muscle layer may be replaced by amyloid. The appearance of the mucosa usually remains normal until massive deposits destroy the glandular structure. A curious feature is a frequently reported band of amyloid found directly under the surface epithelium, creating the appearance of a barrier between the lumen and the bowel wall. Mucosal atrophy and ulceration may be seen owing to secondary amyloid-induced vascular insufficiency. Direct pressure damage to nervous elements in the myenteric plexuses and visceral nerve trunks has been demonstrated.[1]

The extent and location of intestinal involvement is highly variable, and the frequency with which these abnormalities result in intestinal symptoms in patients with amyloidosis is most difficult to determine from published series. In the secondary form, symptoms from amyloid deposition are often difficult to separate from those of the underlying disease.

ROENTGEN APPEARANCE

The principal roentgen finding in amyloidosis of the intestine is conspicuous symmetrical, sharply demarcated thickening of the valvulae conniventes, producing

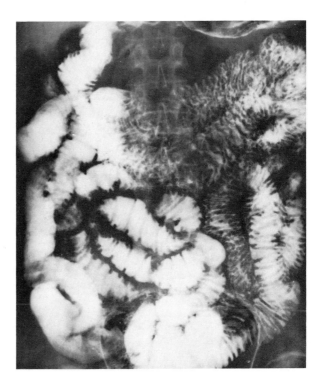

Figure 80-2. Symmetrical, sharply demarcated thickening of the valvulae conniventes throughout the small intestine, producing a uniform appearance characteristic of amyloidosis. (Courtesy of Dr. R. H. Marshak.)

a uniform appearance throughout the entire intestinal tract. The thickening of the folds in the ileum produces an appearance Marshak and Lindner refer to as "jejunization," which is most characteristic of amyloidosis[9] (Fig. 80-2). Segmentation, fragmentation, or any evidence of inflammatory lesion is not seen. The small bowel pattern may be normal, despite significant infiltration with amyloid.[10]

PATHOPHYSIOLOGY OF CLINICAL MANIFESTATIONS

MOTILITY DISTURBANCE

Amyloid deposition in the bowel may severely alter motility, leading to disabling diarrhea or constipation. Diarrhea appears to be the most frequent intestinal manifestation in amyloidosis. Muscle replacement by amyloid or destruction of autonomic innervation of the intestine may be responsible. A patient with primary amyloidosis has been described in whom there was uncontrollable diarrhea and steatorrhea with amyloid involvement primarily of myenteric and submucosal autonomic plexuses, and thoracolumbar autonomic nerves and ganglia, in the absence of direct muscle involvement.[11] Other, similar cases of disabling diarrhea are reported with autonomic dysfunction not unlike that seen in diabetic neuropathy.[12] In the Portuguese type of hereditary amyloidosis, severe diarrhea and peripheral neuropathy are characteristic features. In such cases the disease is predominantly a neuropathy with damage to major nerve trunks.[11] Nevertheless, in most cases of amyloidosis it has not been possible to determine whether muscle replacement or involvement of autonomic innervation is the major cause of impaired motility. In addition, the manner by which amyloid infiltration about nerves and ganglia disturbs function, e.g., irritation or compression and degeneration, is not understood.

A wide spectrum of motor disturbance of the intestine may be seen by X-ray. Decreased propulsive activity with delayed transit, dilatation of the proximal small bowel, segmental dilatation, narrowing, and diffuse distention of loops of small and large bowel have been described.[10] These changes, however, are all nonspecific for amyloidosis.

A clinical picture resembling mechanical obstruction of the bowel with abdominal cramps and active bowel sounds, but with X-ray pattern characteristic of paralytic ileus, frequently referred to as "intestinal pseudo-obstruction," has been described with amyloidosis involving the small bowel.[13] Such manifestations probably result from propulsive activity in portions of the bowel less heavily infiltrated than more distal segments. Similar findings may occur in progressive systemic sclerosis. This paradoxical combination should alert the physician to the possibility of a problem other than typical mechanical obstruction. The recognition of amyloidosis may help avoid surgical treatment which would be ineffectual and fraught with dangerous complications and high mortality.

INTESTINAL ISCHEMIA

Blood supply to the small bowel may be impaired by progressive encroachment upon the lumen of mesenteric and intestinal vessels. Segmental bowel infarction has been reported in amyloidosis.[1, 12] Ischemia may be a significant cause of intestinal symptoms in patients with amyloidosis, but it is not possible to determine the frequency with which this occurs.

HEMORRHAGE

Gastrointestinal bleeding is not infrequently seen in amyloidosis. It may be secondary to discrete ulceration of a markedly infiltrated area of bowel. Often either no lesion is found at laparotomy or autopsy, or diffuse bleeding is encountered. In such cases hemorrhage may result from vascular insufficiency, causing increased permeability of blood vessels or small areas of infarction.[1, 14]

PERFORATION

A well documented case of acute perforation of ileum has been reported.[15] The bowel wall was markedly infiltrated with amyloid, rigid, and very fragile. Rupture of the bowel wall may result from sudden distention of a fragile segment, hemorrhage into the gut wall, or possibly ischemic necrosis. It is a rare but catastrophic complication of amyloidosis.

PROTEIN-LOSING ENTEROPATHY

Increased transudation of protein into the intestinal lumen in amyloidosis has been documented in studies with polyvinyl pyrrolidone-I[131] and radioiodinated serum albumin. Unexplained low serum albumin levels are frequently found in patients with amyloidosis, and these may possibly be due to protein loss into the gut. Vascular insufficiency has been suggested as a possible cause for the protein-losing enteropathy.[14] Lymphatic destruction has not been found, and increased permeability of capillaries is postulated.

MALABSORPTION

Although rare, malabsorption syndrome with steatorrhea has been well documented in amyloidosis.[1, 6, 8, 16, 17] Six cases were found in a recent review of 103 patients with primary or secondary amyloidosis.[16] The pathogenesis of the malabsorption is uncertain, but probably variable, depending on the site of amyloid deposition. Mucosal destruction by massive amyloid deposition, vascular insufficiency, motility disturbance with stasis, and intestinal bacterial overgrowth have been considered. Amyloid may also be massively deposited in the pancreas with marked acinar destruction and must not be overlooked as a potential cause of steatorrhea. Amyloid infiltration in the tips of villi and lamina propria has been found in patients with malabsorption, but its significance is questionable. In patients studied by peroral jejunal biopsy, no correlation between intensity of amyloid infiltration and diarrhea or steatorrhea was found.[7] The amyloid band, found beneath the surface epithelium in some cases, may present a barrier to lipid absorption, but this has yet to be demonstrated. As mucosal cell integrity is usually unaffected, except in extreme cases of massive local deposition, motility disturbance with stasis and bacterial overgrowth may be the major cause of malabsorption in amyloidosis. Although data such as presence of steatorrhea, increased stool nitrogen, vitamin

B_{12} malabsorption without response to intrinsic factor, low calcium and carotene levels, and prolonged prothrombin times have been noted, there is not enough information available in reported cases to characterize specific pathophysiological mechanisms. More comprehensive malabsorption studies and evaluation of response to therapy, including broad-spectrum antibiotics, must be obtained in such patients before special mechanisms can be delineated.

Selective lactose intolerance and lactase deficiency have been documented in three patients with rheumatoid arthritis and secondary amyloidosis by lactose tolerance test and jejunal mucosal assay.[8] A more vigorous search for malabsorption in patients with amyloidosis may reveal a higher incidence of abnormalities than previously anticipated.

TREATMENT

There is no specific treatment for any variety of amyloidosis. Only supportive measures are available. Eradication of predisposing disease may slow the progress of secondary amyloidosis. Diagnosis of intestinal amyloidosis may be helpful in avoiding hazardous and ineffective surgery in some instances. Further elucidation of specific pathophysiological mechanisms causing malabsorption in amyloidosis may assist in the selection of useful supportive therapy.

REFERENCES

1. Gilat, T., and Spiro, H. M.   Amyloidosis and the gut. Amer. J. Dig. Dis. 13:619, 1968.
2. Barth, W. F., Glenner, G. G., Waldmann, T. A., and Zelis, R. F.   Primary amyloidosis. Ann. Intern. Med. 69:787, 1968.
3. Cohen, A. S.   Amyloidosis. Part I. New Eng. J. Med. 277:522, 1967.
4. Cohen, A. S.   Amyloidosis. Part II. New Eng. J. Med. 277:628, 1967.
5. Gilat, T., Revach, M., and Sohar, E.   Deposition of amyloid in the gastrointestinal tract. Gut 10:98, 1969.
6. Levinson, J. D., and Kirsner, J. B. Infiltrative diseases of the small bowel and malabsorption. Amer. J. Dig. Dis. 15:741, 1970.
7. Green, P. A., Higgins, J. A., Brown, A. L., Jr., and Hoffman, H. N., II   Amyloidosis: Appraisal of intubation biopsy of the small intestine in diagnosis. Gastroenterology 41:452, 1961.
8. Pettersson, T., and Wegelius, O.   Biopsy diagnosis of amyloidosis in rheumatoid arthritis. Gastroenterology 62:22, 1972.
9. Marshak, R. H., and Lindner, A. E. Amyloidosis. In Radiology of the Small Intestine, Philadelphia, W. B. Saunders Co., 1970, p. 62.
10. Legge, D. A., Carlson, H. C., and Wollaeger, E. E.   Roentgenologic appearance of systemic amyloidosis involving the gastrointestinal tract. Amer. J. Roent. Radium Ther. Nuc. Med. 110:406, 1970.
11. French, J. M., Hall, G., Parish, D. J., and Smith, T. W.   Peripheral and autonomic nerve involvement in primary amyloidosis associated with uncontrollable diarrhea and steatorrhea. Amer. J. Med. 39:277, 1965.
12. Brody, I. A., Wertlake, P. J., and Laster, L. Causes of intestinal symptoms in primary amyloidosis. Arch. Intern. Med. 113:512, 1964.
13. Legge, D. A., Wollaeger, E. E., and Carlson, H. C.   Intestinal pseudo-obstruction in systemic amyloidosis. Gut 11:764, 1970.
14. Jarnum, S. Gastrointestinal hemorrhage and protein loss in primary amyloidosis. Gut 6:14, 1965.
15. Akbarian, M., and Fenton, J. Perforation of small bowel in amyloidosis. Arch. Intern. Med. 114:815, 1964.
16. Herskovic, T., Bartholomew, L. G., and Green, P. A.   Amyloidosis and malabsorption syndrome. Arch. Intern. Med. 114:629, 1964.
17. Beddow, R. M., and Tildon, I. L.   Malabsorption syndrome due to amyloidosis of the intestine secondary to lepromatous leprosy: Report of a case. Ann. Intern. Med. 53:1027, 1960.

Chapter 81

Allergic Disorders of the Intestine and Eosinophilic Gastroenteritis

Norton Greenberger, Joyce D. Gryboski

INTRODUCTION

In recent years there have been several reports describing patients with gastrointestinal intolerance to specific foods, milk protein intolerance in children, eosinophilic gastroenteritis, eosinophilic granuloma of the stomach or intestine, and allergic gastroenteropathy. From what was at one time a large number of confusing and incomplete clinical reports, a clearer picture has gradually emerged, suggesting that some of these disorders are distinct clinical entities. A classification of allergic diseases of the intestine and of eosinophilic gastroenteritis is listed in Table 81–1.

For a number of reasons the spontaneous occurrence of gastrointestinal allergy in man is still regarded as an uncertain entity. In particular, it should be emphasized that specific skin tests are highly variable and frequently unreliable. In addition, symptoms claimed to be specific or characteristic of gastrointestinal allergy are in fact nonspecific and highly variable. Further, the occurrence of abdominal complaints in patients with other allergic manifestations, such as rhinitis, asthma, hives, and eczema, has led to the tendency to diagnose such complaints as a gastrointestinal allergy, whereas in actuality there may be little objective evidence on which to base such a diagnosis. Last, except for a relatively small number of cases, no lesions in the gut or abnormalities in intestinal absorptive function have been demonstrated in patients with other symptoms and findings which suggest the diagnosis of gastrointestinal allergy.[1-4]

In 1949, Ingelfinger and his colleagues[5] listed the criteria that would have to be fulfilled before a diagnosis of gastrointestinal allergy could be seriously considered. These requirements were as follows: (1) the symptoms should be caused by specific substances that are innocuous when given to the bulk of the population; (2) lesions or functional changes in the gut should be demonstrated; (3) emotional and mechanical factors should be excluded; and (4) the role of subjective attitudes should be minimized by testing various substances under carefully controlled conditions. Specific foods should be given in such a manner that the patient is unaware of the administered food. Reproducible symptoms, signs, or X-rays findings should consistently follow administration of the

TABLE 81–1.   EOSINOPHILIC GASTROENTERITIS AND ALLERGIC DISEASES OF THE INTESTINE

I. *Eosinophilic Gastroenteritis*
   A. Criteria for diagnosis
      1. Infiltration of gut wall with eosinophils
      2. Increased number of eosinophils in peripheral blood
      3. Abnormal symptoms or signs following ingestion of specific foods
   B. Clinical patterns
      1. Predominant mucosal disease
         a. Iron deficiency anemia
         b. Increased fecal blood loss
         c. Hypoproteinemia due to protein-losing enteropathy
         d. Malabsorption
      2. Predominant muscle layer disease
         a. Pyloric narrowing and obstruction
         b. Incomplete small bowel obstruction
         c. Differentiation from eosinophilic granuloma
            (1) Localized polypoid lesions of stomach, small bowel, or colon
      3. Predominant subserosal disease
         a. Eosinophilic ascites

II. *Allergic Gastroenteritis in Childhood*
   A. Milk intolerance in infancy and childhood
      1. Clinical features similar to eosinophilic gastroenteritis with predominant mucosal disease
      2. Chronic diarrhea with coproantibodies in stool
      3. Milk sensitivity with rapid onset of symptoms
         a. Asthma
         b. Urticaria
         c. Angioedema
      4. Differentiation from syndrome of iron deficiency anemia, hypoferremia, and hypocupremia of infants fed milk exclusively
   B. Soy protein allergy
   C. Gluten enteropathy

III. *Gastrointestinal Food Intolerance with Systemic Allergic Reactions*
   A. Anaphylactic reactions

disguised food at a more or less constant interval not greater than two hours. Other innocuous foods given in the same manner should not produce symptoms or functional changes.

Only a small number of reported cases of eosinophilic gastroenteritis appear to have met the criteria set forth by Ingelfinger. Yet, even in these cases, the question arises as to whether an allergic process alone can account for the manifestations of the disease. In this regard, it has been suggested that "eosinophilic gastroenteritis is not a simple, reversible allergic reaction to specific foods but rather a self-perpetuating process which may be symptomatically aggravated by different foods."[3] It seems clear that institution of more rational therapy in eosinophilic gastroenteritis with predominantly mucosal disease will require a clearer definition of the cause and pathogenesis of this disorder.

Marked changes in the gastroscopic appearance of the stomach are noted in patients with specific food intolerances after the administration of offending foods.[6] However, the significance of these observations is uncertain, because the studies were not carried out in a double-blind controlled manner, and the mucosa was not examined histologically. Infants and children with protein-losing enteropathy may have gastrointestinal sensitivity to milk.[7] Because of its complexity and the lack of clear evidence that reactions to milk are allergic, this topic will be discussed separately later.

Recently, severe gastrointestinal symptoms caused by soy protein, including villous atrophy of jejunum, have been reported.[4, 8] Although eosinophilic infiltration of the gut and eosinophilia are absent, these cases appear to represent a gut allergy as defined by Ingelfinger et al.[5] The question of the allergic nature of the toxic effect of gluten in patients with celiac sprue is unanswered in immunological terms; however, in the terms defined above, it must clinically be considered an allergic enteritis (see pp. 864 to 884).

EOSINOPHILIC GASTROENTERITIS

DEFINITION

Eosinophilic gastroenteritis refers to a disorder of the stomach and/or small bowel characterized by infiltration of some part of the gastrointestinal tract or gut wall with eosinophilic leukocytes; increase in the number of eosinophils in the peripheral blood; and development of gastrointestinal symptoms, signs, or abnormal laboratory studies following ingestion of specific foods. As indicated in Table 81–1, the clinical manifestations of eosinophilic gastroenteritis are protean. For the purpose of classification, three major clinical patterns can be identified. These include primary mucosal disease with enteric protein loss and malabsorption, predominant muscle layer disease with obstructive symptoms, and primary subserosal disease with eosinophilic ascites.

PATHOGENESIS

The pathogenesis of eosinophilic gastroenteritis is not clearly understood. Several lines of evidence, however, support the concept of an allergic or immunological etiology in this group of disorders. These include the following: (1) A greatly increased number of eosinophils in the peripheral blood. (2) Infiltration of some part of the gastrointestinal tract by increased numbers of eosinophilic leukocytes. (3) A greatly increased incidence of allergic disorders such as seasonal rhinitis, asthma, eczema, and urticaria. (4) The demonstration that specific foods consistently precipitate gastrointestinal symptoms, whereas foods of which the patients are tolerant cause no adverse symptoms

when administered in the same manner. In a few instances, dramatic signs and symptoms such as severe abdominal pain, diarrhea, tachycardia, and leukocytosis have developed within one to two hours after challenge with a food historically incriminated as causing symptoms.[1-3] (5) The documentation of rapid amelioration of symptoms after initiation of therapy with corticosteroids. (6) The demonstration that both direct skin tests and indirect tests for skin sensitizing antibody (Prausnitz-Kustner or P-K test) may correlate well with the patient's food sensitivities.

Despite this seemingly clear picture, major questions concerning gastrointestinal allergy remain unresolved in these and similar patients.

First, why do these patients develop gastrointestinal symptoms when challenged with specific foods that are innocuous when given to the bulk of the population? Second, what is the relationship between peripheral blood eosinophilia along with eosinophilic-leukocyte infiltration of the gut wall and the *intermittent* gastrointestinal symptoms and abnormal tests of intestinal absorptive function? Third, what is the explanation for the frequent occurrence of extensive infiltration of eosinophils in the deeper muscular layers, subserosa, and mesenteric lymph nodes in the absence of mucosal involvement? Fourth, what is the mechanism by which presumed antigen-antibody reactions in the gastrointestinal mucosa result in eosinophilic infiltration in the gut wall as well as peripheral blood eosinophilia? In this regard, it has been suggested that direct contact of sensitized tissue with allergen results in an antigen-antibody reaction with the liberation of substances such as histamine, which might be chemotactic for eosinophils.[2, 9] It is also possible that immunoglobulins elaborated by the intestinal mucosa in response to antigens are chemotactic. There is preliminary in vitro evidence indicating that certain immunoglobulins are chemotactic for eosinophils.[10, 11] Further studies are needed on (1) humoral antibody responses to specific antigens; (2) delayed hypersensitivity responses and the relationship between such responses and the development of eosinophilia and tissue infiltration with eosinophils; and (3) intestinal secretion of immunoglobulins in response to specific antigens. Such studies might clarify the nature of the presumed immunological abnormalities in patients meeting the criteria for a diagnosis of gastrointestinal allergy.

CLINICAL PICTURE

Patients with eosinophilic gastroenteritis have all the following general clinical findings: specific food intolerances, eosinophilia, increased eosinophils in the small bowel mucosa, abnormal tests of intestinal absorptive function, induction of gastrointestinal symptoms after blind challenge with an "offending food," and amelioration of symptoms with corticosteroids alone or in combination with food-elimination diets.[1-3] A more complete description for each of the categories follows.

EOSINOPHILIC GASTROENTERITIS WITH PREDOMINANT MUCOSAL DISEASE

The clinical features are summarized in Table 81–2. Patients in this group frequently complain of intermittent nausea, emesis, and abdominal pain, which

may be exacerbated by eating specific foods. A history of weight loss and sporadic diarrhea is not uncommon, and prior asthma and allergic rhinitis are frequently noted. Physical examination may reveal evidence of atopic eczema, urticaria, and pedal edema. Laboratory studies usually reveal a moderate to marked eosinophilia, a low erythrocyte sedimentation rate, and iron deficiency anemia. Stool specimens are negative for ova and parasites, but are frequently positive for occult blood and Charcot-Leyden crystals (presumably derived from eosinophils). Tests of intestinal absorptive function may be abnormal, with evidence of mild steatorrhea and impaired absorption of D-xylose. Serum albumin, IgG, IgA, and IgM levels are often decreased owing to excessive enteric loss of protein, which can be demonstrated by excessive fecal loss of Cr^{51}-labeled albumin or $Cr^{51}Cl_3$. Jejunal biopsy specimens characteristically reveal infiltration of eosinophils, which may vary from a slight increase (Fig. 81–1) to massive infiltration with marked epithelial abnormalities and complete loss of villi (Fig. 81–2). It should be pointed out that the lesions are often patchy, and biopsies from several

TABLE 81–2. CLINICAL FEATURES OF EOSINOPHILIC GASTROENTERITIS WITH PREDOMINANT MUCOSAL DISEASE

1. History	Intermittent nausea, emesis, abdominal pain, specific food intolerances
	Occasional diarrhea and weight loss; high incidence of prior asthma, allergic rhinitis
2. Physical examination	Atopic eczema, urticaria, pedal edema
3. Laboratory studies	Iron deficiency anemia
	Stool specimens positive for occult blood
	Stool specimens positive for Charcot-Leyden crystals
	Eosinophilia with low erythrocyte sedimentation rate
	Steatorrhea, often mild
	Impaired absorption of D-xylose
	Decreased serum albumin
	Decreased levels of serum immunoglobulins IgG, IgA, IgM
	Increased enteric protein loss by Cr^{51}-labeled albumin test
	Small bowel X-rays may be normal or show evidence of mucosal edema
	Abnormal jejunal biopsy with increased infiltration or eosinophils
4. Diagnosis	Peripheral blood eosinophilia
	Increased eosinophils in intestinal mucosa
	Gastrointestinal symptoms or signs after food ingestion
5. Therapy	Avoidance of offending foods
	Corticosteroids in intermittent courses as needed

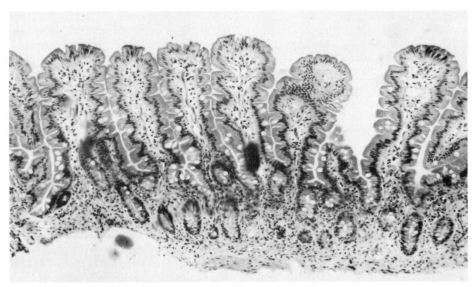

Figure 81–1. Jejunal biopsy specimen, revealing normal villous structure. Hematoxylin and eosin stain. Original magnification × 130.

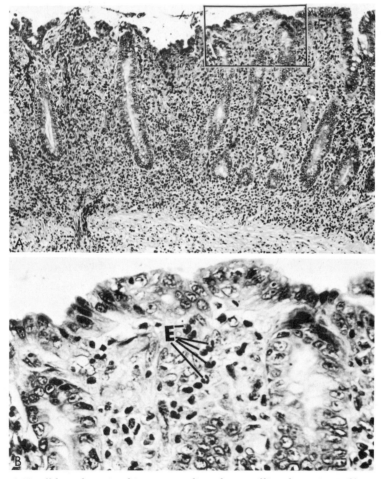

Figure 81–2. *A,* Small bowel suction biopsy, revealing absent villi and massive infiltration of the lamina propria with eosinophilic leukocytes. Hematoxylin and eosin stain × 100. *B,* Enlargement of boxed area in *A.* Note the surface epithelial abnormalities and the eosinophils (E). (From Leinbach, G. E., and Rubin, C. E.: Gastroenterology 59:874, 1970.)

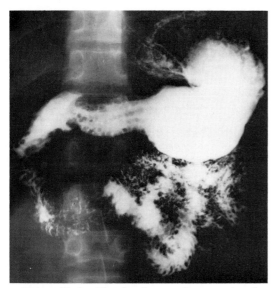

Figure 81-3. The distal stomach is noted to be cobblestoned with multiple polypoid filling defects. Similar defects are noted in the upper duodenum with coarsening of folds in the upper small intestine. (Courtesy of Dr. M. H. Sleisenger.)

sites may be required to establish the diagnosis. Small intestinal roentgenograms may be normal or may show nonspecific changes such as a mucosal edema and coarsening and nodularity of the folds (Figs. 81–3 and 81–4). Direct skin tests and passive transfer studies (P-K test) are often positive. Challenge studies with foods of which the patient states he is intolerant often result in the abrupt onset of gastroin-

testinal symptoms, but there are only a small number of reports[1-3] in which this has been done in a double-blind manner. The diagnosis is established by the three criteria cited earlier and listed in Table 81–2. It should be emphasized that patients may exhibit some, but not necessarily all, of the manifestations listed in the table. A history of recurrent symptoms dating over many years, associated with a history of allergic diathesis and specific food intolerances, should prompt serious consideration of the diagnosis. The differential diagnosis should include malabsorptive disorders such as nontropical sprue, other causes of protein-losing enteropathy such as intestinal lymphangiectasia, neoplastic diseases such as visceral lymphoma, connective tissue disorders such as polyarteritis nodosa, parasitic infestations, and regional enteritis (see the appropriate chapters of this text for complete discussions of these disorders).

Since many patients with eosinophilic gastroenteritis may associate exacerbation of symptoms with specific foods, it appears reasonable to try elimination diets as an initial mode of therapy. However, review of cases reported in the literature suggests that elimination diets are not consistently effective in bringing about amelioration of symptoms.[2, 3] The lack of effectiveness of dietotherapy seems to be due to several factors: (1) The precipitating events in acute flare-ups remain largely unknown and in all likelihood include factors other

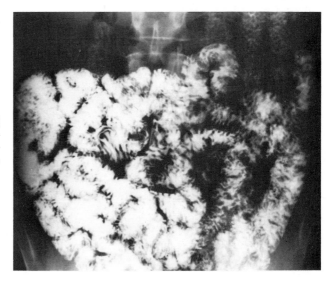

Figure 81-4. Coarsening of the small intestinal folds in eosinophilic gastroenteritis. Abnormality due to edema and infiltration of cells. (Courtesy of Dr. M. H. Sleisenger.)

than food allergies alone. (2) The course of the illness varies considerably, and careful, long-term objective evaluation of elimination diets is lacking. (3) Patients may respond initially to dietotherapy, but the effect is not permanent and corticosteroids frequently have to be added to sustain the patient in remission. (4) Elimination diets may be impractical. Despite these limitations, a trial of an elimination diet should be considered, because occasional patients respond dramatically and for long periods of time.[1] Acute exacerbation of symptoms usually responds promptly to short-term corticosteroid therapy (prednisone in a dosage of 20 to 30 mg per day for seven to ten days). Some patients, however, require treatment with corticosteroids on a prolonged basis. The majority of patients with eosinophilic gastroenteritis and mucosal disease improve or become asymptomatic on corticosteroid therapy. Antihistamines and antispasmodic drugs have not been reported to be beneficial.

Representative Case Study of Eosinophilic Gastroenteritis with Predominant Mucosal Disease. A 22-year-old white male student was admitted to the hospital in December 1965 for evaluation of abdominal pain and eosinophilia of many years' duration. He had been hospitalized previously on three occasions for similar complaints, but no diagnosis had been established. Since the age of 13, the patient had experienced recurrent episodes of abdominal pain. The pain was crampy in nature, epigastric, and periumbilical in location, occurred 30 to 60 minutes after meals, and was frequently associated with diarrhea. The episodes of pain occurred at least once to twice per week. The patient usually had one to two stools per day, but with attacks of pain he had up to 12 to 15 watery stools per day. Several stool examinations failed to reveal ova and parasites, but because of persistent abdominal symptoms and eosinophilia he had received two courses of therapy with Delvex without effect. The patient had also been treated with iron tablets for an iron deficiency anemia while in his teens. There was no history of febrile episodes, melena, joint symptoms, or perirectal disease.

In 1962, the patient was found to have mild atopic dermatitis. In 1964, he was hospitalized with acute bronchitis. There was no history of asthma, seasonal rhinitis, hives, or urticaria. However, he had previously noted intermittent pedal edema. The patient stated that he was intolerant of many foods, including meat products (beef, pork, veal, lamb), oats, wheat products (pastries, cakes), and eggs. Ingestion of red meats in particular would consistently precipitate episodes of abdominal pain, and accordingly he had not eaten any meat products for five years. He was not intolerant of alcohol and milk products. A trial on a gluten-free diet in 1964 did not appreciably alter his symptoms.

Physical examination on admission revealed a thin, well developed young man in no distress. The temperature was 99° F, pulse 80 per minute, respiration 16, and blood pressure 140 systolic and 60 diastolic. There were eczematous and lichenified lesions present on both antecubital fossae, the left wrist, and both ankles. There was no lymphadenopathy. The heart and lungs were normal. No abdominal organs or masses were palpable. There was mild pedal and pretibial edema. Sigmoidoscopic examination was entirely normal.

Initial laboratory studies revealed a hematocrit of 39 per cent, a hemoglobin of 12.2 g per 100 ml, a white cell count of 11,500 with 32 per cent eosinophils, and an erythrocyte sedimentation rate of 2 mm per hour. The urinalysis was normal. Urinary excretion of D-xylose after a 25-g oral dose was 11.2 g. Quantitative stool fat excretion was 6.8 g in 24 hours, with a coefficient of fat absorption of 91.5 per cent. The serum albumin was 3.2 g per 100 ml and the serum globulin 1.7 g per 100 ml. The serum immunoglobulins were as follows: IgG, 410 mg per 100 ml; IgA, 105 mg. per 100 ml; and IgM, 25 mg per 100 ml. The serum cholesterol was 160 mg per 100 ml and the serum calcium 9.2 mg per 100 ml. The serum iron was 35 μg per 100 ml, and the iron binding capacity was 366 μg per 100 ml. A small bowel biopsy revealed minimal eosinophilic infiltration but otherwise was interpreted as normal (Fig. 81–1). Roentgenographic examinations of the upper gastrointestinal tract, small bowel, and colon were interpreted as being normal. An augmented histamine gastric analysis was within normal limits, with a maximal acid output of 7 mEq in one hour. The 24-hour urinary excretion of 5 HIAA was 5.0 mg. A lactose tolerance test was normal. An oral iron tolerance test was also normal, the serum iron level increasing from a fasting value of 50 μg per 100 ml to 360 μg per 100 ml in three hours. The patient also ingested 25 g of a gluten solution without any untoward effects. A Cr^{51}-albumin test performed while the patient was in relapse resulted in fecal excretion of 6.6 per cent (normal = <1.0 per cent) (see pp. 35 to 48) and urinary excretion of 20 per cent of the given dose.

Cutaneous scratch tests with 84 common food extracts revealed positive responses to eggs, oats, wheat, pork, corn, and rice. However, cutaneous intradermal tests with the common inhalant allergens and yeasts were negative. Direct skin reactivity to bovine, gamma globulin, porcine serum, porcine serum albumin, and porcine gamma globulin was quite marked in dilutions of 1:1000 to 1:50,000. The patient's serum was assayed for skin sensitizing antibody by the P-K test and was positive for porcine serum.

The patient was challenged with various foods in a manner in which he could not identify the food being administered. A bland food produced no symptoms. However, after a challenge with a food to which he was intolerant, the patient developed tachycardia, nausea, emesis, abdominal cramps, diarrhea, leukocytosis, and increased eosinophilia. Small intestinal biopsies obtained after challenge demonstrated a slightly increased infiltration of eosinophils of uncertain significance and no change in jejunal histamine or serotonin concentrations.

After the challenge studies the patient received a seven-day course of prednisone in a dosage of 20 mg per day with complete cessation of symptoms. He has remained largely asymptomatic on a diet free of meat and wheat products. Infrequent exacerbations of abdominal cramps and diarrhea have responded dramatically to four- to seven-day courses of prednisone therapy. One year after the diagnosis, the serum albumin level was 3.8 g per 100 ml, the serum IgG was 370 mg per 100 ml, the serum IgA was 80 mg per 100 ml, and the serum IgM was 20 mg per 100 ml.

COMMENT. This patient with atopic eczema had a nine-year history of specific food intolerances, intermittent abdominal pain, and diarrhea and was found to have eosinophilia, minimal steatorrhea, hypoalbuminemia, hypoglobulinemia, and a protein-losing enteropathy. A small bowel biopsy revealed eosinophilic infiltration of the jejunal mucosa. After challenge with a specific foodstuff, the patient developed nausea, emesis, abdominal cramps, diarrhea, and tachycardia, all of which dramatically subsided after corticosteroid therapy. A cause-and-effect relationship is strongly suggested by the marked clinical symptoms in response to a food historically incriminated as causing similar symptoms. The slight increase in eosinophilia noted in serial jejunal biospy specimens is open to question, because Leinbach and Rubin have recently emphasized the spotty nature of the intestinal lesion necessitating the evaluation of many control and test biopsies.[3]

EOSINOPHILIC GASTROENTERITIS WITH PREDOMINANT MUSCLE LAYER DISEASE

Patients in this group usually have marked thickening and rigidity of the stomach, as well as of the small bowel,

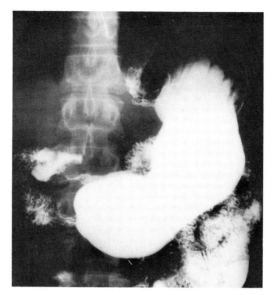

Figure 81–5. Narrowing of distal antrum in eosinophilic gastroenteritis due to hypertrophy of the muscle layer and eosinophilic infiltration. (Courtesy of Dr. M. H. Sleisenger.)

manifested by symptoms of pyloric outlet obstruction or incomplete small bowel obstruction (Fig. 81–5). The terms "polyenteric" and "monoenteric" have been proposed to describe a diffuse form and localized form of the disease process, respectively.[12] In the polyenteric type there is extensive thickening and induration of the stomach, duodenum, and small bowel with some areas appearing firm and cartilaginous. Hyperplastic nodes in the mesentery along with the aforementioned gross picture simulate regional enteritis. Histological examination reveals diffuse infiltration of sheets of mature eosinophilic leukocytes in the submucosa, extending through the muscular layers to the serosa (Fig. 81–6). In the monoenteric form the process is usually confined to the pylorus and antrum of the stomach. The majority of the patients with predominantly muscle layer disease reported in the literature[2, 12] have had involvement of the stomach alone, whereas approximately 30 per cent have had stomach and small bowel involvement.

Clinical Picture and Diagnosis. The diagnosis of eosinophilic gastroenteritis with muscle layer disease is usually established between the second and fifth decades. The patients frequently complain of nausea, emesis, and crampy abdominal

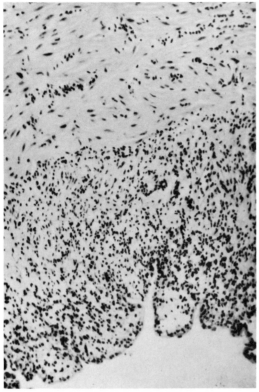

Figure 81–6. This histologic section of the upper small intestines shows infiltration with eosinophils in a thickened serosa and also in the muscle layer. Hematoxylin and eosin stain. × 200. (Courtesy of Dr. M. H. Sleisenger.)

pain not relieved by antacids or anticholinergic drugs. Approximately half of them have a prior allergic history, and an indeterminate number have had specific food intolerances. Eosinophilia is usually present. Gastrointestinal X-ray studies may show a smooth concentric narrowing of the antrum, with decreased peristalsis or multiple polypoid filling defects in the distal stomach (Fig. 81–5). The roentgenographic abnormalities may simulate an infiltrating gastric carcinoma, antral gastritis caused by acid peptic disease, and regional enteritis involving the stomach. Blood loss anemia and hypoproteinemia caused by excessive enteric protein loss have been described in patients with stomach involvement alone, as well as in those with stomach and small bowel involvement. The diagnosis is established by histological examination of full thickness biopsies of stomach and/or small bowel. The differential diagnosis includes gastric carcinoma, lymphosarcoma, gastric polyps, polyarteritis nodosa, regional enteritis, and eosinophilic granuloma. The clinical features of eosinophilic granuloma are summarized in Table 81–3. Briefly, eosinophilic granulomas are localized lesions not associated with specific food intolerances or peripheral blood eosinophilia.[13, 14] They are usually firm, smooth, sessile, pedunculated polypoid lesions located at or near the pylorus. In addition to pyloric outlet obstruction, polypoid granulomata of small gut may present as acute intussusception or acute abdominal pain, and ileal lesions may mimic acute appendicitis.[14] After surgical excision there are no reported recurrences.

TABLE 81–3. CLINICAL FEATURES OF GASTROINTESTINAL EOSINOPHILIC GRANULOMA

		No.	%
1. Onset	Most frequently fourth to sixth decade		
2. Allergic history	Infrequent history of hay fever, asthma, urticaria, eczema		
3. Eosinophilia	Usually absent		
4. Leukocytosis	Usually absent		
5. Sites of involvement in 32 cases[14]	Pharynx	1	3
	Stomach	17	53
	Small bowel	5	16
	Colon and rectum	9	28
6. Gastrointestinal X-rays	Circumscribed polypoid lesions, most frequent in stomach, causing pyloric outlet obstruction and simulating gastric carcinoma; lesions may also occur in small bowel and colon		
7. Pathology	Sharply localized eosinophilic granuloma admixed in connective tissue stroma		

In earlier reports which have been summarized,[12] the usual recommended treatment for eosinophilic gastroenteritis localized to the stomach was subtotal gastrectomy and gastroenterostomy or gastroenterostomy alone. However, after such surgical procedures, patients have developed recurrent symptoms requiring corticosteroid therapy. In a review of the more recent literature, evidence has been presented suggesting that continuous or intermittent corticosteroid therapy will frequently result in dramatic relief of obstructive symptoms.[2]

EOSINOPHILIC GASTROENTERITIS WITH PREDOMINANTLY SUBSEROSAL DISEASE

Patients with this form of eosinophilic gastroenteritis develop ascites with marked eosinophilia in the ascitic fluid. Laparotomy usually reveals thickened serosa of the small bowel with subserosal eosinophilic infiltration (Fig. 81–6). Not infrequently there is also involvement of the stomach. It has been demonstrated that corticosteroid therapy results in prompt diuresis and clearing of ascites.[2] Improvement may persist despite discontinuation of corticosteroid therapy.

MILK-RELATED GASTROINTESTINAL DISEASE IN CHILDREN

Intolerance to milk in the neonate who presents with vomiting and diarrhea or diarrhea alone may be a manifestation of protein allergy, lactose intolerance, monosaccharide malabsorption, or galactosemia. The last disease, although not primarily gastrointestinal, is to be suspected always in the infant who develops vomiting and diarrhea during the first few days of life while taking a lactose-containing formula. Eventually jaundice, cataracts, hepatosplenomegaly and mental retardation develop if it remains undiagnosed and untreated. There is an absence or severe reduction of galactose-1-phosphate uridyl transferase in the liver, kidney, brain, lens, and red blood cells, leading to an accumulation of galactose-1-phosphate. The urine is positive to Clinitest (Benedict's) but negative to Clinistix (glucose oxidase). The disease may be definitively diagnosed by demonstration of very low enzyme activity in the peripheral erythrocytes.

Milk and Milk Formulas. A brief comment should be made about the variations between human milk and the different formula preparations. One hundred ml of human milk contains 7 g of lactose, 1.1 g of protein, and 3.8 g of fat. The same quantity of cow's milk contains 4.8 g of lactose, 3.3 g of protein, and the same quantity of fat. Although the fat content is similar, there is a qualitative difference, for human milk contains far greater quantities of unsaturated fatty acids and linoleic and oleic acids but less of the shorter chain fatty acids than cow's milk. There is four times the calcium but six times the phosphorus in cow's milk as in human milk. This is important because the high phosphorus intake in the presence of neonatal renal immaturity may cause a high serum phosphorus level and precipitate neonatal tetany. Many synthetic formulas attempt to simulate the composition of breast milk and contain a higher lactose composition, but the amount of protein is the same as cow's milk. Nutramigen is considered nonallergenic and contains the protein hydrolysate products of casein. Sucrose is the sugar. The synthetic soy or meat-based formulas use sucrose or maltose as the carbohydrate. These formulas eliminate milk sugar as well as protein from their composition.

All the commercial formulas are adequate for the nutrition of the normal full-term infant. The demands for feeding of the premature infant, however, require a diet high in protein (at least 4 g per kilogram per day), calcium, and phosphorus, and low in fat and solute. Increased fecal fat has been noted in the premature;[15] the percentage of this varies directly with the type of dietary fat—greater with animal and less with vegetable fat, indicating the advantage of the latter.

Milk Protein Allergies. Cow's milk allergy may present protean symptoms: vomiting, colic, eczema, diarrhea, thrombocytopenia, or respiratory disease.[16, 17] It is more frequent in males than in females. In healthy children the incidence of such allergy varies from 0.3 to 7 per cent, whereas in allergic children it may be as high as 30 per cent.[18] Most children outgrow allergy to cow's milk protein, but 2 per cent remain allergic after six years of age.

Antibodies to cow's milk proteins may appear in the sera of healthy infants and children.[19] Some antibody may be detected in cord blood owing to passive transfer from the mother. The earliest antibody response to a cow's milk feed is seen at five days, and high titers may develop between seven and ten days and persist for 20 to 30 days after onset of milk feeding.[20] Different methods to determine antibody account for the different results in reported studies; however, the allergic infants generally have the highest antibody titers of circulating antibodies, up to 98 per cent of normal infants studied by the coated tanned red cell techniques.[19] Further, children with antibodies have a higher incidence of anemia, respiratory disease, and poor growth than the group which did not have precipitins.[21] The Ouchterlony or agar-gel technique is less sensitive; thus when precipitins are detected, the antibody is abundantly present.

Milk-allergic children can be classified into two groups: those with allergy involving both the respiratory tract and skin, and those with digestive symptoms alone. Infants who develop severe reactions to milk challenge develop other allergies later in life; those who react more mildly to challenge are not allergic later.[22] In our experience, those with the most severe gastrointestinal symptoms tend to develop allergies which are for the most part respiratory.

In 1960, an association between circulating cow's milk antibodies and chronic pulmonary disease was first reported.[23] This was expanded later into Heiner's syndrome by 1962 (see below). Its postulated basis is delayed hypersensitivity, intravascular precipitation of antigen-antibody complexes, and vascular hypersensitivity in the pathogenesis of the pulmonary lesions. As in pulmonary hemosiderosis, iron-laden macrophages are noted in the gastric or bronchial aspirates. Aspiration of milk with sensitization developing by this route may be another fac-

tor in chronic respiratory disease in infancy. A similar picture may be seen in infants who have had neonatal esophageal anomalies. It is postulated that the IgA protective antibodies in bronchial secretions lag behind several weeks in development after IgG and IgM and that Heiner's syndrome is limited to infancy by the later development of mucosal immunity.[23]

Cow's milk contains at least 20 antigenic protein components, but to date only a few seem to be of clinical importance.[24] Beta-lactoglobulin is considered the most active fraction. Those with lesser antigenic activity are alpha-lactalbumin, casein, and bovine serum albumin. Despite the route of sensitization (oral, intravenous, or subcutaneous), the resultant circulating antibodies are similar.[25] Of therapeutic interest, there is a cross sensitivity between cow and goat milk albumin, alpha-lactalbumin and an immune globulin.[26, 27] A similar situation exists between human and cow's milk, for a small number of cow's milk proteins have partial identity and cross reactivity with human serum proteins. Cow's milk antigen may be transmitted through human milk.

There is evidence that heating milk may modify the proteins and decrease or eliminate their antigenicity.[28] Other data, however, indicate that heating milk may increase its anaphylactogenic properties.[29] The reactions between lactose and the milk proteins during pasteurization, storage, and handling tend to increase milk's allergic potential. These differences may be explained in part by whether the proteins are studied separately or in whole milk preparations where they might combine with lactose.[30, 31]

The mode of milk protein absorption and the stimulation of sensitivity are not fully understood. Large peptides are subjected to extracellular hydrolysis within the lumen of the small bowel; most small peptides are hydrolyzed after contact with the brush border and entry into the cell. For a short period at least the newborn can absorb intact ingested protein and antibody, but cannot absorb significant amounts of the larger molecular weight immune globulins.[32, 33]

Antibodies to ingested antigens may be found in intestinal secretions or in rectal mucus.[34] These have been termed coproantibodies or stool precipitins. These precipitating antibodies are contained in the immunoglobulin A fraction of the intestinal secretions. Most plasma cells of the intestine contain IgA, and unlike serum the intestinal secretions contain IgA combined with transport piece, forming "secretory IgA." The other serum immunoglobulins IgM and IgG are present in lesser quantities. Sensitization to milk proteins usually develops by six weeks of age, which is the time required for the neonate to develop maximal antibody production. It is also the time of appearance of secretory IgA (see pp. 51 to 68).

Cutaneous testing is not always positive in allergic individuals, and the correlations of circulating milk antibodies with gastrointestinal milk allergy have been poor.[35] The establishment of the diagnosis has depended upon the fulfillment of the criteria that the symptoms recur within 48 hours after a trial feeding of milk, that three challenges must be positive and similar, and that the symptoms must subside after each challenge reaction.[36] However, in the young, sensitive infant, challenges may induce anaphylactic shock or severe gastrointestinal hemorrhage. A safe and reliable test has been the examination of the supernatant fluid from a freshly spun stool for the presence of precipitating antibodies against cow's milk and its separate proteins.[37] Although some studies have found false-positive tests from non-immunoglobulin precipitin lines and others have reported precipitins to milk proteins in the stools from breast-fed infants, milk-fed infants, and infants with diarrhea, the test remains of value.[38, 39] In at least 80 per cent of young children with chronic diarrhea and precipitins to cow's milk protein in the stool, the symptoms will be totally alleviated within 48 hours after elimination of milk proteins from the diet.

CLINICAL PICTURE

The most common form of gastrointestinal allergy to cow's milk proteins is chronic diarrhea of infancy.[16] The stools may vary from several soft, semiformed stools to numerous watery, explosive diarrhea stools. Mucus is frequent (80 per cent), and gross blood or blood streaking of the stools may be noted. Occult blood is present in up to 80 per cent of patients. There may occasionally be granular, white, seedy material or even bean-sized white curds in the stool. The age of onset of milk protein allergy may be between two days and four and a half months, but most infants become symptomatic within the first six weeks of life. Colic may precede or accompany changes in bowel habits. A family history of some form of allergy is present in the families of at least half the infants. Those with mild symptoms grow well, but those with severe diarrhea will be retarded in height, weight, and even head circumference growth.

Patients ranging in age from six months to 14 years may exhibit more serious clinical findings believed to be due to gastrointestinal allergy to milk and other specific foods.[7] These patients have a history of eczema, asthma, allergic rhinitis, diarrhea, and vague abdominal discomfort and emesis after ingestion of certain foods. Physical examination reveals pedal edema and evidence of growth retardation. Laboratory abnormalities include peripheral blood eosinophila, hypochromic microcytic anemia, decreased serum iron levels, and stools positive for occult blood and Charcot-Leyden crystals. Hypoalbuminemia and hypoglobulinemia caused by excessive enteric loss of protein are readily documented. There is no laboratory evidence of malabsorption or lactase deficiency, although studies are incomplete in some patients. Upper gastrointestinal roentgenograms are either normal or show nonspecific mucosal edema. Peroral small intestinal mucosal biopsy specimens in a few patients reveal infiltration of eosinophils but are otherwise normal. One of the strongest lines of evidence supporting the concept that these patients have gastrointestinal allergy is the response to elimination diets and milk-challenge studies. Half the patients have precipitating antibodies to whole milk in their serum. Elimination diets ameliorate symptoms immediately, especially milk-free diets, which are associated with a significant elevation of serum albumin levels to normal, decreased fecal excretion of Cr^{51}-labeled albumin, and prolongation of the $T_{1/2}$ for serum albumin toward normal. In addition, stool examinations become negative for occult blood and Charcot-Leyden crystals. On the other hand, challenge studies with milk reintroduced into the diet result in the reappearance of several abnormalities: decreased serum albumin levels, increased fecal excretion of Cr^{51}-labeled albumin, shortened $T_{1/2}$ for serum albumin, stools positive for occult blood and Charcot-Leyden crystals, and increased peripheral blood eosinophilia. A small number of patients treated with corticosteroids showed rapid improvement.[7]

Although there is indisputable evidence that these children have protein-losing enteropathy, the diagnosis of gastrointestinal allergy is less firm. The diagnosis rests on the prior history of other allergic manifestations, and eosinophilic overabundance in the blood, intestinal mucosa, and stools (Charcot-Leyden crystals). As emphasized earlier, such criteria are indirect. Furthermore, the relationship between this syndrome in children and eosinophilic gastroenteritis in adults is not firmly established for several reasons. First, only a small number of challenge studies have been carried out. Second, only a limited number of mucosal biopsies have been obtained and repeat biopsies not done. Third, gastrointestinal symptoms seemed to improve spontaneously with advancing age. Only long-term follow-up studies of larger numbers of similar cases will clarify the nature of this disorder and its relationship to adult forms of eosinophilic gastroenteritis.[7]

Similar findings have been described in infants and children thought to be intolerant of cow's milk (Heiner's syndrome).[40, 41] The patients range from eight months to seven years. Clinical findings include the presence of iron deficiency anemia, occult gastrointestinal bleeding with stools positive for occult blood, decreased serum iron levels, normal serum copper values, minimal hypoalbuminemia, and precipitins to cow's milk in the serum. Evidence of gastrointestinal bleeding stops within two days after milk is withdrawn and reappears within a few days after reintroduction of milk. This picture is probably more frequent than is generally appreciated, because, as noted, it has been estimated that 0.3 to 0.7 per cent of infants and children are sensitive to cow's milk.[41] It should also

be emphasized that there may be considerable variation in symptoms after milk ingestion, ranging from an immediate anaphylactic response (see below) to markedly delayed effects such as the syndromes described above.[40, 41] Delayed reactions after 30 minutes may be difficult to recognize unless accompanied by such obvious findings as asthma, eczema, urticaria, or angioedema.

Precipitating substances or coproantibodies to milk, cereal products (barley, wheat, rye, oats), and soy were present singly or in combination in stools of almost all patients, two and a half weeks to two and a half years, with chronic diarrhea.[42] None of these patients, however, had circulating precipitins to the proteins tested. Diarrhea improved in many patients treated with an elimination diet. The demonstration of stool precipitins against dietary antigens being ingested at the time of the study correlated well with the clinical improvement observed after removal of the offending antigen from the diet. These data suggest that sensitization to certain dietary proteins and the consequent immunological phenomena might be localized to the gastrointestinal tract. The reasons for such apparent sensitization are unknown. Similarly, the precise mechanism for the presumed allergic reaction in the gut has not been elucidated.

The milk intolerance with iron deficiency anemia and occult gastrointestinal blood loss described above must be differentiated from the syndrome of iron deficiency anemia, hypocupremia, and hypoproteinemia caused by ingestion of a diet almost exclusively milk.[43, 44] Infants with the latter disorder have pallor, edema, hypoproteinemia, anemia, low serum iron, and serum copper values but a *normal* serum iron binding capacity. The cause of this syndrome is thought to be an inadequate dietary intake of both iron and copper. This conclusion is supported by the fact that there is prompt reversal of all abnormalities after administration of oral iron *despite* continued ingestion of milk.

Milk-induced colitis is a distinct entity in infancy and is characterized by chronic diarrhea and the passage of blood, mucus, and, at times, sheets of colonic epithelial cells in the stool.[45] The onset may occur from two days to two months of age. The

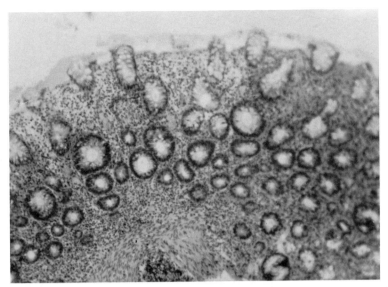

Figure 81-7.   Rectal biopsy from a six-week-old infant with milk-induced colitis. There is a marked round cell infiltrate, and moderate polymorphonuclear infiltrate as well as destruction of normal architecture. × 100.

barium enema is normal, but sigmoidoscopy reveals the changes of ulcerative colitis: a hemorrhagic, friable mucosa which may or may not be covered with a purulent or mucoid exudate. Rectal biopsy is consistent with the changes of nonspecific colitis (Fig. 81-7). There are loss of mucosal architecture, polymorphonuclear cell infiltrate, and crypt abscess formation. Within 48 to 72 hours after the elimination of milk from the diet the symptoms improve or disappear and the pathological changes revert to normal. Because of the dramatic response to milk restriction, this disorder must be considered in no way related to ulcerative colitis.

TREATMENT

Most infants and children sensitive to milk will respond to the elimination of milk from the diet within 24 to 48 hours. Tolerance develops gradually and usually requires one year, although some infants cannot tolerate milk for three to five years. Substitute formulas consist of Nutramigen (protein hydrolysate), soy formulas, or Lambase. The protein hydrolysate formula may cause a green-mucoid diarrhea in some infants. Soy may be tolerated for several days and may then be associated with diarrhea. Up to 40 per cent of infants al-

lergic to milk may become allergic to soy products.

ALLERGY TO SOY PROTEIN

Soy formulas have been recommended increasingly as a cow's milk formula substitute in allergic children or as the initial formula of choice for potentially allergic infants.[4, 46] The antigenicity of soy is significant, and it has been implicated in anaphylaxis, asthma, and gastrointestinal dysfunction.[46] The neonate may develop watery diarrhea and even proctitis with bloody streaking of the stool. The older child may develop recurrent abdominal pain. This is usually not associated with diarrhea or flatulence. The pain occurs during the daytime and early evening. It is not nocturnal, and it is not related to meals or posturing. The diagnosis is confirmed by finding precipitins in the stool to soy, the demonstration of injury to jejunal mucosa, and the relief of symptoms when soy is eliminated from the diet (Fig. 81-8).[4, 46]

CELIAC SPRUE

This disease may or may not be due to an allergy of the intestine to gluten, contained principally in cereals. This disease

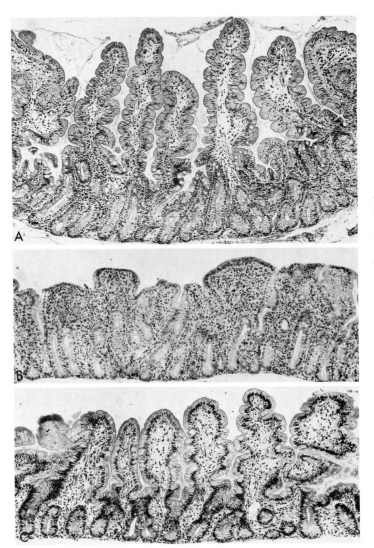

Figure 81–8. Jejunal response to soy proteins in a ten and one-half month infant. *A,* Normal baseline biopsy at the duodenojejunal junction, before challenge. Note normal villi. *B,* Biopsy at the duodenojejunal junction, 24 hours after challenge. Note absence of villi and similarity in appearance to biopsy illustrated in Figure 81–2. *C,* Biopsy at the duodenojejunal junction 96 hours after challenge. Note return of villi. Hematoxylin and eosin stain. × 115. (From Ament, M. E., and Rubin, C. E.: Gastroenterology 62:227, 1972.)

is discussed on pages 864 to 884. It suffices here to state that withdrawal of gluten from the diet brings about nearly complete to complete remission of the disease. In this clinical sense, then, it may be viewed as an allergic gastroenteritis.

Approximately 40 per cent of milk-sensitive infants develop gluten sensitivity. Small bowel biopsies in this group of children have been normal, and, as in pure milk-protein allergy, tolerance to gluten products develops by one to two years of age.

GASTROINTESTINAL FOOD INTOLERANCE WITH SYSTEMIC ALLERGIC REACTIONS

Although anaphylaxis to ingested antigens is rare, it is very important to identify the causative antigen in order to prevent a subsequent lethal reaction. Cases have recently been reported of systemic allergic reactions to ingested antigens.[47] These patients have potentially fatal reactions with cutaneous, respiratory, gastrointestinal, and hypotensive manifestations.

In all cases, an explosive allergic reaction follows a meal. The patients present with hypotension, urticaria, angioedema, dyspnea, cyanosis, syncope, and crampy abdominal pain with nausea and emesis. A few patients have laryngeal stridor, requiring tracheal intubation.

The aforementioned abnormalities clear rapidly after treatment with sympathomimetic and antihistaminic drugs. None of the patients demonstrated peripheral blood eosinophilia, but the reactions may well have been too brief for eosinophilia to develop. The causative antigens may be identified through a careful exploration of historical details; they include foods such as halibut, rice, shrimp, and a cereal mix and drugs such as penicillin, acetylsalicylic acid, and demethylchlortetracycline. In some patients, the cause is considered proved when repeated inadvertent ingestion of the offending food causes a recurrent anaphylactic reaction. About 60 per cent have a positive P-K test. Further, in the majority of such patients tested, histamine is released from leukocytes challenged with specific antigen; no histamine is released from leukocytes obtained from normal donors treated in an identical manner. These provocative observations clearly indicate that systemic allergic reactions can occur following ingestion of specific antigens, but shed little light on the pathogenetic mechanisms involved.

REFERENCES

1. Greenberger, N. J., Tennenbaum, J. I., and Ruppert, R. Protein-losing enteropathy associated with gastrointestinal allergy. Amer. J. Med. 43:777, 1967.
2. Klein, N. C., Hargrove, M. D., Sleisenger, M. H., and Jeffries, G. H. Eosinophilic gastroenteritis. Medicine 49:299, 1970.
3. Leinbach, G. E., and Rubin, C. E. Eosinophilic gastroenteritis: A simple reaction to food allergens. Gastroenterology 59:874, 1970.
4. Ament, M. E., and Rubin, C. E. Soy protein—another cause of the flat intestinal lesion. Gastroenterology 62:227, 1972.
5. Ingelfinger, F. J., Lowell, F. C., and Franklin, W. Gastrointestinal allergy. New Eng. J. Med. 241:303, 337, 1949.
6. Pollard, H. M., and Stuart, G. H. Experimental reproduction of gastric allergy in human beings with controlled observations on the mucosa. J. Allergy 13:467, 1942.
7. Waldmann, T. A., Wochner, R. D., Laster, L., and

Gordon, R. S. Allergy gastroenteropathy. New Eng. J. Med. 276:761, 1967.
8. Mendoza, J., Meyers, J., and Snyder, R. Soybean sensitivity: A case report. Pediatrics 46:774, 1970.
9. Archer, R. K. The Eosinophil Leukocytes, Oxford, Blackwell Scientific Publications, 1963, p. 205.
10. Kay, A. B., Stechschulte, D. J., and Austen, K. F. Eosinophil leukocyte chemotactic factors. J. Allergy 47:118, 1971.
11. Laster, C. E., and Gleich, G. J. Chemotaxis of eosinophils and neutrophils by aggregated immunoglobulins. J. Allergy Clin. Immunol. 48:297, 1971.
12. Ureles, A. L., Alschibaja, T., Lodico, D., and Stabins, S. J. Idiopathic eosinophilic infiltration of the gastrointestinal tract, diffuse and circumscribed. Amer. J. Med. 30:899, 1961.
13. Swartz, J. M., and Young, J. M. Primary infiltrative eosinophilic gastritis, enteritis, and peritonitis. Gastroenterology 28:431, 1955.
14. Salmon, P. R., and Paulley, J. W. Eosinophilic granuloma of the gastrointestinal tract. Gut 8:8, 1967.
15. Davidson, M., Levine, S. A., Bauer, C. H., et al. Feeding studies in low birth weight infants. J. Pediat. 70:691, 1967.
16. Gryboski, J. D. Gastrointestinal milk allergy in infants. Pediatrics 40:354, 1967.
17. Stanfield, J. P. A review of cow's milk allergy in infancy. Acta Paediat. 48:85, 1959.
18. Bachman, K. D., and Dees, S. Milk allergy. II. Observations on incidence and symptoms of allergy to milk in allergic infants. Pediatrics 20:400, 1957.
19. Gunther, M., Aschaffenburg, R., Matthews, R. H., et al. The level of antibodies to the proteins of cow's milk in the serum of normal human infants. Immunology 3:296, 1960.
20. Lippard, V. W., Schloss, O. M., and Johnson, P. H. Immune reactions induced in infants by intestinal absorption of incompletely digested cow's milk. Amer. J. Dis. Child. 51:562, 1936.
21. Holland, N., Hong, K., Davis, C. N., et al. Significance of precipitating antibodies to milk proteins in the serum of infants and children. J. Pediat. 61:181, 1962.
22. Von Sydow, S. Some cases of cow's milk idiosyncrasy. Acta Paediat. Scand. 23:383, 1939.
23. Heiner, D. C., Sears, J. W., and Kniker, W. T. Multiple precipitins to cow's milk in chronic respiratory disease. Amer. J. Dis. Child. 103:634, 1962.
24. Bleumink, E., and Young, E. Identification of the atopic allergen in cow's milk. Int. Arch. Allergy 34:521, 1968.
25. Rothberg, R., Kraft, S., and Farr, R. S. Similarities between rabbit antibodies produced following ingestion of bovine serum albumin and following parenteral administration. J. Immunol. 98:386, 1967.
26. Hanson, L. A., and Anderson, H. J. A comparison of the antigenic relations of human milk and goat's milk to bovine milk. Acta Paediat. Scand. 51:509, 1962.
27. Lee, M. Human serum precipitins to goat's milk

proteins and to cow's milk proteins. Pediatrics 35:247, 1965.

28. Ratner, B., and Dworetzky, M. Studies on the allergenicity of cow's milk. II. Effect of heat treatment on the allergenicity of milk and protein fractions from milk tested in guinea pigs by parenteral milk sensitization and challenge. Pediatrics 22:648, 1958.

29. Bertok, E. J., and Baker, B. E. Anaphylactoid shock in guinea pigs produced by casein degradation products. J. Sci. Food. Agric. 12:852, 1961.

30. Luz, A. Q., and Todd, R. H. Antigenicity of heated milk proteins. Amer. J. Dis. Child. 108:478, 1964.

31. Marquand, T. C., and Hedler, L. Anaphylotoxin und DAS (Frügift) Wirkung in Milch. Arzneimittelforsch 16:831, 1966.

32. Matthews, D. M., and Laster, L. Absorption of protein digestion products: A review. Gut 6:411, 1965.

33. Gunther, M., Cheek, E., Matthews, R. H., et al. Immune responses in infants to cow's milk proteins taken by mouth. Int. Arch. Allergy 21:257, 1962.

34. Plaut, A. G., and Keonil, P. Immunoglobulins in human small intestinal fluid. Gastroenterology 56:522, 1969.

35. Buckley, R. H., and Dees, S. Nutritional and antigenic effects of two bovine milk preparations in infants. J. Pediat. 69:238, 1966.

36. Goldman, A. S., Anderson, D. W., Seller, W. A., et al. Milk allergy. I. Oral challenge with milk and isolated proteins in allergic children. Pediatrics 32:425, 1963.

37. Gryboski, J. D., Katz, J., Reynolds, D., et al. Gluten intolerance following cow's milk sensitivity: Two cases with coproantibodies to milk and wheat proteins. Ann. Allergy 26:33, 1968.

38. Kraft, S., Rathberg, R. M., and Kriebel, G. W. Nonimmunologic precipitin lines between serum and enteric contents giving false positive evidence of local antibody production. J. Immunol. 104:528, 1970.

39. Davis, S. D., Bierman, C. W., Peirson, W. E., et al. Clinical nonspecificity of milk coproantibodies in diarrheal stools. New Eng. J. Med. 282:612, 1970.

40. Wilson, J. F., Heiner, D. C., and Lahey, M. E. Studies on iron metabolism; evidence of gastrointestinal dysfunction in infants in the iron deficiency anemia: A preliminary report. J. Pediat. 60:787, 1962.

41. Heiner, D. C., Wilson, J. F., and Lahey, M. E. Sensitivity to cow's milk. J.A.M.A. 189:563, 1964.

42. Self, T. W., Herskovic, T., Dzapak, E., Caplan, D., Schonberger, T., and Gryboski, J. D. Gastrointestinal protein allergy: Immunologic considerations. J.A.M.A. 207:2393, 1969.

43. Sturgeon, P., and Brubaker, C. Cooper deficiency in infants: A syndrome characterized by hypocupremia, iron deficiency anemia, and hypoproteinemia. Amer. J. Dis. Child. 92:254, 1956.

44. Zipursky, A., Dempsey, H., Markowitz, H., Cartwright, G., and Wintrobe, M. Studies in copper metabolism. XXIV. Hypocupremia in infants. Amer. J. Dis. Child. 96:148, 1958.

45. Gryboski, J. D., Burkle, F., and Hillman, R. Milk-induced colitis in an infant. Pediatrics 38:299, 1966.

46. Fries, J. Experiences with allergy to soybean in the United States. J. Asthma Res. 3:209, 1966.

47. Golbert, T. M., Patterson, R., and Pruzansky, J. J. Systemic allergic reactions to ingested antigens. J. Allergy 44:96, 1969.

THE BILIARY TRACT

Chapter 82

Anatomy and Embryology

M. Michael Thaler, Lawrence W. Way

Knowledge of the anatomy and embryology of the biliary tract is important not only for surgeons but also for those who wish to understand congenital lesions of the biliary tract caused by abnormal organogenesis.

Early in development a diverticulum capped by a cluster of cells appears on the ventral surface of the primitive foregut near the yolk stalk. This is the anlage of the liver, bile ducts, gallbladder, and primitive ventral pancreas. At four weeks of gestation, three separate buds can be recognized on the original diverticulum: the cranial bud gives rise to the liver, the caudal bud becomes the gallbladder, and a smaller basal segment develops into the ventral pancreas (Fig. 82–1). The cells

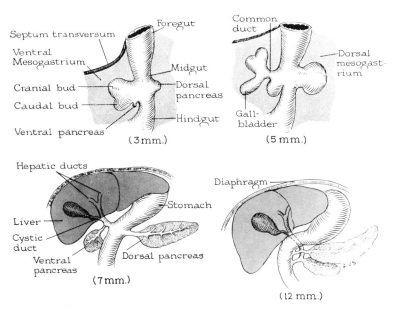

Figure 82–1. Stages in the embryological development of the extrahepatic biliary tree and pancreas. (Courtesy of Dr. Harold Lindner.)

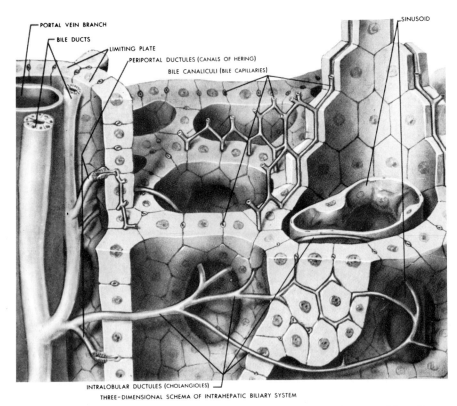

PORTAL VEIN BRANCH
BILE DUCTS
LIMITING PLATE
PERIPORTAL DUCTULES (CANALS OF HERING)
BILE CANALICULI (BILE CAPILLARIES)
SINUSOID
INTRALOBULAR DUCTULES (CHOLANGIOLES)
THREE-DIMENSIONAL SCHEMA OF INTRAHEPATIC BILIARY SYSTEM

Figure 82-2. Three-dimensional schema of intrahepatic biliary system. (After Hans Elias. Courtesy of Ciba Pharmaceutical Company.)

forming the cranial bud invade the septum transversum whose mesenchymal tissue contributes to the hepatic vasculature. The intrahepatic bile ducts arise as tributaries of the hepatic duct after eight weeks, differentiating into interlobular ducts at points of contact with connective tissue investing the branching portal vein.

Canaliculi possess a lumen from their earliest appearance as small vesicles between hepatic cells of the six-week embryo. Interlobular ducts and ductules develop from epithelial vesicles which appear in hepatocytes of the limiting plate surrounding the terminal branches of the portal vein. Bile is secreted in fetuses about four months old, enters the intestine, and colors the meconium. The gallbladder originates from the caudal portion of the hepatic diverticulum, and elongates to form the cystic duct at four weeks' gestation. Initially, the gallbladder and the hepatic ducts are hollow structures, but proliferation of the epithelial lining temporarily converts them into solid cords.

Recanalization occurs around the seventh week by vacuolization of the epithelial cords. The common bile duct acquires its lumen first, followed by the cystic duct, which expands at its distal end to form the definitive gallbladder.

The hepatic terminal of the fully developed biliary system consists of intercellular canaliculi which empty into the smallest ductules. These unite to form interlobular bile ducts which follow the terminal branches of the portal vein (Fig. 82–2). Larger ducts arise from the converging interlobular ducts. In the hilar region, where the intrahepatic and extrahepatic bile ducts meet, their coordination with the branches of the portal vein is lost. The right and left lobar ducts continue outside the liver as the corresponding hepatic ducts, joining to form the common hepatic bile duct in front of the portal vein. The gallbladder is drained by the cystic duct, which usually enters the common hepatic bile duct from the right side, 1 to 2 inches below its origin to form the common bile

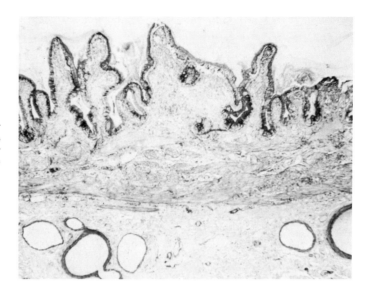

Figure 82–3. Full-thickness photomicrograph of the gallbladder wall, showing the mucosal folds, submucosa, muscular layer, and serosa. × 100.

duct. Variations in the length and course of the cystic duct and its site of anastomosis with the common hepatic duct occur relatively frequently.

The common bile duct has an average length of 3 inches; it runs distally along the right edge of the lesser omentum, behind the duodenum, and between the pancreas and the inferior vena cava, and terminates as an intramural structure (papilla of Vater) on the left side of the duodenum where it unites with the major pancreatic duct. The common ductal segment within the papilla has been called the ampulla of Vater, although the name implies an enlargement of the channel which does not exist. The sphincter of Oddi is a complex of smooth muscle fibers which invests the intraduodenal portion of the common bile duct, the pancreatic duct in 80 per cent of individuals, and the ampulla. It regulates the flow of bile into the intestine, inhibits entry of bile into the pancreatic duct, and prevents reflux of intestinal contents into the ducts. The remainder of the common bile duct and the hepatic ducts contain small amounts of smooth muscle which appear to be of no physiological importance in biliary dynamics.

The gallbladder is a distensible sac 3 by 1.5 inches in size, with a normal capacity of 30 to 50 ml. Its usual position marks the division between the right and left hepatic lobes. Its infundibulum curves anteriorly to form the cystic duct. Columnar cells line the mucosa which is thrown into numerous folds, increasing the surface area for absorption (Figs. 82–3 and 82–4). The

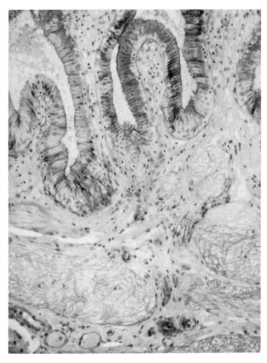

Figure 82–4. High-power photomicrograph of mucosal epithelium. × 320.

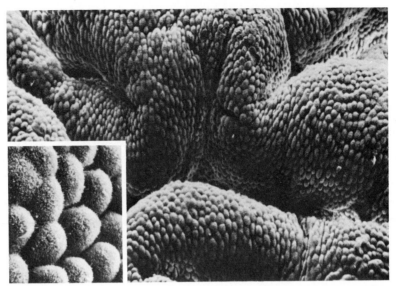

Figure 82–5.   Scanning electron micrograph of unfilled gallbladder mucosa, showing bulging cell surfaces. × 520. Inset is a higher magnification of individual cell surfaces covered with microvilli. × 3200. (Courtesy of Drs. John Mueller and Albert L. Jones.)

gross anatomical arrangement of mucosa is beautifully demonstrated in Figure 82–5, a scanning electromicrograph. As in the intestine, submucosal, muscularis, and serosal layers are present. The well developed layer of smooth muscle is located in the wall of the gallbladder in an interlocking pattern of longitudinal and spirally arranged fibers.

Chapter 83

Biliary Disease in Infancy and Childhood

M. Michael Thaler

Disorders of the biliary tract are relatively common in newborn and very young infants compared with children and adolescents. The main cause of persistent cholestasis in infancy is structural abnormality of the bile ducts.[1] Extrahepatic atresia of the major bile ducts accounts for at least 90 per cent of *obstructive* lesions. Other biliary malformations include intrahepatic bile duct hypoplasia or atresia, choledochal cyst, congenital hepatic fibrosis, and congenital dilatation of the intrahepatic bile ducts. The differentiation of these lesions from each other and from hepatocellular disease in young infants is a most challenging diagnostic problem.

NEONATAL ABNORMALITIES

The shrunken gallbladder and narrow fibrous cords which replace the biliary system in patients with extrahepatic biliary atresia may represent failure of the lumen to reopen completely in the course of embryonic differentiation. However, the processes which interfere with normal biliary development are not understood. With one exception (dilatation of the intrahepatic bile ducts),[2] congenital biliary malformations do not follow recognizable patterns of genetic inheritance. Hays et al.[3] have recently emphasized that biliary atresia is not present in association with other congenital defects. Bile duct malformations are seen rarely in aborted or stillborn infants who display other anomalies. Many physicians have hypothesized that biliary atresia and neonatal hepatitis represent different phases of the same pathological process. However, clear-cut concurrence of biliary and *extensive* hepatocellular disease is relatively uncommon in the neonatal period. Intrauterine infections with cytomegalic inclusion virus, rubella virus, herpes simplex virus, toxoplasmosis, and syphilis produce hepatocellular disease in the newborn without associated bile duct malformations. Despite these considerations, it is possible that a teratogenic factor, e.g., an infectious agent or a drug, may interfere with the formation of biliary structures early in pregnancy, whereas later in gestation the same agent may cause parenchymal disease.

In most infants with extrahepatic biliary atresia, clinical evidence of cholestasis appears soon after birth. However, occasional babies with atretic ducts remain anicteric for several weeks. In such "late-blooming" patients, and in others biopsied during the first month of life, the histopathological features characteristic of extrahepatic biliary obstruction are frequently accompanied by giant-cell transformation of hepatocytes and randomly distributed inflammatory infiltrates. It is usually assumed that these parenchymal changes are secondary to obstruction. In some cases, however, sclerosis of the bile ducts may be part of a generalized hepatobiliary disease process. We have investigated jaundiced infants in whom biliary excretory deficiency developed gradually until sclerosis of the extrahepatic bile ducts was complete, in agreement with findings described by Holder.[4] Similarly, the postnatal evolution of *intrahepatic* bile duct hypoplasia or atresia has been recognized by several authors.[1] Consequently, it cannot be assumed that all extrahepatic and intrahepatic atretic lesions of the biliary system are congenital.

DIAGNOSTIC CONSIDERATIONS IN PEDIATRIC BILIARY DISEASE

Most malformations of the bile ducts require surgical repair. For this reason, biliary lesions must be distinguished from

hepatocellular disease in early infancy. Extrahepatic biliary atresia accounts for at least 50 per cent of all instances of persistent cholestasis during the first four months of life. The remainder, with relatively few exceptions, are due to idiopathic parenchymal disease processes collectively referred to as neonatal hepatitis. There are no biochemical findings which serve to distinguish extrahepatic biliary atresia from other causes of cholestasis in the newborn period. The serum alkaline phosphatase and leucine aminopeptidase activities are consistently elevated as they are in hepatitis; the transaminases (SGOT and SGPT) and lactate dehydrogenase exhibit considerable variability.

The diagnostic management of infants with persistent "obstructive" jaundice has stimulated considerable debate. The differentiation between biliary atresia and neonatal hepatitis can be extremely difficult; both conditions may exhibit nearly total biliary excretory failure (see Fig. 83–1).[5] For this reason, many experienced clinicians resort to exploratory laparotomy

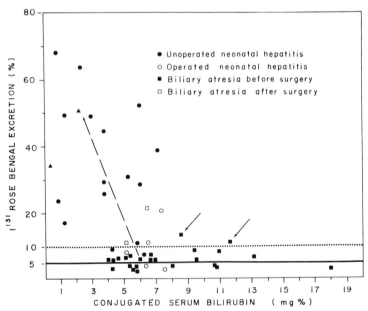

Figure 83–1. Fecal excretion of I[131]-rose bengal and conjugated serum bilirubin in patients with biliary atresia and neonatal hepatitis (72 hours). In every instance of extrahepatic atresia, excretion was less than 10 per cent of the dose administered, with the majority clustered around 5 per cent. Improved excretion is shown in three infants with atresia repaired surgically, including one tested before and after surgery. (Broken arrow leads to postoperative value, denoted with a triangle). Two patients with intrahepatic biliary atresia, denoted by short arrows, excreted more than 10 per cent of the radioactive dye. Approximately 20 per cent of cases of neonatal hepatitis excreted less than 10 per cent of the dose, revealing nearly complete biliary deficiency at the time of testing. Note the poor correlation between extrahepatic biliary obstruction and conjugated serum bilirubin concentrations.

early in the development of cholestasis. The use of surgical means for rapid diagnosis, rather than for repair of atretic ducts documented with medical studies, rests upon two assumptions: (1) that the presence and type of the extrahepatic biliary lesion can be determined with certainty only by direct inspection; and (2) that delay in relieving obstructed bile flow may lead to irreversible liver damage in infants with *operable* biliary malformations, unless surgical repair is performed during the first two months of life. On the other hand, growing experience with the interpretation of percutaneous liver biopsies and the introduction of isotopic procedures in the investigation of neonatal liver disease may provide valid alternatives to diagnosis by exploratory surgery.

The physician who deals with infants with persistent idiopathic cholestasis must therefore weigh the risks of surgery in infants with hepatitis against the chances of successful repair of biliary malformations. Although bile-duct-to-bowel anastomoses can be performed in up to 20 per cent of patients with extrahepatic biliary atresia, bile flow is successfully restored in less than 5 per cent. Although the rarity of correctible malformations (Fig. 83–2) is primarily responsible for these discouraging results, the disparity between attempts and successes is usually attributed to advanced cirrhosis at the time of operation. Pre-existing liver disease may contribute to the poor outcome of surgical repair, but neither age[6] nor the histological appearance of the liver at the time of operation[7, 8] correlates with the prognosis in infants with functioning biliary anastomoses. In addition, hepatocellular lesions develop relatively slowly in biliary atresia during the first year[9] and may regress after biliary flow is restored. Striking functional and histological improvement from the effects of biliary obstruction has been reported in infants in whom advanced intrahepatic bile duct proliferation and fibrosis were present at operation.[7, 8]

Another important factor in choosing the appropriate diagnostic approach in such cases is the mortality and morbidity associated with abdominal surgery performed on infants with hepatocellular disease.[10] Long-term follow-up data from 62 infants with neonatal hepatitis revealed a three-fold incidence of progressive liver disease in those who underwent laparotomy in the first three months of life, compared with those who were not operated on.[11] In view of the low salvage rates in biliary atresia, the deleterious effects of exploratory surgery on infants with liver disease, and the additional possibility that potentially operable biliary malformations may be missed if explored prematurely,[12, 13] we use percutaneous liver biopsies and radioactive rose bengal excretion tests as the primary diagnostic means for differentiating biliary obstruction from parenchymal disease during the first three months of life.

LIVER BIOPSY

The percutaneous liver biopsy is a valuable diagnostic tool in infants with persistent cholestasis. At minimal risk to the patient, a core of liver tissue can be obtained with a Menghini biopsy needle which usually provides sufficient tissue for diagnostic examination. In addition to hematoxylin and eosin stains, a connective tissue stain is especially useful in outlining areas of maximal involvement.

The typical biopsy taken from the liver of an infant with extrahepatic biliary obstruction reveals a pathological process which involves every periportal lobular zone. The hallmarks of extrahepatic obstruction are extensive proliferation of lobular bile ducts and periportal fibrosis

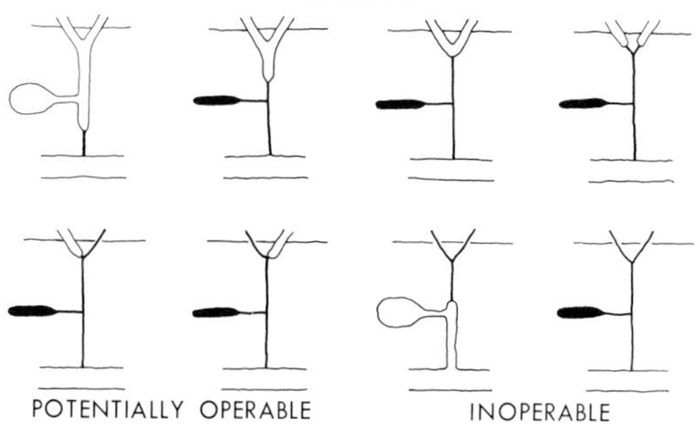

Figure 83–2. Atretic lesions of the extrahepatic bile ducts. Patency of both hepatic bile ducts is required for operability, because each hepatic bile duct drains only the major lobe from which it originates. The proximal (hepatic) end of the extrahepatic biliary system is usually atretic, rendering most cases of biliary atresia inoperable.

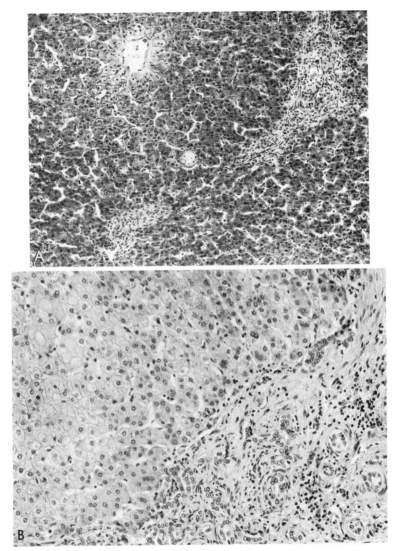

Figure 83–3. Extrahepatic biliary atresia. *A,* Appearance of hepatic parenchyma early in the course. Islands of fibrous tissue are confined to portal areas, in which proliferating interlobular bile ducts are the most prominent feature. The lobular architecture and sinusoidal pattern are well preserved at this stage. Masson's trichrome stain. × 180. *B,* Higher magnification of periportal region (lower right), showing sharply demarcated fibrous tissue, proliferating atypical bile ducts, and inflammatory cells. Occasional parenchymal cells containing inspissated bile. Hepatic cells are otherwise unremarkable. Hematoxylin and eosin. × 250.

(Fig. 83–3). Severe cholestasis, predominantly in the form of canalicular bile plugs, varying degrees of periportal inflammation, and occasional giant cells complete the histological picture. Formation of bile lakes is rare. In expert hands, the predictive value of this procedure probably approaches that of open liver biopsy.[2, 14] Experience with percutaneous liver biopsies at the University of California in San Francisco indicates that accurate diagnostic predictions can be expected in approximately three of four patients with postnatal cholestatic jaundice.

I^{131}-ROSE BENGAL EXCRETION

The quantitative I^{131}-rose bengal excretion test is a useful physiological procedure for the investigation of infants with obstructive jaundice. Stools and urine are collected separately 72 hours after intravenous injection of 3 μc of I^{131}-rose bengal per kilogram of body weight. Fecal

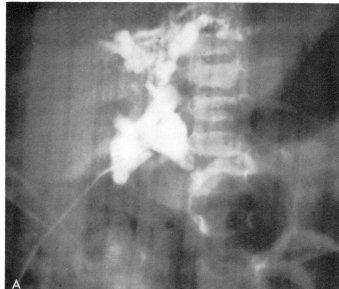

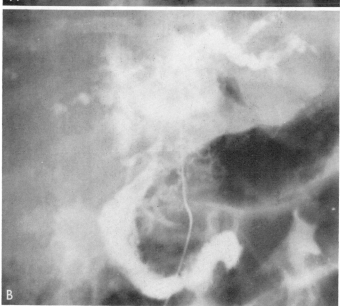

Figure 83–4. Operative cholangiograms in extrahepatic biliary atresia. A, Dye injected into a malformed gallbladder reveals irregular, segmentally dilated extra- and intrahepatic bile ducts above the junction of the cystic and common hepatic ducts. Ducts do not drain to the intestine. B, Flow of bile from liver to intestine re-established by anastomosis of hepatic duct and jejunum.

excretion of less than 5 per cent of the dose during the three-day test period indicates essentially complete absence of biliary drainage, and is consistent with the diagnosis of extrahepatic biliary atresia (Fig. 83–1). It should be re-emphasized, however, that this degree of excretory deficiency may also occur in approximately 20 per cent of patients with neonatal hepatitis. During the "obstructive" phase, hepatocellular disease is impossible to distinguish from extrahepatic biliary obstruction using the rose bengal test alone.

The percutaneous liver biopsy, in combination with the quantitative I^{131}-rose bengal test, reveals the diagnosis in nearly 90 per cent of cases, a figure which compares favorably with the results of operative cholangiography.[3, 15]

OPERATIVE CHOLANGIOGRAPHY

Operative cholangiography through a limited incision is indicated in infants in whom findings of biopsy and rose bengal indicate atresia. Demonstration of continuity of the biliary system from the major intrahepatic ducts to the duodenum rules out the possibility of extrahepatic biliary atresia. When a cholangiogram cannot be performed owing to malformations of the gallbladder, the incision is extended and the porta hepatis is explored carefully. Choledochal cysts or bile-containing remnants of the biliary system are anastomosed to the small intestine, preferably the jejunum (Fig. 83–4).

Other surgical procedures, designed to facilitate the passage of bile from liver to intestine, have been uniformly unsuccessful. Very recently, a novel approach has been proposed in Japan, where malformations of the extrahepatic biliary tree are relatively common. A segment of jejunum is anastomosed to a decapsulated area of liver in the porta hepatis region, and to the duodenum. A conduit for bile is thus established between the major intrahepatic bile ducts and the intestine. The results of this approach in inoperable situations appear promising, but its ultimate usefulness will become apparent only after sufficient follow-up data are available.

CLINICAL CONDITIONS ASSOCIATED WITH BILIARY OBSTRUCTION IN INFANCY

EXTRAHEPATIC BILIARY ATRESIA

With the exception of nonpatency of a single branch of the hepatic duct or absence of the gallbladder and cystic duct, structural discontinuity of any portion of the extrahepatic biliary duct system results in permanent interruption of bile flow to the intestine (Fig. 83–2). Conjugated hyperbilirubinemia, pale stools, dark urine, and hepatomegaly are noted soon after birth. Splenomegaly develops in most patients.

The diagnosis of extrahepatic biliary obstruction can usually be made with the aid of percutaneous biopsy and I^{131}-rose bengal excretion tests.

Infants with inoperable extrahepatic biliary malformations eventually develop portal hypertension, ascites, or gastrointestinal hemorrhage. Treatment is aimed at prevention of these complications and at maintenance of adequate nutrition.[16] Dietary supplements of medium-chain triglycerides and fat-soluble vitamins (especially K and D) are helpful in counteracting the effects of malabsorption, whereas low sodium diets and antidiuretics temporarily retard the growth of ascites. Despite these measures, survival rarely extends beyond two years.

INTRAHEPATIC BILIARY ATRESIA, OR HYPOPLASIA OF THE INTERLOBULAR BILE DUCTS

The pathogenesis of these conditions is unclear. Certain cases begin with a clinical and histological picture indistinguishable from neonatal hepatitis. As the disease progresses, the parenchyma reverts to a near-normal appearance, whereas the interlobular bile ducts decrease in number until few, or none, are identifiable in liver biopsies. In others, paucity of intrahepatic bile ducts in the absence of other histological changes may be observed soon after birth. Evidence of parenchymal disease is confined to intracanalicular bile plugs, occasional giant cells, and isolated hepatocytes containing inspissated bile. The unremarkable appearance of parenchyma, coupled with a striking absence of periportal ductular structures, stands in marked contrast to the proliferating ductules and periportal fibrosis of extrahepatic biliary obstruction (compare Figs. 83–3 and 83–5).

The extent of biliary excretory deficiency varies considerably from patient to patient, but is seldom complete (Fig. 83–6). The 72-hour rose bengal fecal excretion is usually above 5 per cent of the dose, although nearly complete excretory failure may also occur.[17]

Cholestatic jaundice develops during the first month of life in most instances. Characteristic findings are rapidly rising serum cholesterol and triglyceride concentrations and serum alkaline phosphatase values which may be five to twenty times normal. Xanthomata eventually develop over extensor surfaces, in palmar creases, or imbedded in scratch marks. Generalized arteriosclerotic changes and fatty deposits in the heart, kidneys, and pancreas occur later in the course.

Severe pruritus, steatorrhea, and bleeding tendency are the most common clinical

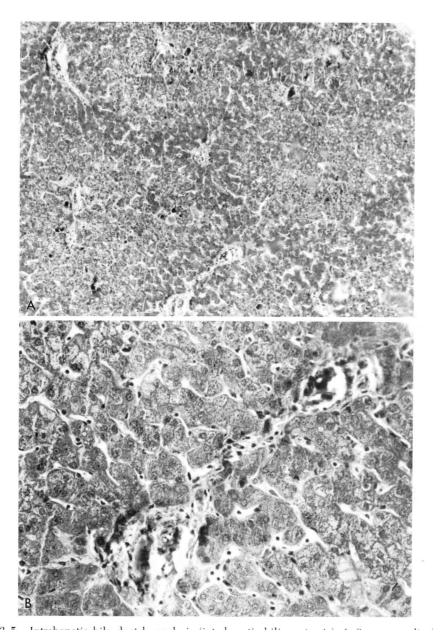

Figure 83-5. Intrahepatic bile duct hypoplasia (intrahepatic biliary atresia). *A,* Severe canalicular chole-stasis and absence of recognizable interlobular bile ducts in portal areas are the most prominent features in liver biopsies. Note the absence of fibrosis and inflammatory cells. Masson's trichrome stain. ×80. *B,* Higher magnification of portal area in lower center of *A.* Branches of hepatic artery and portal vein and dilated lymphatic channels are clearly visible; bile ducts are absent. ×300.

problems encountered in children with intrahepatic biliary atresia. Treatment includes low-fat, high-protein diets, supplemented with medium chain triglycerides, and fat-soluble vitamins, including vitamin K. Cholestyramine feedings usually improve pruritus and may correct abnormalities in liver function tests in cases with partial rather than complete biliary deficiency (hypoplasia versus atresia).[18]

Treatment with phenobarbital has recently been introduced into the clinical management of intrahepatic biliary atresia.[18, 19] The use of this drug is based on its ability to stimulate biliary excretion in animals.[20] Phenobarbital in daily doses of 5 to 10 mg per kilogram has eliminated or reduced pruritus, decreased the serum bilirubin concentration, and reduced xanthoma formation in children in whom cho-

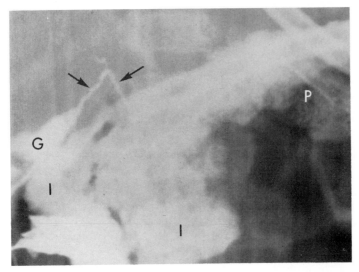

Figure 83–6. Intrahepatic biliary atresia. Operative cholangiogram, showing shrunken gallbladder (G) and hypoplastic extrahepatic bile ducts (arrows). Note opacification of pancreas and pancreatic duct (P) and large collections of dye in the upper intestine (I).

lestyramine therapy was relatively unsuccessful. Recent studies suggest that the mechanisms of action include enhancement of bile flow, improved biliary excretion of bile salts and bilirubin,[19] and a rapid reduction of the extrahepatic bile salt pool.[21] Occasional patients treated with phenobarbital may benefit from concurrent cholestyramine therapy to prevent intestinal reabsorption of biliary components. Although these measures improve the well being of children with intrahepatic biliary atresia, longer follow-up studies will be required to determine whether survival can be prolonged beyond the five to ten years currently expected.

CHOLEDOCHAL CYST

This developmental abnormality of the bile duct wall occurs most frequently as a dilatation of the common bile duct, with a slightly expanded segment of the duct above, and a narrowed duct below the cyst. Other types of cystic dilatation include diverticulum of the common bile duct, and choledochocele of the intraduodenal portion of the common duct. Associated dilatation of the intrahepatic bile ducts has been reported in Japanese patients, among whom choledochal cysts occur relatively frequently. Cholangitis may develop in infancy or childhood, or may be delayed for two or three decades. In nonjaundiced patients, intravenous cholangiography may reveal the cystic lesion in the subhepatic region (Fig. 83–7). Visualization by means of I[131]-rose bengal

scintiphotography has also been reported.[23] However, we find that operative cholangiograms are necessary to confirm the diagnosis. The recommended treatment is Roux-en-Y choledochocystojejunostomy with cholecystotomy, or primary excision of the cyst. Long-term complications, found in 65 per cent of operated patients reviewed recently, include ascending cholangitis, stricture at the site of anastomosis, residual biliary tract disease, cirrhosis, intestinal obstruction caused by adhesions, and steatorrhea attributed to distal displacement of bile drainage.[24] Patients with choledochal cysts who are not treated surgically suffer from

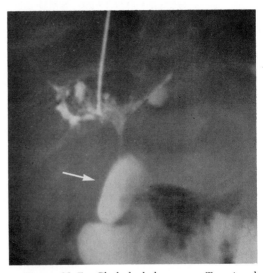

Figure 83–7. Choledochal cyst. Transjugular cholangiogram in a seven-month old infant. (Courtesy of Dr. H. Goldberg, Department of Radiology, University of California, San Francisco.)

recurrent bouts of cholecystitis and cholelithiasis.

CYSTIC DILATATION OF THE INTRAHEPATIC BILE DUCTS (CAROLI'S DISEASE)

This familial disease is characterized by
saccular dilatation of the right and left
hepatic bile ducts and their main branches
(Fig. 83–8). It is frequently associated
with cystic disease of the kidneys.[25]
Cholangitis, cholelithiasis, and liver abscesses are commonly present, caused by
bile stasis. Crampy abdominal pain and
fever may develop at any time after birth.
However, 22 years has been reported to be
the average age at onset.[26] Symptoms subside temporarily after passage of calculi
and control of infection, but invariably
recur until the anomaly is finally diagnosed by operative cholangiography.
Liver function is generally unimpaired,
and cirrhosis or portal hypertension does
not develop. Temporary palliation can be

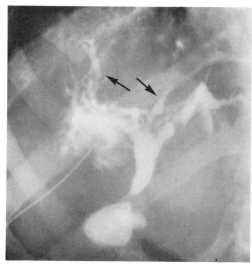

Figure 83–8. Cystic dilatation of intrahepatic
bile ducts (Caroli's disease). Operative cholangiogram. (Courtesy of Dr. H. Goldberg, Department of
Radiology, University of California, San Francisco.)

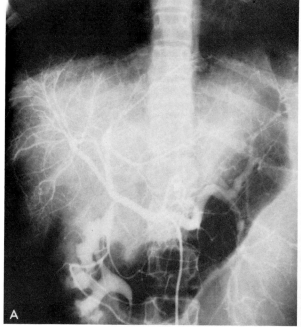

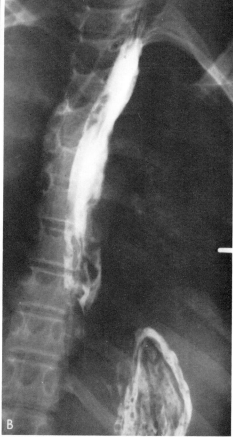

Figure 83–9. Congenital hepatic fibrosis. A, Selective
celiac arteriogram, showing curvilinearity of intrahepatic
arteries. Several areas of hypovascularity are seen during
the parenchymal phase of the study. Urogram (right kidney
is visible) outlines dilated end tubules in papillae, characteristic of renal tubular ectasia. B, Esophagram demonstrates voluminous varices in the lower esophagus.
(Courtesy of Dr. M. T. Korobkin, Department of Radiology, University of California, San Francisco.)

achieved by surgical removal of stones and relief of biliary obstruction. After cholangitis becomes established, liver abscesses and septicemia contribute to an extremely grave prognosis.

CONGENITAL HEPATIC FIBROSIS

Congenital hepatic fibrosis is a developmental anomaly characterized by excessive numbers of disordered terminal interlobular bile ducts, which form multiple microscopic and macroscopic bile-containing cysts inbedded within wide bands of fibrous tissue. Renal cysts are usually associated (Fig. 83–9). In contrast to Caroli's disease, portal hypertension may develop relatively early, and may progress to a fatal termination caused by gastrointestinal hemorrhage.[27]

BILIARY DISEASE IN CHILDHOOD AND ADOLESCENCE

Biliary pathology in children is most commonly a continuation of conditions apparent from early infancy. Diseases of the biliary system which originate in the pediatric population after the first two years of life are relatively rare. The gallbladder is the usual focus of involvement in such cases.

ACUTE CHOLECYSTITIS

Acute inflammation of the gallbladder in children is usually idiopathic. The common acute viral diseases of childhood, such as gastroenteritis, and upper respiratory infections have been associated with cholecystitis. Rarely, parasitic infestation with *Giardia lamblia* or Ascaris, typhoid fever, shigellosis, or streptococcal infections can be documented by means of cultures of bile or fluid recovered from the gallbladder at laparotomy. Gallstones occur much less frequently than in adult cholecystitis. For example, at the Mayo Clinic, children represented a bare 0.13 per cent of all instances of cholelithiasis.[28] A survey of 620 consecutive cholecystectomies performed for calculous cholecystitis revealed 33 (5.3 per cent) patients under 21, all of whom were female.[29] Ex-

cept for one ten-year-old, all were between 16 and 20 years of age. Formation of gallstones in this group of patients was associated with pregnancy in 84 per cent, suggesting a close relationship between childbearing and calculous cholecystitis in adolescent girls.

The clinical features of cholecystitis are similar to those in adults. Right upper quadrant pain and guarding, nausea, and vomiting occur in most cases. Jaundice develops in approximately one-fourth of patients, and may suggest the correct diagnosis. Despite this relatively clear-cut clinical picture, the fact that the diagnosis is usually made at exploratory laparotomy probably reflects the rarity of gallbladder disease in children. Operative cholangiography may reveal the presence of gallstones in the common duct or gallbladder. Cholecystectomy is generally performed in patients with cholelithiasis.

CHOLELITHIASIS

Cholelithiasis in children is confined to the gallbladder in over 90 per cent of cases. Pigmented stones and cholesterol stones are found with approximately equal frequency. Pigmented gallstones occur in children with hemolytic diseases, the most common being congenital spherocytosis in Caucasians and sickle cell anemia in Negroes. Other hemolytic conditions associated with cholelithiasis include the thalassemias, red cell enzymopathies, Wilson's disease, and erythroblastosis fetalis in newborn infants. Cholesterol gallstones occur in acute cholecystitis. As with childhood cholecystitis generally, the cause for cholecystitis associated with stones is unclear in nearly half of the patients. Obesity and a family history of gallbladder disease are present in a small number of these patients.[30, 31] Cholelithiasis may also be a complication of biliary malformations, cystic fibrosis, pancreatitis, portal hypertension, neonatal sepsis, and chronic gastrointestinal infections.

As mentioned previously, cholelithiasis over the age of ten and not associated with an obvious cause is noted predominantly in females. Thus constitutional factors which predispose adult females to biliary disease appear to operate occasionally in childhood. The treatment of cholelithiasis includes measures directed toward the underlying disease and cholecystectomy.

ACUTE HYDROPS OF THE GALLBLADDER

This idiopathic distention of the gallbladder appears in the absence of obvious obstructive or inflammatory disease. Gallstones are not found. In contrast to cholelithiasis, a predominance of males is apparent among the reported cases, which range in onset from early infancy to early adolescence.

Generalized abdominal tenderness and a mass in the right upper quadrant are the typical clinical features. Surgery reveals an edematous gallbladder and, in most instances, hypertrophied mesenteric lymph nodes. Drainage of the gallbladder is usually followed by full recovery.

REFERENCES

1. Brent, R. L. Persistent jaundice in infancy. J. Pediat. 61:111, 1962.
2. Kerr, D. N. S., Harrison, C. V., Sherlock, S., and Walker, R. M. Congenital hepatic fibrosis. Quart. J. Med. 30:91, 1961.
3. Hays, D. M., Woolley, M. M., Snyder, W. H., Jr, Reed, G. B., Gwinn, J. L., and Landing, B. H. Diagnosis of biliary atresia: relative accuracy of percutaneous liver biopsy, open liver biopsy, and operative cholangiography. J. Pediat. 71:598, 1967.
4. Holder, T. M. Atresia of the extrahepatic bile duct. Amer. J. Surg. 107:458, 1964.
5. Thaler, M. M. and Gellis, S. S. Studies in neonatal hepatitis and biliary atresia. IV. Diagnosis. Amer. J. Dis. Child. 116:280, 1968.
6. Thaler, M. M., and Gellis, S. S. III. Progression and regression of cirrhosis in biliary atresia. Amer. J. Dis. Child. 116:271, 1968.
7. Krovetz, L. J. Congenital biliary atresia. II. Analysis of the therapeutic problem. Surgery 47:468, 1960.
8. Cameron, R., and Bunton, G. L. Congenital biliary atresia. Brit. Med. J. 2:1253, 1960.
9. Hollander, M., and Schaffner, F. Electron microscopic studies in biliary atresia. Amer. J. Dis. Child. 116:49, 1968.
10. Gellis, S. S., Craig, J. M., and Hsia, D. Y. Y.: Prolonged obstructive jaundice in infancy. IV. Neonatal hepatitis. Amer. J. Dis. Child. 88:285, 1954.
11. Thaler, M. M., and Gellis, S. S. II. The effect of diagnostic laparotomy on long-term prognosis of neonatal hepatitis. Amer. J. Dis. Child. 116:262, 1968.
12. Carlson, E. Salvage of the "noncorrectable" case of congenital extrahepatic biliary atresia. Arch. Surg. 81:893, 1960.
13. Zeyer, J., and Schärli, A. Die Bedeutung der Relaparatomie bei totaler extrahepatischer Gallengangsatresie. Z. Kinderchir. 2:364, 1965.
14. Brough, A. J., and Bernstein, J. Liver biopsy in the diagnosis of infantile obstructive jaundice. Pediatrics 43:519, 1969.
15. Danks, D. M., and Campbell, P. E. Extrahepatic biliary atresia: Comments on the frequency of potentially operable cases. J. Pediat. 69:21, 1966.
16. Thaler, M. M. Cirrhosis, massive hepatic necrosis and tumors of the liver. In Current Pediatric Therapy, S. Gellis, and B. Kagan (eds.). Philadelphia, W. B. Saunders Co., 1970, pp. 355–360.
17. Thaler, M. M. Effect of phenobarbital on hepatic transport and excretion of ^{131}I-rose bengal in children with cholestasis. Pediat. Res., 6:100, 1972.
18. Sharp, H. L., Carey, J. B., Jr., White, J. G., and Krivit, W. Cholestyramine therapy in patients with a paucity of intrahepatic bile ducts. J. Pediat. 71:723, 1967.
19. Stiehl, A., Thaler, M. M., and Admirand, W. H. The effects of phenobarbital on bile salts and bilirubin in patients with intra- and extra-hepatic cholestasis. New Eng. J. Med. 286:858, 1972.
20. Klaassen, C. D., and Plaa, G. L. Studies on the mechanism of phenobarbital-enhanced sulfobromophthalein disappearance. Amer. J. Physiol. 213:1322, 1967.
21. Stiehl, A., Thaler, M. M., and Admirand, W. H. Effects of phenobarbital on bile salts in cholestasis. Pediat. Res. 5:391, 1971.
22. Tsuchida, Y., and Ishida, M. Dilatation of the intrahepatic bile ducts in congenital cystic dilatation of the common bile duct. Surgery 69:776, 1971.
23. Williams, L. E., Fisher, J. H., Courtney, R. A., and Darling, D. B. Preoperative diagnosis of choledochal cyst by hepatoscintigraphy. New Eng. J. Med. 283:85, 1970.
24. Trout, H. H., and Longmire, W. P., Jr. Long-term follow-up study of patients with congenital cystic dilatation of the common bile duct. Amer. J. Surg. 121:68, 1971.
25. Caroli, J., and Corcos, V. La dilatation congenitale des voies biliaires intrahepatiques. Rev. Medicochir. Mal. Foie 39:1, 1964.
26. Mujahed, Z., Glenn, F., and Evans, J. A. Communicating cavernous ectasia of the intrahepatic ducts (Caroli's disease). Amer. J. Roent. Radium Ther. Nuc. Med. 113:21, 1971.
27. Kerr, D. N. S., Harrison, C. V., Sherlock, S., and Walker, R. M. Congenital hepatic fibrosis. Quart. J. Med. 30:91, 1961.
28. Brenner, R. W., and Stewart, C. F. Cholecystitis in children. Rev. Surg. 21:327, 1964.
29. Calabrese, C., and Pearlman, D. M. Gallbladder disease below the age of 21 years. Surgery 70:413, 1971.
30. Seiler, I. Gallbladder disease in children: Cases illustrating familial predisposition. Amer. J. Dis. Child. 99:662, 1960.
31. Hagberg, B., Svennerholm, L., and Thoren, L. Cholelithiasis in childhood. A follow-up study with special reference to heredity, constitutional factors and serum lipids. Acta Chir. Scand. 123:307, 1962.

Chapter 84

Radiography of the Biliary Tract

John Amberg

As with gastrointestinal disease in general, radiography plays a large part in the diagnosis of disease of the biliary tract. This chapter presents the important techniques for demonstration of the clinical disorders of the gallbladder and ductal system.

ABDOMINAL PLAIN FILM

The plain film of the abdomen is the simplest radiological examination of the biliary tract. Calcium which has been deposited either within the gallbladder wall, within gallstones, or concentrated in the bile ("milk of calcium bile") may be seen (Fig. 84–1).

Similarly, gas may appear as an abnormality within the biliary tract. A fistula between the gallbladder or common duct and the gut results in air-contrast views of these structures (Fig. 84–2). Cholecystitis caused by gas-forming bacteria results in gas in the lumen of the gallbladder and the gallbladder wall (Fig. 84–3). On plain films, a distended gallbladder may appear as a soft tissue mass, particularly if it indents a gas-filled hepatic flexure of the colon. Usually the plain film alone does not suffice. In nonacute conditions, oral cholecystography is usually necessary. In the face of an urgent problem or the ab-

sence of the gallbladder, intravenous cholangiography is a logical second step. The management of the patient with jaundice requires an entirely separate approach (see pp. 1107 to 1109).

ORAL CHOLECYSTOGRAPHY

PHARMACOKINETICS OF MEDIA

All current compounds used for gallbladder visualization are chemically similar, each having three iodine atoms attached to the benzene ring of the anionic portion of the molecule (Fig. 84–4). The usual dose of these compounds in adults is 2 to 3 g in tablet form, given in the evening. Absorption, excretion by the liver, and concentration by the gallbladder proceed over the next 12 hours prior to radiography.

Various oral cholecystographic agents have been in use for almost 30 years. Despite this long use, the knowledge of the pharmacokinetics of the compounds is limited. The first step in satisfactory cholecystography is normal intestinal absorption; it is also the rate-limiting step in the appearance of these media in the bile.[1, 2] In patients with gastric outlet obstruction the gallbladder will not visualize because

1098

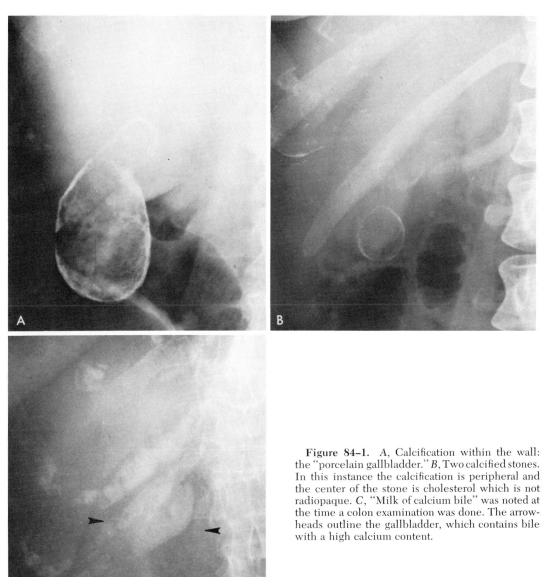

Figure 84–1. *A*, Calcification within the wall: the "porcelain gallbladder." *B*, Two calcified stones. In this instance the calcification is peripheral and the center of the stone is cholesterol which is not radiopaque. *C*, "Milk of calcium bile" was noted at the time a colon examination was done. The arrowheads outline the gallbladder, which contains bile with a high calcium content.

these substances are not absorbed from the stomach. If the contrast material reaches the small bowel and the anionic absorptive mechanisms are intact, the contrast material will pass into the portal circulation. Absorption by the colon has also been demonstrated. The comparative rate of absorption in various segments of the small bowel in man is not known. Experimental

studies of one contrast medium, iopanoic acid, have shown a similar rate of absorption throughout the small bowel and colon. Experimental studies done with the cannulation of the thoracic duct show no evidence that iopanoic acid is absorbed into the lymphatic system. pH is another variable experimental factor which influences absorption. If the iopanoate is infused into

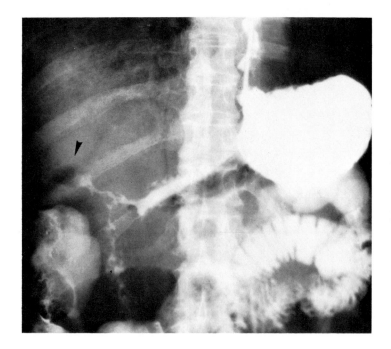

Figure 84–2. Barium given orally is seen in a fistulous tract extending to the gallbladder. The arrowhead points to air within the gallbladder lumen. Usually this situation occurs when a stone erodes from the gallbladder into the duodenum.

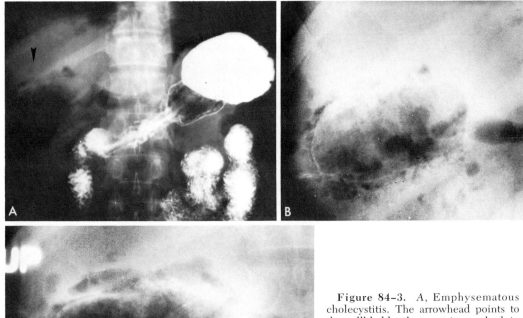

Figure 84–3. *A*, Emphysematous cholecystitis. The arrowhead points to the gallbladder that contains gas both in its wall and its lumen. This is caused by an infection with a gas-forming organism. *B*, Close-up of gallbladder. *C*, Upright film, showing gas-bile level.

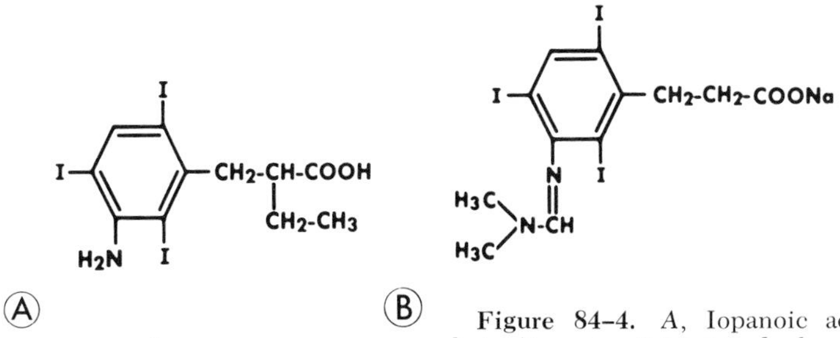

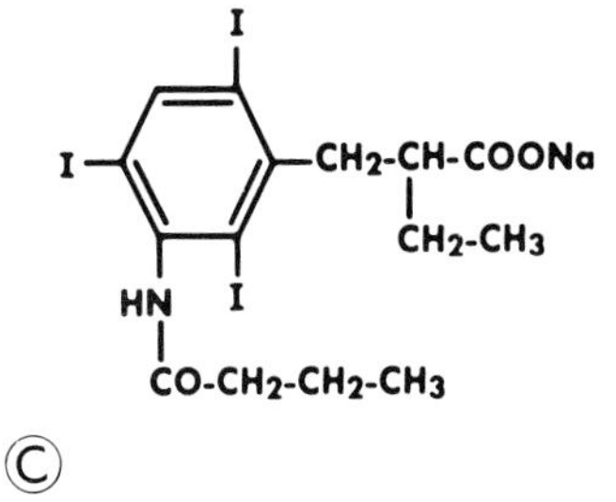

Figure 84–4. *A*, Iopanoic acid, beta-(3-amino-2,4,6-triiodophenyl)-alpha-ethylpropionic acid (66.7 per cent I); 0.5 g tablets. *B*, Sodium o ipodate, 3-(dimethylamino-methyleneamino)-2,4,6-triiodohydrocinnamic acid sodium salt (61.4 per cent I); 0.5 g capsules. *C*, Sodium tyropanoate, beta-(3-butyramido-2,4,6-triiodophenyl)-alpha-ethylpropionic acid sodium salt (57.5 per cent I); 0.75 g capsules.

the small bowel of the dog at pH 9.5 instead of 7.0, its excretion rate by the liver is increased tenfold. It seems likely that the pKa of the compound and the intraluminal pH may both be expected to influence absorption in man.

Cholecystopaques are bound to serum albumin for transfer to the hepatocyte. A fraction is excreted by the kidney, occasionally associated with burning on urination and a false-positive test for albumin in the urine (pseudoalbuminuria).

Within the hepatocyte, the metabolic pathways of these agents are probably similar to those of bilirubin. It has been found that they are then bound to the so-called Y and Z proteins.[3] Further, some are conjugated with glucuronic acid, a routine that depends upon glucuronyl transferase. This hypothesis is supported somewhat by the increase in jaundice in patients with unconjugated hyperbilirubinemia after ingesting iopanoic acid, an observation which indicates that bilirubin and these contrast materials compete for enzymes and binders. This hypothesis is contradicted, however, by studies in the Gunn rat, which neither conjugates nor excretes bilirubin, but excretes iopanoic acid.[4]

Very little is known about the factors that influence excretion of these substances into the bile. Experimental studies have shown that the excretion of iopanoic acid depends upon the presence of bile salts.[5, 6] It is also known that transport

through the liver is a very rapid process, with contrast material appearing in the bile within 15 minutes after contact with the small bowel mucosa. It is conventional to relate the degree of visualization of the gallbladder to the concentration of the hepatic bile in the gallbladder. Because of relatively slow absorption and consequent slow excretion into the bile, contrast media are not ordinarily sufficiently concentrated in the ductal system to opacify it. Indeed, visualization of the intrahepatic ducts and common bile duct by oral administration of this material is unusual. It is of interest, however, that when sodium iopanoate (pH 9.5) is placed directly into the jejunum of the dog, absorption and excretion are sufficient to radiographically demonstrate not only the gallbladder immediately, but also the common bile duct.[2]

INDICATION AND TECHNIQUE

The prime indication for doing oral cholecystography is the clinical suspicion of gallstones. Its use in preventive medicine in detecting asymptomatic gallstones has as yet not gained favor, but it does seem worthy of serious consideration in certain high risk groups, i. e., diabetics, American Indian women, patients with hemolytic disease or stable cirrhosis, patients with ileal disease, or patients with ileal resection. Anomalies and other abnormalities demonstrated by cholecystography usually

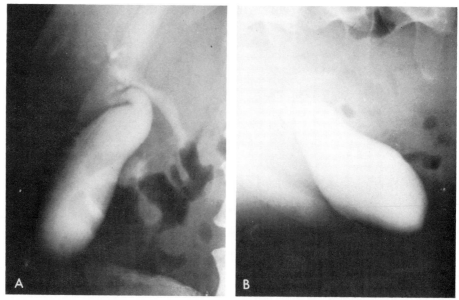

Figure 84–5. *A,* Upright film of the gallbladder. In this instance, there is unusually good visualization of cystic duct, hepatic ducts, and common bile duct for an oral study. Note intestinal gas over the gallbladder. *B,* A right lateral decubitus film of the gallbladder. Intestinal gas has risen and the gallbladder is shown to be free of calculi.

represent radiological curiosities rather than clinically significant disorders.

Since the advent of cholecystography, preventing contraction of the gallbladder after ingestion of the contrast material has been regarded as important. Current evidence, however, suggests that this belief is unfounded; on the contrary, intermittent contraction of the gallbladder during the long absorptive phase appears to enhance visualization by ridding the gallbladder of noncontrast-containing bile. Thus the interdiction of the use of fats in the evening meal the night before cholecystography seems unnecessary.[7]

The roentgen technique for gallbladder filming is quite simple. Ordinarily, straight posteroanterior and oblique films of the gallbladder are made with the patient supine. The patient may then be put either in an upright position or in a right lateral decubitus position for films taken with a horizontally directed X-ray beam (Fig. 84–5). These last films are important, because they permit evaluation of whether defects seen within the gallbladder are fixed to its wall. They also occasionally allow one to see stratification of stones that is visible only in the upright or the decubitus positions.

Repeating the films 20 to 30 minutes following ingestion of a fatty meal has been recommended as being helpful in searching for small stones. This technique also has the advantage of frequently visualizing the cystic and common bile ducts. The lack of contraction of the gallbladder cannot be considered significant, as the ingested fat may not have reached the duodenum to release cholecystokinin prior to taking this second set of films.

Gallbladder contrast material eventually reaches the intestinal lumen, but it is not reabsorbable in its conjugated form. Recirculation of a significant extent can be expected only if the contrast material is deconjugated, as for example by bacterial beta-glucuronidase present in large amounts in diseases of bacterial overgrowth (see pp. 927 to 936).

TOXICITY

Oral cholecystographic media are rarely responsible for significant side effects. Diarrhea and dysuria often follow ingestion of iopanoic acid, but are mild and brief. The incidence of diarrhea is diminished with sodium ipodate or sodium tyropanoate. Serious complications from these biliary contrast materials relate primarily to renal toxicity.[8] Usually this phenomenon is transient, but it may cause a severe azotemia. In the reported cases of this complication, usually more than 3.0 g per day of contrast material has been given. Of considerable interest is the recent observation that iopanoic acid is uricosuric.

The main contraindication to oral cholecystography is the knowledge that either absorption of the material or its excretion by the liver might be expected to be impaired, as in patients with gastric outlet obstruction or atony or hepatocellular damage or bile duct obstruction, respectively. If serum bilirubin is greater than 3 mg per 100 ml, the chance for visualization is virtually nil.

DIAGNOSIS OF GALLBLADDER CALCULI

Movable filling defects within an opacified gallbladder are gallstones. False-positive errors are rare. The most serious problem is the reverse, i.e., false-negative cholecystography. A certain number of gallbladders that appear radiologically normal contain gallstones. The reasons for such false-negative studies are as follows: (1) The stones may be too small in size and too few in number to be detected. (2) Poor opacification of the gallbladder may hinder detection. (3) Technical factors, such as the patient's obesity, may make the detection difficult. Since small stones passing through the biliary duct may be responsible for severe symptoms, special efforts should be expended to detect stones in patients with histories of classic cholecystitis or biliary colic. All studies should include an upright or lateral decubitus film to allow for layering of stones. Occasionally this maneuver is the only way in which the stones can be seen. Films taken after a fatty meal or tomography of the gallbladder in the upright position may also help to visualize small stones.

RADIOGRAPHY OF HYPERPLASTIC CHOLECYSTOSES

This group is composed of a variety of abnormalities of the gallbladder.[9] They are the subject of controversy, particularly when found in patients suffering from vague postprandial and intermittent right upper quadrant discomfort. The majority opinion favors regarding these as variations in anatomy of the gallbladder which are not responsible for symptoms. In addition to the anatomic changes, it has been

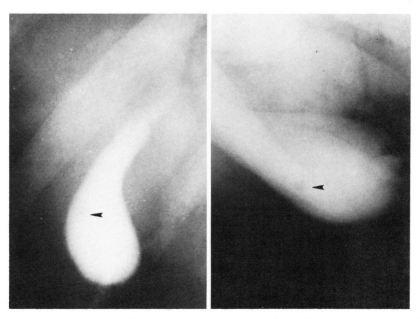

Figure 84–6.   Cholesterol deposit. The arrowhead points to small fixed filling defect attached to the gallbladder wall. No change in position occurs in comparing the supine film (right) with the lateral decubitus film (left).

suggested that these conditions may be associated with hyperconcentration of the contrast medium within the gallbladder and hypercontraction of the gallbladder. Evidence to support these contentions is at the moment quite weak.

CHOLESTEROSIS

Deposits of cholesterol in the gallbladder wall (the so-called strawberry gallbladder) may not be visible radiographically when they are slight. However, when the deposition of cholesterol is more marked, an irregularity of the gallbladder contour or multiple polypoid-like projections in the gallbladder may be seen. On changing the patient's position during examination, these defects are seen to be fixed to the gallbladder wall. Occasionally, only a single cholesterol deposit, frequently incor-

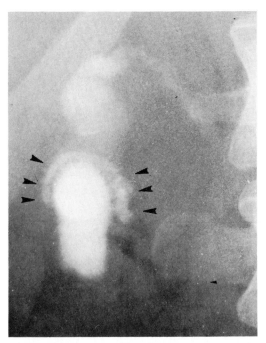

Figure 84–8. Aschoff-Rokitansky sinuses. Multiple diverticula of the gallbladder wall exist. Because the necks of the diverticula are narrow, the pouches themselves create a halo effect (arrowheads).

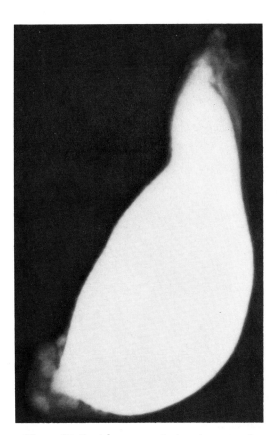

Figure 84–7. Adenomyomatosis. An operative specimen filled with contrast material and radiographed. The fundic deformity with crypt-like spaces within it is shown.

rectly called a polyp, will be noted (Fig. 84–6).

ADENOMYOMATOSIS

Hamartomas of the gallbladder wall are most often solitary and characteristically involve the fundus. They may be almost entirely muscular tissue, or may have tubules, crypts, and saccules with epithelial linings (Fig. 84–7).

ASCHOFF-ROKITANSKY SINUSES

A rather frequent histological finding but an unusual radiological finding is diverticulosis of the gallbladder. These diverticula may appear as small specks or range up to 1 cm in size (Fig. 84–8). They can be seen projecting from the gallbladder lumen as a string of beads. Occasionally the sinuses will be filled with mucus or nonopaque bile, and may only be visible after a fatty meal. Muscular function of the gallbladder is normal, and it is not known whether this condition predisposes to cholecystitis or cholelithiasis.

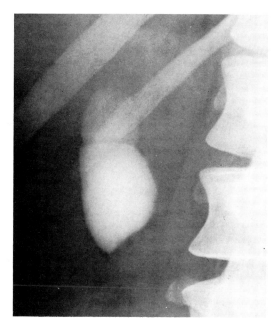

Figure 84–9. Septate gallbladder. In this instance the septum is quite incomplete.

COMPARTMENTALIZED GALLBLADDER

The septate gallbladder is a very unusual condition (Fig. 84–9). There may be two or more communicating segments. Occasionally gallstones and/or Aschoff-Rokitansky sinuses will be seen in the fundal compartment. Because of the high frequency of gallstones in the general population, it is not known if this condition predisposes to cholelithiasis.

INTRAVENOUS CHOLANGIOGRAPHY

PHARMACOKINETICS

After cholecystectomy, the common duct can be visualized by intravenous cholangiography (IVC). Since excretion of contrast material into the common duct is sufficiently concentrated to visualize it radiographically, contrast material will also appear in the gallbladder rapidly, provided the cystic duct is not obstructed.

The only approved compounds for intravenous cholangiography in the United States are sodium or methylglucamine io-

dipamide (MGI) (Fig. 84–10). As with oral agents, the iodine atoms are bound to the benzene rings in the 2, 4, and 6 positions. The rapid intravenous administration of this compound is frequently associated with nausea, vomiting, and a fall in the systemic blood pressure. For this reason, slow injection over five to 20 minutes is recommended. The usual dose is 20 ml of a solution containing 52 per cent iodine. A 40 ml dose infused over a longer period has been reported as being advantageous, particularly in the presence of hyperbilirubinemia.[10] Data to support this position, however, are not conclusive.

MGI binds with albumin in the plasma and is transported to the liver. Some MGI is excreted by the kidney, and this alternate route of elimination is very important in the presence of liver damage.

The MGI is excreted rapidly by the liver without chemical change. One of the serious problems with this contrast material is that it reaches the hepatic bile in a concentration that is on the borderline of roentgenographic visibility. For this reason, many efforts have been made to enhance biliary concentration by pharmacological means.[11] Unfortunately, neither an increased dose nor addition of other drugs has proved helpful. Although excretion of MGI is similar to bile salt excretion, it is not dependent upon it. MGI is a choleretic, so that with increased dose

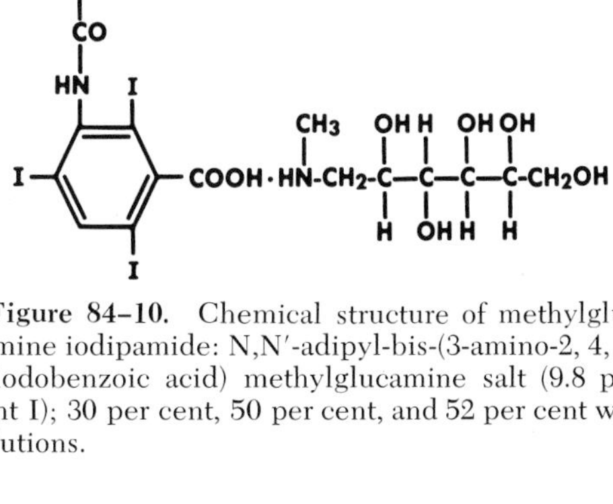

Figure 84–10. Chemical structure of methylglucamine iodipamide: N,N′-adipyl-bis-(3-amino-2, 4, 6-triiodobenzoic acid) methylglucamine salt (9.8 per cent I); 30 per cent, 50 per cent, and 52 per cent w/v solutions.

there is increased bile flow without a consequent increase of MGI concentration within the bile. The hypothesis that dextrose, sorbitol, or bile salts would increase its concentration in bile has not been substantiated by experimental studies.[12] Also, the combination of oral contrast agents such as iopanoic acid with MGI appears to reduce the concentration of iodine in the bile in experimental animals.

MGI is not reabsorbed by the normal mucosal membrane of either the biliary tract or the gut, so that it is eliminated in the feces following biliary excretion.

CLINICAL APPLICATION

There are three well accepted clinical uses of intravenous cholangiography. The most common indication is the study of patients who have had a cholecystectomy and who present with right upper quadrant pain or with clinical or chemical evidence of partial biliary tract obstruction. Common bile duct stones, stones within a cystic duct stump, or a stricture of the common bile duct may be found by this examination. This procedure is also employed to exclude biliary tract disease in the patient with acute abdominal pain. Although visualization of a normal gallbladder and common bile duct virtually excludes cholecystitis, an occasional patient with a rather classic clinical picture of either cholecystitis or common duct stone will have a normal examination. Visualization of the common bile duct without visualization of the gallbladder suggests acute cystic duct obstruction and/or cholelithiasis.

A third indication for intravenous cholangiography is to study the gallbladder of patients in whom malabsorption of the oral contrast material is suspected. It is less clear that all patients with nonvisualization of the gallbladder on oral studies should have IVC. The reliability of properly performed oral cholecystography is so high that there is little information to be obtained about the gallbladder from IVC. Since patients with nonvisualization by oral cholecystography have a relatively high incidence of common bile duct stones, IVC may be useful by demonstrating these stones.[13] Preoperative demonstration of common duct stones, indicating to the surgeon the need for exploration of the duct, is sufficient reason to justify this procedure. Opponents of this view, perhaps the majority, maintain that operative cholangiography should routinely be done, because it is quicker and is undeniably more accurate than the preoperative IVC. The roentgen techniques in in-

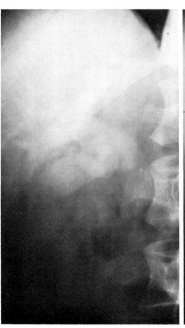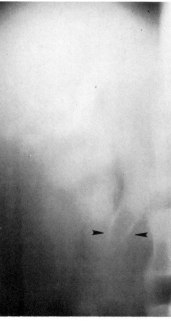

Figure 84-11. Choledocholithiasis. The value of tomography (right) demonstrated when compared with the plain film (left). The arrowheads show the stone impacted in the distal common bile duct.

travenous cholangiography are similar to oral studies; however, tomography is absolutely essential. The generally poor opacification of the bile and the superimposed intestinal gas can be serious hindrances to diagnostic accuracy if tomography is not used (Fig. 84–11). The filming sequence depends on whether the objective is to obtain only general anatomic information about the ducts or to define specific causes for partial obstruction. Some investigators feel that partial obstruction of the common bile duct, whether by a stone, a stricture in the mid-duct, or ampullary stenosis, causes the radiographic density in the bile duct to be greater at 120 minutes after injection than it was at 60 minutes.[14] Others have been highly critical of this concept, and feel that the IVC can yield only anatomic information.[15]

The interpretation of anatomic information is often difficult. Because of the poor concentration of the iodine, small stones may be easily missed. Stones within the hepatic duct are rarely seen. An awareness of the frequency of false-negative studies is important in evaluating patients after cholecystectomy. Common duct size has also proved to be unreliable as absolute evidence of bile duct obstruction. If the bile duct measures above 15 mm in size or has increased its preoperative size, it can

be considered suggestive of obstruction, but the diagnosis is better made when the anatomic cause of the obstruction is seen (Fig. 84–12).

Intravenous cholangiography is contraindicated in those with known idiosyncrasy to the contrast material, and is not helpful in patients with impaired excretory function of the liver. Indeed, an increased serum bilirubin above 4 mg per 100 ml reduces virtually to zero the chances of opacifying the common bile duct. When the bilirubin level is between 3 and 4 mg per 100 ml, only about one-third of the studies will be successful. It is extremely important to delay the IVC if the bilirubin level is diminishing, because delay will enhance the opportunity to opacify the common bile duct. If the bilirubin level is rising rapidly, there is little point in trying intravenous cholangiography.

PERCUTANEOUS TRANSHEPATIC CHOLANGIOGRAPHY

The failure of both oral and intravenous cholangiography in the jaundiced patient led to a more direct technique for visualizing the hepatic ducts. The usual reason for the study is to aid in distinguishing jaun-

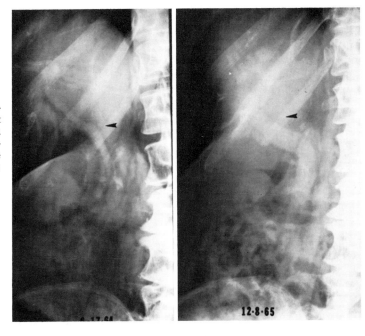

Figure 84–12. Choledocholithiasis. Change in common bile duct size over an 18-month period. A common bile duct stone was removed in January 1966. The stone itself cannot be seen on the films of December 8, 1965.

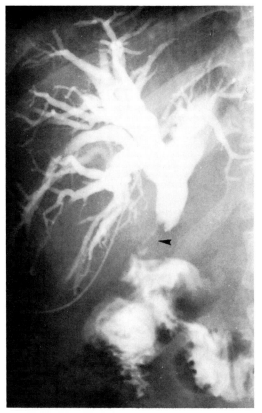

Figure 84–13. Recurrent stricture (arrowhead) of the common bile duct following choledocho-jejunostomy. Percutaneous transhepatic cholangiography is technically easy to do when this degree of hydrohepatosis exists.

dice of extrahepatic obstruction from that of intrahepatic cholestasis. It is also helpful in locating the site of obstruction and perhaps in delineating the pathological anatomy (Fig. 84–13).

The basic technique of percutaneous transhepatic cholangiography (PTC) is similar to a liver biopsy. Either an anterior subcostal or a lateral intercostal approach is used. A 6- to 8-inch plastic sheathed needle is used. The liver is punctured under fluoroscopic control. The metal core of the needle is removed, leaving only the plastic sheath in the liver. Aspiration of the sheath is done while the sheath is slowly withdrawn. When bile is aspirated, withdrawal is stopped and water-soluble, sterile, radiopaque material is injected under fluoroscopic control. Successful studies are directly correlated with the degree of hydrohepatosis. If on three or four passes into the liver no bile is aspirated, it

is fairly accurate to conclude that the bile ducts are not dilated. This finding is most common in patients with intrahepatic jaundice.

Filming techniques are similar to other biliary tract procedures. It is, however, quite important to shift the patient successively to the prone and upright positions, if possible, before films are taken. In this way, thick bile in the distal common bile duct can then be displaced by the contrast material and the site of obstruction outlined.

Fairly characteristic appearances exist for biliary tract carcinoma, pancreatic carcinoma, bile duct stricture, and choledocholithiasis. The nature of the disorder is usually less important than its location.

The main contraindication to this procedure is inadequate blood coagulation. Suppurative cholangitis increases the hazard of injecting contrast material into the ductal system. Complications of the study, in addition to bleeding, are bile peritonitis and, occasionally, cholemia. Since the study is ordinarily done immediately preoperatively, bleeding and bile peritonitis may be dealt with at laparotomy.

There has been a recent interest in percutaneous puncture of the gallbladder.[16] If experience shows this to be a procedure that can be done without an unacceptable incidence of bile peritonitis, it will provide a back-up method for PTC.

OTHER TECHNIQUES

Endoscopic Transampullary Catheterization. This technique is now possible with fiberoptic systems.[17] Successful entrance is far from 100 per cent, but when it is achieved it yields much valuable information. Retrograde injection into the pancreatic duct system may result in pancreatitis. The technical problems of visualizing both the pancreatic and biliary duct system without overdistention of either are not yet solved.

Operative Cholangiography. The direct approach with injection either into the cystic duct or directly into the common bile duct at laparotomy results in excellent visualization of the duct system. A T-tube left in postoperatively is valuable for detection of stones that might have been missed at the time of operation or that might not have been extractable.

Arteriography. Selective hepatic arteriography will result in filling of the cystic artery and opacification of the gallbladder wall. There have been some enthusiastic reports of the use of this modality in the diagnosis of both inflammatory and neoplastic diseases. The radiographic visualization of the branches of the cystic artery allows a judgment to be made regarding the size of the gallbladder. At the present time, however, arteriography does not appear clearly to be of diagnostic value in regard to gallbladder disease except in unusual circumstances.

MOTILITY DISORDERS OF THE GALLBLADDER

The concept that incoordination of the gallbladder and the cystic duct sphincter might be responsible for clinical symptoms is not new. However, it has never been held in much favor, as reliable diagnostic criteria for its support have not emerged. The appearance of symptoms or of cholecystographic abnormalities after a fatty meal as criteria for gallbladder contraction has led to reinvestigation of this concept. Patients with chronic symptoms referable to the right upper quadrant and normal conventional oral cholecystograms who are given a dose of cholecystokinin of approximately 1 unit per kilogram intravenously may suffer right upper quadrant pain; cholecystographic abnormalities may be seen in a number of these patients.[18] Cholecystectomy is alleged to relieve symptoms in most of these patients.

REFERENCES

1. Taketa, R. M., Berk, R. N., Dunn, C. R., and Larry, J. H. The effective pH on the intestinal absorption of Telepaque. Invest. Radiol. 6:399, 1971.
2. Nelson, J. A., Moss, A. A., Goldberg, H. I., Benet, L. C., and Amberg, J. R. Gastro- intestinal absorption of iopanoic acid. Invest. Radiol. 8:1, 1973.
3. Sokoloff, J., Farr, R. S., and Lasser, E. C. Intracellular protein binding of cholecystographic media in the hepatocyte. Radiology 106:519, 1973.
4. Schmid, R., Axelrod, J., Hammaker, L., and Swarm, R. L. Congenital jaundice in rats due to a defect in glucuronide formation. J. Clin. Invest. 37:1123, 1958.
5. Moss, A. A., Amberg, J. R., and Jones, R. S. The relationship of bile salts and bile flow to the biliary excretion of iopanoic acid. Invest. Radiol. 7:11, 1972.
6. Dunn, C. R., and Berk, R. N. The pharmacokinetics of Telepaque metabolism. The relation of blood concentration and bile flow to the rate of hepatic excretion. Amer. J. Roent. 114:758, 1972.
7. Gasparini, G., and Accomazzi, F. La colecistografia orale "ripetuta" nel soggeto normale. Radiol. Med. 48:460, 1962.
8. Canales, C. O., Smith, G. H., Robinson, J. C., Remmers, A. R., Jr., and Sarles, H. E. Acute renal failure after the administration of iopanoic acid as a cholecystographic agent. New Eng. J. Med. 281:89, 1964.
9. Jutras, J. A., and Levesque, H. Adenomyoma and adenomyomatosis of the gallbladder. Radiol. Clin. N. Amer. 4:483, 1966.
10. McNulty, J. G. Drip infusion cholecystocholangiography. Radiology 90:570, 1968.
11. Fischer, H. W. Attempts to improve iodipamide intravenous cholangiography. Amer. J. Roent. 96:477, 1966.
12. Moss, A. A., Nelson, J., and Amberg, J. R. Intravenous cholangiography. An experimental evaluation. Amer. J. Roent. In press.
13. Wollam, G. L., Freeman, F. J., and Priestly, J. J. Relationship of cholecystographic visualization of the gallbladder to incidence of choledocholithiasis. Surgery 61:669, 1967.
14. Wise, R. E. Current concepts of intravenous cholangiography. Radiol. Clin. N. Amer. 4:521, 1966.
15. Bornhurst, R. A., Eitzman, E. R., and McAfee, J. G. Double-dose drip infusion cholangiography. An analysis of 107 consecutive cases. J.A.M.A. 206:1489, 1968.
16. Demasi, C. J., Adkamar, K., Sparks, R. D., and Hunter, F. M. Puncture of the gallbladder during percutaneous transhepatic cholangiography. J.A.M.A. 201:225, 1967.
17. Cotton, P. B., Blumgart, L. H., Davies, G. T., Pierce, J. W., Samen, P. R., Burwood, R. J., Lawrie, B. W., and Read, A. E. Cannulation of papilla of Vater via fiberduodenoscope. Lancet 1:53, 1972.
18. Nathan, M. H., Newman, A., Murray, J. D., and Camponovo, R. Cholecystokinin cholecystography. Amer. J. Roent. 110:240, 1970.

Chapter 85

The Pathogenesis of Gallstones

William Admirand

INTRODUCTION

Gallstones are a major health problem. It is estimated that in the United States 10 per cent of men and 20 per cent of women between the ages of 55 and 65 years have gallstones and that the overall total exceeds 15 million people.[1] The American Indian has the highest incidence of gallstones of any racial or ethnic group within this population. On the basis of epidemiological studies, it has been estimated that 70 per cent of Pima Indian women over the age of 25 have cholelithiasis. The reason for this high incidence in the American Indian has not been determined, but does not appear to be related to abnormal levels of serum cholesterol, to diet, to parity, to an abnormal incidence of diabetes, to obesity, or to infection.[2]

The incidence of gallstones is high among patients with certain diseases. As many as 30 per cent of patients with regional enteritis develop cholesterol gallstones.[3, 4] In these individuals, it is assumed that malabsorption of bile salts caused by disease or resection of the terminal ileum leads to a decrease in the total bile salt pool, lowering concentration of bile acids relative to cholesterol in bile (see below), and favoring precipitation of

cholesterol crystals and the formation of cholesterol gallstones. In particular, an increased incidence of stones may be expected in those who have undergone distal ileal resection.[3, 4] There is also an increased incidence of gallstones in patients with diabetes mellitus, although the reason for this increase has not been established. Nonetheless, age and sex influence the incidence of cholelithiasis in nondiabetics in the Caucasian and Negro races. The disease is more common in women over age 40 than in males of any age or in women under 40. Stasis of gallbladder bile is presumed during pregnancy, perhaps facilitating precipitation of cholesterol crystals—the initiating event for cholelithiasis; however, data to substantiate the hypothesis are not available. Indeed, of the classic "5 F's" of cholelithiasis (fair, fat, forty, fertile, and female), only the last of these is clearly associated with increased incidence of gallstones.

Pigmented gallstones are rare in the United States, but the incidence is increased in patients with hemolytic disease such as sickle cell anemia or thalassemia. In addition, the incidence of pigmented gallstones in patients with cirrhosis of the liver is increased, the reasons for which are unknown.[5]

TYPES OF STONES

A discussion of the pathogenesis of gallstones requires first that gallstones be classified according to their composition. The simplest classification proposes two groups: stones containing predominantly cholesterol, and stones containing predominantly bilirubinate. It is doubtful that pure cholesterol stones exist, because most stones have at least a small nidus of calcium bilirubinate. However, the total content of calcium bilirubinate rarely exceeds 5 per cent of the weight of the stone. In contrast, pigmented stones contain 50 to 70 per cent calcium bilirubinate and only trace amounts of cholesterol. This classification may be an oversimplification, but it is practical for the discussion of the etiology of gallstones.

CHOLESTEROL GALLSTONES

The formation of cholesterol gallstones can be separated into two steps. In the first step, the capacity of bile to solubilize cholesterol is exceeded and insoluble cholesterol microscrystals precipitate from solution. The second step of gallstone formation is the union of these individual microcrystals of cholesterol to form a macroscopic gallstone. It is likely that both these processes proceed simultaneously.

SOLUBILITY OF CHOLESTEROL

Normal bile is a single-phase aqueous solution. Three compounds comprise 80 to 95 per cent of the total solids dissolved in bile: conjugated bile salts, lecithin, and cholesterol. Cholesterol is a neutral sterol; lecithin is a phospholipid; both are almost completely insoluble in water. However, bile salts are able to form multimolecular aggregates or micelles which solubilize lecithin and cholesterol in an aqueous solution. This function of bile salts is related to their structure. The bile salt molecule can be divided into two parts: the steroid nucleus which is nonpolar and water insoluble, and the hydroxyls and terminal carboxyl which are polar and water soluble. Such molecules that possess both water-soluble and water-insoluble portions are called amphipaths; in addition to the bile salts, detergents and certain dyes also possess the unique ability to form multimolecular aggregates or micelles when placed in aqueous solution.[6]

In very dilute solutions, the individual bile salt molecules are freely dispersed throughout the solution, thus forming an ideal solution. Attractive forces (Van der Waal's forces) between the steroid portions of the individual bile salt molecules are strong, but are effective only over short distances. Therefore in dilute solutions the molecules are sufficiently far apart that Van der Waal's forces are ineffective. However, as more and more bile salts are added to the solution, the molecules become closer together and Van der Waal's forces become important. First, dimers and then trimers form, and then, at a finite concentration termed the critical micellar concentration, the individual bile salt molecules coalesce, with the polar portions of the molecule facing the solution and the steroid portion of the molecules facing the center of the aggregate. These molecular clusters are called micelles. The bile salt molecules within the micelles remain in equilibrium with other bile salt molecules in solution. The critical concentration for conjugated bile salts to form micelles in bile is approximately 2 to 4 mM per liter.

An aqueous micellar solution of bile salts is able to solubilize cholesterol by incorporating it within the substance of the micelle; however, bile salts alone are relatively inefficient, because approximately 50 molecules of bile salt is necessary to solubilize one molecule of cholesterol. Lecithin is also solubilized in micellar bile salt solutions, probably interdigitated between the bile salt molecules. The resulting mixed micelle, containing both bile salt and lecithin, has an increased capacity to solubilize cholesterol as compared to the pure bile salt micelle. Thus in a mixed micellar solution of bile salt and lecithin, only seven molecules of bile salt is needed to solubilize one molecule of cholesterol.[6]

From the preceding physicochemical considerations, it is apparent that insoluble cholesterol microcrystals might precipitate from bile because of an absolute increase in the concentration of cholesterol, an absolute decrease in the concentration of bile salts or of lecithin, or some combination of these three factors. This hypothesis for the pathogenesis of stones is logical, and numerous studies have attempted to show differences in the concentrations of bile salt, lecithin, and cholesterol between normal bile and that from patients with cholesterol gallstones. Consistent differences have been difficult to demonstrate, in fact, because of differences in the analytical methods employed as well as in the manner in which the data have been expressed. Thus if the quantities of bile salt, lecithin, and cholesterol per 100 ml of bile are compared, no significant differences in the concentrations of any of these substances in gallbladder bile from normal subjects and from patients with cholesterol gallstones are found. This method of expressing the data, however, does not account for the degree to which the bile has been concentrated in the gallbladder at the time the sample was obtained. Furthermore, the quantity of any single component has little meaning unless expressed in relationship to the quantities of the other two major components. The use of binary ratios such as cholesterol : bile salt or cholesterol : lecithin also fails to show consistent differences between normal bile and bile from patients with cholesterol gallstones. Obviously, this method of expressing data is unsatisfactory, because it omits one of the three components.

Some years ago, Isaksson found that when the ratio of cholesterol to bile salts plus lecithin in an in vitro system was above a critical 1 : 11 level, cholesterol precipitated from solution. Applying these results to the clinical situation, he found that 70 to 95 per cent of patients with cholesterol gallstones had a ratio above the 1 : 11.[7] The method was not entirely satisfactory, because occasionally bile from a normal subject had high ratios, whereas bile from some of the patients with cholesterol gallstones had normal ratios. The difficulty with expressing the data as cholesterol : bile salt plus lecithin is that it does not distinguish between the individual effects of bile salt and lecithin.

More recently, bile composition has been displayed on triangular coordinates whereby any bile which contains bile salt, lecithin, and cholesterol can be plotted as

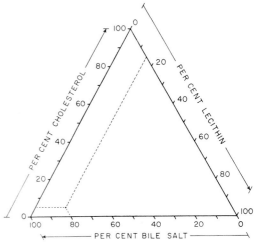

Figure 85-1. The method of representing bile composition on triangular coordinates. The percentage of the total moles of bile salt, lecithin, and cholesterol constituted by each of these components is shown on the scales along the sides of the triangle. Since the sum of bile salt, lecithin, and cholesterol equals 100 per cent, the composition of any bile containing these components can be represented as a single point within triangular coordinates. Thus a bile containing 80 per cent bile salt, 15 per cent lecithin, and 5 per cent cholesterol is represented by a single point formed at the intersection of the dashed lines extended from the 80 per cent level on the bile salt scale at the base of the triangle, the 15 per cent level on the lecithin scale at the right of the triangle, and the 5 per cent level on the cholesterol scale at the left of the triangle. (From Admirand, W. H., and Small, D. M.: J. Clin. Invest. 47:1043, 1968.)

a single point within the triangle, and its position will be determined by the relative molar quantities of the three components (Fig. 85-1).[6] By this method it was found that the relative composition of bile salts and lecithin was decreased, whereas the relative concentration of cholesterol was increased in samples of bile obtained from patients with cholesterol gallstones compared with normal bile (Fig. 85-2). Thus the abnormality in gallstone formation is the result of changes in all three major components rather than a change in any one.

Construction of a model system which represents the physical state of all possible mixtures of bile salt, lecithin, and cholesterol in water defines the limits of cholesterol solubility in bile (Fig. 85-3). When the results of this in vitro system were applied to human bile samples, it was

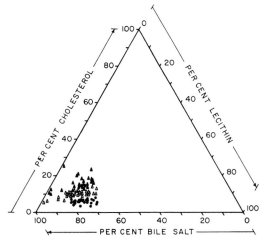

Figure 85–2. The composition of gallbladder bile from normal subjects and patients with gallstones. The composition of gallbladder bile, in terms of bile salts, phospholipids, and cholesterol from each of 25 normal subjects and 66 patients with cholesterol or mixed gallstones is plotted on triangular coordinates. The closed circles represent bile from normal subjects. The triangles represent bile from gallstone patients. The closed triangles indicate the presence of cholesterol microcrystals; the open triangles represent biles without microcrystals of cholesterol. (From Admirand, W. H., and Small, D. M.: J. Clin. Invest. 47:1043, 1968.)

found that the bile from patients with cholesterol gallstones was either saturated or supersaturated with cholesterol (Fig. 85–4).

Subsequently, the same defect was demonstrated in hepatic bile, i.e., in bile before it had reached the gallbladder (Fig. 85–5).[8] From these studies, the concept has been proposed that gallstones are not the result of disease of the gallbladder but reflect a primary fault in bile formation by the liver. The hepatocytes in patients with gallstones produce bile, which is either saturated or supersaturated with cholesterol. In the gallbladder the individual microcrystals of cholesterol usually unite around a pigmented nidus and grow to form a macroscopic stone. Therefore the gallbladder seems to provide a reservoir or a relatively stagnant pool which facilitates the growth of a macroscopic gallstone.

The mechanism for the production of abnormal bile in patients with cholesterol gallstones is not fully understood. The total bile salt pool and daily bile salt excretion are significantly decreased in patients with cholesterol gallstones, and it is possi-

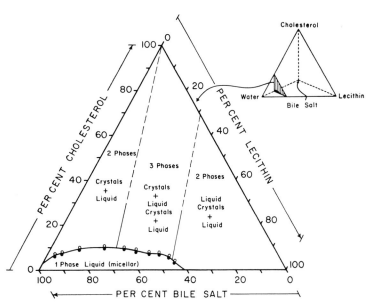

Figure 85–3. The model system. The tetrahedron shown in the upper right corner has been used to represent the physical state of all possible combinations of bile salt, lecithin, cholesterol, and water. The section in the tetrahedron taken at 90 per cent water results in a triangular phase diagram which has been enlarged and is shown on the left. This diagram shows the physical state of all possible combinations of bile salts, lecithin, and cholesterol in aqueous solutions containing a total of 10 per cent solids and 90 per cent water. Closed circles represent mixtures forming one liquid phase. Open circles represent mixtures forming two- or three-phase systems (clear liquid plus cholesterol crystals and [or] islets of lamellar liquid crystal). The line separating the open and closed circles indicates the maximal amount of cholesterol solubilized by any mixture of lecithin and bile salt. (From Admirand, W. H., and Small, D. J.: J. Clin. Invest. 47:1043, 1968.)

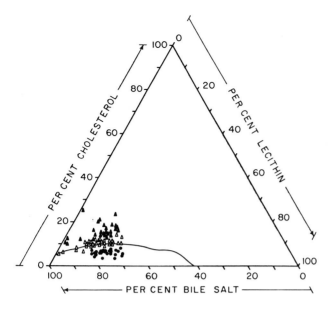

Figure 85–4. The composition of gallbladder bile from normal subjects and patients with gallstones compared with the limits of cholesterol solubility as determined from a model system. The diagram is the same as Figure 85–2 except that the line representing maximal cholesterol solubilization, as defined by Figure 85–3, has been superimposed. The composition of bile from normal subjects (closed circles) is such that all circles fall within the micellar zone. The bile samples from patients with cholesterol or mixed gallstones in which no microcrystals were present (open triangles) fall on or very near the line, indicating maximal cholesterol solubilization. The biles from gallstone patients, which contain microcrystals of cholesterol (closed triangles), fall well above the line of maximal saturation. (From Admirand, W. H., and Small, D. M.: J. Clin. Invest. 47:1043, 1968.)

ble that this is the underlying defect in patients who form stones.[9] Since all lecithin and most cholesterol excreted by liver are linked to the excretion of the bile salts, it follows that lecithin excretion will be decreased in this situation.[10] In addition, although the bile salt-dependent fraction of cholesterol excretion would decrease, the bile salt-independent fraction would be unchanged. Thus bile produced under these circumstances might be saturated or supersaturated with cholesterol owing to the relatively greater decrease in bile salt and lecithin excretion than in cholesterol excretion. Although this theory of cholesterol gallstone formation fits the presently available evidence, additional data are needed to establish its validity in man.

STONE GROWTH

Although much is known about the formation of abnormal bile, relatively little is known about the process by which individual microcrystals of cholesterol unite and grow to form a macroscopic stone. To date it has not been possible to grow cholesterol gallstones in vitro. It has been shown that prior to the formation of gallstones in experimental animals, a mucous substance appears in the mucosa of the gallbladder.[11] The exact nature of this substance or its role in gallstone formation has not been determined. However, it is possible that it acts as a coagulating agent for cholesterol microcrystals, leading to the formation of macroscopic gallstones. This

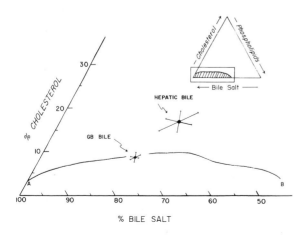

Figure 85–5. The triangle at the upper right represents the three-component system: bile salt, phospholipid, cholesterol. The hatched area represents those mixtures forming one liquid (micellar) phase. The box shows the representative part of the triangle given in the rest of the figure. Line AB indicates the maximal solubility of cholesterol. The mean compositions of hepatic and gallbladder bile from 29 patients with cholesterol gallstones are represented by the black dots. The lines passing through the dots indicate ± 2 SE. (From Small, D. M., and Rapo, S.: New Eng. J. Med. 283:53, 1970.)

mechanism may be similar to the effect of high molecular weight organic compounds in the formation of calcium bilirubinate calculi.[12]

CALCIUM BILIRUBINATE GALLSTONES

Calcium bilirubinate stones are extremely prevalent in Asia but comprise less than 5 per cent of the total stones found in Europe or the United States. It is estimated that approximately 30 to 40 per cent of all the gallstones in Japan are composed of calcium bilirubinate. These stones usually have a dark brown or reddish color and are fragile. The cut surface is sometimes amorphous and sometimes layered. The bilirubin content of calcium bilirubinate stones varies from 40 to 60 per cent of the stone weight. Cholesterol content is 3 to 25 per cent, in contrast to cholesterol gallstones which contain 70 to 95 per cent cholesterol and 0.2 to 5 per cent bilirubin. In the United States, calcium bilirubinate stones are often found in association with hemolytic anemia such as sickle cell anemia or thalassemia. Cultures of bile from patients with calcium bilirubinate stones in Japan have almost invariably grown *Escherichia coli*.[12] In addition, eggs or fragments of cuticles of *Ascaris lumbricoides* have also been identified in approximately half these patients, prompting the suggestion that invasion of the duodenum or biliary tree by parasites leads to an ascending cholangitis. Furthermore, the high incidence of atrophic gastritis with hypo- or achlorhydria in Asia may allow bacterial growth in the duodenum and thus facilitate ascending infection in the biliary tree. Finally, *Ascaris* eggs have frequently been shown to serve as a nidus for calcium bilirubinate stone formation.[12]

The bilirubin moiety of calcium bilirubinate stones has been identified as free, nonesterified bilirubin. Since most of the bilirubin excreted by the liver is conjugated, the bilirubin present in stones must undergo deconjugation in the biliary tree. Bilirubin glucuronide can be hydrolyzed to free bilirubin and glucuronic acid by the enzyme β-glucuronidase. Although normal bile is virtually free of this enzyme, bile infected with *E. coli* has considerable β-glucuronidase activity. Further, the pH

optimum for activity of the β-glucuronidase contained in *E. coli* is approximately the same as the pH of bile. From such data the suggestion has come that inflammation of the biliary tree with *E. coli* leads to the release of free bilirubin, the carboxyl radical of which combines with calcium to form insoluble calcium bilirubinate. Indeed, a series of elegant experiments has demonstrated that calcium bilirubinate stones could be formed in vitro from normal bile incubated with *E. coli* after the addition of calcium carbonate, calcium chloride, and high molecular weight organic compounds.[12] The importance of infected bile in the production of calcium bilirubinate stones in the United States has not been investigated.

REFERENCES

1. Friedman, D. K., Kannel W. B., and Dawber, T. R. Epidemiology of gallbladder disease: Observations in Framingham study. J. Chronic Dis. 19:273, 1966.
2. Sampliner, R. E., Bennett, P. H., and Comess, L. J. Gallbladder disease in Pima Indians: Demonstration of high prevalence and early onset by cholecystography. New Eng. J. Med. 283:1358, 1970.
3. Cohen, S., Kaplan, M., Gottlieb, L., and Paterson, J. Liver disease and gallstones in regional enteritis. Gastroenterology 60:237, 1971.
4. Heaton, K. W., and Read, A. E. Gall stones in patients with disorders of the terminal ileum and disturbed bile salt metabolism. Brit. Med. J. 3:494, 1969.
5. Bouchier, I. A. D. Postmortem study of the frequency of gallstones in patients with cirrhosis of the liver. Gut 10:705, 1969.
6. Admirand, W. H., and Small, D. M. The physicochemical basis of cholesterol gallstone formation in man. J. Clin. Invest. 47:1043, 1968.
7. Isaksson, B. On the lipid constituents of bile from human gallbladder containing cholesterol gallstones. Acta Soc. Med. Upsalien 59:277, 1953.
8. Small, D. M., and Rapo, S. Source of abnormal bile in patients with cholesterol gallstone. New Eng. J. Med. 283:53, 1970.
9. Vlahcevic, Z. R., Bell, C. C., Buhac, I., Farrar, J. T., and Swell, L. Diminished bile acid pool size in patients with gallstones. Gastroenterology 59:165, 1970.
10. Nilsson, S., and Schersten, T. Importance of bile acids for phospholipid secretion into human bile. Gastroenterology 57:525, 1969.
11. Freston, J. W., Bouchier, I. A. D., and Newman, J. Biliary mucous substances in dihydrocholesterol-induced cholelithiasis. Gastroenterology 57:670, 1969.
12. Maki, T. Pathogenesis of calcium bilirubinate gallstone: Role of E. coli, β-glucuronidase and coagulation by inorganic ions, polyelectrolytes and agitation. Ann. Surg. 164:90, 1966.

Chapter 86

Cholelithiasis and Chronic Cholecystitis

Lawrence W. Way, Marvin H. Sleisenger

Cholelithiasis may express itself clinically in a variety of ways, depending to some degree upon the behavior of the stones. Obstruction of the cystic duct may lead to a dramatic attack of acute gallbladder inflammation, or repeated episodes of mild degree may be noted; in turn, obstruction of the common duct or of the ileum by stone leads to distinct clinical pictures. Finally, cholelithiasis is associated in some with *carcinoma of the gallbladder.*

CHRONIC CHOLECYSTITIS

The most common disability that results from cholelithiasis is *chronic cholecystitis.* This is characterized pathologically by various degrees of chronic inflammation on gross or microscopic examination of the gallbladder.[1] Stones are present in most of the patients, but the gallbladder may or may not visualize on cholecystography.

PATHOLOGY

The term *chronic cholecystitis* is used to refer to the stone-containing gallbladder whose wall may demonstrate any of a wide range of histological changes, from essentially no signs of chronic inflammation to a

situation in which the gallbladder wall is reduced to a dense scar contracted over calculi. There is a general correlation between the extent of chronic inflammatory changes and the clinical severity of the disease, but many exceptions to this rule are encountered.

CLINICAL MANIFESTATIONS

Chronic cholecystitis is associated with discrete attacks of epigastric or right upper quadrant pain, either steady or intermittent, and sometimes associated with tenderness to palpation in the right upper quadrant. The term gallbladder or biliary colic is something of a misnomer, because the pain is usually persistent, and, if intermittent, the peaks of pain are usually separated by 15- to 60-minute intervals, unlike the colic of intestinal obstruction.[2]

Usually the onset of pain is abrupt, and its intensity reaches a plateau within 15 minutes to an hour. Attacks of biliary colic may last for as little as 15 minutes or as long as several hours, the average being about one hour. Typically, symptoms subside more gradually than they began. The pain is characteristically felt in the epigastrium or right upper quadrant of the abdomen, although left-sided epigastric pain and even anterior chest pain are not rare.

1116

Referred pain is sometimes noted between the scapulae, or over the tip of the right scapula. If *fever, dark urine* and/or *icterus* accompany the episode, they indicate common duct obstruction caused by a calculus. Gradually gallbladder function is lost.

Symptoms described as indigestion, dyspepsia, flatulence, intolerance to fatty or spicy foods, or discomfort relieved by belching have been shown to be randomly distributed in regard to the presence or absence of chronic cholecystitis.[3] If cholecystectomy is performed for a patient with cholelithiasis whose only symptoms consist of these, a high incidence of persistent discomfort can be predicted after surgery. On the other hand, it appears that some patients with dyspepsia alone experience relief after the gallbladder has been removed, so that the clinician must evaluate the patient's complaints individually in relation to his total physical and emotional makeup.[4] Although the attacks may not be so clear cut, recurrent pain, often with mild nausea or vomiting and right upper quadrant tenderness with episodes occasionally related to ingestion of large meals, strongly suggests the diagnosis.

Obviously, a spectrum of chronic recurrent symptoms is associated with chronic cholecystitis. Symptoms do not always correlate well with either the degree of pathological change in the wall of the gallbladder or the number or type of gallstones. Although cholelithiasis may be found in some persons with postprandial symptoms, one cannot assume that it necessarily underlies such complaints. In fact, it has been shown that the diagnosis of cholelithiasis and chronic cholecystitis cannot be made reliably on the basis of symptoms alone; some patients with apparently typical attacks will be found to have normal gallbladders, and others with unusual pain patterns will be relieved by removal of a small scarred gallbladder. X-ray verification must be sought whenever feasible.

The only *physical sign* present during biliary colic is right subcostal tenderness in the gallbladder area. It is not usually marked, and the organ is rarely palpable.

DIAGNOSIS

Radiological examination of the gallbladder and biliary tract is the principal

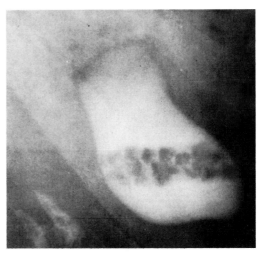

Figure 86–1.   Gallstones floating in a layer in the gallbladder shown by oral cholecystogram.

means of diagnosing cholelithiasis and cholecystitis. Calculi may be demonstrated by plain film of the abdomen or by oral cholecystography with iodopanoic acid (Fig. 86–1). Sometimes cholangiography will be required (see Fig. 84–12, p. 1107). Often the diseased gallbladder is not visualized after ingestion or injection of dye, indicating either cystic duct obstruction or advanced disease with impairment of its ability to concentrate.[5] Occasionally, the gallbladder will opacify, obscuring small stones, which, however, become visible when the patient is in the erect or decubitus position. With careful and proper evaluation, chronic cholecystitis and cholelithiasis may be accurately diagnosed in more than 95 per cent of the patients. Chronic cholecystitis without cholelithiasis may be more difficult to diagnose. (For details, see pp. 1098 to 1109).

The nature of the obstructing lesion may possibly be defined by duodenal drainage. Presence of cholesterol crystals in the absence of jaundice indicates cholelithiasis. Bilirubinate crystals may indicate either stasis or stones. This test is now reserved for those who are sensitive to the organic dyes given orally or intravenously to diagnose biliary tract disease.

DIFFERENTIAL DIAGNOSIS

In view of the lack of specificity of the symptoms suggesting chronic cholecystitis, the patient's history, the findings on physical examination, and the laboratory data must be carefully evaluated. An upper gastrointestinal barium examination is indicated in nearly every patient before the physician can be satisfied that previously demonstrated gallstones were responsible for the symptoms. In many instances, a barium enema and an intravenous pyelogram are necessary to exclude disease in these organs which might give rise to similar complaints. The demonstration of gallbladder disease by cholecystography does not exclude the possibility that other conditions have caused the symptoms. The most common of these are *gastritis, irritable colon, peptic ulcer, diaphragmatic hernia, pancreatitis, renal disease,* and *lesions of the colon (diverticulitis* and *carcinoma).*

Causes of *radiculitis,* such as osteoarthritis or peripheral nerve tumors, are notorious for their ability to mimic gallbladder disease when they create pain in the right upper quadrant. Thoracic spine films and occasionally myelograms should be performed in selected cases when radicular pain cannot be excluded. *Gallstones* and *coronary insufficiency* may coexist, and cholecystectomy may reduce symptoms caused by coronary disease.

TREATMENT

The treatment of chronic cholecystitis with cholelithiasis is surgical, and in most cases cholecystectomy is the procedure of choice.[6-8] If stones are simply removed from a gallbladder and the organ is left intact, stones re-form within several years in the majority of patients.

Patients who complain only of "dyspeptic" symptoms often have normal cholecystograms. These persons often experience fullness, nausea, anorexia, and diffuse epigastric heaviness, caused by motility disturbances of the upper gastrointestinal tract or an irritable colon syndrome. Those in whom a cholecystogram has revealed nothing more than reduced gallbladder function, i.e., faint opacification and impaired emptying, are difficult clinical problems. If operated upon, some of these patients may have calculi with gross and microscopic changes and evidence of inflammation within the gallbladder wall. Some of these patients are relieved of their symptoms after cholecystectomy. Others appear at operation to have a normal extrahepatic biliary system. For these, the results following cholecystectomy are often unsatisfactory.

CHOLESTEROSIS[9, 10]

Occasionally, upper abdominal distress may be associated with deposits of cholesterol in epithelial cells and in macrophages within the mucosa of the gallbladder. Although the distress is more likely to be low-grade and chronic, occasionally episodes of acute cholecystitis may be experienced. In most instances, however, the condition is asymptomatic. Nevertheless, numerous deposits of lipid may be found scattered within the lamina propria. Occasionally the mucosa surrounding the lipid deposits may become inflamed, and in this instance the mucosa of the gallbladder looks like a ripe strawberry. Rarely the collections of lipids in the macrophages of the mucosal folds may appear as lucent defects in the cholecystogram. The cholecystogram in this instance may reveal numerous very tiny radiolucent areas. The gallbladder usually functions normally. Indeed, it has often been noted that the dye is "hyperconcentrated." Occasionally patients with cholesterosis become asymptomatic after cholecystectomy. However, the role of surgery in the treatment of cholesterosis of the gallbladder has not yet been firmly established.

THE "SILENT STONE" PROBLEM[11, 12]

The question arises as to how to advise a patient with truly asymptomatic cholelithiasis. It is a difficult question, and one for which no all-encompassing answer may be given. Within five years of discovery, about 30 per cent of patients with asymptomatic cholelithiasis develop symptoms, and a few of these experience acute cholecystitis, obstructive jaundice, or pancreatitis as the initial manifestation. For this reason it appears wise to recommend cholecystectomy to all patients under age 50 with silent stones. For those between 50 and 60, the problem is especially knotty, because the morbidity and mortality of elective surgery are higher, and many in this age group will eventually die of other causes before symptoms develop from the stones. It appears wise, on balance, to recommend cholecystectomy only for those in good health, for those who have large stones (greater than 2.0 cm in diameter), and for diabetics who are in a state of good control.[13] In anyone who shows evidence of disease in the cardiac, arterial, renal, or pulmonary systems or who may have some liver disease, operation should not be carried out. Operation is not recommended for those in the over-60 age group. The life expectancy in this group appears greater if elective surgery is not performed.

Recently, it has been shown that oral administration of bile salts (chenodeoxycholic acid) over many months results in dissolution of gallstones located in the gallbladder.[14] This exciting observation is still experimental, but it may offer a rational approach to the treatment of so-called silent stone. Possibly, if proved safe on a long-term basis, it may be used in those individuals with symptomatic gallstone disease who are poor operative risks.

REFERENCES

1. Edlund, Y., and Zettergren, L. Histopathology of the gallbladder in gallstone disease related to clinical data. Acta Chir. Scand. 116:450, 1959.
2. French, E. B., and Robb, W. A. T. Biliary and renal colic. Brit. Med. J. 3:121, 1963.
3. Price, W. H. Gall-bladder dyspepsia. Brit. Med. J. 3:138, 1963.
4. Gunn, A., and Keddie, N. Some clinical observations on patients with gallstones. Lancet 2:239, 1972.
5. Higgins, J. A. Nonfunctioning gallbladder. Modern Treatment 5:500, 1968.
6. Haff, R. C., et al. Biliary tract operations. A review of 1000 patients. Arch. Surg. 98:428, 1969.
7. Boquist, L., et al. Mortality following gallbladder surgery: A study of 3257 cholecystectomies. Surgery 71:616, 1972.
8. Dowdy, G. S., Jr., and Waldron, G. W. Importance of coexistent factors in biliary tract surgery. Arch. Surg. 88:178, 1964.
9. Andersson, A., and Bergdahl, L. Acalculous cholesterosis of the gallbladder. Arch. Surg. 103:342, 1971.
10. Salmenkivi, K. Cholesterosis of the gallbladder. Acta Chir. Scand. Suppl. 324, 1964.
11. Carey, J. B., Jr. Natural history of gallstone disease. Modern Treatment 5:493, 1968.
12. Wenckert, A., and Robertson, B. The natural course of gallstone disease. Eleven-year review of 781 nonoperated cases. Gastroenterology 50:376, 1966.
13. Schein, C. J. Acute cholecystitis in the diabetic. Amer. J. Gastroent. 51:511, 1969.
14. Danzinger, R. G., et al. Dissolution of cholesterol gallstones by chenodeoxycholic acid. New Eng. J. Med. 286:1, 1972.

Chapter 87

Acute Cholecystitis

Lawrence W. Way, Marvin H. Sleisenger

ETIOLOGY

Acute cholecystitis is usually a complication of cholelithiasis, and the symptoms result from obstruction of the cystic duct by a gallstone. Although the acute attack frequently subsides spontaneously, it may progress to localized perforation with abscess formation or to generalized peritonitis. Usually the gallbladder bile in patients with acute cholecystitis is initially sterile, but as the attack continues the bile becomes infected in an increasing portion, and septic complications may develop in severe cases.[1] Rarely, repeated attacks of acute cholecystitis, particularly when associated with jaundice, may result in liver damage.

About 5 per cent of cases of acute cholecystitis occur in the absence of gallstones.[2,3] Some cases of acute acalculous cholecystitis have appeared as complications during convalescence from surgery unrelated to the biliary tree;[4] numerous such examples have recently been reported among battle casualties.[5] Bacterial infection of the gallbladder in the absence of gallstones or systemic infections may occasionally cause acute cholecystitis, but one can never exclude the possibility that the patient had passed a gallstone before surgery. In the past, infection of the gallbladder with *Salmonella typhosa* was a rare cause of acute cholecystitis. In elderly patients, an attack of acute cholecystitis may be precipitated by gallbladder carcinoma obstructing the cystic duct.

PATHOLOGY

In the initial few days of an attack of acute cholecystitis the changes in the gallbladder consist principally of hyperemia and edema.[6-8] The cystic duct is nearly always obstructed by a gallstone, and the gallbladder becomes distended with bile, inflammatory exudate, or rarely pus. The histological changes in the mucosa and underlying fibromuscular layers range from mild acute inflammation with edema and cellular infiltration to necrosis and perforation of the gallbladder wall. Early, the bile in the gallbladder is normal in appearance and consistency. Inflammation leads to absorption of bile salts and pigments, and the contents may then become replaced with thin, mucoid material, pus, or even blood. At the beginning of an acute attack, the contents of the gallbladder are usually sterile, but by the second week after the onset of symptoms they have usually become infected with enteric bacteria.[1]

After the initial attack subsides, the mucosal surface heals and the wall becomes scarred. Depending upon the amount of tissue destroyed by the infection, the absorptive capacity of the gallbladder mucosa may be damaged. The impairment may be so slight that it is of no functional importance, or it may be so severe that the gallbladder cannot be demonstrated by oral cholecystography. If the inflammation subsides but the cystic duct remains obstructed, the lumen may become distended with clear mucoid fluid (*hydrops of the gallbladder*).[9] The initial attack of acute cholecystitis may be only the first of a long series of repeated episodes of cystic duct obstruction and inflammation. Recurrent attacks in the presence of stones and infection lead to progressive scarring of the gallbladder with loss of function and further gallstone formation.

CLINICAL MANIFESTATIONS

The manifestations of acute cholecystitis loosely parallel the degree of cystic duct obstruction and mucosal inflammation, but great discrepancies are frequently observed between the clinical and pathological findings. With mild inflammation the patient may complain only of indigestion and moderate pain and tenderness in the right upper quadrant.[10, 11] With more severe inflammation, pain and tenderness increase, muscle spasm appears, and the patient becomes febrile. Murphy's sign, which consists of pain elicited upon inspiration during gentle palpation in the right subcostal region, can be demonstrated in most patients with acute cholecystitis. Localized rebound tenderness owing to peritoneal inflammation is common. Spread of pain, tenderness, and rebound tenderness throughout the rest of the abdomen may indicate perforation or an associated pancreatitis. In about one-third of patients the gallbladder is palpable in acute cholecystitis.[8] If so, it presents as a tender, sausage-like mass, extending below the right costal margin, slightly lateral to its normal location in the midclavicular line. It is more often palpable in patients suffering their first attack of cholecystitis in whom there had been no prior thickening of the gallbladder wall. In more than half of patients, the gallbladder cannot be distinguished on physical examination, principally because of tenderness and voluntary guarding. Emphysematous cholecystitis, acute cholecystitis with pericholecystic abscess, and carcinoma of the gallbladder are other conditions associated with a palpable gallbladder during an acute attack.

Marked toxicity results from acute suppurative cholecystitis. The temperature exceeds 102° F, except occasionally in the elderly. Nausea, vomiting, and abdominal distention with decreased or absent bowel sounds are common. If jaundice is present, it may indicate calculous obstruction of the common bile duct, but mild jaundice is also seen in the absence of choledocholithiasis.[12] In the latter cases the cause may be edema of the extrahepatic bile ducts or direct involvement of the liver by the adjacent inflammation. The urine commonly contains increased amounts of urobilinogen, which usually disappears within 24 to 48 hours after the infection subsides.

As a rule, an attack of cholecystitis is relatively short, lasting about a week or ten days.[8] If infection within the gallbladder continues, the organ may become filled with pus. This condition, called *empyema of the gallbladder,* may produce persistent pain and tenderness for weeks. A somewhat vague, tender mass representing the subacutely inflamed gallbladder may remain palpable for days, gradually becoming smaller and less tender until finally it can no longer be felt.

During the acute attack, the leukocyte count averages 12,000 to 15,000 mm³ with a neutrophilic leukocytosis and an increase in band forms. Serum transaminases, SGOT and SGPT, and alkaline phosphatase may be mildly elevated in the absence of intrahepatic infection or common bile duct obstruction.

Sometimes the serum amylase may exceed 1000μ per 100 ml. This does not warrant a diagnosis of acute pancreatitis in the absence of additional clinical signs or symptoms, because amylase elevations in this range may be seen in acute cholecystitis without any changes in the pancreas.

Fever of unknown origin may rarely be due to subacute or chronic cholecystitis in patients without specific symptoms or abnormal physical findings. These patients are often elderly or otherwise debilitated. In some cases this is due to a slowly resolving perforation. Rarely, fever may be secondary to a subhepatic abscess which follows an earlier attack of cholecystitis. Residual typhoid infection in the gallbladder may be the cause of mysterious fevers in some areas of the world.

DIAGNOSIS

Since acute cholecystitis is a common disease, the sudden onset of pain and tenderness in the right subcostal region should always suggest this diagnosis. In about 15 per cent of cases the gallstones can be seen on plain X-rays of the abdomen. Oral cholecystograms are unreliable during any acute abdominal illness; since nonvisualization of the gallbladder cannot be used to support the diagnosis, the test should not be ordered. On the other hand, intravenous cholangiography will usually outline the gallbladder if it is normal and fail to visualize it during acute cholecystitis.[13, 14] Intravenous cholangiograms should be ordered if the results are expected to enter into treatment decisions. However, they are superfluous in mild cases of acute cholecystitis. Regardless of the cause, if the patient is jaundiced (bilirubin > 3.0 mg per 100 ml), the gallbladder cannot be outlined by cholangiograms.

EMPHYSEMATOUS CHOLECYSTITIS

Emphysematous cholecystitis is a form of acute cholecystitis in which the gallbladder, its wall, and sometimes even the bile ducts or pericholecystic area contain gas.[15, 16] It is the manifestation of infection by gas-producing bacteria. *Clostridium welchii* has been cultured most often, but *Escherichia coli*, anerobic streptococci, and other clostridial species have been found in some patients (Fig. 84–3). Clinically the patients resemble the usual type of acute cholecystitis except that pain may be more severe and the patient more toxic. A mass is often palpable in the region of the gallbladder. About 20 per cent of these patients have diabetes mellitus; unlike other forms of acute cholecystitis, men outnumber women by a ratio of three to one. A substantial number of patients are discovered to have no stones in their gallbladders. The preponderance of men, lack of gallstones, anerobic infection, and frequency of diabetes mellitus have suggested obstruction of the cystic artery as the cause of emphysematous cholecystitis. The dif-

ferential diagnosis must consider other causes of gas in the gallbladder, principally cholecystenteric fistula. Lipomatosis of the gallbladder, a rare condition, may give a similar X-ray picture. Initial therapy should consist of high doses of antibiotics as outlined below (see pp. 1123 to 1125), in addition to other general supportive measures. Laparotomy and cholecystectomy should be performed after preoperative preparation is accomplished; cholecystostomy may be preferable to cholecystectomy in some cases. True gas gangrene of the abdominal wall (clostridial myositis) is a rare complication of emphysematous cholecystitis. The morbidity and mortality of emphysematous cholecystitis is greater than for acute cholecystitis.

DIFFERENTIAL DIAGNOSIS

If the common duct is partially obstructed, the serum transaminases, SGOT and SGPT, may be moderately elevated (200 to 500 units); however, the levels are not usually so high as in acute viral hepatitis. Very rarely, serum transaminase values may exceed 1000 units during the initial 24 to 48 hours, but thereafter they return to normal in the absence of hepatic disease. The location and character of the pain and the history of previous attacks of gallstone colic or jaundice are helpful in distinguishing cholecystitis from peptic ulcer. Free perforation of a duodenal ulcer may produce identical symptoms and findings. However, demonstration of free air in the peritoneal cavity by abdominal X-rays indicates perforated ulcer. Acute appendicitis may sometimes be mistaken for cholecystitis, particularly in patients with a high-lying cecum. The more rapid and steadily progressive symptoms in acute appendicitis may serve to distinguish the two. Sometimes the pain of pyelonephritis of the right kidney simulates cholecystitis. In pyelonephritis the maximal tenderness is usually in the loin; the presence of coexistent urinary symptoms and abnormal urinalysis also aid differentiation. A diagnosis of acute pancreatitis might be suggested by elevated amylase levels in serum or urine, but high amylase levels are sometimes seen in acute cholecystitis in the absence of pathological changes in the pancreas. It should also be remembered that cholelithiasis is an important cause of acute pancreatitis and that the two diseases may appear simultaneously (see pp. 1158 to 1183). Even a normal gallbladder may not opacify on oral or intravenous cholecystography during an attack of acute pancreatitis and often for many weeks after it subsides. An oral study will not visualize if the patient has gastric obstruction or ileus.

In all patients with right upper abdominal pain, a chest roentgenogram and an electrocardiogram should be taken to exclude right lower lobe pneumonia, pulmonary infarction, or acute myocardial infarction. Emergency lung scan may be helpful in patients in whom pulmonary embolism is likely. It is well to keep in mind that distention of the common bile duct may cause T-wave inversions in the electrocardiogram. Also, biliary tract infection and obstruction, as any intercurrent illness, may precipitate myocardial infarction. The SGOT may be elevated in both cholecystitis and myocardial infarction. However, the SGPT does not rise in myocardial disease if the patient is not in congestive failure. Occasionally cholecystitis causes cardiac arrhythmias. The most important distinguishing features are the clinical course over a 48- to 72-hour period and the pattern of serial electrocardiograms.

Rarely, patients with acute hepatitis may present with severe right upper quadrant and epigastric pain and exquisite direct and rebound abdominal tenderness. However, the white blood count is not elevated in viral hepatitis, and abnormal lymphocytes may be noted on blood smear. Serum SGOT and SGPT levels would be markedly elevated if the patient had hepatitis, the SGOT being greater than 1000 units. Patients with acute cardiac decompensation may complain of severe epigastric pain caused by acute hepatic distention; this may be accompanied by icterus. Appropriate X-rays of the biliary tract may be required to rule out acute biliary disease.

Often patients with acute alcoholic hepatitis present with fever, right upper quadrant pain, nausea, vomiting, jaundice, leukocytosis, and moderate elevations of serum transaminase. Sometimes the clinical picture may strikingly resemble cholecystitis. Although the diagnosis can usually be made by observing the patient for several days, the severity of the symptoms may suggest the need for early laparotomy. Diagnosis may be especially difficult in a cirrhotic patient with acute jaundice, upper abdominal pain, tenderness, and fever whose previously anicteric cirrhosis had been stable before a recent drinking binge. If the evidence indicates little or no change in liver function, acute cholecystitis is likely in view of the increased incidence of cholelithiasis in patients with chronic liver disease. Liver biopsy may help in differentiation in selected cases.

TREATMENT

The patient with acute cholecystitis should be admitted to the hospital for observation and treatment. Dehydration from lack of oral intake and vomiting should be corrected by intravenous administration of fluids and electrolytes to ensure adequate urinary output and normal plasma electrolytes. Oral feeding should be stopped temporarily and a nasogastric tube inserted and connected to low pressure suction. The volume aspirated must be replaced intravenously and attention paid to maintenance of plasma sodium and potassium concentrations.

Pentazocine has a theoretical advantage over morphine and meperidine for relief of pain, because it does not elevate biliary pressure. However, no clear-cut differences have yet been demonstrated, and the other drugs should be used if pentazocine provides insufficient comfort.

The earliest symptoms in biliary disease usually follow obstruction of the gallbladder or bile ducts. Ultimately bacterial infection may become superimposed and produce serious morbidity. Antibiotics should be prescribed when secondary bacterial invasion has developed, but they are of no therapeutic value before this stage. For example, the initial picture of acute cholecystitis may consist of no more than persistent severe biliary colic and right subcostal tenderness, and antibiotics need not be given. If the attack has been present for four to five days without improvement or if the clinical picture worsens, antibiotic therapy would be recommended. Ampicillin, tetracycline, cephaloridine, and chloramphenicol have been advocated for the treatment of biliary infections, because they are excreted in the bile of normal subjects. However, biliary excretion of these drugs may be impaired during acute biliary disease, and the practical significance of selecting drugs on this basis has not been established.[17, 18] In mild to moderate infections, such as the average case of acute cholecystitis, parenteral ampicillin (4 g daily) or cephaloridine (2 to 4 g daily) is recommended as an antibiotic regimen. For more advanced cases, such as perforated cholecystitis or severe cholangitis, penicillin (20 million units) with either kanamycin, (15 mg per kilogram) or gentamicin, (2.0 to 4.0 mg per kilogram) should be given parenterally in divided doses.

If the patient is critically ill with signs of generalized peritonitis, laparotomy must be performed as soon as initial resuscitative measures have been accomplished. In the toxic patient, when free perforation of the gallbladder is suspected, high doses of antibiotics should be given, as outlined above. Abdominal exploration should be deferred only until infusion of fluids has replenished volume deficits. This can usually be accomplished within a few hours after admission.

However, the average patient with acute cholecystitis does not present as a surgical emergency. Although fever and mild leukocytosis are common, the pain is usually localized, and systemic toxicity is not present. After admission to the hospital the supportive measures listed above should be instituted, but antimicrobial drugs may be withheld. During the first 12 hours of treatment, as rehydration is being accomplished, some patients will note mitigation of their symptoms. If the patient continues to improve this rapidly, the physician may allow the attack to resolve completely before performing cholecystectomy.

In most cases, the attack evolves somewhat slower, and after rehydration is satisfactory the patient will still exhibit the signs and symptoms of a continuing attack. Most surgeons prefer to schedule the patient for cholecystectomy at this point rather than to allow the attack to subside, even though the patient does not appear to be in imminent danger of complications. The technical performance of cholecystectomy during acute cholecystitis is facilitated by the pathology, which consists in the early period of edema with little in the way of fibrosis. Fibrosis becomes prominent late in the second week, at which time the operation may be more difficult, although this is not invariably true. It should be emphasized, however, that early surgery in uncomplicated acute cholecystitis does not imply that an emergency operation is required. Rather, when the decision to operate has been made, the procedure should be scheduled in the next available opening in the operating schedule during regular working hours with adequate preparations for operative cholangiography. Since about a 5 per cent incidence of false-positive diagnosis of acute cholecystitis results from considering clinical data alone, patients who are being prepared for cholecystectomy during an acute attack should have a preoperative intravenous cholangiogram. In the absence of jaundice, nonvisualization of the gallbladder further substantiates the clinical impression; visualization would rule out acute cholecystitis.

The spectrum of severity of acute cholecystitis is so broad that the attitudes of clinicians vary widely toward surgery in the acute stage. Some surgeons operate on few patients during an acute attack, choosing to perform cholecystectomy after six to 12 weeks; others operate on most patients within the first few days of hospitalization. The available evidence suggests that early operation maximizes benefit to the patient by avoiding the complications of delay and by reducing total hospitalization and length of incapacity.[8, 19-22] Obviously, individual factors may enter into many of these decisions.

When surgery is performed for acute cholecystitis, cholecystectomy will be possible in most cases. Exploration of the common bile duct is done for the same indications as in elective cholecystectomy. Sometimes the general condition of the patient is so precarious that cholecystostomy is a better choice than cholecystectomy.[23-25] This procedure consists of evacuating the gallbladder of its gallstones and infected bile and inserting a rubber tube (for example, a large Foley catheter) which is then brought out through the abdominal wall and allowed to drain by gravity. Cholecystostomy is simpler and less time consuming than cholecystectomy and solves the problem of acute cholecystitis with lower immediate morbidity and mortality in the critically ill patient. It is not adequate therapy in the presence of common duct obstruction and acute cholangitis. The incidence of cholecystostomy in an institution generally reflects the number of elderly patients who are treated for acute cholecystitis, because it is indicated mainly for those over 60 years.

After cholecystostomy, a cholangiogram should be made through the tube when the patient has fully recovered from the acute attack. If stones are seen in the gallbladder or bile ducts, cholecystectomy must be scheduled for the near future. Even in the absence of residual stones cholecystectomy should be performed to prevent recurrent symptoms in patients who regain good health. However, in elderly patients with relative contraindications to surgery whose biliary tree is clear, the cholecystostomy tube may be withdrawn and no further therapy planned unless symptoms return. More than half of such patients will develop symptomatic gallstones or biliary pain without stones within five years.

COMPLICATIONS

Perforation of the gallbladder is the most serious complication of acute cholecystitis. It may occur without a preliminary course of severe symptoms or may be the product of delay in treatment of a patient whose clinical condition gradually deteriorated. Three types of perforation occur: localized perforation with abscess formation; free perforation into the peritoneal cavity with generalized peritonitis; and perforation into an adjacent hollow viscus with formation of a cholecystenteric fistula. Surgical intervention is indicated for all three types.

LOCALIZED PERFORATION

Pericholecystic abscess is the most common type of perforation from acute chole-

cystitis.[26, 27] The initial stages of acute cholecystitis consist of cystic duct obstruction, gallbladder distention, and secondary inflammation, but the luminal contents are usually sterile. Bacterial proliferation becomes prominent after several days have elapsed, and progression to the stage of perforation may consume several days more. During this process adjacent viscera become firmly adherent to the inflamed gallbladder, and if perforation occurs it often remains localized by these adhesions. Thus the relatively slow evolution of acute cholecystitis probably accounts for the high frequency of contained perforations. High fever, right upper quadrant pain with direct and rebound tenderness, and the presence of a palpable mass all indicate this complication. Surgery must be performed to halt progression of the infection. Preoperative therapy consists of nasogastric suction, intravenous fluids, electrolytes, and potent antibiotics. If the abscess is small and the patient in good condition, the surgeon may elect to perform a cholecystectomy. However, some patients are better treated by cholecystostomy and drainage of the abscess.

FREE PERFORATION[28, 29]

Generalized bile peritonitis is associated with about a 30 per cent mortality and fortunately is seen in only 1 to 2 per cent of patients with acute cholecystitis. The disruption of the wall of the gallbladder is usually in the fundus as the result of progressive inflammation and distention. Sometimes a patient with acute cholecystitis will experience transient relief from severe pain coincident with perforation and decompression of the gallbladder into the peritoneal cavity. Then more serious symptoms evolve as purulent peritonitis becomes established. Antimicrobial drugs must be given, and abdominal exploration must be performed as an emergency. Cholecystostomy with peritoneal lavage should be carried out at the time of laparotomy.

CHOLECYSTENTERIC FISTULA

During acute cholecystitis the gallbladder may perforate into the lumen of an adjacent organ.[30-36] The duodenum is the most common site for spontaneous biliary-intestinal fistula, and the hepatic flexure of the colon is next. Fistulas to the stomach and jejunum are less common, and instances of perforation into the thoracic cavity and renal pelvis are rare. When perforation decompresses the contents of the inflamed gallbladder into the intestine, the attack of acute cholecystitis often subsides. Chronic symptoms may develop later, particularly if gallstones remain in the gallbladder. Oral cholecystography visualizes neither the gallbladder nor the fistula. In some cases a preoperative diagnosis of chronic cholecystitis has been made, and the presence of the fistula is unsuspected. If an upper gastrointestinal barium X-ray is done, it may demonstrate a cholecystoduodenal fistula; a barium enema must be performed to demonstrate chronic perforation into the colon. Uncomplicated cholecystenteric fistulas rarely produce significant morbidity. In fact, deliberate surgical anastomosis of the gallbladder to the intestine is performed frequently to bypass an obstructed common bile duct. Partial obstruction by gallstones in the gallbladder or common duct is usually present if the patient has persistent complaints. Cholecystectomy and closure of the affected bowel are curative. Exploration of the common duct will be indicated in many of these patients.

GALLSTONE ILEUS[37, 38]

This form of mechanical intestinal obstruction is caused by a gallstone impacted in the intestinal lumen which entered the bowel through a cholecystenteric fistula. The stone is nearly always 2.5 cm or greater in diameter. Most occur in elderly women, and the diagnosis should always be considered in patients over 70 years with intestinal obstruction. The absence of an external hernia or scars from a previous laparotomy would place gallstone ileus high on the list of possible causes of small bowel obstruction in this age group. Although some patients relate a history compatible with recent acute cholecystitis, the majority do not. It has been suggested that the fistula formation in patients with gallstone ileus is often caused by gradual pressure leading to erosion through the fundus by the large heavy stone instead of cystic

duct obstruction, inflammation, and perforation.

Usually the gallstone enters the bowel through a cholecystoduodenal fistula and travels a varying length aborally before stopping. It may temporarily occlude the lumen in one spot and then dislodge and move further along. This results in intermittency of the patient's symptoms and may lead the physician to think that the obstruction is partial and likely to resolve. Then complete obstruction appears when the stone finally reaches bowel too narrow to allow further progression.

Most gallstone obstructions occur in the ileum, because the diameter of the bowel diminishes from the jejunum toward the ileocecal valve. Less commonly the stone may enter the colon either after negotiating the entire small intestine or by direct passage through a cholecystocolonic fistula. Gallstone obstruction of the colon is uncommon because of the large size of its lumen. When it does occur, the obstructing stone has usually lodged in a segment narrowed by another disease process, usually chronic sigmoid diverticulitis.

The diagnosis of gallstone ileus may be suspected from clinical data such as coincidental acute cholecystitis, intermittent bowel obstruction, or age of the patient. Abdominal X-rays will show the typical findings of mechanical small bowel obstruction (see pp. 338 to 351). Air is present in the biliary tree on plain films, but it may be difficult to detect unless carefully sought. Sometimes the gallstone is radiopaque and the diagnosis is obvious. The intermittency of the obstruction occasionally leads the clinician to order an upper gastrointestinal series which visualizes an unsuspected cholecystoduodenal fistula. The delay necessary to confirm the diagnosis by barium studies is contraindicated if gallstone ileus is suspected on the basis of other data.

The mortality of gallstone ileus is high, about 15 to 20 per cent, and can be attributed mainly to delay in surgical treatment. Typically the patient has been symptomatic for several days before seeking medical care, and further delay is incurred during diagnostic efforts in a puzzling clinical situation. These elderly patients do not tolerate acute illness of this duration, and pneumonitis or cardiovascular complications are frequent.

Gallstone ileus should be treated by emergency laparotomy. The obstructing stone should be removed through a small enterotomy which is then closed. The intestine proximal to the obstruction must be carefully palpated for a second stone which could cause an immediate recurrence postoperatively. Surgical treatment of the cholecystoduodenal fistula is almost never indicated acutely. Many of these fistulas will close spontaneously, because the gallbladder has discharged its only stone.

After recovery from the operation, cholecystectomy is indicated only if chronic symptoms of gallbladder disease are present, a finding in less than half the patients. The incidence of recurrent gallstone ileus is about 2 per cent and should not be considered a factor demanding cholecystectomy.

PROGNOSIS

The overall mortality of acute cholecystitis is under 5 per cent, but several factors distinguish classes of patients in whom the death rate is high. Age is the major variable affecting mortality; nearly all patients who succumb to complications are over 60 years, and those over 70 have an even higher mortality. Most deaths are due to uncontrolled sepsis, pneumonitis, or cardiovascular complications. Acute cholecystitis is particularly lethal in patients with diabetes mellitus.[39] A high incidence of suppurative complications accounts for a mortality rate of about 20 per cent. The diabetic with acute cholecystitis should have cholecystectomy performed as soon as he can be prepared for operation. It is also wise to recommend cholecystectomy in diabetics with cholelithiasis, even in the absence of symptoms.

Common duct stones are not considered a direct complication of acute cholecystitis, but they coexist in about 15 per cent of patients. If acute cholecystitis is accompanied by jaundice and cholangitis, the morbidity increases significantly. Pancreatitis is also thought to be more a complication of choledocholithiasis than of acute cholecystitis, but patients simultaneously afflicted by both have a worse prognosis.

The stage of the pathology in the gallbladder influences the outcome substantially, as mentioned previously. Empyema, gangrene, and localized or diffuse peritonitis progressively diminish the chances of recovery. Since cholecystostomy must be done in most of these critically ill patients, clinical reports note mortality rates of about 20 per cent for this procedure.

Carcinoma of the gallbladder is found in a small percentage of patients with acute cholecystitis. Although the immediate mortality is not excessive, nearly all are dead within one year.

REFERENCES

1. Edlund, Y. A., Mollstedt, B. O., and Ouchterlony, O. Bacteriological investigation of the biliary system and liver in biliary tract disease correlated to clinical data and microstructure of the gallbladder and liver. Acta Chir. Scand. 116:461, 1959.
2. Hoerr, S. O., and Hazard, J. B. Acute cholecystitis without gallbladder stones. Amer. J. Surg. 111:47, 1966.
3. Andersson, A., Bergdahl, L., and Bonquist, L. Acalculous cholecystitis. Amer. J. Surg. 122:3, 1971.
4. Knudson, R. J., and Zuber, W. F. Acute cholecystitis in the postoperative period. New Eng. J. Med. 269:289, 1963.
5. Lindberg, E. F., Grinnan, G. L. B., and Smith, L. Acalculous cholecystitis in Viet Nam casualties. Ann. Surg. 171:152, 1970.
6. Edlund, Y., and Zettergren, L. Histopathology of the gallbladder in gallstone disease related to clinical data. Acta Chir. Scand. 116:450, 1959.
7. Edlund, Y., Lanner, O., and Olsson, O. Cholecystography and cholegraphy in gallstone disease (with notes on the causation and course of acute cholecystitis). Acta Chir. Scand. 120:366, 1961.
8. Edlund, Y., and Olsson, O. Acute cholecystitis; its aetiology and course, with special reference to the timing of cholecystectomy. Acta Chir. Scand. 120:479, 1961.
9. Gambill, E. E., Hodgson, J. R., and Priestly, J. T. Painless obstructive cholecystopathy. Arch. Intern. Med. 110:442, 1962.
10. French, E. G., and Robb, W. A. T. Biliary and renal colic. Brit. Med. J. 3:121, 1963.
11. Glenn, F. Pain in biliary tract disease. Surg. Gynec. Obstet. 122:495, 1966.
12. Fish, J. C., Williams, D. D., and Williams, R. D. Jaundice with cholecystitis. Arch. Surg. 96:875, 1968.
13. Chang, F. C. Intravenous cholangiography in the diagnosis of acute cholecystitis. Amer. J. Surg. 120:567, 1970.
14. Harrington, O. B., Beall, A. C., Jr., Noon, G., and DeBakey, M. E. Intravenous cholangiography in acute cholecystitis. Arch. Surg. 88:585, 1964.

15. May, R. E., and Strong, R.   Acute emphysematous cholecystitis. Brit. J. Surg. 58:453, 1971.
16. Rosoff, L., and Meyers, H.   Acute emphysematous cholecystitis. Amer. J. Surg. 111:410, 1966.
17. Schoenfield, L. J.   Biliary excretion of antibiotics. New Eng. J. Med. 284:1213, 1971.
18. Mortimer, P. R., Mackie, D. B., and Haynes, S.   Ampicillin levels in human bile in the presence of biliary tract disease. Brit. Med. J. 3:88, 1969.
19. Cafferata, H. T., Stallone, R. J., and Mathewson, C. W.   Acute cholecystitis in a municipal hospital. Arch. Surg. 98:435, 1969.
20. Lindahl, F., and Cederqvist, C. S.   The treatment of acute cholecystitis. Acta Chir. Scand. Suppl. 396:9, 1969.
21. van der Linden, W., and Sunzel, H.   Early versus delayed operation for acute cholecystitis. A controlled clinical trial. Amer. J. Surg. 120:7, 1970.
22. Wenckert, A., and Hallgren, T.   Evaluation of conservative treatment of acute cholecystitis. Acta Chir. Scand. 135:701, 1969.
23. Ross, F. P., and Dunphy, J. E.   Studies in acute cholecystitis. II Cholecystostomy: Indications and technique. New Eng. J. Med. 242:359, 1950.
24. Gingrich, R. A., Aew, W. C., Boyden, A. M., and Peterson, C. G.   Cholecystostomy in acute cholecystitis. Amer. J. Surg. 116:310, 1968.
25. Crosby, V. G., and Ziffren, S. E.   Cholecystostomy as definitive therapy in the aged with acute cholecystitis. J. Amer. Geriat. Soc. 13:496, 1965.
26. Essenhigh, D. M.   Perforation of the gallbladder. Brit. J. Surg. 55:175, 1968.
27. MacDonald, J. A.   Perforation of the gallbladder associated with acute cholecystitis. Ann. Surg. 164:849, 1966.
28. Abu-Dalu, J., and Urca, I.   Acute cholecystitis with perforation into the peritoneal cavity. Arch. Surg. 102:108, 1971.
29. McCarthy, J. D., and Picazo, J. G.   Bile peritonitis. Amer, J. Surg. 116:664, 1968.
30. Haff, R. C., Wise, L., and Ballinger, W. F.   Biliary-enteric fistulas. Surg. Gynec. Obstet. 133:84, 1971.
31. Piedad, O. H., and Wells, P. B.   Spontaneous internal biliary fistula, obstructive and nonobstructive types. Ann. Surg. 175:75, 1971.
32. Porter, J. M., Mullen, D. C., and Silver, D.   Spontaneous biliary-enteric fistulas. Surgery 68:597, 1970.
33. Zatzkin, H. R., Tugendhaft, R. I., and Curran, H. P.   Roentgen diagnosis of spontaneous internal biliary fistulas and gallstone ileus. Surg. Gynec. Obstet. 102:234, 1956.
34. Stull, J. R., and Thomford, N. R.   Biliary intestinal fistula. Amer. J. Surg. 120:27, 1970.
35. Sedlack, R. E., Hodgson, J. R., Butt, H. R., Stobie, G. H. C., and Judd, E. S.   Gas in the biliary tract. Gastroenterology 41:551, 1961.
36. Elsas, L. J., and Gilat, T.   Cholecystocolonic fistula with malabsorption. Ann. Intern. Med. 63:481, 1965.
37. Andersson, A. and Zederfeldt, B.   Gallstone ileus. Acta Chir. Scand. 135:713, 1969.
38. Raiford, T. S.   Intestinal obstruction caused by gallstones. Amer. J. Surg. 104:383, 1962.
39. Schein, C. J.   Acute cholecystitis in the diabetic. Amer. J. Gastroenterol. 51:511, 1969.

Chapter 88

Choledocholithiasis and Cholangitis

Lawrence W. Way, Marvin H. Sleisenger

Gallstones frequently pass from the gallbladder into the common bile duct where they remain and give rise to complications by causing biliary obstruction. About 15 per cent of patients with cholelithiasis are found to have concomitant choledocholithiasis; the association increases with the aging of the patients. Although the great majority of ductal stones originate in the gallbladder, stones may form in the intrahepatic biliary or common bile duct in special circumstances. Spontaneous passage of common duct stones into the duodenum has been well documented and may even be common with small stones. However, information on the incidence of this event is not available, and in handling clinical problems one rarely observes passage of a stone into the intestine.

PATHOLOGY AND PATHOPHYSIOLOGY

Choledocholithiasis may cause four types of complications: (1) cholangitis, (2) hepatic abscesses, (3) secondary biliary cirrhosis with hepatic failure, or (4) portal hypertension with bleeding esophageal varices. These complications also follow other causes of biliary obstruction such as biliary stricture and malignant tumors, although secondary bacterial invasion is considerably less common with malignant obstruction.

The morbidity of choledocholithiasis can be almost entirely explained on the basis of the functional obstruction to bile flow. Obstruction increases biliary pressure and diminishes the flow of bile. If bacteria enter the duct proximal to the obstruction, the clinical picture of cholangitis may result. Although obstruction does not always cause cholangitis, cholangitis requires at least some degree of obstruction. The rate of onset of obstruction, its degree, and the amount of bacterial contamination of the bile are the major additional factors which determine the type of complications caused by obstructing lesions of the bile ducts. Thus acute obstruction usually causes severe biliary colic and jaundice, whereas obstruction which has developed gradually over several months may present at first with only pruritus and without pain or even jaundice. If bacteria proliferate in the ducts, fever and chills accompany the jaundice.

Obstruction without cholangitis, seen most commonly in periampullary malignancy, creates marked dilatation of the intrahepatic bile ducts. If infection com-

1129

plicates obstruction, proximal dilatation is restricted by scarring and edema, and the caliber of the ducts may be completely normal despite nearly total occlusion.

The chills and fever of cholangitis are due to bacteremia caused by regurgitation of bacteria from the bile ducts into the bloodstream.[1, 2] Experimental studies have shown that regurgitation of particles of various sizes from bile (including bacteria) into the circulatory system is directly proportional to the height of biliary pressure and hence the degree of obstruction.[3] Multiple intrahepatic abscesses may develop after prolonged or severe cholangitis. Once multiple abscesses become established, neither antibiotics nor surgery are very successful in reversing a persistent septic course ending in death.

Secondary biliary cirrhosis may result from any lesion causing extrahepatic biliary obstruction. The rate of production of cirrhosis varies directly with the duration and extent of obstruction. The earliest that it has been reported is after three to four months of severe obstruction, but the average duration of symptoms in the few patients with choledocholithiasis who progress to cirrhosis is about five years. Once substantial hepatic damage has developed, it tends to progress slowly to biliary cirrhosis even after the cause has been removed. Hepatic failure may appear as the terminal complication in progressive biliary cirrhosis. Its evolution may be rapid in high grade obstruction such as that seen with malignancies.

Bleeding esophageal varices caused by portal hypertension is the other major end result of prolonged biliary obstruction and cirrhosis. Varices seem to be more common after prolonged incomplete obstruction, in contrast to complete blockage which tends to create hepatic failure.

CLINICAL PICTURE

There is a considerable range of clinical manifestations in choledocholithiasis. Indeed, many patients harbor stones in the bile ducts for long periods without developing symptoms.

The less severely ill patients may experience biliary colic, jaundice, or, less often, fever as an isolated symptom. Frequently these are present simultaneously. Charcot's triad consists of pain, jaundice, and fever (and chills), and comprises the classic definition of clinical cholangitis.

Patients with cholangitis fall into four groups:

1. In *acute cholecystitis with cholangitis* the jaundice, chills, and fever arise from the effects on the bile ducts of the inflamed gallbladder. Biliary duct obstruction is due to pressure from the adjacent gallbladder and reactive swelling in the periductal tissues. The degree of obstruction is usually mild and self-limited.

2. *Nonsuppurative cholangitis* is the most common type of cholangitis caused by calculous biliary obstruction, biliary stricture, and periampullary malignancy. Chills, fever, jaundice, and abdominal pain are present. Blood cultures are frequently positive during the onset of a rapid rise in temperature, but the patient is not toxic and the severe symptoms subside spontaneously or under antibiotic treatment within 24 to 48 hours.

3. *Acute suppurative (obstructive) cholangitis* consists of unremitting severe cholangitis accompanied by pus in the obstructed duct. Often these patients display mental confusion, lethargy, or septic shock. Acute suppurative cholangitis is a surgical emergency.

4. *Cholangitis with hepatic abscess*, consisting of unrelieved biliary obstruction complicated by infection, is probably the most common cause of hepatic abscess formation. Typically the abscesses are multiple and are scattered throughout the liver parenchyma. The usual course is progressively downhill, ending in a septic death.

Biliary colic in choledocholithiasis seems to be caused by rapidly increasing biliary presure owing to sudden obstruction to the flow of bile. The site, intensity, and time course of biliary colic in choledocholithiasis closely resembles cholecystolithiasis. Nausea and vomiting are more commonly associated with biliary colic produced by obstruction of the common bile duct than with blockage of the cystic duct. Also, radiation of the pain to the region of the scapula more often distinguishes common bile duct obstruction. However, these generalizations by themselves are insufficiently reliable to permit an accurate estimate of whether the symptoms originate from a stone in the cystic or the common duct.

Jaundice and dark urine usually appear within 24 hours of the onset of an attack of cholangitis. Considerable variability in the rate of appearance of jaundice may exist, depending on the site and degree of obstruction and the presence and functional condition of the gallbladder. If obstruction occurs in the common duct distal to a functioning gallbladder, the latter may dilate, concentrate bile, and delay the appearance of jaundice for a day or two. In the absence of a gallbladder, jaundice develops quickly. If obstruction is complete or nearly so, lack of bilirubin in the intestine causes the stools to become light. However, continued pigmentation of the stools cannot be used to infer the absence of an obstructive cause for the jaundice.

Fever and chills usually accompany sudden calculous obstruction, and leukocytosis parallels the febrile exacerbations. As mentioned, these symptoms are due to bacteremia from inoculation of biliary organisms into the bloodstream and signify elevated biliary pressure in the obstructed duct.

The time course of cholangitis varies in relation to the pattern of obstruction. Both transient, self-limited, mild attacks and the more severe ones causing toxicity are commonly seen in choledocholithiasis. *Once cholangitis has developed, biliary obstruction must be assumed to be present and the diagnostic process should not be concluded before a cause is found.*

An enlarged and palpable gallbladder is unusual in patients with common duct obstruction caused by a stone.[4] The gallbladder in these patients is usually scarred and nondistensible, because it has been the site of chronic cholecystitis for many years. An unscarred, pliable gallbladder in the presence of common duct obstruction may become a large, palpable mass in the right subcostal region. This finding is most frequent in obstructing malignancies and forms the basis of Courvoisier's law: in a jaundiced patient the presence of a palpable, nontender gallbladder suggests that the biliary obstruction is due to malignancy.

Hepatic enlargement may be detected in calculous biliary obstruction, and tenderness is often present in the right upper quadrant during an attack of cholangitis.

DIAGNOSTIC TESTS

Intravenous Cholangiography. Intravenous cholangiography and transhepatic cholangiography are often useful to demonstrate the site and cause of the obstruction. The intravenous administration of sodium iodopamide (Biligrafin or Cholegrafin) visualizes the common and hepatic bile ducts and demonstrates calculi in patients with incomplete obstruction without jaundice. Delineation of the common duct can be improved by tomography. Dilatation of the common bile duct may be seen after cholecystectomy, and may erroneously suggest the presence of common duct stone. Dilatation of the cystic duct stump also may be seen with this technique. As already noted, the ducts will not opacify if serum bilirubin is greater than about 3.0 mg per 100 ml or if the liver is diseased, or both (see pp. 1098 to 1109).

Percutaneous Transhepatic Cholangiography. During the past few years, the diagnosis of biliary tract obstruction by stone, stricture, or tumor has been facilitated by the ability to outline it with radiopaque dye that is injected through a needle inserted percutaneously into the parenchyma of the liver. If technically successful, the procedure may localize an obstruction or, occasionally, demonstrate a normal biliary tract, excluding extrahepatic obstruction. Usually the biliary tract cannot be visualized unless it is dilated. Bile may leak into the peritoneal cavity from the puncture site in the liver when obstruction is marked and cause bile peritonitis, for which immediate laparotomy is imperative. Transhepatic cholangiography should not be performed in the presence of active untreated cholangitis because of the serious risk of causing septicemia and septic shock.

Serum Enzymes and Tests of Liver Function. Choledocholithiasis is commonly accompanied by an elevation of the serum alkaline phosphatase. The rise may be transient in the presence of transient obstruction, and its degree is no indication of the nature or site of the obstructing lesion. Parallel elevations of the serum enzymes *5'- nucleotidase and leucine-aminopeptidase* result from ductal obstruction. All these enzymes may be significantly elevated, even when serum bilirubin is only slightly abnormal. However, the levels do not clearly differentiate extrahepatic obstructive jaundice from intrahepatic cholestasis.

Rarely in patients with cholangitis accompanying common duct obstruction, there may be transient elevation of the serum transaminases, SGOT and SGPT, in the range of 200 to 500 units. A few patients will have SGOT values greater than 1000 units. These very high elevations last for only 24 to 48 hours and are accompanied by increased LDH levels seven to ten times above normal (higher than those found in acute viral hepatitis). Liver biopsy permits differentiation from viral hepatitis in instances in which this procedure can be performed without excessive risk.

DIFFERENTIAL DIAGNOSIS[4-7]

Biliary colic can usually be identified from the patient's description. If the patient has not had a previous cholecystectomy, pain or cholangitis from choledocholithiasis must be differentiated from biliary colic caused by obstruction of the cystic duct. Sometimes acute cholecystitis without choledocholithiasis can cause cholangitis, but it is neither practical nor important to determine immediately whether or not a common duct stone is present if the patient's condition is satisfactory. After the acute attack of cholangitis has passed, an oral cholecystogram may demonstrate either the absence of gallbladder filling or the presence of stones in the gallbladder. An intravenous cholangiogram may be performed to search for common duct stones, but it is not really essential if gallbladder disease has been documented, because examination of the duct can be easily and accurately done during laparotomy for cholecystectomy. If the oral cholecystogram shows no stones in the gallbladder, an intravenous cholangiogram should be obtained, because sometimes stones are present only in the duct. In the latter situation the oral study should be repeated.

Renal and intestinal colic are rarely confused with biliary pain. The pain of renal colic starts in the flank and often radiates downward, especially to the inner surface of the thigh, or to the genitalia; dysuria and hematuria ae often present.

The pain of intestinal colic is usually generalized and crampy and is often felt somewhat more severely below the level of the umbilicus. If it is due to intestinal obstruction, there are increasing emesis, distention of the abdomen, and the auscultatory finding of high-pitched borborygmi in association with the waves of colic.

The pain of acute intermittent porphyria may closely simulate biliary colic; the presence of dark urine from uroporphyrin or of urine that becomes dark on exposure to light is of decisive importance. The presence of central or peripheral neurological findings should suggest this condition. The Ehrlich aldehyde test for porphobilinogen will be diagnostic.

An hepatic abscess, either pyogenic or amebic, may closely simulate cholangitis caused by choledocholithiasis. Patients with solitary abscesses experience right upper quadrant pain which often has an acute onset. Chills and fever are characteristic, but jaundice will be either absent or faint. Subcostal tenderness is usually present, and the liver may be palpable. An important clue to differentiation in a difficult case may be the detection of pleural fluid on the right side in patients with an abscess. Hepatic scanning should be performed if an abscess is suspected (see pp. 1392 to 1396).

The pain of acute coronary thrombosis and of choledocholithiasis may be confused. In some instances coronary thrombosis causes abdominal distress which may be localized to the right upper quadrant or epigastrium. The electrocardiogram helps in clarifying this problem. The presence of a pericardial friction rub is distinctive for myocardial infarction. Slight jaundice may follow an attack of coronary thrombosis, but it is less common than with biliary calculus, and it usually does not appear until several days after the attack. Although SGOT may be elevated in both myocardial infarction and choledocholithiasis with cholangitis, it is rare for the former to have levels higher than 100 to 150 units except in very severe cases; elevation of the SGPT will be noted in the latter but not in the former condition.

Jaundice resulting from calculous obstruction of the common bile duct must be differentiated from extrahepatic bile duct obstruction resulting from other causes (usually carcinoma of the head of the pancreas or carcinoma of the bile duct) and from intrahepatic cholestasis.

The differentiation of intrahepatic cholestasis caused by viral or toxic hepatitis from extrahepatic obstructive jaundice is the most difficult diagnostic problem in patients with disease of the liver and bile ducts. Tests of liver function, including serum enzymes, serum levels of conjugated or unconjugated bilirubin, cholesterol, and sulfobromophthalein excretion, may not be helpful in this differential diagnosis. Sometimes the liver biopsy may show histological changes that help differentiate intrahepatic from extrahepatic cholestasis. Often a percutaneous cholangiogram is necessary to exclude extrahepatic biliary obstruction (see p. 1107).

Rarely, acute viral hepatitis may be associated not only with severe right upper quadrant pain but also with exquisite tenderness, rigidity, and even rebound tenderness. The differential diagnosis may be difficult. A low or normal white blood count and particularly the presence of an abnormal number of mononuclear cells may be extremely helpful. Likewise, acute congestion of the liver, associated with cardiac decompensation, may cause intense right upper quadrant pain and even jaundice. In this condition, however, the temperature is normal, and the white blood cell count is normal or only slightly elevated. The patient has other obvious signs of cardiac decompensation, of which the enlarged tender liver may be only one feature.

The palpation of a smooth, nontender gallbladder, in association with complete biliary obstruction, indicates the possibility of carcinoma of the pancreas, common bile duct, or ampulla of Vater. Complete biliary obstruction is accompanied by the finding of less than 5 mg of fecal urobilinogen per day over a four-day period, with less than 0.3 mg of urobilinogen in the 24-hour urine. It is much more frequently associated with malignant conditions than with choledocholithiasis. Also, occult blood in the stool is often found with these diseases. Malignant obstruction of the common bile duct, pancreas, and ampulla is rarely accompanied by febrile cholangitis, which is characteristic of choledocholithiasis and biliary stricture.

TREATMENT[5, 8]

An acute attack of cholangitis should be treated with systemic antibiotics chosen for their effectiveness against enteric organisms. Ampicillin, tetracycline, chloramphenicol, and cephaloridine may have an advantage, because these drugs are excreted in bile, although on the other hand hepatic excretion is impaired in biliary obstruction. Recommended antibiotic regimens are discussed in detail on page 1123. In the majority of cases the attack can be brought under control within a day or two of the onset of treatment. If substantial improvement is not achieved within this interval, surgical therapy should be considered to abort the acute attack. If symptoms of acute suppurative cholangitis (vide infra) supervene, surgical intervention becomes a life-saving measure.

If cholangitis has resolved under medical therapy, additional diagnostic studies may be scheduled to verify the nature of the obstruction. It is important to appreciate that episodic cholangitis is always a symptom of an underlying mechanical block to biliary flow and that antibiotic treatment cannot be considered definitive. Intravenous cholangiography will be helpful if the bilirubin is dropping rapidly or is under the absolute value of 3.0 mg per 100 ml. Percutaneous transhepatic cholangiography can be dangerous in the patient whose acute cholangitis has recently subsided. In this situation injection of contrast media into the partially obstructed duct has caused reactivation of the infection and even septic shock. If the preceding acute attack was mild, this test may be carried out if appropriate systemic antibiotics are being given and if the injection into the bile ducts is made slowly. Transhepatic cholangiography should not be done in the midst of a full-blown attack of cholangitis.

After the investigations have been accomplished and choledocholithiasis is known or presumed to have caused the symptoms, the earliest possible surgical removal of the stones should be recommended. Preoperative correction of possible vitamin K deficiency is most important. If the liver is not diseased, the elevated prothrombin time will rapidly return to normal after intramuscular injection of 5 to 10 mg of vitamin K.

Many patients with common duct stones will come to treatment having suffered nothing more serious than an occasional attack of biliary colic. An oral cholecystogram will have demonstrated a gallbladder containing stones, but precise information on the status of the common duct is not available. Under these circumstances laparotomy and cholecystectomy may be performed with or without a preoperative intravenous cholangiogram. If at surgery there is reason to suspect the presence of stones in the common duct, the surgeon will either perform an operative cholangiogram or proceed directly with exploration of the duct after cholecystectomy. Pre-exploratory operative cholangiography is simple, safe, and reliable. Many surgeons advocate its use as a routine accompaniment to cholecystectomy; others restrict it to patients who have isolated minor indications for exploration which have a low yield of stones (e.g., small stones in the gall bladder). Then the decision regarding exploration is based upon the cholangiographic interpretation. If attacks of typical cholangitis have occurred or if stones can be palpated in the common bile duct, exploration may be done without preliminary operative cholangiograms.

After the common bile duct has been opened and explored and any stones removed, a T-tube is inserted and the incision in the duct is closed tightly around it. This technique provides a vent to decompress biliary pressure which could possibly cause a bile leak from the suture line. The tube can be pulled a week after surgery, and the tract from the duct through the abdominal wall closes within about 24 hours. In most cases, before extracting the T-tube a cholangiogram should be made by injecting contrast medium directly into the ducts through the tube. In spite of meticulous surgical technique about 2 per cent of patients undergoing choledochotomy are discovered to have a residual stone by the postoperative cholangiogram. Recently several methods have been devised to remove retained stones by nonsurgical means. It has been shown that by slowly infusing a solution of sodium cholate, 100 mM per liter, into the T-tube, the majority of these stones will dissolve and disappear within two weeks of start of treatment.[5] Another way to treat retained stones is to pass a ureteral stone basket into the duct under radiological control. Small to moderate-sized stones can sometimes be pulled out this

way without another laparotomy. If these indirect methods fail, re-exploration should be performed unless there are overriding contraindications to further surgery.

COMPLICATIONS

Acute cholangitis frequently accompanies ductal obstruction by stone. Suppurative cholangitis and focal hepatic abscesses may result from the presence of pathogenic organisms, and may threaten the life of the patient. Chronic obstruction with infection may lead to secondary biliary cirrhosis.

Acute, recurrent, and chronic pancreatitis is often related to calculous biliary tract disease (see pp. 1158 to 1197).

ACUTE SUPPURATIVE (OBSTRUCTIVE) CHOLANGITIS

Acute suppurative cholangitis[9, 10] is a severe type of biliary infection in which pus is found in the obstructed bile ducts and persistent septicemia is present. The obstruction is usually caused by stones in the common bile duct, but may be secondary to a stricture or rarely a periampullary carcinoma.

PATHOLOGY

The bile ducts, both intrahepatic and extrahepatic, are dilated above the site of obstruction, which is usually in the common bile duct. There is inflammatory thickening of the wall of the ducts. The liver is enlarged, and in fatal cases there may be multiple abscess cavities in the hepatic parenchyma. Microscopic examination of a liver biopsy specimen reveals *pericholangitis* with acute and chronic inflammatory cells (neutrophils, lymphocytes, and plasma cells) within and adjacent to the portal spaces. Occasionally polymorphonuclear leukocytes may be visualized within small bile ducts. Necrosis of hepatic parenchymal cells may occur in periportal areas; occasionally microabscesses will be formed. With prolonged obstruction there may be large areas of parenchymal necrosis with extravasation of bile (bile infarcts or bile lakes).

The term *cholangitis lenta* signifies a rare hematogenous form of suppurative cholangitis in the absence of biliary obstruction with which secondary endocarditis may be associated. The blood stream is probably seeded in most patients, but bacteremia is not always demonstrable by blood culture.

CLINICAL MANIFESTATIONS

Acute suppurative cholangitis results from the same pathophysiological processes as nonsuppurative cholangitis. However, it is worthwhile to separate this condition as a distinct clinical entity, because it is characterized by distinct clincal manifestations, and, if unrecognized, it will be rapidly fatal in the absence of surgical therapy.

The clinical counterparts of biliary obstruction and infection are usually present. The attack begins with biliary colic, chills, high fever, and jaundice. Hepatic enlargement and tenderness are noted on physical examination.

In acute suppurative cholangitis optimal conditions for progressive biliary infection result in actual pus formation proximal to the obstruction. Persistent systemic sepsis is present and the patient becomes toxic. Mental confusion, lethargy, and drowsiness are ominous signs of toxicity whose clinical significance must not be overlooked, for they herald approaching septic death. Unremitting high fever, leukocytosis, and clinical toxicity with altered mentation comprise the usual manifestations of suppurative cholangitis. Although jaundice of some degree is nearly always present, the level is under 5 mg per 100 ml in many. Unfortunately for the clinician, suppurative cholangitis may also be present in elderly patients in the absence of high or sustained fever or leukocytosis, in which case the patient's confusion may be the principal clue to the seriousness of the condition.

In the course of suppurative cholangitis with high grade or complete obstruction, septicemia may cause instability of the blood pressure or bona fide shock. Obviously when septicemia has created lability of the circulatory system, the outlook is grave, but prompt resuscitation and choledochotomy can be expected to save about two-thirds of the patients.

DIAGNOSIS

Suppurative cholangitis should be suspected in any patient with right upper quadrant pain, chills, fever, jaundice, leukocytosis, and subcostal tenderness. A previous history of biliary colic, cholecystectomy, or proved cholelithiasis should enhance suspicion. Failure of apparent nonsuppurative cholangitis to improve after treatment with antibiotics for a day or two signifies the possibility that suppurative cholangitis is present. Mental confusion and an unstable blood pressure are signs of clinical deterioration.

Blood cultures should be taken; they usually reveal the same organisms that are present in the bile ducts. White blood cell counts range from 5000 to 30,000 mm,[3] but more commonly they are 15,000 or above. Depending upon the duration of obstruction, the bilirubin varies from being slightly elevated to about 15 mg per 100 ml. A substantial percentage of patients will have values in the range of 3 to 5 mg per 100 ml. Thrombocytopenia is characteristic of the most acute phase; it has not been reported to lead to hemorrhagic complications during laparotomy and need not be treated. Hypoglycemia often accompanies the presence of mental changes such as lethargy and confusion. Treatment with hypertonic glucose solutions is said to be of therapeutic value.

Amebic or cryptogenic bacterial hepatic abscess may present with a similar clinical picture. Radiological demonstration of reactive fluid in the pleural cavity may suggest these entities. However, suppurative cholangitis sometimes presents with intrahepatic abscesses as a complication. Toxic patients in whom the distinction cannot be made should be treated surgically.

Pylephlebitis resulting from septic foci elsewhere in the abdomen might be confused with suppurative cholangitis. Knowledge of the presence of a source for the metastatic infection would aid diagnosis. In any case pylephlebitis has become quite uncommon in recent years.

TREATMENT

The patient with suppurative cholangitis may improve spontaneously but temporarily if the obstruction is partially relieved by movement of calculi in the common duct, but this event is infrequent and unpredictable. Surgery should be considered mandatory as an emergency procedure unless there is sudden subsidence of symptoms during preoperative preparation.

Preoperative treatment should consist of immediate systemic administration of antibiotics and institution of measures designed to restore circulatory homeostasis. Antibiotic solutions, plasma, or whole blood should be given as necessary for the treatment of septic shock. Simultaneous measurement of central venous pressure, arterial blood pressure, and urinary output via a Foley catheter must be carried out when judging the adequacy of volume replacement. Pharmacological doses of corticosteroid drugs have an uncertain role in treatment of septic shock. Digitalis or isoproterenol may be indicated for its inotropic effect on the heart if restitution of circulatory volume does not lead to improvement in blood pressure and urinary output.

The blood sugar should be measured at intervals and sufficient hypertonic glucose solution given to restore values to the normal range.

Laparotomy should be performed as soon as these resuscitative measures have been accomplished. It is paradoxical to conclude that the patient is too sick for surgery, because relief of the biliary obstruction has been shown to be the only chance for survival for the sickest of these patients. The surgical treatment consists first of opening the common bile duct. Often the purulent bile will escape as if trapped under considerable pressure. If the patient is critically ill, choledochotomy and insertion of a T-tube are the simplest measures that can be counted on to relieve the sepsis. If, on the other hand, the patient's condition is relatively good and is stable, common duct exploration with extraction of stones or the correction of an obstructing stricture may be advisable, and cholecystectomy could be performed if the gallbladder is still present.

When bile flow has been re-established by surgical drainage of the common bile duct, the full effectiveness of antimicrobial therapy can then be attained.

ORIENTAL CHOLANGIOHEPATITIS

Oriental cholangiohepatitis[11, 12] is a chronic recurrent pyogenic cholangitis which affects mainly Chinese and is most prevalent in the south of China. In Hong Kong it is the most common disease of the biliary tract and is the third most frequent cause of acute abdominal pain requiring surgical intervention. In Western countries cholangiohepatitis must be considered as a cause of cholangitis in immigrants from Asia.

ETIOLOGY AND PATHOLOGY

A close but inexact correlation exists between the distribution of cholangiohepatitis and infestation with *Clonorchis sinensis*. This parasitic fluke is acquired by ingesting raw fresh-water fish. The parasite migrates from the duodenum into the biliary tree where it takes up prolonged residence. Inflammation of the ductal epithelium occurs at focal points throughout the intra- and extrahepatic biliary tree. Stone formation is facilitated by the inflammation and scarring and may be further enhanced by excessive excretion of bilirubin in patients also suffering from malaria. Secondary bacterial infection becomes established when sludge and stones cause obstruction to the duct. The process primarily affects the bile ducts, but in 15 per cent of patients stones are present in the gallbladder.

CLINICAL MANIFESTATIONS

The patient suffers from recurrent attacks of abdominal pain and cholangitis. Pain either in the epigastrium or right upper abdominal quadrant is the first symptom. Nausea and vomiting are usually present. Chills, fever, and jaundice appear as an attack progresses, but subclinical elevations of bilirubin are common even in severely toxic patients.

Since the gallbladder is spared from the

major effects of the disease, it is usually palpable when the subcostal region is examined during an acute attack. Occasionally pronounced distention of the organ leads to tenderness, and in a few patients free perforation and bile peritonitis have occurred.

DIAGNOSIS

Cholangiohepatitis must be considered in Chinese patients with right upper quadrant pain who have spent prolonged periods of time in the Orient. *Clonorchis sinensis* ova can be demonstrated in the stools of most patients, but this by itself is not diagnostic because many people of similar background without clinical disease have positive stool examinations.

Oral or intravenous cholangiograms will not visualize the bile ducts during an acute attack.

The presence of a palpable gallbladder in this disease during an acute attack of cholangitis allows differentiation from cholangitis caused by cholesterol gallstones. Empyema of the gallbladder, carcinoma of the gallbladder, emphysematous cholecystitis, and an occasional case of cholangitis complicating periampullary malignancy would be other causes of a right subcostal tender mass in a patient with acute cholangitis.

TREATMENT

Antibiotics should be given parenterally. If the attack is severe, laparotomy should be performed. The common duct will usually contain multiple palpable stones. An enlarged, tense gallbladder which is secondarily inflamed is usually encountered. Choledochotomy must be performed and the common duct cleared of stones and debris. Operative cholangiography may reveal multiple strictures of the biliary ducts with proximal obstruction and stone formation. It may be impossible to entirely rid the ducts of stones. A side-to-side choledochoduodenostomy seems to be the surgical treatment most likely to provide drainage of the large common duct which is usually encountered. Cholecystectomy should be performed as well.

If abscesses have formed in the liver, they may be drained, but the prognosis at this stage is poor. For some reason there is a predilection for abscesses to affect the left lobe of the liver more often than the right.

SCLEROSING CHOLANGITIS

Sclerosing cholangitis[13-15] is a rare condition in which the bile ducts are involved by a stenosing inflammatory process of unknown origin. Patients generally present with jaundice or pruritus. Initially the degree of obstruction may fluctuate, but later it becomes constant and severe. Attacks of fever and chills are uncommon in the absence of previous surgery on the biliary system.

Many of these patients have ulcerative colitis, and a few others have been reported with regional enteritis, retroperitoneal fibrosis, mediastinal fibrosis, or retroorbital tumors. Diagnostic tests reveal changes typical of extrahepatic obstruction of the ducts. Antimitochondrial antibodies are usually absent from the serum. Intravenous and oral cholangiography rarely visualize the pathological ducts because of obstruction. The diagnosis is usually made only at laparotomy.

The operative findings consist of marked thickening of the entire extrahepatic bile ducts and sometimes edema of the adjacent tissues. It is often difficult for the surgeon to find the tiny lumen in the common duct. Indeed, it may even be totally obliterated. The wall of the duct is thickened and is comprised mainly of collagen scar with generally few inflammatory cells. In most cases the process has been confined to the extrahepatic ducts, but total ductal involvement and isolated stenosis of the intrahepatic system have also been reported.

Certain malignancies of the bile ducts present as strictures. Biopsies of the stenotic duct must be taken during laparotomy to differentiate between these desmoplastic tumors and sclerosing cholangitis.

At surgery the ducts should be dilated and a T-tube inserted. Prompt symptomatic improvement can be expected if the T-tube provides significant drainage. The tube should be left in place for six months or more if it has not become obstructed. Since the largest tube that the lumen of the duct will accommodate is about No. 10 or 12 French, it tends to become obstructed from precipitated debris rather early. A number of patients have been treated with systemic steroids with apparent good response, so this therapy is recommended to be started postoperatively.

The outcome is unpredictable. A rare patient may appear to recover completely; others progress to secondary biliary cirrhosis and its complications. Improvement is common enough that no patient should be deprived of the potential benefit of treatment. When sclerosing cholangitis and ulcerative colitis appear together, treatment of the colonic disease is thought not to affect the cholangitis.

REFERENCES

1. Williams, R. D., Fish, J. C., and Williams, D. C. The significance of biliary pressure. Arch Surg. 95:374, 1967.
2. Huang, T., Bass, J. A., and Williams, R. D. The significance of biliary pressure in cholangitis. Arch. Surg. 98:629, 1969.
3. Jacobsson, B., Kjellander, J., and Rosengren, B. Cholangiovenous reflux. Acta Chir. Scand. 123:316, 1962.
4. Schenker, S., Balint, J., and Schiff, L. Differential diagnosis of jaundice: Report of a prospective study of 61 proved cases. Amer. J. Dis. 7:449, 1968.
5. Way, L. W., Admirand, W. H., and Dunphy, J. E. Management of choledocholithiasis. Ann. Surg. 176:347, 1972.
6. Almersjo, O., Hultborn, K. A., and Jensen, C. Diagnosis of choledocholithiasis. Acta Chir. Scand. 141:112, 1966.
7. Madden, J. L., Vanderheyden, L., and Kandalaft, S. The nature and surgical significance of common duct stones. Surg. Gynec. Obstet. 126:3, 1968.
8. Smith, R. B., Conklin, E. F. and Porter, M. R. A five-year study of choledocholithiasis. Surg. Gynec. Obstet. 116:731, 1963.
9. Hinchey, E. J., and Couper, C. E. Acute obstructive suppurative cholangitis. Amer. J. Surg. 117:62, 1969.
10. Dow, R. W., and Linderauer, S. M. Acute obstructive suppurative cholangitis. Ann. Surg. 169:272, 1969.
11. Ong, G. B. A study of recurrent pyogenic cholangitis. Arch. Surg. 84:199, 1962.
12. Stock, F. E., and Fung, J. H. Y. Oriental cholangiohepatitis. Arch. Surg. 84:409, 1962.
13. Warren, K. W., Athanassiades, S., and Monge, J. I. Primary sclerosing cholangitis. Amer. J. Surg. 111:23, 1966.
14. Thorpe, M. E. C., Scheuer, P. J., and Sherlock, S. Primary sclerosing cholangitis, the biliary tree, and ulcerative colitis. Gut 8:435, 1967.
15. Bhathal, P. S., and Powell, L. W. Primary intrahepatic obliterating cholangitis: A possible variant of sclerosing cholangitis. Gut 10:886, 1969.

Chapter 89

Neoplasms of the Gallbladder and Bile Ducts

Lawrence W. Way, Marvin H. Sleisenger

CARCINOMA OF THE GALLBLADDER

ETIOLOGY AND INCIDENCE

Carcinoma of the gallbladder[1-3] is an uncommon neoplasm which occurs mainly in elderly patients. About 80 per cent of patients have coexisting gallstones, which strongly suggests an etiological relationship between stones and subsequent malignant degeneration. The incidence in females is about four times greater than that in males and corresponds to the relative frequency of gallstones in the two sexes.

PATHOLOGY

Both adenocarcinomas and squamous cell carcinomas arise in the gallbladder, but the latter are rare. The adenocarcinomas can be divided into those with a scirrhous pattern (55 per cent), papillary adenocarcinomas (25 per cent), and mucinous or colloid tumors (15 per cent). Growth of the tumors is rapid, and spread outside the gallbladder is virtually certain by the time symptoms have appeared. The cancer invades the liver and other adjacent structures and extends as well by metastasis. Both types of spread are generally present. Regional lymph nodes in the hilum of the liver are involved early, and abdominal carcinomatosis develops in many patients. Pulmonary metastases are common, and secondary pulmonary complications often lead to the patient's death.

Obstruction of the cystic duct or common bile duct by the enlarging growth may cause acute cholecystitis or obstructive jaundice with or without cholangitis (see pp. 1120 to 1127).

CLINICAL MANIFESTATIONS

Most patients with carcinoma of the gallbladder previously have had intermittent symptoms of chronic cholecystitis. They often report having experienced symptoms similar to those which had been noted before, but with increased intensity and persistence for the past several months. Abdominal pain is common and, as noted, may be part of an attack of acute cholecystitis. The presence of a palpable mass in the region of the gallbladder in an

1139

elderly patient with acute or chronic cholecystitis should strongly suggest the diagnosis.

If obstructive jaundice is present, it will usually be associated with a mass which can be felt. Cholangitis may appear and provide conditions favorable for intrahepatic abscess formation. Local abscesses may also develop adjacent to the gallbladder or in areas of the liver involved by direct invasion.

Death is usually a complication of malnutrition and bronchopneumonia or uncontrolled sepsis in the liver.

TREATMENT

There is no effective treatment for carcinoma of the gallbladder. The great majority of these tumors have spread beyond the scope of surgical resection by the time the diagnosis is made. Neither radiotherapy nor chemotherapy has much beneficial effect. The handful of survivors of this disease consist for the most part of patients in whom the tumor was an incidental finding when the gallbladder was examined after cholecystectomy for cholelithiasis. In the absence of obvious distant spread, laparotomy is indicated despite the poor prognosis, because resectability of the tumor should be judged by direct inspection. Rarely radical excision of the gallbladder and an adjacent portion of liver may be warranted but only if it appears to offer chance for cure. Unfortunately, about 90 per cent of such patients are dead within one year of diagnosis.

Since somewhat more than half of those who die of this disease have been known for some time to harbor symptomatic gallstones, these patients theoretically could have been saved by performing cholecystectomy before the tumor arose. The possibility of future development of cancer of the gallbladder is probably a valid argument for elective cholecystectomy, particularly if confined to young patients with asymptomatic stones.

CARCINOMA OF THE EXTRAHEPATIC BILE DUCTS

Malignant tumors of the extrahepatic bile ducts[4-6] are less common than primary gallbladder carcinoma, but are not rare in afebrile patients with cholestatic jaundice. The association of carcinoma of the extrahepatic bile ducts with cholelithiasis is less (40 to 50 per cent) than for gallbladder carcinoma, and the incidence is about equal for males and females. Thus cholelithiasis seems less likely to play a causative role in bile duct tumors. There appears to be an increased incidence of bile duct malignancy in patients with chronic ulcerative colitis, and the tumor presents at an earlier age in these patients. The greater incidence of biliary carcinoma in the Orient is at least in part due to the chronic effects of *Clonorchis sinensis* infestation.

PATHOLOGY

The tumors arise principally from the common hepatic duct or common bile duct and less often from the cystic duct. By the time laparotomy is performed it may be impossible to pinpoint the origin of the tumor because of extension and invasion of much of the space in the liver hilum. The cell type is nearly always an adenocarcinoma, but there is a wide range in the histological appearance, depending on the amount of fibrous stroma present between cells. In fact, some of these tumors are so acellular that a histological diagnosis may be difficult unless several biopsy specimens are taken from differing sites.

Jaundice develops early because of the strategic location of bile duct cancers, so they are frequently small when initially discovered. Unfortunately many have already metastasized, and invasion of contiguous structures has rendered most of the remainder incurable by the time surgical exploration is performed.

Secondary complications of biliary obstruction are the cause of death in most cases.

CLINICAL MANIFESTATIONS

Obstructive jaundice is usually the first clinical manifestation, although it is occasionally preceded by pruritus. Weight loss appears in most patients. Cholangitis and biliary colic are distinctly uncommon, and the bile has been sterile in most patients in whom it has been cultured. A deeply felt abdominal pain unlike that in biliary colic is reported by many of these patients. The course may be painless.

The liver becomes enlarged and firm; the spleen is not enlarged unless obstruction has been present long enough to produce biliary cirrhosis. A palpable gallbladder is present if the obstruction is confined to the common bile duct, leaving the cystic duct uninvolved. If the cystic duct is obstructed, the gallbladder usually becomes collapsed and contains only a small volume of clear, thin fluid. Gallbladder distention is also absent when the tumor arises from or involves the common hepatic duct.

DIAGNOSIS

Primary biliary tumors should be considered in the differential diagnosis of any case of obstructive jaundice. Malignant obstruction generally produces higher levels of bilirubin than are seen in choledocholithiasis, with a mean value being about 18 mg per 100 ml.

Tumors of the common bile duct produce a clinical picture similar to that of carcinoma of the head of the pancreas, carcinoma of the ampulla of Vater, and primary adenocarcinoma of the duodenum. Collectively these four lesions are termed *periampullary carcinomas*, and it may be impossible to distinguish between them on the basis of information available before surgical exploration. Typically, the gallbladder is prominent as a palpable mass emerging beneath an enlarged liver. The presence of a nontender palpable gallbladder in obstructive jaundice is a highly reliable indication that the cause of the obstruction is neoplastic (Courvoisier's law). However, failure to detect an enlarged gallbladder by physical examination does not have similar significance, and cannot be held to rule out obstruction by tumor, because (1) the hepatic enlargement may override a distended gallbladder and shield it from the examiner's hand, or (2) concomitant cystic duct obstruction in the absence of cholelithiasis may prevent the gallbladder from distending with bile, and (3) the tumor may be located in the common hepatic duct.

An upper gastrointestinal X-ray exami-

nation may suggest that a suspected periampullary tumor has arisen from the ampulla of Vater or head of the pancreas. In the early stages the jaundice may fluctuate in intensity with tumors of the ampulla and of the bile ducts, but this is uncommon for lesions in the head of the pancreas. Examination of the stool for occult blood is most often positive in ampullary tumors, but repeated testing in pancreatic tumors will usually demonstrate blood, and biliary tumors may occasionally cause the same reaction.

Transhepatic cholangiography is of great value in demonstrating malignant obstruction of the biliary tree (Fig. 89-1). Technically the study can be done successfully in the majority of patients. The intrahepatic bile ducts are nearly always greatly distended, and injection of the contrast agent delineates the site of obstruction in the hepatic hilum.

The most difficult diagnostic problem for the clinician occurs in patients without a palpable gallbladder. The gradual onset of jaundice or pruritus with little pain and no fever resembles intrahepatic cholestasis. Often these patients have been followed for months and even years with a presumptive diagnosis of primary biliary cirrhosis or toxic (drug) hepatitis with cholestasis. Since nausea and anxiety are early reactions by the patient to the illness,

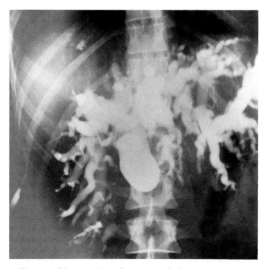

Figure 89-1. Transhepatic cholangiogram in a patient with adenocarcinoma of the bile duct. Since the tumor involved the cystic duct, the gallbladder was not distended and was not visualized on the X-ray.

drugs such as chlorpromazine or prochlorperazine have often been prescribed at some point for symptomatic purposes and then later become considered as causative agents when jaundice develops.

Primary biliary cirrhosis occurs mainly in women between the ages of 40 and 60 years. Demonstration of antibodies reactive against mitochondrial membranes is positive in about 90 per cent of patients with primary biliary cirrhosis. Recent reports indicate a high incidence of mitochondrial antibodies in patients with long-standing extrahepatic biliary obstructions such as occurs with malignant tumors. Thus one must not rely entirely on this test for distinguishing primary biliary cirrhosis from surgical jaundice.

HAA antigen titers have been reported to be positive in some patients with hepatic tumors, and we have seen a positive reaction in a patient with a primary biliary carcinoma in whom no other cause was evident.

Liver biopsy may at times permit differentiation of intrahepatic from extrahepatic cholestasis, but the diagnostician must appreciate the imperfect reliability of this and other tests. A wise approach is to assume an extrahepatic obstructive cause for cholestatic jaundice until it has been eliminated as a possibility. This course will lead to diagnostic laparotomy or transhepatic cholangiography as definitive examinations in many patients and should obviate the many instances of excessive delay in discovering these biliary tumors.

It has been pointed out by several physicians that *adenocarcinoma of the junction of the hepatic ducts* presents as a distinct clinical entity. Usually the tumors in this location are slow growing, and they rarely metastasize early. Morbidity is essentially that of biliary obstruction, and the indolent growth characteristics of the tumor create a clinical picture resembling diseases with intrahepatic cholestasis. Minimal elevation of bilirubin and a moderately to markedly raised level of alkaline phosphatase and leucine amino peptidase are early findings of obstruction of only one hepatic duct. As the tumor grows, biliary flow is obstructed by occlusion of the junction of the right and left hepatic ducts.

These tumors present a diagnostic trap for the unwary surgeon. When laparotomy is performed a small common bile duct and a collapsed gallbladder may be noted. The tumor itself, high in the hilum, may be entirely hidden from view; indeed, there may be no more than a focal stricture of the common hepatic duct by tumor with no hint of neoplasm in external tissues. Exploration of the common bile duct must be carried out, and attempts should be made to pass probes into the intrahepatic bile ducts. Obstruction to passage of the probe indicates the presence of a tumor. Operative cholangiograms must be sufficient to outline the bifurcation of the common hepatic duct. Although these tumors are usually unresectable, considerable palliation can be expected in some patients by inserting a rubber stent across the obstructing tumor to re-establish biliary flow. Survival with such treatment has been reported for as long as five years in some patients.

TREATMENT

Surgical treatment has more to offer the patient with primary carcinoma of the bile ducts than those with gallbladder malignancy. Although cure is still uncommon, resection may be accomplished in some patients. Radical pancreaticoduodenectomy (Whipple procedure) may be performed for tumors of the distal common bile duct if the resected specimen is likely to encompass all the gross tumor. However, this procedure is too extensive and the morbidity is too high for palliation. Often involvement of the portal vein or other nearby structures excludes the possibility of resection for cure. In these cases some procedure should be performed to facilitate entry of bile into the intestine. Usually, either a cholecystojejunostomy or choledochoduodenostomy will relieve jaundice and pruritus.

Tumors of the proximal extrahepatic bile ducts should be removed if this is technically feasible. The extensive fibrous stroma and the localized involvement of some of these tumors may suggest the presence of sclerosing cholangitis or a benign post-traumatic stricture and lead to inadequate therapy. *It is a useful clinical axiom to consider any focal stricture which develops in the absence of previous biliary surgery to be malignant until proved otherwise.*

The palliative value of placing a stent across unresectable tumors of the bile ducts has been mentioned above. Even in incurable cases the relief of symptoms is sufficiently great to emphasize the need for accurately diagnosing these tumors.

BENIGN TUMORS AND PSEUDOTUMORS OF THE GALLBLADDER[7, 8]

A variety of rare conditions may produce polypoid projections on cholecystograms or may be discovered by examining the specimen after cholecystectomy. The literature on this topic is confusing because of the lack of a common nomenclature. It has been difficult to establish whether these lesions are truly responsible for producing symptoms, partly because of their scarcity. Physicians who have studied these conditions most carefully have generally concluded that each may be symptomatic, but that they also exist many times in patients who are free of complaints. This is not difficult to accept, because it is the same situation that gallstones have relative to symptom production (see pp. 1103 to 1105).

POLYPS

These entities are not true neoplasms. Cholesterol "polyps" are the most common type. They are often noted on the cholecystogram as single or multiple small intraluminal projections. Histologically they consist of localized aggregations of lipid-filled histiocytes within the lamina propria. They are easily detached from the epithelial surface when the gallbladder is manipulated, and then they may be found floating free in the bile. Cholesterol polyps seem to be due to a process closely related to cholesterosis of the gallbladder. The two conditions differ only in extent, with the former consisting of focal and the latter, diffuse involvement of the wall. It seems likely that at least some patients with cholesterol "polyps" have symptoms which originate from the gallbladder, but whether this is directly due to the "polyps" themselves is unclear.

Inflammatory polyps are much less common than cholesterol polyps.

ADENOMATOUS HYPERPLASIA

Adenomatous hyperplasia is probably a developmental defect of the gallbladder wall. In any case, it, too, is non-neoplastic. It consists of hyperplastic smooth muscle intermingled with epithelial-lined sinuses. Adenomatous hyperplasia has been called a number of different things, among which are adenomyomatosis, cholecystitis glandularis proliferans, and diverticulosis. Most occur as localized patches in the fundus of the organ. Radiologically there may be nothing abnormal seen on the cholecystogram, or there may be an impression into the contour of the lumen punctuated by a central umbilication. There is nothing to suggest that adenomatous hyperplasia predisposes to malignancy. There are a number of well documented instances in which cholecystectomy relieved postprandial right upper quadrant pain which had been present for many years.

ADENOMAS

Adenomas are true neoplasms of the mucosa which usually have a pedunculated configuration. Histologically, they may be papillary or nonpapillary. This is the most common benign neoplasm of the gallbladder. Although several have been found in association with carcinoma in situ, the relationship is infrequent.

MISCELLANEOUS

Other rare benign lesions are hemangiomas, granular cell tumors, fibroxanthogranulomas, and gastric heterotopic cell rest.

BENIGN TUMORS OF THE EXTRAHEPATIC BILE DUCTS[9]

About 90 cases of benign tumors of the extrahepatic bile ducts have been reported, making them a rare cause of obstructive jaundice. Histologically they consist of papillomas and adenomas. Some of the patients have developed occult blood in their stools from bleeding by the tumors (hematobilia). Operative cholangiography usually depicts the site of the lesion, and common duct exploration uncovers the cause. Local excision is satisfactory treatment for those that arise from the papilla of Vater, but benign tumors of the ducts themselves must be radically excised. If they are not, the recurrence rates are unacceptably high.

REFERENCES

1. Appleman, R. M., Morlock, C. G., Dahlin, D. C., and Adson, M. A. Long-term survival in carcinoma of the gallbladder. Surg. Gynec. Obstet. *117*:459, 1963.
2. Pemberton, L. B., Diffenbaugh, W. F., and Strohl, E. L. The surgical significance of carcinoma of the gallbladder. Amer. J. Surg. *122*:381, 1971.
3. Solan, M. J., and Jackson, B. T. Carcinoma of the gallbladder. A clinical appraisal and review of 57 cases. Brit. J. Surg. *58*:593, 1971.
4. Altemeier, W. A., Gall, E. A., Zinninger, M. M., and Hoxworth, P. I. Sclerosing carcinoma of the major intrahepatic bile ducts. Arch. Surg. *75*:450, 1957.
5. Klatskin, G. Adenocarcinoma of the hepatic duct at its bifurcation within the porta hepatis. Amer. J. Med. *38*:241, 1965.
6. Van Heerden, J. A., Judd, E. S., and Dockerty, M. B. Carcinoma of the extrahepatic bile ducts. A clinicopathologic study. Amer. J. Surg. *113*: 49, 1967.
7. Christensen, A. H., and Ishak, K. G. Benign tumors and pseudotumors of the gallbladder. Report of 180 cases. Arch. Path. *90*:423, 1970.
8. Selzer, D. W., Dockerty, M. B., Stauffer, M. H., and Priestley, J. T. Papillomas (so-called) in the non-calculous gallbladder. Amer. J. Surg. *103*:472, 1962.
9. Burhans, R., and Myers, R. T. Benign neoplasms of the extrahepatic biliary ducts. Amer. Surg. *37*:161, 1971.

Chapter 90

Postoperative Syndromes

Lawrence W. Way, Marvin H. Sleisenger

BILIARY STRICTURE

Benign biliary strictures[1-5] are caused by surgical trauma in about 95 per cent of cases. The remainder are the result of external abdominal trauma or, rarely, are from erosion of the duct by a gallstone. Biliary stricture was more frequent in the past when many cholecystectomies were performed by incompletely trained surgeons. This aspect of the problem has not yet been eliminated, but improvement is continuing. Operations in the hilum of the liver require not only technical skill and experience but also a thorough knowledge of the normal anatomy and its variations in order to avoid the technical pitfalls that result in inadvertent injury to the ducts. However, after all preventive measures have been exhausted, iatrogenic trauma will still be seen occasionally, because operations on the gallbladder are so common.

The surgeon may or may not recognize at the operation that the duct has been damaged. If the duct has been transected, it should be repaired and a T-tube inserted through a nearby choledochotomy. Just as often, the event goes unnoticed. The varieties of injury consist of transection, incision, excision of a segment, or occlusion of the duct by a ligature. Sometimes the accident can be attributed to technical difficulties resulting from advanced pathology.

Signs of an injury to the duct may or may not be evident in the postoperative period. If complete occlusion has been produced, jaundice will develop rapidly; but more often a rent has been made in the duct, and the earliest sign may be excessive or prolonged drainage of bile from the drains after surgery. The leak contributes to the development of localized infection which accentuates scar formation and development of a fibrous stricture.

CLINICAL FINDINGS

Depending on the severity of the trauma and the amount of aggravating infection, symptoms may be produced within two weeks or as late as a year or more after the operation. However, it is rare that more than two years separate the trauma and its initial symptoms. Cholangitis which appears after this period would more likely be due to common duct stones than to stricture.

Cholangitis is the most common syndrome produced by stricture. In the typical case the patient notices episodes of pain, fever, chills, and mild jaundice within a few weeks to months after cholecystectomy. Antibiotics are usually suc-

1145

cessful in controlling the symptoms, but additional attacks occur at irregular intervals. The pattern of symptoms varies between patients, from mild transient attacks to severe toxicity with suppurative cholangitis.

Sometimes documentation of an operative injury is available, and other patients present with a history of previous operative procedures for stricture repair. When cholangitis develops in either of these types of patients, a diagnosis of recurrence of the stricture is virtually certain.

Physical findings are not distinctive. The right upper quadrant may be tender, but it usually is not. Jaundice can usually be detected during an attack of cholangitis.

LABORATORY FINDINGS

An intravenous cholangiogram may outline the stricture if the study can be done at a time when the bilirubin is normal. In other cases transhepatic cholangiograms have been invaluable.[6] Failure to enter the intrahepatic bile ducts when attempting a transhepatic cholangiogram does not rule against stricture as the cause of symptoms. In some patients the stricture can be outlined by refluxing barium into the biliary tree during an upper gastrointestinal X-ray series.[7]

The alkaline phosphatase, leucine aminopeptidase, and 5'nucleotidase are elevated in most cases. The bilirubin may fluctuate in relation to symptoms. Usually it remains below 10 mg per 100 ml.

Blood cultures may be positive during an acute attack.

DIFFERENTIAL DIAGNOSIS

Choledocholithiasis is the condition which will have to be differentiated most often. The clinical and laboratory findings may be identical. A history of trauma to the duct may point toward stricture as the proper diagnosis. The final distinction must await radiological or surgical findings in many instances. An intravenous cholangiogram or, if that fails, transhepatic cholangiogram may answer the question. If not, a laparotomy would probably be indicated once episodic cholangitis had been verified.

Other causes of cholestatic jaundice may have to be ruled out in some cases.

TREATMENT

Strictures of the bile duct should be surgically repaired in all but a few patients whose general condition dictates a nonoperative approach.[1] Symptomatic treatment with antibiotics should be used to control acute attacks of cholangitis, but long-term antibiotic treatment is not recommended as a definitive regimen. Although attacks of cholangitis may regularly respond to antibiotics, this therapy does not relieve the liver of the damaging effects of the partial obstruction to the flow of bile. If the stricture is left uncorrected, secondary biliary cirrhosis or hepatic failure will gradually develop.

The surgical procedure should be selected on the basis of technical considerations presented by the individual patient. The general goals of the repair should be to re-establish biliary flow by anastomosing normal duct from the hepatic side of the stricture to either the intestine or normal duct below the stricture. Conceptually, excision of the strictured segment with end-to-end repair seems the simplest solution, but frequently this entails greater technical difficulties than connecting the proximal duct directly to the intestine. The duct can be reimplanted into the duodenum or a Roux-en-Y loop of jejunum. In the average case Roux-en-Y hepaticojejunostomy is most likely to provide a suitable anastomosis without tension.[1]

COMPLICATIONS

Complications are usually the result of delay in surgical correction of the stricture or technical failure. In these situations persistent cholangitis may progress to multiple intrahepatic abscesses. When this stage has been reached, it is usually impossible to save the patient from a septic death.

Other patients develop portal hypertension and esophageal varices over symptomatic periods which usually exceed five years.[8] When portal hypertension has developed, operations in the hilum of the liver may be bloody, and technical problems are often insurmountable. A prophylactic splenorenal shunt should be performed and the stricture repair scheduled for several months later.

PROGNOSIS

The death rate from biliary stricture is about 10 to 15 per cent, and the morbidity is high. If the stricture is not repaired, episodic cholangitis and secondary liver disease are inevitable.

Surgical correction of the stricture is successful in about 75 per cent of attempts. Experience at centers with a special interest in this problem indicates that good results can be obtained even if several previous attempts did not relieve the obstruction. Therefore, in general, if a stricture is present, the patient should be considered for correction despite a previous history of surgical failure.

POSTCHOLECYSTECTOMY SYNDROME

This term has been used to designate the heterogeneous group of patients who continue to complain of symptoms after cholecystectomy. It is not really a syndrome, and the term is confusing.

The usual reason why relief is incomplete after cholecystectomy is that the preoperative diagnosis of chronic cholecystitis was incorrect. The only symptom entirely characteristic of chronic cholecystitis is biliary colic. When a calculous gallbladder is removed in the hope that patients will gain relief from dyspepsia, fatty food intolerance, and belching, the operation will often leave the symptoms unchanged. The amount of scarring in the gallbladder wall correlates fairly well with the symptomatic improvement after cholecystectomy, and patients with vague postoperative complaints are more likely to have had a thin-walled, unscarred organ.

In other cases another diagnosis has been overlooked during the preoperative evaluation. Pancreatitis, peptic ulcer, irritable colon, gastritis, or esophagitis may have actually been the origin of symptoms attributed to the gallstones. These possibilities should be reinvestigated when symptoms persist.

Choledocholithiasis or biliary stricture is sometimes responsible for abdominal pain after cholecystectomy. Liver function studies and an intravenous cholangiogram should be obtained. One normal intravenous cholangiogram does not eliminate the possibility of a common duct stone; in suspicious cases the aforementioned studies should be repeated, and in some cases a transhepatic cholangiogram is indicated.

REFERENCES

1. Way, L. W., and Dunphy, J. E. Biliary stricture. Amer. J. Surg. *124*:287, 1972.
2. Aust, J. B., Root, H. D., Urdaneta, L., and Varco, R. L. Biliary stricture. Surgery *62*:601, 1967.
3. Smith, R. Strictures of the bile ducts. Progr. Surg. *9*:157, 1971.
4. Cole, W. H., Ireneus, C., Jr., and Reynolds, J. T. Strictures of the common bile duct. Ann. Surg. *142*:537, 1955.
5. Warren, K. W., Mountains, J. C., and Midell, A. I. Management of strictures of the biliary tract. Surg. Clin. N. Amer. *51*:711, 1971.
6. Walker, J. G., Young, W. B., George, P., and Sherlock, S. Percutaneous cholangiography in the management of biliary stricture. Gut *7*:164, 1966.
7. Wise, R. E., and Keefe, J. P. Radiologic evaluation of hepaticojejunal anastomoses. Surg. Clin. N. Amer. *48*:579, 1968.
8. Sedgwick, C. E., Poulantzas, J. K., and Kune, G. A. Management of portal hypertension secondary to bile duct strictures. Ann. Surg. *163*:949, 1966.
9. Longmire, W. P., Jr. Early management of injury to the extrahepatic biliary tract. J.A.M.A. *195*:111, 1966.

THE PANCREAS

Chapter 91

Anatomy and Embryology

Lloyd L. Brandborg

HISTORY

The pancreas was one of the last organs in the abdomen to receive the critical attention of anatomists, physiologists, physicians, and surgeons.[1-3] It was first referred to as the "finger of the liver" in the Talmud, written between 200 B.C. and 200 A.D. Galen, who named it (Ruphos, ca. 100 A.D., should probably be credited[3]), thought the pancreas served to support and protect blood vessels. Vesalius considered it a cushion for the stomach. Little further information was available until the reports of Wirsung, who demonstrated the pancreatic ducts in man in 1642, and de Graaf, who discovered pancreatic secretion from the pancreatic fistula in dogs in 1664.

Almost 200 years later, Eberle in 1834, Purkinje and Pappenheim in 1836, and Valentin in 1844 observed the emulsification of fat, proteolytic activity, and digestion of starch, respectively, by pancreatic juice and extracts. Claude Bernard subsequently proved the digestive action of pancreatic juice on sugar, fats, and proteins, using secretions from pancreatic fistula preparations.

Kühne isolated trypsin and introduced the term enzyme in 1876, following investigations which spanned ten years. The concept of enzymes led shortly to the identification of pancreatic amylase and lipase. In 1899, Chepovalnikoff, a student of Pavlov, discovered enterokinase in the duodenal mucosa which is essential for activation of the proteolytic enzymes. Another of Pavlov's students, Dolinsky, stimulated pancreatic secretion by instilling acid into the duodenum in 1895. This led to the discovery, by Bayliss and Starling, of secretin, which proved to be not an enzyme but the first hormone.

The pancreas was the last gland to be described histologically by Langerhans, in 1869. Pancreatic disease was rarely recorded prior to the nineteenth century. Friedreich wrote the first systematic description of pancreatic diseases in 1875. The classification of acute pancreatitis by Fitz in 1889 remains a classic. Although Fitz suggested operation for pancreatitis, surgery of pancreatic neoplasms and diseases was not popular until the 1930's, resulting mostly from the work of Whipple and Brunschwig. Brunner had successfully extirpated the pancreas in dogs in 1683.

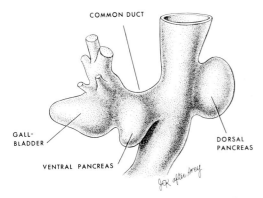

Figure 91–1. Pancreas at approximately four weeks of gestation. (Modified after Arey.)

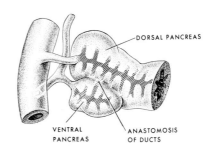

Figure 91–3. Pancreas at approximately seven weeks. Fusion has occurred, and ductular anastomosis is beginning. (Modified after Arey.)

EMBRYOLOGY

The pancreas first appears in embryos of approximately 4 mm size in the fourth week of gestation.[4, 5] Two outpouches from the entodermal lining of the duodenum develop at this time: the ventral pancreas and the dorsal pancreas (Fig. 91–1). The dorsal anlage grows more rapidly, and by the sixth week it is an elongated nodular structure extending into the dorsal mesentery within which its growth continues (Fig. 91–2). The ventral pancreas remains smaller and is carried away from the duodenum by its connection with the common bile duct. The two primordia are brought into apposition by the uneven growth of the duodenum and fuse by the seventh week (Fig. 91–3). The tail, body, and part of the head of the pancreas are formed by the dorsal component whereas the remainder of the head and the uncinate process arise from the ventral pancreas.

These primitive relationships are still distinguishable in the adult pancreas.[5]

Both the primitive pancreases contain an axial duct. The dorsal duct arises directly from the duodenal wall and the ventral duct from the common bile duct. On fusion of the ventral and dorsal pancreas, the ventral duct anastomoses with the dorsal one, forming the main pancreatic duct (Fig. 91–4). The proximal end of the dorsal duct becomes the accessory duct in the adult and is patent in 70 per cent of specimens.[6] The common outlet of the bile duct and pancreatic duct observed in most adults is the result of the common origin of the bile duct and the ventral pancreas.

The pancreatic acini appear in the third month as derivatives of the side ducts and termini of the primitive ducts. The acini remain connected to the larger pancreatic ducts by small secretory ductules. At the same time the islets of Langerhans are differentiating from the ducts of the dorsal pancreas. The dorsal pancreas also contributes acini and is probably the sole

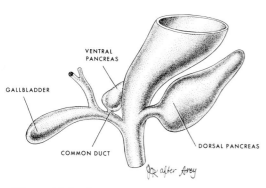

Figure 91–2. Pancreas at approximately six weeks of gestation, (Modified after Arey.)

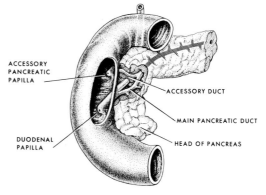

Figure 91–4. Pancreas at birth. (Modified after Arey.)

source of the islet cells,[4] which are most numerous in the tail. Although tubular structures occasionally connect the islets to the larger pancreatic ducts, they are vestigial and do not contain a lumen.

No morphological or functional differences exist between the acini derived from the dorsal and the ventral pancreas. The fetal pancreas has been shown to contain trypsinogen at 16 weeks, amylase at 24 weeks, and lipase at 32 weeks. The alpha and beta cells of the islets begin to function relatively early in fetal development. Insulin has been identified prior to the appearance of trypsinogen. The mesenchymal tissue in which the gland grows provides the connective tissue capsule and divides the gland into lobes and lobules.

CONGENITAL ANOMALIES

Accessory pancreases and ectopic pancreatic tissue are common and occur at diverse areas throughout the gastrointestinal tract. One report described an incidence of 13.7 per cent in 410 autopsies.[7] Usually they are found within the wall of the stomach, particularly the distal greater curvature, and in the wall of the duodenum. Foci of pancreatic tissue may occur in the gallbladder, the spleen, the omentum, and occasionally Meckel's diverticula. The ventral pancreas may not migrate to the right of the duodenum. When it divides and encircles the duodenum, an annular pancreas is formed. Failure of union of the primitive anlage, independent duct systems, and single ducts are all reported; these anomalies are of no clinical consequence.

Annular pancreas is the most common anomaly obstructing the duodenum in infancy; it is best treated by surgical bypass. It is frequently associated with other congenital anomalies, including atresia of the duodenum. The most common association is with Down's syndrome.[8] Conversely, an annular pancreas may be present without producing symptoms and may be only an incidental finding at surgery or autopsy, or symptoms may appear in adult life.

It has been suggested that ectopic pancreatic tissue is more prone to malignant degeneration than pancreas in the normal location. Functioning non-beta cell tumors, characteristic of the Zollinger-Ellison syndrome, commonly occur in the wall of the duodenum,[9] as well as in the pancreas, possibly arising from ectopic pancreatic tissue.

The finding of immunoreactive gastrin in the duodenal and jejunal mucosa[10] raises the possibility that these gastrin-producing cells may be the cells of origin of these functioning tumors. They are morphologically and functionally indistinguishable from those occurring in the pancreas. They are often malignant.

NORMAL ANATOMY

The pancreas is an elongated, flattened, somewhat prismatic gland, 12 to 15 cm in length.[11-13] The adult gland weighs between 70 and approximately 110 g. The head lies within the curve of the duodenum and in intimate apposition with it. The right border is grooved, and the pancreas overlaps the duodenum anteriorly and posteriorly to a variable extent. The neck, body, and tail of the pancreas lie obliquely in the posterior abdomen, with the tail extending as far as the gastric surface of the spleen (Figs. 91–5 and 91–6).

The pancreas has a rich circulation derived from branches of the celiac artery and the superior mesenteric artery. The anterior and posterior superior pancreaticoduodenal arteries arise as branches of the gastroduodenal artery, a branch of the celiac artery. The anterior and posterior inferior pancreaticoduodenal arteries arise from the superior mesenteric artery. These vessels usually lie in a groove between the head of the pancreas and the duodenum and supply branches to both organs. The other major arterial supply of the pancreas is derived from the splenic artery, which gives off numerous small branches and usually three larger ones: the dorsal pancreatic, the pancreatica magna, and the cauda pancreatis.

The venous drainage all flows into the portal venous system. The pancreatic veins drain the tail and body of the pancreas and join the splenic vein. The pancreaticoduodenal veins lie close to their corresponding arteries and empty either into the splenic vein or directly into the portal vein.

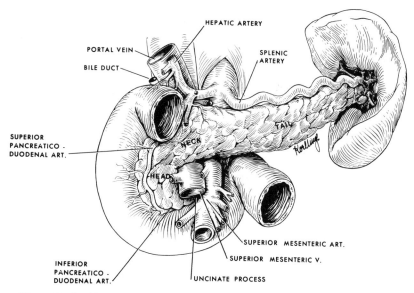

HEPATIC ARTERY

PORTAL VEIN

BILE DUCT

SPLENIC ARTERY

SUPERIOR PANCREATICO - DUODENAL ART.

NECK

TAIL

HEAD

SUPERIOR MESENTERIC ART.

SUPERIOR MESENTERIC V.

INFERIOR PANCREATICO - DUODENAL ART.

UNCINATE PROCESS

Figure 91–5. Diagrammatic representation of an anterior view of the pancreas.

The lymphatics of the pancreas are in the vicinity of the accompanying arteries and veins. Most of the lymphatics terminate in the pancreaticosplenic lymph nodes. Some end in the pancreaticoduodenal nodes and some in the preaortic nodes near the origin of the superior mesenteric artery.

The visceral efferent innervation of the pancreas is through the vagi and splanchnic nerves via the hepatic and celiac plexuses. The efferent fibers of the vagi pass through these plexuses without synapsing and terminate in parasympathetic ganglia found in the interlobular septa of the pancreas. The postganglionic fibers innervate acini, islets, and ducts. The bodies of the neurons of the sympathetic efferent nerves originate in the lateral gray matter of the thoracic and lumbar spinal cord. The bodies of the postganglionic sympathic neurons are located in the great plexuses of the abdomen. Their postganglionic fibers innervate only blood vessels. The autonomic fibers, both efferent and afferent, are located in proximity to the blood vessels of the pancreas. Little is known about the distribution of the visceral afferent fibers in man. They probably run through the splanchnic nerves to the sympathetic trunks and rami communicantes and through spinal nerves and ganglia. The vagi are thought to carry some visceral afferent fibers.

Figure 91–6. Diagrammatic representation of a posterior view of the pancreas.

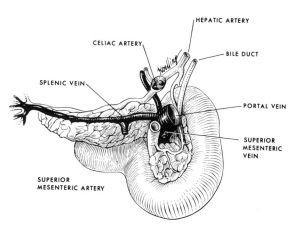

HEPATIC ARTERY

CELIAC ARTERY

BILE DUCT

SPLENIC VEIN

PORTAL VEIN

SUPERIOR MESENTERIC VEIN

SUPERIOR MESENTERIC ARTERY

RELATION TO OTHER ORGANS

The pancreas is strategically situated close to a number of important structures in the posterior abdomen. Beginning at the head of the gland and progressing toward the tail, the pancreas has the following relationships with adjacent structures. The posterior surfaces of the head and body are devoid of peritoneum. The inferior vena cava runs behind the head of the pancreas. This surface also overlies the terminal parts of the right renal veins and the right crus of the diaphragm. The common bile duct is situated either in a groove in the upper lateral surface or in the substance of the gland. The posterior surface of the neck overlies the superior mesenteric vein and the origins of the portal vein. The body is in contact with the aorta and the origin of the superior mesenteric artery, the left crus of the diaphragm, the left adrenal gland, and the left kidney and its vasculature. The splenic vein courses between the pancreas and the preceding structures. The kidney is separated from the pancreas by the perirenal fat and fascia. The tail of the pancreas is located within the two layers of the splenorenal ligament along with the splenic vessels.

The anterior surface of the head is separated from the transverse colon only by areolar tissue. The caudal surface of the gland is covered with peritoneum which is continuous with the transverse mesocolon and lies close to a coil of jejunum. The uncinate process of the head is anterior to the aorta and is traversed by the superior mesenteric vessels which pass between the pancreas and duodenum. The anterior surface of the neck is covered with peritoneum and abuts the pylorus, separated by a part of the lesser sac of the peritoneum. The anterior surface of the body is separated from the stomach by the lesser sac. The inferior surface of the body is also peritonealized and is close to the duodenojejunal junction and the splenic flexure of the colon. The superior border of the body is in contact with the posterior aspect of the lesser omentum. The splenic artery has its tortuous course along this border. The superior mesenteric arteries and veins pass under the body at its junction with the uncinate process.

The pancreatic duct (duct of Wirsung) begins near the tail and is formed from anastomosing ductules draining the lobules of the gland. It courses from left to right and is enlarged by additional ducts of various sizes until it reaches the neck, where it turns caudal and posterior and where it usually joins the common bile duct. The short common segment is the ampulla of the bile duct which terminates in the duodenal papilla. An accessory pancreatic duct (duct of Santorini) is frequently present; it may terminate in the main pancreatic duct or separately in the accessory pancreatic papilla. The accessory duct is patent in 70 per cent of autopsy specimens.[14] In 10 per cent the main duct drains into the accessory papilla and has no connection with the common bile duct.[14]

CORRELATION WITH DISEASES

Because of the strategic location of the pancreas, disease processes of adjacent organs frequently involve it, and diseases of the pancreas often affect its neighboring structures. Peptic ulcers of the stomach and duodenum may penetrate into the pancreas, resulting in pancreatitis and, rarely, abscess. Carcinomas of the stomach may involve the pancreas by direct extension or by metastasis to the pancreaticoduodenal lymph nodes. Occasionally, the pancreas is invaded by lymphoma of the adjacent lymphatics. Pancreatic arteries are frequently affected in arteritis of the abdominal vasculature. Aneurysm of the aorta may encroach upon the pancreas, and it is not rare to confuse expanding aneurysm with pancreatitis or tumor, as well as other abdominal pain syndromes.

Few observations are available, in man, on the effects of occlusion or stenosis of the superior mesenteric artery and celiac axis on the pancreas. Experimental occlusion results in infarction but not in pancreatitis. In intestinal ischemia or infarction of the intestine, the attention of the surgeon is directed to removing infarcted intestine or to revascularizing the bowel. Since much of the circulation of the pancreas is derived from branches of the celiac axis and superior mesenteric artery, it is probable that it is also infarcted or ischemic in arterial occlusion. No data are available concerning pancreatic function subsequent to massive small bowel resection for infarction in man. Theoretically, pancreatic insufficiency could result from pancreatic infarction or excision of the small intestinal sites of secretin and cholecystokinin elaboration, depriving the pancreas of some of its physiological stimuli.

Aneurysm of the splenic artery may encroach upon the pancreas and even be embedded in its substance. These aneurysms can rupture into the main pancreatic duct as well as into the gut and be the source of serious upper gastrointestinal hemorrhage. Tumors and cysts of the kidney may encroach upon the pancreas and simulate pancreatic disease.

Pancreatitis regularly involves adjacent tissues. Fat necrosis is frequently present and may be widely disseminated. Ordinarily it is confined to the peripancreatic fat and to the fat of the mesenteries and omentum. Pylephlebitis is a rare complication of pancreatitis. Phlebothrombosis has been observed to occur in the splenic vein, the superior and inferior mesenteric veins, and the portal vein. Arterial thrombosis is much less common, although intestinal infarction has accompanied pancreatitis. Obstruction of the transverse colon or the duodenum may occur from compression of the intestine by pancreatic pseudocysts, from surrounding inflammatory masses, or, with recovery, from adhesions and scarring. It may simulate carcinoma of the transverse colon. Ileus is frequent in pancreatitis. The entire intestine may be affected. Most often it is segmental and apparent on plain roentgenograms of the abdomen as a loop of small intestine, containing air, in the midabdomen—the so-called sentinel loop. The presence of a sentinel loop, although noted with other intra-abdominal inflammatory lesions, suggests pancreatitis if it is in the vicinity of the pancreas.

Acute pancreatitis commonly results in mild and transient obstructive jaundice caused by edema and compression of the common bile duct or, perhaps, by spasm of the sphincter of Oddi. Chronic and relapsing pancreatitis may result in cholestasis, with or without jaundice, owing to the gradual compression of the common bile duct, and, rarely in chronic cases, in biliary cirrhosis. Obstructive jaundice often results from compression of the biliary tree

by cysts, pseudocysts, and tumors of the pancreas located near the head. Pancreatic cancer regularly involves adjacent organs and lymphatics and invades the stomach, duodenum, and common bile duct. Pseudocysts and tumors of the body may compress the splenic vein and result in gastric and esophageal varices via collaterals through the short gastric veins and the hilar veins of the spleen. Large pseudocysts regularly displace the stomach anteriorly and compress and may even obstruct the duodenum. Pseudocysts of the tail have produced symptoms suggestive of renal colic, with roentgen findings suggesting primary cyst or tumor of the kidney. Acute pancreatitis, particularly with pseudocyst formation, may produce ascites which occasionally is intractable. Pleural effusions are common, especially in the left thorax, and may be bilateral. Pseudocysts may rupture into the gastrointestinal tract, the free abdominal cavity, or the retroperitoneum. They may present in unusual sites, such as the mediastinum or pleural space.

NORMAL HISTOLOGY, HISTOCHEMISTRY, AND ULTRASTRUCTURE

The pancreas is a compound, racemose, finely nodular gland which is grossly similar to but less compact than the salivary glands. It is surrounded by fine connective tissue but does not have a fibrous tissue capsule. The lobules are visible upon gross examination.

The exocrine acini consist of single rows of pyramidal epithelial cells with their broad bases on a basal lamina and their apices converging on a central lumen[15] (Fig. 91-7). The nuclei are located at the bases of these cells. The acini are rounded or short tubular structures which are the subunit of the lobule. The lobules are connected by loose connective tissue which contains the blood vessels, nerves, lymphatics, and excretory ducts. Small secretory capillaries between each row of acinar cells drain into the central lumen of the acinus. This lumen is inconspicuous when the gland is at rest but becomes distended during secretion.

The morphology of acinar cells is de-

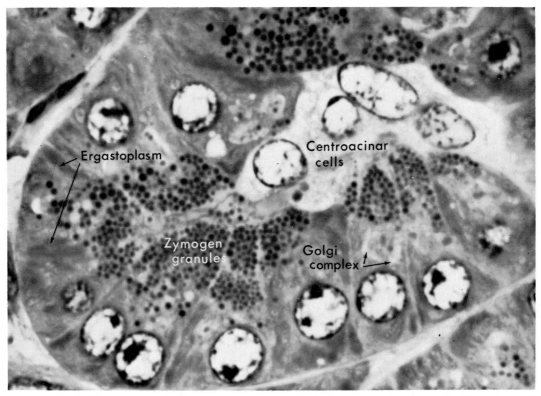

Figure 91-7. Photomicrograph of a human acinus, showing acinar and centroacinar cells. The acinar cell ergastoplasm, Golgi complex, and zymogen granules are easily identifiable. Formalin, osmium fixation. Epon-embedded section. Toluidine blue stained. × 3200. (From Bloom, W., and Fawcett, D. W.: A Textbook of Histology. Philadelphia, W. B. Saunders Co., 1968. With the kind permission of Dr. Susumu Ito.)

pendent on many factors. It is difficult to procure well-preserved tissue from man because of rapid autolysis after death and the danger of biopsying the pancreas at surgery. The state of preservation of the specimen, functional status, and fixative used are all critical. For most histological purposes, Zenker-formol fixation and hematoxylin and eosin staining are suitable. Under these conditions, the basilar parts of the acinar cells are usually a dark purple and the secretory granules appear bright orangish red. With stains for ribonuclear protein, the basal cytoplasm is darkly basophilic. Often this basophilic material, called the ergastoplasm, appears laminar or filamentous.

The Golgi apparatus is in the supranuclear aspect of the cell and is variable in size and location, depending upon the secretory state and other physiological factors. The zymogen granules appear first in the region of the Golgi apparatus, although enzyme synthesis probably occurs in the basal cytoplasm. In the resting state they are extremely numerous and are rapidly depleted after pilocarpine injection or a large meal. This reduction in zymogen granules occurs with a substantial increase in pancreatic enzyme secretion. The Golgi apparatus enlarges with the appearance of the new zymogen droplets.

The lumen of the acinus connects with a small duct surrounded by centroacinar cells. These cells are pale staining in histological sections and are easily recognizable. The part of the duct which they surround drains into the intralobular ducts. The intralobular ducts are covered by low columnar epithelium similar in appearance to the centroacinar cells. These ducts anastomose and form the interlobular ducts, which are lined by a columnar epithelium. Goblet cells and occasional argentaffin cells are also present. An occasional small mucous gland is seen. The interlobular ducts anastomose to become the main pancreatic duct. The larger ducts have a somewhat thick wall, consisting of connective tissue and elastic fibers.

In addition to the exocrine ducts, a system of anastomosing small tubules arising from large ducts and coursing in the connective tissue is present in the guinea pig and probably also in man. Their diameters range from 12 to 27 μ. They are connected to the islets of Langerhans and small mucous glands and possibly to the acini. The lining epithelium is a low irregular cuboidal type with occasional mitoses. Occasional goblet cells are present. These tubules connect by one or more short stalks to the large islets. They are composed of undifferentiated epithelium and are thought to be the source of new islet and possibly acinar cells. Secretion has never been identified within them.[15]

The pancreas' also contains numerous endocrine cells, the islets of Langerhans, which number about a million in man. These are usually separated from the sur-

rounding acinar tissue by fine reticular fibers. Very little reticulum is present within the islet. The islets do not connect with the lumen of the pancreatic ducts by any functional connections. Granules are not visible with hematoxylin and eosin staining. By Mallory-azan staining three types of granular cells are present: the alpha cell, the beta cell, and the delta cell. The alpha cells contain relatively large granules which are stained a brilliant red and tend to be located around the periphery of the islet. The beta cell granules are smaller, stain a brownish orange, and are in the center of the islet. The delta cells are relatively few in number; they contain small, blue-staining granules. The alpha cell secretes glucagon, the beta cell, insulin; the product of the delta cell is unknown.

The pancreas has long been an object of histochemical investigation.[16] It is particularly suitable for the demonstration of nu-

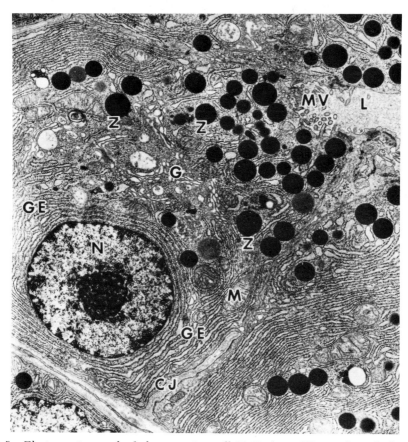

Figure 91–8. Electron micrograph of a human acinar cell. N, Nucleus; GE, granular endoplasmic reticulum; G, Golgi complex; Z, zymogen granules; MV, microvilli; L, lumen of acinus; M, mitochondria; CJ, cell junction. × 15,000. (Kindly provided by Dr. Susumu Ito.)

cleic acid by various techniques such as the Feulgen reaction, methyl-green pyronin, and galocyanin staining. This is due to the large nucleic acid content which is related to enzyme synthesis. Alcian blue and periodic acid–Schiff staining have long been used to demonstrate mucopolysaccharides in the pancreas as well as in other tissues. Carbonic anhydrase has been demonstrated only in the ductular epithelium.[16] The acinar cells do not contain this enzyme, although small amounts are observed in the basal membranes of the capillaries.

The intracellular localization of proenzymes in acinar cells in man is unknown. No histochemical techniques are available for their demonstration. They have been identified in other species by fluorescent conjugated specific antibodies against proenzymes. Unfortunately, there is some cross-reactivity among these enzymes, and the technique is not entirely specific.[17] Procarboxypeptidase and chymotrypsinogen are found in zymogen granules, and ribonuclease is found both in the granules and in the cytoplasm in the pig.[18] In bovine pancreas chymotrypsinogen and procarboxypeptidase were in the apex of the acinar cells, in zymogen granules, and in the matrix around the granules. Zymogen granules also contain deoxyribonuclease and ribonuclease. Alpha amylase occurs in almost every acinar cell in the pig. It is located largely in the base of the cell, with some activity in the zymogen granules around the nucleus, and is visible in the Golgi apparatus. Trypsinogen and chymotrypsinogen stain in the zymogen granules near the nucleus

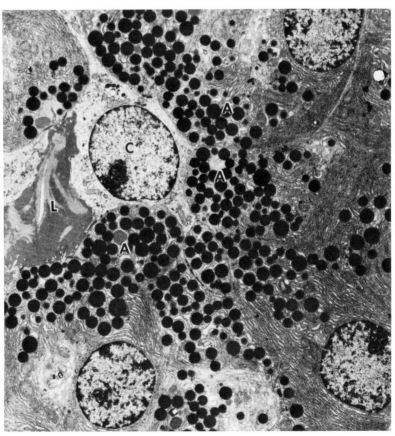

Figure 91–9. Electron micrograph of a centroacinar cell, C, and several acinar cells, A. Note the pale appearance, scanty numbers of mitochondria, and paucity of membrane structures. L is the lumen of the acinus. × 9000. (Kindly provided by Dr. Susumu Ito.)

but not in apical granules. Lipase activity is found throughout the acinar cell.[19] There is intense activity in the apex of the cell, even more in the region of the Golgi apparatus, and less in the base of the cell. Little or no lipase activity is found within zymogen granules, and most of it surrounds the granule in the dog pancreas.[19]

Although the pancreas contains only one morphological type of acinar cell, synthetic products may differ from cell to cell as well as from granule to granule. It is not known whether individual zymogen granules contain more than one proenzyme. Amylases and lipases may be cytoplasmic enzymes. The failure of the apical cells to react to specific fluorescent antibody may be due to an increasing impermeability of the membrane surrounding the granule as it approaches the lumen of the acinus.

The ultrastructure of the pancreatic acinar cell has been intensively studied.[15] An extensive granular endoplasmic reticulum arranged in parallel cisternae is found in the basilar aspects of the cell. There are abundant free ribosomes in the cytoplasm. The mitochondria in most species are elongated and contain well developed cristae and many matrix granules. The Golgi apparatus consists of closely approximated parallel cisternae, numerous small vesicles, and condensing vacuoles which may contain a relatively low density secretory substance. The mature zymogen granules, which are very electron opaque, are found close to the Golgi apparatus and are distributed to the apex of the cell. Lysosomes and lipid droplets are occasionally observed in the region of the Golgi apparatus. The apices of the acinar cell usually have a few short microvilli (Fig. 91–8). The intracellular zymogen particles are discrete, although they may fuse with one another at the apex of the cell, particularly during active secretion. Zymogen granules, which are liquid, may be seen discharging into the lumen of the acinus. Ordinarily, zymogen droplets are not seen within the endoplasmic reticulum.

The centroacinar cells (Fig. 91–9) have virtually no endoplasmic reticulum and are probably not active in protein synthesis. They have variable number of mitochondria.

REFERENCES

1. Clarke, E. S. History of gastroenterology. *In* Gastroenterologic Medicine, M. Paulson (ed.). Philadelphia, Lea and Febiger, 1969.
2. Garrison, F. H. An Introduction to the History of Medicine. 2nd ed. Philadelphia, W. B. Saunders Co., 1917.
3. Major, R. H. A History of Medicine. Springfield, Ill., Charles C Thomas, 1954.
4. Arey, L. B. Developmental Anatomy. A Textbook and Laboratory Manual of Embryology. 7th ed. Philadelphia, W. B. Saunders Co., 1965.
5. Patten, B. M. Human Embryology. 3rd ed. New York, The Blakiston Division, McGraw-Hill Book Co., 1968.
6. Kleitsch, W. P. Anatomy of the pancreas. A study with special reference to the duct system. Arch. Surg. 71:795, 1955.
7. Feldman, M., and Weinberg, T. Abberant pancreas, a cause of duodenal syndrome. J.A.M.A. 148:893, 1952.
8. Silverberg, M., and Davidson, M. Pediatric gastroenterology. A review. Gastroenterology 58:229, 1970.
9. Oberhelman, H. A., Jr., Nelsen, T. S., Johnson, A. N., Jr., and Dragstedt, L. R., II. Ulcerogenic tumors of the duodenum. Ann. Surg. 153:214, 1961.
10. Berson, S., A., and Yalow, R. S. Nature of immunoreactive gastrin extracted from tissues of gastrointestinal tract. Gastroenterology 60:215, 1971.
11. Johnston, T. B., and Willis, J. R. Gray's Anatomy, Descriptive and Applied. 29th ed. London, Longmans, Green & Co., 1946.
12. Grant, J. C. B. A Method of Anatomy, Descriptive and Deductive. 4th ed. Baltimore, The Williams and Wilkins Co., 1948.
13. Goss, C. M. Gray's Anatomy. 28th ed. Philadelphia, Lea and Febiger, 1966.
14. Kleitsch, W. P. Anatomy of the pancreas. A study with special reference to the duct system. Arch. Surg. 71:795, 1955.
15. Bloom, W., and Fawcett, D. W. A Textbook of Histology. Philadelphia, W. B. Saunders Co., 1968.
16. Becker, V. Histochemistry of the exocrine pancreas. *In* The Exocrine Pancreas, A. V. S. de Reuck and M. P. Cameron (eds.). Boston, Little, Brown and Co., 1961.
17. Yasuda, I. C., and Coons, A. H. Localization by immunofluorescence of amylase, trypsinogen and chymotrypsinogen in acinar cells of the pig pancreas. J. Histochem. Cytochem. 14:303, 1966.
18. Marshall, J. M., Jr. Distributions of chymotrypsinogen, procarboxypeptidase, deoxyribonuclease and ribonuclease in bovine pancreas. Exp. Cell Res. 6:240, 1954.
19. Abe, M., Kramer, S. P., and Seligman, A. M. The histochemical demonstration of Pancreatic-like lipase and comparison with the distribution of esterase. J. Histochem. Cytochem. 12:364, 1964.

Chapter 92

Acute Pancreatitis

Lloyd L. Brandborg

INTRODUCTION

"Inflammatory pancreatic disease of all forms continues to be an ill-defined collection of puzzling entities. No perfect etiological or clinical separation has yet been obtained. Different investigators have devised various experimental methods of inducing pancreatitis. Bile reflux, biliary tract disease, and alcoholism as associated findings have previously been documented and continue to be investigated."[1] Subsequent to this statement, little has been added to change this opinion. Bile reflux in man is only assumed and not proved.

PATHOLOGY

The pathologic findings in pancreatitis, regardless of the clinical causes, are similar and represent a spectrum of damage. The following classification, which includes the possibility that the initiating factor may be vascular disease, has been proposed.[2] Pancreatitis is either nonhemorrhagic or hemorrhagic. Nonhemorrhagic pancreatitis includes acute edematous, acute suppurative, and acute necrotizing pancreatitis, and pancreatic infarction caused by primary arterial disease, with or without the presence of fat necrosis. Hemorrhagic pancreatitis has the same classification with superimposed hemorrhage. Pancreatic apoplexy supposedly caused by primary arterial disease with superimposed pancreatitis is included in this classification.

Acute Edematous Pancreatitis. Acute edematous pancreatitis is ordinarily not fatal. The gland is two or three times normal size, indurated, edematous, and paler than normal. Microscopic examination discloses intralobular and acinar edema. A mild to moderate polymorphonuclear leukocyte infiltration is present. The ductular cells and glandular cells do not appear to be damaged by light microscopy. The adjacent lymph nodes often have a reactive hyperplasia.

Acute Suppurative Pancreatitis. Acute suppurative pancreatitis may result from progression of the acute edematous form or may represent an initial lesion. Experimentally, the gland at first swells and becomes hyperemic. Pus is found in dilated pancreatic ducts, and small abscesses develop which may coalesce and extend to involve surrounding structures. Liquefaction of the pancreas and fat necrosis are present. Cultures of such lesions at surgery or postmortem examination are often sterile. An identical morbid anatomy may develop during septicemia or septic embolization from other sites. The microscopic appearance is characterized by large collections of polymorphonuclear leukocytes within the ducts, abscesses, and extensive necrosis of the acini, ducts, and islets.

Acute Necrotizing Pancreatitis. Acute necrotizing pancreatitis is also characterized by an enlarged gland, containing soft, grayish to black areas of necrosis. Extensive fat necrosis is usually present. As the necrotic areas grow older, liquefaction and cyst formation occur. On microscopic examination extensive destruction of all elements of the gland is present. Leukocyte infiltration is a "late" event in this form of pancreatitis. Suppurative and necrotic pancreatitis may progress to gangrene with total destruction of the gland.

Infarction. Diagnosis of infarction of the pancreas is rare. When infarction is observed, it resembles infarction in any other organ and is usually without evidence of associated pancreatitis. If observed early enough, the infarction is confined to the area of the terminal arterial supply and on microscopic examination coagulation necrosis with ghost cells is present.

Hemorrhagic Pancreatitis. Hemorrhagic pancreatitis is similar, with variable amounts of interstitial hemorrhage. Usually, hemorrhage is not massive and is confined to the interstitial areas. Microscopically, hemorrhagic pancreatitis resembles the other forms. Cystic areas filled with erythrocytes or hemolyzed blood and extensive areas of necrosis may be noted.

Hemorrhage within the pancreas may, however, be a feature of pancreatitis, the result of trauma, aneurysmal rupture, erosion of the pancreatic arterial supply by neoplasm, or thrombophlebitis of either the pancreatic veins or the portal vein. It has been observed in severe congestive heart failure. Pancreatic hemorrhage may be manifested by the spread of blood throughout the abdominal cavity and retroperitoneum. Ecchymoses in the flanks or around the umbilicus are clinical signs of pancreatic hemorrhage.

Fat Necrosis. Fat necrosis is common. Grossly it is dull, opaque, and usually yellowish white in color. Necrotic fat stained with bilirubin or biliverdin is yellow to dark green. Fat necrosis may be found in adjacent adipose tissue and at distant areas such as subcutaneous tissues, bone marrow, and central nervous system. Early fat necrosis, by hematoxylin and eosin staining, is characterized by necrotic spaces filled with an eosinophilic, granular material. On precipitation with calcium this substance becomes deeply basophilic.

As the lesion progresses, an inflammatory reaction and migrating macrophages surround the area. Subsequently the necrotic area liquefies and is encapsulated by connective tissue. Cysts may develop. Some areas may contain foreign body–type giant cells.

Acinar Necrosis. Acinar cell necrosis is either coagulative or cytolytic in type and is likely to be part of a continuum. The distinguishing features are that in coagulation necrosis ghost structures of the cells remain, whereas in cytolytic necrosis only debris without recognizable cellular elements is present. In severe and extensive pancreatitis the islet cells undergo the same changes.

Nonspecific Pathology. Squamous or goblet cell metaplasia of the ductal epithelium has been observed in association with pancreatitis. These findings are incidental, because the same changes have been found in autopsy specimens in patients without pancreatitis.

The blood vessels of the pancreas are often affected in patients with vasculitis, thrombosis, or thrombophlebitis. There may be extensive necrosis of the vessel walls. Arteritis, atherosclerosis, and thrombotic thrombocytopenic purpura have been observed in association with pancreatitis. The same lesions are observed in patients with a similar age distribution who do not have pancreatitis.

ETIOLOGY AND PATHOGENESIS

EXPERIMENTAL PANCREATITIS

A vast, confusing, and inconclusive literature exists concerning experimental pancreatitis. An almost unimaginable variety of experiments designed to injure the pancreas have been applied to a large number of species to produce pancreatitis. Often the experiments seem to have been designed to support the investigator's preconceived conclusions. Unfortunately, none of the models resemble de novo human pancreatitis, regardless of etiology.

A possible exception is the recent observation of a patchy lesion similar to chronic pancreatitis in man, resulting from administration of ethanol to rats for 30 months.[3] The pathology included protein precipitates in the ducts with focal calcification, reduced acinar cells which were replaced with dilated ducts, and sclerosis. The ultrastructural changes were nonspecific, with little resemblance to human pancreatitis.

There are two possible criticisms of this experiment. One is that young, growing rats weighing 100 to 120 g at the beginning and 400 g at the end of the experiment were used. (The control rats, given water, grew at the same rate.) Most patients with pancreatitis associated with alcohol do not begin drinking in childhood. The other is the amount of ethanol ingested, 4 g per rat daily. Although one cannot extrapolate directly on a weight basis to man, one can speculate that a 70-kg human subject would have to ingest between 700 and 2800 g of ethanol daily to produce this kind of pancreatitis. This amounts to 1400 to 5600 ml of 50 per cent ethanol or 3500 to 14,000 ml of "dessert" wine daily. The rats were also maintained on normal diets, whereas many alcoholic patients with pancreatitis are malnourished.

Perhaps the vast body of data on experimental pancreatitis contains hints as to the etiology and pathogenesis of human pancreatitis. However, to date no one has been astute enough to extract these clues from the morass. Perhaps it is time to call a moratorium on experimental pancreatitis and to analyze the existing data. This may be the only way to determine whether this tremendous effort has been worthwhile.

ETIOLOGICAL HYPOTHESES

It is still not established that acute and chronic pancreatitis are different stages of the same disease. The most important product of the symposium in Marseilles held in 1963[4] was a clinical classification which is simple and reflects the state of knowledge of human pancreatitis. This classification is as follows: (1) acute pancreatitis and relapsing acute pancreatitis, and (2) chronic pancreatitis and relapsing chronic pancreatitis, i.e., chronic pancreatitis with acute relapses. The difference between these two is residual permanent damage in the chronic varieties. Duration of the disease is not implied in this classification. It has the advantages of being simple, easily understood, and universally applicable (see pp. 1185 to 1197).

OBSTRUCTION-SECRETION THEORY

A widely held opinion is that acute pancreatitis results from obstruction of the pancreatic duct in an actively secreting gland.[5] The preponderance of experimental and clinical evidence is against this theory. In most patients with pancreatitis organic obstruction of the ducts is not present. Duct obstruction was found in only 3 of 100 fatal cases of pancreatitis in one series.[6] Ligation of the pancreatic duct in several species leads to atrophy and not pancreatitis. Patients with obstructing carcinomas of the head of the pancreas do not often have associated acute pancreatitis. Ligation of the pancreatic duct in animals followed by secretin stimulation results in reversible edema without pancreatitis. Stimulation with secretin in patients with acute pancreatitis does not exacerbate or aggravate the disease. Although dilated ducts are frequently found in patients with chronic pancreatitis, obstruction is infrequent. The calculi which are often present may be the result of ductal damage. This ductal ectasia may be caused by destruction of supporting tissues. This explanation draws on the analogy to the dilated bronchi seen in bronchiectasis.

COMMON CHANNEL THEORY

Another theory which has a large number of adherents is the common channel theory first advanced in 1901.[7] This theory assumes a common channel between the biliary tract and the pancreatic duct. Pancreatic juice is considered to enter the common bile duct and be activated, whence bile and activated enzymes regurgitate up the pancreatic duct, at low pressure, causing hemorrhagic pancreatitis. Evidence of a functional common channel in vivo is not present in the majority of patients with pancreatitis. The physiological pressures within the pancreatic duct are substantially higher than those within the common bile duct. Increasing bile duct pressure artificially does not result in regurgitation of fluid up the pancreatic duct. Performance of T-tube cholangiograms, a nonphysiological situation, often results in reflux up the pancreatic duct without harmful sequelae. The pancreatic duct is rarely visualized during intravenous cholangiography. Diversion of biliary flow through the pancreatic duct at physiological pressures does not result in pancreatitis. Lipase is the only pancreatic enzyme activated by bile. Spasm of the duodenal papilla has been shown to close both ducts. A number of bacteria and bacterial toxins, when forcefully injected into the duct and, occasionally, when allowed to enter under low pressure, result in experimental pancreatitis. Infection has not been proved to be a significant factor in the etiology or pathogenesis of human pancreatitis.

DUODENAL REGURGITATION THEORY

Reflux of duodenal contents into the pancreatic duct has been proposed as being largely responsible for pancreatitis.[5] This theory is based upon the observations that active pancreatic enzymes can produce experimental acute hemorrhagic pancreatitis and that the pancreatic proteolytic enzymes are activated only on contact with duodenal contents. Creation of a closed duodenal loop in dogs results in hemorrhagic pancreatitis which is prevented by ligation of the pancreatic ducts. The same experimental technique applied to germ-free dogs leads to hemorrhagic pancreatitis, excluding infection as a factor in this model.

In support of this theory is an apparent increase in deaths from acute pancreatitis following gastrojejunostomy, a situation which may predispose to regurgitation of duodenal contents, whereas gastroduodenostomy is attended by a lower mortality from pancreatitis. Although duodenal regurgitation may be a factor in some patients with pancreatitis, little or no real evidence exists to support this assumption in most cases. Further arguments against this hypothesis are that active pancreatic enzymes do not digest healthy living tissue. Even if materials refluxed up the pancreatic duct, including duodenal contents, no explanation has been offered as to how this material penetrates the ductal epithelium and initiates the process of pancreatitis. The ducts are permeable to many substances in the presence of pancreatitis. No substance within the lumen of the duct has been shown to cause this permeability. Free bile acids, which may be cytotoxic, have been found in gallbladder bile or duodenal contents in a few but not in most patients with "gallstone" pancreatitis.[8] No free bile acids were found in patients with alcoholic pancreatitis. The ductal epithelium is not an absorptive epithelium morphologically. Even if it were, whole proteins, such as enzymes, could not cross it.

PATHOGENESIS

Virtually all the enzymes synthesized by the pancreas have been incriminated in the pathogenesis of pancreatitis.[9] Although it is generally held that acute pancreatitis is due to autodigestion of the gland, this has not been proved. The proteolytic enzymes, especially trypsin, have received the most attention, but observations in recent years have cast doubt on their role.

PROTEOLYTIC ENZYMES

Active trypsin has not been found in the pancreas during acute pancreatitis. Clinical experience with treatment with trypsin inhibitors is, at best, controversial. The production of experimental acute or hemorrhagic pancreatitis by injection of trypsin into the pancreatic duct depends on species, the amount given, and the pressure with which it is administered. Injected trypsin is rapidly inactivated by endogenous trypsin inhibitor. The animal models exhibit extensive vascular damage, hemorrhage, and edema, with thrombosis in vessels but relatively little acinar necrosis.

The effect of chymotrypsin is similar, whereas the carboxypeptidases produce no lesions. It has been concluded that "autodigestion" is not the effect of trypsin. It has been suggested that minute, unmeasurable amounts of trypsin activate other proenzymes which are not inhibited by trypsin inhibitor and which thus are responsible for pancreatitis (elastase, kallikrein and phospholipase).[9]

Elastase. Elastase probably has a role in the vascular lesions in pancreatitis.[10] Proelastase requires trypsin for activation.

It has the specific property of digesting elastic fibers, as well as a nonspecific proteolytic effect. Intrapancreatic injection of elastase results in a histology similar to that produced by trypsin. Most of the damage occurs in the walls of blood vessels which contain most of the elastic fibers within the pancreas. Decreased proelastase has been observed in dogs with induced pancreatitis and in specimens from human pancreatitis secured at autopsy.

Kallikrein. The kallikrein-kinin mechanisms have been postulated as being important in the pathogenesis of pancreatitis, but their role is as yet undetermined.[11] Kallikreinogen may be activated by trypsin. The active bradykinin and kallidin produce vasodilation, vascular permeability, diapedesis of leukocytes, and pain. Pancreatic rather than systemic kinins released during pancreatitis may be important in pathogenesis. Injection of kallikrein into the pancreatic ducts in rats results in extensive, transitory edema, but no pancreatitis.

Lipase. The possible role of lipolytic enzymes in the pathogenesis of pancreatitis has been largely neglected.[9] If reflux of duodenal contents into the pancreatic duct occurs, lipolytic enzymes may be important, because they require bile acids for enzymatic activity. The experimental observations on injection of lipase into the pancreatic ducts have been controversial. Some have reported chronic pancreatitis similar to that noted in man. Others have observed no effect, when highly purified pancreatic lipase activated by bile acids is injected. Lipase injected into adipose tissue does not produce fat necrosis. If the lipase and bile acids are injected intraperitoneally, typical fat necrosis ensues.

Phospholipase A. A strong argument for the role of phospholipase A in the pathogenesis of pancreatitis has been advanced.[9] It has been identified as a digestive enzyme in the human pancreas. The products resulting from the activity of phospholipase A, lysolecithin, and lysocephalin are cytotoxic to red cells as a result of their incorporation into cell membranes, leading to dissolution or damage of the plasma membrane.

Lysolecithin prepared from purified egg lecithin and phospholipase A from *Naja naja* (hooded cobra) have been shown to break the mucosal barrier in the vagally denervated canine gastric pouch. However, human pancreatic juice containing phospholipase A, with and without added taurocholate, had no effect. Neither did phospholipase A contained in venom from Russell's viper.[12]

Injection of 2 per cent lysolecithin into the pancreatic duct under "slight pressure" in ether-anesthetized rats produces extensive necrosis in the entire pancreas which progresses to involve all the adipose tissue within the abdominal cavity.[9] The effect of 0.2 per cent lysolecithin, a more physiological concentration, was "markedly less." Injection into the pancreatic duct with purified phospholipase A obtained from bee venom does not produce necrosis in the rat pancreas. Addition of small amounts of bile acids to phospholipase A, in this experiment, led to the same lesion that lysolecithin produces. It is unclear whether in these experiments sufficient pressure was used to damage the ducts.

The phospholipid composition of necrotic pancreas is changed in these experiments and in human specimens. Lecithin and cephalin are greatly reduced, and lysolecithin, which occurs in trace amounts in the normal pancreas, is markedly increased. Increased activity of phospholipase A has been observed in the plasma and ascitic fluid of dogs during experimental pancreatitis. Free trypsin was not detectable.

The pathology of necrotic pancreas in human pancreatitis is similar to that of experimental pancreatitis in the rat after injection of phospholipase. Phospholipase A is activated by trypsin and bile acids. The intestinal contents and bile contain the precursors required for synthesis of lysolecithin and lysocephalin following action by phospholipase A. This scheme also requires minute quantities of trypsin and postulates reflux up the pancreatic duct.[9]

Although suggestive, this hypothesis has unproved assumptions and cannot be extrapolated to human pancreatitis. It is apparent that phospholipase A from different sources has different activities. Until it can be shown that endogenous phospholipase A and lysolecithin are cytotoxic, their role in the pathogenesis of pancreatitis must remain speculative. Furthermore, the human small intestine contains considerable lysolecithin during fat digestion,[13] but mucosal damage does not result from its presence. The observed phenomena could be the result and not the cause of pancreatitis in man.

VASCULAR AND IMMUNOLOGICAL THEORIES

Possible vascular and immune causes of pancreatitis have received substantial attention.[14, 15] Pancreatitis has been produced by the intra-arterial injection of inert beads into the pancreas. Beads injected up the pancreatic duct resulted in the highest amylase in these experiments but did not result in significant pancreatitis.

Antisera against pancreas have been prepared in a large number of species. These antibodies appear to be organ and species specific. Antipancreas antibodies appear following injection of staphylococcal exotoxin into the pancreas. Circulating antipancreas antibodies have been detected in patients with pancreatic disease, particularly chronic pancreatitis (chronic relapsing pancreatitis). The percentage of false-positive reactions in patients with nonpancreatic disease or in normals is small. As with many other autoimmune diseases, the significance of the antipancreatic antibodies is not known. Cytotoxicity studies of these antibodies or of circulating lymphocytes have not been performed. The most reasonable explanation is that the antibodies result from the disease and are not the cause of it.

ALCOHOL

Regarding alcoholic pancreatitis, it has recently been suggested that the direct effect of alcohol on the acinar cell be re-examined.[16] It is well established that alcohol damages hematopoietic tissue and the liver. Perhaps one does not have to invoke bile reflux or obstruction to the pancreatic duct in the pathogenesis of alcoholic pancreatitis. Nor would direct damage to acinar cells exclude a possible role of proteolytic and lipolytic enzymes released or activated by injury in the pathogenesis of pancreatitis.

CONCLUSIONS

Much experimental pancreatitis is hemorrhagic, suppurative, or necrotic pancreatitis. Many of the speculations regarding human pancreatitis have been concerned with these varieties. Yet in fatal human edematous pancreatitis little acinar necrosis is present. Thus autodigestion in its pathogenesis cannot be invoked. If endogenous lysolecithin in physiological amounts produces membrane damage, leakage of cell contents out of, or other substances into the cell could explain some of the features of acute pancreatitis. However, to date this has not been proved.

ETIOLOGIC ASSOCIATIONS OBSERVED CLINICALLY

BILIARY TRACT DISEASE

The most common associated clinical entity in acute pancreatitis is biliary tract disease, particularly cholelithiasis.[17-19] Untreated biliary tract disease associated with pancreatitis often leads to relapsing acute pancreatitis. Chronic pancreatitis and chronic relapsing pancreatitis are rather uncommon sequelae if the biliary tract disease is adequately treated surgically.

It has been stated that there is no conceivable mechanism by which cholelithiasis could cause pancreatitis and that this group should be considered "idiopathic."[5] However, the association is much more than chance. The incidence of pancreatitis among 17,717 patients, in four large series, operated for gallstones was 4.8 per cent.[17] Further evidence that cholelithiasis has some etiological role in acute pancreatitis is its higher incidence in females at an older age than pancreatitis associated with other possible causes. These populations have more gallbladder disease than males or younger females.

How cholelithiasis causes pancreatitis is unknown. One may speculate on several possible mechanisms. It is clear that common duct stones per se are not the major cause of pancreatitis.[17] In one collected series, only 118 of 2653 patients with gallstones and pancreatitis had stones impacted in the ampulla of Vater. There were

813 of these patients who had a stone in either the bile ducts or the ampulla.[17] Two clues provide possible explanations. It has been shown that patients with gallstones have abnormal bile acid metabolism. Perhaps the individual with pancreatitis produces excessive amounts of toxic bile acids. The finding of free bile acids in the gallbladder or duodenal contents in a few patients with gallstone pancreatitis[8] has not been confirmed. Another possibility is that gallstones often contain enteric bacteria. Numerous experimental models have shown that bacterial toxins in the pancreatic duct are capable of producing pancreatitis. It is well established that several species of enteric bacteria deconjugate bile salts. Perhaps these unconjugated bile acids in the presence of phospholipase A, if they refluxed up the pancreatic duct, could release lysolecithin and initiate pancreatitis.

It has recently been observed that experimental cholecystitis in the dog also causes pancreatitis. When India ink was injected into the gallbladder lymphatics, it arrived at subacinar pancreatic locations through anastomotic lymph channels.[20] Perhaps some toxic factors such as free bile acids or microbial toxins arrive at the pancreas through these channels in gallbladder disease.

Gallstones occurring with metabolic abnormalities, such as hemoglobinopathies, resection of the distal small intestine, inflammatory disease of the ileum, and the strikingly high incidence of gallstones among female American Indians, are not associated with a high incidence of pancreatitis (see pp. 1116 to 1119). Patients with cirrhosis of the liver caused by alcoholism have an increased incidence of gallstones, but acute pancreatitis is rare in these patients. Postmortem studies have shown, however, that many of these cirrhotic patients do have focal histological pancreatic damage suggestive of previous pancreatitis.

ALCOHOL

The role of alcohol as an etiological agent in pancreatitis is well documented. It is most important in association with chronic and chronic relapsing pancreatitis. A single episode of acute alcoholic pancreatitis with complete recovery is rare without abstinence from alcohol. In cultures in which alcoholism is rare, chronic pancreatitis and chronic relapsing pancreatitis are rare. The mechanism by which alcohol produces pancreatitis is unknown. An alleged irritant effect of alcohol on the duodenal mucosa, alteration in sphincter function, and increase in intraduodenal pressure with vomiting and retching, resulting in reflux of duodenal contents up the pancreatic duct, has been suggested.[5, 9] This hypothesis would appear tenable if such reflux up the pancreatic duct could be established as a pathogenetic mechanism in the development of human pancreatitis, but satisfactory data to support this concept in man have not been produced. It does not explain why symptoms often begin 24 to 48 hours after the patient has stopped drinking and why acute pancreatitis rarely appears during alcoholic debauches.

PEPTIC ULCER

Peptic ulcer of the stomach or duodenum which penetrates into the pancreas may result in clinical pancreatitis. There is often a local, histological pancreatitis in the vicinity of these ulcers. Overt clinical pancreatitis is the exception rather than the rule in penetrating peptic ulcers. If the ulcer should penetrate deep enough to cause obstruction of the common pancreatic duct, the serum enzymes, e.g., amylase and lipase, may be elevated to the levels observed in acute pancreatitis.

TRAUMA AND SURGERY

Pancreatic trauma accounts for a small but important proportion of pancreatitis,[17, 19] and is probably the most common cause of pancreatitis in childhood. The abdominal trauma is usually blunt, e.g., "steering wheel" types of injury, but pancreatitis may follow penetrating wounds of the abdomen, such as knife wounds or bullet wounds. Fistulas and cysts are more usual sequelae of penetrating injuries. Traumatic pancreatitis may result in cysts which are due to rupture of the pancreas or pancreatic ducts. Infarction results, of course, if the pancreas is avulsed from its vascular supply. Pancreatitis also appears postoperatively (see p. 1197).

VASCULAR DISEASES

Vascular diseases have been suggested as causes of pancreatitis, but it is more likely that the association is coincidental. Pancreatitis has been described in small numbers of patients in association with malignant hypertension, vasculitis, and other vascular diseases. It is possible that some of the pharmacological agents used to treat these entities are responsible for pancreatitis. Arterial occlusion results in pancreatic infarction and not pancreatitis; however, other viscera within the abdomen are also infarcted. In the presence of atherosclerosis, small pancreatic infarcts are not uncommon in autopsy specimens without histological evidence of acute or previous pancreatitis.

HYPERLIPOPROTEINEMIAS

Some metabolic disorders are associated with pancreatitis.[21, 22] Types 1, 4, and 5 hyperlipoproteinemia have all been associated with pancreatitis. The pathogenesis of pancreatitis in these disorders is completely obscure. Hypotheses such as hypoxia caused by sludging, poor circulation, xanthoma in the pancreas, and fat embolization from other sites have been advanced. However, most patients with these disorders do not have associated pancreatitis. Hypertriglyceridemia may also result from acute pancreatitis and, on recovery, may clear completely. A defect in fat metabolism in some patients can be demonstrated by a fat challenge during asymptomatic intervals.[22] The abnormality in hyperchylomicronemia (type 1) appears to be an abnormal or deficient activity of lipoprotein lipase. In hyperprebetalipoproteinemia (type 4) the defect may be excessive release from the liver or deficient removal from the plasma.

HYPERCALCEMIA

Pancreatitis occurs in from 7 to 19 per cent of patients with hyperparathyroidism,[21] as well as in patients with hypercalcemia from other causes, including multiple myeloma, sarcoidosis, and excessive ingestion of vitamin D. The pathogenesis of pancreatitis in hypercalcemia is unknown. Precipitation of calcium in the ducts, conversion of trypsinogen to trypsin, and thrombotic vascular damage have been suggested as explanations. However, experimental calciphylactic pancreatitis which is associated with extreme hypercalcemia has interstitial sclerosis and calcification without necrosis, different from the histology observed in hypercalcemia-associated pancreatitis.

HEREDITARY PANCREATITIS

A number of kindreds are described in which the incidence of pancreatitis is extremely high.[23, 24] This hereditary pancreatitis is of unknown cause and without explanation. A high proportion of the various kindreds appears to be affected, and although the transmission is not known, it appears to be non-X-linked autosomal dominant. The amino aciduria in some of these patients appears to be a coincidental and unrelated metabolic defect. Most of these patients do not have any other associated clinical factors and are not alcoholics. The incidence of carcinoma of the pancreas appears to be higher than predicted in this group (see p. 1233).

INFECTIOUS PANCREATITIS

A number of infectious agents may cause pancreatitis.[18] The most usual in adults is the mumps virus. Others include hemolytic streptococci, *Salmonella typhosa,* Coxsackie virus, and *Candida albicans* and perhaps other pancreatotrophic viruses, e.g., infectious hepatitis, which has been associated with hemorrhagic pancreatitis. Infectious pancreatitis is ordinarily self-limited, does not result in complications, and does not lead to chronic pancreatitis.

MISCELLANEOUS

A small proportion of pancreatitis has been associated with parasitic infections such as hydatid disease, *Clonorchis sinensis,* and *Ascaris lumbricoides.*

Another small category includes drug- or toxin-associated pancreatitis. Some of the incriminated substances are corticosteroids, anticoagulants, methyl alcohol, chlorothiazide, and isoniazid.

A final category is the interesting association of acute pancreatitis and the bite of the scorpion *T. trinitatis* in Trinidad.[25] Twenty-four of 30 patients (80 per cent) bitten by this insect had a self-limited acute pancreatitis. Nine of the patients had no abdominal pain.

Despite the large list of clinical causes, most pancreatitis occurs in patients with biliary tract disease and alcoholism. A large group must be called idiopathic. It is still unclear whether all pancreatitis is the same or different diseases. The pancreas, like other highly specialized tissues, has a limited number of ways to react to injury. The failure of the damage to progress in most cases of biliary-associated pancreatitis, in most infectious varieties, and in those associated with venom suggests that the development of chronic pancreatitis and chronic relapsing pancreatitis requires continuous or frequent insults to the gland whatever the etiological agent may be.

SYMPTOMS AND SIGNS OF PANCREATIC INFLAMMATION

PAIN

Pain is present in 95 per cent of patients and is the cardinal symptom of pancreatitis. It may vary from mild, tolerable distress to a severe, incapacitating pain.[17] Both acute and chronic pancreatitis may be painless. The pain characteristically is initially located in or near the midepigastrium; because of the retroperitoneal location of the pancreas it tends to bore directly through to the back. Variability in pain distribution depends upon whether the disease is confined largely to the head of the pancreas, which is most common, involves the entire gland, or is focal in the tail. As the disease progresses, pain may become generalized and involve the entire abdomen. The pain results from stretching of the pancreatic capsule owing to edema and inflammation; extravasation of blood, inflammatory exudates, and pancreatic products into the retroperitoneal area; chemical peritonitis; and obstruction and distention of the pancreatic ducts.

NAUSEA AND VOMITING

Nausea and vomiting are the next most common symptoms, occurring in 84 per cent of patients.[17] They are nonspecific symptoms. When a patient has severe abdominal pain, gastric motility decreases, pyloric spasm occurs, the distal esophageal sphincter relaxes, and, on contraction of the abdominal musculature, vomiting ensues.

FEVER

Sixty per cent of patients with acute pancreatitis have fever, rare in chronic pancreatitis.[17] The pathogenesis of fever is almost certainly due to tissue injury whether infection is present or not. Although injection of etiocholanolone and progesterone produces fever in man, no evidence exists for action of steroids in febrile states in man.[26] Products of tissue injury, whether from infection or other causes, gain access to the circulation and cause fever by their effects on cerebral thermoregulatory centers. These pyrogens are thought to come from polymorphonuclear leukocytes.[26] In the majority of patients with pancreatitis, infection cannot be demonstrated. Prolonged fever in pancreatitis, however, is strongly indicative of pancreatic abscess.

SHOCK

The fourth most common symptom of acute pancreatitis is shock, which is noted in 44 per cent of patients.[17] The pathogenetic mechanisms of shock in pancreatitis are complex. These include hypovolemia caused by exudation of plasma into the retroperitoneal space, i.e., a retroperitoneal "burn" and activation of the kallikrein-kinin systems. The hypovolemia, together with peripheral vasodilatation resulting from excessive release of, or insufficient inhibition of kinin activity, can account for the shock in acute pancreatitis. Circulating blood volume is also decreased by the accumulation of fluid in dilated, atonic intestine, the so-called third space effect. Hemorrhage and loss of protein into tissues and the gut further contribute to this loss. However, volume deficits of up to 30 per cent may occur in the absence of hemorrhage.[18] The kinin effects of vasodilatation, the change in vascular permeability, and the diapedesis of leukocytes may also contribute to the pain of pancreatitis.

ILEUS

Ileus frequently accompanies pancreatitis. Initially, it may be just a dilated air-filled loop of gut in the upper abdomen in the vicinity of the pancreas. Often it involves the entire intestine, particularly in severe pancreatitis. The pathogenesis of ileus in pancreatitis, as in other intra-abdominal diseases, is not entirely clear. Clearly, it is a response of the gut to an inflammation of the peritoneum. In addition to direct effects of inflammation, other contributing factors may be reflexes within the gut itself, vascular or circulatory abnormalities, and, in the presence of diarrhea, hyponatremia and hypokalemia. Hypocalcemia, on the other hand, would tend to cause diarrhea.

COAGULATION ABNORMALITIES

Thrombophlebitis and phlebothrombosis have been associated with carcinoma in diverse organs but appear to be more common in carcinoma of the pancreas.[27] The association of thrombophlebitis with acute pancreatitis is less common. A striking and consistent elevation of thromboplastic component (factor VIII) and fibrinogen has been observed in acute pancreatitis. In this small series factor V activity was definitely increased. Thromboplastic component, released from erythrocytes and platelets, was suggestively increased in the plasma.[27]

PSEUDOCYST

A pseudocyst of the pancreas is a variably sized, nonepithelial lined cavity containing plasma, blood, pancreatic products, and inflammatory exudate; it develops most often in alcoholic pancreatitis. It is assumed that the pathogenesis includes obstruction of the pancreatic duct with acinar tissue that is still capable of secreting pancreatic juice. Pseudocysts may be small and nonpalpable on physical examination or large enough to fill the entire abdomen. They may present in the mediastinum, in the chest, or even in the neck.

HEMORRHAGE

Rarely, acute pancreatitis is manifested by gastrointestinal hemorrhage with hematemesis and melena. Hemorrhage associated with pancreatitis may result from associated peptic ulcer disease, from hematobilia, or directly from involvement of contiguous organs by hemorrhagic necrosis of the pancreas. Rarely, a pseudocyst will rupture into the gastrointestinal tract or erode into a major artery and result in massive, even exsanguinating hemorrhage. Esophageal and gastric varices may result from obstruction of the splenic vein by masses or pseudocysts of the pancreas. Variceal hemorrhage is a rare sign of pancreatitis.

EFFUSIONS

A small amount of ascites is common in pancreatitis, resulting from exudation and transudation of fluid from the pancreas and serous surfaces caused by the inflammatory process. Some degree of lymphatic obstruction also accounts for some of the effusion. Small pleural effusions are common, especially so in the left thorax; they are thought to result from fluid entering pleural spaces by way of pores in the diaphragm. Occasionally, pancreatic ascites is massive and intractable. Most of these patients have a large pseudocyst which may or may not be leaking fluid. Analysis of these effusions is useful in diagnosis, because they tend to have high amylase and lipase content.

FAT NECROSIS

Other rare symptoms and signs include fat necrosis at distant areas[28] in the subcutaneous adipose tissue, bone marrow, joints, mediastinum, pleura, and nervous system. When the skin is involved, the lesions resemble erythema nodosum, nonsuppurative panniculitis, vasculitis, or granulomatous lesions. The diagnosis is established by finding typical fat necrosis on examination of an appropriate biopsy specimen. The pathogenesis of distant fat necrosis is obscure. Circulating lipase has been proposed as the cause; but in one case at least, serum lipase levels were normal.[28]

DIABETIC COMA

Patients with fulminant hemorrhagic, necrotic, or suppurative pancreatitis may present in diabetic coma. Patients with diabetic coma with no history of diabetes should always be suspected of having severe pancreatitis.

HYPOCALCEMIA

Hypocalcemia, with or without tetany, is frequently present in patients with acute and, particularly, severe pancreatitis. It is peculiarly resistant to the administration of exogenous calcium. In the past, it had been thought that the depression in calcium was due to precipitation of calcium with fatty acids. The data do not indicate that sufficient calcium is precipitated by this mechanism to account for the severe and resistant hypocalcemia. Severe hypocalcemia induced experimentally by infusion of sodium ethylenediaminetetraacetic acid returns to normal in about one hour.[29] Two patients with pancreatitis have been described who had high serum glucagon levels associated with hyperparathyroidism.[30] Serum glucagon increases in dogs with hypocalcemia induced with nonlethal pancreatitis, and infusion of glucagon induces hypocalcemia in dogs which is prevented by thyroidectomy.[31] Thus the hypocalcemia[4] of pancreatitis could be due to an increased glucagon secretion, stimulating release of thyrocalcitonin and leading to inhibition of bone resorption. Patients with normal calcium levels during pancreatitis should have calcium determinations after recovery, because they may have been hypercalcemic—perhaps as a result of hyperparathyroidism—prior to the onset of their illness.

INFECTIONS

Secondary infections are not particularly common in pancreatitis. Most superinfections are due to streptococci or staphylococci.[17] Pancreatic abscesses may contain enteric flora. It is presumed that these organisms gain access to the vicinity of the pancreas through an increased permeability of the gut, particularly the colon. Injudicious use of broad-spectrum antibiotics in the absence of infection, particularly to treat fever, may result in superinfection with resistant organisms.

EFFECTS OF PANCREATITIS ON CONTIGUOUS ORGANS

Mild jaundice is common in acute pancreatitis owing to compression of the common duct as a result of edema and inflammation of the head, to which it is closely proximate or through which it passes. Other causes of jaundice in pancreatitis are common duct stones and, perhaps, spasm of the sphincter of Oddi. Deep jaundice solely as a result of pancreatitis is rare and suggests common duct obstruction by stones or tumor or associated hepatic disease.

On roentgenographic examination of the upper gastrointestinal tract, the duodenal loop is often "widened" in the presence of acute pancreatitis. "Irritability" and an edematous, coarse appearance of the folds of the duodenum may also be apparent. If a large inflammatory mass or pseudocyst is present, the stomach and duodenum are displaced anteriorly, a finding particularly evident on lateral projections. Rarely, the duodenum may be completely obstructed by encroachment of the inflammatory process.

Spasm and edema of the transverse colon is often seen because of its close proximity to the pancreas, and the gas in the colon may appear simply to be cut off. Occasionally, carcinoma of the colon may be simulated. Pseudocysts may rupture into the colon as well as into the stomach and duodenum.

Pancreatic pseudocysts and inflammatory masses occasionally impress upon the kidney, particularly the left. They may simulate tumors or cysts within the kidney on intravenous pyelography. Microscopic hematuria is not rare in association with pancreatitis and may not betoken kidney disease. Mild or minimal pyuria is common.

Pleuritic chest pain is frequent in pancreatitis. It is often associated with pleural effusions in the left thorax. Atelectasis is often present. Patients often have painful, jerky breathing with this diaphragmatic involvement. Inflammation of the diaphragm may also be associated with hiccups and may be a contributing factor to cyanosis.

DIAGNOSIS

CLINICAL FEATURES

Acute pancreatitis has a wide gamut of manifestations, and often the diagnosis is not considered. Most pancreatitis seen by physicians presents a problem in differential diagnosis of abdominal pain. If the pain happens to be rather mild and tolerable, the patient is likely to be dismissed as having psychophysiological symptoms.[32] On the other hand, the disease may be fulminant and rapidly fatal.

The diagnosis of pancreatitis in many patients is not difficult. Although the pain may be rather innocuous in many, in most it tends to have a characteristic knife-like or boring quality, localized in the upper abdomen and boring directly through to the back. The diagnosis is probably often missed in patients whose pain is less severe. Characteristically, the patient is uncomfortable and the pain is aggravated when he lies on his back. Some pain relief is obtained sitting with the trunk flexed and the arms pressed against the abdomen. The pain is continuous in nature, lasting usually for days; it rarely waxes and wanes and is not colicky. It is particularly resistant to relief by narcotics.

A history of recent heavy alcohol ingestion or gluttony will often suggest that the pain is due to pancreatitis. The occurrence of pancreatitis is increased around holidays which are characterized by ingestion of more than usual amounts of food and drink. A past history of biliary colic with the subsequent development of pain

which is typical of pancreatitis should also arouse suspicion of pancreatitis.

PHYSICAL EXAMINATION

The patient often appears acutely ill, restless, and uncomfortable, and prefers not to lie supine. Mild scleral icterus may be present. If he is not in shock, the skin is slightly flushed; occasionally excessive perspiration is present. With shock, the skin is cold and clammy and often has a livid, cyanotic appearance; the patient is listless and confused. Shock suggests hemorrhagic, suppurative, or necrotic pancreatitis. Rarely, in hemorrhagic pancreatitis a bluish discoloration is present in the flanks or around the umbilicus and indicates intra-abdominal hemorrhage.

Fever does not usually exceed 1 to 2° C of normal; occasionally body temperature is subnormal. Higher fever suggests pancreatic abscess, ascending cholangitis, or other complicating infection. Mild systolic hypertension and tachycardia are frequent. In patients with shock, a rapid, feeble pulse and hypotension are present.

Patients with pulmonary complications may have restricted thoracic expansion. Often the patient has painful, jerky respiration. Dullness to percussion is found in the presence of effusions. Pleural friction rubs are not uncommon. Rales, which are usually heard in the lower halves of the lung fields, suggest atelectasis or associated pneumonitis.

The abdomen is often distended owing to ileus. Ascites in most patients is not prominent. Bowel sounds are decreased; hyperactive bowel sounds suggest disease other than pancreatitis. Early in the course of the disease, the discrepancy between the severity of the patient's pain and the paucity of physical findings is sharp. Initially, he may only have some mild voluntary guarding localized to the epigastrium. With progression, guarding becomes generalized, distention increases, and rebound pain suggesting peritoneal irritation appears. These findings create a difficult problem in differentiating pancreatitis from perforated viscus, intestinal infarction, and strangulation of the intestine. With increasing ileus fecal vomiting may occur. Pseudocysts are usually not palpable. Even large pseudocysts may be difficult to detect by palpation because of abdominal guarding and rigidity.

Severe hypocalcemia is manifested by a positive Chvostek sign (a brisk contraction of the facial muscles elicited by a light tap over the facial neves in front of the external auditory meatus) and a positive Trousseau sign (carpal or pedal spasm induced by inflation of the sphygmomanometer cuff on the limb). Rarely, patients with tetany may have epileptiform convulsions. Rare patients have bilateral posterior cutaneous hyperesthesia in the fifth to ninth thoracic dermatomes as a sign of pancreatitis.[32]

LABORATORY STUDIES

AMYLASE

The laboratory confirmation of pancreatitis is imprecise.[33, 34] The determination of the serum amylase in acute pancreatitis has had the most extensive clinical application. The finding of an elevated serum amylase in the presence of acute pancreatitis has been so useful that clinicians have often ignored the limitations of this test. In acute pancreatitis the serum amylase is ordinarily elevated two to 12 hours after the onset of acute pancreatitis and returns to normal within three to four days in most cases. In many patients, the serum amylase is not elevated when the patients are first seen.

An increased renal clearance of amylase during acute pancreatitis is well documented. The determination of the rate of urinary amylase excretion has been useful in confirming pancreatitis when the serum levels of amylase are normal.

Early in acute pancreatitis the ratio of renal clearance of amylase to creatinine clearance is elevated to three times normal.[35] Determination of this ratio appears to be more sensitive than serum or urinary amylase in differentiating renal insufficiency from acute pancreatitis. When the creatinine clearance is less than one-third normal, the urinary amylase alone is of little diagnostic value. Correcting the urinary amylase clearance for creatinine clearance eliminates renal factors as a cause of elevated serum amylase and obviates errors caused by incomplete urine collection. Elevated urinary amylase or the ratio of renal clearance of amylase to creatinine clearance would not distinguish pancreatitis from most other diseases causing an elevated serum amylase.

An occasional patient will have an elevated serum amylase caused by the recently described occurrence of macroamylase.[36] These individuals have two types of amylase in their serum, one that is filtered normally by the kidney, and the other, larger than normal, which is not filtered. Some of these patients have had abdominal pain; although an elevated serum amylase points toward pancreatitis, normal or low urinary amylase suggests macroamylasemia if renal function is normal. These patients also have a very low ratio of renal amylase clearance to creatinine clearance.[35] Some of these patients have had normal secretin tests during episodes of abdominal pain.

Since significant amounts of amylase activity are present in tissues other than the pancreas (salivary glands, liver, kidney, heart, intestine, muscle, adipose), diseases of other organs may result in elevated serum amylases. The liver is the primary source of the serum amylase normally, whereas the pancreas is the source of the elevated serum amylase caused by pancreatitis. It reaches the circulation first through venous routes and later through lymphatics and by absorption from the peritoneum.

Other diseases which may be associated with elevated serum amylase are parotitis, hepatitis, renal insufficiency, cholecystitis, perforated duodenal ulcer, strangulation obstruction of the intestine, mesenteric thrombosis, and ruptured aortic aneurysm. This overlap of abdominal catastrophes, of which only pancreatitis, acute cholecystitis, and hepatitis may be managed conservatively, presents a difficult problem in differential diagnosis. Parotitis should not be difficult to diagnose on physical examination. Even with salivary duct stones the gland is enlarged. Obstruction of an afferent loop following a gastrojejunostomy may create a syndrome that is not distinguishable from acute pancreatitis and which is invariably fatal if not treated surgically.[37]

LIPASE

The serum lipase has long been used as a test of acute pancreatitis. Its application has not been as wide as the serum amylase because of technical difficulties and, until recently, the lack of a rapid sensitive assay technique. With a more sensitive technique which uses an emulsion-type substrate, 90 per cent of patients with acute pancreatitis had elevated serum lipase levels.[38] The determination of urinary lipase is not widely used. Elevated lipase activity in serum tends to occur in the same situations as hyperamylasemia, except for parotitis, hepatitis, and macroamylasemia.

ANALYSIS OF EFFUSIONS

A diagnostic paracentesis or thoracentesis is useful in the presence of suspected pancreatitis associated with ascites and pleural effusions. The fluid may be hemorrhagic or nonhemorrhagic. In the presence of pancreatitis it may contain very high concentrations of amylase and lipase, even with normal serum levels of these enzymes. High amylase and lipase activity in these fluids, of course, has the same limitations as high serum activities. If the concentrations are lower than the serum, pancreatitis is virtually excluded as the cause. Effusions should also be examined for malignant cells, because unsuspected cancer may be detected. Pleural effusions were reported in 15 of 228 patients in one series with pancreatitis.[39] In nine of these patients, it was in the left thorax, in six it was bilateral, and in one, right-sided. Culture of the fluid may reveal aerobic or anerobic organisms, because the effusion may be secondarily infected.

JAUNDICE

Jaundice occurs in approximately 15 to 17 per cent of patients with acute pancreatitis and ordinarily is not severe.[17] The bilirubin rarely exceeds 4 mg per 100 ml in serum. More severe jaundice suggests a possible associated extrahepatic obstructive lesion, such as a common bile duct stone, or an associated hepatitis or other decompensated liver disease. No systematic studies of BSP excretion in acute pancreatitis are available.

OTHER ENZYMES

Phospholipase A has been measured in the serum and is elevated in the presence of acute pancreatitis.[40] The elevation correlates well with elevations of lipase and amylase. Estimation of this enzyme is still investigational and not available in most clinical laboratories.

The proteolytic enzymes have been measured during pancreatitis, utilizing synthetic substrates such as benzoylarginine amide. There is suggestive evidence that this hydrolysis represents tryptic activity.[41] These observations have not been confirmed, and the procedure is not available generally for clinical application.

An elevated leucine aminopeptidase along with the various transaminases usually implies an associated hepatic or biliary disease; isolated, high leucine aminopeptidase activity suggests obstructive jaundice. A mild elevation of alkaline phosphotase in the absence of jaundice or bone disease may be seen in acute pancreatitis.[18]

ABNORMAL PROTEIN

Methemalbumin may be present in serum in acute hemorrhagic pancreatitis and not in nonhemorrhagic pancreatitis. The value of this determination is limited, because this protein may be found in the serum associated with any hemorrhagic or necrotizing lesion within the abdomen.[34]

GLUCOSE

Transient hyperglycemia is not rare in acute pancreatitis. It has been suggested that glucagon release from alpha cells may contribute to this elevation of the blood glucose. Indeed the intravenous tolbutamide test has been suggested to aid in the differential diagnosis of pancreatitis.[42] In one study, 14 of 17 patients (78 per cent) with acute pancreatitis had a diabetic response. The presence of glycosuria and an elevated blood glucose when associated with elevated serum amylase adds support to the diagnosis of acute pancreatitis. Some caution must be used in interpreting these findings, because patients with diabetes are as susceptible as nondiabetics to the diseases other than pancreatitis which cause elevated serum levels of pancreatic enzymes.

OTHER LABORATORY FINDINGS

Hypocalcemia is common in acute pancreatitis, but levels are usually not lower than 8.5 mg per 100 ml.[2, 17, 18] Calcium levels below 7.0 mg per 100 ml are seen only in those with severe pancreatitis; they are associated with tetany and an ominous prognosis. Hypocalcemia may persist for two weeks after clinical recovery. An elevated level is found in pancreatitis associated with hypercalcemia. Patients with normal serum calciums during pancreatitis should always be examined for hypercalcemia after recovery. Decreased serum magnesium levels[2] have been observed in a few patients with acute pancreatitis and could partly account for the failure of hypocalcemia to respond to exogenous calcium.

Serum potassium is usually normal or only slightly depressed. Levels greater than 5.0 mEq per liter have been seen in fulminant pancreatitis.[2]

Anemia is common and it may be severe in acute hemorrhagic pancreatitis.[2, 17, 18] Leukocytosis of from 10,000 to 30,000 per cubic millimeter is common. Rarely, a leukemoid reaction with white blood counts of 60,000 per cubic millimeter is seen.[2] The sedimentation rate is increased in more than half the patients with acute pancreatitis.

Hyperlipoproteinemia may be present as a result of pancreatitis or may be due to an antecedent metabolic abnormality.[21, 22]

Patients with acute pancreatitis caused by alcohol may exhibit "milky serum" as a result of marked elevation of lipids. The cause for this finding is not clear; however, lipoprotein lipase activity is diminished. This defect does not seem to represent an underlying abnormality of lipoprotein metabolism in the majority. Presumably, injury to the pancreas by alcohol interferes with lipoprotein lipase ("clearing factor") activity. Serum triglycerides may reach 1000 mg or higher. (These levels may interfere with accurate amylase determinations.) Additional contributing factors include a rise in serum lipids which accompanies the alcohol-induced rise in liver triglycerides. The lactescence slowly clears over a five- to seven-day period.[21]

Some of these patients may have evidence of acute alcoholic hepatitis with jaundice and abdominal pain as well as an acute hemolytic anemia. The cause for the hemolysis is uncertain. It is important in patients with alcoholic hepatitis to determine whether or not pancreatitis is present, because nasogastric suction, in contrast to high protein feedings, is an important pillar of therapy.

RADIOLOGIC FEATURES

CHEST FILMS

There are often pulmonary complications of pancreatitis which occasionally

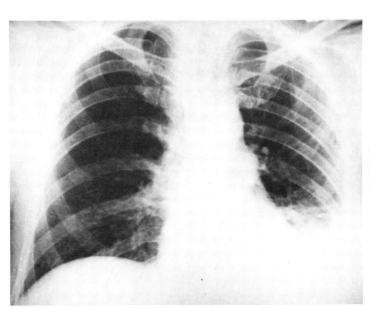

Figure 92–1. Left-sided pleural effusion and basilar atelectasis (or infiltrate) in acute pancreatitis. (Kindly provided by Dr. M. H. Sleisenger.)

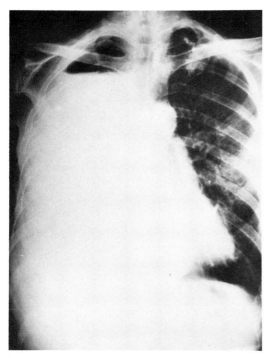

Figure 92-2. Massive right-sided pleural effusion with fistula and air-fluid level in acute pancreatitis. (Kindly provided by Dr. M. H. Sleisenger.)

ficity of the findings.[43, 44] Gas abscess in the region of the pancreas (Fig. 92-3) and pancreatic calcifications are practically the only certain roentgenographic findings on plain films of pancreatic disease. Calculi are infrequent in acute pancreatitis but may be seen in chronic pancreatitis and chronic relapsing pancreatitis. An occasional pancreatic cyst may have calcification within the wall (Fig. 92-4). When ascites is present, the plain film of the abdomen has a hazy, ground glass appearance, with obliteration of the psoas margins. An air-filled loop of small bowel in the region of the pancreas, the "sentinel loop" (Fig. 92-5), is found in from 10 to 55 per cent of patients with acute pancreatitis. Unfortunately, it occurs with equal frequency in other inflammatory diseases in the abdomen. If all or virtually all the intestine is involved with ileus (Fig. 92-6), a difficult differential diagnosis exists between intestinal obstruction, ischemia, or infarction. The colon cut-off sign, absence

may be the first clue to the diagnosis (Figs. 92-1 and 92-2). One retrospective study found 45 instances of pulmonary complications in 228 episodes of pancreatitis.[39] In addition to effusions, the diaphragm was elevated in 20 patients; in nine the left leaf alone was elevated, in six the right leaf, and in five both leaves. Parenchymal infiltrates were common in these patients. An associated pneumonitis could not be excluded. Twenty patients had disc atelectasis in one or both lungs. The pulmonary manifestations of pancreatitis tend to be restricted to the lower part of the thorax. Mediastinal abscesses and pseudocysts have been described with pancreatitis. If the abscess is due to gas-producing organisms, an overpenetrated chest film may demonstrate gas and fluid in the mediastinum. The radiographic findings are not specific for pancreatitis.

ABDOMINAL FILMS

Plain films of the abdomen in the presence of acute pancreatitis have a limited role owing to the complete lack of speci-

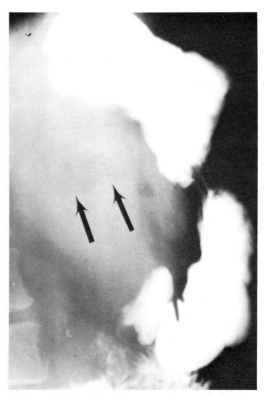

Figure 92-3. Erect film; gas abscess of pancreas with air-fluid level (arrows). (Kindly provided by Dr. Henry I. Goldberg.)

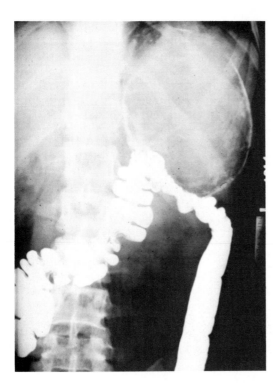

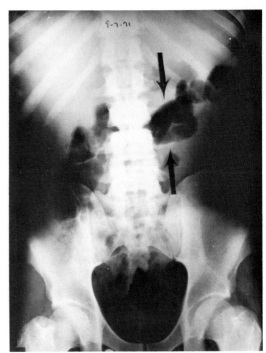

Figure 92-4. Pancreatic cyst with a calcified wall. (Kindly provided by Dr. Henry I. Goldberg.)

Figure 92-5. "Sentinel loop" in the left upper quadrant of the abdomen (arrows).

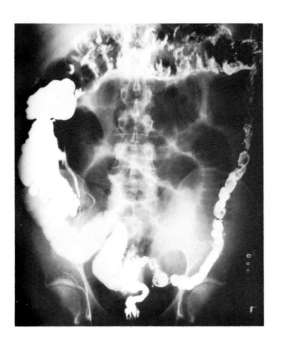

Figure 92-6. Extensive ileus as the presenting finding in acute pancreatitis. The normal barium enema eliminates obstruction. Pancreatitis proved at laparotomy.

of gas from the transverse colon, is so non-specific as to have little diagnostic validity.

BILIARY TRACT ROENTGENOGRAPHY

Oral cholecystography is useful in differentiating acute cholecystitis from acute pancreatitis.[43, 44] A normally visualizing gallbladder excludes a diagnosis of cholecystitis; however, nonvisualization does not imply that cholecystitis is present, because in about half the patients with pancreatitis and normal gallbladders, the gallbladder is not visualized. Repeat examination several weeks after convalescence, however, will often demonstrate a normally functioning gallbladder. Such delayed visualization of the gallbladder does not exclude the possibility that small stones may have been passed or that the patient may have had cholecystitis. Intravenous cholangiography should be performed if biliary tract disease is suspected or if there is spiking or persistent fever or persisting amylase or alkaline phosphatase elevation without jaundice. If the bilirubin is 1.0 mg per 100 ml or less, visualization of the common duct may be expected in 92 per cent of patients. With bilirubins greater than 4.0 mg per 100 ml, visualization is seen in 9 per cent of patients.[45] If it demonstrates a normal gallbladder and common duct, biliary tract disease is excluded. Nonvisualization if liver disease is not present indicates that the underlying difficulty is in this system. Of course, demonstration of cholelithiasis or common duct stone establishes a possible basis for the pancreatitis. In the presence of obstructive jaundice, the percutaneous cholangiogram may disclose the site and cause of the obstruction (see pp. 1107 to 1108).

UPPER GASTROINTESTINAL SERIES

Despite the lack of sensitivity, the upper gastrointestinal series is among the most useful roentgenographic techniques for detection of pancreatic disease.[43, 44] The frequency with which pancreatic disease may be diagnosed is in the order of 50 per cent. It is useful in detecting evidence of pancreatic enlargement from any cause. Pancreatic enlargement occurs with or without the presence of a pseudocyst. The abnormality most often seen with contrast

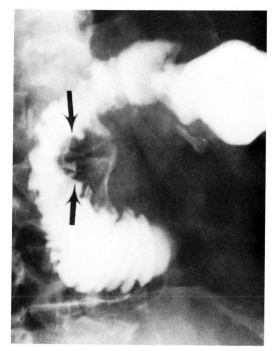

Figure 92–7. Duodenal paresis, swollen papilla (arrows), and mucosal edema.

examinations in acute pancreatitis is duodenal paresis (Fig. 92–7), if the patient is examined within 24 to 48 hours of the onset of symptoms. Irritability and spasm of the duodenum are frequent; these signs are nonspecific. A swollen duodenal papilla (Fig. 92–7), although nonspecific, is an important sign of pancreatitis. The range of normal is relatively great, and minor enlargement may be difficult to detect. Edema of the duodenal mucosa and other segments of the gastrointestinal tract is a common feature of pancreatitis. A swollen pancreas or pseudocyst (Fig. 92–8) tends to adhere to the stomach and displace it anteriorly. Gastric mucosal edema is also a common finding.

Hypotonic duodenography (Fig. 92–9) permits a more detailed examination of the duodenum than do conventional upper gastrointestinal examinations.[43, 44, 46] Usually, the duodenum is intubated and the patient given either 30 mg intravenously or 60 mg intramuscularly of propantheline bromide (Pro-Banthine). Barium is then injected through the tube, and several filled views of the duodenum are obtained in various projections. The

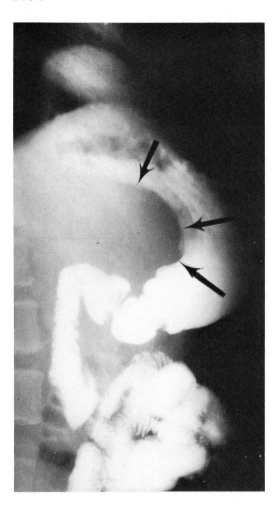

Figure 92–8. Large retrogastric mass (arrows) caused by pancreatic pseudocyst.

Figure 92–9. Normal hypotonic duodenogram. (Kindly provided by Dr. Henry I. Goldberg.)

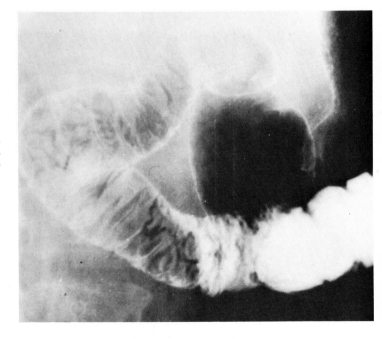

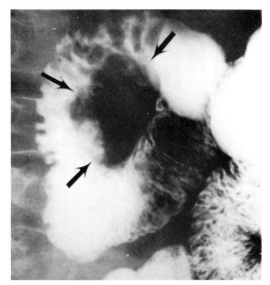

Figure 92-10. Hypotonic duodenography in acute pancreatitis. Mass in head of pancreas (arrows).

barium is then aspirated and air introduced so as to obtain double contrast views. It is useful in diagnosing lesions of the head of the pancreas (Fig. 92-10), but is not sensitive in distinguishing between pancreatitis and cancer of the gland.

Direct pancreatography has not been widely used in the presence of acute pancreatitis but is indicated during surgical therapy of chronic pancreatitis. If acute pancreatitis is present, the pancreatic parenchyma is characteristically opacified (Fig. 92-11). Some caution must be used in interpreting this finding, because injection of the pancreatic duct under excessive pressure will produce opacification of a normal pancreas.

Arteriography has not been widely applied in acute pancreatitis and has an undetermined role. The potential complications of the procedure may outweigh its usefulness. Because of the wide variability of the "normal" pancreatic arterial supply, interpretation is difficult. Arteriography may be useful in detecting masses within the pancreas, but because of failure of many carcinomas to have a "tumor blush" it may not distinguish between cancer and cysts in the absence of vascular invasion.

Barium enema performed during acute pancreatitis and convalescence may demonstrate segmental spasm, edema of the mucosa caused by contiguous inflammation and stricture, or narrowing owing to pericolonic fibrosis and adhesions.

Intravenous pyelography in patients with pancreatic tumors or pseudocysts (Fig. 92-12) may reveal compression, distortion, or displacement of the left kidney, sufficiently marked to be interpreted as primary renal disease.

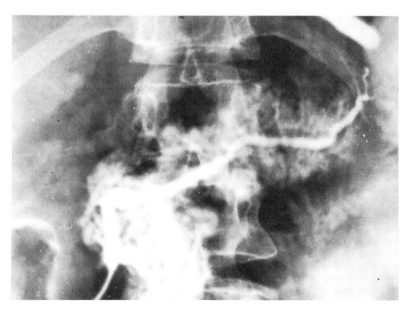

Figure 92-11. Pancreatogram in acute pancreatitis, illustrating opacification of the entire gland. (From White, T. T.: Pancreatitis. London, Edward Arnold, Ltd., 1966.)

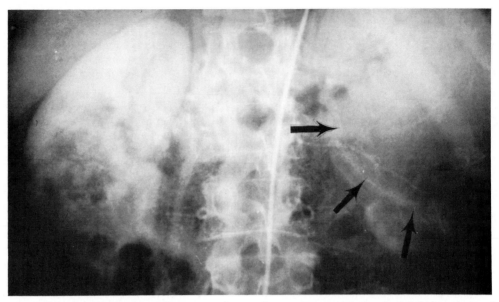

Figure 92–12.   Renal arteriogram. Large pseudocyst of pancreas compressing the left kidney (arrows). Interpreted on IVP as a primary renal lesion. (From Gorder, J. L., and Stargardter, F. L.: Amer. J. Roent. Radium Ther. Nuc. Med. *107*:65, 1969.)

PANCREATIC SCANNING

Pancreatic scanning has been directed mainly to the detection of neoplasms of the pancreas. Most reports suggest that the investigators are more enchanted with instrumentation than with the possible clinical usefulness of the procedure. Since the visualization of the gland in these studies depends not only on anatomic variations but also on cellular function, it is not unexpected that varying degrees of "visualization" of the organ would be obtained in different disease states.

One extensive, carefully conceived and executed prospective study[47] utilized a standard technique with the intent of determining the variations between normal and abnormal. Se[75]-Selenomethionine was used, the investigator recognizing that it is not a pancreas-specific substance. The conclusion was that the scan alone cannot be relied upon, and that it is critical in pancreatitis to utilize all the available clinical information before arriving at a final diagnosis.

A normal scan was found in 43 per cent of patients with acute pancreatitis and in 29 per cent of patients with acute relapsing pancreatitis. Abnormal scans consisted mainly of decreased activity of isotope over the pancreas. In the presence of a large pseudocyst, activity was less than background. No patient with chronic pancreatitis or chronic relapsing pancreatitis had a normal scan. It is not possible to differentiate diseases causing an abnormal scan with any degree of certainty. After recovery from acute pancreatitis the scan may return to normal. An abnormal scan of the pancreas was never seen in an unequivocally normal subject.[47]

There was a reasonably good correlation between the estimation of tryptic activity, by the Lundh test, in duodenal contents and the pancreatic scan. Many individuals with normal scans during acute pancreatitis had normal tryptic activity in their duodenal contents.[47]

A relatively large list of "nonpancreatic diseases" resulted in abnormal scans. Most often the abnormality was reduced uptake over the gland. Some of these entities include diabetes mellitus, alcoholic cirrhosis, infectious hepatitis, peptic ulcer, starvation, gross hepatomegaly obscuring the pancreas, vascular diseases of the abdomen, vagotomy and gastric resection, and a variety of patients studied during the immediate postoperative period.[47]

Placed in its proper context, scanning can be of substantial clinical help. It should be related to all the other clinical information available on the patient, and should never be relied upon alone for diagnosis. More attention should be paid to clinical application than to the instrumentation.

DIFFERENTIAL DIAGNOSIS

As recounted in the section on laboratory diagnosis, elevated serum, urine, and fluid amylases and lipases do not distinguish among a large number of entities. Also many other diseases of the abdomen and thorax may refer pain to the midepigastrium and be confused with acute pancreatitis. In acute cholecystitis, a previous history of biliary colic is of use in differentiating the pain from that of pancreatitis. In noncalculous cholecystitis the differential diagnosis becomes more difficult. Nonvisualization of the gallbladder during oral or intravenous cholecystography is of little use in the differential diagnosis because of the high incidence of failure to visualize the gallbladder in pancreatitis in persons with normal gallbladders. The finding of calcified gallstones in the region of the gallbladder on plain roentgenograms of the abdomen helps but does not exclude a diagnosis of pancreatitis. The tendencies of the pain of cholecystitis to localize to the right upper quadrant and to be referred to the right subscapular area and shoulder are important clinical findings. But it must be stressed that pancreatitis may be associated with acute cholecystitis or choledocholithiasis. In the latter instance correct differentiation of the cause of the upper abdominal pain is most difficult (see pp. 1116 to 1127).

Penetrating or perforated peptic ulcer, particularly posterior ulcers, may clinically mimic pancreatitis. If the pancreas is sufficiently involved to elevate serum amylase and lipase, the differential diagnosis becomes exceedingly difficult. Upper gastrointestinal roentgenograms and gastroscopy may be of great use in detecting the presence of peptic ulcer, but not necessarily excluding pancreatitis. With the current fiberoptic endoscopes it is possible in most patients to enter the duodenum and directly visualize ulcers which are not demonstrable on roentgeno-

logic examination. If there is free air within the peritoneal cavity on upright films and lateral decubitus films, the diagnosis is perforated viscus; however, two-thirds of patients with perforated ulcers do not have free air within the abdomen at the time of examination. The history is also important; the onset of pain in perforated ulcer is frequently abrupt, whereas in pancreatitis it is more gradual. Finally, many patients with peptic ulcer have a history of symptoms typical for this disease prior to perforation (see pp. 759 to 762).

Occasionally, patients with angina pectoris or myocardial infarction may refer part or most of their pain to the midepigastrium. The pain may bore through to the back and resemble pancreatitis; however, unless relatively severe congestive heart failure is present, serum and urinary amylases are not elevated. Electrocardiographic evidence of ischemia or myocardial infarction aids in the differential diagnosis. Other cardiogenic signs such as arrhythmias and pleuropericardial friction rubs suggest cardiac disease. Serum enzymes such as CPK, SGOT, and LDH are much less likely to be elevated in pancreatitis than in myocardial infarction. A history of anginal pain, particularly with exercise, would, of course, point toward heart disease, although patients with coronary artery disease are not immune to pancreatitis.

Pneumonia, caused by any agent, with diaphragmatic pleurisy is often referred to the upper abdomen and may be confused with pancreatitis; again, however, the serum amylase and lipase are not elevated. The finding of a pleural fluid amylase concentration that is lower than that in serum excludes pancreatitis.[39] Radiological study will not differentiate pneumonia from pulmonary complications of pancreatitis; further, pleural fluid may be infected in pancreatitis as well as pneumonia.[39]

A number of the other entities in which the serum and urinary amylase and lipase are elevated are discussed in the section on laboratory diagnosis. Renal insufficiency may be distinguished by the simultaneous determination of creatinine clearance and amylase clearance. The problem is complicated by the occasional presentation of acute hemorrhagic pancreatitis as acute renal failure caused by acute tubular necrosis (see below).

The recent administration of narcotics, particularly morphine and codeine, will also frequently result in an elevated serum amylase, even in individuals who do not have any evidence of pancreatic disease. Thus it is important to obtain a history of analgesic medication given by another physician or emergency room before ascribing an elevated amylase to pancreatitis.

MANAGEMENT

MEDICAL THERAPY

Medical therapy of acute pancreatitis is empiric, although based on theoretical considerations. Most regimens are instituted with the intent of "putting the gland to rest." Controlled data proving the efficacy of the various regimens are unavailable. Despite this empiric approach, most patients recover.

GASTRIC SUCTION

Gastric suction, which has long been used in the therapy of pancreatitis,[34] is best accomplished with a sump tube which is self-tending and does not require frequent attention to maintaining its patency. Theoretically, gastric suction has two important benefits: (1) To reduce or entirely prevent entry of acid gastric contents into the small intestine with a consequent decrease in the release of secretin and cholecystokinin. It is possible that decreased pancreatic stimulation from these physiological stimulants results in a more rapid convalescence. (2) To prevent the passage of swallowed air into the intestine with a reduction in the accumulation of gas within bowel affected by ileus. Regardless of the mechanisms, the patient with pancreatitis frequently obtains pain relief with the simple measure of gastric suction.

ANTICHOLINERGIC DRUGS

Anticholinergic drugs, e.g., atropine and propantheline bromide, have enjoyed wide popularity in acute pancreatitis.[34] Their efficacy remains in doubt. The amount of pancreatic secretion during acute pancreatitis is unknown. Although anticholinergic drugs have been shown to reduce basal pancreatic secretion in experimental models, their effect on the pancreas in pancreatitis is virtually unknown. These agents do reduce basal gastric acid secretion and may thereby be beneficial. Whether they reduce pancreatic metabolic activity in dosages clinically administered is not known. Clinically, these agents appear to be useful. Patients receiving anticholinergic drugs should be carefully observed for ileus, urinary retention, tachycardia, arrhythmias, and glaucoma, particularly when they are given parenterally. They are best withheld during therapy for shock, when ileus is present, and in all patients with lower urinary tract problems.

ANALGESIA

Patients with acute pancreatitis should receive sufficient medication to relieve pain. Because of the observation of elevated serum amylase and lipase in association with the administration of narcotics, physicians have been reluctant to provide adequate analgesia for pancreatitis. Elevations of serum amylase are noted in normal persons given various narcotics. There are no data to show that the administration of narcotics is deleterious to patients with pancreatitis, and narcotics should not be withheld for this possibility. Stimulation of the pancreas with cholinergic drugs and secretin after the administration of morphine does not result in deterioration of the patient with pancreatitis.[48] If gastric suction and anticholinergic drugs do not relieve pain, meperidine hydrochloride (Demerol) may be given in doses of 50 to 100 mg intramuscularly as required.

MAINTENANCE OF CIRCULATION AND RENAL FUNCTION

Fluid replacement is essential in the treatment of patients with pancreatitis. The amount of fluid replaced should be equal to the observed output from all sources plus the anticipated insensible loss. Patients with shock or hypovolemia, as indicated by either the central venous pressure determination or postural hypotension and tachycardia, require more vigorous administration of fluid. Circulating volume must be maintained by the administration of plasma, dextran, or whole blood.[34] The administration of low molecular weight dextran significantly improves survival in experimental fatal pancreatitis.[49] Therapy with low molecular weight dextran in one clinical report suggests a beneficial effect.[50] It is thought to decrease blood viscosity and to have antithrombic activity in addition to expansion of plasma volume and improvement of peripheral blood flow.

Patients who are still hypotensive or in shock after adequate volume replacement require intravenous vasopressor substances, e.g., levarterenol bitartrate (Levophed) or isoproterenol hydrochloride (Isuprel). Such patients may also require endotracheal intubation or tracheostomy and assisted respiration.

Low urinary output (10 to 20 ml per hour or less) is associated with hypotension caused by diminished blood volume. The efficacy of infusions of blood, plasma, dextran, fluids, and pressors must be gauged by urine flow and central venous pressure as well as by blood pressure. Although flow often rises to greater than 50 to 60 ml per hour with restoration of blood volume and pressure, oliguria persists in an unfortunate few. These patients must be considered to have acute tubular necrosis (ATN), chronic renal disease, or, rarely, renal vein thrombosis. It is crucial that ATN be recognized (high urine Na^+, low urine osmolarity, low U/P creatinine) and appropriate measures taken. Early in ATN these measures include intravenous "pushes" of diuretics (up to 480 mg furosemide) and of mannitol (25 g). If unsuccessful, and blood volume has been restored, the volume of daily intravenous fluid must equal gastric aspirate, urine output, and calculated insensible loss. If severe oliguria persists and K^+ continues dangerously to rise, hemodialysis may be required.

Patients who are deteriorating after gastric suction, anticholinergic drugs, adequate fluid and blood, vasopressors, and assisted respiration, particularly if the serum calcium is 7.0 mg per 100 ml or less, almost certainly have hemorrhagic, suppurative, or necrotic pancreatitis. They should be considered for possible surgical therapy.

Administration of heparin or fibrinolysin and postganglionic sympathectomy have been observed to maintain the microcirculation in experimental pancreatitis. Few clinical data regarding these measures are available. Controlled studies are required to determine the role of these measures before they are introduced into practice.

ANTIBIOTICS

Although fever is frequent in pancreatitis, the majority of patients do not have detectable bacterial infections. If the temperature is more than 2° C above normal, infection is more probable. After appropriate cultures of blood, urine, sputum, and effusions, therapy may be initiated with intramuscular ampicillin, 500 mg, and kanamycin, 250 mg, every six hours. This combination of antibiotics is effective against gram-negative organisms, streptococci, and nonpenicillinase-producing staphylococci.

Prolonged or high fever (greater than 40° C) in patients with pancreatitis strongly suggests either pancreatic abscess or cholangitis, particularly if the serum bilirubin is greater than 4 to 6 mg per 100 ml. Antibiotics are ineffective, and surgical drainage or relief of duct obstruction followed by appropriate antibiotic therapy is the treatment of choice (see p. 416).

MISCELLANEOUS

A beneficial effect of therapy with enzyme inhibitors in human pancreatitis has not been demonstrated. Their value has been shown only in the dog and other species with induced pancreatitis. Bovine kallikrein-trypsin inhibitor (Trasylol) has not been effective in treating pancreatitis, preventing postoperative pancreatitis when given prophylactically, or altering the clinical course of pancreatitis.[51] Other measures such as peritoneal dialysis, administration of glucagon, and generalized hypothermia are unproved, and require further controlled study.

SURGICAL THERAPY

A widely held opinion among internists and surgeons is that acute pancreatitis is best treated medically. This approach evolved as a result of a marked surgical mortality during times when abdominal surgery was considerably more hazardous than it is presently. Recent reports have suggested that operation in the presence of severe pancreatitis is not excessively dangerous and, in some instances, may even improve prognosis.[52-54] Surgery may be indicated when the diagnosis is in doubt.[53]

A major indication for surgical intervention is infection in the biliary tract, particularly cholangitis, which is a dire surgical emergency. Relief of biliary obstruction and appropriate drainage are mandatory, even if the pancreatitis appears to be fulminant. An elevated serum amylase level in the presence of acute biliary tract disease does not necessarily imply an associated acute pancreatitis. If pancreatitis is associated with asymptomatic cholelithiasis, surgery can be deferred for four to six weeks.

Surgical consultation should be obtained for acute pancreatitis, particularly if the amylase is greater than 1000. In one series, 60 of 86 patients with amylase levels greater than 1000 had acute or chronic cholecystitis and cholelithiasis. Fourteen of 33 coming to surgery or autopsy had no associated pancreatitis.[53] Afferent loop obstruction is particularly lethal when treated medically.[37]

COMPLICATIONS WHICH MAY REQUIRE SURGERY

Patients with pancreatitis who are deteriorating despite apparent adequate vigorous medical therapy or in whom the diagnosis is in doubt should be considered for surgical exploration.[17, 19, 52, 54] If abscess or pseudocysts are discovered, they can be drained. The biliary tract must be carefully examined for stones. If hemorrhagic, necrotic, or suppurative pancreatitis is found, it has been suggested that aggressive drainage of the pancreatic bed may improve prognosis.[55] Fifteen highly selected patients with severe, fulminant pancreatitis, as judged by shock after adequate fluid, blood, and vasopressor treatment, and requiring assisted respiration were treated surgically. Thirteen of the 15 had hypocalcemia. In seven, the serum calcium was below 7 mg per 100 ml, and in one, less than 6 mg. Eleven of these patients recovered. The four deaths were due to sepsis and severe bilateral pneumonia.[55]

Apparent beneficial results in some patients have been reported following sphincteroplasty, not sphincterotomy, for recurring episodes of both alcoholic and "idiopathic" acute pancreatitis.[56] The procedure consisted of a sphincterotomy and a plastic repair of stenotic or narrowed ducts of Wirsung. The pathology in the pancreatic ducts included varying degrees of inflammation and fibrosis.

Pancreatography should be performed on patients who are operated upon for pancreatitis to ascertain the presence or absence of ductal obstruction. The recurrence of pancreatitis following adequate treatment of biliary tract and pancreatic ductal disease suggests that the pancreatitis may be just coincidental.

Surgical intervention for pancreatic pseudocyst per se is not indicated, because many pseudocysts will spontaneously reabsorb with time, and some spontaneously rupture into the intestinal tract. For those pseudocysts which do not resolve spontaneously, drainage of the pseudocyst is indicated four to six weeks after detection. This interval is suggested to allow the wall of the pseudocyst to "ripen," and to provide a tissue which will retain sutures and reduce fistula formation. Pseudocysts which obstruct the splenic vein may require earlier surgical intervention because of their predisposition to cause the development of esophagogastric varices.

HEMODIALYSIS

As noted above, acute and persistent renal failure, not obviously caused by continuing hypovolemia (ATN), must be recognized and treated. Hemodialysis may be required.

MORTALITY

Acute pancreatitis is a serious disease. The reported mortality in hemorrhagic, suppurative, or necrotic pancreatitis is from 50 to 90 per cent.[34, 55] Acute edematous pancreatitis is attended with a lower mortality in the order of 5 per cent.[34] Death is most often due to severe shock and its complications; occasionally it results from superimposed sepsis. No controlled clinical data are available to indicate a superiority of either aggressive medical or aggressive surgical treatment in severe pancreatitis. These data are mandatory before surgery can be routinely recommended in acute or acute relapsing pancreatitis. Surgery is not indicated for acute edematous pancreatitis.

CONVALESCENT MANAGEMENT

Most patients with acute uncomplicated pancreatitis treated with gastric suction, parenteral anticholinergic drugs, adequate analgesia, and fluid and blood replacement will be pain free in four to five days. Intestinal ileus will have resolved, bowel sounds will be present with passage of gas and feces, and fever will resolve in three to four days. The serum amylase and lipase will also have returned to normal. At this point, the patient may be started on a clear liquid diet. If he tolerates this diet for 24 hours, it may be liberalized to full liquids and, in another 24 hours, to a regular diet. Empirically, the patient should be treated with hourly, effective antacids while awake (liquid aluminum hydroxides with magnesium in dosages of 30 ml or calcium carbonate tablets or powder in dosages of 2 g per hour). An anticholinergic drug given to the point of mild side effects, e.g., buccal mucosal dryness, should be added to the regimen. Most patients will not have a recurrence of symptoms on this regimen. Elective surgery of uncomplicated cholelithiasis and unresolved pseudocysts should be deferred for four to six weeks.

A difficult decision faces the clinician when the asymptomatic patient still has an elevated serum amylase or lipase. If he has been pain free for four to five days, the preceding regimen should be instituted. Some patients may require several days or even weeks before the enzymes return to normal. Continued high serum levels are suggestive of pancreatic pseudocyst, pancreatic duct obstruction, partial common duct obstruction, or macroamylasemia. If the patient remains pain free, reinstitution of gastric suction and other measures are not indicated to treat high serum or urinary enzymes. If he does relapse, an abbreviated two- to three-day reinstitution of therapy is warranted.

When the patient is asymptomatic, the other diseases associated with pancreatitis should be sought. Care must be taken in interpreting a nonvisualizing gallbladder soon after pancreatitis, because it may not visualize even if it is normal. If hypercalcemia is found, the causes, particularly hyperparathyroidism, must be determined and appropriately treated. Hyperlipoproteinemias must be treated as indicated. The patient must be advised to discontinue all alcohol intake if the pancreatitis is associated with alcohol ingestion.

REFERENCES

1. Zimmerman, M. J., and Janowitz, H. D. The pancreas. Gastroenterology 51:242, 1966.
2. Blumenthal, H. T., and Probstein, J. G. Pancreatitis. Springfield, Ill., Charles C. Thomas, 1959.
3. Sarles, H., Lebreuil, G., Tusso, F., Figarella, C., Clemente, F., Devaux, M. A., Fagone, B., and Payan, H. A comparison of alcoholic pancreatitis in rat and man. Gut 12:377, 1971.
4. Symposium of Marseilles, April 1963. Etiology and pathological anatomy of chronic pancreatitis. Bibl. Gastroent., 1965.
5. McCutcheon, A. D. A fresh approach to the pathogenesis of pancreatitis. Gut 9:296, 1968.
6. Shader, A. E., and Paxton, J. R. Fatal pancreatitis. Amer. J. Surg. 111:369, 1966.
7. Opie, E. L. The etiology of acute hemorrhagic pancreatitis. Bull. Johns Hopkins Hosp. 12:182, 1901.
8. Hansson, K. Experimental and clinical studies in aetiologic role of bile reflux in acute pancreatitis. Acta Chir. Scand. Suppl. 375, 1967.
9. Creutzfeldt, W., and Schmidt, H. Aetiology and pathogenesis of pancreatitis. Scand. J. Gastroent. 5:Suppl. 6, 1970.
10. Geokas, M. C., Rinderknect, H., Swanson, V., and Haverback, B. J. The role of elastase in acute hemorrhagic pancreatitis in man. Lab. Invest. 19:235, 1968.
11. Papp, M., Fedor, J., and Makara, G. B. Bradykinin-induced histological changes in the pancreas. Z. Ges. Exp. Med. 147:264, 1968.
12. Davenport, H. W. Effect of lysolecithin, digitonin, and phospholipase A upon the dog's gastric mucosal barrier. Gastroenterology 59:505, 1970.
13. Borgstrom, B. Studies of the phospholipids of human bile and small intestinal content. Acta Chem. Scand. 11:749, 1957.
14. Perrier, C. V., and Janowitz, H. D. The pancreas. Gastroenterology 42:481, 1962.
15. Perrier, C. V., and Janowitz, H. D. The pancreas. II. Gastroenterology 44:493, 1963.
16. Janowitz, H. D., and Bayer, M. Alcohol and pancreatitis. Ann. Intern. Med. 74:444, 1971.
17. White, T. T. Pancreatitis. Baltimore, Williams and Wilkins Co., 1966.
18. Dreiling, D. A., Janowitz, H. D., and Perrier, C. V. Pancreatic Inflammatory Disease. A Physiologic Approach. New York, Hoeber Medical Division, Harper and Row, Publishers, 1964.
19. White, T. T., Murat, J. E., and Morgan, A. Pancreatitis. I. Review of 733 cases of pancreatitis from three Seattle hospitals. Northwest Med. 67:374, 1968. II. Management of patients with acute and recurrent acute pancreatitis. Northwest Med. 67:470, 1968. III. Pancreatitis related to trauma, duodenal ulcer and surgery. Northwest Med. 67:557, 1968. IV. Management of patients with chronic pancreatitis. Northwest Med. 67:643, 1968. V. The immediate surgical manage-

ment of a mass in the head of the pancreas, Northwest Med. 67:731, 1968.

20. Weiner, S., Gramatica, L., Voegle, L. D., Hauman, R. L., and Anderson, M. C. The role of the lymphatic system in the pathogenesis of inflammatory disease of the biliary tract and pancreas. Amer. J. Surg. 119:55, 1970.

21. Banks, P. A., and Janowitz, H. D. Some metabolic aspects of exocrine pancreatic disease. Gastroenterology 56:601, 1969.

22. Greenberger, N. J., Hatch, F. T., Drummey, G. D., and Isselbacher, K. J. Pancreatitis and hyperlipemia. Medicine 45:161, 1966.

23. Comfort, M. W., and Steinberg, A. G. Pedigree of a family with hereditary chronic relapsing pancreatitis. Gastroenterology 21:54, 1952.

24. Davidson, P., Costanza, D., Swieconek, J. A., and Harris, J. B. Hereditary pancreatitis. A kindred without gross aminoaciduria. Ann. Intern. Med. 68:88, 1968.

25. Bartholomew, C. Acute scorpion pancreatitis in Trinidad. Brit. Med. J. 1:666, 1970.

26. Petersdorf, R. G. The physiology, pathogenesis and diagnosis of fever. Med. Times 96:50, 1968.

27. Shinowara, G. Y., Stutman, L. J., Walters, M. I., Ruth, M. G., and Walker, G. J. Hypercoagulability in acute pancreatitis. Amer. J. Surg. 105:714, 1963.

28. Schrier, R. W., Melmon, K. L., and Fenster, L. F. Subcutaneous nodular fat necrosis in pancreatitis. Arch. Intern, Med. 116:832, 1965.

29. Holland, J. F., Danielson, E., and Sahagian-Edwards, A. Use of ethylene diamine tetra-acetic acid in hypercalcemic patients. Proc. Soc. Exp. Biol. Med. 84:359, 1953.

30. Paloyan, E., Lawrence, A., Straus, F., Paloyan, D., Harper, P. V., and Cummings, D. Alpha cell hyperplasia in calcific pancreatitis associated with hyperparathyroidism. J.A.M.A. 200:757, 1967.

31. Avioli, L., Birge, S., Scott, S., and Shieber, W. Role of the thyroid gland during glucagon-induced hypocalcemia in the dog. Amer. J. Physiol. 216:939, 1969.

32. Hanscom, D. H. Diagnostic tests in pancreatic disease. Med. Clin. N. Amer. 52:1483, 1968.

33. Zieve, L. Clinical value of determinations of various pancreatic enzymes in serum. Gastroenterology 46:62, 1964.

34. Banks, P. A. Acute pancreatitis. Gastroenterology 61:382, 1971.

35. Levitt, M. D., Rapoport, M., and Cooperband, S. R. The renal clearance of amylase in renal insufficiency, acute pancreatitis, and macroamylasemia. Ann. Intern. Med. 71:919, 1969.

36. Berk, J. E., Kizu, H., Wilding, P., and Searcy, R. L. Macroamylasemia: A newly recognized cause for elevated serum amylase activity. New Eng. J. Med. 277:941, 1967.

37. Everett, W. G., and Sampson, D. Afferent-loop obstruction mimicking acute pancreatitis. Brit. J. Surg. 56:843, 1969.

38. Song, H., Tietz, N. W., and Tan, C. Usefulness of serum lipase, esterase, and amylase estimation in the diagnosis of pancreatitis—a comparison. Clin. Chem. 16:264, 1970.

39. Roseman, D. M., Kowlessar, O. D., and Slei-

senger, M. H. Pulmonary manifestations of pancreatitis. New. Eng. J. Med. 263:294, 1960.

40. Zieve, L., and Vogel, W. C. Measurement of lecithinase A in serum and other body fluids. J. Lab. Clin. Med. 57:586, 1961.

41. Gullick, H. D. Increased plasma proteolytic activity due to arginine amidase in patients with pancreatitis. New Eng. J. Med. 268:851, 1963.

42. Berkowitz, D., and Glassman, S. The intravenous tolbutamide test as a diagnostic aid in acute pancreatitis. Amer. J. Med. Sci. 246:439, 1963.

43. Clement, A. R. Examination of the pancreas. In Alimentary Tract Roentgenology, A. R. Margulis and H. J. Burhenne (eds.). St. Louis, C. V. Mosby Co., 1967, Chapter 32.

44. Clement, A. R.: Non-neoplastic disease of the pancreas. In Alimentary Tract Roentgenology, A. R. Margulis and H. J. Burhenne (eds.), St. Louis, C. V. Mosby Co., Chapter 33.

45. Wise, R. E.: Intravenous cholangiography. In Alimentary Tract Roentgenology, A. R. Margulis and H. J. Burhenne (eds.), St. Louis, C. V. Mosby Co. 1967, Chapter 38.

46. Eaton, S. B., Fleischli, D. J., Pollard, J. J., Nesebar, R. A., and Potsaid, M. S. Comparison of current radiologic approaches to the diagnosis of pancreatic disease. New Eng. J. Med. 279:389, 1968.

47. McCarthy, D. M. Pancreatic scanning. A thesis on the clinical use of the amino acid Se^{75}-1-selenomethionine in scintigraphic visualization of the human pancreas in health and disease. Dublin, University College, National University of Ireland, 1970.

48. Dreling, R. A., and Richman, A. Evaluation of provocative blood enzyme tests employed in diagnosis of pancreatic diseases. Arch. Intern. Med. 94:197, 1954.

49. Wright, P. W., and Goodhead, B. Low molecular weight dextran in experimental pancreatitis. Surgery 67:807, 1970.

50. Goodhead, B. Vascular factors in the pathogenesis of acute hemorrhagic pancreatitis. Ann. Roy. Coll. Surg. Eng. 45:80, 1969.

51. Boden, H., Jordal, K., Lund, F., and Zachariae, F. Prophylactic and curative action of Trasylol in pancreatitis. A double-blind trial. Scand. J. Gastroenterol. 4:291, 1967.

52. Cohen, R., Priestly, J. T., and Gross, J. B. Abdominal surgery in the presence of acute pancreatitis. Mayo Clin. Proc. 44:309, 1969.

53. Adams, J. T., Libertino, J. A., and Schwartz, S. I. Significance of an elevated serum amylase. Surgery 63:877, 1968.

54. Diaco, J. F., Miller, L. D., and Copeland, E. M. The role of diagnostic laparotomy in acute pancreatitis. Surg. Gynec. Obstet. 129:263, 1969.

55. Lawson, D. W., Daggett, W. M., Civetta, J. M., Corry, R. J., and Bartlett, M. K. Surgical treatment of acute necrotizing pancreatitis. Ann. Surg. 172:605, 1970.

56. Acosta, J. M., Nardi, G. L., and Civantos, F. Distal pancreatic duct inflammation. Ann. Surg. 172:256, 1970.

Chapter 93

Chronic Pancreatitis

John A. Benson, Jr.

Chronic pancreatitis is an irreversible inflammatory disease of the pancreas associated with a number of predisposing factors; it is of long duration and is often characterized by recurrent acute episodes of pain and disability.[1-3] Occasionally discomfort is chronic; regardless of the character and duration of the pain, nutrition becomes progressively impaired. The most common clinical form of chronic pancreatitis is termed chronic relapsing pancreatitis, signifying exacerbations of acute disease superimposed upon a previously injured gland. Although acute pancreatitis may recur frequently and not progress to chronic pancreatitis, such attacks often irreparably and progressively damage the pancreas. Whether a given episode of pancreatitis arises de novo or is the consequence of a chronic silent pancreatitis may be difficult to determine; recurrent attacks, however, are very likely to be part of the clinical spectrum of chronic pancreatitis. When such episodes are frequent and the underlying pathological changes in the gland are chronic and irreversible — having been present frequently for indeterminate periods of time — the best descriptive term for the condition is chronic relapsing pancreatitis. Occasionally chronic pancreatitis is painless and is discovered on radiographs of the abdomen showing calcification. Some patients with painless chronic pancreatitis present with the metabolic consequences of pancreatic insufficiency.

ETIOLOGY

Chronic relapsing pancreatitis may be caused by a variety of insults to the gland,[4,5] the principal one of which is a toxic effect of alcohol. The mechanism of the toxicity, however, is not yet known. That the association between alcoholism and chronic relapsing pancreatitis is common is attested to by the fact that one in eight autopsies on alcoholic individuals discloses clinically unsuspected pancreatitis, frequently including calcification of the gland. A second common cause in temperate zones of the world, albeit far less frequent than alcoholism, is untreated biliary tract disease (gallstones), particularly in women. Inflammatory disease of the biliary tract associated with stones may underlie a sporadic attack or attacks of acute pancreatitis (see pp. 1158 to 1183). Since the majority of these individuals are operated upon with resultant cholecystectomy and ductal exploration, the damage to the pancreas is not progressive, and therefore chronic relapsing pancreatitis caused by gallstones or common duct obstruction is relatively rare. Indeed, successful surgery for biliary tract disease almost always prevents further attacks of acute pancreatitis in such nonalcoholic individuals. On the other hand, patients with chronic relapsing pancreatitis with coincidental biliary tract disease are not relieved of their pancreatic problem despite successful surgical management of the biliary tract disease. The same might be said for treatment or management of any other suspected predisposing cause of chronic relapsing pancreatitis once the disease is established. The process is peculiarly inexorable and is especially notable and severe in alcoholism despite marked reduction of alcohol intake or even abstinence. Abstinence is often associated with a decrease in the frequency and severity of pain, although the progressive destruction and calcification of the gland continue. This course of progressive relentless inflammatory change and fibrosis in the pancreas is explained in part by the pathological changes wrought by successive attacks, creating conditions which cause frequent and recurrent bouts of inflammation.

Trauma may also be an important cause of chronic relapsing pancreatitis,[6] because the initial event may seriously disrupt the ductal system in the gland, providing the basis for future inflammatory attacks and progressive insufficiency of the organ. Often traumatic pancreatitis leads to pseudocyst formation as well; if extensive enough, the associated inflammatory change may progress into a chronic process. With the increasing use of the automobile and the high accident rate, this cause of chronic relapsing pancreatitis assumes greater importance.

Familial hypertrophy of the sphincter of Oddi provides a rare but another correctable cause. Either atheromatous obstruction of the lumen or extrinsic compression of the orifices of the celiac axis and superior mesenteric artery fails to lead to chronic pancreatitis. Occlusion of smaller pancreatic vessels by atheromatous emboli, periarteritis nodosa, and thrombotic thrombocytopenic purpura is more apt to cause pancreatic infarcts than a progressive pancreatitis. Chronic relapsing pancreatitis is difficult to associate with pregnancy, hyperlipemia, hypercalcemia, drug ingestion (including corticosteroids), penetrating peptic ulcer, "postoperative" pancreatitis, diabetes, or infections. Although cystic fibrosis rarely produces the clinical picture of relapsing pancreatitis, hemochromatosis causes a painless fibrosis with pancreatic insufficiency. Instances of hereditary pancreatitis, usually beginning

in childhood, number about 100.[7] It is probably transmitted as a non-X-linked autosomal dominant trait. Half these patients have aminoaciduria, probably an unrelated metabolic defect, excreting excessive quantities of arginine, lysine, and cystine. Painless pancreatitis, apparently in nonalcoholics, has also been reported in the United States, but is more common in Asia, particularly in young adults who present with diabetes and have pancreatic calcification. Atrophy, acinar ectasia, inspissated secretion, epithelial metaplasia, and fibrosis may follow upon chronic protein malnutrition, whether caused by starvation or malabsorptive syndromes. Finally, in 10 to 25 per cent of cases, no cause for chronic relapsing pancreatitis can be detected.

Alcoholism is a complicating feature of many cases of chronic relapsing pancreatitis, no matter what the original cause. Numbers of individuals who have had trauma, biliary tract disease, or postoperative pancreatitis also imbibe large amounts of alcohol. Undoubtedly, it contributes to the progression of the disease to the point of chronic relapsing pancreatitis in many and enormously complicates the problem of management.

ROLE OF ALCOHOL

In the United States chronic relapsing pancreatitis is associated in 75 per cent of patients with chronic alcoholism. Recurrent pain syndromes usually begin after an average of ten years of enthusiastic consumption of alcoholic beverages, further suggesting that the first manifestations of this chronic relapsing inflammatory disease follow upon much earlier injury. The lack of reasonable, safe indications for biopsy of the gland in a prospective clinical study inhibits proof of this notion. In a series of alcoholic veterans in Atlanta,[8] a typically male (4 to 6 : 1) population with this disease, pain ensued on the average at age 33 years, calcification at age 39, diabetes at age 39, steatorrhea at age 41, and death at age 48, 24 years after the start of heavy drinking. Thus it is not a disease of young adults. Chronic pancreatitis is uncommon in countries such as Israel where alcoholism is unusual. Pancreatitis is not uncommon after intermittent but heavy drinking, in contrast to the steady and prolonged drinking which leads to chronic liver disease. It is also noteworthy that clinically advanced septal cirrhosis caused by alcoholism is not often seen in individuals with chronic relapsing pancreatitis, although nearly half of those autopsied have some cirrhosis. Susceptible populations have not been identified, with the possible exception of the predilection of colorblind men to develop alcoholic cirrhosis. This association has not been studied in patients with alcoholic pancreatitis. Alcohol also tends to aggravate the disease and its pain by leading to relapses even though relatively small quantities are imbibed.

The pathogenesis of chronic relapsing pancreatitis caused by alcoholism is poorly understood. If an adequate diet is given, alcohol has no proved harmful effect on the normal human pancreas. Chronic pancreatitis with calcification is common in populations taking protein-deficient diets, suggesting that associated malnutrition, if present, may contribute to the damaging effect of alcohol. The conjecture that alcohol stimulates the pancreas to secrete against ductal obstruction from spasm or edema of the papilla of Vater with "duodenitis" is not substantiated. Biliary tract obstruction does not always accompany recurrent attacks of pancreatitis. Malnutrition associated with chronic alcoholism may initiate the disease, much as with the fatty liver. To continue the analogy, bouts of chronic relapsing pancreatitis may not ensue until some unknown intermediate step, akin to acute alcoholic hepatitis, has developed in the course of susceptible alcoholics. The final disease, with squamous metaplasia of plugged and ectatic ducts, diffuse fibrosis, and lobular destruction, may resemble the end-stage pathology of the liver as seen in septal cirrhosis.

Ductal obstruction, presumably the most important factor in pathogenesis, is caused by proteinaceous plugs, diffuse intraductal epithelial squamous metaplasia, pasty intraductal calcium carbonate deposits without definite stony structure, bands of fibrous septa disrupting normal lobular and acinar architecture, and sheer ductal destruction. The role of ductal obstruction is speculative. All the preceding phenomena could be the result of more obscure pathogenetic processes. Ligation of the ducts leads to acinar atrophy and not to chronic pancreatitis. At times of more acute inflammation, abscesses, edema, hemorrhage, and pseudocysts may also compress and destroy the peripheral arborization of the main pancreatic ducts.

PATHOLOGY

As in acute pancreatitis, there may be any combination of edema, necrosis, fibrosis, pseudocysts, abscesses, and calcification.[9,10] The glassy edema has been attributed to the action of kinins on small vessels. Trypsin and phospholipase A play a central role in the necrosis and activation of other enzymes such as elastase, which is felt to be responsible for the vascular injury (see pp. 1158 to 1183). The hydrophilic effect of hypertonic necrotic tissue leads to the development of cystic structures bounded by adjacent tissue rather than by secretory epithelium. These pseudocysts may expand after acute episodes or trauma and displace adjacent organs, maintain elevated serum and urinary amylase, and underlie continuing pain. Spontaneous resorption is common. In early stages occult and limited inflammation and spotty periductal and interlobular fibrosis lead to an enlarged gland.[11] Diffuse ductal obstruction, already described, explains the poor results which follow surgical drainage of major pancreatic ducts. Gradually ducts dilate and contain in their lining and within the lumen calcified cellular and mucous debris. Recurrent destruction of acinar tissue leads to a fatty gland with regenerative proliferation of terminal intralobular ductules and islands of Langerhans scattered among broad bands of fat and interlobular fibrosis. Neural elements seem to collapse together with ductal structures and reticulum and are often encased in fibrosis and calcification. Calcium is deposited in the parenchyma in areas of fat necrosis as a hydroxyapatite and within ducts, especially obstructed ducts, as calcium carbonate. The development of calcification leads to a small, hard gland. Such pathology is not seen after simple obstruction of the duct of Wirsung. The total pathological picture is similar in its final stages, whatever the etiology.

CLINICAL PICTURE

PAIN

Severe abdominal pain most commonly calls attention to chronic relapsing pancreatitis.[2-4] This pain is frequently so incapacitating and prolonged that the patient's misery has promoted diverse surgical approaches. It usually appears as a discrete attack of transepigastric pain associated with vomiting and usually lasting two to seven days, in contrast to the briefer pain of uncomplicated gallstones.

The pain is generally transmitted over sympathetic splanchnic fibers, and cerebral spinal segmental nerves (T7 to T9) are involved. The sympathetic supply emerges in the anterior spinal nerve roots as preganglionic fibers which pass via rami communicantes to adjacent parts of the sympathetic ganglionated trunks and then into the thoracic-splanchnic nerves to the celiac plexus and ganglia. The axons of celiac and superior mesenteric ganglia, the postganglionic fibers, follow arterial branches of the celiac and superior mesenteric arteries to the pancreas.

The pain is presumably due to irritation by the products of inflammation, perhaps kinins, of the exposed rich neural plexus in the pancreas, inflammatory reactions of the parietal peritoneum, tonic contraction of adjacent skeletal muscle through viscerosomatic reflexes with resulting painful muscle ischemia, and probably true visceral pain from ductal obstruction. The central upper abdominal location suggests a frequent component of the last-named cause. Hyperalgesia and referred pain are not common.

The pain is of a boring, poorly localized variety, tends to radiate to the midback bilaterally at about the T10 to T12 level, and is sometimes partially relieved when the patient sits up and leans forward. Patients are apt therefore to seek sleep in a bedside chair, bent across the bed. The pain is sometimes asymmetrical and is frequently aggravated by jarring, walking, riding on a rough road, or descending stairs. The pain is incessant, and seems to be both relieved by and precipitated by small amounts of alcohol. It is generally agreed, however, that total abstinence significantly reduces the frequency of recurrent attacks of pain.

The constancy of the pain, its nocturnal curse, and the frequent incidence of addiction to narcotic analgesics bespeak its prominence and organic quality and the attendant behavioral decompensation. Pain may be suffered for prolonged periods—weeks or even months—by patients with chronic relapsing pancreatitis. A rare patient may have pain constantly. In such individuals it is difficult to ascribe the pain to continuing inflammation.

OTHER SIGNS AND SYMPTOMS

The attack of pain, often occurring several hours after a drinking bout, is usually associated with vomiting, and transient jaundice appears in about 10 per cent of the patients. The patient has low-grade fever, anorexia, and, rarely, chills. The physical examination may disclose mild icterus, mild tachycardia, emaciation, or a limp from a form of aseptic necrosis of the hips. Retinopathy and peripheral vascular complications of diabetes are rare but occur with long-standing disease. The abdomen contains the key findings. Except during the ileus of acute flare-ups, abdominal gaseous distention is less common than in malabsorption syndromes caused by primary small intestinal diseases. There are often a diminution or absence of bowel sounds and diffuse tenderness to percussion and palpation in the upper abdomen. Friction rubs may be present with acute inflammation, and a soft venous hum may be heard when the splenic vein is partially obstructed. Splenomegaly and ascites are unusual. A tender mass with overlying voluntary spasm and involuntary guarding in the upper abdomen signals a pseudocyst. If cirrhosis is also present, appropriate signs are found.

Since hydrolysis of fat in the intestinal lumen is compromised, unabsorbed oil may provide a clue to the pancreatic insufficiency. It may take the form of oil droplets on the toilet water or anal seepage, soiling undergarments. Steatorrhea caused by pancreatic exocrine insufficiency signifies destruction of at least 80 per cent of the gland. Fecal fat losses in excess of 50 per cent of oral intake may result from deficient pancreatic lipase.

Deficiencies of fat-soluble vitamins may lead to tetany, a hemorrhagic tendency, night blindness, and coarse skin. Between attacks of pain the patient may eat voraciously to overcome caloric loss in the stool; during attacks eating ordinarily aggravates the pain, and the patient is often content to ingest his calories as alcohol. The result is progressive diarrhea, steatorrhea, and weight loss, often despite a reasonable, albeit intermittent, dietary intake.

Diabetes caused by insulin deficiency, both fasting and in response to oral or intravenous glucose, is another result of pancreatic destruction. The glucose intolerance infrequently is brittle with insulin reactions. Complications such as retinopathy, glomerulosclerosis, peripheral vascular disease, and skin necrosis are uncommon, perhaps because of insufficient duration of the diabetic state in chronic relapsing pancreatitis, but diabetic acidosis may be life threatening.

Other symptoms are worthy of note. During attacks there may be bone pain from fat necrosis in the marrow, subcutaneous tender nodules resembling the panniculitis of the Weber-Christian syndrome, frank pancreatic abscess, pericardial and pleural effusions, mediastinal and pulmonary infiltrates, and hemorrhages. Ascites may be bloody or even chylous. Indeed, patients with chronic relapsing pancreatitis may present with nonbloody ascites as the principal finding. It is often associated with an inflammatory pseudocyst. Laboratory examination of this fluid shows it to be an exudate with elevated amylase (see p. 1584).

The patients often have serious personality disorders. Delirium may follow alcohol withdrawal or result from the scopolamine-like effects of atropine therapy. Besides narcotic addiction (10 per cent), they demonstrate other evidences of dependence on sedatives, physicians, and, of course, alcohol. A peculiar depression, sometimes suicidal, often outlasts the acute episodes.

COMPLICATIONS

The unusual instance of chronic relapsing pancreatitis leads to splenic vein obstruction caused by either thrombosis and fibrosis or compression of the splenic vein by a pseudocyst, with resulting splenomegaly, splenic hypertension, esophageal varices, and gastrointestinal bleeding.

Perhaps because of reduced bicarbonate secretion by the pancreas, peptic ulcer is thought to be high in these patients; however, increased incidence is unproved, and gastric secretion is lower than average in chronic pancreatitis.

Obstructive jaundice, sometimes with cholangitis, may develop secondary to a pseudocyst, scarring at the sphincter of Oddi, peripancreatic abscess, and associated biliary tract disease. Other infrequent complications include intraperitoneal hemorrhage, gallstones, septicemia, ruptured pseudocysts, pancreatic abscesses infected with combinations of aerobic and anaerobic bacteria, postoperative sepsis and hemorrhage, and other operative deaths. Hemorrhage into a pseudocyst may follow rupture of a contained false aneurysm. Malnutrition may result from the steatorrhea and creatorrhea. Whether cancer is a complication of relapsing pancreatitis is moot; the diagnosis would be difficult and therapy even more desperate.

CLINICAL DIAGNOSIS

Tests affording help in the diagnosis of chronic relapsing pancreatitis are of four general types: tests revealing inflammation, tests of assimilation, tests of secretory capacity, and tests presenting miscellaneous circumstantial evidence.

Tests for Inflammation. The serum amylase is increased by stimulation of pancreatic secretion in the face of obstruction of the pancreatic ducts or is due to increased vascular permeability, permitting regurgitation of enzyme into the blood. This phenomenon is the common denominator of the pathophysiology of pancreatitis no matter what the course, and serves as a major laboratory aid in diagnosis. Enzymes leak into the lymph, peritoneal cavity, and bloodstream, with either necrosis of acinar cells and rupture of ductules or changes in membrane permeability. Acute inflammation floods the blood with amylase, lipase, and "trypsin" before these substances can be eliminated. The renal threshold for amylase is low, so increased serum levels are ordinarily short lived unless continuing inflammation recharges the blood.

Serum amylase activity (α-1,4-glucosidase) is found in the albumin and gamma globulin fractions; three serum isoenzymes derive from pancreas and three others from salivary glands. Isoenzymes from the fallopian tubes or ovary may also appear in the blood, bound to beta globulins, but α-amylases from liver and intestinal mucosa have not been isolated from plasma. In chronic pancreatitis the serum amylase exceeds normal only when the degree of acute necrosis is sufficient to overcome renal clearance of amylase (1 to 4 ml of plasma per minute).

Often levels are normal during acute attacks in those with chronic relapsing disease. This lack of elevation is explained by marked destruction of glandular cells. Amylase activity in the urine remains elevated despite return of the plasma level to normal because of increased amylase clearance; a timed (two-, 12-, or 24-hour) urine output is a sensitive method of detecting a pseudocyst, recurrent mild attacks, or even cancer, particularly when serial tests are performed. Elevations caused by renal insufficiency or macroamylasemia (polymers of amylase molecules bound to IgG or IgA molecules too large to be filtered by glomeruli) must be excluded. Serum increases may be prevented when destruction of the gland reduces secretory capacity sufficiently.

In early stages of chronic pancreatitis provocative tests employing morphine and prostigmine or secretin and pancreozymin have been employed. The increase in serum amylase in the four hours following such stimulation is related to ductal obstruction by inflammation, stones, hyperplasia of duct epithelium, or strictures. In nondiabetic patients with good exocrine secretory capacity in terms of duodenal flow there may be small but definite increases in the serum amylase. Such tests, however, are not very reliable; an increased serum amylase after morphine and prostigmine administration is a normal response in many healthy persons.

Serum lipase is seldom valuable in the diagnosis of recurrent attacks of chronic pancreatitis. Provocative tests may cause increases in serum lipase in nondiabetics. Serum proteases have not enjoyed popular use despite the development of synthetic substrates because they have not added significantly to diagnosis.

Tests of Secretory Capacity. These tests most closely quantitate the magnitude of the pancreatic defect.[12] The time-honored secretin test involves collection by gentle suction or siphonage of duodenal content through a double-lumen tube which prevents gastric acid from entering the duodenum where it can affect bicarbonate by dilution, neutralization, or endogenous secretin stimulation. Fluoroscopic placement of the duodenal tube is required, so the openings are beyond the ampulla of Vater, permitting continuous recovery of secretions. A 20-minute basal specimen is collected. Secretin (1 unit per kilogram of body weight in 10 to 20 ml), after appropriate intravenous (0.1 to 0.5 unit) testing for animal protein allergy, is injected intravenously, and four 20-minute collections made after stimulation. This dose of the more purified preparations of secretin produces near maximal stimulation. Data are fewer regarding the gain in diagnostic information from adding pancreozymin (1.7 units per kilogram intravenously, 30 minutes after the secretin), with the intention of determining enzyme deficiency. Ninety-five per cent of normal individuals secrete at least 2 ml of water per kilogram of body weight in the 80 minutes, show an increase in duodenal bicarbonate concentration to at least 85 mEq per liter, secrete 6 units of amylase per kilogram in the 80 minutes (the most variable parameter), and show bile staining of duodenal content, indicating gallbladder emptying. Patients with chronic pancreatitis early in the disease and particularly after painful attacks fail to produce a normal rise in bicarbonate concentration. Late in the disease the volume flow may also fall off. The mean normal volume is 3.2 ml per kilogram for 80 minutes, with a rise in bicarbonate to 108 mEq per liter. In chronic pancreatitis the mean rise is 2.7 ml per kilogram for 80 minutes and to 57 mEq per liter bicarbonate. Patients with cancer of the head of the pancreas tend to exhibit normal ductal secretion of bicarbonate in response to secretin but show reduced flow (1.3 ml per kilogram) caused by ducts obstructed by the neoplasm. The secretin test is of considerable value in diagnosing abnormal pancreatic secretion. It may be of little value in establishing a precise diagnosis of the etiology of the abnormal response. The pancreatic fluid collected after secretin administration should also be studied with cytological techniques. The study of feces for enzyme deficiency (less than 20 μg trypsin per gram or less than 74 μg chymotrypsin per gram) is a research tool.

The response to a Lundh test meal of trypsin in jejunal aspirate is another approach to estimating secretory capacity.

Tests of Assimilation. These depend upon studies of fecal fat and nitrogen. The simple microscopic examination of a random stool specimen passed during a normal oral intake of fat and red meat affords a good screening test. The patient with the reduced hydrolysis of chronic pancreatitis exhibits excessive, large droplets of triglyceride oil when feces are stained at a neutral stool pH with alcoholic Sudan III. Normally one sees no such "neutral fat." When representative portions of stool are carefully mixed on a glass slide with 36 per cent acetic acid and Sudan III and the covered slide is warmed gently over an alcohol lamp or lighter, the soaps of the hydrolyzed fatty acids are dissociated and the fatty acids melt into oil globules into which the Sudan stain dissolves. As the slide cools, sheaths of crystals of fatty acid snap tangentially off the stained globules. Normally less than 100 tiny (less than 4 μ) droplets are seen in a high-power field. Patients with pancreatic insufficiency show neutral oil in their stools and also excessive fatty acids, which have been hydrolyzed by bacterial lipases, particularly in the colon.

Patients who have absorptive rather than digestive disorders have no neutral fat in the feces. Undigested meat fibers with squared-off ends and cross-striations easily stain with 2 per cent eosin on a microscopic slide and indicate a deficiency of tryptic activity. Microscopic estimation of fatty acids in the stools correlates well with chemical fat analyses, particularly when the steatorrhea exceeds 10 per cent of the oral fat intake. The chemical determination of fecal fatty acids (van de Kamer method) is expensive but, when carefully done, is the most accurate estimate of the magnitude of defective lipolysis. Measurement of fecal fat does not discriminate between steatorrhea caused by pancreatic exocrine insufficiency and other causes of steatorrhea. A three-day fecal collection on an oral fat intake of 70 to 100 g per day, carefully measured by the dietician, permits reference of the daily fecal output to the daily oral intake. Normally less than 7 per cent of such oral intake is lost. A particularly useful diagnostic maneuver in patients with chronic pancreatitis is to correct this steatorrhea with a potent oral pancreatic extract taken with each feeding during a second three-day stool collection.

Isotopic estimates of steatorrhea with carrier meals and distinctions between labeled triolein and -oleic acid absorption are unreliable.

Normally with 70 g of protein intake by mouth, daily fecal nitrogen (Kjeldahl) is less than 1.5 g. Grossly negative nitrogen balances with stool losses of greater than 2 g per day are seen in chronic pancreatitis and may be largely corrected by oral pancreatic extracts. Nitrogen losses in pancreatic insufficiency are not as prominent as steatorrhea because of the numerous proteolytic enzymes and peptidases in the intestinal mucosa.

Oral tolerance tests are not quantitative. Diabetes is present in about 33 per cent of patients with pancreatic insufficiency. Flat blood curves of fat, protein, or carbohydrate are sometimes observed after test ingestion of vitamin A, labeled triolein, butter fat, gelatin, casein, or starch. If the response is an abnormally flat curve, the patient can be fed the corresponding product of hydrolysis, such as oleic acid, a 1-amino acid, or glucose, to prove with a normal tolerance curve that the defect is digestive rather than absorptive.

Miscellaneous Procedures. Miscellaneous diagnostic procedures include the elevated sweat chloride of cystic fibrosis and improved absorption of cobalt[57]-labeled vitamin B_{12} when fed with sodium bicarbonate and pancreatic extract. A prolonged Q-T interval on the electrocardiogram may reflect a low serum calcium concentration. Associated biliary tract disease may be disclosed by elevated levels of serum alkaline phosphatase, conjugated bilirubin, and transaminases or sulfobromophthalein retention; cholesterol and calcium bilirubinate crystals may be

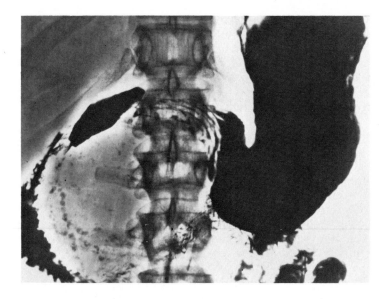

Figure 93-1. The upper gastrointestinal series, demonstrating a pseudocyst in the head of the pancreas causing peripheral displacement of pancreatic calcification and upward and medial deviation of the gastric antrum. Note the flattened mucosal folds of the antrum.

seen on microscopic study of the centrifuged sediment of duodenal drainage after emptying the gallbladder with 60 ml of 25 per cent magnesium sulfate solution instilled through an intraduodenal tube.

The X-ray diagnosis of chronic pancreatitis is improving rapidly.[13] There may be a cut-off sign with gas built up behind spasm in the transverse colon caused by irritation from adjacent pancreatitis. After appropriate plain films for calcification of the gland have been obtained, barium studies are indicated in patients with recurrent attacks of pain and vomiting. Forward and upward displacement of the stomach by masses, particularly lifting the antrum, may be seen, along with widening of the loop of the duodenal sweep (Figs. 93-1, 93-2, and 93-3). More important, the medial aspect of this duodenal sweep may be flattened by an expanding mass or tented by adhesions outlined by hypotonic duodenography (Fig. 93-4). The latter procedure involves instilling air and barium into the second portion of the duodenum after it has been rendered flaccid by large doses of anticholinergic (45 to 60 mg propantheline intramuscularly). Selective (gastroduodenal, pancreaticoduodenal, and splenic) arteriography has disclosed both enlargement in early phases and later contraction in the size of the pancreas, filling defects against the capillary phase with or without magnification techniques, and large avascular collections with hyper-

vascularity of the walls (Fig. 93-5). The splenic vein may be displaced or occluded with thrombosis on such angiography or splenoportography (Fig. 93-6).

In the future, one may expect demon-

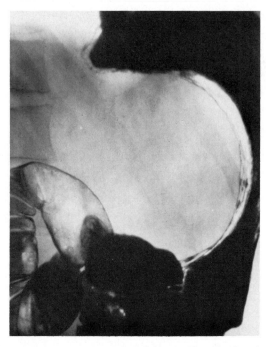

Figure 93-2. Barium in the stomach is displaced forward by a retrogastric pseudocyst in the body of the pancreas which smoothes but does not invade the gastric wall draped over it. Note that the vertebral-gastric distance exceeds the normal limit of approximately one A-P width of a vertebral body.

Figure 93–3. This pseudocyst of the tail of the pancreas displaces the greater curvature of the stomach up and medially and depresses the ligament of Treitz and splenic flexure. (From Rösch, J.: Roentgenology of the Spleen and Pancreas. Springfield, Ill., Charles C Thomas, 1967.)

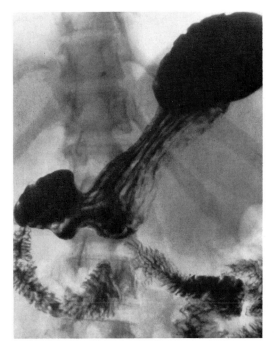

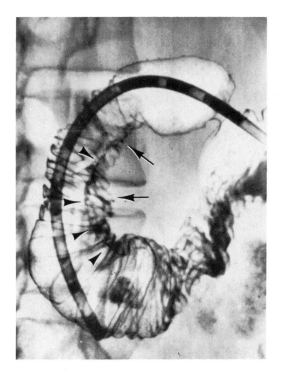

Figure 93–4. Hypotonic duodenography, demonstrating minimal changes in chronic pancreatitis. The duodenal sweep is not widened, nor is its mucosal pattern effaced, but a double contour of its medial wall delineates (arrowheads) the swollen head of the pancreas. Spiculations (arrows) result from slender adhesions tenting the duodenal wall.

Figure 93–5. Angiography of the celiac axis opacifies the splenic (S), gastroduodenal (GD), gastroepiploic (GE), and various pancreatic (P) arteries. In the head of the enlarged pancreas both calcification and arteries are displaced around and straightened by a hypovascular mass. In the tail of the pancreas arteries are spare and tortuous but not encased or cut off abruptly as in cancer.

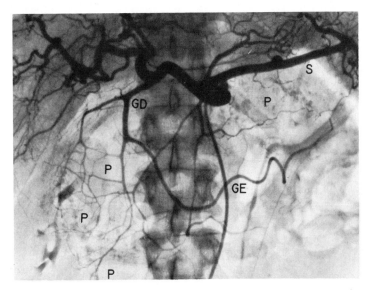

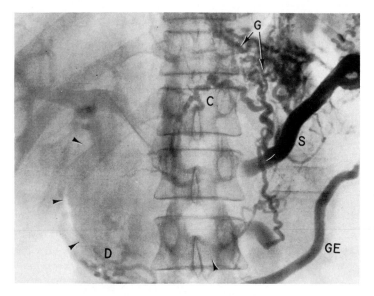

Figure 93-6. Splenoportog-raphy film, showing obstruction of the splenic vein (S) by a pseudo-cyst (arrows). The resulting collat-erals have created gastric varices (G) and hepatopedal portal flow via these varices, the coronary vein (C), the gastroepiploic vein (GE), and duodenal varices (D). (From Rösch, J.: Roentgenology of the Spleen and Pancreas. Springfield, Ill., Charles C Thomas, 1967.)

stration of the pancreatic duct by contrast agent instilled by cannulating the sphincter with the aid of side-viewing fiberoptic duodenoscopes (Fig. 93–7); strictures, stones, and other obstructions have been demonstrated in pancreatitis.[14] The procedure is technically difficult. Expert endoscopists are successful in obtaining endoscopic pancreatocholangiograms in approximately 75 per cent of patients.[14] The role of the procedure in clinical practice is not yet defined. Data are unavailable regarding the incidence of false-positive and false-negative diagnoses. Nor is any information available as to how often the

procedure has resulted in a change of therapy or the selection of therapy which would not have been indicated by the less specialized diagnostic methods. A disadvantage is the high expense of the instruments which have little or no application for other endoscopic examination.

Enthusiasts claim that Se[75]-methionine scintiscans of the pancreas show poor or patchy opacification or localized defects in the image in 75 per cent with chronic pancreatitis. Cost, liver uptake, and relatively gross definition detract from the benefit of this relatively unavailable procedure.

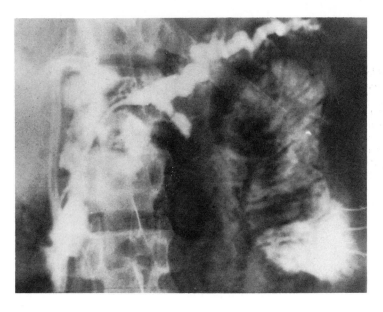

Figure 93-7. Operative pancreatogram, illustrating a markedly dilated, tortuous main pancreatic duct. This patient also had a pseudocyst obstructing the common bile duct. (From White, T. T.: Pancreatitis. London, Edward Arnold, Ltd., 1966.)

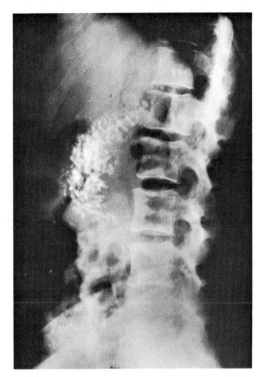

Figure 93–8. Lateral plain film of abdomen, demonstrating diffuse pancreatic calcification seen in chronic pancreatitis. (Courtesy of Dr. O. D. Kowlessar.)

To distinguish pancreatic from small intestinal insufficiency the following tests may be helpful. In digestive pancreatic disorders the oral glucose tolerance test may be diabetic rather than flat, the five-hour urine xylose excretion usually exceeds 6 g and may be even 8 or 9 g after a 25-g dose, and the jejunal biopsy is normal. Urinary serotonin metabolites are not elevated. The serum cholesterol may be increased, and anemia is unusual. A simple flat film may be adequate (Fig. 93–8). Secretin tests, sweat chloride, and response of steatorrhea to pancreatic extract also help to discriminate with a high degree of accuracy.

TREATMENT

MEDICAL

Since alcoholism is associated with three-quarters of patients, its treatment is crucial. Unfortunately, it is spectacularly unsuccessful. Successful treatment is further limited because of dependence upon alcohol for pain as well as for personal inadequacies. The use of psychotherapy, support by lay alcoholic societies, and a positive, firm approach by an available sympathetic physician may help.

Nutritional replacement takes many forms (see Table 20–4, p. 276). Pancreatic extract (Pancreatin, Viokase, or Cotazym) should be given in generous doses during each meal and nourishment. Sodium bicarbonate makes the pancreatic extract more effective. Enteric coating may reduce the availability of enzyme from the extract, particularly in the upper small intestine. Pancreatic extract, useful only when there is measurable steatorrhea, permits an increase in dietary fat and therefore in caloric intake. Added bile salts are probably ineffective; most are also cathartics. Nutritional replacement should include folic acid, vitamin B_{12}, calcium, and vitamin K if serum deficiencies are established. Since amino acids are particularly potent in stimulating and perpetuating pancreozymin release, an elemental diet is not indicated. Medium-chain triglyceride (Portagen) also reduces fecal fat.

The insulin deficiency imposes a therapeutic requirement in half the patients. Initially, oral hypoglycemic agents may function well, but in advanced disease insulin will be required; however, hypoglycemia is not uncommon, particularly in the malnourished patient.

Pain occurring with acute exacerbations requires careful treatment. The danger of addiction is great, so administration of narcotics should be avoided as much as possible. Nasogastric suction, avoidance of oral feedings, particularly protein, and antacids when the gastric tube is withdrawn combine to reduce secretion against obstruction. Aspirin should be given first for pain. All narcotics increase intraductal pressure, especially after meals, but Demerol may be the least troublesome. When feeding can be resumed, small frequent meals may minimize the physiological stimulation of the pancreas. Abstinence from alcohol leads to fewer, less severe pain attacks. Surgical division of afferent pain fibers from the pancreas (bilateral thoracolumbar sympathectomy, splanchnicectomy) generally offers only temporary and/or incomplete relief.[3,15]

Antacids may be useful in curbing a tendency toward peptic ulcer, even though alcoholic gastritis reduces acid secretion.

SURGICAL

Surgical treatment is successful in only a limited number of cases. Relief of biliary tract obstruction by common duct exploration and cholecystectomy to remove gallstones or by sphincteroplasty (Oddi) offers the most help, especially in nonalcoholics whose attacks have not led to measurable damage. Long-armed T-tubes should be avoided. Relief of pressure in larger pseudocysts in alcoholics by internal marsupialization is frequently helpful. The possibilities of failure to resorb and rupture are thereby averted. When hyperparathyroidism is responsible for attacks of pancreatitis, neck dissection is indicated. Surgery is sometimes indicated, particularly in the nonalcoholic, to distinguish pancreatitis from cancer or gallstones.

The usual indication for surgery is intractable pain. The necessity for narcotics, the frequency of hospitalization, and personality and nutritional deterioration are major factors which press the surgeon. Unfortunately, most approaches to draining the major pancreatic ducts, including sphincteroplasty, stone removal, retrograde (Roux-en-Y) drainage by laying a jejunal loop over the filleted pancreatic duct,[16] and resection have not proved very satisfactory in the experience of most surgeons. Operative pancreatography may afford the surgeon an opportunity to correct ampullary obstruction not apparent by inspection or palpation. This procedure may also convince him of the futility of attempts at drainage procedures. Perhaps radical resection (total, with a Whipple reconstruction, or 95 per cent) should be performed earlier in hopes of greater rehabilitation if the patient does not continue to drink alcohol.[17] Such extirpation, it is reasoned, recognizes the random, diffuse obstruction of many tiny ducts, which cannot be surgically drained. Indiscriminate use of sphincteroplasty and mere removal of ductal stones are to be condemned. The

partial gastrectomy and gastrojejunostomy inherent in the radical Whipple procedure add to difficulties in digestion and nutritional control. Ninety per cent of such patients become insulin dependent, aggravating the condition and increasing morbidity in an unreliable patient or one unable to manage the acquired diabetes. Splanchnicectomy is of greatest value in patients in whom nonextirpative procedures have failed to control pain and there is some contraindication to pancreatectomy,[15] a technically difficult operation. Pancreatic cysts should be drained.[18] Large, thin-walled infected cysts in very ill patients should be evacuated and drained externally with sump tubes. Cysts with well developed walls or those adherent to the posterior stomach wall may be drained into the stomach. Distal pancreatectomy is indicated in spontaneous or traumatic cysts confined to the distal segment of the pancreas.

TRAUMATIC PANCREATITIS

Acute pancreatitis may follow abdominal injuries.[6] The problem may not be suspected because the pancreas is uncommonly injured, the severity of the trauma seems insufficient to account for pancreatic injury, and the onset of complaints frequently follows injury by weeks. In one series in Georgia, one-third of pancreatic pseudocysts resulted from trauma. Trauma was also the third most common cause of pancreatitis in patients reported from community hospitals in Seattle. Handlebars on bicycles or tricycles were implicated in pancreatitis in children, in whom 72 per cent of pseudocysts are caused by trauma. Trauma in automobile accidents, especially from steering wheels, compressed air drills, stomping, kicks, punches, falls on railings or furniture, and other blunt injury have caused pancreatitis. Sometimes blunt injury can shear the main pancreatic duct and common bile duct off the duodenum and lead to a slowly developing collection and late symptoms. The pancreas may fracture where it passes over the spine, in association with duodenal rupture, in automobile accidents. Penetrating wounds, biopsies, and instrumentation of the pancreatic ducts or ampulla have all resulted in pancreatitis.

Postoperative pancreatitis may result from trauma, but is also felt to stem from a compromise in pancreatic circulation. Most such cases follow surgery on the stomach or biliary tract. Pancreatitis has also followed transurethral prostatectomy, renal transplantation, extracorporeal circulation, mastectomy, and other surgery remote from the upper abdomen. Often masked by postoperative vomiting, abdominal pain, and tenderness attributed to ileus and other causes, the first indication of this complication is apt to be an abdominal mass, the onset of jaundice, or vascular collapse with oliguria. Besides the development of pseudocyst, subdiaphragmatic abscess, massive gastrointestinal hemorrhage, mediastinal fat necrosis, ascites, intra-abdominal hemorrhage, and infection all may complicate traumatic pancreatitis. Most patients will have an elevated serum amylase and leukocytosis. Abdominal pain, weight loss, nausea and vomiting, abdominal tenderness, and an abdominal mass and ascites are frequently found. The surgeon's diagnostic maneuver, the four-quadrant tap, will reveal blood in the peritoneal cavity and a peritoneal fluid amylase concentration higher than that in the serum. Other diagnostic help is afforded by films showing soft tissue masses, ascites, anterior and lateral displacement of the stomach, widening of the duodenal loop, normal gallbladder visualization, and pleural effusion.

Early laparotomy is indicated, sometimes after diagnostic arteriography. Treatment consists of repair of plasma and blood volume deficits, appropriate antibiotics, and surgical drainage with debridement of necrotic abdominal tissue. Internal drainage of resulting pseudocysts is more effective if the cyst wall is well developed and strong enough to retain sutures. External drainage has been complicated by maceration of wound margins, poor nutrition, and slow recovery. Hyperalimentation by subclavian vein catheter or feeding jejunostomy may provide critical support (see Table 73–1, p. 975).

REFERENCES

1. Sarles, H.   Pancreatitis symposium, Marseilles, April 25-26, 1963. Basel, S. Karger, 1965.
2. Gross, J. B., and Comfort, M. W.   Chronic pancreatitis. Amer. J. Med. 21:596, 1956.
3. Strum, W. B., and Spiro, H. M.   Chronic pancreatitis. Ann. Intern. Med. 74:264, 1971.
4. Gambill, E. E., Bagenstoss, A. H., and Priestley, J. T.   Chronic relapsing pancreatitis. Gastroenterology 39:404, 1960.
5. Howard, J. M., and Ehrlich, E. W.   The etiology of pancreatitis: A review of clinical experience. Ann. Surg. 152:135, 1960.
6. Tucker, P. C., and Webster, P. D.   Traumatic pseudocysts of the pancreas. Arch. Intern. Med. 129:583, 1972.
7. Gross, J. B., Gambill, E. E., and Ulrich, J. A.   Hereditary pancreatitis. Description of a fifth kindred and summary of clinical features. Amer. J. Med. 33:358, 1962.
8. Owens, J. L., Jr., and Howard, J. M.   Pancreatic calcification: A late sequel in the natural history of chronic alcoholism and alcoholic pancreatitis. Ann. Surg. 147:326, 1958.
9. Howards, J. M., and Nedwich, A.   Correlation of the histological and operative findings in patients with chronic (nonbiliary) pancreatitis. Surg. Gynec. Obstet. 132:387, 1971.
10. Sarles, H. M., Muratore, R., and Sarles, J. C.   Anatomical study of chronic pancreatitis of the adult. Semaine Hôp. Paris 37:1507, 1961.
11. Sarles, H., Sarles, J. C., Camatte, R., et al.   Observations on 205 confirmed cases of acute pancreatitis, recurring pancreatitis, and chronic pancreatitis. Gut 6:545, 1965.
12. Dreiling, D. A., Janowitz, H. D., and Perrier, C. V.   Pancreatic Inflammatory Disease. A Physiologic Approach. New York, Paul B. Hoeber, Inc., 1964.
13. Rösch, J.   Roentgenology of the Spleen and Pancreas. Springfield, Ill., Charles C Thomas, 1967.
14. Kasugai, T., Kuno, N., Kizu, M., et al. Endoscopic pancreatocholangiography. II. The pathological endoscopic pancreatocholangiogram. Gastroenterology 63:227, 1972.
15. White, T. T., Lawinski, M., Stacher, G., et al.   Treatment of pancreatitis by left splanchnicectomy and coeliac ganglionectomy. An analysis of 146 cases. Amer. J. Surg. 112:195, 1966.
16. Gillesby, W. J., II, and Puestow, C. B.   Pancreatico-jejunostomy for chronic relapsing pancreatitis: An evaluation. Surgery 50:859, 1961.
17. Child, C. G., Frey, C. F., and Fry, W. J.   A reappraisal of removal of 95 percent of the distal portion of the pancreas. Surg. Gynec. Obstet. 129:49, 1969.
18. Warren, K. W., Athanassiades, S., Frederick, P., and Kune, G. A.   Surgical treatment of pancreatic cysts: Review of 183 cases. Ann. Surg. 163:886, 1966.

Chapter 94

Carcinoma of the Pancreas

Clifford S. Melnyk

The inaccessibility of the pancreas to palpation and radiological examination combined with its location near vital structures results in considerable difficulty in diagnosis and treatment of pancreatic neoplasms. Emphasis must be placed on key clinical symptoms and selective diagnostic techniques to improve early diagnosis and ultimate survival rate of this catastrophic disease.

The classification of exocrine neoplasms of the pancreas[1] is listed in Table 94–1. Neoplasms may originate in acinar or duct cells. Most of the neoplasms are rare except for the solid adenocarcinoma of ductal origin. The incidence of pancreatic carcinoma is 2 to 4 per cent of all types of carcinoma.

TABLE 94–1. CLASSIFICATION OF
EXOCRINE PANCREATIC TUMORS

I. Acinar cell
  A. Adenoma
  B. Adenocarcinoma
II. Ductal cell
  A. Benign
    1. Solid adenoma
    2. Cystadenoma
  B. Malignant
    1. Solid carcinoma
      a. Adenocarcinoma
      b. Anaplastic carcinoma
      c. Squamous cell carcinoma
    2. Cystadenocarcinoma

CYSTADENOMA AND CYSTADENOCARCINOMA

The cystadenoma and cystadenocarcinoma are uncommon, but present with certain clinical features which differ from the solid neoplasms.[2] They occur at an earlier age, with one-third of the patients being less than 50 years of age. There is female predominance in a ratio of 9:1; solid tumors are more frequent in males. The patients have few symptoms and present with poorly defined upper abdominal masses which are nontender (Fig. 94–1). A neoplastic cyst is suggested when pancreatitis induced by alcohol or trauma is excluded. Total excision of the cystic neoplasm is the ideal treatment rather than marsupialization. The tumor generally can be removed with ease, because it is frequently derived from the distal portion of the gland and has minimal surrounding inflammatory and fibrous reaction.

SOLID ADENOCARCINOMA

The most common neoplasm of the pancreas is the solid adenocarcinoma of duct cell origin. The mean age of onset of symptoms is 55 years. The male:female ratio is 2:1. The neoplasm occurs in the head of the gland in 70 per cent, the body in 20 per cent, and the tail in 10 per cent of patients. Predisposing factors which have been cited in the development of pancreatic neoplasms are chronic pancreatitis, heavy

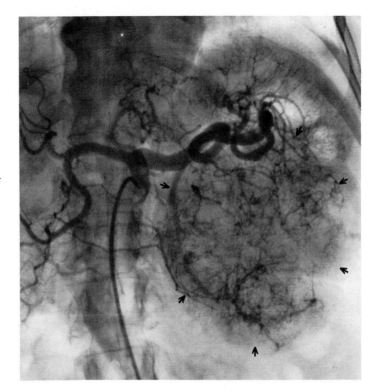

Figure 94-1. Angiogram of cystadenoma of distal pancreas shown as a large, circular, hypervascular mass (outlined by arrows).

alcohol intake,[3] and diabetes mellitus.[4] However, in the majority of patients such factors are absent. Diabetes mellitus is particularly illustrative of the problem, because it is difficult to discern whether the abnormality in glucose tolerance preceded or occurred as a result of the tumor. At present the relationship of these three factors to the development of carcinoma of the pancreas is not established.

CLINICAL PICTURE

The initial symptoms are generally vague and ill defined, and do not concern the patient or arouse suspicion in the physician that organic disease exists. Difficulty in diagnosis is further compounded by the frequent lack of findings on standard gastrointestinal X-rays when symptoms have abdominal localization. This combination usually prompts a diagnosis of neurotic or functional disorder. Only 15 per cent of the patients with early symptoms consult a physician within the first month after the onset of symptoms, and only 65 per cent do so within six months. The significance of this delay was high-lighted in one study[5] in which 56 per cent of the carcinomas of the head of the pancreas were resectable when symptoms were present for less than three months but only 13 per cent were resectable when symptoms had existed for a greater length of time.

The classic triad of pain, weight loss, and jaundice unfortunately appears relatively late in patients with pancreatic carcinoma, and usually portends an early death.

Pain at first is dull and vague, sometimes localized to the epigastrium, often extending to the left and right upper quadrants or to the back. The pain may be initially episodic and related to meals, but later becomes persistent and severe and radiates through to the back. Severe pain suggests malignant infiltration into the retroperitoneal area around the celiac axis with invasion of its associated neural plexus. A characteristic feature of the tumor is direct nerve and vessel invasion or encasement rather than displacement combined with an associated fibrotic reaction. This may explain the occurrence of severe and unremitting pain. Pancreatic pain has some anatomical localization:

tumors in the head of the pancreas produce more intense pain in the right epigastrium, whereas those located in the body will tend to localize in the midline, and those occurring in the tail may refer to the left upper quadrant. The pain is ameliorated by the sitting position, particularly by leaning forward.

Weight loss invariably occurs and results in a mean loss of 15 to 20 pounds. The loss is dramatic and progressive. It often precedes all other symptoms and occurs while the tumor is still resectable. This may result from what is considered a distinctive feature of pancreatic carcinoma, an aversion to food rather than true anorexia. Pain induced by eating, diabetes, and malabsorption from pancreatic insufficiency may all contribute to the weight loss.

Indeed, malabsorption may dominate the clinical picture for as long as nine months to a year or so; its basis becomes clear when jaundice supervenes. Thus the tumor has marched from tail-body to head.

Jaundice occurs in 75 per cent of the patients with pancreatic carcinoma. The jaundice is usually deep and progressive. The patient complains of pruritus, dark urine, and light-colored stools. An enlarged and palpable gallbladder is certainly strongly suggestive of a pancreatic carcinoma. The absence of a palpable gallbladder in a jaundiced patient does not exclude a pancreatic carcinoma. Since the laboratory studies of the jaundice demonstrate an obstructive pattern, a palpable gallbladder facilitates the clinical distinction between an intrahepatic and an extrahepatic obstruction.

Diabetes mellitus occurs in 25 to 50 per cent of cases and is manifest most frequently as an abnormal glucose tolerance test rather than overt glucosuria or fasting hyperglycemia. This abnormality in any person over the age of 40 without a genetic predisposition for diabetes, along with abdominal complaints, particularly with diarrhea and steatorrhea, warrants a complete evaluation of the possibility of pancreatic carcinoma. An unexplained increase in severity of established diabetes with abdominal complaints should prompt similar consideration. Although complications of diabetes are uncommon, retinopathy has been noted in pancreatic carcinoma with neither pre-existing nor familial diabetes.

Gastrointestinal bleeding may be massive or occult and may result from a variety of causes. The tumor may invade the stomach or duodenum directly, producing an ulceration; obstruct the outlet of the stomach, inducing a benign gastric ulceration; or compress the portal venous system, producing portal hypertension and esophagogastric varices.

Thrombophlebitis of the migratory type and resistant to anticoagulants is seen with pancreatic carcinoma, but also occurs in association with other neoplasms. Multiple venous thromboses occur most frequently when the tumor involves the body or tail of the pancreas.

Mental symptoms of depression, premonition of illness, and anxiety occur in 76 per cent of the patients with pancreatic carcinoma.[6] Nearly 50 per cent of the patients report mental symptoms as the first indication of the disease. Similar symptoms may occur with involutional depression in this age group. The presence of these symptoms in conjunction with abdominal complaints should prompt concern regarding the pancreas.

Subcutaneous fat necrosis and polyarthralgia occur principally in association with acinar-cell carcinomas,[7] which are uncommon. The fat necrosis presents as tender subcutaneous nodules, involving first the lower extremities and then spreading over the body. A possible mechanism for the fat necrosis is excessive production of lipase by the tumor.[7] These nodules must be differentiated from tumor metastases which may appear in the skin and scalp.

Uncommon clinical features which have been reported in association with pancreatic carcinoma are hypoglycemia,[8] hypercalcemia,[9] carcinoid syndrome, excessive adrenocorticotropic hormone (ACTH)[10] production by the tumor, and inappropriate antidiuretic hormone (ADH) secretion.[11]

Physical findings are variable, depending on the location and extent of the neoplasm, whether it involves the head, body, tail, or contiguous structures. The findings consist of altered mental status, jaundice, emaciation, epigastric tenderness and spasm, palpable pancreatic mass, palpable gallbladder in 50 per cent of jaundiced patients, and enlarged, hard liver. Signs of portal hypertension, i.e., splenomegaly, prominent abdominal wall veins, upper abdominal venous "hums," and hemorrhoids, may result from compression, invasion, or thrombosis of the portal venous system, especially the splenic vein. A systolic bruit in the left upper quadrant may result from splenic artery compression by tumor. However, a similar bruit can result from other arterial alterations, i.e., aneurysm, arteritis, or arteriovenous malformation. Ascites may appear.

DIAGNOSIS

The *clinical laboratory* is of minimal value in establishing a diagnosis of pancreatic neoplasm. The serum or urinary *amylase* may be mildly elevated in a few patients as a result of pancreatitis secondary to an obstructing tumor. The *glucose tolerance test* is abnormal in 25 to 50 per cent of the patients. This is more frequent than frank glucosuria or fasting hyperglycemia. The reason for the glucose intolerance is unknown and cannot be attributed to replacement of the normal islet cell mass by tumor.

The *secretin-pancreozymin test* is a means of measuring the functional capacity of the exocrine pancreas. The significance of the test for assessing the functional pancreatic reserve is discussed on pages 1190 to 1191. In pancreatic carcinoma the typical test results in a greatly diminished volume flow but a normal bicarbonate concentration and amylase secretion. In contrast, in chronic pancreatitis the volume flow is normal but the bicarbonate concentration and amylase secretion are reduced. Although there is good physiological basis for this stimulation test, the results are frequently conflicting and the procedure is time consuming; therefore, it has not been universally utilized.

Cytological examination of the pancreatic secretions obtained simultaneously with the secretin stimulation test may yield positive results in 30 to 70 per cent of cases with carcinoma.[12] The results, however, are not consistent enough to depend upon cytology for diagnosis.

Photoscanning of the pancreas utilizing Se[75]-selenomethionine results in decreased uptake of radioactive material in pancreatic tumors and pseudocysts. The inability to differentiate benign from malignant processes, the inaccuracy produced by the uptake of the liver, and the complexity and cost of the procedure have limited the value and availability of this technique in evaluating pancreatic disorders.

Roentgenographic studies provide the most useful information in establishing a diagnosis of pancreatic carcinoma. The techniques available consist of barium contrast study of the stomach and duodenum, selective arteriography, and cholangiography. The standard upper gastrointestinal series in pancreatic carcinoma may show mucosal flattening, rigidity, and widening of the duodenal loop and incomplete filling of the gastric antrum (Fig. 94-2). Direct invasion of the duodenal wall may create the "inverted 3" sign of Frostberg. In less advanced cases, the ability to detect early changes is improved by *hypotonic duodenography*, performed with either anticholinergic agents or secretin. Spiculation, flattening of folds, and nodular indentation along the inner aspect of the duodenal loop are the most reliable signs.[13] Similar changes, however, may occur in patients with chronic pancreatitis and collateral circulation second-

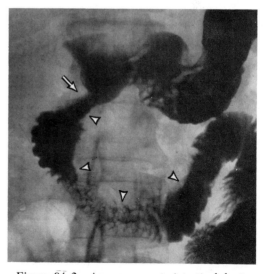

Figure 94-2. An upper gastrointestinal barium study, demonstrating displacement and infiltration of the medial aspect of the duodenal loop by pancreatic adenocarcinoma (arrowheads) and compression of the lateral aspect of the upper duodenum by an enlarged gallbladder (arrow).

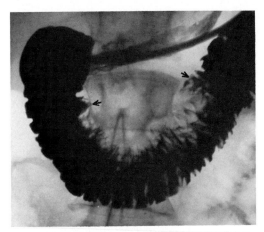

Figure 94–3. Hypotonic duodenography, demonstrating spiculation and nodularity (between arrows) of the medial aspect of the duodenal loop produced by a pancreatic adenocarcinoma. (From Rösch, J.: Roentgenology of the Spleen and Pancreas. Springfield, Ill., Charles C Thomas, 1967.)

ary to portal hypertension. The presence of fine, sharply pointed serrations along the inner aspect of the duodenal loop is strongly suggestive of carcinoma (Fig. 94–3). Disadvantages of the technique are that it provides little information on the body and tail of the pancreas and has limited accuracy in distinguishing cancer from pancreatitis.

Selective or superselective angiography is of considerable value in defining pancreatic carcinoma. Malignant neoplasms of the pancreas are usually hypovascular tumors, and detection depends on demonstration of vascular deviation of pancreatic or peripancreatic vessels. The most reliable angiographic signs are irregular arterial or venous encasement, abrupt cut-off or occlusion of vessels, and occasional neovascular vessels (Fig. 94–4). For the best interpretation of these findings, superselective injection into the dorsal pancreatic, inferior pancreaticoduodenal, and gastroduodenal arteries combined with magnification is invaluable. Venous changes, consisting of occlusion or encasement of the splenic and superior mesenteric veins and their branches, are best demonstrated in the late phase of selective angiography. Angiography provides additional information regarding gallbladder size, the presence of metastases in the liver, and enlarged intrahepatic bile ducts. The accuracy in prospective diagnosis of

pancreatic carcinoma utilizing this technique is at least 75 per cent[14] and may approach 90 per cent at some centers. The presence of chronic pancreatitis can make the distinction from carcinoma much more difficult. Operability is not compromised by mass lesions demonstrated on angiography, but the prospects of resection are diminished in the presence of encasement of the hepatic, gastroduodenal, splenic, and superior mesenteric arteries.[5] The disadvantages of angiography are the limited availability, the cost, and occasional complications such as arterial thrombosis or injury.

In the severely jaundiced patient in whom intrahepatic cholestasis (drug-induced) and extrahepatic obstruction cannot be clinically distinguished, selective angiography and *cholangiography* are helpful. A transhepatic (percutaneous or transjugular) cholangiogram can be performed to confirm an extrahepatic block (Fig. 94–5). Contrast agent can be injected

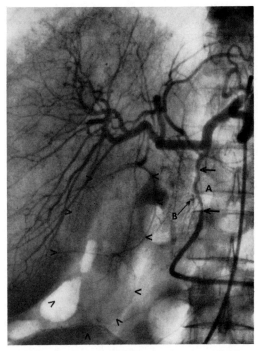

Figure 94–4. Angiogram of pancreatic adenocarcinoma, showing tumor encasement of gastroduodenal artery (A, between arrows), increased and abnormal vascularity in the head of the pancreas (B), and enlarged gallbladder manifest by elongation and displacement of cystic artery branches (outlined by open arrows).

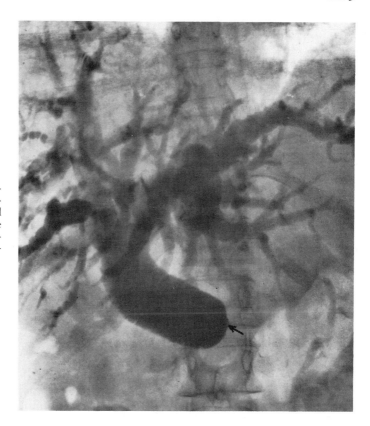

Figure 94–5. Percutaneous cholangiogram, showing massively dilated and completely obstructed common bile duct by pancreatic adenocarcinoma (arrow). Note degree of intrahepatic bile duct dilatation.

after decompression of biliary pressure. A carcinoma involving the head of the pancreas will produce a tapered obstruction of the common bile duct. With demonstration of a dilated ductal system, the patient should have surgery for biliary tract decompression. In the absence of a dilated ductal system the patient can undergo a percutaneous liver biopsy with lessened concern over a bile leak into the peritoneal cavity (see pp. 1105 to 1109).

The possibility of an immunological screening test for pancreatic carcinoma is being evaluated. In preliminary trials, the *carcinoembryonic antigen* has been reported positive in 90 per cent of patients with proved pancreatic carcinoma and 30 to 70 per cent positive in other digestive tract tumors.[15] However, the significance of this immunological assay awaits further standardization of technique and clinical assessment.

Direct catheterization of the ampulla of Vater via a fiberoptic duodenoscope is being evaluated.[16] This procedure provides a means of obtaining secretory, cytological, and roentgenographic data directly which may improve our ability to diagnose pancreatic neoplasm. A hazard of the procedure is the precipitation of acute pancreatitis secondary to the intraductal injection under pressure of contrast material.

Definitive diagnosis or strong clinical suspicion of pancreatic carcinoma requires surgical exploration. Tissue diagnosis is obtained by lymph node biopsy or resection of the lesion. Surgeons are reluctant to biopsy the suspected tumor mass directly because of the possibility of spreading the tumor or producing serious complications such as fistulas. We recommend that if biopsy is performed, a transduodenal needle approach be utilized. The difficulty of pathological interpretation of this biopsy material is compounded by the frequent occurrence of a surrounding inflammatory reaction and an associated distal pancreatitis. Because of these findings, it is not uncommon that a firm tissue diagnosis of carcinoma cannot be established by needle biopsy and the final impression depends upon the surgeon's discriminating palpation of the pancreatic mass.

SQUAMOUS CELL CARCINOMA

Squamous cell carcinoma of the pancreas has similar clinical features to the more common solid adenocarcinoma of the pancreas. The significance of squamous cell carcinoma of the pancreas is that it may present as a pulmonary metastasis and thereby simulate a bronchogenic carcinoma. This is particularly of concern when the carcinoma occurs in the tail of the pancreas where it remains silent for a long period of time and has a greater tendency to metastasize to the lung. The lesion in the lung can produce all the clinical manifestations of bronchogenic carcinoma, including radiological findings, cervical adenopathy, Horner's syndrome, and superior vena cava obstruction.[17] The tumor may permeate the lymphatics of the lung, producing an alveolar capillary block resulting in progressive dyspnea. Because of the similar histological picture of the tumors, a postmortem examination may be required to confirm the diagnosis. The importance of this presentation is that the clinician consider the pancreas as a possible primary site.

PROGNOSIS AND TREATMENT

Pancreatic carcinoma is a progressive, relentless neoplastic process for which there is no satisfactory treatment. Major emphasis must be placed on early diagnosis because surgical extirpation of small, localized lesions is presently the only hope. Unfortunately, the overall resectability rate for adenocarcinoma of the head does not exceed 25 per cent, and it is even less for the tumors of the body and tail.[1] The five-year survival rate for solid adenocarcinoma of the pancreas, whether resectable or not, is less than 1 per cent. When pancreaticoduodenectomy is performed, the five-year survival is 0 to 15 per cent.[18] Surgical exploration in patients with suspected localized pancreatic carcinoma is of value in determining the size and spread of the tumor because radical resection of periampullary tumors has a five-year survival rate of 35 to 40 per cent[18] (see pp. 1139 to 1144). In terms of palliation for relief of pruritus or vomiting, radical resection provides a mean survival of six months, whereas bypassing cholecystojejunostomy provides an average survival of 12 months.[19] Chemotherapy with 5-fluorouracil has little or no effect in prolonging survival or palliating inoperable pancreatic carcinoma.

Medical therapy is directed at maintenance of good nutrition to delay clinical deterioration. The diabetes mellitus initially present as an abnormal glucose tolerance generally progresses to an unstable diabetic state, requiring insulin replacement. This transition may occur in a period of a few months. The development of pancreatic insufficiency can be treated by administering exogenous pancreatic powdered extract with meals, medium-chain triglycerides as multiple doses daily, and antacids to diminish the increased acid secretion. Pain initially responds to nonnarcotic analgesics but may progress in severity, requiring narcotics. With severe pain, serious consideration should be given to nerve blocks, rhizotomy, or cordotomy for the patient's comfort. In the presence of pruritus from obstructive jaundice some relief can be obtained from cholestyramine therapy. The major task and real challenge are to provide comfort, understanding, and reassurance to the patient and his family despite the ominous outcome.

REFERENCES

1. Watson, D. W. Pancreatic carcinoma. Amer. J. Dig. Dis. 15:767, 1970.
2. Becker, W. F., Welsh, R. A. and Pratt, H. S. Cystadenoma and cystadenocarcinoma of the pancreas. Ann. Surg. 161:845, 1965.
3. Burch, G. E., and Ansari, A. Chronic alcoholism and carcinoma of the pancreas. Arch. Intern. Med. 122:273, 1968.
4. Karmody, A. J., and Kyle, J. The association between carcinoma of the pancreas and diabetes mellitus. Brit. J. Surg. 56:362, 1969.
5. Sato, T., Saitoh, Y., Koyama, K., et al. Preoperative determination of operability in carcinomas of the pancreas and the periampullary region. Ann. Surg. 168:876, 1968.
6. Fras, I., Litin, E. M., and Bartholomew, L. G. Mental symptoms as an aid in the early diagnosis of carcinoma of the pancreas. Gastroenterology 55:191, 1968.
7. MacMahon, H. E., Brown, P. A., and Shen, E. M. Acinar cell carcinoma of the pancreas with subcutaneous fat necrosis. Gastroenterology 49:555, 1965.

8. McBee, J. W., Lanza, F. L., and Erickson, E. E. Hypoglycemia due to obstruction of pancreatic excretory ducts by carcinoma. Arch. Path. 81:287, 1966.

9. Marks, C. Hypercalcemia in malignant nonparathyroid disease. Amer. Surg. 31:254, 1965.

10. Meador, C. K., Liddle, G. W., Island, D. P., et al. Cause of Cushing's syndrome in patients with tumors arising from "nonendocrine" tissue. J. Clin. Endocrinol. 22:693, 1962.

11. Marks, L. J., Berde, B., Klein, L. A., et al. Inappropriate vasopressin secretion and carcinoma of the pancreas. Amer. J. Med. 45:967, 1968.

12. Goldstein, H., and Ventzke, L. E. Value of exfoliative cytology in pancreatic carcinoma. Gut 9:316, 1968.

13. Eaton, S. B., Fleischli, D. J., Pollard, J. J., et al. Comparison of current radiologic approaches to the diagnosis of pancreatic disease. New Eng. J. Med. 279:389, 1968.

14. Bookstein, J. J., Reuter, S. R., and Martel, W. Angiographic evaluation of pancreatic carcinoma. Radiology 93:757, 1969.

15. Moore, T. L., Kupchik, H. Z., Marcon, N., et al. Carcinoembryonic antigen assay in cancer of the colon and pancreas and other digestive tract disorders. Amer. J. Dig. Dis. 16:1, 1971.

16. Cotton, P. B., Salmon, P. R., Blumgart, L. H., et al. Cannulation of papilla of Vater via fiber-duodenoscope. Lancet 1:53, 1972.

17. Lisa, J. A., Trinidad, S., and Rosenblatt, M. B. Pulmonary manifestations of carcinoma of the pancreas. Cancer 17:395, 1964.

18. Warren, K. W., Braasch, J. W., and Thum, C. W. Carcinoma of the pancreas. Surg. Clin. N. Amer. 48:601, 1968.

19. Crile, G. The advantages of bypass operations over radical pancreatoduodenectomy in the treatment of pancreatic carcinoma. Surg. Gynec. Obstet. 130:1049, 1970.

Chapter 95

Cystic Fibrosis

Harry Shwachman, Richard J. Grand

INTRODUCTION

Cystic fibrosis was first reported in 1936. Although initially believed to be an uncommon pancreatic disorder, usually fatal in infancy, it is now appreciated that it is a common disease, that it can occur in adults,[1] and that it is not limited to the pancreas.[2] A variety of names have been used to designate this entity. However, none is satisfactory. Since initial emphasis was placed on the pancreas, this disorder was designated pancreatic infantilism, fibrocystic disease of the pancreas, pancreatic fibrosis, or cystic fibrosis of the pancreas. Farber[3] was the first to indicate the generalized nature of this disease and pointed to the multiglandular involvement. He coined the name mucoviscidosis, a name which is still used in Europe but was dropped in the United States many years ago. The observation by di Sant 'Agnese and his group in 1952[4] that the eccrine sweat glands are functionally disturbed and produce a sweat with a high concentration of sodium, chloride, and potassium indicated multiorgan involvement in cystic fibrosis.

DEFINITION

Cystic fibrosis is an autosomal recessive disease characterized by exocrine gland dysfunction and by altered function of mucous glands. It is manifested clinically by pancreatic insufficiency in 80 per cent of patients, diffuse pulmonary obstructive phenomena and infection in almost all cases, and in males by an abnormality in the normal development of Wolffian duct derivatives. The presence of persistently normal sweat electrolyte concentrations (sodium and chloride below 60 mEq per liter) militates against the diagnosis of cystic fibrosis. At present, the heterozygote cannot be identified with certainty.

Cystic fibrosis is at least ten times as common as phenylketonuria. It may occur without evidence of pancreatic insufficiency in life, or by the finding, in exceptional cases, of a normal pancreas at postmortem examination. The diagnosis can be made very readily even in the neonatal period by the pilocarpine iontophoresis quantitative sweat test. There are great natural variations in the severity of this disease, some patients surviving to adulthood and even motherhood. All males with few exceptions are born with a defect in the Wolffian duct derivatives, i.e., the epididymis, vas deferens, and seminal vesicles, which leads to sterility in adulthood. In most instances, death is related to the pulmonary lesion, which eventually leads to ventilatory insufficiency.

INCIDENCE AND GENETICS

The only population survey to determine the incidence of cystic fibrosis was carried out on Prince Edward Island.

1206

Nearly 40,000 children were subjected to the sweat test, and the figures derived from this study indicated that the incidence of cystic fibrosis was approximately 1:1000 live births. Other estimates range from 1:600 to 1:3500 live births. Estimates of incidence derived from the number of known patients in a given area or population are usually low, because all cases are not diagnosed, in part owing to a failure of recognition of mild cases as well as to the inaccuracies of diagnostic testing in some hands. That some patients escape recognition during childhood is supported by the fact that 11 patients were diagnosed after 15 years of age in our clinic in the past two years. Accurate incidence figures might be obtained by testing all newborns for cystic fibrosis. Unfortunately, there is no simple screening test that could be applied on a large-scale basis. Procedures under investigation include testing of individual infants with a chloride electrode applied to the skin after pilocarpine iontophoresis. Other methods include nail and hair assay for sodium concentration, and the testing of meconium for the presence of serum proteins. The incidence in the United States indicates a preponderance of cases in the northeast, probably a reflection of the number of clinics in this area. In a recent survey, 9 per cent of all patients registered in the National Cystic Fibrosis Research Foundation Centers were seen in our clinic.

Cystic fibrosis occurs in families without regard to economic, social, or intellectual status. It is much more common among the Caucasian than the Negro or Oriental races. It has been reported in the American Indian, in the Japanese, and in the African Negro. It occurs equally in both sexes and in the many ethnic groups that are found in our large American cities. In children's hospitals in this country, approximately 3 per cent of the postmortem examinations are performed on children who succumb to cystic fibrosis.

Cystic fibrosis is transmitted as an autosomal recessive disorder. The frequency of the gene in the population is derived from an estimate of the incidence. If we assume an incidence of the disease as 1 to 1600, then the frequency of the gene would be 1 in 20. This means that the chances of being a heterozygote or carrier is 1 in 20. Should two heterozygotes mate, a likelihood of 1 in 400, they would run the risk of having a child with cystic fibrosis in 25 per cent of their offspring.

A number of clinical observations suggest that cystic fibrosis may be a polygenic disorder or a single gene defect with marked allelic heterogeneity. However, there is no sound laboratory evidence to support such a contention. For example, in the earliest clinical manifestation of cystic fibrosis, meconium ileus, there appears to be a familial aggregation of cases. There are other family pedigrees in which the predominant manifestations are pulmonary with little pancreatic involvement. Still another small group can be segregated because of the atypical response of the sweat glands to pilocarpine iontophoresis, inconsistently yielding elevated concentrations of sweat sodium and chloride.

Genetic counseling is a service provided by many of the cystic fibrosis clinics. All siblings of newly diagnosed patients should have sweat tests to determine their status. Many children with mild forms of the disease have been detected and have been placed on prophylactic and therapeutic programs. One should also test all babies born into cystic fibrosis families at birth. A positive sweat test identifies such individuals as having the disease. One may hold the view that the success of counseling can be measured in terms of the decreasing family size of affected families. At present, we cannot identify the heterozygote or the affected fetus in utero. The composition of amniotic fluid bathing affected fetuses does not differ chemically from that of healthy control subjects, nor do the cultured cells exhibit a recognizable morphologic difference.

ETIOLOGY

Cystic fibrosis has been classified as an inborn error of metabolism, although the nature of the primary defect is unknown, and no single biochemical aberration has been detected which accounts for the varied manifestations of the disease. As with other genetic diseases, the application of tissue culture techniques may provide new insights into the nature of the basic defect.

Conflicting hypotheses have incriminated autonomic dysfunction, defects in glycoprotein biochemistry (perhaps reflected in altered membrane structure or permeability), structural aberrations in mucosubstances, or abnormalities in a variety of regulatory factors: hormones, antibodies, neurohumoral transmitters, and kallikreins. However, none of these yet reconcile the unique sweat gland defect with the abnormal characteristics of mucous secretion. Environmental and exogenous influences, such as climate, altitude, and diet, and familial patterns of response to infection, as well as intrauterine insults and vitamin deficiencies, have all been discarded as causative factors in the disease. At present, cystic fibrosis cannot be reproduced in animals.

PATHOGENESIS

Important observations have been made concerning the pathogenesis of some of the manifestations of this disease.[5] Widespread involvement of the exocrine and mucus-secreting glands has been demonstrated, but the relationship between abnormal electrolyte secretion and mucus production remains unexplained. The pathogenetic mechanisms in the various organ systems involved are summarized in Table 95-1.

GLYCOPROTEINS AND MUCOUS SUBSTANCES

Excessive accumulation of mucus has been demonstrated histologically in almost all organs studied. However, histochemical techniques have failed to reveal any unique characteristics which would differentiate mucus of patients with cystic fibrosis from those with other conditions associated with mucus hypersecretion. The elevations in the cellular content of acidic and sulfomucins seen in many organs of patients with cystic fibrosis are nonspecific.

By contrast, it has been possible to dem-

TABLE 95-1. PATHOGENESIS OF CYSTIC FIBROSIS

Viscid secretions ———→ Small duct obstruction		
Respiratory	Upper	Sinusitis
		Mucous membrane hypertrophy — Nasal polyposis
	Lower	Atelectasis
		Emphysema
		Infection — Bronchitis
		Bronchopneumonia
		Bronchiectasis — Respiratory failure
		Right heart failure — Death
Intestinal	Meconium ileus	Volvulus
		Peritonitis
		Ileal atresia
	Meconium ileus equivalent	Fecal masses
		Obstruction
	Pancreas	Nutritional failure due to pancreatic insufficiency
		Diabetes
	Mucus hypersecretion	
Hepatobiliary	Atrophic gallbladder	
	Focal biliary cirrhosis	
	Cirrhosis	
	Hepar lobatum	
	Portal hypertension	
	Esophageal varices	
	Hypersplenism	
Reproductive system	Females — Increased viscosity of vaginal mucus and decreased fertility	
	Males — Failure of Wolffian duct development — sterility	
	Absent vas deferens, epididymis, and seminal vesicles	
Other	Salt depletion through excessive loss of salt through skin	
	Heat stroke	
	Salivary gland hypertrophy	
	Hypertrophy of apocrine glands	

onstrate the differences in the chemical composition between glycoprotein fractions obtained from the secretions of patients with cystic fibrosis and normal subjects. In duodenal fluid, urine, sweat, and submaxillary saliva, as well as tracheobronchial and rectal mucus, the fucose content is increased by comparison to the other organic constituents, especially sialic acid; however, in some studies the fucose-to-sialic-acid ratio in urinary and tracheobronchial glycoproteins is normal.

Calcium concentration in submaxillary saliva is frequently, but not uniformly, elevated and may be associated with an increase in the turbidity of the fluid. As the disease progresses, the calcium content of the gland rises further, and glycoprotein material precipitates within the secretory duct. Since this finding is not uniform in cystic fibrosis and has been demonstrated in apparently normal adults, its significance is not yet clear. Equally elusive is the significance of other possible roles of calcium in this disease; i.e., it may bring about an increase in the permeability of mucus to other ions and water, and its binding to the keratins of hair in patients with cystic fibrosis is loose in contrast to the firm binding noted in healthy subjects.

ELECTROLYTE SECRETION

Abnormal electrolyte secretion in the exocrine glands, present from birth, is the most characteristic and constant finding in this disease. Elevation of sodium and chloride concentrations in the sweat is most common, although the potassium concentration is also elevated, but less consistently. All patients with clinical manifestations of the disease show the sweat abnormality.

Micropuncture studies of individual sweat glands have revealed that the osmolarity and sodium content of the fluid elaborated by the secretory coil is normal, although the sweat obtained from the ducts shows the characteristic electrolyte elevations. Since the sweat rate is probably not abnormal in affected patients, although an increase in sweating at night has been observed, a defect in the reabsorption of sodium and chloride in the sweat ducts of patients is likely.

Sodium-retaining steroids, aldosterone, deoxycorticosterone, or 9-alpha-fluorohydrocortisone, decrease the concentration of sodium and increase the concentration of potassium in sweat less dramatically in patients with cystic fibrosis than in normal control subjects and the sodium concentration remains above normal range. Sodium-to-potassium ratios, however, are similar to values for normal subjects. Thus these hormones or a low-salt diet will not help distinguish patients with cystic fibrosis.

The sodium and chloride concentrations of mixed saliva are also elevated, as they are in submaxillary saliva. They are either normal or only slightly elevated in parotid saliva and normal in duodenal fluid and tears. Hair and nails also show elevated electrolyte concentrations.

Abnormalities in water and electrolyte secretion by the pancreas after stimulation with pancreozymin and secretin have been observed in children with pulmonary disease but without pancreatic enzyme. In these patients a normal output of pancreatic enzymes follows injection of pancreozymin, but volume and bicarbonate output fail to rise above basal levels, and chloride concentrations do not fall after secretin administration. How this defect relates to those found in other organs affected in cystic fibrosis is not clear, especially because sodium, potassium, and basal chloride levels in pancreatic secretions in these patients are normal.

HUMORAL FACTORS

Approximately 70 to 90 per cent of patients with cystic fibrosis, a large number (but not all) of heterozygous parents and 10 per cent of a "control" adult population in one study contain serum factors, not yet completely characterized, which produce dyskinesia of beating cilia in explants of rabbit trachea or oyster gills. The factors are nondialyzable and heat labile, and have a molecular weight of between 75,000 and 180,000; a similar nondialyzable, heat-labile, factor has also been isolated from the sweat, submaxillary saliva, and parotid saliva of patients with this disease. These materials, when perfused retrograde into the parotid duct of the rat or into normal human sweat glands, lead to an inhibition of sodium reabsorption.

The clinical significance of these various factors is not clear, and much work is necessary before they can be related to the primary defect.

CELL CULTURES

Both long- and short-term cultures of leukocytes and fibroblasts obtained from patients with cystic fibrosis and their heterozygous parents have been extensively studied. Isolated observations exist, but the findings are largely unconfirmed: (1) Abnormal metachromasia with toluidine blue staining, a nonspecific phenomenon, is seen in fibroblast cultures of homozygotes and heterozygotes.[6] (2) The activity of the lysozomal enzyme, alpha-glucosidase, is elevated in leukocyte cultures from patients, whereas cell cultures obtained from heterozygous parents show levels of this enzyme intermediate between those of the homozygote and the normal control subjects. (3) Acid mucopolysaccharides, not specific for cystic fibrosis, are elevated in skin fibroblasts cultured from patients with cystic fibrosis.

PATHOLOGY

The name of the disease is derived from the initial description of the changes observed in the pancreas. Farber[3] and Anderson[7] independently pointed out that the morphological changes in this disease are not limited to the pancreas and occur in many mucus-secreting cells in the body. The main sites affected are in the gastrointestinal tract and appendages as well as in the upper and lower respiratory tract. Neither intestinal mucosal biopsy specimens obtained from the duodenum nor those from the rectum have unequivocal diagnostic value. On the other hand, the appendix may provide a diagnostic clue, as the secretory cells usually show hyperactivity, with mucus secretions extruding into the wide, gaping glandular orifices. The frequent occurrence of nasal polyposis in this disease is one of the many manifestations of hyperactivity of the mucous cells. There is no characteristic chemical staining quality of the mucus; no anatomical, histological, or histochemical change in eccrine sweat glands has been described.

PANCREAS

Grossly, the pancreas is small, firm, and irregular, and feels gritty. The character-

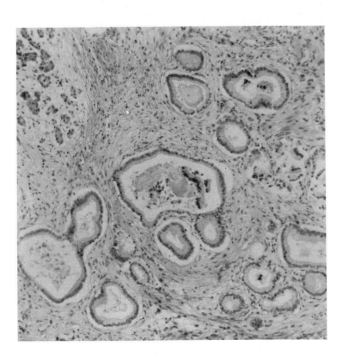

Figure 95–1. Pancreas from patient with cystic fibrosis, showing characteristic histological changes. Hematoxylin and eosin. × 150.

istic histological findings in the pancreas (Fig. 95–1) consist of a dilatation of the ducts, a flattening of the epithelium, enlargement of the acini which may be filled with eosinophilic concretions, and a diffuse fibrosis with varying degrees of leukocytic infiltration. The lesion need not be uniform in all areas. In exceptional cases, the acini become enlarged to form cysts which can be seen grossly. The lesion in the pancreas is not fixed; it is often very minimal during the first months of life, and the changes are more pronounced later on. The end-stage of the pancreatic lesion may be replacement by fat and fibrous tissue, leaving only a few clusters of islet cells, perhaps causing diabetes seen in such patients. Indeed, nearly 80 per cent of the acini and ducts may be affected before clinical evidence of exocrine insufficiency is noted. It is most difficult to establish the diagnosis of cystic fibrosis both in the presence of minimal lesions or at its end-stage.

LIVER

At autopsy 15 to 20 per cent of patients with cystic fibrosis show alterations in the liver. Three stages have been described.[8] The earliest lesion, termed focal biliary cirrhosis (Fig. 95–2), is characterized by plugging of bile ducts with inspissated mucus, increase in inflammatory cells, both polymorphonuclear leukocytes and lymphocytes, bile duct proliferation and dilatation, and focal fibrosis without evidence of bile stasis. Entirely normal liver lobules may exist between affected foci. Fatty infiltration may be present to a varying degree, and probably reflects nutritional status. Grossly, there is irregular and diffuse pitting of the liver capsule.

As the lesion progresses, portal areas coalesce; with collapse of lobules, fibrosis markedly increases and multiple regenerative nodules appear. On occasion, the intrahepatic biliary concretions become calcified, although stone formation is rare and the large biliary radicles are normal. In its final stage, the lesion grossly resembles severe postnecrotic cirrhosis. The liver is deep green. Extensive distortion of liver lobules occurs, and broad bands of fibrous tissue span many lobules. This multilobular biliary cirrhosis occurs in less than 5 per cent of patients and may result in the production of the clinical manifestations of portal hypertension: hypersplenism, hem-

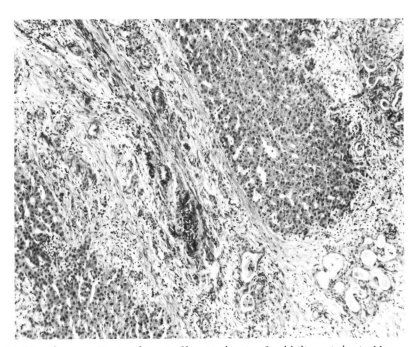

Figure 95–2. Liver from a patient with cystic fibrosis, showing focal biliary cirrhosis. Masson stain. × 250.

orrhage from esophageal and gastric varices, ascites, and hepatic coma.

GALLBLADDER

An atrophic or a hypoplastic gallbladder, filled with thick gelatinous bile, may be found at autopsy. It rarely contains stones.

RESPIRATORY TRACT

Since most deaths are due to respiratory failure attributed to the severe, extensive chronic pulmonary infection, autopsy usually reveals the trachea and bronchi to be filled with tenacious mucopurulent material from which *Pseudomonas aeruginosa* or *Staphylococcus aureus* may be cultured. The thorax is rounded and the lungs are voluminous. Pleural adhesions, emphysematous blebs, hemorrhage, areas of consolidation, abscesses of varying sizes, and massive lung destruction are often noted. When dissected, the bronchi may be found to be dilated and filled with purulent exudate, often appearing as a cast of the peripheral airways. Histologically, there are areas of bronchopneumonia, emphysema, and atelectasis, with widespread, thick, dilated bronchi. The bronchiectasis is usually tubular and generally involves all lobes; often the upper lobes show greater changes than the lower. The hilar lymph nodes are enlarged.

The initial lesion in the lung is bronchial obstruction which results in collapse or overdistention of the alveoli, depending upon whether the obstruction is complete or partial. Infection supervenes and a chronic inflammatory process occurs in which *Staphylococcus aureus* predominates. The bronchial and tracheal mucus-secreting cells appear active and secrete a viscid material. This sputum or mucopurulent secretion is the combined product of the glandular secretions and the infectious process. The bronchial walls become thick, and focal areas of atelectasis appear. Larger segments of the bronchial tree may also become obstructed and cause segmental and even lobar collapse. The atelectatic segment may become the site of abscess cavities. The persistence of the bronchial infection leads to bronchiectasis.

The upper respiratory tract is usually affected. Chronic sinus infection is present in the majority of patients. The mucus-secreting cells may be hyperactive. Nasal polyposis is of frequent occurrence and is present in approximately 10 per cent of patients over ten years of age. It may be noted as early as two years. Often polyps are bilateral and cause nasal obstruction. They may be multiple, requiring surgical removal, and frequently recur.

GENITAL ABNORMALITIES IN MALE PATIENTS

A recent observation indicated that adult males with cystic fibrosis are sterile.[9] The ejaculum was found to be reduced in volume and contained no spermatozoa. Chemical assay of the ejaculum revealed reduced concentration of fructose, whereas the concentration of citric acid and acid phosphatase activity was increased. Anatomical studies revealed normal or slightly smaller testes, and in postpubertal patients there was active spermatogenesis with occasional abnormal forms. The most striking changes occur in the Wolffian duct derivatives, namely, the epididymis, the vas deferens, and the seminal vesicles. The epididymides are poorly developed, and the body and tail are rudimentary or absent. Upon dissection, the efferent ductules of the head end blindly. The rete testes are intact. The vas deferens in most cases cannot be identified. Sometimes a solid smooth muscle cord of varying thickness is found in place of the vas. Multiple sections of spermatic cords rarely show histological patency at more than one level. Seminal vesicles cannot be positively identified. In addition to these defects, there is a striking increase in abnormalities associated with testicular descent, such as inguinal hernia, hydrocele, and undescended testes.

These abnormalities are unique; they have not been noted in any other genetic disease. These defects may be found in male infants shortly after birth and are prenatal in origin. The anatomical changes are responsible for sterility and aspermia. However, testicular hormonal function and male sexual activity are not necessarily impaired.

CLINICAL PICTURE

GENERAL FEATURES

The general appearance of the cystic fibrosis patient may vary considerably from the severely malnourished, stunted individual to one who appears healthy. The disease should be suspected in any child having chronic or recurrent symptoms involving the upper or lower respiratory tract. The complaints may include chronic cough, recurrent pneumonitis, bronchitis or pneumonia, and asthma-like symptoms in infancy. At times, complications of the pulmonary manifestations, such as bronchiectasis, emphysema, or, more frequently, atelectasis, either focal or lobular, may provide the indications for diagnostic sweat testing. In view of the frequency of nasal polyposis in this disease, all children with nasal polyposis should have the sweat test. In spite of the presence of a clear-cut history of allergy, cystic fibrosis may also occur. On the other hand, not all patients with cystic fibrosis and nasal polyps manifest evidences of allergy. Well over 90 per cent of patients show respiratory tract involvement during childhood, and the majority of patients have evidences of pulmonary disease during infancy. The gastrointestinal symptoms are primarily those of malabsorption and maldigestion caused by exocrine pancreatic insufficiency (see p. 260). Bulky and frequent stools may be a minor complaint. In small infants diarrhea and failure to gain weight in spite of a good appetite are often noted. The appetite may be huge, enormous, or expressed by parents in other terms, such as, "He eats like a horse," or "He eats more than I do." However, unless one probes carefully into the dietary history, such revealing information is not obtained. The stools are usually described as large, light, poorly formed, oily, and foul smelling. The odor is often so pungent that an undiagnosed child may be suspected on this account. In small infants, especially if this is the first child, parents are not aware of stool abnormalities, and the physician should examine a specimen himself. A simple diagnostic clue is the detection of excess neutral fat or of decreased stool trypsin or chymotrypsin (see pp. 284 to 285). The development of a pot belly is common in untreated patients, as is the occurrence of rectal prolapse.

By the age of three years, approximately 20 per cent of untreated children have a history of rectal prolapse, a symptom easily avoided by medical therapy. The prolapse may indeed be the initial complaint in some patients. Although this entity is also seen in patients with other intestinal disorders, such as celiac disease, infectious enteritis, kwashiorkor, and severe functional chronic constipation, its occurrence in infancy in the United States is highly suggestive of cystic fibrosis. The cause for this abnormality is related to poor nutrition, frequent voluminous bowel movements, and increased intra-abdominal pressure associated with chronic cough. Prolapse rarely requires surgery. Proper dietary management with pancreatic supplementation usually leads to rapid improvement and prevents recurrences.

The diagnosis of cystic fibrosis should also be suspected in infants with hypoproteinemic edema. This condition often develops because of the early onset of diarrhea and is wrongly attributed to a milk allergy (see pp. 1075 to 1079). A soy preparation is generally substituted for the milk formula. In the absence of pancreatic enzymes the soy protein is not digested, which is equivalent to protein starvation. The feeding of amino acid formulas can alleviate as well as prevent this condition.

Another condition which may lead to the diagnosis of cystic fibrosis is vitamin K deficiency in infancy, in which the initial manifestation may be hemorrhage into the skin. All patients suspected of having celiac disease should have sweat tests. The concurrence of these two diseases is indeed rare. However, a number of patients with cystic fibrosis have been misdiagnosed as having celiac disease and have responded very satisfactorily to dietary therapy at first, with the subsequent discovery, a number of years later, when irreversible pulmonary lesions appeared, that the original diagnosis was incorrect. The diagnosis of celiac disease is established when a mucosal biopsy of the small intestine reveals flattening of villi and the enzyme assays reveal secondary disaccharidase deficiencies (see p. 272).

Infrequently the child presents with signs and symptoms of cirrhosis of the liver and portal hypertension, often with associated hypersplenism. All children with unexplained cirrhosis of the liver should be investigated for cystic fibrosis, and a diagnostic sweat test should be performed. The pulmonary changes may be minimal when the patient is first seen.

During warm weather and during febrile episodes some patients will suffer from heat exhaustion. All such individuals should have sweat tests. The loss of water and electrolytes through excessive sweating results in hypovolemia and shock. Although this condition is easily corrected, it is more important to prevent it by providing adequate dietary salt and fluid.

The symptoms of cystic fibrosis may begin in the first few months or much later, and severity also varies considerably. Some infants have severe manifestations, run a rapidly deteriorating course, and succumb in the first year of life. However, the majority of patients have a milder course and, with early recognition and constant medical supervision, may reach adulthood. Still others, a smaller group, have their first symptoms after four or five years of age. In approximately 15 to 20 per cent of patients, the pulmonary disease predominates in the clinical picture at the time the diagnosis of cystic fibrosis is made, and there are no signs or symptoms of pancreatic involvement. On the other hand, the gastrointestinal manifestations may antedate chronic pulmonary disease for months or years. By far the largest number of infants and children with this disease have both pulmonary and pancreatic involvement. In recent years most of the newly diagnosed older patients appear to have predominantly the respiratory features with little evidence of pancreatic insufficiency.

MECONIUM ILEUS

The earliest manifestation of cystic fibrosis is a form of intestinal obstruction of the newborn, known as meconium ileus. This disorder underlies presentation in 15 per cent of patients with this disease. It appears in utero and is characterized by complete obstruction of a portion of the small intestine, usually the terminal ileum, by tenacious inspissated meconium. Distal to

the obstruction the small intestine is narrowed, whereas the proximal segment is usually markedly distended by meconium. The colon is small, but attains normal size after relief of the obstruction. Failure to recognize this condition within a few hours of birth may lead to perforation or ischemia with death from peritonitis. Approximately 30 per cent of infants with meconium ileus have volvulus, and 6 per cent have intestinal atresia (usually ileal).

The precise pathogenesis of meconium ileus in cystic fibrosis is unknown. It is certainly related to the increased viscosity of meconium, related, perhaps, to the abnormality of the mucosubstances secreted by the intestine, possibly to pancreatic insufficiency, and to increased concentrations of serum proteins.

CLINICAL PICTURE

The clinical picture is intestinal obstruction of the newborn. The infant presents with abdominal distention, and may have bile-stained vomitus; no meconium is passed per rectum. Air has normally passed into the colon by three hours of age, but in meconium ileus the supine roentgenogram of the abdomen shows no gas in the colon. Dilated loops of small bowel are present, but often without air-fluid levels, probably because the intraluminal thick secretions prevent sufficient passage of air to make the appropriate radiological signs. Rounded air bubbles may be seen intraluminally, suggesting an admixture of meconium and air. If meconium peritonitis has occurred in utero, extraluminal calcification may be present, and intraluminal calcifications may be seen occasionally in the meconium.

DIFFERENTIAL DIAGNOSIS

Without a positive family history or knowledge of the sweat electrolyte concentrations, differential diagnosis from other forms of neonatal intestinal obstruction can be difficult. Clinical and roentgenological features considered typical for meconium ileus have been noted also in patients with imperforate anus, Hirschsprung's disease, occasionally in small intestinal atresia without meconium ileus, and in the meconium plug syndrome. Because of the importance of early diagnosis, it is mandatory that a sweat test be performed as soon as possible in such situations. The sweat test can be performed easily during preparation for surgery, and knowledge of the presence of cystic fibrosis aids immeasurably in managing anesthesia and prescribing postoperative care. If the infant's clinical course is stable and diagnosis is difficult, a warm saline enema with dilute barium may be performed. An unexpanded colon is well demonstrated by this procedure, although differentiation from Hirschsprung's disease is not necessarily achieved.

TREATMENT

Intestinal obstruction of this type in the newborn is usually a surgical emergency. Many surgical procedures are available for the management of such patients, but historically either a Bishop-Koop type of end-to-side ileoileostomy with resection of the affected segment or a Mikulicz ileostomy has been preferred. Both allow irrigation of the distal segment with pancreatic enzymes and n-acetylcysteine.

Recently, Gastrografin enemas have been used for the treatment of uncomplicated meconium ileus. Performed in the correct manner and with properly screened patients, this technique may obviate the necessity for surgery. The first criterion for its use must be the presence of uncomplicated meconium ileus, without the possibility of volvulus or peritonitis being present. If the differential diagnosis includes only intestinal atresia, the Gastrografin enema is not contraindicated. When the enema is performed, it must be done under fluoroscopic control, and the infant must be receiving plasma intravenously during the procedure to avoid hypotension.

The current surgical survival rate in patients with meconium ileus is greater than 70 per cent; however, postoperative morbidity is high, with only approximately 30 per cent survival at one year. Survivors of meconium ileus exhibit other symptoms of cystic fibrosis, and their subsequent course depends upon the same factors that determine survival in any other child with the disease. The oldest patients are now young adults, many of them gainfully employed.[1] There is a high incidence of meconium ileus in certain families, and there appears to be a higher incidence of prematurity in patients with meconium ileus than in children with cystic fibrosis born without any complications.

In a number of infants who later develop cystic fibrosis, the meconium may be delayed in passing and an operation to relieve the obstruction is not necessary. Those in charge of newborn nurseries are fully aware of the possibility of this disease in babies who first pass their meconium after 24 hours of age. The presence of serum protein in the meconium may suggest the diagnosis of cystic fibrosis. Tests for stool trypsin after the second day and the application of the sweat test in such babies are advisable. This condition must be differentiated from that of babies with a meconium plug syndrome, which is unrelated to cystic fibrosis.

INTESTINAL OBSTRUCTION IN THE OLDER CHILD OR YOUNG ADULT ("MECONIUM ILEUS EQUIVALENT")

Because of the prolonged survival achieved by patients with cystic fibrosis, older children, teenagers, and young adults are increasingly susceptible to intraluminal intestinal obstruction from fecal impactions. Such patients have been demonstrated to have significant hyperplasia of the mucus-secreting glands in the intestine, and obstruction probably represents the combined effects of pancreatic insufficiency and abnormal mucopolysaccharides. Semisolid or solid fecal material obstructs the lumen, where, under normal circumstances, the fecal stream is liquid.

In its mildest form this obstruction is transient and often asymptomatic. A painless mass in the right lower quadrant may be found during routine examination, which on repeat examination may no longer be palpable. Some patients have more marked intestinal symptoms with anorexia, crampy abdominal pains, and abdominal distention. There may be tenderness over a mass in the right lower quadrant. The barium enema may show an intraluminal filling defect in the colon, suggestive of carcinoma, but the differential diagnosis is rarely difficult. Many operations have been performed for the relief of obstructed ileum in older patients with cystic fibrosis, but a trial of conservative medical management is indicated if the obstruction is uncomplicated. Relief of obstruction has been reported following large quantities, i.e., 200 ml, of a 10 per cent solution of n-acetylcysteine taken by mouth. We usually recommend this therapy accompanied by the instillation of pancreatic enzymes and n-acetylcysteine by rectum and by large doses of Colace and 90 ml of mineral oil by mouth. Patients are encouraged to increase their doses of pancreatic enzymes and fluid. On this regimen surgery is usually unnecessary for simple impaction.

Many complications have been reported in association with fecal impactions, the most common being intussusception[10] and volvulus. The large majority of intussusceptions are ileocolic, and the lead point is frequently a dense accumulation of thick inspissated material in the terminal ileum

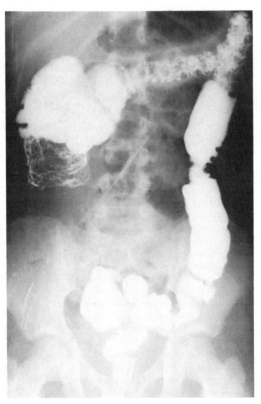

Figure 95-3. X-ray: barium enema in a patient with intussusception.

(Fig. 95–3). A majority of patients have episodes with an acute onset, although an occasional patient will have long-standing crampy abdominal pain or a painless mass. Many patients with intussusception ultimately require surgery for reduction, but in uncomplicated intussusception reduction by means of a judiciously performed barium enema should always be attempted. Intussusception has been the presenting symptom of cystic fibrosis in a few previously undiagnosed cases. Volvulus around the site of impaction can occur at any time, and is always a surgical emergency.

PULMONARY MANIFESTATIONS

One of the earliest symptoms is cough. At first it may attract little attention, but it soon becomes chronic and more frequent, results in vomiting, and may even become paroxysmal, suggesting pertussis. Symptoms may be present at two or three months of age. An observant mother may detect the presence of thick mucus which the baby is unable to expel. An increase in the respiratory rate is common, but very few parents are aware of it. At times noisy respirations or wheezing appear. By two years of age over 75 per cent of children with cystic fibrosis have had the aforementioned symptoms. The physical findings may be minimal. The X-ray of the chest may reveal evidence of irregular aeration and scattered areas of segmental or lobar atelectasis. The lungs are hyperinflated and the diaphragm may be depressed. The peribronchial markings become pronounced. Later in the disease the bronchi become plugged. The diagnosis of cystic fibrosis can be strongly suspected from the X-ray at this time. A characteristic roentgenogram with moderately advanced disease is shown in Figure 95–4.

The earliest functional changes may be reflected in a lowered pO_2 and a prolongation of the expiratory flow rate (FEV). Other changes include decreased vital capacity and an increase in residual volume and in airway resistance. The physical findings may often be minimal despite the presence of widespread pulmonary lesions noted by X-ray. The chest becomes rounded and fixed, with intercostal retrac-

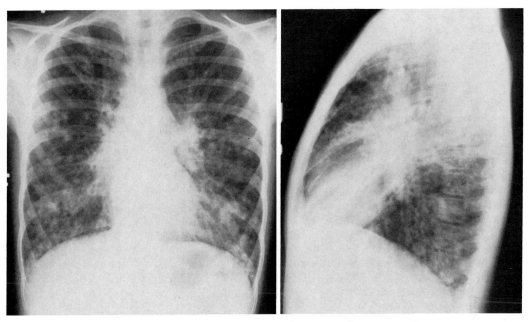

Figure 95–4. Chest X-rays of a patient with severe pulmonary involvement.

tion and very little excursion. Digital clubbing and cyanosis are often present. Fever is usually absent in the early stages of the disease and, when present, generally indicates widespread infection. Persistent rales confirm the impression of bronchiectasis. The right side of the heart may fail. Some of the serious complications include pneumothorax, hemoptysis, and cor pulmonale. The chronic infection may at times produce a granulomatous lesion which has been known as botryomycosis. The cause of death is usually respiratory failure accompanied by a fall in pO_2 and a rise in pCO_2.

The severity of the disease has been determined by a scoring system which takes into account the general activity of the patient, the physical findings, the nutritional status, and the findings on chest roentgenograms. Each of these categories is given equal weight, 25 points. The scoring system is as follows: excellent, over 85; good, between 71 and 85; mild, between 56 and 70; moderate, between 41 and 55; and severe, 40 or below. This useful system permits evaluation of therapeutic programs and comparison of patients, and provides prognostic information. It is based not on laboratory findings but on careful clinical examination.[1]

HEPATOBILIARY SYSTEM

Although the incidence of symptoms caused by involvement of the liver and biliary tree in cystic fibrosis is low, a characteristic form of biliary cirrhosis is frequently found at postmortem examination. The pathology of this lesion is discussed above. Patients with the Stage 1 lesion, termed focal biliary cirrhosis, usually do not show any signs of clinical liver disease. In the small number of patients in whom there is progressive cirrhosis, clinically apparent disease depends upon the degree of liver damage.

Many of the liver function tests may be normal. The earliest change may be an increase in the alkaline phophatase, decreased sulfobromophthalein excretion, or a prolongation of the prothrombin time, followed by an increase in the globulins and lowering of the albumin. The transaminases usually show no changes early in the course of liver involvement. The bilirubin is rarely elevated, and jaundice is an unusual feature.

The end-stage lesion is a multilobular biliary cirrhosis, which occurs in 4 to 5 per cent of patients with cystic fibrosis and leads to the well recognized complications of long-standing liver disease: hypersplenism, esophageal varices, ascites, and hepatic coma and its complications. The clinical appearance of significant liver disease in a patient with cystic fibrosis signifies a very poor prognosis. The elevation of the serum alkaline phosphatase activity often precedes the onset of portal hypertension. Portacaval shunts in patients with symptomatic hypersplenism or bleeding varices have had variable results. The postoperative course is complicated by severe pulmonary disease. Controlled studies of the role of prophylactic shunting procedures in cystic fibrosis are unavailable, but in our patients the long-term management has been considerably simplified by the early treatment of portal hypertension. Twenty-nine patients with cystic fibrosis have had either splenorenal or portacaval shunts in our clinic. Approximately 70 per cent have survived for over a three-year period after surgery. Criteria for surgery have been the presence of documented portal hypertension with esophageal varices and progressive hypersplenism, usually heralded by an elevation in the serum alkaline phosphatase value. In these patients pulmonary drainage has been considerably facilitated by elective tracheostomy five to seven days prior to the shunt operation. At an appropriate time after surgery, the tracheostomy can be removed.

DIAGNOSIS AND DIFFERENTIAL DIAGNOSIS

A high degree of clinical suspicion is essential in making the diagnosis of cystic fibrosis. A positive family history is helpful. A diagnostic sweat test should be performed without delay, and, if positive, a therapeutic program should be begun immediately. The conditions or complaints for which the sweat test should be performed are listed in Table 95–2. It may uncover one patient with cystic fibrosis for every 12 or 13 tested.

The great majority of children with pancreatic insufficiency have cystic fibrosis, and the remaining few have either a congenital anomaly or the Shwachman syndrome. The latter condition is rare. Fewer than 100 cases have been reported, and 18 patients have been seen in our clinic. The

TABLE 95–2. INDICATIONS FOR THE SWEAT TEST (QUANTITATIVE PILOCARPINE IONTOPHORESIS)

Siblings having cystic fibrosis
Chronic cough
Chronic recurrent respiratory infections or
  pneumonia
Chronic or asthmatic bronchitis
Failure to thrive (stunting of growth)
Abnormal stools
Possibility of celiac disease
Rectal prolapse
Nasal polyposis
Hypoproteinemia
Hypoprothrombinemia
Intestinal obstruction of newborn
Bronchiectasis
Lobar atelectasis
Cirrhosis of liver in childhood or adolescence
Portal hypertension
Adult males with aspermia
Heat stroke

TABLE 95–3. DIFFERENTIAL DIAGNOSIS

Pulmonary
  Asthma
  Recurrent respiratory infection
  Recurrent pneumonia
  Chronic bronchitis or sinusitis
  Staphylococcal empyema
  Bronchiectasis
  Recurrent nasal polyposis
  Pertussis
  Pulmonary tuberculosis
  Histoplasmosis
  Ascariasis
Gastrointestinal
  Diarrhea
  Milk allergy in early infancy
  Celiac disease
  Disaccharidase deficiency
  Protein-losing enteropathy
  Meconium plug syndrome
  Intestinal atresia, volvulus
  Hirschsprung's disease
  Shwachman syndrome—pancreatic insufficiency
    and bone marrow hypoplasia
  Enterokinase deficiency
  Trypsinogen deficiency
  Cirrhosis of the liver
  Portal hypertension
  Abdominal masses, especially in right lower
    quadrant
  Intussusception in children over three years
    of age
Other
  Agammaglobulinemia
  Familial dysautonomia
  Heat stroke
  Aspermia

typical features are pancreatic insufficiency, failure to thrive, bone marrow hypoplasia, neutropenia, and, at times, anemia, thrombocytopenia, and metaphyseal dysplasia. This is a familial disorder, and patients have been described from Australia, England, Switzerland, and various parts of the United States (see p. 1227).

The conditions to be considered in the differential diagnosis are listed in Table 95–3.

DIAGNOSTIC TESTS

SWEAT ELECTROLYTES

The best single test for the diagnosis of cystic fibrosis is the quantitative analysis of eccrine sweat for the concentration of sodium and chloride.[11] The elevation of Na+ and Cl− is so characteristic that over 99 per cent of patients with cystic fibrosis show this feature. In no disease that can be confused with cystic fibrosis is there a consistent elevation of sweat electrolyte levels. The elevation is very striking and is approximately four to five times the normal values (see Fig. 95–5). The most practical method of obtaining sweat is to induce sweating in a localized area, the forearm, by pilocarpine iontophoresis. Unfortunately, there are many variations in performing the sweat test. One must scrutinize this procedure very carefully in order to avoid misleading results. We strongly urge that one person, usually a trained technician, be responsible for the entire procedure and that each laboratory use a standard method which yields reliable and reproducible results and establish a range of values for healthy and sick children. A positive sweat test in the absence of symptoms does not establish the diagnosis, except in infants during the first few weeks of life, when the clinical manifestations may not yet have developed.

We prefer to obtain sweat by pilocarpine iontophoresis and collect a sample from both forearms for separate analysis. The sweat glands should be stimulated with a current of 3 ma for five minutes. Sweat is collected for 30 minutes on gauze pads which have been previously weighed. Concentrations of sodium, potassium, and chloride in the sweat collected from each forearm are measured. A simple, homemade apparatus may be used for the iontophoresis, instead of the very costly commercial equipment which is not always properly standardized. Many of the instruments on the market measure conductivity, and this reading is in turn converted into milliequivalents per liter of chloride; it is a procedure of dubious reliability. Clinical laboratories should not undertake to perform this procedure unless they are

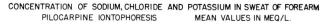
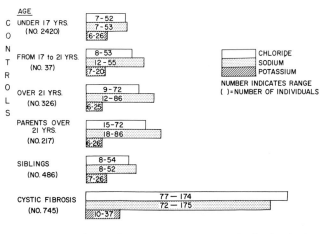

Figure 95–5. Sweat test results: pilocarpine iontophoresis.

properly and fully capable of performing it accurately. Incorrect false-positive diagnosis may result in limitation of family size, family disruption, emotional trauma, and unnecessary and costly treatment for a condition that does not exist. A false-negative diagnosis may result in early death. Some of the factors that influence the level of sweat electrolytes are listed in Table 95–4.

The results of a large number of sweat tests are shown in Figure 95–5. Generally, the electrolyte concentration increases after adolescence and the normal values in adults may be nearly twice as high as in childhood. At times the sweat tests are difficult to interpret in adults, because many in good health have values which exceed the upper limits of normal for children. Parents of children with cystic fibrosis have the same values as a control population. The levels of electrolytes do not in any way indicate the severity of disease. Fortunately, borderline values are uncommon in childhood. Repeat sweat tests as well as careful clinical follow-up observa-

TABLE 95–4. FACTORS INFLUENCING LEVELS OF ELECTROLYTES IN ECCRINE SWEAT

The patient
  Nature of disease
  Genetic stock
  Age
  Sex
  Condition of patient
  Dietary habits
  Acclimatization
Sweat induction and collection
  Drug-induced vs. thermal sweat
  Rate of sweating
  Total body vs. local collection
  Area of body from which sweat collected
  Environmental temperature and humidity
  Time of collection
Drugs used and how given
  Intradermal
  Intramuscular
  By pilocarpine iontophoresis
  Type of drug and vehicle
Analytical factors
  Size of sample
  Weight or volume of sample
  Method of analysis of chloride, sodium, and
    potassium
  Dilution factor
  Contamination, inherent and introduced
  Personal factor

tions are indicated when equivocal results are obtained.

Screening tests for sweat chloride levels are useful when performed properly. These include the hand plate test as well as the application of the chloride electrode to the skin. However, a diagnosis of cystic fibrosis should not be made on the basis of a screening test.

PANCREATIC FUNCTION

The most direct method for studying pancreatic function is to obtain serial samples of duodenal fluid following intravenous administration of secretin and pancreozymin. The volume, pH, and electrolyte, bicarbonate, and enzyme concentrations are determined. In approximately 80 per cent of patients with cystic fibrosis the fasting duodenal specimens will show reduced volume, increased viscosity, reduction in pH, and absent pancreatic enzymes: lipase, amylase, trypsin, chymotrypsin, and carboxypeptidase. In such individuals secretin and pancreozymin fail to increase flow, bicarbonate concentration, or enzyme activity (see pp. 359 to 364). In the remaining 20 per cent of patients the enzyme activity is normal or only partially disturbed. Some of these patients may exhibit a dissociation between changes in lipase, trypsin, and amylase, and pancreatic stimulation may result in an enhancement of enzyme activity.

In addition to direct laboratory measurements, pancreatic function may be assessed clinically and indirectly in a variety of ways. In infants and young children the stool trypsin test is very helpful. Normal stools contain considerable proteolytic activity, in contrast to those with pancreatic insufficiency. A simple gelatin film test or a quantitative trypsin and chymotrypsin assay can be readily done by the physician using synthetic substrates. Tests for stool trypsin are more reliable in infants or small children than in older patients. The measurement of fecal fat by the van de Kamer method is practical and can be performed in most clinical laboratories. Patients with cystic fibrosis may excrete as much as 30 per cent or more of ingested fat per day. They also excrete an excess amount of nitrogen, unlike patients with malabsorption secondary to celiac sprue.

Tests of absorption relating to pancreatic function are discussed on pages 262 and 285. It should be noted that glucose tolerance may be diabetic in type in some patients. This test should be carried out in patients with cystic fibrosis, particularly adolescents. Nearly one-third of patients with cystic fibrosis demonstrate reduced lactase activity on direct measurement of intestinal biopsies, although this finding and the symptoms do not correlate. Also the lactose tolerance test is flat in these patients.

The number of cystic fibrosis patients who develop clinical diabetes requiring insulin therapy is increasing. Thirty such patients have been seen in our clinic. In some patients, glucose intolerance is noted as long as ten to twelve years before insulin-requiring diabetes appears. When tested with intravenous tolbutamide they respond in a manner similar to other diabetics; i.e., there is a relatively small drop in the blood sugar at 20 to 30 minutes. In contrast to childhood diabetics, patients with cystic fibrosis and diabetes rarely develop ketosis. Insulin radioimmunoassays indicate reduced levels of insulin following intravenous glucose stimulation in these older patients. Human growth hormone response is normal or delayed. Measurements of glucagon have not yet been recorded in patients with cystic fibrosis and diabetes. If the diabetes is due to encroachment or destruction of islet tissue, one might expect a diminution in the glucagon level as well as a reduction in insulin. The majority of these patients do not have a family history of diabetes.

TREATMENT

Therapy in cystic fibrosis is designed essentially for both prophylaxis and clinical symptoms, because the basic nature of the disorder is unknown. It is also individualized because of the wide range of clinical manifestations and the varying degrees of involvement of affected organs. Since the disease is life long, therapy must be continuous and comprehensive. Such care is presently best offered by highly specialized clinics in many of our major medical institutions. For children, particularly infants, in whom the diagnosis is strongly suspected but not confirmed, treatment should not wait until clear-cut clinical evidence appears. Such delay could result in the premature development of advanced or irreversible changes.

PULMONARY SYSTEM

The main considerations are twofold: the relief or prevention of bronchial obstruction, and the treatment of the pulmonary infection.

OBSTRUCTION

A variety of measures are employed to remove viscid secretions, which include postural drainage, mucolytic agents, bronchodilators, and expectorant drugs. Some also employ mist-tent therapy in the belief that this will aid in mobilizing secretions and prevent drying and plugging. There is considerable controversy as to the effectiveness of many of the modes of therapy, with the exception of physical therapy, which includes not only postural drainage but also breathing exercises. Parents are taught the technique so that they can do this at home on a regular daily schedule, at least once a day in patients with mild disease and as often as three or more times when there is considerable involvement. The technique involves proper positioning of the child and clapping and vibrating over the affected areas. Mechanical vibrators have been developed to assist older patients so that they can perform this treatment unaided.

The most widely used mucolytic agent is n-acetylcysteine. Approximately 2 to 5 ml may be given from one to four times a day by aerosol in a 10 or 20 per cent solution. It is most effective in patients with moderate amounts of thick secretions. Most patients with advanced pulmonary lesions should receive this therapy, whereas all patients receive physiotherapy. Of the expectorant drugs, iodides in various forms have been used, and their effectiveness is difficult to ascertain. Isoproterenol given by aerosol along with bactericidal antibiotics, e.g., neomycin, colistimethate, or gentamicin, is used in patients with moderately severe disease. Corticosteroids have a limited use, namely, in treating the acutely ill infant with severe bronchospasm.

Pulmonary resection has been carried out in carefully selected patients with long-standing areas of persistent atelectasis and underlying abscess formation or bronchiectasis, and in whom the remainder of the lungs are reasonably free of serious disease. Patients with cor pulmonale are effectively treated with digitalis and, if necessary, restriction of salt and fluid, diuretics, and spironolactone. Other modes of therapy include tracheostomy and bronchial lavage; however, the beneficial effects of lavage are usually of short duration.

INFECTION

One of the greatest advances in the treatment of pulmonary infection dates from late 1948 when Aureomycin was introduced.[12] The remarkable improvement with daily administration in small doses of this broad-spectrum agent marked the first significant advance in therapy. Initially, the microorganism most commonly recovered in the sputum or nasopharynx was the penicillin-resistant *Staphylococcus aureus*. At present a great variety of antibiotics are effective against the Staphylococcus and include oxytetracycline, erythromycin, lincomycin, clindamycin, oxacillin and cephalosporin. The dose of these agents varies from approximately 15 to 50 mg per kilogram per day, administered orally in two or three divided doses. In addition Gantrisin may also be given. Since gram-negative bacteria are often present, broad-spectrum agents are frequently used. *Pseudomonas aeruginosa* and *Klebsiella pneumoniae* may be the predominant bacteria in the sputum, and efforts to eradicate these strains have not been successful. We have found chloramphenicol a very effective agent in spite of the failure to demonstrate in vitro sensitivity by the microorganisms isolated from the sputum.

In patients with persistent infection, continuous antibiotic therapy may be necessary. In patients with moderate pulmonary infections we frequently use a combination of chloramphenicol and oxacillin for prolonged periods. Use of chloramphenicol requires that the patient be observed closely for the development of hematological, ophthalmological and neurotoxic complications. In patients with minimal pulmonary disease, continuous antibiotic therapy is not necessary. Aerosol antibiotics are also used as an adjunct to oral systemic therapy; those most often used in this fashion are neomycin, colistin, and gentamicin in a concentration of 5 mg per milliliter. In patients with extensive disease harboring the mucoid strains of *Pseudomonas*, intravenous gentamicin alone or in combination with intravenous carbenicillin is recommended.

DIGESTIVE SYSTEM

The regimen for the patient with pancreatic insufficiency is relatively simple: a low-fat diet and the prescription of a potent pancreatic preparation with each meal. Since many patients have good to voracious appetites, hunger must be satisfied. The total caloric intake for an infant is as high as 150 cal per kilogram. As soon as more effective digestion is achieved, the appetite may become normal. Individuals vary considerably in their ability to tolerate fats and their response to pancreatic extract. Each patient should receive individual dietary instructions. Some patients, especially those with minimal pancreatic involvement, may tolerate a normal diet. Whenever possible, high protein intake is encouraged. Those with no evidence of pancreatic insufficiency (as determined by assay of their duodenal fluid and by stool trypsin tests in infancy) do not require pancreatin with meals. In general, fats are less well tolerated than proteins or carbohydrates. Multiple vitamin preparations are usually given in twice the recommended dose, and infants and those with liver disease get added vitamin K. Many of our patients also get vitamin E, the dose ranging from 50 to 200 IU per day, depending on age and weight. The majority of our patients receive Viokase, which is a defatted pancreatic preparation and not a pancreatic extract. However, Cotazym has also proved effective. The amount given may vary, depending on size and nature of the meal, from three to ten Viokase tablets or three to five capsules of Cotazym. Powdered preparations are available for infants. One teaspoon of Viokase powder or the contents of one packet of Cotazym given in applesauce or some other fruit with each feeding may suffice. The effective dose may vary, and the proper dose is determined by the response. A small number of patients are allergic to the pork product, and for these individuals a beef preparation is available from the Viobin Corporation.

The recent introduction of medium-chain triglycerides (MCT) as a replacement for fat has brought about an improvement in the nutrition of a number of infants with cystic fibrosis. Various commercial preparations are available, such as Portagen. This is a powdered, milk-based dietary product in which medium-chain triglycerides supply 95 per cent of the fat. MCT have also been used in various recipes and dietary supplements for the older child. A newer formula, Pregestimil, has, in addition to MCT, amino acids and glucose, which makes this a unique formula to be used in babies with milk sensitivity, disacchari-

dase deficiency, and pancreatic insufficiency. It is useful also in the management of babies with meconium ileus.

A patient diagnosed and photographed at the age of one and one-half years and again at three and one-half years following therapy is shown in Figure 95-6.

TREATMENT OF COEXISTING CONDITIONS

Patients with cystic fibrosis are subject to the usual conditions encountered in childhood. There is no evidence that gamma globulins are of special benefit. Patients with cystic fibrosis produce adequate and appropriate antibodies when stimulated. Preventive inoculations are given as provided to all children, but especially against measles and influenza. Congenital anomalies should be corrected appropriately. Except for the high incidence of inguinal hernia and undescended testes in male patients, no increased incidence of other defects has been observed. The incidence of allergic disorders is the same in patients with cystic fibrosis as in the general population; i.e., from 15 to 20 per cent.

COMPLICATIONS

One might consider cystic fibrosis a disease recognized chiefly by its complications. Excluding meconium ileus, a newborn with cystic fibrosis appears just as healthy as a "normal" newborn. At variable periods after birth the child begins to show evidence of pancreatic insufficiency or the effects of the viscid secretions in the respiratory tract. In reality many of the symptoms we recognize are actually the complications listed in Table 95-5. Some complications are iatrogenic; these are listed in Table 95-6. No attempt is made here to list the psychological, emotional, and other life problems that patients encounter as they grow into adulthood.

The aim is to establish the diagnosis very early in life and to attempt to prevent the complications. This approach, which has been practiced for over 25 years, may

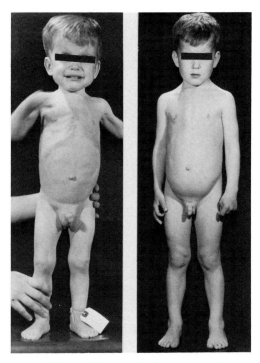

Figure 95-6. Photograph of patient with cystic fibrosis taken at the time of diagnosis when one and one-half years of age and three and one-half years later, following treatment.

TABLE 95–5. COMPLICATIONS NOTED IN CYSTIC FIBROSIS

Common
  Growth retardation
  Intestinal obstruction
  Inguinal hernia
  Undescended testicle
  Rectal prolapse
  Sterility in male
  Delayed sex development
  Glucose intolerance
  Atelectasis

  Irregular aeration with
    increased residual
    volume
  Bronchiectasis
  Sinusitis
  Nasal polyposis
  Digital clubbing
  Emphysema

Occasional
  Duodenitis
  Diabetes
  Cirrhosis
  Portal hypertension
  Osteoporosis
  Vitamin deficiencies–
    A, E, K

  Pneumothorax
  Hemoptysis
  Pulmonary hyperten-
    sion
  Scoliosis
  Arthritis

Rare
  Empyema
  Osteomyelitis
  Botryomycosis
  Hyperglobulinemia
  Hypoproteinemia
  Gynecomastia
  Macrocytic anemia
  Ocular changes
  Amyloidosis
  Parotitis

  Pancreatitis
  Calcification of
    pancreas
  Hypersplenism
  Intussusception
  Salt depletion
    syndrome
  Duodenal ulcer
  Pneumatosis
    intestinalis

TABLE 95–6. IATROGENIC COMPLICATIONS – EFFECTS OF DRUGS

Pancreatin
  Allergy to pork
  Diarrhea
Iodides
  Goiter
  Hypothyroidism
Antibiotics
  Tetracycline
    Dental staining
    Deposition in bone
    Photosensitivity
    Bulging fontanel
    Diarrhea
    Vomiting
  Chloramphenicol
    Ocular changes with visual loss
    Toxic neuritis
    Pancytopenia
  Other antibiotics in some individuals
    Diarrhea
    Vomiting
    Fever
    Rash
    Riboflavin deficiency
Anabolic agents
  Androgenic effects
IPPB
  Many produce pneumothorax and spread
    pulmonary infection

yield a survival rate of over 70 per cent to age 20 years when the diagnosis is established under three months of age.[13] Patients with meconium ileus are excluded, because the long-term prognosis is not so good. Effective screening tests for the newborn are badly needed so that we can effectively identify those with cystic fibrosis prior to their appearance in medical clinics with clinically significant disease. This can be done in high-risk families but not as yet in the general population. Clearly, the identification of heterozygous carriers would aid genetic counseling immeasurably.

PROGNOSIS

The outlook for patients with cystic fibrosis has improved considerably over the past 25 years. Prior to 1945, over 80 per cent of the diagnosed patients died within two years. The exceptional patient survived. A number of factors have changed this dim outlook. These include the following: (1) Increased clinical awareness of the disease and the detection of patients with varying degrees of severity, owing in measure to better diagnostic procedures, particularly the sweat test. (2) Early detection of this disease and early treatment. (3) The advent of antibiotics as a mode of therapy for pulmonary disease. (4) The introduction of improved pancreatic extracts. (5) The concept of preventive and continuous care, owing in large measure to the development of special centers and clinics for diagnosis and treatment. (6) The advent of parents' groups, local chapters and the educational activities and support of research provided by the National Cystic Fibrosis Research Foundation. Beginning in 1960, the National Institutes of Health have also provided research facilities for the study of cystic fibrosis.

REFERENCES

1. Shwachman, H., and Kulczycki, L. L. A report of 105 patients with cystic fibrosis of the pancreas studied over a five to fourteen year period. Amer. J. Dis. Child. 96:6, 1958.

2. Shwachman, H. Cystic fibrosis. *In* Respiratory Disease in Children, E. Kendig (ed.). Philadelphia, W. B. Saunders Co., 1967, pp. 541-564.

3. Farber, S. Pancreatic function and disease in early life. V. Pathologic changes associated with pancreatic insufficiency in early life. Arch. Path. 37:238, 1944.

4. di Sant'Agnese, P. A., Darling, R. C., Perera, G., and Shea, E. Abnormal electrolyte composition of sweat in cystic fibrosis of the pancreas. Clinical significance and relationship to disease. Pediatrics 12:549, 1953.

5. di Sant'Agnese, P. A., and Talamo, R. C. Pathogenesis and physiopathology of cystic fibrosis of the pancreas. New Eng. J. Med. 277:1287, 1344, 1399, 1967.

6. Kraus, I., Antonowicz, I., Shah, H., Lazarus, H., and Shwachman, H. Metachromasia and assay for lysosomal enzymes in skin fibroblasts cultured from patients with cystic fibrosis and controls. Pediatrics 47:1010, 1971.

7. Anderson, D. H. Cystic fibrosis of the pancreas and its relation to celiac disease. Amer. J. Dis. Child. 56:344, 1938.

8. Craig, J. M., Haddad, H., and Shwachman, H. The pathological changes in the liver in cystic fibrosis of the pancreas. Amer. J. Dis. Child. 93:357, 1957.

9. Kaplan, E., Shwachman, H., Perlmutter, A. D., Rule, A., Khaw, K. T., and Holsclaw, D. S. Reproductive failure in males with cystic fibrosis. New Eng. J. Med. 279:65, 1968.

10. Holsclaw, D. S., Rocmans, C., and Shwachman, H. Intussusception in patients with cystic fibrosis. Pediatrics 48:51, 1971.

11. Shwachman, H., and Mahmoodian, A. Pilocarpine iontophoresis sweat testing. Results of seven years' experience. Fourth International Conference on Cystic Fibrosis of the Pancreas (Mucoviscidosis). Berne, Grindelwald, 1966, Part I. Mod. Probl. Pediat. 10:158, 1967.

12. Shwachman, H., Crocker, A. C., Foley, G. E., and Patterson, P. R. Aureomycin therapy in the pulmonary involvement of pancreatic fibrosis (mucoviscidosis). New Eng. J. Med. 241:185, 1949.

13. Shwachman, H., Redmond, A., and Khaw, K. T. Studies in cystic fibrosis: Report of 130 patients diagnosed under 3 months of age and over a 20-year period. Pediatrics 46:335, 1970.

Chapter 96

Diseases of the Pancreas in Childhood

Hans-Béat Hadorn, M. Michael Thaler

Diseases of the exocrine pancreas are rare in childhood; alcoholism is not a problem, and cholelithiasis is uncommon. Fibrocystic disease, the most important cause of pancreatic insufficiency among children, is discussed fully on pages 1206 to 1224. Other causes of pancreatic pathology include congenital structural anomalies of the pancreas, congenital hypoplasia of the pancreas, selective pancreatic enzyme deficiencies, infections, trauma, and hereditary pancreatitis.

CONGENITAL MALFORMATIONS

Annular pancreas is a ring of pancreatic tissue encircling the descending portion of the duodenum. During embryonic development, two separate outpouchings of the primitive duodenum form the dorsal and ventral pancreatic anlage. The ventral anlage rotates around the gut and fuses with the dorsal anlage between the sixth and seventh weeks of gestation. The left portion of the ventral anlage normally atrophies; when it persists, a ring of pancreatic tissue may encircle the descending part of the duodenum.

Symptoms referable to upper intestinal obstruction may develop rapidly after

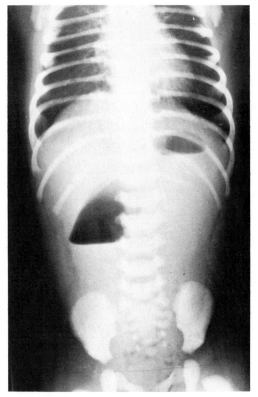

Figure 96–1. Duodenal stenosis in a newborn with annular pancreas. Plain film without contrast material. Note double-bubble sign and no air in the remaining intestine. (Courtesy of Prof. M. Bettex, Department of Pediatric Surgery, University of Berne.)

1226

birth. The upper abdomen is distended, and prominent peristaltic waves are visible. The infants may vomit bile-stained fluid. Radiographs of the abdomen reveal dilatation of the upper portion of the duodenum and the double-bubble sign (fluid levels in the stomach and duodenum). The remaining small bowel is nearly or completely free of air (Fig. 96–1).

Other congenital anomalies, e.g., mongolism, cleft palate, imperforate anus, and colonic malrotation, are frequently found in association with annular pancreas.[1] As with other obstructive malformations of the fetal gut, pregnancy may be complicated by polyhydramnios.

The condition represents a surgical emergency. Obstruction is relieved by retrocolic isoperistaltic duodenojejunostomy, and the pancreas is left undivided to prevent formation of fistulas. Pancreatic function is normal and prognosis excellent, provided corrective surgery is prompt.

Ectopic pancreatic tissue can be located in the mucosa of the stomach, or anywhere in the small intestine. Gastrointestinal obstruction, bleeding, and intussusception may develop, but the condition is usually asymptomatic.

CONGENITAL EXOCRINE PANCREATIC INSUFFICIENCY

After cystic fibrosis, congenital hypoplasia of the exocrine pancreas with neutropenia or pancytopenia may be the most common cause of pancreatic insufficiency in children.[2, 3] Frequency has been estimated at about 1 per cent of cystic fibrosis, i.e., 1 in 20,000 live births, and may be even more frequent. An autosomal recessive pattern of inheritance is suggested by cases reported in families.

Pancreatic biopsy samples, obtained in two patients,[2] showed complete replacement of exocrine tissue with fat (Fig. 96–2). Metaphyseal dysostosis and dwarfism are also recognized as regular features of the syndrome.[4, 5]

Congenital hypoplasia of the pancreas is usually differentiated from cystic fibrosis on the basis of normal sweat electrolytes and absence of chronic pulmonary infections. Hadorn demonstrated gross reduction in all pancreatic enzymes and bicar-

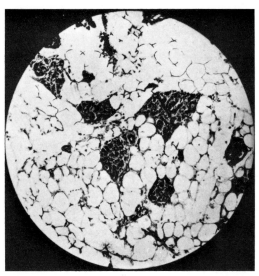

Figure 96–2. Lipomatosis of the exocrine pancreas in a patient with congenital hypoplasia of the exocrine pancreas. The exocrine tissue is completely replaced by fat. Only a few ductules remain. The islets of Langerhans are unaffected. (From Bodian, M.: Fibrocystic Disease of the Pancreas. London, William Heinemann, 1952.)

bonate secretion in this condition (Table 96–1).[6] The neutropenia is usually continuous, but may be cyclic. Hypoplastic anemia and thrombocytopenia are commonly present. The relationship between the myeloid and pancreatic features of the disease is not understood. Recently, immunoglobulin deficiency has been reported in a single patient with this syndrome.[7]

Steatorrhea and retarded growth are the main clinical problems. The steatorrhea usually responds to replacement therapy with pancreatic extracts, but the growth retardation and neutropenia appear to be irreversible. Recurrent upper respiratory and skin infections occur frequently, and are an important cause of mortality in this disease. Infections must be treated aggressively with antibiotics to prevent a deteriorating course similar to that of cystic fibrosis. The metaphyseal dysostosis requires orthopedic corrective measures (Fig. 96–3).

PANCREATIC ENZYME DEFICIENCIES
(Table 96–2)

Isolated lipase deficiency is an extremely rare autosomal recessive disease.[8]

TABLE 96–1. PANCREOZYMIN-SECRETIN TEST* IN FIVE CHILDREN WITH EXOCRINE PANCREATIC INSUFFICIENCY (SHWACHMAN SYNDROME)—TOTAL OUTPUT OF VOLUME, BICARBONATE, AND ENZYMES PER KILOGRAM BODY WEIGHT AND PER 50 MINUTES, COMPARED WITH THE VALUES OF THE CONTROL GROUP†

No.	Sex	Age (yr.)	CLINICAL DIAGNOSIS	VOL. (ML)	BICAR-BONATE (MEQ)	CHYMO-TRYPSIN (μG)	TRYPSIN (μG)	CARBOXY-PEPTIDASE A (IU 10³)ᶜ	AMYLASE (IU)— ONLY CHIL-DREN OVER 1 YR.	LIPASE
1.	M	17	EPI§, neutropenia, metaphyseal dysostosis, dwarfism	3.9	0.04	0.0	2.8	0.0	0.0	0.0
2.	F	1	EPI, neutropenia, rib changes	3.2	0.017	15.0	4.2	–	0.0	0.0
3.	M	3	EPI, neutropenia ⎫	3.6	0.02	0.0	25.5	1149.0	31.0	68.0
4.	F	10	EPI, neutropenia ⎬ S§	1.5	0.03	66.0	321.0	130.0	12.4	0.0
5.	F	13	EPI, neutropenia ⎭	1.7	0.04	105.0	28.0	239.0	10.0	0.0
Controls¶			Mean	3.7 (n=43)	0.17 (n=36)	797 (n=50)	841 (n=46)	730 (n=38)	437 (n=43)	1381 (n=42)
			Range	1.8–6.3	0.08–0.36	262–1862	300–2170	236–2480	139–1000	305–3525

*Two units per kilogram of pancreozymin (Boots) (p), followed by 2 units per kilogram of secretin (Boots) (s) was given intravenously. The duodenal contents were collected during 20 minutes after p and during 30 minutes after s as described by Hadorn et al.[14]

†From Hadorn, B.: Clin. Gastroent. *1*:125, 1972.

‡Case 1 is patient M. A.; cases 2 to 5 are the patients described by Burke et al.[4]

§EPI = Exocrine pancreatic insufficiency; S = siblings; IU = international units.

¶Children with digestive complaints but no malabsorption or maldigestion (age 3 months to 16 years).

Severe steatorrhea and diarrhea begin shortly after birth and require treatment with supplements of pancreatic enzymes. Growth and development are normal. The duodenal juice contains normal amounts of amylase and proteolytic activity, whereas pancreatic lipase is deficient. Prognosis is favorable.

Isolated amylase deficiency is usually not apparent before one year of age, because pancreatic amylase is normally low in young infants.[9] Extreme intolerance to starches causes diarrhea associated with low fecal *p*H. The diagnosis can be established with a starch loading test. When the test is positive, blood glucose concen-

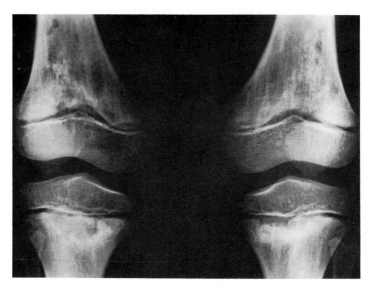

Figure 96–3. Roentgenogram of knees of a ten-year-old boy with neutropenia and pancreatic insufficiency. Irregular rarefied areas are seen in the metaphyses. (Courtesy of Dr. J. R. Hamilton.)

TABLE 96–2. ISOLATED PANCREATIC ENZYME DEFICIENCIES AND DISTURBANCES OF ZYMOGEN ACTIVATION IN CHILDREN*

		CLINICAL FEATURES			DIAGNOSTIC TESTS	TREATMENT	PROGNOSIS	
	Age of Onset	Steatorrhea	Failure to Thrive	Other			Without Treatment	With Treatment
1. Lipase deficiency	At birth	Yes (+++)	No	Other	Lipase in duodenal fluid	Pancreatic extracts by mouth	Fair	Good
2. Amylase deficiency	Variable after introduction of starch in diet	No	Rarely	Fermentative diarrhea	Amylase in duodenal fluid†	Elimination of starch from diet	Good	Good
3. Disturbances of proteolytic zymogen activation								
a. Trypsinogen deficiency	At birth	Yes (+) if secondary pancreatic insufficiency is present	Yes	Diarrhea, hypoproteinemia, edema, anemia, rapid improvement with protein hydrolysates by mouth	Zymogen‡ activation test	Protein hydrolysates, pancreatic extracts	Poor	Good
b. Intestinal enterokinase deficiency	At birth	Yes (+) if secondary pancreatic insufficiency is present	Yes	Same as 3a; in addition, growth retardation, fatty degeneration of liver (older patients)	Zymogen‡	Protein hydrolysates, pancreatic extracts	Poor	Good

*From Hadorn, B.: Clin. Gastroent. 1:125, 1972.

†Diagnostic only if over one year of age.

‡The zymogen activation test is carried out by adding enterokinase to the patient's duodenal juice in vitro. In trypsinogen deficiency no trypsin should appear in the juice after the addition of enterokinase (lack of trypsinogen). By contrast in intestinal enterokinase deficiency, the addition of enterokinase to the juice results in rapid activation of trypsinogen to trypsin, and this is followed by the activation of the other proteolytic zymogens. Although exogenous trypsin, under certain conditions, may activate human trypsinogen, enterokinase is much more efficient in activating trypsinogen and should therefore be used in the "zymogen activation test."

trations remain at basal levels after an oral dose of 50 g starch per square meter. Treatment consists of a starch elimination diet, supplemented with disaccharides. Prognosis is excellent, and growth is unimpaired.

The genetic inheritance patterns of *pancreatic enzyme deficiencies* have not been clarified.

Trypsin deficiency must be extremely rare, a single patient having been reported to date.[10]

Deficiency of trypsinogen results in deficiency of proteolytic enzymes.[11] In this condition, administration of trypsin triggers chymotrypsin and carboxypeptidase activity while trypsin itself remains inactive. Newborn infants develop diarrhea and anemia, and fail to thrive. Severe hypoproteinemia often leads to edema. Treatment consists of frequent feedings of mixtures of amino acids.

Intestinal enterokinase deficiency[12] causes complete absence of pancreatic proteolytic activity in duodenal fluid. Enterokinase is essential for activating zymogen, and addition of enterokinase restores normal proteolytic activity in these patients (Fig. 96–4). Enterokinase can also be assayed in intestinal biopsy specimens. Severe illness occurs soon after

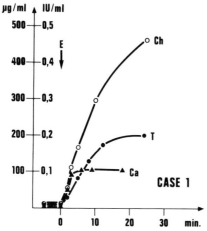

Figure 96–4. Zymogen activation test in one patient with intestinal enterokinase deficiency. One mg of purified human enterokinase was added to 1 ml of the patient's duodenal contents in vitro, and the activation of trypsinogen, chymotrypsinogen, and procarboxypeptidase was followed during incubation of the juice at pH 7.5 and 37° C. T = Trypsin activity (μg per ml). Ch = Chymotrypsin activity (μg per ml). Ca = Carboxypeptidase activity (IU per ml). E = Enterokinase added.

birth, and may lead to dwarfism. Treatment with pancreatic extracts results in rapid improvement.

PANCREATIC INVOLVEMENT IN SYSTEMIC DISEASE

CYSTIC FIBROSIS OF THE PANCREAS

Cystic fibrosis is the most common cause of congenital pancreatic disease in childhood. Although all exocrine glands are involved, only the pancreatic aspects of the disease will be discussed here (see pp. 1206 to 1224).

Pancreatic involvement in cystic fibrosis is extremely variable. Approximately 20 per cent of the children suffering from this disease do not have overt pancreatic insufficiency or steatorrhea.[13] Tests of exocrine pancreatic function performed with secretin and pancreozymin stimulation usually show an extreme reduction of the output of fluid bicarbonate and enzymes. The age of onset of pancreatic symptoms is also variable; maldigestion with steatorrhea may become manifest later in childhood or may be present from infancy. In patients who do not have clinical symptoms of malabsorption, pancreatic function is nevertheless abnormal, because the volume of secretion and the bicarbonate output are reduced in response to secretin.[14] The decrease in volume results in abnormally high pancreatic enzyme concentrations in the lumen of the duodenum under the conditions of this test.

The pancreatic insufficiency should be treated with high doses of pancreatic extracts (Cotazym, Viokase), which are increased until significant improvement or correction of the steatorrhea is observed. Dietary supplements of medium-chain triglycerides may reduce stool fat excretion in patients with severe steatorrhea. The malabsorption syndrome is probably more complex and not entirely due to pancreatic insufficiency. For example, increased fecal amino acid excretion has been reported,[15] which cannot be explained on the basis of pancreatic insufficiency alone.

The course of this severe and chronic illness is not greatly influenced by pancreatic insufficiency. The prognosis—which is still relatively poor—depends largely upon the degree of permanent pulmonary damage caused by frequent and resistant bronchial and pulmonary infections.

THE EXOCRINE PANCREAS IN PROTEIN-CALORIE MALNUTRITION

Atrophy of the pancreas in kwashiorkor was first described in 1926.[16] Loss and vacuolization of the acinar cytoplasm with fibrosis of the entire organ were observed. Epithelial metaplasia and cystic dilatation of the ducts have been described in malnourished children.[17] Pancreozymin and secretin stimulation tests revealed that enzyme output was grossly deficient but not entirely absent in South African children with protein-calorie malnutrition. However, the volume and pH responses of duodenal juice to secretin were unimpaired.[18] Normal pancreatic function was restored upon feeding adequate amounts of protein. It is not clear at which stage of protein-calorie malnutrition damage to the pancreas becomes irreversible.

PANCREATITIS

Acute pancreatitis is usually associated with mumps. Severe epigastric pain, vomiting, and diarrhea develop several days after parotid swelling and persist for about one week. Fever and bradycardia inter-

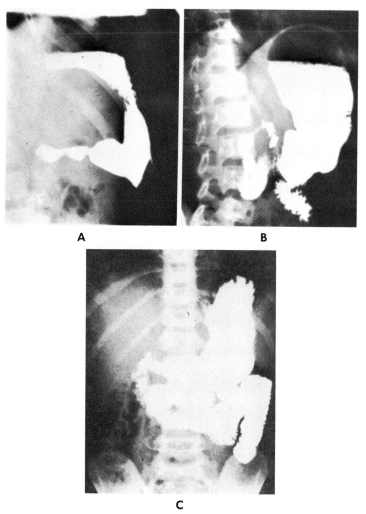

Figure 96–5. Traumatic pancreatic pseudocyst in a boy aged five years, eight months. Upper gastrointestinal radiograph before operation. *A*, The stomach appears to be compressed by the tumor. *B*, The lateral view shows displacement of the stomach. The radiographs are typical of a tumor in the area of the bursa omentalis after drainage. *C*, Upper gastrointestinal radiograph three months after Redon-drainage of the pseudocyst. Complete normalization of the radiological appearance. (From Bettex, M., Küffer, F., and Schärli, A.: Schweiz. Med. Wschr. 96:342, 1966.)

vene. Serum amylase is usually elevated even when the pancreas is not involved, whereas lipase activity may be elevated when symptoms develop. Although transient diabetes develops occasionally, complete recovery of pancreatic functions is the general rule.

Acute hemorrhagic pancreatitis is much rarer in children than in adults. Glucocorticoid therapy is probably the most common cause,[19] and this diagnosis should be considered in children on steroid therapy who suddenly develop severe abdominal pain, nausea, vomiting, abdominal distention, a doughy consistency of the abdominal wall, and signs of shock. Abdominal guarding, epigastric tenderness, and absent bowel sounds may also be present. Ascites, acute vascular collapse, and renal failure are grave complications. Laboratory tests may reveal elevation of serum amylase, hyperglycemia, leukocytosis, glycosuria, and albuminuria. Hypocalcemia may become apparent on the second or third day. Fat necrosis of the peripheral long bones may occur, resembling osteomyelitis. Prognosis is grave, only four of 21 reported patients having recovered.[19]

Acute hemorrhagic pancreatitis was ob-

served in three children who died from acute encephalitis, suggesting a common viral etiology or an immune reaction to the infection.[20]

Acute hemorrhagic pancreatitis has also been a problem in patients with graft-versus-host reactions after receiving organ transplants.

Obstruction of the pancreatic duct caused by infestation with *Ascaris lumbricoides* was a leading cause of acute pancreatitis in the past, but appears to be disappearing. Pancreatic duct obstruction associated with malformations of the common bile duct has been the cause of pancreatitis in a small number of cases.

Blunt trauma caused by a fall, contact sports, or car accidents is a relatively common cause of pancreatitis in older children and adolescents (*traumatic pancreatitis*). After the signs of acute pancreatic inflammation subside, a pseudocyst may develop, formed by entry of pancreatic fluid into the lesser sac of omentum. The abdomen becomes painfully distended, and a tumor may be palpable in the left upper quadrant. Serum amylase and lipase values are usually extremely high. Radiographic studies of the upper gastrointestinal tract with contrast medium reveal

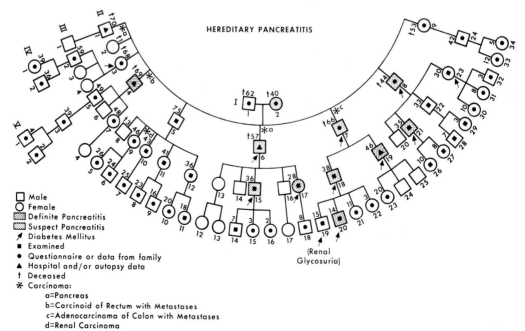

Figure 96–6. Report of a kindred with hereditary pancreatitis. (From Davidson, P., Costanza, D., Swieconek, J. A., and Harris, J. B.: Ann. Intern. Med. 68:88, 1968.)

displacement of the stomach by the cyst (Fig. 96–5).

Pseudocysts of the pancreas should be surgically drained as soon as the diagnosis is established. The chances for full recovery are good.

CHRONIC RELAPSING PANCREATITIS

Chronic relapsing pancreatitis in children is usually an inherited problem. Genetic pedigrees reveal an autosomal dominant pattern of transmission (Fig. 96–6). The disease begins in childhood with recurrent attacks of abdominal pain, associated in some cases with lysinuria and cystinuria. Most families, however, do not exhibit aminoaciduria.[21, 22] Upper gastrointestinal bleeding and pancreatic pseudocysts may develop in the course of the disease, and pancreatic lithiasis complicates the latter stages of the disorder. Most cases of hereditary pancreatitis require surgical removal of all pancreatic tissue. The prognosis is guarded, and death may come quickly.[22] Recurrent pancreatitis has also been observed in familial hyperlipemia[23] and in hyperparathyroidism.[24]

REFERENCES

1. Salzer, G., Stur, O., and Zweymüller, E. Erfolgreich operiertes Pankreas annulare bei einem neugeborenen Mongoloid *Arch. Kinderheilk.* 164:152, 1961.
2. Bodian, M., Sheldon, W., and Lightwood, R. Congenital hypoplasia of the exocrine pancreas. Acta Pediat. 53:282, 1964.
3. Shwachman, H., Diamond, L. K., Oski, F. A., and Khaw, K. T. The syndrome of pancreatic insufficiency and bone marrow dysfunction. J. Pediat. 65:645, 1964.
4. Burke, V., Colebatch, J. H., Anderson, C. M., and Simons, M. J. Association of pancreatic insufficiency and chronic neutropenia in childhood. Arch. Dis. Child. 42:147, 1967.
5. Giedion, A., Prader, A., Hadorn, B., Shmerling, D. H., and Auricchio, S. Metaphysase Dysostose und angeboren Pankreasinsuffizienz. Fortschr. Bebiet Roentgen. 108:51, 1968.
6. Hadorn, B. Diseases of the pancreas in children. Clin. Gastroent. 1:125, 1972.
7. Hudson, E., and Aldor, T. Pancreatic insufficiency and neutropenia with associated immunoglobulin deficit. Arch. Intern. Med. 125:314, 1970.
8. Sheldon, W. Congenital pancreatic lipase deficiency. Arch. Dis. Child. 39:268, 1964.
9. Delachaume-Salem, E., and Sarles, H. Evolution en fonction de l'age de la secretion pancreatique humaine normale. Biol. Gastro-Enterol. 2:135, 1970.
10. Farber, S., Shwachman, H., and Maddock, C. Pancreatic function and disease in early life. I. Pancreatic enzyme activity and celiac syndrome. J. Clin. Invest. 22:827, 1943.
11. Townes, P. L. Trypsinogen deficiency disease. J. Pediat. 66:275, 1965.
12. Haworth, J. C., Gourley, B., Hadorn, B., and Sumida, C. Malabsorption and growth failure due to intestinal enterokinase deficiency. J. Pediat. 78:481, 1971.
13. Farber, S., Shwachman, H., and Maddock, C. Pancreatic function and disease in early life. II. Pathological changes associated with pancreatic insufficiency in early life. *Arch. Path.* 37:238, 1944.
14. Hadorn, B., Johansen, P. G., and Anderson, C. M. Pancreozymin secretin test of exocrine pancreatic function in cystic fibrosis and the significance of the result for the pathogenesis of the disease. Canad. Med. Assn. J. 98:377, 1968.
15. Gibbons, I. S. E., Seakins, J. W. T., and Ersser, R. S. Tyrosine metabolism and fecal amino acids in cystic fibrosis of the pancreas. Lancet 1:877, 1967.
16. Normet, L. Memoire. La boufissure d'Assam. Bull. Soc. Path. Exotique Filiat. 19:207, 1926.
17. Gillman, J., and Gillman, T. Methionine and the fatty liver of infant pellagrins. Nature 155:634, 1945.
18. Barbezat, G. O., and Hansen, J. D. L. The exocrine pancreas and protein caloric malnutrition. Pediatrics 42:77, 1968.
19. Riemenschneider, T., Wilson, J. F., and Vernier, R. L. Glucocorticoid-induced pancreatitis in children. Pediatrics 41:428, 1968.
20. Stofer, S. L., Wanglee, P., and Kennedy, C. Acute hemorrhagic pancreatitis and other visceral changes associated with acute encephalopathy. J. Pediat. 73:235, 1968.
21. Davidson, P., Costanza, D., Swieconek, J. A., and Harris, J. B. Hereditary pancreatitis: A kindred without gross aminoaciduria. Ann. Intern. Med. 68:88, 1968.
22. McElroy, R., and Christiansen, P. A. Hereditary pancreatitis in a kinship associated with portal vein thrombosis. Amer. J. Med. 52:228, 1972.
23. Collet, R. W., and Kennedy, R. L. J. Chronic relapsing pancreatitis associated with hyperlipemia in an eight-year-old boy. Proc. Mayo Clin. 23:158, 1948.
24. Casey, M. L., and Fitzgerald, O. Hyperparathyroidism associated with chronic pancreatitis in a family. Gut 9:700, 1968.

Section 14

THE COLON

Chapter 97

Anatomy

Marvin H. Sleisenger

GROSS CHARACTERISTICS

The proximal part of the colon, concerned with absorption of water and electrolytes and, to a lesser extent, of conjugated and unconjugated bile acids, is derived from the embryonal midgut and is nourished by the superior mesenteric artery. The distal colon springs from the hindgut and receives the greater part of its blood supply from the inferior mesenteric artery and its branches.

The length of the colon varies between 2.54 and 3.69 times the body height. As might be expected, accurate estimation of the length of the colon in vivo is difficult, and nearest approximations to it have been made by ingenious intubation studies.[1] The diameter of the colon diminishes from cecum to anus. The colon is characterized grossly by some tortuosity and redundancy of the sigmoid and by two sharp angulations, the splenic and hepatic flexures, the former situated superior to the latter (see Figs. 97–1 and 97–2).

The wall of the colon contains essentially the same muscular coats as in the small bowel except that the longitudinal muscle forms three separate bands, the *taeniae coli,* about 0.6 to 1.0 cm in width, which run from the tip of the cecum to the

rectum and converge at the base of the appendix. Between the taeniae are outpouchings, which are called haustra, separated by folds. The size and shape of the haustra are determined by the state of contraction of the smooth and longitudinal muscle layers. Covering the serosal surface of the colon are the appendices epiploicae, which are fatty structures attached to the peritoneum. In contrast to the small bowel, the colon does not have a mesentery for its entire length, containing a structure of this sort for a short distance along the transverse colon and the sigmoid.

On plain films of the abdomen, the colon is frequently seen to contain some air, whereas the small bowel normally has little if any gas. The course of the colon can often be traced by identification of haustra, the relatively high position of the splenic flexure, and often partially gas-filled rectum and rectosigmoid (Fig. 97–3). In contrast, the small intestine, often overlying or underlying the colon in many areas, appears normally only as radiolucent spots scattered about the abdomen. When the small intestine is more clearly outlined, the characteristic valvulae conniventes may be noted which traverse the entire diameter of the segment in contrast to the

1234

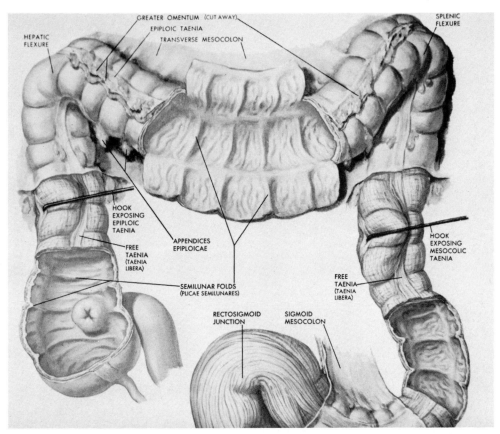

Figure 97–1. Contour and gross anatomy of the colon. Note the ileocecal junction, which is not labeled. (From Netter, F.: Ciba Collection of Medical Illustrations, Volume 3, Section X.)

haustra of the colon which only partially encircle the colon because they do not extend across the midline of the lumen (Fig. 97–4).

The mucosa of the colon is flat. However, it is thrown into some folds, the plicae semilunares (Fig. 97–1). It is highlighted by the presence of epithelial crypts forming the glands of Lieberkühn. These glands open all along the mucosa into the lumen and secrete the mucus which allegedly helps to lubricate the passage of stool (Fig. 97–5).

HISTOLOGY

The wall of the large intestine, like that of the small intestine, consists of four distinct layers. The outermost layer, the serosa, is composed of mesothelial cells to which are attached fatty appendices epi-ploicae, which are extensions of peritoneal fat. The serosa covers only the portions of the large bowel which lie within the peritoneal cavity; thus it is not found in the rectum.

The muscle coat, found immediately beneath the serosa, is composed of an inner circular muscular layer forming a tight spiral circumferentially along the course of the colon and an outer longitudinal muscle layer which is distinctive because it is composed of three separate longitudinal strips (taeniae coli) which run from the rectum to the cecum. The ganglion cells of the myenteric plexus of Auerbach may be found between the circular and longitudinal muscle layers, with the majority being located along the external surface of the circular muscle coat. Unmyelinated postganglionic fibers are also found in the circular muscle layer and communicate with the submucosal plexus of the nerves.

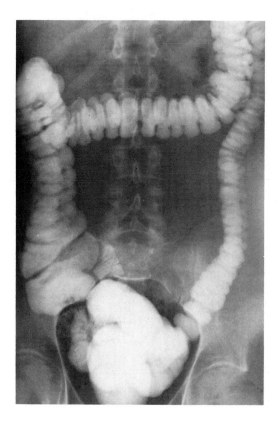

Figure 97–2. Barium enema of the colon. Note tortuosity of sigmoid, the flexures, haustral markings, and ileal reflux.

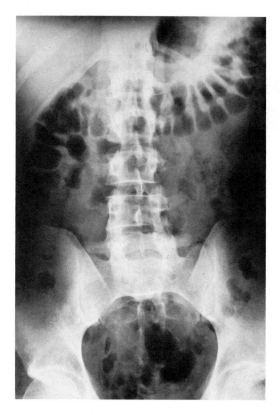

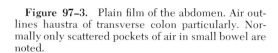

Figure 97–3. Plain film of the abdomen. Air outlines haustra of transverse colon particularly. Normally only scattered pockets of air in small bowel are noted.

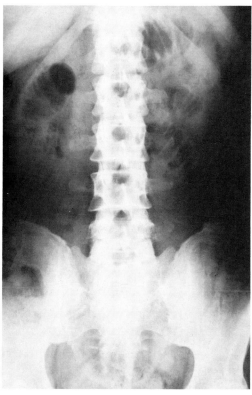

Figure 97-4. Plain film of the abdomen in early small bowel obstruction, showing valvulae conniventes which traverse the diameter, distinguishing small bowel from colon.

The submucosa of the colon resembles the submucosa of the other tubular digestive organs. It contains many blood and lymph vesicles, dense connective tissue

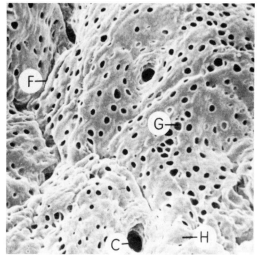

Figure 97-5. Scanning electron micrograph of a control rectal biopsy. The mouths of the crypts (C) are surrounded by numerous goblet cells which have discharged their contents (G). H, Hemispherical projections; F, furrow. × 500. (From Kavin, H., et al.: Gastroenterology 59:426, 1970.)

sparsely infiltrated by cells (lymphocytes, plasma cells, mast cells, macrophages, and eosinophils), and the unmyelinated nerve fibers and ganglion cells that form the submucosal or Meissner's plexus.

The innermost layer of the mucosa is separated from the submucosa by the muscularis mucosae, a layer of smooth muscle cells roughly eight to 12 cells thick. The mucosa of the large intestine differs from that of the small intestine in that villi are absent; instead, the absorptive surface it-

Figure 97-6. Biopsy of normal adult human rectum, showing rectal mucosa. C.E. = Columnar epithelium; L.P. = lamina propria; Cr = crypt; M.M. = muscularis mucosae. × 100.

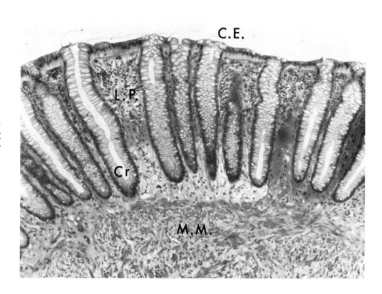

self is flat. However, numerous straight tubular crypts up to 0.7 mm in length are normally present and extend from the muscularis mucosae to the flat absorptive surface (Fig. 97–6). The crypts and the absorptive surface are lined by a continuous sheet of columnar epithelial cells which are separated from mesenchymal tissue of the lamina propria by a well defined, continuous basal lamina applied to the basal plasma membrane of the epithelial cells.

The crypt epithelium in the lower half of the crypts is composed of proliferating undifferentiated cells, mucus-secreting goblet cells, and abundant endocrine epithelial cells. The epithelium of the upper half of the crypts consists of differentiating absorptive cells, goblet cells, and a few endocrine cells. The flat absorptive surface is lined by many absorptive cells as well as a moderate number of goblet cells, most of which are virtually depleted of their mucous granules.

The morphology of the absorptive cells of the large intestine differs significantly from that of absorptive cells in the small intestine. Although the absorptive surface of both cell types is lined by microvilli, the microvilli on colonic absorptive cells are less abundant (Fig. 97–7). However, as in the small intestine, an elaborate fibrillar glycoprotein surface coat is applied directly to the apical plasma membrane which delineates the microvilli (Fig. 97–7). Numerous membrane-bounded, glycoprotein-containing vesicles 0.1 to 1μ in diameter are present in the apical cytoplasm of colonic and rectal absorptive cells (Fig.

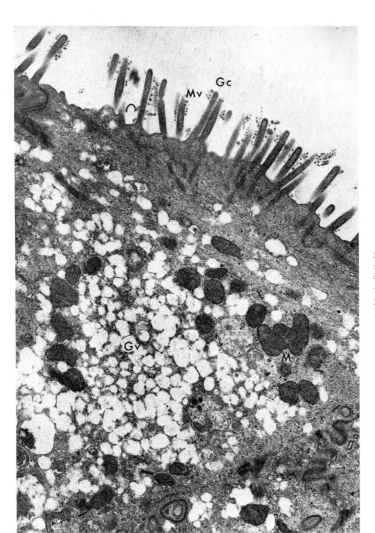

Figure 97–7. Electron micrograph of a normal human rectal absorptive cell. Gc = Glycocalyx; Mv = microvilli; Gv = glycoprotein vesicles; M = mitochondria. × 20,000. (Courtesy of Dr. Gregory Eastwood.)

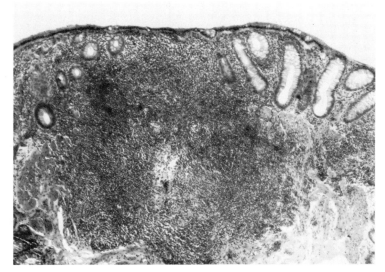

Figure 97–8. Large lymph follicle of lamina propria of normal human rectum. × 75.

97–7). Although their function is unknown, these vesicles are distinctive and they are not found in the cytoplasm of absorptive cells of the small intestine. Unlike the absorptive cells, the morphology of the goblet and endocrine cells of the large intestine resembles closely that of goblet and endocrine cells in the small intestine.

The cellular elements of the lamina propria of the large bowel resemble closely those seen in the small intestine and include lymphocytes, many plasma cells, mast cells, macrophages, eosinophils, and fibroblasts. In addition, there are blood and lymph vessels and unmyelinated nerve fibers in the lamina. Large lymph follicles with typical germinal centers are often seen in the lamina propria of the colon and the rectum, especially in young persons. These frequently extend through the muscularis mucosae into the submucosa. When present, the follicles may markedly distort mucosal architecture and thus make biopsy interpretation difficult (Fig. 97–8).

VASCULATURE OF COLON AND RECTUM

The arterial blood supply and venous drainage of the colon and rectum are described on pages 378 to 383.

LYMPHATIC DRAINAGE

The colon is drained by a vast network of lymphatics (Fig. 97–9) which flow into three groups of lymph nodes: the paracolic nodes along the course of the marginal artery, to which the vessels from the colon wall connect; the intermediate nodes along the major colic vessels; and the central nodes located at the roots of the vessels near the aorta. These pathways intersect at a number of points.

The lymph channels begin in the intramural capillaries associated with lymph follicles; the smaller vessels merge, and the large channels, containing valves, fol-

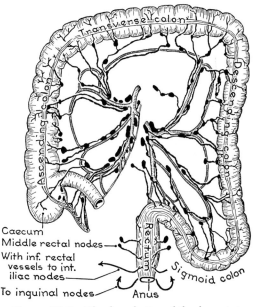

Figure 97–9. The lymphatics of the large intestine. (From Grant's Method of Anatomy. 7th ed. Baltimore, Williams and Wilkins Co., 1965.)

low the course of the superior and inferior
mesenteric arteries. Segments of colon
which have a mesentery contain the lymphatics; drainage for those without these
supporting structures is retroperitoneal.

A major juncture for colonic lymphatics
is at the cysterna chyli, a sac between the
aorta and right crus of the diaphragm; here
they converge with corresponding vessels
from other viscera, the abdominal wall and
lower extremities. From it the thoracic
duct ascends through the diaphragm to
empty into the left subclavian vein at the
jugulo-subclavian angle.

The importance of the colonic lymphatics lies in their involvement in both
inflammatory—particularly granulomatous
—and neoplastic disease of the colon and
rectum. Further discussion of the lymphatics in these diseases of the colon will
be found on pages 1353 to 1354 and 1447
to 1448.

INNERVATION OF THE COLON

The nerve supply of the colon is entirely
autonomic, with a network of ganglia,

plexuses, and fibers which are extracolonic
and another composed of myelinated and
nonmyelinated fibers along with ganglion
cells of nerve plexuses in the submucosa
and between the two layers of smooth
muscle (Fig. 97–10).

The parasympathetic system is composed of the vagus nerve (cranial outflow)
and the sacral nerve, the nervi erigentes,
from the sacral spinal cord. The latter
consists of long, preganglionic fibers
which terminate at synapses within the
myenteric and submucosal plexuses. The
sympathetic division, on the other hand,
has nerves which emerge as splanchnic
nerves from the thoracic spinal cord as
preganglionic sympathetic fibers and synapse in the preaortic ganglia (celiac ganglia, superior mesenteric ganglia, inferior
mesenteric plexus, and hypogastric ganglia). For the ganglia, postganglionic
fibers then follow the blood vessels to the
colon wall.

The splanchnic nerves, which are the effector or efferent nerves of the sympathetic
system, pass through the chain of paravertebral sympathetic ganglia; only rarely,

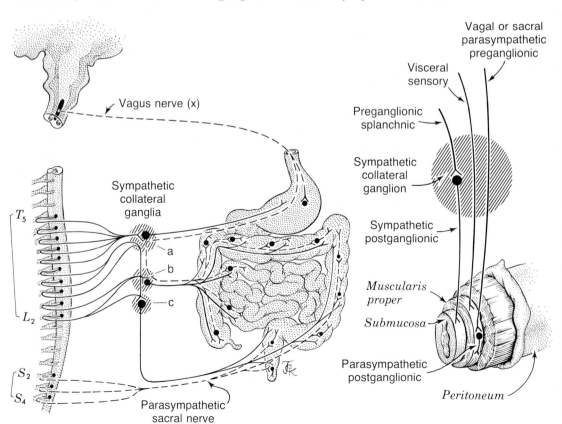

Figure 97–10.   Autonomic innervation of the colon and rectum. (Courtesy of Dr. Albert L. Jones.)

however, do they synapse here; they usually synapse in the preaortic sympathetic ganglion chains. In their course from the spinal cord to these chains they pass through the white ramus, where they join company with the nerve fibers from the dorsal root ganglion cells which are the afferents providing the sensory innervation of the colon. Fibers of these sympathetic sensory afferents terminate in the plexuses of the submucosa and intermuscular layers (pp. 326 to 337).

In view of their importance in transit and defecation, special emphasis on innervation of the cecum and rectum is warranted. The extrinsic nerve supply to the cecum and part of the transverse colon is via the superior mesenteric plexus which sends out both vagal and sympathetic nerve fibers to the colon. From a point in the distal transverse colon down to the rectum, the innervation is derived from the thoracolumbar outflow via the inferior mesenteric plexus. Some vagal fibers, however, are also derived from the celiac and aortic plexuses.

The sympathetic supply of the rectum is from the upper and lower divisions of the hypogastric nerves; the parasympathetic supply is derived from the sacral outflow of the cord contained in the pelvic nerves. The extrinsic supply functions as a modifier, controlling to some extent the intrinsic behavior of the bowel, which is more directly under the influence of local reflex activity mediated by the intramural nerve plexuses. For example, despite transection of the cord, colonic and rectal function continue because of the intrinsic innervation, and greater local activity of the rectum is noted.

The parasympathetic innervation is composed of fibers from the vagus nerve and from the nervi erigentes which arise from cells in the anterior horn of the second, third, and fourth sacral segments of the spinal cord (sacral outflow). The myelinated preganglionic fibers of the vagus ramify profusely at the level of the celiac plexus and intermingle indistinguishably with the pre- and postganglionic sympathetic fibers as they pass down through the preaortic plexuses. They then proceed to the colon, coursing through the mesentery in company with the colonic branches of the superior mesenteric artery. The nervi erigentes are a bundle of myelinated

nerves intermingled with sympathetic nerves of the hypogastric plexuses. The parasympathetic fibers of the sacral outflow enter the colon in its distal portion and may be found as high as the middle of the descending colon; some investigators have found them to proceed as far as the splenic flexure. The preponderant opinion, however, is that they reach as far proximally as a point in the distal transverse colon (Cannon's point). As noted, these fibers from the vagus and nervi erigentes are preganglionic myelinated fibers which synapse in ganglia of the submucosal plexuses of Meissner. This network of myenteric plexuses is the intrinsic innervation of the intestine which may function independent of external stimulation and connections. The levator ani, coccygeus, and external anal sphincter muscles are supplied by motor fibers from the fourth sacral segment of the spinal cord which emerges with the root of the pudendal nerve.

The afferent impulses which respond to stretch and spasm of the colonic musculature are mediated by autonomic afferent fibers which are sympathetic in origin. They pass from the bowel wall through the sympathetic ganglia (preaortic and prevertebral) to the white ramus and into the posterior root ganglion where their nerve cell is located, and thence into the dorsal horns and posterior columns of the spinal cord where they synapse. The anal epithelium, composed of skin as well as mucous membrane, has extremely sensitive receptors which are responsive to stimuli which produce itch as well as pain. These impulses, in contrast to those of the colonic wall, are carried by somatic afferent pathways.

SEGMENTAL CHARACTERISTICS OF THE COLON

The most proximal segment of the colon is the cecum. The terminal segment of ileum enters the cecum at its posterior medial aspect in a horizontal and often slightly downward-directed fashion. The distal aspect of the ileal lumen and the proximal aspect of the cecal lumen are defined by the ileocecal valve (Figs. 97–11 and 97–12). Its distal-most segment may

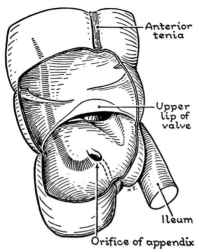

Figure 97–11. Diagram of ileocecal junction. (From Grant's Method of Anatomy. 7th ed. Baltimore, Williams and Wilkins Co., 1965.)

be fixed in part by fusion to the medial wall of the cecum and in part by Lane's membrane, which attaches its antimesenteric border to the parietal peritoneum in the right iliac fossa.

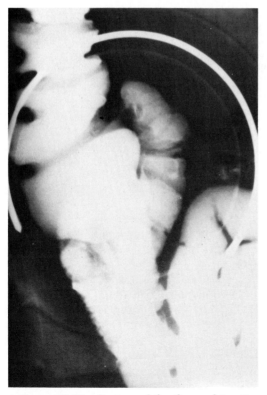

Figure 97–12. Contour of the ileocecal junction as seen on X-ray. Note the "bird beak" appearance.

ILEOCECAL VALVE

Recent studies indicate that the ileocecal valve behaves like a sphincter.[2] Anatomically, it is composed of an upper and lower lip; at their corners of fusion they taper to form transverse folds which are part of the cecal wall (Fig. 97–12). Functionally, the sphincter behaves to prevent reflux of material from the cecal lumen back into the distal ileum; however, if sufficient pressure is exerted, as, for example, during a barium enema X-ray examination, the material will reflux into the terminal ileum (Fig. 97–12). Although thickness of the musculature of the lips at the ileocecal orifice is not strikingly larger than the similar structure in the cecal wall itself, recent motility studies indicate that the ileocecal valve behaves like a sphincter, permitting the delivery of ileal content into the cecum in an intermittent, discontinuous, but orderly fashion.

Although the anatomy of the ileocecal valve is not exactly the same in all individuals, certain features are rather constant: the terminal ileum is directed horizontally and slightly downward; it forms a slot-like orifice in the cecum, the "lips" of which, however, do not contain a specially developed musculature; they are often thicker in children because of the presence of lymphoid tissue; the terminal few centimeters of ileum are usually fixed either by fusion to the cecal wall or by Lane's membrane to the posterior parietal peritoneum. The X-ray appearance of this structure is depicted in Figure 97–12.

THE CECUM

The cecum is the most proximal and widest segment of the colon, occupying the right iliac fossa by virtue of rotation of the intestine during a later embryonic stage. Occasionally it may be noted a bit more toward the midline, particularly in an individual whose colon is somewhat long and redundant. When intestinal rotation has been incomplete, the cecum may be found in the right upper quadrant and in extreme instances in the midline or in the left side of the abdominal cavity. This abnormality is clinically important because it is the basis for cecal volvulus (see pp. 1487 to 1489). Also, the cecum possesses no mesentery, because it is an out-pouching of the antimesenteric border of the gut and is "fixed" posteriorly in only a small percentage of individuals; therefore it has a certain degree of mobility and in extreme instances may actually become twisted, in part owing to excessive mobility. When fully matured, the cecum is somewhat eccentric in shape because of the greater growth of the lateral than the medial sacculation. The appendix is located along its medial aspect and can be located by tracing the convergence of the taeniae.

Attached to the cecum is the *vermiform appendix;* originally it is found at the apex of the cecum, but with full development it is attached to the medial aspect. It is located below the ileocecal junction, varies from a little over 2 cm to over 20 cm in length, and averages about 0.8 cm in diameter. It may be located behind the cecum (over 50 per cent of dissections); downward and to the right of the cecum; pointed over the brim of the pelvis; or anterior or posterior to the ileum (less than 1 per cent of dissections). The appendix is attached to the posterior parietal wall by a triangular fold of mesoappendix. Frequently, however, when the appendix is located behind the cecum, this fold is not present, and it adheres to the colon or to the posterior abdominal wall.

ASCENDING COLON

An approximately 20-cm segment distal to the cecum, between it and the lower pole of the right kidney, is known as the ascending colon. This is located below the undersurface of the right lobe of the liver, at which point it turns toward the midline and downward rather sharply, forming the hepatic flexure. It is usually fixed to the posterior peritoneum. Occasionally, the hepatic flexure containing gas may be interposed between the liver and the diaphragm, obscuring liver dullness on physical examination. Thus it is not a fixed segment of colon, although it is sometimes supported by a fold extending from the hepatorenal ligament. The ascending colon is active in the transport of fluid and electrolytes, and this particular function is discussed more fully on pages 229 and 296.

TRANSVERSE COLON

The transverse colon lies between the hepatic flexure and the splenic flexure, traversing the abdomen from right to left; it is quite mobile, often descending into the pelvis in the upright position. It is located anteriorly and is suspended by the transverse mesocolon which originates from the posterior peritoneum. This latter structure is a fold; its upper part is continuous posteriorly with the lesser peritoneal sac, and its lower portion forms a part of the wall of the greater omentum.

The splenic flexure marks the junction between the transverse and descending colon, and it is attached to the diaphragm at about the level of the tenth to eleventh ribs by phrenicocolic ligaments. At the flexure the colon is directed posteriorly so that the distal transverse colon lies in front of the proximal descending colon in the lateral view. The location and configuration plus fixation of the splenic flexure may be the basis for the discomfort noted in some patients with the irritable colon syndrome; a special entity known as the "splenic flexure syndrome" (see p. 1279) may be noted in an occasional patient in whom an inordinate amount of gas is trapped at this juncture.

DESCENDING COLON

The descending colon descends inferiorly between the psoas and quadratus lumborum muscles and is joined to the sigmoid colon at the pelvic brim; it is only partially peritonealized and usually has no mesentery. Although this segment of the colon is capable of absorbing water, electrolytes, and glucose, the degree of this function is small. Its main purposes are temporary storage and, presumably, mucous secretion to facilitate movement of fecal contents into the rectum to initiate the defecation reflex. The muscular function of the descending colon is extremely important in the pathogenesis of the irritable colon syndrome and of diverticula of the colon.

SIGMOID COLON

From the pelvic brim to the rectum, the upper border of which is at the peritoneal reflection, lies the sigmoid colon, a redundant loop of large bowel with the characteristic sigma shape. Its length varies considerably, the longer ones being coiled to variable degrees. In most individuals it has a mesentery, which explains much of its mobility and winding course. Because of its twists and curves, adjacent loops are superimposed on each other and anteroposterior projections and the loops can be seen separately only by special maneu-

vers in the lateral position. This approach is especially important in individuals suspected of having tumors in the "blind alleys" of the rectosigmoid curve as well as in more superior segments which are partly obscured by the turns of this portion of the colon as it courses superiorly to join the descending colon. The sharpest angulation is at the rectosigmoid junction, the point at which the bowel becomes peritonealized. This is approximately 15 to 18

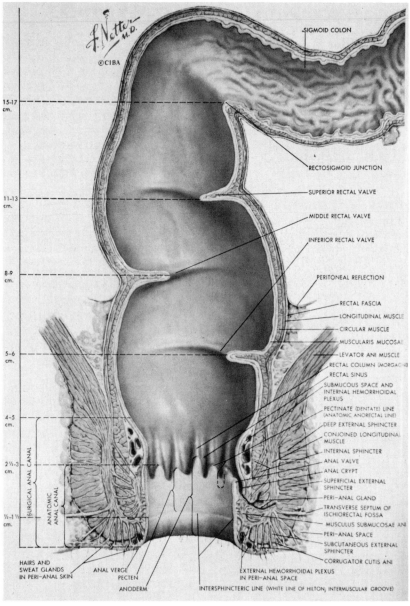

Figure 97–13. Sagittal section of rectum and anus. (From Netter, F.: Ciba Collection of Medical Illustrations, Volume 3, Section X.)

cm from the anus; thus a small portion of the distal sigmoid may be visualized through a sigmoidoscope.

RECTUM

From above downward the rectum begins at the termination of the pelvic mesocolon. At the rectosigmoid junction the mucosa changes in appearance, being smoother in the rectum. The rectum follows the curve of the sacrum and, although not fixed, does not have a great degree of mobility as noted during sigmoidoscopy; anteriorly, it may be impinged upon by the uterus or the cervix uteri in the female.

From below upward, the rectum rapidly becomes capacious and the enlarged fusiform-shaped segment is known as the ampulla; it begins a few centimeters beyond the pectinate line (see Fig. 97–13); its upper portion gradually merges into the segment which is the upper rectum, which, in turn, joins the sigmoid at the peritoneal reflection.

The rectal mucosa has the three valves of Houston, generally two on the left and one on the right. These are shelf-like folds, the most superior one being about 10 to 11 cm from the anus. A detailed anatomical description of the anus and of muscle support and sphincters of the rectum and anus will be found below and on page 242.

EXAMINATION OF THE RECTUM

Examination of the rectum is extremely important and is an integral part of every physical examination. It must be done with the greatest care, particularly in patients in whom one has reason to believe a tumor exists in the lower bowel, or in whom other evidence suggests the possibility of tumor with possible extension into the pelvis. The examining finger can detect much; for example, the tone of the sphincter (internal sphincter), the feel of the mucosa, and the presence or absence of strictures, mucosal tumors, or metastatic tumors impinging on the anterior wall of the rectum, including a ridge-like deformity known as Blumer's shelf. In the male, the prostate and retrovesical and retroprostatic spaces may be palpated as well as the seminal vesicles. In the female, anteriorly

one may feel the cervix of the uterus and posterior vaginal wall. Laterally, the examiner may palpate the ischiorectal space on each side, an important area for abscess formation.

THE ANAL CANAL

The terminal 3 cm of rectum is the anus or anal canal. The separation between rectum and anal canal is marked by longitudinal folds called the columns of Morgagni, which terminate in the anal papillae. These papillae may be quite accentuated in some individuals; they appear whitish and are sometimes sufficiently thickened to look polypoid. The distal two-thirds of the anal canal is extremely short and terminates at the mucocutaneous junction. At this point, the lining of the canal changes from columnar epithelium to stratified squamous epithelium identical with skin. The transition is not sudden but is a rather gradual blending, with an intermediary cuboidal type of epithelium frequently noted. Several plexuses of veins may be found in the anus — the internal hemorrhoidal plexus in the submucosal space at the level of the columns of Morgagni and the anal papillae, and the external hemorrhoidal plexus in the subcutaneous base near the anal verge (Fig. 97–13).

On page 242, a full description is given of the muscular pelvic diaphragm and its function with regard to the defecation reflex and the function of the sphincters. Components of the levator ani muscles—puborectalis, pubococcygeus, and ileococcygeus—make up this pelvic diaphragm which is joined in its posteriormost portion by the small coccygeus muscle. The fibers of the levator ani form a puborectal sling within which the lower rectum turns posteriorly. Contraction of the levator ani raises the pelvic diaphragm, the rectum, and the anus and narrows the anal-rectal angle, contributing to anal continence which is maintained principally by the contraction of the external sphincter (Fig. 97–14).

The internal sphincter of the anal canal is part of the smooth muscle of the rectum. It extends from the distal tip of the rectum to within 1 cm of the anal orifice. The external sphincter circumscribes the anal

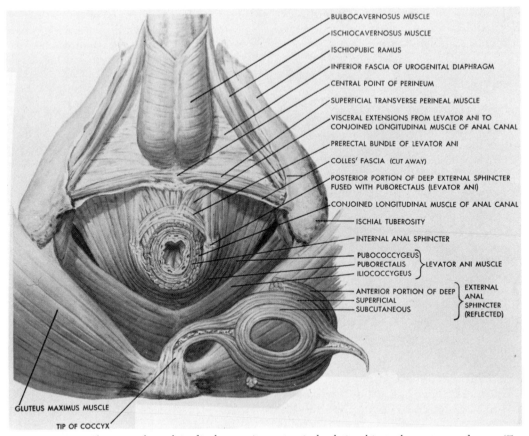

Figure 97–14. The muscular pelvic diaphragm; its anatomical relationship to the rectum and anus. (From Netter, F.: Ciba Collection of Medical Illustrations, Volume 3, Section X.)

canal and is separated from the internal sphincter by a thin layer of elastic fibers and longitudinal muscle which represents an extension of the outer longitudinal muscle coat of the rectum. Superiorly, its fibers blend with those of the levator ani muscle; it is attached posteriorly to the coccyx and anteriorly to the peritoneal body (Fig. 97–14). Distally, the external sphincter ends subcutaneously at the anal margin.

CELL RENEWAL IN THE COLON AND RECTUM

As in the stomach and small intestine, the colon has progenitor cells at the base of the crypts which give birth to other cells. A number of factors determine whether the daughter cells leave the base of the crypt and ascend toward the lumen. These include nutrition and state of function of the proximal intestine.

Proliferation of cells can be considered in terms of phases: M, cells in mitosis; S, cells during DNA synthesis; G_1, postmitotic presynthetic period; G_2, postsynthetic premitotic period; the cycle = $M + G_1 + S + G_2$. By appropriate labeling techniques, the times of each of the phases can be determined as well as number of cells passing a particular boundary in a particular direction per unit of time; finally proliferative rate or birth rate can be calculated (Fig. 97–15).

Microautoradiography of tritium-labeled thymidine identifies the phases of the proliferative cycle.[3, 4] Those cells which synthesize at the full rate, doubling the DNA content and then dividing, may be noted, as well as those which synthesize at a full rate without rapid cell division, and those that do not incorporate the precursor at all. Thus the fraction of mitoses labeled at various times may be calculated. Figure 97–16 demonstrates the technique of mi-

Figure 97–15. Fraction of mitoses labeled at various times between labeling and biopsy, in histologically normal colonic tissue of a 50-year-old male patient. Specimens obtained through a colostomy opening. An inoperable adenocarcinoma of the rectum was present distal to the colostomy site. Inset in upper right corner indicates phases of proliferative cell cycle. Cells become labeled during S phase, proceed through G_2 to mitosis (M), then to G_1 or G_0. After mitosis, cells may also leave the proliferative cycle, and undergo maturation. Vertical bars indicate the limits of a 95 per cent confidence interval. (From Lipkin, P.: *In* Handbook of Physiology, Sect. 6, Vol. V, C. F. Code and W. Heidel (eds.). Baltimore, Williams and Wilkins Co., 1968.)

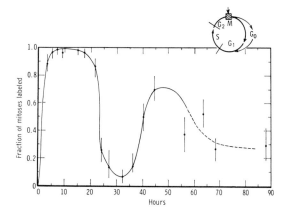

croautoradiography used. The cycle of proliferation is as follows: S phase (cells become labeled)—G_2, M, G_1, or G_0 (fertile cells not actually proliferating). Calculations have indicated that the S phase is about 20 hours, G_2 six hours, and G_1 about 14 hours, totaling 40 hours for the average duration of a cell cycle in the colon (Fig. 97–15).

In rectal tissue a diurnal inhibition in mitotic activity has been noted and may be related to the effect of epinephrine, glucocorticoid hormones, or heparin. Other influences on the cycle include infection,

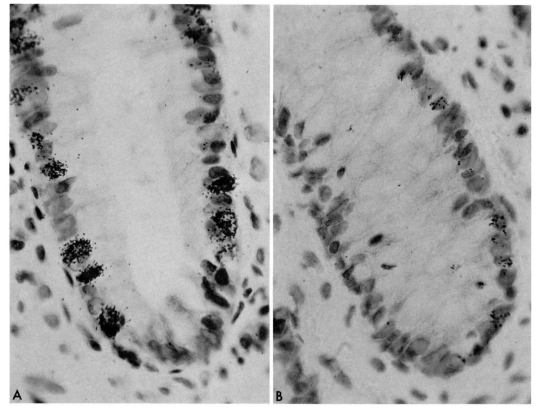

Figure 97–16. Microautoradiograph of the human colon crypt with newly labeled DNA in basal cells. *A*, Two hours, and *B*, eight days after injection of H³-thymidine. Hematoxylin and eosin stain. × 550. (From Lipkin, P.: *In* Handbook of Physiology, Sec. 6, Vol. V, C. F. Code and W. Heidel (eds.). Baltimore, Williams and Wilkins Co., 1968.)

partial small bowel resection, and hypophysectomy. As detailed on page 1407, radiation, of course, will also decrease the rate of cell proliferation.

Some cells in the crypts are labeled at one hour after injection of thymidine, and the time of migration from crypt to surface has been calculated to be about five to six days in the normal human rectum (Fig. 97–16). At 14 days, only a small number of well labeled crypt and surface cells remain. Curiously, although goblet cells are very prominent in the upper crypt regions, they are greatly outnumbered on the surface by columnar cells. A small number of goblet cells in the rectum are initially labeled, but it is difficult to be certain that the radioactive material is not in an adjacent columnar cell. Later, labeled goblet cells are found, indicating, but not proving, that these cells divide. Apparently cells are lost from the surface.

Thus the rectal mucosa is metabolically active, accounting for the ease of damage by noxious agents such as X-irradiation, antimetabolites, and infection, but also for its expediency of repair. The latter quality is notable, for example, in mild ulcerative colitis.

THE COLONIC PERICRYPTAL FIBROBLASTIC SHEATH

Recent detailed histological studies of colonic and rectal tissue in man in which both light and electron microscopy were employed indicate the presence of a so-called pericryptal fibroblast sheath.[5] Fibroblasts of this sheath separate, migrate, and differentiate in a special relationship to the overlying epithelium, indicating a well ordered system of epithelial mesenchymal interaction which is involved in maintaining the normal structure, renewal, and function of the colonic mucosa.[5]

This sheath is composed of specialized populations of fibroblasts which are self-renewing and which migrate from the germinative region at the lower third of the crypt to the collagen stratum beneath the epithelium at the surface of the colonic crypt. The sheath also contains collagen fibers, thus making it a distinct mesenchymal structure. The fibroblasts in the germinative region are undifferentiated, forming a sheath around the crypt. With migration to the upper third of the crypt they become single layered, become differentiated, and lay down collagen.

The exact functional significance of the anatomical relationship of the sheath to epithelium is not yet known. The pericryptal fibroblast sheath is fully differentiated and excessively developed when the mucosa is grossly hyperplastic; however, in adenomatous polyps the sheath cells are immature, showing continued fibroblast division at all levels, failure of morphological differentiation of fibroblasts, and the apparent inability of these cells to secrete their products, collagen and mucopolysaccharides. Their immaturity seems to parallel that of the adenomatous epithelium (see pp. 1432 to 1443).

REFERENCES

1. Blankenhorn, D. H., Hirsch, J., Ahrens, E. H., Jr. Transintestinal intubation; technique for measurement of gut length and physiologic sampling at known loci. Proc. Soc. Exp. Biol. Med. 88:356, 1955.
2. Cohen, S., Harris, L. D., and Levitan, R. Manometric characteristics of the human ileocecal junctional zone. Gastroenterology 54:72, 1968.
3. Lipkin, M. Cell proliferation of the gut. In Handbook of Physiology, Sect. 6, Vol. V, C. F. Code and W. Heidel (eds.), Baltimore, Williams and Wilkins Co., 1968.
4. MacDonald, W. C., Trier, J. S., and Everett, N. B. Cell proliferation and migration in the stomach, duodenum, and rectum in man: Radioautographic studies. Gastroenterology 46:405, 1964.
5. Kaye, G. I., Pascal, R. R., and Lane, N. The colonic pericryptal fibroblast sheath. Gastroenterology 60:515, 1971.

Chapter 98

Developmental Anomalies of the Colon and Rectum

Mervin Silverberg

INCIDENCE AND ETIOLOGY

Clinically, congenital anomalies of the colon consist principally of megacolon caused by aganglionosis and a group of anorectal anomalies. Congenital aganglionosis (Hirschsprung's disease) is discussed on pages 1463 to 1472.

INCIDENCE AND ETIOLOGY

Malformations of the anus and rectum are among the most common congenital abnormalities found in infants. They occur with a frequency ranging between 1:1500 and 1:5000 live births.[1] Embryologically, these anomalies result from arrests or abnormalities in the development of the fetal caudal region between the first and sixth months of intrauterine life. A family history is uncommon, and there is no racial predilection; however, a slight preponderance of affected males is reported.[2]

CLASSIFICATION

There are considerable confusion and lack of uniformity in the various published classifications.[3] Most are modifications of the anorectal malformation classification described by Ladd and Gross in 1934,[4] which still provides a clear basis for understanding the lesions. The recently introduced International Classification, although detailed, has gained wide acceptance.[3] Essentially, 90 per cent of cases are of the two major types, the *low* or translevator, and the *high* or supralevator (see Figs. 98–1 and 98–2 and Table 98–1). Anal agenesis and stenosis are considered *intermediate* types, whereas the rare imperforate anal membrane and cloacal exstrophy are relegated to a *miscellaneous* group. Fistula formation is mainly associated with the high and low lesions and involves the urethra, bladder, vagina, or perineum. Most fistulas in females communicate with the perineum or vagina, and rarely with the urinary tract. In contrast, three-fourths of the fistulas in males communicate with the urinary tract. These "fistulas" actually represent ectopic openings of the distal bowel, which develop with a migration arrest of the normal orifice. The high rectal atresia is considered by some investigators to result from gestational vascular ischemia.[5]

As a rule, those infants in whom the terminal portion of the colon passes through the puborectalis muscle sling of the levator ani (translevator) demonstrate less morbidity and fewer associated anomalies and have a much better prognosis than those in whom the colonic tip ends proximally (supralevator). Abnormalities of the lumbosacral spine, such as sacral agenesis, hemiagenesis, or errors in lumbar segmen-

FISTULAS IN MALE

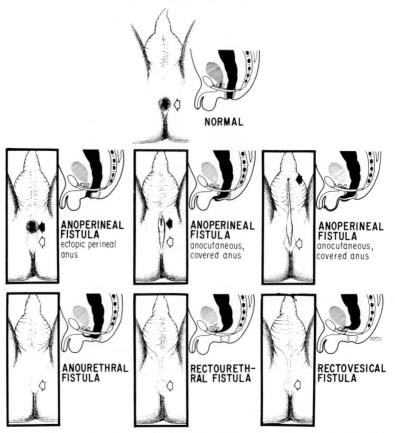

Figure 98–1.   Anorectal anomalies in the male with fistula formation. Note relationship of the rectum to the puborectalis sling of the levator ani muscle. Anoperineal fistulas may be located anywhere between the perineoscrotal junction and the anal dimple. In the ectopic perineal anus, the opening resembles a normal anus. In the anocutaneous fistula or covered anus, the orifice is usually small and is anterior to a thickened median band. Anourethral fistulas are rare and open into the bulbar or membranous urethra. The common rectourethral and the rare rectovesical fistulas represent high anomalies in which the bowel has not traversed the sling. (From Santulli, T. V., et al., J. Pediat. Surg. 5:28, 1970.)

tation, occur in 50 per cent of the high lesions. Seventy per cent of the patients with vertebral abnormalities additionally demonstrate urological anomalies, particularly hydronephrosis or a double collecting system.

At least one-third of patients with any type of anorectal anomaly have developmental malformations involving areas other than the vertebral column and urinary tract.[6] The most significant of these are congenital heart disease and esophageal atresia. Less commonly we may find small and large intestinal atresias, annular pancreas, intestinal malrotation and duplication, bicornuate uterus, vaginal atresia, septate vagina, absence of the rectus ab-dominis muscle, Down's syndrome, anomalies of the fingers and hands, omphalocele, and exstrophy of the bladder and ileocecal area of the intestine.

DIAGNOSIS

A careful perineal inspection of the infant with problems of micturition or defecation or unusual external perineal structures will often reveal the anomaly. Anorectal stenoses and anal membranes have orifices in normal locations and can be diagnosed by digital examination. In the supralevator anomalies, the normal ori-

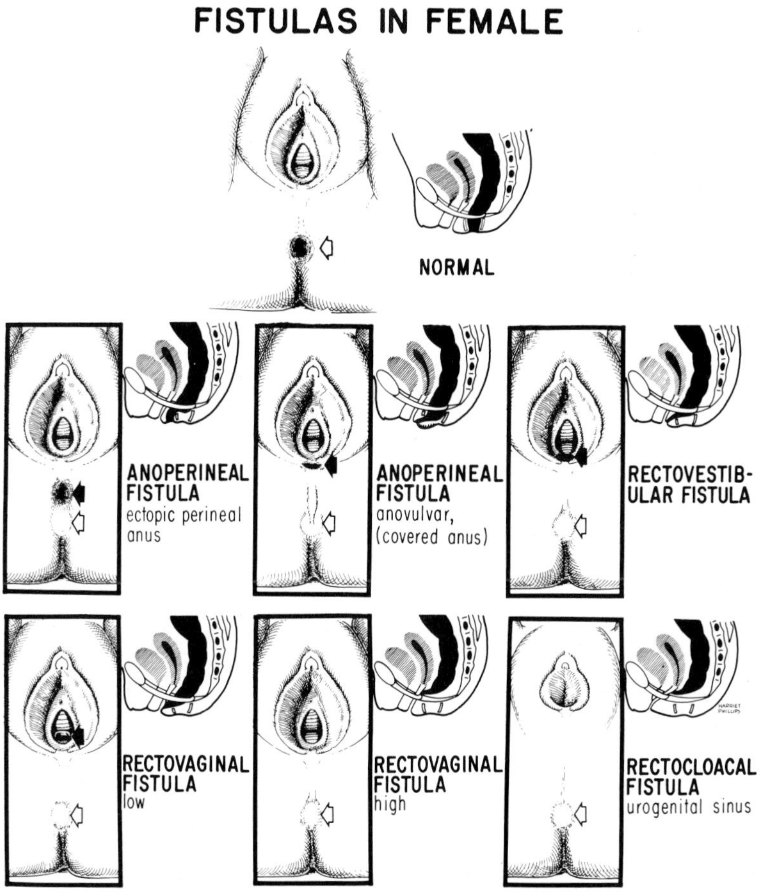

FISTULAS IN FEMALE

Figure 98–2.   Anorectal anomalies in the female with anoperineal fistulas, which may be either an ectopic perineal anus, or an anovulvar fistula, which is in the fourchette. The rectovestibular fistula lies within the vestibule of the vagina and courses cephalad, paralleling the posterior vaginal wall. The anovulvar fistula is directed posteriorly, and is relatively superficial to the skin. Rectovaginal fistulas are usually low, but may be located high in the posterior vaginal wall. The rectocloacal fistula occurs as a high communication in a urogenital sinus. The bowel traverses the sling in all but the last two malformations. (From Santulli, T. V., et al.: J. Pediat. Surg. 5:281, 1970.)

fice, although imperforated, can usually be detected as a pigmented depression (anal dimple) or elevation of thickened skin. Puckering may be noted at this site when the sphincter is stimulated to contract. Occasionally the ectopic perineal anus may be adequate for stool evacuation, and the definitive anomaly may be overlooked for many months or years.

Roentgenographic studies to outline the distal intestinal pouch are adequately achieved by cinefluoroscopy or radiocontrast studies. Adding indigo carmine as a marker will demonstrate rectourinary communications. The traditional plain film with the baby held in an upside down position is now known to be inaccurate in many cases.[7]

TREATMENT

Anal stenosis is easily treated with daily dilatations, using bougies or a finger. The parents should subsequently be taught the procedure in order to continue treatment for a total period of three to six months. The thin, bulging anorectal membrane is easily excised or incised with subsequent dilatations as in anal stenosis.

In lower lesions with fistulous formation, the orifice may be enlarged by a simple "cutback" procedure in the newborn period and continence is invariably uncompromised. A daily digital dilatation program is necessary during follow-up.

In high lesions a more extensive surgical procedure is indicated. A preliminary di-

**TABLE 98–1.   ANORECTAL ANOMALIES:
A SUGGESTED INTERNATIONAL CLASSIFICATION***

MALE	FEMALE
A. Low (translevator)	
1. At normal anal site	1. Same
a. Anal stenosis	a. Same
b. Covered anus — complete	b. Same
2. At perineal site	2. Same
a. Anocutaneous fistula (covered anus — incomplete)	a. Same
b. Anterior perineal anus	b. Same
	3. At vulvar site
	a. Anovulvar fistula
	b. Anovestibular fistula
	c. Vestibular anus
B. Intermediate	
1. Anal agenesis	1. Same
a. Without fistula	a. Without fistula
b. With fistula	b. With fistula
Rectobulbar	(1) Rectovestibular
	(2) Rectovaginal — low
2. Anorectal stenosis	2. Same
C. High (supralevator)	
1. Anorectal agenesis	1. Same
a. Without fistula	a. Without fistula
b. With fistula	b. With fistula
(1) Rectourethral	(1) Rectovaginal — high
(2) Rectovesical	(2) Rectocloacal
	(3) Rectovesical
2. Rectal atresia	2. Same
D. Miscellaneous	
Imperforate anal membrane	
Cloacal exstrophy	
Others	

*From Santulli, T. V., et al.: J. Pediat. Surg. 5:281, 1970.

vided sigmoid colostomy is recommended to decompress the bowel, followed by an appropriate abdominoperineal operation at about one year of age. In selected cases, the colostomy may be avoided and dilatation or cutback of the fistula may suffice as a temporizing measure. For the rectal atresias, a preliminary sigmoid colostomy in the newborn is performed. This is followed at one year of age by a pull-through procedure similar to that utilized in patients with aganglionic megacolon.

Patients of all types are followed closely for many years, because they are more vulnerable to impactions, strictures, rectal inertia, and anal incontinence. In addition, a cryptic fistulous tract, missed at first, may be detected at a later date.

In general, the best surgical results are achieved with lower anomalies and the poorest prognosis with high lesions associated with severe sacral agenesis.

REFERENCES

1. Santulli, T. V.   Malformations of the anus and rectum. *In* Pediatric Surgery, 2nd Ed., W. T. Mustard, et al. (eds.). Chicago, Year Book Medical Publishers, 1969, pp. 983–1007.
2. Weinstein, E. D.   Sex-linked imperforate anus. Pediatrics 35:715, 1965.
3. Santulli, T. V., Kiesewetter, W. B., and Bill, Jr., A. H.   Anorectal anomalies: A suggested international classification. J. Pediat. Surg. 5:281, 1970.
4. Ladd, W. E., and Gross, R. E.   Congenital malformations of the anus and rectum: Report of 162 cases. Amer. J. Surg. 23:167, 1934.
5. Santulli, T. V., and Blanc, W. A.   Congenital atresia of the intestine: Pathogenesis and treatment. Ann. Surg. 154:939, 1961.
6. Moore, T. C., and Lawrence, E. A.   Congenital malformation of the rectum and anus: 11 associated anomalies encountered in a series of 120 cases. Surg. Gynec. Obstet. 95:281, 1952.
7. Berdon, W. E., and Baker, D. H.   The inherent errors in measurements of inverted films in patients with imperforate anus. Ann. Radiol. 10:235, 1967.

Chapter 99

Roentgenographic Methods of Colonic Examination

Henry I. Goldberg, Albert A. Moss

THE USE AND INTERPRETATION OF PLAIN ABDOMINAL ROENTGENOGRAMS IN EXAMINATION OF THE COLON

The roentgenographic study of the colon begins with supine and erect plain films of the abdomen. The demonstration of air, fluid, and fecal material present in the colon provides valuable information about the size, location, and status of the colon.

The colon ordinarily contains an average of 100 ml of gas,[1] although this amount varies with colonic content and extent of air swallowing. In the supine position air rises into the transverse colon, thereby outlining the width and contour of that structure. Normally, gas is noted in a pattern of saclike outpouchings or haustra, representing the normal bulge of colonic wall between longitudinal muscle bands, or taeniae. When the nondistended colon shows loss of the haustral pattern on plain roentgenograms, inflammatory disease must be suspected (Fig. 99–1). In chronic ulcerative colitis, for example, air reveals the wall of the transverse colon to be stiff, and haustra are not seen.[2]

Abdominal films obtained on normal patients in an erect position ordinarily do not demonstrate colonic air-fluid levels, and colonic dilatation may be seen (Fig. 99–2). Colonic air-fluid levels may also be seen in patients with acute diarrheal states and those with paralytic ileus complicated by peritonitis. Although adhesions, post-inflammatory stenosis, and colonic or pericolonic abscess may all cause left colonic obstruction, any patient over age 40 with abdominal distention and plain abdomen films showing colonic dilatation with air-fluid levels should be considered to have a left colonic neoplasm until

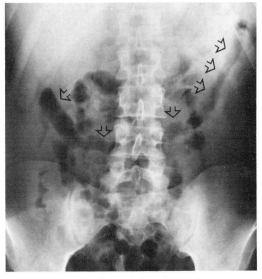

Figure 99–1. The plain abdominal roentgenogram in this patient with chronic ulcerative colitis demonstrates air in a thin, tubular, narrowed transverse colon (arrows).

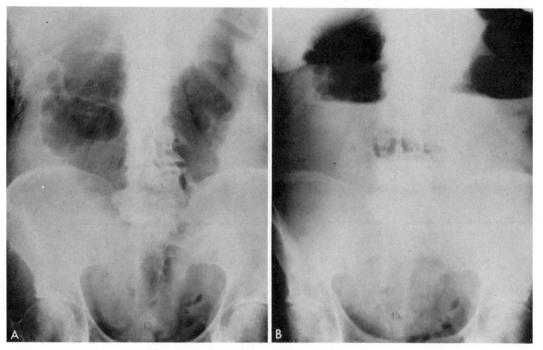

Figure 99–2. Supine (*A*) and erect (*B*) abdominal roentgenograms demonstrate an enlarged gas-filled transverse colon containing air-fluid levels. This megacolon was caused by an obstructing sigmoid carcinoma.

proved otherwise. In one series, 40 per cent of carcinomas of the left colon presented as acute colonic obstruction.[3] It is necessary to perform a barium enema in such patients to confirm a diagnosis of mechanical obstruction.

Simple colonic dilatation without air-fluid levels may result from many different local or systemic disease processes which may cause a paralytic or reflex ileus. Colonic dilatation, or megacolon, has been defined as transverse colonic width of greater than 5.5 cm on the supine abdominal film at standard tube-film distance (36 to 40 inches in United States).[4, 5] However, the presence of a megacolon is a nonspecific roentgenographic finding. It may be a manifestation of serum electrolyte abnormalities, endocrine disorders (Fig. 99–3), vascular insufficiency, drug ingestion, collagen disease, abnormal bowel habits, inflammatory bowel disease, or simply reflex dilatation caused by some form of systemic trauma. If the contour of the dilated colon is nodular, such diseases as ulcerative colitis or colonic ischemia are suggested. In most cases, however, the

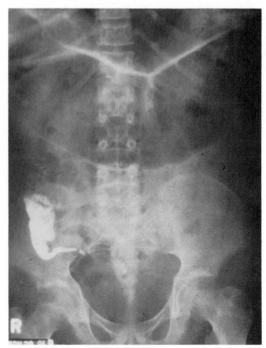

Figure 99–3. The supine abdomen film of this patient with myxedema demonstrates a megacolon. The barium present in the appendix and cecum is residual material from a prior barium enema.

finding of a dilated colon with a smooth internal contour does not suggest a specific cause (see pp. 1463 to 1480).

The plain abdominal roentgenogram also provides information about the nature of extraluminal gas or air. Air in the wall of the colon appears either as lucent streaks parallel to the lumen or as bubbles indenting the lumen. The finding of air in the bowel wall, or pneumatosis cystoides intestinalis, may represent a benign, spontaneously occurring condition, or one associated with lung or collagen disease.[6] The presence of pneumatosis cystoides intestinalis should, however, alert the radiologist to the possibility of underlying bowel necrosis caused by inflammation or ischemia[7] (see pp. 1514 to 1519).

The presence of pericolonic abscess resulting from diverticulitis, tumor, Crohn's disease, or other inflammatory conditions may be determined on a plain abdominal film by the demonstration of a mass in the flank area which displaces colon away from the properitoneal fat line. The area of

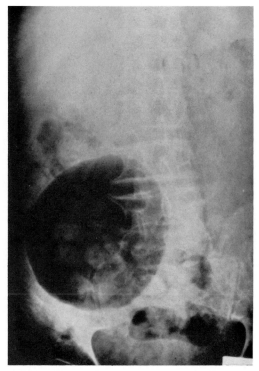

Figure 99–5. The large cystic lucency in the right lower quadrant is a giant sigmoid diverticulum or gas cyst. Fecal material can be seen within this cyst.

the abscess often appears as a conglomerate of mottled lucencies in a mass, representing gas mixed with inflammatory tissue (Fig. 99–4). When the pericolonic abscess abuts upon the peritoneal surfaces, it induces an inflammatory cellular infiltrate which invades the properitoneal fat, thereby locally obliterating the lucent properitoneal stripe, or fat line.

Large, cystic collections of gas adjacent to the sigmoid colon have been noted on plain films of the abdomen. These represent giant gas cysts or diverticula, many centimeters in diameter (Fig. 99–5). These true diverticula are found most frequently in the aged or in those patients with many colonic diverticula.[8]

The plain abdominal roentgenogram may also detect calcifications of colonic origin. Round or oval laminated calcifications in the right lower quadrant may be due to appendicoliths. In a patient with fever, leukocytosis, and abdominal pain, the roentgenographic demonstration of an appendicolith is highly suggestive of acute appendicitis. Larger, crescent-shaped or

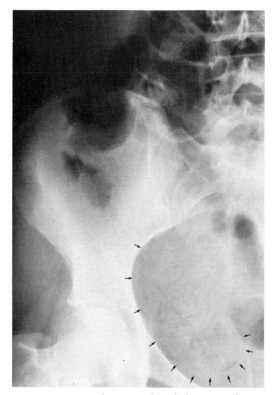

Figure 99–4. This appendiceal abscess is characterized by mottled lucencies forming a mass in the right side of the pelvis (arrows). Cecum and terminal ileum are distended with air above the abscess.

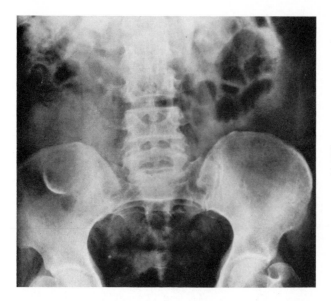

Figure 99–6. A partially calcified muco-cele of the appendix is present in the right lower quadrant. The crescent-like calcification is characteristic of this lesion.

circular calcifications in the right lower quadrant may be produced by a calcified mucocele of the appendix (Fig. 99–6). Occasionally, the fatty excrescences along the taenia of the colon—appendices epiploicae—may infarct and calcify. These produce cyst-like calcific densities adjacent to the air-filled colon, usually the ascending colon. Calcified enteroliths provide roentgenographic evidence of impacted feces, either in the lumen of the colon or in colonic diverticula. Rectal stones, calcified enteroliths in the rectum, may produce fecal impaction. Calcified seeds and pits may also be demonstrated (Fig. 99–7). Mucinous adenocarcinoma of the colon occasionally produces fine, punctate calcification within the tumor or its metastases, which may be demonstrated on the plain abdominal roentgenogram (Fig. 99–8).

Extracolonic masses which displace or indent the colon may occasionally be detected on the plain abdominal roentgenogram. Pelvic masses, such as ovarian cysts or pelvic abscesses, elevate the air-filled

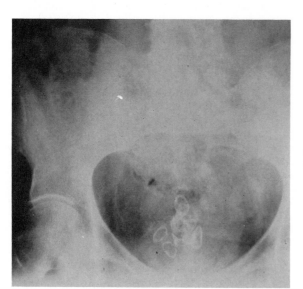

Figure 99–7. Calcified prune pits in the rectum of a 60-year-old female with a congenital rectal stricture.

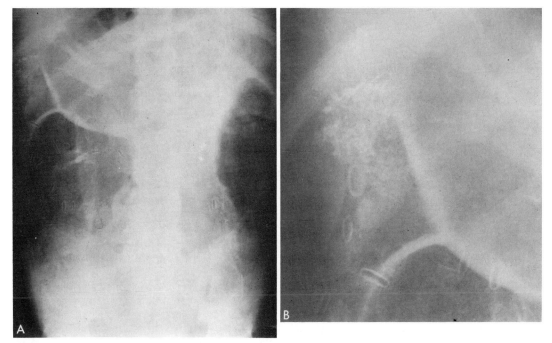

Figure 99–8. *A,* Massive dilatation of small bowel and ascending colon. The extremely large loop of bowel located transversely in the midabdomen was found to be jejunum. Note the multiple disc-like calcifications, caused by inspissated, calcified watermelon seeds. *B,* Close-up of right upper quadrant, demonstrating stippled, punctate calcification in a mucinous adenocarcinoma. This tumor had obstructed the ascending colon.

sigmoid colon. Fluid and infiltrate in the pericolic gutters may displace air-filled cecum and left colon medially. The hepatic and splenic flexures of the colon may be depressed by hepatosplenomegaly. Conversely, the hepatic flexure of the colon may be interposed between liver and diaphragm—a congenital anomaly which may be confused with subdiaphragmatic air or abscess.

BARIUM ENEMA

COLONIC CLEANSING IN PREPARATION FOR BARIUM ENEMA

The usefulness of the barium enema as a diagnostic tool for detecting colonic disease is related to the degree of colonic cleansing obtained prior to the roentgenographic study. Residual colonic fecal material caused by inadequate patient preparation interferes with a complete roentgenographic evaluation of colonic contour and mucosal pattern. The physician requesting a barium enema for a pa-

tient must be familiar with the type of colonic cleansing recommended by the radiologist and must tell the patient of its importance.

A variety of diets, laxatives, and preparatory enemas are used for colon cleansing.[9] Most teaching hospitals recommend a clear liquid or low residue diet 24 to 72 hours before a barium enema.[9] Patients should drink at least six 8-oz glasses of water on the day before the examination to assure that they are adequately hydrated. Many different laxatives, enemas, and combinations of both have been championed by radiologists.[9-11] The regimen most commonly used for preparing patients for a barium enema is castor oil, 2 oz given orally the afternoon prior to the day of the examination, followed by a water enema in the evening or early the next morning.[9] Recently, a new technique for colonic cleansing, the hydration technique, has been tested.[9, 12] This regimen includes a liquid diet on the day before the barium enema examination, including multiple glasses of water, 10 to 12 oz of magnesium citrate laxative, and four bisacodyl tablets in the evening, followed by a bisacodyl suppository on the morning of the examination. Enemas are not used with this cleansing technique. At present there appears to be no difference between all these methods in the rate of successful preparation.[11] The adequacy of colonic cleansing depends upon the diligence of the patient or the hospital nursing staff in fulfilling their instructions. (Unpublished data, Subcommittee on Colon Preparation, American College of Radiology Committee on Cancer Detection, 1969.)

Perhaps the most successful method of colon cleansing is one in which the cleansing is performed by the radiologist—the Malmo technique.[13] Patients are placed on liquid diets two days prior to the examination, given 2 oz of castor oil the evening before, and given preparatory water enemas containing 1 per cent tannic acid in the radiology department on the day of the examination. Tannic acid is not only a colonic irritant but also a mucolytic agent. Although colonic cleansing is probably best with the Malmo technique, most radiology departments do not have the space or personnel to administer preparatory enemas.

COLONIC CLEANSING IN PATIENTS WITH COLITIS AND OBSTRUCTION

Patients with bloody diarrhea, tachycardia, profound weakness as a result of severe ulcerative colitis, or other forms of colitis probably should not be subjected to a barium enema during this phase of their disease. Only if information on the distribution of the colitis and the severity of ulceration is crucial to the immediate man-

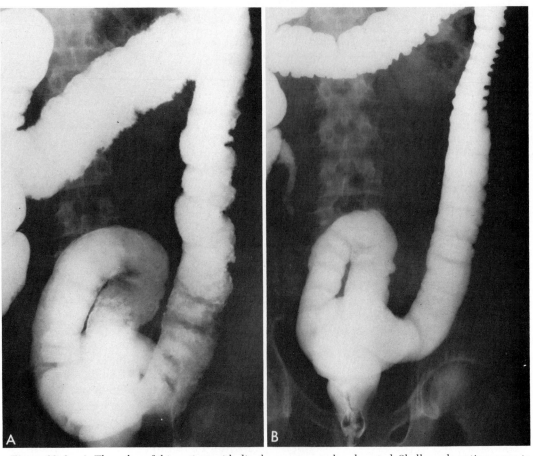

Figure 99–9. *A*, The colon of this patient with diarrhea appears to be ulcerated. Shallow ulcerations seen to the entire left and transverse colon. The patient had received no colon cleansing prior to the barium enema. *B*, The barium enema, repeated one week later, after the patient had been given tap water cleansing enemas, demonstrates a normal colon.

agement of the patient should a barium enema be performed in these extremely ill patients. Colonic cleansing is not a necessity in studying these patients, and laxatives should be avoided; however, patients whose colitis is not very active and who require a barium enema examination should be given a liquid diet for 24 to 48 hours before the examination and given gentle tap water enemas to remove stool, mucus, and food fibers just prior to the procedure. Laxatives should not be used. It is important that the colon be cleansed prior to roentgenographic examination, because an adequate barium-mucosal interface is necessary to accurately outline the mucosal contour of the colon. Fine ulcerations and small pseudopolyps may be obscured or even mimicked by mucus and stool, rendering evaluation of the extent and severity of colitis inadequate (Fig. 99–9).

Patients whose clinical picture and plain abdominal film indicate small or large bowel obstruction or diverticulitis need not undergo colonic cleansing or preliminary dietary restrictions prior to a barium enema examination.

THE TECHNIQUE OF BARIUM ENEMA EXAMINATIONS

Relationship of Barium Enema to Proctoscopy and Rectal Biopsy. It is not desirable to perform a barium enema immediately after proctoscopy, because (1) rectal spasm resulting from proctoscopy may result in difficulty in filling the colon and early evacuation of barium; (2) mucus secretion is often increased; (3) large amounts of air may be introduced into the colon, producing air-locks and causing inadequate distribution of barium; and (4) barium may extravasate intra- or extraperitoneally during a barium enema if a traumatic sigmoidoscopic examination had produced a small rent in the colonic wall.[14] The barium enema should be performed before or one day after proctoscopy.[9, 10]

The time interval between rectal biopsy and barium enema is controversial. In a recent study of 79 radiology departments, 56 delayed performing the barium enema for at least 48 hours after a rectal biopsy was performed, and 48 waited at least one week.[9] Perforations have been reported in patients having had a rectal biopsy within one day of the barium enema examination.[14] On the other hand, 23 of the 79 institutions surveyed reported that barium enemas are performed within one day of rectal biopsy.[9] The hydrostatic pressure developed by the instillation of barium in the rectum is normally well below that required to rupture the colon.[14] However, a rectal biopsy through an area of diseased bowel (carcinoma, colitis), or a deep biopsy of a nondiseased rectum may make a rupture at the biopsy site more likely when the rectum is distended by barium. In addition, the inflation of a balloon catheter in the rectum to prevent barium leakage may inadvertently rupture the colonic wall at the biopsy site. It is important therefore that a barium enema not be performed immediately after biopsy of a diseased rectum. A two- to four-week delay between biopsy and barium enema is necessary if granulation and healing of the biopsy are required. Such delay, however, is often impractical, especially because information is more immediately required for the patient's management. A reasonable approach to this problem is to delay the barium enema for at least 48 hours, during which time the patient is likely to have one or two bowel movements, which may indicate perforation because of attendant pain or recurrent bleeding. Also, clinical evidence of perforation, such as fever, lower abdominal pain, and leukocytosis, is likely to become manifest. Administration of laxatives and enemas in preparation for the barium enema may also unmask underlying perforation.

If barium enema must be performed after the 48-hour delay, it should be done without the use of a firm enema tip or balloon catheter and with extreme caution. The barium container should be raised only 2 to 3 feet above the table top, barium flow rigorously controlled to prevent rapid colonic distention and resultant rectal spasm, and the patient positioned to move barium suspensions into the right colon. Adequate roentgenographic information about the colon may be gained in spite of these precautions. If at all possible, the barium enema should be performed *before* rectal biopsy, or one or two weeks after.

Shallow biopsy of rectal valves and of normal-appearing mucosa or biopsies of polyps do not carry the same risk of complication as biopsy of a diseased rectal wall.[1] Although care must be exercised in examining such patients, the time interval between biopsy and barium enema is less critical and may be selected according to the type and site of biopsy. But unless the radiologist is clearly informed of the exact nature of the biopsy, he must consider all biopsies as potential sites of perforation and counsel delay in the examination.

Technical Considerations. Although many barium sulfate mixtures are available for barium enema radiography, a satisfactory mixture should (1) contain a suspending agent such as carboxymethylcellulose to aid in keeping barium sulfate particles (4 to 20 μ) in suspension; (2) flow through enema tubing easily, without requiring pressure to push it through; and (3) have a viscosity and adhesiveness sufficient to produce good coating of the colonic mucosa. If these properties are present, even dispersal of barium sulfate particles in the lumen and along the colonic mucosa will be obtained, providing high quality roentgenograms of the filled and collapsed colon.[15]

The optimal radiographic technique utilizes high kilovoltage exposures (120 kv) and low density barium sulfate (usually 12 to 15 per cent weight per volume mixture). By means of this technique, the colonic contour is adequately outlined, but the column of barium is translucent enough to permit evaluation of intraluminal masses or overlying loops of barium-filled bowel (Fig. 99–10).

The fluoroscopic examination of the colon varies with the individual radiologist. Some perform only a cursory inspection of the flow of barium through the colon to the cecum, whereas others obtain multiple compression spot films of every segment of colon. The more careful and thorough the fluoroscopic examination, the greater the likelihood of demonstrating colonic abnormalities. In order for a fluoroscopic examination to be considered adequate, all areas of colon redundancy (sigmoid, splenic flexure, hepatic flexure) should be radiographed by proper positioning of the patient. Pressure spot films of the cecal tip and ileocecal valve should be obtained. The observation that barium refluxed into the terminal ileum not only provides an opportunity for radiographing the terminal ileum, but also provides evi-

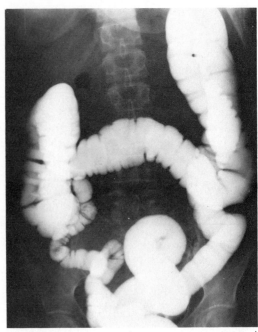

Figure 99–10. The use of high kilovoltage (120 kv) in obtaining roentgenograms of the barium-filled colon permits interpretation of overlying loops of bowel, because high kilovolt exposures result in better X-ray penetration of the barium column. In this roentgenogram of a normal colon, the barium sulfate suspension is of low enough density (15 per cent weight per volume) and the kv high enough to allow appreciation of contour and contents of overlapping loops of sigmoid and transverse colon.

dence of filling of the colon at least to the level of the ileocecal valve. Filling of the appendix with barium is further evidence of complete cecal filling.

After the colon has been filled with barium under fluoroscopic observation, the patient should be placed in the supine, prone, and left posterior oblique positions, and standard overhead-tube radiographs obtained. In addition, many radiologists obtain a lateral view of the rectum in order to monitor the contour of the posterior wall of the rectum, and evaluate the presacral space.[9] In instances when the sigmoid colon is so redundant that all loops cannot be roentgenographed in standard positions, a roentgenogram of the rectum with the tube angled 35 degrees toward the feet while the patient is prone will uncoil redundant loops (Fig. 99–11).

The final roentgenogram of the barium enema examination should be obtained after the patient has evacuated the enema. The postevacuation roentgenogram pro-

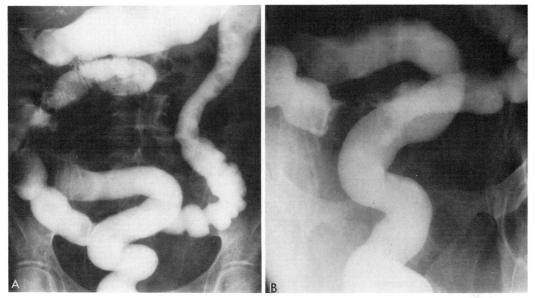

Figure 99–11. *A*, The barium-filled rectosigmoid obscures a carcinoma of the sigmoid on this routine anteroposterior roentgenogram of the barium filled colon. *B*, An angled view of the rectum (patient is prone, with X-ray tube angled 35 degrees caudally) discloses the underlying constricting adenocarcinoma of the sigmoid.

vides information about mucosal pattern and collapsability of the colon. Shallow mucosal ulcerations, particularly long linear ulcers, may be seen best on the postevacuation film; it is also best for detecting edema of the colon. The normal postevacuation mucosal pattern is fine and feathery in nature, with folds usually only a few millimeters wide (Fig. 99–12, *A*). When edema is present, the mucosal pattern is much coarser, the folds wider, and the colon less collapsable (Fig. 99–12, *B*).

Drugs and Additives. Tannic acid has, until recently, been used extensively as an additive to preparatory cleansing enemas and barium enemas.[10, 13] It is a mucolytic agent, as well as a topical astringent which stimulates colonic muscle contraction and evacuation. When added to preparatory water enemas, tannic acid induces thorough evacuation, providing a colon free of fecal material. Its addition to the barium sulfate mixture results in improved mucosal coating and more complete evacuation of barium so that the postevacuation mucosal coating is of excellent quality.[16]

The first reports of the hepatotoxicity of tannic acid administered to patients in a barium enema mixture were in patients who died, presumably as a result of tannic acid absorption.[17, 18] Centrilobular hepatic

necrosis was noted in these patients. The drug was subsequently withdrawn from use until studies on the safety and efficacy of tannic acid enemas could be performed.[19] As of 1972, tannic acid in concentrations of 0.25 to 0.50 per cent may be used as a tannic acid–bisacodyl additive to promote colonic contraction and mucosal coating. At these dose levels, no experimental or clinical toxicity has been shown.[19, 20] However, repeated enemas containing tannic acid and retention of enemas for periods up to one hour are to be avoided. The use of tannic acid in enemas should be avoided in the study of patients with hepatic parenchymal disease and ulcerative colitis because of the increased likelihood of colonic absorption and hepatic damage.

Anticholinergic drugs such as atropine and propantheline bromide have frequently been used as an adjunct to the barium enema to decrease secretions and to produce colonic dilatation and hypotonia during the examination.[9] Atropine in oral doses of 0.25 to 1.0 mg has been used extensively to facilitate high quality roentgenograms of air-barium double-contrast enemas (the Malmo technique.)[13] Although the quality is enhanced by hypotonia, evacuation of barium is often

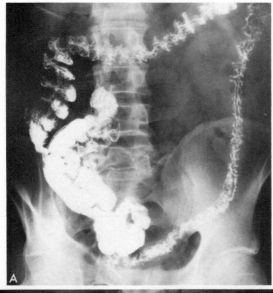

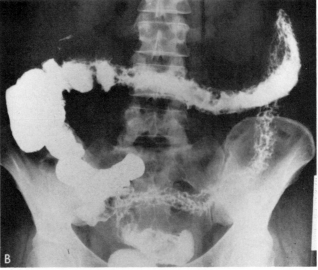

Figure 99–12. *A,* The postevacuation roentgenogram best demonstrates the mucosal folds. Normally, these mucosal folds form the delicate, feathery pattern shown above. *B,* The mucosal pattern in this patient with active ulcerative colitis is coarse and thickened—evidence of mucosal edema. Occasionally the postevacuation mucosal pattern may be the only roentgenographic evidence of inflammation.

inadequate to provide a good postevacuation roentgenogram of the collapsed, emptied colon.

Propantheline bromide (Pro-Banthine), administered intramuscularly or intravenously, may be used to produce colonic relaxation during a barium enema examination. In doses of 15 mg or less it acts as an anticholinergic agent, but at levels of 30 mg or greater it is also a ganglionic blocking agent, relaxing sphincters.[21]

Propantheline is helpful in the differen-

tial diagnosis of colonic lesions detected on barium enema in several instances.[21, 22] If spasm causes complete block to the retrograde flow of barium, parenterally administered Pro-Banthine will relieve the spasm and permit continuation of the study. Failure to reverse a colonic block by means of Pro-Banthine injection is generally considered to be evidence of an organic constricting or space-occupying lesion.[21] The same observation holds for differentiating narrowing of stricture from

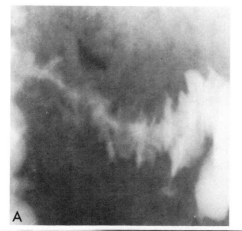

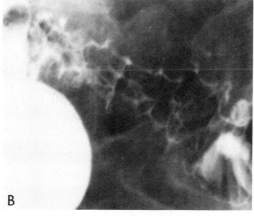

Figure 99–13. *A*, Acute sigmoid diverticulitis produced the appearance of luminal irregularity and narrowing on the spot film of the sigmoid colon. *B*, The caliber and contour of the lumen changed considerably after the administration of 30 mg of propantheline intramuscularly. The reversal of colonic spasm permitted a more accurate roentgenographic appraisal of the inflammatory changes in the sigmoid. (From Margulis, A. R., and Goldberg, H. I.: Radiol. Clin. N. Amer. 7:27, 1969.)

spasm. Segmental colonic inflammation, as in idiopathic ulcerative colitis, granulomatous colitis, and diverticulitis, causes spasm. Propantheline injection may distinguish colonic narrowing caused by diverticulitis from carcinoma roentgenographically, either by abolishing it or by providing a clearer picture of the relationship of the narrowing to diverticulitis (Fig. 99–13). In patients with ulcerative colitis, Pro-Banthine injection has aided in better roentgenographic delineation of narrowed segments and aids in differentiating spasm from stricture or cancer.[21,22] It should not be given, however, to patients with clinically active disease, particularly

if the colon is universally involved, because of the possibility of inducing a megacolon.

Air-Barium Double-Contrast Enemas. The air-barium double-contrast enema may be indicated in a variety of situations, either as an adjunct to a standard barium enema or as the initial roentgenographic study of the colon. Although the standard barium enema provides a roentgenographic outline of the colonic contour in profile, both profile and en face views of the barium-coated, air-distended colonic mucosa can be obtained by using the double-contrast technique. The contour of small mucosal lesions such as adenomatous polyps, particularly those under 5 mm in diameter, is best outlined by the double-contrast enema (Fig. 99–14). In addition, longitudinal shallow ulcers are best demonstrated en face by the double-contrast technique, with barium coating the ulcer trough, and air distention allowing an unobstructed en face view of the extent of the ulcer. The use of the double-contrast technique has increased in the past decade in the United States.[9] The main indications

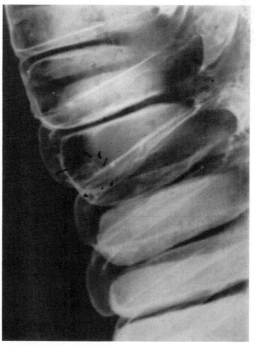

Figure 99–14. This 4-mm benign sessile polyp in the ascending colon was seen on the air-barium double-contrast enema but not on the routine barium enema.

for its use are suspicion of polyps and rectal bleeding whose source has not been determined by standard barium enema. Most radiologists in the United States perform the standard barium enema first. The air-barium study is therefore used as an adjunct to better define abnormalities detected on the barium enema. Perhaps the major reason that air-barium double-contrast enemas are not more often performed initially here is that most preparations for colonic cleansing are inadequate for an air-contrast study. In Sweden, however, this problem does not exist, and so double-contrast study is readily done.[13]

Three different techniques may be used to administer barium and air to obtain a double-contrast enema. Dense, viscous barium may be slowly instilled into the colon up to the splenic flexure, and then maneuvered into the right colon by positioning of the patient and air insufflation so that the barium column always precedes the air. Another method is to fill the colon with barium suspension, have the patient evacuate the enema, and then refill with a barium and air mixture. A third method utilizes the superior mucosal coating of some micropulverized barium mixtures or barium–tannic acid mixtures. Called a

"jiffy" enema, this technique employs air insufflation into the collapsed but barium-coated colon after the patient has evacuated a standard barium sulfate enema. Any of these methods of performing a double-contrast enema may provide roentgenograms of excellent quality.

SPECIAL TECHNIQUES FOR COLONIC EXAMINATION

BARIUM ENEMA VIA COLOSTOMY

Frequently, barium enemas are required after colostomies or ileostomies have been performed to exclude a part or all of the colon from the fecal stream (diverticulitis with abscess, Crohn's disease, unresectable tumor) in order to evaluate the state of the disease in the colon. If the rectum is intact, it may be possible to study the colon in the normal fashion by rectal instillation of barium. Often, however, this is not possible, and the colon must be evaluated by barium instilled via the colostomy opening. This situation presents special problems, because barium solutions instilled via a catheter in-

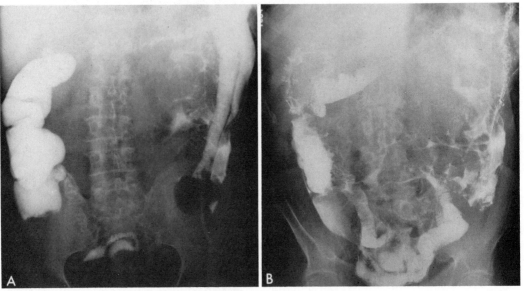

Figure 99–15. *A,* Perforation of the descending colon at the colostomy site caused by inflation of a balloon catheter within the colostomy. Barium is free in the left colonic gutter. *B,* The postevacuation film demonstrates free intraperitoneal extravasation of barium. This complication may be avoided by placing the balloon catheter against the colostomy stoma rather than inflating it inside the bowel. (From Margulis, A. R., and Goldberg, H. I.: Radiol. Clin. N. Amer. 7:27, 1969.)

serted through a colostomy tend to leak onto the abdominal wall. The most common method of preventing barium leakage out of a colostomy stoma is by occluding the stoma, usually with a balloon catheter inflated with 30 ml of air. The catheter tip distal to the balloon is placed in the colon; the balloon is inflated on the outside and held tightly against the stoma, not inside the bowel, because such distention can perforate the bowel (Fig. 99–15).[9, 14]

Special suction devices have been developed which attach to the abdominal wall around an ileostomy or colostomy and allow barium to be instilled into the bowel without leaking onto the abdominal wall.[23, 24]

COLONIC EXAMINATION WITH WATER-SOLUBLE CONTRAST MATERIAL

Although roentgenographic studies of the colon are frequently performed with water-soluble iodinated contrast material (sodium or methylglucamine diatrizoate), the indications for its use are limited to a few specific instances.[9] Because water-soluble contrast enemas fail to coat the mucosal wall, both in the filled and post-evacuation colon, and are more expensive than standard barium sulfate suspensions, they are not used routinely in radiography of the colon. In addition, the hypertonicity of the water-soluble material often results in an influx of fluid into the colon, not only distending and increasing tone in the colon but also aggravating electrolyte imbalances.

Water-soluble contrast enemas are preferable to barium enemas when perforation is present or suspected or the plain film shows evidence of pericolic abscess. Water-soluble contrast material, rather than barium, should be used to demonstrate the course and extent of enterocutaneous and enterovesical fistulas.

THE WATER ENEMA FOR DETECTION OF LIPOMAS

At low kilovoltage ranges (50 kv) the differential photon absorption between fat and water density is enhanced. Based on this observation, the water enema has been employed to delineate colonic lipomas.[25] When a standard barium enema demonstrates a smooth, round mass protruding into the lumen, the colon may be filled with water in order to determine whether the mass is of fat density. If the mass appears lucent when surrounded by water, it is composed of fat, for all other lesions of equal or greater density than water will not be delineated by this technique.

PERORAL AIR CONTRAST ENEMA OF THE CECUM AND RIGHT COLON

When redundant barium-filled loops of sigmoid colon overlie the cecum and terminal ileum, the right colon may be outlined by injecting air via the rectum into the right colon to provide double contrast after barium has been given orally.[10, 26] This examination is performed separately, and requires the regimen for colonic cleansing which precedes an air-barium double-contrast enema. The patient swallows 6 to 10 oz of barium, and the progress

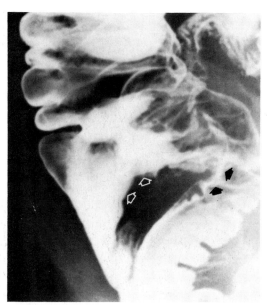

Figure 99–16. Peroral pneumocolon, demonstrating carcinoma of the cecal tip (open arrows) with mucosal invasion of the terminal ileum (closed arrows). The routine barium enema demonstrated neither of the lesions, because redundant loops of barium-filled sigmoid obscured this region. (From Margulis, A. R., and Goldberg, H. I.: Radiol. Clin. N. Amer. 7:27, 1969.)

of barium through the small bowel is followed fluoroscopically. When most of the barium has reached the cecum and ascending colon, air is insufflated into the colon to distend and outline the barium-coated cecum and ascending colon. The roentgenograms obtained by this method are particularly useful in outlining lesions on and around the ileocecal valve, as well as cecal tip deformities. They also provide a good means of evaluating simultaneous involvement of cecum and terminal ileum (Fig. 99–16).

SLOW-FRAME CINE-EVACUATION STUDIES

In 1963, cineradiographic studies were first used to study evacuation in normal and diseased states.[27] Cineradiographic demonstration of evacuation of a barium sulfate enema is still in an experimental stage, although cineradiography of esophageal, gastric, and small bowel motility has been used more extensively. Recently, slow-frame cineradiography has been coupled with radiotelemetric capsule sensing of right colonic pressures and balloon or open-tipped catheter recordings of left colonic pressures.[28] This technique is potentially useful, because simultaneous cineradiography and manometry may provide information about abnormal evacuation patterns, as noted in functional constipation, after spinal cord injury, and, occasionally, in patients with chronic ulcerative colitis.

The proper technique is as follows: The patient swallows a directional radiotelemetric capsule; when it reaches the right colon, as determined by fluoroscopy, open-tipped, perfused, pressure-sensing catheters are placed into the rectum or sigmoid, and barium is instilled into the colon. The patient must then evacuate, in the sitting position, while cineradiographs obtained at 1 to 5 frames per second are obtained simultaneously with pressure recordings.

USE OF ARTERIOGRAPHY IN ROENTGEN EXAMINATION OF THE COLON

The angiographic features of various gastrointestinal diseases are discussed in the chapters dealing with the specific disease entities. However, a few general indications for the use of angiography in the diagnosis of colonic disease are applicable to the scope of this present discussion. The technique of percutaneous transfemoral selective superior and inferior mesenteric arteriography is a well established and successful method of demonstrating colonic vasculature.[29-32] Thus the diagnosis of chronic melena or bright red rectal bleeding from an unknown source may be accomplished by adding to routine barium enema studies a selective superior and inferior mesenteric arteriogram[30] (see pp. 206 to 207).

The major indication for angiography of the colon is to aid in diagnosing the cause of chronic bleeding of undetermined origin. This has been demonstrated in the successful diagnosis of bleeding colonic diverticula, ulcerative or granulomatous colitis, ischemia, neoplasm, arteriovenous malformations, and juvenile polyps.

Although some arteriographic differences have been noted between chronic ulcerative colitis and advanced Crohn's disease,[33] it is somewhat premature to base a radiographic differentiation on arteriographic findings.

COMPLICATIONS OF BARIUM ENEMAS

PERFORATION

Intraperitoneal and extraperitoneal extravasation of barium sulfate suspensions is the most serious complication of the barium enema examination. It is difficult to determine the exact incidence, because it is not often reported. From several survey studies, however, a general incidence may be determined.[14, 34, 35]

Two perforations in 10,000 barium enemas indicate the rarity of this complication.[35] In a large survey from Australia, 15 intraperitoneal perforations and six extraperitoneal perforations[34] were reported in 250,000 barium enema examinations. At the University of California, over an eight-year period during which approximately 20,000 barium enemas were performed, the colon perforated in six patients.

There are several causes for perforation of the colon during the barium enema examination.

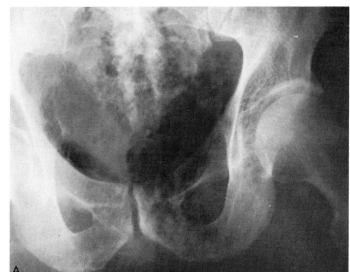

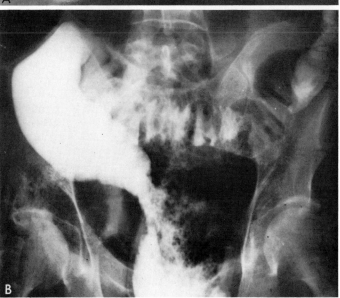

Figure 99–17. *A,* Perforation of rectum by traumatic insertion of the plastic tip of the enema tube prior to barium enema examination. The patient had administered the cleansing enema to himself and had inadvertently produced a rectal perforation. The area of irregular mottled lucency in the left pelvis is due to the perirectal abscess. The contrast-filled rectum is displaced slightly to the right by this abscess *(B).*

1. Perforation by an enema tip through pre-existing colonic disease. This is particularly likely when a carcinoma of the rectum or significant ulcerative proctitis is present.

2. Perforation by the enema tip without pre-existing disease, caused by trauma to the rectal wall during insertion of the tube (Fig. 99–17). The sensory innervation of the rectum ends at the dentate line, so that it is possible to perforate the rectum without the patient feeling pain.[14]

3. Perforation caused by overinflation of the balloon catheter.[10, 14] When pre-existing rectal disease, such as rectosigmoid colitis, diverticulitis, or carcinoma, is present, overinflation is dangerous; however, even a normal bowel may rupture, as noted by extravasation of barium through a rent in the rectum. Included in the group of perforations caused by overinflation are those which occur at a colostomy site as a result of inflation of the balloon catheter inside the colostomy stoma. Perforation is most common near the peritoneal reflection at the level of the pouch of Douglas.[14] To minimize the danger, it is best not to inflate the rectal balloon until some barium has first been placed into the rectum to outline the rectal ampulla and to

determine whether an ulcerative or constricting lesion is present. Further, the balloon should always be inflated under fluoroscopic control by the radiologist.

4. Perforation that follows sigmoidoscopy and rectal biopsy. This is noted particularly after a biopsy has been taken from pathological tissue,[14, 34] but occasionally from normal colon as well, especially if the site is deep, as when searching for ganglia in a suspected case of Hirschsprung's disease or in removing a sessile polyp.

5. Spontaneous rupture during the barium enema without antecedent disease or rectal trauma. Included in this group are those instances of perforation during attempted reduction of a sigmoid volvulus.[10]

Intraperitoneal leakage of barium and fecal content carries with it a higher mortality than does extraperitoneal leakage.[14, 34] Immediate surgical repair of an intraperitoneal leak, discovered by fluoroscopy and plain film radiography, is essential for survival; otherwise the mortality is 67 to 75 per cent.[34]

BARIUM GRANULOMA

The inadvertent instillation of barium sulfate beneath the rectal mucosa during the performance of a barium enema may result in a chronic inflammatory reaction with foreign body granuloma formation.[36,37] These submucosal barium masses appear as polypoid, sometimes ulcerating rectal lesions on roentgenograms and at sigmoidoscopic examination. They vary in size from 0.5 to 10 cm. Laceration of rectal mucosa by the enema tip or the proctoscope provides the barium sulfate suspension with access to the colon wall. Overinflation of a rectal balloon catheter may also produce mucosal tears which lead to granuloma formation. Most often, granuloma formation is limited to the submucosa and muscularis, and spontaneous healing occurs over a three-week to two-month period. Occasionally, extensive barium sulfate infiltration may result in perirectal extravasation with concomitant mass, pain, and tenesmus, requiring debridement.[38]

Histologically, the chronic barium granuloma may appear much like granuloma in Crohn's disease and tuberculosis. Careful inspection of histological sections ob-

tained from biopsy of the rectal mass will reveal barium sulfate crystals in macrophages or surrounding them, a finding enhanced by the use of polarized light.

BARIUM EMBOLISM

Venous embolization of barium sulfate particles is an extremely rare but often fatal complication of a barium enema. Only a few cases have been reviewed,[14, 34] and these seem to be related to tear or rupture of rectal or vaginal tissue with the exit of barium into the pelvic venous system and subsequent hepatic and pulmonary embolization.

TOXIC DILATATION OF THE COLON

A few reports have documented a temporal relationship between the performance of a barium enema in patients with active colitis and the subsequent rapid development of megacolon and systemic toxicity in patients with inactive or quiescent ulcerative colitis; however, the mechanism is obscure.[39, 40] Although the rapid rise in intraluminal colonic pressure caused by rapid distention may cause a dilatation in patients with quiescent colitis, it appears to be harmless in the vast majority of such patients. Thus the procedure should be performed when indicated in quiescent disease; it should be avoided, if at all possible, in those whose colitis is active. Care should be taken, however, to instruct the patient with ulcerative colitis to continue a high liquid intake for 24 hours after the barium enema, and to use rectal suppositories to stimulate emptying if the barium has not been passed. These measures prevent barium inspissation in the colon with subsequent barolith formation, a cause of partial colon obstruction particularly deleterious to patients with this disease.

BARIUM ENEMA EXAMINATION IN SPECIFIC DISEASES

ACUTE AND CHRONIC ULCERATIVE COLITIS

Consultation between the radiologist and the patient's physician is of extreme

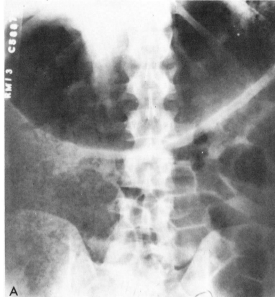
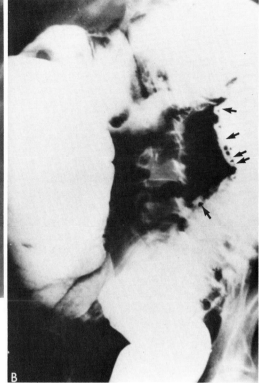

Figure 99–18. *A*, A megacolon in a patient with perfuse bloody diarrhea, fever, anemia, leukocytosis, and tachycardia. The luminal contour of the air-filled transverse colon is irregular, suggesting ulceration or pseudopolyps. *B*, A barium enema, mistakenly performed on the same patient, demonstrates local pericolonic perforations (arrows). A barium enema is contraindicated in toxic megacolon. (Courtesy of Dr. Joachim Burhenne, Childrens Hospital, San Francisco.)

importance for the proper management of active colitis. Only when the radiologist is aware of the patient's history and present status can he plan the proper radiographic approach. In patients with acute ulcerative colitis, interpretation of the plain abdominal roentgenogram is essential to determine the presence of megacolon. Patients with fulminant ulcerative colitis who have findings of systemic toxicity and a plain abdominal roentgenogram showing megacolon must not be subjected to barium enema because of the high risk of colon perforation with spillage of barium contents into the abdomen (Fig. 99–18).

In a very rare instance, in a patient with long-standing quiescent ulcerative colitis with clinical and roentgenographic evidence of megacolon, a limited radiographic examination may be required in order to exclude an obstructing rectosigmoid or sigmoid carcinoma. In the vast majority of patients, malignancy in this situation may be excluded by plain abdominal films alone. When, however, air does not outline the left colon and sigmoid, it may be necessary to gently instill a water-soluble contrast medium far enough into the rectosigmoid to rule out possible rectosigmoid carcinoma. Under no circumstances should the water-soluble enema be given forcefully. A rubber-tipped catheter, *not* a plastic enema tip, should be used. A rectal balloon catheter should not be inflated in the rectum.

Thus in the special instance of differentiating between rectosigmoid carcinoma in long-standing ulcerative colitis and an acute nonobstructive toxic megacolon, the placement of contrast within the colon may be justified. But in all other instances, barium enemas are contraindicated in patients with toxic megacolon.

Barium enema examinations are not recommended for patients with acute fulminant bloody diarrhea, even though plain films of the abdomen may not show toxic megacolon. In patients ill with active disease, with diarrhea and severe bleeding, barium enema examination may further

1270 THE COLON

exacerbate the disease and lead to megacolon or even perforation (see pp. 1326 to 1330). The risk of performing a barium enema in such patients must be balanced against the need for information on the diagnosis and on the extent of disease. Under no circumstances, however, should these patients be subjected to any form of colonic cleansing preparation.

Barium enema examination in patients with active or quiescent ulcerative colitis who are not severely ill should also be performed without submitting the colon to cleansing by laxatives. However, a preliminary liquid diet of 24 to 48 hours' duration and tap water cleansing enemas are necessary preparations in such patients if roentgenograms of adequate diagnostic quality are to be obtained. It must be noted that the colon in a patient with profuse diarrhea is not necessarily clean. Fecal debris, undigested food particles, and mucoid secretions may effectively interfere with a normal barium-mucosa interface and thereby hide valuable diagnostic information.

The barium enema examination is a useful means of following the progress of medical therapy for active ulcerative colitis. Although clinical symptoms and sigmoidoscopy are both important methods of judging therapy for ulcerative colitis, barium enema examination is the only means of determining the appearance of the colon proximal to the sigmoid. The response of the inflamed colon to steroid retention enemas has been monitored in children by barium enema examination. During the initial few months of therapy with steroid retention enemas, one or two barium enemas were performed without complication.[4] Reversibility of the radiographic signs of ulcerative colitis may be noted in many of these children, with complete reversibility of the radiographic findings on the average of five months after treatment is begun (Fig. 99–19). It is often useful to add some barium early in the course of treatment with steroid enemas to determine roentgenographically whether the patient is bathing his entire colon topically.

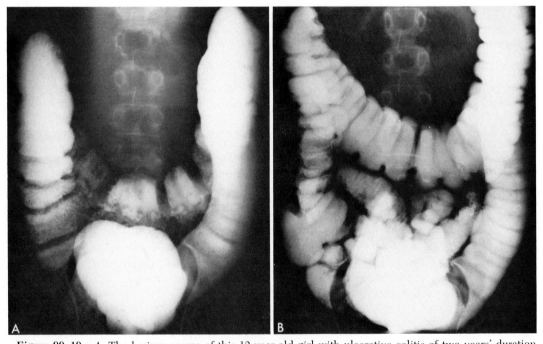

Figure 99–19. *A,* The barium enema of this 12-year-old girl with ulcerative colitis of two years' duration demonstrated deep, irregular, confluent collarbutton abscesses along the border of the transverse colon. Generalized haustral thickening and shallow ulcerations involve the entire colon. A bleeding, friable, ulcerative mucosa was noted at sigmoidoscopy. *B,* After nine months of daily hydrocortisone–safflower oil retention enemas, the colon appears normal roentgenographically, and sigmoidoscopic examination was normal. (From Goldberg, H. I., Carbone, J. V., and Margulis, A. R.: Amer. J. Roent. *103:*365, 1968.)

In view of the known increase in incidence of adenocarcinoma of the colon in patients with chronic ulcerative colitis of ten years or longer, a routine barium enema yearly is reasonable for detecting neoplasm. Certainly, in patients who have had chronic ulcerative colitis for 20 years or longer, annual barium enema examinations are necessary because of the very high likelihood of intercurrent neoplasm.[42]

COLONIC OBSTRUCTION

Supine and upright films of the abdomen alert the radiologist to the possibility of colonic obstruction. In addition to these routine radiographic views, left and right decubitus films may also be important in localizing the site of obstruction. Although plain films of the abdomen may suggest colonic obstruction because of colonic dilatation and air-fluid levels in the colon and sometimes in the small bowel, the diagnosis can only be confirmed by either sigmoidoscopy (if the lesion is in the distal colon) or barium enema examination (see pp. 1483 to 1484).

The exact nature of the obstructive lesion, be it carcinoma, diverticulitis, intussusception, or adhesions, must also be elucidated by a barium enema examination. A few specific rules apply to the roentgenographic examination of patients with colonic obstruction, particularly left colonic obstruction. Barium enemas must be performed without inflation of a rectal balloon catheter. The enema tip should not be placed in the rectum until after digital examination or sigmoidoscopy has been performed, in order to avoid inadvertent trauma to a rectal lesion. The barium enema is instilled under low pressure with slow flow. In a patient with partial colonic obstruction, but with no clinical signs or roentgenographic evidence of fecal impaction proximal to the obstruction, the barium may be instilled proximal to the point of obstruction to allow visualization of the entire colon. The examination stops if a point of high-grade obstruction is seen, because very little detail of the colonic wall is possible in this situation and proximal inspissation of barium is likely. When obstruction is encountered but small amounts of barium pass the site at irregular intervals, colonic spasm is suggested. In such an instance, intravenous or intramuscular Pro-Banthine may be given.[43]

SIGMOID VOLVULUS

The roentgenographic findings of sigmoid volvulus have been amply described, and are illustrated in Figure 99–20. The typical massive dilatation of twisted sigmoid poses no diagnostic problem for the radiologist. However, the diagnosis of distal colonic obstruction caused by sigmoid volvulus should be confirmed by barium enema examination. The differentiation between sigmoid torsion (up to 180-degree turn of the sigmoid) and obstructing volvulus (360-degree turn or greater) can only be made by barium enema. The completely obstructing volvulus will result in a tapered narrowing of the retrograde barium column. The tapered end is often asymmetrical, and the mucosal folds may appear twisted as they converge on the point of obstruction. This type of volvulus is rarely reduced by the barium enema. However, incomplete volvulus, or torsion, is more amenable to reduction by barium enema. In such cases, the areas of sigmoid narrowing at the site of torsion are frequently outlined by barium, as is the dilated sigmoid loop. Torsion may sometimes be reduced on the fluoroscopic table by the barium enema itself, or by positioning and palpating the patient. Such efforts, however, should not be vigorous. Placement of a decompressing rectal tube during sigmoidoscopy still remains the major nonsurgical mode of treatment.

INTUSSUSCEPTION

The ileum is the most common site of gastrointestinal intussusception. Ileoileal and ileocolic intussusception account for the great majority of cases, and these are almost always in infants and children. Intussusception is a much rarer condition in adults, and about one-third of the intussusceptions are colocolic.[44] Although intussusception in infants often has no specific cause, in adults a mucosal or mural colonic lesion, such as a fibroma, polyp, or carcinoma, may frequently be found at the leading edge or at the base of the intussusception.[44, 45]

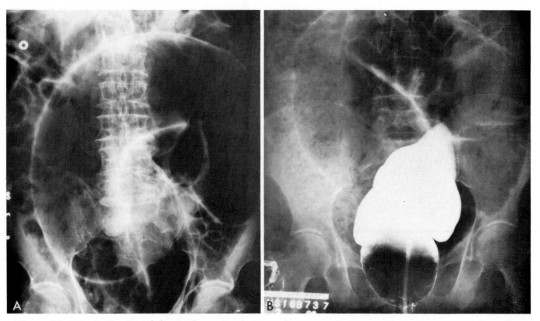

Figure 99–20. *A,* Supine abdominal roentgenogram, demonstrating the typical appearance of a sigmoid volvulus—a massively distended sigmoid forming an inverted "U" owing to torsion. *B,* Barium enema examination on the same patient, demonstrating the funneled narrowing of the barium column with an eccentric tapering, appearing as a "bird's beak" at the site of volvulus.

Acute intussusception in infants may produce pain and bloody diarrhea, whereas in adults colonic intussusception may produce symptoms indistinguishable from those of colonic obstruction caused by carcinoma: change in stool caliber, abdominal distention and cramps, occasional diarrhea, and melena.[44] Plain abdominal roentgenograms may demonstrate small bowel distention with prominent air-fluid levels—a roentgen finding of mechanical small bowel obstruction. If the intussusception is located in the left colon, colonic distention and air-fluid levels may also be seen. As in any patient with suspected ileal or colonic mechanical obstruction, a barium enema examination is commonly performed to define the character of the obstruction. A forceful barium enema which utilizes an inflated rectal balloon and a 4- to 5-foot height to the enema bag is to be avoided, because colonic or ileal perforation may result.[10] This catastrophic event is particularly likely if the intussusception has been present for 48 hours or more, with intercurrent vascular compromise of the invaginated loop of bowel. However, in patients with a more acute onset of distal small bowel or colonic obstruction in which a typical bowel-within-

bowel appearance is demonstrated on barium enema, reduction of the intussusception may be attempted (Fig. 99–21). Great care is exercised by the radiologist

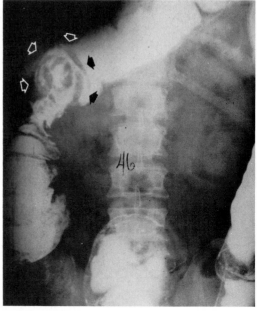

Figure 99–21. Intussusception of an hepatic flexure carcinoma in an adult. The whorled appearance (arrows) of intussuscepting colon is a characteristic roentgenographic finding.

when attempting to reduce an intussusception; the flow of barium is slow, the barium bag is not raised above a 3-foot height from the table top, and the appearance of the invaginated bowel is watched closely during attempted reduction. In infants reduction of intussusception by hydrostatic pressure has proved successful. Most acute intussusceptions in children did not recur after barium enema reduction.[46] However, in adults, less success has been encountered in reducing intussusception by barium enema. If an intussusception is reduced in an adult, great care must be taken to re-examine the colon by barium enema in order to ascertain whether an underlying polyp or tumor is present. This is particularly important in adults, because definitive therapy depends upon discovering underlying colonic pathology.

DIVERTICULITIS

Plain abdominal roentgenograms in patients with clinical symptoms suggestive of diverticulitis may occasionally show a mottled appearance of air and fecal material in the left lower quadrant. However, this finding per se is not specific of diverticulitis with abscess formation. The plain films of the abdomen almost never demonstrate free air beneath the diaphragm caused by ruptured diverticula.

In a patient with left lower quadrant tenderness, fever, leukocytosis, and changing bowel habits, the suspected diagnosis of diverticulitis is not a contraindication for barium enema examination. Indeed, barium enema examination, done with proper precautions, is a valuable adjunct to the diagnosis of diverticulitis, in demonstrating the site of the disease process, outlining the extent of the disease and fistulas or abscesses, and evaluating the colon for concurrent presence of carcinoma (see pp. 1425 to 1426).

The precautions taken during barium enema examination of a patient with suspected diverticulitis include instillation of the barium sulfate suspension under low hydrostatic pressure and slow flow rate to avoid rapid colonic distention. Undue compression of the left lower quadrant is avoided, and a rectal balloon catheter is not used as part of the study. Laxative preparations are strictly interdicted.[47]

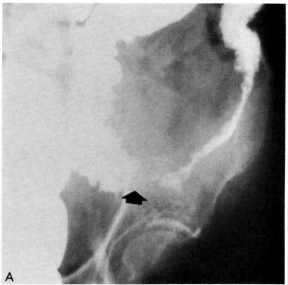 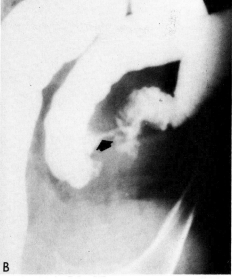

Figure 99–22. *A,* Narrowing and irregularity of a 10-cm segment of distal descending colon in a 60-year-old male with one week's history of left lower quadrant abdominal pain and tenderness, fever, leukocytosis and a palpable mass. In addition to the apparent mass adjacent to and narrowing the colon, an area of pronounced narrowing is noted at the sigmoid–descending colon junction (arrow). Clinical and roentgenographic diagnosis: acute diverticulitis with large pericolonic abscess. *B,* A repeat barium enema, after three weeks of intensive antibiotic therapy, demonstrates disappearance of the inflammatory mass. The underlying constricting carcinoma is now apparent (arrow).

Since diverticulitis is a disease characterized by microperforation of diverticula, the roentgenographic finding of extravasation of barium sulfate into the colonic wall or a pericolonic abscess is neither a surprising nor a catastrophic finding.[47] Once extravasation has been noted, however, the barium enema should be stopped. Free extravasation of barium sulfate into the peritoneal cavity is a rare occurrence in sigmoid diverticulitis, because even extensive diverticular perforations are usually walled off. Therefore unless free perforation with peritonitis is suspected, barium sulfate suspension may be used to examine the colon. However, water-soluble contrast media should be used wherever peritoneal signs are present or a sigmoid-vesical fistula is suspected. Once the diagnosis of diverticulitis is made clinically and radiographically and the patient is placed on antibiotic therapy, a repeat barium examination should be performed within a week after the resolution of symptoms, in order to rule out the possibility of colonic cancer in the same segment. Resolution of the inflammatory process associated with diverticulitis may allow radiographic demonstration of an underlying carcinoma (Fig. 99–22).

In addition, the patient with sigmoid diverticulitis should also be evaluated roentgenographically for evidence of small bowel disease, because Crohn's disease of the colon and sigmoid diverticulitis may be difficult to distinguish roentgenographically.[48] The finding of a small bowel involvement typical of Crohn's disease is suggestive that the colonic lesion is also Crohn's disease.

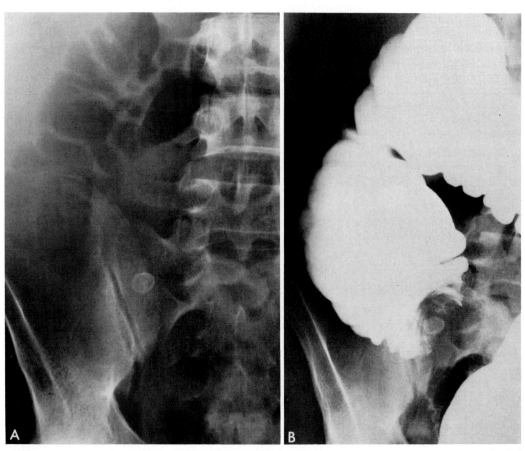

Figure 99–23. A, The cyst-like calcification overlying the right sacral wing is a calcified appendicolith, producing acute appendicitis in this young man. B, The barium enema outlines the appendiceal abscess as it indents the cecal tip. The appendicolith appears to be within the center of the abscess.

ACUTE APPENDICITIS

Although the clinical diagnosis of acute appendicitis is often obvious and does not require radiographic confirmation, diagnosis is difficult in some patients. In these instances, a plain film of the abdomen may reveal nonspecific findings but may also demonstrate appendicoliths appearing either as dense calcifications or as laminated concretions in about 10 per cent of patients with acute appendicitis (Fig. 99–23).[49] The presence of these stones, or of inspissated barium (barolith) in the appendiceal lumen in the appropriate clinical setting strongly supports the diagnosis. The finding of barium in the appendix in asymptomatic patients is of no significance. Roentgenographic findings of small bowel obstruction, gas in the appendiceal lumen, or free air in the peritoneal cavity are all extremely rare in acute appendicitis (pp. 1494 to 1499).

Acute appendicitis does not contraindicate a barium enema examination, because the appendiceal lumen is obstructed; likewise, even the likelihood of appendiceal perforation does not interdict the procedure, because it is always distal to the obstruction and is walled off by mesentery. Indentation on the cecal tip associated with edema of the terminal ileum or barium enemas indicates the probability of acute appendicitis. The terminal ileum and cecum may be separated as well. These findings may be due also to appendicitis with a walled-off abscess, Crohn's disease, tuberculosis, lymphosarcoma, metastatic tumor, and mucocele of the appendix; however, in the clinical setting of acute abdominal pain, acute appendicitis and Crohn's disease are the two major diagnostic considerations.

PNEUMATOSIS CYSTOIDES INTESTINALIS

Air in the wall of the colon, colonic pneumatosis cystoides intestinalis, may be detected on abdominal roentgenograms by the presence of linear streaks of air paralleling the lumen of the bowel, bubble-like cysts of air in the bowel wall, or irregular beaded streaks of air in the mesentery (Fig. 99–24). The finding of air in the wall

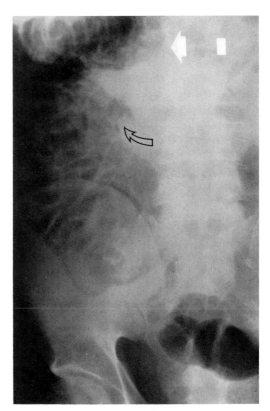

Figure 99–24. Air in the wall of the cecum and ascending colon (pneumatosis cystoides intestinalis) outlines this structure on the plain abdominal roentgenogram. Intramural air is present up to the proximal transverse colon (closed arrow). Streaks of air may be seen in the mesentery as well (open arrow). The ascending colon and proximal transverse colon were found to be necrotic owing to irreversible ischemia.

of the bowel should be considered a serious, possibly life-threatening abnormality, reflecting underlying intestinal necrosis.[6, 7, 50] Although approximately 15 per cent of patients with pneumatosis cystoides intestinalis have no underlying bowel disease, the majority of patients with this finding do have associated large and small bowel disease; the most common is vascular insufficiency with intestinal necrosis, although necrotizing enterocolitis, enteritis with abnormal gas-forming organisms, and intestinal obstruction may all produce air in the bowel wall. The idiopathic form of pneumatosis cystoides intestinalis is sometimes associated with pulmonary fibrosis with alveolar rupture, silent pneumomediastinum, and dissection of air retroperitoneally into the abdominal mesentery and subsequently into the small bowel[6] (see pp. 1514 to 1519).

The radiologist must consider the finding of intramural air or intramesenteric air as a manifestation of underlying intestinal disease until proved otherwise. Under these circumstances, a barium enema must not be done until the patient's clinical situation is fully evaluated. This is particularly true of patients who are receiving systemic steroids, because underlying abdominal symptomatology may be masked. Necrotic colon caused by irreversible ischemic necrosis may perforate during a barium enema examination. Therefore contrast examinations of the colon must be done with the greatest caution, using only a water-soluble material.

REFERENCES

1. Davenport, H. W. Physiology of the Digestive Tract. Chicago, Year Book Medical Publishers Inc., p. 207.
2. Rice, R. P. Plain abdominal film roentgenographic diagnosis of ulcerative diseases of the colon. Amer. J. Roent. 104:544, 1968.
3. Frimann-Dahl, J. Roentgen Examinations in Acute Abdominal Diseases. 2nd ed. Springfield, Ill., Charles C Thomas, 1960.
4. Jones, J. H., and Chapman, M. Definition of megacolon in colitis. Gut 10:562, 1969.
5. Neschis, M., et al.: Diagnosis and management of megacolon in ulcerative colitis. Gastroenterology 55:257, 1968.
6. Seaman, W. B., Fleming, R. J., and Baker, D. H. Pneumatosis intestinalis of the small bowel. Sem. Roent. 1:234, 1966.
7. Rigler, L. G., and Pogue, W. L. Roentgen signs of intestinal necrosis. Amer. J. Roent. 94:402, 1965.
8. Mainzer, F., and Minagi, H. Giant sigmoid diverticulum. Amer. J. Roent. 113:352, 1971.
9. Margulis, A. R., and Goldberg, H. I. The current state of radiologic technique in the examination of the colon: A survey. Radiol, Clin. N. Amer. 7:27, 1969.
10. Margulis, A. R. Examination of the colon. In Alimentary Tract Roentgenology, A. R. Margulis and H. J. Burhenne (eds.). St. Louis, C. V. Mosby Co., 1967, p. 705.
11. Tracht, D. G., and Clemett, A. R. An evaluation of the "clean colon" technique. Radiology 99:69, 1971.
12. Baines, M. R. How to get a cleaner colon with less effort. Radiology 91:948, 1968.
13. Welin, S. Results of the Malmo Technique of colon examination. J.A.M.A. 199:369, 1967.
14. Seaman, W. B. and Wells, J. Complications of the barium enema. Gastroenterology 48:728, 1965.

15. Miller, R. E. Barium sulfate suspensions. Radiology 84:241, 1965.
16. Christie, A. C., Coe, F. O., Hampton, A. O., and Wyatt, G. M. Value of tannic acid enema and post-evacuation roentgenograms in examinations of the colon. Amer. J. Roent. 63:657, 1950.
17. McAlister, W. H., Anderson, M. S., Bloomberg, G. R., and Margulis, A. R. Lethal effects of tannic acid in barium enemas: Report of three fatalities and experimental studies. Radiology 80:765, 1963.
18. Lucke, H. H., Hodge, K. E., and Patt, N. L. Fatal liver damage after barium enemas containing tannic acid. Canad. Med. Assoc. J. 89:1111, 1963.
19. Zboralske, F. F., Harris, P. A., Riegelman, S., Rambo, O. N., and Margulis, A. R. Toxicity studies on tannic acid administered by enema. III. Studies on the retention of enemas in humans. IV. Review and conclusions. Amer. J. Roent. 96:505, 1966.
20. Burhenne, H. J., Vogelaar, P., and Arkoff, R. S. Liver function studies in patients receiving enemas containing tannic acid. Amer. J. Roent. 96:510, 1966.
21. Lumsden, K., and Truelove, S. C. Intravenous Pro-Banthine in diagnostic radiology of the gastrointestinal tract. Brit. J. Radiol. 32:517, 1959.
22. Sheft, D. J. Pharmacoradiology. Advan. Surg. 5:69, 1971.
23. Waldron, R. L., and Seaman, W. B. Roentgenographic examination of patients with colostomies, enterostomies and large fistulous and sinus tracts. Amer. J. Roent. 113:297, 1971.
24. Burhenne, H. J. Technique of colostomy examination. Radiology 97:183, 1970.
25. Margulis, A. R., and Jovanovich, A. Roentgen diagnosis of submucous lipomas of the colon. Amer. J. Roent. 84:1114, 1960.
26. Heitzman, E. R., and Berne, A. S. Roentgen examination of the cecum and proximal ascending colon with ingested barium. Radiology 76:415, 1961.
27. Burhenne, H. J. Intestinal evacuation study: A new roentgenologic technique. Radiol. Clin. 33:79, 1963.
28. Gramiak, R., Ross, P., and Olmsted, W. W. Normal motor activity of the human colon: Combined radiotelemetric manometry and slow-frame cineroentgenography. Amer. J. Roent. 113:301, 1971.
29. Nusbaum, M., Baum, S., Blakemore, W. S., et al. Demonstration of intra-arterial bleeding by selective arteriography. J.A.M.A. 191:117, 1965.
30. Reuter, S. R., and Bookstein, J. J. Angiographic localization of gastrointestinal bleeding. Gastroenterology 54:876, 1968.
31. Clark, R., and Rosch, J. Arteriography in the diagnosis of large bowel bleeding. Radiology 94:83, 1970.
32. Klein, H. J., Alfidi, R. J., Meaney, T. F., and Poirier, V. C. Angiography in the diagnosis of chronic gastrointestinal bleeding. Radiology 98:83, 1971.

33. Brahme, F.   Mesenteric angiography in regional enterocolitis. Radiology 87:1037, 1966.
34. Masel, H., Masel, J. P., and Casey, K. V.   A survey of colon examination techniques in Australia and New Zealand with a review of complications. Australas. Radiol. 15:140, 1971.
35. Lorinc, P., and Brahme, F.   Perforation of the colon during examination by the double contrast method. Gastroenterology 37:770, 1959.
36. Weitzner, S., and Law, D.   Barium granuloma of the rectum. Amer. J. Dig. Dis. 17:17, 1972.
37. Carter, R. W.   Barium granuloma of the rectum: A complication of diagnostic barium enema examinations. Amer. J. Roent. 89:880, 1963.
38. Burnikel, R. H.   Barium granuloma: An anorectal complication of barium enema X-ray studies. Dis. Colon Rectum 5:224, 1962.
39. Wruble, L. D., and Bronstein, M. W.   Toxic dilatation of the colon following barium enema examination during the quiescent stage of chronic ulcerative colitis. Amer. J. Dig. Dis. 13:918, 1968.
40. Smith, F. W., Law, D. H., Nickel, W. F., and Sleisenger, M. H.   Fulminant ulcerative colitis with toxic dilatation of the colon: Medical and surgical management of eleven cases with observations regarding etiology. Gastroenterology 42:233, 1962.
41. Goldberg, H. I., Carbone, J. V., and Margulis, A. R.   Roentgenographic reversibility of ulcerative colitis in children treated with steroid enemas. Amer. J. Roent. 103:365, 1968.
42. Devroede, G. J., Taylor, W. F., Sauer, W. G., Jackman, R. J., and Stickler, G. B.   Cancer risk and life expectancy of children with ulcerative colitis. New Eng. J. Med. 285:17, 1971.
43. Lumsden, K., and Truelove, S. C.   Radiology of the Digestive System. Oxford, Blackwell Scientific Publications, 1965, Chapter 9.
44. Dean, D. L., Ellis, F. H., and Sauer, W. G.   Intussusception in adults. Arch. Surg. 73:6, 1956.
45. Tumen, H. J.   Intestinal obstruction. In Gastroenterology, Vol. II, H. Bockus (ed.). Philadelphia, W. B. Saunders Co., 1964, Chapter 52.
46. Ravitch, M. W.   Intussusception in infancy and childhood. An analysis of 77 cases treated by barium enema. New Eng. J. Med. 259:1058, 1958.
47. Fleischner, F. G.   Diverticular disease and the irritable colon syndrome. In Alimentary Tract Roentgenology, Vol. 2, A. R. Margulis and H. J. Burhenne (eds.). St. Louis, C. V. Mosby Co., 1967, Chapter 29.
48. Marshak, R. H., Janowitz, H. D., and Present, D. H.   Granulomatous colitis in association with diverticula. New Eng. J. Med. 283:1080, 1970.
49. Soter, C. S.   The contribution of the radiologist to the diagnosis of acute appendiceal disease. Med. Radiog. Photog. 45:2, 1969.
50. Scott, J. R., Miller, W. T., Urso, M., and Stadalnik, R. C.   Acute mesenteric infarction. Amer. J. Roent. 113:269, 1971.

Chapter 100

Irritable Colon

Thomas P. Almy

The term irritable colon denotes a variety of disorders of colonic function which occur in chronic or recurrent fashion at times of life stress and emotional tension. Other common terms having a similar meaning are unstable colon, spastic colitis, mucous colitis, colonic neurosis, and dyssynergia of the colon. All these are misleading, because they suggest that the disorder is confined to the colon, when it is clear that the affected patient commonly exhibits dysfunction of other regions of the gut as well as other organ systems. Further, these terms suggest that the colon itself is intrinsically abnormal, whereas no qualitatively abnormal structural or functional pattern has been found. As the symptoms resulting from this disorder, both individually and in combination, are observed in many diseases and disorders of varying etiology, the term irritable colon syndrome is meaningless, except as the starting point of an exhaustive differential diagnosis. When all those cases with etiologically or pathologically specific entities have been excluded, there remains a group whose disorders appear to be part of the bodily adaptation to nonspecific stress; to these the term irritable colon is properly applied.

PREVALENCE

Irritable colon is nowhere a reportable condition, and cannot be diagnosed with accuracy by a simple objective test; hence its true prevalence can only be roughly estimated. It is probably the most common chronic gastrointestinal disorder in developed countries well provided with medical care, and has been considered to account for 30 to 50 per cent of all digestive conditions seen in clinic or private practice. It ranks almost equally with the common cold as a leading cause of industrial absenteeism owing to illness.[1]

Even these statements, nevertheless, constitute an underestimate. It is probable that qualitatively similar disturbances, differing only in intensity and in duration, occur from time to time in the vast majority of human beings as they adapt themselves to their environment. It is clear that these are not always accompanied by symptoms; but clinically evident disturbances in otherwise healthy people commonly occur at times of military action, critical examinations in a university career, change of employment, or contemplation of marriage or divorce. That proportion of the total group affected who present themselves for medical care is determined not only by the intensity of the disorder but also by the availability of medical services and the attitude of the individual toward illness in general and digestive disturbances in particular.

SYMPTOMS AND THEIR INTERPRETATION

Although the clinical picture is highly variable, it usually can be described as some combination of the symptoms listed below. Their mechanisms are visualized by inference from clinical and experimental observation.

Abdominal pain is present at times in most patients. Its location is most commonly in the hypogastrium and left lower quadrant, less often in the other quadrants of the abdomen, and very rarely in the periumbilical area. Its time of onset and its duration are variable; but it may be sharply aggravated by intake of food or of cold liquids, and it usually is relieved by a bowel movement, the passage of flatus, or particularly an enema.[2, 3] It is griping, rather than cramplike or colicky. It varies widely in intensity, but rarely awakens the patient from sleep. Since it can be reproduced by balloon distention of the distal colon or by the spasmogenic effect of morphine or codeine sulfate, it is thought to be due to tension within the muscular coats of the bowel produced either by gaseous distention or sustained spontaneous contraction.

In certain instances, especially in individuals with a high, redundant splenic flexure, the pain may be felt chiefly at the left costal margin in the anterior axillary line, with prominent radiation to the lower substernal region, to the left shoulder, and down the inner aspect of the left arm to the elbow. This pattern, reproducible by balloon distention of the splenic flexure, has been named the *splenic flexure syndrome*.[4] Its importance lies in its resemblance to the symptoms of hiatus hernia, of disease of the gallbladder, or of the coronary arteries, and in its ready relief by thorough evacuation of the left colon.

Constipation, described as the infrequent passage of extremely small, dry, hard stools, often associated with a sense of abdominal distention and/or the excessive passage of flatus, is the more common disturbance of stool frequency. On digital examination of such patients the rectum is usually empty, suggesting an arrest of colonic motility at a higher level. On radiological or manometric study of the sigmoid and descending colon these segments show heightened nonpropulsive contractions, often correlated with an apparent diminution of wave-like motility at higher levels, especially in the proximal colon.

In a smaller number of patients *diarrhea* is steadily or intermittently present. The stools are usually only semiliquid or even mushy in consistency; and though often attended by great urgency or even tenesmus, they are nonfatty and may be quite small in volume. The movements rarely awaken the patient at night, and occur most frequently just before and after breakfast, as well as in the early evening. They may contain copious quantities of visible mucus, and some movements appear to consist of mucus alone. (Indeed, some patients may go to stool several times a day, only once passing a small hard pellet of feces and at the other times pouring forth clear mucus. This may lead to a semantic problem: Does the patient have constipation or diarrhea?) True diarrhea and the passage of mucus, nevertheless, have been reproduced by strong cholinergic stimulation of the bowel, during which the proximal colon is seen to contract vigorously while the left colon becomes shorter and wider, with diminished wave-like contractions.

Dyspepsia—postprandial epigastric fullness, together with anorexia, excessive belching, and mild nausea—not uncommonly is associated with the aforementioned symptoms referable to the colon. Rarely, recurrent episodes of severe nausea and bilious vomiting may occur. Although these may be accompanied by and aggravated by clearly visible aerophagia, it appears from laboratory observations that they are related to reduced gastric peristalsis and heightened nonpropulsive contractions of the duodenum. The reproduction of both the symptoms and the gastroduodenal motility disturbance by centrally acting emetic agents makes it likely that these patterns are integrated at or near the vomiting center in the medulla.

Symptoms of *general vasomotor instability* may be more or less prominent accompaniments of the intestinal symptoms in these patients. There may be palpitation, shortness of breath, precordial discomfort, and fatigue on mild exertion. Sweating, flushing, headaches, sighing respirations, and hyperventilation are often seen, indicating a widespread autonomic disturbance.

NATURAL HISTORY AND CLINICAL PATTERNS

As commonly encountered by the physician, the natural history of irritable colon is that of a chronic or irregularly recurring disorder, with its usual onset in late adolescence or early adult life. Careful or repeated history taking often reveals a much earlier onset of characteristic symptoms than was at first apparent, and it is rare for the disorder to appear for the first time after the age of 50. The duration of individual episodes of illness is highly variable. Although pain and diarrhea may be severe enough to disrupt seriously the desired routines of work, travel, or social activity, the patient rarely loses weight or becomes dehydrated. The severity of the illness changes over months and years in irregular fashion, and seems to correlate best with the degree of difficulty with which the patient adapts to the current stress situation.

Despite great variation in the clinical pictures encountered, most cases seem to fit one of the following three patterns:

1. *Spastic colon* (spastic colitis, spastic constipation), in which the leading symptom is lower abdominal pain, especially in the left lower quadrant. The usual bowel habit is constipation, with the characteristic small stools described above. Distention, passage of flatus, and dyspepsia are commonly associated. Many patients have a stubborn, painless constipation. Except for these, the patients with spastic colon are likely to have an episodic disorder, or else symptoms highly variable in severity.

2. *Painless diarrhea* (nervous diarrhea, spasmomyxorrhea, mucous colitis), which characteristically has a persistent, relatively unvarying course.

3. *Alternating diarrhea* and *constipation*, with highly variable duration of each phase.

PATHOGENESIS

Starting from careful clinical observation of patients with irritable colon, a number of investigators have framed hypotheses concerning its pathophysiology, which have been tested in a laboratory setting. Earlier microbiological and morphological studies had revealed no infectious agent and no characteristic morbid anatomy with which the condition could be identified.

Consideration of the symptoms alone

suggested that the most directly relevant function of the bowel is its motility, and this has become the main focus of objective study. The methods used have included (1) the observation of patients with colonic fistulas or exteriorized colonic loops; (2) prolonged sigmoidoscopic examination of intact patients; (3) kymographic recordings of wave-like motility in the colon as registered by large balloons; (4) electromanometric pressure transducers or telemetering capsules; and (5) fluoroscopy and cineradiography. The apparent contradictions in the data from various sources are mainly explained by differences in methodology; difficulties in the recognition and classification of symptom patterns and feeling states have also complicated the interpretation of results.[5-7]

Using such methods, studies of the normal activity of the colon have revealed a low level of resting motility, consisting almost entirely of uncoordinated segmental wave-like contractions, chiefly of circular muscle. Since these contractions are slightly more vigorous in the distal than in the proximal colon, they serve well the apparent purpose of the organ to delay the passage of its contents. After feeding or the injection of neostigmine, the amplitude and frequency of these contractile waves are notably increased. For brief periods and at long intervals, these patterns are abruptly replaced by the appearance of strong contractions of the proximal colon (i.e., anywhere between the cecum and the splenic flexure), which, coincident with the marked suppression of phasic contractions in the more distal bowel, bring about propulsion. The term mass peristalsis, originally applied to this phenomenon by radiologists observing the barium-filled colon, is no longer used because of evidence that the zone of strong contraction usually does not move progressively toward the anus. Such propulsive activity usually follows ingestion of a meal and an earlier period of heightened phasic activity, but has been induced experimentally by injection of acetylcholine or methacholine.[8] Although this has been the only motility pattern consistently identified with the passage of solid or liquid feces, it is apparent from manometric and cineradiographic observations that the passage of flatus requires only minor shifts in wave-like activity resulting in small pressure differentials between adjacent segments of the colon.[9]

Because the proximal colon is inaccessible to most recording procedures, most of the motility records on which our conceptions of disordered motility are based have been obtained from the sigmoid and lower descending colon. In such records, the resting motility of patients with "spastic colon" or "spastic constipation" has been marked by increased amplitude and frequency of contractions, and that of patients with painless diarrhea has shown marked reduction in wave-like motility.[10] These relationships have, for obvious reasons, been summed up in the phrase "paradoxical motility,"[11] although it is clear that these reactions of the sigmoid are well suited to the establishment of gradients of motor activity favorable, respectively, to the retention or propulsion of luminal contents.

Such studies of the motility of the colon have nevertheless failed to reveal a *qualitative* difference from the normal in the patterns of patients with irritable colon. Except for modest differences in the average total amount of wave-like activity in the resting state, and in the amplitude of contractions induced by neostigmine, there has been no indication that the motility is *quantitatively* outside the range of normal. It would appear that the pathophysiology can best be studied in the patient during the actual experience of emotional conflict.

For more than a century the temporal association of the symptoms of irritable colon with periods of emotional conflict has been recorded by numerous clinical observers, and more recently the regularity of these coincidences has been impressively documented. In the last few years, the frequency with which patients with irritable colon have been beset by stressful life situations,[12-14] generally considered to be productive of emotional tension, has been shown to be significantly greater than that of a control population in a well designed epidemiological study.[15]

The clinical hypothesis that these emotionally charged life situations are etiologically related to the disordered function of the colon has been tested in the laboratory by means of the *stress interview* experiment.[5] With suitable methods in use for the continuous recording of colonic motility, patients with irritable colon have been interviewed in the laboratory, first in a pleasant and sympathetic manner on topics believed to be neutral or nonthreatening, and then in a challenging manner on topics considered to be emotionally disturbing in the light of the patient's history. Little attempt is made to judge his subconscious attitudes and feelings; but from his speech, facial expressions, gestures, and visible signs of autonomic stimulation the intensity and quality of emotional reaction are noted and compared from moment to moment with ongoing changes in colonic motility. Correlations of two kinds have been observed:

1. The association of "coping" behavior (with expressed hostility, defensive attitudes, and feelings of self-sufficiency) with heightened sigmoid contractions (Fig. 100–1). These feeling states and this behavior have most often been identified clinically with patients having the symptoms of spastic colon, and the recorded change in motility of the colon is compatible with present conceptions of the mechanisms of constipation and colonic pain.

2. The association of "giving up" behavior (with expressions of helplessness, depression, grief, guilt, and feelings of per-

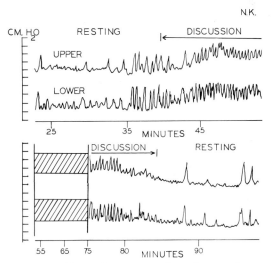

Figure 100–1. During recording of sigmoid motility by tandem balloons, the stress interview gives rise to heightened frequency and amplitude of phasic contractions, in association with expressed feelings of hostility and resentment. (From Almy, T. P., et al.: Proc. Assn. Res. Nerv. Ment. Dis. 29:724, 1950.)

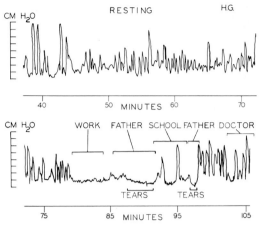

Figure 100–2. Sigmoid motility recording from single balloon. After a baseline period of irregular but continuous phasic contractions, the interview on subjects of personal significance led to suppression of wave-like activity, expressed feelings of depression, guilt, and hopelessness, and two distinct periods of weeping. (From Almy, T. P., et al.: Proc. Assn. Res. Nerv. Ment. Dis. 29:724, 1950.)

sonal inadequacy) with diminution of sigmoid contractions (Fig. 100–2). The most objective and clear-cut correlation, with dramatic implications for the "specificity" of emotional coloring, is that of sigmoid hypomotility with overt weeping. These moods have often been observed clinically in patients with painless diarrhea, and the associated hypomotility of the sigmoid is, of course, compatible with present ideas of the mechanism of diarrhea and the concept of "paradoxical motility" of the distal colon (see above).

These opposite reaction patterns could well be thought of as beyond the range of normal colonic function, each reflecting an inherent potentiality of the individual patient affected, much as grand mal seizures and petit mal seizures are differing products of the cerebral dysrhythmia characteristic of idiopathic epilepsy. Such is not the case; for there are many patients with irritable colon who manifest clinically the rapid alternation of constipation and diarrhea, and in the "stress interview" setting the patterns of "hypermotility" and "hypomotility" of the sigmoid have appeared sequentially in the same patient. In each instance they have seemed to correlate with the mood of the subject at the time, as these moods rapidly fluctuated. Thus it is likely that the disturbances of colonic

function are *bodily reflections of emotional states*, and not ingrained manifestations of a fixed personality type or a disordered nervous system.

This conception is reinforced by a number of observations made on the colonic function of healthy persons under stress. As mentioned above (p. 1278), it is well within the normal experience to have brief periods of constipation, diarrhea, and/or abdominal pain under conditions of special stress; these are perhaps best recognized among military personnel and medical students, because of their readily available medical surveillance. Using at times the same methods of study of sigmoid motility, but more commonly the technique of prolonged proctoscopic observation, the reactions of the normal sigmoid to experimentally induced general stress have been shown to include marked increase in motility (to the point of occlusive spasm), marked hyperemia, and excessive mucous secretion. Although the stresses most commonly applied have been physicochemical (painful stimulation, hypoglycemia), such changes have been shown to accompany spontaneous and experimentally contrived emotional conflict, in which the circumstances were disturbing only because of the attitudes and previous experience of the subject.[5]

The overall conclusion derived from these findings has been that the disturbances of colonic function characteristic of the irritable colon are *normal bodily manifestations of emotional tension*, analogous to sweating, facial flushing, and weeping. The patients with irritable colon thus represent one end of the curve of normal distribution of experiences of this sort, differing from the normal only in the greater intensity or duration of their disorder. The intensification of the disturbance may be due to the now well documented increase in frequency of their life stress experiences,[15] and/or the capacity to be more easily aroused or feel threatened (neurosis). Until recently it has been difficult to suggest how the colon appears to be "selected" as an organ of expression of emotional conflicts in these patients, whereas others react to similar stresses with clinical disorders of the skin, the bronchi, and the vascular system. It now seems at least probable that colonic reactions to threats productive of emotional tension represent an example of the operant conditioning, or "learning," of visceral responses through the neurophysiologic mechanisms of reward (or in clinical terms, secondary gain) dating from early life.[16] Thus a child who obtained sympathy and solicitude from her mother only when her stools were loose may have unconsciously learned to use this mechanism to resolve her emotional conflicts in adult life. At this time the application of these well documented neurophysiological principles to the pathogenesis of irritable colon must be considered tentative, but may serve as a useful guiding hypothesis.

Secondary Factors. It is obvious that the intensity or the time of occurrence of the intestinal symptoms attributed here mainly to psychophysiological mechanisms can be influenced by many other stimuli impinging on the gut. Chemical or physical irritation by laxatives, condiments, seasoned food, or coarse roughage may aggravate or precipitate symptoms, as may ingestion of cold liquids. Fermentation of undigested carbohydrates of milk, beans, and other foods may cause distention or diarrhea. Previous or intercurrent infectious enteritis or colitis may radically alter the reactivity of the colon. The practical aspects of these etiological factors are discussed below.

DIAGNOSIS AND DIFFERENTIAL DIAGNOSIS

The diagnosis of irritable colon and its differentiation from other disorders is one of the most complex clinical problems in gastroenterology. Each of the symptoms and signs can be produced by a variety of other conditions affecting the intestinal tract or other organ systems. A proper diagnosis is based upon three steps:

1. Identification of a symptom complex with a natural history compatible with irritable colon; in view of the great variability of the clinical picture, this requirement is easy to satisfy.

2. Recognition of the coincidence of symptomatic episodes with periods of life stress and emotional tension, a step often performed with insufficient accuracy.

3. A search for other disease processes

which may explain the symptoms; the exclusion of other diagnoses.

In the positive recognition of the syndrome of irritable colon, the three most reliable indices are the presence of lower abdominal pain, small stools, and the variable intensity of symptoms over time; yet the absence even of these features is compatible with the diagnosis. On the other hand, onset of the disorder in old age, the steady progression of symptoms from the time of onset, frequent nocturnal symptoms, fever, weight loss, rectal bleeding, or evident steatorrhea are features which weigh heavily against this diagnosis. Very severe pain, constipation, or distention is *not* incompatible with this diagnosis. The findings of labile pulse and blood pressure; sweating of hands, feet, and axillae; palpable firm sigmoid colon; and abdominal tympany and distention are common.

Sigmoidoscopy often (but not always) reveals moderate to marked engorgement of the mucosa, excessive secretion of mucus, and increased muscular contraction strong enough to occlude the lumen. Bleeding, friability, granularity, and ulceration are absent. The changes seen here may also be found, however, in patients with specific enteric infections, diverticulitis, colonic cancer at a level just above the visualized portion of the bowel, or Crohn's disease of the colon; furthermore, they may be produced in healthy persons by soapsuds enemas, or by the anxiety and embarrassment attending the procedure itself—hence they are by no means diagnostic.

Barium enema X-ray may reveal rapid filling, diffuse narrowing, and increased segmentation or corrugation of the distal colon,[17] or, alternatively, absent haustration in the same area. These findings acquire greater validity if the preparation for the X-rays has involved only saline enemas, as they may be readily produced by laxatives, soapsuds enemas, or instillation of barium at low temperatures or under high pressure.

The search for coincidences between life stress and emotional tension and the colonic symptoms requires that the physician obtain an extensive, painstaking personal history. A simple biographical inquiry, with dates of major life events and

TABLE 100–1. EXAMPLE OF LIFE CHART (E. L. – FEMALE, 36)

AGE	LIFE SITUATION	BOWEL FUNCTION
13–20	Home, father dead, dominating mother	Constipated irregularly, given castor oil
20–23	Nursing training, living near home	Steadily constipated
23–30	Private duty, public health nursing, away from home; 1939 (age 28) mother ill and died	"So regular," except in 1939
30–36	Worked as anesthetist	Severely constipated

changes in social, marital, or economic status, is best, if coupled with the avoidance of leading questions and careful observation for signs of emotion and other nonverbal cues to the significance of matters under discussion. The results are most useful if displayed in the form of a *life chart* (Table 100–1). It must be emphasized that the purpose is not simply to record the time of occurrence of a number of events commonly regarded as stressful (death of father, loss or change of job, divorce, retirement, etc.), but rather to understand which alterations in life status had the most profound meaning *to the patient.* This subjective judgment is at once the most demanding, potentially the most misleading, and by all odds the most *productive* element in the clinical management of the irritable colon. Thus the formulation of the irritable colon as a bodily manifestation of emotional tension has very practical implications for the diagnosis of this condition.

The *differential diagnosis* covers an extremely broad front. So variable is the symptomatology that the full range of possible explanations for *each symptom* should be thought of. Major sources of diagnostic confusion are presented here:

1. Other colonic disorders and diseases: early ulcerative colitis, Crohn's disease, carcinoma, and diverticular disease.

2. Diseases caused by specific microbial agents: shigellosis, salmonellosis, other bacterial enterocolitis (including that caused by *Escherichia coli* producing endotoxin, *Staphylococcus aureus,* and *Proteus* species), amebiasis, giardiasis, strongyloidiasis, and schistosomiasis.

3. Intestinal lactase deficiency.

4. Other causes of abdominal pain, especially intermittent mechanical intestinal obstruction, gallbladder disease, hiatus hernia, angina pectoris, "abdominal an-

gina" (midgut ischemia), porphyria, and tabetic and pseudotabetic crises.

5. Other causes of constipation, such as habitual constipation, fecal impaction, megacolon, hypothyroidism, hyperparathyroidism, scleroderma, and constipating drugs or medications.

6. Other causes for diarrhea, such as steatorrhea, bowel resection, fecal impaction, Addison's disease, Graves' disease, metastatic carcinoid syndrome, and untoward effects of reserpine or other drugs.

A recommended routine for the diagnostic work-up of these patients is included in the section on management (p. 1285). Further details on the diagnosis of the conditions listed above should be sought in appropriate chapters of this and other textbooks.

Since disordered colonic function under stress has been shown to be an apparent characteristic of all human beings, it is not surprising to find the syndrome of irritable colon in association with diseases of the intestinal tract or other organ systems having a totally different etiology. The diagnostic problem then becomes one of assigning to the "functional" and to the "organic" disease their proper respective importance in the total clinical picture, and to each the proper priority in treatment. Illustrative examples follow:

Mrs. T. T., aged 40, had been a disturbed child with persistent enuresis in childhood, and led an emotionally turbulent marital life, during which she was steadily constipated. Dull and persistent pain in the right upper quadrant led to discovery of gallstones by X-ray; but over a five-year period cholecystectomy and two surgical explorations of the common bile duct gave no relief. Sympathetic management of her family problems brought partial relief of both pain and constipation. It seemed likely that the gallstone disease played a minor, and the irritable colon a major, role in her total illness.

Miss E. F., aged 19, had been for a year the mistress of an extremely jealous man who flogged her on slight provocation. Beginning two years earlier, while in a reform school, she had had persistent constipation and pain in the left lower quadrant. Symptomatic and supportive therapy was unavailing. Discovery of *Entamoeba histolytica* cysts in her stools and antiamebic therapy led promptly to relief of her symptoms, despite continued emotional crises. It seemed likely that the irritable colon was a minor, and the amebiasis a major, factor in her colonic disorder.

Thus it is extremely important to consider that more than one condition may be affecting the colon at any one time. Otherwise the patient is exposed to two risks. The more obvious risk is the delayed diagnosis and treatment of a more serious disease, such as carcinoma of the sigmoid colon. Less obvious, but still significant, is the false hope of cure through specific medication or surgical extirpation of various organs in a patient whose psychophysiological disorder goes untreated for too long.

MANAGEMENT

The recognition of the disordered bowel function in irritable colon as a normal bodily accompaniment of emotional tension sets a high priority, in therapy, on helping the patient cope with life stresses. The procedure recommended above for the routine taking of a personal and social history, *beginning with the first visit* and leading to the construction of a life chart, results in a body of specific information by which the effort to assist the patient in his life adjustment can be guided.

The several visits required for the completion of studies necessary in differential diagnosis provide ample opportunity for discussion of these topics, which should never be insisted upon until the patient indicates his confidence in the physician and his willingness to divulge his inner feelings. In nearly all patients it is desirable to perform the following minimum of diagnostic studies, after complete history and physical examination, in the order named:

1. Complete blood count and sedimentation rate.

2. Sigmoidoscopy and anoscopy without preparation, at which time mucus or fecal material adherent to the bowel wall (or any visible exudate) is cultured for pathogenic bacteria and examined for amebae by warm stage examination.

3. One or two stool specimens for culture and examination for amebae and other parasites (using concentration methods for parasites if the stool is formed).

4. Repeat sigmoidoscopy with enema preparation, if on the earlier attempt the view was obscured by feces.

5. Barium enema, including "spot films" of the sigmoid and cecum.

6. In the patient with diarrhea, upper gastrointestinal series, with small bowel films to include the lower ileum.

7. In the patient with diarrhea or bloating as a prominent symptom, lactose tolerance test.

The *critical phase* of the management, which then follows, is the formulation and explanation to the patient of the nature of his disorder, and the projection of a general plan of treatment and of the expected results. To be successful, the physician will have had to indicate by his straightforward and repeated inquiry into the patient's life situations and feeling states that these are a legitimate part of his concern, and that the absence of positive findings diagnostic of other forms of illness will not diminish his therapeutic interest. The patient, after all, cares far less about the diagnosis than the therapy and the prognosis; and those who have already consulted one or several physicians may have been told that "It's only your nerves," or been given simplistic formulations of "mind over matter," together with indications that their doctors are less qualified or interested to help than if some other disorder were found. In other words, the diagnosis of irritable colon must not appear to imply a *rejection* by the physician.

A further prerequisite at this stage is a reasonable estimate of *prognosis* and a clear definition of reasonable goals in therapy. These judgments should be primarily based, as earlier suggested by White and colleagues,[12, 13] on the *natural history* of the disorder. Those patients whose symptoms have shown a close temporal relationship to periods of easily recognizable life stress, such as might be expected to disturb the average individual, and who have been free of bowel symptoms in periods of relative tranquillity, can be considered *less neurotic* and assigned a better long-term prognosis. Although they cannot be assured that the symptoms will not recur, the probability of recurrence will be the likelihood of the return of *major* loss, hardship, or frustration. Those who, on the other hand, have had more continuous symptoms, whose sources of emotional tension lie in situations tolerated quite well by the average individual, or who have shown little or no capacity for improvement when life's challenges abate, can be considered *more neurotic* and as having a poor long-term prognosis.

A secondary indication of prognosis is afforded by the *nature* of the predominant symptoms. As mentioned previously, the observed association of pain and constipation with "coping" behavior of the patient assigns to such symptoms a weight in favor of the less neurotic group, whereas the correlation of diarrhea with "giving up" attitudes and behavior links it generally with the more neurotic group. When the estimates based on the natural history and the nature of the symptoms do not correspond, however, the former should be weighted the more heavily.* Although both groups can be assured of a normal average life span and normal expectation of physical disability, the achievement of complete remission of symptoms, independent of an indefinitely continuing supportive effort by the physician, is generally unattainable in the more neurotic group.

The treatment of a "less neurotic" patient begins with straightforward reassurance as to the absence of potentially disabling or life-threatening disease and a clear explanation of his symptoms as bodily reflections of emotional tension. The common fear of cancer can be met with the statement that after his diagnostic work-up his chances of ever having a neoplasm are *less* than that of the average citizen. He may be confused as to the differences between "mucous colitis" and ulcerative colitis, or he may view his self-awareness of emotional conflicts as a harbinger of insanity or "nervous breakdown." His rejec-

tion of these ideas and his acceptance of a psychophysiological formulation are helped by a careful discussion with him of his life chart, and a review in layman's terms of the evidence indicating that disordered bowel function is a normal bodily accompaniment of emotional tension. The analogy to the meaning of weeping, flushed face, hair standing on end, and so forth is usually not difficult for him to grasp.

The patient can thus be motivated to join his doctor in a search for remedies in (1) the alteration of the stressful environment and (2) the alteration of his attitudes toward this environment. Temporary changes of scene (e.g., vacations, separation from spouse) are advised only when it is clear they are needed to develop constructive long-term solutions; otherwise the end of such a period can be as troublesome as the withdrawal of steroids, opiates, or any other potent therapeutic agent. Complex social problems may call for the interviewing of or correspondence with interested members of the family, employers, or military authorities, all with the understanding and encouragement of the patient, and often with the aid of trained social workers. The patient's attitudes toward current life stresses will have begun to change from the moment he has been relieved of secondary anxieties about disabling illness, has recognized that he can for a time be dependent upon his physician, and has been given the opportunity to ventilate his feelings. This process is extended and reinforced through the scheduling of the next few appointments at relatively short intervals, and the invitation to telephone for advice if symptoms are severe. By continued ventilation to the physician, the patient begins to realize that release of his feelings through discussion with family and friends may be helpful, and it can be suggested that his feelings be sublimated into active sports, games, or avocations appropriate for his physical makeup and social role. Those which symbolize and stylize aggressive behavior or physical assault (golf, squash, bowling, woodchopping, and even bridge!) are most useful. The positive reassurance as to physical health inherent in the encouragement to work for greater physical fitness is itself a major therapeutic

---

*The well documented contrary conclusions of Chaudhary and Truelove[14] are believed to be due to differences in the cultural setting of the patients studied and in the therapeutic methods employed.

measure. All these resources are within the capacity of the primary contact physician and the usual community medical and social agencies. Referral of a patient in the less neurotic group to a psychiatrist is often a disadvantage, unless it is clear to both patient and primary physician that a powerful unconscious motivation exists.

The more neurotic patient also needs strong and continued reassurance as to the absence of potential physical disability; the occurrence of similar psychophysiological reactions in healthy persons should be emphasized. The patient should not be pressed, however, to gain insight into the origin of his critical emotional conflicts, unless and until a long period of marked symptomatic improvement has been obtained. Emphasis is placed instead upon alteration of the environment, most often with the interest and intervention of family and social workers, and on the continued sympathetic, supportive, uncritical attitude of the primary physician. This protective role is enhanced by detailed advice on the temporary relief of symptoms (see below) and by the judicious use of placebos—for most of these patients, the most appropriate placebo is a mild sedative or an anticholinergic drug in minimal doses, e.g., phenobarbital, 15 mg, or tincture of belladonna, 10 drops three times daily. Standard doses of rapidly acting barbiturates (e.g., sodium pentobarbital, 0.050 to 0.100 g) or other sedatives may be required for sleep or at times for urgent daytime sedation, as in other states of emotional tension. Recently, uncontrolled but well conducted studies have indicated the effectiveness of major tranquilizers (such as chlorpromazine) or antidepressant agents (such as amitriptyline) in therapeutically difficult cases of irritable colon.[18] The use of such agents should be guided by balancing the frequency of toxic reactions characteristic of each against the degree of disability experienced by a given patient with this usually benign illness. In most instances the indication for their use will be the degree of anxiety and depression rather than the intensity of the associated intestinal symptoms. On theoretical grounds, centrally acting mood-regulating agents should be the most helpful of all drugs in such cases, and

further research in this area is needed. Referral of the more neurotic patient to a psychiatrist is desirable if feasible, and if accompanied by assurances that either the primary contact physician or the psychiatrist will be prepared to maintain continuing and total responsibility for his care.

Symptomatic relief for the patient, which is usually required prior to the completion of the general measures referred to above, includes attention to the diet, medication, and physical therapy. Detailed instruction in a palatable, moderately restricted, low residue *diet* offers the more neurotic patient a useful ritual, but gives to the less neurotic patient little comfort in exchange for distracting him from more important factors in his illness. In any case it should exclude only strong seasoning and vegetables and fruits known to cause distention and excessive flatus (e.g., onions, cooked cabbage, navy beans, and melons). Other food intolerances reported by the patient should be respected but later subjected to direct testing when symptoms are at a minimum, lest the range of dietary choice be permanently and unnecessarily limited. The testing of milk intolerance, both with whole milk and with the lactose tolerance test, is particularly important. The aim should be a diet which does not prevent the patient from eating easily in restaurants or the homes of friends. Cold liquids and carbonated beverages should be prohibited at times of severe symptoms, and coffee should be disallowed in the presence of diarrhea. Alcoholic drinks at a concentration of 20 per cent or less, taken in moderation, can usually be allowed or even encouraged if they contribute in the overall to the relaxation of emotional tension.

Physical measures, familiar in the ancient armamentarium of psychiatry, may occasionally be employed to advantage. Regular periods of rest during the day, if prescribed by the physician, may not only prevent undue fatigue but also combat the use of compulsive and masochistic behavior in the resolution of guilt feelings. Tepid showers or tubs, swimming, sunbathing, or massage if available may permit relaxation with less or no use of drugs. The application of a hot water bottle or heating pad to the abdomen or the use of a lukewarm tap water enema may give prompt relief from severe colonic pain.

Medication for the direct control of bowel motility has a definite place in therapy, but is best used sparingly and (apart from placebo effects) is not highly effective. Agents useful in the treatment of constipation, along with the general management of that problem, are discussed on pages 323 to 325 and 409 to 410. Pain not responsive to rest, local heat, hydrotherapy, enemas, and sedatives will usually require standard doses of meperidine hydrochloride (Demerol), although an anticholinergic agent, e.g., propantheline (Pro-Banthine), 15 to 30 mg, or tridihexethyl (Pathilon), 25 to 50 mg, may be effective. Opiates should *not* be used, because they are spasmogenic and addictive, two hazards to which these patients are unusually susceptible.

The patient with diarrhea should be advised to avoid cold drinks, to take liquids only before or between meals, and to lie down after meals if possible. The usual binding agents (kaolin, bismuth, pectin, and aluminum hydroxide) are usually ineffective; but *anticholinergics* in the doses recommended above, which should be sufficient to dry the mouth and interfere temporarily with near vision and with emptying of the bladder, commonly afford some relief. More reliably effective is diphenoxylate (Lomotil), 5 to 10 mg, which shares the mechanism of action of opiates but is less addictive. It is wise to limit the use of these agents to the hours of the day when diarrhea will be a particular inconvenience, in order to prevent overuse and tachyphylaxis. The aim should *not* be the *complete* control of loose movements by medication alone.

All measures of treatment of irritable colon have been troublesome to evaluate because of differing criteria for the diagnosis, varying natural history of the disorder in individual patients, and the infrequent and difficult employment of controlled trials. Without discounting in any way the future possibilities of improved pharmacotherapy in this disorder, there are few conditions in medicine so prevalent and so economically important in which the patience and the humanistic interest of the physician count for so much.

REFERENCES

1. Almy, T. P. Digestive disease as a national problem. II. A white paper by the American Gastroenterological Association. Gastroenterology 53:821, 1967.
2. Almy, T. P. Basic considerations in the study of abdominal pain, and medical diseases of the abdomen and its parietes. *In* The Differential Diagnosis of Abdominal Pain, S. M. Mellinkoff (ed.). New York, McGraw-Hill Book Co., 1959.
3. Connell, A. M., Jones, F. A., and Rowlands, E. N. Motility of the pelvic colon. IV. Abdominal pain associated with colonic hypermotility after meals. Gut 6:105, 1965.
4. Dworkin, H., Biel, F. J., and Machella, T. E. Supradiaphragmatic reference of pain from the colon. Gastroenterology 22:222, 1952.
5. Almy, T. P. Experimental studies on the "irritable colon." Amer. J. Med. 10:60, 1951.
6. Chaudhary, N. A., and Truelove, S. C. Human colonic motility: Comparative study of normal subjects, patients with ulcerative colitis and patients with the irritable colon syndrome. Gastroenterology 40:1, 1961.
7. Wangel, A. G., and Deller, D. J. Intestinal motility in man. Gastroenterology 48:69, 1965.
8. Kern, F., and Almy, T. P. The effects of acetylcholine and methacholine upon the human colon. J. Clin. Invest. 31:555, 1952.
9. Ritchie, J. A., Ardran, G. M., and Truelove, S. C. Motor activity of the sigmoid colon of humans; a combined study by intraluminal pressure recording and cineradiography. Gastroenterology 43:642, 1962.
10. Almy, T. P., Kern, F., Jr., and Abbot, F. K. Constipation and diarrhea, as reactions to life stress. Life stress and bodily disease. Proc. Assn. Res. Nerv. Ment. Dis. 29:724, 1950.
11. Connell, A. M. The motility of the pelvic colon. II: Paradoxical motility in diarrhea and constipation. Gut 3:342, 1962.
12. White, B. V., Cobb, S., and Jones, C. M. Mucous colitis. Psychosomatic Med., Monograph No. 1, 1939.
13. White, B. V., and Jones, C. M. Mucous colitis. Ann. Intern. Med. 14:854, 1940.
14. Chaudhary, N. A., and Truelove, S. C. The irritable colon syndrome. Quart. J. Med. 31:307, 1962.
15. Mendeloff, A. I., Monk, M., Siegel, C. I., et al. Illness experience and life stresses in patients with irritable colon and with ulcerative colitis. An epidemiologic study of ulcerative colitis and regional enteritis in Baltimore, 1960-1964. New Eng. J. Med. 282:14, 1970.
16. Miller, N. E. Learning of visceral and glandular responses. Science 163:434, 1969.
17. Lumsden, K., Chaudhary, N. A., and Truelove, S. C. The irritable colon syndrome. Clin. Radiol. 14:54, 1963.
18. Hislop, I. G. Psychological significance of the irritable colon syndrome. Gut 12:452, 1971.

Chapter 101

Irritable Colon in Children

Murray Davidson

INTRODUCTION

The irritable colon syndrome often affects individuals throughout life, beginning at birth. Our experience with longitudinal observation of children indicates that it masquerades under a variety of appellations and that the nature and intensity of symptoms vary at different ages. The newborn with colic, the toddler with nonspecific diarrhea, "pseudoceliac disease," or "starch intolerance," and the older child with recurrent abdominal pain all represent instances of the irritable colon syndrome. Any psychosomatic concept of the genesis of this problem which rests solely on the thesis that only sustained, prolonged, conscious or unconscious unresolved emotional conflict may evoke the colonic symptoms[1, 2] or that functional symptoms are restricted to colons which have undergone prolonged preconditioning[3, 4] could not, on present evidence, constitute a unifying hypothesis for pathogenesis of the disorder in children, certainly during infancy. As noted on page 1281, a good deal more data are available to support a strong role for emotional factors in adults with irritable colon whose periods of conflict are prolonged. Nonetheless, infants may respond to brief, daily conflict with constipation. Familial influences may be both genetic and cultural. It is thus reasonable to propose that the irritable colon syndrome is a lifelong condition, symptoms of which may be manifested at any age.

PATHOPHYSIOLOGY

Irrespective of the net interchanges of fluid resulting from secretion and absorption throughout the gastrointestinal tract, the distal colon receives a relatively fluid residue. Were this not so, material would tend occasionally to become inspissated in the more proximal colon and in the small bowel. Final desiccation of the gastrointestinal contents takes place in the rectum and rectosigmoid segments, wherein the motility patterns demonstrate a predominance of tonus waves. Unreported observations from our laboratory indicate a direct relationship between the incidence of tonus activity in this distal segment and the rate of water absorption. Constipated children consistently demonstrate increased distal colonic tonus activity, and they have been shown to absorb larger than normal amounts of water from the rectum.[5] It is our concept that the individual who is genetically predisposed to the irritable colon is basically one with a tendency to constipation. Childhood constipation is genetic in origin.[6] Studies of children with the irritable colon showed very strong family histories of functional bowel disorders.[7, 8] The question may be raised as to whether these high familial incidences may not point equally to conditioning factors. However, the very early onset of symptoms in some infants tends to militate against this point of view.

Under various conditions, including periods of anxiety and emotional tension,

1289

children with increased tonus of this lower colonic segment, i.e., constipated individuals, may suffer further increase in tonus to the point that the area becomes virtually completely shut and unable to accept material for desiccation from more proximal areas. In this spastic state, colonic contents accumulate more proximally in the descending colon and upper sigmoid. A number of symptoms may result from this condition. The acute colonic distention may induce pain, primarily referable to the periumbilical area, which represents the cutaneous nerve distribution of the colonic embryonic somites. Passage of stool may be difficult, painful, and explosive through the spastic segment. The material passed will reflect rapid passage through the lower segment, consisting of water, mucus, and undigested vegetable fibers. The pathophysiological picture may thus tend to produce different symptoms at different times. Why certain findings predominate at specific ages is not precisely clear. Predisposed children pass through all the clinical pictures at the appropriate ages, although they may not be overly troubled with clinically reportable problems at each stage.

CLINICAL PICTURE

NEONATE

In the young infant, the normal feeding mechanism is associated with swallowing of air. If the air is not raised from the stomach with burping, it usually traverses the gastrointestinal tract and passes as flatus per rectum. Infants suffering from colic have difficulty in passing colonic gas. On rectal examination such babies usually demonstrate a "tight" spastic segment. In a very comprehensive clinical and laboratory study of this subject, Jorup showed that these infants exhibit excessive rectal tonus activity to explain this clinical sign.[9] The finding often presages constipation, which may be symptomatic from birth or which may become apparent later, along with other functional gastrointestinal problems. When the colicky infant is fed in the recumbent position, air traverses the pylorus more easily and greater quantities of intestinal gas accumulate which are not easily discharged through the spastic lower segment. Colonic distention and severe abdominal pain with drawing up of the legs result. Young infants generally relieve discomfort by sucking and feeding, and they are not aware that this "hungry" response to offers of food will be misinterpreted by parents as evidence of need for further feedings. Thus, a vicious symptom cycle is set up in response to crying, and most colicky infants are characterized as being excessively hungry. Frequent feedings with increases in intestinal air and stimulation of the gastrocolic reflex lead to the nightmare which this condition often represents. The appearance of the stools is totally confusing, because they may be alternately infrequent or numerous, vary from small to large, and be hard or watery and explosive as explained by the pathophysiology. With looser stools, multiple formula changes are made to no avail and to the further confusion and anxiety of parents and physicians.

Stress should be laid in treatment on feeding in the upright (sitting) position and on careful burping to prevent as much swallowed air as possible from entering the intestines. Feedings should be limited to no more than 20 minutes of sucking, with frequent interruptions for adequate burping. Once colicky symptoms result the baby should not be fed, but instead should be given aid for removal of accumulated gas by warm baths and rectal insertion of a glycerine suppository or thermometer, the tip of which is well lubricated with Vaseline. Antispasmodic agents and sedatives are of considerably less value than kindness and understanding in support of the worried parents.

The colicky infant usually loses his symptoms by three months of age, although stubborn cases may persist until six months. Infants who have been colicky often pass infrequent, small, scybalum-like stools beyond three months of age, indicating the relationship of the early symptoms to constipation.

LATER INFANCY AND TODDLER PERIOD

Toward the end of the first year of life, children with the irritable colon syndrome develop a different clinical picture.[7, 10]

Alternating with their constipation, they suffer symptoms reminiscent of the adult with the "spastic" colon. Material often fails to enter the lower segment for final desiccation, and there is dyskinesia between the distal descending colon and upper sigmoid, which act as repositories for the residue, and the contracted lower segment. Discomfort may result from the distention, with increase in borborygmi and hyperactive peristalsis. Ultimately, as the pressure head of the trapped material rises, loose stool is forcefully expelled in varying amounts. In addition to the fact that it is unformed, the stool contains mucus and undigested vegetable fibers, is laden with microscopically demonstrable starch, and often has a sickening odor which is more characteristic of upper intestinal contents.

The timing and character of stools which are passed at this time often follow a very characteristic daily pattern. During the relaxed sleep period rectal spasm is usually lessened, and stool which entered the segment would become excessively dry. This material would be passed in the initial movement, which may therefore be entirely formed, or will show formed stool at the head of the column. With subsequent increase in distal colonic spasm, the following bowel movements (often restricted to the earlier part of the day) are more characteristic of the trapped colonic contents, and the amount of formed material expelled with successive bowel movements decreases. If one focuses attention on what is in the diaper or toilet bowl, the condition may be viewed as "diarrhea." If, on the other hand, one focuses on the patient and his difficulty with expelling material and the discomfort he may experience just prior to and during the bowel movement, one might more properly visualize the condition as "constipation." The complex of symptoms is precisely that seen in the adult with the irritable colon.

In the adult with this syndrome there may be a clear-cut relationship between onset of increased spasm, loose stools, and periods of sustained emotional stress.[11] As noted, the applicability of the psychosomatic hypothesis to infants and young children is not so apparent. Young toddlers of the age group in which the irritable colon

of childhood is encountered are generally incapable of sufficient attention span to suffer from sustained emotional stress; however, *prolonged* unresolved conflict may not be necessary for an abnormal bowel habit. Persistent and unremitting physical stresses associated with the pain of teething and ear infections, or the discomfort experienced with other upper respiratory infections and with the mild diseases induced by inoculations, do not require the constant conscious attention of a child to induce states of heightened autonomic nervous system activity.

The pattern of loose stools has led to an alternative name, i.e., chronic nonspecific diarrhea.[12] Episodes are recurrent, lasting for a few days to a few weeks at a time until the child is about three and one-half years of age. During bouts of difficulty the stools range in number approximately from three to five daily. Although the stools usually contain a good deal of mucus, they usually do not contain any pus. Small amounts of rectal blood may occasionally be apparent from the trauma induced by the forceful passage of the stools. As many as 20 per cent of patients experience bleeding at one time or another.[7] The children tend to have a history of constipation prior to the onset of the condition and during the periods between the episodes of loose stools. Many become quite constipated after the problem disappears. There is a strong history of bowel complaints among other members of the family. Although there is often a strong prejudice that these symptoms are related to what is being ingested at the prior suggestion of physicians and others, treatment of the "diarrhea" with various constipating regimens and restrictive diets will not successfully control the symptoms.

Children with persistent irritable colon diarrhea who are ingesting starchy foods usually pass appreciable quantities of extracellular starch which can be demonstrated on microscopic examination of the specimens. Andersen quantitated the examination technique and added the interpretation that the degree of severity of "starch intolerance" was directly related to the amount of starch found.[13] Haas and Andersen and their coworkers therefore introduced the high protein diets which were restriced in starch and fat and which contained a few specific "magic" foods such as bananas that were presumably well tolerated by this group of children.[14-16] The finding of undigested starch in the stool has been demonstrated as not indicative of any disease.[17] Indeed, even normal children without diarrhea may pass appreciable amounts of undigested starch in their stools as do children with celiac disease. For many years a low starch diet was used in treating these children. The increased amount of starch which is demonstrable among patients with loose or frequent stools is of no pathogenetic significance. It is doubtful that such an entity as "starch intolerance" exists, because it has not been established as an identifiable disease by any currently employed laboratory or clinical test.

DIFFERENTIAL DIAGNOSIS

INFANCY AND TODDLER PERIOD

The therapeutic approach to irritable colon is based upon its proper diagnosis, and the physician must therefore be initially satisfied that he has ruled out the principal differential diagnostic possibilities. The two primary types of disorders with which the irritable colon of childhood may be confused are malabsorption syndrome and chronic low-grade enteric infections.

Since the diarrhea of the irritable colon of childhood usually begins at between six and 12 months of age at its earliest, malabsorption should be suspected whenever the history of persistent diarrhea starts earlier. This important feature of history must be ascertained carefully from many mothers who may be seeing a consultant for the first time when the child is one and one-half or two years of age. These women are naturally upset with the chronic difficulties of their children, tending to be impatient to get the history over with and to move on to the business of examination and diagnosis. The physician must therefore be careful in checking the history to ascertain the validity of such statements as: "The diarrhea has always been there."

Another important differential aspect associated with chronic malabsorption is failure to thrive. Many children with the irritable colon of childhood are average or above in weight gain. The weight curves of all patients should therefore be carefully checked. In the face of chronic underachievement or undesirable changes in growth patterns, a sweat test should be performed because the most common malabsorptive condition from which children suffer is cystic fibrosis of the pancreas. In the relatively rare instances in which history suggests significant malabsorption but the sweat electrolyte examination is normal, children should be "screened" with measurements of hematocrit, serum proteins, calcium, phosphate, carotene, and cholesterol concentrations. If any doubt exists, fecal fat must be measured (see p. 281). If these values are normal (including fecal fat), children may not be considered to suffer from fat or protein malabsorption (see pp. 280 to 289).

Primary (congenital) disaccharidase deficiencies may not affect weight gain in all instances, but would be associated with diarrhea. In such patients the diarrhea would be present from early in life, i.e., from the first encounter with ingestion of milk (lactose) or cane sugar (sucrose). A careful history is therefore important. It is doubtful that youngsters with primary lactase deficiency who were continued on mammalian milk formulas from birth could demonstrate normal rates of weight gain or would even survive to the age of onset of the symptoms associated with the irritable colon of childhood. The histories of children with this diagnosis would thus be expected to show that milk had been withdrawn early in life for diarrhea and that the diarrhea recurred when ingestion of lactose-containing materials (milk and milk products) had been restarted. Similarly, in the case of sucrase insufficiency the diarrhea would have begun at the time of introducing sucrose into the diet. This might be at birth from formula additives, or, more frequently, at the time of introduction of solid foods and fruits with added cane sugar. The children with congenital deficiencies of either disaccharidase have one or two explosive (fermentative) bowel movements within one to three hours after ingestion of the offending sugar. Investigation of such symptoms should be carried out as described on pages 1015 to 1028.

Another category of problems which may be confused with the irritable colon of childhood is persistent low grade chronic enteric infection. Low grade infection with salmonella or other chronic dysentery organisms is much more frequently at fault than protozoan parasites. Children are likely not to be suffering from irritable colon if microscopic examination of a smear from their stools reveals many white blood cells. The finding of pus cells is an indication for stool cultures.

LATER CHILDHOOD

Recurrent abdominal pain represents a common complaint among preschool and school age children, and estimates of incidence run as high as one in ten.[8, 18] An organic, treatable cause is infrequently found despite extensive investigation. The pediatrician often assumes therefore that the problem is a psychological one. However, such an attitude often erroneously stigmatizes the child as either a malingerer or one with school phobia, hysteria, or some other emotional aberration, without explaining the basis of the symptoms or offering any substantial therapeutic benefit.[18, 19]

Most physicians who have written on the subject point out that a majority of these children have mainly periumbilical cramping pain. Despite variable severity in different children, there is virtually never a history of being awakened from sleep or of associated systemic symptomatology, such as one might expect with an organic lesion. Frequently the pain is relieved with passage of flatus and/or with bowel movement. A clear history of constipation which would be consistent with these symptoms may be difficult to secure from the mother. Parents are frequently totally unaware of the bowel habits of their children beyond the age at which the children assume responsibility for their own toilet habits, and the children are not very likely to complain of mild degrees of bowel dysfunction to their parents. It is also important to appreciate that the degree of *symptomatic* constipation, i.e., infrequency of stool passage and retention of large amounts of stool, is not an important corollary to development of abdominal pain from trapping of flatus, as some investigators have concluded.[20]

The pain is less related to the amount of stool retained in the rectum at any time than it is to the degree of dyskinesia; i.e., the disproportion between distention of the proximal bowel by trapped material and the resultant involuntary efforts at propulsive activity in the descending colon versus the "cork-in-the-rectum" effect of distal spasm. Associated conditions which increase the amounts of accumulated gas may aggravate the situation to the point that irritable colon may not be considered the primary problem. For example, increased air swallowing associated with the nasal obstruction of an acute upper respiratory infection or chronic allergic state might be considered the principal cause for recurrent or acute abdominal pain. Symptoms may be aggravated by anxiety, which causes not only air swallowing but also greater distal spasm, and thus psychosomatic factors are emphasized. Excessive fermentation from legumes and similar foods, as well as from undigested carbohydrates, might also play a role in increased symptoms.[21]

TREATMENT

INFANCY AND THE TODDLER PERIOD

The most important feature of treatment for a child suffering from the irritable colon syndrome is a reassuring discussion with the parents.[7, 22] The normal physical development of most of these children should be emphasized to help the parents accept the fact that the symptoms do not reflect a malabsorptive state.

Proper management consists of attention to the entire child, not simply to the manner or frequency with which he manages to rid himself of excreta. The problem is not related to kinds of foods ingested and requires no special dietary management. Adherence to the restrictive, high protein, low fat, and simple sugar regimens often recommended imposes unnecessary emotional burdens on child and mother, and tends to be confusing if the symptoms recur despite exact observance of the prescribed regimen. Since patients virtually always come from families in which some other members, parents or siblings, are also affected by functional bowel complaints, acceptance of the explanation is frequently not difficult to achieve. Once reassured that the prognosis is excellent and that the symptoms will wax and wane without regard to food intake, parents are often relieved and content with little else prescribed.

It is our belief that prescription of drugs might minimize the therapeutic advantages gained from frank discussion and reassurance that the condition is not a "disease," and we therefore rarely prescribe them. However, in some instances, administration of sulfisoxazole (Gantrisin), 0.1 to 0.2 g per kilogram per day, has been reported to be of value.[14] Approximately 30 to 50 per cent of patients respond dramatically to 625 to 1875 mg of diiodohydroxyquin (Diodoquin) daily, divided into two or three doses.[12] However, the rationale for giving these drugs is vague, because evidence that enteric infection is the basis for the disorder is nonexistent.

Elimination of chilled fluids is suggested, because laboratory studies indicate that in these children, and in others with diarrheal tendencies, sudden introduction of cold material into the stomach may stimulate colonic propulsion and the urge to defecate.[23]

In virtually all patients the condition clears by three to three and one-half years of age and the children simply remain constipated, without the recurrent diarrheal episodes.

LATER CHILDHOOD

A valid approach to managing this condition in later childhood calls for a therapeutic test if the physician is reasonably certain from his history and examination that the patient suffers from constipation and the irritable colon syndrome. A battery of clinical and laboratory tests are most often not needed. In all instances we offer "excessive" amounts, i.e., 2 to 4 oz per 20 pounds of body weight daily, of an emollient such as mineral oil for a month to ensure adequate emptying of the distal colon. Acute episodes of pain are treated with warm baths or a heating pad. If there

is relief from the symptoms with this therapeutic trial, the youngster is subsequently managed with the stepwise retraining regimen described on page 1475. In addition, gas-producing foods are limited, but not eliminated if strongly desired, from the diet. The quantity of milk intake, if excessive, is curtailed for three reasons: (1) milk per se is a low residue food and may aggravate the tendency to constipation; (2) excessive intakes of this highly caloric food may reduce appetite for a more varied diet; and (3) it is possible that decreased titers of lactase activity may result in colonic fermentation of the undigested lactose.[21] However, it is important to limit intake but not totally to exclude it among those children who like milk and its products and who are not made ill and symptomatic by reasonable intakes.

Since many of these patients are predestined to experience symptoms of this condition during their adult lives, the attitude of the physician who treats them in childhood is an important one. If the doctor is not sufficiently aware and sympathetic to alleviate undue parental concern, or, worse, aggravates fears by excessive stress on either organic or serious psychological causes, the child may neither understand nor accept his symptoms for many decades of adult life. Similarly, if unnecessary dietary restrictions and manipulations are made and their importance emphasized, the physician may be unwittingly converting a potentially mildly symptomatic adult with the irritable colon syndrome who would otherwise function normally into a gastrointestinal neurotic and food faddist.

REFERENCES

1. White, B. V., and Jones, C. M. Mucous colitis: Delineation of syndrome with certain observations on its mechanism and on role of emotional tension as precipitating factor. Ann. Intern. Med. 14:854, 1940.
2. Chaudhary, N. A., and Truelove, S. C. The irritable colon syndrome. A study of the clinical features, predisposing causes and prognosis in 130 cases. Quart. J. Med. 31:307, 1962.
3. Freud, S. Heredity and aetiology of the neuroses. In Collected Papers, Vol. I. London, Hogarth, 1924, Chapters 14 and 16.
4. Prugh, D. H. Childhood experience and colonic disorders. Ann. N.Y. Acad. Sci. 58:355, 1954.
5. Ziskind, A., and Gellis, S. S. Water intoxication following tap-water enemas. A.M.A. J. Dis. Child. 96:699, 1958.

6. Bakwin, H., and Davidson, M. Constipation in twins. Amer. J. Dis. Child. *121*:179, 1971.
7. Davidson, M., and Wasserman, R. The irritable colon syndrome of childhood (chronic nonspecific diarrhea syndrome). Pediatrics *69*:1027, 1966.
8. Stone, R. T., and Barbero, G. J. Recurrent abdominal pain. Pediatrics *45*:732, 1970.
9. Jorup, S. Colonic hyperperistalsis in neurolabile infants; studies in so-called dyspepsia in breast-fed infants. Acta Paediat. Scand. *41*: Suppl. 85, 1952.
10. Davidson, M. Clinical conference: The celiac syndrome. Pediatrics *21*:508, 1958.
11. Prugh, D. H., and Schwachman, H. Observations of "unexplained" chronic diarrhea in early childhood. Amer. J. Dis. Child. *90*:496, 1955.
12. Cohlan, S. Q. Chronic nonspecific diarrhea in infants and children treated with diiodohydroxyquinoline. Pediatrics *18*:424, 1956.
13. Andersen, D. H. Celiac syndrome; relationship of celiac disease, starch intolerance and steatorrhea. J. Pediat. *30*:564, 1947.
14. Andersen, D. H., and Di Sant'Agnese, P. A. Idiopathic celiac disease. I. Mode of onset and diagnosis. Pediatrics *11*:207, 1953.
15. Di Sant'Agnese, P. A. Idiopathic celiac disease. II. Course and prognosis. Pediatrics *11*:224, 1953.
16. Haas, S. V., and Haas, M. P. Management of Celiac Disease. Philadelphia, J. B. Lippincott Co., 1951.
17. Davidson, M., and Bauer, C. H. The value of microscopic examination of the stool for extracellular starch in the diagnosis of starch intolerance. Pediatrics *21*:565, 1958.
18. Apley, J. The Child with Abdominal Pains. Oxford, Blackwell Scientific Publications, 1959.
19. Green, M. Recurrent abdominal pain. *In* Ambulatory Pediatrics, M. Green and R. J. Haggerty (eds.). Philadelphia, W. B. Saunders Co., pp. 225–228.
20. Dimson, S. B. Transit time related to clinical findings in children with recurrent abdominal pain. Pediatrics *47*:666, 1971.
21. Bayless, T. M., and Juang, S. S. Recurrent abdominal pain due to milk and lactose intolerance in school-aged children. Pediatrics *47*:1029, 1971.
22. Davidson, M. Nonspecific diarrhea. *In* Current Pediatric Therapy, Vol. 5, S. S. Gellis and B. M. Kagan (eds.). Philadelphia, W. B. Saunders Co., 1971, pp. 207–210.
23. Davidson, M., Sleisenger, M. H., Almy, T. P., and Levine, S. Z. Studies of distal colonic motility in children. II. Propulsive activity in diarrheal states. Pediatrics *17*:820, 1956.

Chapter 102

Ulcerative Colitis

James H. Meyer

Human ulcerative colitis is an inflammatory disease of unknown and possibly multiple causes, affecting principally the mucosa of the rectum and left colon but in many instances the entire organ; it is a chronic disease with remissions and exacerbations, characterized by rectal bleeding and diarrhea and appearing principally in youth and early middle age. It is a disease with serious local and systemic complications; therapy must be considered nonspecific, and life expectancy is reduced.

HISTORICAL ASPECTS

Ulcerative colitis was first described by Wilks and Moxon in 1875; it has been recognized with increasing frequency, particularly in the past two decades.[1] Its discovery was undoubtedly delayed by the tendency to believe all diarrheal illnesses to be a form of infectious dysentery. Its discoverers were the first therefore to clearly separate it from colitis caused by bacilli or parasites. Interestingly, for many decades it was considered a disease exclusively of Europe and North America; however, its incidence in South and Central America appears to be rising with its increasing recognition. Thus a recent report from Costa Rica indicates a prevalence rate of 1.6 per 100,000. Significantly, Costa Rica is a country with a high standard of living and

an excellent system for providing medical care on a large scale, in which rather complete and accurate epidemiologic data are recorded.

With the description of regional enteritis in the early 1930's by Crohn and his colleagues, separation of mucosal ulcerative colitis from granulomatous disease of the intestine appeared rather clear cut; the two diseases appeared to have distinct pathological features, and each affected a different organ system. Over the past four decades, a marked overlap has become clear not only pathologically but also in anatomic distribution. Thus transmural disease is found in the colon, particularly on the right side, but involving all segments, including the rectum. In many cases resected specimens may show features of both diseases, and in some specimens the findings are completely compatible with either diagnosis. Since etiology in both diseases is an unknown factor, the possibility exists that they share a common cause and result only from a difference of tissue reaction to the noxious agent.

EPIDEMIOLOGY

Earlier studies on the epidemiology of ulcerative colitis suffered from several defects: population areas were poorly defined; incidence and prevalence rates were derived by comparing patients hav-

1296

TABLE 102-1. EPIDEMIOLOGIC STUDIES IN ULCERATIVE COLITIS*

AREA STUDIED	YEARS OF STUDY	NUMBER OF CASES	PREVALENCE†	INCIDENCE†	RATIO, FEMALES: MALES
Copenhagen County	1961–1967	253	44.1	7.3	1.3:1
Oxford area	1951–1960	238	79.9	6.5	1.3:1
Baltimore County	1960–1963	177	–	5.2(female)	1.3:1
				3.9(male)	

*Modified from Bonneure, O., Riis, P., and Anthonsien, P.: Scand. J. Gastroent. 3:432, 1968.
†Per 100,000 general population.

ing ulcerative colitis with other hospitalized patients instead of total populations of the area; data were gathered from selected centers; or socioeconomic or ethnic data were not controlled against the normal population of the area. Impressions gained from these older studies were that the disease seems to be more prevalent in higher socioeconomic groups, among individuals who have positions of greater responsibility or who have achieved a higher degree of education, and among Jews. The disease was thought to be less common in rural than urban areas.

More recent studies (Table 102–1) have avoided the deficiencies of the earlier studies. Both the Oxford and Copenhagen studies attempted to survey both inpatient and outpatient cases within a well defined population area, whereas the Baltimore study identified all hospitalized cases (above age 20) within Baltimore County. Incidence rates (i.e., first diagnosis) from all three studies were comparable. Incidence rates were low below age 20; highest incidence rates were found in those in the third to sixth decades of life. The Oxford study found a bimodal incidence, with peaks in the third and fifth decades; although this was not seen in the other two studies, both also noted a relatively high incidence after age 50 (see p. 1323). Since up to 25 per cent of cases of ulcerative colitis may go undiagnosed for more than two years after the onset of symptoms, the higher prevalence noted in the Oxford study may relate to the longer duration of the study, allowing inclusion of some of the cases with delayed diagnosis.

Both the Oxford and Baltimore studies support the earlier impression of higher incidence among Jews. Incidence among nonwhites was considerably lower than among Caucasians in Baltimore. Although these ethnic-racial differences may partly reflect cultural differences in utilization of medical facilities, their magnitude (twice to four times the incidence in Jews vs. non-Jews, one-fourth the incidence in nonwhites vs. whites) suggests genetic rather than culturally determined differences. Thus, among army personnel in World War II, a situation in which failure to report symptomatic ulcerative colitis would be unlikely, the incidence of reported ulcerative colitis was higher among Jews than non-Jews.[2] No differences were noted in any of these studies in incidence among city vs. country dwellers. In Baltimore, the socioeconomic status of patients with ulcerative colitis was not strikingly different from that of the control population, except that patients' fathers tended to have higher occupational status than in the control sample. In Copenhagen there was a tendency for ulcerative colitis patients to have higher occupational status than the control population: the percentages of patients with ulcerative colitis holding managerial, professional, or farm jobs was about the same as in the control population; but among civil servants and wage earners, the percentage of ulcerative colitis patients holding more skilled positions was higher than the percentage of the control population holding similar types of jobs. Some of these differences may have reflected the fact that the ulcerative colitis population was somewhat older than the control population in this study.

Data obtained from such epidemiological studies obviously cannot account for subclinical ulcerative colitis. The incidence of asymptomatic ulcerative colitis in the general population has been estimated to be about four per 100,000, based upon 50,000 proctoscopies performed for the detection of colonic cancer; only two cases of asymptomatic ulcerative colitis were found in that series of proctoscopies, but again this was a selected population seeking prophylactic medical care.[3]

ETIOLOGY

The cause of ulcerative colitis is not known. For many years it was felt that an infectious agent was responsible, but arguments in favor of an infectious etiology have been discarded for lack of scientific evidence. Other workers have formulated genetic, psychosomatic, or immunological theories of pathogenesis. As yet none of these theories are supported by adequate evidence. They will be briefly reviewed below.

The *infectious* theory of the cause of ulcerative colitis remains attractive because of the inflammatory nature of the disease, which in many respects resembles the tissue reaction in the bowel caused by known pathogens (see pp. 1369 to 1404). Successful microbiological search for bacteria, viruses, or fungi which can be consistently found in ulcerative colitis has not been achieved. Electron microscopy of tissue from diseased colon has not revealed virus particles. Efforts to transmit the disease have failed. The disease is exceedingly rare in unrelated members of the same household (husband and wife), suggesting that environmental or infectious factors are not solely operative.

Data supporting a *genetic* hypothesis are suggestive but far from complete, owing to retrospective analyses of families and incomplete reporting. As noted above, ulcerative colitis has a higher incidence among Jews than non-Jews and a lower incidence among blacks than whites. Additional cases of ulcerative colitis in families of patients with the disease occur with much greater frequency (10 to 15 per cent) than in families of control patients without ulcerative colitis. Some families reported have had up to six members afflicted. The disease has appeared in monozygotic twins. In view of the low prevalence rates of the disease in the general population, such data suggest either a genetic or a common environmental factor, but the rar-

ity of ulcerative colitis in husband and wife and the development of ulcerative colitis in blood relatives long separated from the same environment is evidence in favor of genetic factors. Furthermore, ulcerative colitis has a high association with ankylosing spondylitis, a disease with known genetic transmission. Available family data do not support a mendelian dominant or recessive gene with complete penetrance, but are consistent with any of the following possibilities: (1) simple dominant with low penetrance; (2) polygenic inheritance; (3) genetic predisposition to environmental factor(s); or (4) a spectrum of diseases called ulcerative colitis — some of genetic and some of nongenetic causes.[4] Obviously many more data are needed to clarify the role of genetics in this disease.

Psychosomatic determinants in the pathogenesis of ulcerative colitis have been championed for many years. However, most authors have stressed that psychosomatic factors, rather than being causative, merely facilitate the colonic mucosal reaction to another etiological agent. Exactly how emotional factors may affect the colonic mucosa is not known, but effects mediated via the autonomic nervous system have been postulated. Thus in dogs, acute ulcerative lesions in the colon can be produced by intensive parasympathetic stimulation; however, it is not clear how such lesions may relate to chronic ulcerative colitis in man. Until recently data marshaled to support the psychosomatic theory have been uncontrolled and even anecdotal. For example, basing his conclusions on a retrospective review of 700 cases reported in the psychoanalytic literature and a personal (selected) series of 39 patients, Engle stated that patients with ulcerative colitis tend to be obsessive-compulsive and immature individuals who have difficulty establishing social and sexual relationships and yet are overly dependent on a parent or parent-substitute figure.[5] In most instances, the onset or relapse of ulcerative colitis was traced to emotionally traumatic events in the life of the patient. Again, on the basis of selected patient material, other investigators have suggested that ulcerative colitis patients are characteristically passive, anxious to avoid conflict, and above the norm in intelligence. Because of these personality features, it has been claimed that these patients have not been successful in attaining occupational status commensurate with their educational achievements or intellectual ability.

More recent controlled studies have challenged these views. An extensive psychiatric evaluation of 34 consecutive patients presenting with ulcerative colitis failed to reveal a higher incidence of psychiatric aberration than in a control population similarly examined.[6] Furthermore, emotionally traumatic events preceding the onset of ulcerative colitis could be identified in fewer than 20 per cent of the cases. In the epidemiological studies from Baltimore County (see Table 102–1), surveys were conducted among patients with ulcerative colitis, normal control subjects and control patients with irritable colon in an effort to identify psychosocial factors unique to patients with ulcerative colitis.[7, 8] No precipitating stresses (marital discord, indebtedness, overwork, or physical trauma) could be identified as occurring more frequently in the ulcerative colitis patients than in the control population; in general, the social and occupational background of the ulcerative colitis patients resembled that of the normal population. Occupational status tended to be commensurate with educational achievements, and patients with ulcerative colitis participated in organized social activities (clubs and other social or civic groups) with equal frequency to control subjects. Similarly, in Copenhagen occupational status among ulcerative colitis patients and the control population was not markedly different. Admitting that these demographic surveys are not comparable to extensive psychoanalytic studies, one perceives, nevertheless, that the epidemiological data which include appropriate control material (as well as the psychiatric study cited above) seriously challenge the older concepts of psychosomatic determinants in ulcerative colitis. Thus although psychological factors may influence onset and course of the disease in some patients, until more convincing facts are available it is fair to state that they are not necessarily a major etiological factor.

Immunological mechanisms have been postulated as causative in ulcerative co-

litis.[9] Some support for the concept of ulcerative colitis as an autoimmune disease has come from the clinical association of ulcerative colitis with immunologically related disorders (uveitis, autoimmune hemolytic anemia, erythema nodosum, and systemic lupus erythematosus) and from the demonstration of anticolon antibodies in the sera of patients with ulcerative colitis. Such antibodies, however, are also found in the sera of patients with connective tissue diseases, pernicious anemia, and colonic cancer. They react with antigenic determinants from all organs of the gastrointestinal tract, are not colon specific, and appear to be directed toward carbohydrate antigens probably contained in the gastrointestinal mucin. Furthermore, *Escherichia coli* 014, and probably most other Enterobacteriaceae, contain a lipopolysaccharide with antigenic determinants cross-reacting with anticolon antibodies. It has not been possible to correlate the levels of anticolon antibodies in the sera of patients with ulcerative colitis with severity, duration, course, or extent of the disease. Serum containing anticolon antibodies is not cytotoxic to human fetal colon cells in tissue culture. For all these reasons, the significance of such anticolon antibodies in the pathogenesis of ulcerative colitis remains in doubt. More recently, attention has been directed toward cell-mediated immune responses in ulcerative colitis. Lymphocytes from patients with ulcerative colitis are cytotoxic for colonic epithelial cells in tissue culture.

PATHOPHYSIOLOGY

Ulcerative colitis is not a distinct histopathological entity; most of the histological features of the disease may be seen in other inflammations of the colon of known cause, such as shigellosis. The diagnosis of idiopathic ulcerative colitis therefore rests on a combination of clinical and pathological criteria: the course of the disease, the extent and distribution of the anatomic lesions, and the exclusion of other forms of ulcerating colitis caused by specific infectious agents (shigella, *Entamoeba histolytica,* gonococcus). Before embarking on a detailed account of the clinical features of ulcerative colitis, we shall outline the histopathological findings and briefly attempt to relate these lesions to the clinical and radiographic features of the disease.

Except in rare instances (see below), ulcerative colitis is an inflammatory disease confined to the mucosa and to a lesser extent to the adjacent submucosa. The deeper muscular layers and serosa of the colon are usually not involved, and the process does not extend to the regional lymph nodes, except perhaps as a nonspecific reactive hyperplasia.[10] Many pathologists feel that *cryptitis* or *crypt abscess* involving the crypts of Lieberkühn is the primary lesion. In cryptitis, polymorphonuclear cells accumulate near the tip of the crypt, and the crypt epithelial cells show degenerative changes. On light microscopy poor staining or vacuolization may be seen in these epithelial cells, whereas on electron microscopic examination these cells show shortening of epithelial microvilli, dilatation of the endoplasmic reticulum, swelling of the mitochondria, increased numbers of lysosomes, and widening of the intercellular spaces. In crypt abscess, frank necrosis of the crypt epithelium occurs, with extension of the polymorphonuclear infiltrate into the crypts, the appearance of a more chronic inflammatory infiltrate (lymphocytes, plasma cells, eosinophils, and mast cells), and vascular engorgement in the adjacent submucosa. These microabscesses in the crypts are not visible to the naked eye, but they may coalesce by lateral enlargement to produce shallow ulceration of the mucosa extending down to the lamina propria. Such ulceration may be seen at sigmoidoscopy. Alternatively, lateral extension and coalescence of crypt abscesses may undermine mucosa on three sides, leaving an area of ulceration adjacent to a hanging fragment of the mucosa. Such resulting mucosal excrescences may be seen at sigmoidoscopy as *pseudopolyps*. Concomitant with tissue destruction, the reparative process appears. Highly vascular granulation tissue may develop in denuded areas. Collagen is deposited in the lamina propria, but such fibrosis is patchy and usually minimal and is not a prominent feature in ulcerative colitis. With disease of long duration, the muscularis mucosae may hypertrophy.

None of these changes are specific for ulcerative colitis. Similar epithelial degeneration in the crypts can be seen in postradiation colitis, shigellosis, gonococcal colitis, and Crohn's disease of the colon. Crypt abscess formation may be noted in any infectious colitis. Large ulcerations with overhanging mucosal tags are characteristic of amebic colitis; however, usually the ulcers in amebic colitis are larger than those in ulcerative colitis, and trophozoites of *E. histolytica* can be seen at the edges of the ulcers (see p. 1386).

Although these features are not specific, some are highly characteristic of ulcerative colitis. For example, chronicity of the inflammatory process, the large extent of crypt abscess formation, and the profuse development of granulation tissue repair are more characteristic of ulcerative colitis than of infectious colitis. The disease may smolder, with both destructive and reparative changes continuing simultaneously. Most cases exacerbate intermittently; during remissions the mucosa may heal, often resulting in an atrophic mucosa with decreased numbers of crypts, distortion of crypt architecture, and some irregular thickening of the lamina propria.

The aforementioned histopathological features of ulcerative colitis are helpful in understanding many of the clinical features of the disease which will be discussed in more detail in subsequent paragraphs. The two most prominent symptoms of the disease—hematochezia and diarrhea—relate to extensive colonic mucosal damage. Bleeding results from ulceration, vascular engorgement, and the development of highly vascular, friable granulation tissue; watery diarrhea occurs as mucosa is destroyed or damaged, rendering it less capable of sodium and water reabsorption (see pp. 229 to 230).[11] The confinement of the pathological processes to the mucosa and submucosa accounts for the rarity of sharply localized abdominal pain, well defined peritoneal signs, colonic perforation, and/or fistula formation; further, symptoms of obstruction are rare even when the disease extends to the adjacent ileum ("backwash ileitis"). Although the colon in ulcerative colitis may stenose or the ulceration may occasionally extend beyond the submucosa, such pathological developments are uncommon and do not always underlie radiographic foreshortening and narrowing of the colon, loss of haustral markings, and apparent stricture formation. Indeed, these findings are often reversible, because they are due to hypertrophy and spasm of the muscularis mucosae and not fibrosis.[12] Mucosal changes on barium enema examination (fine serration, frank ulceration, polypoid excrescences) and on sigmoidoscopic examination (friability, granularity, pseudopolyps, and occasional ulceration) are clinical counterparts of the histopathological changes described above.

Although ulcerative colitis is generally confined to the mucosa and submucosa, in the more severe forms of the disease, especially in a condition known as *toxic megacolon*, the disease process may extend through the deeper muscular layers of the colon and even to the serosa. On rare occasions, crypt abscesses penetrate the muscularis, often extending along a blood vessel. When the disease extends to the serosa, the colon may perforate. If the inflammatory process arrests short of perforation, healing may result in fibrosis of the deeper layers of the colon. In toxic megacolon, which occurs in 1 to 3 per cent of all cases of ulcerative colitis, ulcers extend deeply, through the mucosa and submucosa, into the muscular layers of the colon. In addition, vasculitis is often seen, along with swelling and irregularity of the vascular endothelium, inflammatory infiltration into the vessel walls, and thrombosis of small arteries. The extension of ulceration into the muscular layers of the colon and its associated infiltration and vasculitis probably account for the apparent loss of colonic motor tone in this condition, producing colonic dilatation. Deep extension of the inflammatory process, together with dilatation of the colon, predisposes these patients to perforation (see pp. 1326 to 1329).

We have stated that ulcerative colitis may have a variable course (continuous vs. intermittent) and may show varying degrees of histopathologic severity, varying from mild subepithelial inflammation to perforation along the colon. Although ulcerative colitis frequently involves most or all of the organ, it often may affect only the distal colon ("idiopathic proctocolitis") or, even more rarely, may be confined to a proximal segment of the colon ("segmental colitis"). These variations of important features (course, depth of the lesions, distribution along the colon) produce a disease with a highly variable clinical picture.

CLINICAL COURSE

Ulcerative colitis most commonly affects individuals in their second, third, or fourth decades. It is more frequent among females than males, and it appears to be predominantly a disease of Caucasians, with a higher incidence in Jews. Often the patient will associate the onset of symptoms with an upper respiratory infection, a "stomach virus," a trip to a different part of the country, a severe emotional upset, or a period of emotional stress.

Ulcerative colitis is a disease which is highly variable in severity, clinical course, and ultimate prognosis. The onset of the disease, as well as subsequent exacerbations, may be insidious or abrupt. The symptoms may range from small amounts of rectal bleeding, often mistaken for hemorrhoidal bleeding, to fulminant diarrhea with colonic hemorrhage and prostration. Most patients (about 60 to 75 per cent) will have intermittent attacks of symptoms, with complete symptomatic remissions between attacks.[13] A smaller number (about 4 to 10 per cent) will have one attack with no subsequent symptoms for up to 15 years after the initial episode; a few patients (5 to 15 per cent) will be troubled by continuous symptoms without any remission.

The severity of the disease, whether in the initial episode or in a subsequent exacerbation, has important therapeutic and prognostic implications. For example, as seen in Table 102–2, most of the immediate deaths occur in those patients with severe disease, whereas patients with mild disease rarely die. Moreover, as judged by death rates, severe disease has remained refractory to all types of treatment over the last 30 years, but significantly fewer patients with moderate disease now die of ulcerative colitis than was true previously. This improved prognosis for those with moderate disease has probably resulted from several modes of treatment that have been developed by trial and error over the

TABLE 102–2. PERCENTAGE OF PATIENTS DYING FROM AN
ACUTE ATTACK OF ULCERATIVE COLITIS*

YEARS OF STUDY	SEVERITY OF ATTACK		
	Severe	Moderate	Mild
1938–1952	33.8%	19.7%	1.5%
1952–1962	26.8%	2.4%	0.4%

*From Edwards, F. C., and Truelove, S. C.: Gut 4:299, 1964.

last two decades; these treatments will be discussed below.

Because the severity of the disease has these therapeutic and prognostic implications, it is important for the physician to assess the severity of the disease in any given patient. Although in general the intensity of mucosal disease as seen at sigmoidoscopy parallels the severity of the attack, the findings do not always accurately reflect severity, probably because only a small portion of the total colonic mucosa is seen. Likewise, radiographic evaluation does not provide a reliable assessment of severity. Barium enema examination may indicate whether the colitis is localized to the distal colon or whether it involves the entire organ. This type of information is only of limited value in assessing severity; although severe disease almost always involves the whole colon, universal colitis is present in up to 20 per cent of those with mild clinical disease. Other changes seen at barium enema, such as loss of haustral markings and foreshortening or narrowing of the colon, attest as much to chronicity (hypertrophy of the muscularis mucosae or fibrosis) as to severity; usually patients with rapid onset and progression of severe colitis do not show these changes. The best indices of severity, then, are clinical symptoms and signs. Thus large volumes of diarrhea indicate that the colonic mucosa has been involved to such an extent and degree that sodium and water reabsorption are significantly impaired. Frequent bowel movements, on the other hand, may result from either large volume diarrhea or colonic or rectal irritability. Frequency per se, then, is an unreliable indicator of severity.

A large amount of blood in the stools, a fall in blood hemoglobin concentration, and hypoalbuminemia are all signs of widespread and severe mucosal destruction with its attendant significant loss of blood into the colon. Similarly, fever and tachycardia indicate intense or widespread inflammation; rapid weight loss resulting from anorexia and increased catabolism (fever, blood loss) has the same implication. Steady abdominal pain and tenderness point to transmural involvement in the severest forms of the disease.

The classification of ulcerative colitis into three categories of severity is purely arbitrary, but, as noted above, such classification assumes significance because of its prognostic value. The British arbitrarily define mild disease as that associated with fewer than four bowel movements a day and lacking anemia, fever, tachycardia, weight loss, and hypoalbuminemia.[14] Severe disease is defined as that associated with more than six stools a day, with considerable colonic bleeding, anemia, hypoalbuminemia, fever, tachycardia, and weight loss. In the next few paragraphs we will briefly describe the clinical features of mild, moderate, and severe ulcerative colitis and then proceed to consider diagnostic and therapeutic measures in the disease as a whole.

MILD DISEASE

Mild ulcerative colitis is the most common form of the disease, afflicting about 60 per cent of all patients.[15] It may occur in either of two ways: most commonly (80 per cent of the cases), clinically mild ulcerative colitis is segmental in distribution, usually involving just the distal colon; less often, clinically mild ulcerative colitis is seen in patients in whom the whole colon is involved with the disease. The age of onset, sex predilection, and familial incidence of ulcerative colitis are the same in mild disease as in the more severe forms of ulcerative colitis. Similarly, the course of the disease — that is, the percentages of patients having only one attack, intermittent attacks, or chronic continuous disease—is the same for mild ulcerative colitis as for the more severe forms. Anorectal complications as well as extracolonic manifestations of ulcerative colitis (arthritis, pyoderma gangrenosum, uveitis, and erythema nodosum) are noted in mild disease as in more severe forms; sometimes these complications are the chief complaints of the patient rather than diarrhea or rectal bleeding. Because of all these similarities to the more severe forms of ulcerative colitis, mild ulcerative colitis, even when sharply limited to the rectosigmoid colon ("idiopathic proctitis"), is considered to be the same disease as more severe ulcerative colitis. Indeed, a small number (5 to 15 per cent) of patients with disease limited to the rectosigmoid colon will show ultimate progression of their disease to involve a much larger—if not the entire—length of the colon, with the simultaneous development of more severe diarrhea or bleeding.[16]

By definition neither colonic bleeding nor diarrhea is severe in mild ulcerative colitis, and systemic signs and symptoms are absent. Occasionally, patients with mild ulcerative colitis may suffer from short episodes of anorexia and fatigue or mild lower abdominal cramps; but most often hospitalization is not required, and the patient may continue his usual activities. A patient may present with mild rectal bleeding in the absence of diarrhea and be mistakenly diagnosed as suffering from hemorrhoids. Alternatively, some patients have frequent stools, generally small in volume, without apparent bleeding; these patients may be misdiagnosed as having irritable colon syndrome. In either case, the correct diagnosis may be established by sigmoidoscopy. As mentioned above, a few patients with mild ulcerative colitis may present with anorectal or extracolonic complications of ulcerative colitis in the absence of either diarrhea or colonic bleeding. It is not known how often the patient with mild ulcerative colitis may be asymptomatic and/or undiagnosed. Because of the uncertainty as to the incidence of undiagnosed mild ulcerative colitis, available figures on incidence, prevalence, and mortality in ulcerative colitis may be somewhat inaccurate.

The immediate mortality in mild ulcerative colitis (that is, in those patients sick enough to be hospitalized or seen as outpatients) is almost nil (see Table 102-2). Similarly, patients with mild ulcerative colitis have a long-term prognosis little different from a control population. And the development of colonic cancer in mild ulcerative colitis is much rarer, occurring about one-seventh as often as in the more severe forms of the disease.

MODERATE DISEASE

Moderate disease affects about 25 per cent of all patients with ulcerative colitis.[15] In these patients, symptoms are somewhat more intense. During the initial attack or an exacerbation, diarrhea is a major symptom, in contrast to those in the mild category. Stools are frequent, usually numbering four to five per day; they are loose and almost invariably contain blood. Abdominal crampy distress is usually more prominent than in those with the mild form of the disease, although not incapacitating; often, it may wake the patient at night. Usually cramps are relieved by defecation. Many of these patients will have intermittent low-grade fever of 99 to 100° F. Generally the patient is somewhat tired, fatigues easily, and cannot take part normally in all activities. Appetite is usually maintained, but there may be intervals of anorexia and weight loss. The patient may complain of extracolonic symptoms such as low backache or arthritis.

During the initial attack or an exacerbation of ulcerative colitis, the patient with moderate disease may at any time become more severely ill, developing severe or fulminant colitis characterized by high fever and profuse diarrhea. Rapid deterioration may also be manifested by massive bleeding or rapid and progressive dilatation of the colon (toxic megacolon).

Generally it is this moderate category patient who most dramatically responds to treatment with adrenal steroids (see pp. 1314 to 1318). Indeed, since the advent of steroid treatment, the immediate mortality of this type of ulcerative colitis has significantly fallen (see Table 102-2); however, statistically, the long-term prognosis for this category of patient remains poor. Repeated attacks of equal or greater severity are common, and the risk of ultimately developing cancer is appreciable. Long-term prognosis will be discussed in more detail in a subsequent area of this chapter.

SEVERE OR FULMINANT ULCERATIVE COLITIS

This is the rarest form of ulcerative colitis, affecting about 15 per cent of all patients with the disease.[15] Patients with severe ulcerative colitis generally have a rather sudden onset of symptoms which rapidly progress to a point at which the patient is dangerously ill. Occasionally, a less severe attack will progress to this stage. Diarrhea is generally profuse, and rectal bleeding is constant. Fever is high, 101 to 103° F or higher; it may be spiking or sustained. The patient complains of tenesmus with frequent passage of bloody and watery stools. Appetite and weight are quickly lost. Weakness is profound, and pallor is striking to the patient's family and friends.

On physical examination, the patient is acutely ill, febrile, dehydrated, and profoundly weak. Often the patient may draw up his legs in an effort to relieve abdominal cramps. In extreme instances, he may be somewhat obtunded owing to dehydration, fever, and acidosis. The pulse is rapid and blood pressure low because of decreased extracellular fluid volume; if blood volume is sufficiently depleted as the result of profuse colonic bleeding, the patient may be in shock. Abdominal examination usually reveals diffuse abdominal tenderness but no evidence of localized or generalized peritonitis. Frequently the patient has aphthous ulceration of the mouth. The white count is markedly elevated, often in excess of 20,000 per mm^3 and occasionally as high as 50,000 per mm^3, with a high percentage of immature polymorphonuclear cells. Anemia is universally found, and red cells are hypochromic and microcytic. Anemia usually results from a combination of blood loss, iron deficiency, and marrow suppression; occasionally hemolytic anemia develops as a consequence of severe ulcerative colitis. Hypoalbuminemia is the hallmark of severe ulcerative colitis and results from low protein intake (anorexia), together with increased colonic losses of serum albumin. Occasionally, the serum albumin is so low that pretibial or presacral edema appears. Flat films of the abdomen usually reveal some gas in the colon, with minimal colonic distention; the radiolucent intraluminal colonic gas may allow visualization of an irregularly thickened colonic mucosa (see pp. 1308 to 1311).

This type of patient remains most refractory to medical therapy. Death from the acute attack of ulcerative colitis is almost always the result of ulcerative colitis of this degree of severity.

DIAGNOSIS

The diagnosis of ulcerative colitis is usually made on the basis of clinical symptoms and on the demonstration of an abnormal, inflamed colonic mucosa by sigmoidoscopy. Diagnosis may also be supported by barium enema and by rectal biopsy. X-ray examination will often reveal characteristic, although not specific, findings, and rectal biopsy may show crypt abscesses and mucosal inflammation, likewise not specific for ulcerative colitis.

Physical examination is useful in confirming the presence of extracolonic complications (uveitis, aphthous stomatitis, pyoderma gangrenosum, erythema nodosum, arthritis) and in demonstrating the systemic sequelae of severe colitis (tachycardia, fever, dehydration, contracted blood volume). In addition, physical examination can be helpful in detecting the complications of toxic megacolon (increased abdominal girth and tympany) or colonic perforation (direct and rebound abdominal tenderness). Except in detecting these complications of ulcerative colitis, the physical examination is of limited usefulness in establishing the diagnosis. Indeed, in uncomplicated mild and moderate forms of the disease the physical examination is usually normal. Since ulcerative colitis is a disease which predominantly affects the colonic mucosa, the most useful methods of establishing a diagnosis involve procedures which assess the integrity of this mucosa. In 90 to 95 per cent of persons with ulcerative colitis, the mucosa of the rectosigmoid colon is diseased;[17] even cases of localized colitis are most commonly localized in the distal colon. Therefore sigmoidoscopy can be utilized to establish a diagnosis in the majority of patients.

SIGMOIDOSCOPIC FINDINGS

At sigmoidoscopy the normal colonic mucosa appears as a smooth, glistening surface which uniformly reflects the endoscopic light from a broad area. The color of the mucosa is ideally pink, but will depend on a variety of factors, including the color temperature of the endoscopic light and the type of preparation the patient has undergone for the examination. Ramifying superficial submucosal blood vessels may be discerned as a deeper red color reflected through the thin overlying translucent mucosa; however, the distribution of these vessels is quite random, so that their absence from a given area is not in itself abnormal. The normal colonic mucosa may bleed to a small degree after it has been scraped by the rigid sigmoidoscope, but normally the mucosa beyond the tip of the instrument does not spontaneously bleed; nor will the normal mucosa bleed when it is gently massaged with a cotton swab. The rectosigmoid colon is usually easily distensible, although an occasional normal patient, and more often a patient with irritable colon, will evidence a fair amount of spasm during the procedure. The margins of the rectal valves are sharply defined.

The mucosa diseased with ulcerative colitis is markedly altered in many respects. As inflammatory exudate and edema permeate the submucosa, the mucosa becomes less translucent so that ramifying submucosal vessels may no longer be seen. Subepithelial infiltration and edema as well as microscopic mucosal erosions and crypt abscesses make the normally smooth surface irregular in height and depth. Diffusely and uniformly reflected light from the normally smooth surface which gives the impression of a glistening membrane is then replaced by scattered pinpoints of light reflected from these tiny mucosal irregularities; this gives the surface a *granular* appearance. As the mucosa becomes much more irregular with more intense inflammation, this "fine granularity" gives way to "coarse granularity," which greatly scatters the reflected light; as a consequence most of the reflected

light is therefore lost to the eye of the observer, and the mucosa then appears "dry" as opposed to the normal "moist" or glistening surface. If subepithelial and submucosal edema becomes more marked, it may be appreciated by the endoscopist as blunting of the normally sharply angulated rectal valves. Increased vascularity accompanies inflammation in the submucosa and may be appreciated as "hyperemia" of the mucosa. Because of this increased vascularity and because of erosions which undermine the mucosa in some areas and denude it in others, the mucosa becomes friable; that is, it bleeds easily when gently massaged with a cotton swab. With more intense inflammation the mucosa may be seen to bleed spontaneously beyond the leading edge of the scope. In the more severe and chronic forms of the disease, areas of ulceration may become visible in the rectosigmoid, although discrete ulceration is less often seen as a rule in the rectosigmoid than in the more proximal areas of the colon in resected specimens. Similarly, with more severe forms of the disease pseudopolyps can be seen; these are small projections of tissue above the general plane of the surrounding mucosa. They are made up of tags of undermined mucosa or heaped-up granulation tissue or a combination of these abnormalities. Pseudopolyps are usually shallow in depth, but with more chronic disease they may become accentuated by mild submucosal fibrosis and contracture of the colonic surface surrounding them. In active disease, the walls of the rectosigmoid colon may appear "rigid" or nondistensible. Like contractures seen on barium enema, this feature is related more to spasm of the rectosigmoid than to fibrosis; indeed, with healing this rigidity may disappear. Finally, exudate or mucopus—terms which refer to tenacious and discolored (yellow) mucus—may be seen adhering to the mucosa.

These findings vary widely from patient to patient. Thus in the mildest forms of ulcerative colitis changes seen at sigmoidoscopy may be very subtle, consisting only of mild friability, and sometimes in mild disease the sigmoidoscopic examination appears entirely normal. At the other extreme, severe disease floridly displays most of these features which are readily

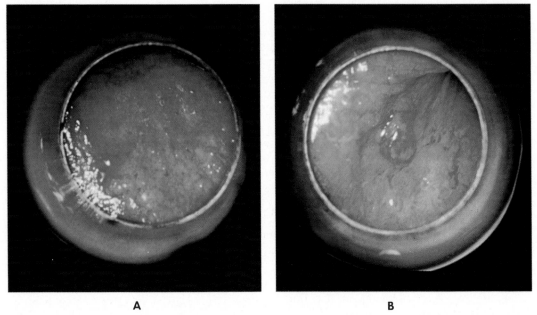

A   **B**

Figure 102–1. Proctoscopic views of colonic mucosa in two patients with ulcerative colitis. *A*, Granularity and minute bleeding mucosal ulcerations. *B*, Minimal granularity, but mucosa is friable and a pseudopolyp can be seen. (Courtesy of Dr. M. H. Sleisenger.)

appreciated: the rectosigmoid is spastic to the point that the scope cannot be passed more than 8 to 10 cm without undue discomfort to the patient; widespread spontaneous mucosal bleeding is present; all light reflex is lost; and pseudopolyps and a few ulcers may be seen (Fig. 102–1).

In addition to the variable appearance of these features, it can be readily appreciated that evaluation of many of these features is subjective. Thus it is not surprising that wide observer variation has been documented among experienced endoscopists regarding the presence or absence of such features as granularity, edema, rigidity, and hyperemia. More uniform agreement is reached over the presence or absence of such features as friability (bleeding on swabbing) or spontaneous bleeding, ramifying blood vessels, and pseudopolyps or ulcers.[18] Despite these difficulties, the overall agreement among observers as to whether the mucosa is normal or abnormal is fairly good, ranging from 70 to 90 per cent.[18, 19]

Nevertheless, the fact that there is observer disagreement at sigmoidoscopy of patients with known ulcerative colitis means that the individual endoscopist may not always feel certain of his findings in any given patient, especially when sigmoidoscopy shows only mild or subtle abnormalities. In such circumstances, rectal

biopsy may be useful in clarifying the diagnosis. Rectal biopsy may be obtained either with a mechanical forceps (usually below the peritoneal reflection and along a rectal valve to minimize the dangers of perforation) or with a suction instrument, which minimizes the dangers of perforation and therefore may safely be used higher in the rectosigmoid colon if desired.

Rectal biopsy may confirm the presence of inflammation in the colonic mucosa and in this way strengthen the endoscopist's impressions. In cases of known ulcerative colitis, rectal biopsies will show a spectrum of findings, according to the severity of the histopathological process, which roughly parallels the clinical status of the patient. These changes range from a mild degree of inflammatory cell (lymphocytes, plasma cells, polymorphonuclear cells, eosinophils) infiltration in the mucosa between the muscularis and the lamina propria, to more pronounced subepithelial infiltration along with epithelial cell degeneration and microscopic erosions of the epithelium, or to the appearance of crypt abscesses (Fig. 102–2). Disease in remission may show some of these inflammatory changes and, in addition, may show atrophic changes in the mucosa (diminution in number of glands with branching of the glands), which is evi-

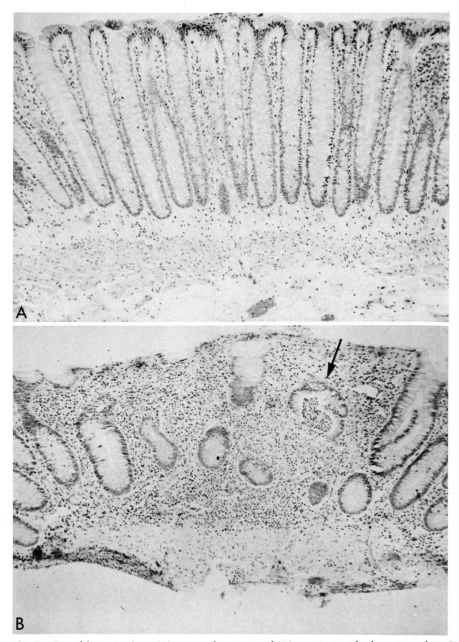

Figure 102–2. Rectal biopsies from (A) a normal patient and (B) a patient with ulcerative colitis. In B, note mucosal atrophy, branching of a gland, cellular infiltration, and crypt abscess (arrow). × 100.

dence of past mucosal destruction and repair. Rectal biopsies from normal patients and patients with irritable colon do not show these inflammatory changes; however, on blind review even the pathologist is not always able to distinguish biopsy specimens of known cases of ulcerative colitis showing only mild subepithelial inflammatory cell infiltration from normal biopsy specimens. Nevertheless, in several series of established cases of ulcerative colitis, rectal biopsy often showed clearly abnormal and significant inflammation in the mucosa when sigmoidoscopy was normal or equivocal.[17, 19] Thus rectal biopsy appears to be more sensitive than sigmoidoscopy in detecting mucosal disease, and may be useful to the clinician when sigmoidoscopic examination is equivocal (see pp. 1501 to 1507).

On the other hand, rectal biopsy is unnecessary when clear-cut mucosal inflammation is demonstrated at endoscopy because unequivocal sigmoidoscopic abnormalities are rarely if ever seen when rectal biopsy is normal. In addition to being an adjunct to the endoscopist, rectal biopsy may be helpful on occasion in establishing the diagnosis of amebic colitis when it is important to distinguish this disease from ulcerative colitis (i.e., if steroid treatment for ulcerative colitis is being contemplated). In amebic colitis trophozoites are usually easily seen in the stools. Occasionally, however, a patient will present for diagnosis after having undergone a barium enema X-ray prematurely. In such a circumstance, the barium remaining in the stools will obscure the trophozoites, and rectal biopsy must be utilized for diagnosis of amebic colitis by showing the presence of *E. histolytica* in the inflamed or ulcerated colonic mucosa (see pp. 1386 to 1392).

RADIOGRAPHY (see pp. 1253 to 1276)

X-ray examination of the colon may be useful in confirming the diagnosis of ulcerative colitis. A plain film of the abdomen may often provide a great deal of information, especially in patients with more severe ulcerative colitis in whom barium enema examination may be contraindicated. Thus the colon may be more or less filled with air so that on plain film features such as foreshortening of the colon and loss of haustration may be appreciated. Many times there is sufficient air in a segment of the colon to silhouette the mucosa, revealing an irregular mucosa caused by pseudopolyps, ulcerations, and mucosal tags (Fig. 102–3). Patients suspected of having toxic megacolon (high fever, abdominal tenderness, and distention) may be seen on plain film to have a colon dilated with air to a diameter of 9 cm or more; in toxic megacolon dissection of gas into deep ulcers may produce a double contour appearance in the wall of the colon.

Barium enema examination may provide information which is useful in several

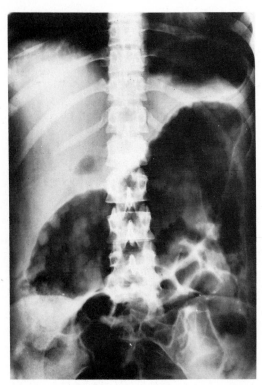

Figure 102–3. Plain film of the abdomen from a patient with ulcerative colitis and toxic megacolon. Note that the air in the colon silhouettes an irregular colonic mucosa.

ways to the clinician. (1) It is at present the best means of diagnosing disease proximal to the sigmoidoscope. When sigmoidoscopic examination confirms the diagnosis of ulcerative colitis, the barium enema examination is useful in determining whether the disease is localized to the rectum or whether it extends proximally in the colon. If the sigmoidoscopic examination is negative, barium enema examination is useful in determining whether the patient's symptoms (bleeding and/or diarrhea) are due to ulcerative colitis or some other disease of the colon (such as tumor, diverticular disease of the colon, ischemic colitis, or granulomatous colitis). In only a small number of patients — probably fewer than 5 per cent — the disease may appear as segmental colitis, involving areas of the colon above the reach of the sigmoidoscope. (2) By demonstrating changes consistent with ulcerative colitis, the barium enema examination may strengthen the diagnosis of ulcerative colitis when sigmoidoscopy and/or rectal biopsy are equivocal. Such findings usually pertain to cases of mild ulcerative colitis or more severe ulcerative colitis in remission. (3) Barium enema examination is helpful in distinguishing ulcerative colitis from granulomatous colitis (see pp. 1350 to 1352). (4) Barium enema examination may be used to detect the development of cancer in the proximal colon in long-standing cases of ulcerative colitis.

It is well to keep these indications clearly in mind when deciding whether to obtain a barium enema examination. This examination is not without hazard to the patient with ulcerative colitis. A vigorous preparation with purgatives and enemas may exacerbate mild ulcerative colitis or moderate ulcerative colitis in remission. In more severe forms of the illness a barium enema may precipitate either dilatation of the colon or perforation; high pressures usually employed to fill the colon with barium may decompensate an already compromised colonic musculature or may cause perforation where inflammation has extended through the muscular walls of the colon. Fortunately, in those patients with more severe disease, barium enema examination is not required for proper management of the patient. In patients with clinically severe colitis characterized by profuse and bloody diarrhea—diagnosis is easily made at proctoscopy. The presence of profuse diarrhea and bleeding invariably signifies widespread colonic mucosal involvement; there is thus no urgent need to confirm the distribution of the colitis in such patients. Obviously the distinction of ulcerative colitis from granulomatous colitis or the detection of cancer is not of immediate concern to the physician trying to manage a patient acutely ill with ulcerative colitis; such information is best obtained at a later time when the patient has recovered from acute illness and is in remission.

Barium enema examination should be performed on all patients with ulcerative colitis, but at a time of the physician's choosing. Under no circumstances should a patient with ulcerative colitis be prepared with cathartics; such treatment may worsen the disease. Preparation for the procedure consists of two to three days of a clear liquid diet and, if the patient has residual material in the rectal ampulla or the rectosigmoid as ascertained by gentle digi-

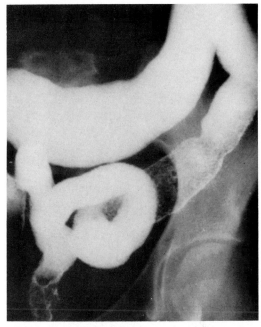

Figure 102–4. Barium enema from a patient with ulcerative colitis, showing fine serrations along edges of the barium column. Serrated appearance is the result of shallow mucosal ulcerations.

tal examination, a gentle cleansing water enema.

The picture on barium enema X-ray varies according to the location and state of the disease. Many patients with early ulcerative colitis will have perfectly normal barium enema X-rays. This point cannot be too heavily emphasized; diagnosis must rest upon the sigmoidoscopic appearance and/or the rectal biopsy. In some patients with early disease, on the other hand, minute ulcerations along the edge of the bowel may be noted (Fig. 102–4); evidence for mucosal disease may better be seen on the evacuation film which reveals denudation of the mucosa with disappearance of its reticulated pattern. Much has been made of the loss of haustra, particularly in the left colon in patients with ulcerative colitis. This sign is nonspecific, for it may be seen in a large number of individuals; however, when taken along with other evidences of colitis, it must be considered as part of the disease.

Usually when haustra have disappeared from the left colon and even the transverse colon, the disease is more advanced and other evidences are noted. These

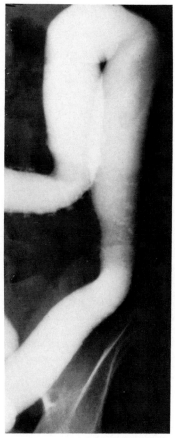

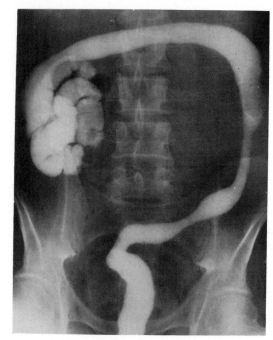

Figure 102–6. Barium enema, showing shortened, narrowed, tubular colon in a patient with chronic ulcerative colitis.

Figure 102–5. Barium enema, showing "collar button" ulcerations in a patient with ulcerative colitis.

include ulceration of the mucosa with further denudation; the ulcers may be particularly accentuated along the margins, where they assume a "collar button" appearance (Fig. 102–5). The bowel progressively shortens, becomes rigid in appearance, and looks like a narrow tube resembling a pipe (Fig. 102–6).

At variable intervals, pseudopolyps make their appearance. These are radiolucent defects which are scattered throughout the bowel but may be localized in certain areas (Fig. 102–7). They may develop in a short period of time. Although they tend to be permanent, they have been noted on occasion to disappear with therapy.

Radiologists pay particular attention to the retrorectal space which is increased as the disease progresses owing to inflammation and spasm or fibrosis. Rather arbitrarily a distance greater than 2 cm is considered by the radiologist to be abnormal

when associated with other findings of ulcerative colitis on the X-ray. It is good evidence that the patient has rather severe inflammatory involvement of the rectum and retrorectal tissues.

What is the correlation between extent of disease on X-ray and the clinical severity of the disease? The correlation appears to be good in patients with mild disease, but among those who have moderate or severe

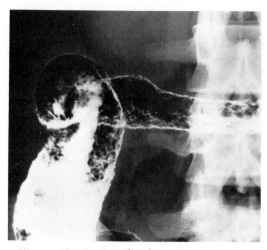

Figure 102–7. Pseudopolyps seen on barium enema examination in a patient with ulcerative colitis.

disease the tendency is for fewer radiological changes than would be anticipated clinically. However, examples of discrepancies at either extreme are common; thus a patient may have a markedly shortened bowel full of pseudopolyps with areas of narrowing and feel perfectly well. Again, he may be ill with bloody stools, abdominal discomfort, and fever, and show a barium enema which at most displays some fine serrations on the margins which are interpreted by the radiologist as ulcers. Recent double-blind studies have indicated that gastrointestinal radiologists may vary widely in their opinion of assessment not only of the severity and extent of ulcerative colitis but also of whether it is present, indicating significant observer variation (see pp. 1361 to 1362).

Frequently on barium enema an area of narrowing which is presumed to be a stricture may be found in patients with ulcerative colitis. Histologically, these areas are often not fibrotic strictures but rather represent segments in which there is marked smooth muscle hypertrophy.[12] Although their presence suggests a napkin ring type of carcinoma, if the lesion is present on the left side they generally represent muscle hypertrophy. In some instances it is merely spasm, because it may disappear with treatment. A full discussion of the comparison between the findings in ulcerative colitis and in granulomatous disease of the colon will be taken up on pages 1350 to 1352.

The use of barium enema X-rays in following the course of a patient should be restricted. Frequently repeated examinations are unjustified; indeed, as noted, the procedure may exacerbate the illness. What, then, are the indications for repeat studies? When the illness recurs after a period of remission or if classic low-grade symptoms dramatically intensify, indicating spread of the disease, repeat barium examination is indicated. The question often arises as to whether or not routine studies should be performed on patients who have long-standing disease in an effort to detect the earliest appearance of carcinoma. This is a difficult question to answer, but we believe that it is wise for every patient who has had the disease longer than ten years to be routinely X-rayed yearly, and whenever bleeding and diarrhea or symptoms of obstruction appear.

During the barium enema X-ray it is important to fill the terminal ileum, because about 10 to 15 per cent of patients with ulcerative colitis who have universal involvement will also have some superficial inflammation of the ileal mucosa associated with edema and possibly some spasm, giving an abnormal appearance to the terminal ileum on X-ray. Often, however, this so-called backwash ileitis can readily be distinguished from granulomatous disease of the terminal ileum by barium enema, because the terminal ileum does not visualize owing to involvement of the ileocecal valve in granulomatous disease.

The incidence of peptic ulcer disease appears to be lower than predicted in patients with ulcerative colitis; however, roentgenographic examination of the upper gastrointestinal tract should be performed in patients with histories suggestive of peptic ulcer.

DIFFERENTIAL DIAGNOSIS

As noted, the typical patient with moderately severe ulcerative colitis presents with chronic watery, large-volume diarrhea, lasting weeks rather than days at a time; there is often some lower abdominal cramping and intermittent low-grade fever. Blood is usually noted in the watery stools from time to time. *Infectious colitis* or *viral enteritis* may present with similar symptoms which, however, are not commonly chronic. *Irritable colon* is characterized by a similar course of chronic, intermittent diarrhea with cramps, but in this disorder stools are usually small in volume, and low-grade fever and hematochezia are not features. Diverticular disease of the colon may also exhibit intermittent attacks of lower abdominal cramping, diarrhea, and fever; although hematochezia appears on occasion, the bleeding from colonic diverticulosis is usually of massive proportions. *Ischemic colitis* may present with hematochezia and diarrhea, but in this disease the course is usually self-limited; *i.e.*, resolution in days to a week or so, laparotomy with resection, or demise from complications. Chronic watery diarrhea may result from a variety of *small bowel diseases* (see pp. 886 to 925). Ulcerative colitis of moderate severity may be easily differentiated from irritable colon, diverticular disease of the colon, and chronic small bowel diarrhea by proctosigmoidoscopy and barium enema examination, which will demonstrate the diagnostic features of ulcerative colitis in almost all cases of moderate and active disease. Differentiation between ulcerative and *granulomatous colitis* is discussed on pages 1350 to 1352.

In mild ulcerative colitis symptoms are more variable. In the patient presenting with recurrent rectal bleeding in the absence of diarrhea, the differential diagnosis includes *hemorrhoids, anal fissure, rectal polyp, carcinoma of the rectum, factitious proctitis* (mechanical trauma to the rectum resulting from insertion of foreign objects), *granulomatous colitis,* and *ulcerative colitis.** Most of these conditions can be diagnosed by proctosigmoidoscopy. If ulcerative colitis is the cause of the rectal bleeding, the rectosigmoid mucosa will invariably show generalized friability and usually many of the other changes consistent with ulcerative colitis. Granulomatous colitis, however, may not always be distinguishable from ulcerative colitis proctoscopically, although the ulcers of this condition are larger, deeper, and more discrete (see pp. 1350 to 1352). Factitious colitis is usually confined to the rectum; granularity, loss of vascular markings, and pseudopolyps are not seen. Whether or not a lesion is found at sigmoidoscopy which can explain the bleeding, barium enema examination is indicated in order to detect polyps, carcinoma, or segments of granulomatous or ulcerative colitis which are beyond the reach of the sigmoidoscope. *Postradiation colitis* may also present with bleeding, usually in women after radium treatment for carcinoma of the cervix. In this situation the diagnosis is made primarily on the basis of history and the distribution of colitis along the colon (see pp. 1406 to 1413).

Patients with mild ulcerative colitis who

---

*We use the term ulcerative colitis synonymously with "idiopathic proctitis," because some cases of idiopathic proctitis may progress to generalized ulcerative colitis or may show other features of ulcerative colitis, and histologically the diseases cannot be differentiated. Whether either term connotes a specific disease entity is uncertain at this time.

do not bleed are misdiagnosed most commonly as having *irritable colon*, because they usually suffer from chronic and intermittent low-volume diarrhea with mild lower abdominal cramps but without systemic symptoms. Although proctosigmoidoscopic and barium enema examinations are normal in patients with irritable colon, they are usually abnormal in those with mild ulcerative colitis; in mild cases the barium enema may be normal and the proctosigmoidoscopic examination may show only minimal or equivocally abnormal findings. In this situation rectal biopsy may be helpful in establishing the correct diagnosis.

In acute severe ulcerative colitis, in which bloody diarrhea, fever, dehydration, and prostration are common, *acute infectious colitis* is the major disease in the differential diagnosis. Sigmoidoscopy will always confirm the presence of colitis, but may not distinguish between idiopathic ulcerative and infectious colitis. Usually acute *salmonellosis, shigellosis,* or acute *amebiasis* may be ruled out within 24 to 48 hours by microscopy of aspirates and stool culture (see pp. 909 to 925, 1373 to 1377, and 1386 to 1392). *Pseudomembranous* and *necrotizing colitis* must also be distinguished from severe ulcerative colitis (see pp. 1369 to 1373).

MEDICAL THERAPY

In recent years several clinics have noted a decline in mortality from the acute attack of moderately severe ulcerative colitis (see Table 102–2). Undoubtedly much of this decrease has resulted from the introduction of corticosteroids in the treatment of this disease in the 1950's; however, other factors have also contributed to this change. In the same decade our understanding of the pathophysiology of ulcerative colitis improved tremendously. Clearer criteria for the diagnosis of the disease emerged. Rational treatment for associated fluid and electrolyte disorders evolved, and blood transfusions became more available and safer. Together all these factors account for the declining mortality in the medical management of acute ulcerative colitis. In addition, there are now better defined indications for colectomy in those patients not responding to medical management; these will be discussed in more detail on pages 1341 to 1343.

GENERAL MEASURES

Those patients having significant diarrhea (moderate and severe ulcerative colitis), particularly when complicated by fever, are prone to dehydration. Colonic losses of sodium and potassium may result in reduced extracellular fluid volume (sodium and water depletion) and hypokalemia. Patients on large doses of corticosteroids may in addition suffer significant renal potassium losses which further contribute to hypokalemia. Fever (increased catabolism), colonic loss of bicarbonate, and decreased extracellular fluid volume which may produce prerenal azotemia together cause metabolic acidosis. Each of these defects should be corrected when it appears. Uncorrected fluid and electrolyte deficits have been incriminated in the development of toxic megacolon and renal calculi (see below).

In the more severe forms of ulcerative colitis, blood loss from the colon is the rule, and patients tend to develop iron deficiency anemia. This may be corrected by oral iron or by parenteral iron in those patients in whom oral iron worsens diarrhea or is otherwise not tolerated. Patients severely ill and showing signs of systemic toxicity may have bone marrow suppression in addition to iron deficiency;[20] such patients are prone to hypoalbuminemia from colonic protein losses, low protein intake (anorexia), and systemic illness. In such patients blood transfusions will be beneficial in restoring hemoglobin concentration, blood volume, and serum albumin concentration toward normal.

Dietary management in ulcerative colitis, as in all gastroenterological disease, has enjoyed its vogue. Most dietary regimens have assumed either (1) allergy (reagin type) to specific dietary protein or (2) mechanical trauma to the damaged colonic mucosa by high residue diets. There is no evidence that the latter plays any role in exacerbations of ulcerative colitis. Evidence in favor of allergy to specific food protein stems largely from the clinical impressions that many patients with ulcerative colitis improve on a diet free of cow's milk, an observation recently documented by a small clinical trial.[21] A few patients with ulcerative colitis have hemagglutinating antibodies to tanned red cells coated with cow's milk proteins; however, normal subjects also have these antibodies, and in patients with ulcerative colitis the titers of such antibodies bear no relation to the state of activity of the disease, the presence or absence of clinical milk sensitivity, or the withdrawal of milk from the diet.[9, 22] Furthermore, passive cutaneous sensitization cannot be demonstrated with sera of patients containing these antibodies. Some patients with ulcerative colitis have intestinal lactase deficiency, which could account for the deleterious effects of cow's milk. The incidence of lactase deficiency in ulcerative colitis has not been well studied (usually only by oral tolerance tests) and varies from 8 to 84 per cent of patients. Jews with ulcerative colitis appear to have a higher incidence than non-Jewish patients, just as they do in control populations. In one study employing both intestinal biopsy and tolerance tests to establish the presence of lactase deficiency, 46 per cent of patients with ulcerative colitis had lactase deficiency as compared to 19 per cent of a normal control population at the same hospital.[23] More than half the patients with biopsy-proved lactase deficiency gave a history that milk worsened their colitis, whereas most of the colitic patients with normal intestinal lactase level did not have an intolerance to milk. Nevertheless, 25.0 g of lactose in water four times a day does not increase diarrhea more than an equivalent amount of glucose in the patients with lactase deficiency.[23] Such data suggest that milk intolerance in patients with ulcerative colitis may indeed be related to substances in milk other than lactose, such as milk proteins.

In general the diet in patients ill with ulcerative colitis should be appealing to the patient in order to overcome anorexia; should contain adequate protein and calories to compensate the patient for enteric protein losses and increased catabolic rates (fever); and should exclude only those substances (such as milk) which careful history indicates may worsen diarrhea. General dietary restrictions cannot be recommended.

The use of opiates (or synthetic derivatives) for symptomatic relief of diarrhea in patients with ulcerative colitis is generally contraindicated. Opiates are effective in diarrheas, such as viral enteritis, because they slow the passage of chyme through the colon, allowing more time for the absorption by the normal colonic mucosa of excessive amounts of sodium and water delivered to the colon from the small bowel. In the more severe forms of ulcerative colitis, profuse diarrhea usually results from widespread destruction of the colonic mucosa (loss of colonic absorptive capacity); in this situation opiates are generally not effective. Furthermore, they may contribute to the development of colonic dilatation (toxic megacolon) and worsen anorexia. For similar reasons anticholinergic drugs are not generally recommended as symptomatic treatment for the diarrhea of ulcerative colitis. Sometimes, however, these agents may be effective in alleviating excessive cramping and nocturnal diarrhea. Likewise, Lomotil (5.0 mg four times daily and at bedtime) may afford some relief. Opiates should be avoided and anticholinergics used sparingly (propantheline, 15 to 30 mg twice a day).

PSYCHOTHERAPY

Just as it is uncertain how often psychosomatic factors play an important role in the development and recrudescence of ulcerative colitis (see p. 1298), it is not clear whether psychotherapy is a useful therapeutic adjunct in most patients with ulcerative colitis. In the best controlled study of the problem, 57 patients were treated with analytically oriented psychotherapy over a seven-year period and matched retrospectively with 57 untreated patients with ulcerative colitis of comparable age, sex, and severity of disease; steroids were given to about an equal number of patients in both groups.[24] The 57 treated patients, however, were referred for psychosis, personality disorders, or psychoneurosis; the control group had a relatively low incidence of psychiatric abnormalities. The mortality and incidence of colectomy (medical failure) in the psychoanalytically treated group was the same as in the control group; however, at the end of eight years clinical and proctoscopic grading of disease was slightly better in the treated group than in the control patients. Those who were not overtly psychotic seemed to benefit the most from psychoanalytic therapy and as a result were much more able to cope with the stresses of their medical disease or social problems. This study as well as several others indicates that psychotic patients (especially schizophrenic patients) have a worse prognosis from ulcerative colitis than controls and are refractory to psychoanalytically oriented therapy.

Such studies do not adequately answer the questions of whether all patients with ulcerative colitis would benefit from psychotherapy, or whether other types of psychotherapy might be more beneficial. Usually supportive therapy from an interested and understanding physician helps most patients with ulcerative colitis.[25] Those patients with personality disorders or severe psychoneuroses may be helped by formal psychiatric treatment. Although psychotic patients may not derive long-term benefits from psychiatric treatment with respect to their ulcerative colitis, the management of a psychotic patient ill with ulcerative colitis is usually improved by the joint care of psychiatrist and physician. Formal psychotherapy, even at a superficial level, is interdicted in a patient who is severely ill with ulcerative colitis.

CORTICOSTEROIDS

Because ulcerative colitis is an inflammatory disease of unknown etiology, ACTH and cortisone, known anti-inflammatory agents, were empirically tried in the treatment of ulcerative colitis in the 1950's. Controlled clinical trials conducted in England quickly demonstrated that a short course of cortisone produced an increased incidence of complete remission in the initial attack or during an acute exacerbation (Table 102–3). Follow-up studies on these patients, however, showed that the benefits of the short course of steroids were transitory: by nine months to two years there was no longer a distinction between the course of the treated patients and the control patients, the numbers of symptomatic patients in each group being equal.[14] Other studies in-

TABLE 102–3.   RESULTS OF CORTISONE TREATMENT AT SIX WEEKS°

RESULT	PATIENTS ON CORTISONE, 100 MG. PO Q.D.	PATIENTS NOT ON CORTISONE
Remission	45 (41%)	16 (16%)
Improvement	30 (28%)	25 (25%)
No change or worse	34 (31%)	60 (59%)
Total	109	101

°From Truelove, S. C., and Witts, L. J.: Brit. Med. J. *1*:387, 1959. Patients in each group had ulcerative colitis of comparable severity, mostly moderate to severe disease.

dicated that maintenance doses of cortisone (50 mg daily) or prednisolone (15 mg daily) after cortisone-induced remissions were not useful in prolonging the remissions.[26, 27] In the years since these studies were completed, newer and more effective cortisone analogues have become available and more experience has been gained with modes of administration and dose schedules. Yet, even though it is clear that corticosteroid therapy may induce remission or improvement in the acute attack, the question of the most effective form of maintenance therapy is still open, and the long-term benefits of steroid treatment have not been adequately assessed.

Dosage and routes of administration of corticosteroid therapy vary with the severity and activity of the disease. In patients with mild disease, especially those with disease limited to the distal colon, rectal instillation of steroids will induce or maintain remission in a high percentage of patients as judged by controlled clinical trials.[28] Dosages usually employed are 50 to 100 mg of hydrocortisone hemisuccinate or 20 to 40 mg of prednisolone phosphate in water; oil-soluble forms may be given in an oil carrier rectally. To induce remission in active disease, the medication may be dripped into the rectum over 20 to 30 minutes or inserted as a bolus nightly and retained during the night. Lower dosages (50 mg of hydrocortisone, 20 mg of prednisolone) several times weekly may be used to maintain remission. The salutary effect seems to be primarily topical, because several studies indicate that the amount of absorption from the large bowel is small (3 to 4 per cent of C^{14}-labeled metabolites of the prednisolone appearing in the urine 24 hours after administration);

more recently this view has been challenged in a study noting a larger percentage of metabolites in the urine and evidence of minor adrenal suppression after steroid enemas. Some authorities maintain that steroid enemas are helpful even in patients with widespread colitis or moderately severe ulcerative colitis. Indeed, rectal steroids appeared to help many patients with moderately severe ulcerative colitis in the initial clinical trials.[28] Efficacy in generalized colitis may, nevertheless, be related to topical effects, because studies in which radiocontrast materials were given with steroid enemas demonstrated movement of the instilled material as far retrograde as the hepatic flexure.

In disease of moderate severity the decision of whether to use systemic or local steroid treatment must be dictated by the clinical status of the patient. The sicker patient—that is, the patient with four to six watery stools daily, low-grade fever, mild constitutional symptoms, ulcerative colitis extending throughout the length of the colon, and perhaps an extracolonic complication such as arthritis—is probably more wisely treated with systemic steroids. In moderate disease the dosage of prednisone or prednisolone given initially is usually 40 to 60 mg daily; this dose is superior to 20 mg in inducing improvement or remission which usually follows within two weeks of the start of steroid treatment.[29] If improvement or remission is induced, the prednisone may be tapered to 10 to 40 mg daily, the speed of steroid withdrawal depending on the status of the patient. If no improvement appears after two to three weeks of oral prednisone treatment, parenteral steroids or ACTH should be given, because either therapy may produce a degree of remission or im-

TABLE 102–4. RESULTS OF TREATMENT IN PATIENTS RANDOMLY ASSIGNED TO ACTH OR ORAL CORTISONE TREATMENT*

RESULT	ACTH (80 UNITS IM/DAY)	CORTISONE (200 MG PO/DAY)
Remission	51 (61%)	33 (39%)
Improvement	12 (14%)	29 (34%)
No change or worse	21 (25%)	23 (27%)
Total (patients)	84	85

*From Truelove, S. C., and Witts, L. J.: Brit. Med. J. *1*:387, 1959.

provement not achieved with orally administered steroids.

The concept that ACTH may be more efficacious than oral prednisone in this situation is based on the subjective impressions of many clinicians and on an older clinical trial which showed that ACTH was somewhat better than oral cortisone in inducing remissions (Table 102–4).[26] The side effects of ACTH in that study were greater than those of the oral cortisone; for this reason the authors recommended ACTH only after a course of oral steroid therapy had failed.

Severe ulcerative colitis is more refractory to corticosteroid treatment, and it is difficult to subject the severely ill patient to prolonged clinical trials of corticosteroids which are relatively unhelpful. Furthermore, the severe form of the disease is the least common, and consequently data accurately defining appropriate dosage, routes of administration, and type or duration of effective cortico-

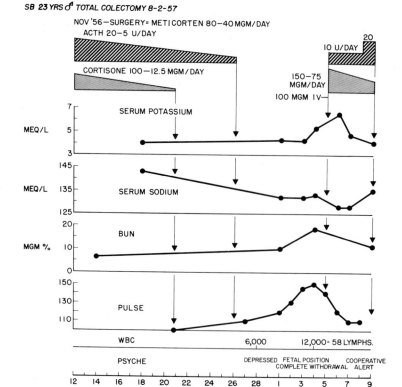

Figure 102–8. Chart illustrating the development of adrenal insufficiency following withdrawal of corticosteroid medication in a patient with ulcerative colitis. (Courtesy of Dr. M. H. Sleisenger.)

steroid therapy in these patients are nearly nonexistent.

In the severely ill patient, either ACTH, 30 to 40 units given intravenously every 12 hours, or a continuous intravenous infusion of 100 mg of prednisolone daily is recommended. The dose is continued for ten to 14 days, by which time sufficient improvement is usually achieved so that oral prednisolone in high dosage (60 to 100 mg per day) may then be substituted. During this period of intensive corticosteroid therapy, the patient should receive antacids (30 ml of aluminum–magnesium hydroxide every two hours) to reduce the possibility of a steroid-induced ulcer, as well as intravenous potassium (40 to 60 mEq per day) to prevent steroid-induced hypokalemia which may contribute to colonic dilatation. High-dose corticosteroid therapy may mask symptoms and signs of sepsis or colonic perforation; for this reason the patient must be carefully examined and his clinical status appraised several times daily during this therapy. Attention to details of fluid and electrolyte management is imperative for a successful outcome of treatment. If no improvement is produced by this treatment in ten to 14 days, the patient should be considered for colectomy (see pp. 1341 to 1343). In case of either medical failure (colectomy) or corticosteroid-induced improvement, signs and symptoms of adrenal insufficiency after withdrawal of corticosteroid therapy must be sought, because adrenal insufficiency is common during withdrawal from high-dose corticosteroids (Fig. 102–8). Another characteristic phenomenon, withdrawal rebound, may be noted in patients with ulcerative colitis who are being weaned from high-dose corticosteroid therapy. In addition to some flare-up in bowel symptoms, patients often complain of fatigability, muscle aches, arthralgias, or arthritis; those patients with associated liver disease are prone to develop an increase in jaundice, and similarly those with uveitis or pyoderma gangrenosum may experience worsening of these complications. Reinstitution of steroid therapy at a higher dose level is often necessary in these patients to alleviate this syndrome.

MAINTENANCE THERAPY

The question of the long-term usefulness of maintenance corticosteroid therapy is unresolved. Existing data suggest that low-dose steroid therapy (50 mg cortisone, 10 to 15 mg prednisone) in the patient in remission will not prevent future exacerbations of ulcerative colitis. For this reason the patient in whom the disease completely remits on treatment should be withdrawn from steroid medication. If the disease remains in remission following steroid withdrawal, no further steroid treatment is indicated until a subsequent exacerbation, when treatment may be reinstituted at a level commensurate with the severity of the exacerbation (steroid enemas for mild to moderate exacerbations; oral steroids for moderate to severe relapse). If on the other hand the patient experiences only partial amelioration of his symptoms on steroid treatment, long-term steroid therapy may be continued until the patient experiences remission. However, the continued use of relatively high doses of oral steroids over a long period of time to maintain the patient relatively free of symptoms is not recommended in view of the potentially serious complications of such treatment (muscle wasting, osteoporosis, growth retardation in children, moon facies, hypertension, diabetes) (Fig. 102–9). We recommend therefore that if the patient requires more than 15 mg of oral prednisone daily for months to keep his colitis and/or extracolonic complications in control, elective colectomy should be considered as an alternative means of treatment. Lower dose oral steroid therapy or steroid enema treatments may be continued indefinitely at the option of the physician and the patient, because the risk of long-term complications from such treatment is much less. Sometimes the patient may be benefited by the long-term use of steroid enemas together with low-dose oral therapy when only high-dose oral therapy without steroid enemas sufficed to control his disease previously.

LONG-TERM EFFECT ON MORBIDITY AND MORTALITY

Whether corticosteroid therapy has altered the long-term morbidity and mortality of ulcerative colitis cannot be answered from existing data. Evidence from a large number of clinics indicates that the cumulative mortality in ulcerative colitis has

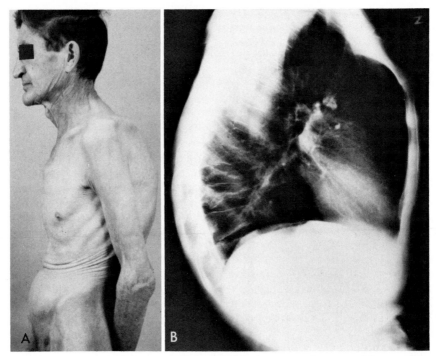

Figure 102–9. *A*, Photograph of a 46-year-old patient with ulcerative colitis treated for six years with cortico-steroids. Note kyphosis, muscle wasting, and atrophy of subcutaneous tissues. *B*, Lateral chest film from the same patient, illustrating kyphosis caused by marked vertebral osteoporosis with collapse of several vertebral bodies.

been reduced by almost 50 per cent since the advent of steroid therapy in the 1950's. Some of this reduction has resulted from decreased mortality in the acute attack of moderate disease, in which situation steroids unquestionably increase the chance of temporary remission or improvement. More liberal use of elective colectomy in clinics with skilled surgeons and anesthetists probably accounts for a significant reduction in long-term mortality in those patients not remitting on steroid treatment. Increasing recognition of complications of long-term disease, together with a vast improvement in general medical treatment of patients ill with ulcerative colitis, has also reduced overall mortality.

SALICYLAZOSULFAPYRIDINE (AZULFIDINE)

This agent was introduced empirically in the treatment of rheumatoid arthritis in the 1940's. Those patients with both arthritis and ulcerative colitis experienced improvement in their colitis when given Azulfidine. Since then, two small controlled trials have been conducted in outpatients with mild to moderate ulcerative colitis localized to the distal colon.[30, 31] The colitis in about one-third of the patients taking Azulfidine remitted within the three- to four-week period of the studies as opposed to remission in about 5 per cent of the control patients receiving placebo tablets. Although there are no controlled trials of the drug in patients with universal colitis or more severe ulcerative colitis, many clinicians have the impression that the drug is beneficial in most forms of ulcerative colitis.

The mode of action of Azulfidine is not known. It is bound to connective tissue throughout the body, slowly breaking down to salicylate + sulfapyridine. It is possible that this property has little to do with the drug's beneficial effects on ulcerative colitis, because other sulfonamides not similarly bound are said to be as effective in the treatment of ulcerative colitis. Azulfidine does not alter the fecal flora; that is, patients taking the drug have the same flora on routine stool culture as ulcerative colitis patients not taking the drug.

Azulfidine has limited usefulness in the treatment of an attack of ulcerative colitis. Although somewhat effective in attacks of mild left-sided colitis, even in this situation Azulfidine produces fewer remissions less promptly than do moderate doses of systemic steroids, and it is not clearly superior to steroid enemas.[32, 33] The drug's benefit in more severe forms of ulcerative colitis or in universal colitis has yet to be documented, but it is probable that Azulfidine is inferior to corticosteroids in the treatment of these forms of the disease. For these reasons we use Azulfidine as an adjunct to corticosteroid therapy, either rectal or systemic, and not as the first line of therapy in the acute attack of ulcerative colitis. Exceptions to this generalization relate to the pediatric or geriatric patient with mild or moderate disease in whom systemic steroids are more hazardous (see pp. 1323 to 1325 and 1345 to 1347, respectively). Doses used are usually 2 to 8 g per day.

Once remission has been induced by corticosteroid therapy, Azulfidine appears to reduce the frequency of subsequent relapse. In a year-long controlled trial of Azulfidine (2 g per day) in patients with mild or moderate ulcerative colitis in remission, relapse appeared in only 21 per cent of patients given Azulfidine as compared with 72 per cent of patients given placebo tablets.[34] Azulfidine thus appears superior to systemic corticosteroids in maintaining remission.

Side effects of Azulfidine are frequent. Malaise, nausea (and/or vomiting), abdominal discomfort, and headache are dose-related side effects appearing in up to 20 per cent of patients given 4 g per day. Like other sulfonamides, Azulfidine also produces idiosyncratic reactions, including skin rash, hemolytic anemia, and aplastic anemia. Because of these side effects, some physicians prefer to use other sulfonamides either in the treatment of acute attacks or as maintenance therapy.

AZATHIOPRINE

For the past five years sporadic reports have appeared concerning the treatment of ulcerative colitis with azathioprine, indicating that remission may be obtained with this agent in patients who have become refractory to steroid therapy or in whom sulfa drugs are not effective either alone or in combination with steroids. The drug is presently indicated for clinical illness which is not so overwhelming, acute, or complicated as to require surgery but which has not responded satisfactorily to steroids.

Preliminary observations from an ongoing controlled clinical trial indicate a more favorable response (fewer relapses per year) in patients receiving azathioprine (1.5 to 2.5 mg per kilogram of body weight daily) than in patients receiving placebo tablets.[35] In this study steroids were used intermittently—that is, during exacerbations. Side effects from the azathioprine were minimal. However, as yet the differences between azathioprine and placebo barely approach significance. Until more data are available from such trials as to the efficacy of azathioprine in ulcerative colitis and until better information is obtained as to risks of long-term treatment with azathioprine, this drug must be considered experimental in the treatment of ulcerative colitis.

OUTCOME

IMMEDIATE PROGNOSIS OF THE FIRST ATTACK

The outlook for recovery from the first attack of ulcerative colitis is very good, but is influenced by a number of factors.[15, 36, 37] Foremost among these is the severity of the initial attack. In all patients suffering from the first attack of ulcerative colitis, whether mild, moderate, or severe,* the mortality rate is 4 to 6 per cent; however, 75 to 90 per cent of those who die have had a clinically severe form of ulcerative colitis. The remainder of deaths result from moderately severe ulcerative colitis, the mortality of mild disease being almost nil (see Table 102–2).

Patients who die of the initial attack

---

*Severe ulcerative colitis: more than six bowel movements daily; significant colonic bleeding, weight loss, fever, tachycardia, anemia, and hypoalbuminemia. Mild disease: less than four bowel movements daily; no fever, anemia, hypoalbuminemia, or weight loss.

most frequently have colitis involving the entire colon, so-called universal colitis. The fact merely reflects the correlation between severity and extent of disease; those patients with severe disease tend to have universal colitis. On the other hand, the correlation between extent and severity is not absolute; about 12 per cent of patients with severe initial attacks have their colitis limited to the left colon, whereas, conversely, nearly 20 per cent of patients with mild disease may have total colonic involvement. The mortality rate among patients with severe colitis is about the same whether the colitis is limited to the left colon or extends throughout the colon. Thus it appears that severity of the illness is the most predictive factor of mortality and that extent of colonic involvement, except as it relates to severity, is not as good an estimate of mortality risk.

In general, patients with short illness prior to hospitalization tend to be more severely ill; this fact is reflected in the relationship between mortality and duration of symptoms; i.e., a short history of symptoms prior to hospitalization for an initial attack is associated with a higher mortality. In fact, the mortality of patients entering the hospital with severe ulcerative colitis of less than one month's duration is two to three times that of the patients who have been ill with severe ulcerative colitis for longer than one month.

A fourth factor in the outcome of the initial attack is the age of the patient at the onset of the illness. All studies of mortality in ulcerative colitis conclude that mortality of the initial attack in patients over 60 years of age is much higher than in younger patients. In part this age factor can be related to severity in that about half of the first episodes of ulcerative colitis in patients over age 60 or under age 20 will be clinically severe, as opposed to about one-fourth of the first episodes in patients between ages 20 and 59. Yet the overall mortality for patients dying of the initial attack below age 20 is close to zero; about 2 per cent of patients who experience the initial attack between ages 20 and 59 die, in contrast to 17 per cent of all patients developing ulcerative colitis over the age of 60. Thus in the two age groups having

severe first attacks (those below age 20 and those over 60), the mortality is much greater in the older age group.

Certain complications affect the prognosis. Principal among these is the development of toxic megacolon, which has a mortality rate of 14 to 30 per cent. Associated liver disease, reflected either by abnormal blood tests of liver function or by a histological abnormality (pericholangitis, cirrhosis, fatty liver), increases mortality. Hypokalemia or hypoalbuminemia also portends a worse prognosis, probably because the degree of these abnormalities parallels clinical severity. On the other hand, ankylosing spondylitis or arthritis does not affect the prognosis.

About half the patients who die of the first attack will have been operated upon for either massive bleeding or perforation, the latter a complication most commonly associated with toxic megacolon. The remainder die from massive hemorrhage, superimposed infection, pulmonary embolism, or cardiac complications.

Fewer patients are dying of the first attack than previously. Mortality is lower as the result of a number of factors. It appears that patients with ulcerative colitis are being diagnosed and successfully treated earlier in the course of their disease, because fewer patients with severe disease are being encountered in most medical centers. Modern medical treatment (corticosteroids, fluid and electrolyte therapy, safe blood transfusions, effective antimicrobials) has sharply reduced the mortality in patients with moderately severe ulcerative colitis (Table 102–2). Earlier recognition of potential candidates for surgery (those with continued brisk colonic bleeding, toxic megacolon not responding to therapy in a few days, or severe disease not responding to treatment in ten to 14 days) and improved anesthetic and surgical techniques have also improved prognosis. In spite of improving medical therapy, mortality from severe disease still remains high—perhaps as high as 30 per cent (see Table 102–2). Many of the referred patients who are presently dying of severe ulcerative colitis in centers did not receive adequate medical treatment at an earlier, less severe stage of their disease.

LONG-TERM OUTLOOK

It is very difficult to make a long-term prognosis for the individual patient with ulcerative colitis. Over a long period of time, the disease may vary in frequency and severity of individual attacks and extent of colonic involvement.[13, 38, 39] Ultimate prognosis is related to each of these factors. However, a few generalizations can be made about groups of patients.

As already noted, about 4 to 6 per cent of patients will be dead within one year of the onset of their disease, either because of a complication of the initial acute episode (including postoperative complications) or because of severe continuing activity of their disease, culminating in a fatal outcome. After the first attack, about 10 per cent of patients will have a remission lasting up to 15 years or more. Their prognosis is therefore good. An additional 10 per cent will experience a continuously active colitis. The sicker ones in this category will invariably undergo colectomy, usually within five years of the onset of their disease. The remaining patients (75 per cent) will experience intermittent remissions and exacerbations of their colitis over the years, whether the initial attack was mild, moderate, or severe, and regardless of the extent of colonic involvement.

Most of those with mild first attacks (80 per cent) will continue to have mild subsequent relapses. Their long-term prognosis is therefore quite good; in fact, their mortality differs little from that of the general population. Particularly fortunate in this group are those with mild colitis limited to the rectum; although they will continue to have relapses, they rarely require hospitalization.[16]

Those with moderately severe first attacks fare less well. Close to half will experience repeated attacks of moderate severity; a few will have severe subsequent attacks, whereas the remainder will have subsequent episodes of a more mild nature. A large percentage of relapses in this group therefore will require subsequent hospitalization. As a result, patients with moderately severe first attacks will have to be hospitalized subsequently about twice as often as the group with mild initial episodes. The mortality in the first five years is between 13 and 20 per cent.

As expected, those with severe first attacks will have the worst long-term outlook. The mortality of this group is 40 per cent in the first five years, about half of whom die during the first attack. After the first severe attack, subsequent relapses are often less severe. This is reflected by the mortality in this group, which after the first five years becomes the same as for patients with moderately severe first attacks; i.e., about 2.5 per cent per annum.

It should be remembered that about 60 per cent of all patients with ulcerative colitis have mild first attacks; about 25 per cent are moderately ill at onset; and only about 15 per cent present with severe colitis. Thus in terms of absolute numbers of patients, both mortality and morbidity from ulcerative colitis are considerably less than might be inferred. It is not surprising therefore that about half of all patients with ulcerative colitis managed medically for a long period of time require no further hospitalizations. Of those who require subsequent hospitalization, about half will be admitted several times. Only about 25 per cent of all patients with ulcerative colitis will come to colectomy within five to ten years after onset of their disease, usually for continuous disease, a severe episode, toxic megacolon, colonic perforation, or colonic stricture. Most patients with ulcerative colitis, including those who require repeated hospitalizations, are not incapacitated by their disease but continue to lead productive lives.

ULCERATIVE COLITIS IN PREGNANCY

A special kind of patient with ulcerative colitis is the female in the child-bearing age. Conflicting reports have indicated different attitudes on the part of knowledgeable physicians concerning the advisability of pregnancy for women with ulcerative colitis. No dogmatic position can be taken on this issue; the evidence makes it clear that each case must be judged individually. The two key questions are (1) what is the effect of pregnancy on the course of ulcerative colitis in a woman afflicted with this disease?, and (2) what is the effect of ulcerative colitis and its treatment on the viability and development of the fetus?

PREVIOUS ULCERATIVE COLITIS QUIESCENT AT THE TIME OF CONCEPTION

About 40 to 50 per cent of women in this category will experience an exacerbation of their colitis during the pregnancy. This overall relapse rate (40 per cent during 37 weeks of gestation) is not too different from the relapse rate of ulcerative colitis in nonpregnant patients, but in the pregnant patient most of these relapses are seen in the first trimester or in the postpartum period.[40] A minority of patients will become ill in the second trimester, and practically none will have a relapse in the third trimester. A past history of an exacerbation of ulcerative colitis during pregnancy is not useful in predicting difficulty during subsequent pregnancies, because only about 25 per cent of the total number of gestations in women in this category are complicated by an exacerbation of ulcerative colitis;[41] that is, many women who relapse during one pregnancy may have an uneventful subsequent pregnancy.

The great majority of patients who have had previous colectomy and ileostomy will experience uncomplicated pregnancies and have normal deliveries and children. Rarely, some prolapse of the ileostomy may be noted during pregnancy.

ULCERATIVE COLITIS ACTIVE AT THE TIME OF CONCEPTION

The likelihood is that the disease may worsen at any time during the pregnancy; indeed, it does so in about 50 per cent of the women in this category. A small percentage of women (about 20 per cent) may experience improvement in their colitis during pregnancy; in the remainder, the disease appears to be unaffected by pregnancy and continues to run an indolent course.

ONSET OF ULCERATIVE COLITIS DURING PREGNANCY

Occasionally ulcerative colitis will begin during pregnancy. Most frequently it will appear during the first trimester and, in a rare instance, may be quite severe. Indeed, fulminant colitis with death has been reported during the first trimester of pregnancy. In comparison with the first two categories, in which ulcerative colitis, quiescent or active, antedates conception, the relative number of individuals in this third category is small—in only one-tenth of pregnancies complicated by ulcerative colitis does the colitis develop after conception.

ONSET OF ULCERATIVE COLITIS IN THE POSTPARTUM OR POSTABORTAL PERIOD

This category also has only one-tenth as many patients as the categories of established disease, either active or quiescent, antedating pregnancy.

The basis for recrudescence of the disease during pregnancy is as mysterious as the etiology of the disease itself. Quiescent disease most commonly exacerbates during the first trimester. One may speculate that somehow levels of endogenous corticosteroids which are high in the second and third trimesters may be responsible for this pattern.[40] Alternatively, much has been made of the possible interrelationships between psychiatric factors in the patient's life, pregnancy, and ulcerative colitis. Some observers feel that the patient's attitude toward the pregnancy, i.e., whether the pregnancy is desired, may affect the subsequent course of the gestation. Others point out that pregnancy may alter interpersonal relationships in the patient's life, thereby influencing the course of the colitis.

EFFECTS ON THE FETUS

About 10 per cent of gestations in women with ulcerative colitis will terminate in spontaneous abortions, an event invariably associated with active colitis. Premature births and cesarean sections are no more common than among the general population. Patients with active disease during pregnancy are frequently treated with sulfonamides and/or corticosteroids. Data are not available as to the efficacy of these agents during pregnancy; however, it is clear that systemically administered steroids do not adversely affect the fetus.

TREATMENT

Treatment for ulcerative colitis during pregnancy is much the same as it is for nonpregnant individuals (see pp. 1312 to 1319); however, there are special considerations. For obvious reasons, a pregnant patient should not have X-ray studies. In the second and third trimesters of pregnancy gentle proctoscopy may be performed in those women whose disease begins during gestation; in the first trimester it is well to avoid the procedure unless the clinical situation is sufficiently unclear to warrant it. In those patients with established disease, proctosigmoidoscopy should be avoided.

The usual indications for steroid therapy may be applied, and the patients can be carried on maintenance doses throughout the gestational period, if need be, without detriment to the fetus. No special attention need be paid to diet except in instances of known sensitivity to milk or other foods. Rectal instillation of steroid in water or oil via catheter may be prescribed, provided that less than 100 ml of fluid is instilled over a 20- to 30-minute period; 60 ml may be instilled gently by syringe as well. Sulfisoxazole, 0.5 to 1.0 g four times daily, may also be given by mouth, or salicylazosulfapyridine (Azulfidine), 1.0 g by mouth four to six times daily, although evidence of superiority over sulfisoxazole is lacking, and toxicity to Azulfidine is greater.

The most important aspect of therapy—indeed, its cornerstone—is the patient-doctor relationship. These young women tend to be apprehensive about all aspects of their experience, particularly the delivery itself. They have self-doubts concerning their ability to care for an infant and manage a household with a child. Therefore the patient must be treated with a great deal of sympathetic understanding and seen at frequent intervals.

Therapeutic abortion has little place in the treatment of pregnant patients with ulcerative colitis. Very low maternal mortality and a low incidence of spontaneous abortion and prematurity indicate that therapeutic abortion should be reserved for the rare case in patients in the first trimester who are desperately ill and very likely to lose the child in any event. Termination transabdominally later in the pregnancy is not indicated inasmuch as unremitting illness usually results in termination of the pregnancy by premature labor. Rarely, a patient with fulminant ulcerative colitis in pregnancy must undergo colectomy and ileostomy as a life-saving measure. The indications for colectomy in the severely ill pregnant patient are the same as in the non-pregnant patient (see pp. 1341 to 1343). Neither spontaneous nor therapeutic abortion in women who are acutely and seriously ill with ulcerative colitis is likely to alter dramatically the severity of the illness.

What advice should be given to a woman with ulcerative colitis regarding childbearing? If the patient's colitis is quiescent and she desires pregnancy, it should be advised. On the other hand, if the patient is ill with colitis, pregnancy should be avoided by the use of appropriate contraceptive measures until the colitis has been controlled and has remained quiescent for a year.

ULCERATIVE COLITIS WITH ONSET AFTER AGE 50

The incidence of ulcerative colitis in individuals over the age of 50 is nearly the same as in younger persons. The disease may be somewhat more severe in these older patients as a group, but generally symptoms of the disease, clinical course, and response to treatment are similar to those of younger patients with ulcerative colitis. About 25 per cent of elderly patients (i.e., over age 50) will have universal colitis, but in the remainder the colitis involves the left colon or the rectosigmoid. Two factors tend to complicate the management of ulcerative colitis in the older age group: (1) failure to diagnose the disease correctly at its onset, and (2) the high incidence of associated disease of the elderly (diabetes, arteriosclerosis, hypertensive cardiovascular disease, emphysema, diverticulosis coli) which complicates the management of the colitis.

CLINICAL PICTURE

Diarrhea and rectal bleeding are the most prominent presenting symptoms, and about half the patients will have significant weight loss for periods of several months to one year, as well as crampy abdominal pain. As in the younger patient, fever is frequently noted, but in the elderly patient fever does not necessarily reflect the severity of the colitis. An older patient may have severe disease with little or no fever, a phenomenon similar to the lack of febrile response to infection frequently noted in the older age group. Extracolonic complications in this age group include erythema nodosum, uveitis, and arthritis, but pyoderma gangrenosum appears to be extremely rare. Since the disease most frequently involves only the distal colon, it is not surprising that the incidence of severe anemia, hypoalbuminemia, and dehydration is on the whole less common than in younger patients.

DIAGNOSIS AND DIFFERENTIAL DIAGNOSIS

The difficulty in correctly diagnosing the disease in many patients lies less with the patient's stoicism or lack of complaints than with the physician's misinterpretation of the findings.[42] In this age group the patient's symptoms (diarrhea and hematochezia) are most frequently seen with either carcinoma or diverticulitis of the colon. Many physicians are not aware of the incidence of ulcerative colitis in the elderly and attribute the patient's complaints to either cancer or diverticulitis. As in the younger age group, the correct diagnosis can most often be established by proctosigmoidoscopy.

Pain, fever, occasionally bleeding, and often diarrhea are prominent symptoms in diverticulitis as in ulcerative colitis. Usually, however, these symptoms are transitory and episodic in diverticulitis, whereas the same symptoms in ulcerative colitis tend to persist for long periods of time. Barium enema examination of the colon usually confirms diverticulosis and/or diverticulitis; but it should be noted that some elderly patients with left-sided colitis may have diverticulosis as well, so that barium enema examination may not differentiate between these two conditions.

The most helpful procedure is a proctosigmoidoscopy. Although bright red blood may be seen coming from above the sigmoidoscope in bleeding diverticulitis, the visible mucosa appears normal and is not friable. By contrast, in ulcerative colitis the mucosa of the rectosigmoid is usually abnormally friable and exhibits other features typical of ulcerative colitis (see pp. 1304 to 1311). Sometimes an episode of diverticulitis, with lower abdominal cramps, fever, diarrhea, and perhaps hematochezia, will culminate in perforation of a sigmoid diverticulum, with the formation of a pericolic abscess and colonic dilatation. Thus severe diverticulitis may rarely be confused with acute toxic dilatation of the colon. The same physical findings—fever, anemia, leukocytosis, localized peritoneal signs, and lower abdominal distention—may be noted in toxic megacolon. Further, onset of symptoms may be acute, and the patient may become critically ill in a few days in both conditions. Here again, proctosigmoidoscopy is essential in distinguishing the two conditions. In toxic megacolon, the flat film of the abdomen may reveal ulceration and serration of the visible colonic mucosa, a feature not seen in diverticulitis.

Since changes in bowel habit, i.e., onset of diarrhea and particularly bleeding, are hallmarks of large bowel cancer, this disease must be carefully excluded by proctosigmoidoscopy and barium enema examination in patients who have these complaints. Both procedures will also establish the diagnosis of ulcerative colitis if this is the cause of the symptoms. Although adenomatous polyps are frequent in older patients with ulcerative colitis (just as they are in older patients in general), colonic cancer complicating ulcerative colitis that begins after age 50 is usual. Presumably, the elderly patient with late-onset ulcerative colitis dies of other causes before his ulcerative colitis evolves into cancer (see below).

The group of patients who are less severely ill with disease confined to the rectosigmoid get along very well with conservative therapy, i.e., topical steroids and in some cases sulfonamides. Systemic corticosteroid treatment should be reserved for those patients who have failed to respond to topical (rectal) steroids and/or oral sulfonamides and are socially and economically handicapped by their symptoms. Although systemic corticosteroids may aggravate pre-existing congestive heart failure, hypertension, diabetes, or osteoporosis in the elderly, adverse reactions to corticosteroids are not as high as one would expect. Lack of adverse effects probably relates to short-term, rather than long-term, use of corticosteroids in these elderly patients. Short-term response has been good on the whole; the majority of elderly patients who respond to systemic corticosteroid treatment no longer require the medication after six to eight weeks. Of the patients who improve on systemic corticosteroids but continue to have symptoms, about half will require surgery, usually on an elective basis.

Surgery for ulcerative colitis in this age group is gratifyingly successful. Providing that the general medical condition of the patient will permit, subtotal colectomy and ileostomy or total colectomy and ileostomy effectively eradicate the disease. Without an ileostomy, patients who are operated upon fare poorly, as in the younger age group. Thus a patient explored for mistakenly diagnosed diverticulitis who is subjected to partial colectomy without ileostomy for ulcerative colitis, or even to simple colostomy, is likely to have a rather stormy course postoperatively. Some may fare well in the postoperative period, but will usually require colectomy and ileostomy within a period of months after the procedure.

As in the younger age group, about 5 to 10 per cent of the elderly will develop fulminant colitis. Treatment for fulminant colitis in this age group is the same as in the younger patients — that is, intravenous ACTH, fluid replacement, blood transfusions, broad-spectrum antimicrobials, and emergency surgery if the patient does not respond to medical management within ten to 14 days (see pp. 1327 to 1329).

COMPLICATIONS

Ulcerative colitis may be complicated by a variety of associated conditions. These most logically fall into two categories: (1) local complications, arising in and around the colon; and (2) systemic complications, affecting sites remote from the colon. The diversity and frequency of the latter have prompted some to consider ulcerative colitis as a systemic disease, for example, an autoimmune disease (see p. 1299). Unfortunately, the pathogenesis of each of the systemic manifestations of ulcerative colitis is not known.

LOCAL COMPLICATIONS

We have chosen to classify these as minor (those which are not life threatening) and major (those which are potentially lethal to the patient). Minor complications include *hemorrhoids* (20 per cent), *pseudopolyps* (15 per cent), *anal fissures* (12 per cent), *anal fistulas* (4 to 5 per cent), *perianal* or *ischiorectal abscess* (4 to 6 per cent), *rectal prolapse* (2 per cent), and *rectovaginal fistulas* (2 to 3 per cent). The percentages indicate the estimated frequency of these lesions among 1089 patients followed for ulcerative colitis.[43,44]

Rectal prolapse, anal fissures, perirectal or ischiorectal abscesses, and rectovaginal fistulas most frequently appear during periods of active colitis when diarrhea is prominent. These lesions are slightly more frequent in patients with universal colitis than in those with proctocolitis, but this may only reflect the more severe diarrhea usually seen in universal colitis as opposed to proctocolitis. Anal fissures heal with control of the colitis and other medical measures. Perirectal abscesses and rectal fistulas heal with conservative surgical treatment, that is, incision and drainage of abscesses and opening of fistulous tracts. Rectovaginal fistulas in ulcerative colitis, on the other hand, rarely heal after local repair and require either colectomy with ileostomy or temporary ileostomy to facilitate successful surgical repair.

Pseudopolyps are either swollen, edematous excrescences of mucosa between ulcerations or heaped-up granulation tissue. They usually appear in patients with severe disease within the first few months to a year after onset; more often, they are seen in patients with universal colitis. Once developed, they tend to persist but occasionally may regress completely when the colitis remits for long periods of time. Contrary to previous widespread beliefs, these islands of tissue are not the seat of future carcinoma which seems to arise more often in atrophic or re-epithelialized mucosa in ulcerative colitis. Therefore the development of pseudopolyps is of no important consequence to the patient.

Enteroenteric fistulas may develop in a very small number of patients with ulcerative colitis — less than 0.5 per cent. It is not clear whether these few patients have ulcerative colitis or granulomatous colitis, which are sometimes difficult to distinguish from each other (see pp. 1350 to 1352). The incidence of enteroenteric fistulas in granulomatous colitis is much higher. Similarly, rectovesical fistula, a fairly common complication of granulomatous colitis, has not been reported in any patient with ulcerative colitis.

Major local complications include *toxic megacolon, colonic perforation, massive colonic hemorrhage, colonic carcinoma,* and *colonic stricture.* Although not usually life threatening, the last has been listed as a major complication because benign stricture cannot always be differentiated from carcinoma. Necrotizing and pseudomembranous colitis may also rarely complicate ulcerative colitis (see pp. 1369 to 1373).

TOXIC MEGACOLON

Definition. As the name implies, this complication is characterized by acute dilatation of all or part of the colon to a diameter greater than 6 cm (occasionally to as much as 17 cm) associated with systemic toxicity. The frequency of toxic megacolon is difficult to estimate; data from retrospective surveys are often incomplete, but two large series of ulcerative colitis patients indicate that toxic megacolon arises in 1 to 2.5 per cent of patients. Most episodes (60 to 75 per cent) develop during a relapse of chronic intermittent ulcerative colitis; yet a substantial proportion (25 to 40 per cent) of attacks constitute the acute initial episode of ulcerative colitis.

Pathogenesis. The pathogenesis of the syndrome is not well understood. As discussed previously (see pp. 1299 to 1301), histological examinations of colons removed at surgery or autopsy from patients with toxic megacolon show extensive deep ulceration and acute inflammation involving all muscle layers of the colon, often with extension of the inflammatory process to the serosa. The depth and extent of the inflammatory process in the colon of patients with toxic megacolon are usually more marked than in the resected colon specimens of patients with severe or ful-

minant ulcerative colitis without colonic dilatation.[45] Presumably, the presence of widespread inflammation involving all layers of the colon in toxic megacolon accounts for both the systemic toxicity (fever, tachycardia, abdominal pain and tenderness, leukocytosis) and the apparent loss of colonic muscular tone, resulting in dilatation of the colon. Evidence of inflammation can be found in small arterioles (vasculitis) and myenteric or submucosal nerve plexuses. However, these latter findings are variable, and so probably vasculitis and inflammation and destruction of myenteric or submucosal plexuses are not responsible for the syndrome. In addition to widespread inflammation and destruction of colonic musculature, other factors which tend to promote high intraluminal pressures or decreased colonic muscular tone are thought to contribute to colonic dilatation; these include barium enema examinations, aerophagia, excessive use of opiates or anticholinergic drugs, and hypokalemia. None of these latter factors individually appear to be causative, because several cases of toxic megacolon have been reported in their absence, and many patients with severe colitis receiving barium enema examinations, opiates, or anticholinergics or having hypokalemia do not develop toxic megacolon. It would appear therefore that the pathogenesis of the syndrome is best explained by widespread inflammation and destruction of colonic musculature, perhaps aggravated by other factors. What is not explained is why relatively few patients with ulcerative colitis (1 to 2.5 per cent) develop the deep ulcerations beneath the submucosa characteristically seen in toxic megacolon. The syndrome may occasionally complicate other forms of infectious colitis, including amebic colitis, bacillary dysentery, and cholera; rarely, granulomatous colitis may evolve into toxic megacolon.

Clinical Picture. The patient with toxic megacolon is usually severely ill with prostration, fever (104 to 105° F), tachycardia, dehydration, and abdominal pain and tenderness as well as distention. Physical examination of the abdomen often reveals diminished or absent sounds, tympany, and mild rebound tenderness. Leukocytosis (often greater than 20,000 per mm³), anemia, and hypoalbuminemia are common. A plain flat film of the abdomen will reveal dilatation of the entire colon or of a segment of colon, most commonly the transverse colon or ascending colon. Some moderate distention of small bowel loops as well as a ragged-appearing, serrated, irregular colonic mucosa silhouetted against the air in the colon may also be discerned on flat film. Upright abdominal films may reveal free air under the diaphragm if the colon has perforated, a common complication of toxic megacolon.

In most instances, toxic megacolon complicates chronic intermittent or chronic continuous ulcerative colitis of long-standing duration. In this setting, the diagnosis of this complication is not difficult. Sudden deterioration of the patient's condition with the development of systemic toxicity (high fever, tachycardia, profound weakness) and abdominal distention point to toxic megacolon and/or colonic perforation. Occasionally, a patient seriously ill with ulcerative colitis and profuse bloody diarrhea will experience a sudden decrease in frequency of bowel movements with the development of toxic megacolon; the decrease in stool frequency reflects diminished colonic evacuation rather than improvement in the patient's status. Misinterpretation may be obviated by examination of the patient's abdomen, which will reveal distention, diminished bowel sounds, and tenderness. The diagnosis may be confirmed by X-ray examination of the abdomen: a plain flat film to confirm colonic dilatation and upright abdominal films to look for perforation (free air).

Diagnosis. When toxic megacolon ushers in ulcerative colitis, the diagnosis is more difficult. Toxic megacolon may supervene so rapidly that a history of rectal bleeding and diarrhea is obscured. In this setting the condition may be confused with acute diverticulitis and pericolic abscess or carcinoma (which is associated with lower quadrant pain, fever, and colonic dilatation), ischemic colitis (which occasionally may be associated with colonic dilatation proximal to the vascular insult), and colonic volvulus. Here the correct diagnosis may be established by flat film of the abdomen and sigmoidoscopy. Often the flat film will reveal a diffusely abnormal and irregular colonic mucosa

(Fig. 102–3). Sigmoidoscopy should be carried out despite the severe illness and the obvious discomfort of the patient. It can be done in the left lateral position in bed if necessary, without colonic preparation. The sigmoidoscope need be inserted only a short distance without air insufflation, for in the vast majority of individuals presenting with toxic megacolon of ulcerative colitis the rectosigmoid mucosa will reveal findings characteristic of ulcerative colitis.

Treatment. Treatment consists of general supportive measures and efforts to arrest the necrotic process in the colon. In the former category is careful correction of fluid and electrolyte deficits, particularly hypokalemia. Fluid and electrolyte deficits may be profound (water deficit may be as great as 10 per cent of body weight) owing to antecedent diarrhea, vomiting, and loss of liters of fluid into the dilated colon. Not uncommonly, 80 to 120 mEq of potassium chloride in the first 24 hours is needed to correct hypokalemia. Blood transfusions should be given when indicated, i.e., with anemia, hypoalbuminemia, evidence of decreased blood volume, and significant colonic bleeding. ACTH, 40 to 60 units, or prednisolone, 100 to 200 mg, should be given by continuous intravenous drip daily. Corticosteroids are given in large dosage in an effort to ameliorate the inflammatory process in the colon. Since many of these patients have been treated previously with corticosteroids for their colitis for weeks, months, or even years, the increased stress of toxic megacolon may precipitate relative adrenal insufficiency. Hence, high-dose corticosteroid therapy may be required. Nasogastric suction should be instituted in an effort to remove swallowed air and thereby to reduce the passage of air and fluid into the colon. The patient should be withdrawn from anticholinergic medicines and opiates if he had been receiving them previously. Usually, abdominal pain is not severe enough to require opiate analgesics. In view of transmural and often serosal inflammation in patients with toxic megacolon, frank perforation is a constant danger; often multiple small, walled-off perforations are found at resection. To help contain the consequences of these perforations should they occur, broad-spectrum antibiotics are recommended. Ampicillin in a dose of 4 to 8 g daily intravenously will be effective against most organisms that can be expected to cause purulent peritonitis or pericolic abscess. In patients who have perforated, kanamycin, 1.0 to 2.0 g daily, should be added.

The patient's response to treatment must be carefully monitored. Abdominal girth should be measured and recorded two or three times daily, and the physician should examine the patient at frequent intervals to ascertain whether bowel sounds are returning, whether an area of localized tenderness or rebound has developed, whether signs of perforation are present, and whether cardiovascular complications associated with falling blood pressure and bacterial sepsis have appeared. In addition, adequacy of fluid and electrolyte repletion must be carefully recorded; in difficult situations close care includes monitoring of central venous pressure in addition to standard intake and output balance sheets.

The first 96 hours of treatment are crucial in determining the future management of the patient. A minority of individuals will experience a rather dramatic decrease in distention with a return of bowel sounds, a drop in temperature, and a slowing of pulse. In these patients a flat film of the abdomen will demonstrate progressive diminution of colonic dilatation which will correlate well with clinical improvement. They should be continued on high-dose ACTH or prednisolone for ten to 14 days and then be gradually tapered off. The patient may be switched to oral prednisolone, 40 to 60 mg per day, at the time he begins to take liquids by mouth, after the removal of the nasogastric tube. Broad-spectrum antimicrobial agents, however, should be continued for several weeks, because intra-abdominal abscess may still complicate the recovery from megacolon in this period of time.

Unfortunately, many individuals do not respond in this fashion; distention and dilatation of the colon persist, although fluid and electrolyte balance is restored and fever may subside in some. The likelihood of perforation of the colon in this situation after four days or so of such intensive treatment remains high—as high as 50 per cent. Thus the risk of continued medical therapy in these patients is great. Ac-

cordingly, the recommended course of action is subtotal colectomy with ileostomy. In the hands of skilled surgeons operative mortality for those treated intensively for four to five days as outlined above is less than 5 to 10 per cent, although postoperative morbidity may be significant. The drop in surgical mortality from over 60 per cent to 5 to 10 per cent in large hospital centers in the past 15 years is due not only to better pre- and postoperative management and surgical technique but also to earlier surgical intervention. During surgery and for three to four days postoperatively the patient is continued on high doses of prednisolone (100 to 200 mg per day, intravenously) to prevent relative adrenal insufficiency. Thereafter the dose is tapered, and the drug may be withdrawn completely by several weeks after surgery if the patient has recovered. At surgery, technical difficulties, as well as the extensively inflamed, dilated, "paper-thin" colonic wall, inevitably result in peritoneal contamination with bacteria; postoperative intra-abdominal abscess formation is common and may be masked by continued administration of corticosteroids. Therefore we recommend that antibiotics be given for two weeks after corticosteroids have been discontinued. If a postoperative intra-abdominal abscess develops, it should be treated by surgical drainage; again, in the event of this complication the patient must be observed carefully for signs of relative adrenal insufficiency.

The most common major complication of toxic megacolon is free perforation of the colon. This event may be dramatic in its suddenness, and shock may be irreversible. With free perforation blood pressure usually falls while pulse rate and temperature rise. On physical examination a marked increase in abdominal distention and obliteration of hepatic dullness by free air may be discerned. Upright abdominal X-ray films will confirm the presence of free air. Multiple walled-off perforations and pericolic abscesses are less serious. Other complications include gram-negative bacteremia, acute renal tubular necrosis (from shock, sepsis, and prolonged fluid and electrolyte depletion), and cardiac arrhythmias (from hypokalemia, acid-base imbalance, and shock). Thrombophlebitis of the leg or pelvic veins may result in pulmonary embolism. Finally, massive colonic hemorrhage may intervene, requiring total colectomy.

Outcome. Overall mortality (in both medically and surgically treated patients) is high, between 12 and 30 per cent. From 14 to 30 per cent of patients require surgery after failure to respond to medical treatment. Of those who respond to medical treatment, with return of the colon to normal caliber, the incidence of further difficulties from colitis is high. About one-third will require subsequent colectomy during the same hospitalization for continued severe colitis. A large number of those who are discharged from the hospital without operations continue to have subsequent problems. A few may redevelop toxic megacolon. Only half will continue to remain well during the first year after the episode of toxic megacolon, and many thus come to eventual elective colectomy within this period of time. Colons removed from these patients within a year of the episode of toxic dilatation reveal fibrosis in the muscular layers of the colon, i.e., scarring in the areas of muscular inflammation and necrosis during the acute episode.

COLONIC PERFORATION

As just noted, colonic perforation may complicate toxic megacolon, but free perforation of the colon also occurs in ulcerative colitis in the absence of toxic dilatation. Most perforations arise in patients with severe disease; a very small percentage of patients with moderately severe colitis perforate, but this complication is not seen in mild disease. Overall, about 3 per cent of patients with ulcerative colitis perforate in the absence of toxic megacolon. For reasons which are not clear, the chance of perforation seems to be greatest in the initial severe attack of ulcerative colitis.[43]

In severe ulcerative colitis the colonic inflammatory process may occasionally extend deep into the colonic wall, just as in toxic megacolon (see pp. 1299 to 1301). However, unlike the situation in toxic megacolon, transmural extension is less common in severe disease; when present, it is often localized at one point in the colon rather than extensively spread along large segments of the colon. Presumably, perforation of the colon in severe colitis arises from such a point of transmural involvement.

Some have claimed that corticosteroid treatment for ulcerative colitis may increase the incidence of perforation by rendering the bowel and surrounding peritoneum less capable of containing transmural inflammation. However, available data do not substantiate this notion, because the incidence of colonic perforation complicating ulcerative colitis has not increased since the introduction of corticosteroid therapy. However, corticosteroids may mask symptoms and signs of perforation. High intraluminal pressures developed in the colon during barium enema examination would theoretically promote perforation through an area of transmural disease. The incidence of perforation in severe disease after barium enema is not well documented, but prudence would dictate that this procedure be deferred until the patient has recovered from the severe attack. Unfortunately, it is the patient most prone to perforate—a severely ill patient seen for the first time with the initial attack of ulcerative colitis—who makes the physician anxious to diagnose the patient's problem quickly by a barium enema. Diagnosis, however, can usually be made with gentle proctoscopy (see p. 1327).

Perforation may be easily diagnosed or strongly suspected in many patients with colitis. Sudden deterioration with increased abdominal pain, tachycardia, fever, increased abdominal girth, and direct and rebound tenderness point to perforation. However, on equally many occasions, these signs and symptoms are not present, often when the patient is receiving high doses of corticosteroid treatment. In this situation perforation may be heralded only by a nonspecific deterioration in the patient's status in the absence of abdominal signs. In either case, diagnosis may be confirmed by the demonstration of free air within the abdominal cavity on upright abdominal X-ray films. Sometimes serial films must be taken daily before free air in the peritoneal cavity is appreciated. Even in centers most experienced in treating ulcerative colitis, colonic perforation may be undiagnosed ante mortem.

Without question, the diagnosis of perforation or indeed of strongly suspected per-

TABLE 102–5. CAUSES OF DEATH IN 137 PATIENTS WITH
ULCERATIVE COLITIS (1930 TO 1966)°

Death as a direct outcome of colitis:		
Colonic perforation		16
Postoperative deaths		16
Postoperative peritonitis	10	
Miscellaneous	6	
Fulminant colitis		12
Colonic hemorrhage		1
Malnutrition		1
		—
		46 patients
Death related to colitis:		
Carcinoma of the colon		16
Deaths related to treatment		15
Transfusion		
Incompatibility	3	
Fulminant hepatitis	2	
Congestive heart failure	2	
Drug-related		
Drug reactions	3	
Steroid ulcers	2	
Crystalluria	1	
Anticoagulation bleeding	1	
Other	1	
Suicide		6
Liver disease		5
Bleeding varices	3	
Hepatic failure	2	
Thromboembolism		2
Renal amyloidosis		1
Pyoderma gangrenosum		1
		—
		46 patients
Deaths not related to colitis:		45 patients

°From Morowitz, D. A., and Kirsner, J. B.: Gastroenterology 57:581, 1969.

foration necessitates laparotomy. Continued medical treatment in the face of recognized or unrecognized perforation results in about an 80 per cent mortality. Even if surgery is performed immediately for suspected perforation, operative mortality may be as high as 50 per cent. Overall, colonic perforation accounts for about one-third of the deaths directly related to colitis (Table 102–5).

CANCER OF THE COLON

Carcinoma of the colon afflicts patients with ulcerative colitis at a much higher rate than would be expected in the general population; the observed incidence in adults with ulcerative colitis is seven to 11 times greater than in a control population. Indeed, one-third of colitis-related deaths are due to cancer of the colon and rectum (Table 102–5).

Both in adults and children the risk of cancer in ulcerative colitis is related to two factors: (1) duration of the colitis, and (2) extent of colonic involvement with colitis. In addition, there is some indication that carcinoma arises more frequently in the chronic continuous form of ulcerative colitis than in the intermittently active disease. Probably related to these factors is a slightly higher incidence in those patients who have severe initial attacks.

Duration of Colitis. Actuarial estimates of cumulative risks of cancer in ulcerative colitis, based on observed cases in two large series of adults, indicate that the risk of cancer rises steadily in all patients with the duration of the colitis.[46, 47] By 15 years, the cumulative risk of cancer is about 5 to 8 per cent. However, after 20 years the cumulative risk of cancer rises at a much steeper rate, so that at 20 years the cumulative risk in all patients is about 12 per cent, and by 25 years, is 25 per cent. Stated in another way, it has been estimated that the cumulative risk of cancer in all patients with ulcerative colitis of more than 20 years' duration is 6 per cent per annum, or 20 times the risk of colonic cancer in a normal population.

In children the data are similar. It is estimated that about 3 per cent of patients who develop ulcerative colitis in childhood will have colonic cancer after ten years of the disease.[48] Thereafter, about 20 per cent of exposed children will develop cancer per decade. Thus in children, as in adults, there is a small but steady rise in cumulative cancer risk over the first decade of colitis. However, in children with colitis the incidence of cancer rises steeply after the first decade of the disease, in contrast to adults, in whom this rise appears after 20 years. Also, the overall risk of cancer with each passing decade of the illness in children is somewhat higher than in adults.

Extent of Colonic Involvement. In examining the differences of risks of carcinoma in children as opposed to adults, it must be remembered that in children ulcerative colitis most often involves the entire colon (see pp. 1345 to 1347), whereas in adults a large number of patients have disease limited to the distal colon. The extent of colonic involvement with colitis greatly influences the risk of cancer. Thus in adults in whom colitis is limited to the rectum, the observed incidence of colonic cancer is one-seventh of that in all patients

with ulcerative colitis, and in fact does not exceed the risk in a normal, age-matched population.[16, 49] Likewise, the incidence of cancer in adults with colitis involving the left colon and rectum is much lower than in those with universal colitis. Actuarial estimates of cumulative risk of cancer in adults with universal colitis indicate a risk of 13 per cent at 15 years, of 23 per cent at 20 years, and of 42 per cent at 25 years of the disease, much higher than the estimates of cancer risk for *all adult patients with colitis* stated above. These estimates in adults with universal colitis, then, are not strikingly different from the estimates of cancer deaths in the series quoted above, in which 80 per cent of the children observed had universal colitis (Fig. 102–10). Conversely, the minority of children in that series who had their colitis limited to the rectum had a much lower incidence of colonic carcinoma—about 10 per cent at 25 years. It would seem therefore that in terms of the development of cancer, ulcerative colitis is the same disease for both children and adults; children differ only in that the majority of them have universal involvement, so that their risk of cancer is therefore higher than in all adult patients with ulcerative colitis.

Site of Colonic Cancer. Most colonic cancers in adults with colitis arise in the rectum and descending colon, even though most patients who develop cancer have universal colitis. (Almost paradoxically, however, most patients with ulcerative colitis limited to the distal segment—so-called proctocolitis—do not develop cancer.) The second most common site of colonic cancer in ulcerative colitis is the transverse colon, but any segment of the colon may give rise to carcinoma. Cancer is multicentric in 15 to 20 per cent of patients with malignancy of the colon associated with ulcerative colitis.

Outcome. Cancer of the colon arising in ulcerative colitis tends to be extremely virulent. The lesions tend to be flat and infiltrative, rather than polypoid, and in most patients metastases are evident at laparotomy. It is noteworthy that in adults with colitis who develop cancer under the age of 45 the cure rate is 8 per cent, whereas it is 40 per cent in those developing cancer over the age of 45. Similarly, death in children or young adults developing cancer from ulcerative colitis is the rule.

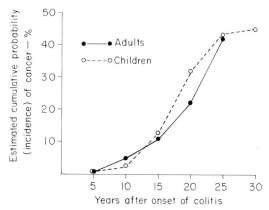

Figure 102–10. Graphs illustrating estimated cumulative incidence with time of cancer complicating ulcerative colitis in adults[47] and children[48] with panproctocolitis.

The Question of Prophylaxis. From the aforementioned data, it appears that the risk of death from colonic cancer complicating ulcerative colitis is formidable in those patients with universal colitis—either adults or children—of more than ten years' duration. Consequently, prophylactic colectomy has been advocated in children and in adults with universal colitis who have had the disease for longer than ten years.[47, 48] An alternative to this mode of treatment for such individuals is annual screening of patients with proctosigmoidoscopy and barium enema. Even with these precautions, however, inoperable cancer may develop. Recently it has been suggested that routine rectal biopsy will reveal precancerous changes in the rectal mucosa that may indicate the presence of noninvasive carcinoma elsewhere in the colon.[50] Such studies have been based on retrospective analyses of resected specimens. Whether routine rectal biopsy will be useful prospectively in identifying those patients with ulcerative colitis who are developing carcinoma of the colon at a curable stage remains to be determined.

COLONIC STRICTURE

Colonic stricture complicates ulcerative colitis in 7 to 11 per cent of cases.[47] Strictures rarely cause symptoms and are often incidental findings on barium enema examination or at colectomy. Occasionally, a stricture in a patient with ulcerative colitis will produce partial colonic obstruction, with lower abdominal cramping unrelieved by defecation.

The most common site of stricture is the rectum, followed next in frequency by the transverse colon. However, strictures may appear anywhere along the colon and are sometimes multiple. Most often they are short (2 to 3 cm) but may extend to 30 cm in length. Strictures are most common in patients with universal colitis (17 per cent), less common in those with subtotal colitis (8 per cent), and least common in those with proctocolitis (4 per cent). The incidence (new cases) of stricture does not increase with the duration of colitis. About one-third of strictures develop within the first five years of colitis; sometimes colonic stricture will appear immediately after a severe first attack of ulcerative colitis.

Strictures most frequently are fibrous—that is, they consist of extensive submucosal fibrosis. It would appear that they arise in patients in whom the colitis extends beneath the submucosa, i.e., a small number of patients usually with more severe forms of colitis. Some strictures result from thickening and muscular hypertrophy of the muscularis mucosae (see above). These latter strictures are potentially reversible on therapy of the colitis. Finally, some strictures arise from mucosal hyperplasia (exuberant granulation tissue and mucosal overgrowth).

Strictures present a difficult clinical problem, because they cannot be readily distinguished from colonic cancer. Like cancer in ulcerative colitis, strictures have a predilection for the rectum and transverse colon, most commonly complicate universal colitis, and can be multiple. Preoperative differentiation between stricture and cancer is usually uncertain. Although radiographic features on barium

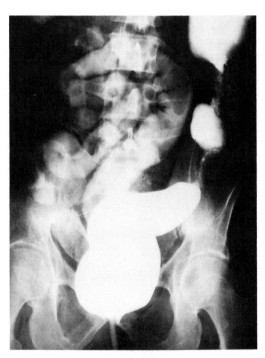

Figure 102–11. Barium enema of a patient with ulcerative colitis of 15 years' duration. The patient had been asymptomatic for ten years and off medication until six weeks prior to this examination. Multiple strictures are evident, and the distal stricture appears smooth in contour, suggesting a benign process. At operation both strictures were found to arise from colonic carcinoma.

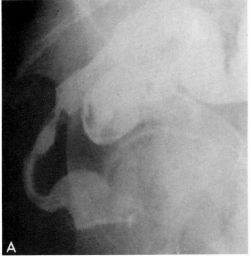

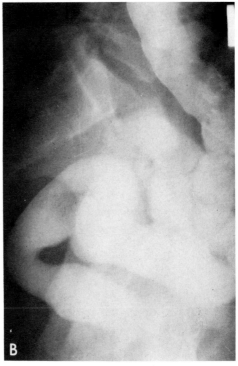

Figure 102-12. *A,* Rectal stricture in an adult with ulcerative colitis of two years' duration. Shelf-like upper margins of the stricture suggest malignancy. *B,* Repeat barium enema examination of the same area in this patient after six months of treatment with steroid enemas shows that stricture has disappeared. Original stricture probably arose from muscular hypertrophy and spasm.

enema examination such as "shelving" and mucosal irregularities along the stricture point to carcinoma rather than benign stricture, the absence of these findings does not exclude cancer as the cause of the colonic narrowing (Figs. 102–11 and 102–12). Therefore patients with ulcerative colitis who develop a fixed colonic stricture should be surgically explored for diagnosis.

MASSIVE HEMORRHAGE

Although rectal bleeding is a common symptom of ulcerative colitis, massive hemorrhage necessitating rapid and frequent blood transfusion to prevent cardiovascular collapse is rare, occurring in only about 4 per cent of patients, usually in those who have severe colitis. It must be considered a medical emergency, the treatment of which is rapid replacement of blood to restore blood volume. Colonic hemorrhage is not well tolerated in patients already compromised with fever, tachycardia, and extracellular fluid volume depletion. Accurate estimation of transfusion requirements is often difficult. As in all forms of acute hemorrhage, the hema-

tocrit does not accurately reflect the magnitude of the blood loss; furthermore, patients with fever from severe colitis may not exhibit signs of peripheral vasoconstriction, although their blood pressures may be at shock levels. In difficult cases careful monitoring of central venous pressure may be helpful in managing this problem. Correction of hypoprothrombinemia, if present (see p. 1336), is indicated. Obviously, anticoagulants should be withdrawn in patients with ulcerative colitis who bleed while receiving these agents for thromboembolism.

Most patients with massive colonic hemorrhage can be managed medically with blood transfusions. Hemorrhage usually subsides spontaneously. A rare patient may require colectomy to control bleeding. Death from colonic hemorrhage in ulcerative colitis is rare (see Table 102–5).

SYSTEMIC COMPLICATIONS

LIVER DISEASE

As noted on page 1320, liver disease associated with ulcerative colitis worsens the prognosis of the colitis; further, a small percentage of patients with ulcerative colitis die of liver disease (cirrhosis) as the result of bleeding esophageal varices or hepatic failure (Table 102–5).

The pathogenesis of liver lesions is not understood, and the incidence of liver disease in colitis is uncertain. Clinically, overt liver disease (jaundice) in patients with ulcerative colitis is uncommon (about 1 to 3 per cent). Minor abnormalities in one or more liver tests (serum alkaline phosphatase, Bromsulphalein retention, serum glutamic oxaloacetic transaminase) are much more common but are not precisely correlated with demonstrable histological lesions.[51] There are large discrepancies in the reported prevalence of various hepatic lesions in ulcerative colitis as determined by needle biopsy, wedge resection (at laparotomy), or autopsy. Many of these discrepancies are related to patient selection: needle biopsies have been performed most frequently in patients with overt jaundice, hepatomegaly, or abnormal liver tests; surgical biopsies have been obtained in patients with more severe and/or chronic forms of colitis requiring colectomy; and postmortem specimens have obviously come from a highly selected minority of patients with ulcerative colitis.

Some of the lesions in the liver in ulcerative colitis have a patchy distribution, raising the possibility of sampling error by needle biopsy. Few patients have been studied over long periods of time by serial needle biopsies; thus the natural history of liver lesions is not well documented. Until needle biopsy examinations are applied prospectively to large numbers of unselected patients with ulcerative colitis and more reports of serial biopsies become available, the prevalence and evolution of liver disease in ulcerative colitis will remain obscure. In spite of these difficulties, it is apparent that four histological liver lesions are seen in patients with ulcerative colitis more frequently than in control populations: pericholangitis, fatty infiltration, chronic acitve hepatitis, and postnecrotic cirrhosis.

Pericholangitis is found in about 30 to 50 per cent of liver biopsies in selected patients with ulcerative colitis. It seems to be more common in patients who have uni-

versal or subtotal colitis than in those with ulcerative colitis limited to the distal colon. This type of liver lesion is characterized by periportal inflammatory infiltrate of variable intensity (round cells, eosinophils, and about 15 per cent polymorphonuclear cells); degenerative changes in the bile ductules (swelling, hyalinization, or slough of ductal epithelium); periportal edema and lymphectasia; periportal fibrosis of varying degrees; and a variable amount of associated intralobular changes (fatty infiltration, hepatocyte drop-out, eosinophilic bodies, and fibrosis).

Attempts have been made to subclassify pericholangitis into "acute" forms (more infiltrate and less fibrosis) and "subacute" and "chronic" forms (more fibrosis, less inflammatory infiltrate).[52] In our opinion, the validity of such a classification, which implies a temporal progression of these lesions, remains in doubt for several reasons. All three subcategories have been seen on biopsy samples from patients in their first attack of ulcerative colitis; a few patients with pericholangitis followed with serial biopsy have shown complete resolution to normal histology. The staging is subjective (quantitative rather than objective qualitative change), and the process involves individual portal triads to different degrees, so that a sampling error on needle biopsy may result in inappropriate staging. In spite of these reservations, serial biopsies have shown evolution of pericholangitis to postnecrotic cirrhosis in a few patients, although it is not clear how often patients follow this course.[51, 52]

The etiology of pericholangitis is not understood. The lesion may appear in patients who have not received blood transfusions and who are negative for hepatitis-associated antigen (HAA). Some have suggested that chronic portal vein bacteremia resulting from colonic inflammation is the cause; however, cultures of liver biopsies from patients with pericholangitis have been negative for bacteria and L-forms, and prolonged treatment with tetracycline in a few patients has not resolved the lesion. Jaundice is rare in patients with pericholangitis uncomplicated by cirrhosis. Minor abnormalities in serum alkaline phosphatase and in

Bromsulphalein retention tests are common, but these tests may be normal in a small but significant number of patients with biopsy-proved pericholangitis.

Fatty infiltration is another common liver lesion in ulcerative colitis. The incidence varies widely, being highest in autopsy material and in wedge resections taken at colectomy; however, as many as 40 per cent of needle biopsy samples from patients with ulcerative colitis may show fatty infiltration, either appearing as the sole abnormality or associated with other histological changes such as pericholangitis. Fat accumulation is heaviest at the periphery of the lobules. Serial biopsies have shown that the lesion is reversible. Although the cause is not known, fatty infiltration is assumed to be due to malnutrition and protein depletion resulting from anorexia, diarrhea, and protein-losing enteropathy. Consistent with this theory is the higher incidence of fatty liver in autopsy material and in patients with low serum albumin.[53]

Some studies have not shown this correlation between fatty infiltration and either the extent of colitis in the colon or the severity of symptoms at the time of biopsy. Liver function tests may be normal or mildly abnormal in patients who have fatty infiltration as the sole lesion demonstrable on biopsy.[51]

Chronic active hepatitis is associated with ulcerative colitis, although this lesion is much less frequently encountered (1 to 16 per cent of biopsy material). Its pathogenesis is not understood. This lesion may appear in patients with ulcerative colitis who have not had blood transfusions. *Cirrhosis*, usually postnecrotic, can be demonstrated in about 3 to 4 per cent of patients with ulcerative colitis selected for biopsy. This lesion may develop from pericholangitis or chronic active hepatitis, but other causes are also probable. Although *amyloidosis* is a complication of chronic ulcerative colitis (see below), hepatic amyloidosis is not common, comprising only about 1 per cent of lesions seen on liver biopsy from patients with colitis. Jaundice, chronic or intermittent, in ulcerative colitis is usually associated with either chronic active hepatitis or cirrhosis; occasionally it may be seen with sclerosing cholangitis (see below) or other causes of extrahepatic obstruction.

A rare patient with ulcerative colitis will develop *sclerosing cholangitis*. In this disorder, the common bile duct becomes severely narrowed to only several millimeters in diameter.[54] The cause is unclear; stenosis may appear without associated gallstones, gallbladder abnormalities, or other evidence of infection in the biliary tree. Patients with this disorder present with recurrent attacks of jaundice, right upper quadrant pain, fever, and leukocytosis. Liver function tests indicate extrahepatic biliary obstruction. Differentiation among common duct stone, obstructing lesion, and sclerosing cholangitis is usually made only with transhepatic cholangiography or at operation (see pp. 1107 to 1108). *Carcinoma of the bile ducts* appears to have a slightly higher prevalence (0.5 per cent) in patients with ulcerative colitis.

An important question which remains unresolved is whether colectomy arrests, ameliorates, or reverses liver disease associated with ulcerative colitis. A recent follow-up study of a large series of patients undergoing panproctocolectomy for ulcerative colitis claimed considerable improvement in liver pathology demonstrated by wedge biopsy at the time of colectomy.[55] In this study, 33 out of 138 patients had a subsequent needle biopsy of the liver from three to seven years after colectomy. Although considerable improvement in liver pathology was noted in this interval, this assessment is clouded by the small numbers of patients examined and the incomparable techniques (needle vs. surgical biopsy) employed in evaluation. Furthermore, abnormal liver function tests persisted in large numbers of the 138 patients during the postoperative follow-up period. Others have reported that colectomy does not reverse pericholangitis.[52] Until more data are available regarding the prevalence and course of specific hepatic lesions associated with ulcerative colitis and the effects of colectomy on these lesions, colectomy cannot be advised solely for the treatment of liver disease in ulcerative colitis.

HEMATOLOGICAL ABNORMALITIES

The most common hematological defect in ulcerative colitis is anemia secondary to colonic blood loss. Its severity varies, depending on the rate and duration of bleeding. The patient is commonly iron deficient. Frequently, even patients who appear clinically asymptomatic during periods of remission will continue to have abnormal blood loss from the colon as measured after injection of Cr^{51}-labeled red cells.[20] Thus a persistent hypochromic anemia despite oral or parenteral iron therapy may indicate continuing activity of colitis in a patient who is little troubled by symptoms of diarrhea or gross hematochezia. Conversely, a normal hemoglobin level maintained without iron therapy or with small doses of oral iron supplements almost always indicates relative quiescence of the ulcerative colitis.

Most patients with mild anemia (hemoglobin about 60 per cent of normal) complicating mild or moderate ulcerative colitis may be treated with iron supplementation. Oral ferrous sulfate (0.1 to 0.2 g orally, three times a day) is effective in many of these patients. Unfortunately, some experience nausea, vomiting, upper abdominal distress, or even worsening of their diarrhea on this medication. Parenteral iron injections (Imferon) may be required in such patients to correct their anemia. During severe episodes of ulcerative colitis the hemoglobin level may fall below 50 per cent of normal and, especially with severe hemorrhage, is often sufficiently depressed to require blood transfusion. In the sickest patients with high fever, malnutrition, and protein depletion, the bone marrow often does not respond to iron supplementation, and these patients may also require transfusion to correct their anemia.

Some patients with ulcerative colitis may develop hemolytic anemia. Mild hemolytic anemia associated with Heinz bodies on peripheral smear is seen in some patients receiving salicylazosulfapyridine (Azulfidine). This type of hemolytic anemia appears to be drug related, and is not seen in patients not receiving Azulfidine. More severe hemolytic anemia may complicate ulcerative colitis. Sometimes this more severe type of hemolytic anemia is associated with nonabsorbable sulfonamide medication, but hemolytic anemia may be "idiopathic." A Coombs-positive, autoimmune hemolytic anemia has been described in ulcerative colitis, as has microangiopathic hemolytic anemia with or without disseminated intravascular coagulation. When ulcerative colitis is complicated by cirrhosis, a megaloblastic anemia may develop, just as in cirrhosis. Rarely, oral sulfonamides will produce aplastic anemia.

Leukocytosis is a common finding associated with the more severe varieties of ulcerative colitis. Sometimes this leukocytosis may be marked, with total white cell counts as high as 40,000 to 50,000 per mm^3 and a predominance of young cell forms, including promyelocytes, on peripheral smear. On such occasions a high leukocyte alkaline phosphatase and bone marrow examination will differentiate between a myelophthisic response and acute myelogenous leukemia. Occasionally, in severe disease circulating leukocyte counts will be low as in severe bacterial infection.

Thrombocytosis may appear in ulcerative colitis, most commonly in those patients having marked leukocytosis. Unlike primary thrombocytosis, the thrombocytosis complicating ulcerative colitis is not associated with coagulation defects.

Deficiencies in coagulation factors may complicate ulcerative colitis. *Hypoprothrombinemia* (prolonged prothrombin time) is a commonly found defect in moderate or severe ulcerative colitis. Advanced liver disease associated with ulcerative colitis (see above) accounts for some cases of hypoprothrombinemia, but this defect is more common than can be accounted for by advanced liver disease. Malnutrition (low vitamin K intake, low protein intake) may be responsible in many of these patients. Most often prolonged prothrombin times in patients with ulcerative colitis can be corrected with parenteral administration of vitamin K. It is important to restore the prothrombin time to normal with vitamin K injections in such patients, because hypoprothrombinemia may in part contribute to profuse colonic bleeding. In patients with inherited coagulation defects (Christmas disease [factor IX deficiency], hemophilia [factor X deficiency]), the course of ulcerative colitis may be stormy, particularly at the onset, which is usually heralded by massive hemorrhage sometimes so severe that emergency colectomy is required. In severe ulcerative colitis and/or after emergency surgery, multiple coagulation defects occasionally arise from disseminated intravascular coagulation (consumption coagulopathy). This process results in bleeding into the skin, soft tissues, or wounds and from mucous membranes. A marked drop in platelet count and fibrinogen with the appearance of fibrin "split products" is good laboratory evidence of this syndrome.

THROMBOEMBOLIC DISEASE

A serious and occasionally fatal complication (Table 102–5) is pulmonary embolism resulting from thrombosis of the leg or pelvic veins. Pulmonary embolism usually complicates the course of those patients with active disease who are moderately or severely ill. As with thromboembolism in the setting of any disease, it must be suspected in those patients who suddenly develop unexplained pulmonary complications or shock. Diligent search will reveal a site of thrombosis in the legs in probably less than 50 per cent of cases. A pelvic locus must be suspected in those individuals who continue to be severely ill with lower abdominal pain and high fever but in whom diarrhea, bleeding, and distention are not prominent.

In rare instances, thromboembolic disease in ulcerative colitis may be accompanied by thrombosis of arteries, particularly in the retina and glans penis. Such patients may also suffer from a kind of nodular vasculitis which takes the form of subcutaneous nodules, especially over the arms. The lesions may be widespread and difficult to distinguish from polyarteritis; they may involve kidneys, retroperitoneal tissues, and brain. Hypercoagulability of the blood has also been described in active ulcerative colitis attributable to accelerated formation of thromboplastin.

Therapy of thromboembolism in ulcerative colitis is complicated by the risks of colonic bleeding during anticoagulation. Heparin is the drug of choice and should be administered intravenously every four hours; the dose must be determined by careful measurement of venous clotting time just prior to the succeeding dose (goal: clotting time two and one-half times normal four hours after last dose). Repeated pulmonary embolism despite adequate anticoagulation therapy or massive colonic hemorrhage during anticoagulation may necessitate vena caval ligation with or without colectomy. The decision regarding colectomy at the time of caval ligation must be dictated by the clinical course and status of the patient.

THE ARTHRITIS OF ULCERATIVE COLITIS

The arthritis of ulcerative colitis is characterized by the following features:[56] (1) It usually appears at the same time that bowel symptoms become prominent, although occasionally it may antedate them. (2) The affliction tends to be migratory and to affect larger joints more than smaller joints; it is often monarticular. (3) Frequently there is synovitis with effusion, and the joint is swollen, often erythematous, and tender. Motion is limited to a varying degree, depending upon the extent of involvement. (4) The joint cartilages and bony appositions, however, are unaffected, and except for involvement of the spinal column (see below), no residual damage is suffered. Thus ankylosing does not result from this type of arthritis. Serum from these patients is usually negative for rheumatoid factors. Rarely, of course, ulcerative colitis may be associated with rheumatoid arthritis. Approximately 6 to 10 per cent of patients with ulcerative colitis will have arthritis at one time or another during their course. It frequently appears in conjunction with skin disorders, particularly erythema nodosum, and is also commonly seen with ocular involvement, particularly iritis. Arthritis usually subsides with control of the colitis.

There is an inordinately high incidence of ankylosing spondylitis in patients with ulcerative colitis. It has been estimated that the incidence of such involvement of the spine is perhaps ten to 20 times as frequent as in the normal population. Conversely, the incidence of inflammatory bowel disease in patients with ankylosing spondylitis is high.[57] Further, it seems to involve women much more frequently than in the population at large, although twice the number of men afflicted with ulcerative colitis have ankylosing spondylitis. An occasional patient may also have aortic valvular disease, as commonly noted in patients with ankylosing spondylitis without inflammatory bowel disease. Of interest, the frequency of ankylosing spondylitis among blood relatives of patients with ulcerative colitis is also increased.

Although the progress of spondylitis in these individuals is rather gradual, it is nonetheless progressive. Occasionally, the onset of arthritis of the spine antedates bowel symptoms; whether or not the bowel is diseased at this time cannot be ascertained, because the colon is not generally investigated in those patients without clinical evidence of an inflamed colon. Generally, the course of the ankylosing spondylitis in ulcerative colitis is identical with the usual form of the disease. It is chronic, progressive, troublesome, deforming, and frequently generalized. It does not seem to respond to corticosteroids — in many instances, the spinal arthritis progresses despite quiescent colitis — and it does not seem to have any better response to X-ray therapy than idiopathic ankylosing spondylitis without colitis.

The incidence of sacroiliitis is higher than ankylosing spondylitis in patients with ulcerative colitis. The disease may be found in many cases only by appropriate X-rays of the pelvis, including oblique views.[58] Many of these patients are asymptomatic. A high percentage of them, however, have evidence of associated spondylitis. As with the latter disease in general, serological tests for rheumatoid factor are negative.

OCULAR LESIONS

Several different eye lesions may arise in patients with ulcerative colitis. The pathogenesis of these lesions is not understood. Some of the rarely occurring lesions may simply be coincidental. *Iritis (uveitis)* is the most common lesion seen with ulcerative colitis, appearing in about 5 to 10 per cent of patients.[58] In the acute phase, the patient experiences blurred vision, eye pain, and photophobia. Physical findings include iridospasm, protein flare and cells in the anterior chamber, and keratitic precipitates. The attack may be followed by atrophy of the iris, anterior and posterior synechiae, and old pigment deposits on the lens. In about half the cases the uveitis will be bilateral. *Episcleritis* is less common. This lesion is characterized by inflammation of the episcleral tissues associated with discomfort but no discharge or infection. It is most commonly bilateral, but usually involves only a small portion of the episcleral area in each eye. Other lesions rarely seen in ulcerative colitis include *superficial keratitis* with *blepharitis, interstitial keratitis, retinitis,* and *retrobulbar neuritis.*

In about one-third of the patients with uveitis, the eye lesion will precede the onset of clinical symptoms of colitis; in another third it will complicate an exacerbation of ulcerative colitis, more commonly a recurrent attack than an initial episode; and in the remainder the uveitis appears while the colitis remains in remission. Eye lesions are most likely to appear in patients with severe and/or universal ulcerative colitis but may be encountered when the disease is limited to the distal colon. Over 75 per cent of patients who have uveitis complicating ulcerative colitis will have other systemic complications of ulcerative colitis as well. These include arthralgias, arthritis, sacroiliitis, spondylitis, erythema nodosum, and aphthous stomatitis. Of these, the most commonly associated systemic complication is arthritis or sacroiliitis. On the other hand, episcleritis is not associated with other systemic complications. Females are more prone to have eye complications than males with ulcerative colitis.

Corticosteroid treatment during periods of colonic disease will usually have a salutary effect on both the colitis and the uveitis. If the colitis is quiescent during an attack of uveitis, the ocular condition will usually respond to local therapy, i.e., cycloplegics, mydriatics, and topical corticosteroids. In more extreme cases, subconjunctival injection of a respository from of corticosteroid may be quite effective. When the uveitis is severe, systemic corticosteroids may be required despite the inactivity of the bowel disease.

The uveitis tends to recur in only about 20 per cent of patients. In a minority of instances it may become chronic; rarely, it leads to blindness. An occasional patient may have to be maintained on low doses of oral steroids for frequent recurrences of the iritis despite inactive bowel disease. Subtotal colectomy will usually ameliorate the uveitis; however, recurrences thereafter may still be noted. Only when the entire diseased colon is resected will the patient be protected against future episodes of uveitis.

The combination of ocular lesions and arthritis appearing just prior to the onset of colonic symptoms may occasionally mislead the physician into making a diagnosis of Reiter's syndrome. However, the other features of Reiter's syndrome (urethritis and keratosis blennorrhagica) are absent. Proctosigmoidoscopy and/or barium enema examination will confirm the diagnosis of ulcerative colitis.

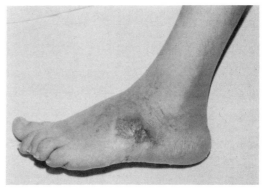

Figure 102–13. Pyoderma gangrenosum of the foot in a patient with ulcerative colitis.

SKIN

About 3 per cent of patients with ulcerative colitis will develop *erythema nodosum*, with raised, tender, erythematous swellings measuring 2 to 5 cm in diameter along the extensor surfaces of the arms and especially the legs. As with erythema nodosum in general, this disorder is more common in women than men with ulcerative colitis. The condition usually appears during an exacerbation of the colitis and is prone to develop when arthritis also accompanies the attack of colitis. Occasionally both arthritis and erythema nodosum may appear just prior to the first attack of overt ulcerative colitis, when bowel symptoms are not as yet prominent; in this situation the patient may be thought to have rheumatic fever. However, the diagnosis of erythema nodosum should always raise suspicion of chronic inflammatory disease of the bowel, because it is seen in both ulcerative colitis and granulomatous disease.

Pyoderma gangrenosum is a much less frequent complication of ulcerative colitis, afflicting about 0.6 per cent of patients. Most commonly this condition complicates severe ulcerative colitis, but it has been seen in a few patients with mild disease. The lesion starts with the appearance of a boil or infected hair follicle. As it grows, it collects purulent-looking material which may drain spontaneously (Fig. 102–13). This material, however, contains few polymorphonuclear cells and no bacteria. Eventually these lesions become gangrenous, resulting in progressive necrosis of the surrounding dermis, with deeply ulcerated areas, often involving underlying soft tissue. When the lesions are widespread, the skin disease can be serious and, on rare occasions, fatal (Table 102–5).

Almost invariably, these lesions appear during a bout of active colitis; healing of skin lesions will usually follow control of the colitis with either corticosteroid therapy or colectomy. Persistent severe pyoderma gangrenosum, involving many areas of the skin and underlying tissues, is an indication for colectomy. In rare instances, however, even panproctocolectomy will not control the skin disease.[59, 60]

Aphthous ulceration of the mouth is a more common but less serious complication of ulcerative colitis, and is seen in about 8 per cent of patients. It is most frequent during severe attacks of colitis, but it occasionally appears even during remissions. It may be complicated by moniliasis, for which specific treatment should be given (Mycostatin or gentian violet mouthwashes). Uncomplicated aphthous ulceration may be treated with hydrocortisone mouthwashes.

Other skin lesions seen in ulcerative colitis are usually drug reactions (maculopapular eruptions, urticaria, erythema multiforme). Rarely, a patient with ulcerative colitis may develop a generalized eczematoid maculopapular eruption unrelated to medication but appearing during exacerbations of colitis.

RENAL DISEASE

Two types of renal disease appear to be associated with ulcerative colitis: pyelonephritis and nephrolithiasis or urolithiasis. The explanation for the former is not clear unless it is related in some way to dehydration and its consequent scanty urine flow with high concentration of solutes and electrolytes.

The increased incidence of nephro- and urolithiasis may be explained by dehydration, inactivity of the patient (calcium mobilization), and changes in the composition of the urine which predispose to stone formation. A significant proportion of the patients with nephrolithiasis and ulcerative colitis have undergone colectomy and have functioning ileostomies (see below). An occasional patient with ulcerative colitis may have involvement of the ureter or the bladder owing to complication of the enteric disease, particularly fistula or abscess, but such involvement is rare and is encountered much more frequently with granulomatous disease of the small and large bowel (Crohn's disease). In some cases glomerulonephritis has been reported in ulcerative colitis, but it is quite rare. Rare individuals with severe diarrhea caused by ulcerative colitis or malfunctioning ileostomy with profuse discharge containing high content of potassium may, over a long period of time, develop renal changes secondary to hypokalemia—so-called hypokalemic nephropathy. This lesion is often not reversible and results in slowly progressive renal dysfunction.

AMYLOIDOSIS AND ULCERATIVE COLITIS

As in any chronic inflammatory disease, amyloidosis may be noted in ulcerative colitis, although it is more common in the granulomatous form of the disease. The amyloid involvement is of the so-called secondary type, affecting primarily liver, kidney, and spleen, although blood vessels in any part of the body, including the gut, may be involved. The disease is usually manifested by hepatosplenomegaly, proteinuria (occasionally severe enough to cause the nephrotic syndrome), and varying degrees of involvement of other organs, including the endocrine system. Its widespread nature explains the protean manifestations of secondary amyloidosis. The question of whether or not excision of the bowel will slow the inexorable course of the amyloid deposition remains to be answered. There is some evidence that in the patients with granulomatous bowel disease the secondary amyloidosis has been halted by resection.

SURGERY IN ULCERATIVE COLITIS

In contrast to surgery in granulomatous disease of the bowel, removal of the colon in ulcerative colitis is curative in most instances. Colectomy removes the primary focus of the disease, usually rids the patient of systemic complications (a rare case of pyoderma gangrenosum will not respond, and the effects on liver disease are not clear), and obviates the risk of future local complications, including carcinoma of the colon. On the other hand, colectomy carries an operative risk; some patients will require further surgery for both early complications (anastomotic leaks, intraperitoneal abscess) and late sequelae (adhesions, mechanical problems with ileostomy, stomal ileitis); and not all patients will accept an ileostomy. It is obvious therefore that colectomy is not indicated in those patients whose disease can be easily controlled by medical measures. However, it is equally obvious that surgery has an important therapeutic role in ulcerative colitis which responds incompletely to medical management, a state of affairs also fraught with complications.

The standard surgical procedure for ulcerative colitis is total colectomy in one or two stages. In the two-stage procedure, the rectum is not removed, and the patient has a functioning ileostomy with a sigmoid mucous fistula after the first stage. Proctectomy is performed at the second stage. Some surgeons advocate ileoproctostomy in the rare circumstance when the rectum is free of disease. Ileoproctostomy in patients in whom the rectum is diseased is not worthwhile; although it spares the inconvenience of ileostomy, it is attended by sufficient diarrhea, bleeding, and perirectal inflammation to discourage its performance. Furthermore, the retained rectum may become a site of future carcinoma.[49]

Postoperative mortality has declined steadily since 1950. At that time mortality was about 10 per cent after elective colectomy in patients not seriously ill; about 50 per cent in chronically ill and debilitated patients with severe ulcerative colitis; and about 70 per cent in patients requiring emergency colectomy for toxic megacolon. At present, postoperative mortality for an elective one-stage colectomy is about 3 per cent; even in patients with acute severe disease, mortality of subtotal colectomy with ileostomy is now only 10 to 15 per cent in skilled hands. This improvement in mortality has resulted from many technical advances, including improved anesthesia, better surgical techniques, efficient blood banking, more skillful management of fluid and electrolyte problems or cardiovascular complications, and better selection of antimicrobial agents for postoperative infections. In addition, many surgeons feel that declining surgical mortality reflects earlier operative intervention in patients with ulcerative colitis before the patient becomes desperately ill or chronically debilitated.

INDICATIONS FOR COLECTOMY

We have alluded to indications for surgery in previous sections of this chapter. There are three general situations in which surgery is contemplated in ulcerative colitis.

1. A complication arises from which the risk of dying is high and for which medical management is known to be ineffective. In this category are suspected or proved colonic perforation and suspected (colonic stricture) or proved colonic cancer.

2. The clinical condition of the patient is grave, but medical management may be effective; however, as time elapses without apparent benefit from medical treatment, the chance of successful outcome as the result of medical therapy diminishes. In this category are severe ulcerative colitis, toxic megacolon, and uncontrolled colonic hemorrhage.

3. There is no immediate threat to life, but cumulative morbidity or mortality is high. This would include morbidity from recurrent and/or intractable moderate or severe colitis; intractable uveitis or pyoderma gangrenosum; ill effects from long-term systemic corticosteroid treatment; growth retardation in pediatric patients; and the ultimate risk of colonic cancer or colitis-related death.

Only indications under the first category are clear. In the second category there is general agreement as to which patients are at risk of dying, but few data indicating how long medical treatment should be tried before being abandoned in favor of surgery. In the third category, cumulative risks or definitions of acceptable morbidity remain poorly defined; only recently have the risks of death from colonic cancer been established.

Acute severe colitis is the form of the disease most often refractory to medical management and most often fatal. Because of this fact, we have categorically recommended that these patients undergo surgery if little or no improvement is induced after ten to 14 days of intensive medical treatment. It must be admitted that the recommended duration of this trial is not based upon well founded empiric data, but is suggested only as a reasonable period beyond which the chance of remission is small and the continued severe morbidity of the patient would probably render him a less favorable candidate for surgery. Recently, this view has been challenged; it has been suggested that the patient with severe acute colitis undergo colectomy after four to five days of medical treatment if remission or improvement has not been induced.[61] The proponents of earlier surgery base their argument on a retrospective analysis of mortality; there was only a 1.3 per cent overall mortality in severe ulcerative colitis in a series of patients seen from 1964 to 1966 in which the policy of earlier surgical intervention (after four to five days of medical trial) was instituted, as opposed to an overall mortality of 11.3 per cent in an earlier series of patients (1952 to 1963) with severe colitis who were operated upon only after ten days of medical therapy had been unsuccessful. The argument is weakened somewhat by the retrospective nature of the study; but this important question, i.e. when should medical therapy be abandoned in favor of surgery, could be adequately answered by a randomized prospective trial of these two policies.

Advocates of early surgery also argue that statistically a large number of patients with acute severe colitis will ultimately undergo colectomy for refractory ulcerative colitis. Although this statement may be true, it is difficult to predict the ultimate outcome of the disease in an individual patient on the basis of the severity of a single episode (see pp. 1319 to 1321). Similarly, we have recommended that the patient with toxic megacolon be operated upon if his condition does not improve after 96 hours of medical therapy. Again, this recommendation is based upon theoretical considerations (the chance of perforation with prolonged colonic dilatation, the poor long-term outlook in patients recovering from toxic megacolon), not objective data. Likewise, the definition of "uncontrolled" colonic hemorrhage remains vague, because it depends on many factors, including how well a particular patient may tolerate acute blood loss. Clearly, more data are needed to define the temporal indications for surgery in patients acutely and seriously ill with ulcerative colitis.

Indications for colectomy based on cumulative long-term morbidity are most difficult to outline and depend upon the clinical judgment of the physician, the overall adjustment of the patient to his disease, and the patient's attitude toward elective colectomy. We can only point out certain general guidelines that we find helpful in making decisions concerning colectomy. First among these are the *functional capacity of the patient;* i.e., how well can the patient carry out his or her chores in the face of continuing disease? Obviously related to this question is *the amount of systemic corticosteroid* needed to maintain the patient at a reasonable functioning level. Together these two considerations make the decision for colectomy a joint undertaking. The patient is usually best able to judge whether he can cope with his colonic disease, and the physician must decide whether the duration and dosage of corticosteroid medication needed is a serious hazard. We feel that the long-term oral administration of more than 15 mg daily of prednisolone to control the colitis at acceptable levels of activity is a cumulative hazard to the patient not justifiable when colectomy is an alternative.

The *long-term course of the colitis* is also important in deciding on elective colectomy. Regardless of the initial severity of the disease, if subsequent attacks are mild, the patient may be managed without surgery. On the other hand, continued exacerbations of moderate severity requiring repeated hospitalizations or even one severe episode complicating an otherwise mild series of attacks of colitis warrant elective colectomy in our opinion. The *age of the patient* is also important. As pointed out below (see pp. 1345 to 1347), the mortality and long-term morbidity in the young patient with ulcerative colitis is forbidding; we feel strongly that colectomy should be entertained early as an effective mode of treatment in these patients. Systemic steroids are less well tolerated in the elderly, whereas colectomy—as in the younger patient—is curative. On the other hand, the decision may be more safely deferred in the older patient who requires 10 mg or less of prednisone daily to control his disease.

A potential threat to many patients with ulcerative colitis is the development of colonic cancer. In addition to severity, *duration and extent* of the disease are important parameters in determining the risk of cancer. Patients with distal colitis and/or mild disease are at little risk. Those with more severe disease, with total colonic involvement, and especially with the continuous form of the disease are at the highest risk. This risk becomes much greater after the first ten years of the disease (see above). Because of this fact, we recommend colectomy to our adult patients who have had universal colitis of more than ten years' duration, when the disease remains active, albeit intermittently. The decision for colectomy in patients in this category who are asymptomatic or who tolerate mild colitis is obviously extremely difficult; in these instances the risks should be explained to the patient, and he should be closely involved in the course to be followed.

Since most patients with ulcerative colitis will continue to have only mild attacks, only a minority of patients will eventually undergo colectomy. Nevertheless, in this minority who have one of the several indications for colectomy (which fall under the general category of more severe long-term disease), the life expectancy under medical management appears considerably reduced. We do not hesitate therefore to recommend colectomy as a potentially curative procedure under these circumstances. Unfortunately, these guidelines have been established only by a retrospective evaluation of the literature and our own experiences with this disease. Many more prospective analyses of indications for surgery are needed.

OUTCOME OF SURGERY

As noted above, postoperative mortality is low (3 per cent) in elective colectomy, but higher (10 to 15 per cent) in patients undergoing emergency surgery for acute severe disease. Surgical mortality is highest in those who are critically ill at the time of operation and approaches 50 per cent in patients who have had colonic perforation.[62] The most frequent cause of postsurgical death is peritonitis secondary to colonic perforation, either preoperatively or during surgery (Table 102–5). Another large percentage of deaths is attributable to extraperitoneal infection (septicemia, bronchopneumonia), followed next in frequency by cardiovascular complications. Death from all causes is about twice as frequent in patients over 50 years of age as in the younger age group.

Nonfatal complications, often requiring subsequent surgery, are frequent, involving about 25 per cent of patients.[60, 62] As with postoperative mortality, complications are least frequent after elective colectomy (14 per cent) and most frequent in critically ill patients (38 per cent). They may arise in the immediate postoperative period or after a long period of time following surgery, but most appear within four years of the original procedure. A frequent complication is small intestinal obstruction (9 per cent), which may result as a consequence of adhesions, intestinal volvulus, or internal herniation of small bowel through a mesenteric defect (the last is now less common because of improved surgical technique). Small intestinal obstruction after colectomy and ileostomy for inflammatory bowel disease is much more common than after the same operation for noninflammatory disease of the colon (familial polyposis, colonic cancer).[63]

A second source of complication arises from problems associated with the ileostomy. In the late 1940's and early 1950's, postoperative ileostomy problems were very common (40 to 60 per cent of cases) and were related to prolapse or retraction of the ileostomy, fistulization from the ileal stoma, or mechanical obstruction at the ileal stoma. Since the late 1950's, these problems have become much less frequent owing to improved surgical techniques. Prolapse or retraction of the ileal stoma has been obviated by suturing the terminal ileal mesentery to the peritoneum and posterior rectus fascia adjacent to the ileostomy site. Fistulization has been reduced by avoiding the placement of sutures through the full thickness of the stoma.

Mechanical obstruction at the ileal stoma is now less frequent because of two technical innovations: (1) the stoma is now brought out through a circle of excised skin instead of a slit incision; and (2) no longer is the serosa of the protruding ileal stoma left exposed, allowing contracture as a result of serosal infection and scarring; instead, the terminal ileum is everted, and the distal end of the everted ileum is sewn to the skin at the ileostomy site. This maneuver leaves a terminal cuff of ileal mucosa covering the protruding stoma and approximates serosa of the everted portion to the serosa of the more proximal protruding ileum. As a result, problems with the ileostomy requiring subsequent ileostomy revision have been reduced to 10 to 14 per cent.[64] Minor problems with the ileostomy arise in an additional 4 per cent of cases (see below).

The third major source of postoperative complication relates to rectal excision. In nearly two-thirds of patients who have had rectal disease at the time of subtotal colectomy with ileostomy, a subsequent rectal excision will have to be performed because of continued activity of the disease in the rectal stump.[60] Furthermore, there is a substantial risk of developing carcinoma in the retained rectal stump.[49] Whether proctectomy is performed as a single stage procedure (panproctocolectomy) or at a second operation, complications arise from removal of the rectum. Chief among these are prolonged perineal drainage and slow healing (requiring more than six months) of the perineal wound, often necessitating a subsequent hospitalization in 12 to 20 per cent of cases.[62, 63] This problem is more common in females or patients with severe rectal and/or perirectal disease at the time of proctectomy.[60] Proctectomy may also result in impotence in males, which, however, may be temporary. Permanent difficulties with sexual function are either failure to obtain erection (presacral nerve damage) or ability to have erection but inability to ejaculate or experience orgasm (parasympathetic nerve injury). The exact incidence of this problem after proctectomy for ulcerative colitis is difficult to estimate because of incomplete reporting, but may be as high as 10 per cent.[60, 63, 65] A few females will experience dyspareunia as the result of excessive scarring during healing of the perineal wound.[60] Infertility in females after panproctocolectomy has also been reported and is believed to be due to either retroflexion of the uterus or blockage of the Fallopian tubes after extensive pelvic inflammation.[65]

LIFE WITH AN ILEOSTOMY

In spite of the aforementioned complications, colectomy with ileostomy restores the majority of patients to excellent health. Among those patients who survive the initial operations, life expectancy remains somewhat below normal for the first few postoperative years, owing to a small but significant mortality (about 3 per cent) associated with complications of intestinal obstruction and mechanical difficulties with the ileostomy (see above).[39, 62] The development of carcinoma in a retained rectal stump also contributes to late mortality in those patients who have not undergone proctectomy. Nevertheless, the long-term mortality in patients with panproctocolectomy and ileostomy who survive the procedure is virtually the same as for a normal population.[66] Furthermore, the quality of life for this group of patients is very good. Ninety per cent of patients with ileostomies who responded to a survey rated the results of their operation as excellent and claimed little inconvenience.[63, 65] Almost all are able to lead normal lives and enjoy normal sexual relationships. Certain activities requiring frequent bending, lifting, or twisting and contact sports cannot be pursued, however, because of the ileostomy.

The normal ileostomy does not cause any major physiological defects. What has been lost by colectomy is simply the sodium and water absorbing capacity of the colon, which in most instances was already impaired by extensive ulcerative colitis prior to surgery. The colon normally reabsorbs about 40 to 60 mEq of sodium and about 400 ml of water daily (see pp. 229 to 248). Unlike the colon and kidney, the small bowel has a minimal ability to conserve sodium during periods of sodium deprivation. On a normal diet, patients will not become sodium depleted because of losses from the ileostomy; however, negative sodium balances may follow periods of sodium deprivation. Moreover, because of their ileal sodium and water losses, ileostomists tend to have lower urine volumes and lower Na^+/K^+ ratios in their urine owing to compensatory renal conservation of sodium and water.[67] In turn, the low urine volume may contribute to the increased incidence of urolithiasis (probably about 5 per cent) in these patients who tend to have urinary tract stones of either urate or calcium salts. Although low urine volume may be offset by increased water intake, high sodium intake usually results in greater output from the ileal stoma and decreased urine volume; this seemingly paradoxical effect reflects the fact that the small bowel cannot efficiently absorb increasing amounts of sodium during a high sodium load.

A well functioning ileostomy discharges about 500 to 600 g of material daily; about 92 per cent of this dejecta is water. High cellulose foods increase the total volume of output by increasing the solid residue in the effluent. Prune juice, which contains a chemical cathartic, diphenylisatin, will increase both the water and residue content of the ileal discharge.[68] Although individual patients may experience increased output and/or cramping with certain foods (rhubarb, alcohol, cabbage, onions and milk give the highest incidence of difficulty), most patients can tolerate a normal diet.[69] Many physicians report anecdotes about ileostomies which have been obstructed by nuts or beans; yet the overall experience of a large number of ileos- tomists and a clinical study have failed to document this impression. Some patients do complain of problems with control of odor from the ileostomy bag. Certain foods, especially onions and beans, seem to increase odor. However, most odor arises from bacterial action on the contents of the bag; this may be offset by frequent emptying of the bag and/or adding sodium benzoate or chlorine tablets to the bag.

In spite of the fact that most ileostomists can lead a normal life and eat a normal diet, a few have minor difficulties. Minor mechanical problems most frequently in- volve skin excoriation around the ileos- tomy site. Impingement of a malfitting ap- pliance on the ileal stoma may eventually erode the stoma and produce fistulization. There is a low incidence of peristomal abscess and peristomal hernia. A small number of pregnant women may develop stomal prolapse.

Major long-term problems relate to mal- functioning ileostomies or prestomal ileitis. If the ileostomy was improperly constructed (with newer techniques this is now a much less frequent problem), the stoma may become obstructed. Such ob- struction produces a syndrome of either continuous or episodic cramping, in- creased ileal discharge (up to 4 liters daily) with fluid and electrolyte depletion, and small bowel dilatation. Excessive ileal out- put probably arises at least in part from increased small bowel secretion as the result of small bowel dilatation proximal to the obstructed stoma. Stomal obstruction can usually be demonstrated either by probing the stoma or by barium enema ex- amination through the stoma which will reveal a dilated ileum proximal to the point of obstruction.[70] Many of these ileos- tomies require reconstruction. At opera- tion punched-out ulcerations are often found in the resected terminal ileum; their pathogenesis is unclear but probably re- lates in some way to the mechanical prob- lem of obstruction.

A much less common problem is pre- stomal ileitis.[71] Patients with this syn- drome exhibit the features of mechanical obstruction but in addition have signs of systemic toxicity (fever, tachycardia, ane- mia). Deeply penetrating punched-out ulcers extending to the serosa are found in the resected specimen of terminal ileum. It is not clear whether prestomal ileitis has a different pathogenesis from simple me- chanical obstruction of the stoma. Both syndromes may arise in a segment of ileum which was histologically normal at the time of colectomy, and the presence of "backwash ileitis" in the ileum at the time of ileostomy does not seem to predispose the patient to the development of either problem. On the other hand, in patients who have had colectomy and ileostomy for granulomatous colitis, subsequent prob- lems with the ileal stoma may arise from spread of the transmural granulomatous disease to the terminal ileum.

ULCERATIVE COLITIS IN CHILDHOOD

William Michener, James H. Meyer

The most perplexing and difficult pa- tients with ulcerative colitis are those in the pediatric age group. The disease tends to be severe and chronic. Chronic diarrhea with nutritional deficiencies, impairment of growth, associated emotional changes, the long-term risk of mortality, and cancer of the colon are all disturbing problems facing the physician caring for the child with colitis.

Ulcerative colitis has been well docu- mented in infants aged two to three months, but most commonly symptoms begin later in life, usually between eight and 15 years of age. Whether the etiology for pediatric patients is different from that for adults with colitis is unknown. In gen- eral, the disease in the young is similar to colitis in the adult with respect to sig- moidoscopic appearances, histopathology, short-term course, response to treatment, and both colonic and extracolonic compli- cations. In the young, however, the dis- ease is more often severe, more often in- volves the entire colon, and more often is complicated by carcinoma (see p. 1331).

In general, the clinical picture in the child is the same as in the adult; the dis- ease may present with anorexia and weight loss, abdominal cramping, diarrhea and/or hematochezia, fever, or extra- colonic symptoms. In addition, growth is significantly retarded in 10 to 20 per cent of children with this disease. The degree of such retardation correlates inversely with the age of onset of the disease. It may result from a combination of malnutrition and secondary hypopituitarism;[72] low urinary gonadotropin levels and depressed growth hormone responses to hypoglycemia have been demonstrated in some of these patients.

Unfortunately, there is often undue delay between the development of symptoms and the diagnosis of the disease. Children do not readily communicate their bowel habits to their parents. Thus a child may be brought to the pediatrician by a parent complaining that the child does not eat, is losing weight, appears anemic, or is not growing. Often parents are completely surprised when the child will admit to three or four bloody bowel movements daily when carefully questioned by the physician. As in the adult, the child may present with an extracolonic manifestation of ulcerative colitis; diarrhea and hematochezia may be mild. Failure of the pediatrician to consider ulcerative colitis in a setting of fever, erythema nodosum, arthritis, iritis, or pyoderma gangrenosum may also delay diagnosis. Finally, even when the history of diarrhea and/or rectal bleeding is elicited, the pediatrician may be reluctant to perform proctosigmoidoscopy or order a barium enema examination. Although these procedures will establish the diagnosis, they are not readily undertaken for fear of emotionally traumatizing the child.

In fact, proctosigmoidoscopy can be performed without significant physical or emotional trauma to the child. The major difference between this examination in the child and in the adult is that it must be performed quickly in children, because they will not tolerate a prolonged examination. Insertion of the proctoscope to 5 to 9 cm is usually sufficient to recognize disease and obtain specimens for microscopic examination and culture. For those patients younger than the age of two, an infant proctoscope should be used. For children older than two years, an adult proctoscope is satisfactory and safe. Children will usually tolerate the procedure without anesthesia if adequate communication has been established between the physician and child. Sedation before the procedure is occasionally indicated (Seconal suppository, 1 mg per pound of body weight, or Thorazine suppository, 0.5 mg per pound of body weight, one hour before proctoscopy); rarely, anesthesia is required. Most often the examination can be performed in the office, outpatient clinic, or hospital bed, and the findings are identical to those in the adult with ulcerative colitis.

TREATMENT

Generally the child with an acute episode of ulcerative colitis responds to medical treatment in the same fashion as the adult. Such a program particularly includes hospitalization for the initial evaluation and institution of a therapeutic program and affords better opportunity for the physician to establish a relationship of mutual trust with both parents and child necessary to explain the illness and the goals of therapy. A few patients may respond to the elimination of milk from the diet, oral sulfonamides (Azulfidine, 2 to 6 g daily), judicious sedation (chlordiazepoxide [Librium], 10 to 25 mg orally, three times a day) and fluid and electrolyte repletion. Psychotherapy has been advocated by many physicians as an important part of the overall medical treatment in the young. The damage to the child's emotions is often more evident and serious than in the adult, in part because the child is less able to understand the physical effects of the disease, and in part because of a dramatic change in normal child-parent interrelationships owing to parental reaction to the illness.

If these measures fail, topical instillation of corticosteroids by enema may control the disease (methylprednisolone acetate, 40 mg in 110 to 150 ml of water). In the more severe cases of ulcerative colitis orally administered corticosteroids (prednisolone, 30 mg per m² of body surface) are often effective. In the very ill juvenile patients high doses of parenteral corticosteroids or ACTH (40 units every 12 hours) may dramatically induce rapid improvement. As in the adult, once remission has been induced by these systemic agents, they must be withdrawn gradually — usually over a six- to eight-week period — to avoid a recrudescence of symptoms. After six to eight weeks of treatment if more than 5 to 10 mg of oral prednisolone daily is needed to control either the colonic or extracolonic manifestations of the disease at a tolerable level, colectomy should be considered as an alternative means of treatment.

Two reasons support this strong attitude. First, the cumulative side effects of long-term corticosteroid therapy in children are more severe than in adults; these include growth retardation, susceptibility to infections (including tuberculosis), osteoporosis, unsightly skin blemishes, and myopathy. Although growth retardation is usually the result of the disease itself, corticosteroid treatment may further aggravate this problem. A program of alternate-day administration of steroids has been advocated to avoid these difficulties.[73] Second, the long-term survival of this group of patients without colectomy is very bad, and roughly only 60 per cent are alive after 20 years. In our opinion therefore it makes little sense to subject these children to the continued ravages of a serious disease and to the risks of prolonged corticosteroid treatment when the chance for an ultimately successful therapeutic outcome is so poor.[74]

Even if the disease remits in childhood and the patient grows normally to adulthood, the incidence of recurrence of the disease in the third and fourth decades is high. Actuarial studies indicate that the life expectancy of such people is considerably reduced, perhaps by as much as 20 years. Recent evidence indicating a remarkably high incidence of subsequent carcinoma of the colon after 20 years of disease in children with ulcerative colitis further supports earlier surgical intervention for children with this disease.[48]

The cumulative risk for developing cancer of the colon is about 40 per cent after 20 years of ulcerative colitis. In fact, this dismal prospect of colonic cancer has prompted one group to advocate prophylactic colectomy regardless of the short-term benefits of corticosteroid treatment.[48] In our opinion, the psychological reaction to colectomy and ileostomy in children is usually less adverse than the severe emotional problems which arise from a chronic and debilitating disease such as ulcerative colitis. Much of the problem in recommending colectomy with ileostomy in children stems from the understandable concern of the parents about this procedure.

REFERENCES

1. Wilks, S., and Moxon, W. Lectures on Pathological Anatomy, 2nd ed. London, J. & A. Churchill, 1875.
2. Acheson, E. D., and Nefzger, M. D. Ulcerative colitis in the United States Army in 1944 – epidemiology. Gastroenterology 44:7, 1963.
3. Almy, T. P., and Sherlock, P. Genetic aspects of ulcerative colitis and regional enteritis. Gastroenterology 51:757, 1966.
4. Sherlock, P., Bell, B. M., Steinberg, H., and Almy, T. P. Familial occurrence of regional enteritis and ulcerative colitis. Gastroenterology 45:413, 1963.
5. Engle, G. L. Studies of ulcerative colitis, III. The nature of the psychological processes. Amer. J. Med. 19:231, 1955.
6. Feldman, F., Cantor, D., Soll, S., and Bachrach, W. Psychiatric study of a consecutive series of 34 patients with ulcerative colitis. Brit. Med. J. 2:14, 1967.
7. Mendeloff, A. I., Monk, M., Siegel, C. I., and Lilienfield, A. Illness experience and life stresses in patients with irritable colon and with ulcerative colitis. New Eng. J. Med. 282:14, 1970.
8. Monk, M., Mendeloff, A. I., Siegel, C. I., and Lilienfield, A. An epidemiological study of ulcerative colitis and regional enteritis among adults in Baltimore – III: Psychological and possible stress-precipitating factors. J. Chron. Dis. 22:565, 1970.
9. Kraft, S. C., and Kirsner, J. B. Immunological apparatus of the gut and inflammatory bowel disease. Gastroenterology 60:922, 1971.
10. Mottet, N. K. Histopathologic Spectrum of Regional Enteritis and Ulcerative Colitis. Philadelphia, W. B. Saunders Co., 1971.
11. Harris, J., and Shields, R. Absorption and secretion of water and electrolytes by the intact human colon in diffuse untreated proctocolitis. Gut 11:27, 1970.
12. Goulston, S. J. M., and McGovern, V. J. The nature of benign strictures in ulcerative colitis. New Eng. J. Med. 281:290, 1969.
13. Edwards, F. C., and Truelove, S. C. The course and prognosis of ulcerative colitis. II. Long-term prognosis. Gut 4:309, 1964.
14. Truelove, S. C., and Witts, L. J. Cortisone in ulcerative colitis. Report on therapeutic trial. Brit. Med. J. 2:375, 1954; 2:1041, 1955.
15. Edwards, F. C., and Truelove, S. C. The course and prognosis of ulcerative colitis. I. Short-term prognosis. Gut 4:299, 1964.
16. Sparberg, M., Fennessy, J., and Kirsner, J. B. Ulcerative proctitis and mild ulcerative colitis: A study of 220 patients. Medicine 45:391, 1966.

17. Matts, S. F. The value of rectal biopsy in the diagnosis of ulcerative colitis. Quart. J. Med. 30:393, 1961.

18. Baron, J. H., Connell, A. M., and Lennard-Jones, J. E. Variation between observers in describing mucosal appearances in proctocolitis. Brit. Med. J. 1:89, 1964.

19. Watts, J. M., Thompson, H., and Goligher, J. C. Sigmoidoscopy and cytology in the detection of microscopic disease of the rectal mucosa in ulcerative colitis. Gut 7:288, 1966.

20. Beal, R. W., Skyring, A. P., McRae, M. B., and Firkin, G. G. The anemia of ulcerative colitis. Gastroenterology 45:589, 1963.

21. Wright, R., and Truelove, S. C. A controlled therapeutic trial of various diets in ulcerative colitis. Brit. Med. J. 2:138, 1965.

22. Wright, R., and Truelove, S. C. Circulating antibodies to dietary protein in ulcerative colitis. Brit. Med. J. 2:142, 1965.

23. Cady, A. B., Rhodes, J. B., Littman, A., and Krane, R. K. Significance of lactase deficit in ulcerative colitis. J. Lab. Clin. Med. 70:279, 1967.

24. O'Connor, J. F., Daniels, G., Flood, C., Karush, A., Moses, L., and Stearn, L. O. An evaluation of the effectiveness of psychotherapy in the treatment of ulcerative colitis. Ann. Intern. Med. 60:587, 1964.

25. Groen, J., and Bastiaans, J. Psychotherapy of ulcerative colitis. Gastroenterology 17:344, 1951.

26. Truelove, S. C., and Witts, L. J. Cortisone and corticotropin in ulcerative colitis. Brit. Med. J. 1:387, 1959.

27. Lennard-Jones, J. E., Misiewicz, J. J., Connell, A. M., Baron, J. H., and Jones, F. A. Prednisone as maintenance treatment for ulcerative colitis in remission. Lancet 1:188, 1965.

28. Truelove, S. C. Treatment of ulcerative colitis with local hydrocortisone hemisuccinate. A report on a controlled therapeutic trial. Brit. Med. J. 2:1072, 1958.

29. Baron, J. H., Connell, A. M., Kanaghinis, T. G., Lennard-Jones, J. E., and Jones, F. A. Outpatient treatment of ulcerative colitis: Comparison between three doses of oral prednisone. Brit. Med. J. 2:441,1962.

30. Baron, J. H., Connell, A. M., Lennard-Jones, J. E., and Jones, F. A. Sulphasalazine and salicylazosulphadimidine in ulcerative colitis. Lancet 1:1094, 1962.

31. Dick, A. P., Grayson, M. J., Carpenter, R. G., and Petrie, A. Controlled trial of sulphasalazine in treatment of ulcerative colitis. Gut 5:437, 1964.

32. Lennard-Jones, J. E., Longmore, A. J., Newell, A. C., Wilson, C. W. F., and Jones, F. A. An assessment of prednisone, salazopyrin, and topical hydrocortisone used as outpatient treatment for ulcerative colitis. Gut 1:217, 1960.

33. Truelove, S. C., Watkinson, G., and Draper, G. Comparison of corticosteroid and sulphasalazine therapy in ulcerative colitis. Brit. Med. J. 2:1708, 1962.

34. Lennard-Jones, J. E., Connell, A. M., Baron, J. H., and Jones, F. A. Controlled trial of sul-

phasalazine in maintenance therapy for ulcerative colitis. Lancet 1:185, 1965.

35. Jewell, D. P., and Truelove, S. C. Azathioprine in ulcerative colitis: An interim report on a controlled therapeutic trial. Brit. Med. J. 1:709, 1972.

36. Watts, J. M., deDombal, F. T., Watkinson, G., and Goligher, J. C. Early course of ulcerative colitis. Gut 7:16, 1966.

37. Jalan, K. N., Prescott, R. J., Sircus, W., et al. An experience with ulcerative colitis. II. Short-term outcome. Gastroenterology 9:589, 1970.

38. Watts, J. M., deDombal, F. T., and Goligher, J. C. Long-term prognosis of ulcerative colitis. Brit. Med. J. 1:1447, 1966.

39. Jalan, K. N., Prescott, R. J., Sircus, W., et al. An experience with ulcerative colitis. III. Long-term outcome. Gastroenterology 59:598, 1970.

40. deDombal, F. T., Watts, J. M., Watkinson, G., and Goligher, J. C. Ulcerative colitis and pregnancy. Lancet 2:599, 1965.

41. Krawitt, E. L. Ulcerative colitis and pregnancy. Obstet. Gynec. 14:354, 361, 1959.

42. Law, D. H., Steinberg, H., and Sleisenger, M. H. Ulcerative colitis with onset after the age of fifty. Gastroenterology 41:457, 1961.

43. Edwards, F. C., and Truelove, S. C. The course and prognosis of ulcerative colitis. III. Complications. Gut 5:1,1964.

44. deDombal, F. T., Watts, M. B., Watkinson, G., and Goligher, J. Incidence and management of anorectal abscess, fistula, and fissure in patients with ulcerative colitis. Dis. Colon Rect. 9:201, 1966.

45. Norland, C. C., and Kirsner, J. B. Toxic dilatation of the colon (toxic megacolon): etiology, treatment, and prognosis in 42 patients. Medicine 48:229, 1969.

46. Edwards, F. C., and Truelove, S. C. The course and prognosis of ulcerative colitis. IV. Carcinoma of the colon. Gut 5:15, 1964.

47. deDombal, F. T., Watts, J. M., Watkinson, G., and Goligher, J. C. Local complications of ulcerative colitis: Stricture, pseudopolyps, and carcinoma of the colon and rectum. Brit. Med. J. 1:1442, 1966.

48. Devrode, G. J., Taylor, W. F., Sauer, W. G., Jackman, R. J., and Stickler, G. B. Cancer risk and life expectancy of children with ulcerative colitis. New Eng. J. Med. 285:17, 1971.

49. MacDougall, I. P. M. The cancer risk in ulcerative colitis. Lancet 1:655, 1964.

50. Morson, B. C., and Pang, L. S. C. Rectal biopsy as an aid to cancer control in ulcerative colitis. Gut 8:423, 1967.

51. Perrett, A. D., Higgins, G., Johnston, H. H., Massarella, G. R., Truelove, S. C., and Wright, R. The liver in ulcerative colitis. Quart. J. Med. 158:211, 1971.

52. Mistillis, S. P. Pericholangitis and ulcerative colitis. I. Pathology, etiology, and pathogenesis. Ann. Intern. Med. 63:1, 1965.

53. Eade, M. N. Liver disease in ulcerative colitis. I. Analysis of operative liver biopsy in 138 consecutive patients. Ann. Intern. Med. 72:475, 1970.

54. Warren, K. W., Athanassiades, S., and Monge,

J. I. Primary sclerosing cholangitis. A study of forty-two cases. Amer. J. Surg. *111*:23, 1966.

55. Eade, M. N. Liver disease in ulcerative colitis. II. The long-term effect of colectomy. Ann. Intern. Med. 72:489, 1970.

56. McEwen, C., Lingg, C., and Kirsner, J. B. Arthritis accompanying ulcerative colitis. Amer. J. Med. 33:923, 1962.

57. Jayson, M. I., Salmon, P. R., and Harrison, W. J. Inflammatory bowel disease in ankylosing spondylitis. Gut *11*:506, 1970.

58. Wright, R., Lumsden, K., Luntz, M. H., Sevel, D., and Truelove, S. C. Abnormalities of the sacro-iliac joints and uveitis in ulcerative colitis. Quart. J. Med. 34:229, 1965.

59. Johnson, M. L., and Wilson, T. H. Skin lesions in ulcerative colitis. Gut *10*:255, 1969.

60. Watts, J. M., deDombal, F. T., and Goligher, J. C. Long-term complications and prognosis following major surgery for ulcerative colitis. Brit. J. Surg. 53:1014, 1966.

61. Goligher, J. C., deDombal, F. T., Graham, R. G., and Watkinson, G. Early surgery in the management of severe ulcerative colitis. Brit. Med. J. 3:193, 1967.

62. Ritchie, J. K. Ileostomy and excisional surgery for chronic inflammatory disease of the colon: A survey of one hospital region. I. Results and complications of surgery. Gut *12*:528, 1971.

63. Roy, P. H., Sauer, W. G., Beahrs, O. H., and Farrow, G. M. Experience with ileostomies: Evaluation of long-term rehabilitation in 497 patients. Amer. J. Surg. *119*:77, 1970.

64. Graham, W. P., Galante, M., Goldman, L., McCorkle, H. J., and Wanebo, H. J. Complications of ileostomy. Amer. J. Surg. *110*:142, 1965.

65. Daly, D. W., and Brooke, B. N. Ileostomy and excision of the large intestine for ulcerative colitis. Lancet 2:62, 1967.

66. Ritchie, J. K. Ileostomy and excisional surgery for chronic inflammatory disease of the colon: II. Health of ileostomists. Gut *12*:536, 1971.

67. Clarke, A. M., and McKenzie, R. G. Ileostomy and the risk of urinary uric acid stones. Lancet 2:395, 1969.

68. Kramer, P., Kearney, M. S., and Ingelfinger, F. J. The effect of specific foods and water loading on the ileal excreta of ileostomized human subjects. Gastroenterology *42*:535, 1962.

69. Thompson, T. J., Runice, J., and Kahn, A. Effect of diet on ileostomy function. Gut *11*:482, 1970.

70. Fleischer, F. G., and Mandelstam, P. Roentgen observations of the ileostomy in patients with idiopathic ulcerative colitis. II. Ileostomy dysfunction. Radiology 70:469, 1958.

71. Knill-Jones, R. P., Morson, B., and Williams, R. Prestomal ileitis: Clinical and pathological findings in five cases. Quart. J. Med. *39*:287, 1970.

72. McCaffery, T. D., Nasr, K., Lawrence, A. M., and Kirsner, J. B. Severe growth retardation in children with inflammatory bowel disease. Pediatrics 45:386, 1970.

73. Sadeghi-Nejad, A., and Senior, J. B. The treatment of ulcerative colitis in children with alternate-day corticosteroids. Pediatrics 43:840, 1969.

74. Korelitz, B. I., and Gribetz, D. Prognosis of ulcerative colitis with onset in childhood. II. Steroid era. Ann. Intern. Med. 57:592, 1962.

Chapter 103

Granulomatous Disease of the Colon

James H. Meyer, Marvin H. Sleisenger

INTRODUCTION

Granulomatous colitis is a chronic inflammatory disease of the colon predominantly occurring in young people (second and third decades) and most often involving the proximal portion of colon and terminal ileum; occasionally it affects isolated or multiple segments, often sparing the rectum. In its pure form, it differs from ulcerative colitis pathologically, but, as will be noted, there is considerable overlap. Its clinical features are more distinctive. Granulomatous disease of ileum and proximal colon as an entity separate from "right-sided ulcerative colitis" has been recognized only in the past decade. Despite its distinctive history, clinical course, characteristic radiological signs, and peculiar anatomical distribution, as well as the frequent presence of granuloma, a complete separation from ulcerative colitis is often impossible.

For the present, however, the difference between the diseases warrants our continued thinking in terms of two entities: such separation may be important not only in management but also in providing clues to etiology.

The disease is complicated by stenosis, perforation, fistulas, abscesses, perianal and perirectal sepsis, multisystemic symptoms, and a distressingly high recurrence rate after surgery for ileocolitis. It differs from ulcerative colitis in that its distribution is segmental, predominantly proximal, and gross rectal bleeding is uncommon.

DISTINCTION FROM ULCERATIVE COLITIS

Granulomatous disease frequently affects the colon in patients with regional enteritis; about 50 per cent of all patients with small bowel disease will exhibit colonic involvement. In this circumstance, the colonic disease resembles the associated disease in the small bowel with the development of skip areas, enteric fistulas, and likewise the same morphological characteristics (transmural inflammation and granuloma formation). The type of inflammatory disease of the colon which exhibits these same characteristics even in the absence of small bowel involvement is therefore considered to be granulomatous disease or regional enteritis of the colon. As can be seen from Tables 103–1 and 103–2, these features of granulomatous colitis are sufficiently characteristic to permit a distinction from ulcerative colitis.

Similarly, certain features of ulcerative colitis (Table 103–1) are not seen in granulomatous disease. These include pseudo-

1350

TABLE 103–1. CLINICAL FEATURES DISTINGUISHING ULCERATIVE COLITIS FROM GRANULOMATOUS COLITIS

	INCIDENCE IN	
	Ulcerative Colitis (per cent)	Granulomatous Colitis (per cent)
Pathognomonic for ulcerative colitis:		
Pseudopolyps	15	0
Disease limited to rectosigmoid	10	0
Free colonic perforation	3	<0.2
Pathognomonic for granulomatous colitis:		
Associated small bowel disease	5	80
Skip areas of colitis	0	50
Enteric fistula	<0.5	10
Nondistinguishing:		
Diarrhea	80	70
Hematochezia	90	50
Rectal involvement	95	50
Rectal sparing	5	50
Perianal disease	25	70
Deep ulcers	25	60
Colonic stricture	11	23
Toxic megacolon	3	0.5
Colonic carcinoma*	3.5	1.2

*Observed incidence in all cases of ulcerative colitis (segmental or universal) and all cases of granulomatous disease of the colon (with or without associated regional enteritis of the small bowel).

polyps and confinement of the pathology to the rectosigmoid. Although free colonic perforation has been reported in granulomatous colitis, it is so rare that it permits a diagnosis of ulcerative colitis in the setting of inflammatory disease of the colon. These pathognomonic features of ulcerative colitis, however, are infrequent. Thus their value in distinguishing the two diseases is very limited.

Both diseases share a wide spectrum of clinical and morphological features (Tables 103–1 and 103–2). These include hematochezia, diarrhea, perianal disease, colonic stricture, toxic megacolon, colonic carcinoma, and crypt abscesses. Similarly, sigmoidoscopic features of the two diseases overlap: although deep ulcers are more characteristic of granulomatous disease involving the rectum (see below),

TABLE 103–2. HISTOPATHOLOGICAL FEATURES DISTINGUISHING ULCERATIVE COLITIS FROM GRANULOMATOUS COLITIS*

	INCIDENCE IN	
	Ulcerative Colitis (per cent)	Granulomatous Colitis (per cent)
Pathognomonic for granulomatous colitis:		
Granuloma (noncaseating)†	0	60–80
Transmural involvement	10	80–100
Pathognomonic for ulcerative colitis		
None		
Nondistinguishing		
Crypt abscess	90	60–80
Lymphectasia	20	90
Lymph node hyperplasia	60	80

*Gross pathological features which can be discerned clinically have not been included in this table. Such features include distribution of the lesions and enteric fistulas (see Table 103–1).
†By accepted definition, colitis showing submucosal granulomas is defined as granulomatous rather than ulcerative colitis.

they are seen often enough in patients with ulcerative colitis that they do not definitely establish the diagnosis of granulomatous colitis. Combinations of these nondistinguishing features, however, often permit a diagnosis; for example, diarrhea in the absence of rectal bleeding, perianal disease with sparing of the rectosigmoid, and stricture in the proximal colon would be encountered 40 times more often in granulomatous colitis than in ulcerative colitis.

In addition to differences in frequency, there are qualitative differences in some of the features shared by these two diseases. About 5 per cent of ulcerative colitis is associated with disease of the small intestine, always confined to the terminal ileum (backwash ileitis); up to 80 per cent[1] of granulomatous colitis is associated with small intestinal disease, nearly always affecting the terminal ileum; in many instances the proximal intestine is affected as well. Furthermore, the disease of the terminal ileum in ulcerative colitis is limited to the mucosa and the submucosa, whereas in granulomatous disease the ileal involvement is transmural. This difference is reflected in radiographic studies of the ileum in these two diseases; in ulcerative colitis the ileum is widely patent, showing mucosal irregularities, whereas in granulomatous colitis the ileum is frequently narrowed by transmural fibrosis and edema. Similarly, rectal bleeding presents differently in the two diseases. It is usually present early and is a constant feature in ulcerative colitis, whereas in granulomatous colitis rectal bleeding is most often a late manifestation and is usually intermittent. Perianal pathology complicates both diseases. However, rectal fissures, fistulas, and abscesses in granulomatous disease are more often multiple and/or extensive, whereas these same lesions in ulcerative colitis are usually single and uncomplicated by extensive undermining of perianal tissue.

It can be seen, then, that in many instances there is a sharp distinction between these two diseases on clinical and pathological grounds. However, sufficient overlap exists that 10 to 20 per cent of the patients in whom inflammatory disease is limited to the colon cannot be classified as having either granulomatous or ulcerative colitis.

ETIOLOGY AND PATHOGENESIS

The same considerations discussed for ulcerative colitis (pp. 1298 to 1301) apply to granulomatous colitis. Because the distinctive pathological feature is the granuloma, a lesion frequently noted with delayed hypersensitivity, recent searches for etiology have concentrated on immunological mechanisms. Although lymphocytes from patients with granulomatous colitis exhibit cytotoxicity for colon epithelial cells, no additional data are available to support this theory. The disease does not appear to be a form of sarcoidosis, if recently reported negative reaction to Kveim antigen is acceptable evidence. Further, patients with granulomatous colitis (and enteritis as well) do not suffer the pulmonary manifestations (X-ray and clinical) noted in 90 per cent or so of patients with sarcoidosis.

At the moment, no scientifically acceptable evidence exists in support of theories that propose the cause of granulomatous bowel disease to be infection (viral or pathogenic *Escherichia coli*), endotoxin, proteolytic enzymes, psychogenic disturbances, metabolic or connective tissue disease, or food allergy. Its incidence in patients with hypogammaglobulinemia is not increased; although some think that the incidence of various allergies such as hay fever and eczema is higher than normal in these patients and in their families, no suitable control data are available. The same considerations apply to the similar claims of an association with periarteritis nodosum, autoimmune hemolytic anemia, Reiter's syndrome, or Behçet's disease.

A possible clue to etiology appears to be in a genetic abnormality, because this disease has a strikingly high familial incidence. A search is underway to find a suitable genetic marker that will permit further epidemiological study as well as investigation of etiology.

EPIDEMIOLOGY

The relative incidence of ulcerative colitis and granulomatous colitis comprising the category of noninfectious chronic inflammatory disease of the colon varies according to the site of the experience. Thus the population at risk influences the data, because certain groups, particularly Jews, are more prone to suffer the granulomatous form of the disease. Also, criteria for diagnosis vary widely from group to group. Available epidemiological information indicates that granulomatous colitis or ileocolitis is less common than ulcerative colitis. Thus the incidence of the disease has been reported to range from 1.4 to 3.4 per 100,000 in the Caucasian population per year, with a slight predominance in females. Exact incidence is difficult to ascertain, because correlation of pathological findings with clinical diagnosis is often difficult. Clear-cut, characteristic histological features of granulomatous disease are more readily found in patients with fistulas, stenosis, and abscesses—hallmarks which clearly distinguish the disease *clinically* from ulcerative colitis. It is not known how many patients with colitis not having these clinical features would be classified by histological criteria as having granulomatous colitis, but it is estimated that 12 to 25 per cent of those with clinical ulcerative colitis would show granulomas and transmural disease on pathological examination.[1-3] As in ulcerative colitis, there appears to be a higher than predicted incidence of associated ankylosing spondylitis.

PATHOLOGY

GROSS AND MICROSCOPIC FEATURES

The pathology of granulomatous colitis is characterized by transmural inflammation and thickening, stenosis, deep linear ulceration, and heaped-up islands of inflammatory tissue surrounded by fibrous scars. Microscopically, granulomas and lymphoid hyperplasia are often noted. Grossly, the fissuring is deep, often longitudinal; progressive fibrosis explains in large part the thickening and stenosis.

The lymphatics are often also involved in granulomatous disease, giving the appearance of lymphangiectasia in contrast to mucosal ulcerative colitis; enlarged mesenteric nodes are almost always found. Fistulas between loops of gut and between involved gut and contiguous organs are common. Scattered deep ulcerations, often circular or oval, are particularly striking in the rectum.

Mucosal ulceration may be (and often is) deep with either normal or inflamed mucosa between the longitudinal fissures, giving the appearance of cobblestones (Fig. 103–1). Areas of ulceration are large; compared with those in mucosal ulcerative colitis, the ulcers are deep and undermined, and frequently extend for long distances along the colon. Although crypt abscesses may be seen, they are not so frequently encountered as in mucosal ulcerative colitis. Likewise, pseudopolyps are not found.

However, only a little more than half the specimens with granulomatous disease will show granuloma on histological examination. Occasionally, perhaps in a third of instances, these granulomas will be widespread; in other instances they will be seen only irregularly after careful search. They are noncaseating, contain small

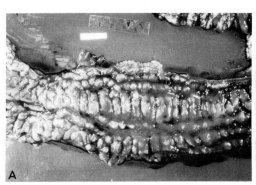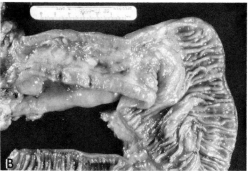

Figure 103–1. Resected specimens of colon from patients with granulomatous colitis. *A*, Note "cobblestone" mucosa formed by protuberant mucosa between confluent linear ulcers. Also note thickened colonic wall. *B*, Note segment of narrowed, thickened bowel giving "hose pipe" appearance on X-ray. Normal bowel (right) is adjacent. (Courtesy of Dr. Carolyn Montgomery.)

TABLE 103–3.   DISTRIBUTION OF COLONIC LESIONS IN CASES OF
HISTOLOGICALLY CONFIRMED GRANULOMATOUS COLITIS*

	PRIMARY CROHN'S COLITIS† (130 CASES) (PER CENT)	ILEOCOLITIS‡ (89 CASES) (PER CENT)
Rectum	58	44
Sigmoid	72	35
Descending colon	59	30
Transverse colon	65	38
Ascending colon	54	26
Cecum	34	38
Ileum	0	100
Total colonic involvement	28	17
Skip areas	22	25

*Data are a composite of cases reported in references 8, 16, 17 and from Lockhart-Mummery, H. E., and Morson, B. C.: Gut 5:493, 1964.
†No small bowel disease demonstrated.
‡Small bowel disease (ileum) together with colitis.

numbers of giant cells, and are formed by epithelioid cells. They are scattered in the lamina propria, submucosa, muscularis, and subserosa (see Fig. 112–3, A).

ANATOMIC DISTRIBUTION

The distribution of the disease is of interest (Table 103–3). It is frequently segmental, and often involves the right side of the colon, including the cecum; in most of these instances, the disease affects the terminal ileum for a variable length, usually for one or more feet. In many patients, the transverse and descending colons are also involved. The rectum is diseased in 50 per cent of cases—either in contiguity with descending colon and sigmoid or as a discrete "skip" area itself. In some patients most of the colon is affected, and half of these also have disease in the rectum. Isolated granulomatous disease in the rectum is rare. The remainder of the cases are made up of segmental disease of right colon (without ileal disease) of the transverse descending colon or sigmoid. The involvement of colon and ileum is four times more common than disease confined to the colon alone.

RECTAL LESIONS

The rectal lesions consist mainly of ulcers, with or without fissures or deep fistulas, arising in the rectal crypts and ending in the perirectal fat, forming abscesses. Occasionally the ulceration will be so severe as to erode into the sphincters and their supporting musculature. Perirectal sepsis with soft-tissue necrosis may be extreme (Fig. 103–2).

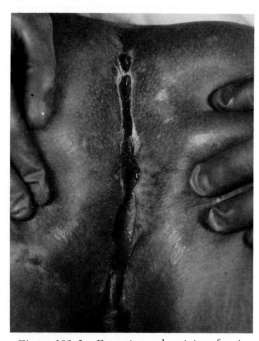

Figure 103–2.   Extensive undermining of perirectal tissue in a patient with granulomatous colitis and perianal abscess. As in this patient, extensive perianal disease complicating granulomatous colitis is frequently indolent, relatively painless, and unaccompanied by extensive erythema.

CLINICAL PICTURE

GENERAL FEATURES

The disease occurs predominantly in persons in the second, third, and fourth decades, but may appear at any age. As with ulcerative colitis, the peak incidence is at age 28 to 30, with a slight predominance of females. However, the clinical picture of granulomatous disease of the colon differs in some important respects from ulcerative colitis. It may present with a distressingly large number of complications: as a perianal and perirectal abscess and fistulas, as intestinal obstruction, or with symptoms of intra-abdominal fistula or abscess. Indeed, these patients are more prone to appear for the first time with local complications of their disease than are patients with ulcerative colitis.

Also, in contrast to patients with mucosal ulcerative colitis, whose symptoms at onset are often dramatic (marked diarrhea, rectal bleeding, high fever, tachycardia, prostration, and dehydration), are the many patients with granulomatous disease of the colon with subtle symptoms, such as low grade fever (99 to 100°F); mild to moderate, nonbloody diarrhea; gradual weight loss; mild to moderate anemia; and slow progression over periods of months or even years. Anemia may be due to occult blood loss and to malabsorption of vitamin B_{12} by a sizable diseased segment of terminal ileum.

Rectal bleeding dominates the course of ulcerative colitis, but in granulomatous colitis gross bleeding early in the course of the disease is rare. Bleeding may be noted later, when about half the patients will have involvement of the rectum and rectosigmoid with some degree of edema and friability of mucosa.

Pain is a notable complaint in over half the patients; it is crampy, colicky, and usually confined to the lower quadrants, particularly on the right side. Insidious weight loss may also be the principal complaint—not dramatic at first but gradually leading to varying degrees of disability. It is frequently associated with diseased contiguous ileum which is unable to resorb bile acids normally. These unabsorbed compounds are deconjugated and metabolized by bacteria to secondary bile acids in the proximal colon where they are only partially absorbed. As a result, the total bile salt pool shrinks, resulting in a reduced concentration of conjugated bile acids in the proximal small bowel with appearance of steatorrhea. Further, unabsorbed bile acids aggravate diarrhea by interfering principally with absorption of sodium and water in the proximal colon (see pp. 229 to 248). Diminished bile salt concentration in bile also leads to cholelithiasis in these patients, particularly after resection of the terminal ileum (see below; see also pp. 1110 to 1115). Edema and hypoproteinemia, caused in part by excess protein loss in a diseased bowel, are frequent findings.

PRESENTATION WITH COMPLICATIONS

Bowel Complications. Since some form of perianal or perirectal disease—such as fissures, hemorrhoids, fistulas in ano, and perianal or perirectal abscesses—appears in half the patients at some time during the course of the disease, it is not surprising that about 10 per cent will present with one or more of these symptoms. In 20 to 30 per cent, a mass will be palpable, the result of adherence of loops of small or large bowel to diseased segments, in some cases caused by fistulas between loops of bowel. Abscess commonly accompanies fistulas between loops of bowel or between bowel and contiguous organs; abscess also forms as the result of perforation into the mesentery. Occasionally patients present with high spiking temperatures (101 to 103°F or higher daily), owing to perforation and abscess. A small fraction of patients will have their diagnosis made as a result of surgery for intestinal obstruction caused by stenosis of an involved segment, usually terminal ileum. However, many such patients relate having had bouts of diarrhea with or without fever for months to many years, apparently insufficient to warrant thorough study. In others, adequate investigations for recurrent diarrhea led to diagnoses of irritable colon, infectious enteritis, or "nonspecific colitis."

Extraenteric Complications. As with ulcerative colitis, extracolonic manifestations of the disease may be the presenting symptoms. Arthritis is reported in about 10 per cent of patients, in many of whom it is an early complaint. About 10 per cent of patients have either spondylitis or serious skin involvement, either erythema nodosum or pyoderma gangrenosum, and, as in mucosal ulcerative colitis, smaller numbers have aphthous stomatitis, iritis, or thrombophlebitis (see pp. 1333 to 1340).

PHYSICAL EXAMINATION

Findings on physical examination depend on the extent and severity of the primary disease as well as the presence or absence of complications. Thus the patient may have no signs of illness except for some pallor and vague lower abdominal tenderness; at the other extreme, he may have a palpable mass, varying in size from an orange to a large grapefruit, often firm to hard and fixed; splenomegaly may be noted in 10 per cent of patients (particularly those with contiguous small bowel involvement); arthritis may be evident, with swollen, tender wrist, knee, or ankle joints and with effusion or limited motion. Also, aphthous ulcers of the mouth and pharynx, iritis, thrombophlebitis, erythema nodosum, and pyoderma gangrenosum may be noted. Those who are extremely ill demonstrate dehydration, hypotension, marked wasting, tachycardia, and fever. Women with enterovaginal fistula may have feculent vaginal discharge. In a high percentage of patients, perirectal or perianal disease may be found on examination. Clubbing of the fingers may also be present in about 10 per cent of patients. In an occasional patient, localized tenderness or limited motion may be evidence of sacroileitis or ankylosing spondylitis.

If the small bowel is extensively diseased, evidence of malabsorption and malnutrition may be present on examination, including muscle wasting, abdominal protuberance, edema, glossitis, and dermal changes, reflecting deficiencies of vitamins A and K as well as of niacin (see pp. 250 to 277). Rarely, one may note carpopedal spasm and positive Chvostek or Trousseau signs caused by hypocalcemia. Muscle weakness and fluidity and abdominal distention may reflect hypokalemia.

LABORATORY FINDINGS

These patients frequently have a moderate anemia, most often because of iron deficiency, but occasionally a macrocytic anemia may be found caused by poor diet (folic acid deficiency) or failure to absorb vitamin B_{12} normally. Polymorphonuclear leukocytosis is common; the white blood count ranges from 10,000 to 15,000 but may be normal in mild cases. The erythrocyte sedimentation is usually elevated. Hypoproteinemia and hypoalbuminemia are often present. These findings are due in some part to diminished intake and possibly to malabsorption, but mainly result from excessive enteric protein loss—so-called protein-losing enteropathy (see pp. 35 to 47).

PROCTOSIGMOIDOSCOPY

As noted, the rectosigmoid colon is spared of disease in up to 50 per cent of patients with granulomatous colitis. Sigmoidoscopic findings are frequently normal in this group of patients. On the other hand, some patients will exhibit indolent but rather advanced anal or perianal disease. These lesions include anal ulceration, frequently multiple anal fissures or rectal fistulas, and perirectal and ischiorectal abscesses (see Fig. 103–2).

When the rectosigmoid colon is involved with disease, a variety of sigmoidoscopic abnormalities are found, some of which are characteristic of granulomatous colitis. In contrast to mucosal ulcerative colitis, granulomatous colitis is a transmural disease. Grossly visible changes in the mucosa are sometimes secondary to underlying inflammation in the wall of the colon. Islands of normal mucosa may protrude into the colonic lumen as the result of submucosal inflammation and edema. In other areas, prolonged and severe submucosal inflammation may produce a slough of overlying mucosa, leaving large areas of ulceration which are sometimes round or punched out in appearance but may be serpiginous or linear in configuration, often extending deeply into the colonic wall. Just as granulomatous disease characteristically involves separate regions along the enteric tract, leaving skip areas of uninvolved bowel between diseased segments, so also on the local level the disease process sometimes affects the rectosigmoid irregularly, leaving areas of relatively uninvolved mucosa amid areas of grossly visible pathology. These pathological processes result in visible changes in the mucosa characteristic of granulomatous colitis. Large ulcerations of varying shape may be seen, sometimes with islands of normal, nonfriable mucosa between the ulcers. In other patients, the rectosigmoid mucosa may take on a cobblestone appearance; that is, islands of normal mucosa protrude into the lumen as the result of submucosal inflammation and edema, and are accentuated and segmented by depressed linear clefts or ulcers. Such findings, when present, differ markedly from the appearance of the mucosa in ulcerative colitis, in which ulcers result from the coalescence of crypt abscesses and thus tend to be small, circular, and shallow. Further, the mucosa in ulcerative colitis is most often uniformly involved with disease, exhibiting generalized friability and edema. Because the mucosa in ulcerative colitis is more uniformly edematous, broad islands of raised mucosa (cobblestoning) are not frequently encountered.

However, it must be emphasized that these frequently described differences in sigmoidoscopic appearances between ulcerative and granulomatous colitis are not always evident.[4] In many of the patients in whom granulomatous colitis involves the rectosigmoid colon, the sigmoidoscopic findings are identical to those of ulcerative colitis. This fact is not unexpected, inasmuch as the same pathological changes—i.e., crypt abscess formation and mucosal inflammation (see Table 103–2)—often affect the mucosa in both diseases. Similarly, many have emphasized that narrowing of the rectosigmoid lumen reflecting transmural disease is more characteristic of granulomatous colitis; yet stricture, as the result of muscular spasm or extension of the inflammatory process to the colonic wall, is also occasionally seen in ulcerative colitis.

RECTAL BIOPSY

Biopsy of sigmoidoscopically abnormal rectosigmoid mucosa may further aid in establishing the diagnosis of granulomatous colitis.[5] Inflammatory changes in the mucosa similar to those of ulcerative colitis are frequently encountered. In the absence of extensive mucosal disease, however, pronounced submucosal inflammation, lymphoid hyperplasia, and/or the presence of a noncaseating granuloma strongly support the diagnosis of granulomatous colitis (see pp. 1501 to 1507). Granulomas are not frequently encountered in biopsy material, so that their absence does not exclude granulomatous colitis. Conversely, the development of granulomas may be incited by a variety of agents (foreign bodies, fungus, tuberculosis, amebiasis, schistosomiasis, syphilis, lymphogranuloma venereum), so that the finding of a granuloma on rectal biopsy is not pathognomonic of granulomatous colitis. Rectal biopsy from patients in whom the rectosigmoid is sigmoidoscopically uninvolved with disease rarely reveals pathology. Biopsies of anal lesions complicating granulomatous disease of the colon or small bowel may support the diagnosis by revealing granulomas.

ROENTGENOGRAPHIC DIAGNOSIS

The clinical diagnosis of granulomatous colitis rests primarily on the findings of barium enema examination. By contrast, the diagnosis of ulcerative colitis is best made by proctosigmoidoscopy. The reasons for this difference are obvious. Ulcerative colitis is primarily a mucosal disease with incidental involvement of the submucosal tissues; it usually affects the rectosigmoid colon. Endoscopy is superior to roentgenography in detecting superficial mucosal changes in the rectum and sigmoid colon. As a result, proctoscopic diagnosis of ulcerative colitis may be made in a significant number of patients in whom the barium enema examination is normal. On the other hand, granulomatous colitis is primarily a disease of the colonic wall with secondary involvement of the mucosa; furthermore, it frequently spares the rectosigmoid mucosa. Diagnosis is more frequently made by barium enema examination, which will detect disease in the colonic wall in all parts of the colon by demonstrating colonic narrowing or sinus formation as well as secondary mucosal abnormalities.

The roentgenographic diagnosis of granulomatous colitis depends on demonstrating the characteristic pathologic features of the disease: (1) evidence of transmural disease (colonic narrowing from fibrosis or edema, sinus, or fistula formation); (2) the peculiar distribution of the inflammatory process (skip areas along the colon, eccentric involvement of the colon, the presence of small bowel disease, or the localized involvement of the ascending or transverse colon); and (3) the less easily detected but nonetheless characteristic mucosal changes (large and deep ulcerations, linear ulcers, cobblestoning). The bases for these findings have been discussed in preceding sections of this chapter (see pp. 1353 to 1354).

Most cases of granulomatous disease in the colon are associated with small bowel involvement, frequently disease of the terminal ileum. Ileal disease may often be seen on barium enema examination, showing a narrowed, thickened ileum, sometimes with fistulization across the ileocecal valve (Fig. 103–3). In cases of suspected granulomatous colitis, a small bowel series

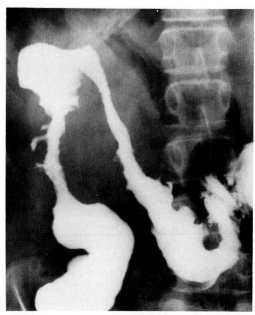

Figure 103–4. Granulomatous colitis producing narrowing of segments of the ascending and transverse colon. Note that the hepatic flexure is not involved so that narrowed segments are "skip areas" of disease. Also note the extension of the barium column through the wall of the ascending colon, demonstrating short sinus tracts.

may also demonstrate regional enteritis in the more proximal intestine. As already noted (see pathology), common sites of localized colonic disease are the ascending colon (including the cecum) or the transverse colon (Fig. 103–4). When the colon is more extensively involved, there may be skip areas of normal colon between diseased segments. A special form of irregular involvement (skip areas) on the local level may be appreciated as eccentric involvement of a segment of colon (Fig. 103–5) in which only one aspect of the colonic wall is involved. A more striking but less common example of the peculiar distribution of this disease is focal involvement. In this situation the area of disease appears as a small tumor-like defect, simulating a sessile intramural, extramucosal mass. It may regress but often progresses to a classic segmental form of colitis with the development of a strictured area in the colon in a short period of time. These types of localized distribution, detected on X-ray examination as mural disease because of stenosis or mural edema, are characteristic of granulomatous colitis.

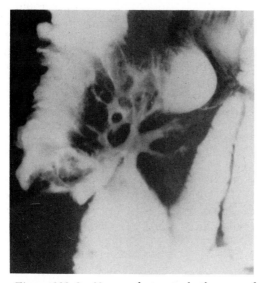

Figure 103–3. Narrowed terminal ileum and ileocecal fistula in a patient with granulomatous colitis. (Courtesy of Dr. H. I. Goldberg.)

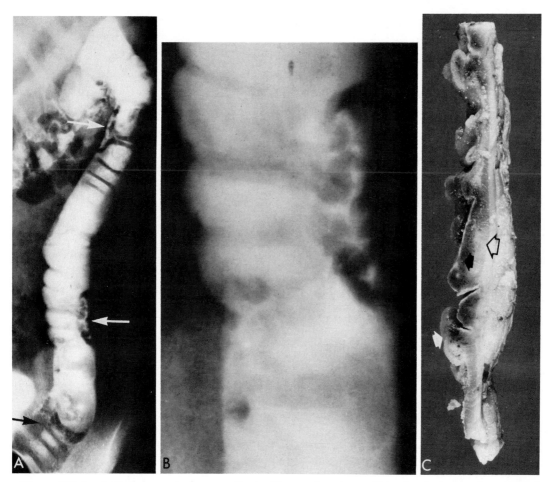

Figure 103-5. *A,* Barium enema from a patient with granulomatous colitis, showing eccentric segmental narrowings of the colonic wall (arrows) with plaque-like ulcerations. *B,* Close-up of middle lesion in *A,* showing a transmural mass with surface ulceration. *C,* Gross pathological specimen of the same lesion, showing transition between normal and diseased mucosa (solid white arrow), extensive submucosal infiltrate (solid black arrow) with denudation of overlying mucosa, and thickened muscularis (open arrow). Note also the penetrating clefts. (From Goldberg, H. I.: Amer. J. Roent. *101*:296, 1967.)

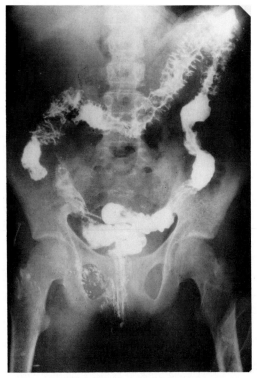

Figure 103–6. Deep transverse ulcers penetrating into the colonic wall along the distal transverse and descending colon in granulomatous colitis.

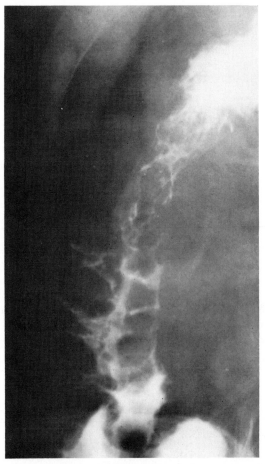

Figure 103–7. Cobblestoning of the mucosa of ascending colon on barium enema examination in a patient with granulomatous colitis. The rectangular areas result from intersections of transverse fissures and deep longitudinal ulcers. (Courtesy of Dr. H. I. Goldberg.)

Mucosal peculiarities of granulomatous colitis are less frequently appreciated because of the limitations of the X-ray techniques. Large and deep ulcerations, linear clefts or ulcers, and cobblestoning of the mucosa are much more characteristic of granulomatous colitis than ulcerative colitis. These lesions may be detected on barium enema examination (Figs. 103–6 and 103–7).

DIFFERENTIAL DIAGNOSIS

The principal diseases from which transmural colitis must be differentiated are ulcerative colitis, tuberculosis of the cecum and terminal ileum, carcinoma of the colon, amebiasis of the colon, segmental ischemic colitis, and diverticulitis of the colon, particularly the sigmoid. (The reader is referred to the appropriate chapters for more detailed discussions of these diseases.)

ULCERATIVE COLITIS

The major features distinguishing granulomatous from ulcerative colitis have been discussed and tabulated in preceding sections of this chapter. These differences have been established by careful retrospective correlation of clinical findings with pathological material obtained at colonic resection or autopsy. The clinician, however, is seldom able to utilize such pathological correlation in a patient who comes to him with inflammatory disease of the colon. There is considerable similarity between these two disorders in terms of presenting colonic symptoms as well as systemic complications. Rectal biopsy seldom provides sufficient material for histological distinction between the two diseases. Essentially the physician has two parameters by which he can distinguish these two diseases of the colon: (1) the distribution of the lesions as determined by barium enema examination and proctosigmoidoscopy; and (2) the character of the demonstrated lesions; i.e., whether they appear to be predominantly confined to the mucosa as in ulcerative colitis, or whether they are mainly transmural as in granulomatous colitis. Proctosigmoidoscopy is important in demonstrating rectal sparing and/or extensive perianal disease, findings more consistent with granulomatous colitis. Occasionally, visible endoscopic lesions are characteristic of granulomatous colitis. However, ulcerative colitis may be complicated by perianal disease, and sigmoidoscopic lesions typical of ulcerative colitis may be seen in granulomatous colitis often enough that this procedure is not definitive in differentiating these types of colitis. Consequently, clinical differentiation depends frequently on the findings of the barium enema examination.

Distribution of the Lesions. Radiographic *sparing of the rectum* is seen roentgenographically nearly twice as often in histologically proved granulomatous colitis as in ulcerative colitis. Nevertheless, by radiographic criteria alone, the rectum is free of disease in about 20 per cent of patients with ulcerative colitis. This overlap can be significantly diminished by proctosigmoidoscopy, which will detect a higher incidence of rectosigmoid disease in those with ulcerative colitis, especially when minimal or equivocal endoscopic findings are corroborated with rectal biopsy. Bona fide rectal sparing—i.e., no rectal disease on barium enema, sigmoidoscopy, and biopsy—is therefore highly suggestive of granulomatous colitis. Even if the initially spared rectal segment later becomes diseased, the subsequent course of the colitis and often the pathological findings at subsequent operation are consistent retrospectively with granulomatous colitis.[6] Conversely, however, granulomatous colitis involves the distal colon often enough (in up to 50 per cent of patients) that demonstrated rectal involvement does not distinguish these two conditions. Segmental colitis of the left colon is seen frequently in both diseases and therefore is not diagnostic. *Segmental involvement of the transverse or the right colon*, however, is virtually diagnostic of granulomatous colitis. Such isolated involvement of the transverse or right colon is seen in only about 15 to 30 per cent of all instances of granulomatous colitis (see Table 103–3), and therefore the value of this criterion is limited. *Terminal ileum* is diseased frequently in both diseases. Radiographically, however, the ileum is more frequently narrowed in granulomatous disease than in ulcerative colitis (see above); fistulization across the ileocecal valve is pathognomonic of granulomatous disease (as is fistulization elsewhere). *Skip areas along the colon* are diagnostic of granulomatous colitis. This finding, however, must be qualified: demonstrable skip areas are evident in a minority (25 per cent) of patients. Eccentric narrowing of the colon is seen often enough in ulcerative colitis that its demonstration alone is not diagnostic of granulomatous disease. *Pathology demonstrated in small bowel* proximal to the ileum by small bowel series in cases of colitis is also presumptive evidence of granulomatous colitis.

Character of the Lesions. Shallow and deep ulcers, "collar button" ulcers, and lesions radiographically resembling cobblestone mucosa or pseudopolyps* are seen in both diseases and are nondiagnostic (see pp. 1308 to 1311). *Linear clefts* penetrating deeply into the colonic wall, when seen, are diagnostic of granulomatous disease. Likewise, *pericolic abscess*, *sinus tracts*, or *fistulas* are characteristic of granulomatous colitis, indicating transmural disease. However, such transmural extension of the disease may be seen in only 50 per cent of patients with granulomatous colitis referred to university centers, and may be even less frequent in the population of patients with this disease at large.

Radiographic diagnosis by these criteria

---

*Pseudopolyps—i.e., polypoid protuberances of undermined mucosa and granulation tissue—are not seen at endoscopy in granulomatous colitis or on examination of resected specimens (see Table 103–1). It would seem therefore that what the radiologist describes as pseudopolyps in persons with granulomatous colitis are probably some other type of mucosal irregularity.

correlates with histopathological diagnosis in about 75 per cent of the patients.[3] Moreover, there is significant observer variation among radiologists as to the probable diagnosis (granulomatous vs. ulcerative colitis). Also, there are a significant number of patients who cannot be classified as having either granulomatous colitis or ulcerative colitis by radiographic criteria; this unclassifiable group corresponds only incompletely with those who cannot be differentiated by histopathological criteria. Nevertheless, radiography is probably the best single method of differentiating these two diseases on clinical grounds.

It is appropriate at this point to ask why such differentiation might be important. Since the etiology of both diseases is unknown, this separation may be purely arbitrary—i.e., the two diseases so recognized may be part of a spectrum of a single disease, or, alternatively, several etiological processes may produce the clinical disease which is classified as either ulcerative or granulomatous colitis by such criteria. The distinction between ulcerative and granulomatous colitis is important only insofar as it aids the clinician in choosing therapy or in assessing prognosis. As will be discussed in subsequent sections of this chapter, many questions remain incompletely resolved concerning the appropriate medical or surgical therapy of the condition termed granulomatous colitis by the aforementioned criteria. In regard to prognosis, separation of colitis into the following two entities at present has clearer utility: (1) colonic cancer appears to be a significant complication of long-standing ulcerative colitis, whereas carcinoma is not clearly a sequel of granulomatous colitis; and (2) there is a greater propensity for granulomatous colitis to form enteric fistulas and to spread to the small bowel. The value of this second prognostic implication, however, is somewhat limited, because the diagnosis of granulomatous colitis often depends upon the demonstration of these complications themselves.

TUBERCULOSIS AND AMEBIASIS

Tuberculosis and amebiasis are difficult differential problems. Tuberculosis may be ruled out by a negative tuberculin skin test, but the converse is not helpful. Clinical pictures, areas of disease, and roentgenographic pictures may be superimposable. Presence or history of active pulmonary tuberculosis makes this disease more likely. In most cases surgery is required (see pp. 1377 to 1381). Likewise, distinguishing localized, multisegmental, or even universal granulomatous disease from amebiasis can be very difficult. When localized to the cecum and terminal ileum or when it affects skip areas, recovery of the parasite from stools is unlikely, because the lesion is chronic, intramural, and inflammatory—an ameboma. In these instances, a hemagglutination test may be very helpful, because it is positive in a high percentage of such patients (see pp. 1386 to 1392).

ISCHEMIC BOWEL DISEASE

Ischemic bowel disease may produce segmental distortion on X-ray of the colon which closely resembles granulomatous disease. In most instances, however, the attack is rather abrupt, significant rectal bleeding is noted, and the patient is acutely ill. In the early stage the characteristic "cat's paw" appearance on barium enema examination points strongly to ischemia as the cause. Sigmoidoscopy is negative (see pp. 1569 to 1571).

DIVERTICULITIS

Diverticulitis is often preceded by a long history of rather benign lower abdominal complaints caused by diverticula. It is generally an acute disease, reflecting perforation of a diverticulum with perirectal sepsis. Sigmoidoscopy is negative.

Since diverticula of the colon are common, localized granulomatous disease of the colon, particularly in the sigmoid and descending colon, may be difficult to distinguish clinically from acute diverticulitis. Diverticulitis of the rectosigmoid colon may be characterized by episodes of cramping left lower abdominal pain, associated with fever, tenderness, and even rebound tenderness. However, certain clinical differences distinguish the two conditions. Patients with localized granu-

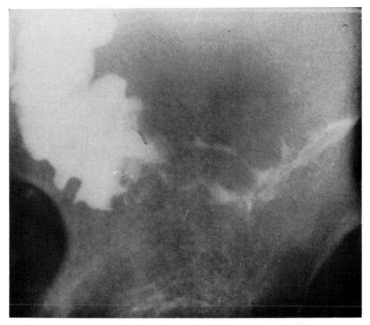

Figure 103–8. A segment of sigmoid colon, demonstrating a lengthy area of narrowing and an irregular, nodular luminal contour. A short fistula tract parallels the lumen and represents typical fistula formation through a segment of transmural granulomatous disease. The irregular ulcerated mucosa, the lack of diverticula, and the fistula aid in differentiating granulomatous colitis from diverticulitis. (Courtesy of Dr. H. I. Goldberg.)

lomatous disease of the left colon will often have histories of perianal or perirectal sepsis or fistula and of bouts of unexplained diarrhea which are difficult to attribute to diverticula. Recurrent fever unassociated with exacerbation of abdominal symptoms or change in bowel habit indicates granulomatous disease rather than diverticulitis.

The barium enema X-ray characteristics of localized granulomatous disease differ sufficiently from diverticulitis to separate the two entities in the majority of cases. Deep longitudinal ulcers characterize localized granulomatous disease. These tracts may be connected by multiple transverse fissures, producing the appearance of a stepladder;[7] although diverticula may also be present on the barium enema, the ulcerated mucosa and thickened folds indicate granulomatous disease. The roentgenographic pictures of localized granulomatous colitis of the sigmoid and of diverticulitis may be similar (compare Fig. 103–8 with Fig. 106–13, p. 1426). Severe mucosal ulceration is often seen in the former condition and not in the latter; also the abscesses associated with diverticulitis appear as an extramural defect which is thought to be distinguishable from perforation and abscess formation of granulomatous disease. In some instances, it must be admitted that differentiation radiographi-

cally before deep longitudinal sinus tracts are noted may be impossible.

ACUTE BACILLARY AND AMEBIC DYSENTERY

As in the differential diagnosis of ulcerative colitis, specific bacterial infection, caused particularly by shigellosis organisms, must be ruled out. The procedure is discussed on page 925. Similarly, acute colonic infection with *Entamoeba histolytica* must be excluded, as outlined in detail on pages 1386 to 1392.

CLINICAL COURSE AND RESPONSE TO TREATMENT

At present it is almost impossible to outline the natural history of granulomatous colitis or to assess the efficacy of various medical and surgical treatments. Distinction of granulomatous from ulcerative colitis has been popular only since about 1960, when distinguishing histopathological and clinical features were described by Lockhart-Mummery and Morson.[8] Most series reported since then are retrospective collections of cases gleaned from all cases of surgically resected colitis which allowed histopathological confirmation of the diagnosis. Such material is obviously unsuited for the appraisal of the natural history of the disease (since only the refractory or complicated cases were referred for surgery) or for the assessment of therapy (almost all case material having been surgically treated). Furthermore, many reported series do not distinguish granulomatous colitis unassociated with small bowel disease from regional enteritis of the small bowel associated with colonic pathology; yet several reports indicate that the prognosis for isolated granulomatous disease of the colon may differ from the outlook for colonic disease complicated by significant enteritis (see below). Because of the many clinical and histopathological similarities between colonic and small bowel Crohn's disease, most workers have assumed that surgical treatment of the colonic disease must adhere to the principle of limited resection with reanastomosis which has proved useful for regional enteritis; only recently has this view been challenged (see below). There are as yet no prospective trials of medical or surgical treatment for granulomatous colitis. Consequently, only limited generalizations can be made from the available material reported in the literature.

MEDICAL TREATMENT

The medical treatment generally prescribed for granulomatous colitis is similar to that used in ulcerative colitis, provided the patient does not have a complication requiring surgery (severe colonic stenosis, colonic fistula, pericolic abscess). These measures include a liberal and nutritious diet, eliminating *only* those foods which the patient says aggravate his symptoms (such as milk), nonabsorbable sulfonamides, and corticosteroids. Dosages of these drugs are the same as those used in ulcerative colitis (see p. 000). Fulminant granulomatous colitis with severe diarrhea, high fever, prostration, marked anemia, and hypoalbuminemia appears to be infrequent, so that high doses of systemic corticosteroids or intravenous ACTH are used less often in granulomatous colitis. However, toxic megacolon is being recognized with increasing frequency in this disease; the same therapeutic consider-

ations apply to this complication as in toxic megacolon associated with ulcerative colitis. Chronic therapy with corticosteroids carries the same hazards as in the treatment of ulcerative colitis; in addition, however, symptoms and signs of colonic fistulization and abscess formation (complicating granulomatous disease) may be masked by corticosteroid therapy. Therefore careful follow-up evaluation is imperative in patients with granulomatous colitis receiving this treatment. Patients who have associated disease of the terminal ileum may require parenteral vitamin B_{12}, and patients who have extensive small bowel disease with steatorrhea may require additional treatment aimed at alleviating the problems associated with small bowel malabsorption (see pp. 886 to 908).

About 60 per cent of patients with granulomatous colitis will improve on this regimen, whether or not the disease is limited to the colon (primary Crohn's disease of the colon) or involves the small bowel as well.[9, 10] The improvement is often only temporary; many will require surgery within the first year of treatment, and most within five years. It is to be emphasized that these data are uncontrolled. It is unknown how many of those patients seemingly improved by corticosteroid treatment would have shown spontaneous improvement without medication. By contrast, empiric treatment of ulcerative colitis with sulfonamides and/or corticosteroids has been shown to be effective by controlled trials (see pp. 1314 to 1319). Such documentation of efficacy is lacking in the medical treatment of granulomatous colitis.

SURGICAL THERAPY

Surgical excision of all or part of the colon is usually undertaken for chronic, persistent, and serious perianal disease; for fistula or abscess formation found elsewhere in the colon; for acute or chronic obstruction secondary to colonic stenosis; or for intractability (i.e., persistent symptoms of diarrhea, abdominal pain, fever, and debilitation). The indications are thus similar to those for surgery in patients with regional enteritis. By these criteria, about 75 per cent of all patients with granulomatous colitis will be operated upon within five years of the onset of their disease.[9, 11] As in Crohn's disease of the small bowel, most physicians prefer to delay surgery as long as possible for fear of recurrent and spreading disease after surgical excision.

Indeed, it appears that the most frequent form of granulomatous colitis—that associated with regional enteritis of the small bowel—does follow a postoperative course similar to that of regional enteritis. Most series report a recurrence rate of 30 to 50 per cent[9, 11, 12] after segmental or colonic resection for granulomatous colitis associated with regional enteritis. Likewise, subtotal resection with ileoproctostomy is attended with recurrent disease within the bowel or in the perirectal tissues in 50 per cent of patients.[13, 14] On the other hand, several reports stress that permanent ileostomy with subtotal or total colectomy reduces the frequency of postoperative recurrence and the extent of postoperative morbidity.[8, 9, 11, 12, 15] Patients with granulomatous colitis treated by ileostomy, however, have a significantly higher postoperative incidence of stomal ileitis than do those with ulcerative colitis similarly operated.[15] These reports notwithstanding, the standard surgical approach to colonic Crohn's disease has been right hemicolectomy with ileotransverse colectomy for segmental colitis of the ascending colon; segmental resection with reanastomosis for localized disease elsewhere in the colon; and total or subtotal colectomy with ileostomy for diffuse granulomatous disease of the colon. Treatment by simple diverting colostomy is unsatisfactory because of continued morbidity in almost all patients after this procedure.[8, 11] Some prefer ileoproctostomy in patients with extensive colonic disease, sparing the rectum despite its attendant loose stools, soiling, and high recurrence rate. When the rectum is involved in diffuse granulomatous colitis, subtotal colectomy with ileostomy is indicated.

For the minority of patients with granulomatous colitis, those with so-called primary Crohn's disease of the colon or granulomatous colitis limited to the colon, the outlook may not be so dismal. In most reported series, only about 10 per cent of this group of patients developed recurrent disease after segmental resection or colectomy.[9, 11, 12, 16] However, this was not the experience of McGovern and Goulston,[17] who noted a very high recurrence rate in these patients (type of initial surgery not stated).

PROGNOSIS

Most patients with this disease will require surgery earlier than patients with ulcerative colitis. Recurrence rates following resection and anastomosis are high, so that total colectomy often becomes necessary. Life expectancy is good, however, and the prognosis for life appears substantially better than for patients with ulcerative colitis, primarily because those with granulomatous colitis do not so frequently develop colonic cancer.

COMPLICATIONS

TOXIC MEGACOLON

This complication, more commonly noted in patients with ulcerative colitis, may occasionally be encountered in granulomatous disease[18] and seems to be confined to those in whom granuloma, sinus tracts, and inflammation extending as far as the subserosa have not been noted.

CANCER OF THE COLON

Colonic cancer has been reported in about 1 per cent of all patients with granulomatous colitis. It is possible that the actual incidence is higher, because granulomatous colitis has been recognized as a clinical entity distinct from ulcerative colitis only in the last decade. Nevertheless, the incidence of cancer associated with this disease appears to be appreciably less than the incidence of carcinoma with ulcerative colitis (Table 103–1). Furthermore, in many of the reported instances, cancer has been discovered at the onset of symptomatic segmental granulomatous colitis.[19] It would appear therefore that the development of colonic cancer is unrelated to either the duration or the extent of the granulomatous colitis, unlike carcinoma in ulcerative colitis, which is related to both of these factors (see pp. 1330 to 1332). From this evidence, colonic cancer cannot be considered an outcome of granulomatous colitis.

HEPATIC DISEASE AND SCLEROSING CHOLANGITIS

Several types of abnormalities of the liver are found in patients with granulomatous disease of the bowel. These are discussed in detail on pages 1333 to 1335, but will be summarized here. The spectrum of disease appears to be the same as in ulcerative colitis, except that hepatic granuloma may rarely be noted and amyloidosis, although rare, is more likely to be associated with granulomatous disease than with ulcerative colitis. Pathologically, the incidence of fatty change and pericholangitis is equal—about 20 per cent in a recent series. These lesions are more commonly noted with small bowel disease alone or with ileocolitis; they are very rarely associated with isolated granulomatous colitis. Chronic active hepatitis is rare. Pathological changes may be found when the liver function tests are normal. Conversely, histology may be normal in the face of mild disturbances in liver function tests. When liver disease is unequivocally noted, however, the BSP test is more frequently abnormal than the alkaline phosphatase. Overall, only 2 per cent of patients have overt liver disease, and these are usually patients with primarily small bowel, not colonic disease.

MALABSORPTION

Malabsorption associated with granulomatous disease of the colon is of two types: (1) failure to absorb H_2O and Na^+ normally in diseased proximal colon; and (2) small intestinal malabsorption because of disease in the terminal ileum (vitamin B_{12} or bile salt malabsorption) or in the more proximal bowel (steatorrhea) (see pp. 259 to 280).

AMYLOIDOSIS

This disease may complicate granulomatous colitis as well as ulcerative colitis. It is not clear whether the incidence varies according to site of granulomatous involvement (see pp. 1061 to 1065).

URINARY TRACT COMPLICATIONS

Nephrolithiasis. The incidence of renal and vesical calculi in chronic inflammatory disease of the bowel is increased; although the incidence of nephrolithiasis among hospitalized patients in general is one per 1000, the corresponding figure for patients with inflammatory bowel disease is approximately six per 100. In granulomatous colitis three factors contribute to urinary stone formation:

1. Loss of fluid and electrolytes from the bowel during episodes of diarrhea results in renal conservation of water with the production of a concentrated urine. When systemic acidosis supervenes (usually less often than in ulcerative colitis, in which diarrhea can be fulminant), a highly acid, concentrated urine predisposes to uric acid precipitation.

2. Uric acid and calcium excretion rates are higher than normal. The mean 24-hour outputs of urinary uric acid are slightly higher than normal in patients with granulomatous or ulcerative colitis treated with corticosteroids.[20] However, about one-sixth of these patients excrete almost twice the normal amount of uric acid—over 700 mg per 24-hour period. Similarly, one-third of patients with inflammatory bowel disease receiving corticosteroid medication excrete more than 250 mg per 24 hours of calcium, the upper limit of normal.[20]

3. Patients with granulomatous colitis associated with extensive disease of the terminal ileum may excrete large amounts of oxalate in their urine, predisposing them to calcium oxalate stone formation. The postulated sequence of events leading to this abnormality is related to the malabsorption of bile salts. Glycocholate, escaping resorption in the ileum, enters the colon, where it is split by bacteria into glycine and cholic acid. The glycine is converted to glyoxalate and, on absorption, to oxalate by the liver; oxalate is then excreted in the urine. Whether a defect in the liver favoring the formation of oxalate or heightened absorption of dietary oxalate also exists in these patients is currently under investigation.

Hydronephrosis. Inflammatory bowel disease may extend through the serosa to involve contiguous organs such as the ureter and urinary bladder.[21] Although the exact incidence of this complication is not known and is undoubtedly rare, it is nonetheless serious. Flank pain with or without fever is a clinical hallmark of urinary tract obstruction. The presence and severity of superimposed infection of the kidney depends upon several factors, principally the rapidity and degree of obstruction. Pyonephrosis is heralded by high fever, often spiking. Examination of the urine may or may not reflect infection (many white cells, white cell casts) or even ureteral irritation (few white and red blood cells). Intravenous pyelography should be done on all patients with granulomatous bowel disease, regardless of the absence of symptoms of urinary tract disease, because the involvement may be sufficiently insidious and chronic to be unassociated with flank pain, dysuria, fever, and abnormal urine.

Cholelithiasis. As noted on pages 1110 to 1115, patients with inflammatory disease or absence of the distal ileum have an inordinately high incidence of cholelithiasis. This complication results directly from the diminished total bile salt pool characteristic of these states. Thus the critical concentration of conjugated bile acids in bile may not be achieved and cholesterol precipitates from its saturated or supersaturated solution.

OTHER COMPLICATIONS

As noted above, *arthritis, sacroiliitis, erythema nodosum, pyoderma gangrenosum, aphthous stomatitis,* and *uveitis* are complications of granulomatous colitis. Their incidence is about the same in this disorder as in ulcerative colitis (see pp. 1337 to 1340).[16]

EPILOGUE

In the past decade, granulomatous colitis has been recognized as a clinical and pathological entity separate from ulcerative colitis. In its most frequent form, it is associated with regional enteritis of the small bowel. In this form, the disease in the colon closely resembles the disease in the small bowel: it is associated with sub-

mucosal granulomas and inflammation, sinus or fistula formation, segmental distribution, and luminal stenosis; it is relatively refractory to corticosteroid therapy, most cases requiring surgical intervention within five years of diagnosis; and it is characterized by a high recurrence rate after segmental colonic resection for localized disease. It does not give rise to colonic cancer.

A second form of granulomatous colitis consists of disease limited to the colon with histopathological lesions of similar nature (granulomas, transmural inflammation). Although this form of the disease may sometimes be recognized clinically by sigmoidoscopic changes, segmental distribution, and fistula formation, in the absence of these clinical features granulomatous colitis cannot be differentiated from ulcerative colitis until pathological material is obtained on resection of the colon. Whether such pathological differentiation will ultimately prove useful to the clinician by allowing him to make a prognosis remains to be verified. It is probable that 12 to 25 per cent of patients diagnosed as having clinical ulcerative colitis would prove to have granulomatous colitis by histopathological criteria.

At this time, most evidence supports the concept that granulomatous colitis isolated to the colon does not frequently recur after surgical extirpation. Moreover, there is some evidence suggesting that total colectomy with ileostomy, as in ulcerative colitis, may be curative. In the coming years it may be ascertained that histopathological distinction of these two isolated colonic diseases is not as predictive of clinical outcome or response to treatment as are the clinical criteria which distinguish them. Thus colonic disease limited to the proximal colon or showing evidence of fistulization may follow a course more like regional enteritis, whereas diffuse disease of the colon or segmental left-sided colitis without fistulization may resemble ulcerative colitis regardless of the histopathological demonstration of granulomas. What is needed at this time is more prospective study of these clinical entities rather than retrospective appraisals based on histopathological definitions.

REFERENCES

1. Zetzel, L. Granulomatous (ileo)colitis. New Eng. J. Med. 282:600, 1970.
2. Lewin, K., and Swales, M. B. Granulomatous colitis and atypical ulcerative colitis. Histoligical features, behavior, and prognosis. Gastroenterology 50:211, 1966.
3. Margulis, A. B., Goldberg, H. I., Lawson, T. L., Montgomery, C. K., et al. The overlapping spectrum of ulcerative and granulomatous colitis: A roentgenographic-pathologic study. Amer. J. Roent. 113:325, 1971.
4. Farmer, R. G., Hawk, W. A., and Turnbull, R. B. Regional enteritis of the colon: A clinical and pathologic comparison with ulcerative colitis. Amer. J. Dig. Dis. 13:501, 1968.
5. Gear, E. V., and Dobbins, W. O. Rectal biopsy. A review of its usefulness. Gastroenterology 55:522, 1968.
6. Korelitz, B. I. Clinical course, late results and pathological nature of inflammatory disease of the colon initially sparing the rectum. Gut 8:281, 1967.
7. Marshak, R. H., Janowitz, H. D., and Present, D. H. Granulomatous colitis in association with diverticula. New Eng. J. Med. 283:1080, 1970.
8. Lockhart-Mummery, H. E., and Morson, B. C. Crohn's disease (regional enteritis) of the large intestine and its distinction from ulcerative colitis. Gut 1:87, 1960.
9. Janowitz, H. D., Lindner, A. E., and Marshak, R. H. Granulomatus colitis. J.A.M.A. 191:825, 1965.
10. Jones, J. H., and Lennard-Jones, J. E. Corticos-

teroids and corticotropin in the treatment of Crohn's disease. Gut 7:181, 1966.
11. Jones, J. H., Lennard-Jones, J. E., and Lockhart-Mummery, H. E. Experience in the treatment of Crohn's disease of the large intestine. Gut 7:448, 1966.
12. deDombal, F. T., Burton, I., and Goligher, J. C. Recurrence of Crohn's disease after primary excisional surgery. Gut 12:519, 1971.
13. Baker, W. N. W. Ileo-rectal anastomosis for Crohn's disease of the colon. Gut 12:432, 1971.14. Burman, J. H., Cooke, W. T., and 1971.
14. Burman, J. H., Cooke, W. T., and Williams, J. A. The fate of ileorectal anastomosis in Crohn's disease. Gut 12:432, 1971.
15. Glotzer, D. J., Gardner, R. C., Goldman, H., et al. Comparative features and course of ulcerative and granulomatous colitis. New Eng. J. Med. 282:582, 1970.
16. Cornes, J. S., and Stecher, M. Primary Crohn's disease of the colon and rectum. Gut 2:189, 1961.
17. McGovern, V. J., and Goulston, S. J. M. Crohn's disease of the colon. Gut 9:164, 1968.
18. Javatt, S. L., and Brooke, B. N. Acute dilatation of the colon in Crohn's disease. Lancet 2:126, 1970.
19. Jones, J. H. Colonic cancer and Crohn's disease. Gut 10:651, 1969.
20. Breuer, R. J., Gelzayd, E. A., and Kirsner, J. K. Urinary crystalloid excretion in patients with inflammatory bowel disease. Gut 11:314, 1970.
21. Enker, M. D., and Block, G. E. Occult obstructive uropathy complicating Crohn's disease. Arch. Surg. 101:319, 1970.

Chapter 104

Infectious and Parasitic Diseases

Kimberly J. Curtis, Marvin H. Sleisenger

PSEUDOMEMBRANOUS ENTEROCOLITIS

Pseudomembranous enterocolitis is a well documented but poorly understood inflammatory disease of the gut characterized by the formation of membranous-like collections of exudate overlying the mucosa. It usually appears in the setting of a variety of acute or chronic illnesses and is also known as necrotizing enterocolitis, diphtheritic enterocolitis, acute postoperative enterocolitis, staphylococcal pseudomembranous enterocolitis, and antibiotic enterocolitis. For purposes of organization its description is included in the section of the colon; but it must be emphasized that although in approximately one-third of the patients it is confined solely to the colon, in the remaining two-thirds the small bowel alone or in combination with the colon may be involved. In the majority of patients, pseudomembranous enterocolitis is a serious disease which is often fatal.

ETIOLOGY

The precise etiology and pathogenesis of pseudomembranous enterocolitis have yet to be defined. The wide variety of clinical circumstances in which it is seen makes difficult the search for its cause, as attested by the large number of theories of etiology which have been invoked.[1] The common denominators in the majority of cases are underlying illnesses, drug therapy, and surgery, usually abdominal. Pseudomembranous enterocolitis was known in the 1800's, and was thought to be an inflammatory reaction to ingested poisons and irritants of undefined nature; however, it has subsequently been described in association with such diverse entities as staphylococcal infection of the bowel, obstruction of the colon, uremia, congestive heart failure, and ischemia of the gut. Bacterial infection with endotoxin release has frequently been incriminated as the main etiological factor in pseudomembranous enterocolitis. In particular, *Staphylococcus aureus* has been often cultured from these patients. However, its recovery has not been consistent.[2] Antimicrobial therapy has been followed closely by the development of pseudomembranous enterocolitis,[3] and it has been postulated that in some patients the growth of resistant organisms is the cause of the disease. Acceptance of this theory is precluded by lack of microbiological confirmation of the pathogenic organisms and the fact that enterocolitis was a well established entity prior to the advent of antibiotics.

Obstruction of the large bowel caused

1369

by either tumor or stricture has been complicated by pseudomembranous enterocolitis, and it has been suggested that there is dilatation of the proximal bowel with a release of a toxin.[4] Others have noted an association with shock and/or ischemia of the bowel; however, there is a serious question as to whether diminished perfusion precipitates or results from pseudomembranous enterocolitis. In summary, then, pseudomembranous enterocolitis has been described in association with a variety of possible etiologies, none of which can be consistently found in all cases, suggesting either multiple causes or an elusive single cause.

PATHOLOGY

Pseudomembranous enterocolitis may affect either the small or large bowel separately, or it may be extensive and involve both.[5] In approximately one-third of patients, it is confined to the colon. Grossly the bowel is dilated and has lost its usual mucosal pattern. The mucosal surface is studded with raised yellow-green membranous plaques which in some areas become confluent, giving the appearance of a membrane; hence its name (Fig. 104–1). The mucosa beneath varies from a surprisingly normal appearance to edema and congestion of the mucosa; in advanced cases there are granularity, friability, and

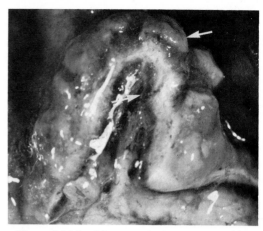

Figure 104–1. Macroscopic appearance of sectioned colon in pseudomembranous colitis. The thickness and edema of the wall and the elevated mucosal plaques are indicated by the arrows. (From Groll, A., et al.: Gastroenterology 58:88, 1970.)

frank ulceration with bleeding. The latter is unusual, however, and its absence serves to alert the sigmoidoscopist of the possibility of pseudomembranous colitis rather than ulcerative colitis.

Microscopically, the exudate is made up of fibrin, mucus, and a varying number of mononuclear and polymorphonuclear leukocytes and necrotic cells (Figs. 104–2 and 104–3). Patients in whom staphylococci are cultured usually have clusters of gram-positive cocci, whereas those with negative cultures show gram-positive and gram-

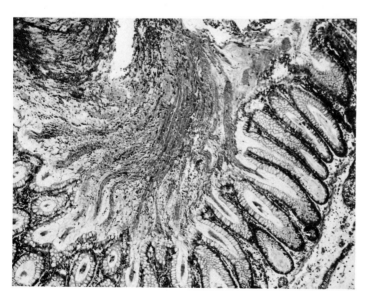

Figure 104–2. Pseudomembranous colitis. Hypersecretory mucous glands with streaming of mucus into lumen. Mucus, admixed with fibrin and blood, is infiltrated with large number of inflammatory cells to form the pseudomembrane. × 50. (From Groll, A., et al.: Gastroenterology 58:88, 1970.)

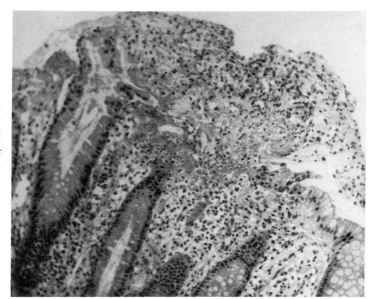

Figure 104–3. Pseudomembranous colitis. Rectal mucosa with adherent fibrinous purulent pseudomembrane, necrosis of superficial epithelium, and inflammation of lamina propria. × 200. (From Gelfand, M. S., and Krone, C. L.: Amer. J. Dig. Dis. *14*:278, 1969.)

negative rods or no bacteria at all. The goblet cells are increased in number and distended with mucus. There are scattered foci of epithelial necrosis and erosion, with adhesion of a fibrinous, purulent exudate to the underlying mucosa. The lamina propria is edematous with a leukocytic infiltrate. The submucosa is congested and edematous, but usually has minimal leukocytic infiltration, although macrophages may be numerous. Small vessels and capillaries are enlarged and congested, but vasculitis is not a feature of the pathology. In the later stages of the disease, the mucosa of the bowel may be covered in its entirety by a pseudomembrane consisting of necrotic mucosa, fibrin, and leukocytes which may be sloughed off in part or even in toto, leaving ulceration with a pyogenic basis which penetrates deep into the wall of the bowel. At this stage, the patient may have a considerable amount of bleeding, friability, and congestion of the edematous, necrotic mucosa.

CLINICAL PICTURE

Pseudomembranous enterocolitis usually appears in the setting of a serious clinical condition such as a postoperative state, colonic obstruction, infection (even mild ones being treated with an-

timicrobials), renal insufficiency, and shock. The clinical picture is usually one of rather abrupt onset of fever, with temperature ranging from 101 to 104° F. This is usually followed by watery diarrhea which varies in color from brown to green, is foul smelling, and contains mucus, pus, and occasionally blood. Fluid loss may be rapid and marked, resulting in oliguria, mental confusion, and shock. Disturbed acid-base balance, particularly metabolic acidosis and loss of sodium and potassium, may result in muscle weakness, abdominal distention, and cardiac arrhythmias. Shock caused by sepsis may also be part of the clinical picture. The prognosis is poor, particularly in view of the fact that this condition usually complicates previous, often serious illness. Mortality was about 75 per cent until about ten years ago; more recently, with earlier recognition and rapid treatment the outlook, although still grave, is somewhat improved.

DIAGNOSIS

This potentially serious disease should be suspected when sudden fever and diarrhea appear in the course of any illness. Apparent relapses after initial improvement in patients being treated with antibiotics should alert the clinician to the possibility of pseudomembranous enterocolitis even in the absence of diarrhea. Examination of a gram stain of the stool may reveal abundant gram-positive cocci, suggesting Staphylococcus. In these cases, culture will usually yield a rich growth of coagulase-positive *S. aureus*. In some cases, however, other organisms such as Proteus, Pseudomonas or even normal fecal flora will predominate.[6]

When the colon is involved, sigmoidoscopy will reveal a hyperemic bowel with a patchy, whitish exudate and moderate friability, with scattered areas of normal-looking mucosa. In severe cases, large, shallow, scattered ulcers may be noted. The hyperemia is due to the marked dilatation and congestion of small vessels of the mucosa, particularly the capillaries, and there is congestion as well in vessels of the submucosa along with marked edema. Rectal biopsy reveals the changes described previously and depicted in Figures 104-2 and 104-3. A flat film of the abdomen will usually reveal ileus and/or minimal to moderate dilatation of the colon generally not so severe as that noted in patients with

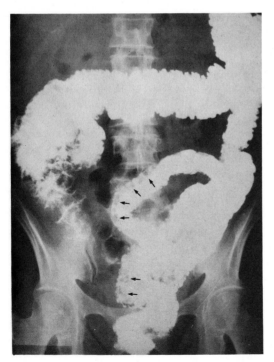

Figure 104-4. Pseudomembranous colitis. There is diffuse ulceration throughout the entire colon. The larger nodular contour defects (arrows) represent collections of necrotic debris and pseudomembrane formations. (Courtesy of Dr. H. I. Goldberg.)

toxic megacolon of ulcerative colitis. Barium enema X-ray examination of these patients reveals nonspecific findings which must sometimes be distinguished from those of ulcerative colitis (Fig. 104-4). Abnormal laboratory data are nonspecific, and include leukocytosis, neutrophilia, rapid sedimentation rate, hemoconcentration, azotemia, metabolic acidosis, electrolyte imbalance, and hypoproteinemia.

TREATMENT

Survival depends upon measures which successfully combat the rapidly developing or existing shock. The tremendous loss of fluid and electrolytes may be associated with oliguria, hyponatremia, and hypokalemia. Vigorous replacement of fluid, electrolytes, and plasma protein is the cornerstone of therapy. Guidelines for such replacement of tremendous losses of fluid isotonic with plasma are contained on pages 301 to 304. It should be re-emphasized here, however, that as much as 10 to 15 liters of fluid containing mainly glucose and saline may be required in less than 48 hours to restore urinary output to normal. Potassium should also be given in this period, albeit cautiously, with constant monitoring of the electrocardiogram and plasma levels of potassium. When adequate urinary output has been achieved (80 to 100 cc per hour), potassium up to 200 mEq in 24 hours may be necessary, along with the daily volume of intravenous fluid necessary to maintain plasma volume. Special attention must be paid to the danger of rapid correction of acidosis by use of bicarbonate intravenously before potassium is infused. It may further lower the level of plasma potassium and lead to fatal cardiac complications; therefore potassium must be given before or with bicarbonate intravenously (see p. 916). (Also rapid infusion of bicarbonate in the presence of severe acidosis may paradoxically further drive down cerebrospinal fluid *p*H akin to the effect noted with such therapy for diabetic acidosis.)

If hypotension in the presence of septicemia is not responsive to antibiotics, intravenous fluids, electrolytes, and pressor agents, corticosteroids (100 mg of prednisone per 24 hours) should be given intravenously. If staphylococci are present, an appropriate antimicrobial therapy such as methicillin (2 to 4 g) or cephalothin (6 to 8 g) per day intravenously, or, if the patient is sensitive to penicillin, erythromycin, 2.0 to 4.0 g intravenously, should be employed. Severe, rapidly developing hypoproteinemia secondary to protein loss in the gut may also complicate the problem, requiring that plasma be given in large amounts (1000 to 2000 ml per day) in order to support plasma oncotic pressure as well as plasma volume. Intravenous supplements of salt-free albumin (50 to 100 g per 24 hours) will be necessary in some cases. Adequate replacement of plasma protein in the early phase of the disease is of definite value in combating the development of intravascular volume depletion and shock.

PROGNOSIS

The course downhill is often rapid and irreversible; mortality is 50 to 75 per cent because of the severity of this complication in patients already seriously ill or severely debilitated. Recovery is heralded by rapid return of blood pressure to normal or near normal levels, with increasing urinary output, gradual cessation of diarrhea, and stabilization of corrected plasma volume and electrolytes. Usually these hopeful signs are noted within 72 hours.

SHIGELLOSIS

Shigellosis, otherwise known as bacillary dysentery, is a gram-negative bacterial infection of the gastrointestinal tract. It primarily involves the colon and is manifested by fever, abdominal cramps, tenesmus, and diarrhea which may contain mucus and blood. Also known as the bloody flux, this clinical entity has been historically recognized for centuries. Its distribution is worldwide, and outbreaks have been associated with unfavorable sanitary conditions, particularly in time of war. In 1896, Shiga first demonstrated the bacterial etiology of the disease by isolating the organism now known as *Sh. dysenteriae*. Subsequently, numerous other strains have been identified, many bearing the discoverer's name.

ETIOLOGY

The Shigella organism is a genus of the family Enterobacteriaceae or enteric bacteria, which are gram-negative, non-spore-forming rods found in the gastrointestinal tract of man and animals. Although some Enterobacteriaceae form the normal flora of the intestine, others are pathogenic for man, and Shigella is an example of the latter.

The Shigella group is comprised of a large number of strains which for simplification have been arbitrarily classified into four subgroups, depending upon their antigenic characteristics and their ability to ferment mannitol.[7]

Subgroup A, *Shigella dysenteriae*, does not ferment mannitol. It is comprised of several antigenic specific types, including Type I (Shiga), Type II (Schmitz), and several other types which are also known as Large-Sachs.

Subgroup B, *Shigella flexneri*, usually ferments mannitol.

Subgroup C, *Shigella boydii*, ferments mannitol.

Subgroup D, *Shigella sonnei*, also ferments mannitol.

All the subgroups are comprised of several different types which are identified antigenically.

EPIDEMIOLOGY

Bacillary dysentery has generally been associated with the tropics; however, its distribution is worldwide. The highest incidence in the United States occurs in lower socioeconomic groups, particularly in the states of California and Texas. Shigella was reported as the most frequent cause of diarrhea among military personnel in Vietnam.[8] The usual source of infection is man, and no animal reservoir has yet been found. Overcrowding and poor sanitary conditions, particularly in warm, humid climates, predispose to the spread of infection. Contamination of the fingers with fecal material is the primary mode of dissemination, and institutions such as asylums and military installations are particularly prone to this type of spread. The handling of food and water by infected, unclean personnel and the mechanical spread of organisms by flies are common routes of infection. The carrier state in man has not been well studied, but it is known to exist in a minority of patients. Persistence of the organism after acute infection has been documented for variable lengths of time, and these individuals are particularly apt to be sources of infection through inadvertent contamination of food.

PATHOGENESIS

The pathogenesis of Shigella infection is poorly understood. It has been suggested that the organism produces a proteolytic enzyme which allows it to penetrate the intestinal mucosa. The Shigella organism elaborates an endotoxin, as do most of the gram-negative enteric flora, and once the mucosa is invaded by the bacteria this endotoxin is absorbed, with resultant local and systemic effects.[9] Patients with widespread involvement have rather abrupt onset of fever, abdominal pain, diarrhea, and the passage of bloody mucus. *Shigella dysenteriae* Type I also elaborates a heat-labile neurotrophic exotoxin which on injection into experimental animals causes paralysis, diarrhea, and death. It has been referred to as the Shiga neurotoxin and is highly antigenic, lending itself to the production of antitoxin. It may also be converted to a toxoid by adding formalin. Despite the demonstration of this substance, its role in the pathogenesis and clinical

picture in human infection is not clear. It may be responsible, in part, for stupor and coma in very serious cases of the disease.

PATHOLOGY

The pathological process of shigellosis is essentially an inflammatory response to the mucosal invasion of the organism. This primarily involves the colon, although the terminal ileum may also occasionally be involved. As seen through the proctoscope, advanced shigellosis can very closely resemble ulcerative colitis. The mucosa is inflamed, granular, edematous, and friable, with variable degrees of bleeding. In more advanced stages, there may be ulceration and necrosis which can penetrate to the muscularis mucosae. Microscopically, the bowel wall is edematous, hemorrhagic, and infiltrated with polymorphonuclear cells (Fig. 104–5).

CLINICAL PICTURE

The spectrum of clinical symptoms is wide, ranging from an insidious, mild chronic diarrhea to an overwhelming toxic process leading to collapse and death. Typically, after a variable incubation period which may be as short as 24 hours, abdominal pain and cramps herald the onset of the disease. This is shortly fol-

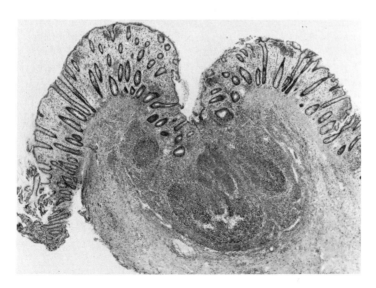

Figure 104–5. Shigellosis. This low-power magnification of the mucosa and submucosa of the colon from a patient with shigellosis shows an ulcer with central necrosis and a polymorphonuclear leukocyte infiltrate.

lowed by fever and diarrhea. In advanced cases, there are straining and tenesmus and the stools contain mucus and blood. The majority of infections are self-limited, and symptoms resolve spontaneously within a week. Occasionally the acute illness may be particularly toxic and severe, with high fever, shaking chills, headaches, and profuse bloody diarrhea, leading to rapid dehydration and electrolyte imbalance, blood loss, shock, and death. Fortunately, this is rare, and it has been thought that the endotoxin plays a major role in this picture.

Complications include the persistence of the organism in the stools despite the subsidence of clinical symptoms. This is unusual; however, as mentioned earlier, such patients have the potential of spreading the disease. Either during the active symptomatic period of the disease or sometimes in the convalescent period, joint effusions may be noted, particularly in the lower extremities. These are usually transient, and permanent disability is rare. Joint aspirations are usually sterile, but on occasion the bacillus may be isolated. Synovial fluid may agglutinate the appropriate dysentery bacillus, indicating the presence of antibodies to the organism. Occasionally surgical intervention is required for severe hemorrhage or perforation with peritonitis which may then be further complicated by localized abscess or liver abscess. Nephritis with hematuria and renal failure, pneumonia, and a variety of purpuric rashes may complicate the illness. A variety of sequelae have been described after attacks of bacillary dysentery, none of which, however, can be related with certainty. These include stenosis of the large intestine (underlying granulomatous disease or ulcerative colitis?), peripheral neuritis, and a variety of infections of the genitourinary tract. At one time Reiter's syndrome was thought to be caused by bacillary dysentery.

DIAGNOSIS

Diagnosis must be suspected in an individual who has a rapid onset of cramping abdominal pain, fever, and diarrhea, rapidly progressing to repeated bloody, mucoid discharges. The history of recent travel may be helpful, as well as the docu-

mentation of the patient's exposure to unsanitary conditions or infected contacts.

Sigmoidoscopic examination will reveal varying grades of mucosal hyperemia, friability, and ulceration. In milder cases the mucosa is granular and somewhat erythematous. With increasing severity, there will be increasing hyperemia with friability and mild bleeding upon wiping the mucosa. In severe cases, superficial ulceration with necrotic exudate is present. Rectal biopsy characteristically shows a nonspecific inflammation with a polymorphonuclear response. Mucosal appearance may be indistinguishable from acute ulcerative colitis or proctitis; until cultures and the clinical course resolve it, the differentiation between the two remains difficult. The radiographic picture of shigellosis may also be similar to that of ulcerative colitis (Fig. 104–6). Shigellosis differs from amebiasis in that the ulcers of acute amebic colitis are classically described as being undermined at the edges and the intervening mucosa is relatively normal. Lack of this appearance does not entirely rule out amebiasis, and smears from the ulcer bases as well as stools should be examined for ova and parasites.

Gram stain of a smear of stool or exudate

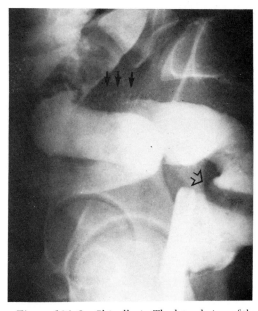

Figure 104–6. Shigellosis. The lateral view of the rectum shows narrowing and mucosal ulceration similar to that seen in ulcerative colitis. (Courtesy of Dr. H. I. Goldberg.)

may be informative in that the presence of polymorphonuclear leukocytes suggests an infection of bacterial origin, in contrast to the predominantly mononuclear response seen in *Entamoeba histolytica* colitis.

The most reliable method of diagnosis in infectious diarrhea is the isolation and identification of the organism with microbiological techniques. The culture of specimens obtained by swabbing the ulcerated lesion during sigmoidoscopy provides the most satisfactory approach; otherwise, discharged mucus and fecal material may be used for culture. Because the Shigella organism tends to be somewhat labile, it is good practice to inoculate culture plates with the specimen as soon as possible. The recommended media are MacConkey's agar which is relatively noninhibitory and a selective medium such as Salmonella Shigella agar which will suppress the growth of coliform bacilli and gram-positive organisms. Subculturing and testing with specific antisera will identify the exact dysenteric bacillus responsible for the disease. In all instances, when positive cultures are obtained, in vitro drug sensitivity should be carried out to guide proper therapy.

Serological diagnosis is theoretically possible because of the formation of specific antibodies against the infecting organism; however, this technique is impractical for the individual case. The multiplicity of strains makes this form of investigation a long and tedious process; the antibodies develop irregularly, and the diagnosis, when obtained, is retrospective. Serological technique is perhaps more useful therefore in special epidemiological studies.

TREATMENT

The treatment of shigellosis is in part dictated by the severity of the clinical picture. The disease is usually self-limited, with symptoms rarely lasting more than seven days.[10] For the most part, mildly ill patients do well with only symptomatic therapy, whereas those with severe infection with toxemia require fluid and electrolyte replacement and antibiotics. At present there is controversy over the use of antibiotics in the treatment of shigellosis.

Few dispute the use of an appropriate drug to which the organism is sensitive, particularly in the case of a severe fulminating attack with complications. However, there are many who feel that antibiotic therapy in mild cases of Shigella infection is not appropriate, because not only is the disease self-limited, but there is evidence of increasing resistance of the organism to a variety of antibiotics, including sulfonamides, ampicillin, tetracycline, neomycin, and streptomycin.[11] It has been suggested that this resistance is transferable among organisms and that unnecessary antibiotic therapy predisposes to the further emergence of drug-resistant strains.

On the other hand, some investigators feel they have shown that antibiotics, specifically ampicillin, significantly abbreviate the clinical course and shorten the duration of the organism in the stool when compared with nontreated control subjects.[12] On this basis, as well as that of alleged reductions of the incidence of complications and of the carrier state, many feel that all patients with Shigella should be treated. The outcome of this controversy and a definitive recommendation for therapy await further studies.

Presently ampicillin is the antibiotic of choice. For children the dosage is 50 mg per kilogram per day parenterally or 100 mg per kilogram per day orally, and for adults 2 g per day orally or parenterally in four divided doses.[13] When ampicillin cannot be used because of hypersensitivity, other antibiotics such as tetracycline, 2.0 g orally, or neomycin, 6.0 to 8.0 g orally, may be employed. Sensitivities of the organism to antibiotics should be determined to help re-evaluate therapy, if symptoms persist. There is no hard and fast rule governing the length of antibiotic treatment, although seven days appears to be a standard recommended course.[14] Several days after completion of therapy, the stool should be recultured to check for persistence of the organism. Failure to eradicate the organism despite antibiotic therapy is found in a minority of patients, but when it occurs, it calls for reassessment of therapy. In many such cases the organism will eventually disappear spontaneously; however, in cooks and food handlers who are likely to spread the disease, repeat sensitivities and retreatment are indicated.

There have been attempts to produce antitoxin and antisera aiming to provide some protection against *Shigella* infection; however, these techniques have been found to be largely ineffectual. At present there is no good prophylaxis against the disease except community cleanliness and good personal hygiene.

TUBERCULOSIS OF THE COLON

Tuberculosis of the colon is a chronic granulomatous infection which may be caused by *Mycobacterium tuberculosis* or *Mycobacterium bovis*. The disease may present in any part of the gastrointestinal tract; in the colon, the ileocecal region is a particular site of frequent involvement. Historically, tuberculosis of the bowel is an ancient disease; it continues to be a common finding in underdeveloped areas of the world where there is a high incidence of human and bovine tuberculosis. In countries with adequate public health techniques and effective tuberculosis control, intestinal tuberculosis has become a rare clinical phenomenon; if present, it is usually associated with infection elsewhere in the body. The diagnosis of isolated colonic tuberculosis is unusual in North America and is not often thought of until the surgical specimen is under the pathologist's microscope.

ETIOLOGY AND PATHOGENESIS

In the United States the majority of cases of tuberculosis of the colon are caused by *Mycobacterium tuberculosis*; however, in areas where cattle are diseased and milk is not pasteurized, *Mycobacterium bovis* may be the etiological agent. At present, there are no good recent epidemiological studies citing the incidence of Mycobacterium infection of the colon. Most of the older studies were carried out before tuberculosis was adequately controlled and incidence figures varied widely. In countries such as India where tuberculosis is prevalent, gastrointestinal tract involvement has been noted in 0.02 to 5.1 per cent of unselected autopsy cases. In other countries where tuberculosis is relatively infrequent, the figure will be much lower. The relative frequencies of involvement with bovine vs. human strains of tubercle bacilli are also unknown, owing in part to the difficulty in isolating the organism from the diseased specimen. At present in the Western Hemisphere, the number of cases of colonic tuberculosis is decreasing along with the incidence of pulmonary and miliary tuberculosis. The segments of the population in North America and Europe now most likely to be afflicted with this entity are patients with untreated cavitary tuberculosis of the lungs and the elderly.[15]

CLASSIFICATION AND DISTRIBUTION OF THE DISEASE

The literature classifies tuberculosis of the intestine into primary and secondary infections. The primary variety is defined as infection of the bowel without evidence of infection elsewhere, in particular, the lungs. The secondary type is defined as infection of the bowel in the presence of disease in other organs such as lungs or genitourinary tract. Possible mechanisms of infection include invasion by ingested organisms, hematogenous seeding, and extension from adjacent diseased organs or lymph nodes. The pathogenesis implied by most authors has been the ingestion of tubercle bacilli by the host with subsequent invasion of the bowel mucosa with the development of localized infection. The increased incidence of gastrointestinal disease in patients with active cavitary tuberculosis with bacilli-laden sputum supports this mechanism. Animal studies have shown that intestinal tuberculosis can result from ingestion of the organism; nevertheless, studies which accurately define modes and mechanisms of gastrointestinal infection are lacking, and the pathogenesis must now be considered as speculative.

It has been stated that the ileocecal area is the most frequent site of tuberculous infection of the gut; this finding may be due to stasis and the abundant lymphoid tissue in this region for which the bacilli have a predilection. Some investigators feel that the incidence of ileocecal involvement may be overestimated because of confusion with Crohn's disease, and they suggest that the cecum alone is the primary site with secondary extension into

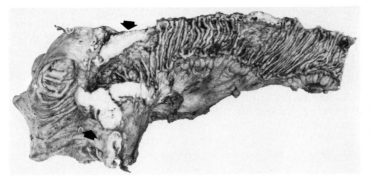

Figure 104–7. Tuberculosis of the ileocecal region and terminal ileum. Note the mucosal destruction and thickening of the bowel wall by multiple discrete and coalescent granulomas (arrows). This ultimately led to stenosis and obstruction in this patient.

the ileum. Less frequently involved are other portions of the colon such as the ascending colon, the sigmoid colon, and the rectum.

PATHOLOGY

A classification has become established in the literature describing the gross appearance of tuberculosis of the gastrointestinal tract. Its varieties include (1) ulcerative, in which ulceration of the mucosa is the predominant lesion; (2) hypertrophic, which is characterized by thickening of the bowel wall; and (3) ulcerohypertrophic, which is a combination of the preceding two.[16] The clinical significance of this classification is due to two important facts about the hypertrophic variety: it is usually a primary lesion and is clinically more benign, in contrast to the ulcerative

and ulcerohypertrophic lesions which are secondary and are associated with higher mortality and morbidity. Whether the lesion is essentially ulcerative or hypertrophic, the bowel wall appears thickened and a mass simulating a tumor is often described (Fig. 104–7). The overlying serosal surface may be dotted with scattered, small, yellow-white tubercles (Fig. 104–8). The mucosa is hyperemic, edematous, and, in both varieties, ulcerated (Fig. 104–9). Occasionally, pseudopolyps form. Adjacent nodes may be involved, and in advanced disease, strictures and fistulas may develop. The intestine may be segmentally involved, with areas of disease separated by normal intervening bowel.

Histologically, the characteristic findings of tuberculosis are present, i.e., fol-

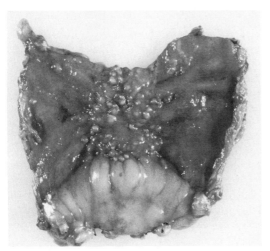

Figure 104–8. Serosal surface of tuberculous small bowel with tubercle formation.

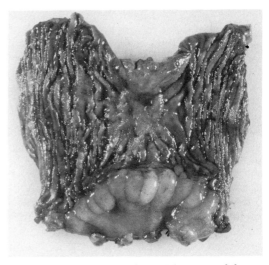

Figure 104–9. Tuberculosis of the terminal ileum. Segmental involvement, mucosal ulceration, and thickening of the bowel wall with stricture formation are apparent.

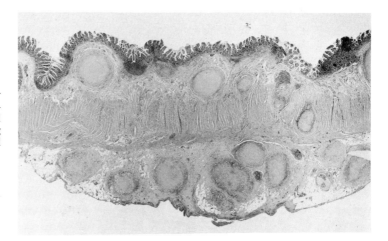

Figure 104–10. Low-power view of tuberculosis of the terminal ileum, showing transmural distribution of multiple caseating granulomas. Hematoxylin and eosin stain. × 10.

licular lesions with epithelioid cells, and Langhans giant cells located predominantly in the submucosal and serosal areas (Figs. 104–10 and 104–11). The submucosa is most predominantly involved with thickening caused by connective tissue proliferation and edema. Ulceration which may be present is usually superficial. The picture is often difficult to distinguish from Crohn's disease, which, however, is usually manifested by a greater degree of bowel wall thickening, deep linear ulceration, and a greater tendency to perforation. The ulcerations of tuberculosis are more superficial and annular. The presence of caseation necrosis is a strong point in favor of tuberculosis; however, it is not pathognomonic, because it may be found in syphilis, beryllium poisoning, and fungal infection. Demonstration of the organism in the histological specimen, using Ziehl-Neelsen staining, or microbiological isolation by guinea pig culture is absolute proof of the presence of tuberculosis. Such evidence is difficult to obtain, however, especially if the patient has received antituberculosis therapy. Overall, the isolation rate is only about 20 per cent. Often when the intestinal findings are equivocal, the adjacent lymph nodes may show characteristic lesions of tuberculosis.

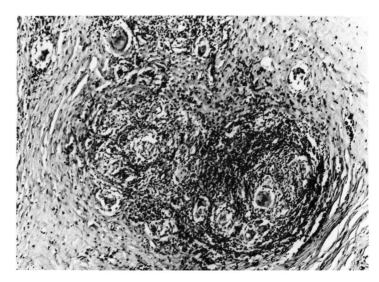

Figure 104–11. High power view of small early miliary sized granuloma with Langhans type giant cells in tuberculosis of the bowel. Hematoxylin and eosin stain. × 100.

CLINICAL FEATURES

The clinical features of intestinal tuberculosis are nonspecific and difficult to distinguish from a number of other conditions with similar clinical presentations. The most important symptoms include cramping, lower quadrant abdominal pain, usually on the right, diarrhea, and occasionally blood in the stool. Symptoms have usually been chronic, months or years in duration, with gradual weight loss and increasing debility. Massive bleeding is rare. Symptoms of obstruction may supervene, with vomiting, abdominal distention, and increasing cramping pain (see p. 346). Since the majority of patients in the Western Hemisphere also have pulmonary tuberculosis, cough, fever, night sweats, hemoptysis, anorexia, and weight loss are also commonly present. Indeed, in many instances intestinal disease is the basis for appearance of abdominal complaints in patients with active pulmonary tuberculosis, particularly if it is cavitary and the patient has positive sputum. A number of clinical variations of the disease result from progressive disease, such as obstruction, massive bleeding, malabsorption or acute perforation caused by stenosis (usually with multiple strictures), deep ulceration, fistulization, and perforation.[17] Malabsorption may also be due to widespread involvement of the mesenteric lymphatic system — tabes mesenterica.[18]

EXAMINATION

A firm, fixed, and nontender mass may frequently be felt, particularly in the right lower quadrant, in about 75 per cent of patients with cecal tuberculosis. Nothing about the characteristics of the mass distinguishes it from a malignancy or nonspecific granulomatous enteritis or enterocolitis. When tuberculosis causes rectal disease, a stricture or mass may be felt on digital examination.[19] Sigmoidoscopy will confirm this finding, and the mucosa may be thickened, edematous, cobblestone-like, and ulcerated. In addition, features of active pulmonary tuberculosis, such as fever, tachycardia, and abnormal auscultatory findings, are commonly present. A few may have evidence of malabsorption if the small bowel is also extensively involved.

DIAGNOSIS AND DIFFERENTIAL DIAGNOSIS

The diagnosis of tuberculosis of the colon is a difficult one, not only because of its infrequency, but also because there is little that is pathognomonic about the clinical, laboratory, and radiological findings. The clinician's suspicion should be aroused when the patient with pulmonary tuberculosis presents with bowel complaints, particularly cramping pain and diarrhea.

Laboratory investigation in patients with intestinal tuberculosis usually reveals a moderate decrease in hematocrit caused principally by occult blood loss and an elevated erythrocyte sedimentation rate. The white blood count is normal or slightly elevated; if the liver is involved, some abnormality of liver function, particularly elevation of the alkaline phosphatase, may be found. Stool examination may show the presence of mucus and blood, but very rarely will acid-fast bacilli be found on smear. When the small bowel is also involved, the manifestations of malabsorption and protein loss may be present (see pp. 259 to 279 and 918 to 919). A positive tuberculin skin test may be helpful in the pediatric and young adult age groups or in patients previously known to have been negative.

Roentgenographic examination of the colon reveals a picture which resembles Crohn's disease of the large bowel and terminal ileum (Fig. 104–12). Ileocecal tuberculosis is the most common form of tuberculosis demonstrable by barium studies, displaying distortions of the mucosal folds, ulcerations, varying degrees of thickening and stenosis of the bowel, and a type of pseudopolyp formation similar to the so-called cobblestoning seen in nontuberculous granulomatous disease (see pp. 1357 to 1360). The cecum is contracted, and there is distortion of the ileocecal valve. In some patients in whom only the cecum is involved, the radiographic findings may be interpreted as consistent with carcinoma. Segmental involvement of the colon demonstrating narrowing or ulcera-

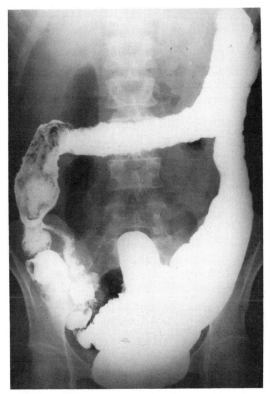

Figure 104–12. A barium enema of tuberculosis of the colon shows extensive involvement of the cecum and ascending and transverse colon. The ulcerated, narrowed, ahaustral appearance is typical of granulomatous infiltration of the bowel. (Courtesy of Dr. H. I. Goldberg.)

tion unfortunately makes the distinction of granulomatous disease even more difficult. Isolated disease in the terminal ileum, similar to regional enteritis, may be the only finding radiographically. Finally, calcified mesenteric lymph nodes, evidence of pulmonary tuberculosis on chest X-ray and positive sputum smear or culture, and positive culture of gastric washings for *M. tuberculosis* all strongly indicate that the bowel lesions in question are tuberculosis.

In many patients (indeed, the majority living in countries with satisfactory sanitation) who have no pulmonary disease, the diagnosis of tuberculosis of the bowel cannot be made with certainty until tissue is obtained for microscopic study either by laparotomy or, in the case of rectal tuberculosis, by biopsy through the sigmoidoscope. The histological picture is characterized by the presence of granulomas with caseation and, in some patients, of acid-fast bacilli in the bowel wall or lymph nodes. Extracts of specimens should be cultured and injected into guinea pigs. These techniques are still necessary to make diagnosis in some cases.

Diseases other than Crohn's disease of the colon to be considered in a differential diagnosis include carcinoma, amebiasis, appendiceal abscess, and occlusive vascular disease. For discussion of the characteristics of these diseases, the reader is referred to appropriate chapters in this section. When the rectum is diseased, syphilis, lymphogranuloma venereum, and mycotic diseases must be considered, as well as Crohn's disease. Syphilis and lymphogranuloma will be ruled out by appropriate serological and pathological studies; Crohn's disease will almost always be associated with proximal segmental involvement of the colon or even small intestine (see pp. 1350 to 1367).

TREATMENT

Tuberculosis of the colon will respond to treatment with the conventional antituberculous agents; i.e., isoniazid (INH), 300 mg per day, and para-amino salicylic acid (PAS), 12 g per day orally; for more seriously ill patients and at the time of surgery in all patients, streptomycin, 20 mg per kilogram per day, should be used. Ethambutol may replace PAS in treatment of this disease. Treatment with INH and PAS should be continued for two years. Approximately 50 per cent of patients with colonic or ileocolonic tuberculosis can be treated with medical therapy alone; the remainder require resection of their disease for a variety of complications, particularly obstruction, perforation, and symptoms caused by fistula formation.[20] The ulcerative type of intestinal tuberculosis probably responds best to medical management, and the hypertrophic form often requires surgery despite drug therapy, because it frequently progresses to stricture formation, increasing compromise of the lumen and, finally, obstruction.[21] Surgery is also indicated in many patients with hypertrophic tuberculosis of the intestine, because the disease clinically and radiographically cannot be distinguished from carcinoma.

LYMPHOGRANULOMA VENEREUM

Lymphogranuloma venereum is an infectious disease caused by an agent belonging to the Bedsoniae group. It is transmitted by sexual contact and chiefly involves the genitalia and regional lymph nodes but may produce significant rectal disease, leading to stricture formation. Synonyms for the disease include lymphogranuloma inguinale, lymphopathia venereum, climatic bubo, and Nicolas-Favre disease. It should not be confused with granuloma inguinale, an ulcerative disease of the skin caused by the gram-negative bacillus *Donovania granulomatis*.

ETIOLOGY

The microbe responsible for lymphogranuloma venereum is related to those producing psittacosis and has been included in the group entitled Bedsoniae. These agents appear as small intracellular bacteria and occupy a position intermediate between the rickettsiae and the viruses. They may be identified in the cytoplasm of affected cells, are transferable to experimental animals, and may be grown in tissue culture and yolk sacs. Lymphogranuloma venereum organisms may be agglutinated by specific antisera and are employed to produce material for complement fixation and intradermal testing.

The incidence of lymphogranuloma venereum is not well known. It is found throughout the world and is most prevalent among Negro populations in tropical areas such as the West Indies. This is probably a reflection of unfavorable socioeconomic conditions. It is said to be uncommon in the United States; however, there has been an increase in the reported incidence recently.[22] The rectal form of the disease is most prevalent in females, one study reporting that of 113 cases of rectal stricture 92 per cent were in women, most of whom had had chronic disease for several years.[23]

PATHOGENESIS

Lymphogranuloma venereum is transmitted primarily through sexual contact. In most cases the genitals and regional lymph nodes are involved; however, in as many as 25 per cent of patients, the rectum is the site of predominant disease. In the former variety, a transient primary genital lesion appears and is subsequently followed by secondary adenitis or inguinal bubo. Inguinal lymphadenopathy may coincide with systemic symptoms of fever, chills, and headache. The lymph nodes may suppurate, ulcerate, and drain. Indeed, elephantiasis of the genitalia has been observed in long-standing disease.

The pathogenesis of rectal disease has been debated. Since it is found mainly in females, one theory suggests that rectal infection occurs as a result of spread to the perirectal lymphatics from a vulval or vaginal lesion. Another possibility is direct invasion from the posterior vaginal wall, sometimes leading to a rectovaginal fistula. More likely, however, is direct infection either through anal intercourse with an infected partner or by contamination from infected vaginal discharge.

PATHOLOGY

The gross pathology of the early rectal lesion reveals a granular proctitis with an edematous and inflamed mucosa, containing scattered punctate superficial hemorrhages. Progression of the disease is reflected by thickening and fibrosis of the bowel wall with luminal narrowing and stricture formation. Condylomas at the anal margin and a rectovaginal fistula may be present.

Microscopically, the acute lesion presents as a nonspecific granulomatous inflammatory process. Mononuclear cells predominate, especially plasma cells, and proliferation of macrophages with giant cell transformation may be seen. Subsequently, there is proliferation of fibrous tissue, which, as noted, often leads to bowel wall thickening and stricture formation.

CLINICAL MANIFESTATIONS

The initial venereal lesion of lymphogranuloma venereum may appear as a small, painless erosion or nodule. It is inconspicuous and frequently goes unnoticed, particularly in women. The lesion is transient, usually lasting a few days, but is followed one or two weeks later by the appearance of inguinal adenopathy. In some cases the nodes resolve spontaneously; however, 60 to 70 per cent suppurate and drain spontaneously. Systemic signs and symptoms most frequently accompany the formation of inguinal lesions and include fever, headache, malaise, arthralgia, meningismus, and conjunctivitis.

Rectal disease is usually independent of the appearance of inguinal buboes. Proctocolitis presents with the passage of mucus, blood, and pus from the rectum in nearly every case. This is usually accompanied by either diarrhea or constipation or both, tenesmus, rectal pain, and weight loss. Low grade fever, perianal fistulas, and recurrent abscesses may also be present. On physical examination, there may be lower abdominal tenderness, particularly on the left. The rectal mucosa feels granular and occasionally nodular on digital examination.

The development of rectal stricture is signified by symptoms of constipation, straining at defecation, and the passage of thin stools. In nearly all instances, the stricture is located 3 to 5 cm from the anal margin and can be felt on rectal examination as a smooth, fibrous structure.

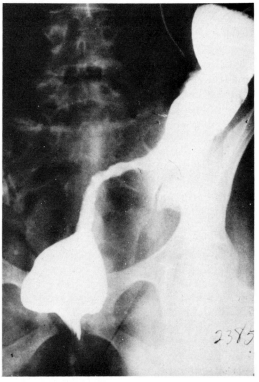

Figure 104–13. Barium enema in a patient with lymphogranuloma venereum, showing extensive stricture formation of the rectum. (Courtesy of Dr. H. I. Goldberg.)

DIAGNOSIS

The appearance of the acute proctocolitis of lymphogranuloma venereum is nonspecific and may be difficult to distinguish from other inflammatory conditions such as ulcerative colitis, granulomatous colitis, and Shigella infection. A high index of suspicion, stricture formation, the presence of discharging sinuses, and inguinal adenopathy all help to make the diagnosis clinically. Sigmoidoscopy reveals blood, pus, and mucus covering the mucosa which is inflamed, edematous, granular, and friable, and bleeds easily with wiping. Involvement is most marked within the first 5 cm but may extend to 25 cm. The bowel wall appears rigid and poorly distensible. Biopsy of the rectum or affected lymph node may reveal a histological picture suggestive of lymphogranuloma venereum.

Radiographically, lymphogranuloma venereum proctocolitis can resemble ulcerative colitis, because there is a similar mucosal pattern with poor distensibility and loss of haustration. The anorectal area usually appears most involved; however, extension through the ascending colon may be present. Barium enema is the best method of evaluating the presence and severity of stricture formation (Fig. 104–13). The lesion may vary in appearance from a short isolated narrowing to a long stenotic segment which has been described as proctitis obliterans. Multiple strictures with normal intervening portions similar to the skip areas of granulomatous colitis have been described, as well as lateral sinuses connecting with abscessed cavities.

Routine blood work is nonspecific in this disease. The complete blood count usually reveals anemia and mild leukocytosis with a relative lymphocytosis or monocytosis. The erythrocyte sedimentation rate is elevated, and there may be a decrease in serum albumin with a rise in serum globulin. Biological false-positive serologic tests for syphilis are not infrequent. The two major diagnostic laboratory tests in use are the complement fixation test and the Frei intradermal skin test. Both are helpful, but may be misleading. The complement fixation test is usually positive in titers of 1 to 40 or more; a rising titer strongly indicates acute disease. The test may remain positive after antimicrobial therapy and an apparent clinical remission; however, a reversion to a negative titer may be taken as presumptive evidence of successful treatment of the disease.

The Frei test consists of an intradermal injection of antigen paired with a control injection. The test usually becomes positive one to six weeks after the onset of adenitis and remains positive for life. If the disease is suspected and the initial skin test is negative, it should be repeated after three weeks. A negative Frei test followed by a positive reaction is highly significant. Both the complement fixation and Frei tests must be interpreted with care as they can reflect past or present disease with any of the psittacosis-like organisms. Neither test correlates significantly with the other, nor with the severity of the disease. In a recent study it was found that the complement fixation test was the most sensitive diagnostic parameter (83 per cent), followed by isolating the agent (55 per cent). The Frei test was the least sensitive (36 per cent).[24]

TREATMENT

Tetracycline has been recommended as the drug of choice for treatment of acute lymphogranuloma venereum.[25] It is usually given in doses of 500 mg every six hours until the desired clinical response has been obtained (usually about two weeks). Sulfadiazine, 4 g daily for 14 days, is also commonly used. Chloramphenicol has been shown to be of value as well in acute disease.

The treatment of rectal stricture can be difficult. Some patients with rectal disease go on to stricture formation despite antibiotic therapy. The conservative approach in these patients consists of periodic rectal dilatation. This treatment can be success-ful if the narrowing is soft and pliable; however, such is frequently not the case. Stretching rigid strictures is hazardous, because the bowel may split or perforate. In patients with chronically symptomatic severe disease, surgical correction may be necessary. Criteria for surgery include (1) stricture leading to obstruction which can be relieved by no other means; (2) infection failing to respond to antibiotic therapy; (3) persistent large rectovaginal fistulas or multiple anal fistulas; and (4) gross destruction of the anal canal and sphincter. Numerous corrective procedures have been described, with preservation of anal sphincter control a primary objective. In far advanced cases, abdominoperitoneal resection with colostomy may be necessary.

RECTAL GONORRHEA

Robert L. Owen

Rectal gonorrhea has been known to occur as a medical oddity since 1884, when the gonococcus was first demonstrated in smears taken from the rectum and stained by the process described in that year.[26] Only in recent years, however, has rectal gonorrhea been recognized as a public health problem. Asymptomatic rectal carriers, both women and homosexual men, have proved a reservoir for perpetuation and spread of gonorrheal urethritis. Carriers not only are a risk to others but are also at risk to develop gonococcal sepsis, endocarditis, myocarditis, meningitis, or arthritis.[27]

Autoinfection of the rectum has occurred in women with genitourinary gonorrhea by the use of contaminated thermometers and enema nozzles or by direct spread from the vagina.[28] Prior to the introduction of antibiotics, rectal infection in men sometimes followed rupture of prostatic gonorrheal abscesses. Today, almost all rectal infections in men and many in women result from rectal sexual exposure.[29] In women, rectal coitus has long been known as a method of contraception. Physicians, however, did not usually recognize rectal coitus in men as a significant possibility prior to Kinsey's report in 1948 of the widespread incidence of male homosexuality. In most urban areas rectal gonorrhea in homosexual men is recognized as a significant reservoir of infection. In women asymptomatic and unrecognized rectal gonorrhea is recognized as an important factor in therapeutic failures in the treatment of genital infections.[29]

CLINICAL PRESENTATION

Unfortunately, there is no characteristic clinical picture. Although some patients will present with rectal burning, itching, a bloody or mucoid discharge, or diarrhea, most people infected with rectal gonorrhea will have no symptoms.[28, 32-34] A recent study of medical complaints in a homosexual population showed that rectal symptoms occurred as frequently in those who were not infected as in those who were, suggesting that symptoms reflect anxiety or sexual trauma rather than infection.[34] Any known or suspected homosexual patient presenting with any rectal complaint should be considered as possibly having gonorrhea.

Sigmoidoscopic examination is unfortunately also not specific. There may be generalized redness and edema of the rectal mucosa with increased mucus on the wall. Ulceration of the mucosa has only rarely been described.[28, 32, 33] Symptomatic patients will often have other rectal pathology such as condylomata acuminata, superficial fissures, fistulas, or inflamed hemorrhoids. Most patients with a positive culture for gonorrhea but no symptoms will show nothing at all or at most increased mucous streaking of the rectal wall.

PATHOLOGY

Punch biopsy samples of rectal mucosa are reported to show degeneration of columnar epithelium on the surface and in the crypts. There are capillary engorgement and infiltration with inflammatory cells. The distinctive feature is the presence of gonococci in the necrosed mucous membrane; they become less frequent at lower levels, and are not seen beyond the muscularis mucosae.[26] In most patients there will be no lesion to biopsy.

CULTURE TECHNIQUE

Formerly, culture was difficult because of overgrowth with normal colonic flora. With the development of Thayer-Martin selective media, containing vancomycin, colistimethate, and nystatin, it is now easier to isolate gonococci from the rectum. Swabbing rectal crypts through an anoscope is preferable, but adequate specimens can usually be obtained with careful blind insertion of swabs into the anal canal. At present, high rates of recovery of the organisms demand streaking swabs directly onto Thayer-Martin plates and storing and transporting plates in a candle jar prior to incubation. Small lots of plates can be purchased from commercial suppliers and refrigerated until needed. They can then be processed by most pathology laboratories. In clinics or private practices in which large numbers of cultures are taken, a small holding incubator will further improve recovery rates. Transgrow, a new transport and holding medium for N. gonorrhoeae, is now available for use when direct culture on plates is not practiced. Transgrow contains the same inhibitory antibiotics as Thayer-Martin medium, with the addition of trimethoprim to inhibit overgrowth of Proteus spreaders. Specimens collected, mailed, and planted 48 to 96 hours later give 80 to 90 per cent positive results, compared with direct plating on Thayer-Martin medium.[30]

TREATMENT

The great variety of treatment regimens reported for rectal gonorrhea is evidence of the ineffectiveness of any of them in producing a sure cure.[31] No regimen is 100 per cent effective, and it is impossible to assess treatment by improvement in symptoms, because symptoms do not correlate with infection. Regimens using readily available drugs with acceptable cure rates are 4.8 million units of procaine penicillin in two equally divided simultaneous intramuscular injections, with 1.0 g of probenecid given orally prior to or at the time of penicillin injection; or 3 g of tetracycline divided into two oral doses one-half hour apart, followed by 500 mg. four times a day for three days or spectinomycin, 4 g in two equally divided simultaneous intramuscular injections. Regardless of which regimen is used, follow-up culture must be done as a test of cure.

AMEBIASIS

Amebiasis is an acute and chronic disease caused by the organism *Entamoeba histolytica*. Although multiple organs may be involved, the colon is the usual site of initial disease. The manifestations of illness may vary from the asymptomatic carrier state to a severe fulminating illness with mucosal inflammation and ulceration, occasionally with a fatal outcome. The disease is worldwide in distribution, but is most prevalent in the tropics and in areas where sanitation and living conditions are suboptimal.

ETIOLOGY

There are numerous species of amebae which inhabit the human intestinal tract, including *Entamoeba coli, E. polecki, Entamoeba buetschlii, Endolimax nana*, and *Dientamoeba fragilis;* however, with rare exceptions *E. histolytica* seems to be the only variety pathogenic for man. Within the *E. histolytica* group there are morphological differences in the size of the organism, and there has been a recent subdivision of this group. The strain characterized by small size and lack of virulence is *E. hartmanni*. True *E. histolytica*, previously known as the large race, is generally recognized as the ameba pathogenic for man.

EPIDEMIOLOGY

The worldwide average incidence of amebiasis has been estimated at 10 per cent. However, there is a wide variation of incidence figures, depending upon the population studied. In the tropics, where the disease is prevalent, 50 to 80 per cent of the population have been reported to harbor the organism.[35] Unsanitary conditions, close living, and poor personal hygiene all contribute to the spread of the disease. In the United States amebiasis is often thought of as a tropical disease to be looked for only in other areas of the world or in travelers returning from abroad. It is estimated, however, that at least 5 per cent of the untraveled population of the United States are infected with *E. histolytica*.[36] Ninety per cent of this group are asymptomatic cyst passers, making detection and accurate epidemiological study difficult.[37]

Asymptomatic patients with no evidence of tissue invasion harbor only cysts in their stools. However, they are of the most concern epidemiologically. The cyst form of the organism can resist the outside environment, whereas the trophozoite, passed by patients with acute or chronic invasive disease, cannot survive outside the host. The disease can therefore be transmitted by individuals who are unaware of their infective potential. On the other hand, there are patients with gastrointestinal complaints of nonamebic origin who harbor cysts in their stools but who are living in a peaceful symbiotic relationship with the organism. These patients are often erroneously diagnosed as having symptomatic amebiasis.

LIFE CYCLE

Entamoeba histolytica exists in the human colon in two forms, the motile trophozoite and the nonmotile cyst. The cyst is the infective form that is ingested, resulting in colonization of the host. Cyst forms predominate in the stools of individuals who are asymptomatic carriers or who have a mild form of the illness. They vary greatly in size, containing refractile masses of chromatin or chromatoid bodies. Early cyst forms contain one nucleus which divides by binary fission to form the mature quadrinucleate cyst; thus cysts found in the stools will contain one to four nuclei. Cysts may survive outside the body for as long as ten days if kept cool and moist. Otherwise they die quickly. The cyst is important because it is the infective stage of the life cycle, and through it infection is conveyed from one host to another. This occurs when food or water is ingested that has been contaminated with fecal material containing *E. histolytica* cysts. Upon entering the bowel there is a division resulting in eight trophozoites from one cyst. On excystation the parasites transform to motile trophozoites, the active, potentially pathogenic stage which causes amebic colitis. They are recognized by their occurrence in clumps or masses and their uneven distribution throughout stool specimens. The trophozoite appears as a clear transparent organism with an eccentric nucleus about three to five times the diameter of a red corpuscle. The presence of trophozoites with intracytoplasmic red cells is pathognomonic for infection by *E. histolytica* and serves to distinguish it from the nonpathogenic amebas, e.g., *E. coli* and *D. fragilis*. Movement is accomplished by pseudopods and is brisk in warm, fresh specimens. Binary fission then produces the precystic forms which develop into fully mature cysts in the period of a few hours in the lumen of the bowel. These are passed out into the stools and are ingested by a new host, and the cycle continues.

PATHOGENESIS OF COLITIS

It has been shown in germ-free animals that the virulence of *E. histolytica* is in some ways dependent upon the presence of bacteria, and this fact is the basis for the rationale of using antibiotic therapy in the early stages of treatment. The majority of individuals who harbor amebae remain asymptomatic carriers of cysts, which, however, may yield invasive trophozoites at any time. The contributing factors leading to emergence of virulence of the organism are not yet fully defined.[38] Some postulate that nonvirulence is due to failure to form trophozoites. Others feel that perhaps an unrecognized virulence factor may be brought into play as a result of the phagocytosis of certain bacteria. Still others suggest that some change in the host allows a trophozoite to assume invasive potential. The mechanism of invasion is also not clearly understood. It is postulated, however, that perhaps a lysozyme situated on the surface of the ameba breaks down the cell wall of the host on contact. With continued destruction the classic ulcer with undermined edges is formed. As amebas move into the bowel wall, they are picked up in the portal circulation and become disseminated systemically. The organ distant from the bowel most frequently involved is the liver, which is often the site of abscess formation. With widespread disease, however-

er, especially in individuals treated with corticosteroids, amebae can be found in virtually every organ of the body, including the brain, lungs, and eyes.

PATHOLOGY

The basic pathological lesions of amebiasis are ulcers which first appear covered with small yellow hemispheric elevations of exudate. These are scattered throughout the large intestine, most frequently involving the cecum and ascending colon, with the descending colon, sigmoid, rectum, and hepatic flexure following in that order. Rarely, the disease may involve the terminal ileum. As the disease progresses, the size of the ulcers may grow to an inch or more in diameter. With increasing size, the edges become more undermined and the base extends from the submucosa into the muscular coat. The craters may be filled by necrotic tissue. On rare occasions, involvement of the blood vessels at the base of the ulcer may produce brisk bleeding. More rarely, the patient may perforate and die of peritonitis. In contrast to bacillary dysentery and ulcerative colitis, the intervening mucosa between ulcers appears relatively normal.

Histologically, the lesion begins at the base of the crypts with necrosis of tissue, presumably caused by cytolysins elaborated by the organism. *E. histolytica* does not stimulate an inflammatory response in the host. The few polymorphonuclear cells, lymphocytes, and plasma cells which may be present are secondary to host tissue necrosis or bacterial infection. The amebae progress to the muscularis mucosae, at which point they spread out laterally, producing an ulcer with undermined edges, classically described as flask shaped. On histological section, the amebae can be seen at the leading edge of the ulceration (Fig. 104–14). Occasionally, an ulcer may penetrate deep enough to involve the circular and longitudinal muscle layers of the bowel. For unknown reasons, a dense, fibrous, and granulomatous reaction may be induced in some cases, leading to the formation of a mass lesion called an ameboma, important clinically because of its resemblance to carcinoma.

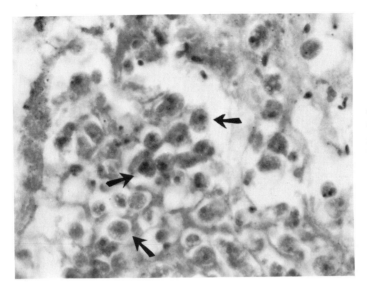

Figure 104-14. *E. histolytica* trophozoites in an ameboma (arrows). The appearance is the same at the edge of amebic ulcers. Note lack of inflammatory response in their immediate vicinity. Hematoxylin and eosin. × 400. (Courtesy of Dr. Frank R. Dutra.)

CLINICAL PICTURE

Patients harboring amebae may vary clinically from being completely asymptomatic to being acutely ill with an ulcerative colitis-type picture. The asymptomatic carrier lives in good relationship with the organism; however, cysts are passed in the stool, and the patient is at risk of infecting others as well as becoming acutely ill himself at any time. The type and severity of complaints in the symptomatic patients vary with the location and extent of bowel pathology. Often there are abdominal pain, intermittent diarrhea, anorexia, and malaise. In the chronic form these symptoms may wax and wane for months or weeks. The acute, fulminant picture is similar to, and must be differentiated from, other acute inflammatory bowel diseases such as ulcerative colitis and bacillary dysentery. Diarrhea is common, containing blood and mucus; the stools number around seven to ten per 24 hours. They are usually associated with cramping abdominal pain; tenesmus is associated with rectal involvement.

On physical examination, tenderness may be localized anywhere in the lower abdomen, but usually over the cecum, transverse colon, or sigmoid. The liver may be slightly enlarged and tender. If untreated, the patient may go on to develop extreme dilatation of the bowel similar to the toxic megacolon of ulcerative colitis, accompanied by high fever,

rapid dehydration, vomiting, and circulatory collapse. One of the most common and grave complications of this state is perforation, leading to peritonitis, overwhelming sepsis, shock, and death. In some areas of the world the mortality of amebic colitis is as high as 3 per cent, and perforation probably accounts for about 30 per cent of these deaths. Other bowel complications include massive hemorrhage, which is rare, ameboma formation in any part of the colon which may lead to obstruction or intussusception, stricture formation during the healing stage, and postdysenteric colitis which usually resolves over a period of weeks or months without specific therapy. The systemic dissemination of infection may involve other organs such as brain, lung, pericardium, and liver. The most common extraintestinal infection by ameba is liver abscess.

DIAGNOSIS

The diagnosis of amebiasis is important, not only because it is readily made in most acute cases, but also because therapy is highly effective. It is also necessary to distinguish amebiasis from inflammatory bowel disease such as ulcerative colitis or granulomatous colitis, because steroids are often prescribed in the latter and these drugs may be lethal in patients with acute invasive amebiasis.

Microscopic examination of repeated (three to six) fresh stool specimens, if done correctly, will reveal trophozoites and establish the diagnosis in 90 per cent of patients with symptomatic amebiasis. In acute infection, trophozoites will be seen to contain ingested red blood cells, making the diagnosis virtually certain. Other amebae, such as *E. hartmanni, E. coli, E. nana, E. buetschlii,* and *D. fragilis,* can be found in the human gastrointestinal tract and are nonpathogenic in most instances, but some experience is necessary to distinguish them from the pathogenic *E. histolytica.*

The traditional method of examining stools is a saline wet-mount preparation, which is satisfactory in most cases. Experienced laboratories use concentration techniques and make permanent mounts using stains such as D'Antoni's or iron hematoxylin for improved identification of cysts. Stool examination should be completed before barium studies are performed, because the yield is markedly decreased for days to weeks after introduction of barium to the colon. Prior treatment with mineral oil or broad-spectrum antimicrobial agents will also hinder the search for the parasite.

Sigmoidoscopy will be helpful in some but not all patients with acute amebiasis, because rectal involvement is less frequent than cecal involvement. The ulcers are small, discrete, flat, and shallow based with undermined edges, and are often covered with an elevated yellow-white collection of exudate. The intervening mucosa is strikingly normal in contrast to that in patients with ulcerative colitis and bacillary dysentery. However, in those with acute fulminant amebiasis, the rectum can become markedly involved and may be easily mistaken for either of the latter two entities. Trophozoites may be obtained from the base of the ulcers by scraping or aspiration of the material into a pipette. A warm saline wet-mount is then made with the specimen and examined microscopically for the parasite. As an adjunct to diagnosis, the indirect hemagglutination test has been found to be of significant value in detecting patients with invasive disease.[39, 40] Asymptomatic cyst passers frequently have low titers. The test is most useful in differentiating amebic colitis from other types of inflammatory bowel disease, or in the evaluation of a hepatic mass. Unfortunately, it is not per-

formed in many areas, and the serum sample has to be sent to the Communicable Disease Center in Atlanta, Georgia, limiting its applicability in acute fulminating disease. However, as the demand for the test grows, it will surely become more widely available.

Barium enema examination usually reveals changes in the shape, size, and distensibility of the cecum in patients with active infection (Figs. 104–15 and 104–16). In chronic amebic colitis, multiple strictures of significant length have been noted, most commonly in the transverse colon and at the hepatic and splenic flexures. Nonspecific mucosal changes with loss of the normal pattern and irregularities giving a granular appearance are also

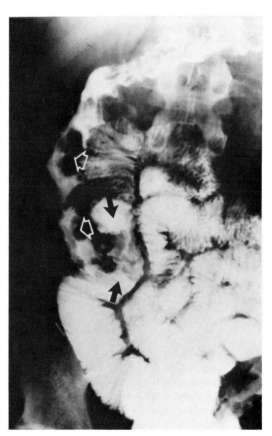

Figure 104–15. Narrowing, ulceration, and nodular contour defects of the cecum and ascending and transverse colon in a patient with amebic colitis. The large filling defects (open arrows) were due to extensive submucosal infiltration and hemorrhage. Note the *relative* sparing of the terminal ileum (closed arrows), although terminal ileal ulceration is present. (Courtesy of Dr. H. I. Goldberg.)

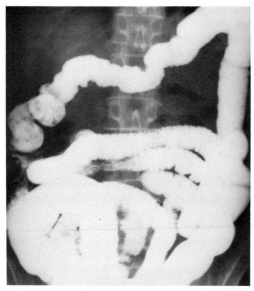

Figure 104-16. Acute amebic colitis of eight days' duration, characterized radiographically by loss of the normal haustral pattern and mucosal ulceration of the right and transverse colon. (Courtesy of Dr. H. I. Goldberg.)

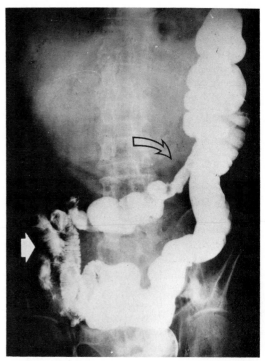

Figure 104-17. Colonic stricture due to ameboma. The midtransverse colon is narrowed secondary to fibrous tissue proliferation induced by chronic amebic infection (open arrow). These lesions can be virtually indistinguishable from carcinoma of the colon. The cecum is also diseased with narrowing and contraction (closed arrow).

present. An ameboma appears as a mass lesion often impossible to distinguish from a neoplasm (Fig. 104-17).

The most important differential diagnosis lies in distinguishing acute amebiasis from ulcerative or granulomatous colitis (see pp. 1296 to 1367). Acute, severe parasitic infection may closely resemble these diseases; on occasion, patients with ulcerative colitis harbor amebae. Another condition to consider in the differential diagnosis is bacillary dysentery, clinically confirmed by an appropriate stool culture. Ischemic colitis and acute diverticulitis usually occur in the older age group and have rather characteristic findings, as does diverticulosis with bleeding (see pp. 1423 to 1424 and 1569 to 1571). Acute appendicitis and carcinoma must also be included in the differential diagnosis (see pp. 1448 to 1453 and 1495 to 1497).

TREATMENT

The recommended treatment of amebiasis has varied considerably over the past ten years, chiefly because numerous drugs have been employed and none has been found to be entirely satisfactory, either because of toxicity or an unacceptably

low cure rate. The emergence of metronidazole (Flagyl) as an antiamebic drug may provide a solution to this problem, because it appears to be highly effective and is less toxic than drugs which have long been given for the disease. The drug is currently under investigation, and optimal dosages as well as therapeutic success rates are still being evaluated. It appears certain that metronidazole will be a potent amebicide in extraluminal disease; however, its efficacy against organisms within the bowel lumen has yet to be proved. With recent FDA approval, metronidazole is now considered to be the drug of choice for invasive amebiasis. The dosage is 750 mg three times daily for ten days. This should be followed by diiodohydroxyquin (Diodoquin), 650 mg three times daily for 21 days, to ensure eradication of intraluminal organisms.[41]

The conventional therapeutic agents hitherto available for treatment of amebiasis act at selected sites: intraluminally, intramurally, or systemically. Diiodohydroxyquin (Diodoquin) is a safe and effective agent that acts against amebae that are located intraluminally. Tetracycline has also been of value and presumably acts by altering the gastrointestinal flora. Since bacteria may facilitate colonization of the gut by *E. histolytica* as well as heighten its invasive potential, an antibiotic may act to depress the overall virulence of the organism. It may also be useful in controlling postulated secondary bacterial invasion of the damaged gut wall. Chloroquine diphosphate (Aralen) is of value primarily in treating amebae in the liver. Emetine hydrochloride is a toxic but effective amebicidal agent which is used in 'severe colitis, amebic-hepatic abscess, or apparent systemic dissemination. The physician and the patient should be aware that all these drugs have a multiplicity of side effects. Emetine, in particular, must be used with caution, because it may be cardiotoxic; fatal myocarditis has been reported with this agent. Although T-wave changes are noted in two-thirds of patients receiving emetine, arrhythmias are the prime indication for withdrawing the drug. Dehydroemetine, an analogue of emetine, has been shown to be effective and is less toxic than emetine. It can be used instead of emetine in equivalent doses. Recommended dosage schedules for treatment of intestinal amebiasis with conventional agents are as follows:[41]

ASYMPTOMATIC INTESTINAL INFECTION

Diiodohydroxyquin (Diodoquin), 650 mg three times daily for 21 days.

MILD INTESTINAL INFECTION

1. Diiodohydroxyquin (Diodoquin), 650 mg three times daily for 21 days, plus
2. Tetracycline, 250 mg every six hours for ten days, plus
3. Chloroquine, 500 mg (salt) twice daily for two days and then 250 mg twice daily for 19 days.

SEVERE INTESTINAL INFECTION

1. Dehydroemetine, 1 to 1.5 mg per kilogram (maximal total dose, 1 g), *or*
    Emetine, 1 mg per kilogram (maximal total dose, 65 mg) intramuscularly or subcutaneously, for the least number of days necessary to control symptoms (usually four to six days, maximum ten days), plus
2. Tetracycline, 250 mg four times daily for ten days, plus
3. Diiodohydroxyquin, 650 mg four times daily for 21 days, followed by
4. Chloroquine, 500 mg (salt) twice daily for two days and then 250 mg twice daily for 19 days.

INTESTINAL COMPLICATIONS

A rare patient with severe diffuse inflammation of the colon may progress to a fulminant condition before antiamebic therapy can take effect. The clinical picture then is virtually indistinguishable from fulminant ulcerative colitis. The bowel is dilated, particularly in its transverse portion, to a diameter greater than 9 cm. The patient is extremely febrile and toxic, manifesting evidence of hypovolemia, electrolyte deficits such as tachycardia, and profound weakness. It is remarkable that despite the severity of the illness, amebae may not be readily recovered from the stools in these individuals. If examination and flat films of the abdomen reveal no change in the degree of distention over a period of several days and if evidence of increasing peritoneal inflammation appears, surgery should be considered. The risk of surgery is high, as in ulcerative colitis; however, in good hands a subtotal colectomy may be carried out as antiamebic therapy is continued.

Another classic indication for surgical intervention in this disease is colonic perforation while the patient is receiving antiamebic therapy. This catastrophe, requiring immediate laparotomy, is very similar to its counterpart in fulminant ulcerative colitis. The patient will suddenly have an increase in abdominal pain, usually generalized, evidence of free air in the peritoneal cavity on flat film of the abdomen, and a rapidly progressing picture of septic peritonitis. In some instances the perforation may not be quite so dramatic and the abdominal signs are more localized. In either event, if it is clinically apparent or justifiably suspicious that the colon has perforated, the abdomen should be explored. Closure of the rent in the colon, drainage of the peritoneal cavity, and exteriorization of the perforated bowel are indicated. With continued antiamebic therapy, these patients will usually recover and the colostomy can be subsequently closed. Alternatively, if the involved segment is irreversibly damaged, exteriorization and colostomy may be followed by a resection and anastomosis.

Another amebic lesion that often requires surgical consideration is ameboma (Fig. 104–17). Every effort should be made to achieve accurate diagnosis before surgery in any patient with a mass lesion of the colon in whom there is historical or other reason to suspect previous or current amebic infection, because ameboma must be treated medically. Surgery for this lesion is usually followed by complications such as perforation, fistula, peritonitis, and death. Although the parasite is usually absent in stools, the indirect hemagglutination test is usually positive in those with amebomas and should be done when the diagnosis is suspected. If ameboma is likely to be present, the patient should be treated with the drugs outlined earlier, and it will resolve the majority of cases. If the lesion does not disappear after a course of such treatment, surgery should then be undertaken under cover of continuing antiamebic therapy.

PROPHYLAXIS OF AMEBIASIS

The best prophylaxis is correction of unsanitary conditions. Houseflies should be eradicated, unboiled water should not be drunk, and raw vegetables or other foods which might have been contaminated by human feces should be avoided. Those who handle food should be carefully studied, and any cyst-passers should be excluded from contact with food and water. Treatment must be administered to them before they are allowed to engage in these activities. If water which is suspected of being contaminated is going to be used on a large scale, measures aside from boiling may be employed, including the addition of aluminum sulfate, 400 to 600 mg per gallon, filtration, and, finally, chlorination. A number of preparations may be used to protect against amebiasis during periods of exposure. Diodoquin (in doses cited above) is a standard preparation and is reported to be highly effective. This medication is usually not given for more than 15 to 20 days and may be suitable for individuals who have spent a period of time in places where amebiasis is endemic.

AMEBIC ABSCESS OF THE LIVER

Although the major manifestations of amebiasis are enteric in location, the pathogenicity of the organism is not limited to the intestinal tract and other anatomic sites may be affected. The liver is the most commonly involved extraintestinal organ, and hepatic abscess is a major complication which, if untreated, often proceeds to a fatal outcome. Amebic abscess of the liver is a well known entity which is frequently observed in many countries of the world. It may present in a variety of ways as well as manifest a number of unusual complications. The prognosis for eradication of the organism with today's drugs is excellent; if amebic abscess of liver is diagnosed while confined, present modes of treatment are curative.

EPIDEMIOLOGY

The incidence of hepatic amebic abscess varies widely according to population and geographic location. It is highest in tropical countries and in areas where sanitary conditions are poor, because these conditions favor a high incidence of intestinal infection. A recent report states that less than 1 per cent of patients with intestinal amebiasis develop amebic abscess of the liver.[43] On the other hand, some institutions are reporting an increasing incidence of amebic abscess of the liver, possibly because of a combination of advanced techniques for scanning the liver in a selected population with high risk of endemic exposure to amebiasis.[44] Thus hospitals which employ up-to-date techniques and which care for Mexican-Americans or military returnees from the tropics may be expected to encounter increasing numbers of patients with amebiasis and liver abscess. There are differing opinions regarding racial susceptibility to amebiasis and liver abscess;

however, no convincing evidence is available on the subject. In general, for unknown reasons males seem to be more frequently afflicted than females, and the peak incidence of the disease is in the third, fourth, and fifth decades of life.

PATHOGENESIS AND PATHOLOGY

Although it is not always possible to consistently document liver involvement in relationship to intestinal infection, presumably it occurs from migration of the organism from the bowel to the liver by way of the portal circulation. The predisposing factors leading to this type of invasion and spread are unknown, as are the pathogenetic mechanisms for abscess formation. The right lobe of the liver is most often involved. Usually the abscess is solitary, but the formation of multiple abscesses in both lobes is not rare. Whether or not abscess formation is preceded by an active phase of amebic hepatitis is debatable.[45, 46] Most observers believe that right upper quadrant pain and slight enlargement of the liver may be seen during the course of acute intestinal amebiasis; however, this clinical event may represent a nonspecfic reaction rather than diffuse dissemination of organisms throughout the liver. In one extensive pathological study of 145 patients with acute or recent amebiasis, no examples of amebic hepatitis were found.[47]

Gross pathological changes include an enlarged liver with an abscess cavity that may be quite large, occupying at times almost an entire lobe. The material from the abscess cavity is typically thick and brown, and is often described as anchovy sauce-like. It is usually sterile, and E. histolytica organisms are absent. Rarely, the abscess may become secondarily infected with bacteria, its content becomes more purulent, and the invading bacterial organism may be cultured. Microscopically the amebae may be seen limited to the outer wall of the abscess as they invade the normal surrounding parenchyma.

CLINICAL FEATURES

Amebic abscess of the liver may present in a variety of ways. It may accompany an acute attack of intestinal amebiasis or may appear weeks to years later. Often there is no clear-cut history of amebiasis or diarrhea, and less than 50 per cent of patients will have E. histolytica in their stools at the time the abscess is diagnosed. The onset of symptoms may be slow and insidious or may be quite rapid. Fever, right upper quadrant pain, and malaise are among the most prominent symptoms. The temperature may vary from low grade elevation to spiking fevers accompanied by chills and diaphoresis. The right upper quadrant pain may be dull and constant, but can also be sharp and stabbing, accentuated by coughing or breathing. Radiation to the right shoulder, aggravated by inspiration, signifies diaphragmatic involvement. Anorexia, weight loss, nausea, vomiting, and fatigue may all be present. Jaundice is rare; it is usually present only in advanced cases.

The most common finding on physical examination is an enlarged tender liver. Splenomegaly is rare; if it is present, other diagnoses must be seriously considered. If the abscess is in the left lobe, tenderness and a palpable liver edge will be felt in the epigastric area. Occasionally a bulge in the abdominal or chest wall will indicate the site of an abscess which is "pointing." The right diaphragm may appear elevated to percussion, and its excursion is poor. A friction rub may also be heard over the pleura and, occasionally, over the liver as well. Some patients may present with complications of hepatic amebic abscess, most of which are manifestations of rupture of the abscess into adjacent structures. Rupture through the diaphragm into the pleural cavity is a common complication and results in empyema. When the process extends into the lung parenchyma, bronchopleural as well as bronchohepatic fistulas may result, the latter manifested by periodic expectoration of thick, dark, anchovy sauce-like material. Rupture into the peritoneal cavity results in peritonitis; it is a most serious complication with a mortality rate of 75 per cent. Abscess of the left hepatic lobe may perforate into the pericardial sac, precipitating sudden tamponade, vascular collapse, and, in most cases, death. Rupture through the abdominal wall may be further complicated by draining fistulous tracts. Other sites of perforation include the stomach, intestine, vena cava, and biliary tree. All these situations require intensive therapy, including rapid evacuation of the abscess.

DIAGNOSIS AND DIFFERENTIAL DIAGNOSIS

The key to diagnosis of amebic abscess of the liver is a high degree of suspicion of the condition, particularly in individuals who have resided in an endemic area and present with fever and an enlarged, tender liver. It should be emphasized that often the patient does not have a prior history of amebic dysentery (or even of diarrhea), and the physician must never dismiss the diagnosis on the basis of absence of diarrhea and E. histolytica in the stools at the time the patient consults him.

Laboratory features include a moderate anemia and polymorphonuclear leukocytosis. Eosinophilia, in contrast to some other parasitic diseases, is not a feature of this disease. Liver function tests in general are nonspecific. The alkaline phosphatase is elevated in 50 per cent of patients, and the serum glutamic oxaloacetic transaminase may also be abnormal (ca. 50 to 100 units).[48] Hyperbilirubinemia is rare. Serum albumin may be depressed and the globulin elevated. If readily available, the indirect hemagglutination determination (IHAA) is helpful, because it is positive in over 95 per cent of cases. However, since this test is performed in only a few centers, in the majority of instances its results are of interest only in a retrospective sense, because treatment must not be withheld pending results in the face of an abundance of clinical evidence which indicates that an abscess is present. Eighty per cent of patients have roentgenographic abnormalities, most commonly elevation and poor mobility of the right diaphragm with obliteration of the right cardiophrenic angle.

Photoscanning techniques developed over the past 15 years have been of major importance in dealing with amebic abscess of the liver (Fig. 104–18). The identification of one or more filling defects with fever and a tender liver is highly suggestive of hepatic abscess. Not only are these studies useful in diagnosing and localizing the site of disease, but they are also valuable in assessing the results of therapy.

Needle aspiration of the abscess has been used as a maneuver to establish the diagnosis of an abscess. The type of material contained within it is noted, and the aspirate should be carefully examined microscopically for E. histolytica. The latter is often unrewarding unless the specimen

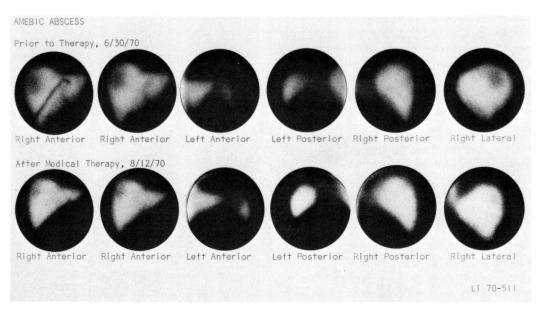

Figure 104–18.   Scintiphotography in amebic abscess of the liver. (Courtesy of Dr. M. Powell.)

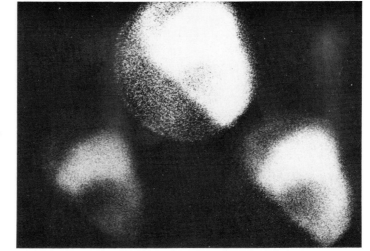

Figure 104–19. Scintiphotograph of the liver, right lateral view. This patient, who presented with fever and hepatomegaly, was first thought to have an hepatic amebic abscess. The final diagnosis was hepatoma.

is from the edge of the abscess, where most of the organisms are concentrated. Biopsy of the edge of the abscess with a Vim-Silverman needle to obtain material with the organism has also been tried unsuccessfully. Attempts to identify the organism through these procedures have become progressively less important because of the availability of serological testing and liver scanning and the effectiveness of a trial of drug therapy. The advantage of aspiration is the detection of superimposed bacterial infection and possibly the prevention of rupture of a large abscess.

Amebic abscess of the liver must be distinguished from pyogenic abscess of the liver, tumors in the liver, biliary tract infection, and subphrenic abscess. Nonamebic hepatic abscesses will usually feature a history of antecedent intra-abdominal septic disease (e.g., ruptured appendix, ulcer, diverticulum) or of biliary tract disease, usually with jaundice (acute cholecystitis and cholangitis), that will point the clinician toward the correct diagnosis.

An interesting condition which enters into the differential diagnosis is carcinoma of the liver, which may present with fever, hepatomegaly, weight loss, and a filling defect on liver scan (Fig. 104–19); usually, however, the patient does not have leukocytosis. Further evaluation by means of ar-

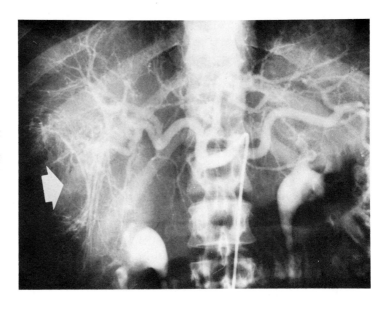

Figure 104–20. Celiac arteriogram in the same patient shown in Figure 104–19. There is a mass displacing and separating the hepatic vasculature in the lateral aspect of the right lobe of the liver (arrow).

teriography is indicated in such cases (Fig. 104–20). Liver biopsy may be helpful but is hazardous. The rapid response to medical therapy for amebic abscess is of great diagnostic value, distinguishing it from tumors. Patients who do not respond to amebicidal drugs should be explored for a diagnosis.

TREATMENT

Amebic abscess of the liver can be treated successfully with drugs alone in the vast majority of patients, providing that it has not ruptured, as previously described. Until recently therapy has consisted of:

1. Emetine hydrochloride, 1 mg per kilogram (maximal dose 65 mg) intramuscularly every day for ten days, plus

2. Chloroquine phosphate, 500 mg twice daily for two days and then 250 mg twice daily for 26 days, plus

3. Diiodohydroxyquin (Diodoquin), 650 mg three times daily for 21 days.[41]

Dehydroemetine, 1 to 1.5 mg per kilogram (maximal dose 1 g), is less toxic and may be used instead of emetine. In order to avoid the prevalent myocardial toxicity of emetine, one clinician has recently advocated giving chloroquine only, 500 mg per day for ten weeks.[44] This regimen has had no complications, and effective resolution of the abscess has been achieved.

Recent trials of metronidazole (Flagyl) have shown it to be useful in treating amebic abscess.[49] It has the advantage of being effective against concurrent intestinal infection as well. Also, toxicity appears slight. Many investigators feel that metronidazole is now the drug of choice for treatment of amebic hepatic abscess. It requires further evaluation, because some experience indicates that amebic abscess appears after an apparently successful course of treatment of amebic colitis with metronidazole.[50] Current recommendation for dosage is 750 mg three times a day for ten days.[51] This should be followed by diiodohydroxyquin (Diodoquin), 650 mg three times daily for 21 days.

Nearly all patients with amebic abscess of the liver will respond to medical therapy with a fall in temperature within 72 hours. Failure of such response demands further diagnostic evaluation to rule out other septic or malignant disease in the liver. Early drug therapy is strongly recommended in suspected patients who are moderately to severely ill, because the danger of rupture and death is real. The trial of therapy is quite safe and, if amebic abscess is present, effective, constituting an attractive mode for simultaneous diagnosis and treatment.

Surgical drainage is no longer indicated in the treatment of uncomplicated hepatic amebic abscess. Neither needle aspiration nor surgery hastens resolution of an abscess; furthermore, surgical intervention may lead to secondary bacterial infection and prolonged drainage. Needle aspiration may be beneficial for a patient with an impending rupture of an abscess, but for the usual patient it is unnecessary.

SCHISTOSOMIASIS (BILHARZIASIS)

Schistosomiasis is a disease produced by trematodes belonging to the family Schistosomatidae. The three principal species affecting man are *Schistosoma mansoni*, *S. japonicum*, and *S. haematobium*. It has been estimated that more than 200 million of the world's population are affected with schistosomiasis.[52] Conditions which contribute to the prevalence of the disease include poor sanitation, contaminated water, and a specific snail host required to complete the life cycle. These requirements are best found in the tropical and subtropical climates. *S. mansoni* is prevalent in Africa, the Arabian peninsula, Brazil, and Puerto Rico. *S. japonicum* is found primarily in the Far Eastern countries: Japan, Taiwan, and the Philippines. *S. haematobium* is centered in the Nile Valley, but also causes disease throughout Africa.

LIFE CYCLE

Man acquires the infection by exposure to water contaminated by the cercaria form of the organism, which emerges in large numbers from the snail host. If they locate a human host within 48 hours, they penetrate the skin and find their way to the peripheral venules. The metacercariae, as they are now termed, are carried to the right heart and lungs where they enter the systemic circulation by an as yet undetermined pathway. They eventually reach the intrahepatic portal bed, where, in four to six weeks, they mature into the adult forms. As fertilization takes place between the male and female, the worms migrate upstream together into the terminal mesenteric vein and venules. Once situated, the female deposits the fertilized eggs. The egg secretes a lytic substance and migrates into the surrounding tissue partly by destroying it. It then erodes through the gut wall into the lumen and is excreted in the feces. If the eggs reach fresh water, they hatch and release miracidia which seek out and then penetrate a specific snail host. Each miracidium develops into a sporocyst, which in turn produces several daughter sporocysts. Within weeks, the sporocysts begin to release thousands of cercariae which escape into the surrounding water to actively seek out a human host and repeat the cycle.

PATHOLOGY

The severity of the disease varies considerably from country to country. This may reflect virulence of the organism or such factors as worm burden, nutrition, or host defense.

As the adult worms traverse the portal system, *S. japonicum* preferentially finds its way into the superior mesenteric veins, *S. mansoni* to the inferior mesenteric veins, and *S. haematobium* to the vesical plexus. Because of this interesting anatomical migration, *S. japonicum* tends to involve the small intestine and ascending colon, *S. mansoni* the descending colon, and *S. haematobium* the bladder, pelvic organs, and rectum.

Pathological changes result from the deposition of large numbers of eggs in the intestinal submucosa (Fig. 104–21). As the eggs enzymatically digest their way through the intestinal mucosa, and as they die and release toxins, they provoke an inflammatory response. Grossly, the mucosal surface appears hyperemic, granular, and friable. Punctate hemorrhages as well as small, shallow ulcerations may be present. In cases of *S. haematobium* infection,

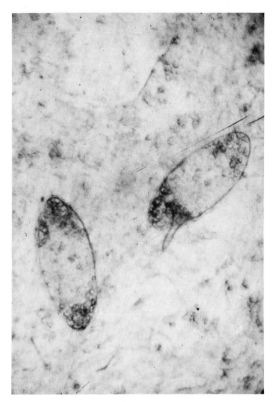

Figure 104–21. *S. mansoni* ovum as it appears microscopically in the bowel wall. × 200. (Courtesy of Dr. C. M. Knauer.)

patchy areas of the rectal mucosal surface may have a sandpaper appearance.[53] In later stages of the disease, papillomas and polyps may develop, which are frequently multiple and most often are found in the rectum. Fistulas have also been described in the advanced disease state. Rarely, acute bilharzial dysentery may be fatal. In these cases the bowel and lumen contain blood and mucus; the mucosal surface is intensely congested, and multiple punctate hemorrhages and small ulcerations are present. Microscopically, the picture varies with the severity of the disease. In many cases of schistosomiasis, there may be ova or their remnants present in the mucosa and submucosa, accompanied by little or no inflammatory or fibroblastic response. In more advanced disease there may be focal areas of mucosal necrosis. Ova in the mucosa and submucosa form the nucleus for a pseudotuberculoid reaction and are surrounded with foreign-body giant cells, epithelial cells, eosinophils,

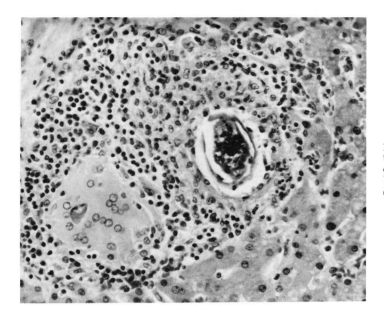

Figure 104-22. Granulomatous pseudotubercle of the liver in a patient with schistosomiasis. Note the ovum on the right and the foreign body giant cell on the left. × 150. (Courtesy of Dr. Jack Choy.)

plasma cells, and lymphocytes. The "sandy patch" lesions of *S. haematobium* appear to be large collections of calcified ova lying in the submucosa. Histology of the polyps reveals large numbers of ova in various stages of degeneration, evoking a hyperplastic, adenomatous response with an inflammatory infiltrate made up of lymphocytes, eosinophils, and plasma cells.

In addition to involving the intestine, the Schistosoma ova are carried by the portal circulation to the liver where they become entrapped in the portal areas. Granu-lomatous pseudotubercles then develop around the ova (Fig. 104–22). With continued deposition of the ova in the portal areas, progressive portal and periportal fibrosis ensues, with relative sparing of hepatic parenchyma. The late stages of the disease were first described in 1904 by Symmers, who described the cut surface of the liver as appearing as though a number of white clay pipe stems had been pushed through the organ at various angles.[54] The severe involvement of the portal areas results in so-called presinusoidal portal hypertension (Fig. 104–23).

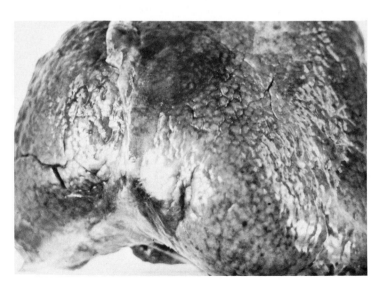

Figure 104-23. Cirrhosis of the liver in a patient with schistosomiasis. Note the coarse nodules. (Courtesy of Dr. Jack Choy.)

CLINICAL PICTURE

The initial clinical picture is associated with penetration of the skin of the host by the cercariae. Most of the cercariae die at this stage, and repeated exposures provoke a hypersensitivity response characterized by pruritus and a papular rash. Approximately four to six weeks after the initial infection, the flukes mature, migrate from the portal area to the bowel, and deposit eggs in the intestinal submucosa. In heavy infestations, the large numbers of eggs will damage the bowel wall, resulting in lower abdominal cramping pain and diarrhea with the passage of bloody mucus. Allergic-type responses such as urticaria, swelling of the face and lips, cough, and fever with a daily spike of temperature to 101 to 102° F may develop. Some patients suffer tenderness and enlargement of the liver as well as the spleen and lymph nodes. Peripheral blood eosinophilia is invariably present. In Japan where S. japonicum is prevalent, a severe form of this reaction is known as Katayama fever. It appears somewhat earlier after cercarial invasion than is noted in S. mansoni infection, and may be fatal, particularly in children with heavy infestations. Many feel that the clinical features of this phase of the illness are consistent with a serum sickness-like response. If the initial exposure is heavy and left untreated, or if there are repeated infections, both acute and chronic intestinal disease may follow. Children in particular may succumb to the acute dysentery. In the chronic form of the illness, the mucous membrane of the colon thickens, sufficiently pronounced and discrete on occasion to give the appearance of a papilloma on sigmoidoscopic examination. Ulcers may also be noted and may be due to the sloughing of these pedunculated papillomas. Polyps in the cecum may lead to intussusception. Occasionally, eggs infiltrate the appendix, causing a syndrome akin to acute appendicitis.[55] If the infection is virulent and widespread in the bowel, the parasite may penetrate the serosa with the formation of multiple nodules resembling tuberculomas, and regional lymph nodes may be infiltrated with Schistosoma eggs. Rectal prolapse and colonic obstruction are also late complications of advanced disease.

Eggs which are laid in the mesenteric venous system can travel through the portal system to the liver. They lodge in the portal areas, forming granuloma-like lesions which with accompanying fibrosis produce presinusoidal obstruction.[56] Thus wedged hepatic vein pressure is normal, as in obstruction or cavernous transformation of the portal vein. The course is slow and progressive, and patients are often asymptomatic. It is characterized by hepatosplenomegaly and, in advanced stages, by portal hypertension with ascites and variceal bleeding. Liver function, despite widespread involvement of the liver, appears to be much better than in most types of cirrhosis. With altered hemodynamics secondary to liver disease, eggs may bypass the liver to lodge in the pulmonary bed, giving rise to pulmonary hypertension. Central nervous system symptoms may also occur with secondary involvement of the brain and spinal cord.

DIAGNOSIS

During the acute stage of the disease, the diagnosis may be readily made by finding ova in freshly passed stools; concentration techniques improve the yield significantly. S. mansoni may be easily recognized by its oval shape and prominent lateral spine. By comparison, S. japonicum is somewhat diminished in size and the spine is small and difficult to see. S. haematobium has a conspicuous terminal spine. Since the eggs are present in the mucosa in a high percentage of patients, a rectal biopsy is often successful in making the diagnosis. This is performed by taking a small mucosal snip from the surface of one of the valves of Houston. This specimen is compressed with a small amount of warm saline between a glass slide and coverslip and examined by light microscopy for ova (Fig. 104–21). Needle biopsy of the liver may be diagnostic in patients with liver involvement. The biopsy may be examined by routine histological techniques; the pathological picture, as previously described, is very characteristic. Part of the specimen should also be crushed between a slide and coverslip and examined for eggs as carried out with the rectal tissue. Characteristically, the

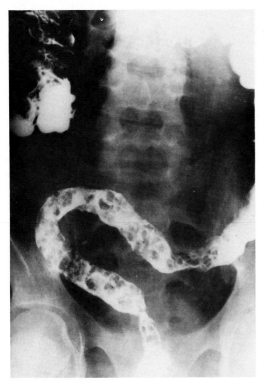

Figure 104–24. *S. mansoni* infestation of the colon in a 20-year-old Egyptian man with bloody diarrhea and tenesmus. Note the multiple polypoid lesions throughout the rectosigmoid colon, which is displaced out of the pelvis by a large pericolic bilharzial abscess. There is a generalized narrowing of the left colon with scattered areas of stricture formation. Note also the spasm, mural spiculation, and loss of haustration in the less involved descending colon, whereas the proximal colon appears relatively normal. (From Reeder, M. M., and Hamilton, L. C.: Radiol. Clin. N. Amer. 7:55, 1969.)

wedged hepatic vein pressure is normal in those patients with portal hypertension and cirrhosis, affording indirect evidence for the diagnosis of schistosomiasis of the liver. A skin test and numerous serological tests are currently available for the diagnosis of schistosomiasis.[57] Probably the best of these is the complement fixation test, although some experienced laboratories find the indirect hemagglutination test useful as well. However, reliance upon serological testing alone to make the diagnosis is hazardous, because false-positive tests may result from cross-reactions with other antibodies generated by other parasitic infections. Also, false-negative reactions may be obtained. The radiological picture of colonic schistosomiasis varies from an edematous mucosal pattern with tiny ulcerations and spasm to loss of haustration and the presence of multiple polyps (Fig. 104–24).

TREATMENT

Treatment of schistosomiasis still requires drugs which are potentially toxic to man; therefore caution must be exercised in their use. Antimony potassium tartrate (tartar emetic) is the drug of choice for *S. japonicum*, the most highly resistant of the three schistosoma species. Tartar emetic should be freshly made up in a 0.5 per cent solution and must be given intravenously to avoid local reaction at the injection site. It is administered on alternate days, beginning with 8 ml and increasing to 12, 16, 20, 24, and 28 ml. Thereafter, 28 ml is continued on alternate days until a total of 360 ml (1.8 g) has been given. It must be given slowly under continuous observation to avoid coughing and vomiting. Rarely, reactions are fatal. The patient should remain at rest for an hour after the injection. Signs of cardiotoxicity, hepatitis, nephritis, encephalitis, and dermatitis must be sought at all times during the course of therapy.

S. mansoni infections may be treated with a less toxic antimony compound, stibophen (Fuaden), that is given intramuscularly in doses of 4 ml every other day for a total of 80 to 100 ml. Side effects are similar to those of antimony potassium tartrate, but are less frequent and less severe. Sodium antimony dimercaptosuccinate (Astiban) may also be used in a total dose of 40 mg per kilogram given in five divided doses intramuscularly once or twice per week. Stibophen and antimony dimercaptosuccinate are contraindicated in the presence of cardiac, renal, and hepatic disease not caused by schistosomiasis. *S. haematobium* and often *S. mansoni* are treated with niridazole (Ambilhar), a new oral drug. In the United States this drug is only available on a clinical investigational basis from the Parasitic Disease Section, Center for Disease Control, Atlanta, Georgia. Niridazole is administered orally to both children and adults in doses of 25 mg per kilogram per day in two divided doses for five to seven days. The total daily dose should not exceed 1500 mg. Side effects include T-wave flattening or inversion on electrocardiogram, central nervous system manifestations, and occasional impairment of spermatogenesis.

Surgery may be considered for advanced cases with portal hypertension and recurrent bleeding varices. In general, patients with schistosomiasis tolerate bleeding better than patients with portal hypertension secondary to cirrhosis. Portal decompression should be reserved for the recurrent bleeder who is difficult to manage conservatively. Although some reports indicate that patients with schistosomiasis may tolerate bypass very well, the preponderant evidence indicates that they often have diminished liver function with encephalopathy after the procedure. Accordingly, great caution should be exerted in selection of cases and type of procedure. A new approach to treatment, currently under evaluation, involves cannulation of the portal vein, followed by trapping of the adult worms in a filter system.[58] Administration of antimony potassium tartrate induces the worms to migrate into the portal circulation, thus increasing the yield. As many as 799 worms have been removed from one patient by this method.[59]

BALANTIDIASIS

Although human infection with the organism Balantidium (*B. coli*) is rare, it is important to recognize, because it is a curable disease which may produce severe intestinal symptoms and even death.

ETIOLOGY

Balantidium coli is a protozoan and the only member of the class Ciliata known to infect man.[60] The trophozoite is quite large, and may occasionally be seen with the naked eye. It averages 50 to 100 μ in length. The organism is oval in shape, and the anterior end contains a funnel-shaped cytosome leading to the cytopharynx. At the posterior end, there is a small, barely visible cytopyge or anal pore. The organism is covered with cilia which act to propel it as well as direct food into its digestive passage. A large, variably shaped macronucleus, an adjacent small micronucleus, and numerous vacuoles which may contain red blood cells, starch granules, and other inert substances may be seen in the cytoplasm. The cyst, which is the infective form, develops when the organism is passed in the feces and is exposed to the outside environment. It is a round, thick-walled, ovoid structure 40 to 65 μ in diameter within which the organism can be seen.

EPIDEMIOLOGY

The majority of reported cases of Balantidium have been found in the tropics; however, the organism is encountered in the United States and has been identified as far north as Sweden and Norway.[61] There are several antigenically distinguishable species of Balantidium, and these may reside in numerous animals, particularly monkeys and hogs.[62] The evidence linking infection in man with exposure to pigs in an unsanitary environment is suggestive but not conclusive. The Balantidium found in hogs is morphologically indistinguishable from the organism in man, but there are antigenic differences; further, the exact mode of transmission remains unclear. Epidemiologically significant outbreaks of Balantidium have occurred in mental institutions where poor sanitation and neglected personal hygiene are prevalent.

PATHOGENESIS AND PATHOLOGY

Infection presumably begins when the Balantidium cyst is ingested. The parasite excysts in the small intestine and the new trophozoite passes into the colon where it penetrates the mucosal epithelium. The organism produces an enzyme, hyaluronidase, which apparently aids invasion of the tissue. The gross pathological appearance is similar to that in amebiasis.[63] Usually only the colon is involved, although rarely the terminal ileum may also be infected. The gross pathological changes consist of multiple superficial ulcers with necrotic bases and undermined edges; the intervening mucosa ranges from normal to hemorrhagic. In some infections, the ulcers are deep and may perforate.

The balantidia may be seen microscopically clustered at the bases of the crypts where they penetrate through the intact mucosal epithelium. They progress through the muscularis mucosae to the submucosa, where they may become lodged in capillaries and dilated lymph channels. The protozoan may also be seen in the bases and edges of the ulcer. Round cells dominate the inflammatory response, and eosinophils may be numerous. Rarely the organism may be seen in the regional lymph nodes.

CLINICAL PICTURE

Generally balantidiasis presents one of three differing clinical states. (1) The patient may be a completely asymptomatic carrier, capable of spreading the infection, particularly in an institutional environment. (2) The patient may have chronic diarrhea with loose, frequent bowel movements alternating with periods of constipation. Mucus may be present, but blood or pus rarely appears. The organism is not easily recovered in this stage, and multiple fresh stool specimens must be examined to make the diagnosis. It may cause appendicitis. (3) The patient may be acutely ill with the sudden onset of frequent stools containing mucus and blood; he complains of epigastric pain, tenesmus, nausea, and abdominal tenderness. Weight loss and dehydration are common. In its extreme form the illness is severe and fulminant with rectal hemorrhage, which, along with rapid dehydration and fever, leads to shock and death within a few days. Extraintestinal involvement in this form may be noted: peritonitis, urinary tract infection, vaginitis, liver abscess, pleuritis, and even pneumonia have been described.[64]

DIAGNOSIS

The sigmoidoscopic picture of B. coli infection may be difficult to distinguish from acute amebiasis or bacillary dysentery. The mucosa is erythematous, and small ulcerations may be seen. The diagnosis is best made by examination of scrapings of the bases of the ulcers for the trophozoites. Rectal biopsy may reveal the organism

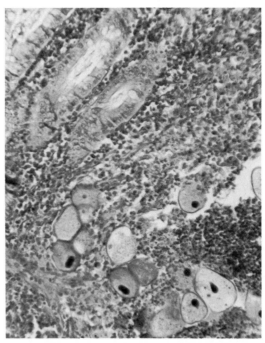

Figure 104-25. *B. coli* parasites in intestinal ulcer. (Photomicrograph by Zane Price. From Markell, E. K., and Voge, M.: Medical Parasitology. 3rd ed. Philadelphia, W. B. Saunders Co., 1971.)

which has penetrated the epithelial surface (Fig. 104-25). Stool examination will also provide the diagnosis; however, it must be emphasized that multiple fresh specimens must be analyzed before the disease can be excluded. *B. coli* may be cultured on certain media, and a fluorescent antibody test has recently been under investigation.[65]

TREATMENT

The drug of choice for treatment of Balantidium infection is tetracycline, 1.0 to 2.0 g given orally in four divided doses for ten to fourteen days. It may be combined with diiodohydroxyquin (Diodoquin), 650 mg three times daily. Carbasone, 200 mg four times a day orally for ten days, is also effective. Ampicillin has been used also, and recent trials of metronidazole (Flagyl) appear promising.[66] Treatment should be directed toward asymptomatic carriers as well as the acutely or chronically ill in order to eradicate the organism and prevent its spread.

WHIPWORM

LIFE CYCLE: EPIDEMIOLOGY

Trichuris trichiura has a worldwide distribution, but is most commonly found in the tropics and in areas with poor sanitary conditions. It belongs to the group Nematoda or roundworms.[60] Although found in other animals, man is the principal host. Commonly referred to as whipworm, the parasite is aptly named. Its whip-like appearance consists of a long, thin anterior segment containing the esophagus and a thick posterior portion harboring the digestive and reproductive organs (Fig. 104–26). Adult worms range from 3 to 5 cm in length. The egg is barrel- or lemon-shaped with a plug at either end, and contains an unsegmented embryo. Infection occurs through the ingestion of stale fecal material, the embryo requiring a period of three to five weeks outside the body to reach the infective stage. Once the egg is ingested, the digestive juices dissolve the shell, releasing larvae in the small intestine. The larvae reside in the small intestinal mucosa for three to ten days and then emerge to relocate in the cecal area. Here they attach themselves to the mucosa with the attenuated anterior end and mature in 30 to 90 days. The adult egg-laying worm may survive in this location for several years. In heavy infestations, the entire colon extending down to the rectum may be involved.

CLINICAL PICTURE

Trichuris infections are quite common in the tropics; the majority of patients are asymptomatic, although an eosinophilia may occur. Heavy infestations may result in right lower quadrant abdominal pain, abdominal distention, blood-streaked stools, diarrhea, weakness, emaciation, and anemia. Appendicitis and rectal prolapse have been described as direct consequences of whipworm infection.

DIAGNOSIS AND TREATMENT

Diagnosis is best made by finding the characteristic barrel-shaped ova in the feces. In severe infections, the clinging, writhing worms may be seen on the rectal mucosa during sigmoidoscopy. Treatment is usually directed toward patients with symptoms of heavy infestation and food handlers. Otherwise, asymptomatic individuals do not require therapy. The infection may be treated with hexylresorcinol 0.2 per cent solution, 500-ml enema retained for one hour. Because of its local irritant effect, this form of treatment should be given in hospital surroundings; it is

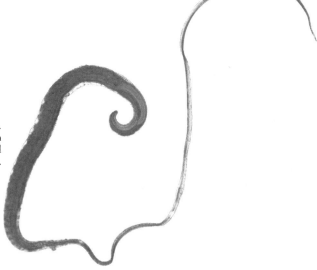

Figure 104–26. *T. trichiura*, adult male. (Photomicrograph by Zane Price. From Markell, E. K., and Voge, M.: Medical Parasitology. 3rd ed. Philadelphia, W. B. Saunders Co., 1971.)

contraindicated in patients with advanced colonic involvement. An alternative drug is thiabendazole, 25 mg per kilogram twice a day for two days; however, cures are reported in only 20 per cent of cases. In general, the present therapy for whipworm infestation is unsatisfactory, and the search for more effective drugs continues.

REFERENCES

1. Birnbaum, D., Laufer, A., and Freund, M. Pseudomembranous enterocolitis, a clinicopathologic study. Gastroenterology 41:345, 1961.
2. Gelfand, M., and Krone, C. L. Nonstaphylococcal pseudomembranous colitis. Amer. J. Dig. Dis. 14:278, 1969.
3. Benner, E. J., and Tellman, W. H. Pseudomembranous colitis as a sequel to oral lincomycin therapy. Amer. J. Gastroent. 54:55, 1970.
4. Goulston, S. J. M., and McGovern, V. J. Pseudomembranous colitis. Gut 6:207, 1965.
5. Newman, C. R. Pseudomembranous enterocolitis and antibiotics. Ann. Intern. Med. 45:409, 1956.
6. Dearing, W. H., Baggenstoss, A. H., and Weed, L. A. Studies on the relationship of Staphylococcus aureus to pseudomembranous enteritis and to postantibiotic enteritis. Gastroenterology 38:441, 1960.
7. Dubos, R. J. Bacterial and Mycotic Infections of Man, 4th ed. Philadelphia, Lippincott Co., 1965.
8. Martin, D. G., Tong, M. J., Ewald, P. E., and Kelly, H. V. Antibiotic sensitivities of Shigella isolates in Vietnam, 1968–1969. Military Med. 135:560, 1970.
9. Grady, G. F., and Keutsh, G. T. Pathogenesis of bacterial diarrheas. New Eng. J. Med. 285:831–891, 1971.
10. DuPont, H. L., Hornick, R. B., Dawkins, A. T., Snyder, M. J., and Formel, S. B. The response of man to virulent Shigella flexneri 2a. J. Infect. Dis. 119:296, 1969.
11. Davies, J. R., Farrant, W. N., and Uttley, A. H. C. Antibiotic resistance of Shigella sonnei. Lancet 2:1157, 1970.
12. Tong, M. J., Martin, D. G., Cunningham, J. J., and Gunning, J. J. Clinical and bacteriological evaluation of antibiotic treatment in shigellosis. J.A.M.A. 214:1841, 1970.
13. On drugs and therapeutics. The Medical Letter 10:38, 1968.
14. Today's drugs. Brit. Med.J. 1:35, 1970.
15. Amerson, J. R., and Martin, J. D. Tuberculosis of the alimentary tract. Amer. J. Surg. 107:340, 1964.
16. Bentley, G., and Webster, J. H. H. Gastrointestinal tuberculosis. A. 10-year review. Brit. J. Surg. 54:90, 1967.
17. Prout, W. G. Multiple tuberculous perforations of ileum. Gut, 9:381, 1968.
18. Fung, W. P., Tan, K. K., Yu, S. F., and Kho, K. M. Malabsorption and subtotal villous atrophy secondary to pulmonary and intestinal tuberculosis. Gut 11:212, 1970.
19. Hawley, P. R., Wolfe, H. R. I., and Fullerton, J. M. Hypertrophic tuberculosis of the rectum. Gut 9:461, 1968.
20. Chuttani, H. K. Intestinal tuberculosis. Modern Trends Gastroent. 309, 1970.
21. Abrams, J. S., and Holden, W. O. Tuberculosis of the gastrointestinal tract. Arch. Surg. 89:282, 1964.
22. Abrams, A. J. Lymphogranuloma venereum. J.A.M.A. 205:199, 1968.
23. Annamunthodo, H. Rectal lymphogranuloma venereum in Jamaica. Dis. Colon Rectum 4:17, 1961.
24. Schacter, J. Lymphogranuloma venereum. I. Comparison of the Frei test, complement fixation test and isolation of the agent. J. Infect. Dis. 120:372, 1969.
25. The choice of systemic antimicrobial drugs. The Medical Letter 14:8, 1972.
26. Harkness, A. H. The pathology of gonorrhea. Brit. J. Vener. Dis. 24:137, 1948.
27. Holmes, K. K., Counts, G. W., and Beaty, H. N. Disseminated gonococcal infection. Ann. Intern. Med. 74:979, 1971.
28. Nicol, C. S. Some aspects of gonorrhea in the female – with special reference to infection of the rectum. Br. J. Vener. Dis. 24:26, 1948.
29. Pariser, H., and Marino, A. F. Gonorrhea – frequently unrecognized reservoirs. South. Med. J. 63:198, 1970.
30. Martin, J. E., and Lester, A. Transgrow, a medium for transport and growth of Neisseria gonorrhoeae and Neisseria meningitidis. HSMHA Health Reports 86:30, 1971.
31. Phillips, I., Ridley, M., Rimmer, D., Lynn, R., and Warren, C. In vitro activity of twelve antibacterial agents against Neisseria gonorrhoeae. Lancet 1:263, 1970.
32. Catterall, R. D. The complications of homosexuality (abridged). Proc. Roy. Soc. Med. 55:871, 1962.
33. Harkness, A. H. Anorectal gonorrhea. Proc. Roy. Soc. Med. 47:476, 1948.
34. Owen, R. L., and Hill, J. L. Rectal and pharyngeal gonorrhea in homosexual men. J.A.M.A. 220:1315, 1972.
35. Markell, E. K., and Voge, M. Medical Parisitology. 3rd ed. Philadelphia, W. B. Saunders Co., 1971, Chapter 5.
36. Brooke, M. M. Epidemiology of amebiasis in the U.S. J.A.M.A. 188:519, 1964.
37. Barrett-Conner, E. Amebiasis, today, in the United States. Calif. Med. 114:1, 1971.
38. Neal, R. A. Pathogenesis of amoebiasis. Gut, 12:483, 1971.
39. Turner, J. A., Lewis, W. P., Hayes, M., and Ziment, I. Amebiasis – a symposium. Calif. Med., 114:44, 1971.
40. Kagan, I. Serologic diagnosis of parasitic diseases. New Eng. J. Med. 282:685, 1970.
41. Catchpool, J. F. Antiprotozoal drugs. In Review of Medical Pharmacology, F. H. Meyers, E. Jawetz, and A. Goldfein, eds. Los Altos, California, Lange Medical Publications, 1972.
42. Levine, S. M., Stover, J. F., Warren, J. G., Chappelka, A. R., and Burke, E. L. Ameboma,

the forgotten granuloma. J.A.M.A. *215*:1461, 1971.

43. Barrett-Conner, E. Amebiasis, today, in the United States. Calif. Med. *114*:1, 1971.

44. Reynolds, T. B. Amoebic abscess of the liver. Gastroenterology *60*:952, 1971.

45. Elsdon-Dew, R. Amoebiasis: Its meaning and diagnosis. S. A. Med. J. *43*:483, 1969.

46. Doxiades, T. Chronic amoebic hepatitis. Brit. Med. J. *44*:831, 1956.

47. Kean, B. H., Gilmore, H. R., Jr., and Van Stone, W. W. Fatal ambebiasis: Report of 148 fatal cases from the Armed Forces Institute of Pathology. Ann. Intern. Med. *44*:831, 1956.

48. Viranuvatti, V., Harinasuta, T., Pienguanit, U., et al.: Liver function tests in hepatic amebiasis based on 274 clinical cases. Amer. J. Gastroent. *39*:345, 1963.

49. Powell, S. J. Drug therapy in amoebiasis. Bull. WHO. *40*:953, 1969.

50. Weber, D. M. Amebic abscess of liver following metronidazole therapy. J.A.M.A. *216*:1339, 1971.

51. Drugs for parasitic infections. The Medical Letter *14*:54, 1972.

52. Jordan, P. Chemotherapy of schistosomiasis. Bull. N.Y. Acad. Med. *44*:245, 1968.

53. Bhagwandeen, S. B. The clinico-pathological manifestations of schistosomiasis in the African and the Indian in Durban. Pietermaritzburg, University of Natal Press, 1968.

54. Symmers, W. St. C. Note on a new form of liver cirrhosis due to the presence of the ova of *Bilharzia hematobia*. J. Path. Bact. *9*:237, 1904.

55. Cowper, S. G. A Synopsis of African Bilharziasis. London, H. K. Lewis and Co., Ltd., 1971.

56. Hidayst, M. A., and Wanid, H. A. A study of the vascular changes in bilharzic hepatic fibrosis and their significance. Surg. Gynec. Obstet. *132*:997, 1971.

57. Kagan, I. G. Serologic diagnosis of schistosomiasis. Bull. N.Y. Acad. Med. *44*:262, 1968.

58. Kessler, R. E., Amadoo, J. H., Tice, D. A., and Zimmon, D. S. Filtration of schistosomes in unanesthetized man. J.A.M.A. *214*:519, 1970.

59. Goldsmith, E. I., Carvalholuz, F. F., Prata, A., and Kean, B. H. Surgical recovery of schistosomes from the portal blood. J.A.M.A. *199*:235, 1967.

60. Markell, E. K., and Voge, M. Medical Parasitology. 3rd ed. Philadelphia, W. B. Saunders Co., 1971, pp. 78–81.

61. Arean, V. M., and Koppish, E. Balantidiasis, a review and report of cases. Amer. J. Path. *32*:1089, 1956.

62. Biagi, F. Unusual isolates from clinical material. Balantidium coli. Ann. N.Y. Acad. Sci. *174*:1023, 1970.

63. Baskerville, L. Balantidium colitis. Report of a case. Amer. J. Dig. Dis. *15*:727, 1970.

64. Marsden, P. D., and Schultz, M. G. Intestinal parasites. Gastroenterology *57*:724, 1969.

65. Dzbenshi, T. M. Immunofluorescent studies on *Balantidium coli*. Trans. Roy. Soc. Trop. Med. Hyg. *60*:387, 1966.

66. Zamar, V. In vitro trials of metronidazole against *Balantidium coli*. Trans. Roy. Soc. Trop. Med. Hyg. *63*:152, 1969.

Chapter 105

Radiation Enteritis and Colitis

David L. Earnest, Jerry S. Trier

Damage to the intestine resulting from radiation therapy for abdominal and pelvic malignancy is well known. Although symptoms caused by radiation of the colon and small intestine may appear at different times, they frequently occur in concert. Therefore coexistent small bowel involvement should be considered when radiation damage to the colon is suspected and vice versa.

Although the damaging effect of radiation on intestinal tissue had been demonstrated years before in experimental animals, the first clinical report of intestinal radiation injury after radiotherapy for malignant disease appeared in 1917.[1] Since then, there have been numerous reports of radiation damage to the small intestine, colon, and rectum after treatment with externally administered X-rays and with internally placed cobalt, radium, or radioactive gold. The development of modern supervoltage technique has permitted delivery of doses of radiation to pelvic and abdominal viscera with little or no warning skin injury. Such radiation therapy of lymphomas and carcinomas involving a variety of pelvic, intra-abdominal and retroperitoneal structures has resulted in radiation enteritis and colitis in many patients.[2]

INCIDENCE

The incidence of radiation injury to the small bowel and colon has been reported to vary between 2.4 and 25 per cent of patients treated for pelvic and intra-abdominal malignancies with radiotherapy.[3, 4] A review of patients treated at a large medical center for carcinoma of the cervix with radium implantation and external orthovoltage, with a total dose of about 5000 rads delivered over five weeks, shows that approximately 8 per cent of all patients developed serious sequelae of radiation colitis.[5] This is similar to the reported incidence from other centers using comparable techniques.[3, 4]

The threshold radiation dose necessary to produce lasting intestinal injury in a clinical situation varies considerably, but basically depends upon the intensity and duration of the radiation reaching the bowel wall and its sensitivity to irradiation. Although patients have developed chronic radiation damage after tissue doses below 4000 rads,[6] the incidence of significant radiation damage to the bowel rises sharply when the dose exceeds 5000 rads.[4-6] Previous abdominal or pelvic surgery or pelvic inflammatory disease which might cause fixation by adhesions of

1406

normally mobile portions of small bowel or colon has been associated with more frequent gross evidence of radiation damage to the bowel.[6] The true incidence of radiation enterocolitis is probably underestimated in most older, retrospective studies, but available evidence suggests that clinically apparent disease is greatest in the rectum and less common in the small intestine. A recent prospective analysis reported symptomatic sigmoiditis in 75 per cent and abnormal rectal biopsy samples in all of eleven patients undergoing radiotherapy for pelvic malignancy.[7]

PATHOGENESIS

Interest in the mechanism of bowel injury after controlled radiation therapy and in the so-called intestinal deaths after total body irradiation has prompted numerous studies of the effects of radiation on the intestine. The intestinal epithelium is most sensitive to radiation damage. Cell renewal studies with tritiated thymidine have shown that the mucosa is populated by a proliferating pool of undifferentiated cells located in the intestinal crypts.[8] As these cells differentiate, they lose the capacity to divide. In addition, they migrate to the mucosal surface, mature, and are eventually extruded into the lumen. Radiation results in a suppression of cell proliferation in the crypts which leads to a characteristic acute lesion.[9] Although rapid denudation of the mucosa might be expected to result from a reduction of mucosal cell repopulation, the existing cells usually maintain the integrity of the mucosal surface unless radiation exposure is prolonged or sufficiently great to destroy irreparably the proliferating cell population. If the radiation dose is not excessive, prompt recovery of epithelial cell proliferation and repair of the mucosal lesion occur within a week or two after cessation of irradiation.[9] Recent evidence demonstrates that the effect of repeated radiation doses depends on the stage in the cell cycle of the crypt cells at the time of exposure (see pp. 1246 to 1248). Those cells in the G1-postmitotic phase of the cell cycle have been shown to be the most radiosensitive, whereas those cells in the late S-synthetic phase are the most resistant.[10, 11] Only a fraction of the total proliferating crypt cell population is in a given stage of cell proliferation at any specific time. This helps explain why only some of the dividing cells die after a single, substantial, but

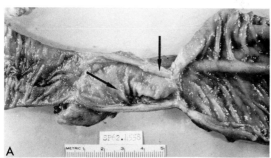
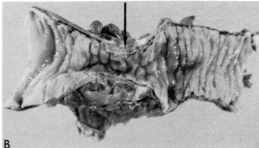
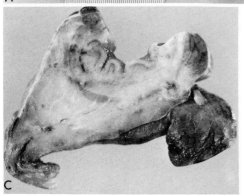

Figure 105–1. Postirradiation bowel strictures. A, Narrow stricture of the ileum one year after radiation therapy for carcinoma of the urinary bladder. Note the pale granular mucosa overlying the fibrotic area. B, Radiation fibrosis, producing stricture of the colon. C, A sagittal view of the colonic stricture shows the extreme bulky fibrosis.

known lethal dose of irradiation, and why mitotic activity again reaches normal levels a few days after radiation exposure.

The endothelial cells of the small submucosal arterioles are exceedingly radiosensitive and respond to large doses or radiation with swelling and proliferation. It must be emphasized that these vascular changes usually develop weeks after the acute mucosal changes. Eventually the vessel wall may undergo fibrinoid degeneration, and subsequent fibrin deposition facilitates vascular thrombosis. Thus an obliterative endarteritis and endophlebitis develop, producing graded ischemic changes in the intestinal wall and contributing to mucosal ulceration and necrosis.[12] If mucosal integrity is lost owing to the compromised blood supply, intestinal bacteria probably contribute to further damage (see p. 382).

After extensive radiation, the bowel wall becomes edematous, and bizarre fibroblasts are evident in all layers of the bowel wall. The connective tissue and smooth muscle undergo hyaline degeneration. Eventually, extensive fibrosis results, which may lead to stricture, as well as to distortion and disruption of the mucosal surface (Fig. 105–1).[12] Thus radiation may produce changes in the intestine, ranging from a reversible transitory disturbance of the architecture of the mucosa to a chronically inflamed, thickened, ulcerated, and fibrotic bowel.

PATHOLOGY

The gross pathological changes induced in the bowel by irradiation have been amply reviewed in a number of good monographs.[7, 12] These changes can be conveniently divided into acute, subacute, and chronic or latent periods. Acute changes which occur during and immediately after irradiation involve abnormal epithelial cell proliferation and maturation with a decrease in crypt cell mitosis, as discussed above. In the small bowel, a distinctive architectural lesion of the mucosa develops, characterized by a marked decrease in mucosal thickness caused by villous shortening (Fig. 105–2).[9] In addition, there are hyperemia, edema formation, and extensive inflammatory cell infil-

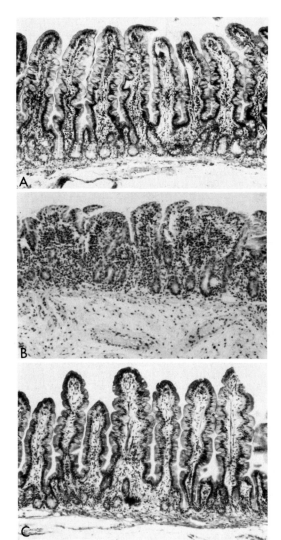

Figure 105–2. Three biopsies from the duodenojejunal junction of a patient undergoing abdominal X-ray therapy. *A*, Before treatment, the villous architecture is normal. *B*, After 3300 rads of X-ray therapy, the villi are shortened, there is increased infiltration of the lamina propria with inflammatory cells, and submucosal edema is present. *C*, Twelve days after cessation of therapy, villous architecture has returned to normal. Hematoxylin and eosin stain. × 75. (From Trier, J. S., and Browning, T. H.: J. Clin. Invest. *45*:194, 1966.)

tration of the mucosa.[9] Crypt abscesses, consisting of acute inflammatory cells, eosinophils, and sloughed epithelial cells, may be present (Fig. 105–3).[7, 9] If the dose of radiation is high or radiation exposure is prolonged, the mucosa may ulcerate owing to failure of epithelial regeneration. Such ulceration may be diffuse or localized, de-

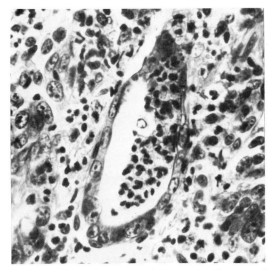

Figure 105-3. A crypt abscess in a biopsy of small bowel exposed to 3300 rads X-ray. The surrounding epithelial cells are flattened and contain megaloblastic nuclei. The crypt abscess is composed primarily of polymorphonuclear leukocytes, which are also seen in the lamina propria. Hematoxylin and eosin stain. × 500. (From Trier, J. S., and Browning, T. H.: J. Clin. Invest. 45:194, 1966.)

pending upon the area of exposure and extent of exposure.

In the subacute period, which begins two to 12 months after radiotherapy, the mucosa has regenerated and healed to a variable extent. However, during this period, the endothelial cells of the small arterioles in the bowel submucosa may undergo swelling, detachment from their basement membrane, and ultimately degeneration.[13] Fibrin plugs and thrombosis may form in the lumen. In some instances, recanalization may occur. Large foam cells are seen beneath the intima; these are claimed to be diagnostic of radiation vascular injury in man (Fig. 105-4). The result of these obliterative changes in the small arterioles is progressive ischemia. The submucosa becomes thickened and fibrotic, and often contains large and bizarre fibroblasts.[13] This vascular damage and ischemic fibrosis may progress at different rates, and in the subacute period bowel circulation is often adequate. However, with the presence or onset of hypertension, diabetes mellitus, generalized atherosclerosis, or coronary insufficiency and heart failure, the splanchnic circulation may become progressively compromised, and areas of microvascular insufficiency from radiation vasculitis then acquire dangerous significance.[2] Ulceration on an ischemic basis is particularly prone to develop in the sigmoid and rectum. Abscess and fistula formation may occur, with sinus tracts connecting the involved bowel and the vagina, bladder, or ileum. Late carcinomatous degeneration has been reported as a late complication, but this is rare.[14]

CLINICAL PICTURE

The setting for symptomatic presentation of radiation enterocolitis is a patient

Figure 105-4. Characteristic radiation-induced change in a small submucosal arteriole. There are marked thickening of the vessel wall (arrows) and hydropic change of the subintimal cells. Luminal occlusion, thrombosis, and recanalization may occur. Hematoxylin and eosin stain. × 100.

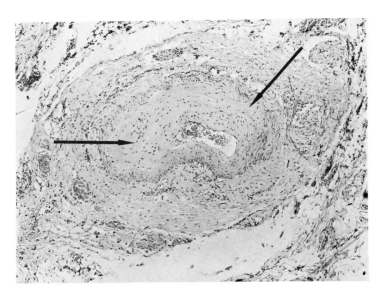

with an intra-abdominal, most often pelvic, malignancy who has either just begun or may have in years past completed radiotherapy for this tumor, with a totaled tumor dose in excess of 4000 rads. Symptoms may appear early during therapy, shortly after therapy has been completed, or months to many years after treatment has ended.

EARLY SYMPTOMS

Frequently gastrointestinal symptoms occur during the first or second week of radiation therapy. Nausea and vomiting are common, but their cause is not clear. Indeed, it has been suggested that the nausea originates from a central nervous system response to any major dose of irradiation, because it also occurs when the gastrointestinal tract is not directly exposed to X-ray (i.e., during irradiation of the chest or neck). The patient may develop altered bowel habits with the onset of diarrhea or, occasionally, constipation. A mucoid rectal discharge may develop. A sensation of incomplete rectal evacuation is common, and suggests involvement of the rectum. Cramping lower abdominal pain may suggest concomitant small bowel involvement. Rectal bleeding from the radiation may appear during this acute stage if there is mucosal ulceration.[2, 7, 14] In many instances, the picture resembles the acute onset of idiopathic ulcerative colitis of the distal colon. Sigmoidoscopy at this time reveals a dusky, edematous mucosa. The mucosal edema obscures the mucosal vascular pattern which is normally visible. Friability is usually not marked, and ulcers are infrequent in the early stages. However, with excessive doses of irradiation, mucosal necrosis may occur. This is usually accompanied by marked tenesmus and significant rectal bleeding. In such patients, sigmoidoscopy reveals a markedly hyperemic and occasionally necrotic mucosa with patchy areas of superficial ulceration.

LATE SYMPTOMS

Many of these patients are not seen by the gastroenterologist until six months to many years after completion of radiation therapy. With rectal and colonic involvement, either gross rectal bleeding or blood-streaked stools are a frequent complaint. Excessive mucus, frequently mixed with blood, may be passed, closely resembling the rectal discharge seen in chronic ulcerative colitis. A history of colicky abdominal pain, a decrease in stool caliber, increasing difficulty in defecation, tenesmus, and progressive obstipation may herald the development of a colonic or rectal stricture. An ileal stricture should be suspected when there is colicky abdominal pain associated with evidence of small intestinal obstruction. Fistulization with other pelvic or abdominal organs may produce such symptoms as a feculent vaginal discharge, pneumaturia, and the rapid passage of undigested food in the stool. Intra-abdominal abscesses, usually pelvic, may also develop, producing signs of sepsis. If such abscesses are not localized by fibrosis, frank peritonitis may develop. Free perforations of the involved ileum and colon are uncommon, but do occur, and may produce acute and fulminant peritonitis. Rarely, massive intestinal bleeding develops from ileal or colonic ulcerations.

If the small intestine and the ileum in particular are affected, signs and symptoms of malabsorption, especially of fat, may be prominent.[15, 16] Therefore patients with known radiation involvement of the small intestine, especially if they have a history of weight loss, should have intestinal absorptive function evaluated by such tests as stool fat, vitamin B_{12} absorption, or xylose absorption (see pp. 260 to 267). With extensive ileal submucosal fibrosis and mucosal involvement, bile salt malabsorption may contribute to both the diarrhea and the steatorrhea observed (see p. 269). If the small bowel is strictured, stasis may predispose to intraluminal bacterial overgrowth of the small intestine, contributing to malabsorption. In addition, enterocolonic fistulas, if present, may cause massive intraluminal bacterial overgrowth of the small intestine and result in severe steatorrhea and malabsorption of vitamin B_{12} (see pp. 927 to 937).

If the rectum is involved at this stage, changes in the mucosa are usually seen at sigmoidoscopy. The mucosa appears granular and is friable. Multiple telangiectases are characteristic and are usually most prominent around ulcerated necrotic areas. Ulcerations may be quite variable in size, are frequently transverse in orientation, and are most often seen on the anterior rectal wall about 4 to 6 cm above the pectinate line adjacent to the area of the cervical cuff, especially in patients who received radiation therapy for cervical carcinoma. Occasionally these ulcers may have a neoplastic appearance. Rectal strictures tend to be located higher than the ulceration and are usually 8 to 12 cm above the anal verge.[2] Biopsy of the ulcer or strictured area may be helpful but should be performed with caution, because bleeding and perforation of the necrotic bowel have been reported.

RADIOLOGICAL EXAMINATION

Barium contrast examinations are often helpful in assessing the extent of radiation damage to the intestine, but the abnormalities present are not specific for the diagnosis of radiation enterocolitis.[17] In the early postirradiation period, the barium enema may reveal segmental changes with irregularity, spasm, and fine serrations of the bowel wall, much as is seen in other inflammatory disease of the colon such as ulcerative colitis. If an acute ulcerative lesion has developed on the anterior rectal wall, its appearance with raised mucosal margins may resemble carcinoma.

The appearance of small intestinal le-

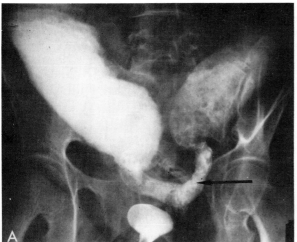

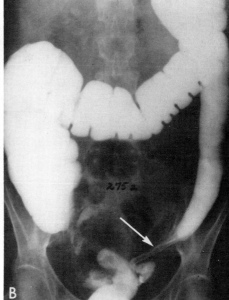

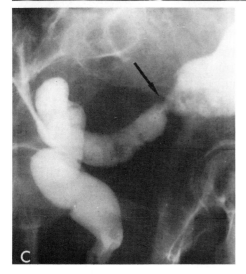

Figure 105–5. Late radiation change in the colon after approximately 5500 rads. *A,* Long stricture of rectum and sigmoid colon with symmetrical concentric luminal narrowing. There is large bowel dilatation proximal to the stricture. *B,* The mucosal pattern is generally intact throughout this long radiation stricture of the descending and proximal sigmoid colon. Note the smooth tapered proximal margins of the stricture. *C,* Short postradiation strictures such as this one in the proximal sigmoid colon may be difficult to differentiate radiologically from malignancy.

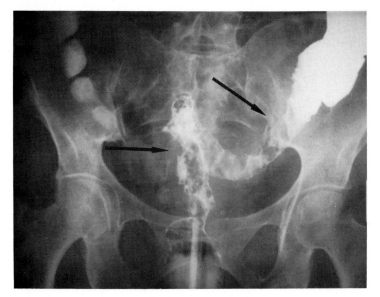

Figure 105–6. Severe recto-sigmoid radiological abnormalities are present on this barium enema performed two months after the patient underwent radiation therapy for cervical carcinoma. Subacute radiation injury of the colon may present radiologically as edematous, occasionally ulcerated, mucosa, with asymmetrical areas of narrowing suggestive of granulomatous colitis (arrows).

sions on barium contrast studies, especially the ileal lesions, may closely resemble other inflammatory disease of the small bowel such as regional enteritis. The mucosal pattern may be distorted, the bowel wall thickened, and the lumen narrowed. X-rays may be helpful in documenting the presence of fistulas or sinus tracts; multiple views should be taken when this complication is suspected. Fibrosis of the colon or the small bowel may result in long narrowed areas which are smooth and symmetrical with tapered edges (Fig. 105–5). However, short areas of radiation stricture with overhanging margins indistinguishable from carcinoma have also been reported.[17] Occasionally a stricture may represent invasion of the intestinal wall by recurrent extraintestinal neoplasm. In addition, the strictured area may resemble and must be distinguished from those which may occur in chronic ulcerative colitis and granulomatous disease of the small and large intestine (Fig. 105–6). A history of previous radiation therapy and the absence of other radiological changes of idiopathic inflammatory bowel disease suggest radiation damage as the cause of the observed X-ray changes.

Some help in the dilemma created by lack of diagnostically characteristic barium contrast findings in radiation enterocolitis may eventually come from recent advances in mesenteric angiography. Since arteriolar damage with bowel ischemia is

the pathological process which leads to formation of strictures, it is not surprising that abnormalities in the smaller branches of the mesenteric vasculature have been found.[18] However, their differential diagnostic usefulness awaits further clinical experience.

MANAGEMENT

Modern radiotherapy techniques directed at minimizing complications should include careful planning, detailed calculation of radiation dose, proper techniques, and in vivo monitoring of the delivered radiation.[19] Measurements of radiation delivered to the pelvic organs can be accomplished by means of various types of radiosensitive probes inserted into the rectum, bladder, and paracervical areas.[4, 19] Careful monitoring of the dose and delivery in small increments at definitely spaced intervals tend to reduce colonic complications.

During the period of acute reaction, conservative measures will usually suffice to treat the mild diarrhea and discomfort of proctitis and sigmoiditis. Sedation, antispasmodics, stool softeners, local analgesics, warm sitz baths, adequate nutrition, and careful surveillance are the principal components of therapy at this stage. More severe injury with rectal bleeding tends to occur weeks, months, or years after therapy and may be treated with steroid retention enemas and oral sulfonamide preparations, although firm data documenting their efficacy are not available.[2] The rectal bleeding is usually not severe, but occasionally it may require administration of oral or parenteral iron or transfusion of whole blood. Rarely, massive and unrelenting hemorrhage may occur. In such patients a direct surgical approach is indicated, with ligation of the bleeding site if it is localized. A colostomy or ileostomy to divert the fecal stream may be required if the bleeding is due to generalized colonic involvement.

As the disease progresses, symptomatic strictures or fistulas may develop. Mild and short strictures of the distal colon can be dilated manually. Attempts at dilatation of long and well established strictures may be hazardous, and mild symptoms of partial sigmoid or rectal obstruction may be temporarily helped by administration of mineral oil or stool softeners. Progression of strictures to significant obstruction, regardless of their location in the large or small intestine, obviously necessitates surgery. Occasionally, rectovaginal fistulas may close either spontaneously or after diversion of the fecal stream with a transverse colostomy. On the other hand, enterocolic, enterovesical, rectovesical, and some rectosigmoid fistulas must be treated surgically. Intra-abdominal and pelvic abscesses should be drained promptly, and free perforations are, of course, a surgical emergency. Presacral sympathectomy has been recommended by some for severe pelvic pain which is resistant to medical management, but long-term results are uncertain.

Surgical therapy in patients with radiation disease of the bowel has significant morbidity and should be reserved for definite indications as outlined above. The vascular supply of the bowel is already compromised by radiation change, and healing is often severely impaired. Progressive ischemic necrosis in the remaining adjacent bowel segments may occur. For distal colonic disease, a colostomy, preferably placed in the transverse colon near the hepatic flexure, is often helpful as the initial procedure unless an abscess which requires drainage is present. This may subsequently allow a long, mobile segment for a pull-through operation if

rectal resection is ultimately necessary. Once a colostomy has been established, its closure should not be attempted in less than six to twelve months to allow adequate time for healing of the defunctionalized bowel.

In patients with malabsorption resulting from intestinal involvement, the cause of the malabsorption must be treated. If there is stasis with bacterial overgrowth caused by stricture, broad-spectrum antibiotics should be administered, or, if necessary, the stricture resected. Bacterial overgrowth caused by enterocolonic fistulas will require surgery, either resection or bypass. If there is sufficient ileal mucosal involvement to compromise bile salt absorption but no major obstruction, administration of cholestyramine may reduce diarrhea by binding bile salts.[20] If malabsorption is severe, dietary supplementation with medium-chain triglycerides or amino acid and simple sugar supplements is now available in the newer elemental diet preparations.

If treatment of the basic underlying neoplastic process has been successful and systemic vascular disease is absent, most patients will not experience lasting or persistent morbidity from radiation damage to the intestine. It should be stressed that in the majority of instances in which the colon is seriously involved, the small bowel is likewise frequently affected, and the overall management and prognosis for the patient's bowel-related symptoms will be in large part determined by the extent and severity of the damage to the small intestine. In most cases, the ultimate outcome of radiotherapy will depend on the response of the underlying malignancy. The onset of symptomatic radiation enteritis and colitis, however, may present the physician with yet another complicated therapeutic challenge.

REFERENCES

1. Franz, K., and Orth, J.   Fall einer Röntgenschadingung. Berl. Klin. Wschr. 45:662, 1917.
2. DeCosse, J. J., Rhodes, R. S., Wentz, W. B., Reagan, J. W., Dwarken, H. J., and Holden, W. D.   The natural history and management of radiation-induced injury of the gastrointestinal tract. Ann. Surg. 170:369, 1969.
3. Manson, G. R., Guernsey, J. M., Hanks, G. E.,

and Nelson, T. S. Surgical therapy for radiation enteritis. Oncology 22:241, 1968.

4. Roswit, B., Malsky, S. J., and Reid, C. B. Severe radiation injuries of the stomach, small intestine, colon and rectum. Amer. J. Roent. 157:62, 1963.

5. Fletcher, G. H., Brown, T. C., and Rutledge, S. N. Clinical significance of rectal and bladder dose measurements in radium therapy of cancer of the uterine cervix. Amer. J. Roent. 79:421, 1958.

6. Strockbine, M. F., Hancock, J. E., and Fletcher, G. H. Complications in 831 patients with squamous cell carcinoma of the intact uterine cervix treated with 3000 rads or more whole pelvis radiation. Amer. J. Roent. 108:293, 1970.

7. Gelfand, M. D., Tepper, M., Katz, L. A., Binder, H. J., Yesner, R., and Floch, M. H. Acute irradiation proctitis in man. Gastroenterology 54:401, 1968.

8. Bertalanffy, F. D., and Lau, C. Cell renewal. Int. Rev. Cytol. 13:357, 1962.

9. Trier, J. S., and Browning, T. H. Morphologic response of human small intestine to X-ray exposure. J. Clin. Invest. 45:194, 1966.

10. Hagemann, R. F., Sigvestad, C. P., and Lesher, S. Intestinal crypt survival and total crypt levels of proliferating cellularity following irradiation; fractionated X-ray exposure. Rad. Res. 47:149, 1971.

11. Hagemann, R. F., and Lesher, S. Intestinal crypt survival and total and per crypt levels of proliferative cellularity following irradia-

tion; age response and animal lethality. Radiat. Res. 47:159, 1971.

12. Warren, S., and Friedman, N. B. Pathology and pathologic diagnosis of radiation lesions in the gastrointestinal tract. Amer. J. Path. 18:499, 1942.

13. Ackerman, L. V. The pathology of radiation effect of normal and neoplastic tissue. Amer. J. Roent. 114:447, 1972.

14. Black, W. C., and Ackerman, L. V. Carcinoma of the large intestine as a late complication of pelvic radiotherapy. Clin. Radiol. 16:278, 1965.

15. Greenberger, N. J., and Isselbacher, K. J. Malabsorption following radiation injury to the gastrointestinal tract. Amer. J. Med. 36:450, 1964.

16. Tankel, H. I., Clark, D. H., and Lee, F. D. Radiation enteritis with malabsorption. Gut 6:560, 1965.

17. Mason, G. R., Dietrich, P., Friedland, G. W., and Hanks, G. E. The radiological findings in radiation-induced enteritis and colitis. A review of 30 cases. Clin. Radiol. 21:232, 1970.

18. Dencker, H., Holindahl, K. H., Lunderquist, A., Olivecrona, H., and Tylen, U. Mesenteric angiography in patients with radiation injury of the bowel after pelvis irradiation. Amer. J. Roent. 114:476, 1972.

19. Fletcher, G. H. Radiation Therapy. Philadelphia, Lea and Febiger, 1966, p. 580.

20. Hofmann, A. F., and Poley, J. R. Cholestyramine treatment of diarrhea associated with ileal resection. New Eng. J. Med. 281:397, 1969.

Chapter 106

Diverticular Disease
of the Colon

Peter M. Loeb, Marvin H. Sleisenger

INTRODUCTION

Diverticula of the colon are acquired herniations of mucosa through the muscular layers of the bowel wall and are thus false diverticula. The phrase diverticular disease of the colon has been used to emphasize three overlapping stages of the condition which may often be distinguished by clinical, radiological, and pathological criteria: the prediverticular state, diverticulosis, and diverticulitis.[1, 2]

The prediverticular state has many features of diverticulosis without grossly visible diverticula. Diverticulosis is the most commonly identified category of diverticular disease and is the presence of diverticula which are not inflamed.[3, 4] Diverticulitis is the presence of inflamed diverticula and most probably means that a diverticulum has perforated.[5-7]

INCIDENCE AND EPIDEMIOLOGY

Virtually all studies indicate that the incidence of diverticular disease of the colon increases with age.[8-11] Radiological surveys on healthy subjects demonstrate diverticula in about 8 per cent of the adult population under age 60 and in 40 per cent of individuals over age 70.[9] They are rarely found in individuals who are less than 30 years of age. The overall incidence of diverticula in necropsy series ranges from 20 to 43 per cent and as high as 50 per cent in patients over 60 years of age.[8, 11] Pathological evidence of diverticulitis is found in as many as 12 per cent of patients with diverticulosis, although the majority of them have no prior history suggestive of an attack of diverticulitis.[8] Conversely, one-third of patients with a prior clinical diagnosis of diverticulitis have no pathological evidence of inflammation.[12] The incidence of diverticulitis is proportional to the extent of colonic involvement by diverticula. Up to 50 per cent of patients with diverticulosis of the entire colon have evidence of diverticulitis.[13]

Diverticular disease is reported to be rare in the so-called underdeveloped countries but has been increasing in incidence since 1900 in the Western world.[14-16] Its incidence is higher in urban than in rural areas in both the West and Africa. A racial predilection cannot be implicated, because the incidence in the urban black American is much greater than in the rural black African and equal to that in the white American.[17, 18]

PATHOLOGY

Diverticulosis. Diverticula of the colon are pulsion or false diverticula, because the mucosa herniates between muscle fibers of the inner circular muscle. The outpouchings usually appear between the mesenteric and lateral taeniae where the largest nutrient vessels penetrate the inner circular muscle. The best studies indicate that the mucosal protrusions occur adjacent to these vessels and suggest that the course of the penetrating vessels provides a pathway for the diverticula.[1, 19-21]

Careful dissections in many resected and necropsy specimens of colon containing diverticula with and without inflammatory changes demonstrate that there is a high incidence of thickening or enlargement of both the circular and longitudinal muscles.[1, 4, 8, 12, 14, 22, 23] The taeniae coli are often thick and appear shortened; the circular muscle may appear corrugated.[15] In some instances, the mucosa is "thrown up into folds" or seems reduplicated (Fig. 106–1). The results of studies performed to determine whether this muscular enlargement is due to hyperplasia or hypertrophy are conflicting.[1, 23, 24] It is certain, however, that the colonic muscular enlargement is present without associated pathological evidence of inflammation and in patients who have had no clinical history of diverticulitis.[1, 8, 12, 23] Diverticula may also be present in great numbers without smooth muscle thickening.[8, 14] As will be discussed under the section on pathogenesis, Fleischner has coined the terms spastic colon diverticulosis or myochosis when diverticula are associated with muscular enlargement and simple massed diverticulosis when multiple diverticula are present and there is no muscular enlargement.[25]

Ninety-five per cent of patients with colonic diverticula have involvement of at least the sigmoid colon; the prevalence of diverticula in the more proximal colon is progressively less but increases with the duration of the disease.[8, 13] The diverticula vary in size from 1 to 2 mm up to 7 cm, and in any patient there may be a few or hundreds of diverticula. Rarely an isolated diverticulum may be found, particularly in the cecum or sigmoid colon, and occasionally a giant diverticulum is present in the sigmoid.

Many patients who have had previous radiological demonstration of diverticula are found to have no diverticula when careful

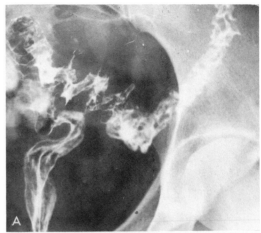

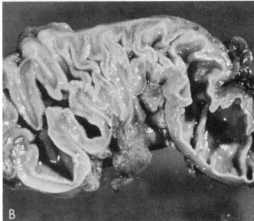

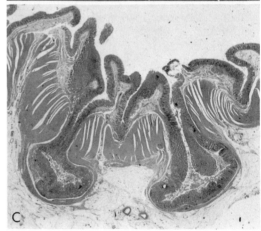

Figure 106–1. Spastic colon diverticulosis. *A,* Diverticula and interhaustral folds are demonstrated on the postevacuation film of a barium enema. *B,* The gross surgical specimen of the sigmoid colon reveals the corrugated thickened muscles, luminal narrowing, and "chamber formation" (see section on pathogenesis). *C,* A histological section shows thickened circular muscles, redundant mucosa, and two diverticula which have herniated between the enlarged muscles. (From Fleischner, F. G.: Gastroenterology 60:316, 1971.)

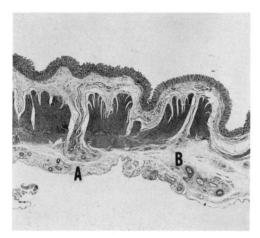

Figure 106–2. Gaps between the enlarged circular muscle are indicated at A and B where herniations of the mucosa have previously occurred but are now reduced. (From Fleischner, F. G.: Gastroenterology 60:316, 1971.)

dissections are performed at postmortem examination.[15] Careful histological studies in the colons of these patients sometimes demonstrate gaps in the muscular wall through which the reducible herniations have passed (Fig. 106–2). Thus diverticula may not be fixed. Conversely, the diverticula may burrow along the wall of the colon intramuscularly, making them difficult to demonstrate at operation and often impossible to visualize by barium enema. In the prediverticular state diverticula are not seen radiographically; at necropsy there is thickening of the colonic musculature, but no diverticula are present.

Diverticulitis. The correlation of clinical, radiological, and pathological studies has revised the classic concept of an inflamed diverticulum. Diverticulitis has been equated with appendicitis, in that it was assumed that narrowing of the neck of a diverticulum with subsequent retention of inspissated fecal material resulted in ulceration, inflammation, and formation of a retention abscess. However, if radiological and pathological studies are performed on patients who have had clinical evidence of diverticulitis (fever, elevated white blood count, and localized tenderness in the abdomen), it is apparent that clinical diverticulitis is the result of a perforation of diverticulum, not merely inflammation within a diverticulum.[5, 7, 14] Pathological studies therefore reveal not only acute and

chronic inflammation in the mucosa of the diverticulum, but also evidence of suppuration in the serosa, the pericolic fat, or the adjacent peritoneum. The residue may be a focus of granulation tissue, inflammatory cells, or fibrous tissue, indicating that a microperforation had occurred in the past which was localized and resolved spontaneously (Fig. 106–3). At the other end of the spectrum, one or more large peridiverticular abscesses may form. With a macroperforation, a perisigmoid abscess may be present which often surrounds the colon and occludes the lumen. Sometimes several points of communication can be demonstrated between diverticula and multiple abscesses, forming a long multiloculated channel parallel to the bowel wall.

A free perforation into the peritoneal cavity may also occur with resultant generalized peritonitis if the perforation is large enough. A peridiverticular abscess may also burrow and drain into adjacent organs (for example, the ureter, vagina, large or small intestine, bladder, or abdominal wall and cutaneous tissue), forming a fistula.

Muscular enlargement and thickening are present in up to 95 per cent of the involved colons of patients with diverticulitis.[8, 26] With recurrent or chronic diverticulitis, fibrosis of the colonic wall will

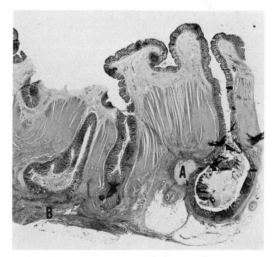

Figure 106–3. A ruptured diverticulum is present at A, where there is a small abscess adjacent to the diverticulum. At B there is extensive fibrosis beneath the diverticulum, the residue of a prior rupture of the diverticulum. (From Fleischner, F. G.: Gastroenterology 60:316, 1971.)

even develop. However, it must be re-emphasized that muscular enlargement also occurs without pathological or prior clinical evidence of inflammation.

MANOMETRIC STUDIES

Measurements of intraluminal segmental pressure of the sigmoid colon in response to certain stimuli in both normal subjects and patients with diverticula of the colon have revealed some interesting differences. In general, patients with diverticulosis have elevated intraluminal pressure responses. Using open-ended water-filled catheters placed in the sigmoid colon, Arfwidsson found that the phasic or segmental pressure waves in patients with diverticula, when recorded in the fasting state, are more frequent and have greater amplitude and duration than those of the control group.[1] Painter and Truelove performed similar measurements in the resting colon and reported that the differences between normal subjects and patients with diverticulosis were not striking (Fig. 106–4).[27, 28] There was general agreement that patients with diverticulosis generated high segmental pressures in response to certain stimuli.

After normal subjects and patients with diverticulosis ingested food, the total intraluminal sigmoid pressure (derived from the amplitude and duration of pressure waves) and the frequency of high pressure waves were increased. This increase in frequency of high pressure waves and in total intraluminal sigmoid pressure was

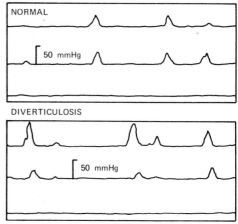

Figure 106–4. Simultaneous pressure tracings from three water-filled catheters 7.5 cm apart in the sigmoid colon in a normal subject and in a patient with diverticulosis in the fasting state. Low pressure segmental, nonpropulsive waves are seen in the normal sigmoid colon. In the tracing recorded from the patient with diverticulosis, occasional segmental pressure waves of greater than 60 mm Hg are seen, but the differences between the normal subject and the patient with diverticulosis are not significant. (Adapted from Painter, N. S., and Truelove, S. C.: Gut 5:201, 365, 1964.)

much greater in patients with diverticulosis.[1] A similar increased pressure response was demonstrated after the injection of morphine and neostigmine (prostigmin), a parasympathomimetic agent.[1, 28] As indicated in Figures 106–5 and 106–6, patients with diverticulosis developed higher segmental pressure responses than normals. It is of considerable importance that these segmental contractions could be dampened by the administration of

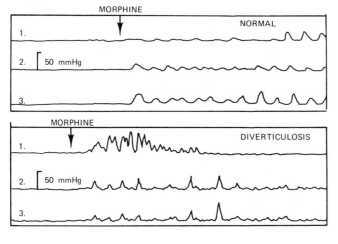

Figure 106–5. Pressure recording similar to Figure 106–4. When intravenous morphine is administered, there is an increase in the pressure of segmental waves in the sigmoid colon in a normal subject. In a patient with diverticulosis, the frequency of high pressure waves and the total pressure are much greater, especially in the first lead which is taken in the sigmoid segment containing diverticula. (Adapted from Painter, N. S., and Truelove, S. C.: Gut 5:201, 365, 1964.)

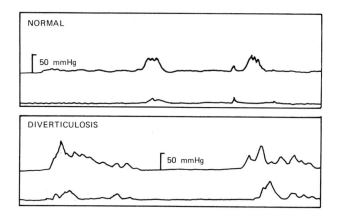

Figure 106–6. Pressure tracings recorded in a normal subject and in a patient with diverticulosis after the administration of neostigmine reveal greater segmental responses in diverticulosis. (Adapted from Painter, N. S., and Truelove, S. C.: Gut 5:201, 365, 1964.)

Demerol or an anticholinergic agent (Fig. 106–7).

Painter pointed out that these exaggerated segmental contractions were localized to certain segments of the colon (Fig. 106–5). By combining the pressure measurements with cineradiography, he found that the excessive pressure responses occurred when the tips of the catheters were located in segments of colon which contained diverticula. After the injection of morphine, the diverticula became distended with barium to an alarming degree.

Pressure studies in patients with prediverticular disease demonstrated similar elevated segmental responses.[1] These changes are very much like those recorded in patients with irritable colon[29] (p. 1281).

PATHOGENESIS

Although the pathogenesis of diverticular disease of the colon has not been elucidated, epidemiological, pathological, and

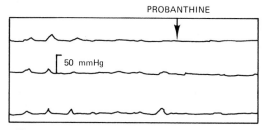

Figure 106–7. When propantheline (an anticholinergic agent) is given, the segmental response produced by intravenous morphine is inhibited. (Adapted from Painter, N. S., and Truelove, S. C.: Gut 5:201, 365, 1964.)

radiographic as well as manometric studies have provided a framework upon which several interesting theories have been constructed. Any theory must take into account several outstanding features of the disease: (1) its predominance in the sigmoid colon; (2) the muscular thickening found in many patients; (3) the abnormal pressure responses in the sigmoid colon; (4) the increasing incidence with age; and (5) the increasing incidence in Western society and rarity in underdeveloped areas of the world.

PRESSURE

In order for a herniation to occur, there must be weakness of the colonic wall and increased intraluminal pressure or a combination of the two.[4] As previously stated, diverticula appear to occur at a presumed site of weakness adjacent to the penetrating vessels between the lateral and mesenteric taeniae. This, however, does not explain why the mucosa herniates in the sigmoid colon in certain populations, or why the incidence of the disease is increasing.

The findings of muscular enlargement and elevated segmental pressure responses in the sigmoid colon strongly suggest that the factor altered is the intraluminal pressure. There is indirect evidence that both muscle and motor abnormalities precede the development of the mucosal herniations. In the prediverticular state muscular thickening and elevated segmental pressure responses are present, but the mucosa has not yet been forced through the colonic wall. Furthermore, there is the condition which might be considered intermediate between the prediverticular state and diverticulosis in which diverticula are present when intraluminal pressure is increased but disappear when the colon is not contracted. It might follow then that diverticulitis occurs when a diverticulum ruptures as a result of increased pressure. It must be pointed out that there is no evidence to support the theory that the abnormal motor pattern precedes the muscular enlargement, and whether the muscular abnormality represents true muscular hypertrophy has not yet been resolved.

If elevated intraluminal segmental pressure is the force producing herniations in the colon, then one must explain why diverticula occur most frequently in the sigmoid colon. Almy suggested that if the colon behaves like a cylinder, one might invoke Laplace's law to account for elevated intraluminal pressure in the sigmoid colon.[30] In the sigmoid colon fecal residue has been reduced to a minimum and the

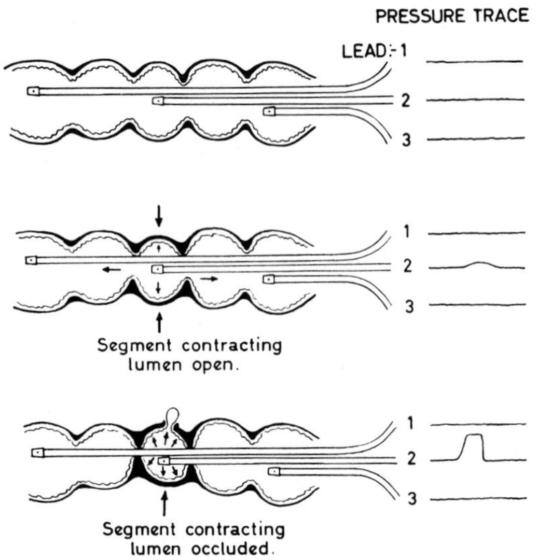

lumen is more narrow than in the proximal colon. According to Laplace's law, with a given tension (T) in the wall of a cylinder, pressure (P) is inversely related to the radius (R) of the cylinder, $P = T/R$. Therefore in the sigmoid colon with its narrow lumen, a given tension produced by the circular muscle contractions will generate higher intraluminal pressures than in the proximal colon which has a wider lumen. Herniations would then be expected to occur predominantly in the sigmoid where higher intraluminal pressures could be generated.

On the basis of pathological and radiological studies, Painter has constructed a more elaborate explanation.[27, 28] He emphasizes that the sigmoid colon normally functions in part to halt the fecal stream, thereby preserving continence and preventing constant distention of the rectum. Abnormalities in the fecal stream might require excessive segmentation in the sigmoid colon to halt the fecal stream. This segmentation, if strong enough, could isolate a segment of the colon by occluding its outflow both proximally and distally. "Little bladders" or chambers would be formed in which much higher pressures may be localized and result in mucosal herniations (Figs. 106–1 and 106–8).

DIET

In either case, there must be some factor which is altered that produces further luminal narrowing or excessive segmentation. Epidemiological and experimental data suggest that an abnormal diet is this factor.[15, 17, 27] In the United States and parts of Europe, natural fiber, roughage, has been removed from foodstuffs as a result of technological advances in food processing. This is most noticeable in food made from sugar and wheat in which the nonabsorbable cellulose component is discarded. The refined food is absorbed in large part, and a reduced fecal bulk or abnormal fecal stream enters the colon. This could cause further narrowing of the colonic lumen, excessive segmentation, a corresponding increase in intraluminal pressure, and perhaps even "work hypertrophy"[23] of smooth muscle with a resultant cycle of additional segmentation, narrowing, and elevated pressures.

The increasing incidence of diverticula in Western society therefore could be re-

Figure 106–8. Painter's diagram illustrating how excessive segmentation might produce a diverticulum. Three open-ended recording tubes in the sigmoid colon are diagrammed with the corresponding pressure tracing on the right. The upper panel illustrates that when the lumen is open, there is no increase in pressure. The middle panel reveals that partial segmentation around the second catheter causes a slight rise in pressure. In the lower panel, complete segmentation occludes the proximal and distal lumen around the second catheter, creating a "little bladder" and a greater rise in pressure and herniation of the mucosa. (From Painter, N. S.: Ann. Roy. Coll. Surg. 34:98, 1964.)

lated to the continuing refinement of foods and elimination of nonabsorbable residue. The diverticula which eventually develop proximal to the sigmoid colon could be due to attempts of the proximal colon to overcome the obstruction caused by the segmented and narrowed sigmoid. The increasing incidence with age might reflect the ravages of the low residue diets on the colon in persons between 50 and 70 years of age. The lower incidence of diverticula in underdeveloped areas of the world, particularly Africa, could be explained by the fact that the diets in these areas have a high fiber content. In fact, some of these people have colons which are large and tend to develop volvulus rather than diverticula.[15, 18]

These theories are supported by data from experiments performed in rats in which feeding of low residue diets produced narrow colons and diverticula.[31] Conversely, animals fed high residue diets did not develop herniations. However, it must be pointed out that these diverticula were single and occurred in the cecum proximal to an acute angulation in the colon. Their development may not be comparable to processes which occur in man.

EMOTION

A second possible factor which might explain the altered pressure responses is emotional tension. Increased sigmoid contractions do occur in response to psychological stress, and, as will be mentioned below, there is a striking similarity between irritable colon disease and prediverticular disease. Whatever the initiating factor, the postulated sequence of events—elevated segmental pressure, muscular enlargement, and mucosa herniation—does not take into account the substantial number of patients who have diverticulosis without muscular enlargement. In addition, there is no evidence that abnormal segmental pressures precede the muscular enlargement.

TYPES

Fleischner has proposed that diverticulosis be classified into two types on the basis of clinical, radiographic, and pathological criteria.[14, 25, 32] Spastic colon diverticulosis or myochosis refers to that category in which there is muscular thickening

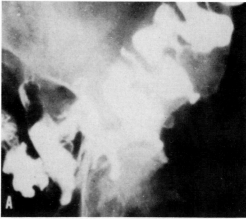

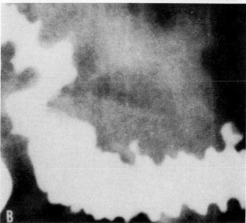

Figure 106–9. Contrast studies in two patients with spastic colon diverticulosis reveal thickened interhaustral folds, mucosal irregularity, and a sawtoothed deformity in A. In B, the muscular thickening has resulted in a serrated pattern proximally and thickened interhaustral folds distally in the sigmoid colon. (From Fleischner, F. G.: Gastroenterology 60:316, 1971.)

associated with the diverticula; irregularity, narrowing, and even a sawtoothed appearance of the bowel are often demonstrated with a barium enema examination (Fig. 106–9). A second form is called simple massed diverticulosis in which no muscular enlargement is present and radiological features consist of colonic narrowing, thin haustral folds, and frequently multiple diverticula of the descending and sigmoid colon (Fig. 106–10). Abnormalities of pressure responses in the sigmoid colon are well documented in the spastic form of the irritable colon, and radiographic and clinical features are similar to those described for diverticulosis.[4, 5, 14, 29, 33] Fleischner therefore concludes that spastic colon diverticulosis is the end re-

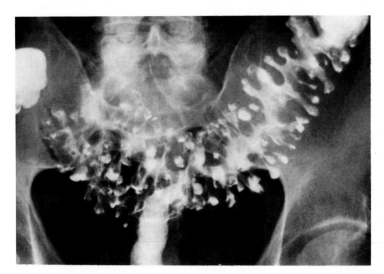

Figure 106–10. Simple massed diverticulosis. Multiple grape-like diverticula are present and the sigmoid lumen is narrow. Pathological studies in this type of diverticulosis reveal no muscular enlargement. (Courtesy of Dr. Robert Berk, Department of Radiology, University of California at San Diego.)

sult of the "spastic" variety of irritable colon.[25] It becomes apparent that this form of the irritable colon syndrome is clinically indistinguishable from the prediverticular state; only pathological studies of the colonic smooth musculature are needed to confirm this theory. Simple massed diverticulosis which is found in a substantial number of patients is considered by Fleischner to be a late sequel of the "painless diarrhea" variety of irritable colon, although there is very little evidence as yet to support this notion.

It appears that when an isolated diverticulum or many diverticula occur without associated muscle enlargement, it may be the result of an entirely different process. These herniations could develop without elevated segmental pressures. Certainly, the segmental pressure responses in this type of diverticulosis have not been studied. The enlargement of the herniations during radiographic examination when the bowel contracts suggests that increases in intraluminal pressure play some role in simple massed diverticulosis. A further definition of diverticular disease of the colon awaits the results of manometric studies in patients with diverticulosis with no muscular enlargement.

CLINICAL FEATURES

DIVERTICULOSIS

Although the majority of patients with diverticulosis have no symptoms, severe symptoms can occur in patients with diverticula which are not inflamed.[5, 12, 23] A large percentage of patients who were thought to have diverticulitis by clinical and radiological criteria were found to have no evidence of diverticulitis when the colon was examined pathologically. As a result, clinical and radiographical features previously attributed to the presence of diverticulitis have been revised (Fig. 106–9).

A patient with diverticulosis may have slight lower abdominal distress and distention or episodic and severe cramping abdominal pain. These severe symptoms are usually seen in those with spastic colon diverticulosis, and the degree of discomfort may relate to the intensity of segmentation and presence of partial obstruction of the sigmoid colon. Constipation or alternating diarrhea and constipation may accompany this pain, and the passage of stool may alleviate the lower abdominal discomfort. These symptoms are quite similar to those seen in patients with the irritable colon syndrome and are probably due to abnormalities of the colon rather than the diverticula (see pp. 1278 to 1288).

Physical examination may reveal tenderness or a loop of sigmoid in the left lower quadrant. Evidence of localized or generalized peritonitis is absent. Fever and leukocytosis do not occur in diverticulosis. Although distention may be present, there is no evidence of total colonic obstruction. Stool is usually present in the rectal ampulla, bowel sounds are active, and roentgenograms do not reveal dilated loops of small and large bowel.

When severe symptoms are associated with diverticulosis, it is termed, appropriately, painful diverticular disease. Yet this diagnosis can be made with assurance *only* when careful clinical, sigmoidoscopic and radiological examinations have excluded other diseases that could produce these symptoms.

Bleeding in Diverticulosis. Bleeding of varying degrees may occur from diverticula, particularly in elderly patients. Although it probably results from erosion of penetrating vessels adjacent to a diverticulum, it is unusual to document bleeding coming from a diverticulum either at laparotomy or by pathological study.[11, 34-36] On rare occasions, sigmoidoscopic examination will reveal bleeding from a hernia sac low in the sigmoid, but the expected finding is fresh blood coming from the more proximal colon.[36] No predisposing factors for these episodes have been identified. Gross bleeding in small quantities may frequently be associated with diverticulitis. In such cases blood loss is usually minimal, and the signs and symptoms of intra-abdominal inflammation are the predominant symptoms.

Treatment of Diverticulosis. In the past, the classic measures for management of diverticulosis have been the low residue diet and mineral oil. Present evidence indicates that neither of these measures has any theoretical basis to support its use and certainly neither has been demonstrated to be clinically efficacious. Instead, our understanding of the pathogenesis dictates that treatment should be directed toward increasing the bulk in the diet so that a greater residue reaches the distal colon. In this manner, it is hoped that further narrowing of the colon and excessive segmentation with abnormal rises in intraluminal pressures can be prevented. This objective may be accomplished with the institution of high residue diets containing fruits and vegetables and with the administration of other substances which increase the bulk of the stools such as products containing hemicellulose or psyllium seeds. By this means, the stools will become not only larger and formed, but soft and easily passed. Because of the folklore and tradition surrounding the injurious effect of high residue diets, many physicians and patients are loath to recommend or accept such a program. It is very important, when one initiates a high residue regimen, that the physician explain to the patient how a large fecal bulk widens the colon and could prevent the further development of diverticula and its complications. Indeed, no matter how forcefully and positively a physician institutes such a diet, prior conditioning of the patient may be such that foods containing high fiber content may cause discomfort. This reaction may be due to intolerances to specific ingredients of the diet, or, more likely, to a psychologically conditioned response. Some physicians find that a modification of such a program, with exclusion of foods containing seeds and the interdiction of uncooked fruits and vegetables, is more acceptable to the patient and yet perhaps less efficacious. Certainly purgatives, medication such as mineral oil, bile salt derivatives, other colonic irritants, and foods which cause watery diarrhea should be avoided.

Treatment of Painful Diverticular Disease. As mentioned previously, anticholinergics inhibit segmental contractions in the sigmoid colon and therefore may reduce the severe cramping pain which can occur in diverticulosis. Belladonna, atropine, or a synthetic agent like propantheline may be given by mouth two or three times a day, just before or with meals. Caution should be observed when the patient has constipation; glaucoma and prostatism are contraindications to their usage. Frequently, administration of phenobarbital, 32 to 64 mg two or three times a day, or Valium or Librium, 5 mg two or three times a day, will be helpful in the anxious patient, although these agents have no specific pharmacological action on the bowel itself and should not be used routinely. Morphine should be avoided even when the patient complains of severe pain, because it increases segmental pressures and might aggravate the clinical situation. Demerol is more acceptable, because studies of colonic pressures show that it inhibits segmental contractions. Initially the patient may have to be given nothing by mouth, because feeding, like morphine, stimulates increased segmental pressures. Within a few days the patient's symptoms generally subside and a high residue diet should be instituted.

Surgery for Diverticular Disease. In the past several years sigmoid colectomy has been utilized for the treatment of intractable, painful diverticular disease with satisfactory results.[1] More recently, a myotomy over the affected area of the colon has been advocated.[37] The reported results are good to excellent, with a low operative mortality and a follow-up period of satisfactory duration. Surgery, however, is rarely required for this condition, because it is well managed in the vast majority of patients with the medical and dietary approach outlined above.

Treatment of Bleeding in Diverticulosis. Bleeding from a diverticulum is usually mild; in 95 per cent of patients it stops spontaneously even when it is massive.[38] With laparotomy, the likelihood of finding the bleeding site is small, the mortality rate is high, and the incidence of recurrent hemorrhage is not significantly reduced unless a subtotal colectomy is performed. Therefore when confronted with a patient with rectal bleeding and known diverticulosis, one should transfuse the patient to maintain adequate circulating volumes, perform a sigmoidoscopy and barium enema to ensure that another lesion is not the source of hemorrhage, and wait for the bleeding to stop. Surgery should be reserved for that small group of patients who have significant bleeding which persists, or those patients who have recurrent life-threatening hemorrhage.

Selective visceral angiography has been used to localize bleeding in patients with diverticulosis (Fig. 106–11).[39] It has been estimated that bleeding of the rate of 0.5 ml per minute is necessary in order for contrast material to be visualized in the lumen of the gastrointestinal tract.[40] It is likely that in the hands of an experienced angiographer, selective arteriography will be the most accurate and successful method of localizing bleeding in patients with diverticulosis, and will allow the surgeon to perform a more limited resection without fear of recurrent bleeding. Casarella, Kanter, and Seaman were successful in demonstrating the bleeding point in 18 of 27 patients with acute rectal bleeding with emergency selective arteriography. It is important to note that 12 of the 13 that were secondary to diverticulosis were located to the right of the splenic flexure.[24a]

DIVERTICULITIS

As mentioned previously, diverticulitis is a complication of diverticulosis in which micro- or macroperforation of a diverticu-

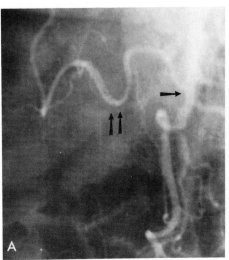
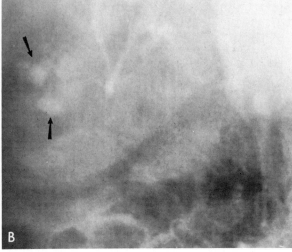

Figure 106–11. Angiographic localization of bleeding from a diverticulum. A superior mesenteric arteriogram in a patient with rectal bleeding. In *A*, the early arterial phase, the right colic branch is seen coming off the superior mesenteric artery (arrows). In the venous phase, *B*, several collections of contrast media are present in the ascending colon near the hepatic flexure (arrows). (From Reuter, S. R., and Bookstein, J. J.: Gastroenterology *54*:876, 1968.)

lum has taken place. The clinical symptoms which result from this pericolitis or peridiverticulitis are predominantly pain and fever. Pain is usually the most prominent symptom and is most frequently constant and localized in the lower abdomen, particularly in the left lower quadrant — so-called left-sided appendicitis. The patient may complain of fever or even chills. In fact, fever may be the only clinical manifestation of diverticulitis. The pericolitis or a pericolonic abscess frequently causes ileus or partial or complete colonic obstruction, with secondary abdominal distention, anorexia, and nausea.

The severity of the clinical symptoms and physical signs is influenced by the length of the colon involved and the extent of the peridiverticular inflammation. Since the process may quickly involve the serosal surface and its peritoneal cover, the patient is usually found to have marked tenderness, both direct and rebound, even without widespread peritonitis. Palpation of the abdomen may often reveal a tender mass. Rectal examination will often be painful if a loop of inflamed bowel is reached or if the patient has developed a pelvic abscess.

The results of laboratory examination almost invariably reveal a leukocytosis with an increase in polymorphonuclear leukocytes. Frequently these patients have red cells or white cells in the urine owing to contiguous involvement of the bladder or left ureter by a pericolic abscess. This may result in ureteral obstruction and signs and symptoms of left hydronephrosis and pyelonephritis. In older individuals and patients receiving steroids, many of these signs, symptoms, and laboratory values may be normal.

The diagnosis of diverticulitis is strongly suspected when a patient with known diverticulosis has fever, leukocytosis, and signs of pericolic and peritoneal inflammation in the left lower quadrant, particularly if a mass is palpated. However, despite the discomfort to the patient, sigmoidoscopy should be performed, using no air, to rule out other conditions as discussed below. Usually a normal rectum and sigmoid are visualized. Roentgenograms of the abdomen may be normal. With complete sigmoid obstruction, air may be absent in the rectum and the proximal colon may be distended with air. If the small bowel is directly involved, a characteristic picture of small bowel obstruction may be seen. Air under the diaphragm or free air in the abdominal cavity indicates a rupture of the diverticulum into the peritoneal cavity without localization.

Most experienced clinicians and radiologists advise that a barium enema is contraindicated in the acute phase of diverticulitis, because the increased intraluminal pressure exerted by the barium column may further complicate the perforated diverticulum. The signs and symptoms of inflammation will usually subside in a few days with treatment, and a

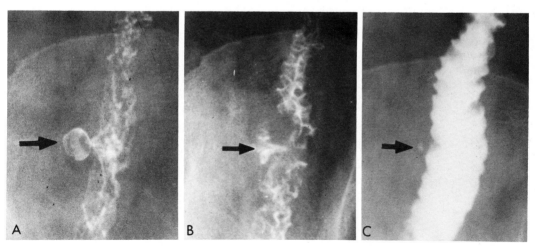

Figure 106–12. A diverticulum is present in the descending colon (A); eight months later (B), during an attack of diverticulitis, barium is demonstrated outside the diverticulum. After recovery (C), a persistent fleck of barium is seen. (From Fleischner, F. G.: Gastroenterology 60:316, 1971.)

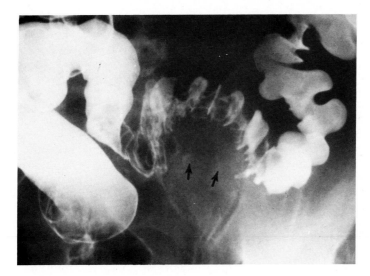

Figure 106–13. A paracolic mass which deforms and displaces the sigmoid lumen is delineated in a patient with diverticulitis and a palpable left lower quadrant mass. (Courtesy of Dr. Robert Berk, Department of Radiology, University of California at San Diego.)

barium enema can then be performed safely. As previously noted, features such as irregularity, thickening, and even a saw-toothed appearance of the bowel contour can be seen in the spastic type of diverticulosis and are not diagnostic of diverticulitis (Fig. 106–9). The only roentgenographic features characteristic of diverticulitis are the presence of barium outside a diverticulum (Fig. 106–12), the delineation of a paracolic mass (Fig. 106–13), or the demonstration of a fistula originating in the colon. The latter two abnormalities can also be seen with other entities such as carcinoma or inflammatory bowel disease. In all patients with diverticulitis it is wise to evaluate the urinary tract by intravenous pyelography in order to discover asymptomatic urinary tract obstruction.

COMPLICATIONS OF DIVERTICULITIS

Fistulas. Pericolic abscesses may burrow or rupture into neighboring organs, i.e., the urinary tract, vagina, adjacent bowel, and even the abdominal wall and skin. Thus symptoms which occur will depend upon which organ is affected. Vesicocolic fistula occurs primarily in men, because there are no intervening vagina and uterus. Recurrent urinary tract infections, chronic cystitis, and pneumaturia are the hallmarks of this complication. Intravenous pyelography, cystoscopy, or a

barium enema may confirm the presence of a vesicocolic fistula (Fig. 106–14). It may be difficult to distinguish this fistula from one which occurs secondary to a rectal carcinoma, because inflammation may render the bowel wall rigid. A colovaginal fistula results in the passage of air or feces through the vagina and may be diagnosed with rectal or vaginal examination or sometimes with a barium enema. An enterocolonic fistula may result in diarrhea or steatorrhea if significant absorbing surface of the small bowel is bypassed, if bile salt depletion results from terminal ileal bypass, or if significant anaerobic colonic bacteria colonize the upper small intestine.

Intra-abdominal Abscess. Diverticulitis may lead to large collections of pus adjacent to the bowel, in the pelvis, or under the diaphragm. Persistent temperature elevation in patients whose acute episode has subsided should immediately raise the possibility of an unresolved intra-abdominal abscess. Frequently, careful evaluation will reveal the site of the abscess, e.g., a high fixed diaphragm with a subdiaphragmatic abscess, a tender mass felt on rectal or vaginal examination with a pelvic abscess.

Generalized Peritonitis. Perforation of a diverticulum which is not promptly sealed off may cause generalized peritonitis. When there is diffuse spread of bacteria and other fecal material the symptoms are usually dramatic. Diffuse abdominal pain and distention are the usual

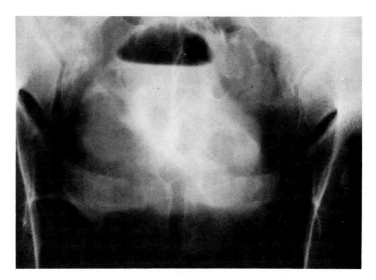

Figure 106–14. An upright film of the bladder made during an intravenous pyelogram performed in a patient with pneumaturia reveals air in the bladder and confirms the presence of a vesicocolic fistula. (Courtesy of Dr. Robert Berk, Department of Radiology, University of California at San Diego.)

presenting complaints. The diagnosis of peritonitis is confirmed by the finding on physical examination of fever and diffuse rebound tenderness, the absence of bowel sounds, boardlike rigidity, and often shock. Radiographically, one may find ileus or free air. Any elderly individual who is known to have diverticulosis and develops peritonitis should be suspected of having a ruptured diverticulum.

DIFFERENTIAL DIAGNOSIS OF DIVERTICULOSIS AND DIVERTICULITIS

Diverticulosis and Diverticulitis. Episodes of pain caused by diverticulosis may be difficult to distinguish from those of diverticulitis. When abdominal distention, marked local tenderness, and a palpable sigmoid loop are present in diverticulosis (painful diverticular disease), they can be mistaken for an inflammatory mass secondary to diverticulitis. As previously noted, the demonstration by barium enema of an irregular luminal contour, a narrowed sigmoid, and even a sawtoothed appearance of the mucosa can occur in diverticulosis; the presence of barium outside a diverticulum, a fistula, and evidence of a mass are the features seen only in diverticulitis. The presence of fever, leukocytosis, and signs of peritoneal irritation should exclude the possibility of uncomplicated diverticulosis.

Carcinoma of the Colon. Since diverticulitis often causes luminal narrowing with partial or complete bowel obstruction and is frequently associated with mild rectal bleeding, it is often difficult to distinguish diverticulitis from carcinoma of the colon. In addition, perforation may also occur with colonic malignancies, and the roentgenographic appearance may be identical to diverticulitis. The presence of localized tenderness, leukocytosis, and fever supports the diagnosis of diverticulitis, whereas chronic rectal bleeding and weight loss more often accompany a carcinoma. This distinction is obscured when diverticulitis develops in a patient with colonic carcinoma. A tumor may sometimes be diagnosed by biopsy through a sigmoidoscope. A barium enema examination may reveal a mass, luminal irregularities, and partial obstruction in both carcinoma and diverticulitis (Fig. 106–15).

Once the signs and symptoms of obstruction and inflammation subside, a repeat barium enema may reveal marked improvement in a patient with only diverticulitis. Should a suspicious defect persist, even in the presence of diverticulitis, exploration and resection will be necessary to differentiate carcinoma from diverticulitis.

Granulomatous Colitis. Differentiating diverticulitis from granulomatous colitis when there are marked luminal narrowing or multiloculated channels parallel to the bowel wall may be difficult (pp. 1362 to

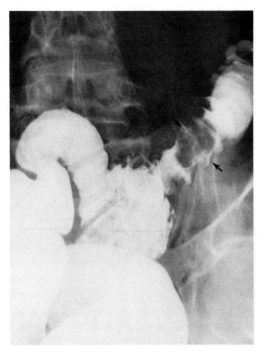

Figure 106–15. A mass is seen in the sigmoid colon of a patient recovering from an attack of acute diverticulitis. Radiographically, a tumor could not be excluded. This mass subsequently was found to be a mural abscess secondary to a perforated diverticulum. (Courtesy of Dr. Robert Berk, Department of Radiology, University of California at San Diego.)

1363).[41, 42] Clinically both may manifest pain, partial obstruction, a lower abdominal mass, rectal bleeding, fever, and leukocytosis. Sigmoidoscopic and barium enema examinations are quite helpful in making the distinction, but, as with carcinoma, diverticulitis may occur in association with granulomatous colitis. The principal radiographic features which distinguish granulomatous colitis are cobblestoning, long intramucosal sinus tracts, and skip areas (see Figs. 103–5, 103–6, and 103–7).

Ulcerative Colitis. Severe bleeding from diverticulosis can be distinguished from ulcerative colitis by the finding of a normal mucosa on sigmoidoscopy and the absence of the typical features of ulcerative colitis on barium enema.

Ischemic Colitis. Severe rectal bleeding in the elderly may result from ischemic colitis. In addition, signs and symptoms of bowel necrosis with peritonitis and sepsis may simulate diverticulitis. The characteristic finding with a barium enema of thumbprinting, especially in the area of the splenic flexure, is often critical for this diagnosis. Since ischemic colitis and diverticulitis occur in the aged, concomitant evidence of vascular disease may not be helpful in distinguishing the two. However, a hypercoagulable state or evidence of prior hypotension or decreased cardiac output may predispose to bowel ischemia (pp. 1569 to 1571).

TREATMENT OF DIVERTICULITIS

Uncomplicated Diverticulitis. Therapeutic maneuvers for acute diverticulitis are directed toward "resting" the colon and combating infection so that inflammation, edema, and spasm will subside and obstruction, if present, will be relieved. The patient is given nothing orally. If nausea, vomiting, and abdominal distention are present, nasogastric suction is instituted. An appropriate combination of parenteral antibiotics must be administered to cover the normal bowel flora, including gram-positive cocci, *Escherichia coli,* and anaerobic Bacteroides. Penicillin, ampicillin or cephalothin, and tetracycline are usually adequate with a localized infection, but in cases of peritonitis or septicemia, kanamycin or gentamicin should be added. Tetracycline or chloramphenicol is necessary in either case to cover Bacteroides (p. 416). Appropriate intravenous replacement therapy is given to maintain intravascular volume, urine output, electrolyte balance, and caloric requirements.

An intravenous pyelogram should be performed early if there is clinical or laboratory evidence of urinary tract infection or left ureteral obstruction. The patient should be observed carefully with frequent abdominal examinations and appropriate roentgenograms of the abdomen so that complications such as peritonitis or an enlarging abscess can be detected early. In all instances, surgical consultation should be obtained early, because surgical intervention may be required at any time, and the surgeon's evaluation will be vital in future decisions of therapy.

As the diverticulitis subsides in response to therapy, local peritoneal signs will recede, distention will lessen, and fever and leukocytosis will abate. Long-term therapy is identical to that outlined for diverticulosis, i.e., it should be directed toward increasing the residue in the diet, because there is no evidence that various nonabsorbable substances irritate or obstruct diverticula and result in inflammation.

Surgical Therapy. Surgical intervention will be necessary if initially there is evidence of generalized peritonitis or in the course of treatment there is evidence of failure of medical therapy.[43, 44] Failure of medical therapy is signaled by the enlargement of a previously noted mass, the development of a tender mass, increasing or persistent intestinal obstruction, the development of a fistula, or generalized peritonitis. Since the most dreaded complication is septic peritonitis caused by rupture of a pericolic abscess, medical management of such an abscess is justified only as long as there is prompt and progressive resolution. If an intra-abdominal abscess progresses rapidly to generalized peritonitis with septic shock, surgical drainage should await only rapid attempts to stabilize the patient's condition. However, if peritonitis is confined to the left lower quadrant, some patients can be managed with medical therapy for 24 to 48 hours, and if definite evidence of resolution occurs, emergency surgery can be avoided.

Indications for elective surgery are recurrent attacks of diverticulitis and the inability to exclude a carcinoma as the cause of narrowing or deformity of the colon. Some authorities suggest that elective surgery be performed in patients younger than 50 years old with diverticulitis and in any patients with dysuria.[44]

An increasing number of surgeons advocate primary resection of the inflamed sigmoid and an end-to-end anastomosis of the colon in a one-stage procedure.[22, 45] A high rate of significant complications, severe peritonitis, and difficulty in detecting the presence of a carcinoma limit the applicability of this approach to patients in whom there is no significant obstruction and the inflammatory process is confined.[44, 46] The safest surgical approach is the three-stage procedure: (1) proximal colostomy, drainage of abscesses, and closure of perforations; (2) resection of diseased colon after inflammation has subsided; and (3) closure of the colostomy at a later date.[44]

The mortality rate of surgical intervention for diverticulitis varies according to the age group, associated illnesses, and, most important, the point in the course of the disease at which surgery is performed. Overall surgical mortality is reported to be 5 to 6 per cent.[43, 44] Seventy-five per cent of those who die during or after surgery are over the age of 60. Elective surgery is attended by a lower mortality rate. It is no higher than for most other major abdominal procedures and is therefore advised for patients with recurrent attacks of diverticulitis or persistent symptoms which do not respond to medical management.

GIANT SIGMOID DIVERTICULA

Rarely, giant sigmoid diverticula develop and may be as large as 25 cm in diameter.[47-49] They are acquired diverticula of the pulsion type, because they contain no muscle in their wall. They are usually discovered on a plain film of the abdomen because they frequently fill with air or by barium enema examination, although they may not fill with barium. Physical examination may reveal a soft, occasionally tender lower abdominal mass which may be palpable only intermittently. Volvulus of the diverticulum with acute pain and signs of inflammation may develop. If the patient has symptoms referable to the giant diverticulum, sigmoid resection is indicated and pathological studies may reveal that fibrous and granulation tissue have replaced normal mucosa.

CECAL DIVERTICULA

One or more diverticula are found in the cecum in 2 to 12 per cent of colons examined.[26, 32, 50] Only about 5 per cent of these cecal diverticula occur as isolated abnormalities; the remaining 95 per cent occur in association with left-sided diverticulosis or only muscular enlargement of the sigmoid colon. The vast majority of cecal diverticula are false diverticula, because they do not contain the outer muscular layers in their walls. When isolated cecal diverticula are found in the absence of abnormalities of the left colon, it is possible that motor abnormalities in the sigmoid colon are not related to their formation.

Clinically, the majority of cecal diverticula are asymptomatic. However, they can masquerade as acute appendicitis when diverticulitis develops; in some instances, melena or even massive hemorrhage can occur from a cecal diverticulum. When cecal diverticulitis ensues, it is difficult to treat the patient medically, because the possibility of acute appendicitis cannot be excluded. At laparotomy, when cecal diverticulitis is found, abscesses should be drained and usually a right hemicolectomy performed.[5]

REFERENCES

1. Arfwidsson, F.   Pathogenesis of multiple diverticula of the sigmoid colon in diverticular disease. Acta Chir. Scand. (Suppl.) *342*:1, 1964.
2. Spriggs, E. I., and Marxer, O. A.   Multiple diverticula of colon. Lancet 2:1067, 1927.
3. Case, J. T.   Diagnosis and treatment of colonic diverticula. Amer. J. Surg. *4*:573, 1928.
4. Edwards, H.   Diverticula and Diverticulitis of the Intestine. Bristol, John Wright and Sons, Ltd., 1939.
5. Fleischner, F. G.   Diverticular disease and the irritable colon syndrome. *In* Alimentary Tract Roentgenology, Vol. 2, A. R. Margulis and H. J. Burhenne (eds.). St. Louis, C. V. Mosby Co., 1967, p. 784.
6. Fleischner, F. G., and Ming, S. C.   Revised concepts of diverticular disease of colon. II. So-called diverticulitis: Diverticular sigmoiditis and perisigmoiditis; diverticular abscess, fistula and frank peritonitis. Radiology *84*:599, 1965.
7. Wolf, B. S., Khilnani, M., and Marshak, R. H.   Diverticulosis and diverticulitis: Roentgen findings and their interpretation. Amer. J. Roent. *177*:726, 1957.
8. Hughes, L. E.   Postmortem survey of diverticular disease of the colon. I. Diverticulosis and diverticulitis. II. The muscular abnormality in the sigmoid colon. Gut *10*:336, 344, 1969.
9. Manousos, O. N., Truelove, S. C., and Lumsden, K.   Prevalence of colonic diverticulosis in the general population of Oxford area. Brit. Med. J. *3*:762, 1967.
10. Parks, T. G.   Natural history of diverticular disease of the colon: A review of 521 cases. Brit. Med. J. *4*:639, 1969.
11. Slack, W. W.   The anatomy, pathology and some clinical features of diverticulitis of the colon. Brit. J. Surg. *50*:185, 1962.
12. Morson, B. C.   The muscle abnormality in diverticular disease of the sigmoid colon. Brit. J. Radiol. *36*:385, 1963.
13. Horner, J. L.   Natural history of diverticulosis of the colon. Amer. J. Dig. Dis. *3*:343, 1958.
14. Fleischner, F. G., Ming, S. C., and Henken, E. M.   Revised concepts of diverticular disease of colon. I. Diverticulosis: Emphasis on tissue derangement and its relation to irritable colon syndrome. Radiology *83*:859, 1964.
15. Painter, N. S.   Diverticular disease of the colon – a disease of Western civilization. Disease-A-Month. Chicago, Year Book Medical Publishers, June 1970.
16. Reilly, M.   The surgical treatment of diverticulitis. Hosp. Med., 1088, September 1967.
17. Cleave, T. L., Campbell, G. D., and Painter, N. S.   Diabetes, Coronary Thrombosis, and the Saccharine Diseases, 2nd ed. Bristol, John Wright and Sons, Ltd., 1969.
18. Wells, C.   Diverticula of the colon. Brit. J. Radiol. *22*:449, 1949.
19. Drummond, H.   Sacculi of the large intestine, with special reference to their relations to the blood vessel of the bowel wall. Brit. J. Surg. *4*:407, 1917.
20. Noer, R. J.   Hemorrhage as a complication of diverticulitis. Ann. Surg. *141*:674, 1955.
21. Slack, W. W.   Diverticula of the colon and their relation to the muscular layers and blood vessels. Gastroenterology *39*:708, 1960.
22. Keith, A.   Diverticula of the alimentary tract of congenital or of obscure origin. Brit. Med. J. *1*:376, 1910.
23. Morson, B. C.   The muscle abnormality in diverticular disease of the colon. Proc. Roy. Soc. Med. *56*:798, 1963.
24. Slack, W. W.   Bowel muscle in diverticular disease. Gut *7*:668, 1966.
24a. Casarella, W. J., Kanter, I. E., and Seaman, W. B.   Right-sided colonic diverticula as a cause of acute rectal hemorrhage. New Eng. J. Med. *286*:450, 1972.
25. Fleischner, F. G.   Diverticular disease of the colon. New observations and revised concepts. Gastroenterology *60*:316, 1971.
26. Miangolarra, C. J.   Diverticulitis of the right colon. Ann. Surg. *153*:861,1961.
27. Painter, N. S.   The etiology of diverticulosis of the colon with special reference to the action of certain drugs on behavior of the colon. Ann. Roy. Coll. Surg. *34*:98, 1964.
28. Painter, N. S., and Truelove, S. C.   Potential dangers of morphine in acute diverticulitis of the colon. Brit. Med. J. *2*:33, 1963.
29. Chaudhary, H. A., and Truelove, S. C.   Human colonic motility: A comparative study of normal subjects, patients with ulcerative colitis, and patients with the irritable colon syndrome. Gastroenterology *40*:1, 1961.
30. Almy, T. P.   Diverticular disease of the colon: The new look. Gastroenterology *49*:109, 1965.
31. Carlson, A. J., and Hoelzel, F.   Relation of diet to diverticulosis of the colon in rats. Gastroenterology *12*:108, 1949.
32. Smithwick, R. H.   Experiences with the surgical management of diverticulitis of the sigmoid. Ann. Surg. *115*:969, 1942.
33. Williams, I.   Changing emphasis in diverticular disease of the colon. Brit. J. Radiol. *36*:393, 1963.

34. Quinn, W. C. Gross hemorrhage from presumed diverticulosis of the colon. Ann. Surg. *153*:851, 1961.

35. Rosenberg, I. K., and Rosenberg, B. F. Massive hemorrhage from diverticula of the colon with demonstration of the source of bleeding. Ann. Surg. *159*:570, 1964.

36. Smith, N. D. Diverticulosis and diverticulitis. Amer. J. Surg. *82*:585, 1951.

37. Reilly, M. Sigmoidmyotomy. Brit. J. Surg. *53*:859, 1966.

38. Rigg, B. M., and Ewing, M. R. Current attitudes on diverticulitis with particular reference to colonic bleeding. Arch. Surg. *92*:321, 1966.

39. Reuter, S. R., and Bookstein, J. J. Angiographic localization of gastrointestinal bleeding. Gastroenterology *54*:876, 1968.

40. Nusbaum, M., and Baum, S. Radiographic demonstration of unknown sites of gastrointestinal bleeding. Surg. Forum *14*:374, 1963.

41. Schmidt, G. T., Lennard-Jones, J. E., Morson, B. C., and Young, A. C. Crohn's disease of the colon and its distinction from diverticulitis. Gut *9*:7, 1968.

42. Marshak, R., Janowitz, H. O., and Present, D. Granulomatous colitis in association with diverticulitis. New Eng. J. Med. *283*:1080, 1970.

43. Asch, M. J., and Markowitz, A. M. Diverticulosis coli: A surgical appraisal. Surgery *62*:239, 1967.

44. Rodkey, G. V., and Welch, C. E. Diverticulitis of the colon. Evolution in concept and therapy. Surg. Clin. N. Amer. *45*:1231, 1965.

45. Ryan, P. Acute diverticulitis and diverticulitis with perforation. Med. J. Austral. *2*:51, 1964.

46. Smithwick, R. H. Surgical treatment of diverticulitis of the sigmoid. Amer. J. Surg. *99*:192, 1960.

47. Bergeron, R. B., and Hanley, P. H. Giant sigmoid diverticulum. Amer. J. Surg. *109*:5, 1965.

48. Massachusetts General Hospital. Case 43402. New Eng. J. Med. *257*:677, 1957.

49. Silberman, E. L., and Thorner, M. C. Volvulus of giant sigmoidal diverticulum. J.A.M.A. *177*:782, 1961.

50. Goligher, J. C. Surgery of the Anus, Rectum, and Colon, 2nd ed. London, Cassell and Co., Ltd., 1967.

51. Reid, D. R. K. Acute diverticulitis of the caecum and ascending colon. Brit. J. Surg. *39*:76, 1957.

52. Painter, N. S., and Truelove, S. C. The intraluminal pressure patterns in diverticulosis of the colon. Gut *5*:201, 365, 1964.

Chapter 107

Polypoid Tumors of the Colon

John Q. Stauffer

INTRODUCTION

Tumors of the colon are extremely important in the morbidity and mortality of colonic disease.[1,2] Carcinoma of the colon continues to be the most commonly occurring carcinoma in the United States,[1,2] and has been responsible for more deaths during the past half century than any other visceral neoplasm. The physician must be alert to the signs and symptoms of colonic neoplasms, as well as to disease entities which may predispose to the development of colonic carcinoma, if progress is to be made in improving the rather dismal five-year survival rate for this disease.

This chapter will be concerned with polypoid tumors of the colon, with emphasis on the commonly occurring epithelial tumors. A distinction will be made between "glandular" adenomas and "villous" adenomas. The relationship of both these neoplasms to the pathogenesis of adenocarcinoma will be considered in detail. Whether epithelial polyps consistently undergo malignant transformation remains controversial. In patients with familial polyposis and Gardner's syndrome, the presence of multiple polyps clearly augurs the development of colonic adenocarcinoma. These entities are discussed on pages 1051 to 1059. Sufficient evidence is available, however, to provide the clinician with some guidelines for the management of patients with single or multiple epithelial polyps.

Malignant neoplasms of the rectum and colon are discussed on pages 1445 to 1461. Polypoid lesions such as hemangiomas, neurofibromas, lipomas, and leiomyomas will be mentioned briefly in this discussion. The so-called hyperplastic mucosa is included in the differential diagnosis of epithelial polyps. The hamartomas of the familial-hereditary syndromes such as generalized juvenile polyposis, the Peutz-Jeghers syndrome, and the Cronkhite-Canada syndrome are discussed on pages 1051 to 1059.

POLYPS

Epithelial tumors of the colon have been collectively called polyps, a rather imprecise term. Broadly defined, a polyp is any mass of tissue which protrudes into the lumen of the bowel; it may originate from either the mucosa or the submucosa. The adenomatous polyp or epithelial tumor, which is a localized proliferation of the colonic mucosa, is a distinct entity, neoplastic in nature, and must be distinguished from either inflammatory or hamartomatous polyps. Hamartomas are tumor-like malformations composed of an abnormal mixture of the normal constituents of an organ or tissue. Thus a variety of mesenchymal elements may be present, including fibrous, adipose, myxomatous, and muscle tissues (Table 107–1). Inflammatory and hamartomatous polyps do not have any malignant potential.

1432

TABLE 107–1. POLYPOID LESIONS OF THE COLON AND RECTUM

A. Neoplastic
   1. Epithelial
      a. Adenomatous
      b. Villous
B. Hamartomas (mixed mesodermal tumor, including fibrous, adipose, myxomatous muscle, etc.)
   1. Juvenile polyps (retention polyps, congenital polyps)
   2. Peutz-Jeghers polyps
   3. Hemangiomas
      Neurofibromas
      Lipomas   } ?Neoplastic
      Leiomyomas
C. Inflammatory
   1. Ulcerative colitis or regional enteritis
   2. Dysenteries   } Have no malignant potential
   3. Benign lymphomas
D. Unclassified
   1. Hyperplastic
   2. Cystic pneumatosis

Approximately 5 per cent of the adult population have one or more polypoid lesions,[3-6] which may range in size from less than 1 cm to over 10 cm in diameter. Depending upon the histological structure of the polyp, the gross appearance ranges from smooth-surfaced to corrugated. The polyps may be sessile, separated from the mucosa by a stalk (pedunculated), or intramural. Over 80 per cent of the polyps are of epithelial origin, and most of these are located in the rectum or sigmoid colon. The vast majority of these polyps are asymptomatic.

ADENOMATOUS POLYPS

HISTOLOGY

Adenomatous polyps are localized, benign tumors of the colonic mucosa.[5, 6] Histologically, these polyps differ markedly and are considered either as predominantly glandular (Fig. 107–1) or villous (Fig. 107–2) in overall structure.

The glandular adenomas are composed of rounded masses of branching glandular tubules lined by mature, mucus-secreting goblet cells. The proliferation appears to begin in the crypts where actively dividing columnar cells form the characteristic glandular appearance. These polyps are commonly pedunculated (Fig. 107–3), al-

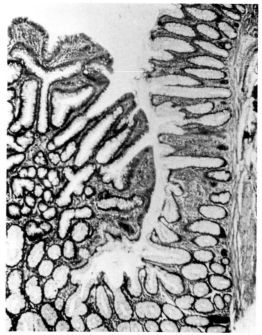

Figure 107–1. Adenomatous polyp. The glandular adenomas are composed of rounded masses of branching glandular tubules lined by mature mucus-secreting goblet cells. Occasionally, there are atypical or abnormal-appearing columnar epithelial cells which may resemble malignant cells. However, these polyps rarely undergo malignant transformation.

though they may be sessile (Fig. 107–4). Occasionally there are atypical or abnormal-appearing columnar epithelial cells which may resemble malignant cells. There may also be some dedifferentiation; for example, cessation of mucus production. However, these adenomatous polyps rarely if ever undergo malignant transformation (see below) if invasion of the stalk or bowel wall is the criterion for malignancy.

RELATIONSHIP OF ADENOMATOUS POLYPS TO CARCINOMA

For decades a rather heated debate has raged concerning the malignant potential of adenomatous polyps.[6-10] Although the question is still not completely settled,[11-14] sufficient experience has been gained to formulate a workable policy with regard to their management. The most important principle of this approach is not affected by the argument; that is, all polyps within

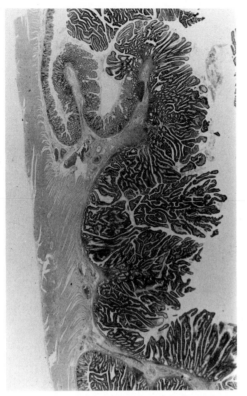

Figure 107–2. Villous adenomas consist of a loose vascular stroma covered by a single layer of epithelial cells that are taller and more basophilic than normal cells. No glands are seen. These sessile tumors have a strong tendency to undergo malignant transformation.

reach of the sigmoidoscope must be removed in toto, if possible. Since the vast majority of polyps are located in this segment of the large bowel, the question of management concerns only the remaining 20 per cent. Hence in all patients the pros and cons of removal of these proximal polyps, no matter what the size or appearance, must be critically reviewed.

The Adenoma as a Premalignant Lesion. The argument for the premalignant potential of an adenomatous polyp attached to the mucosa by a stalk is based primarily upon circumstantial evidence on the one hand and unacceptable pathological criteria on the other. The proponents for malignant potential[9, 10, 12] point to the following facts:

1. Foci of atypia in the body of the polyp are not uncommon, and atypical cells are considered by some to be a transition stage between benign and unequivocally malignant tissue.

2. Direct transformation of a benign adenomatous polyp to a malignancy often cannot be demonstrated, because with malignant degeneration the head of the polyp containing the glandular structure of the originally benign tumor has sloughed off, leaving only malignant tissue.

3. Residual benign adenomatous tissue is allegedly occasionally found around the margins of colonic and rectal cancers.

4. Second or metachronous carcinomas are found twice as frequently in specimens of carcinoma of the colon which also contain adenomatous polyps.[4, 16] Polyps adjacent to carcinomas are called sentinel polyps.

5. Some heredofamilial syndromes characterized by gastrointestinal polyposis

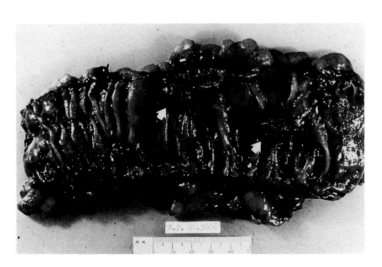

Figure 107–3. Benign adenomas are commonly pedunculated. The presence of a well defined stalk is often used as a criterion of benignancy.

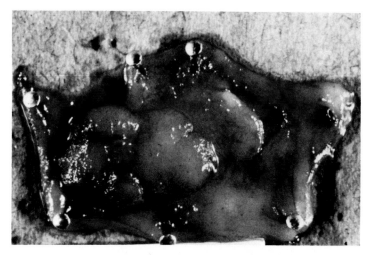

Figure 107-4. Gross specimen of a sessile adenoma. When sessile polyps are found, it is difficult clinically to decide whether or not they are malignant. The question should be settled by the pathologist, even though sessile glandular adenomas rarely undergo malignant transformation.

have a high incidence of carcinoma of the gastrointestinal tract (see pp. 1051 to 1059).[17]

6. Benign adenomatous polyps and carcinoma of the colon have been thought to have a similar anatomical distribution.

The Adenoma as a Benign Lesion. Many pathologists maintain that adenomatous polyps of the glandular type are not premalignant.[11, 13, 14] The evidence is based upon the following considerations:

1. Polyps less than 1 cm in diameter with stalks have been shown to have a less than 1 per cent possibility of containing an invasive carcinoma.[15]

2. Atypia cannot be considered to be a criterion of malignant transformation. Most pathologists agree that only invasion of the stalk by carcinoma cells can be accepted as the basis for malignant transformation. In instances in which invasion is noted, it appears that the polyp is a villous adenoma or at least a mixed villous and glandular type of polyp and not a "pure" glandular adenoma (Fig. 107-5).[12-14]

3. The anatomic distribution of adenomatous polyps and of carcinoma of the colon have not been confirmed as being the same, according to more recent and thorough studies of the subject.[11]

4. The finding of sentinel polyps and of an increased incidence of carcinoma in patients whose resected specimens contain polyps is no more than circumstantial evidence for a relationship between adenomatous polyps and carcinoma.

5. Careful reviews of small carcinomas of the sigmoid and rectum discovered incidentally reveal no evidence for the prior existence of a benign adenoma in these lesions; hence it is very likely that such polyps are polypoid carcinomas from the outset.[18] Since these cancers were un-

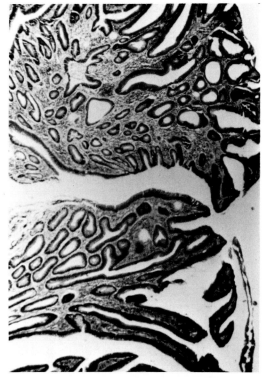

Figure 107-5. If a villous adenoma is tangentially sectioned it may have areas that have a glandular appearance. In this section there are areas that appear glandular; however, the predominant pattern is that of a villous adenoma. Perhaps it is in these so-called "mixed tumors" that confusion has arisen in attempting to define the malignant potential of epithelial tumors. Villous adenomas clearly have a strong tendency to undergo malignant degeneration.

TABLE 107–2. CHANGING CONCEPTS IN THE HISTOLOGIC DIAGNOSIS OF CANCER IN POLYPS[12-14]

1952 (WELCH ET AL.)	DIAGNOSIS	NUMBER OF PATIENTS
	Carcinoma in situ	18
	Adenocarcinoma, Grade I	18
	Adenocarcinoma, Grade II	22
	Adenocarcinoma, Grade III	1
	Colloid carcinoma	1
		60

1962 (CASTLEMAN AND KRICKSTEIN)	REVISED DIAGNOSIS	NUMBER OF PATIENTS
	Adenomatous polyp	33
	Adenomatous polyp with carcinoma	1
	Villous adenoma	4
	Villous adenocarcinoma	5
	Polypoid adenocarcinoma	14
	Not available for review	3
		60

doubtedly in various stages of their growth, and since the calculated doubling time for carcinoma of the colon varies from 34 to 210 days, it would have been reasonable to expect some residual benign tissue in some of the specimens; however, none was found.

6. Castleman and Krickstein reviewed a series of 57 cases previously reported by Welch et al.[12] as examples of the malignant transformation of benign adenomas. Thirty-three of these patients had benign adenomas without evidence of malignancy; fourteen had polypoid adenocarcinomas with no benign tissue present, even with multiple resectioning of the tissue blocks; four had villous adenomas; and five had villous adenomas containing foci of invasive carcinoma. Only one case was confirmed as a "benign glandular adenoma" with a focus of invasive carcinoma. Of the nine patients with metastatic disease, all had either villous adenomas or polypoid adenocarcinomas (Table 107–2).

As indicated at the outset of this discussion, despite disagreement and confusion, a sensible attitude can be formulated for polyps above the range of the sigmoidoscope. When larger than 1 cm in diameter, or if sessile (without regard to the size) or multiple, surgical removal is indicated. The size of the adenoma is important, because 5 per cent of those between 1 and 2 cm in diameter contain an invasive carcinoma; for those between 2 and 2.5 cm, the corresponding incidence of malignancy is approximately 10 per cent. Since the clinical distinction between benign adenomatous polyps and polypoid carcinoma can be extremely difficult if not impossible at times, all questionable lesions should be removed and the argument settled by the pathologist. This course is particularly important for the individual who has a family history of carcinoma of the colon.

As screening techniques, particularly radiographic, improve in accuracy, the incidence of asymptomatic polypoid tumors of the large bowel continues to rise. Indeed, some reports within the past decade indicate that 12.5 per cent of patients examined by barium enema with air contrast study have polyps. This coincides with an equal figure obtained from over 3000 consecutive autopsies at the same institution. This high yield, however, is probably due to the use of tannic acid in the enemas employed by these investigators.[19, 20] Reevaluation of the anatomic distribution is also in order, because some studies indicate that almost 40 per cent of polyps are located in the cecum, transverse colon, and descending colon.

VILLOUS ADENOMAS

HISTOLOGY

Villous adenomas, also known as papillary adenomas, are benign tumors which

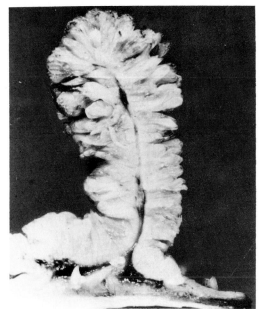

Figure 107–6. Gross specimen of a villous adenoma. Villous adenomas are rather large tumors, frequently over 6 cm. The majority are located in the rectum or sigmoid and have a rather typical cauliflower appearance. These tumors are soft and may not be detected on a routine rectal examination.

transformation is based not upon the appearance of atypical cells, but upon evidence of invasion of the bowel by tumor cells. Villous adenomas are rather large tumors, frequently over 6 cm in diameter. They are shaggy, soft, and usually sessile, although on occasion they may have well-formed stalks. The majority are located in the rectum or sigmoid and have a rather typical cauliflower-like appearance with an irregular vascular surface. Villous adenomas comprise about 5 per cent of all polyps found in the large bowel and occur equally among both sexes. Patients presenting with these tumors may be somewhat older, on the average, than those with benign adenomas. Frequently, polyps may contain elements of both benign and villous adenomas. On occasion the villous adenoma may surround the lumen of the bowel in an eccentric or circumferential manner.

Microscopically, the frond-like surface of the villous adenoma is seen to consist of projections of loose vascular stroma covered by a single layer of epithelial cells

have a strong tendency to develop into malignancies. The reported incidence of such transformation ranges from 40 to 60 per cent.[21] The diagnosis of malignant

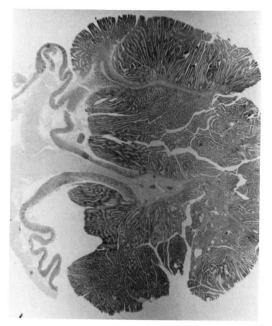

Figure 107–7. Villous adenomas, although usually sessile, may have well defined stalks.

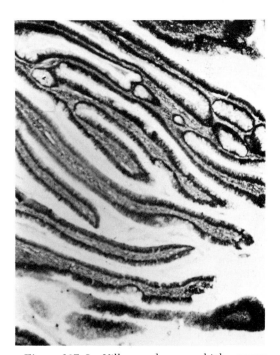

Figure 107–8. Villous adenoma, high power magnification. This specimen emphasizes the frond-like appearance of these tumors. There is a single layer of epithelial cells covering a loose vascular stroma. These cells also have an "atypical" appearance owing to the increased basophilic staining.

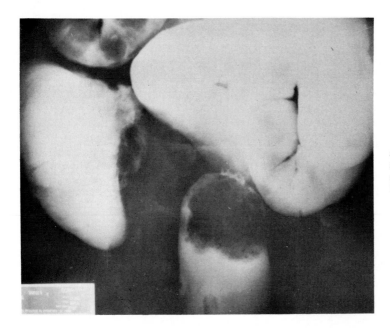

Figure 107–9. A large villous adenoma seen in the rectum. The surface is seen to be coarse and shaggy. (Courtesy of D. J. Sheft, M. D., and A. R. Margulis, M. D.)

that are taller and more basophilic than normal cells. No glands are present, and cells contain little or no mucus (Figs. 107–2 and 107–6 to 107–9).

CLINICAL PICTURE ASSOCIATED WITH POLYPS

In the majority of instances, the patient is asymptomatic when harboring benign adenomatous polyps. Vague abdominal discomfort, flatulence, or a change in bowel habits should not necessarily be attributed to polypoid lesions unless removal of the polyp eliminates these symptoms. However, a large polyp with a stalk may be the leading point for intussusception which may be transient and recurrent in the colon. The most common symptom of benign adenomas is rectal bleeding. The appearance of blood in the stool is dependent upon the distance of the polyp from the anus, the rate of bleeding, and colonic motility. Usually the blood is rather bright red and fresh in appearance; it may or may not be associated with bowel movements.

In patients with villous adenomas, additional symptoms may be noted.[21, 22] These include a rather remarkable amount of mucus passed per rectum, often unassociated with bowel movements, and occasionally sufficiently severe to lead to hypo-proteinemia, particularly hypoalbuminemia (see pp. 35 to 48). Since the mucus has a high content of protein, in effect the villous adenoma is responsible for protein-losing enteropathy. In addition, the mucus secretion contains a sufficient amount of potassium to cause hypokalemia. Rarely the patient may have sufficient diarrhea with profuse discharge of mucus that hypovolemia may result. Thus it is important that these symptoms which are associated with villous adenomas be detected and corrected by adequate replacement of fluid, protein, and electrolytes preoperatively. Since villous adenomas tend to be large, they are more prone to cause mild recurrent obstructive symptoms. However, complete obstruction or episodes sufficiently severe to necessitate laparotomy are rare.

There is no disagreement as to the malignant potential of villous adenomas. The incidence of invasive carcinoma in villous adenomas has been reported to be as high as 60 per cent.[21] A diagnosis of malignancy, however, may depend upon the number of sections examined.

DIAGNOSTIC EVALUATION OF POLYPOID LESIONS

The diagnosis of colonic polyps is made by sigmoidoscopy and barium enema with

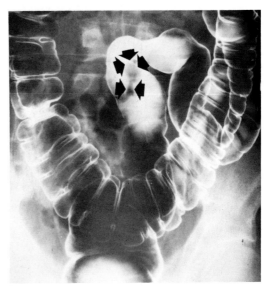

Figure 107–10. Barium enema, showing a glandular adenomatous polyp with a well defined stalk. Free movement of the polyp on the pedicle is an important sign of benignancy. A polyp should be seen on at least two studies before surgical intervention is considered. (Courtesy of D. J. Sheft, M.D., and A. R. Margulis, M.D.)

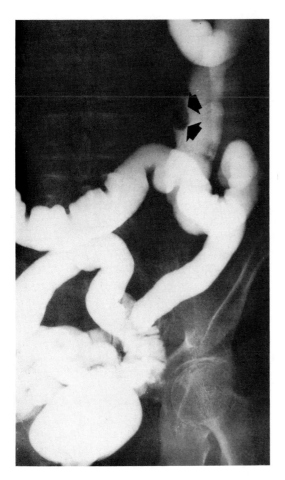

Figure 107–11. Adenomatous polyp. This barium enema X-ray should be compared with Figures 107–14, 107–15, and 107–16. This adenoma is sessile and smooth; although histologically it proved to be benign, it is difficult to be sure that it is not an adenocarcinoma. (Courtesy of D. J. Sheft, M.D., and A. R. Margulis, M.D.)

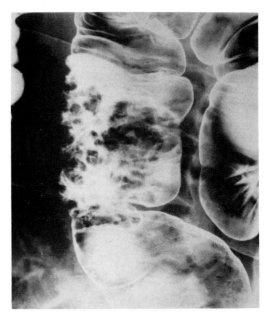

Figure 107–12. An example of the corrugated surface appearance of the villous adenoma. It is apparent that these tumors may cover a large area of bowel. (Courtesy of D. J. Sheft, M.D., and A. R. Margulis, M.D.)

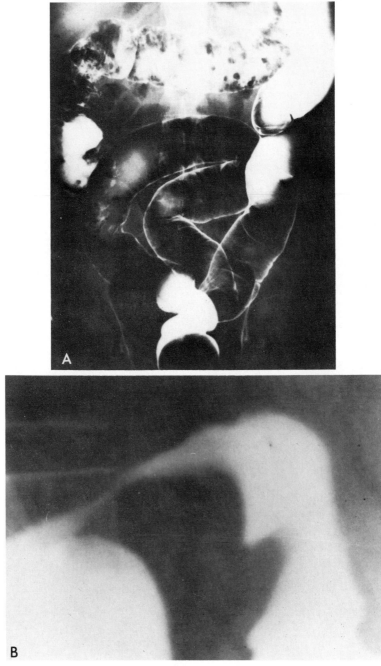

Figure 107–13.   The inflammatory polyps of ulcerative colitis may be indistinguishable from the polyps in familial polyposis. These polyps are not premalignant. In ulcerative colitis the adenocarcinomas seem to arise from atrophic mucosa and not from the inflammatory polyps. Multiple inflammatory polyps in the transverse colon are shown in A, whereas an adenocarcinoma in the splenic flexure of a patient with chronic ulcerative colitis is shown in B. The mucosal surface around the carcinoma in this case appeared atrophic, when the tumor was examined histologically.

appropriate air insufflation. Although the reported figures on the distribution of polyps in the large bowel may vary somewhat, the majority seem to be within reach of the sigmoidoscope. They are readily identified as discrete structures slightly more red or purplish-red than the underlying mucosa, often with a stalk. Frequently, benign adenomatous polyps are smooth and range from 1 to 4 cm in diameter (see Figs. 107–10 and 107–11), whereas villous adenomas tend to have a corrugated surface and to be larger (Figs. 107–9 and 107–12). Grossly benign adenomas cannot be differentiated from pseudopolyps of ulcerative colitis except that the latter do not have well defined stalks. The differential diagnosis rests upon the finding of diffuse disease of the mucosa compatible with ulcerative colitis and ultimately upon histological examination after excision (see Fig. 107–13).

Barium enema X-rays with air contrast studies will reveal the majority of polyps 1 cm or larger in diameter. Since the majority of polyps are smaller than 1 cm, it can safely be assumed that a large number are not visualized unless intensive cleansing of the colon precedes expert examination. The presence of a polyp should be confirmed on two barium enemas before surgical intervention.

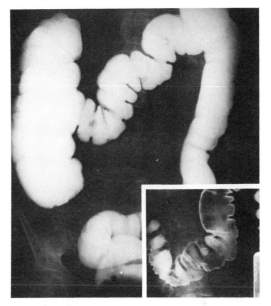

Figure 107–14. This study demonstrates a smooth, small, round polypoid lesion which appears to have a short stalk. Histologically this proved to be an adenocarcinoma. (Courtesy of D. J. Sheft, M.D., and A. R. Margulis, M.D.)

DIFFERENTIAL DIAGNOSIS

Benign adenomas and villous adenomas must be distinguished primarily from polypoid carcinomas of the colon and rectum. This differentiation is often very difficult, because polypoid adenocarcinomas may be round and smooth in appearance, and have no evidence of local invasion on X-ray and sigmoidoscopy. The principal difference between this type of malignancy and the benign adenoma is the presence of a stalk in the case of the benign adenoma, although this may also be misleading (compare Figs. 107–10 and 107–14). Differentiation between villous adenoma and carcinoma is academic, because all villous adenomas must be removed when identified. An example of the difficulty in differentiation is noted in Figure 107–15, in which a smooth, flat, polypoid tumor of the colon proved to be an adenocarcinoma on

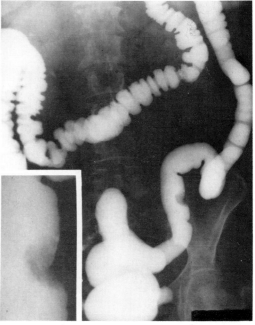

Figure 107–15. This smooth-surfaced polypoid lesion proved to be an adenocarcinoma. Compare with Figure 107–11. (Courtesy of D. J. Sheft, M.D., and A. R. Margulis, M.D.)

resection. Adenomas which are less than 1 cm in diameter and have stalks are most probably benign. Tumors with well defined stalks between 1 and 2 cm have a less than 5 per cent chance of containing an invasive carcinoma. The incidence of a polyp containing an invasive carcinoma rises to about 10 per cent for adenomas which are larger than 2 cm in diameter.

Differentiation of benign adenomas from lipomas, carcinoid tumors, circumscribed lymphoma, leiomyomas, so-called benign lymphoma, lymphangiomas, and metastatic implants of the colon from ovarian carcinomas, gastric carcinomas, or malignant melanomas may be extremely difficult, if not impossible (Fig. 107–16). The question is usually settled by surgical exploration and excision, because these tumors often tend to be large.

Differentiation of benign adenomas from so-called hyperplastic polyps of the colon and from pseudopolyps may be difficult at times. This differentiation, fortunately, is necessary only for extremely small

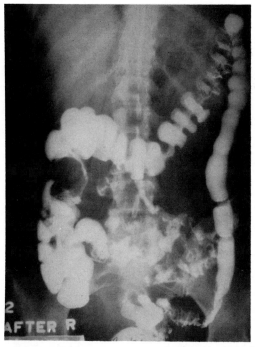

Figure 107–16. Metastatic implants in the bowel wall may look like polypoid lesions. The size of these lesions makes an extensive evaluation necessary. This is an example of an ovarian carcinoma metastatic to the colon. (Courtesy of D. J. Sheft, M. D., and A. R. Margulis, M.D.)

tumors, generally less than 5 mm in diameter. The hyperplastic polyp is not neoplastic, that is, it is not truly an adenoma or a structure in which epithelial cells have proliferated. These hyperplastic polyps have epithelial and mesenchymal characteristics of extremely well differentiated tissue, and no transition from hyperplastic to adenomatous mucosa has been found.[7, 8] The distinguishing feature is that these minute polyps have the same surface appearances as the normal adjacent mucosa; a line of demarcation between the hyperplastic polyp and its adjacent mucosa can generally be noted. The mucosa surrounding the pseudopolyps of ulcerative colitis is usually diagnostic of ulcerative colitis.

MANAGEMENT OF COLONIC AND RECTAL POLYPS

As indicated, a great debate continues to rage over guiding principles for the management of benign epithelial tumors of the colon. Despite strong convictions regarding the advisability of excision of all polyps regardless of location, shape, or attachment, general agreement is possible on many points.

Polyps greater than 1 cm in diameter, regardless of location or the presence of a stalk, should be removed if the patient's age and general condition are satisfactory for laparotomy. Since many patients, particularly in the older age groups, have benign adenomatous polyps and since the total operative mortality for what are probably benign tumors in the vast majority of instances would be higher than the currently reported mortality from carcinoma, surgical candidates must be carefully selected. Obviously, an isolated smooth polyp slightly larger than 1 cm in diameter with a stalk or even two such adenomas located above the peritoneal reflection in patients in the seventh or eighth decades of life should be managed by careful check for change in size at six-month intervals. Enlargement of the polyps would then be an indication for exploration. Each patient in the older age group must be treated individually, because the number and severity of associated medical conditions vary. A family history of carcinoma of the colon or a history of previous removal of polyps through the sigmoidoscope, particularly if they were "mixed" adenomas or villous adenomas, would certainly influence the decision.

Patients with polyps who previously have had resections for carcinoma of the colon should be subjected to polypectomy no matter what the location, because studies indicate that such individuals have a risk of a second primary carcinoma of the colon which is double that of a control population.

Polyps over 2 cm in diameter should be removed no matter what the location, because the risk of invasive carcinoma in these tumors is about 10 per cent. This dictum applies even to those polyps which have well defined stalks, unless the clinical risk for exploratory laparotomy is great.

Villous adenomas should be removed regardless of location. Even the smaller ones carry a high risk of malignancy.

All polyps within range of the sigmoidoscope, no matter what their size or appearance, should be removed.

Excision of multiple (more than two) adenomatous polyps 1 cm or less in diameter on stalks above the reach of the sigmoidoscope is recommended, although each patient must be considered individually. The question of simple removal of polyps vs. resection of colon must be settled by the attending surgeon. It is his judgment whether or not he is dealing with carcinoma, and he must often resort to the use of frozen sections. Extensive colectomy for scattered polyps is probably not a good approach; individual colotomies, with excision of polyps found, are preferable. It is not necessary to perform radical surgery for the benign, glandular type of adenoma.

It is well to remember that in older persons laparotomy and multiple colotomies increase the operative morbidity and mortality. Mortality may be as high as 5 per cent, and an equal number of patients may suffer from wound infection or postoperative complications related to associated diseases of advanced age, including particularly atherosclerosis, hypertension, and pulmonary disease.

One or two discrete adenomatous polyps with well defined stalks 1 cm or less in diameter may be followed by periodic barium enema examinations, because the likelihood of carcinoma developing in them is extremely low, less than the mortality and morbidity from laparotomy.

All patients who have had polyps removed previously should have repeat X-ray studies with air contrast at six-month to yearly intervals, because this group has a higher incidence of appearance of new polyps. In those individuals who have previously had carcinomas resected, the evidence indicates that the risk of a second malignancy is considerably higher than in control populations, and therefore removal of the newly found tumors should be undertaken if the patient's condition permits.

Polyps 1 to 2 cm in size in patients under age 50 should be excised even though they may be isolated.

HAMARTOMAS

These mixed mesodermal tumors which include fibrous, adipose, and muscle tissue are found primarily in heredofamilial syndromes, including multiple juvenile polyposis and Peutz-Jeghers polyposis; they are discussed on pages 1051 to 1059.

INFLAMMATORY AND UNCLASSIFIED POLYPS

The inflammatory pseudopolyp of ulcerative colitis or granulomatous colitis which has no malignant potential is discussed on pages 1310 and 1311. So-called benign lymphomas are mentioned briefly above. Hyperplastic polyps are considered in the discussion on adenomatous polyps. Cystic pneumatosis is treated separately on pages 1514 to 1519.

REFERENCES

1. Gilbertsen, V. A.   The earlier diagnosis of adenocarcinoma of the large intestine. Cancer 27: 143, 1971.
2. Galante, M., Dunghy, J. E., and Fletcher, W. S. Cancer of the colon. Ann. Surg. 157:732, 1967.
3. Morson, B. D. Precancerous lesions of the colon and rectum. J.A.M.A. 170:316, 1962.
4. Rider, J. A., Kirsner, J. B., Moeller, H. C., and Palmer, W. L. Polyps of the colon and rectum. Amer. J. Med. 16:555, 1954.
5. Blatt, L. J. Polyps of the colon and rectum:

Incidence and distribution. Dis. Colon
Rectum 4:277, 1961.

6. Potet, F., and Soullard, J. Polyps of the rectum
and colon. Gut 12:468, 1971.

7. Kaye, G. I., Pascal, R. R., and Lane, N. The
colonic pericryptal fibroblast sheath: Replication, migration, and cytodifferentiation of
a mesenchymal cell system in adult tissue.
Gastroenterology 60:515, 1971.

8. Lane, N., Kaplan, H., and Pascal, R. R. Minute
adenomatous and hyperplastic polyps of
the colon. Divergent patterns of epithelial
growth with specific associated mesenchymal changes. Gastroenterology 60:537, 1971.

9. Morson, B. D. Precancerous and early malignant lesions of the large intestine. Brit. J.
Surg. 55:725, 1968.

10. Enterline, H. T., Evans, G. W., Mercado-Lugo,
R., and Miller, R. Malignant potential
of adenomas of the colon and rectum.
J.A.M.A. 179:322, 1962.

11. Spratt, J. S., Ackerman, L. V., and Moyer, C. Relationship of polyps of the colon to colonic
cancer. Ann. Surg. 148:682, 1958.

12. Welch, C. E., McKittrick, J., and Behringer, G.
Polyps of the rectum and colon and their
relation to cancer. New Eng. J. Med. 247:
959, 1952.

13. Castleman, B., and Krickstein, H. Do adenomatous polyps of the colon become malignant? New Eng. J. Med. 267:469, 1962.

14. Castleman, B. Current approach to the polyp-
cancer controversy. Gastroenterology 51:
108, 1966.

15. Grinnel, R., and Lane, N. Benign and malignant adenomatous polyps and papillary
adenomas of colon and rectum: Analysis of
1856 tumors in 1335 patients. Int. Abstr.
Surg. 106:519, 1953.

16. Copeland, E. M., and Jones, R. S. Multiple
colonic neoplasms. Arch. Surg. 98:141, 1969.

17. Calabro, J. J. Hereditable multiple polyposis
syndromes of the gastrointestinal tract.
Amer. J. Med. 33:276, 1962.

18. Spratt, J. S., and Ackerman, L. V. Small primary
adenocarcinomas of the colon and rectum.
J.A.M.A. 179:125, 1962.

19. Welin, S., and Youker, J. E. Colonic polyps.
In Alimentary Tract Roentgenology, Vol. 2,
A. R. Margulis and H. J. Burhenne (eds.).
St. Louis, C. V. Mosby Co., 1967, pp. 811–
833.

20. Ekelund, G. On cancer and polyps of the colon
and rectum. Acta Path. Microbiol. Scand.
59:165, 1963.

21. Nicoloff, D. M., Ellis, C. M., and Humphrey,
E. W. Management of villous adenomas of
the colon and rectum. Arch. Surg. 97:254,
1968.

22. Eisenberg, H. L., Kolb, L. H., Yam, L. T., and
Godt, R. Villous adenoma of the rectum
associated with electrolyte disturbance.
Ann. Surg. 159:604, 1964.

Chapter 108

Cancer of the Colon and Rectum

R. Scott Jones, Marvin H. Sleisenger

BACKGROUND AND EPIDEMIOLOGY

Cancer of the colon and rectum is a frequent and at times lethal disease confronting the gastroenterologist. An estimated 46,000 persons died of cancer of the colon or rectum in 1969. The occurrence of 73,000 new cases of colonic or rectal cancer in 1969 also emphasizes further the importance of this disease, because it is now the most common malignant disease in the United States after skin cancer.[1] The malignant tumors of the colon or rectum are adenocarcinoma, lymphoma, sarcoma, and carcinoid. Over 95 per cent of malignant colonic or rectal lesions are adenocarcinomas. Although adenocarcinoma of the colon and rectum occasionally appears in young persons, colonic cancer occurs with increasing frequency in older age groups.[2] Most patients treated for carcinoma of the colon and rectum are in the sixth and seventh decades of life (Fig. 108–1). Carcinoma of the rectum tends to occur more frequently in men than in women, with a ratio of about 2:1; however, the incidence of colonic cancer is approximately the same in each sex.

The populations of Northwest Europe and North America have a much higher incidence of cancer of the large bowel than do those of East Africa, Asia, and South America. Japan, likewise, has a low incidence of this disease. With the exception of Japan, carcinoma of the colon tends to occur in countries where there is a higher standard of living. The differences in the geographic occurrence of bowel cancer have led to speculation regarding the factors involved in this phenomenon.[3-5] There are dietary differences between countries having high and low incidences of colonic cancer. In countries having a high incidence, there is a generally higher fat composition in the diet; in addition, some have speculated that food additives in the Western world may have some carcinogenic effect. Also, in the industrialized societies, the population may be exposed to carcinogenic pollutants.[3]

There are differences in bowel function between Western populations and certain

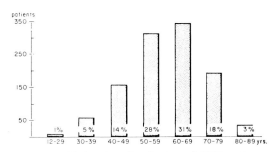

Figure 108–1. Age distribution of 1084 patients with carcinoma of the colon or rectum. (From Copeland, E. M., et al.: Amer. J. Surg. *116*:875, 1968.)

more primitive African populations. For example, the South African Bantu may evacuate his colon three or four times a day, compared with once a day for a Caucasian. The travel time of digesta may therefore be much faster through the colon of the Bantu than of the Caucasian, and perhaps exposure of the bowel mucosa to certain carcinogens may be less in the less industrialized person.[5]

The colonic bacterial flora has been studied in different populations. Persons in Britain and the United States of America, where the incidence of colonic cancer is high, have higher counts of Bacteroides and lower counts of enterococci and other aerobic bacteria than do people in Africa, India, or Japan where the incidence of colonic cancer is low. In addition, the feces of the people in the Western countries contain higher concentrations of degraded steroids than do those of peoples in the African and Eastern countries. This led to the additional hypothesis that the geographic differences in colonic cancer may be due to differences in bacterial flora and that certain bacteria may be capable of altering steroids to render them carcinogenic. It must be emphasized that these possible explanations for the geographic distribution of colonic cancer, although very interesting, are as yet purely hypothetical suggestions.[4]

GENETIC CONSIDERATIONS

Hereditary factors are undoubtedly important in many instances of colonic cancer.[6] The following observations suggest a hereditary role in this disease. First, some studies suggest an increased incidence of colonic or rectal cancer in relatives of probands with the disease. In addition, there are at least two diseases in which there is a definite hereditary relationship in the development of colonic and rectal cancer. Familial polyposis is characterized by the presence of myriads of adenomatous polyps throughout the colon and rectum. Familial polyposis is usually detected in childhood or adolescence as a result of symptoms related to the presence of the polyps, commonly rectal bleeding. Patients with familial polyposis develop adenocarcinoma of the colon, and their risk of developing cancer increases with the duration of the polyposis. Available evidence suggests that this disease is transmitted by a single dominant autosomal gene. Another syndrome revealing inheritance of colonic or rectal cancer is Gardner's syndrome, which is manifested by epidermoid cysts, osteomas of the skull, polyps of the small and large bowel, and adenocarcinoma of the colon and rectum. Colonic cancer may occur somewhat later in life in Gardner's syndrome than in familial polyposis, but the risk, nonetheless, increases with aging. Pedigrees also suggest that Gardner's syndrome is transmitted by a single autosomal dominant gene. A cancer-family syndrome has been described in which adenocarcinoma of the colon may occur in many members of a pedigree.[7] Some of these colonic cancers may be associated in some persons with cancers of other parts of the alimentary tract or, in some instances, carcinoma of the uterus. Examples such as these provide striking evidence supporting hereditary factors in many instances of colonic and rectal cancer (see pp. 1051 to 1059).

Studies of cell renewal and biochemical changes in normal colon and colonic cancer may provide some insight into the development of cancer and provide avenues for further study. The proliferating cells in the human colon are in the lower two-thirds of the crypt cell column below the luminal surface. Newly formed cells migrate from the crypts toward the surface as they differentiate. Normally most DNA synthesis occurs in the lower portion of the crypts and stops as the cells migrate toward the surface and mature. As the colonic cells migrate toward the surface, the activity of the enzymes for DNA synthesis (thymidine kinase) is lost, and as the colonic mucosal cells differentiate, they develop higher concentrations of adenine phosphoribosyl transferase and hypoxanthine ribosyl transferase. Recent studies show that cells on the surface of colonic cancers have high thymidine kinase activity similar to the immature cells proliferating in the crypts. Also, the surface cells of colonic cancer have low levels of adenine phosphoribosyl transferase and hypoxanthine ribosyl transferase. These studies suggest that the mechanism for "turning off" DNA synthesis, usually present in normal colonic cells, is lost in colonic cancer and that the developing colonic cells fail to differentiate into mature cells; that is, the cells in colonic cancer biochemically resemble the cells normally seen deep in the crypts.[8]

PATHOLOGY OF COLONIC AND RECTAL CANCER

LOCATION

Adenocarcinoma may develop in any portion of the colon or rectum. Seventy per cent of these tumors occur in the rectum, rectosigmoid, or sigmoid colon, whereas 3 to 6.9 per cent of colonic cancers occur in each of the remaining anatomical portions of the colon (Fig. 108–2).

TYPES OF CANCER

There are four types of adenocarcinoma of the colon: ulcerating, polypoid, colloid, and scirrhous.[9]

Generally, right colon lesions are likely to be polypoid; ulcerating or scirrhous lesions are more frequent in the left colon. Ulcerating carcinoma is the most common form of colonic cancer and is often associated with obstruction. This type of tumor

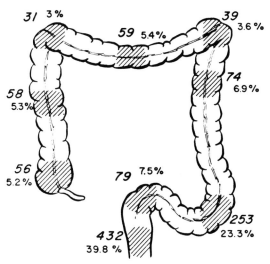

Figure 108–2. Anatomic distribution of lesions in 1084 patients with carcinoma of the colon or rectum. (From Copeland, E. M., et al.: Amer. J. Surg. *116*:875, 1968.)

may infiltrate along the bowel wall. Polypoid colonic cancer ranks second in frequency behind ulcerating tumors. Polypoid cancers are usually well differentiated and slower growing. Colloid carcinoma is characterized by an abundance of mucus-secreting cells. Scirrhous carcinoma is uncommon and occurs most often in the rectum or rectosigmoid. These lesions feel leathery or rubbery and have been called the "linitis plastica type" of colonic cancer. Histologically, scirrhous adenocarcinoma of the colon and rectum exhibits a preponderance of fibroplasia with scant glands.

MODES OF SPREAD

After arising in the mucosa, adenocarcinomas of the large bowel may extend proximally or distally in the bowel wall. Some cancers extend directly from the mucosa through the bowel wall and through the serosa of the bowel. Thus they may invade adjacent organs or seed peritoneal surfaces with tumor implants. Another important route of spread is via regional lymphatics draining the colon. The lymphatic drainage of the colon characteristically accompanies the blood supply and drains into the mesenteric nodes and later into the preaortic nodes. Lymphatic drainage of the left transverse colon, descending colon, sigmoid colon, and rectum is into the nodes about the inferior mesenteric artery from the left colonic, sigmoidal, or superior hemorrhoidal nodes, whereas the lymphatic drainage of the cecum, ascending colon, and right transverse colon is into the nodes about the superior mesenteric artery from the ileocolonic and right colonic nodes. Lymphatic drainage of the anus is usually into the inguinal nodes; however, the proximal anus may drain into the groin, so that for some anorectal lesions there may be bidirectional lymphatic drainage. Some colonic and rectal cancers spread by venous invasion; invasion of the tributaries of the portal vein probably accounts for hepatic metastasis from colonic and rectal cancer. In a smaller number of cases, distant metastases occur from colonic cancer in the lung, bone, brain, and occasionally the adrenal glands.

PRECANCEROUS LESIONS

There are several diseases which may be associated with an increased risk of colonic cancer.

Villous Adenomas. Villous adenomas are usually large, sessile, soft tumors which occur with greater frequency in the rectum and distal sigmoid colon. An estimated 85 per cent of villous adenomas are benign; however, about 15 per cent may show varying degrees of malignancy.[9] Because of the high incidence of malignancy in villous adenomas, these tumors are generally regarded as being premalignant.

Ulcerative Colitis. It is now widely accepted that there is an increased risk of carcinoma of the colon and rectum in patients with ulcerative colitis. De Dombal and coworkers[10] have reported that the fatality rate from carcinoma of the colon developing in patients with ulcerative colitis is 11 times greater than the expected rate in a matched sample of the general population. The development of carcinoma in patients with ulcerative colitis, however, seems related to the duration of the symptoms of colitis as well as to the extent of the involvement of the colon and rectum. The cumulative incidence of carcinoma of the colon in those patients with total involvement of the colon by ulcerative colitis rises after 30 years' duration to approximately 56 per cent. Of further interest in that study is that none of the 218 patients with ulcerative colitis limited to the rectum or to the left side of the colon had developed carcinoma at the time of the report.

Familial Polyposis. Familial polyposis has been discussed previously and is definitely regarded as a precancerous lesion (see pp. 1052 to 1054).

Gardner's Syndrome. Gardner's syndrome is also considered to be associated with the development of colonic cancer. Patients with Gardner's syndrome tend to develop colonic cancer later in life than do patients with familial polyposis (see p. 1055).

CLINICAL PICTURE OF CANCER OF THE COLON AND RECTUM

SYMPTOMS

Most patients with adenocarcinoma of the colon or rectum have symptoms, and the symptoms depend upon the site of the lesion to a certain extent (Table 108-1). Some of the factors responsible for the manifestations of colonic cancers, depending upon anatomic site of the tumor, are (1) the gross features of the tumor, i.e., polypoid tumors are more common in right colon; (2) the caliber of the bowel, and (3) the consistency of feces, i.e., more liquid in the right colon. Abdominal pain is one of the most common complaints, occurring in half to three-fourths of patients with tumors of the colon proximal to the sigmoid, but is a less frequent symptom in those with carcinoma of the rectum and distal sigmoid. Anemia occurs with much greater frequency in patients with cancer of the cecum or ascending colon. About 37

TABLE 108-1. SIGNS AND SYMPTOMS OF COLONIC OR RECTAL CARCINOMA RELATIVE TO SITE OF ORIGIN*

	RECTUM	RECTO-SIGMOID	SIGMOID	DESCEND-ING COLON	SPLENIC FLEXURE	TRANS-VERSE COLON	HEPATIC FLEXURE	ASCENDING COLON	CECUM
Patients in series	432	79	253	74	39	59	32	58	55
Asymptomatic	5.3%	2.5%	4.4%	0	2.6%	5.1%	9.4%	0	1.8%
Abdominal pain	24.4%	45.6%	60.5%	77.0%	77.0%	74.5%	78.0%	76.0%	54.5%
Anemia	22.2%	22.8%	21.3%	27.0%	33.3%	35.6%	31.2%	77.8%	74.6%
Weight loss	36.0%	30.4%	28.8%	28.4%	38.5%	40.5%	40.5%	40.0%	47.4%
Change in bowel habits	45.5%	49.5%	48.0%	55.5%	38.5%	34.0%	34.4%	19.0%	18.0%
Diarrhea	16.3%	25.4%	12.7%	4.0%	11.0%	6.8%	9.4%	13.8%	16.4%
Blood in stool	77.2%	73.5%	48.5%	33.8%	36.0%	29.0%	22.0%	25.5%	23.6%
Hemorrhoids	27.4%	10.1%	5.5%	8.1%	2.5%	3.4%	3.1%	1.7%	0
Abdominal mass	4.2%	15.2%	24.2%	32.5%	18.0%	37.4%	44.0%	62.0%	58.0%
Rectal mass	65.6%	28.0%	7.9%	0	0	0	0	0	0
Obstruction	2.3%	10.1%	17.0%	28.4%	41.0%	29.0%	12.5%	13.8%	16.4%
Appendicitis	0.5%	1.3%	0.8%	1.4%	5.1%	0	6.2%	3.5%	5.5%

*From unpublished observations of E. M. Copeland, L. B. Miller and R. S. Jones.

per cent of anemic patients exhibited symptoms of the anemia, such as shortness of breath, weakness, easy fatigability, or cardiac symptoms. Weight loss occurs in one-fourth to one-half of patients. A recent change in bowel habits, either increasing constipation or alternating constipation and diarrhea, occurs very commonly, particularly in those with cancer of the rectum, sigmoid, and descending colon. Diarrhea occurs frequently in patients with distal colonic lesions, but it is interesting that only about 16 per cent of patients with cecal tumors have diarrhea. Gross blood in the stool occurs in over three-fourths of the patients with rectal cancer. Blood in the stool must be considered to be due to rectal cancer in an adult until proved otherwise. No patient should receive treatment for hemorrhoids until sigmoidoscopy and barium enema have excluded the possibility of colonic or rectal cancer. Despite the fact that rectal bleeding is a common symptom of rectal cancer, about one-fourth of the patients with rectal cancer have had some form of treatment for hemorrhoids before being treated for rectal cancer.

PHYSICAL FINDINGS

The physical findings depend upon the site and extent of the cancer. Anemia may be detected by pallor of the skin and mucous membranes. Recent weight loss is usually evidenced by redundant skin or ill-fitting clothing. Jaundice occurs in the latest stages of the disease, usually owing to hepatic metastases or to invasion of the bile ducts. Signs of ascites are occasionally seen in persons who fail to notice earlier symptoms or who are reluctant to seek medical attention. Abdominal masses are very common, and the examiner may feel the primary tumor. Multiple masses or an enlarged nodular liver are ominous physical findings. A mass may be felt on rectal digital examination of many patients with cancer of the rectum, rectosigmoid, or sigmoid. Rectal lesions may be felt directly in the lumen of the bowel, and occasionally a sigmoid tumor can be felt in the cul-de-sac through the rectal wall. Patients suspected of having rectal lesions should have rectal examinations performed in the supine position with the legs drawn up or even in a squatting position to facilitate palpation of high rectal lesions. Metastases to the peritoneal floor by direct extension or by implantation can be felt and are called Blumer's shelf. Following rectal examination, any feces on the examining finger should be tested for occult blood, using the guaiac test. With females, a careful pelvic examination is necessary; it may reveal involvement of the uterus, ovaries, or vagina.

OBSTRUCTION

Ten to 41 per cent of adenocarcinomas of the colon occurring proximal to the rectum may produce intestinal obstruction, the incidence varying with the site of the tumor. Any patient with abdominal distention, abdominal pain, and failure to pass gas or feces per rectum should be suspected of having intestinal obstruction. The most common cause of colonic obstruction in the adult is adenocarcinoma.

PERFORATION

Perforation may occur in association with colonic cancer as result of two processes: (1) the tumor may penetrate the bowel wall, producing perforation at the site of the tumor; and (2) some patients with colonic cancer will develop perforation of the colon as the result of obstruction, with the colon becoming gangrenous proximal to the obstructing tumor. The cecum may burst in patients with obstruction of the left colon.

ENDOSCOPY

Sigmoidoscopy is an essential examination in all patients with rectal bleeding or any of the other signs and symptoms suggesting colon or rectal malignancy. Approximately 60 per cent of patients have large bowel cancers within reach of the conventional 25-cm sigmoidoscope. In these patients, a diagnosis can be made and confirmed histologically by biopsy before any surgical procedure is initiated. Before performing a sigmoidoscopic biopsy of a rectal lesion, the operator must be satisfied that the patient does not have a bleeding tendency. It is appropriate to determine the patient's prothrombin, bleeding, and clotting times before performing a sigmoidoscopic biopsy. In addition, an electrocautery unit should be available in order to secure hemostasis after the biopsy. Large polypoid tumors or ulcerating tumors can be biopsied through the sigmoidoscope, using the biopsy punch forceps. Smaller polypoid lesions are usually best removed by using the cautery snare. The complications of sigmoidoscopic biopsies are hemorrhage, bowel perforation, and, rarely, explosion of flammable bowel gases. The recent development of a fiberoptic colonoscope has added a new dimension to the direct inspection and histological examination of colonic tumors. In some instances, the fiberoptic colonoscope will allow direct inspection of the bowel as far proximal as the ascending colon or cecum, and this instrument may allow removal or biopsy of tumors as far proximal as the right colon. The use of this new instrument will certainly increase the accuracy in diagnosis of colonic lesions.

X-RAY DIAGNOSIS

Plain films of the abdomen are particularly useful in patients suspected of having intestinal obstruction. In most instances, plain abdominal X-rays will permit differentiation between colonic and small intestinal obstruction. In some patients this distinction is not possible, so barium enema may be necessary. All patients who exhibit the aforementioned signs and symptoms of colonic cancer should be examined by both proctosigmoidoscopy and barium enema. In patients suspected of having obstruction or partial obstruction on the basis of history, physical examination, and sigmoidoscopy, barium enema should be performed carefully, using fluoroscopic monitoring to prevent filling of the colon with barium proximal to the lesion. In some patients with large partial obstructing lesions the barium cannot be emptied from the colon proximal to the lesion, and it is possible that the barium may increase the degree of obstruction. A barium enema should be performed on patients in whom the diagnosis of colonic or rectal cancer has already been made on the basis of sigmoidoscopy, if there is no obstruction, because approximately 3 per

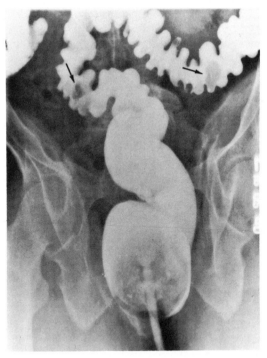

Figure 108–3. This barium enema demonstrates two polypoid lesions in the sigmoid colon. The distal lesion was an adenocarcinoma of the colon, whereas the proximal lesion was an adenomatous polyp. This X-ray points out the difficulty in differentiating between benign and malignant polyps seen on barium enema. (Courtesy of R. W. Postlethwait, Professor of Surgery, Duke University.)

cent of patients will have a second simultaneous colonic cancer which may be detected by the barium enema study.

Several radiographic signs suggest colonic neoplasm.[11] An intraluminal radiolucent mass seen in the same location on repeated exposures is a polypoid lesion (Fig. 108–3). When such a finding occurs, one must decide whether the lesion is a polypoid adenocarcinoma or a benign polyp. Criteria most helpful in making this decision are the size of the lesion and the presence or absence of a stalk. There is increasing risk of cancer with increasing size of a polypoid lesion. If a stalk is present, the lesion is probably benign; sessile lesions are more apt to be malignant. A classic X-ray sign of colonic cancer is stenosis of the colon, producing the appearance of an apple core (Fig. 108–4). This sign is due to narrowing of the colonic lumen by a tumor mass. Other signs of cancer of the colon include distortion or loss of mucosal pat-

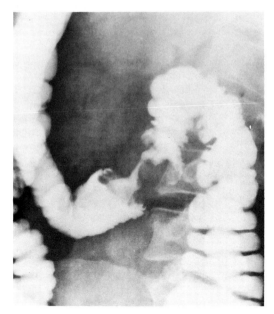

Figure 108–4. This barium enema demonstrates an apple core lesion of the right transverse colon. Notice the narrowing of the bowel lumen, the loss of mucosal detail at the site of the lesion, and the overhanging edge on either end of the lesion, which is caused by the tumor. (Courtesy of R. W. Postlethwait.)

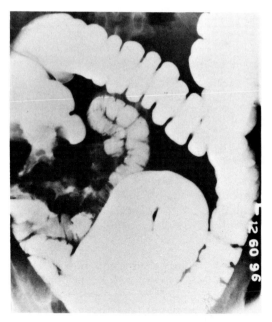

Figure 108–5. Barium enema demonstration of a carcinoma of the cecum and proximal ascending colon. (Courtesy of R. W. Postlethwait.)

tern, stiffness or rigidity of the bowel wall, and evidence of invasion of adjacent structures. Occasionally, adjacent structures can be seen by additional studies; for example, an upper gastrointestinal series may reveal deformity of the stomach or duodenum secondary to colonic cancer.

The accuracy of barium enema diagnosis of cancer of the colon is excellent, except at the extreme ends of the organ. Detection of rectal carcinoma is complicated by the fact that the balloon through which the barium is administered may obscure a low rectal lesion. This problem is surmountable, because those lesions are usually readily demonstrated by sigmoidoscopy. Redundant loops of sigmoid colon may hamper examination, but by careful positioning of the patient and repeated exposures, satisfactory films are usually obtained. The cecum is often difficult to examine accurately; it is difficult to empty the cecum of feces and keep it empty, and any amount of nonopaque residue in the bowel complicates the examination. It is sometimes difficult to determine whether the ileocecal valve is normal or enlarged, or whether the shadow in fact

represents cancer (Fig. 108–5). In addition, previous lesions or surgery, such as appendicitis with appendectomy, may produce cecal abnormalities which are difficult to distinguish from cancer.

Patients being evaluated for colonic and rectal tumors should usually have X-ray examination of the urinary tract by intravenous pyelograms and occasionally by cystography. Since carcinomas of the pelvic colon may involve the distal ureter or the bladder, any patient being considered for surgery of the pelvic colon should have an intravenous pyelogram in order to ascertain renal function and ureteral integrity. Defining the anatomy of the ureter also helps to avoid injury of that structure during the surgical procedure.

LABORATORY AIDS IN THE DIAGNOSIS OF CANCER OF THE COLON AND RECTUM

The most important laboratory determinations are hemoglobin, hematocrit, and blood smear. Evidence for iron deficiency anemia is common in this disease, because of either gross or occult bleeding. Many patients will have chronic iron deficiency anemia characterized by hypochromic microcytic red cells in the blood smear. The diagnosis of iron deficiency anemia may be confirmed by measurement of plasma iron. Examination of the feces for gross and occult blood is very important. In the anemic patient, or patients with other symptoms of colonic cancer, repeated examinations of the stool for occult blood should be carried out. Plasma protein concentrations may be lower than normal in patients with carcinoma of the colon. Leukocytosis may be noted in patients with inflammatory complications of their carcinoma, such as necrosis of tumor, or local colonic perforation. Urinalysis may reveal leukocytes or erythrocytes, which would suggest involvement of the bladder, ureters, or kidneys by the tumor. Hepatic function tests should be performed to seek evidence of hepatic metastases. The BSP retention is likely to be over 5 per cent at 45 minutes in patients with hepatic metastases. Serum alkaline phosphatase measurement is also likely to be elevated. Recent studies have revealed that many malignant tumors, including colonic cancer, may produce an isoenzyme of alkaline phosphatase, which may contribute to the elevated alkaline phosphatase levels in some of these patients.[12] In patients with advanced hepatic metastases, elevation of serum bilirubin usually occurs. Percutaneous needle biopsy of the liver may be useful in documenting hepatic metastases from the colon or rectum.

CARCINOEMBRYONIC ANTIGEN (CEA)

Carcinoembryonic antigen is a glycoprotein found in the digestive organs of two- to six-month-old fetuses. This antigen has been found in the blood of most of the patients with carcinoma of the colon or rectum tested.[13] Initial reports indicated specificity of this antigen for colonic and rectal cancer. Subsequently, however, carcinoembryonic antigen has been found in the blood of persons with other gastrointestinal malignancies, such as carcinoma of the pancreas; also it may be positive in nonmalignant diseases of colon, lung, and liver.[14] Further work is needed to define the role of the carcinoembryonic antigen in the diagnosis of gastrointestinal malignancy. In addition to aiding in the evaluation of patients with symptoms of colonic cancer, the carcinoembryonic antigen would be very helpful in the follow-up of patients to detect recurrence after surgical excision of their tumor. Also, this technique may provide great help in decisions regarding patients with premalignant lesions, such as ulcerative colitis. Management of patients with colonic polyps would also be aided by cancer-specific tests to aid in the discrimination between benign and malignant polyps.

DIFFERENTIAL DIAGNOSIS OF COLONIC CANCER

Colonic cancer is an extremely common disease, and in most instances the diagnosis can be determined accurately. There are occasional patients with inflammatory disease mimicking the picture of colonic cancer. One instance in which it may be difficult to distinguish between benign and malignant disease is in the patient with chronic ulcerative colitis who develops a stricture of the colon. Because patients with ulcerative colitis have an increased risk of developing colonic cancer, the presence of a colonic stricture in such a patient may present a difficult differential diagnostic problem. Approximately 11 per cent of patients with ulcerative colitis will develop a colonic stricture; in some instances colonic strictures will be multiple (Fig. 108–6). Benign strictures in patients with ulcerative colitis are usually produced by hypertrophy and contraction of the muscularis mucosae of the colon; in some instances these strictures have been observed to be reversible.[15] If the stricture in the ulcerative colitis patient appears benign, that is, if it possesses a concentric lumen, fusiform tapering margins, and a smooth contour, then a repeat barium enema after a short period of therapy would be appropriate. If the stricture remains unchanged, then surgical exploration should be performed. If, however, the deformed area of the colon is not apparent on repeat study, it is likely that the defect was produced by benign stricture.

Granulomatous colitis may produce multiple strictures of the colon which are difficult to distinguish from carcinoma. Although adenocarcinoma of the colon may occur in patients with granulomatous colitis, it has not been demonstrated that there is an increased risk of cancer in this disease. The risk of cancer notwithstanding, the appearance of strictures of the colon in patients with granulomatous disease may be an indication for surgery, particularly if there is symptomatic or radiographic evidence of obstruction.

Diverticulitis is a disease which is easily confused with carcinoma, because it may present with a pelvic mass associated with abdominal pain and X-rays may reveal narrowing of the sigmoid colon. The syndrome of diverticulitis may be characterized by exacerbations and remissions. Fever and tenderness are usually characteristic of diverticulitis, but it must be emphasized that it may be difficult to distinguish these conditions on this basis, because signs of inflammation are present with a locally perforated tumor. The radiographic evidence of diverticulosis and diverticulitis assists further in differentiating between tumor and inflammation. However, occasionally one will encounter patients who have carcinoma of the colon and diverticulosis or whose X-ray cannot distinguish diverticulitis from cancer. If there is uncertainty of the differential diagnosis of diverticulitis and sigmoid colon cancer, then surgical intervention should be considered, provided the patient's general health and condition do not prohibit surgery.

Other inflammatory diseases may mimic carcinoma of the colon, particularly the granulomatous diseases. Tuberculosis of the cecum may be difficult to differentiate from carcinoma. Amebic granuloma may mimic carcinoma of the cecum, and a fungus infection of the cecum, particularly actinomycosis, may be difficult to diagnose; however, these lesions are unusual when compared with the incidence of colonic cancer (see pp. 1377 to 1381 and 1386 to 1392). Also ischemic vascular disease may cause narrowing which may be difficult to distinguish from cancer (see pp. 1569 to 1571).

TREATMENT OF CARCINOMA OF THE COLON AND RECTUM

SURGICAL TREATMENT

After the diagnosis of carcinoma of the colon has been made on the basis of history, physical findings, and X-ray examination, perhaps with histological confirmation by a specimen obtained by procto-

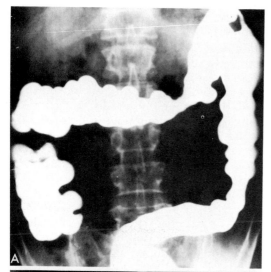

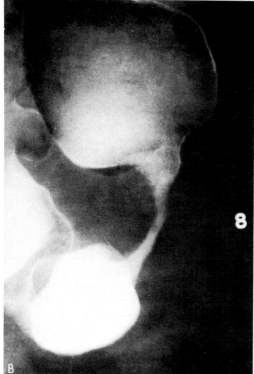

Figure 108–6. *A*, A representative film from a barium enema examination performed on a patient with chronic ulcerative colitis. This patient was operated upon because of stricture at the hepatic flexure, and was found to have an adenocarcinoma of the colon. *B*, A spot film of the stenosing cancer. (Courtesy of A. D. Hall, Associate Professor of Surgery, University of California Medical School.)

scopic biopsy, and the anatomic extent of the disease has been evaluated (by pelvic examination in the female, by intravenous urography, and by photoscanning as well as by physical and chemical examination of the liver), then surgical treatment of the disease can be planned. One important step in the preparation of the patient for therapy involves a discussion with the patient regarding the plan for therapy. If a histological diagnosis has been obtained, in most instances it is appropriate to discuss it with the patient and his family. Statements regarding prognosis, however, are best reserved until the tumor has been removed surgically. If it is likely that the treatment of the disease will necessitate a colostomy, this possibility should be discussed with the patient as frankly as possible; in many instances it is quite helpful to provide the patient an opportunity to speak with a person who has had a colostomy. If the patient has a pelvic tumor or rectal tumor, certain of the more common complications of such surgery should be mentioned to the patient, such as the risk of impotence and of urinary tract complications.

In elective cases, several days may be required to prepare a patient for colonic surgery. Such preparation should include correction of anemia and hypoproteinemia when possible. The patient's cardiovascular, pulmonary, renal, and hepatic status should be analyzed, and any remediable problems corrected; for example, elderly patients in congestive heart failure may require digitalization.

Generally, preparation of a patient for colonic surgery would involve mechanical cleansing of the colon as well as the reduction of bacterial flora with nonabsorbable antibiotics. This bowel preparation usually requires three to five days and is performed by the administration of a cathartic, usually castor oil or magnesium sulfate each morning, and the administration of saline enemas until clear each evening. Optimal bowel cleansing will be achieved if the patient is placed on a clear liquid diet for at least 48 hours before operation. Nonabsorbable sulfa drugs such as Sulfasuxidine are usually administered for three to four days before surgery, and either kanamycin or neomycin may be administered by mouth during the 24 hours

preceding surgery. The objectives of such a regimen are to clean the colon mechanically and reduce the numbers of enteric flora in order to minimize contamination of the peritoneal cavity when the colon is opened at the time of surgery.

There are two complications to be avoided in such a bowel preparation regimen. One is fluid and electrolyte imbalance caused by repeated enemas and purgation. The patient's serum electrolytes should be monitored during this period. Another, more serious complication is pseudomembranous enterocolitis, which is thought to be related to the reduction in the enteric flora, allowing establishment and overgrowth by virulent staphylococcal organisms (see pp. 1369 to 1373).

The most effective therapy for colonic cancer is surgical excision. The effectiveness of surgical treatment of colonic cancer depends upon removal of the primary tumor and upon an adequate margin of bowel proximal and distal to the tumor and the lymph nodes draining the tumor. For tumors of the cecum, ascending colon, hepatic flexure, and right transverse colon, right hemicolectomy is usually employed. After right hemicolectomy, intestinal continuity is usually restored by ileotransverse colostomy, i.e., an anastomosis between the terminal ileum and the transverse colon. Tumors of the central transverse colon are excised by transverse colectomy, and the resulting defect is repaired by colocolostomy. Tumors of the left transverse colon, splenic flexure, and proximal descending colon are usually treated by left colectomy. Anterior resection of the sigmoid colon is employed for lesions of the distal descending colon, sigmoid colon, and, in some instances, the rectosigmoid. Abdominoperineal excision of the rectum is the usual treatment for rectal cancer and by definition results in a permanent colostomy. This operation is carried out by transabdominal mobilization of the sigmoid colon and rectum down to the levator ani muscles. At that point in the operation, the bowel is transected proximal to the tumor, and a permanent colostomy is fashioned before the abdominal wound is closed. The abdominoperineal resection is then completed by making a perianal skin incision and removing the mobilized rectum through a perineal dissection.

Because an appreciable incidence of recurrence of tumor occurs at the suture line when an anastomosis is performed, it is believed that malignant cells from the tumor in the bowel lumen become implanted in the wound when the bowel is transected. Some surgeons suggest ligating the bowel proximal and distal to the tumor before any operative manipulation to endeavor to minimize the intraluminal dissemination of cancer cells. Other surgeons advocate a "no-touch" technique in which the blood supply of the segment of colon to be removed is ligated and divided as the first step in the operation to prevent vascular dissemination of malignant cells.

In addition to the anatomic and pathological factors concerning the spread and recurrence of tumors, two other very important technical factors in colon surgery are (1) ensuring an adequate blood supply to the portion of the bowel involved in the anastomosis or colostomy, and (2) avoiding tension at the suture line. Attention to these factors is essential to ensure proper healing of the bowel. At the time of surgery, the tumor must be evaluated as to whether it is confined to the bowel or whether it has extended either into regional lymph nodes or into adjacent organs. The liver should be inspected and palpated carefully to determine whether it contains hepatic metastasis and of course the surgeon must decide whether the primary tumor can be excised. If it is technically possible to remove the lesion, this should generally be done, even if metastases are found. In some instances, the primary tumor cannot be removed because of fixation to adjacent structures; if this is the case, one must consider some palliative procedure such as colostomy proximal to the tumor or a bypass operation to short-circuit the alimentary stream about the tumor. The overall operative mortality of surgery for colonic cancer varies from 3 to 7 per cent; however, the mortality for surgical emergencies related to colonic cancer may have mortality rates in excess of 30 per cent.

Tumors between 5 and 20 cm from the dentate line deserve special mention because of the possibility of removing such tumors by one of two operations. Cancers of the distal rectum are generally removed by a combined abdominoperineal resection of the rectum. Sigmoid colon tumors, on the other hand, are conventionally removed by transecting the colon proximal and distal to the tumor and rejoining the bowel, thus avoiding a colostomy. With tumors of the rectosigmoid or proximal rectum, the surgeon must decide whether to perform an anterior resection, thus avoiding a colostomy and sparing the rectum, or to excise the rectum and perform a permanent colostomy. Several factors must be considered in making this decision.[16, 17] In order to perform a so-called low anterior resection, the lesion should be proximal enough in the rectum or rectosigmoid that approximately 5 cm of bowel distal to the tumor may be removed and sufficient distal bowel remains for an anastomosis. This principle of adequate margin for anastomosis may be compromised in patients who already have hepatic metastases. The cancer cannot be cured and a colostomy will be avoided. A low anterior resection may be technically difficult, particularly in the very obese patient or the patient with a long narrow pelvis in whom exposure of the depths of the pelvis would be difficult.

EMERGENCY SURGERY FOR PATIENTS WITH COLONIC CANCER

Obstruction. One of the common manifestations of colonic carcinoma is complete intestinal obstruction. All colonic cancers may produce the syndrome of colonic obstruction except tumors of the cecum, which usually cause small bowel obstruction. When tumors of the transverse, descending, or sigmoid colon or rectum produce obstruction, the preferred surgical treatment is the creation of a colostomy proximal to the obstructing tumor to relieve the obstruction. In elderly, poor risk patients with massive colonic distention, tube cecostomy may be performed under local anesthesia. After the patient has recovered from the obstruction, it is appropriate to resect the tumor as outlined previously. Carcinomas of the cecum or ascending colon may be treated best by right colectomy and anastomosis of the ileum to the right transverse colon in one stage. If the patient is particularly ill, a bypass operation, usually an ileotransverse colostomy, may be carried out and the tumor may be resected after the patient has recovered from the ill effects of the intestinal obstruction. The operative mortality in patients with intestinal obstruction caused by colonic cancer is about 13 per cent and the five-year survival rate is approximately 20 per cent.[18]

Perforation. Colonic carcinomas may perforate; about half these perforations will be contained or localized, and the rest will be free perforations. The surgical treatment of perforated colonic cancers may include resection of the tumor; however, in general, a colostomy should be performed because of the increased risk of disruption of colon anastomoses performed in the presence of infection. The operative mortality in colon perforation is about 15 per cent and the five-year survival rate in patients in whom perforation has occurred is about 28 per cent.[18]

A smaller portion of patients may experience both obstruction and perforation. In most patients, the obstruction and perforation are at the site of the tumor; however, occasionally a patient with an obstructing tumor distal to a competent ileocecal valve will have a ruptured cecum. Patients with perforation and obstruction have an operative mortality of 31 per cent, and a five-year survival rate of 7 per cent.[18]

PROGNOSIS AFTER SURGICAL TREATMENT OF COLONIC CANCER

The overall five-year survival rate in one series of patients with colonic and rectal cancer after surgical therapy was 37.3 per cent (Table 108–2). Several factors are important in predicting survival of patients after surgery for colonic cancer. Complications of obstruction and perforation have already been discussed. The anatomic site of cancer seems to be a factor in survival, with lesions of the rectum and rectosigmoid tending to be less favorable than more proximal lesions (Fig. 108–7). When the number of lymph node metastases is related to prognosis, it is apparent that one metastatic node in the specimen indicates a materially less favorable prognosis and that increasing numbers of positive nodes generally indicate declining chances of cure. If five or more lymph node metastases are detected in a surgical specimen, the five-year survival rate is about 10

TABLE 108–2. STATUS AT FIVE YEARS AFTER TREATMENT*

STATUS	GROSS SURVIVAL (1084 PATIENTS)	ESTIMATED CURABLE (826 PATIENTS)
Alive; no details available	0.0%	4.1%
Alive with no carcinoma	34.4%	40.6%
Alive with carcinoma	2.9%	3.4%
Dead with no carcinoma	11.5%	13.9%
Dead with carcinoma	51.2%	38.0%

*These figures represent the status of 1084 patients treated for carcinoma of the colon and rectum at five years following surgery. The column of figures on the right depicts the data for those patients who were estimated curable by the operating surgeon for comparison with the gross overall survival rate. (From Copeland, E. M., et al.: Amer. J. Surg. *116*:875, 1968.)

per cent, as indicated in Table 108–3. The degree of penetration of the bowel wall by the tumor is related to prognosis, as indicated in Table 108–4. The presence of venous invasion indicates a decreased chance for five-year survival, as indicated in Table 108–5. The histological appearance of the tumor regarding cellular differentiation may be an indicator of prognosis; the five-year survival in patients with well differentiated tumors was 57 per cent, whereas for poorly differentiated lesions

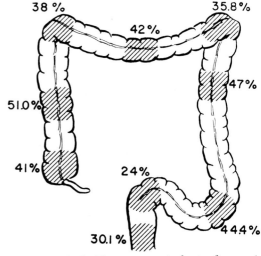

Figure 108–7. Five-year survival rate after surgical treatment of carcinoma of the large bowel according to anatomic site. (From Copeland, E. M., et al.: Amer. J. Surg. *116*:875, 1968.)

TABLE 108–3. CORRELATION OF NODAL INVOLVEMENT AND FIVE-YEAR SURVIVAL OF PATIENTS WITH CARCINOMA OF THE COLON*

STATUS	NO NODES INVOLVED (584 PATIENTS)	ONE NODE INVOLVED (112 PATIENTS)	TWO NODES INVOLVED (68 PATIENTS)	THREE NODES INVOLVED (40 PATIENTS)	FOUR NODES INVOLVED (24 PATIENTS)	FIVE OR MORE NODES INVOLVED (110 PATIENTS)
Alive with no carcinoma	48.5%	26.8%	25.0%	15.0%	29.1%	9.1%
Alive with carcinoma	3.0%	3.5%	2.9%	2.5%	4.2%	0.9%
Dead with no carcinoma	17.6%	6.2%	5.9%	2.5%	4.2%	4.5%
Dead with carcinoma	31.9%	63.5%	66.2%	80.0%	62.5%	85.5%

*From Copeland, E. M., et al.: Amer. J. Surg. *116*:875, 1968.

TABLE 108–4. BOWEL WALL INVOLVEMENT WITH AND WITHOUT NODAL METASTASIS AS RELATED TO FIVE-YEAR SURVIVAL*

STATUS AT FIVE YEARS	INVOLVEMENT OF MUCOSA WITHOUT NODES (66 PATIENTS)	INVOLVEMENT OF MUCOSA WITH NODES (3 PATIENTS)	INVOLVEMENT INTO BUT NOT THROUGH MUSCLE WITHOUT NODES (150 PATIENTS)	INVOLVEMENT INTO BUT NOT THROUGH MUSCLE WITH NODES (58 PATIENTS)	INVOLVEMENT THROUGH MUSCLE WITHOUT NODES (379 PATIENTS)	INVOLVEMENT THROUGH MUSCLE WITH NODES (329 PATIENTS)
Alive; no details available	0	0	1%	0	1%	0
Alive with no carcinoma	71%	67%	61%	48%	39%	13%
Alive with carcinoma	3%	0	3%	5%	3%	2%
Dead; no details available	0	0	0	0	1%	2%
Dead with no carcinoma	20%	33%	16%	0	16%	3%
Dead with carcinoma	6%	0	18%	47%	40%	80%

*From Copeland, E. M., et al.: Amer. J. Surg. *116*:875, 1968.

TABLE 108–5. FIVE-YEAR SURVIVAL RELATED TO VEIN INVASION*

STATUS	WITHOUT VEIN INVASION (482 PATIENTS)	WITH VEIN INVASION (115 PATIENTS)
Alive with no carcinoma	40%	19%
Alive with carcinoma	3%	3%
Dead with no carcinoma	12%	3%
Dead with carcinoma	45%	75%

*From Copeland, E. M., et al.: Amer. J. Surg. *116*:875, 1968.

TABLE 108–6. FIVE-YEAR SURVIVAL BASED ON THE PATHOLOGIC DIFFERENTIATION OF LESION FOUND AT SURGERY*

STATUS	LESION		
	Well Differentiated (33 Cases)	Moderately Well Differentiated (462 Cases)	Poorly Differentiated (159 Cases)
Alive with no carcinoma	51.5%	39.4%	20.1%
Alive with carcinoma	6.1%	3.0%	1.3%
Dead with no carcinoma	15.2%	12.3%	9.4%
Dead with carcinoma	27.2%	45.3%	69.2%

*From Copeland, E. M., et al.: Amer. J. Surg. *116*:875, 1968.

TABLE 108–7. FIVE-YEAR FOLLOW-UP DATA IN PATIENTS UNDERGOING LOCAL RESECTION FOR LESIONS ESTIMATED CURABLE*

STATUS	LOCAL RESECTION MARGIN GREATER THAN 5 CM. (141 PATIENTS)	LOCAL RESECTION MARGIN LESS THAN 5 CM. (206 PATIENTS)
Alive with no carcinoma	51.1%	38.4%
Alive with carcinoma	5.7%	2.4%
Dead with no carcinoma	10.6%	17.4%
Dead with carcinoma	32.6%	41.8%

*From Copeland, E. M., et al.: Amer. J. Surg. *116*:875, 1968.

it was 21 per cent (Table 108–6). Also, the data in Table 108–7 indicate the importance of removing an adequate segment of bowel proximal and distal to the tumor.

FOLLOW-UP CARE

After surgery for colonic cancer, the great majority of patients can promptly return to normal dietary and living habits. Occasionally patients will have transient diarrhea following right colectomy; this is usually a minor problem that subsides spontaneously, provided excessive amounts of terminal ileum have not been resected. If the patient's surgery has ne-

cessitated a permanent colostomy, a training program in colostomy care should begin early in the postoperative period when the patient's wounds are healing and he is fully ambulatory. He should be instructed in the use of colostomy irrigation apparatus while still in the hospital. By using systematic colostomy irrigations, most patients will achieve a regular schedule of colonic evacuation and have minimal, if any, colostomy discharge between irrigations. Some patients achieve such regular colonic evacuation that they do not need to wear a colostomy bag but can simply place a gauze dressing over the colostomy stoma. Most patients, however, feel more comfortable with the use of a colostomy appliance which is changed daily. The one hazard that exists for the patient who irrigates his colostomy is the possibility of perforation of the colon; all patients should be warned about this and instructed to irrigate their colostomy with devices which do not have to be inserted fully into the colon.

Because a majority of patients having colonic surgery will experience a recurrence within five years after the surgical excision of their tumor, some program of follow-up visits should be instituted by a physician and a physical examination and laboratory tests, such as chest X-ray, barium enema, and liver function tests, performed when indicated. Approximately 3 per cent of patients undergoing surgery for colonic cancer will develop a second primary colonic cancer,[19] and a much larger percentage will develop evidence of ei-

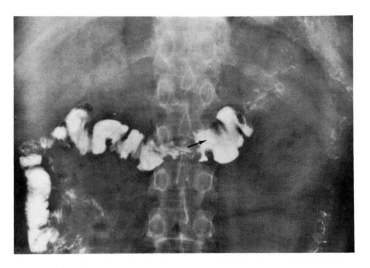

Figure 108–8. This is a follow-up barium enema on an asymptomatic 49-year-old man who underwent a right colectomy for adenocarcinoma of the cecum five years previously and excision of a rectal polyp three years previously. He had a family history of colonic cancer. This study shows a polypoid lesion in the transverse colon just distal to the ileotransverse colostomy (arrow), which was adenocarcinoma of the colon. This is an example of a patient developing a resectable metachronous second colonic cancer. (Courtesy of R. W. Postlethwait.)

ther local recurrence or metastasis. In some instances, further palliation can be achieved by medical or surgical treatment of these recurrent tumors (Fig. 108–8).[20]

NONOPERATIVE TREATMENT OF RECTAL CANCER

Conservative treatment of rectal cancer may be considered for several reasons.[9] First, some patients may refuse radical surgical treatment. In addition, because of age or other concomitant diseases, the patient may not be considered suitable for radical excision of the rectum, and an alternative form of treatment may be necessary. In such patients, particularly those with polypoid carcinoma involving only a portion of the rectal wall, fulguration may provide acceptable palliation by maintaining bowel lumen, and thus preventing obstruction and the necessity for colostomy, and by reducing the local symptoms of the tumor, such as tenesmus, bleeding, and mucous discharge. Fulguration of large rectal tumors may be accomplished best by several staged treatments. When the tumor recurs locally after fulguration, additional fulguration may be helpful, so that frequent follow-up visits for proctoscopy are important in the management of rectal tumors treated by this method. Local excision of rectal cancers may be appropriate in some patients not suitable for radical surgery.

CHEMOTHERAPY FOR COLONIC CANCER

The most extensively investigated chemotherapeutic agent used in treating cancer of the alimentary tract has been 5-fluorouracil (5-FU).[21] The reported rates of objective regression of advanced adenocarcinoma of the large bowel range from 8 to 85 per cent. Although the range responsiveness is great, it seems clear that many tumors regress after administration of 5-FU. The difficulty in objectively assessing response probably accounts for the varied response rate. The toxicity of 5-FU is manifested in several ways. Nausea and vomiting occur in half to three-fourths of the patients treated, but may be ameliorated to a certain extent by treatment with antiemetic drugs. Stomatitis may be first detected on the mucosa of the lower lip, but may occur on the palate, pharynx, or buccal mucosa. Diarrhea appears in more than half the patients. Dermatitis, esophagopharyngitis, and alopecia are infrequently noted. Leukopenia occurs in over 70 per cent of patients treated, usually affecting the granulocytes. Granulocytopenia may last two to three weeks; it is the most serious complication of 5-FU therapy and may result in death from infection.

Although tumor regression may be observed in many patients treated for advanced colonic or rectal cancer, a very important question is: will treatment with 5-FU increase survival rates in patients treated surgically? A recent preliminary report of a prospective randomized study of the use of 5-FU in patients treated surgically for colonic cancer indicated no statistically significant difference between treatment and control groups.[22] In that study, however, in all three groups of patients—those resected for cure, those having palliative resection with a single treatment of 5-FU, and those having palliative resection with multiple treatments with 5-FU—survivals were insignificantly greater than in the control groups. Further follow-up is necessary before any conclusion can be reached concerning the effectiveness of 5-FU in increasing the five-year survival rate in patients treated surgically for colonic cancer.

RADIATION

A retrospective study performed at Memorial Hospital in New York City indicated an increased survival rate in patients receiving preoperative X-ray therapy for lymph node metastasis from carcinoma of the rectum when compared with a group of patients receiving no X-ray therapy preoperatively.[23] Other authors have suggested that X-ray treatment may occasionally render an unresectable rectal cancer resectable.[24] A recent prospective randomized study failed to demonstrate any significant difference in the survival rates in patients treated preoperatively by X-ray therapy as compared with controls.[25] Examination of the available evidence, therefore, does not permit a confident conclusion regarding the efficacy of such X-ray treatment in colonic and rectal cancer at present.

Combined 5-FU and supervoltage radiation therapy of locally unresectable gastrointestinal cancer has been investigated in the treatment of gastric, pancreatic, and large bowel tumors in a prospective controlled double-blind study. The addition of 5-FU significantly augmented the effectiveness of the X-ray therapy.[26] This finding should stimulate further study of the effectiveness of combined 5-FU and radiation therapy in the treatment of colonic cancer.

OTHER MALIGNANT DISEASES OF THE COLON, RECTUM, OR ANUS

SQUAMOUS CELL CARCINOMA

Squamous cell carcinoma of the anus or distal rectum usually arises from the perianal skin or from the anal canal. It is infrequent when compared with adenocarcinoma of the rectum, comprising only 3.9 per cent of patients treated for cancer of the anorectal region. This disease tends to appear earlier in life than adenocarcinoma. Symptoms may be bleeding, a noticeable lump or nodule, anorectal discomfort, or anal drainage. Physical examination may reveal an ulcer on the perianal skin or in the anal canal. Some tumors may invade the distal rectum. Anal tumors spread via the lymphatics to the groin, or upward along the rectum into the drainage about the superior hemorrhoidal vessels. Any perianal or anal ulcer should be biopsied. Because squamous cell carcinoma of the anus and rectum is infrequent, its treatment has not been evaluated as well as the treatment of adenocarcinoma. Treatments have consisted of abdominoperineal excision of the rectum, wide local excision, or radiation. Also, the question of whether to remove inguinal lymph nodes must be considered. Stearns and Quan,[27] reporting the experience from Memorial Hospital in New York, have suggested the following approach: If the tumor arises from the anal skin and is small and clearly mobile, wide local excision should be performed. If the lesion is large, is fixed, or involves the anal sphincter, then abdominoperineal excision is the choice. Radical groin dissection should not be done un-

less there is clinical evidence of inguinal metastasis. After treatment of the primary tumor careful follow-up is necessary to detect inguinal metastasis, and radical groin dissection should be considered in patients who develop clinical evidence of lymph node metastasis in this region. The overall five-year survival rate after surgical treatment of squamous cell carcinoma of the anus is about 57 per cent.

MALIGNANT MELANOMA

Malignant melanoma rarely arises in the perianal area. Abdominoperineal resection of the anus and rectum is the most common form of surgical therapy in this disease; however, even with radical excision, prognosis is very poor in patients with this malignant melanoma. The mean survival time in one series of patients treated with radical surgery was 30 months[28] (see p. 1557).

CARCINOID TUMORS

Carcinoid tumors arise from the enterochromaffin cells in the crypts of Lieberkühn and are generally regarded as slowly growing, low-grade malignant tumors.[29] These tumors occur in the stomach, small intestine, appendix, and large bowel. Large bowel carcinoids are probably more common in the rectum. Rectal carcinoids appear as rounded, yellowish nodules which are submucosal or intramural, giving a smooth appearance. Although carcinoid tumors arising in other parts of the alimentary tract may produce the carcinoid syndrome (see pp. 1031 to 1041), this syndrome is rarely caused by rectal carcinoid tumors. Most patients with rectal carcinoids are reported to be asymptomatic. These tumors may be treated by local excision. In some patients in whom a small carcinoid tumor may be located in a site inaccessible for local excision, fulguration may be appropriate after establishing the diagnosis. Jackman and Beahrs[9] recommend radical excision of carcinoid tumors only if they are extremely large or if deep invasion is demonstrable.

LEIOMYOSARCOMA

Leiomyosarcomas are rare rectal tumors comprising 0.01 to 0.1 per cent of rectal malignancies. These tumors arise from the rectal smooth muscle and histologically appear as interlacing spindle cells. It may be difficult to decide whether the lesion is benign or malignant. Rectal leiomyosarcoma causes rectal pain, bleeding, and constipation. These tumors spread mainly by local extension and by hepatic metastasis. Treatment is controversial. If the lesion is confidently thought to be a sarcoma, abdominoperineal resection of the rectum is appropriate.[30]

LYMPHOMAS

Lymphomas rarely arise in the colon or rectum. All gastrointestinal lymphomas comprise about 1.7 per cent of malignant disease of the alimentary tract. Common symptoms of large bowel lymphomas are abdominal pain and rectal bleeding.[31] A recent report suggests that lymphomas of the large bowel may mimic ulcerative colitis (Fig. 108–9).[32] Recommended treat-

ment of large bowel lymphomas consists of surgical excision when possible, associated with X-ray therapy.

CLOACOGENIC CARCINOMA

Cloacogenic carcinoma may develop in a small zone of transitional epithelium at the anorectal junction. The cloacogenic zone consists of mucosa and glandular structures identical to those of the bladder neck and posterior urethral mucosa, and in the adult this zone is about 0.3 to 1.1 cm. long. It is situated between the rectal mucosa and the anal skin in the distal anal canal. The histologic appearance of these tumors generally suggests transitional cell carcinoma. The symptoms associated with these tumors are generally bleeding, pain, sensation of a mass, or change in bowel habits. The treatment is usually abdominoperineal resection of the rectum.[33]

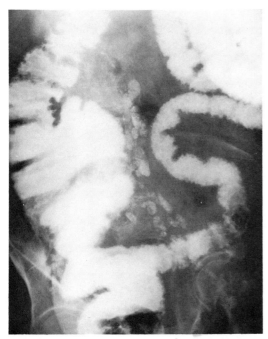

Figure 108–9. Barium enema demonstrating malignant lymphoma, lymphocytic type, of colon, in a 73-year-old woman with no bowel symptoms except "irritation." Biopsy of rectal nodule revealed a poorly differentiated tumor. X-ray shows many such shallow polypoid lesions. The film suggests possible ulcerative colitis. (Courtesy of Dr. Kevin Ryan, Woodland Medical Clinic, Woodland, California.)

REFERENCES

1. American Cancer Society. Cancer Facts and Figures. New York, 1969.
2. Copeland, E. M., Miller, L. D., and Jones, R. S. Prognostic factors in carcinoma of the colon and rectum. Amer. J. Surg. 116:875, 1968.
3. Wynder, E. L., and Shigematsu, T. Environmental factors of cancer of the colon and rectum. Cancer 20:1520, 1967.
4. Hill, M. J., Drasar, B. S., Aries, V., et al. Bacteria and aetiology of cancer of the small bowel. Lancet 1:95, 1971.
5. Walker, A. R. P. Diet, bowel motility, faeces composition and colonic cancer. S. African Med. J. 45:377, 1971.
6. Burdette, W. J. Carcinoma of the Colon and Antecedent Epithelium. Springfield, Ill., Charles C Thomas, 1970.
7. Smith, W. G. The cancer-family syndrome and heritable solitary colonic polyps. Dis. Colon Rectum 13:362, 1970.
8. Troncale, F., Hertz, R., and Lipkin, M. Nucleic acid metabolism in proliferating and differentiating colonic cells of man and in neoplastic lesions of the colon. Cancer Res. 31:463, 1971.
9. Jackman, R. J., and Beahrs, O. H. Tumors of the Large Bowel. Philadelphia, W. B. Saunders Co., 1968.
10. De Dombal, F. T., Watts, J. M., Watkinson, G., et al. Local complications of ulcerative colitis: stricture, pseudopolyposis, and carcinoma of colon and rectum. Brit. Med. J. 1:1442, 1966.
11. Steinbach, H. L. Colonic malignancy. In Alimentary Tract Roentgenology, A. R. Margulis and H. J. Burhenne (eds.). St. Louis, C. V. Mosby Co., 1967.
12. Stolbach, L. L., Krant, M. J., and Fishman, W. H.

Ectopic production of an alkaline phosphatase isoenzyme in patients with cancer. New Eng. J. Med. *281*:757, 1969.

13. Gold, P., and Freedman, S. O.   Specific carcinoembryonic antigens of the human digestive system. J. Exp. Med. *122*:467, 1965.

14. Lo Gerfo, P., Krupey, J., and Hansen, H. J. Demonstration of an antigen common to several varieties of neoplasia. New Eng. J. Med. *285*:138, 1971.

15. Goulston, S. J., and McGovern, V. J.   The nature of benign strictures in ulcerative colitis. New Eng. J. Med. *281*:290, 1969.

16. Dunphy, J. E., and Broderick, E. G.   A critique of anterior resection in the treatment of cancer of the rectum and pelvic colon. Surgery *30*:106, 1951.

17. Postlethwait, R. W.   An appraisal of operations for rectal carcinoma. *In* Monographs in the Surgical Sciences, Vol. 4, Baltimore, Williams and Wilkins Co., 1967, pp. 217-242.

18. Glenn, F., and McSherry, C. K.   Obstruction and perforation in colo-rectal cancer. Ann. Surg. *173*:983, 1971.

19. Copeland, E. M., Jones, R. S., and Miller, L. D. Multiple colon neoplasms. Arch. Surg. *98*:141, 1969.

20. Polk, H. C., and Spratt, J. S.   Recurrent colo-rectal carcinoma: Detection, treatment, and other considerations. Surgery *69*:9, 1971.

21. Moertel, C. G., and Reitemeier, R. J. Chemotherapy of gastrointestinal cancer. Surg. Clin. N. Amer. *47*:929, 1967.

22. Higgins, G. A., Dwight, R. W., Smith, J. V., and Keehn, R. J.   Fluorouracil as an adjuvant to surgery in carcinoma of the colon. Arch. Surg. *102*:339, 1971.

23. Quan, S. H., Deddish, M. R., and Stearns, M. W.   The effect of preoperative roentgen therapy upon the 10- and 5-year results of the surgical treatment of cancer of the rectum. Surg. Gynec. Obstet. *111*:507, 1960.

24. Fletcher, W. S., Allen, C. V., and Dunphy, J. E. Preoperative irradiation for carcinoma of the colon and rectum. Amer. J. Surg. *109*:76, 1964.

25. Roswit, B., Higgins, G. A., and Keehn, R. J.   A controlled study of preoperative irradiation in cancer of the sigmoid colon and rectum. Radiology 97:133, 1970.

26. Moertel, C. G., Reitemeier, R. J., Childs, D. S., et al.   Combined 5-fluorouracil and supervoltage radiation therapy of locally unresectable gastrointestinal cancer. Lancet 2:865, 1969.

27. Stearns, M. W., and Quan, S. H.   Epidermoid carcinoma of the anorectum. Surg. Gynec. Obstet. *131*:953, 1970.

28. Sinclair, D. M., Hannah, G., McLaughlin, I. S., et al.   Malignant melanoma of the anal canal. Brit. J. Surg. 57:808, 1970.

29. Ponka, J. L., and Walke, L.   Carcinoid tumors of the rectum. Dis. Colon Rectum *14*:46, 1971.

30. Somervell, J. L., and Mayer, P. F.   Leiomyosarcoma of the rectum. Brit. J. Surg. 58:144, 1971.

31. Loehr, W. J., Mujahed, Z., Zahn, F. D., et al. Primary lymphoma of the gastrointestinal tract: A review of 100 cases. Ann. Surg. 170:232, 1969.

32. Friedman, H. B., Silver, G. M., and Brown, C. H. Lymphoma of the colon simulating ulcerative colitis. Amer. J. Dig. Dis. *13*:911, 1968.

33. Glickman, M. G., and Margulis, A. R.   Cloacogenic carcinoma. Amer. J. Roent. *107*:175, 1969.

Chapter 109

Megacolon

Murray Davidson, Marvin H. Sleisenger

DEFINITION AND CLASSIFICATION

Megacolon—enlarged or giant colon—is a clinical disorder of the large intestine characterized by marked dilatation and severe constipation or obstipation. The condition may be congenital or acquired (Table 109–1). In the congenital form the dilated bowel is proximal to a "narrowed" segment in which intramural ganglion cells are absent in the submucosal (Meissner's) and myenteric (Auerbach's) plexuses. This aganglionic intestine does not enter into normal propulsion of colonic contents, and the dilatation of the normally innervated areas is secondary to the distal obstruction. The extent of distal colon which is aganglionic ranges from short segments of rectum to the entire colon and, rarely, includes all the small intestine as well.

In acquired forms of megacolon dilatation extends through the whole colon, including the distal rectum.

CONGENITAL MEGACOLON

AGANGLIONIC MEGACOLON (HIRSCHSPRUNG'S DISEASE)

This form of megacolon usually becomes apparent shortly after birth when the infant passes scant or no meconium and becomes distended (Fig. 109–1). Digi-tal examination of the rectum, insertion of a rectal tube, or administration of a small enema may result in a gush of retained fecal material with apparent relief of the symptoms. If a long segment of aganglionosis exists, these measures may not relieve the symptoms and emergency decompression by colostomy is required to forestall perforation of a dilated portion of proximal colon, cecum, or appendix. More frequently the initial maneuvers are successful in inducing passage of meconium, but this respite is short lived. Signs of partial obstruction return, with persistent vomiting and distention as the major symptoms. If the presence of the condition is not suspected during the early weeks of life, about 20 per cent of patients develop persistent diarrhea caused by development of pseudomembranous enterocolitis, secondary to the obstruction. Mortality is about 75 per cent with this lesion, despite vigorous attempts to replace fluid and electrolyte losses. Decompression by performance of a colostomy in the more proximal bowel *after* enterocolitis has developed is also not helpful.

Infants who escape this extreme picture may, with help of frequent enemas and laxatives, survive to present the more characteristic symptoms of later childhood, i.e., obstipation and distention. Among these children growth and maturation are usually retarded; they frequently show evidence of anemia, malnutrition, and hypoproteinemia from protein-losing enter-

1463

TABLE 109–1. CLINICAL CLASSIFICATION OF MEGACOLON

I. Congenital Megacolon
  A. Aganglionosis (Hirschsprung's disease)
  B. Ganglionated
      Achalasia of distal rectal segment
      Segmental dilatation of the colon
II. Acquired Megacolon
  A. Psychogenic (abnormal bowel habit)
      Childhood psychogenic megacolon
      Psychosis
      Cathartic abuse
  B. Smooth muscle atrophy
      Scleroderma
      Myotonia dystrophica
      Congenital myotonia (Thomsen's disease)
  C. Metabolic disease
      Myxedema
      Porphyria
      Lead poisoning
      Hypokalemia
      Amyloidosis
  D. Neurological disease
      Chagas' disease
      Cerebral atrophy
      Parkinsonism
      Diabetic neuropathy
      Paraplegia
      Drug Toxicity
  E. Infection and inflammation
      Lymphogranuloma venereum
      Granulomatous colitis
      Pelvic irradiation
  F. Other obstructive lesions
      Rectal strictures
      Rectum and sigmoid tumors
      Extracolonic compression (endometriosis; carcinomatosis; adhesions)
  G. Toxic megacolon of ulcerative colitis
  H. Pseudo-obstruction of the colon

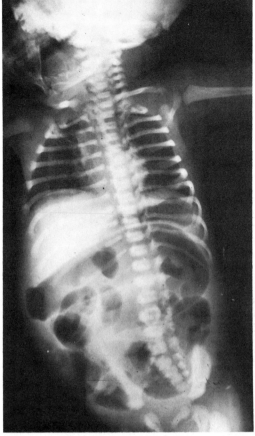

Figure 109–1. Plain film of abdomen in a neonate with colonic distention of meconum ileus caused by aganglionosis of the colon (Hirschsprung's disease). (Courtesy of Dr. H. I. Goldberg.)

opathy, and difficulty with resistance to recurrent infections.

INCIDENCE AND GENETICS

The defect occurs in approximately one of each 5000 live births and is a familial disease.[1] Seventeen of 326 index cases in males (2.6 per cent) and 13 of 88 index cases in females (7.2 per cent) had affected siblings, with an overall incidence of 3.6 per cent among siblings of all index cases. Since the disease was highly lethal until recent years, accurate assessment of the incidence in offspring of successfully treated patients is still impossible. Consanguinity of parents is exceptional, and only three such instances have been reported in a study of 326 families. The disease is dis-cordant in dizygotic twins and appears to be concordant in monozygotes.

Association of congenital aganglionosis of the colon with Down's syndrome (mongolism) is ten times more frequent than would be expected by chance.[2] Approximately 2 per cent of the patients with congenital megacolon have Down's syndrome. Other anomalies which have been reported to be associated with congenital megacolon include megacystis and mega-ureter, hydrocephalus, ventricular septal defect, cystic deformities of the kidney, cryptorchidism, diverticulum of the urinary bladder, imperforate anus, Meckel's diverticulum, hypoplastic uterus, polyposis of the colon, ependymoma of the fourth ventricle, and the Laurence-Moon-Biedl-Bardet syndrome.

PATHOLOGY AND PATHOPHYSIOLOGY

Normal investment of the submucosal and myenteric plexuses with ganglion cells proceeds from the cephalic to the caudal end in embryonic development. Arrest of this process presumably accounts for the fact that in virtually all reported patients with congenital megacolon the aganglionic area extends proximally from the internal anal sphincter for varying distances. In the vast majority of patients, the proximal border of the aganglionic segment is located within the rectum or sigmoid colon.[1] In only 10 to 20 per cent of individuals is there a longer segment

involvement. Involvement of the entire colon is rare, and in only seven patients has aganglionosis been reported to extend proximally throughout the entire small intestine.

The mechanism of disease consists of failure of the abnormally innervated distal segment to permit entry of proximal colonic contents and to carry them along in peristalsis.[3] Motility studies indicate that phasic (nonpropulsive) activity is normal in both the proximally dilated and distal narrowed segments.[4] However, the abnormally innervated segment does not relax after subcutaneous administration of methacholine (Fig. 109–2). Such relaxation is

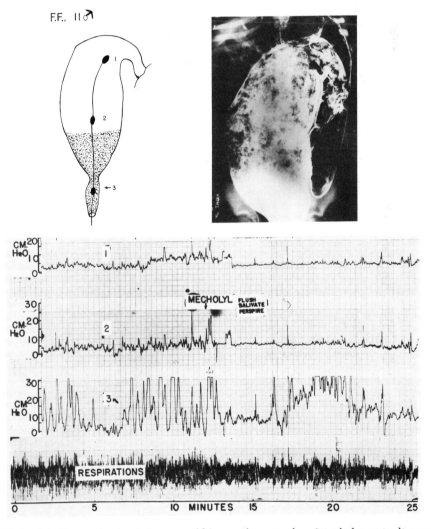

Figure 109–2. Motility tracing in eleven-year-old boy with megacolon. Stippled area in diagram at upper left shows extent of aganglionosis. Positions of catheter tips referred to in motility tracing shown in diagram. Following intramuscular injection of Mecholyl, there was diminution of phasic activity in normally innervated segments, but no relaxation in aganglionic area. (From Davidson, M., et al.: Gastroenterology 29:803, 1955.)

noted in *all* segments of the distal colon in 50 per cent of normal people after injection of methacholine.[4] This consistent pattern of response indicates that abolition of resting activity and onset of propulsion are coordinated via the autonomic nervous system. However, relaxation of only the normally innervated colon with failure to achieve any effect of methacholine in the distal aganglionic segment of the same individual may be interpreted as evidence for defective intrinsic autonomic innervation of this segment.[5] Other techniques of motility study involve observations on the behavior of the internal and external anal sphincters in response to rectal distention; disturbances of these responses are also found among patients with congenital aganglionosis of the colon. These various motor abnormalities may be utilized for diagnostic tests in cases of doubtful diagnosis (see below).

CLINICAL PICTURE

Although the characteristic clinical picture of congenital aganglionosis of the colon involves difficulty with innervation dating from birth, the presenting symptoms may be variable. In most instances, regardless of the eventual severity of the clinical picture, meconium is passed after a delay of 48 hours or more after birth or is not passed at all. Vomiting ensues if there is no relief after 48 to 72 hours; however, this symptom does not distinguish between small and large bowel obstruction in infants. It is sufficient that the physician appreciate that the symptoms in these infants are not functional; the precise level of neonatal obstruction need not be fixed. Plain films demonstrate dilated gas and fluid-filled loops, although delineation of small and large bowels is virtually impossible in the newborn and the films are therefore not diagnostic (Fig. 109–1). Digital examination usually reveals no stool in the rectum, but withdrawal of the finger or of a rectal tube may lead to a gush of meconium and to decompression. Barium enema is also not likely to be diagnostic, because sufficient time has not elapsed in a newborn for the transition zone to be developed. However, slow and poor evacuation of the contrast medium is common.

Among infants presenting with this picture, the subsequent clinical course varies. Some infants continue with complete obstruction, do not pass any meconium, and require surgery in the first few days of life. In others there is recurrent or delayed incomplete obstruction, usually relieved by repeated enemas after the second or third day of life. As a rule, these patients fare poorly unless surgery is performed. In a third group the successful management of the initial neonatal obstruction by conservative means with subsequent repeated enemas for the continuing partial obstruction is suddenly, and often unexpectedly, thwarted by development of fulminant enterocolitis with bloody diarrhea.[6, 7] The mortality with this condition is very high. The problem requires vigorous fluid and electrolyte replacement; antimicrobial drugs are not of proved value in treatment, and decompression by colostomy or ileostomy after the condition has appeared is not very useful.

The disease picture among older infants and children is not as variable as in the newborn period. The common symptoms are persistent abdominal distention and stool retention. Malnutrition, anemia, rectal bleeding caused by ulcers from colonic stasis, protein-losing enteropathy, and recurrent systemic infections are regular complicating features of the disease in older children.

In those instances in which the entire colon is aganglionic, whether or not the small bowel is also involved, the extensive defect represents a serious neonatal problem.[2] The initial presentation is generally the same in this condition as in the more usual instance of distal colonic aganglionosis; i.e., the infant shows signs of intestinal obstruction within the first 24 to 48 hours of life. The abdomen is not likely to be as distended in these patients with long segments of disease, especially if much of the small intestine is aganglionic. Barium enema reveals a true microcolon throughout. Since enterocolitis commonly arises among infants with long segments of aganglionic bowel, this lethal complication is especially likely in this group of patients and the infants must therefore be operated on immediately to relieve the obstruction. The level at which the intestine is normally innervated should be ascertained by frozen section examinations prior to performance of a decompressing ileostomy.

COMPLICATIONS

Patients with congenital megacolon are prone to certain complications. One of the most common is neonatal bowel obstruction by a meconium plug. One of four patients with meconium plugs will ultimately prove to have congenital megacolon, including those with minimal as well as those with extensive aganglionosis.

Patients with congenital megacolon also suffer *neonatal perforation of the appendix*. At surgery, an uninflamed but perforated appendix is found which, on histological examination, may show diminution or absence of ganglion cells.

The most common and least serious complication in older children and young adults is *recurrent fecal impaction* and low bowel obstruction. Large quantities of inspissated feces collect at the upper border of the aganglionic segment, progressively distending the bowel and slowly obstructing the more proximal small bowel. If unrelieved, vomiting and dehydration result.

Stercoral ulcers caused by pressure of the fecal mass upon the bowel wall may be noted in patients with congenital megacolon. Rarely, these ulcers bleed or perforate. *Perforation of the colon* is a rare but serious complication. Patients may be undernourished, with subnormal response to antimicrobial therapy for peritonitis; shock is common. The mortality—even with early surgical decompression, antimicrobials, fluid and electrolyte replacement, and blood transfusions—is high.

Urinary tract infection, particularly of the lower tract, may occasionally complicate the course of patients with associated megacystis; the kidneys may also be infected if megaureter is present. Fortunately, this condition is rarely associated with congenital aganglionosis of the colon.

DIFFERENTIAL DIAGNOSIS

Congenital aganglionosis of the colon (Hirschsprung's disease) must be distinguished in the neonate from other causes of intestinal obstruction. Later, it must be distinguished from secondary megacolon caused by an associated condition (e.g., anal stricture, myxedema, or psychogenic problems; see below). The diagnosis of congenital aganglionosis of the colon beyond the neonatal period is usually not too difficult. Obstipation with infrequent spontaneous passage of stool dating from infancy is an important part of the history. Enemas and laxatives to facilitate bowel movements are frequently required. The patients are virtually all children; undiagnosed cases among young adults (second and third decades) are rare. Rectal examination usually reveals an empty ampulla. In extreme instances, the abdominal wall is stretched so that the skin is shiny and the venous pattern is prominent; large fecal masses may be felt over the left colon; in some instances, nutrition is obviously poor.

Barium enema X-ray will usually confirm the diagnosis because of the characteristic transition from the normal caliber

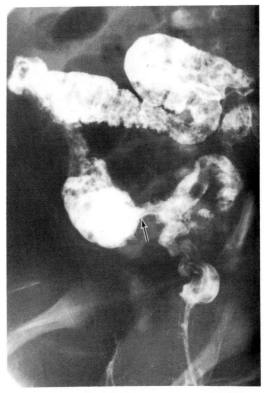

Figure 109–3. Barium enema in eleven-month-old child with Hirschsprung's disease, showing transition zone (arrow) between dilated proximal and narrowed distal segments.

or "narrowed" distal rectal or rectosigmoid segment to the more dilated proximal colon (Figs. 109–3 and 109–4). This finding is usually best demonstrated in a lateral view. It is not useful in infants with meconium retention, because sufficient time will not have elapsed for the differences in caliber to become prominent. In adults, however, the narrowed segment is still readily noted (Fig. 109–4). Among patients with acquired megacolon, dilatation extends all the way to the anus and a transition zone is not seen (Fig. 109–5, *A* and *B*). X-ray findings on barium enema in acquired megacolon caused by organic disease involving the rectum vary, depending on the underlying cause. Careful search for narrowing of the rectum or rectosigmoid by tumor or stricture is made; however, the degree of proximal dilatation is usually not nearly so pronounced as in congenital aganglionosis of the colon.

Proctosigmoidoscopy reveals a normal

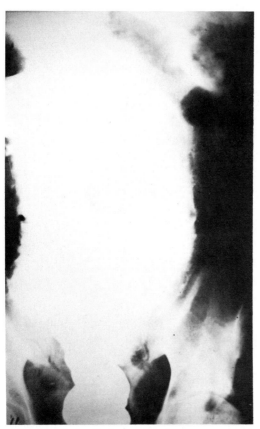

Figure 109–4. Barium enema in a teenager with congenital aganglionosis; note relatively "narrowed" distal rectal segment in contrast to Figure 109–5.

but empty rectum. The dilated proximal bowel, if within range of the scope, is easily traversed except for enormous fecal retention in the dilated lumen; occasionally, stercoral ulcers may be noted. The important differential diagnostic findings are the empty lower segment with no evidence of organic obstruction.

In doubtful cases the diagnosis may be aided by examination of a full thickness biopsy specimen of the rectum (Fig. 109–6, *A* and *B*). The tissue is examined histologically for ganglion cells. Their presence in normal number effectively rules out the diagnosis. More recently, experience with mucosal biopsy has proved equally satisfactory in many instances.[8] It is the initial procedure of choice for diagnosis, because it is performed easily and it requires no anesthesia. The depth of the examination is sufficient to show the presence of ganglia in a number of cases, and thus excludes the diagnosis of Hirschsprung's disease. Absence of ganglion cells in a specimen obtained by suction biopsy at about 5 to 6 cm above the valves of Houston does not establish the diagnosis. In order to be perfectly certain that the aganglionosis demonstrated on a particular biopsy is of diagnostic significance, it should be full thickness and obtained at least 3 cm within or proximal to the pectinate line. Diminution or absence of ganglion cells distal to this point is difficult to interpret, and their absence does not establish Hirschsprung's disease. Careful measurements proximal to the internal sphincter indicate that no ganglia may be found in the normal infant in the myenteric plexuses over a distance of 4 mm in this segment; none will be seen in the deep submucosal layer for 7 mm and in the superficial submucosal layer for 10 mm.

Physiological tests, believed to be based upon the abnormalities of parasympathetic innervation, may be used for diagnosis in doubtful cases.[4, 5] In addition to their usefulness as screening procedures, such measurements may also detect short segment congenital megacolon undetectable by X-ray or inadvertently missed by biopsy. One such test is the abnormal response of the rectum to injection of acetylcholine or methacholine parenterally. In 50 per cent of patients this segment does not relax despite relaxation of the normally innervated colon (Fig. 109–2).

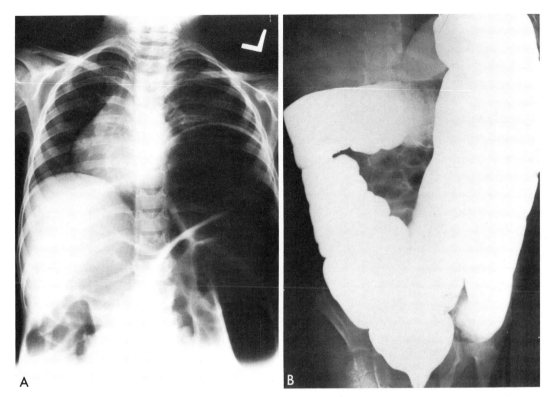

Figure 109–5. *A,* Plain film in seven-year-old boy with acquired megacolon and severe obstipation, showing enormous enlargement of colon with elevation of left hemidiaphragm and mediastinal shift. *B,* Barium enema in same patient, showing marked dilatation of entire colon, including rectal segment.

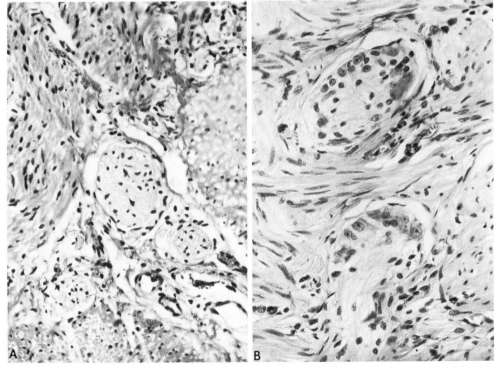

Figure 109–6. *A,* Biopsy of rectum in a patient with Hirschsprung's disease, showing Auerbach's plexus at center with neural elements but absence of ganglion cells. Hematoxylin and eosin stain. × 200. *B,* Normal specimen at same magnification and staining techniques, showing ganglion cells within plexus.

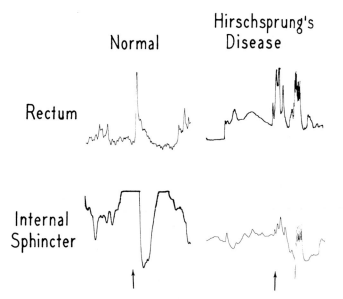

Figure 109-7. Response of rectum and internal sphincter to distention (arrows) of rectal balloon (at anus) in normal control subject and in infant with Hirschsprung's disease.

Another physiological test is based on the response to distention of the rectum rather than to injection of parasympathomimetic agents. In contrast to normal individuals and to patients with acquired megacolon, the internal sphincter in patients with congenital aganglionosis contracts rather than relaxes after distention of the rectum (Fig. 109–7).[9, 10] In addition, about half the individuals with this disease also show contraction of the rectal segment itself, rather than the more usual relaxation which follows distention of the segment.

Although the precise roles of the sympathetic and parasympathetic systems in these various pathophysiological findings are not clear, the internal sphincter abnormality may possibly contribute to the continuing obstruction which creates problems in some patients during the postoperative period after resection of the involved segment. It has now become standard to divide the sphincter.

SURGICAL AND MEDICAL TREATMENT

Once the diagnosis is established, definitive cure via surgery is the treatment of choice. Preliminary decompression via colostomy may be necessary to relieve obstruction in infants in whom it is decided to postpone definitive correction for a later time, or in older individuals in whom diversion of the fecal stream may be necessary to provide a grace period in which nutritional status is improved.

In general, many patients whose aganglionic segments do not extend above the sigmoid segment are maintained in a relatively decompressed state with regular enemas prior to surgery. Serious complications of this medical treatment may result from the use of the evacuating enemas.[11] Large amounts of plain tap water (greater than 2.0 liters) are readily absorbed by the dilated, hypertrophied colon, and serious symptoms of water intoxication may result.[12] Dilution of essential plasma electrolytes, particularly sodium, results in weakness, nausea, headache, vomiting, muscle cramps, polyuria, and, in extreme instances, convulsions and death associated terminally with refractory shock. However, use of saline enemas is no guarantee against these serious complications, because shock has also been reported from the absorption of water with excessive quantities of isotonic saline.

The recent more frequent use of hypertonic phosphate enemas is also attended by complications, particularly in infants and young children. With these preparations, large quantities of water move into the colon while sodium and/or phosphate are absorbed. The potential is great for damage of the central nervous system from the increased extra- and intracellular sodium concentration in the face of decreased blood volume. Hyperphosphatemia and hypocalcemia with tetany may also occur in some instances after administration of hypertonic sodium phosphate enemas.

The main goals of surgery are to establish regular and spontaneous defecation, to maintain normal continence, and to avoid interference with sexual potency. The procedure employed should have essentially no mortality and a minimal morbidity. A number of procedures are available, and surgeons differ in their opinions as to the superior method. The choice of procedure should be left to the surgeon who is asked to repair the defect; if he is experienced with whatever procedure he uses and his results are good, it is best to permit him to handle the situation without interference.[13]

The original standard procedure for correction of congenital megacolon is the Swenson pull-through operation in which normally innervated colon is brought through the denervated segment and anastomosed to the seromuscular coat of the distal rectum above the internal sphincter.[14, 15] Because of the pull-through, the proximal colon is anastomosed to the distal rectum extracorporeally. Sometimes the patient develops a form of colitis postoperatively because of the retention of material proximal to a "spastic" internal sphincter. Leakage and breakdown at the anastomotic site have also been attributed to back pressure from the tightness of this sphincter so that most surgeons now advocate incision of the internal sphincter as part of the procedure.

In the Duhamel procedure, normally innervated colon is anastomosed side-to-side to the posterior wall of the distal rectal segment which is retained as a blind pouch to avoid the potentially dangerous dissection of the nerves adjacent to the serosa of the anterior rectal wall.[16] This advantage of the operation is often offset by the retention of fecal material in the rectal redundant pouch and retention of significant lengths of the colonic and rectal septum created by the anastomosis. Modifications of the basic procedure have been proposd which eliminate the pouch and the septum as well as their complications.

In the Soave technique, the mucosa of the aganglionic rectum is stripped off; the surrounding muscular coat with its sensory reflexes is retained.[17] Normally innervated propulsive colon is pulled through this cuff down to the mucocutaneous junction. The internal sphincter remains intact for continence but is bypassed from within by the placement of the normal bowel. This procedure minimizes damage to the pelvic nerves, a danger in other procedures, and it also obviates the problem of a "spastic" internal sphincter present after either the Swenson or Duhamel operations. These infants are able to develop voluntary control of defecation despite the absence of rectal mucosa, indicating that the sensory receptors are probably located in the muscular layers rather than in the mucosal.

CONGENITAL MOTOR DISTURBANCES IN GANGLIONATED BOWEL

This group of disorders deals with megacolon which develops in infants and young children and with clinical pictures and barium enema X-rays which may be confused with those associated with aganglionosis (Hirschsprung's disease). However, in these conditions the distal colon may be shown on histological study to be normally innervated.

Achalasia of Distal Rectal Segment. In this entity children experience constipation or obstipation dating from birth; on X-ray studies there is proximal dilatation with a short distal narrow segment of rectum.[18] The histories and clinical pictures simulate aganglionosis of the colon, and motility studies may demonstrate abnormal behavior of the distal rectal segment akin to that of an aganglionic segment. However, histological examination of a biopsy specimen from this segment will reveal normal ganglion cells. The same type of surgical correction is indicated as for a patient with aganglionosis of the distal segment.

Segmental Dilatation of the Colon. This entity is also characterized by severe constipation from birth; however, the colon is segmentally dilated proximal to a nondilated distal segment. Although the proximal dilated bowel has the characteristic hypertrophy of the muscle layers seen in congenital aganglionosis of the colon, normal ganglion cells are found both in the dilated bowel and in the distal narrowed segment, and it is assumed that the lesion may be secondary to a vascular accident.

ACQUIRED MEGACOLON

This category of megacolon may be either of psychogenic origin or secondary to an associated disease (Table 109–1). This category is also called acquired because neither aganglionosis nor any other congenital motor abnormality is present. A major distinguishing feature is that in congenital megacolon difficulty with bowel movement dates from early infancy in most individuals. In acquired megacolon, evidence for other causes, ranging from "stool holding" in childhood to symptoms of severe inflammation with stricture of the anus or rectum or of malignancy of the rectum or rectosigmoid (low grade obstruction), is readily noted. Whether associated with organic disease or related to psychogenic factors, these patients do not have aganglionosis or hypoganglionosis, except in Chagas' disease in which degeneration of ganglia results from acquired infection.

Patients with psychogenic megacolon of childhood (and in some instances, adulthood) have severe dilatation of the rectum as well as the colon on barium enema. These patients have a history of encopresis, and almost always have had an obvious long-standing disturbance in bowel habit. Other underlying causes range from neuroses to psychoses, particularly depression; indeed, this type of megacolon is often encountered in patients in mental hospitals. On physical examination, in contrast to congenital megacolon, fecal impactions are common. In addition, patients with these types of psychogenic megacolon have no history of meconium ileus.

Adult patients with megacolon caused by organic disease, metabolic disturbances, or neurological disease will have features consistent with their underlying disorder (myxedema, porphyria, lead poisoning, parkinsonism), or histories of increasing constipation caused by irradiation to the pelvis, annular carcinoma, strictures of chronic granulomatous disease of the rectum or anus, or ingestion of anticholinergics or opiates. In certain areas of the world, particularly Central and South America, infection with *Trypanosoma cruzi* (Chagas' disease) (see below) will cause megacolon as well as megaesophagus. Extrinsic pressure on the sigmoid or rectum by extracolonic tumor, endometrial implants, or adhesions may slowly and chronically obstruct the distal bowel with an appearance of marked proximal dilatation. Acquired megacolon may result from strictures after surgery to correct imperforate anus, fissures, or fistulas, to evacuate perirectal abscesses, or to remove hemorrhoids.

Appropriate studies will, of course, clearly indicate the role of these diseases in the patient's megacolon. Patients with serious spinal cord disease such as transverse myelitis, spinal cord transection, and compression caused by tumor, abscess, multiple sclerosis, or spina bifida will not have normal bowel or bladder function. The defecation reflex, dependent upon impulses to the anus from the rectum in response to distention, is impaired in patients with spinal cord disease but may be restored by early enemas. Most paraplegics will regain some function based on intrinsic innervation and spinal cord reflexes below the site of cord damage. The megacolon of ulcerative colitis is discussed in detail on pages 1326 to 1329.

For convenience the causes of acquired megacolon may be divided into the following groups (Table 109–1: psychogenic disease, smooth muscle disease, metabolic disease, neurological disease, infection and inflammation, and other obstructive lesions. Although constipation accompanies acquired megacolon, it is not present in all instances. Megacolon in these categories is defined as dilatation of the transverse diameter of the colon to greater than 5.5 cm as measured on plain roentgenograms of the supine abdomen, or 6.5 cm on air-contact barium enema studies.

Radiographic Features. The colon responds by dilatation to many different stimuli, producing a megacolon (Table 109–1). Careful attention to specific roentgenographic findings allows the diagnostic possibilities to be narrowed considerably, but further clinical information is required for a precise diagnosis.

In adynamic ileus, pronounced colonic

distention and elongation are frequently observed, with a smooth, regular luminal contour and loss of most haustra. When haustra or septa are identified, they are of normal thickness and are frequently associated with dilatation of the small bowel. Dilatation of the colon resulting from chronic obstruction usually causes thickening of haustra and irregularity of the contour of the dilated colon because of muscular hypertrophy. Air-fluid levels are seen frequently.

A careful analysis of the clinical history is necessary to reduce to a reasonable number the list of possible causes of megacolon.

Proctosigmoidoscopy. This procedure is obviously valuable in the differential diagnosis of megacolon. A capacious rectum with normal mucosa may be noted in the disorders of categories II A, B, C and D in Table 109–1. Such findings are not found in patients with megacolon secondary to inflammatory disease of the anus and rectum, with stricture or tumor of the distal segment (easily visualized or felt in most cases), with aganglionosis of the colon, or with chronic obstruction resulting from torsion, adhesions, or extrinsic pressure on the colon. The most capacious rectums (often with impacted feces) are associated with psychogenic and neurological disorders. On the other hand, a spastic or stenotic sphincter, often with perirectal sepsis and severe inflammation of the anorectal segment, is typical of chronic inflammatory disease.

Biopsy is important in establishing diagnosis in some of the diseases which may cause megacolon, particularly granulomatous disease, amyloidosis, tumor, and, as noted, aganglionosis.

PSYCHOGENIC MEGACOLON

One form of acquired megacolon, particularly among children, which may be difficult to distinguish from Hirschsprung's disease is so-called psychogenic megacolon.[19, 20] The suggestion from the name of the disease that the child has a psychological basis for willfully withholding stool is usually somewhat incorrect. However, the lack of appreciation by many physicians and parents of the pathophysiology of this problem in most children generates further unhealthy emotional interaction between mothers and children. This complication contributes considerably to the child's abnormal behavior when the clinical picture is full blown, at which time the psychogenic aspects of the problem act to prevent appreciation of the fundamental physiological basis for the condition.

Under normal circumstances, the urge to pass stool is perceived after the distal colonic (rectal and rectosigmoid) musculature has sufficiently squeezed the luminal contents into a bolus of a particular size and consistency. Activation of this urge to defecate is actually less dependent upon the characteristics of the bolus than upon the state of tone of the surrounding distal colonic musculature. Among constipated individuals the urge to defecate is perceived only when there is a relatively heightened state of tone, which in fact means that the stools of such individuals have been dried to smaller size and firmer consistency than that of "average" individuals. In some instances this difficulty with expelling of the firm stools will be encountered early, and, in extreme cases, in the newborn period. Generally, however, the difficulty becomes clinically more apparent as the child passes beyond the first months of life and the number of stools tends to decrease. When the average number usually becomes once or twice daily (at six months to one year), the constipated infant may begin to skip days and the stools may become so firm that they cause pain with passage. The child tends then, often as early as six to eight months of age, but more frequently and characteristically at between one and two years of age, voluntarily to hold back stool to avoid pain. This is evidenced by the child's stiffening up, crying at the time of bowel movement, and refusing to get into a squatting position; i.e., the urge passes off within a short period of time and he is no longer "troubled" by the need to defecate. As this pattern becomes fixed, the intervals between bowel movements become longer. In addition, development of a more patulous distal colon makes it necessary for larger amounts to accumulate before sufficient stretch of the musculature takes place to create the urge. Although the disturbance of the regularity of bowel movement is initially voluntary, it quickly becomes perpetuated involuntarily as the urges to defecate are diminished with increasing intervals between them. Thus a conscious act develops into a "habit" over which less and less control is exerted.

Following build-up of material in the distal colon of a child with psychogenic obstipation, he may pass a massive stool. Once achieved, a period follows during which he is relatively more comfortable and will not have the urge to defecate until the large ampulla which has developed becomes filled again. In addition, as the situation progresses and as larger fecal impactions are encountered, overflow tends involuntarily to leak around the impactions and the patient exhibits encopresis, or paradoxical soiling. When this situation supervenes there is further attempt in many instances to pinpoint this as a psychological problem, because the act of soiling oneself, presumably voluntarily, is difficult to understand on any basis other than emotional. By the time such children present for differential diagnosis of significant obstipation at two to four years of age, a number of features will have developed which confuse the picture with congenital megacolon.

Diagnosis. History in these patients differs from aganglionosis in that the problem usually does not date from birth or early infancy. There is evidence of a prior strong urge to defecate, and encopresis is common. Occasionally severely affected patients with psychogenic megacolon may be constipated from birth; however, there are other reliable diagnostic features of this condition. The anal sphincter is normal to the examining finger, to neurological examination, and to motility techniques. The ampulla is ample and patulous, without any evidence for a cause of obstruction such as a stricture. Stool is usually palpable in the ampulla in large amounts, in contrast to congenital megacolon. Often these children will have perianal irritation and fissures. One of the most important historical features for distinguishing these patients from those with Hirschsprung's disease is the fact that these children still appreciate an urge to defecate, a sensation that can be perceived when stool is regularly delivered to the distal colon. Among many patients with Hirschsprung's disease, despite enormous degrees of obstipa-

tion and fecal retention, the urge to defecate has not regularly been felt because their distal segment remains empty.

The barium enema helps enormously in establishing the diagnosis and may be performed if the picture is not clear (Figs. 109–5 and 109–8). A trial of therapy may aid in differential diagnosis and will usually obviate the need for X-rays. Should a trial of therapy fail in a patient with no narrowed segment or a questionably narrowed segment, repeat barium enema must be performed along with motility studies and biopsy (see pp. 1467 to 1470).

Treatment. The condition should not be treated surgically, although some authors have advocated removal of the distal portion of the dilated colon. In those instances stools are passed normally imme-

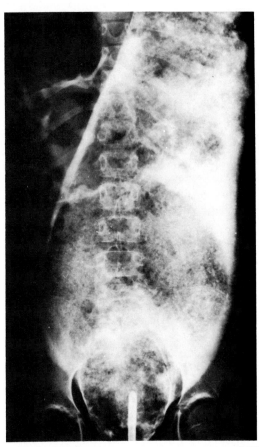

Figure 109–8. Barium enema in a young child with acquired (psychogenic) megacolon. Entire rectum is markedly dilated. (Courtesy of Dr. H. I. Goldberg.)

diately after surgery; but as withholding reappears, so does massive secondary colonic dilatation.

On the other hand, if one treats medically and keeps the rectum empty most of the time, the large patulous ampulla gradually shrinks and as the musculature becomes more normal permanent cure becomes possible. Administration of five cleansing enemas daily for a period of two to three months will decompress the distal colon considerably; however, it is an extremely difficult and ill-advised treatment for children. Prescription of sufficient amounts of light mineral oil to achieve four to five bowel movements daily is preferred. Initially one to two ounces for every 10 pounds of body weight is recommended in the early morning and at bedtime. The dose is gradually increased by $1/2$ to 1 ounce daily as needed. Indeed, in some instaces it is necessary to give as much as one quart daily for older children in whom this habit has been present for many years before the four to five bowel movements daily are achieved. Commercially flavored mineral oils are too thick to use at these dosages. Patients may leak oil between bowel movements as a result of continuing attempts to withhold stool, with failure of thorough mixing of oil and stool. Leakage of oil is common with physical activity by the patient. In these instances the dose is raised until four to five daily stools result and leakage disappears. Since the oil is not given with food, no deficiency of fat-soluble vitamins is noted. The regimen is continued for three months.

Interestingly, this technique of treatment also results in retraining the child. Ultimately he ceases to resist the urge to defecate, because the bowel movements are being passed with ease and without pain. In children under four years of age no effort is made to force them to the toilet during this period. However, older children are usually quite accepting of toileting if they have been previously resistant, once the bowel movements become relatively painless, and especially if they become disturbed by the multiple times daily that large volumes of loose stool are passed into their undergarments.

If it is desired that the underlying constipation be managed on a more compulsive basis with development of a regular toileting habit, the oil may be continued in smaller dosage for a number of weeks after this treatment has been carried out. No attempt should be made to develop regular bowel habits during the first three months, but continuation of oil beyond that point may make it somewhat easier to motivate a child to develop a regular daily bowel habit.

This regimen may also be used as a diagnostic test to avoid repeated X-ray studies and biopsy in children with this problem. It is not likely that any patients with true Hirschsprung's disease will ever develop a consistent bowel pattern of four to five movements daily after administration of large doses of mineral oil. Usually, such patients may appear to be successful for a few days at a time but will then become obstipated while the medication is continued. If patients are refractory to an adequate dosage of mineral oil given for three to four weeks, the diagnosis of Hirschsprung's disease becomes more likely, and further diagnostic studies, including biopsy and motility, should then be conducted. Usually, this approach prevents unnecessary diagnostic maneuvers among most young children who present with severe abdominal distention and obstipation but who have no narrowed segment on barium enema. Since so-called psychogenic megacolon is at least 20 times as frequent as congenital megacolon in patients beyond infancy, such a plan appears wise.

PSYCHOSIS

This group of adult patients should be distinguished from those with the psychogenic megacolon of childhood, which is associated with disturbed parental relationships or failure to establish normal bowel habits. Although some adults with psychological problems and megacolon may suffer these symptoms as a continuation of problems that began in childhood, a larger group will have onset of obstipation and megacolon in young adulthood or middle age. Most of these patients suffer from serious mental disorders, particularly schizophrenia and depression. Frequently, they are institutionalized; they become constipated because their mental disorder somehow blunts the defecatory urge or

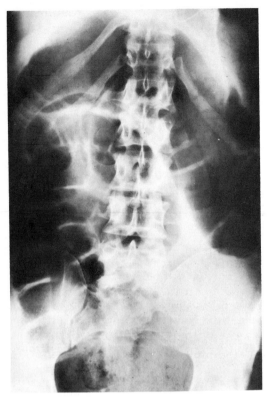

Figure 109–9. Plain film of abdomen in an adult male with megacolon associated with psychosis treated with chlorpromazine. He was obstipated. Note marked distention of transverse colon. (Courtesy of Dr. H. I. Goldberg.)

causes them to ignore it and, in part, because of neglect by those caring for them. The constipation progresses insidiously to obstipation, and the colon dilates (Fig. 109–9). Indeed, such individuals may not have spontaneous bowel movements for weeks. Vigorous efforts are required to evacuate their colons, and much attention must be given to re-establish a normal bowel habit (Fig. 109–10). The etiologic role of the so-called psychopharmacological agents with which these patients are often treated is not clear at this time; however, some evidence exists that these agents (e.g., phenothiazines, Valium, Librium) inhibit gut motility, most likely by way of a central effect, and may contribute to the constipation. It must be stressed, however, that unquestionably the major factor in the appearance of this picture is the underlying mental disorder itself, which probably dulls the stimulus for def-

ecation. Barium enema reveals unusual distention (Fig. 109–11).

Management depends upon the alleviation of fecal impaction, evacuation of the colon by carefully administered saline enemas or hypertonic phosphate preparations, and the re-establishment of normal bowel habits in these patients by prescribing the same regimen outlined for psychogenic megacolon in children.

CHRONIC CATHARTIC USE

Lifelong and frequent (daily or even more often) resort to irritant cathartics may be associated with marked dilatation of the colon on barium enema X-ray examination (Fig. 109–12). Dilatation generally involves the entire colon down to the anal canal; in this way the condition also may be distinguished from congenital aganglionosis. The right and transverse colons are most often enlarged. More important in differential diagnosis, however, is the ab-

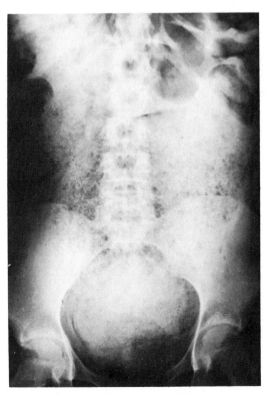

Figure 109–10. Plain film of abdomen in a patient with psychogenic megacolon. Note the enormous amount of fecal material extending down into the rectum. (Courtesy of Dr. H. I. Goldberg.)

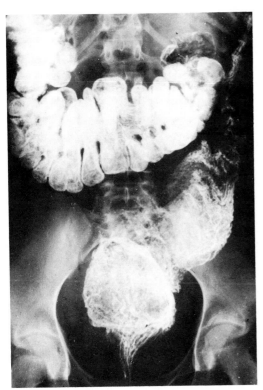

Figure 109–11. Barium enema, demonstrating megacolon in a psychotic patient with obstipation. (Courtesy of Dr. H. I. Goldberg.)

serious disease of the small intestine and esophagus; also, these patients will very likely have involvement of skin, joints, and other evidences of the systemic nature of the disease. Much like those with so-called pseudo-obstruction of the colon, they suffer a generalized type of ileus with vomiting, distention, and, in some instances, passage of small amounts of liquid stool several times daily. A characteristic feature of the barium enema is the "sacculation" of the colon (Figs. 109–13 and 109–14) which may be seen; however, it appears in a minority of instances.

Myotonia dystrophica, like scleroderma and Chagas' disease, is also characterized by a dilated esophagus and delayed emptying; however, the distal segment is not narrowed, and response to methacholine is normal. This disease, which affects striated and smooth muscle alike, is characterized principally by weakness and atrophy of skeletal muscle associated with inability of skeletal muscles to relax after

sence of a history of severe constipation from infancy which would indicate congenital aganglionosis. Conversely, the positive history of a long-time use of laxative substances is striking. Chief among the ingredients of such mixtures are irritant compounds containing aloin, podophyllum, cascara sagrada, or castor oil. Mineral oil and bulk laxatives rarely cause megacolon.

Although the predominant roentgenographic feature of irritant cathartic colon is loss of haustration and effacement of the normal mucosal pattern, giving the bowel an appearance of "burnt-out" ulcerative colitis, marked distensibility of the colon may also be noted (Fig. 109–12). It is this marked distention which qualifies it to be classified as a form of megacolon.

SMOOTH MUSCLE ATROPHY

In the category of smooth muscle disease, scleroderma may be recognized because it is nearly always associated with

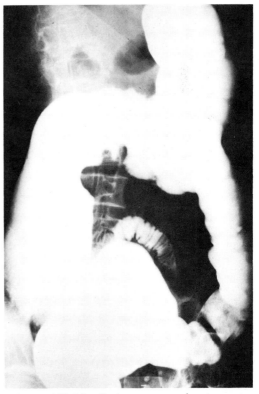

Figure 109–12. Barium enema, showing somewhat dilated colon with absent haustra simulating ulcerative colitis caused by lifelong cathartic abuse (cascara sagrada). (Courtesy of Dr. H. I. Goldberg.)

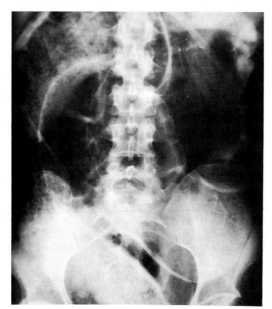

Figure 109–13. Plain film of abdomen in a patient with scleroderma and obstipation. Note large dilatation of the colon. (Courtesy of Dr. H. I. Goldberg.)

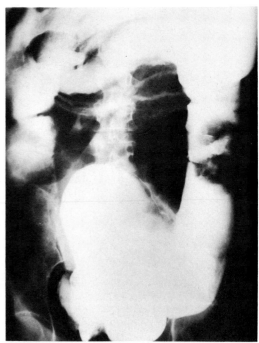

Figure 109–14. Barium enema in a patient with scleroderma. Haustra are absent; colon is slightly dilated. Note sacculation of hepatic flexure and stercoral ulcer in descending colon. (Courtesy of Dr. H. I. Goldberg.)

forceful contraction; frontal baldness, and testicular atrophy may also be noted. The family history is strong, because it is a hereditary disease, and the defect appears to be transmitted in a dominant fashion. Colonic dilatation in this disease extends down to the anus (Fig. 109–15).

Congenital myotonia (Thomsen's disease) likewise causes smooth muscle atrophy and may be the basis for megacolon. Other features of this disease include difficulty in initiating movement combined with slowness of relaxation of skeletal muscles and skeletal muscular hypertrophy during the early years of life.

METABOLIC AND NEUROLOGICAL DISEASE, INCLUDING DRUG TOXICITY

Metabolic diseases such as myxedema and porphyria have rather characteristic clinical pictures. Some individuals with porphyria may have chronic constipation with dilatation of the colon; severe constipation and even obstipation are not uncommon in myxedema, the clinical features of which should be readily apparent to the physician (Figs. 109–16 and 109–

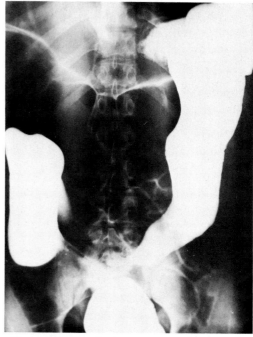

Figure 109–15. Barium enema demonstrating megacolon in myotonia dystrophica. (Courtesy of Dr. H. I. Goldberg.)

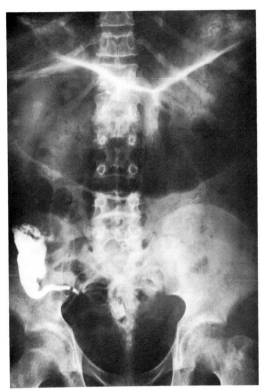

Figure 109–16. Plain film of abdomen showing megacolon in severe myxedema. Transverse colon is hugely dilated. (Courtesy of Dr. H. I. Goldberg.)

similar to congenital aganglionosis. Radiologically, the colon is markedly dilated and the picture closely resembles congenital aganglionosis of the colon (Hirschsprung's disease). The left colon is often the only portion demonstrating dilatation.

Other neurological diseases and dysfunction are readily diagnosed, particularly cerebral atrophy, diabetic neuropathy, parkinsonism, and paraplegia. The mechanisms are not known, but involvement of the visceral autonomic innervation is presumed in diabetes. The megacolon seen in patients with Parkinson's disease may, to some degree, be due to use of long-term anticholinergic-type medications such as Artane and Cogentin (Fig. 109–18). Withdrawal of these drugs in some patients has been associated with alleviation of constipation and megacolon. Severe spinal cord disease or compression may also cause constipation and megacolon until the patient overcomes the loss of the defecation reflex. Lack of attention to

17). Hypokalemia may be responsible for transient megacolon (see p. 1326). Lead poisoning must be considered in the differential diagnosis of constipation and acquired megacolon, particularly in children. Recently, amyloidosis has been described as a cause of megacolon.

Chagas' disease, caused by the parasite *Trypanosoma cruzi*, involves the gastrointestinal tract and the heart.[21] In the former system, the esophagus and colon are the organs principally affected. Disease of the esophagus results in a clinical picture which closely resembles North American and European achalasia of the esophagus; Chagas' disease of the colon causes marked dilatation proximal to a distal segment of variable length of aganglionic colon. These patients are severely symptomatic with obstipation for many years and require periodic enemas for relief.

The ganglion cells of the myenteric plexuses of the esophagus and colon appear to be destroyed by a neurotoxin released by the parasite. The effect is very

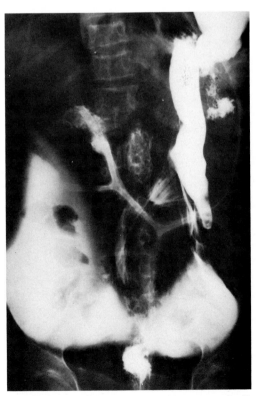

Figure 109–17. Barium enema, showing markedly dilated colon in severe myxedema. (Courtesy of Dr. H. I. Goldberg.)

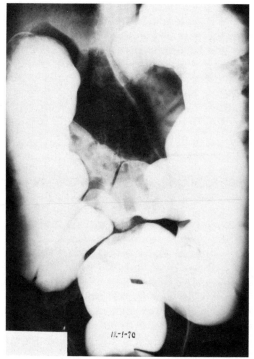

Figure 109–18. Barium enema in a patient with parkinsonism on Artane, demonstrating megacolon. Patient was obstipated. (Courtesy of Dr. H. I. Goldberg.)

the need for regularly evacuating these patients also contributes to this complication.

Drug intoxication, often subtle, may lead to megacolon with severe constipation. Good examples are found in individuals who are addicted to opium or who are taking excessive amounts of anticholinergic or other antidiarrheal agents. (The megacolon to which such practices may contribute in patients with ulcerative colitis is toxic megacolon; see pp. 1326 to 1329). Drug addicts thus may be severely constipated.

INFECTION AND INFLAMMATION; OTHER OBSTRUCTIVE LESIONS

Inflammatory strictures of the rectum caused by lymphogranuloma venereum, granulomatous colitis, or irradiation may also gradually cause megacolon. Likewise, a gradually progressive stenosing carcinoma of the rectum or rectosigmoid will lead to dilatation. (The reader is referred to more detailed descriptions of these dis-

ease states in the appropriate chapters.) Narrowing of the anorectal or rectosigmoid lumen caused by strictures which follow surgery for fissures, fistula, or abscesses may underlie acquired megacolon, usually associated with frequency of constipation and, in many cases, complete obstruction. Extracolonic compression by tumor or endometrial implant may rarely result in such a clinical picture.

Toxic megacolon of ulcerative colitis and pseudo-obstruction of the colon are discussed on pages 1326 to 1329 and 1484 to 1487.

TREATMENT OF ACQUIRED MEGACOLON

The treatment of acquired megacolon is directed toward the underlying disease or disorder. Simple therapy may be dramatic, as in withdrawal of drugs which exacerbate porphyria, cessation of lead intake in those poisoned by it, or discontinuance of constipating drugs.

Treatment is symptomatic for neurological diseases and is generally much less satisfactory, although return of spontaneous defecation in those individuals with spinal cord damage may be helped by repeated enemas early in the course of the disease. Unfortunately therapy for diabetic neuropathy and scleroderma is symptomatic, consisting mainly of prescribing gentle laxatives. Certainly surgical intervention for lesions compressing the cord is indicated, as it is for low-lying tumors and strictures which cause megacolon while progressively obstructing the colon. Surgical management of diseases causing extrinsic compression may also be successful in alleviating acquired megacolon.

REFERENCES

1. Ehrenpreis, T. Hirschsprung's Disease. Chicago, Year Book Medical Publishers, 1970.
2. Bowden, D. H., Goodfellow, A. M., and Munn, N. D. Hirschsprung's disease in the neonatal period; a report of five cases, four of which involved the small intestine. J. Pediat. 50:321, 1957.
3. Bowden, D. H., Neuhauser, E. B. D., and Picket, L. K. New concepts of the etiology, diagnosis and treatment of congenital megacolon (Hirschsprung's disease). Pediatrics 4:201, 1949.
4. Davidson, M., Sleisenger, M. H., Steinberg, H.,

and Almy, T. P. Studies of distal colonic motility in children. III. The pathologic physiology of congenital megacolon (Hirschsprung's disease). Gastroenterology 29:803, 1955.

5. Davidson, M. Congenital aganglionosis. *In* Handbook of Physiology, C. F. Code (ed.), Sect. 6, Vol. 5. Washington, D.C., American Physiological Society, 1968, p. 2783.

6. Bill, A. J., Jr., and Chapman, N. D. The enterocolitis of Hirschsprung's disease. Its natural history and treatment. Amer. J. Surg. 103:70, 1962.

7. Fraser, G. C., and Berry, C. Mortality in neonatal Hirschsprung's disease: With particular reference to enterocolitis. J. Pediat. Surg. 2:205, 1967.

8. Dobbins, W. O., and Bill, A. H., Jr. Diagnosis of Hirschsprung's disease excluded by rectal suction biopsy. New Eng. J. Med. 272:990, 1965.

9. Lawson, J. O. N., and Nixon, H. H. Anal canal pressures in the diagnosis of Hirschsprung's disease. J. Pediat. Surg. 2:544, 1967.

10. Tobon, F., Rein, N. C. R. W., Talbert, J. L., and Schuster, M. M. Nonsurgical test for the diagnosis of Hirschsprung's disease. New Eng. J. Med. 278:188, 1968.

11. Moseley, P. K., and Segar, W. E. Fluid and serum electrolyte disturbances as a complication of enemas in Hirschsprung's disease. Amer. J. Dis. Child. 115:714, 1969.

12. Hiatt, R. B. The pathologic physiology of congenital megacolon. Ann. Surg. 133:313, 1951.

13. Koop, C. E. The choice of surgical procedures in Hirschsprung's disease. J. Pediat. Surg. 1:523, 1966.

14. Swenson, O. A new surgical treatment for Hirschsprung's disease. Surgery 28:371, 1950.

15. Swenson, O. Follow-up on 200 patients treated for Hirschsprung's disease during a ten-year period. Ann. Surg. 146:706, 1957.

16. Duhamel, B. New operation for treatment of Hirschsprung's disease. Arch. Dis. Child. 35:38, 1960.

17. Soave, F. Hirschsprung's disease: A new surgical technique. Arch. Dis. Child. 39:116, 1964.

18. Davidson, M., and Bauer, C. H. Studies of distal colonic motility in children. IV. Achalasia of the distal rectal segment despite presence of ganglia in the myenteric plexuses of this area. Pediatrics 21:746, 1958.

19. Davidson, M., Kugler, M. M., and Bauer, C. H. Diagnosis and management in children with severe and protracted constipation and obstipation. J. Pediat. 62:261, 1963.

20. Davidson, M. Constipation, ulcerative colitis and regional enteritis. *In* Ambulatory Pediatrics, M. Green and R. J. Haggerty (eds.). Philadelphia, W. B. Saunders Co., 1968, pp. 220-225, 696-706.

21. Atias, A., Neghme, A., Mackay, L. A., and Jarpa, S. Megaesophagus, megacolon, and Chagas' disease in Chile. Gastroenterology 44:432, 1963.

Chapter 110

Obstruction and Pseudo-Obstruction

Steven Jacobsohn, Marvin H. Sleisenger

Large bowel obstruction may be defined as a clinical state in which the patient cannot evacuate colonic luminal contents because of compromise of the lumen by either organic disease or other disorders. In this sense, it differs from ileus of the colon in which the failure of colon function is due to systemic illness, intoxication, or motor disorder or represents a response to bowel ischemia or intraperitoneal sepsis. The contents distal to the point of obstruction may be evacuated after the onset of the problem; thus passage of formed or even loose stools, especially early in the course, is not inconsistent with total large bowel obstruction. Colonic obstruction may be acute, subacute, or chronic, depending on the rapidity and completeness of luminal compromise (see pp. 338 to 351).

SUBACUTE AND CHRONIC OBSTRUCTION OF THE COLON

ETIOLOGY

The most common cause of subacute and chronic large bowel obstruction is carcinoma (see pp. 1445 to 1461). Other important conditions include fecal impaction, particularly rectal; motility disturbances

such as those noted in myotonia congenita, congenital aganglionosis, and scleroderma (see also pp. 1463 to 1480); adhesive bands; strictures caused by granulomatous disease of the colon; and diverticular disease of the colon.[1] Acute obstruction is usually due to volvulus, intussusception, or herniation into the inguinal canals.

CLINICAL PICTURE

Pain is the most characteristic finding. It may be sudden in onset, as in volvulus, but is usually more insidious. Periods between pain are longer than in small bowel obstruction, but the crampy character of the distress is similar. The pain caused by obstruction of the cecum, ascending colon, and right transverse colon is usually referred to the midepigastrium, and that of left colon obstruction usually to a site below the umbilicus. The more distal the obstruction, the less discomfort suffered by the patient; indeed, slowly progressive constipation may be the only symptom, especially when the ileocecal valve is incompetent.

Nausea and frequently vomiting generally accompany the abdominal cramps. The latter may simply be a response to the abdominal pain or it may be feculent. It does not necessarily imply ileocecal valve incompetence, but may simply reflect stasis proximal to the point of obstruction with secondary bacterial overgrowth.

Constipation and/or obstipation are always seen as part of large bowel obstruction. Failure to pass flatus accompanies the constipation.

PHYSICAL FINDINGS

Abdominal examination reveals a distended abdomen; tympany is a physical sign only early after onset. Dullness and fluid waves are more commonly present in long-standing obstruction because of a massive shift of fluid into the lumen. Peristalsis may be visible, but it is more common in small bowel obstruction. Some tenderness, albeit slight, is almost always present; when it is marked and associated with muscular rigidity and rebound, compromise of the blood supply is suggested. Auscultation usually reveals high-pitched, tinkling bowel sounds, whereas absence of bowel sounds is ominous, suggesting strangulation. The rectal examination is crucial, because many obstructing lesions are in the lower sigmoid colon and a mass or marked narrowing may be felt on digital examination. A grossly bloody stool reflects possible gangrene of the colon and may make differential diagnosis of ischemic colitis difficult (see below). Sigmoidoscopy is essential to determine the possible presence of an intraluminal lesion and, as discussed under volvulus, may be therapeutic.

DIAGNOSIS AND DIFFERENTIAL DIAGNOSIS

Routine laboratory studies may reveal normal, elevated, or depressed hematocrit, depending upon whether the underlying lesion has bled and upon the state of hydration. The white blood count may be normal or elevated if necrotic tumor or infarcted or inflamed bowel is the cause of obstruction. The urine is generally negative unless tumor or infection has secondarily involved the uterus or bladder.

Plain roentgenograms of the abdomen, taken with the patient in supine, lateral, and upright positions, are important. Gas-filled loops at the lateral margins of the abdomen, characterized by haustral markings, place the likely site of obstruction in the colon; dilated large bowel and small bowel loops with a cut-off in the colon likewise indicate the probable site of the block. In patients with small bowel obstruction little or no gas may be seen in the colon, and a distinct pattern of "laddering" of the small bowel loops with air-fluid levels is characteristic. Small bowel obstruction, pancreatitis, pseudo-obstruction, and ileus must be considered in the differential diagnosis. Differentiation from ileus is discussed on page 348.

Definitive diagnosis of long-standing organic obstruction is made by barium enema, cautiously performed. When due to neoplasm the cause is usually visualized. Examples of obstructing cancers are presented on pages 1254 and 1261 (Figs. 99–2 and 99–11).

Small Bowel Obstruction. The pain of small bowel obstruction is generally more severe than that of large bowel obstruction. This fact, however, is of little help in acute obstruction, except that the cycles of colic in large bowel obstruction are at greater intervals than those in small bowel obstruction. The site of pain, likewise in the acute situation, often does not distinguish between these conditions. A previous history of surgery, other than pelvic surgery, favors small bowel obstruction, as adhesions infrequently obstruct the colon. Other points in the history, however, are helpful in predicting large bowel obstruction. Thus progressive symptoms over a period of weeks or months, reflected in a change in bowel habit, either constipation or diarrhea, favor large bowel obstruction. Findings such as cachexia, an abdominal mass, or hepatomegaly point to cancer of the colon as the cause for the obstruction. Vomiting is common in small bowel obstruction but is seen only irregularly in large bowel obstruction; it is not unusual to find it in advanced stages of the process. As noted, fecal material in the vomitus makes colonic obstruction more likely, but prolonged stasis in small bowel obstruction leads to bacterial overgrowth and feculent vomiting. Distention, on the other hand, is more characteristic of large bowel obstruction because of its more insidious onset; however, small bowel obstruction, depending on the cause, may lead secondarily to large bowel ileus. In patients who have had symptoms for weeks or months, marked distention of the abdomen certainly favors large bowel obstruction.

Acute Pancreatitis. This condition may be difficult to distinguish from bowel obstruction without vascular compromise. In general, the pain is more constant and more localized, with radiation into the back. Often, however, the physical findings are not proportional to the severity of pain in acute pancreatitis; the degree of tenderness, distention, and rigidity is disproportionately slight. Also, borborygmi are frequently found in bowel obstruction (except very late), whereas ileus is more common in pancreatitis. In advanced bowel obstruction with strangulation, the patterns of abdominal pain change from rhythmic to those of peritoneal irritation, making the distinction from hemorrhagic pancreatitis impossible. High levels of serum and peritoneal fluid amylase are helpful, because mild elevations may be seen in intestinal obstruction. Pseudo-obstruction is discussed below.

TREATMENT

Since fluid losses into the gut lumen may be marked, large quantities of sodium, chloride, and potassium may have to be given. Metabolic acidosis is usually present, and, if severe, must be corrected with intravenously administered sodium bicarbonate. The rate of fluid replacement, particularly in the elderly, should be monitored by continuous measurement of central venous pressure by an appropriate line. Decompression via nasogastric tube is usually adequate; however, a longer tube might be required if small bowel distention is marked.

When fluid and electrolyte balance is restored, the patient with demonstrated organic obstruction must be operated upon, as discussed on pages 1453 to 1459.

FECAL IMPACTION

Debilitated, elderly, or depressed patients may suffer obstruction of the large bowel caused by fecal impaction. Repeated failure to observe the defecation reflex because of depression, senility, or medications such as sedatives, tranquil-izers, or Artane is common in the older age group. Illness with confinement to bed and dehydration will often lead to this complication, particularly in the elderly, but in any age group if the patient has a history of constipation. It may often follow a barium meal if laxatives are not given when the barium has not passed spontaneously 24 hours after the examination. Patients who have had previous rectal or anal surgery with residual strictures and those with distal luminal narrowing caused by inflammatory disease are likewise prone to impaction. (For details, see pp. 1531 to 1534).

PSEUDO-OBSTRUCTION OF THE COLON

Clinically, obstruction of the large bowel may rarely be noted without organic occlusion. It is a recurrent, serious condition which may or may not be associated with disorders of other organs. It is currently known as idiopathic pseudo-obstruction, and it appears to involve small bowel as well as colon.[2-4]

ETIOLOGY AND PATHOGENESIS

The cause of so-called pseudo-obstruction is not known; studies of bowel motility in these patients have indicated some decreased incidence of contractions in the colon with an increased frequency of low pressure waves, with, however, normal response to intravenous neostigmine. Upper small bowel motility, particularly duodenal, is also abnormal, but the abnormality cannot be clearly related to disturbed physiological function.

PATHOLOGY

The findings are not dramatic and are certainly not specific for any disease. They consist of minimal local infiltration with round cells and some submucosal fibrosis; in no instance has there been evidence of atrophy of muscle coats, arteritis, or endothelial proliferation. Ganglion cells are present in adequate numbers in all parts of the gastrointestinal tract.

Since the condition is reminiscent of the pseudo-obstruction often seen in patients with advanced scleroderma of the intestinal tract, it is not surprising that culture of upper intestinal contents may reveal anaerobic organisms (see pp. 70 to 82).

CLINICAL PICTURE

Most patients with intestinal pseudo-obstruction have their first episode early in life; characteristically, the episodes are recurrent. Because the picture is virtually indistinguishable from obstruction of organic cause in some instances, operation is often performed. Unfortunately, since no cause is obvious, no rational surgical procedure can be offered to alleviate the disorder.

The principal symptoms of the syndrome are abdominal pain of cramping nature, generalized in the abdominal cavity, associated with vomiting, progressive distention, and in some instances up to six loose, often light colored bowel movements per day. Fecal fat may be increased; other evidence of malabsorption during bouts of pseudo-obstruction, such as macrocytic anemia, low serum carotene, and markedly disturbed serum electrolyte patterns, have been documented. Characteristic of diarrheal states, acidosis is frequently noted in

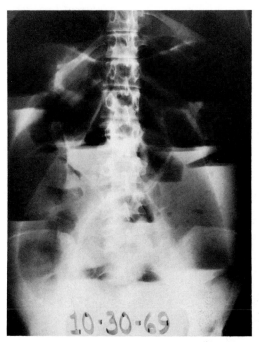

Figure 110–2. Patient shown in Figure 110–1, during another episode two months later. (Courtesy of Dr. H. I. Goldberg.)

these patients, associated with slight hyponatremia, hyperchloridemia, and hypokalemia (see pp. 291 to 316).

The symptoms last for several days to as long as a week or more. During this time the abdomen is distended and the patient is anorectic, may vomit small amounts of liquid which are fed, and has a variable degree of abdominal discomfort.

On physical examination the temperature is usually normal; it has been reported, in fact, to be subnormal. The abdomen is distended with mild generalized tenderness but betrays no evidence of peritoneal irritation. Bowel sounds are diminished and high pitched; frequently, they are absent for long periods of time.

Roentgenographic examination of the abdomen on flat film reveals distended loops of small and large bowel (Figs. 110–1 and 110–2). On barium film examination, the small bowel reveals markedly dilated loops and delay in transit; in some instances, the dilatation is localized to the duodenum and upper jejunum, reminiscent of scleroderma of the intestine.

Barium enema X-ray may be normal (Fig. 110–3), but it may also show suffi-

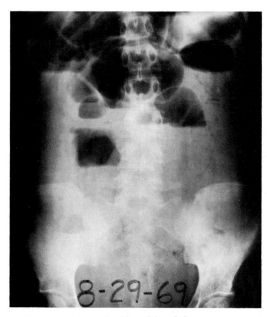

Figure 110–1. Flat film of the abdomen in patient with pseudo-obstruction of the large bowel, with air fluid levels. Small bowel distention is evident. (Courtesy of Dr. H. I. Goldberg.)

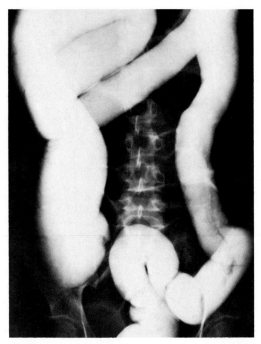

Figure 110-3. Barium enema in the patient shown in Figures 110-1 and 110-2, after the episode filmed in Figure 110-2, revealed no obstruction. (Courtesy of Dr. H. I. Goldberg.)

cient distention to meet the radiological criteria for megacolon. Technically, then, this disorder is a cause of megacolon.

ASSOCIATED DISEASES

Idiopathic pseudo-obstruction of the colon is associated with a number of diseases, including cardiovascular disease, retroperitoneal disease, and systemic infection.[2-4]

Congestive heart failure or other vascular disease may be the setting in which massive large bowel distention appears. It is thought that somehow hypoxia associated with this condition interferes with motor function of the large bowel. It is not known whether diuretics play a role in the genesis of pseudo-obstruction, perhaps because of hypokalemia. Similar marked distention of the colon has been rarely noted after myocardial infarction and is apparently not due to administration of opiates for relief of pain.

Retroperitoneal disease has been associated with idiopathic pseudo-obstruction of the colon. It is thought that these tumors

interfere with the intrinsic autonomic nerve supply to the bowel wall. This supposition has been based on the finding of malignancy in the region of the celiac plexuses.

Systemic infection has also been associated with this condition, particularly pneumonia and bacteremia of any cause. The manner by which systemic infection affects large bowel motility is unknown at this time.

DIAGNOSIS AND DIFFERENTIAL DIAGNOSIS

Pseudo-obstruction of the intestine is distinguished from mechanical small bowel obstruction by the more insidious onset of symptoms, the absence of a cut-off of gas in the bowel on plain film of the abdomen, and failure of clinical and radiographic progression of the condition which indicates organic obstructions; i.e., rising pulse, temperature, and white blood cell count; abdominal signs indicating compromise of circulation of a portion of the intestine; and clear evidence of obstruction (laddering, separation of loops, absence of gas in large bowel) on successive flat films of the abdomen.

Pseudo-obstruction in the colon is distinguished from large bowel obstruction of organic cause (stricture, carcinoma, volvulus), because gas is found in the loops of colon all the way down to the anal canal; in addition, the barium enema X-ray reveals no point of obstruction.[5] In addition, in contrast to patients with organic obstruction of the large bowel, the history is neither one of insidious decrease in size and number of stools per day with gradual abdominal distention nor one of sudden, dramatic obstruction of the colon associated with either volvulus of a loop of colon or intussusception.

In some instances, the key to the diagnosis is a history of undiagnosed recurrent episodes of the same type in a patient in whom discernible causes often have previously been excluded. Sometimes it is difficult to distinguish idiopathic pseudo-obstruction from the generalized ileus or pseudo-obstruction of advanced intestinal scleroderma. However, some important differences are apparent. The principal distinguishing feature is the absence in idiopathic pseudo-obstruction of the physical changes or symptoms of disease in other organs which are characteristic of scleroderma, i.e., skin disease, arthritis, or Raynaud's phenomenon. The history of obstructive symptoms associated with diarrhea appears much earlier in life in patients with pseudo-obstruction than in those with scleroderma. Finally, in contrast to scleroderma, lasting response to broad-spectrum antimicrobial drugs is generally ineffective in idiopathic pseudo-obstruction.

TREATMENT

The treatment for this condition is conservative, i.e., nasogastric suction, and intravenous fluids to replace electrolytes and correct acidosis. Broad-spectrum antimicrobial drugs are given during episodes of obstruction, e.g., ampicillin, 4.0 g intravenously per day. Long-term oral antimicrobial therapy may be tried to facilitate decrease in diarrhea, decrease in distention, and gain in weight. Beneficial long-term results of such therapy, however, have not been realized. Treatment with cholinergic drugs, based on the possibility of a parasympathetic insufficiency of the intestine, is ineffective. Likewise, corticosteroids appear to have no place in the treatment of this disorder.

Multiple resection of segments of bowel or various bypass procedures have not alleviated the problem. Indeed, surgery should be avoided in these patients.

CLINICAL COURSE AND PROGNOSIS

The disorder may last for many years, with recurrences at unpredictable intervals. The prognosis is poor. Life expectancy from onset ranges from a few years to 18 or more years. Patients will often have continuing low grade activity of the disease—mild diarrhea, difficulty maintaining weight, slight distention, and abnormal vomiting.

In terms of prognosis, two different categories of pseudo-obstruction of the colon have been described. One is the type which is chronic and recurrent and resembles in many respects scleroderma of the intestine. The other is an acute pseudo-ob-

struction of the colon; these cases appear not to be associated with other conditions such as congestive heart failure, myocardial infarction, or infection,

Those who have pseudo-obstruction of the colon associated with other diseases usually recover when the underlying or associated condition has been successfully treated. Thus the idiopathic variety tends to have the worst prognosis on a long-term basis; those with pseudo-obstruction associated other serious medical illnesses, however, may suffer a 25 per cent mortality during the acute episode of colonic ileus.

ACUTE OBSTRUCTION OF THE COLON

VOLVULUS OF THE CECUM

Volvulus or torsion of the colon involves two sites: the sigmoid and the cecum. The latter is less common, but no less serious. The term cecal volvulus is inaccurate, because the ascending colon and terminal ileum are also involved. The term cecal volvulus, however, will be used in this discussion.

Pathogenesis. The twist of the cecum is associated with both prior failure of its fixation and the disappearance of its mesentery—events which ordinarily take place during the third stage of embryological rotation. Thus the patient has an abnormally long and mobile mesentery of the cecum and ascending colon. An association of cecal volvulus with adhesions has also been noted. In some instances, however, it may be associated with a distal obstructing lesion of the colon. Somehow, in this situation the accumulation of fluid and gas in the proximal colon secondary to the distal obstruction causes the twist. In practically all instances the degree of rotation of the bowel in volvulus is 360 degrees or more around the ileocolic artery and is more common in the clockwise direction.

Males are more commonly affected than females. The majority of patients are in the third, fourth, and fifth decades; however, volvulus may be noted at any age and must not be ruled out as a cause of acute large bowel obstruction in the elderly.

Nutrition and geographic location influence the incidence of cecal and sigmoid volvulus; thus it is most common in areas of the world where the population is undernourished and also in areas of the world where there is a high fiber content in the diet.[6]

Clinical Picture. When the process is acute, pain is the predominant symptom. It is severe, intermittent, and colicky, and is appreciated by the patient in the right lower quadrant but may be generalized. The waves of colic appear at progressively longer intervals after onset of the twist, but it is rare for discomfort to disappear entirely. As in many other inflammatory and obstructive processes in the intestine, the patient frequently is nauseated and vomits, presumably owing to stimulation of sympathetic afferents. The vomitus is not feculent and is usually composed of gastric contents, with or without some bile. The abdomen gradually becomes distended over the first day or so.

If the patient is not given fluids, he will become progressively dehydrated. This complication is more likely in acutely ill patients in whom the twist is complete, vomiting is more profuse, and the possibility of a "closed-loop obstruction" with cecal perforation is the greatest.

Some cases are more gradual in onset, with intermittent episodes of cramping pain and only occasional vomiting. The abdomen distends either minimally or not at all. The patient, in contrast to patients with the acute or complete type of obstruction caused by volvulus, may continue to pass gas and have some small amount of feces, indicating that the obstruction is only partial and the condition is not so serious. Constipation often leading to obstipation is more common.[7] Such episodes may subside spontaneously or after the patient has been given an enema and may recur at unpredictable intervals over a period of many years.

The danger of the acute, complete twist is the closed-loop obstruction that results, stressing the relatively thin walls of the cecum to the extreme. Whether or not perforation occurs is a function of how much gas and fluid are trapped, how complete the obstruction is, and how much the blood supply of the cecum is impaired in the process. Obviously, the acute form is very serious and requires immediate attention. The three most common physical findings are abdominal distention, a palpable mass, and temperature elevation.[7]

Diagnosis and Differential Diagnosis of Cecal Volvulus. The diagnosis depends to some extent upon the history and physical findings, but more often it is made by the characteristic findings on flat film of the abdomen and barium enema examination. The cecum is usually distended and displaced (Figs. 110–4 and 110–5); in addition, the ascending colon is markedly dilated, and this rather large loop may be seen in the middle or upper abdomen and no gas noted in the normal location of the cecum. In some instances, proximal dilatation of small bowel loops may be noted which in a matter of hours may be filled with fluid as well as air. Little or no gas is seen in the remainder of the colon; however, it is difficult to make this determination in some patients in whom the cecum and ascending colon are tremendously distended and fill a large part of the abdominal cavity.

Barium enema examination will reveal filling of the colon distal to the loop of cecum and ascending colon involved; if such obstruction is demonstrated, along with the appearance of the dilated segment of large bowel on flat film of the ab-

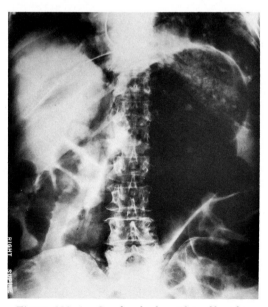

Figure 110–4. Cecal volvulus. Plain film showing markedly distended viscus in the left upper quadrant. There is a dilated loop of small bowel in the right lower quadrant, but no cecal gas. (Courtesy of Dr. H. I. Goldberg.)

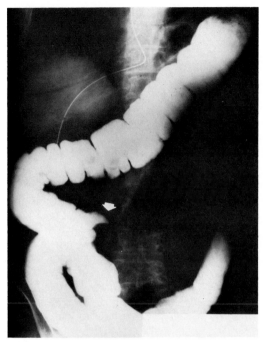

Figure 110–5. Bird's beak appearance at the site of cecal volvulus in a patient with acute obstruction of the colon. (Courtesy of Dr. H. I. Goldberg.)

domen in a patient whose history is consistent with the diagnosis, volvulus must be considered a likely diagnosis and surgery undertaken.

Treatment. The general principles for management of intestinal obstruction are detailed on pages 348 to 351. The treatment for cecal volvulus is surgical decompression; the cecum is also fixed to the posterior parietes in the right lower quadrant by cecopexy. In those instances in which strangulation has occurred, resection may be necessary. If so, diverting ileostomy must be done and reanastomosis carried out at a later stage.

If not diagnosed and not operated upon, cecal as well as sigmoid volvulus may progress to strangulation of the twisted loop of bowel with ischemia, perforation, and peritonitis. In such cases, the white blood count is elevated, the abdomen is diffusely tender with rebound tenderness, and the patient has a tachycardia and all the classic signs and symptoms of intestinal gangrene and perforation. This complication is especially treacherous in older persons, because it may not be accompanied by dramatic physical findings. In this instance, the white blood count and tem-

perature may be either normal or minimally elevated.

With gangrene a right hemicolectomy is the most satisfactory procedure. Exteriorization has been recommended for late cases but is probably not a better procedure. If the bowel is grossly distended, a double-barreled ileocolostomy can be used to provide decompression. The mortality ranges from 10 to 40 per cent, depending to a large extent upon time of diagnosis, age of the patient, and associated complications.

VOLVULUS OF SIGMOID

Sigmoid volvulus is due to a 180 to 360 degree twist of the sigmoid in a counterclockwise direction around the axis of its mesentery, accompanied by a torsion about the axis of the bowel itself. It is classically associated with a long, redundant sigmoid and mesentery, but may also result from adhesions. The degree of obstruction depends upon the extent of torsion; the degree of dilatation and the consequences of the twist, in turn, depend on whether or not proximal bowel contents can gain access to the involved segment of sigmoid. Usually peristalsis will push fluid, gas, and feces into this segment, from which there is no egress; rapid distention of the sigmoid volvulus ensues. With greater degrees of torsion, strangulation is more likely, because venous and arterial tunnels are inevitably compromised, resulting in infarction of a twisted loop of bowel; perforation and peritonitis follow infarction.

The bases for an abnormally long sigmoid mesentery and for the redundant loops of sigmoid which characterize this condition are not clear; however, a clue to the situation may be gained from the fact that it is commonly seen in patients with schizophrenia who are institutionalized and whose bowel habits are bizarre. Indeed, as noted on page 1475, these individuals often have an acquired megacolon, not having spontaneous bowel movements for days or weeks. Perhaps the accumulation of feces produces elongation and stretching of the sigmoid mesentery. That the abnormality of the mesentery is probably acquired is attested to by the fact that only rarely is this condition noted in patients under 40 years of age; approximately three-quarters of the cases are males. Volvulus complicating pregnancy, however, is a well known entity.[8]

A remarkable feature of sigmoid volvulus is the considerable geographical variation in its incidence. Volvulus of the sigmoid is a comparatively rare disease in Britain, Western Europe, and North America. In contrast, it is one of the most common causes of acute intestinal obstruction in Eastern Europe, Scandinavia, the Ukraine and India, as well as among the black population of Africa and the West Indies. Volvulus of the sigmoid also appears to be more common in American blacks than whites. These interesting geographical variations are probably related to several factors, including bowel habits, diet, and anatomical differences.[9, 10]

Clinical Picture. Frequently the onset of this disorder is abrupt and is characterized by rather severe colicky abdominal pain in the lower abdomen which gradually becomes steady and localizes in the left lower quadrant. Although a small bowel movement may be noted after the onset, thereafter the patient passes no gas or feces.

In a number of patients the attacks are recurrent and not so severe, although at any time a single episode may be dramatic. Some patients have chronic symptoms caused by volvulus, and these are the individuals who are in psychiatric institutions, have neurological problems, or are in nursing homes or homes for the aged. These patients have extreme constipation and marked abdominal distention with little or no pain or discomfort.

On physical examination the abdomen is generally found to be distended, usually markedly so; early in the episode bowel sounds may be noted, and on palpation only rarely are there marked tenderness and muscular rigidity. When the tenderness is extreme and accompanied by rebound, peritonitis must be suspected owing to strangulation with or without perforation. On rectal examination nothing is felt in the ampulla. The temperature and the white blood count are normal unless strangulation has supervened, in which case they are elevated to varying degrees, depending upon duration, severity, or age.

Diagnosis and Treatment. The diag-

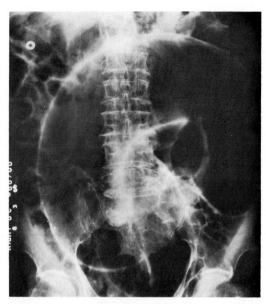

Figure 110–6. Plain film, showing inverted "U" of markedly dilated, twisted sigmoid colon in a patient with sigmoid volvulus. Obstruction is not complete, because the transverse colon and right colon are not dilated. (Courtesy of Dr. H. I. Goldberg.)

nosis of sigmoid volvulus is made by X-ray examinations, including both plain film of the abdomen and barium enema examination. The former indicates a marked distention of the sigmoid which is displaced to the right side of the abdomen and contains fluid and gas. In contrast to cecal volvulus, the remainder of the colon is found to be filled with air (Figs. 110–6 and 110–7).

Barium enema X-ray reveals a characteristic picture of the so-called "ace of spades" appearance (Fig. 110–7). The proximal rectum is markedly narrowed, appearing as a beak-like projection at the site of obstruction. Some patients, particularly children, are relieved completely by this examination.

It is extremely important that these patients undergo a proctoscopic examination in the knee-chest position before barium enema or conservative therapy is employed, because proctoscopy may reveal changes in the upper rectal mucosa which indicate early gangrene of the bowel. In such instances, it is not wise to proceed with barium instillation or with intubation of the colon in an effort to deflate the twisted loop. This is done if the mucous membranes on proctoscopy look good; the

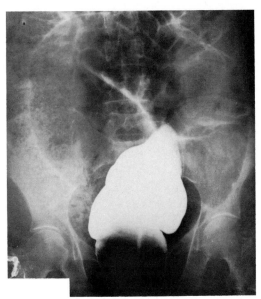

Figure 110–7. A patient with sigmoid volvulus, with complete obstruction to retrograde flow of barium. Note the typical tapered narrowing at the site of torsion ("ace of spades"). (Courtesy of Dr. H. I. Goldberg.)

technique is to pass a rubber rectal tube past the site of obstruction under direct vision. If the tube gains access to the involved loop, violent expulsion of gas and fluid usually promptly relieves the patient's symptoms. If the obstruction cannot be relieved or if the mucosa looks compromised or the clinical picture indicates that strangulation of the loop is taking place as evidenced by elevated temperature, white blood count, and pulse, in addition to abdominal signs indicating peritoneal irritation, then operation must be carried out immediately. In those instances in which relief is obtained by passage of the proctoscope or tube or the barium enema examination itself, elective surgery should be carried out at the earliest possible moment.[11, 12]

The surgical technique employed depends upon the situation encountered. The object is to resect that segment of the bowel which has become twisted and perform an end-to-end anastomosis. Obviously, this cannot be carried out if the patient has compromised circulation of the bowel or if perforation has taken place, in which case a diverting colostomy and a staged procedure must be undertaken thereafter.

VOLVULUS OF THE TRANSVERSE COLON

This type of volvulus is extremely rare. It gives the same kind of clinical picture in its acute form as do cecal and sigmoid volvulus, and diagnosis is established by barium enema examination. The treatment is surgical.

INTUSSUSCEPTION

Intussusception is the invagination of one part of the bowel into the lumen of a distal adjacent section. It is one of the most frequent acute abdominal conditions seen in children after the first month of life. It ranks second only to appendicitis as the most common acute abdominal emergency in children and is the most frequent cause of intestinal obstruction in the pediatric age group.

INCIDENCE

Less than 10 per cent of intussusceptions are in adults.[13-19] Any hospital of 100 or more surgical beds should admit one adult with intussusception every 12 to 18 months.[18] For some unexplained reason, there seems to be an increased incidence between June and September.[15] In contrast to the situation in children, intussusception in adults is usually secondary to some pre-existing disease or lesion involving the bowel wall. In over 90 per cent of cases in children, no underlying pathological condition is found.

Review of the literature from 1900 to 1947 revealed nearly 67 per cent males in 685 patients with adult intussusception.[19] In 158 cases there was no known cause; 213 were secondary to benign tumors, and 123 were secondary to malignant tumors. The remainder were due to lesions that included Meckel's diverticula, gastroenterostomies with herniation, typhoid ulcers, and appendiceal invaginations.

Roper reviewed 134 of 144 cases of adult intussusception between 1947 and 1952. Eighteen were idiopathic; seven were due to Meckel's diverticula; 42 were due to benign tumors; and 49 were due to malignant tumors.[18]

PATHOLOGY

The pathophysiology is the same in both infants and adults. Two factors seem necessary for production of intussusception: a relatively rigid segment of bowel such as a tumor mass or inflammatory mass, and a mobile segment long enough to permit telescoping. As one section of bowel (intussusceptum) moves into the adjacent bowel (intussuscipiens), there is a constriction of this area, leading to the characteristic symptoms of partial obstruction. By its normal physiological action, the bowel tends to move the intussusceptum along, with increasing amounts of bowel being involved, along with associated mesentery and vessels; complete obstruction ensues with interruption of the vascular supply with or without gangrene.[17]

Polypoid and pedunculated tumors are particularly inclined to intussuscept. One out of nine small bowel tumors presents as an intussusception.[16] The lesion in the adult is in the small bowel one-third of the time, ileocecal one-third of the time, and colonic one-third of the time.[14]

CLINICAL PICTURE

Symptoms in the adult are quite different from those in the child in that most adults have a history of chronic gastrointestinal symptoms, occasionally spanning several years. The most frequently noted symptom at the time of the first examination is intermittent colicky abdominal pain that may be located anywhere, but is usually in the right lower quadrant with frequent radiation to the back and is increased by eating. Vomiting is present in 70 per cent of patients.[15] Diarrhea is more common than constipation. Roper found that only one-third of the patients had blood in the stool; this contrasts with the situation in infants in whom blood is one of the key findings in diagnosis.[18] Weight loss is frequent, regardless of whether carcinoma is the cause of the intussusception; indeed, it is more pronounced with benign lesions, perhaps because eating induces pain.

PHYSICAL FINDINGS

Patients frequently do not appear to be ill. The most prominent physical sign is moderate tenderness of the abdomen; sometimes the abdomen is slightly distended. A palpable mass is not as frequently found in adults as in children. Burmeister found a mass in 66 per cent with ileocecal conditions, in 43 per cent with small bowel intussusception and in 33 per cent of those with colonic intussusception. An inconsistent or changing mass reflects fluctuation in the degree of intussusception but is not always found. Bowel sounds may range from normal to accentuated (rushes), depending on the degree and duration of the intestinal obstruction. In advanced cases, of course, signs and symptoms of strangulation supervene.

LABORATORY DATA

Laboratory findings are of little value. The findings on flat film of the abdomen are those of an acute large bowel obstruction (see pp. 339 to 343). It is frequently difficult to pick up the lesion with contrast examination, because the barium may fail to enter the intussusception. Barium enema may reveal no more than the level of obstruction, but there are three signs which are diagnostic: (1) the "coiled spring" appearance (Fig. 110–8), (2) the

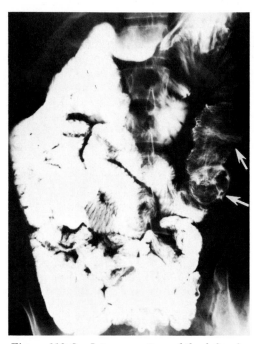

Figure 110–8. Intussusception of the left colon. Note tumor (intussusceptum, lower arrow) and "coiled spring" appearance of the bowel through which it has moved (intussuscipiens, upper arrow). (Courtesy of Dr. J. Fenlon.)

crescentic edge, and (3) the "pitchfork" sign.[18] The danger in performing a barium enema examination is perforation; also, residual barium in the colon may subsequently cause difficulty at the time of surgery. Barium by mouth is not contraindicated in bowel obstruction and occasionally will reveal the diagnosis by outlining either the tumor or the intussusception or both.

TREATMENT

Surgical intervention, unless absolutely medically contraindicated, should always be performed in adults with intussusception. The reason is obvious; there is almost always underlying pathology which must be treated along with the intussusception. Intussusception in the colon almost always signifies cancer. This contrasts with the situation in children, in whom barium enema reduction is usually adequate, because there is usually no remediable precipitating cause. Barium enema reduction should not be attempted in adults. Unfortunately, because of the vagueness of symptoms and paucity of physical findings, the correct diagnosis is often not made until gangrene is present.

REFERENCES

1. Compton, R. Scleroderma with diverticulosis and colonic obstruction. Amer. J. Surg. *118*: 602, 1969.
2. Caves, P. K., and Crockard, H. A. Pseudo-obstruction of the large bowel. Brit. Med. J. *2*: 583, 1970.
3. Maldonado, J. E., Gregg, J. A., Green, P. A., and Brown, A. L., Jr. Chronic idiopathic intestinal pseudo-obstruction. Amer. J. Med. *49*: 203, 1970.
4. Stephens, F. O. Intestinal pseudo-obstruction. Med. J. Austral. *1*:1026, 1966.
5. Morton, J. H., Schwartz, S. I., and Gramiak, R. Ileus of the colon. Arch. Surg. *81*:425, 1960.
6. Dowling, B. L., and Gunning, A. J. Caecalvolvulus. Brit. J. Surg. *56*:124, 1969.
7. Kerry, R. L., and Ransom, H. Volvulus of the colon. Arch. Surg. *99*:215, 1969.
8. Lazarro, E. J., Das, P. B., and Abraham, P. V. Volvulus of the sigmoid colon complicating pregnancy. Obstet. Gynec. *33*:553, 1969.
9. Volvulus of the sigmoid colon. Brit. Med. J. *1*:264, 1968.
10. Shepherd, J. J. The epidemiology and clinical presentation of sigmoid volvulus. Brit. J. Surg. *56*:353, 1969.
11. Shepherd, J. J. Treatment of volvulus of sigmoid colon: A review of 425 cases. Brit. Med. J. *1*:280, 1968.
12. Sutcliffe, M. M. Volvulus of the sigmoid colon. Brit. J. Surg. *55*:903. 1968.
13. Coran, A. G. Intussusception in adults. Amer. J. Surg. *117*:735, 1969.
14. Steckler, R. J., et al. Intussusception in adults. Calif. Med. *109*:291, 1968.
15. Cotler, A. M., and Cohn, I., Jr. Intussusception in adults. Amer. J. Surg. *101*:114, 1961.
16. Bond, M. R., and Roberts, J. B. Intussusception in the adult. Brit. J. Surg. *51*:818, 1964.
17. Burmeister, R. W. Intussusception in the adult. Amer. J. Dig. Dis. *7*:360, 1962.
18. Roper, A. Intussusception in adults. Surg. Gynec. Obstet. *103*:267, 1956.
19. Donhauser, J. L., and Kelly, E. C. Intussusception in the adult. Amer. J. Surg. *79*:673, 1950.

Chapter 111

Acute Appendicitis

Davey Ronald Deal

Appendicitis, or acute inflammation of the vermiform appendix, is the most common acute surgical condition affecting the abdomen. The incidence of primary appendectomies in a large city is about 16 per cent for males and 20 per cent for females.[1] The annual incidence of surgery for appendicitis among employees of a large insurance corporation was found to be 1.5 per thousand for males and 1.9 per thousand for females between the ages of 17 and 64.[2] There is a strikingly lower incidence of appendectomies among black men as compared with white men; the same comparison is true for women, but it is not so marked.[1]

Acute appendicitis is rare before age two and increases thereafter to a peak incidence in the second and third decades of life. In a series from Cook County Hospital, almost half the patients were between five and 15 years of age.[3] Other experience indicates that over half the patients are age 11 to 30.[4] Beyond age 40 the disease decreases in frequency. At all ages, however, it is frequent enough to be considered of utmost importance in the differential diagnosis of acute abdominal symptoms.

PATHOLOGY

On gross inspection, the acutely inflamed appendix can vary from appearing near-normal to being discolored and gangrenous with a distal perforation. Classi-

cally, it is swollen, reddened, warm, and covered with a fibrin exudate. Microscopically, the complete picture consists of polymorphonuclear leukocytes in the lumen and extending from the mucosa to the serosa. Superficial mucosal ulcerations are common.[5] The minimal criterion for the histological diagnosis of appendicitis is acute inflammatory cells in the lumen and mucosa with tracking of the polymorphonuclear cells into the submucosa.[6]

If the inflamed appendix is not removed soon enough, or if the process is especially virulent, as in older persons, the appendix may perforate. This is found at the time of surgery in slightly less than 30 per cent of all cases.[4, 7-9] In patients over age 60, the incidence is about 70 per cent.[7, 10, 11] Perforation leads to either localized or generalized peritonitis, depending upon the response of the patient to the insult. From a clinical standpoint, the disease is usually considered either as acute simple (unruptured) appendicitis or as appendicitis with rupture. The two categories differ considerably with regard to both morbidity and mortality.

ETIOLOGY AND PATHOGENESIS

Early experiments in dogs demonstrated that obstruction plus infection causes acute appendicitis.[12] Neither obstruction alone nor infection alone results in inflammation. Since bacteria are always present in the human appendix, obstruction may

1494

be the most important factor in the human disease. The obstructed human appendix can secrete fluid into the lumen at pressures high enough to compromise mucosal integrity and lead to acute appendicitis.[13] The postulated sequence of events is obstruction leading to an increase in intraluminal pressure which interferes with venous outflow, resulting in thrombosis, hemorrhage, edema, and bacterial invasion of the wall. Edema increases with bacterial invasion, aggravating the tissue anoxia, and a vicious cycle becomes established. Obstruction is undoubtedly an important factor in many patients with appendicitis.

Calculi are the most extensively investigated of the possible obstructive mechanisms. There is some debate over what constitutes an appendiceal calculus. Any calcium-containing body in the appendix is considered a calculus by some.[14] Calculi usually have a radiolucent center and laminated structure and contain a high percentage of water and organic material in addition to calcium phosphate salts. The nidus of the calculus is thought to be inspissated fecal material which causes mucosal irritation and secretion of calcium phosphate–rich mucus. Under conditions of stasis, the inorganic salts precipitate on the organic nidus. Although radiopaque, appendiceal calculi are not usually hard and often can be cut with a knife. Thirty-three per cent of inflamed appendices have a radiologically demonstrable calculus, as compared with 2.7 per cent of normals.[14, 15] Plain films of the abdomen reveal stones in 12 per cent of those with inflamed appendices and in only 1 per cent of normal persons.[16] Appendiceal calculi therefore are more common in inflamed organs. When calculous disease is present, the incidence of gangrene and rupture is significantly increased.[15-17]

Although calculi are important in the pathogenesis of a proportion of cases of appendicitis, they are absent in between 67 and 80 per cent of cases, indicating that some other pathogenetic factors must be sought. Kinking caused by adhesions, parasites, and lymphoid hyperplasia have all been incriminated. In addition, functional obstruction resulting from a valve system at the entrance of the appendix may have etiological importance.[12]

There are some who feel that the primary lesion is not obstruction but superficial mucosal ulceration.[5] Indeed, well defined, superficial mucosal ulcers have been found in 75 per cent of inflamed appendices. Such ulceration precedes dilatation, which is more apt to be present in advanced disease of the appendiceal wall. Such data support the hypothesis that appendicitis begins with mucosal ulceration which might result from a viral infection. The process is then advanced by the invasion of enteric bacteria.

Most likely, acute appendicitis is caused by several possible mechanisms. Once inflamed, the appendix is liable to progress to gangrene and perforation, because the arteries at its tip act as end arteries.[18] This is especially true in older persons and probably helps to account for the high incidence of perforation in the elderly.

CLINICAL PICTURE AND DIAGNOSIS

The majority of patients with acute appendicitis present to the hospital within 12 to 48 hours of the onset of symptoms. From 95 to 97 per cent complain of abdominal pain which most commonly is well localized to the right lower quadrant.[3, 7] Classically, the pain of acute appendicitis is first referred to the epigastric or periumbilical areas, and then later localizes to its usual position where it persists as a steady although sometimes colicky pain. The history of migrating pain can be obtained in only about 50 per cent of patients.[8] Although most patients have right lower quadrant pain, a significant number will have either diffuse or crampy generalized lower abdominal pain. Rarely, the pain may radiate down to the right testicle, simulating ureteral pain, or localize in the left lower quadrant. Anorexia is the second most frequent symptom, followed by nausea, often accompanied by vomiting. These three complaints are found in nearly 90 per cent of patients.[3, 7] Constipation is present in about 10 per cent, whereas diarrhea is encountered less often.[3] The temperature is typically low grade (38 to 38.6° C) unless the patient has a perforation with peritonitis, which can result in temperatures averaging 39° C.[8]

The order of symptoms is important in diagnosis. Pain comes before anorexia, nausea, or vomiting, all of which precede fever.[19]

The findings on physical examination depend somewhat on the stage of the appendiceal pathology. Abdominal tenderness is the single most important and consistent finding in all age groups.[3, 7, 8, 20, 21] If an attack of pain lasts for two hours without abdominal tenderness, the diagnosis of acute appendicitis must be in doubt. Tenderness is usually well localized in the right lower quadrant at McBurney's point but may vary, depending upon the location of the appendix. Rectal tenderness is found in about one-third of patients.[8] Severe or diffuse rectal tenderness indicates pelvic peritonitis. A palpable mass is present in some individuals, and represents perforation of the appendix with a localized abscess. Localized guarding and rebound tenderness may be present in up to 70 per cent of cases even without perforation,[8] but are usually absent in the earlier stage and are occasionally absent even with pelvic peritonitis.[20] Rebound tenderness is invariable only with perforation and generalized peritonitis.[8] Presence or absence of bowel sounds is of no aid in the diagnosis of acute appendicitis.

An appreciable rise in the total white blood cell count and in the percentage of polymorphonuclear cells is encountered in most patients with acute appendicitis. About 90 per cent will have white blood cell counts over 10,000 per mm^3; greater than 75 per cent polymorphonuclear cells will be found in 80 per cent of patients.[22] Regardless of age, fewer than 4 per cent will have a normal leukocyte profile.[10, 11, 20, 22] The urinalysis will be normal in most patients, but 10 to 20 per cent will have minor degrees of proteinuria, pyuria, or hematuria.[8] Pyuria or hematuria of more than minor degree or the presence of white blood cell casts should direct attention toward the urinary tract. As noted, from 10 to 12 per cent of patients will have demonstrable fecaliths on plain films of the abdomen,[23, 24] but a negative film is not significant. A positive film combined with clinical symptoms virtually assures the diagnosis. Other radiographic findings which can be seen in acute appendicitis

are a sentinel loop ileus (gas or fluid filled) in the right lower quadrant, obliteration of the right psoas density, especially in its lower half, gas bubbles in the right lower quadrant (found with perforated appendix), a right lower quadrant soft tissue mass which suggests perforation, gas in the appendix (which may be noted rarely in a normal person), pneumoperitoneum (rare), and fluid in the peritoneal cavity (with perforation and generalized peritonitis).[25] Recently, fluid interposed between the colonic contents and the fat flank stripe in the right lower quadrant has been emphasized as a finding in appendicitis.[26] It must be stressed, however, that in the great majority of instances, abdominal roentgenological studies will be nondiagnostic.

Acute appendicitis is much more difficult to diagnose at both age extremes than in the middle years. Fortunately, it is relatively uncommon in the very young and over age 60. Diagnostic accuracy for all patients operated upon for appendicitis is slightly over 80 per cent in most centers.[8, 27] When only patients over 60 years of age are considered, however, accuracy falls to below 70 per cent.[10, 21] This is not because these individuals differ with regard to specific symptoms or physical findings, but because their presentation is more subtle. Elderly patients tend to complain less of their symptoms and to exhibit less tenderness on abdominal examination. At surgery, they have much more advanced disease than their younger counterparts. The incidence of perforation with either localized or spreading peritonitis at surgery is nearly 70 per cent in the group over age 60,[7, 10, 11] compared with below 30 per cent in all age groups combined.[4, 7-9] Delay in seeking medical attention and difficulty in making the diagnosis are the stated reasons for this high incidence of advanced disease. The evidence indicates that perforation of the inflamed appendix probably occurs earlier in the elderly.[10, 11]

Accurate early diagnosis of appendicitis in children is likewise a major problem. In one study only 53 per cent of patients were admitted to the hospital on the first visit to the physician.[28] This delay in surgical treatment was associated with an increased incidence of complications. As many as 68 per cent of patients below age six and 87 per cent of those below age two may rupture before surgery.[20] Such figures stress the need for earlier diagnosis in young children who often are unable to give an adequate history. Vomiting is quite frequent in children and is apt to precede the parental awareness of any abdominal discomfort in the child. Abdominal tenderness is invariably present and is the single most important finding. Since the appendix is longer in relationship to the body in children, tenderness is more variable in location than in adults.[28] Rectal examination may be positive in up to three-fourths of patients, and must be performed. The triad of vomiting, fever, and abdominal tenderness strongly suggests the diagnosis. If there is doubt, the child should be admitted to the hospital for observation; if doubt persists after a few hours in the hospital, surgery should be advised.

DIFFERENTIAL DIAGNOSIS

The conditions simulating acute appendicitis include almost all intra-abdominal diseases, as well as some in the chest. A detailed description of the differential diagnosis is offered on pages 338 to 343. (See also the book by Cope.[19]) The most common childhood diseases mimicking acute appendicitis are viral gastroenteritis and mesenteric adenitis. Although the history is usually one of pain *after* the onset of nausea and vomiting, other family members may be similarly affected, and tenderness is usually diffuse without associated spasm; the exclusion of appendicitis may be impossible without surgery. In the child-bearing ages, the diagnosis of appendicitis is more easily missed in the female, owing to confusion with various diseases of the reproductive system. Acute pelvic inflammatory disease, ruptured graafian follicle, twisted ovarian cyst, ectopic pregnancy, dysmenorrhea, and ruptured endometrioma are only some of the diseases that may resemble appendicitis. A careful history, especially with regard to the menstrual cycle, and adequate pelvic examination are mandatory in female patients. Acute urinary tract infection, especially in young females, must be excluded. If any doubt remains, operative intervention

is indicated, because the complications of a ruptured appendix are much more severe than the morbidity associated with laparotomy for a normal appendix.

In elderly patients, there is usually no problem with mesenteric adenitis or gynecological disease. Cholecystitis, diverticulitis, mesenteric thrombosis, intestinal obstruction, incarcerated hernia, and perforated ulcer with spillage down the right gutter are some of the conditions that present difficult problems in diagnosis.[10, 11, 21] The recognition of a surgical abdomen is more important than a correct preoperative diagnosis. One should be careful not to subject elderly patients, who often have complicating medical problems, to the risk of surgery for medical problems such as myocardial infarction or pneumonia, both of which may cause abdominal symptoms. Careful examination of the chest, chest X-rays, electrocardiogram, abdominal X-rays, and a careful urinalysis will help to avoid such mistakes.

TREATMENT

With rare exceptions, the only acceptable therapy for acute appendicitis is the earliest possible removal of the appendix. The overall mortality and morbidity in appendicitis depends upon the severity of the disease at the time of operation; i.e., whether the appendix has perforated.[8, 9] Except for elderly patients who may perforate earlier in the course of the disease,[10, 11] the incidence of perforation is directly related to the duration of symptoms.[4, 8] Therefore mortality correlates with delay in surgery, ranging from a figure only slightly above that of general anesthesia to levels associated with surgery for generalized peritonitis. Early surgical intervention is crucial. Since the diagnosis of acute appendicitis is often difficult to make with certainty early in the course of the disease, a certain number of normal appendices will have to be removed. An acceptable figure for this necessary evil is 20 to 25 per cent.[9]

It is beyond the scope of this presentation to discuss surgical technique. There are certain general principles in management that should be observed. Once the diagnosis is considered, the patient should have the head of his bed elevated, unless contraindicated by hypotension. In case of rupture, this allows the appendiceal contents to collect in the pelvis where abscess formation is easiest to manage.[28] Dehydrated patients, especially children, should receive adequate intravenous fluid therapy even if it means a slight delay in surgery.[20, 28] Fever should be reduced preoperatively in children to prevent febrile convulsions.[20, 28] If the patient has eaten within the past eight hours, a nasogastric tube should be passed and the gastric contents aspirated. If perforation is suspected by findings of localized or generalized peritonitis, continuous nasogastric suction is instituted. Antibiotics are not indicated in uncomplicated cases.[9, 28] They should be reserved for patients suspected of having gangrenous or perforated appendix. Such patients can often be differentiated by higher temperatures (often greater than 102° F), symptoms of greater than 36 hours' duration, and definite signs of peritonitis.[8, 20, 28] Broad-spectrum antibiotics, usually high dose penicillin and streptomycin or high dose ampicillin, are administered to combat the enteric organisms involved, the most common of which is *Escherichia coli*.[8]

For patients with findings indicative of appendiceal abscess, or with a clinical history of perforation five or more days prior to admission to the hospital, management consists of nasogastric decompression, continuous broad-spectrum antibiotics, intravenous fluid therapy, and bedrest.[28] Once a localized area of sepsis has been identified, it can be drained retroperitoneally, preferably through the rectum. After the inflammation has subsided, the appendix should be removed at the earliest possible time.

Occasionally, an episode of acute appendicitis develops when there is no one adequately trained to perform surgery. In such situations, it is wiser to treat the patient medically than to perform unskilled surgery. In 1946, Crile treated 50 patients with ruptured appendices and peritonitis with antibiotics and supportive care.[29] He had only one death, and that was due to mesenteric vein thrombosis. Twenty-six of his patients had no surgery. Fifteen of this group developed an abdominal or pelvic mass. Although some were large enough to

occlude the rectum, none required drainage and all eventually disappeared. The average febrile period was eight days, but over half the patients were afebrile by the third day. These results indicate that although surgical treatment is the preferred mode of therapy, medical therapy is a surprisingly good second choice (see pp. 408 to 420).

MORBIDITY AND MORTALITY

As previously mentioned, postoperative morbidity depends almost entirely upon the stage of the disease at the time for surgery.[7, 8, 10, 20, 28] In patients without perforation, the overall complication rate is about 14 per cent.[8] In those with perforation and localized peritonitis, this increases to 35.6 per cent; with perforation and generalized peritonitis, it reaches 70 per cent. In spite of liberal pre- and postoperative antibiotics, the most common postoperative complication is wound infection, which complicates from 3 to 15 per cent of cases.[7, 28] As expected, this range more than doubles if the appendix has perforated, in which case intra-abdominal abscesses are found in 15 per cent of patients.[8, 28] Mechanical small bowel obstruction, fecal fistula, and intraperitoneal hemorrhage are occasional complications. Pyelophlebitis must be kept in mind as a possible complication, but is rare (seen in about one patient in 1000).[7] In addition, the usual postoperative pulmonary, cardiac, and cerebral problems may be encountered, especially in the elderly.

The overall mortality of acute appendicitis has been steadily decreasing until it is now less than one per 100,000 population per year.[2] This favorable trend can be attributed to overall improved surgical care, not to earlier presentation of the disease. The mortality of unruptured appendicitis very nearly equals that of general anesthesia alone.[9, 27] Theoretically therefore, if perforation can be prevented, mortality could be almost entirely eliminated. Still, mortality ranges from 0.18 to 1.6 per cent.[3, 7, 8] This residual mortality can be attributed to the interrelated factors of age and perforation. Thus the mortality over age 50 ranges from 3.8 to 5 per cent.[3, 7, 30] The mortality rate in series limited to patients over age 60 has ranged from 6.4 to 14 per cent.[7, 11, 21] This high mortality is more related to the extremely high percentage of perforation than to any other single factor.[10, 11] Causes of death in acute appendicitis may be attributed equally to the septic and nonseptic complications.

SPECIAL CONSIDERATIONS

INCIDENTAL APPENDECTOMY

Whether or not to remove a normal appendix routinely during any abdominal operation is still an unanswered question. The answer depends upon the immediate additional risk, the risk of future acute appendicitis, and the possibility of long-term hazards of appendectomy. Additional immediate risk can be estimated only by the surgeon at the operating table. Since the risk of future appendicitis decreases with advancing age, the ideal candidates for incidental appendectomy are children and youths. The setting for this procedure, however, is usually elective surgery in an adult whose risk of developing acute appendicitis in the future is on the wane. Such risk after age 37.5, the median age for incidental appendectomy, has been computed to be 0.0431 for men and 0.369 for women. The risk of dying from appendicitis for men of age 40 is about one in 800.[31] In light of these figures, it is difficult to make a strong case for or against incidental appendectomy. With regard to hazards to future health, a higher prevalence of primary appendectomy has been found in male patients with Hodgkin's disease than in control subjects. Women with breast or large bowel cancers have also been found to have a higher prevalence rate when compared with some control groups, but not when compared with others.[1] The actual significance of these observations remains to be determined. If they turn out to be of importance in themselves, rather than as indicators of other factors leading to abdominal surgery, they will discourage incidental appendectomy. One thing is certain: if the patient has had an incidental appendectomy, it is important that he be made aware of it.

PROPHYLACTIC APPENDECTOMY

In general, there is no place in medicine for elective prophylactic appendectomy. The only possible exception is the presence of an appendiceal fecalith in an individual going into a region without adequate medical facilities. Otherwise, the risk of developing appendicitis is not sufficient to warrant prophylactic appendectomy.[31, 32]

REFERENCES

1. Hyams, L., and Winder, E. L. Appendectomy and cancer risk: An epidemiologic evaluation. J. Chronic Dis. 21:391, 1968.
2. Appendicitis in recent years. Statistical Bulletin of the Metropolitan Life Insurance Company 50:4, 1969.
3. Sethi, S. M., Matsuda, T., Pemberton, B., and Stroltz, E. L. An analysis of 500 consecutive cases of acute appendicitis in a metropolitan charity hospital. Ill. Med. J. 138:147, 1970.
4. Babcock, J. R., and McKinley, W. M. Acute appendicitis: An analysis of 1662 consecutive cases. Ann. Surg. 150:131, 1959.
5. Sisson, R. G., Ahlvin, R. C., and Harlow, M. C. Superficial mucosal ulcerations in the pathogenesis of acute appendicitis. Amer. J. Surg. 122:378, 1971.
6. Howie, J. G. R. Too few appendectomies. Lancet 1:1240, 1964.
7. Mittelpunkt, A., and Nora, P. F. Current features in the treatment of acute appendicitis: An analysis of 1000 consecutive cases. Surgery 60:971, 1966.
8. Kazarian, K. K., Roeder, W. J., and Mersheimer, W. L. Decreasing mortality and increasing morbidity from acute appendicitis. Amer. J. Surg. 119:681, 1970.
9. Cantrell, J. R., and Stafford, E. S. The diminishing mortality from appendicitis. Ann. Surg. 141:749, 1955.
10. Coran, A. G., and Wheeler, H. B. Early perforation in appendicitis after age 60. J.A.M.A. 197:745, 1966.
11. Thorbjarnarson, B., and Loehr, W. J. Acute appendicitis in patients over the age of 60. Surg. Gynec. Obstet. 125:1277, 1967.
12. Wagensteen, O. H., and Bowers, W. F. Significance of the obstructive factor in the genesis of acute appendicitis. Arch. Surg. 34:496, 1937.
13. Wagensteen, O. H., and Dennis, C. Experimental proof of the obstructive origin of appendicitis in man. Ann. Surg. 110:629, 1939.
14. Shaw, R. E. Appendix calculi in acute appendicitis. Brit. J. Surg. 52:451, 1965.
15. Felson, B. Appendiceal calculi; incidence and clinical significance. Surgery 25:434, 1949.
16. Faegenburg, D. Fecaliths of the appendix: Incidence and significance. Amer. J. Roent. 89:752, 1963.
17. Forbes, G. B., and Lloyd-Davies, R. W. Calculous disease of the vermiform appendix. Gut 7:583, 1966.
18. Lindgren, I., and Aho, A. J. Microangiopathic

investigations in acute appendicitis. Acta Chir. Scand. 135:77, 1969.

19. Cope, Z.   The early diagnosis of the acute abdomen. London, Oxford University Press, 1968.

20. Longino, L. A., Holder, T. M., and Gross, R. E. Appendicitis in childhood. A study of 1358 cases. Pediatrics 22:238, 1958.

21. Williams, J. S., and Hale, H. W.   Acute appendicitis in the elderly—a review of 83 cases. Ann. Surg. 162:208, 1964.

22. Sasso, R. D., Hanna, E. A., and Moore, D. L. Leukocytic and neutrophilic counts in acute appendicitis. Amer. J. Surg. 120:563, 1970.

23. Steinert, R., Harcide, I., and Christiansen, T. Roentgenologic examination of acute appendicitis. Acta Radiol. 24:13, 1943.

24. Faegenburg, D.   Fecaliths of the appendix. Amer. J. Roent. 89:752, 1963.

25. Beneventano, T. C., Schein, C. J., and Jacobson, H. G.   The roentgen aspects of some appendiceal abnormalities. Amer. J. Roent. Med. 96:344, 1966.

26. Casper, R. V.   Fluid in the right flank as a roentgenographic sign of acute appendicitis. Amer. J. Roent. 110:352, 1970.

27. Barnes, B. A., Behringer, G. E., Wheelock, F. C., and Wilkins, E. W.   Treatment of appendicitis at the Massachusetts General Hospital (1937-1959). J.A.M.A. 180:122, 1962.

28. Stone, H. H., Sanders, S. L., and Martin, J. D. Perforated appendicitis in children. Surgery 69:673, 1971.

29. Crile, G.   Peritonitis of appendiceal origin treated with massive does of penicillin. Surg. Obstet. Gynec. 83:150, 1946.

30. Ross, F. P., Zarem, H. A., and Morgan, A. P. Appendicitis in a community hospital. Arch. Surg. 85:1036, 1965.

31. Hewitt, D., Milner, J., and LeRiche, W. H. Incidental appendectomy—a statistical appraisal. Canad. Med. Assoc. J. 100:1075, 1969.

32. Leedbrook, J., and Spears, G. F.   The risk of developing appendicitis. Brit. J. Surg. 52:856, 1965.

Chapter 112

Other Diseases of the Colon and Rectum

David L. Earnest, Marvin H. Sleisenger

Frequently encountered diseases of the colon as well as colonic involvement in generalized or systemic illness are extensively discussed elsewhere in this section and in Part I. There are, however, certain diseases of the colon which cannot be conveniently classified with other inflammatory, vascular, motor, or malignant conditions and are therefore discussed in this chapter. These miscellaneous diseases of the colon are for the most part uncommon, often of uncertain etiology, occasionally of questionable significance to the patient, and frequently perplexing to diagnose and treat.

The current state of knowledge about most of these miscellaneous diseases is less than desirable. In order adequately to diagnose their presence, the physician must employ radiologic, sigmoidoscopic, and biopsy techniques. Of the three, sigmoidoscopy and rectal biopsy offer the greatest possibility for a precise diagnosis. Sigmoidoscopy is discussed on pages 1543 to 1547. Rectal biopsy is discussed in the first part of this chapter, with comments regarding specific diseases in which it is helpful. Histological abnormalities characteristic of a particular disease are found in the general discussion of that entity elsewhere in this text.

RECTAL BIOPSY

During anoscopy or sigmoidoscopy the physician should be prepared to obtain biopsy specimens of rectal or lower sigmoid lesions in order to obtain objective histological evidence pertaining to the observed abnormality. Rectal biopsy must always be done under direct vision with optimal lighting except when a suction-type instrument is used. There are at least four types of biopsy instruments: a suction biopsy tube, cutting forceps, punch biopsy forceps, and snares (Fig. 112–1). It is not necessary to have all these available, although certain instruments may facilitate biopsy of a particular lesion.

INDICATIONS AND TECHNIQUES

Pedunculated polyps on a narrow, well defined stalk can be easily removed at the base by either cold or electrothermic snares or by cutting forceps. The entire polyp, including the stalk, must be removed in order that a thorough search for malignant change can be made. Partial excision of adenomas, which usually consists of removal of pieces of tissue from the rounded

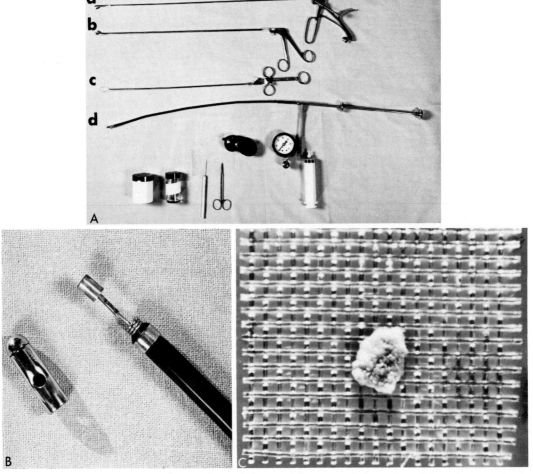

Figure 112–1. *A,* Instruments frequently used for rectal biopsy include (a) straight cutting forceps, (b) angled cutting forceps, (c) polyp snare, and (d) suction biopsy tube. *B,* The disassembled tip of the suction biopsy tube shows the biopsy port into which the mucosa is sucked and the guillotine-type cutting blade. *C,* Using a dissecting needle and hand lens, the biopsy specimen is transferred mucosal side up to a small piece of monofilament mesh before being placed in fixing solution. Rectal biopsy samples should be handled similarly to the jejunal biopsy sample shown here.

top, is to be condemned. If a broad base is present or complete removal of the polyp would produce a sizable mucosal defect, surface abrasion for cytology should be carried out and surgical consultation obtained.

Biopsy specimens of ulcerating lesions should be taken at their margin and include some surrounding normal mucosa. If the biopsy is taken directly from the ulcer base, only nondiagnostic necrotic debris will be obtained. A cutting forceps with angulated jaws is the most convenient instrument to biopsy this lesion. If small, superficial, and discrete ulcerations are to be

biopsied, one low in the rectum should be chosen. This is because of the danger of bowel perforation when biopsies are taken above the peritoneal reflection which is approximately 12 cm above the pectinate line. If the mucosal lesion is high in the rectum, forceps with short angulated jaws should be used, and the grasped mucosa gently tented up by the forceps before the final cut is made. If this cannot be done, the biopsy should not be completed, because a good possibility exists that too deep a cut will be made. Biopsy of large mucosal tumors may be made by either punch or cutting forceps.

In situations in which apparent diffuse mucosal disease exists, rectal biopsy can be accomplished easily and safely either with cutting forceps, if only the valve is biopsied, or with a suction biopsy tube. When biopsying a valve of Houston with cutting forceps, one can easily take an excessively large bite, causing a disconcerting amount of bleeding. This complication can be avoided by being certain to biopsy only the valve tip or by taking the specimen from one surface of the valve. The biopsy site should always be inspected after the specimen is taken. Excessive bleeding is not common, but, if present, it can be managed by local tamponade, application of epinephrine solution, or cauterization.

The multipurpose suction biopsy tube is especially well suited for obtaining mucosal biopsies when diffuse mucosal disease is present. Specimens adequate for interpretation can be easily obtained with minimal patient discomfort and risk. A detailed description regarding the use of this tube is available.[1, 2] Briefly, the tube is lubricated and, with the cutting blade closed, is inserted 7 to 10 cm proximal to the anus. If desired, biopsies may be taken above the peritoneal reflection, because bowel perforation with the suction biopsy tube does not occur.[3] To obtain a specimen from the proximal rectum or sigmoid colon, the biopsy tube is inserted under direct vision through a sigmoidoscope and maintained in place while the sigmoidoscope is removed. A small rubber catheter is then inserted into the rectum to remove excess air and then withdrawn so that the necessary vacuum can be achieved. The knife blade is opened and a vacuum of 5 to 10 inches of mercury is produced for three seconds by aspiration with a syringe. The guillotine biopsy knife is closed and the tube removed. The procedure should be painless.

Proper handling of the biopsy specimen is as necessary as proper technique in obtaining it. The specimen is blown out of the tube and onto a clean surface and unfolded; then, with the use of a dissecting needle, it is mounted mucosal side up on a monofilament mesh similar to that shown in Figure 112–1, C. Correct mounting on the mesh is of utmost importance in order to obtain a flat specimen rather than a curled one. This orientation and mounting procedure should be accomplished quickly and should be applied to all biopsy specimens regardless of the instrument used to obtain them. After fixation and embedding, sections should be cut perpendicular to the mucosal surface. Proper orientation for sectioning is more difficult to achieve if the specimen was not

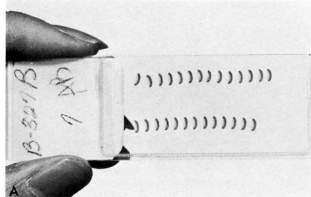

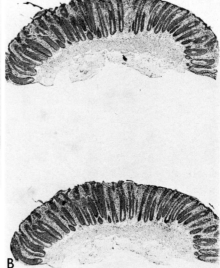

Figure 112–2. *A*, Multiple sections made perpendicular to the mucosa of a properly oriented biopsy specimen can be mounted on the same slide for review. *B*, If staining is adequate, a properly oriented, sectioned, and mounted specimen will provide optimal material for interpretation. The crypts should be long and parallel, and should end perpendicular to the muscularis mucosae. Improper mounting and tangential sectioning will produce an artifact similar to that at the right side of this biopsy specimen.

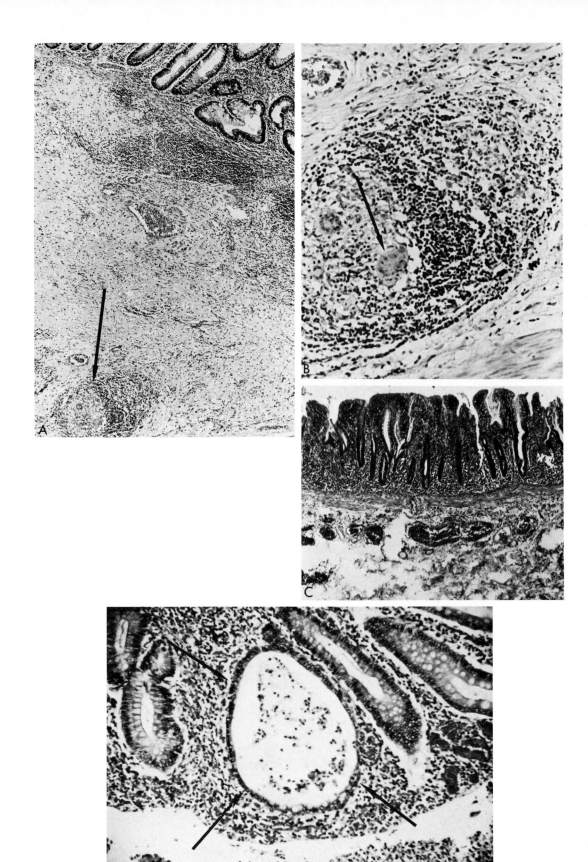

Figure 112-3. *See opposite page for legend.*

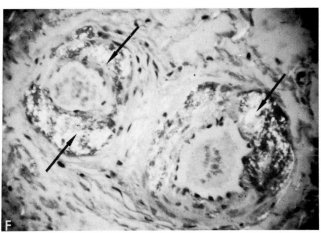

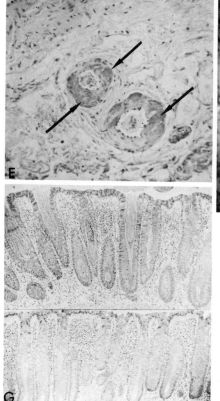

Figure 112–3. *A*, Forceps biopsy from a rectal valve in a patient with granulomatous colitis. Chronic inflammatory cells are present beneath the muscularis mucosae and throughout the submucosa. A granuloma (arrow), seen here in the deep submucosa, is not always present in superficial mucosal biopsies. Hematoxylin and eosin stain × 50. *B*, A higher power view of the granuloma in *A* shows lymphocytes surrounding the typical epithelioid cells. Two large giant cells are present in the center (arrow). × 250. *C*, Forceps biopsy from a rectal valve in a patient with acute ulcerative colitis. Acute and chronic inflammatory cells fill the mucosa and appear to "push apart" the crypts, but do not extend below the muscularis mucosae. Hematoxylin and eosin stain. × 25. *D*, A typical crypt abscess (arrows) from another area of the same rectal biopsy specimen in *C*. Note the markedly dilated crypt with polymorphonuclear leukocytes in the lumen. Serial sections may show inflammatory necrosis of the crypt wall. Hematoxylin and eosin stain. × 250. *E*, Rectal biopsy from a patient with massive proteinuria. Amorphous deposits (arrows), causing irregular thickening of the walls of submucosal arterioles, are present and are suggestive of amyloid. Hematoxylin and eosin stain. × 250. *F*, A Congo red stain of the tissue in *E*, viewed with polarized light, demonstrated a shiny green birefringence in the area of the deposits (arrows), which is characteristic of amyloid. × 600. *G*, Rectal suction biopsies. *Top*, Cystic fibrosis, characterized by dilated rectal glands or crypts filled with thick, viscous mucus. *Bottom*, normal control. Hematoxylin, eosin, and alcian blue stain. × 100. (Courtesy of Dr. Cyrus E. Rubin.)

fixed in a flattened state. Multiple sections can be mounted on the same slide, as shown in Figure 112–2. For thorough histological evaluation, it is usually desirable to examine multiple levels of the biopsy specimen. Preparing and mounting the tissue in this manner will practically assure one of an interpretable specimen.

To perform rectal biopsy safely, it is necessary to have excellent illumination and clear visualization of the tissue to be removed. The two main complications of the procedure are excessive bleeding and perforation. Bleeding usually results from taking a large biopsy, especially from a valve or from a highly vascular tumor. Although this complication is usually easily managed, transfusions may be required. Prolonged rectal pain and tenesmus after the procedure may be due to the development of pneumatosis cystoides intestinalis. Fever with more generalized abdominal pain should prompt evaluation for a bowel perforation, which, fortunately, is rare. It must be remembered that perforation of the bowel at the site of rectal biopsy can be precipitated by a barium enema performed shortly after the biopsy.[4] Thus the X-ray procedure should either be done before rectal biopsy or be delayed for three to five days after it.

DIAGNOSES

Rectal biopsy is useful in diagnosing many varied disease processes. It is most commonly used for histological evaluation of a mass lesion. However, the following entities, as emphasized in a recent review, can be conveniently diagnosed and followed by this examination.[3] Some examples are seen in Figure 112–3.

PARASITIC DISEASE

Diagnosis of parasitic disease of the colon may occasionally be facilitated by rectal biopsy. This is especially true for schistosomiasis in which infestation with S. mansoni and S. japonicum can be easily identified in a squash preparation of the specimen. One half of the biopsy is placed in saline for a few minutes and then pressed between a glass slide and coverslip before microscopic examination under low magnification[5] (Fig. 104–21). This is

the preferred method for demonstrating the ova, because viability can also be assessed. In addition, rectal biopsy from an area of mucosal ulceration will occasionally make the diagnosis of amebiasis even when repeated stool examinations are negative (see pp. 1387 to 1388). Special stains should be made and serial sections examined for ameba with close attention given to any clumps of exudate on the mucosa.[6] If amebiasis is suspected, enemas which might remove exudate containing the parasite should never be given before the biopsy procedure.

CHRONIC INFLAMMATORY DISEASES

Rectal biopsy is especially useful in inflammatory bowel disease and may aid in differentiating Crohn's disease of the colon from idiopathic ulcerative colitis. The finding of epithelioid granulomas in the mucosa or submucosa strongly suggests Crohn's disease, but is not diagnostic; their absence does not exclude the diagnosis (Fig. 112–3, A and B).[6] The hallmark of active ulcerative colitis is the presence of polymorphonuclear leukocytes in the lamina propria, especially with microabscesses of the crypts. This is also by no means absolutely diagnostic of idiopathic ulcerative colitis, because crypt abscesses have been demonstrated in many inflammatory disorders of the colon, including amebiasis, bacillary dysentery, and Crohn's disease (Fig. 112–3, C and D).[2, 6–8] However, rectal biopsy is more sensitive than barium enema or sigmoidoscopy in diagnosing early or quiescent ulcerative colitis and can also be used successfully to follow activity of the disease during treatment.[9, 10] The usefulness of rectal biopsy in detecting premalignant changes in ulcerative colitis has been suggested, but needs further evaluation.[11] Demonstration of typical histological changes in the rectal biopsy specimen is not essential for diagnosis of ulcerative colitis, but is useful to confirm the diagnosis when classic features of the disease are not present.

INFILTRATIVE AND OTHER DISEASES

Rectal biopsy can also be helpful in diagnosing diseases characterized by abnormality in specific tissues. Congo red stains will demonstrate the green bi-refringence of amyloid deposits in walls of small arterioles in the submucosa and muscularis mucosae (Fig. 112–3, E and F). In one study, only renal biopsy gave more frequent positive results than rectal biopsy in proved cases of amyloidosis.[12] Diagnostic rectal biopsy in Hirschsprung's disease can be obtained by a punch or cutting forceps biopsy of rectal valves or by a suction biopsy taken at least 3 cm above the pectinate line (see p. 1468). Serial sections should be made to ascertain the absence of ganglion cells and the presence of hypertrophied and disorganized non-myelinated nerve fibers in the submucosa.[13] Abnormalities in the rectal mucosa, including widely dilated and gaping crypts packed with mucus and with prominent goblet cells, are often found in patients with cystic fibrosis (Fig. 112–3, G). However, these changes are not pathognomonic.[14] Unfortunately, rectal biopsy is not as accurate as small bowel biopsy in diagnosing Whipple's disease. Typical cases of Whipple's disease have been described in which no periodic acid–Schiff (PAS) positive macrophages were observed in the lamina propria of the rectal biopsy tissue. Conversely, PAS positive histiocytes are frequently seen in rectal biopsies from patients who do not have Whipple's disease.[3] In pediatric neurology the value of rectal biopsy as it relates to diagnosis of various storage diseases has been emphasized.[3, 15] This is especially true for Tay-Sachs disease in which diagnostic ganglion cell abnormalities may be readily seen in the rectal mucosal specimen.[16]

Other systemic diseases can produce abnormalities in rectal tissue, including focal arteritis in patients with rheumatoid arthritis; absence of plasma cells in the lamina propria in some patients with agammaglobulinemia; cytomegalic cells with inclusion bodies in specimens from patients with systemic disease; and anorectal tuberculosis, histoplasmosis, and granulomatous fibrosis in patients with lymphogranuloma venereum. Biopsy features of radiation damage to the colon are discussed on pages 1408 to 1409.

Finally, diagnosis of certain miscellaneous diseases of the colon is often facilitated by rectal biopsy examination. These diseases include pneumatosis cystoides intestinalis, stercoral ulcer, colitis cystica profunda, nonspecific ulcer of the colon, melanosis coli, malakoplakia, and colonic endometriosis. They are considered in detail in the remainder of this chapter.

COLITIS CYSTICA PROFUNDA

Benign, mucus-filled lesions of the colon are of two main types: (1) colitis cystica profunda, with discrete, mucus-filled cystic spaces below the muscularis mucosae and primarily located in the distal colon; and (2) colitis cystica superficialis, in which the cysts are entirely superficial to the muscularis mucosae and are present throughout the colon. The superficialis type appears grossly as thousands of barely visible, minute gray blebs on the mucosal surface and from which mucus can be expressed. Colitis cystica superficialis occurs mainly in association with pellagra and may even be present in the absence of typical skin lesions. It has also been uncommonly associated with adult celiac disease.[17–20] Unfortunately, little attention has been given to this lesion in the literature in the past quarter century, and the reader therefore is referred to older references. In this section we will not be concerned further with the superficialis type, because it is the cystica profunda variant that usually presents a diagnostic problem.

PATHOLOGY

There are a number of good reports of the gross and histological findings in colitis cystica profunda.[17, 20, 21] These should be consulted for evaluation of tissue from any suspected patient, because most standard pathology textbooks omit the entity. Inspection of resected surgical specimens has revealed that the bowel wall is usually thickened and occasionally edematous. The thickening is most often due to the submucosal cysts which vary from 0.1 to 1.5 cm in diameter. Incision into and compression of the cystic area will usually produce a thick, gelatinous material. The overlying mucosa may grossly appear normal or may either be ulcerated or contain a small umbilication.

On microscopic examination, cysts are seen below the muscularis mucosae and may even penetrate into the muscularis

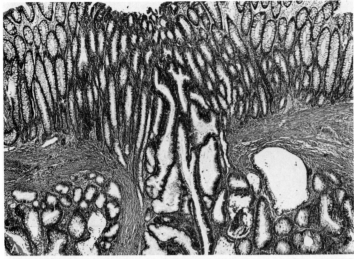

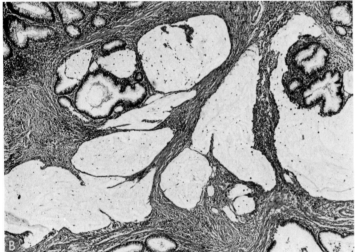

Figure 112–4. Biopsy of the polypoid sigmoid mass shown in Figure 112–5. *A*, Communication between the submucosal cysts and the bowel lumen through a defect in the muscularis mucosae may occasionally be demonstrated by serial sections. Hematoxylin and eosin stain. × 345. (From Fechner, R. F. Dis. Colon Rectum *10*:359, 1967). *B*, Pools of mucin without epithelial lining as well as epithelially lined cysts are present in the submucosa. Although the cyst epithelium is benign, this appearance has occasionally resulted in misdiagnosis of mucus-producing carcinoma. Hematoxylin and eosin stain. × 64.

propria. The cysts are filled with basophilic staining mucoid material and are lined by colonic epithelium showing varying degrees of pressure atrophy. Communications between the cyst and bowel lumen may occasionally be demonstrated by serial sections (Fig. 112–4, *A*).[17, 22, 23] The submucosa surrounding the epithelium-lined cysts and unlined mucous collections may have evidence of chronic inflammation with infiltration of lymphocytes, plasma cells, and occasionally fibrosis. It is this picture of aberrant gland forming colonic epithelium with acellular mucous lakes that has led to misdiagnoses of a mucus-producing carcinoma (Fig. 112–4, *B*). Non-neoplastic glands deep in the submucosa should raise the possibility of colitis cystica profunda.

PATHOGENESIS

The variability in reported cases does not give a clinical basis for postulation of a cause for the submucosal cysts. Therefore reconstruction of events from studies of pathological material has given rise to current theories of etiology. Variation in the types of cases reflects differences in the theories advanced to explain development of cysts. Early reports attributed the cyst to changes produced by the inflammation and scarring of chronic dysentery.[22] More recently, support for an inflammatory cause has again been offered, but with emphasis on the "follicular" ulcers present in some cases.[17] According to this theory, necrotizing lesions develop in the colonic lymphoid follicles which are intimately associated with the base of the mucosal crypts. When the necrosis connects the base of the crypt and the follicle, a narrow "follicular" ulcer develops with its base below the muscularis mucosae. Healing occurs with downgrowth of colonic epithelium, and a narrow-mouthed mucus-filled cystic area is produced. Against this theory have been (1) the reports of colitis cystica profunda in persons with no apparent inflammatory disease of the colon and (2) the absence of typical colitis cystica profunda in a large number of specimens of resected bowel from chronic ulcerative colitis patients.[20]

Congenitally ectopic colonic mucosa has also been postulated as a cause. However, the absence of colonic submucosal cysts in autopsies of pediatric patients is evidence against this theory.[20] Finally, it has been suggested that the lesion of colitis cystica profunda is acquired and develops from a basic "weakness" in the muscularis mucosae which allows herniation of the mucosal epithelium into the submucosa.[20] This theory seems to be supported by those cases with no evidence of inflammation. However, the occurrence of a previously subclinical and localized inflammatory process remains a possibility. Whatever mechanism is responsible, it is evident that colitis cystica profunda is seen under a variety of clinical situations. Awareness of its histological features is crucial in avoiding a mistaken diagnosis of malignancy.

CLINICAL PICTURE AND DIAGNOSIS

Early reports of colitis cystica profunda emphasize the occurrence of mucus-filled cystic lesions of the rectosigmoid colon during and after severe dysentery.[22] In more recent years and unrelated to acute diarrheal illness, patients have been described with symptomatic polypoid cystic lesions in the rectosigmoid colon. There has been no consistent sex distribution. Although cases have been reported in patients from nine to 63 years of age, the majority are young adults.[20] Symptoms of systemic illness such as fever, weight loss, and severe malaise are usually absent. Cramping lower abdominal pain, however, may be present. Partial obstruction of the colon may be caused by large or fibro-

tic lesions. The most consistent symptoms are mild diarrhea and rectal tenesmus and the occasional passage of blood and mucus with the stool. It is usually these symptoms which prompt evaluation.

Digital rectal examination may reveal one or more smooth, rubbery-firm masses which are easily movable and nonadherent to either the overlying mucosa or surrounding tissue. Because of the variability of the lesion, sigmoidoscopy may show sessile or polypoid lesions covered by normal mucosa, edematous congested mucosa, or even areas of ulceration or umbilication at the top of the intraluminal protrusion. When the lesion is massive or scarred, it may be impossible to advance the sigmoidoscope through the strictured area. Some patients with long-standing colitis symptoms before operative diagnosis of colitis cystica profunda were previously found to have sigmoidoscopic changes compatible with ulcerative colitis or nonspecific proctitis.[17, 22] This has certainly not been true in a majority of cases. Although the cystic process is usually limited to an area within reach of the sigmoidoscope, the transverse and upper descending colon may be the only area involved.[24]

Radiological examination is not diagnostic. The barium enema may show only a nodular irregularity of the bowel wall. However, larger cysts may present as an intraluminal nodular space-occupying lesion or lesions (Fig. 112–5). Small outpouchings of barium in the wall of the mass may suggest ulceration.[25] Therefore barium enema frequently raises the differential possibilities of polypoid bowel lesions, but does not help greatly in diagnosis.

The radiological differential diagnosis usually includes adenocarcinoma or lymphoma, benign adenomatous polyps, villous adenoma, submucosal lipoma, pneumatosis cystoides intestinalis, endometriosis of the bowel, pseudopolyps of ulcerative and granulomatous colitis, and a polypoid granulomatous reaction of schistosomiasis. Radiologically, lesions similar to those of colitis cystica profunda have also recently been reported in patients with obliterative arteriosclerosis and focal colonic mucosal necrosis.[26, 27] Tissue obtained from biopsy of one of the cystic nodules may give adequate information to

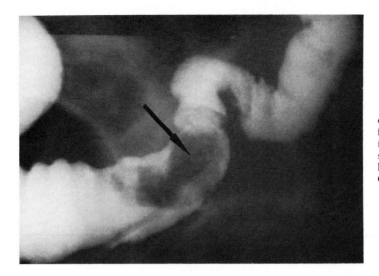

Figure 112–5. Barium enema examination in colitis cystica profunda may disclose small nodular irregularities of bowel wall or large space-occupying lesions, as shown here. (From Fechner, R. F.: Dis. Colon Rectum 10:359, 1967.)

settle the dilemma posed by this extensive differential diagnosis.

MANAGEMENT

The paucity of reported cases makes a firm statement regarding management difficult. Misdiagnosis has often led to radical cancer operations. An inadequate biopsy may be nondiagnostic and still lead to extensive surgery with colitis cystica profunda as an unsure choice in the differential diagnosis. However, a movable submucosal lesion can often be fully excised, and the correct diagnosis should then be possible. Excisional biopsy of a small lesion is usually adequate therapy.

Large bulky lesions or those producing severe bowel obstruction may require more radical excision. If metabolic abnormality occurs, such as recurrent iron deficiency from chronic blood loss or hypokalemia or hypoalbuminemia from excessive colonic mucous secretion,[25, 28] excision of the entire involved area is indicated. To date, surgical excision has been the only reported effective treatment. There are no reports of recurrence in uninvolved intestine after the primary excision.

The rule of therapy therefore is to perform the most conservative excision possible for the individual case. More reported experience with the entity and a better understanding of its pathogenesis may alter this view.

NONSPECIFIC ULCER OF THE COLON

The occurrence of solitary nonspecific ulcers in the colon was first described in 1832[29] and for a number of years remained only an interesting observation usually made at postmortem examination. In the past four decades, the lesion has been documented to be a definite clinical and pathological entity.[30-35] However, the frequency of this nonspecific ulceration is unknown, and the paucity of cases reported in the past 140 years suggests either that it is an uncommon entity or that many cases resolve without diagnosis. Against the latter possibility are reports documenting extreme chronicity, even exceeding 30 years in isolated cases of rectal ulceration.[30]

Although nonspecific ulceration of the colon was initially described as a single process involving different segments of the colon, review of more recent reports suggests that it should be divided into different clinical syndromes, depending upon the location of the colonic ulceration. Acute inflammation with perforation tends to complicate cecal location, whereas a chronic process frustratingly resistant to therapy characterizes the rectosigmoid lesion.[30-33] This variability in clinical presentation may not reflect a different cause but instead only anatomical variation between colonic segments, such as thickness of the muscularis propria or proximity of peri-colic supporting tissue. Because the exact cause of the ulceration is unknown, in the following discussion nonspecific ulcer of the colon will be treated as a single entity but with emphasis on the differences in presentation both clinically and patholog-ically when the disease occurs in different segments of the colon.

ETIOLOGY

Theories advanced to explain an iso-lated ulceration of the colon have been varied and often stimulated by the specific case involved. Ulceration in the cecum has usually been located near the ileocecal valve. A comparison has been drawn be-tween this lesion and ulceration in the duodenum,[30, 31] because both ulcers de-velop distal to a sphincter in an area with possibly marginal blood supply and occa-sionally acid luminal contents. However, evaluation of these factors revealed that the cecal fluid of cecostomy patients was usually neutral or only slightly acid, and vascular injection studies did not demon-strate a specific cecal area with poor blood supply.[32] Other authors have considered ischemia to be important, but have not been able to find convincing proof for this hypothesis regardless of location of the ul-ceration in the bowel.[36]

Some instances of cecal ulceration were shown to result from extensive inflamma-tion in a cecal diverticulum.[35] An obstruct-ing fecalith seemed to be a likely initiating factor. Nevertheless, isolated cecal diver-ticula are uncommon, and reported histol-ogy does not suggest for the majority of cases that the ulceration began in a true diverticulum. Other postulated causes for colon ulcers include drugs,[37] mechanical trauma caused by fecal roughage[38] or digi-tal trauma,[34] and viral and bacterial infec-tion.[39]

Until recently, pathological studies of the ulcer and adjacent bowel have not sup-ported more than one cause to explain the variable location of the ulcer in the colon.[40] However, in 1969, submucosal lesions similar to those of colitis cystica profunda were found in association with the ulcer-ation in some patients with solitary ulcer of the rectum.[34] It was suggested that in pa-tients with rectal involvement, the mucosa ulcerates over a localized area of hetero-topia or congenital duplication of the rec-tal mucosa. The opposite view could be taken, i.e., that the cystic process results from previous inflammation, as discussed above. In addition, the absence of submu-cosal islands of colonic mucosa adjacent to nonspecific ulcers in other locations in the large bowel is evidence against this etio-logical theory.

PATHOLOGY

The ulceration is usually single or soli-tary, but more than one ulcer may be present. All segments of the colon have been involved. The cecum, ascending colon, and rectosigmoid area are the most common sites, with the transverse colon the least frequently involved.[30, 32] Most au-thors comment that the ulcer is located on the antimesenteric bowel wall, in contrast

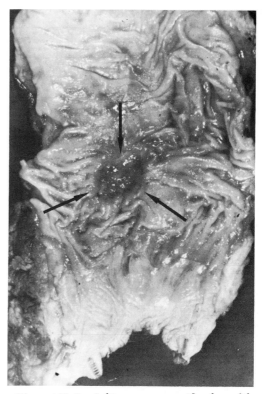

Figure 112–6.   Solitary or nonspecific ulcer of the sigmoid colon. Note sharp demarcation of the mucosal ulceration from the surrounding normal tissue (arrows).

to diverticula which occur along the mesenteric border.

The ulceration may vary in size from 5 mm to 4 or 5 cm. The edges are usually slightly raised and edematous, and the margin is sharply demarcated from the surrounding normal mucosa (Fig. 112–6). If the ulcer is chronic, some increase in connective tissue with fibrotic scarring and contracture may be evident. There may be a considerable inflammatory response with enough cellular reaction to produce a pseudotumor-like lesion.

Microscopically, there is nothing characteristic about the ulcer. The base is covered by a layer of necrotic granulation tissue with lymphocytes, plasma cells, and fibroblasts. Regenerative activity is evident in adjacent mucosa. There may be thickening of the walls of the small blood vessels near the ulcer with occasional thrombosis and recanalization.[36] If the ulcer extends transmurally and bowel has perforated, the expected changes of peritonitis will also be present.

The histological picture in nonspecific ulcer of the rectum varies slightly. The most characteristic feature is obliteration of the lamina propria in the region of the ulcer by fibroblasts and muscular fibers derived from the muscularis mucosae. These stream up between the mucosal crypts and appear to spread them apart. This appearance is not specific, because it is also seen in prolapse of the rectum.[34] In one series 10 per cent of the biopsy specimens contained small areas of ectopic mucosa located in the submucosa at the margin of the ulceration.[34] This constellation of histological findings is characteristic of nonspecific ulcer of the rectum (in the absence of rectal prolapse).

CLINICAL PICTURE

Nonspecific ulcers of the colon can have an extremely varied clinical presentation. They mainly affect persons in the fourth and fifth decades of life, although some patients in their teens have been reported. Incidence in males is higher. In contrast, solitary ulcer of the rectum may be a slightly different disease, because it is found predominantly in a younger age group (20 to 40 years) and without a difference in sex incidence.[34]

CECAL ULCER

Patients with ulceration in the cecum or ascending colon usually present with right lower quadrant abdominal pain and nausea but without vomiting. Fever and leukocytosis may be present. There are no pathognomonic signs to aid in diagnosis of cecal ulcer.[35] The pain is variable and may be acute or chronic. A history of constipation has been noted in many patients, but this is usually not helpful. In contrast to nonspecific ulcer of the left colon, the presence of gross blood in the stool is uncommon in patients with cecal involvement. The usual initial diagnosis is appendicitis, although pelvic inflammatory disease, ovarian disease, regional enteritis, and tuberculous enteritis may be considered. A palpable, tender, right lower quadrant abdominal mass is often present, however, in the latter two conditions. Perforation of the cecum with peritonitis is not uncommon (Fig. 112–7).

Nonspecific ulceration is less common in the colonic flexures, transverse colon, and descending colon. With ulceration in these locations, vague abdominal pain is frequent and perforation with peritonitis is a common complication. Although profuse

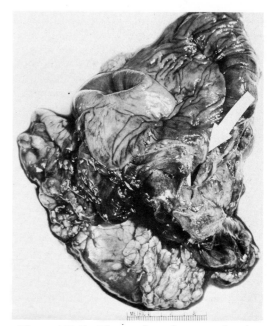

Figure 112–7. This perforated nonspecific ulcer (arrow) of the cecum was found at surgery in a patient suspected to have acute appendicitis. No cause for the ulceration was apparent.

rectal bleeding has been reported with nonspecific ulcers of the transverse colon,[41] this symptom is more common with more distant ulcers.

SIGMOID ULCER

The sigmoid colon is the second most common site of nonspecific ulcer, and diagnosis is seldom made prior to surgery. The most common symptom is constipation.[42] Chronic lower abdominal pain may be present, but it is not common until the bowel has perforated. Recurrent rectal bleeding is frequently encountered; its conjunction with pain usually stimulates clinical evaluation.[42, 43] The ulcer is often beyond the reach of the sigmoidoscope. On sigmoidoscopy, a bloody flux may be seen coming from above a normal rectal mucosa. Lower abdominal pain and, occasionally, fever may prompt a tentative diagnosis of diverticulitis. With sigmoid ulceration there is also a high incidence of perforation, and the diagnosis becomes evident at the time of surgery.[42]

RECTAL ULCER

In contrast to the acute symptoms of nonspecific ulceration in the more proximal bowel, solitary ulcer of the rectum is a chronic condition which can be diagnosed by sigmoidoscopy and biopsy and may require prolonged care. Two current reviews more extensively cover the clinical aspects of the disease than can be included here and should be consulted.[34, 44] Frequently there is dull pain in the rectum or left iliac fossa which is increased during defecation. Passage of blood or bloody mucus with the stool is common, but massive bleeding is unusual. At least half the patients have no history of abnormality of stool frequency or consistency. Although the duration of symptoms before physician evaluation is relatively short for ulceration in other areas of the colon, it averages around five years for rectal ulceration.[34] The diagnosis can be suspected from findings at sigmoidoscopy. A shallow ulcer with flat edges, clearly demarcated from normal mucosa by a thin line of hyperemia, is usually seen 7 to 10 cm from the anal margin and often on a valve of Hous-

ton. The ulcer may have an irregular outline or may be round or even linear. The base can be white, gray, or yellow and is said to look like "wash leather."[34] The surrounding mucosa may be slightly nodular. A preulcer, hyperemic, or "granular" phase can antedate the actual crater. Because of its flat margin, the ulcer is difficult to biopsy. Biopsy of the lesion to help rule out malignancy should be done initially unless barium enema is planned; otherwise it should follow the X-ray examination.

DIAGNOSIS

Unfortunately, with the exception of the rectal lesion, diagnosis is usually made at laparotomy. Physical examination is not too helpful and may be negative until perforation with peritonitis has developed. When the disease involves the rectum, an area of induration may be felt preceding ulceration. When benign ulcers are present, no fixation of the bowel wall to adjacent structures should be present. With the exception of solitary ulcerations in the rectum, sigmoidoscopy and biopsy are not helpful in diagnosis except to help exclude idiopathic inflammatory bowel disease as a cause of the symptoms.

The changes on barium enema examination produced by solitary ulcer of the colon have been described.[45] These consist mainly of a visible ulcer defect with nodular swelling caused by edema around the ulcer; however, the ulcer may not be seen. Colonic motility may be increased adjacent to the ulcer, and localized spasm or actual fibrotic change may produce a strictured appearance. Radiologic signs of bowel perforation may be present. The large inflammatory mass can simulate carcinoma, especially if it is ulcerated. Therefore the barium enema findings are usually nonspecific and stimulate an extensive differential diagnosis. The yield of positive radiological findings, even if an unequivocal ulcer is present, decreases as one goes from the right to the left colon, and X-ray is usually not helpful in diagnosis of rectal ulcer.[34, 32] Diagnosis, however, is facilitated by the use of air contrast studies.

Since cancer is usually a leading differential possibility, surgery is recommended to establish the diagnosis except for ulcer of the lower rectum which is unquestionably benign on biopsy. The more widespread use of fiberoptic colonoscopy may change this diagnostic problem for more proximal locations of the ulceration.

TREATMENT

Except when it is located in the rectum, the appropriate management for patients with nonspecific ulcer of the colon is surgical excision. Laparotomy is required for correct diagnosis or to treat a perforated viscus. Many surgeons will perform a hemicolectomy for an ulcerated mass which grossly resembles carcinoma. Patients, however, may recover uneventfully without surgery.[46, 47] Some instances of right abdominal pain which resolve spontaneously may represent transient ulceration. The use of modern antibiotic agents has apparently lowered the previously high mortality rate from perforation.

Nonspecific ulcers of the rectum are remarkably static for years.[34] This extreme chronicity is matched by an equal resistance to treatment. Many forms of therapy, including local electrocautery, caustic agents, antibiotics, steroid retention enemas, and partial excisional biopsy, have failed to alter the course of the disease. The only certain cure is total excision of the ulceration. However, since perforation is not the rule and symptoms may be mild and only intermittent, treatment with stool softeners, local analgesics, and periodic examinations seem warranted unless excessive bleeding or discomfort forces a more drastic approach. The ulcer may spontaneously heal even after many years.[44]

PNEUMATOSIS CYSTOIDES INTESTINALIS

Pneumatosis cystoides intestinalis is a benign, relatively rare condition affecting both the large and small intestine and characterized pathologically by multiple gas-filled cysts in the subserosal or submucosal tissue. In the majority of instances, it is an unexpected finding on plain abdominal film or during a barium study. However, its appearance is occasionally associated with other diseases, particularly of the gastrointestinal and respiratory tracts.

ETIOLOGY AND PATHOGENESIS

Although people of any age may be affected, pneumatosis cystoides intestinalis is most common in those between the ages of 25 and 50 years, with no difference in sex incidence.[48, 49] The majority of cases are in patients with either pulmonary or pyloroduodenal disease, with almost 60 per cent having some degree of pyloric obstruction resulting from peptic ulcer disease.[50, 51] Patients with scleroderma of the intestine may develop pneumatosis cystoides intestinalis as well, as do a small minority of patients with inflammatory or ischemic bowel disease.[52-54] Other patients appear to have developed gas cysts in the rectum and sigmoid after traumatic sigmoidoscopy or excision of a polyp.[55, 56] Approximately 30 per cent of patients with pneumatosis have no apparent coexisting gastrointestinal pathology, but do have acute or chronic obstructive pulmonary disease.[51, 57] In this latter group, the cysts most frequently involve only the small intestine. Only about 2 per cent of patients with pneumatosis cystoides intestinalis have no other abnormality.

The exact cause of the gas-filled cysts remains unknown. One current theory suggests that air is forced into the tissue spaces around an obstructing pyloric ulcer crater during repeated vomiting.[58] The air or gas then dissects through the bowel wall and finally reaches the subserosal space. The gas-filled intestinal cysts associated with obstructive lung disease are thought to result primarily from rupture of pulmonary blebs and infiltration of air into the subpleural space. Since this space is continuous with the retroperitoneal space, the theory holds that air could dissect infradiaphragmatically along facial planes, proceed out along blood vessels into the mesentery, and thereby gain entrance to the subserosa of the gut.[51, 59, 60] This latter mechanism is supported by animal studies in which air injected into the mediastinum was shown to dissect down along the aorta and eventually out the mesenteric vascular tree to the bowel wall, producing a picture

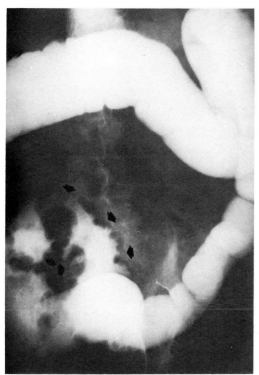

Figure 112–8. The spiculated appearance of the sigmoid colon on this barium enema was produced by multiple air-filled cysts (arrows) in the bowel wall which developed after sigmoidoscopy. They were absent on a similar X-ray a few months earlier.

similar to that of pneumatosis cystoides intestinalis.[51]

Another theory explains the gas cysts by tissue invasion of gas-producing bacteria.[54] In the majority of cases, however, there is no clinical support for this mechanism. Cyst rupture usually does not produce peritonitis, and signs suggesting bacterial invasion of the bowel wall are rare. Nevertheless, there may be a bacterial cause for the pneumatosis which develops in some patients with severe ischemic colitis. In this situation, colonic bacteria may invade the damaged bowel wall and produce gas which becomes entrapped to form cysts. Pneumatosis cystoides intestinalis associated with ischemic colitis is a serious complication, because cyst rupture in this situation is equivalent to perforation of the bowel with its high risk of peritonitis.

It has been suggested also (especially in children) that bacterial enteritis may produce changes in mucosal permeability, permitting entry of intestinal gas into submucosal lymphatics.[61] Obstruction of these lymphatics by inflammation at the base of the mesentery would trap the gas in the bowel wall.

Analysis of the gas in the intestinal cysts neither gives support to any specific theory of cyst formation nor suggests its source. Although there is considerable variation in the exact percentage of the various gases present, in general the composition has been similar to that of atmospheric air: 70 to 90 per cent nitrogen; 3 to 20 per cent oxygen; 0 to 15 per cent carbon dioxide; and traces of methane.[58] The only condition in which submucosal cysts appear to contain luminal gas is when pneumatosis of the rectosigmoid colon develops following sigmoidoscopy (Fig. 112–8).

PATHOLOGY OF GAS CYSTS

Grossly, the gas-filled cysts vary in size from a few millimeters to several centimeters and may give a bubbly appearance to the bowel wall. They may look like multiple lymphangiomas or even multiple sessile polyps (Fig. 112–9). On cross-section the cystic area has a honeycomb appearance. No communication of the cysts with the bowel lumen is apparent.

Microscopically, the cysts occasionally suggest massively dilated lymphatic channels (Fig. 112–10) and are usually lined by a layer of endothelial cells which have eosinophilic cytoplasm. These cells have a tendency to coalesce and form giant cells.[50] It is unknown whether the formation of giant cells in pneumatosis cystoides intestinalis is related to the primary process or is secondary to the presence of the gas itself. A foreign body type of giant cell reaction has been reported after subcutaneous injection of various gases.[62] Instead of endothelial cells, some cysts are lined by simple cuboidal epithelium and giant cells are usually absent. The connective tissue around the cysts often contains evidence of inflammation with eosinophilic leukocytes, plasma cells, lymphocytes, and, occasionally, well developed granulomas.[50] A progressive fibrotic reaction develops and may ultimately obliterate the cysts. This would explain the spontaneous disappearance of the cysts which is occasionally noted.

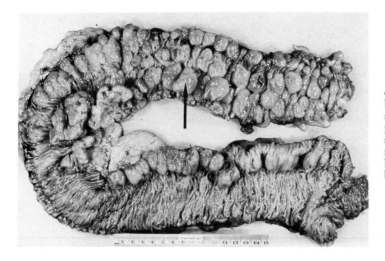

Figure 112–9. Pneumatosis cystoides intestinalis of the small bowel. The gross appearance may suggest lymphangiomas or polyps. Involvement of the rectosigmoid may be diagnosed sigmoidoscopically. The cysts collapse without sequelae if biopsied.

CLINICAL PICTURE

There is no definite clinical syndrome produced by pneumatosis cystoides intestinalis.[48, 56, 63, 64] It is usually discovered during X-ray examination of the abdomen or intestine which is being performed for unrelated symptoms. Patients with pneumatosis cystoides intestinalis may complain of lower abdominal cramping pain. Rectal bleeding, tenesmus, and recurrent diarrhea are also noted in these patients with no other apparent cause. Several patients with pneumatosis have been alleged to have mild steatorrhea; however, since one of these patients also had intestinal scleroderma and the steatorrhea in the others is not well documented, it is unlikely that pneumatosis per se causes malabsorption. Pneumatosis and malabsorption have been reported in association with lymphosarcoma involving the small intestine. It is likely in this instance that the pneumatosis is somehow secondary to the malignancy of the bowel, which, by obstruction of the lymphatics, is also responsible for malabsorption.

Intestinal obstruction may rarely complicate pneumatosis cystoides intestinalis. This is probably due to adhesions between intestinal loops or to volvulus or intussusception. Other mechanisms include direct obstruction of the lumen by the cyst or external luminal compression from cysts in adjacent intestine.[63] Ischemia of the colon may be followed by formation of gas-filled cysts in the bowel wall which can lead to serious complications, as discussed above. If the rectal mucosa tears during sigmoidoscopy or polypectomy, intraluminal gas can dissect into the bowel wall and produce vague abdominal pain and mild ten-

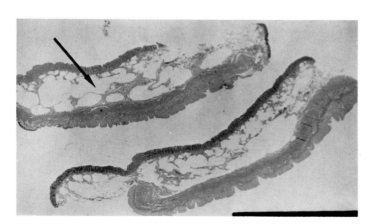

Figure 112–10. A cross-section of colon with pneumatosis cystoides intestinalis shows the honeycomb-like air spaces (arrow) suggestive of dilated lymphatics. Hematoxylin and eosin stain. × 5.

esmus. Pneumatosis cystoides intestinalis, as well as bowel perforation, should be considered in patients who continue to have rectal discomfort after sigmoidoscopy. Finally, pneumatosis cystoides intestinalis must be considered in patients who present with vague abdominal complaints and who are found on X-ray to have free air beneath the diaphragm and no other evidence of a perforated viscus.

DIAGNOSIS AND DIFFERENTIAL DIAGNOSIS

General physical examination yields no specific information suggestive of pneumatosis. Nontender, movable abdominal masses may occasionally be palpated if the cysts are large. Rarely, with left colon involvement a sponge rubber-like resistance can be felt in the left lower quadrant.

When the rectosigmoid is involved, pneumatosis may be diagnosed or its presence confirmed by sigmoidoscopy.[49, 65] The cysts appear as pale or bluish, rounded, soft masses protruding into the lumen and are often mistaken for sessile polyps. Biopsy will help establish the correct diagnosis, because puncture, usually innocuous, will collapse the "polyp."

X-ray findings contribute most to correct diagnosis. Plain films of the abdomen will show localized collections of air in a scattered and often linear fashion or clustered in segments along the wall of the small or large intestine.[66] Pneumoperitoneum may be suggested when a single gas cyst is very large or may, in fact, be produced from cyst rupture. Occasionally gas may be seen between the layers of mesentery. Lateral decubitus films are helpful in demonstrating that the air is not free in the peritoneal cavity.

Barium X-ray examination of the small or large bowel can be striking in appearance and is the most useful aid in establishing the diagnosis.[54, 56] Small radiolucent areas of air density are seen lining the bowel wall and indent the barium column (Fig. 112–11). The base of the filling defect caused by the cyst is wide in contrast to that produced by polyps, and the margin is smooth, unlike that of carcinoma. The extreme lucency of the air cysts also helps to differentiate them from more dense masses produced by soft tissue other than

fat. In addition, the configuration of the filling defects caused by air cysts may be altered by abdominal compression.

Radiological differential diagnosis should not be difficult. Pneumatosis cystoides intestinalis should be considered in any patient who has free air under the diaphragm but no clinical peritonitis. Enterogenous cysts are usually single, whereas bowel involvement with pneumatosis is more extensive. Infection of the gut wall by gas-forming organisms such as clostridia is a rather rare condition complicating ischemic necrosis, and signs of sepsis are usually present. Ulcerative, granulomatous, and ischemic bowel disease may produce polypoid mucosal irregularities on barium enema, but they do not have the marked lucency of air cysts as outlined by adjacent bowel.

TREATMENT

No treatment except that for the underlying or primary disease is necessary in the majority of patients with small intestinal pneumatosis. Few bowel complications result when the pneumatosis accompanies chronic pulmonary disease. Surgery directed toward small bowel cysts is contraindicated even when pneumoperitoneum develops, because its course is benign.[51] The value of a correct diagnosis is mainly in preventing unnecessary surgery and in directing therapy toward underlying conditions.

When pneumatosis involves mainly the left colon, therapy must be individualized, depending upon the severity of symptoms and the underlying cause of the disease. Although pneumatosis is usually asymptomatic and frequently resolves spontaneously, perforation, severe tenesmus, bleeding, pain, and even partial obstruction may necessitate surgery.[50, 56] Unfortunately, surgery is not always successful, because the pneumatosis occasionally becomes more extensive after resection.[67]

If surgery is required and the rectum is involved, it should be spared, because regression of the process in the rectum usually occurs following resection of involved proximal segments.[65] In general, bowel resection for pneumatosis should be reserved for those patients in whom the aforementioned symptoms or complica-

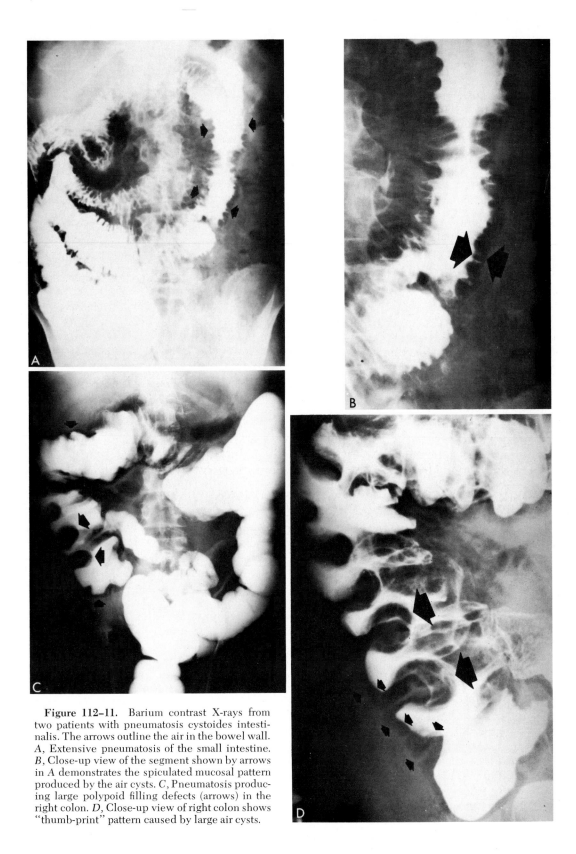

Figure 112–11. Barium contrast X-rays from two patients with pneumatosis cystoides intestinalis. The arrows outline the air in the bowel wall. *A*, Extensive pneumatosis of the small intestine. *B*, Close-up view of the segment shown by arrows in *A* demonstrates the spiculated mucosal pattern produced by the air cysts. *C*, Pneumatosis producing large polypoid filling defects (arrows) in the right colon. *D*, Close-up view of right colon shows "thumb-print" pattern caused by large air cysts.

tions can be attributed to no other cause. Although the etiology and natural course of the disease are poorly understood, the prognosis for the cystic process is usually favorable, with less than 5 per cent of patients developing complications necessitating resection.[48]

ENDOMETRIOSIS

Endometriosis is a fascinating disease of importance to the gastroenterologist as well as the gynecologist. It affects many women during their middle and later reproductive years and may produce a wide spectrum of symptoms. In simplest terms, endometriosis refers to heterotopic endometrium. When the abnormally located endometrium is restricted to invasion of the uterine myometrium, the process is referred to as adenomyosis. The term endometriosis therefore is reserved for extrauterine endometrial tissue and the clinical sequelae produced by its normal function in an abnormal site.

Tissues in proximity to the uterus such as the ovaries, uterine ligaments, rectovaginal septum, and pelvic peritoneum are most commonly involved. However, the frequent involvement of the colon and even the small intestine in endometriosis makes its consideration pertinent for the gastroenterologist, especially when bowel symptoms are related temporally to the menstrual cycle.

PATHOGENESIS

Various theories have been advanced to explain how isolated segments of endometrial tissue become implanted outside the uterus. Although not the first to describe the condition, Sampson in 1921 established endometriosis as a distinct clinical entity and postulated that extrauterine endometrial implants were the result of reflux of endometrial tissue through the fallopian tubes during menstruation.[68] In addition, endometrium present in menses has been demonstrated to be capable of implantation and growth on peritoneum.[69, 70] Other theories include origin from celomic epithelium and both lymphatic and hematologic dissemination of endometrial

cells capable of heterotopic growth and survival.[71, 72] The latter explanation seems almost necessary to explain the rare cases of endometriosis involving the lungs, pleura, arms, and legs.

PATHOLOGY

Intestinal involvement with endometriosis is usually greatest in those parts of the bowel that are pelvic. The rectosigmoid colon has been reported to be involved in 16 to 25 per cent of cases.[73, 74] Less frequently, endometrial implants are found in the appendix, cecum, ileum, and even jejunum.[75, 76]

Initially, the heterotopic endometrium invades the subserosa of the bowel. Under hormonal influence, there are maturation and finally slough of the surface epithelium, with bleeding as in the uterine cavity. If this takes place in an enclosed cystic area, expansion from the blood may cause necrosis of adjacent tissue. Cyclic repetition results in dissection of the process through the subserosa and the muscularis to the submucosa (Fig. 112–12). The advancing endometriosis almost never "invades" the mucosa, a fact which helps in clinical differential diagnosis of endometriosis and malignancy, and explains why cyclical intestinal bleeding is a rare part of the clinical picture.

Progressive involvement of the small intestine, usually the ileum, may cause obstruction. Such obstruction, however, usually results from dense adhesive bands which have developed after repeated shedding of endometrium and blood into the peritoneal cavity.

In the colon, particularly the sigmoid area, dissection of small endometrial nodules along the bowel wall may progress to almost encircle the colon and cause obstruction. The rectum may be densely adherent to the posterior wall of the uterus owing to endometriosis of the rectovaginal septum; however, because of the large diameter of the rectum, obstructive symptoms are often minimal.

Some difference of opinion exists regarding the pathological sequelae of endometriosis in the colonic wall. The frequently described bulky lesions have been attributed mainly to fibrosis, but also to smooth muscle hyperplasia.[77-79] Usually both processes coexist, making up the largest part of the mass, with actual endometrial tissue being less prominent.

In patients with advanced pelvic endometriosis, fibrotic adhesions may be quite extensive, matting together the uterus, bladder, rectosigmoid colon, and loops of small bowel which lie on these pelvic organs.

CLINICAL PICTURE

Endometriosis is usually a disease of the reproductive period, with peak incidence between the ages of 30 and 40 years. It is uncommon in the 20's and, although rare, has been reported to produce symptoms as long as 14 years after menopause.[73, 80] It has the greatest incidence in white females seen in private clinics. This has been explained both by later onset of the first pregnancy and by less total parity of this group.[81]

The severity of symptoms may not correlate with the extent of involvement. Although some clinical and nonoperative studies suggest that as many as 27 per cent of women with symptomatic endometriosis have rectosigmoid involvement, it is often difficult in many cases to attribute symptoms primarily to intestinal endometrial implants.[74, 77] Also, small endometriomas may frequently be present on the intestinal wall with no symptoms.

The symptoms of endometriosis are well known, and include mainly dysmenorrhea, menometrorrhagia, intermenstrual pelvic pain, sterility, dyspareunia, and low backache. When significant rectosigmoid involvement is present, cramping pain in the rectum and occasionally mild tenesmus may be present in addition to the aforementioned complaints. When the lesion progresses to an obstructing state, the patient experiences progressive constipation with lower abdominal and rectal discomfort during defecation. Stool caliber may be diminished owing to narrowing of the rectosigmoid lumen. Less frequently, diarrhea or rectal bleeding may be present. However, subsequent surgery usually reveals intact mucosa over the endometrial implant, and the exact source of bleeding remains undetermined (Fig. 112–13). Intraluminal hemorrhage caused by an endometrioma is exceedingly rare, because implants seldom if ever invade the mucosa. Rectal bleeding should therefore alert the clinician to the possibility of another disease.[71, 74] The cyclical nature of these symptoms, preceding and during menstruation, in the absence of weight loss or cachexia should suggest symptomatic rectosigmoid endometriosis.

The more proximal colon may be involved, but it usually is asymptomatic unless obstruction develops. Endometriosis of the appendix occurs rather commonly, but symptoms are rare and usually inconsequential. Nevertheless, some patients have typical symptoms and signs of acute appendicitis owing to endometriosis

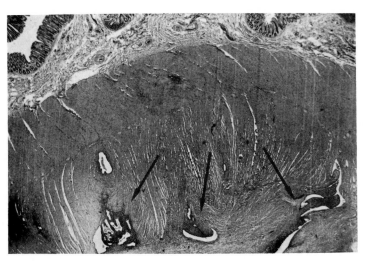

Figure 112–12. Both glandular and stromal endometrial tissue (arrows) are present, "dissecting" between the hypertrophied muscle of the intestinal wall. Hematoxylin and eosin stain. × 40.

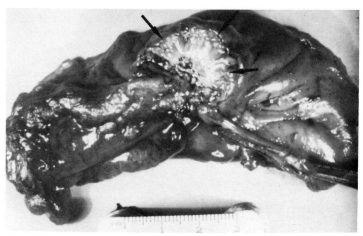

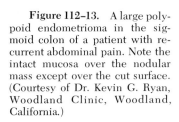

Figure 112–13. A large polypoid endometrioma in the sigmoid colon of a patient with recurrent abdominal pain. Note the intact mucosa over the nodular mass except over the cut surface. (Courtesy of Dr. Kevin G. Ryan, Woodland Clinic, Woodland, California.)

of the appendix.[82] Regardless of known coexisting endometriosis, the clinical picture compatible with acute appendicitis requires laparotomy.

Endometrial implants on the small intestine are usually an incidental finding during abdominal surgery. The lesions are most often limited to the serosa and, unless adhesions develop or deeper layers of the bowel are penetrated, remain asymptomatic. Cramping abdominal pain with nausea, especially postprandial, may be prominent symptoms when the small bowel is extensively diseased. These symptoms also tend to be more severe just before and during menstruation. With endometriosis, obstruction of the small intestine may result from (1) kinking of the small bowel caused by fibrous adhesions, (2) stenosis resulting from fibrosis, (3) volvulus, and intussusception.[76, 83] With any of these initiating mechanisms, the usual symptoms and signs of small bowel obstruction will follow.

DIAGNOSIS

Clinical diagnosis of endometriosis involving the bowel requires a high index of suspicion. The diagnostic approach should begin with a thorough pelvic examination which includes combined rectovaginal palpation. The finding of tender nodules and an irregular induration in the cul-de-sac, especially when palpating anteriorly in the rectum, is strong evidence for endometriosis involving the rectosigmoid area. Since the character of these lesions often changes during the menstrual cycle, pelvic examination should be done before and after menstruation. When a lesion is palpable in a free portion of the sigmoid and none in the cul-de-sac, the diagnosis of endometriosis is much less certain.

Unfortunately, sigmoidoscopy may not contribute to the diagnosis. The rectal lumen may be markedly narrowed. The mucosa is usually intact, but may be puckered over a firm, indurated, tender, and occasionally bluish submucosal mass. The indurated area may be quite tender, in contrast to carcinomatous stricture which characteristically is painless. If stricture caused by endometriosis is suspected, a repeat sigmoidoscopy ten to 14 days later should be performed, looking for a noticeable increase in luminal size accompanying cyclical change in the endometrial tissue. Mucosal biopsy is frequently unhelpful.

Radiological examination of the colon or small intestine is also usually not diagnostic of endometriosis. The important diseases of the colon to be considered in differential diagnosis include carcinoma, diverticulitis, ameboma, chronic inflammatory diseases with stricture such as ulcerative colitis and granulomatous colitis, benign tumors, and polyps, as well as pelvic and mesenteric tumors and cysts.[75]

Radiological findings that favor endometriosis are (1) an intact mucosa, (2) a long lesion or area of constriction, (3) tapered margins suggestive of an intramural lesion rather than acutely angulated overhanging margins of a mucosal lesion, and (4) the absence of ulceration in the mass.[77, 84, 85]

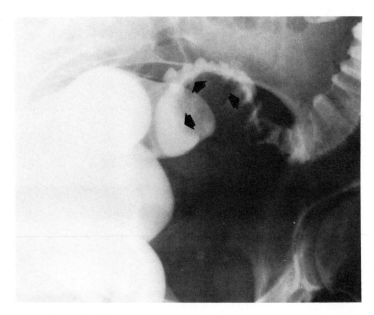

Figure 112–14. Spot film of a filling defect produced by the large polypoid endometrioma shown in Figure 112–13 demonstrates an intact mucosa (arrows). Note the angle between the "tumor" and the bowel wall, suggestive of an intramural lesion. (Courtesy of Dr. Kevin G. Ryan, Woodland Clinic, Woodland, California.)

Polypoid "intramural" lesions are occasionally seen, especially in the sigmoid colon (Fig. 112–14). Tenderness of the involved area of palpation at the time of fluoroscopy is also suggestive of endometriosis. If the lesion is more proximal than midsigmoid, roentgenographic diagnosis of a constricting endometrioma is hazardous, because endometrial implants on portions of bowel which are freely suspended on a mesentery are less likely to produce obstruction than when they involve a segment of bowel which is partially extraperitoneal and more firmly fixed, such as the rectosigmoid.

After complete diagnostic evaluation, uncertainty frequently exists about the nature of a constricting rectosigmoid lesion, especially in older women. If the lesion is low, persistently enlarges, and involves the cul-de-sac area, even though the diagnosis of endometriosis seems certain, a direct needle biopsy should be attempted, because primary adenocarcinoma of the rectovaginal septum arising from endometrial tissue has been reported.[86, 87]

A small bowel series should be performed when periumbilical or right lower quadrant cramping abdominal pain is present, especially if pelvic examination reveals endometriosis involving the ovary and cul-de-sac. A positive radiological examination may be facilitated by arranging the study to be done just before or during the menstrual period. With fixation of the cecum and terminal ileum by adhesions, the X-ray picture may be compatible with partial small bowel obstruction. A pattern suggesting disordered motility with segmentation of the barium in the distal small bowel may be all that is seen in some cases without obvious evidence of ileal obstruction.[75] A general haziness of the abdomen may suggest the presence of ascites, a rare finding in endometriosis.[75, 88]

TREATMENT

The therapy of symptomatic endometriosis is difficult. Choices lie between watchful waiting, hormone therapy, surgical excision, and castration. Gynecological texts or reviews should be consulted for management of symptomatic endometriosis without significant bowel involvement. For these patients initial treatment usually includes only analgesics, antispasmodics, and sedatives. Further therapy is best undertaken with gynecological consultation.

Although approximately 25 per cent of women with endometriosis will have rectosigmoid involvement, less than half of them will have severe bowel symptoms.[77] Symptoms from appendiceal, cecal, or small bowel endometriosis are even less frequent. More than routine therapy is usually necessitated by symptoms of intestinal obstruction. Treatment may be approached by three methods.[74, 75]

In the first method of treatment, the localized lesion or a segment of bowel may be excised with concomitant lysis of adhesions. If intestinal endometriosis is localized or is only an incidental finding at laparotomy, the surgeon can dissect implants from the bowel wall without entering the lumen. If a large constricting adenofibromuscular lesion is present, especially in the rectosigmoid area, simple removal of the lesion is usually impossible and the involved segment of bowel must be excised with an end-to-end anastomosis. A proximal colostomy may be necessary for a short period postoperatively. Because carcinoma is the most serious disease in the differential diagnosis of an obstructing lesion, pathological interpretation of frozen sections should be obtained before abdominal closure. This procedure may prevent an extensive abdominal perineal resection for endometriosis mistaken for carcinoma. It may also, of course, reveal carcinoma admixed with endometrial tissue.

In addition to the intestinal surgery, a hysterectomy, excision of other peritoneal implants, or even oophorectomy may be done. Castration has been reported to result in regression of colonic endometriosis.[89] Such treatment may be too extreme, especially for young women. Furthermore, if the lesion is annular or large enough to produce obstruction, castration will usually not be effective, and the treatment of choice remains primary excision.[90] As mentioned, exploratory surgery is occasionally necessary for right lower quadrant abdominal pain simulating acute appendicitis. Also, about 4 per cent of women with endometriosis who undergo emergency surgery will present with an acute abdomen and hemoperitoneum.[91] This complication is most commonly suffered during the premenstrual, menstrual, or decidual phase of the menstrual cycle when softening and engorgement of the endometrial implant occur. For the same reasons the incidence of hemoperitoneum is increased in women receiving progesterone as treatment for their endometriosis.

A second form of treatment for endometriosis is hormonal therapy, which may produce dramatic and long-lasting improvement. Androgens have been reported to relieve painful symptoms of endometriosis and to produce regression of partially obstructing rectosigmoid lesions.[92] However, their effect is unpredictable, and the resulting masculinizing side effects are undesirable. More recently, progestin agents have been shown to be an effective form of therapy.[93, 94] Their beneficial effects on endometriosis are thought to be secondary to anovulation, amenorrhea, and a persisting decidual reaction in the areas of endometriosis which eventually undergo necrobiosis and subsequent absorption.[94] Also, progestin therapy may occasionally be associated with regression and even disappearance of symptomatic colonic endometriosis. Since this result is inconstant, and in view of the possible increased danger of hemoperitoneum from progestin therapy, a conservative primary resection is still recommended.[93, 94] It would seem prudent, however, to try progestin therapy if the bowel is only minimally involved. Unless symptoms are promptly alleviated, obstructing lesions should be excised.

Finally, castration by surgical excision or radiation will lead to regression of endometriosis. This radical therapy should be reserved for the older woman in whom a total abdominal hysterectomy is also performed, or for the younger woman who is incapacitated by disease and in whom conservative medical or previous surgical therapy has not been successful.

Treatment of endometriosis must therefore be individualized and be flexible during the course of the disease. Patience will be needed to forestall early radical therapy for recurrent monthly symptoms. The many beneficial extragenital effects of estrogens make gonadal preservation an aim of successful therapy. Coordination of the efforts of the gastroenterologist and gynecologist will usually yield a satisfactory result.

MALAKOPLAKIA

Malakoplakia is a rare granulomatous disease of unknown cause which until recently was reported only in the urinary tract.[95, 96] The term malakoplakia is derived from the Greek, meaning soft plaque, and was introduced to describe the gross appearance of the lesion in the urinary bladder.[97] In the last two decades, the condition has been described in the kidneys and ureter,[96, 98] the testicle,[99] and the prostate gland;[100] it also affects the colon.[101, 102] It now appears that lesions previously considered to be nonspecific granulomatous inflammatory reactions may actually be malakoplakia.[100-107]

ETIOLOGY

Theories regarding the cause of malakoplakia relate to coexistent disease such as neoplasia, tuberculosis, sarcoidosis, and fungal and viral infections.[100, 102, 104] Uri-

nary tract disease was initially thought to be a necessary antecedent of the bowel lesion, but more recent studies as well as the reported cases involving the gastrointestinal tract do not support this concept.[99] The frequent occurrence of *Escherichia coli* and other coliform organisms in the urologic form of the disease has led to their incrimination as the etiologic agent. However, the frequency of *E. coli* urinary tract infections and the rarity of malakoplakia make a direct causal relationship unlikely.[104]

The most typical and diagnostic finding in malakoplakia is the presence of peculiar intracytoplasmic, round, dark, laminated inclusion bodies in histiocytes. These are called Michaelis-Gutmann bodies, after the authors who originally described the disease. Characteristically, these bodies

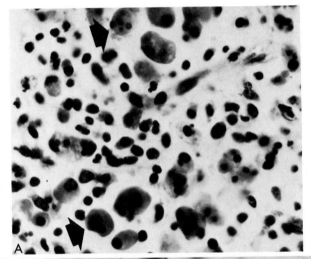

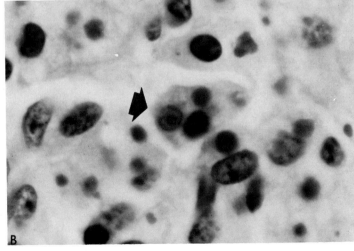

Figure 112–15. *A,* Sheets of large pale histiocytes containing Michaelis-Gutmann bodies (arrows) characterize the histological change in malakoplakia. *B,* High power view of one of these histiocytes (arrow) containing the dark, concentrically laminated Michaelis-Gutmann bodies. Hematoxylin and eosin stain. × 2000. (Courtesy of Dr. R. L. Goldman, Mount Zion Hospital, San Francisco.)

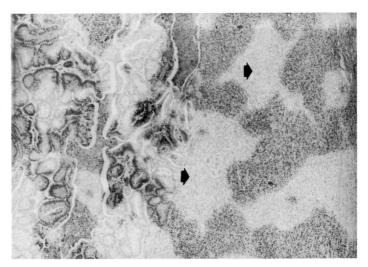

Figure 112-16. Invasion of the submucosa by adenocarcinoma of the colon with coexistent malakoplakia. The dense collections of the pale histiocytes (arrows) are characteristic of malakoplakia. Hematoxylin and eosin stain. × 40.

are PAS positive and stain for both calcium and iron (Fig. 112–15). The Michaelis-Gutmann bodies are composed of a glycolipid matrix probably from a specific microorganism and coated by a layer of calcium and iron.[102]

Electron microscopic studies of malakoplakia from the intestine have demonstrated ultrastructural details similar to those found in studies of urinary tract malakoplakia.[106] Both histochemical and electron microscopic findings are compatible with malakoplakia being a cellular reaction to breakdown products of bacteria. A particular physico-chemical environment may be necessary for the development of the lesion. The exact cause of the process and the origin of the Michaelis-Gutmann inclusion bodies, however, remain unknown.

CLINICAL PICTURE

Too few cases of malakoplakia of the gastrointestinal tract have been reported to allow formulation of a specific clinical syndrome. With the exception of one case in a five-year-old male,[100] all patients with gastrointestinal malakoplakia have been over 50 years of age. Intestinal malakoplakia has most often been an incidental finding in elderly, debilitated patients associated symptomatically and histologically with adenocarcinoma of the rectosigmoid colon (Fig. 112–16). However, in a few instances, symptoms and even death were directly attributed to the malakoplakia.

With colonic malakoplakia, the clinical presentations have included the following: (1) Fever and hematochezia with isolated sessile polypoid masses in the rectosigmoid colon on digital examination and sigmoidoscopy. The mucosa overlying the polypoid masses may appear normal or ulcerated. Involvement of the mesenteric lymph nodes may produce narrowing of the bowel lumen suggestive of malignant stricture. (2) Diffuse involvement of the entire colon, with the gross appearance varying from soft, grayish-tan confluent lesions with serpiginous borders to confluent superficial ulcerations. (3) A mass-like lesion with abdominal pain, local tenderness, and fever. The process may also extend to the retroperitoneum with abscess formation. In association with colonic involvement, gastric malakoplakia may occur with tannish-yellow, irregular, partially ulcerated mucosal plaques.[104]

DIAGNOSIS

Radiological examination has not been helpful in diagnosis. Barium enema has only documented changes consistent with carcinoma in those patients in whom malakoplakia was a secondary diagnosis to the tumor. In one case of isolated colonic malakoplakia, polypoid rectosigmoid lesions were seen on barium enema but without any differentiating feature.[100] Involvement of mesenteric lymph nodes may externally compress the bowel lumen, creating a strictured appearance. A single large mass lesion radiologically suggesting carcinoma may also result from the extensive granulomatous reaction. Fixation of the bowel to adjacent tissue may produce the radiological picture of local extension of a malignant process.

Correct diagnosis is possible from histological examination of biopsy specimens, although unfamiliarity with the process has led to misdiagnosis of polyp of the colon.[100] Grossly, the lesions are usually soft and tan-gray and have irregular margins. The mucosa may be intact over the lesion. If the mucosa is absent, the specimen may then have a red-tan granular appearance and be covered with necrotic material. The cut surface is usually dull gray and flecked with yellow areas.[102] Microscopically, a clue to the correct diagnosis comes from the sheets of large, pale monocytic cells or histiocytes with eosinophilic cytoplasm, many of which contain the dark, concentrically laminated Michaelis-Gutmann bodies. Stains for calcium and iron should be done to confirm that these spherules are not just artifacts of hematoxylin and eosin preparation. Unless the typical inclusion bodies are noted, the appearance of the histiocytes may initially suggest reticulum cell sarcoma.[107] Also, the inclusion-filled histiocytes might be confused with Whipple's disease, fungal disease, or ceroid-like colonic histiocytes.[104] Appropriate stains will exclude these differential possibilities.[104, 108]

TREATMENT

The small number and dissimilarity of reported cases of malakoplakia involving the gastrointestinal tract give no specific direction for planning treatment. In addition, its association with malignancy and extensive multiorgan disease has resulted in few attempts at specific therapy. The overall rarity of the lesion regardless of location has prevented real evaluation of any form of treatment. Although malakoplakia of the urinary bladder has been successfully treated by streptomycin, paraaminosalicylic acid, and isoniazid therapy,

this therapy was not successful in a patient with polypoid malakoplakia of the colon.[100, 109] Many patients with malakoplakia, including those reported in the urological literature, have had some other systemic disease with debilitation. Therefore any patient with biopsy-proved malakoplakia should have full general medical evaluation. If no specific abnormality is found, localized intestinal malakoplakia can be treated by excisional biopsy or fulguration. For more diffuse gastrointestinal involvement, a trial of antituberculous therapy or antibiotics may be considered with limited expectation of favorable results. More general awareness of this apparently rare colonic lesion should result in better definition of its clinical presentation, course, and management.

MELANOSIS COLI, CATHARTIC COLON, AND SOAP COLITIS

"Irritant" purgatives have been incriminated as the causative factor in at least three colonic abnormalities: melanosis coli, cathartic colon, and soap colitis. Of the three, only melanosis coli has received extensive clinical and pathological study. In the past few years, the availability of newer bulk-forming laxative preparations has seemed to correspond to an apparent decrease in the number of cases of melanosis coli encountered in a large medical center. Although only sporadic reports of cathartic colon and soap colitis have appeared, the entities may produce problems in both diagnosis and management which should be appreciated by physicians. Each of these conditions will be discussed separately because of variability in the clinical pictures.

MELANOSIS COLI

The appearance of an abnormal brown or black pigment in the colonic mucosa has captured the attention of investigators for years. It was first described over 140 years ago by Cruveilhier, who referred to a person with chronic diarrhea in whom "the inner surface of the large intestine was as black as Chinese ink."[110] Rudolf Virchow later microscopically demonstrated the black pigment in the colon of an autopsy case and termed the condition melanosis coli.[111] Since that time, melanosis coli has remained something of a medical curiosity. In the past 40 years, several excellent papers have appeared which document the historical evolution of concepts regarding the etiology of the condition and also report clinical observations in large numbers of patients with melanosis coli.[112-116] These and many other smaller studies have contributed to the current concept that melanosis coli is a benign condition found in some persons who use cathartics of the anthracene type, including cascara sagrada, senna, aloe, rhubarb, and frangula. In almost all cases it is completely reversible. The age distribution of reported patients varies, but in general the condition occurs in adults or older persons, with a tendency for higher frequency among females.[113, 114] This may represent patient selection bias, because the sex incidence determined by analysis of autopsy material shows either no difference or a slight predominance of males.[112, 116]

The cause of the condition appears to be use of anthracene carthartics in the presence of fecal stasis. This seems adequately documented by clinical and experimental evidence.[113, 114] The shortest time observed for the appearance of melanosis coli in patients taking a cascara preparation is four months and the longest was 13 months (mean, nine months). After stopping the cascara, the melanosis disappeared in five to 11 months (mean, nine months).[114]

In addition to laxative abuse, melanosis coli has been reported in about half of two series of patients with carcinoma of the colon.[112] It is uncertain how many of these persons really took laxatives. However, the incidence of bowel carcinoma in patients with known melanosis coli is low, and most authors deny a direct relationship.

The incidence of macroscopic melanosis coli varies tremendously. Incidence data obtained from autopsy studies range from 0.04 to 11.2 per cent, whereas those obtained from sigmoidoscopic evaluation of patients with symptomatic colon stasis are approximately 5 per cent.[113]

The pigment may be distributed over the entire colon, but it is found mainly in the cecum and rectum.[112, 113] When melanosis occurs in association with a partially obstructing colonic carcinoma, the pigmentation is usually more intense proximal to the tumor. Melanosis specifically related to laxative abuse is most intense just inside the anal sphincter and less dark higher in the sigmoid.

Although the melanosis pigment was classically described in the colon, it has also been found in the appendix, in mesenteric lymph nodes, and in the terminal ileum.[116, 117] A similar dark pigment has also been reported in the esophagus in association with esophagitis but may be only lipofuscin.[118]

Various picturesque descriptions have been applied to the gross appearance of melanosis coli pigment. It has been compared with the appearance of tiger or crocodile skin, a toad's back, and a cross-section of nutmeg.[113] The color varies from a light brown or buff to very dark brown or black. Excessive mucus over the mucosa may cause it to appear blue-black. The darker areas are divided into a polyhedral design by fine striae of lighter color. These unpigmented reticular areas are not due to the presence of mucosal blood vessels, but to variation in degree of pigment deposition. Submucosal lymphoid follicles are not pigmented and therefore appear as light dots on the dark surface.[116] Mucosal polyps in areas of melanosis do not grossly contain the pigment and may present a striking pink appearance against the dark background.[112, 116]

Routine microscopy demonstrates that the epithelial cells of the mucosa are normal. The submucosa, however, may have a thickened and edematous appearance with increased numbers of plasma cells. The most striking finding is the presence of large mononuclear cells or macrophages in the lamina propria of the mucosa which contain a brownish-black pigment (Fig. 112–17). Four histological grades have been defined. These vary from Grade 1 with few cells in the lamina propria containing pigment granules to Grade 4 in which the pigmented cells are extensive and found below the muscularis mucosae, in lymph vessels, and in regional lymph nodes.[115] No significance for this classification seems to exist except for descriptive purposes. It should be recognized that the pigment-laden cells may be present micro-

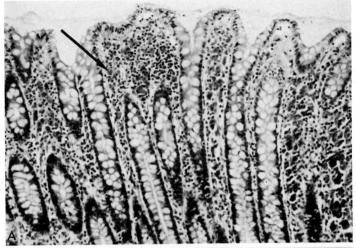

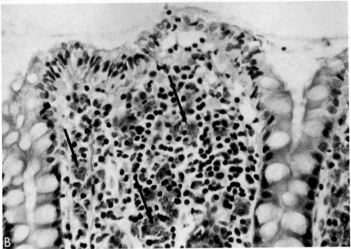

Figure 112–17. *A,* Rectal biopsy from a patient with melanosis coli. The dark mucosal coloration is due to pigment granules in large submucosal macrophages (arrow). Hematoxylin and eosin stain. × 250. *B,* A higher magnification of the area shown by the arrow in *A.* × 500.

scopically in the absence of gross melanosis.

In recent years, investigators have attempted to better characterize the pigment in order to define more precisely its origin. Histochemical studies have contributed little more than confirmation that the pigment gives many of the reactions for both melanin and lipofuscin.[117, 119-121] Electron microscopic findings, however, have permitted some speculation on the origin of the pigment granules; they may originate in degenerating mitochondria, endoplasmic reticulum, and glycogen.[120, 121]

The discovery of melanosis coli in a patient should prompt questioning about laxative use and symptoms of fecal stasis. In the absence of a history of anthracene laxative abuse, melanosis coli warrants radiological evaluation for an occult colonic

malignancy. Per se it has no known long-term prognostic meaning, but only continues to perplex those who ponder the origin of the pigment.

CATHARTIC COLON

In 1943, attention was first drawn to the fact that chronic laxative abuse could produce severe radiological abnormalities of the colon.[122, 123] The subsequent three decades have witnessed validation of this fact but with almost no contribution to our understanding of the genesis of the pathology involved.[124-126] The exact functional significance of cathartic colon is unknown, and the entity remains for the most part a radiological diagnosis.

Almost all reported cases have occurred

in women who have taken "irritant" laxatives over a period of at least 15 years.[123] The medications incriminated contained varying amounts of the following laxative groups: emodin (cascara segrada, senna, rhubarb, aloe), resinous (jalap, elaterin, podophyllin), irritant oil (castor oil, croton oil), and miscellaneous (phenolphthalein, calomel). The clinical histories contain nonspecific abdominal complaints led by chronic constipation. Vague bloating discomfort and ill-defined lower abdominal pain are often present. Of utmost importance is the absence of fever, recurrent diarrhea, or the passage of mucus or blood in the stool. If a history of the latter is obtained, either the diagnosis of cathartic colon should not be made or the presence of coexistent disease must be assumed.

DIAGNOSIS

No abnormality in the general physical examination has been correlated with cathartic colon. Sigmoidoscopy is usually normal, although the mucosa has been described as edematous but never friable. If the laxative preparation contained cascara, melanosis coli may be present.

The diagnosis therefore is radiological. The earliest or mildest changes are limited to the cecum and ileocecal valve. On barium enema, the cecum appears shortened and may become conical. When the changes become more extensive, the colon distal to the cecum often becomes tubular, with diminished or completely absent haustrations. The ascending colon appears shortened, and the hepatic flexure may not be definable as the colon sweeps toward the left upper quadrant of the abdomen. The mucosal pattern is linear or smooth, especially in the constricted segments, and ulcerations are not seen. In most cases, these colonic changes extend no farther than the mid-transverse colon, although the abnormality may reach the lower descending colon.[123] Distensibility remains, and although certain segments of the colon appear tonic, no rigidity is demonstrated. Inconstant areas of constriction with long, tapering margins may be seen (Fig. 112–18). At fluoroscopy, colonic distensibility is evident as well as the long, bizarre, and inconstant areas of contraction. These narrowed segments might pos-

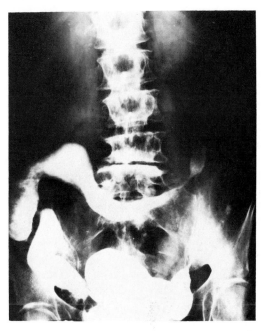

Figure 112–18. Barium enema examination of a patient with severe cathartic colon. The bowel appears shortened with long, tapered areas of narrowing. Haustrations and normal mucosal pattern are absent. The terminal ileum is also dilated. At fluoroscopy the colon distended normally. The barium enema findings may be strikingly similar to advanced ulcerative colitis if only part of the roentgenograms are reviewed.

sibly be interpreted as strictures if they are not repeatedly observed throughout the period of fluoroscopy. Evacuation of the barium is often incomplete.

It is also important to note that even in mild cases there is abnormality of the ileocecal valve, which becomes flattened and gaping. A similar abnormality has recently been emphasized as being present in ulcerative colitis.[127] Radiographic changes similar to those in the right colon are also frequently present in the terminal ileum. The ileum may be tubular, slightly narrowed, and without a normal mucosal pattern. The extent of terminal ileal and colonic abnormality tends to correlate. In severely ill patients a plain film of the abdomen may show a tubular outline of these gas-filled intestinal segments.

The differential diagnosis of the radiological abnormality includes chronic ulcerative colitis, granulomatous colitis, and amebic colitis.[123, 125, 126] An adequate medical history will usually solve the problem. Unlike ulcerative colitis, the process is more marked in the right colon, and significant shortening of the bowel is lacking. Luminal narrowing is inconstant, thickness and stiffness of the bowel wall are absent, and ulceration is not seen. Ileal changes are unlike those of granulomatous bowel disease, fistula formation is never present, and there are no longitudinal ulcerations or transverse fissures of the colonic mucosa. The stool should be examined for amebae. However, distensibility of a conical cecum at fluoroscopy and the described ileal changes should not strongly suggest amebiasis.

POSSIBLE EXPLANATIONS

Very little is known about the abnormal pathophysiology resulting from chronic laxative abuse which may produce cathartic colon. The few reported descriptions of involved bowel at laparotomy vary from thickening of the terminal ileum and cecum to no gross pathology.[122, 123] Reports of histopathological examination of resected or postmortem tissue specimens are rare. In the one extensively studied case, the mucosa was described grossly as dark brown, suggesting melanosis coli, the submucosa was infiltrated by excessive fat, and the muscular layers were atrophic. Silver impregnation stain of the myenteric plexus revealed abnormalities similar to those produced in experimental animals given senna.[128] Recent evidence suggests that activated senna produces colonic contraction by contact stimulation of the submucosal or Meissner's plexus, which in turn stimulates the deeper intermuscular myenteric plexus.[129, 130] Therefore it is possible that prolonged cathartic use may produce abnormality in the neural pathways regulating colonic motor activity and lead to the observed pathological and functional changes.

The exact pathological significance and sequelae of cathartic colon remain unknown. In some patients the radiological abnormality has shown improvement as early as one month after discontinuing the irritant laxative and, in rare instances, has returned to normal after approximately a year.[122-124] The main problem is usually management of the constipation which prompted the drug use initially. Bulk and emollient laxatives have not been reported

to cause similar roentgenologic changes even after prolonged use, and may offer an alternative if laxative therapy remains necessary (see pp. 409 to 410).

SOAP COLITIS

In contrast to melanosis coli and cathartic colon, which are associated with chronic oral laxative abuse and which may have no immediate significance to the patient, soap colitis is an acute inflammatory reaction of the colon with significant morbidity. It usually follows within hours the administration of a "cleansing" soapsuds enema and encompasses a spectrum of responses, varying from slight discomfort to severe prostration. Although severe reactions to soapsuds enemas are rare, mild sequelae are more common in these patients than is generally appreciated. One combined hospital study in a large city revealed that 10 to 30 per cent of hospitalized patients were given soapsuds enemas.[131] Another study employing questionnaires found that 30 per cent of patients receiving such enemas experienced irritative effects, producing abnormal bowel function for up to three months.[132]

Colonic reaction to the soapsuds enema probably results from a direct irritant effect of the soap on the mucosa, and its severity is related to the concentration of the soap solution. The mucosal reaction may vary from mild irritation to frank necrosis. Sigmoidoscopy performed shortly after a soapsuds enema will usually demonstrate hyperemic and often mildly edematous rectal mucosa with excessive mucus production. Colonic irritability and marked spasm may make sigmoidoscopy more difficult. Mucosal friability, however, should not be attributed to the irritant effects of the soap. Barium enema examination is also much more uncomfortable for the patient who has been "prepared" by means of soap-containing enemas.

Serious concern over the widespread use of soap enemas is generated by the well documented possibility of severe adverse reactions, including anaphylaxis, rectal gangrene, acute hemorrhagic colitis, acute renal failure, and even death.[133-136] Symptoms begin within hours after the enema and may include severe abdominal cramps, distention, mucorrhea, serosanguineous diarrhea, hypovolemia, and acute hemoconcentration resulting from rapid exudation of fluid into the colon. Hypokalemia may also develop during massive production of mucus by the colon. The transverse and descending colon are usually tender and may be felt as a painful tubular mass. Sigmoidoscopy reveals markedly hyperemic to hemorrhagic mucosa. Barium enema may rarely show marked spasm, abnormal massive propulsive movements, and submucosal edema of the colon.[135, 136]

Treatment consists of close observation, careful replacement of fluid and electrolytes, and possible administration of broad-spectrum antibiotics. Use of corticosteroid therapy has not been reported. Most patients recover completely from this frightening, painful, and serious iatrogenic illness.

Thorough cleansing of the bowel, especially in a hospital setting, is necessary in modern medical practice. The ingestion of a low bulk diet (for a few days before a planned procedure) and a mild oral laxative will usually produce a colon free of large, bulky feces. If more thorough cleansing is still necessary, a warm water or saline enema should be sufficient. The recent condemnation of soapsuds enemas is clearly justified.[131, 136]

FECAL IMPACTION AND STERCORAL ULCER

Incomplete evacuation of feces over an extended period may lead to the formation of a large, firm, immovable mass of stool in the rectum, a fecal impaction. The rectosigmoid becomes dilated, and the firm, irregular mass (fecaloma or stercoroma) is not plastic enough to be expelled through the disproportionately small anal canal by the patient's often weak defecatory effort. A smaller, rounded, smooth hard mass of stool which cannot be expelled is called a stercolith or enterolith; a scybalum is a mass composed of small particles.[137]

PREDISPOSING CONDITIONS

Fecal impactions are most often noted in children who have undiagnosed megaco-

lon or psychogenic problems, or in elderly debilitated and sedentary persons. The frequency of impactions is highest among institutionalized geriatric patients and those in mental institutions, and the need for preventive measures is great.[138] Patients who are inactive for long periods (e.g., with myocardial infarction or orthopedic problems) tend to develop fecal impaction if mild laxatives are not given for constipation. Gentle rectal examination is not harmful in these patients, and should be done early as well as when indicated in these illnesses in order to prevent impaction.[139] Diseases such as hemorrhoids, fissures, and cryptitis, which involve the anal area, cause chronic stool retention because defecation is painful. Bismuth, barium, and kaolin may form a hard nidus around which a fecaloma develops. Elderly patients with a history of constipation are especially at risk for development of a "concretion" in the colon after a barium examination of the upper digestive tract. Obstipation and impaction are also common in patients with megacolon (see pp. 1463 to 1480).

CLINICAL PICTURE

Multiple small fecaliths or calculi may cause lower abdominal pain. These are discrete, smooth, often faceted stones which have radiopaque calcific laminations.[140] They are usually proximal to an area of stricture in the colon or the terminal ileum and are thought to result from stasis. These "stones" are not expelled with the fecal stream and may remain in place for years. Mucosal ulceration is the most common complication unless they are sufficiently numerous to cause obstruction. A small fecalith may obstruct the appendix and predispose to appendicitis. Since these masses are visible on plain film of the abdomen, they should be looked for in patients with lower abdominal pain.

A fecal impaction is formed of firm, compacted stool and may be putty-like in consistency. It is usually located in the rectum or rectosigmoid but may extend proximally to the cecum.

The symptoms of fecal impaction are usually vague and nonspecific. Uncommonly, a sensation of rectal fullness and tenesmus or colicky lower abdominal pain may be present. More often, vague abdominal discomfort is noted, especially after meals. Weight loss resulting from voluntary decrease in food intake is reported. Nausea and vomiting may appear, and dehydration is frequent. Headache and a general sense of ill being are common.[137]

Frequently the patient suffers from uncontrolled passage of small amounts of watery and semiformed stool. This symptom is an "overflow" phenomenon of a large impaction and must not be interpreted as evidence against obstruction. Fecal incontinence in children unaccompanied by urinary incontinence warrants prompt rectal examination for fecal impaction.[141] As liquid from the proximal colon is forced around the impacted mass, it elevates the mass like a ball-valve and a small amount of liquid stool escapes, thus preventing complete obstruction. This mechanism is common in elderly bedridden patients; too often its significance is missed to the extent that the patient may be treated for diarrhea. Also, soft, semiformed stool can be passed because of a similar mechanism in a large impaction.

On physical examination, the large firm mass of stool is usually palpated in the left lower quadrant. Bimanual abdominorectal examination should be done in both males and females to diagnose fecal impaction. The impaction may not be located in the rectal ampulla but lodged in the sigmoid colon above the examining finger and feel like a smooth but irregular mass in the intestinal wall. Firm pressure against the mass with the finger will produce a persistent indentation which will not occur with a polyp or carcinoma. A variety of unusual physical findings have been described for large fecalomas, but are nonspecific.[137] Sigmoidoscopy will usually clarify the nature of the rectosigmoid mass, and X-rays should be diagnostic. If a large fecaloma is suspected, a small amount of hypertonic, water-soluble upper gastrointestinal contrast media should be used for the enema instead of barium, because it may aid in breaking up the mass.

TREATMENT

Treatment of large fecal impactions may be difficult. Enemas usually will not be successful. Removal of the impaction should be done by the physician. A low-lying mass should be broken up with the finger and as much stool removed manually as possible. Frequently the anal sphincter will relax and dilate as the procedure is carried out. Occasionally systemic sedation and analgesia are necessary. More proximal sigmoid masses can be broken up through the sigmoidoscope, although extreme care must be taken not to perforate the bowel wall with the instruments used. A large rubber tube is recommended for this purpose. The tube is advanced through the sigmoidoscope into the fecal mass, and the stool bolus is broken up by flushing small amounts of water through the tube. Once the large mass has been softened and broken up, warm water or saline enemas may be given as well as mineral oil orally. Occasionally, a water-soluble X-ray contrast material enema is helpful at this point to further fragment the stool. Warm oil enemas are unnecessary and may be dangerous, causing burns of the heat-insensitive colonic mucosa. Dilute (5 to 10 per cent) solutions of hydrogen peroxide as an enema have also been used to break up the fecal mass, but this method risks rupture of an already distended colon by the liberated gas.[142] Newer papain and cellulase preparations as enemas may also help in breaking up the nondigestible cellulose and nitrogenous waste products in stool, but their evaluation is incomplete. Dilatation of the anus under anesthesia will be required for some patients who have painful anal disease or other medical problems and cannot tolerate the aforementioned procedures. In extreme cases, laparotomy has been necessary for removal of the fecal mass.

COMPLICATIONS

A number of interesting but uncommon complications or accompaniments of fecal impaction have recently been summarized.[143] These include hernia, recurrent volvulus, megacolon, rectal prolapse, dystocia, and intestinal obstruction. More common complications include urinary tract obstruction, spontaneous perforation of the colon, and stercoral ulceration.

Marked enlargement of the rectosigmoid colon resulting from fecal impaction can produce urinary tract obstruction by compression of the ureters near the ureterovesical junction or, more commonly, by elevation of the bladder, producing marked angulation of the urethra.[144] Intracystic voiding pressure eventually becomes incapable of overcoming the increased urethral outflow resistance, and hydroureter and hydronephrosis result. The possibility of chronic fecal impaction should be evaluated when recurrent urinary tract infection occurs without obvious cause, especially in children. Urinary tract obstruction from this mechanism may occur at any age, and is more common in females than in males.[143, 145]

Spontaneous perforation of the colon has occurred in association with large fecal impactions. The patient's history is typical, with constipation almost invariably present.[145] There are few if any warning symptoms. The onset is acute, often after straining. Only a few hours of left lower abdominal pain precede shock and the physical findings of a perforated viscus. The misdiagnosis of a perforated duodenal ulcer is common, because many of these patients have been treated previously for peptic disease. At laparotomy the peritoneal fluid has a foul smell. There is often little generalized inflammatory response, and small pieces of stool are free in the peritoneal cavity. A small colonic tear is usually present on the antimesenteric border at the rectosigmoid junction. The adjacent bowel appears normal. Rectal examination before laparotomy may disclose a large fecal impaction. This finding should suggest the possibility of colonic rupture and lead to an adequate exploratory incision. The condition is not benign, and mortality may reach 31 per cent.[146]

STERCORAL ULCERS

Stercoral ulcers are lesions of the mucous membrane of the colon and rectum most certainly produced by pressure necrosis. They have been called decubitus ulcers of the colon and usually appear in elderly, debilitated patients who have a large, firm fecal impaction. Because a long rectal stump is often left at autopsy and not fully examined, the true incidence of this lesion is unknown. One carefully done prospective study found the incidence to be 4.6 per cent in 175 consecutive adult autopsies, with the average age of the patient being 68.6 years.[147]

The ulcers are most often confined to the rectosigmoid colon, although the transverse colon may be affected.[148] The size of these ulcers varies remarkably; they usually have an irregular or geographic outline conforming to the surface of the adjacent fecal mass. The surface of the ulcerated area is characteristic, with dark, yellow-gray to greenish-purple discoloration. Thinning and stretching of the involved segment of bowel is evident, with depression of the ulcer surface below the adjacent mucosa. The site of perforation is the central portion of this area where thinning is maximal.

Microscopic examination shows denuding of the mucosa and ischemic pressure necrosis of deeper layers. An interesting and characteristic phenomenon is the presence of minimal inflammatory change with few polymorphonuclear leukocytes unless the process has extended to the adventitia.[147] Small pieces of fecal material may be embedded in the base of the ulcer, and bacteria line the necrotic surface but do not invade the adjacent bowel wall. Vascular changes are not striking, although thrombi may be present in the small compressed vessels. Suppurative peritonitis usually follows perforation.

Chronic stercoral ulceration of the colon may be asymptomatic. It has been postulated that some patients die undiagnosed from complications, especially in hospitals for mentally and chronically ill patients.[149] Minor bleeding may be an early sign. Severe, even exsanguinating rectal bleeding and perforation with peritonitis are the most serious sequelae.[150, 151] Treatment for this complication is obviously surgical. Removal of the fecal mass should relieve the precipitating cause. However, the thinned and ulcerated bowel is fragile and may perforate during attempts to relieve impaction. The onset of abdominal pain and fever after disimpaction should suggest the possibility of perforation.

PROPHYLAXIS

Fecal impaction most frequently complicates other illness and may eventually itself create serious problems in clinical management. Preventive therapy consists of careful recording of bowel movements, periodic examinations of the rectum, administration of stool bulk-former or mild laxatives or stool wetting agents, or, if necessary, periodic enemas. This program will usually prevent impaction in patients who are candidates for it. Also, awareness of subtlety of onset and symptoms of fecal impaction and the willingness to perform a rectal examination are important in preventing a serious problem. Special attention must be given to those patients receiving drugs which may cause constipation (including tranquilizers), patients with myxedema and neurological disorders, and those who are elderly, debilitated, or psychotic.

NONSPECIFIC ULCERATIVE PROCTITIS

Patients may present with rectal bleeding, tenesmus, and occasionally a mucopurulent rectal discharge, who at proctosigmoidoscopy are found to have an inflammatory process of the rectal mucosa with a clearly demarcated upper border above which the mucosa is normal. No specific cause such as trauma or infection is apparent. Subsequent X-ray examination of the colon also reveals the process to be restricted to the rectum and possibly the distal sigmoid colon. With continued observation, the disease does not progress to involve the remainder of the colon or ileum.

This disease, nonspecific ulcerative proctitis, is most probably a variant of diffuse ulcerative colitis but with a markedly different clinical course and prognosis. The reader should also refer to the chapters on ulcerative colitis and other inflammatory diseases of the colon for discussion of this entity (see pp. 1296 to 1347).

CLINICAL PICTURE

Although any age group may be affected, the age of onset parallels typical ulcerative colitis, with a sharp increase in incidence in the late 20's. Large series report conflicting sex incidence; probably there is little difference.[152-154]

Typically, the patient presents with rec-

tal bleeding. It is seldom severe, but may be moderate or scant with only blood staining of the toilet paper. Initially the blood may be attributed by the patient and physician to hemorrhoids. A change in bowel habit is common, with both diarrhea and constipation being frequent complaints. Patients with diarrhea will often describe normal stool volume but frequent passage of a mucoid or mucosanguineous discharge. Rectal tenesmus is a common complaint among these patients. Although vague abdominal discomfort is occasionally present, systemic symptoms such as fever, severe malaise, and weight loss are usually absent. The history of a similar symptom complex with apparent spontaneous resolution is frequently obtained.

DIAGNOSIS

Diagnosis is made by the finding of the typical changes of nonspecific ulcerative colitis on proctosigmoidoscopy, biopsy, and, occasionally, barium enema examination. During the acute phase, sigmoidoscopy reveals a glistening edematous mucosa covered by streaks of a gray mucosanguineous exudate. Although the mucosa bleeds easily after it is touched, definite mucosal ulcerations are very uncommon. The rectal valves are edematous and blunted, and the normal submucosal vascular network is obscured by the edema and hyperemia present.

As symptoms improve or as the inflammatory process becomes chronic, the mucosa appears drier with a rough or granular surface; there is no spontaneous bleeding. Abrasion with a cotton swab will demonstrate pinpoint bleeding as evidence of continued friability. Eventually, in late stages of healing, friability is lost and the submucosal vascular pattern may reappear.[152]

The inflammatory process may be localized to only the distal 3 or 4 cm of the rectum or may extend up to the sigmoid flexure. The sigmoidoscopic finding which suggests the diagnosis of ulcerative proctitis is a sharp line of demarcation between the distal inflammatory process and proximal normal rectal or lower sigmoid mucosa. Ulcerative proctitis is a good example of a disease that is best diagnosed and followed by sigmoidoscopy.

Biopsy of the rectal mucosa will reveal changes indistinguishable from those found in typical ulcerative colitis (Fig. 112–3, *C* and *D*). The findings are discussed above and in the chapter dealing with that entity (pp. 1306 to 1308). Barium enema examination should be done without an occlusive balloon on the rectal enema catheter. It commonly demonstrates no abnormality in the lower rectum, but may show typical mucosal changes of ulcerative colitis when the proximal rectum or distal sigmoid is involved. The important finding on the barium enema is the absence of radiological evidence for disease in the remainder of the colon and terminal ileum.

The differential diagnosis includes radiation proctitis, bacillary dysentery, amebiasis, lymphogranuloma venereum, gonorrheal proctitis, chemical or mechanical irritation, and proctitis resulting from gold therapy for rheumatoid arthritis.[152, 155] Appropriate history, cultures, examination of the mucoid discharge, biopsy, and the Frei test should help exclude these differential possibilities (see pp. 1373 to 1401).

TREATMENT

The general approach to treatment of ulcerative proctitis is the same as that outlined for mild ulcerative colitis. However, the evaluation of any treatment for nonspecific ulcerative proctitis must be judged with knowledge of the natural history of the disease, which includes spontaneous periods of remission. Since severe complications of the disease are uncommon, therapy is directed mainly at treating the symptomatic rectal mucosal lesion. In mild cases, therapy can be limited to sedatives and stool softeners. Troublesome rectal bleeding and tenesmus usually respond to nonabsorbable sulfur preparations orally and rectal administration of adrenocorticosteroids either in solution or suppository form.[153, 154] Since the severity and duration of symptoms can be markedly reduced by these simple measures, systemic corticosteroid administration is not indicated.

COURSE OF THE DISEASE AND COMPLICATIONS

Most patients with ulcerative proctitis will experience three or four symptomatic episodes a year similar to those of more generalized ulcerative colitis. Ulcerative proctitis differs, however, in that it tends to remain localized to the rectum and lower sigmoid colon. It extends proximally to a more generalized form of ulcerative colitis in less than 15 per cent of patients.[152, 154] Also, in contrast to diffuse ulcerative colitis, the complications of arthritis, uveitis, and pyoderma gangrenosum are not seen. Carcinoma of the rectum or sigmoid colon complicating long-standing cases is rare.[153] When the inflammation is chronic, a rectal stricture may occasionally develop.

Coexisting local diseases of the anus, such as fissures, fistulas, and abscesses, will require specific treatment (see pp. 1540 to 1558). Iron deficiency anemia can result if rectal bleeding is excessive and prolonged but is uncommon after diagnosis and proper management.

In summary, ulcerative proctitis appears to be a localized, milder form of generalized ulcerative colitis but with a better prognosis. Periodic recurrences of rectal tenesmus and bleeding are common, and good response to conservative therapy can be anticipated. Less than 15 per cent of patients with the disease progress to develop diffuse ulcerative colitis. Toxic episodes, the need for surgical resection, and the development of bowel carcinoma are rare.

REFERENCES

1. Brandborg, L. L., Rubin, C. E., and Quinton, W. E. A multipurpose instrument for suction biopsy of the esophagus, stomach, small bowel, and colon. Gastroenterology *37*:1, 1959.
2. Flick, A. L., Quinton, W. E., and Rubin, C. E. A peroral hydraulic biopsy tube for multiple sampling of any level of the gastrointestinal tract. Gastroenterology *40*:120, 1961.
3. Gear, E. V., and Dobbins, W. O., III. Rectal biopsy. A review of its diagnostic usefulness. Gastroenterology *55*:522, 1968.
4. Hemley, S. D., and Kanick, V. Perforation of the rectum: A complication of barium enema following rectal biopsy. Report of two cases. Amer. J. Dig. Dis. *8*:882, 1963.
5. Spingarn, C. L., Edelman, M. H., Gold, T., Yarnis, H., and Turell, R. Value of rectal biopsies in the diagnosis and treatment of *Schistosoma mansoni* infection. New Eng. J. Med. *256*:290, 1957.
6. Hawk, W. A., Turnbull, R. B., and Farmer, R. G. Regional enteritis of the colon. Distinctive features of the entity. J.A.M.A. *201*:738, 1967.

7. Juniper, R., Steele, V. W., and Chester, C. L. Rectal biopsy in the diagnosis of amebic colitis. South. Med. J. 51:545, 1958.

8. Tandon, H. D., Prakash, O., and Tandon, B. N. A study of chronic colonic diarrhea and dysentery. Part II. Rectal biopsy study. Indian J. Med. Res. 54:629, 1966.

9. Dick, A. P., Holt, L. P., and Dalton, E. R. Persistence of mucosal abnormality in ulcerative colitis. Gut 7:355, 1966.

10. Edling, N. P. G., Eklöf, O., Kistner, S., and Lagarlöf, B. Correlation of findings at barium enema examination, rectoscopy and biopsy of rectum. Acta Radiol. 4:536, 1966.

11. Morson, B. C., and Pang, L. S. C. Rectal biopsy as an aid to cancer control in ulcerative colitis. Gut 8:423, 1967.

12. Blum, A., and Sohar, E. The diagnosis of amyloidosis. Lancet 1:721, 1962.

13. Dobbins, W. O., and Bill, A. H. Diagnosis of Hirschsprung's disease excluded by rectal suction biopsy. New Eng. J. Med. 272:990, 1965.

14. Parkins, R. A., Eidelman, S., Rubin, C. E., Dobbins, W. O., III, and Phelps, P. C. The diagnosis of cystic fibrosis by rectal suction biopsy. Lancet 2:851, 1963.

15. Britt, E. M., and Berry, C. L. Value of rectal biopsy in paediatric neurology: Report of 165 biopsies. Brit. Med. J. 2:400, 1967.

16. Bodian, M., and Lake, B. O. The rectal approach to neuropathology. Brit. J. Surg. 50:702, 1963.

17. Goodall, H. B., and Sinclair, I. S. R. Colitis cystica profunda. J. Path. Bact. 73:33, 1957.

18. Denton, J. The pathology of pellagra. Amer. J. Trop. Med. 5:173, 1925.

19. Herzenberg, N. Pellagra (pathologisch-anatomische Studie). Beitr. Path. Anat. 97, 1935.

20. Epstein, S. E., Ascari, W. A., Ablow, R. C., Seaman, W. B., and Lattis, R. Colitis cystica profunda. Amer. J. Clin. Path. 45:186, 1966.

21. Allen, M. S. Hamartomatous inverted polyps of the rectum. Cancer 19:257, 1966.

22. Manson-Bahr. P., and Gregg, A. L. The surgical treatment of chronic bacillary dysentery. Brit. J. Surg. 13:701, 1926.

23. Fechner, R. E. Polyp of the colon possessing features of colitis cystica profunda. Dis. Colon Rectum 10:359, 1967.

24. Barner, J. L. Colitis cystica profunda. Radiology 89:435, 1967.

25. Salzman, E. W., and Castleman, B. Rectal lesion associated with diarrhea and hypoproteinemia: Case record, Massachusetts General Hospital. New Eng. J. Med. 275:608, 1966.

26. Brock, D. R., and Suckow, E. E. Obliterative arteriolosclerosis of the colon with focal mucosal necrosis. Gastroenterology 44:190, 1963.

27. Sternlieb, I. Brock-Suckow polyposis of the colon (obliterative arteriolosclerosis of the colon?). Gastroenterology 46:193, 1964.

28. Crane, C. W. Observations on sodium and potassium content of mucus from the large intestine. Gut 6:439, 1965.

29. Cruveilhier, J. Un beau cas de cicatrisation d'un ulcère de l'intestine gaele datant d'une douzine d'armées. Bull. Soc. Anat. 7:1, 1832.

30. Barron, M. E. Simple nonspecific ulcer of the colon. Arch. Surg. 17:355, 1928.

31. Cameron, J. R. Simple nonspecific ulcer of the caecum. Brit. J. Surg. 26:526, 1939.

32. Barlow, D. Simple ulcer of the cecum, colon and rectum. Brit. J. Surg. 28:575, 1941.

33. Williams, K. L. Acute solitary ulcers and acute diverticulitis of the cecum and ascending colon. Brit. J. Surg. 47:351, 1960.

34. Madigan, M. R., and Morson, B. C. Solitary ulcer of the rectum. Gut 10:871, 1969.

35. Benninger, G. W., Honig, L. J., and Fine, H. D. Nonspecific ulceration of the cecum. Amer. J. Gastroent. 55:594, 1971.

36. Butsch, J. L., Dockerty, M. B., McGill, D. B., and Judd, E. S. Solitary nonspecific ulcer of the colon. Arch. Surg. 98:171, 1969.

37. Debenham, G. P. Ulcer of the cecum during oxyphenbutazone therapy. Canad. Med. Assoc. J. 94:1182, 1966.

38. Parker, R. A., and Sergeant, J. C. B. Acute solitary ulcer and diverticulitis of the caecum. Brit. J. Surg. 45:29, 1957.

39. Miller, S. M., and Juhl, J. H. Nonspecific ulcers of the colon. Minn. Med. 50:1327, 1967.

40. Friedman, M. H., and MacKenzie, W. C. Simple ulcer of the colon. Canad. J. Surg. 2:279, 1959.

41. Wright, H. H. Simple ulcer of transverse colon: Report of a case. Wisc. Med. J. 48:801, 1947.

42. Yates, J. N., and Clausen, E. G. Simple nonspecific ulcers of the sigmoid colon. Arch. Surg. 81:535, 1960.

43. Bosien, W. R., and Crandell, W. B. Hemorrhage from a benign ulcer of the sigmoid colon. New Eng. J. Med. 251:944, 1954.

44. Jalay, K. N., Brunt, P. W., Maclean, N., and Sircus, W. Benign solitary ulcer of the rectum—a report of five cases. Scand. J. Gastroent. 5:143, 1970.

45. Feldman, N. Clinical Roentgenology of the Digestive Tract. p. 901. Baltimore, Williams and Wilkins Co., 1948.

46. Tagart, R. E. B. Acute phlegmonous caecitis. Brit. J. Surg. 40:437, 1953.

47. DeCamp, P. I., and Penick, R. M. Acute nonspecific inflammatory lesions of the cecum. Ann. Surg. 143:665, 1956.

48. Andrade, S., and Andrade, V. H. Intestinal pneumatosis. Presentation of five cases. Amer. J. Proctol. 19:39, 1968.

49. Smith, W. G., Anderson, M. J., and Pemberton, H. W. Pneumatosis cystoides intestinalis involving left portion of colon. Report of four cases diagnosed at sigmoidoscopy. Gastroenterology 35:528, 1958.

50. Ross, L. G. Abdominal gas cysts (pneumatosis cystoides intestinorum hominis). Arch. Path. 53:523, 1952.

51. Keyting, W. S., McCarver, R. R., Kovarik, J. L., and Daywitt, A. L. Pneumatosis intestinalis: A new concept. Radiology 76:733, 1961.

52. Rienhoff, W. F., and Collins, N. D. Pneumocystoides intestinalis and regional enteritis. Ann. Surg. 149:593, 1959.

53. Merhoff, W. E., Hirschfield, J. S., and Kern, F. Small intestinal scleroderma with malabsorption and pneumatosis cystoides intestinalis. J.A.M.A. 204:854, 1968.

54. Nelson, S. W. Extraluminal gas collections due to diseases of the gastrointestinal tract. Amer. J. Roent. 115:225, 1972.

55. Neumeister, C. A. Left sided pneumatosis coli. Minn. Med. 42:407, 1959.

56. Marshak, R. H., Blum, S. D., and Eliasoph, J. Pneumatosis involving the left side of the colon. J.A.M.A. 161:1626, 1956.

57. Doub, H. P., and Shea, J. J. Pneumatosis cystoides intestinalis. J.A.M.A. 172:1238, 1960.

58. McGregor, J. K., and McKinnon, D. A. Intestinal interstitial emphysema. Gastroenterology 35:206, 1958.

59. Botsford, T. W., and Krakover, C. Pneumatosis of intestine in infancy. J. Pediat. 13:185, 1938.

60. Yunich, A. M., and Fredkin, N. F. Fatal sprue (malabsorption) syndrome secondary to extensive pneumatosis cystoides intestinalis. Gastroenterology 35:212, 1958.

61. Paris, L. Pneumatosis cystoides intestinalis in infancy. J. Pediat. 46:1, 1955.

62. Wright, A. W. Local effect of injection of gases into the subcutaneous tissue. Amer. J. Path. 6:87, 1930.

63. Mujahed, A., and Evans, J. A. Gas cysts of the intestine (pneumatosis intestinalis). Surg. Gynec. Obstet. 107:151, 1958.

64. Kushlan, S. D. Pneumatosis cystoides intestinalis. Report of a case mimicking the irritable bowel syndrome with X-ray diagnosis of resolution. J.A.M.A. 179:699, 1962.

65. Pemberton, H. W., Smith, W. G., and Holman, C. B. Pneumatosis cystoides intestinalis diagnosed sigmoidoscopically. Report of a case and review of literature. Amer. J. Surg. 94:472, 1957.

66. Lerner, H. H., and Gazin, A. L. Pneumatosis intestinalis. Its roentgenologic diagnosis. Amer. J. Roent. 56:464, 1946.

67. Witkowski, L. J., Pontius, G. V., and Anderson, R. E. Gas cysts of the intestine. Surgery 37:959, 1955.

68. Sampson, J. A. Development of implantation theory for origin of peritoneal endometriosis. Amer. J. Obstet. Gynec. 40:549, 1940.

69. TeLinde, R. W., and Scott, R. B. Experimental endometriosis. Amer. J. Obstet. Gynec. 60:1147, 1950.

70. Scott, R. B., TeLinde, R. W., and Wharton, L. R., Jr. Further studies on experimental endometriosis. Amer. J. Obstet. Gynec. 66:1082, 1953.

71. Novak, E. R., and Woodruff, J. D. (eds). Gynecologic and Obstetric Pathology, 5th ed. Philadelphia, W. B. Saunders Co., 1962, pp. 470–491.

72. Javert, C. T. Observations on the pathology and spread of endometriosis based on the theory of benign metastases. Amer. J. Obstet. Gynec. 62:477, 1951.

73. Colcock, B. P., and Lamphier, T. A. Endome-

triosis of the large and small intestine. Surgery 28:997, 1950.

74. Gray, L. A. The management of endometriosis involving the bowel. Clin. Obstet. Gynec. 9:309, 1966.

75. Boles, R. S., and Hodes, P. J. Endometriosis of the small and large intestine. Gastroenterology 34:367, 1958.

76. Rio, F. W., Edwards, D. L., Regan, J. F., and Schmutzer, K. J. Endometriosis of the small bowel. Arch. Surg. 101:403, 1970.

77. Jenkinson, E. L., and Brown, W. H. Endometriosis—a study of 117 cases with special reference to constricting lesions of the rectum and sigmoid colon. J.A.M.A. 122:349, 1943.

77. McGuff, P., Dockerty, M. B., Waugh, J. M., and Randall, L. M. Endometriosis as a cause of intestinal obstruction. Surg. Gynec. Obstet. 86:273, 1948.

79. Valdes-Dapena, A. "Organizer" effect as a pathogenetic mechanism of obstruction and intestinal endometriosis. J. Indian Med. Prof. 13:5985, 1967.

80. Kempers, R. D., Dockerty, M. B., Hunt, A. B., and Symmonds, R. E. Postmenopausal endometriosis. Surg. Gynec. Obstet. 111:348, 1960.

81. Meigs, J. V. Endometriosis. Ann. Surg. 127:795, 1948.

82. Heupel, H. W., Reece, R. L., and Pincus, M. Stromal endometrioma mimicking acute appendicitis. Minn. Med. 53:153, 1970.

83. Bose, A., and Davson, J. Endometriosis of the small intestine. Brit. J. Surg. 56:109, 1969.

84. Spjut, H. J., and Perkins, D. E. Endometriosis of the sigmoid colon and rectum. Amer. J. Roent. 82:1070, 1959.

85. Theauder, G. Deformity of the rectosigmoid junction in pelvic endometriosis. Acta Radiol. 55:241, 1961.

86. Ferreira, H. P., and Clayton, S. G. Three cases of malignant change in endometriosis, including two cases arising in the rectovaginal septum. J. Obstet. Gynec. Brit. Empire 65:41, 1958.

87. Beyoung, E. E., and Gamble, C. N. Primary adenocarcinoma of the rectovaginal septum arising from endometriosis. Report of a case. Cancer 24:597, 1969.

88. Bernstein, J. S., Perlow, V., and Brenner, J. J. Massive ascites due to endometriosis. Amer. J. Dig. Dis. 6:1, 1961.

89. Goligher, J. C. Surgery of the Anus, Rectum and Colon. London, Cassel and Co., Ltd., 1961, pp. 644–646.

90. Parsons, L. Conservative surgical management of external endometriosis. Obstet. Gynec. 32:576, 1968.

91. Ranney, B. Endometriosis. II. Emergency operations due to hemoperitoneum. Obstet. Gynec. 36:437, 1970.

92. Marshak, R. H., and Friedman, A. I. Endometriosis of the large bowel treated with testosterone. Gastroenterology 14:576, 1950.

93. Williams, B. F. P. Conservative management of endometriosis: Follow-up observations of progestin therapy. Obstet. Gynec. 30:76, 1967.

94. Kourides, I. A., and Kistner, R. W. Three new

synthetic progestins in the treatment of endometriosis. Obstet. Gynec. 31:821, 1968.

95. Melicow, M. M. Malakoplakia. J. Urol. 78:33, 1957.

96. Nation, E. F. Malakoplakia of the urinary tract. J. Urol. 76:576, 1956.

97. von Hansemann, D. Ueber Malakoplakia der Harnblase. Arch. Path. Anat. 173:302, 1903.

98. Purpon, I., and Perez-Tamayo, R. Malakoplakia of the kidney. J. Urol. 84:231, 1960.

99. Blackwell, G. J., and Finlay-Jones, L. R. Malakoplakia of the testis. J. Path. Bact. 78:571, 1959.

100. Gonzales-Angulo, A., Corral, E., Garcia-Torres, R., and Quijano, M. Malakoplakia of the colon. Gastroenterology 48:383, 1965.

101. Terner, J. Y., and Lattes, R. Malakoplakia of the colon. Fed. Proc. 22:572, 1963.

102. Terner, J. Y., and Lattes, R. Malakoplakia of colon and retroperitoneum. Amer. J. Clin. Path. 44:20, 1965.

103. Goldman, R. L. A case of malakoplakia with involvement of the prostate gland. J. Urol. 93.:407, 1965.

104. Yunis, E. J., Estevez, J. M., Pinzon, G. J., and Moran, T. J. Malakoplakia. Arch. Path. 83:180, 1967.

105. Kuzman, J. P. Polypoid lymphoid hyperplasia of the colon with malakoplakia. In Proceedings of the Thirty-Second Seminar on Gastrointestinal Diseases, M. Swerdlow (ed.). Chicago, American Society of Clinical Pathology, 1967, pp. 9-13.

106. Finlay-Jones, M. B., Blackwell, J. B., and Papadimitriou, J. M. Malakoplakia of the colon. Amer. J. Clin. Path. 50:320, 1968.

107. Dockerty, M. B. Primary malakoplakia of the colon. Mayo Clin. Proc. 47:114, 1972.

108. Fisher, E. R., and Hellstrom, H. R. Ceroid-like colonic histiocytosis. Amer. J. Clin. Path. 42:581, 1964.

109. Curtis, W. R., Bozzell, J. D., and Green, C. L. Malakoplakia of bladder: Report of a case successfully treated with antituberculosis medical therapy. J. Urol. 86:78, 1961.

110. Cruveilhier, J. Cancer avec melanose. In Anatomie Pathologique du Corps Humain, J. B. Bailliere (ed.) Paris, 1829, p. 6.

111. Virchow, R. Die pathologischen Pigmente. Virchow Arch. Path. Anat. 1:379, 1931.

112. Stewart, N. J., and Hickman, E. M. Observations on melanosis coli. J. Path. Bact. 34:61, 1931.

113. Bockus, H. L., Willard, J. H., and Bank, J. Melanosis coli. J.A.M.A. 101:1, 1933.

114. Speare, G. S. Melanosis coli. Experimental observations on its production and elimination in 23 cases. Amer. J. Surg. 82:631, 1951.

115. Wittoesch, J. H., Jackman, R. J., and McDonald, J. R. Melanosis coli: General review and a study of 887 cases. J. Dis. Colon Rectum 1:172, 1958.

116. Roden, B. Melanosis coli. A pathological study: Its experimental production in monkeys. J. Med. Sci. 6:654, 1940.

117. Won, K. H. and Ramchand, S. Melanosis of the ileum. Case report and electron microscopic study. Amer. J. Dig. Dis. 15:57, 1940.

118. Andrejauskas, G. Rare case of esophagitis with melanosis. Medicina 18:13, 1937.

119. Lillie, R. D. Histopathologic Technique and Practical Histochemistry, 2nd ed. Boston, Little, Brown and Co., 1961, p. 998.

120. Schrodt, R. G. Melanosis coli: A study with the electron microscope. Dis. Colon Rectum 6:277, 1963.

121. Ghadially, F. N., and Parry, E. W. An electron-microscope and histochemical study of melanosis coli. J. Path. Bact. 92:313, 1966.

122. Heilbrun, N. Roentgen evidence suggesting enterocolitis associated with prolonged cathartic abuse. Radiology 41:486, 1943.

123. Heilbrun, N., and Bernstein, C. Roentgen abnormalities of the large and small intestine associated with prolonged cathartic ingestion. Radiology 65:549, 1955.

124. Jewell, F. C., and Kline, J. R. The purged colon. Radiology 62:368, 1954.

125. Plum, G. E., Weber, H. M., and Sauer, W. G. Prolonged cathartic abuse resulting in roentgen evidence suggestive of enterocolitis. Amer. J. Roent. 83:919, 1960.

126. Ziter, F. M. Cathartic colon. New York State J. Med. 67:546, 1967.

127. Margulis, A. R., Goldberg, H. I., Lawson, T. L., Montgomery, C. K., Rambo, O. N., Noonan, C. D., and Amberg J. R. The overlapping spectrum of ulcerative and granulomatous colitis: A roentgenographic pathologic study. Amer. J. Roent. 113:325, 1971.

128. Smith, B. Effect of irritant purgatives on the myenteric plexus in man and the mouse. Gut 9:139, 1968.

129. Hardcastle, J. D. and Mann, C. V. Study of large bowel peristalsis. Gut 9:512, 1968.

130. Hardcastle, J. D., and Wilkins, J. L. The action of sennosides and related compounds on human colon and rectum. Gut 11:1038, 1970.

131. Lewis, A. E. Dangers inherent in soap enemas. Pacific Med. Surg. 73:131, 1965.

132. Hicks, E. S. Observations regarding enemas. Canad. Med. Assoc. J. 51:358, 1944.

133. Smith, D. Severe anaphylactic reaction after a soap enema. Brit. Med. J. 4:215, 1967.

134. Bendit, M. Gangrene of the rectum as a complication of an enema. Brit. Med. J. 1:664, 1945.

135. Barker, C. S. Acute colitis resulting from soap suds enema. Canad. Med. Assoc. J. 52:285, 1945.

136. Pike, B. F., Phillippi, P. J., and Lawson, E. H. Soap colitis. New Eng. J. Med. 285:217, 1971.

137. Abilla, M. E., and Fernandez, A. T. Large fecalomas. Dis. Colon Rectum 10:401, 1967.

138. Smith, C. W., and Evans, P. R. Bowel motility, a problem in institutionalized geriatric care. Geriatrics 16:189, 1961.

139. Earnest, D. L., and Fletcher, G. F. Danger of rectal examination in patients with acute myocardial infarction—fact or fiction? New Eng. J. Med. 281:238, 1969.

140. Harland, D. A case of multiple calculi in the large intestine with a review of the subject of intestinal calculi. Brit. J. Surg. 41:209, 1953.

141. Suckling, P. V. The ball-valve rectum due to impacted feces. Lancet 2:1147, 1962.

142. Andrews, N. L. Impactions of the rectum and colon. Amer. Surgeon 21:693, 1955.

143. Lal, S., and Brown, G. N. Some unusual complications of fecal impaction. Amer. J. Proct. 18:226, 1967.

144. Ravich, L., Lerman, T. H., and Schell, N. B. Urinary retention due to fecal impaction. New York State J. Med. 63:3289, 1963.

145. Grunberg, A. Acute urinary retention due to fecal impaction. J. Urol. 83:301, 1960.

146. Berger, P. L., and Shaw, R. E. Spontaneous rupture of the colon. Brit. Med. J. 1:1422, 1961.

147. Grinvalsky, H. T. and Bowerman, C. I. Stercoraceous ulcers of the colon. Relatively neglected medical and surgical problem. J.A.M.A. 171:1941, 1959.

148. O'Reilly, J. J., and Belf, M. B. Death following perforation of a stercoraceous ulcer. Lancet 2:1175, 1935.

149. Liedberg, G. Stercoraceous perforations of the colon. Acta Chir. Scand. 135 552, 1969.

150. Milliser, R. V., Greenberg, S. R., and Neiman, B. H. Exsanguinating stercoral ulceration. Amer. J. Dig. Dis. 15:485, 1970.

151. Printz, J. H., Hoffman, J. S., and Khazei, H. Multiple stercoraceous ulcers of the colon associated with huge fecalomas and perforation; case report. Amer. Surgeon 27:714, 1961.

152. Lennard-Jones, J. E., Cooper, G. W., Newell, A. C., Wilson, C. W., and Jones, F. A. Observations on idiopathic proctitis. Gut 3:201, 1962.

153. Farmer, R. G., and Brown, C. H. Ulcerative proctitis; course and prognosis. Gastroenterology 51:219, 1966.

154. Sparberg, M., Gennessy, J., and Kirsner, J. B. Ulcerative proctitis and mild ulcerative colitis: A study of 220 patients. Medicine 45:391, 1966.

155. Folley, J. H. Ulcerative proctitis. New Eng. J. Med. 282:1362, 1970.

Chapter 113

Diseases of the Anus

David L. Earnest

The anal canal, a short passage, usually only 1¼ to 1½ inches long, is a site of discomfort to most persons at some time in their lives. Because of its being prone to certain diseases and because of its key function in maintaining rectal continence, familiarity with anal and perianal disease is of importance to both the internist and the surgeon. This chapter briefly outlines anatomy, technique of examination, and certain frequently encountered diseases of the anus.

ANATOMICAL DESCRIPTION

The anatomy of the anal canal is described in detail on pages 1245 to 1246. Briefly, the anal canal is lined by an upper mucosal and a lower cutaneous type of epithelium. These two meet about ½ to 1 inch inside the anal orifice at the level of the anal valves. These valves give a serrated appearance to the mucocutaneous junction and form what is called the pectinate or dentate line (see Fig. 97–13, p. 1244). Below the pectinate line, the anal canal is lined by squamous epithelium which appears thin and stretched. However, within an inch distal to the pectinate line it becomes thicker, and outside the anal orifice it contains histological features of normal skin. Above the pectinate line there are longitudinal folds in the mucosa called rectal columns or columns of Morgagni. At the pectinate line these col-

umns meet to form the small anal valves. Behind each valve is a small pit called the anal sinus. Small bits of tissue at the pectinate line between the valves form the anal papillae. The mucosa just above the valves is cuboidal, but it rapidly changes to columnar.

Probably the most important part of the anus is the musculature comprising the internal and external anal sphincters. The terminal muscle fibers of the rectum pass down through the levator ani muscles and become the walls of the anal canal. Their termination forms the internal anal sphincter. The inferior edge of this internal sphincter is rounded and is well defined about ⅓ inch above the anal orifice and ⅓ inch below the level of the anal valves. The lower end of the internal sphincter can easily be recognized as the superior margin of a distinct groove palpated just inside the anal orifice. The inferior border of this groove is formed by the lower part of the external anal sphincter. The fibers of this external sphincter extend up and over the lateral margins of the internal sphincter and ultimately end in the puborectalis part of the levator ani muscles.

The internal sphincter is an involuntary muscle, and its surgical disruption does not result in incontinence. However, the external sphincter and puborectalis muscles are voluntary, playing a role in anal control. Indeed, complete transection will usually cause rectal incontinence. Therefore the anorectal ring, composed of the upper border of the external and internal anal sphincters, is an important landmark in proctological surgery for abscesses and fistulas in the anal region. Its complete transection must be avoided.

The nerve supply to the anal canal is also detailed on pages 1240 to 1241. A few points deserve special emphasis. The pectinate line marks the point of division between the autonomic nerve supply to the rectum (pain fibers sensitive mainly to stretch but not to heat or touch) and the sensory innervation of the anus which is somatic and contains nerve endings for normal dermal sensitivity. These sensory fibers are carried by the inferior hemorrhoidal nerves and are extremely sensitive to the slightest irritation of the anal canal. Even very small lesions in this area can produce a great deal of local discomfort. Much less intense sensory phenomena arise from stimulation of the rectum above the pectinate line. This is usually felt as a dull sensation which is occasionally painful. This visceral pain sensation is probably mediated by parasympathetic afferent nerves.

The nerve supply to the internal anal sphincter is from the splanchnic nerves and contains both sympathetic fibers which are stimulatory and parasympathetic ones which are inhibitory. Parasympathetic impulses may be stimulated by distention of the rectum. Their inhibitory action causes reflex relaxation of the internal anal sphincter. Basal sympathetic stimulation maintains internal sphincter tone.

The external anal sphincter is under voluntary control. The somatic supply is from branches of the internal pudendal and fourth sacral nerves. Sympathetic preganglionic fibers also pass from the splanchnic nerves through the white ramus into the chain that connects with the dorsal motor root ganglion of nerves to the external sphincter. This nerve supply is primarily responsible for reflex action of the anorectal musculature (see Fig. 97–10, p. 1240).

The vasculature of the colon and rectum is described on pages 378 to 381. Briefly, the anus receives its blood supply from three major arterial branches: (1) the superior hemorrhoidal artery, which descends on the rectum from the inferior mesenteric artery; (2) the middle hemorrhoidal artery, which traverses the lateral rectal ligaments from the internal iliac artery; and (3) the inferior hemorrhoidal artery from the internal pudendal artery. Of these three, the main arterial supply comes from the superior hemorrhoidal vessels; however, the remaining blood supply is adequate when this vessel is compromised.

Venous drainage of the anal canal closely follows the arteries. The superior hemorrhoidal venous plexus lies in the submucosa of the upper part of the anal canal and in general drains blood above the pectinate line into the inferior mesenteric vein of the portal system. The middle hemorrhoidal vein drains into the internal iliac vessels and ultimately into the vena cava, as does the more important inferior hemorrhoidal vein which drains the veins under the skin of the external anal orifice. There are extensive anastomoses between these three venous pathways.

The veins of the portal system do not have valves; thus the connections of the superior hemorrhoidal veins with the portal system involve the entire anorectal venous plexus in patients with portal hypertension. Special mention will be made later of the problem of internal hemorrhoids associated with portal hypertension resulting from this anastomotic relationship.

Lymphatics draining the anus also follow the blood supply and therefore drain upward along the superior hemorrhoidal and inferior mesenteric vessels to the preaortic nodes, laterally to the inferior iliac nodes, and downward across the perineum to the inguinal nodes. The latter pathway explains why perianal disease may occasionally present with tender inguinal lymphadenopathy.

The ischiorectal and perirectal spaces are important. Infections in the anal area, especially small abscesses, are prone to rupture into these spaces and produce serious deep infection requiring extensive surgical drainage.

EXAMINATION OF THE ANUS

The patient may be examined in any one of a number of positions, but most examiners prefer the knee-elbow or knee-chest position, preferably on a proctosig-moidoscopy table. The Sims left lateral position is also quite acceptable for a debilitated patient.

DIGITAL EXAMINATION

It is important to begin the examination by separating the buttocks and making a close inspection of the perianal skin for skin disease, tumors, scars, fistulous openings, and hemorrhoids. The patient should be instructed to bear down as if he were going to defecate in order to demonstrate prolapsing mucosa and hemorrhoids. With a gloved finger, the anal and perianal area should be palpated for tenderness or masses. A well lubricated index finger (little finger for small children or infants) should then be placed against the anal opening and, with the thumb pointed toward the coccyx, be introduced slowly. Rapid insertion of the finger may cause painful reflex sphincter spasm and destroy the patient's confidence. The patient should then be asked to relax and take a few deep breaths if still anxious. To maintain relaxation, it is often helpful to talk reassuringly to the patient while the examination is in progress.

Pain produced by introduction of the finger may indicate the possibility of an anal fissure or a localized inflammatory process. Discovery of a fissure is facilitated by turning the finger around and pressing against all four quadrants. Abnormal sphincter tone may also be indicative of anal or perianal disease. For example, a lax sphincter may indicate a neuropathic process, damage to the internal musculature, or, as is alleged by some, possibly a carcinoma of the rectum or rectosigmoid. Sphincters are more commonly spastic than lax; spasticity may reflect either heightened tension on the part of the patient or inadequate reassurance and poor technique on the part of the physician; or it may reflect an inflammatory or irritative process involving the anal canal which prevents satisfactory sphincter relaxation. If the procedure is very uncomfortable for the patient, it should be terminated at this point, the anal canal lubricated with a topical anesthetic ointment, and, after a short wait, the examination repeated. Persistence of severe pain may require several

injections of local anesthetic into the perianal tissue. In those instances in which extensive inflammatory disease is obviously present (usually associated with granulomatous disease of the intestine), intramuscular injection of 50 to 100 mg of meperidine before the procedure may be quite helpful. Local anesthetic injections in the area of obvious or possible perianal and perirectal inflammation or infections should be avoided.

Once the examining finger has been introduced fully into the rectum, it should sweep circumferentially around the anal canal and the rectal ampulla, feeling for induration, intrinsic and extrinsic masses, and the status of the prostate and seminal vesicles in the male and the pelvic organs in the female. Palpation of the coccyx, the sacrospinal ligaments, and the piriform muscles may reveal musculoskeletal causes of pain. The patient should be asked to bear down once more as if going to defecate while the examiner advances the finger as far cephalad as possible. This will allow digital examination of higher portions of the rectum. During this maneuver, masses in the more proximal sigmoid colon may be felt through loops of rectal mucosa. Small lumps of stool often feel like polypoid masses. Firm pressure with the examining finger against the mass will usually produce a persistent indentation if it is due to feces.

After this part of the examination and with the index finger still in the anal canal and rectum, a bidigital examination of the perianal tissue should be done by palpating the entire circumference of the anus between the thumb externally and the index finger. This maneuver can reveal small areas of tenderness from deep and localized inflammation which may otherwise be undetected.

A rectovaginal examination should next be done in a nonvirginal female by inserting the second finger into the vagina and palpating the rectovaginal septum between the two fingers.

A bimanual rectoabdominal or rectovaginal examination should be performed last. It is helpful to take a minute to reassure the patient about the examination while he or she is turning over into a supine position with knees bent for the bimanual examination.

ANOSCOPY

Anoscopy should be performed routinely after digital examination. Results of the rectal examination should allow the examiner to decide whether a proctoscope of normal diameter can be passed without excessive discomfort. The instrument is inserted with its obturator in place and the handle pointing toward the sacrum. The anal sphincter will usually relax with gentle pressure against it. With a posterior direction, the proctoscope should be passed to its hilt. The obturator is then removed and an external light source employed to illuminate one quadrant of the anal canal and the distal rectum. The presence of blood, pus, or mucus should be noted on the proctoscope obturator or in stool in the rectum. Feces and rectal discharge should be swabbed away to allow clear inspection of the mucosa which is normally a pale pink. Submucosal vessels should be visible as a purplish-pink network on the rectal wall. In some patients with proctitis, particularly those with ulcerative colitis, the papillae of the columns of Morgagni will be inflamed and edematous. The distal rectal mucosa likewise may be erythematous, thickened, hemorrhagic, and granular in appearance. In this case, the submucosal vessels are no longer apparent. Mild abrasion of the mucosa with a cotton swab will produce punctate areas of bleeding if the mucosa is friable, as in ulcerative colitis. Occasionally, deep anal ulcers may be noted in patients with granulomatous disease. These ulcers may extend to involve the sphincteric musculature. Low rectal tumors may also be encountered. Internal openings of fistulae in ano may also be seen, usually in the area of the anal crypts.

In attempting to demonstrate internal hemorrhoids, the examiner should carefully inspect the anal canal at the 9, l, and 5 o'clock positions. In the knee-chest position, hemorrhoids may not be prominent because of positional drainage; this phenomenon is support for the use of Sims' position for digital and anoscopic examination when hemorrhoids are suspected. Asking the patient to "bear down" while the proctoscope is being withdrawn will also make internal hemorrhoids more apparent. In addition, during withdrawal of the instrument, inspection at the 12 and 6 o'clock positions may demonstrate anal fissures which appear as slightly excavated raw areas and which occasionally bleed.

The sphincteric musculature gives the anal canal an anterior-posterior elliptical shape, and rotation of a conventional anoscope in the anal canal may be difficult as well as uncomfortable to the patient. This is especially true when the lateral anal wall is being examined. Therefore the examiner should withdraw the proctoscope, replace the obturator, and reinsert the instrument on four occasions in order to examine each quadrant if any difficulty in turning the instrument is encountered. Biopsy of any anal nonvascular lesion should be made after the full examination is completed.

SIGMOIDOSCOPY

Sigmoidoscopy is an indispensable part of adequate examination of the rectum and colon for patients of any age, and is an integral part of the complete physical examination for individuals over age 40. When combined with biopsy, sigmoidoscopy is the best single diagnostic procedure for disorders of the rectum and lower sigmoid colon. The high incidence of carcinoma of the colon in the United States and the fact that approximately 70 per cent of these tumors are within reach of the sigmoidoscope make the importance of this procedure quite clear.

INDICATIONS AND INSTRUMENTS

Indications for sigmoidoscopy are many and varied. Some obvious ones include local anal or rectal discomfort, change in bowel pattern or stool character, weight loss, lower abdominal pain, rectal tenesmus, overt rectal bleeding or melena, unexplained iron deficiency anemia, and fever of unknown origin. It is useful for diagnosis of bacterial or parasitic diarrheas, as a gauge of therapeutic effectiveness in the treatment of ulcerative colitis or proctitis, and in reduction of sigmoid volvulus. The only real contraindication to sigmoidoscopy is rectal obstruction near the anus, although an uncooperative patient may make the procedure inadvisable. The consideration of need for a barium enema examination should simultaneously prompt plans for an antecedent sigmoidoscopy.

Most adult sigmoidoscopes are cylindrical, rigid instruments 25 cm long and 1.6 cm wide. Small diameter instruments are available for infants and persons with severe anal disease or low rectal strictures. Sigmoidoscopes differ mainly in whether the light is located at the tip of the instrument or near the proximal end. Those sigmoidoscopes with a proximal light source are less likely to have the illumination obscured by liquid or stool during insertion of the instrument, but they do not illuminate mucosa quite so well as instruments with the light placed distally. The proximal light source, nevertheless, is usually sufficient unless subtle changes in the mucosa are being sought. Newer, flexible fiberoptic sigmoidoscopes and longer colonoscopes are becoming more generally available and should dramatically increase the diagnostic ability of the endoscopist.

PREPARATION AND POSITIONING

An equally good case can be made either for no bowel-cleansing preparation before sigmoidoscopy or for the routine use of an enema prior to sigmoidoscopy to assure a feces-free rectosigmoid. Irritant enemas tend to cause mild mucosal hyperemia and increase colonic mucus production. A reasonable course to follow would seem to be avoidance of preparative enemas in those patients who have diarrhea as their major complaint or who are suspected of having primarily diffuse mucosal disease. In the remainder of patients or in those in whom presigmoidoscopic rectal examination reveals firm stool in the ampulla, a preparative enema or laxative suppository may be used. The sigmoidoscopist should take careful note of changes induced by such preparations in otherwise normal persons in order to properly evaluate subsequent patients having mucosal disease.

The procedure should begin with a brief explanation to the patient of what will be done, being certain to clarify that some degree of discomfort will occur but that pain should not be severe if relaxation is good. Many patients experience an intense sensation of need to defecate when the rectum is instrumented. A brief forewarning will contribute much toward alleviating such anxiety. The examiner should maintain a reassuring conversation throughout the procedure, explaining what is going on and what will happen next. Adults should be examined in the knee-chest or knee-elbow position or on a special inverting sigmoidoscopy table. Debilitated patients may have sigmoidoscopy in Sims' position with the hips close to the edge of the bed or table and the foot of the support elevated.

TECHNIQUE

At least monodigital rectal examination must always precede sigmoidoscopy in order to exclude low rectal strictures, to give warning of a low rectal mass, and also to promote sphincter relaxation. Following rectal examination and with the obturator in place, a well lubricated and warm sigmoidoscope should be placed against the anal sphincter and firm but gentle pressure applied. The patient may be asked to "bear down" against the tip, a maneuver which usually results in easy passage of the instrument through the anal sphincter. As the tip of the sigmoidoscope is introduced, it should be turned upward or posteriorly toward the sacrum and the instrument advanced blindly for only 2 or 3 inches. The sigmoidoscope should never be passed blindly until an obstruction is reached. The obturator is removed and any adherent stool or mucus examined for blood and pus. After adjustment of the light source, excessive liquid or stool in the rectal ampulla should be aspirated or removed, the glass window closed, and the insufflation bulb attached. Fastidious cleansing of the mucosal wall is not indicated at this point, because the sigmoidoscope should be inserted to its full length as early in the procedure as possible. Some insufflation of air may be required to visualize the distal lumen to be traversed; however, the sigmoidoscope can usually be passed with little or no air being used. "Pumping up" the colon in attempts to pass the sigmoidoscope will only produce patient discomfort, and may lead to cardiac arrhythmias in patients with cardiovascular disease.[1]

During passage of the sigmoidoscope through the rectum, side-to-side movement of the tip is occasionally necessary if the valves of Houston are quite prominent. The tip of the instrument is initially directed posteriorly as the rectum follows the hollow of the sacrum. The direction is then changed to slightly anterior toward the umbilicus as the rectum rises out of the pelvis. The first major difficulty is usually encountered at the rectosigmoid junction, or at about 15 cm from the pectinate line. Here the sigmoid flexure begins and the bowel lumen turns more anteriorly and may go either briefly to the right or directly to the left. Often the bowel wall on the inner side of the curve will appear as a semilunar ring of tissue beyond which a blind pouch exists. If the side of the sigmoidoscope is placed against this "rim" and the tip of the instrument swung laterally and anteriorly to that side while being slowly advanced, the distal lumen may then become visible. It is at this point that colicky pain is likely to be felt by the patient, and subsequent passage of the instrument may be difficult because of the spasm produced. Under no circumstances should the sigmoidoscope be forcefully pushed against the mucosa with the hope that the bowel will eventually slide along the instrument. Such action may perforate the rectum. Continued insufflation with air will not make the lumen visible and will only increase difficulty of passage. The patient should be reassured and attempts at passage repeated with extreme gentleness. If the head of the sigmoidoscope is held firmly and the shaft maneuvered in such a manner that the angle of movement is at the anus, the tip can usually be directed without excessive pulling on pain-sensitive anal tissue and sphincter musculature. Occasionally the rectosigmoid flexure cannot be passed, even by experienced sigmoidoscopists. Barium enema examination in these cases is adequate above this point unless biopsy of a known lesion is desired. Once the rectosigmoid curve is negotiated, the instrument can usually be passed to its hilt with ease and inspection to 25 or 30 cm accomplished by insufflation of small amounts of air.

After insertion to the greatest depth possible, the sigmoidoscope should be withdrawn slowly and close inspection made of the mucosa. During this procedure intermittent air insufflation is helpful in "ironing out" the mucosa for a complete 360-degree inspection of the lumen. A circular corkscrew-like motion of the tip of the sigmoidoscope will facilitate visualization of the entire lumen. Sharp angulation of the instrument with the perineum may be necessary to inspect the entire rectal ampulla. Anoscopy should be done to inspect anal lesions or those in the lower part of the ampulla, because their evaluation with the sigmoidoscope is usually unsatisfactory.

Specific notation should be made of the content of the sigmoid colon and rectum, including character of the stool, location of mucus or pus, and, if blood is present, its source, i.e., the proximal lumen, a specific lesion, or a diffuse mucosal disease. Any change in luminal size or contour such as might be produced by stricture or external compression is important. Local mucosal disease such as polyps or tumors should be described not only by appearance but also by location on the bowel wall and depth of insertion of the sigmoidoscope.

EVALUATION OF THE MUCOSA

Finally, close attention must be given to the appearance of the mucosa. The normal rectal mucosa is smooth, pale salmon pink and glistening; through it the submucosal blood vessels should be visible as a bluish-purple network. This vascular pattern is most prominent in the rectal ampulla and becomes less visible or even absent in the lower sigmoid colon. Inflammation of the mucosa produces hyperemia and edema, with the earliest sign usually being loss of this vascular pattern. The mucosa may also lose its glistening appearance and will later appear thickened and granular. A characteristic finding in persons with proctocolitis is mucosal friability. This refers to the occurrence of minute mucosal bleeding points or petechiae after the mucosa is mildly abraded with a cotton-tip swab. The blunt end of a biopsy forceps may also be used, if a swab is not available.

Apparent mucosal ulceration should be closely evaluated. Small patches of whitish mucus on the mucosa may give the appearance of discrete ulcers, but the differentiation should be easily made. Rectal ulceration is uncommon in idiopathic proctocolitis and, if definitely present, should suggest the possibility of another diagnosis such as amebiasis (see pp. 1386 to 1392).

Any lesion projecting into the lumen should be carefully described. It is important to note not only size and location but also whether it is sessile or pedunculated, whether it is single or multiple, and whether the overlying mucosa is intact or ulcerated (Fig. 113–1). (The typical sigmoidoscopic features of polyps are also discussed on pages 1438 to 1441.) A carcinoma either may be exophytic and cauliflower-like in shape or may be an ulcerating lesion with raised margins (Fig. 113–2).

Biopsy of a lesion or of a suspicious-looking mucosa during sigmoidoscopy should be accomplished as soon as possible, because it may be difficult to visualize later if the lesion is small or excess stool or blood is present (see pp. 1501 to 1507).

COMPLICATIONS

Complications of sigmoidoscopy should be minimal if good technique has been used. A sensation of abdominal fullness and "gas pains" are sequelae of excessive use of air insufflation. Occasionally vague lower abdominal pain may represent peritoneal irritation from ill-defined causes, although compression of the bowel wall

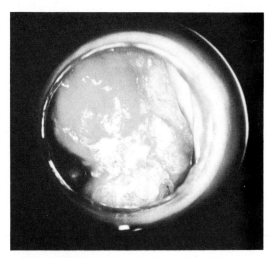

Figure 113–2.   An exophytic cancer of the rectum seen on sigmoidoscopy.

between the sigmoidoscope and the promontory of the sacrum, as well as excess traction on the mesentery, may be contributory factors. Bleeding from a biopsied lesion or rectal valve is usually not excessive. More extensive intestinal trauma must always be considered in the patient who develops increasing abdominal discomfort or fever after the procedure. Mild tenesmus which begins during sigmoidoscopy should disappear after the instrument is removed. Its persistence may result from blood or air in the bowel wall which has dissected there during the procedure through a small mucosal tear. The tip of the sigmoidoscope may perforate the bowel. A tear in the rectum below the peritoneal reflection is usually extraperitoneal, and a localized abscess may develop. The most frequent site of bowel perforation during sigmoidoscopy, however, is on the anterior intestinal wall just above the peritoneal reflection. This almost always occurs while the operator is attempting to traverse the rectosigmoid flexure and produces a free communication of the bowel lumen with the peritoneal cavity. Aggressive surgical therapy is indicated as soon as an intra-abdominal perforation is recognized, because any delay increases mortality.

In patients with profuse rectal bleeding, sigmoidoscopy is rightly considered an early diagnostic procedure. However, initial correction of blood volume should precede the procedure, and the use of Sims'

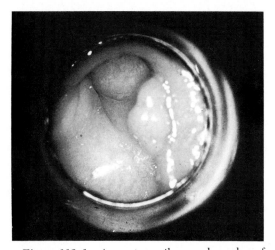

Figure 113–1.   A squat, sessile vascular polyp of the rectum seen on sigmoidoscopy.

position instead of the classic head-down position should be considered. Acute pulmonary edema, shock, and cardiac arrhythmias may result from failure to consider cardiovascular hemodynamics. Cardiac arrhythmias and even death have occurred during sigmoidoscopy in patients with advanced heart disease. In these patients, the procedure should be as brief as possible, and excessive air insufflation and traction on the intestine should be avoided.

With experience, the sigmoidoscopist can usually complete the procedure with minimal discomfort to the patient. Avoidance of mucosal biopsies above the peritoneal reflection and awareness of the aforementioned complications will concontribute safety to the known value of sigmoidoscopy in diagnosing and following anorectal disease.

HEMORRHOIDS

Hemorrhoids or piles are varicosities of the veins comprising the hemorrhoidal venous plexus. When they are below the anorectal line, covered by anal skin, and involve only the inferior venous plexus, they are termed external hemorrhoids. Those from the superior plexus above the dentate line and covered by mucous membrane are called internal hemorrhoids. Mixed hemorrhoids exist because of the free anastomosis of these two plexuses. It is important to differentiate the location involved, because symptoms, treatment, and clinical course differ. The following discussion will outline some essential clinical points regarding hemorrhoids. Communications in proctology journals detailing special modes of surgical treatment are frequent, and therefore are only briefly mentioned here. Proctology texts should be consulted for a more detailed discussion.[2, 3]

Although the terms *hemorrhoid* and *pile* are both used, they have different meanings; hemorrhoid is derived from the Greek and means bleeding, whereas pile is of Latin origin and means a ball. They both refer to common presentations of the condition. The incidence of hemorrhoids or piles is difficult to determine. They are rare in children but become progressively more frequent after age 20 and tend to occur in active persons whose occupations entail muscular straining or prolonged standing or sitting in one position.

PATHOGENESIS

Pressure in the hemorrhoidal veins has been shown to increase threefold when the erect posture is assumed.[4] The absence of valves in the portal venous system makes hydrostatic pressure of the superior hemorrhoidal veins the likely cause for this increase in pressure and explains why man's erect posture makes him uniquely susceptible to hemorrhoid formation and why recumbency has an ameliorating effect. During the straining which occurs with defecation, the hydrostatic pressure in the superior hemorrhoidal veins is increased by the increased intra-abdominal pressure with some degree of distention of the hemorrhoidal plexus in the anal canal. Over the years, repetition of minor distention of these veins may result in internal hemorrhoid formation. This phenomenon, associated with weakness of the anal paravenous supporting tissue, may explain why about 70 per cent of persons over 40 years of age have hemorrhoids.[5] In addition this concept helps to explain why certain clinical situations or activities have been associated with the development of symptomatic hemorrhoids. Examples of these include cirrhosis of the liver with portal hypertension, thrombosis of the portal vein, excessive straining at stool, both constipation and diarrhea, chronic heart failure or constrictive pericarditis, chronic coughing or recurrent vomiting, and occupations requiring prolonged straining.

Intra-abdominal or pelvic tumors are also frequently associated with the development of hemorrhoids. Pregnancy is the prime example, and is the most common cause of hemorrhoids in young women. Carcinoma of the rectum may contribute to hemorrhoid formation both directly, by compromising venous drainage, and indirectly, by straining during defecation. This straining may occur in association with the characteristic alternating constipation and diarrhea of carcinoma of the left colon or in attempts to relieve the sensation of incomplete rectal emptying.

EXTERNAL HEMORRHOIDS

Varicosities of the external hemorrhoidal plexus are usually properly referred to as piles, because excessive bleeding is usually not a major symptom. These piles form just outside the anal orifice, often develop during straining at stool, and are covered by anal skin rather than mucosa; therefore pain is the major symptom. The acute pile develops because of venous thrombosis or, probably more commonly, from rupture of the vein and formation of a subcutaneous hematoma. The patient suddenly develops a lump on the anus which is painful and which is worsened by defecation. Examination reveals a rounded, bluish, very tender mass covered by tense skin. Spontaneous resolution usually occurs in four or five days with either complete disappearance or the formation of a small, loose anal tag. Occasionally ulceration of the skin overlying the acute pile develops. Infection may occur if the clot is not completely expressed.

In general, treatment is conservative and consists mainly of maintaining a recumbent position as much as is practical, systemic and local analgesics, hot sitz baths, stool softeners, and the avoidance of straining or strenuous work. If rupture of the pile occurs, the clot must be completely expressed or extracted, or the complete hemorrhoid excised. If small anal skin tags form after resolution, no specific therapy for them is indicated. The finding of anal tags on physical examination suggests former active piles. These primary skin tags are to be differentiated, however, from a secondary skin tag which is often found at the external end of a fissure in ano or in association with pruritus ani.

INTERNAL HEMORRHOIDS

Varicosities of the superior hemorrhoidal veins may be properly referred to as either piles or hemorrhoids, because their main symptoms are prolapse with formation of an anal mass and bleeding. Internal hemorrhoids protrude during defecation but retract above the dentate line early in the course of the disease. Later prolape is more complete but is still transient and is associated with increased intra-abdominal pressure. Eventually, the hemorrhoids may be more or less permanently prolapsed. In the moderately advanced stage, a mucoid anal discharge is common and worsens with increasing prolapse. Anal irritation from the discharge often produces intense pruritus and may contribute to maceration of the tissue overlying the hemorrhoid. This, combined with excessive tissue thinning from stretching and abrasion caused by firm stool, may result in bleeding. Bleeding from hemorrhoids is usually intermittent, occurs with defecation, is usually of a small amount, and is seen as bright red streaks on the outside of the stool or on toilet paper. Recurrent hemorrhoidal bleeding may produce iron deficiency and even severe anemia. Therefore inquiry about hemorrhoidal symptoms and anoscopy should be part of any evaluation for occult blood loss or iron deficiency anemia. Occasionally bleeding is severe, and its volume tends to be exaggerated by the patient. True acute massive bleeding is uncommon unless portal hypertension is present.

OTHER COMPLICATIONS

In contradistinction to external hemorrhoids, true internal hemorrhoids are covered by mucosa rather than skin and are not painful, even with prolapse and bleeding. Protruding, bleeding hemorrhoids which become extremely painful are probably a mixed type. Nevertheless, the physician should always consider the possibility that a severely prolapsed internal hemorrhoid has acutely thrombosed. In this situation, the hemorrhoid becomes hard, tender, and nonreducible. Some edema of the perianal skin may develop. The patient usually becomes aware of a painful swelling at the anus which makes sitting uncomfortable. The onset is not so dramatic as occlusion of an external hemorrhoid; if the thrombosed vessel is completely above the pectinate line, it is possible that the process will be painless. In addition to local edema, examination of the anus usually reveals the purplish-red skin or mucosa overlying the prolapsed thrombosed hemorrhoid. Digital examination of the anal canal is very painful, and anoscopy may be impossible in the acute stage.

Similar to the course of external hemorrhoids, the condition usually resolves spontaneously over a few days. A fibrotic mass may persist on the anal wall which is easily palpable during subsequent digital rectal examinations. Occasionally ulceration of the overlying mucosa develops, leading to abscess formation in either the perianal or ischiorectal areas. Finally, although rare, dislodgment of infected clots into the superior hemorrhoidal vein and portal tributaries can produce septic emboli to the liver.[6]

DIAGNOSIS AND TREATMENT

The diagnosis of internal hemorrhoids is usually easy if careful proctoscopy is performed. Using Sims' position as well as having the patient strain down intermittently while the anal canal is visualized will facilitate demonstration of internal hemorrhoids. Particular attention should be directed to the right anterior, right posterior, and left lateral anal wall, because the majority of patients will have internal hemorrhoids located only in these positions.[2]

Conservative treatment for internal hemorrhoids is similar to that outlined above for external piles. The use of astringent preparations may diminish bleeding. The only definitive treatments are injection therapy or surgical removal. Because symptomatic hemorrhoids tend to be a cyclical problem, many patients do not require either of these procedures. However, when persistent severe prolapse or recurrent significant bleeding develops, definitive therapy is indicated.

Surgical therapy for hemorrhoids may be indicated for bleeding, protrusion, thrombosis, ulceration, infection, or coexistent severe pruritus ani. The exact time to resort to surgery will vary from patient to patient. Acute thrombosis of internal hemorrhoids is best treated by early surgical referral.

Injection therapy is applicable only for uncomplicated internal hemorrhoids, and is performed most commonly for troublesome bleeding which occurs with defecation. A solution which provokes an inflammatory response and subsequent fibrosis is injected directly into the hemorrhoid or into the submucosal tissue above it, with the purpose of both obliterating the hemorrhoid and removing its communication with the hydrostatic pressure in the portal system. If done properly, results can be satisfactory. This procedure should be considered for severe cardiac patients in whom rectal bleeding is a significant problem and in whom anesthesia and painful surgery are best avoided. Injection treatments should not be done when there is a coexistent abscess, fistula, fissure, cryptitis, or anal stenosis.

Internal hemorrhoids may also be treated by ligation with small rubber bands applied with special instruments. After ischemic necrosis, the hemorrhoid sloughs off the mucosa. Patients selected for this procedure are similar to those in whom surgical excision would otherwise be done. Bleeding and thrombosis of the perianal veins are the main complications. Because it is a relatively painless procedure and can be accomplished on an outpatient basis, this treatment is a reasonable approach for a single, moderate-sized internal hemorrhoid.

SPECIAL CONSIDERATIONS IN TREATMENT

Three situations require comment. Hemorrhoids appearing during pregnancy should not be considered for surgical treatment for at least six months after pregnancy is terminated unless severe complications develop. Even the largest hemorrhoids can recede after delivery. Close attention to stool consistency, avoidance of prolonged periods of straining with defecation, and lubrication of the anal canal if necessary prior to defecation will usually help the situation to remain uncomplicated.

Secondly, the hemorrhoidal anastomosis of the portal vein with the systemic venous system can provide significant decompression of the portal system in patients with advanced cirrhosis and portal hypertension. Removal of this collateral pathway may elevate portal pressure and precipitate esophageal variceal bleeding. In general, if patients with portal hypertension develop excessive bleeding from internal hemorrhoids, the exact hemorrhoid which is bleeding should be located. If it is low in the anal canal, a Foley catheter with a large balloon may be placed in the rectum, the balloon inflated, and tamponade effected by pulling down gently on the catheter. Hemostatic surgical foams can be interposed between the balloon and the anal mucosa. If this fails or if the hemorrhoid is higher in the rectal ampulla, a hemostatic suture will be necessary. In these patients, elective hemorrhoidectomy and injection therapy should be avoided.

Finally, symptomatic hemorrhoids in persons with leukemia, incurable cancer, or intractable heart disease should have the most minimal therapy which is effective.

ANORECTAL ABSCESS AND FISTULA IN ANO

ANORECTAL ABSCESS

Patients who present with a rapidly developing painful anal mass should be examined for the possibility of an anorectal abscess as well as for hemorrhoids. Abscess formation is relatively common in perianal and perirectal tissues and, after an acute period, may persist as a chronic infection. Awareness by internists of the condition and its sequelae is necessary for proper diagnosis; however, the correct treatment is surgical.

Abscesses which develop in potential spaces surrounding the anus and rectum are named by their location. Most common are *perianal abscesses.* These superficial abscesses are immediately adjacent to the anal opening, and may extend up between the external and internal sphincters to the level of the anal valves. They can become quite large and contain thick pus. Severe, often throbbing pain is the major symptom; it is aggravated by pressure on the area either during sitting or from stool passage. The patient may notice a swelling adjacent to the anus. Occasionally the abscess drains spontaneously, with concomitant relief of the intense pain. Examination reveals a painful red swollen area adjacent to the anus with little or no tenderness of surrounding tissues. Digital examination of the anus should demonstrate pain and induration only below the level of the anorectal ring. Treatment is surgical drainage.

The *ischiorectal fossa* is the second most common location for an anorectal abscess. This abscess involves deep tissues in the buttocks. Although it lies outside the external anal sphincter and below the levator ani muscles, it may extend through both these muscular barriers. In addition, it is not uncommon for the abscess to be bilateral, encircling the posterior part of the rectum. Instead of pain, toxic symptoms, including fever and malaise, are most prominent. Perirectal discomfort deep in the buttocks and fever may be the only findings. Fever with no spontaneous pain is encountered frequently enough to make careful anorectal examination part of any evaluation of fever of unknown origin. Inspection reveals a diffuse swelling of the perianal region, usually only on the one side which is tender. On rectal examination there is a large tender mass which may bulge into the anal canal either on one side or bilaterally and posteriorly when both ischiorectal fossae are involved. Patients in whom fever is the only manifestation usually have an abscess high in the ischiorectal fossa. Often these may be diagnosed only by firm palpation of the deep perirectal tissue between a finger in the rectum and the thumb placed externally. A deep postanal abscess can extend to become an ischiorectal abscess and also present only with toxic symptoms. This location for the abscess is palpated posterior to the anus as a midline lump. Treatment in each instance is again surgical drainage.

Toxic symptoms are also prominent in submucous and pelvirectal abscesses. *Submucous abscesses* are located in the submucous space of the anal canal above the anal valves and may extend superiorly above the anorectal ring into the rectal submucosa. The abscess may cause fever and a dull pain in the rectum but occasionally presents with only a purulent rectal discharge. Usually there is no visible perianal abnormality. Digital rectal examination reveals a smooth tender swelling on the upper wall of the anal canal or lower rectum. Pus can occasionally be expressed from the indurated area during proctoscopic examination if spontaneous damage has occurred.

A *pelvirectal abscess* may appear "spontaneously" or can develop from infections elsewhere in the pelvis. Minimal local anorectal discomfort is present in this situation, and toxic symptoms again predominate. Rectal examination will demonstrate a tender mass high in the pelvis, with the rectal mucous membrane seemingly involved in the inflammatory process. Surgical drainage is the only proper treatment.

Anorectal abscesses may develop as a complication of ruptured acute hemorrhoids; secondary to anal fissures; after anal injections for hemorrhoids, fissures, or pruritus ani; or from direct trauma to the anorectal area, such as in improper use of enema nozzles. Hard objects in the feces may abrade the anal canal, and infection may develop. However, there is often no obvious history to incriminate any of the aforementioned states. Extension of infection into the anal glands from anal cryptitis and subsequently into the perianal and perirectal spaces has been a popular etiological theory for abscess formation.[7] However, its merit continues to be debated.[2] The exact causal relationship between inflammatory bowel disease, especially granulomatous colitis, and anorectal abscess is not known. The association occurs so frequently, however, that recurrent anorectal abscesses should prompt evaluation for more generalized bowel disease.[8]

A *tuberculous anorectal abscess* often presents with a gradually enlarging perianal or ischiorectal mass. Frequently, the mass ruptures spontaneously and drains a watery discharge. Fortunately, tuberculous abscesses are now rare in this country. Periurethral abscess in the male and infection in Bartholin's glands in the female may be confused with an anterior perirectal abscess. Acute early hidradenitis, which is an inflammation in the perianal apocrine sweat glands, may also be mistaken for a more typical perianal abscess.

FISTULA IN ANO

After an acute infection in the anorectal area, a chronic suppurative process frequently develops in the form of an anal fistula. This fistula is a tract of chronic granulation tissue which connects two epithelial surfaces, either cutaneous or mucosal, and may have several external openings. The wall of the tract is usually thick fibrous tissue lined by granulation tissue. It can frequently be palpated as a tubular mass. If the chronic granulating tract is only open at one end, it is referred to as a sinus. Therefore a fistula in ano which follows an anorectal abscess usually has one internal opening to the mucosa of the anal or rectal canal and one or more external openings draining to the perianal skin. Any of the anorectal abscesses just discussed may lead to a chronic fistula, especially if spontaneous rupture occurs or drainage has been incomplete.

Treatment of a fistula in ano is an incision along the length of the fistulous tract with excision of its fibrous wall. The course of the fistula tract must be determined with localization of both internal and external openings.

The location of the internal fistula opening tends to follow Goodsall's rule; i.e., fistulas with their external openings anterior to a line drawn across the midportion of the anus will run directly to the adjacent anal wall, whereas fistulous openings posterior to this line will curve around the anal wall and have their opening in the posterior midline. The vertical extension of the tract is also important, because hospitalization is prolonged if the tract involves the levator ani muscles. In addition, rectal incontinence may develop if the therapeutic incision must cut across the anorectal line.

Usually symptoms of a fistula follow those of an abscess, but occasionally no history of an acute infection can be obtained. Occasionally there may be a history of one or more surgical procedures for the original abscess. When it follows a perianal abscess, the anal fistula is usually painless unless its drainage has been blocked. The main symptom is a persistent or intermittent discharge from the opening which soils the patient's clothes and leads to soreness and itching of the perianal skin. If the fistula is from an ischiorectal abscess, the patient may continue to have discomfort in the region. The external opening is usually quite a distance from the anus. When a fistula develops after a submucous abscess, the patient may have persistent anal discomfort with a troublesome anal discharge but no apparent external fistulous opening. Digital rectal examination will reveal a firm cord on the anorectal wall extending up from the pectinate line.

Full examination of the external anal skin, anal canal, and lower rectal lumen will be necessary by inspection, palpation, and anoscopy if symptoms suggest a fistula. If the diagnosis is unsure, proctological consultation is indicated, because conservative treatment is rarely successful. Although a perianal sinus tract may appear to be only a typical fistula in ano, other possibilities may exist. Anterior "fistulas" may result from chronically infected periurethral or Bartholin's glands, and multiple fistulous openings may develop in patients with chronic hidradenitis. Other possibilities which can produce chronic perianal fistulous tracts include tuberculosis, rectal lymphogranuloma venereum, actinomycosis, colloid carcinoma of the anorectal area, and, most important, both ulcerative colitis and regional enteritis.

ANAL FISSURE

Fissure in ano or anal fissure refers to a painful ulcer at the anal orifice which is elliptical in shape and extends from the anal verge into the anal canal as far as the pectinate line. It is a common condition and produces severe anal pain of a far greater degree than its size suggests.

An acute anal fissure is usually located in the midline posteriorly and appears as a simple split in the skin. Secondary changes soon develop, the most striking of which is swelling of the anal skin at the lower end of the fissure. This tag-like swelling, called a sentinel pile, is often very inflamed, and may later undergo fibrosis and persist as a permanent skin tag even after the fissure has healed. The anal valve above the fissure may become swollen and form a hypertrophied anal papilla. This is smaller than the sentinel pile. The fissure may "erode" down to the internal sphincter musculature which then becomes visible as whitish strands in the ulcer base. In a chronic fissure, fibrous induration develops in the lateral margin of the fissure. At any stage, the process may suppurate and lead to formation of a perianal abscess. Of special concern is the persistent spasm of the internal anal sphincter. After several months fibrosis

may occur, and a fibrotic, tightly contracted internal sphincter may result.

The exact cause of an anal fissure is unknown. Many patients date the onset of symptoms to passage of a large bolus of hard stool. This may suggest that anal trauma, overstretching of the anal canal, or distention of hemorrhoidal veins produces excessive thinning of the overlying mucosa, making it more susceptible to trauma. Infection may be contributory, but it seems unlikely as a primary cause. Sphincter spasm has been incriminated as contributing to chronicity, it being suggested that spasm keeps the edges of the fissure together, preventing adequate drainage.

SYMPTOMS AND DIAGNOSIS

The main symptom of anal fissure is a sharp, very painful cutting or tearing sensation in the anus which occurs during passage of stool and which may be followed for a few hours by severe burning pain. Although common, bleeding is not always present and usually limited to staining the toilet tissue. The sentinel pile may be interpreted by persons with previous symptomatic hemorrhoids or piles as a recurrence of former disease, but persistence of symptoms and the painful sphincter spasm will cause the patient to seek assistance. A copious amount of anal discharge may be present and contribute to the development of pruritus ani which compounds the problem.

Diagnosis can be made by the typical history and during physical examination often by inspection alone. However, anal spasm may tightly close the anal orifice and conceal the fissure. A gradual lateral pull on the edges of the anus may overcome the spasm. Local application of a topical anesthetic ointment may be necessary. The sentinel pile and vertical elliptical ulcer should be easily seen. Insertion of the finger for digital examination produces much pain, with most tenderness elicited from pressure on the fissure itself. Induration lateral to the fissure as well as the presence of the hypertrophied anal papilla at the superior margin may be felt. Because of the pain, proctoscopy is often not possible during the acute stage but should be done eventually to look for other lesions.

The diagnosis should be readily made. However, differential possibilities must be considered, especially in chronic fissures and in those involving the lateral or anterior anal walls. Broad fissures with marked surrounding inflammation may be seen with ulcerative colitis or ulcerative proctitis, and if there is extensive fissuring, coexistent Crohn's disease should be considered. Pruritus ani may develop secondary to anal fissures or vice versa. In the latter case true anal spasm is absent, and there are often other cracks in the anal skin. A chancre of primary anal syphilis may resemble a typical anal fissure, but there is often a lesion on the opposite anal wall. In seven to ten days, marked induration around the apparent fissure and enlargement of inguinal nodes may develop. In questionable cases, a dark-field examination of material from the ulcer and serological tests for syphilis should be done. Tuberculous ulcers and erosions occurring with squamous cell carcinoma of the anus may occasionally produce changes similar to a chronic fissure. Biopsy should be done if the fissure appears abnormal.

TREATMENT

Most fissures probably heal spontaneously after a relatively short history of pain. Initial conservative treatment includes hot sitz baths, stool softeners, and topical anesthetic ointment before stool passage. Dilatation of the spastic sphincter has been shown to give good results in many cases.[9, 10] The simplest method is to stretch the anus with the finger during digital examination after adequate anesthesia. This procedure is most useful when the fissure complicates inflammatory bowel disease and any surgery seems best avoided. When there is recurrence of the fissure after sphincter stretching and especially if there is extensive exposure of fibers of the internal sphincter muscles in the base of the fissure, surgical therapy will usually be required.

CRYPTITIS AND PAPILLITIS

Cryptitis refers to a local infection in a crypt of Morgagni behind an anal valve. If it is associated with persistent occlusion of a duct of the anal gland, the inflammatory process may become an abscess in the connective tissue of the anal canal or in the perianal and ischiorectal spaces. Papillitis is inflammation of a papilla manifested by mild anal discomfort, usually worsened during defecation. Digital examination of the rectum often demonstrates a small area of induration and tenderness below the anorectal ring at the level of the pectinate line. An enlarged anal papilla is easily felt as a movable nodule on the anal wall. During anoscopy, an area of redness on the anal wall at the pectinate line and enlargement of the adjacent papilla can be seen. Occasionally, a small amount of pus can be expressed by pressing at the edge of the indurated area.

The crypts should be explored with a curved tip probe and any obstructing fecal particles removed. Usually no specific treatment is needed. If symptoms persist, the affected crypt can be cauterized. However, the main concern is extension of the process with abscess formation. If a large area of induration persists, pain intensifies, or a sinus tract seems to be present, the patient should be referred to a proctologist.

A large edematous anal papilla will usually disappear as the inflammation subsides. Occasionally fibrosis causes an enlarged anal papilla to persist. Usually no therapy is indicated. However, with time some enlarged papillae elongate, undergo considerable fibrous thickening, and may produce symptoms by projecting through the anus during defecation. In this situation, surgical removal of the papillae may be required. A fibrosed hypertrophied anal papilla may also be present at the upper end of a chronic anal fissure. Careful inspection for a fissure should be made, because treatment for it is indicated.

PRURITUS ANI

Pruritis ani is a term used to describe intense, perianal itching. In some instances it refers to a symptom which accompanies another well defined disease involving the anus; however, in the majority of patients it represents the primary manifestation of a disease process having intense anal pruritus as its main symptom and no obvious cause.

Anal pruritus from any cause may begin with slight itching in only one part of the anus. Later it may become more severe and spread to involve not only the entire perianal skin but also the vulva and posterior scrotum; however it is most marked around the anus and the median raphe. Many patients experience most intense symptoms at night and during warm weather. A maddening desire to scratch the perianal area almost incessantly develops, and the relief achieved thereby is short lived. In severe cases the itching becomes almost intolerable, and exhaustion caused by inability to sleep at night and constant anxiety during the day may become a major problem.

TYPES

General examination of the patient as well as complete examination of the anus will usually immediately help to determine whether the condition is primary or secondary to another disease. In the latter group are a number of skin diseases which may involve the anus and the so-called surgical lesions of the anus with associated pruritus. This latter group includes prolapsing hemorrhoids, prolapse of the rectum, benign or malignant tumors of the rectum, chronic anal fissure and anal fistula, diarrhea with colitis or proctitis, and, possibly, extreme hypertrophy of an anal papilla. Nevertheless, even if one of these is present, it may not be the cause of the patient's pruritus.

In early cases, the secondary skin folds are less prominent and the primary rugae may be quite edematous and red. Regardless of the cause, chronic scratching of the perianal area in advanced pruritus will cause the anal skin to be moist and macerated with multiple excoriations. Later the skin is usually thickened or lichenified with increased pigmentation. Superficial traumatic ulcers may be present. With extreme chronicity, leukoplakia of the anus may develop, with pale white areas of skin contained within hyperpigmented patches.

SKIN DISORDERS

Dermatological abnormalities must be closely evaluated. Seborrheic dermatitis, atopic eczema, psoriasis, lichen planus, neurodermatitis, and contact dermatitis may all produce severe itching when the perianal area is involved. Although anal psoriasis may not have the typical red plaque with a shiny scale, the adjacent buttocks are often involved and more typical lesions are often present on the elbows, knees, and scalp. Anal seborrheic dermatitis can occasionally be difficult to distinguish from psoriasis, but the finding of seborrheic lesions on the scalp and trunk may help. Lichen planus presents with violaceous flat-topped papules and is usually present elsewhere on the body. Atopic eczema frequently occurs in the flexor surface of the elbows and knees and should be present in these areas if the anal lesion is also present. Neurodermatitis tends to occur in patients with a history of psychiatric problems, but evidence of the same process elsewhere on the skin should be found to secure this diagnosis. Allergic or contact dermatitis may result from soaps or ointments used by the patient in an attempt to alleviate the initial mild symptoms. Ointments containing topical anesthetics are notorious offenders in this regard. Any medication used topically or as a suppository by the patient for the pruritus must be suspected as contributing to the process on an atopic basis and should therefore be temporarily discontinued.

INFECTION

Inspection of the perianal area may also suggest a parasitic or fungal cause. Scabies should certainly be considered as a cause if the characteristic lesions are also present between the fingers and on the volar surface of the wrist. The findings of nits or the parasite itself may lead to a diagnosis of pediculosis pubis with extension to the perianal region. However, in both these conditions, an area larger than perianal skin is involved. In children, pinworm infestation is a common cause of pruritus ani. The adult female worms migrate out of the anus at night to lay eggs. Occasionally, the small hair-like white adult worms can be seen on proctoscopy. The diagnosis is better and more easily made by finding the typical *Enterobius vermicularis* eggs (eliptical, with one side flattened) on a piece of transparent adhesive tape pressed against the anus in the early morning (sticky side out on a tongue-blade as support) and then placed on a microscope slide for later examination.

Both fungi (Epidermophyton or Trichophyton) and yeast, usually *Candida albicans*, may produce pruritus ani. This diagnosis should be suspected when there is a well defined lateral border of an area of abnormal perianal skin.

Monilial infection may be the cause of pruritus ani in patients with diabetes mellitus. Epidermophyton infection is often desquamative and may be wet or dry. It may even present with vesicles or pustules. Typical lesions of tinea pedis or tinea cruris establish these parasites as the cause of pruritus ani. In monilial infection, the lesions tend to be pustular and the skin redder and more moist with an almost succulent appearance. Scrapings from the surface of the lesion should be mixed with a 10 per cent potassium hydroxide solution, warmed, and examined microscopically. Coccoid refractile bodies occurring in chains suggest yeast or monilia, whereas branching mycelia are present in epidermophytosis. Cultures should be taken for further substantiation. Antibiotics, such as the tetracyclines, have also been incriminated in producing pruritus. A monilial infection should be considered but frequently cannot be found as the explanation.

OTHER CAUSES

In women, excessive vaginal discharge and urinary incontinence may contribute to the maintenance of abnormal perianal moisture. The seemingly greater incidence of pruritus in hot weather has been explained by excessive sweating. The use of mineral oil as a cathartic also may produce increased anal moisture owing to its tendency to leak from the anus. In all these moisture-producing states, poor anal hygiene seems to be a necessary concomitant factor.

As with other diseases of unclear cause,

a psychological basis for many cases of idiopathic pruritus ani has been postulated.[11] Sexual and gastrointestinal complaints are common in these patients. If no other specific cause can be found, the possibility of psychological disturbance should be evaluated.

Finally, many patients with idiopathic pruritus ani have been shown to have a very alkaline anal discharge, with a pH of 9 or 10 in contrast to the usual 6 or 7.[12] This change in pH has been suggested to result at least in part from putrefactive action of gram-negative colonic flora on ingested protein, especially meat. The alkaline fluid then supposedly produces a chemical dermatitis or alters skin resistance to the normal superficial skin bacteria. In support of this theory, surprisingly good results have been obtained in cases of resistant pruritus ani by measures which change the colonic flora.

TREATMENT

Treatment of pruritus ani should begin with an accurate diagnosis of the underlying cause. It is not our purpose to describe the treatment of the various dermatologic, fungal, and surgical factors which may be causative. Decision as to when to resort to surgery for correction of the aforementioned "surgically correctable" causes is also a difficult question, because repair of co-existing hemorrhoids occasionally does not produce relief of pruritus ani.

A large number of cases are cured by the patient's adopting strict anal hygiene. The anal area should be washed with plain white soap each morning and evening and, if possible, after each bowel movement. Occasionally, patients with pruritus ani do not empty the rectal ampulla completely, contributing to excessive anal soilage.[13] If this is found to be the case, a small amount of warm water instilled in the rectum by hand syringe after each bowel movement and then expelled may be helpful. After drying with a soft towel or gauze, the anus can be powdered with a zinc, starch, or boric acid dusting powder. Harsh toilet paper should be avoided, and clothing which provides good ventilation should be worn (avoiding tight, thin mesh nylon underwear). Severe pruritus may be greatly

helped by local application of hydrocortisone or betamethasone cream. The patient
should be instructed to apply this to the
anus instead of scratching.

Both constipation and diarrhea should
be avoided. Any attempt to alter stool consistency should not employ irritant laxatives such as saline purgatives, phenolphthalein, aloes, or mineral oil. Newer
bulk-forming laxatives are preferred.

Older textbooks give great emphasis to
dietary factors as being important in the
control of pruritus ani. Highly spiced
foods, shellfish, coffee, and alcohol are
commonly mentioned. It seems most
reasonable to advise avoidance of only
those dietary items which aggravate symptoms. It also seems reasonable to attempt to
reduce flatus by decreasing intake of foods
known to lead to increased intestinal gas
such as onions, bean products, and those
high in carbohydrates.[14] If colonic bacterial fermentation indeed plays a role, diminishing dietary protein intake, especially meat, for a period is indicated.
Decreasing dietary sugar has also been
recommended.

In a direct attempt to alter the rectal bacterial flora and subsequently the pH of the
incriminated alkaline anal discharge, rectal lavage with dilute solutions of lactic
acid, insertion of gelatin suppositories
containing betalactose, oral administration
of capsules of *Lactobacillus acidophilus*,
and oral administration of malt soup extract have all been recommended. The latter has been most recently popularized.
Reported results testify to its effectiveness, although strict anal hygiene is also
a part of the program recommended.[15] One
or two tablespoonfuls of malt soup extract
(Maltsupex) are administered twice a day.
In the reported patients, severe symptoms
were relieved in two or three days and
perianal skin returned to normal by ten
days. Periodic administration was continued thereafter as necessary. Stool pH returned to normal. This change in stool pH
and beneficial effect are reportedly due to
stimulation of growth of a gram-positive
bacterial flora which replaces the normal
predominantly gram-negative organisms
of the colon.

Regardless of other treatment employed,
the temporary use of sedatives and tranquilizers is often helpful for the very uncomfortable patient fatigued yet agitated
with his symptoms. Antihistamines such as
Benadryl or Temaril should be given systemically, not topically.

When all these approaches to therapy
have failed, the patient with intractable
pruritus ani may be considered a candidate for more drastic therapy. Radiotherapy, used in the past, has no place in modern treatment. Various surgical techniques
may be of some help. These include (1) injections into the anal and perianal skin of
various agents to produce obliteration of
the sensory nerve supply, (2) tattooing of
the perianal skin with mercuric sulfide to
change dermal sensitivity, and (3) under-
cutting operations or primary excision of
portions of the anal skin. The value of
these techniques is debatable, and proc-
tologists' opinions differ. Fortunately, only
a few patients with pruritus ani ever reach
a stage at which consideration of these
procedures becomes necessary.

CARCINOMA OF THE ANUS

Malignant growths in the anal region
may vary from an indolent, usually localized process to an aggressive cancer with
wide metastases. All suspicious, particularly ulcerating, lesions should be immediately biopsied and subjected to pathological examination. A large tumor projecting
into the anal canal is often a downward extension of an adenocarcinoma of the rectum. Anoscopy and biopsy will rapidly
substantiate this diagnosis.

BASAL CELL CANCER

In an elderly patient, a small anal nodule which ulcerates with rolled edges as it
enlarges may be a basal cell carcinoma.
Since it does not metastasize widely, excisional biopsy is usually adequate. Also,
in older patients, an irregular reddish
plaque with a weeping crust or an ulcerated center may represent intraepithe-
lial squamous cell carcinoma or Bowen's
disease. Wide local excision is the therapy
of choice. Paget's disease may involve the

perianal dermal apocrine sweat glands. This is more common in females and usually presents with itching and an elevated weeping red lesion which occasionally ulcerates. Diagnosis is made by finding typical clear, vacuolated Paget's cells in the biopsy specimen. Again, wide local excision is the recommended treatment.

MELANOMA

Fortunately rare, malignant melanomas of the anus are highly lethal. They metastasize quickly, and they may have disseminated widely by both blood and lymphatics at the time of diagnosis. A small melanoma is often interpreted as a pile by the patient as well as the physician, and the true diagnosis is made only after pathological examination of the "hemorrhoid." An early melanoma appears as a bluish-black polypoid lesion projecting into the anal lumen. Larger lesions become more polypoid and tend to ulcerate, at which time their appearance suggests their true malignant nature. Diagnostic excisional biopsy of the primary lesion should be carried out as soon as possible. Although radical excision of the rectum and extensive abdominoperitoneal resections have been recommended in the past, survival is insufficiently improved to warrant the increased morbidity.

SQUAMOUS CELL CANCER

The most common malignant tumor of the anus and anal canal is squamous cell carcinoma. However, its incidence is far less than that of adenocarcinoma of the rectum. Opinions regarding treatment differ. Although once recommended, irradiation for lesions confined to the anal canal has fallen into disfavor. Radical excision of the anus and rectum by the abdominoperineal method is the operation commonly performed (see p. 1460).

PROCTALGIA

There are several conditions in which the main symptom is pain in the anorectal area, but which have no evidence of any recognizable cause such as a fissure or abscess. All patients presenting with pain in the anus should have full proctological evaluation, including sigmoidoscopy.

COCCYGODYNIA

Coccygodynia is a term used to designate pain in and around the coccyx. Initially the patient may complain of pain in the rectum, but the pain later localizes in the area of the coccyx. Severe shooting pain involving the anorectal area occurs superimposed on chronic aching pain. Coccygodynia may develop in persons experiencing trauma to the coccyx or in persons with poor or slouched sitting posture; it may also appear to develop spontaneously. It occasionally plagues women who at some previous time experienced fracture-dislocation of the coccyx, often during childbirth. Tonic spasm of the levator ani, coccygeal, and piriform muscles is thought to be the main pathogenetic mechanism.[16] Diagnosis is made during digital rectal examination by pain being produced by pressure on the anterior surface of the coccyx, with movement of the coccyx, or by deliberate stroking of the spastic muscles. Treatment consists of improved sitting posture, warm sitz baths, and, during rectal examinations, repeated massage of the spastic muscles in the direction of the muscle fibers. Diathermy treatment to the anal and coccygeal area and tranquilizers with a muscle relaxant property, such as diazepam, may be helpful.

PROCTALGIA FUGAX

Proctalgia fugax is an obscure yet severe type of rectal pain of adults. It is similar to the severe pain of the very rare rectal crisis of tabes dorsalis, but can be immediately differentiated from it by absence of the associated straining efforts and typically lax sphincter muscles as well as by absence of other typical neuropathic changes of tabes dorsalis. The pain of proctalgia fugax is quite severe. It is more common in young men and is described as a spasmodic or cramplike pain in the anus or lower rectum. It frequently occurs in tense individuals and typically awakens them at night. In females it is noted most frequently after intercourse.

As the name implies, the pain is of short duration, lasting only 30 to 45 minutes. Therefore few people are examined during an attack. However, a group of physicians has been reported who digitally examined their anal canals during attacks and found a tender muscle band on one side of the lower rectum.[17] Therefore, although spasm of a segment of the levator ani muscle seems a likely cause of this symptom, the specific cause is unknown.

Treatment is unsatisfactory. Occasionally, hot sitz baths, defecation, warm water enemas, passing flatus, sublingual nitroglycerin, or firm upward pressure on the anus will help shorten the duration of an attack.[17, 18]

OTHER CAUSES OF RECTAL PAIN

A number of other uncommon conditions may present with mainly anorectal pain. In some patients with carcinoma of the prostate, there may be a tubular rectal stricture at the level of the prostate or a mucosal ulcer with pain as a prominent symptom. Tumor of the cauda equina of the spinal cord may also produce anorectal pain. Examination of the anus will show a slight weakness of the external sphincter and a small area of diminished cutaneous sensation in the perianal region. Transient sigmoidorectal intussusception or procidentia causes brief pain, tenesmus, and a heavy sensation in the anorectal area. However, chronic intussusception of the sigmoid colon into the rectum is not rare in older persons, and usually has a carcinoma at the leading edge of the intussusceptum.

Finally, pain during and after defecation, tenesmus, and chronic constipation have been termed the puborectalis syndrome.[19] Pain occurs only with attempted defecation and is the result of spasm of the puborectalis muscle sling. Hypertrophy and spasm of this muscle pull the anorectal angulation forward, lengthen the anal

canal, and constrict the inlet. The diagnosis is made on digital examination by finding at the upper end of the anal canal a constricted ring which is tender to palpation. Use of a topical anesthetic may allow passage of the finger into the rectum.

Conservative treatment should be tried initially, including the use of bulk-forming stool softeners and anal dilatation with either the gloved finger or a dilator just prior to defecation.[3] If unsuccessful, surgical resection of a small segment of the puborectalis sling usually cures the condition without producing rectal incontinence.

It should be emphasized again that the diagnosis in any of these vague and uncommon causes of anorectal discomfort cannot be made until all other more common disorders have been excluded by complete examination.

REFERENCES

1. Fletcher, G. F., Earnest, D. L., Shuford, W. F., and Wenger, N. K. Electrocardiographic changes during routine sigmoidoscopy. Arch. Intern. Med. 122:483, 1968.
2. Goligher, J. C. Surgery of the Anus, Rectum and Colon, 2nd ed. London, Bailliere, Tindall and Cassell, 1967, pp. 111–167.
3. Turell, R. Diseases of the Colon and Rectum, 2nd ed. Vol. 2. Philadelphia, W. B. Saunders Co., 1969, pp. 895–954, 1072–1085, 1295–1296.
4. Taylor, F. W., and Egbert, H. L. Portal tension. Surg. Gynec. Obstet. 92:64, 1951.
5. Miles, W. E. Observations upon internal piles. Surg. Gynec. Obstet. 29:497, 1919.
6. Gabriel, W. B. The Principles and Practice of Rectal Surgery, 5th ed. London, H. K. Lewis and Co. 1963, pp. 118–119.
7. Kratzer, G. L. Anal ducts and their clinical significance. Amer. J. Surg. 79:32, 1950.
8. Atwell, J. B., Duthie, H. L., and Goligher, J. C. The outcome of Crohn's disease. Brit. J. Surg. 52:966, 1965.
9. Moore, H. D. Treatment of fissure-in-ano. Lancet 1:909, 1964.
10. Watts, J. M., Bennett, R. C., and Goligher, J. C. Stretching of anal sphincters in the treatment of fissure-in-ano. Brit. Med. J. 2:342, 1965.
11. Macalpine, I. Pruritus ani, a psychiatric study. Psychosomat. Med. 15:499, 1953.
12. Granet, E. Pruritus ani: The etiologic factors and treatment in 100 cases. New Eng. J. Med. 223:1015, 1940.
13. Henley, F. A. Primary pruritus ani. Proc. Roy. Soc. Med. 52:390, 1959.
14. Calloway, D. H. Respiratory hydrogen and

methane as affected by constipation of gas-forming foods. Gastroenterology *51*:383, 1966.

15. Brooks, L. H.   Further studies on the management of pruritus ani. Dis. Colon Rectum *12*:193, 1968.

16. Thiele, F. H.   Coccygodynia: The mechanism of its production and its relation to anorectal disease. Amer. J. Surg. *79*:110, 1950.

17. Douthwaite, A.   Proctalgia fugax. Brit. Med. J. *2*:164, 1962.

18. Granet, E.   Proctalgias and allied noninflammatory perianal dyscrasias: Coccygodynia, proctalgia fugax, neurogenic pruritus ani. Amer. J. Dig. Dis. *13*:330, 1946.

19. Wasserman, I. F.   Puborectalis syndrome: Rectal stenosis due to anorectal spasm. Dis. Colon Rectum *7*:87, 1964.

DISEASES OF THE INTRA-ABDOMINAL VASCULATURE AND SUPPORTIVE STRUCTURES

Chapter 114

Vascular Diseases of the Bowel

Robert K. Ockner

In this chapter, the clinical features of certain splanchnic vascular syndromes will be considered. For a general discussion of the blood supply of the abdominal viscera, and of the anatomic and physiological factors involved in the pathogenesis of ischemia, the reader is referred to pages 381 to 383.

CHRONIC INTESTINAL ISCHEMIC SYNDROMES

Most patients with clinically significant occlusive disease of the mesenteric vasculature present with one of the acute syndromes to be described in the following section. "Chronic" (actually, recurrent acute) ischemia is uncommon, but is represented by two clinical entities which differ greatly in virtually every respect, but which between them illustrate most of the principles and problems with which the clinician must deal in approaching the patient with suspected mesenteric vascular disease.

ABDOMINAL ANGINA

Occlusive vascular disease, usually atherosclerotic and affecting at least two of the three major splanchnic vessels, may uncommonly be associated with a characteristic syndrome of intermittent dull or cramping midabdominal pain, or abdominal angina.[1,2] The pain classically occurs from 15 to 30 minutes after a meal and lasts for up to a few hours. It is during this period that nutrients are undergoing digestion and absorption in the small intestine, and adequate vascular perfusion is essential to provide for the concomitant increase in intestinal blood flow and oxygen consumption. Because of the extensive occlusive disease, however (affecting not only the superior mesenteric artery but also other vascular channels which might provide effective collateral supply), this period constitutes one of relative ischemia, and the patient has pain. It is reasonable to regard this type of abdominal pain as the intestinal counterpart of angina pectoris in patients with coronary artery disease under conditions of myocardial ischemia.

Clinical Picture. In addition to the complaint of pain, patients with this syndrome quickly discover the importance of eating in the initiation or aggravation of their pain. As a result, they develop a fear of eating and tend to decrease both the size of individual meals and their total food intake. Consequently, marked weight loss is the general rule in this condition. (Weight loss in these patients may be aggravated to some degree by mild to moderate steatorrhea.) Other digestive symptoms such as diarrhea, constipation, nausea, vomiting, and abdominal bloating may be reported, but are less constant. The duration of the symptoms from onset to diagnosis may vary considerably, depending upon the severity of the symptoms and the awareness of the physician. Retrospectively, however, it is clear that many patients who present with frank infarction of the intestine have had antecedent symptoms suggestive of abdominal angina for periods of weeks to months.[1] Accordingly, the syndrome of abdominal angina assumes major clinical significance, not only for the disability and discomfort which it causes but also because it may be a harbinger of imminent catastrophe.

Physical examination in these patients, in addition to showing evidence of marked weight loss, will as a rule disclose other findings consistent with advanced atherosclerotic disease, with or without hypertension or diabetes mellitus. Consistent with this common association, patients with abdominal angina tend to be in the older age group. An abdominal bruit may be detectable, but neither its presence nor its absence carries major diagnostic weight, because many patients with advanced mesenteric vascular disease have no bruits, and totally insignificant abdominal bruits are well described in normal individuals.

Laboratory findings are generally nonspecific. In a number of patients, however, steatorrhea has been well documented. As a rule, it is mild to moderate, up to about 20 g fecal fat per day;[3] in the case of atherosclerotic mesenteric insufficiency it is almost always associated with pain.[4] Although the steatorrhea may contribute to the malnutrition which such patients exhibit, diminished food intake is usually the major factor, and malabsorption is ordinarily not an important clinical problem. The cause for the malabsorption is not well understood, but presumably reflects reduced mesenteric blood flow,[5] and specific alterations in mucosal morphology have been described in such patients.[3] It is of interest, however, that steatorrhea may persist after revascularization, even though bowel morphology is normal.[6] Possibly, ischemic injury to autonomic nerves or stricture formation may alter intestinal motility and lead to bacterial overgrowth.

Diagnosis and Treatment. The presentation of an older patient with recurrent severe abdominal pain and progressive weight loss may suggest a diagnosis of intra-abdominal malignancy. However, on careful questioning it is usually possible to elicit the fact that it has been *fear of eating* rather than lack of appetite that accounts for the patient's decreased food intake. Advanced atherosclerotic vascular disease may be present, but its absence (in weighing against the diagnosis) is of greater diagnostic significance. A systolic abdominal bruit may be heard, but most often this clinical sign (or its absence) is of no help. Barium contrast studies do not usually disclose abnormalities sufficient to account for the clinical picture. If the diagnosis of abdominal angina is suspected, and if the patient's condition is such that corrective surgery would be undertaken were the diagnosis to be established, then angiographic study of the splanchnic circulation is indicated. A positive study will disclose significant (>50 per cent) narrowing in at least two of the three major arteries, and often evidence for collateral flow (Figs. 114–1 and 114–2). Unfortunately, generally available tech-

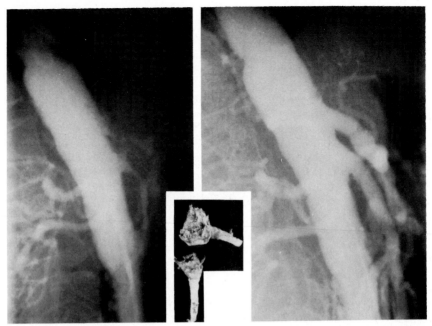

Figure 114-1. Diffuse atherosclerosis of splanchnic vessels in a patient with abdominal angina. Lateral aortogram, before and after endarterectomy, demonstrating the virtually complete occlusion of both the celiac and superior mesenteric arteries at their takeoff. The inset shows the atherosclerotic plaques which were removed at surgery. (Courtesy of Dr. William Ehrenfeld, Department of Surgery, University of California, San Francisco.)

niques permit an accurate evaluation of *vessel diameter* but not of *blood flow.*[7] Since it is blood flow rather than vessel caliber that determines the adequacy of tissue oxygenation, it is understandable why many patients with apparently severe mesenteric vascular disease (as judged by angiography) have no clinical evidence of vascular insufficiency, and why others with both clinical and radiographic evidence suggestive of mesenteric ischemia do not respond to corrective vascular

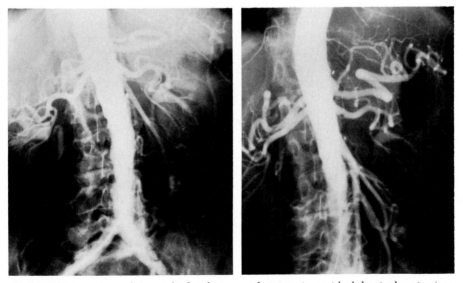

Figure 114-2. Diffuse atherosclerosis of splanchnic vessels in a patient with abdominal angina (same case as shown in Fig. 114-1). Anteroposterior projection of aortogram, before and after surgery, shows improved filling of the superior mesenteric artery. (Courtesy of Dr. William K. Ehrenfeld.)

surgery. Because of these considerations, one cannot look to angiography as a means of positively establishing the diagnosis of abdominal angina. Rather, the diagnosis must be made clinically; the angiogram may be interpreted as consistent with that diagnosis, or may show normal splanchnic vessels, thereby excluding it. If there is serious doubt that the clinical story is consistent with abdominal angina, then angiography will be helpful (negatively) only if normal.

The decision to operate on a patient for abdominal angina should be made only when other significant and potentially contributing abdominal pathology has been excluded, and when angiography shows significant narrowing near the ostia (i.e., in a surgically accessible area) of at least two major vessels. Even with these preconditions, however, errors in diagnosis must be anticipated. At surgery a gradient of more than 35 mm Hg across a stenotic area will confirm the significance of the block.[1] Bypass, endarterectomy, and reimplantation procedures have all been effective. The general experience has been that results are favorable, especially in regard to relief of pain and correction of malabsorption.[1] However, it should be noted that, as yet, long-term follow-up statistics are not adequate to establish conclusively that surgical correction protects against subsequent acute intestinal infarction.[1, 8]

CELIAC COMPRESSION SYNDROME

A number of well documented cases have been reported, in which recurrent abdominal pain is associated with narrowing of the celiac axis alone.[9-13] This disorder is an apparent exception to the general rule that at least two major visceral arteries must be occluded before symptoms occur, and for this reason there was initially considerable skepticism as to its validity. However, several rather constant clinical and anatomic features have been noted, and the syndrome is gaining general acceptance as an uncommon but correctable cause of otherwise unexplained abdominal pain.

Clinically, most patients are women, younger than those expected to have significant atherosclerotic disease, who describe epigastric pain of variable

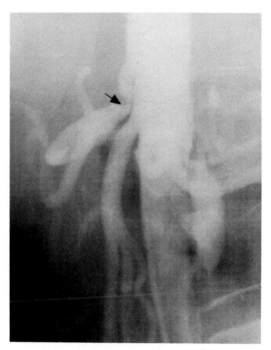

Figure 114–3. The lateral aortogram in a patient with celiac compression syndrome shows marked stenosis of the celiac axis near its take-off from the aorta (arrow), together with a normal superior mesenteric artery. (Courtesy of Dr. Henry I. Goldberg, Department of Radiology, University of California, San Francisco.)

frequency and duration. The pain may or may not be related to meals, but only infrequently is it associated with nausea and vomiting. The only physical finding noted with regularity is an epigastric bruit which does not radiate to the lower abdomen. Other gastrointestinal pathology has not been demonstrable in most cases.

The diagnosis requires abdominal angiography, with lateral views of the celiac axis (Fig. 114–3). This vessel is narrowed near its origin, with poststenotic dilatation. Other vessels are normal.

At surgery, the celiac axis is often found to have a high take-off (Fig. 114–4) and to be compressed by the median arcuate ligament of the diaphragm or by neurofibrous tissue of the celiac ganglion. Occasionally, fibromuscular hyperplasia of the vessel itself has been found. The structure(s) causing extrinsic compression should be divided. In some cases, stenosis ascribed to intimal fibrosis will persist, and bypass graft may be necessary.[14] By these techniques, the pre-existing pressure gradient across the obstruction[10] should be greatly

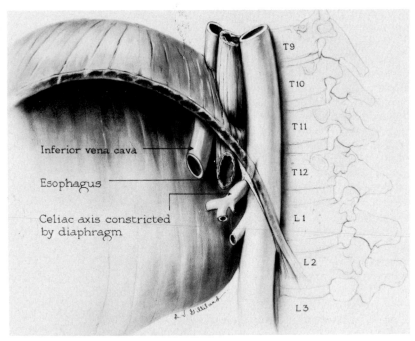

Figure 114-4. This diagram illustrates the anatomical features found in many patients with the celiac compression syndrome. The celiac axis has a high take-off, and in its downward course is compressed by the adjacent median arcuate ligament of the diaphragm. (From Stoney, R. J., and Wylie, E. J.: Ann. Surg. *164*:714, 1966.)

reduced or eliminated. Follow-up results have generally been quite satisfactory, with relief of pain in about 80 per cent of reported cases.[13]

Two major problems remain to be clarified before this syndrome can be placed in proper perspective. First, the cause of the pain remains obscure, because it is clear that in most patients the pancreaticoduodenal arcades are adequately functioning as a collateral route for supply of blood in the distribution of the celiac axis. Possibly, it is this diversion leading to a decreased flow with resulting ischemia in areas normally supplied by the superior mesenteric artery, that accounts for the pain.[13] It has also been suggested that the celiac ganglion itself may be the source of the pain.[11, 12] A second unresolved and possibly related problem is that significant stenosis of the celiac axis may be found incidentally at autopsy,[15] or on abdominal angiography,[10, 16] indicating that this lesion may be asymptomatic in many if not most individuals, although pain may well depend upon the degree of narrowing.

These unresolved problems are cited in order to serve as a precautionary note against overenthusiastic diagnosis of celiac compression syndrome.[12, 13] The fact remains, however, that enough patients with disabling and otherwise unexplained abdominal pain have benefited from correction of this lesion to make it worthy of consideration in selected patients.

ACUTE INTESTINAL ISCHEMIC SYNDROMES

Most patients with ischemic disease of the bowel present with an acute episode. Because of the various anatomical, temporal, physiological, and etiological factors which may be operating, these acute syndromes may differ greatly, and may present quite different challenges to the clinician in his evaluation and management of the problem patient. Among these, several more or less well defined entities are characterized by certain specific clinical features. In addition, the section dealing with acute mesenteric arterial thrombosis includes a discussion of the assessment and management of patients with bowel infarction.

ACUTE MESENTERIC ARTERIAL THROMBOSIS

When intrinsic disease of the splanchnic arterial tree compromises blood flow to below a critical level, ischemic necrosis of the supplied areas of bowel will result. Most commonly, this is due to advanced atherosclerotic disease affecting at least two of the major visceral branches of the aorta. In atherosclerosis, it is usually the first segment of the artery, near its take-off from the aorta, that is most severely involved, and this is advantageous not only in angiographic diagnosis but also in surgical reconstruction. Atherosclerotic occlusion, however, may involve more distal segments of the arteries or their branches. Other disease processes may also cause occlusion of the splanchnic arteries, including dissecting aortic aneurysm, thromboangiitis obliterans, fibromuscular hyperplasia, and systemic vasculitis. Thrombosis has also been reported in patients taking oral contraceptive agents.[17] Systemic diseases associated with vasculitis may involve the splanchnic arterial tree at any or all of several points, including major arterial trunks at the one extreme and intramural arterioles at the other. Vasculitis in general, as it affects the bowel, is considered separately below, and on pages 396 to 399.

Clinical Presentation. Acute infarction of the small intestine is dominated clinically by severe abdominal pain, which initially may be colicky in nature and periumbilical in location. In this phase of the disease bowel sounds may not only be intermittently heard, but may even be hyperactive. In fact, there is often a striking paucity of abdominal findings relative to the systemic manifestations, which may be severe and may include tachycardia, hypotension, fever, hemoconcentration, and marked leukocytosis (often in excess of 30,000 with a left shift). Hemoconcentration reflects loss of extracellular fluid into the bowel lumen; as ileus becomes manifest, vomiting and a picture of intestinal obstruction may supervene. Blood may be absent from both vomitus and stool early in the course, but almost invariably appears with time. As ischemia progresses, pain becomes constant and poorly localized. Ultimately, when ischemic necrosis becomes transmural, signs of generalized peritonitis appear. At this point, in the patient with signs of intestinal obstruction, peritonitis, and gastrointestinal bleeding, the diagnosis of bowel infarction is almost inescapable, but the prognosis at this advanced state (with or without surgery) is extremely poor. Accordingly, the chances for the patient's survival will be maximized if the diagnosis of bowel ischemia is considered and established early in the course.

Diagnosis. The history and physical examination are often of little help in arriving at a specific diagnosis. Significant clues may include a history or physical findings of occlusive vascular disease elsewhere in the body, recurrent postprandial abdominal pain suggestive of abdominal angina (as many as 50 per cent of patients presenting with acute thrombotic infarction have given such a history),[1] recent episodes of significant hypotension or anoxia, or predisposition to, or other peripheral evidence of, arterial embolization (see below). As with the history and physical findings, laboratory studies are of little help early in the course. Serum amylase may be elevated. In general, however, in addition to the findings of hemoconcentration and leukocytosis as noted above, the presence of blood in nasogastric aspirate or vomitus or in the stool, together with the clinical and radiographic picture of ileus (including distended loops of bowel with air-fluid levels), is most helpful (Fig. 114–5). Plain and erect films of the abdomen may also show thickening of the bowel wall itself, reflecting the intramural hemorrhage and edema which accompany infarction. Other radiographic changes, such as the early absence of small bowel gas or the later appearance of gas in the portal vein (Fig. 114–6) are less frequently seen, but are helpful when present.

The decision to undertake additional raidographic studies in patients with suspected bowel infarction is a difficult one and must be individualized. In the patient in whom signs of peritonitis are already present, further examination may not only delay appropriate management but may also be deleterious in itself. In regard to

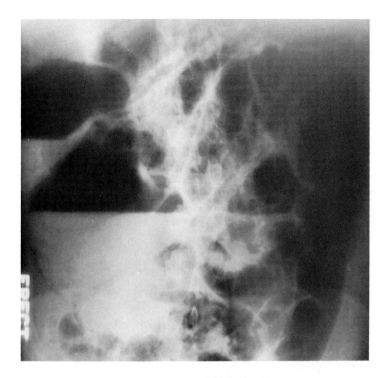

Figure 114–5. This upright film of the abdomen shows marked dilatation of loops of small and large intestine in a patient with acute bowel infarction. Air-fluid levels are present both in small intestine and cecum (which is also outlined by intramural gas). These radiographic findings should suggest the diagnosis of bowel infarction, but may be seen with intestinal obstruction of other causes. (Courtesy of Dr. Henry I. Goldberg.)

Figure 114–6. In this plain film of the right upper quadrant, gas may be seen in the portal vein and its intrahepatic radicles (arrows). This phenomenon does not occur until an advanced stage of acute bowel infarction is reached, and represents extensive loss of epithelial and vascular integrity with invasion of gas-forming organisms. (Courtesy of Dr. Henry I. Goldberg.)

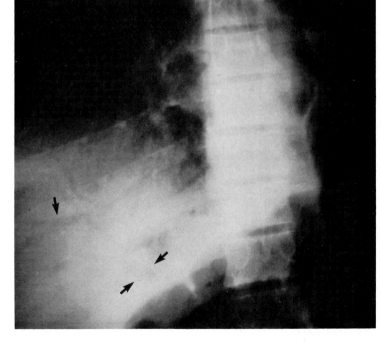

angiography, it is clear that all the difficulties in the interpretation of demonstrated arterial occlusive disease which pertain to the patient who has chronic abdominal symptoms but is not at the moment acutely ill are further compounded in the unstable, acutely ill patient who may have gangrenous bowel in his abdomen. It has been suggested that angiography, if it fails to disclose significant major arterial occlusions, may be used as evidence in support of the diagnosis of nonocclusive infarction (see below), and that this might modify the therapeutic approach. Although it is possible that, in time, methods will be developed to permit the nonoperative management of such patients if diagnosed early in the course, at present such treatment must be regarded as experimental, and not yet established for routine clinical use.[1] Therefore abdominal angiography, although useful in selected cases, probably should not be considered to be a *routine* procedure in the acutely ill patient with suspected bowel infarction.

Treatment. The management of patients with bowel infarction can be divided into two major categories: supportive and operative. Supportive management includes nasogastric suction, appropriate fluid and electrolyte replacement (including albumin, fresh frozen plasma, or blood) and administration of antibiotics after cultures have been obtained. Fluid balance must be carefully monitored. Because many patients with this disease will be in the older age group and already have evidence of vascular disease affecting other organs, including the heart, parenteral fluid administration must be carried out with extreme care in order to avoid precipitation of acute congestive cardiac failure. The administration of digitalis to patients not already receiving it, but who are at risk for developing congestive failure, is somewhat controversial in view of evidence that cardiac glycosides cause splanchnic vasoconstriction, thus potentially compounding the visceral ischemia. If failure supervenes, however, digitalis should not be withheld. In the management of a falling blood pressure not correctable by appropriate volume replacement, isoproterenol is preferable to other sympathomimetic amines (e.g., norepinephrine), because it both exerts a positive

inotropic effect on the heart and causes splanchnic vasodilatation. In general, however, in the presence of bowel infarction, significant congestive heart failure and/or uncorrectable shock carry an extremely unfavorable prognosis, and the prime objective of initial management should be to prepare the patient for surgery before these complications arise.

At surgery, necrotic bowel is resected and efforts are made to re-establish mesenteric arterial flow by means of bypass graft, embolectomy, or endarterectomy. At the time of the initial exploration, it may not be possible for the surgeon to conclusively identify the limits of viable bowel. Accordingly, it may be desirable to undertake a "second look" operation 12 to 36 hours after the initial exploration, in order to identify and resect any additional bowel which in the interim has declared itself to be nonviable.[18-20]

Prognosis. Under the best of circumstances, spontaneous thrombotic intestinal infarction carries with it a grave prognosis, and the mortality rate is in the vicinity of 60 to 70 per cent. This poor outlook results from several factors which include (1) the fact that the patients in general are in an older age group, with other clinically significant and potentially life-threatening cardiac, pulmonary, renal, or cerebral disorders; (2) the nonspecific nature of the early presentation of the acute process, leading to delays in diagnosis and operative intervention; and (3) the complications related to one or two major surgical procedures in these severely ill and elderly patients.

ACUTE ARTERIAL EMBOLIZATION

When arterial emboli interfere with the blood supply to the abdominal viscera, they most commonly lodge in the superior mesenteric artery. As noted earlier, the caliber of this vessel and the obliquity of its take-off from the abdominal aorta account for this predisposition. Emboli to the celiac axis and particularly to the inferior mesenteric artery are most uncommon. The vast majority of mesenteric emboli occur in patients who have rheumatic or atherosclerotic heart disease with mural thrombi in the heart. Emboli may also arise from vegetations of bacterial endocarditis or from atherosclerotic plaques in the thoracic or upper abdominal aorta. Patients may give a history of previous embolic episodes, or there may be evidence of simultaneous peripheral embolization (brain or extremities). Typically, the event is signaled by the abrupt onset of severe midabdominal cramping pain, accompanied by vomiting or diarrhea. Bleeding and evidence of intestinal obstruction are absent initially, and although the subjective impression of severe illness is obvious both to patient and physician, objective findings are deceptively sparse, because the abdomen is soft and bowel sounds are active. If the process is not recognized and treated properly, mesenteric embolus will lead to bowel infarction and the clinical manifestations described in the preceding section.

On the other hand, the characteristic clinical setting (a patient with atrial fibrillation or other known heart disease) of this condition and its abrupt, almost unmistakable onset offer a greater opportunity for early diagnosis and operative treatment. For these reasons, as well as the fact that the patients are on the average younger, the prognosis is generally more favorable than with nonembolic causes of bowel infarction.

As soon as the diagnosis is apparent and the patient's condition suitable, laparotomy with embolectomy should be carried out. Preoperative angiography, if performed, will confirm the presence of an occluded vessel and the absence of collateral flow (indicating the acute nature of the process). Fortunately, the majority of emboli lodge within the proximal few centimeters of the superior mesenteric artery and are accessible to the surgeon at the time of surgery. As is the case with thrombotic infarction, it may not be possible to define initially the extent of viable bowel, and a "second look" operation may be necessary. However, early operation (e.g. within 30 hours) after superior mesenteric embolization may often result in complete recovery of the intestine with no resection being required.[21] In regard to subsequent bowel function, such patients generally fare quite well, although a transient but self-limited malabsorption syndrome may persist for a period of several months.

NONTHROMBOTIC INTESTINAL INFARCTION

In approximately 12 to 50 per cent[1, 19, 20] or more of patients with intestinal infarction, significant occlusion of the mesenteric arteries cannot be demonstrated. This phenomenon of "nonthrombotic infarction" has gained increasing recognition as an important cause of abdominal catastrophe. In most cases, these patients have exhibited severe congestive cardiac failure, shock, or anoxia,[22] but occasionally a precipitating event is not identifiable.[23] In the presence of inadequate cardiac output and generally poor tissue perfusion, blood flow distribution favors the brain and other vital organs, and splanchnic flow falls disproportionately. The use of pharmacological vasoconstrictors in such patients with shock adds to the effect of already increased secretion of endogenous catecholamines, further reducing splanchnic flow because of mesenteric arteriolar constriction. As perfusion pressure falls in the splanchnic bed to below a critical level (closing pressure), tension in the arteriole walls may exceed hydrostatic pressure in the lumen, leading to collapse of the vessel. Many patients with this syndrome have been receiving digitalis glycosides as well; although it has been shown that these agents cause splanchnic vasoconstriction, their role in the pathogenesis of nonthrombotic infarction remains uncertain. Some patients with this disorder may have evidence of occlusive disease in the smaller splanchnic vessels, and these lesions may contribute to the ischemia.[24]

Of the various layers of the intestinal wall, the mucosa is most sensitive to anoxia, and in some patients only this portion of the bowel will undergo hemorrhagic necrosis.[22] In others, infarction is transmural, resulting in a clinical picture indistinguishable from that of mesenteric artery thrombosis.

The diagnosis of nonthrombotic intestinal infarction should be suspected in patients with congestive cardiac failure, shock, or anoxia who develop signs of intestinal infarction, with or without bleeding. If angiography is performed acutely, absence of occlusive disease in the major visceral arteries will add support to, but will not conclusively establish, the diagnosis. At surgery or autopsy, it may be observed that areas of infarction are patchy and irregular in distribution, and do not necessarily conform to the area supplied by a major vessel.[22]

Although various nonoperative therapeutic manuevers intended specifically to improve splanchnic blood flow (e.g., ganglion blockade, or intra-arterial infusion of vasodilator substances) in nonthrombotic infarction are being evaluated,[23] no form of therapy has been shown definitely to be effective in this syndrome. As with thrombotic infarction, supportive management is directed at maintaining blood pressure and cardiac output, treating infection, and replacing fluid and electrolytes. A major dilemma arises in weighing the decision to operate on a patient with cardiac failure and signs suggestive of bowel infarction. It is clear that, unoperated, this situation is attended by an exceedingly high mortality. Conversely, however, the surgical procedure itself may prove fatal in patients with advanced decompensated heart disease. Although generalizations are difficult in such matters, the presumptive diagnosis of intestinal infarction should be considered as an indication for surgical exploration as soon as the patient's overall condition permits, so that frankly necrotic areas of bowel may be resected. With or without surgery, however, survival after nonthrombotic intestinal infarction is unusual.

ISCHEMIC COLITIS

As with the small intestine, the response of the colon to vascular insufficiency depends upon several factors, including the location and extent of an occlusive process, and possible associated systemic disorders.[25] Thus extensive gangrene of the colon may accompany nonthrombotic infarction of the small intestine in patients with cardiac disease, may result from interruption of the inferior mesenteric artery during removal of an abdominal aortic aneurysm, or may follow localized occlusive disease in the inferior mesenteric artery or in its critical collateral channels.[23, 25] Uncommonly, the syndrome is associated with hypercoagulable states, use of oral contraceptives,[26] amyloid, and vasculitis. The clinical picture is similar to that of gangrene of the small intestine, and it is approached similarly.

More recently, a number of less catastrophic variants of ischemic disease of the colon have been recognized, which seem to be associated with more localized areas of ischemia. Particularly vulnerable are those areas of the colon which lie on the "watershed" between two adjacent arterial supplies, i.e. the splenic flexure (superior and inferior mesenteric arteries) and the rectosigmoid area (inferior mesenteric and internal iliac arteries).[27, 28]

In general most patients with ischemic disease of the colon are over 50 years of age, and have evidence of vascular disease, usually atherosclerotic. They characteristically present with abrupt onset of lower abdominal cramping pain, rectal bleeding, and variable degrees of vomiting and fever. Physical and laboratory findings of left-sided peritonitis may suggest a diagnosis of acute diverticulitis. Some patients give a history of similar symptoms several weeks to months prior to presentation.

Initial therapy consists of general supportive measures and antibiotics.[25, 27, 29, 30] Because the severity of the clinical picture may suggest local or generalized peritonitis and therefore the possibility of a perforated or infarcted viscus, clinical judgment often dictates surgical exploration shortly after the time the patient is seen. In a significant number of these patients, ischemic bowel will require resection and reanastomosis or, preferably, resection and temporary colostomy with subsequent reanastomosis when the patient's condition improves. In a substantial group of patients, however, although the process appears acute in onset, clinical signs do not indicate a present peritonitis, and such patients may be closely watched. Many will stabilize, and pain, distention, and fever may subside without surgical intervention. Subsequent barium enema examination usually shows a stricture of variable length, often associated with the characteristic picture of intramural hemorrhage and edema, including "thumbprinting," tubular narrowing, "saw tooth" irregularity, and sacculations (Figs. 114–7 and 114–8,

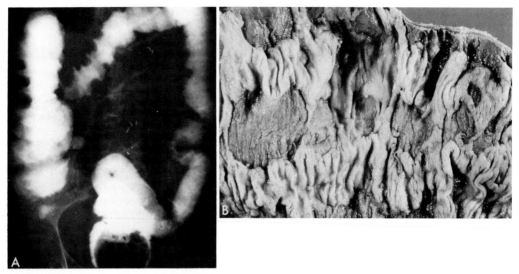

Figure 114–7. *A*, Barium enema, showing large nodular impressions (thumbprinting) in ascending and transverse colon of a patient with ischemic colitis, with ulcerations in the descending colon *(B)*. (Courtesy of Dr. Henry I. Goldberg.)

A). In some patients, the clinical process may subside completely, with disappearance of symptoms and return of X-rays to normal.[27, 29] In most patients, however, a residual stricture will remain (Fig. 114–8, *B*) and often requires resection.

As noted, ischemic disease may also affect the rectosigmoid area.[25, 28] These pa-

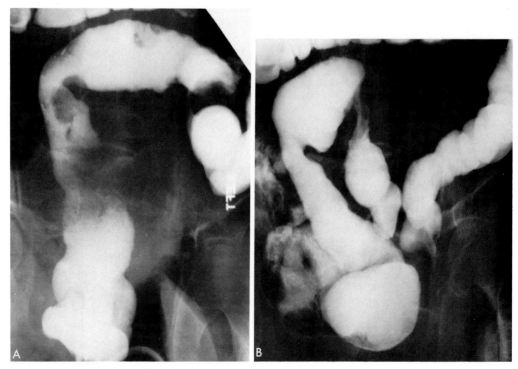

Figure 114–8. Ischemic colitis secondary to amyloid disease. *A*, Large impressions in the sigmoid colon reflect intramural hemorrhage. Sigmoidoscopy showed blue nodular masses. *B*, Follow-up study, three weeks later, shows healing with two strictures present in sigmoid colon. (Courtesy of Dr. Henry I. Goldberg.)

tients, also in the older age group, present with abdominal pain, rectal bleeding, and change in bowel habits. Unlike those with more proximal involvement, however, signs of peritonitis are unusual. Sigmoidoscopic findings are variable, and include a picture suggestive of nonspecific proctitis, multiple discrete ulcers, polypoid or nodular lesions which occasionally are blueblack (reflecting underlying hemorrhage), or an adherent membrane.[28] Rectal biopsy may show ischemic necrosis, but in most patients the histological picture is nonspecific, with variable ulceration, crypt abscesses, submucosal inflammation and fibrosis, and thrombosis in small vessels.[25, 28] Radiographic changes, if present, are similar to those noted above; i.e., thumbprinting early and, perhaps, smooth narrowing after recovery.[28]

The differentiation of ischemic colitis from nonspecific ulcerative colitis or proctitis, infections of the colon, Crohn's disease of the colon, or other forms of colitis may be difficult, if not impossible, on the basis of clinical evidence alone. Furthermore, ischemic colitis has even been reported to cause a picture of "toxic dilatation."[31] Histological examination may also fail to differentiate these various diseases. However, it is important to consider the diagnosis of ischemic colitis in patients in the older age group who present with what appears to be an initial episode of acute ulcerative colitis. Arteriography may be helpful in establishing the presence of vascular disease, but occlusions may be localized to smaller vessels and therefore not be detectable. Moreover, as noted, the presence of mesenteric vascular disease does not by itself establish the diagnosis of ischemic bowel disease. Although steroid enemas have been suggested as a form of therapy for ischemic proctitis, their efficacy has not been conclusively established. Surgical therapy, if necessary, is aimed primarily at resection of areas of infarction and stricture. Reconstructive surgery of the inferior mesenteric artery has not been generally successful.

MESENTERIC VENOUS OCCLUSION

Acute thrombosis in the mesenteric venous system occurs less frequently than arterial occlusion, accounting for approximately 10 to 45 per cent of mesenteric vascular accidents.[1, 32] Within this group, thrombosis of the superior mesenteric vein is far more common than that of the inferior mesenteric vein, but incidence figures may only reflect the fact that disease in the latter vessel may be more difficult to recognize clinically.

Mesenteric thrombosis occurs in patients with hypercoagulable states such as polycythemia, venous congestion, and stasis (e.g., cardiac failure, portal hypertension), and secondary to tumor infiltration, sepsis, and trauma. It has also been reported to occur in association with the use of oral contraceptives,[33] and may develop spontaneously without any evident predisposing cause.[1, 32]

Clinically, the disease may present as a fulminating abdominal catastrophe, similar to that observed in acute infarction secondary to arterial insufficiency. In some cases, however, especially those occurring spontaneously, the process may be a more gradual one, with development of progressive abdominal discomfort, anoxia, and change in bowel habit over a period of one to two weeks.[32] Hematemesis and melena are uncommon early, but serosanguineous ascites may occur in up to 80 per cent of patients.[32] Physical findings are nonspecific.

The diagnosis may be established at the time of surgical exploration for presumed peritonitis or other abdominal catastrophe. It may also be suspected preoperatively if selective superior mesenteric arteriography shows a prolonged arterial phase and failure to opacify the venous system.[1]

Treatment, as with other forms of bowel infarction, is supportive and operative. Infarcted bowel, evident grossly from the congestion, is resected along with its mesentery. Reconstructive venous surgery is not generally practical. Because up to 25 per cent of patients may experience a recurrence within the first several weeks postoperatively,[32] anticoagulation has been recommended for these patients.[1, 32]

In general, the overall prognosis of mesenteric venous occlusion is more favorable than that of arterial disease, and mortality, reported earlier to be from 50 to 80 per cent,[32] may now be as low as 20 per cent,[1] but remains higher in some series.[34]

OTHER DISORDERS AFFECTING THE SPLANCHNIC CIRCULATION

VASCULITIS

Occlusive disease of the visceral arteries may result from a variety of systemic conditions associated with vasculitis. The process may involve the larger main arterial trunks, the smaller vasa recta and intramural vessels, or both. When the larger vessels are involved, as in polyarteritis nodosa or the vasculitis associated with rheumatoid arthritis,[35] the patient may present with symptoms and signs of massive acute intestinal infarction with gangrene and perforation. Although the abdominal findings may be indistinguishable from those of atherosclerotic or embolic infarction, these disorders can usually be recognized by other evidence of systemic disease, such as renal involvement, eosinophilia, and hypertension in the case of polyarteritis, or rheumatoid nodules and a very high serum titer of rheumatoid factor in rheumatoid vasculitis. Involvement of major arteries by vasculitis may also lead

to the formation of aneurysms, the rupture of which results in gastrointestinal or intra-abdominal hemorrhage.

Vasculitis may affect primarily the vasa recta and intramural arteries and arterioles in virtually all the disorders associated with systemic vasculitis, including lupus erythematosus,[26, 37] dermatomyositis, polyarteritis,[37] Henoch-Schönlein purpura ("allergic vasculitis"), and rheumatoid vasculitis.[37] Patients present with abdominal pain, fever, gastrointestinal bleeding (usually, but not invariably occult), and variable evidence of intestinal obstruction; they may develop signs of frank perforation or infarction. Barium contrast studies may show a segment of variable length which is marked by ulceration or a spiculated or thumbprint appearance, reflecting submucosal hemorrhage and edema (Fig. 114–9). This picture may not be distinguishable radiographically from that of regional enteritis.

In *polyarteritis nodosa*, abdominal pain and other gastrointestinal symptoms have been reported in up to 65 per cent of cases. Moreover, about 50 per cent of autopsied cases show vasculitis involving the intestinal tract and liver. Although clinically sig-

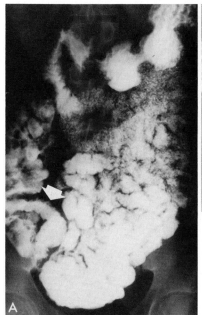
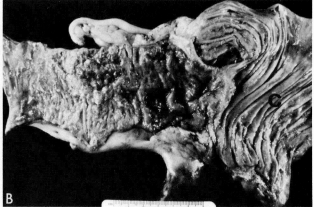

Figure 114–9. Vasculitis affecting the terminal ileum. A, The terminal ileum is ulcerated, and separation of bowel loops reflects a thickened mesentery. This patient presented with abdominal pain and diarrhea, and was treated with corticosteroids for a diagnosis of regional enteritis. Several months later significant lower gastrointestinal bleeding occurred, requiring surgery. The terminal ileum was found to be involved by a diffuse vasculitis, affecting the intramural arteries and arterioles. B, This is the resected specimen from the case described in A; it shows the extensive ischemic ulceration, hemorrhage, and necrosis caused by the vasculitis, involving terminal ileum but not cecum (C). (Courtesy of Dr. Henry I. Goldberg.)

nificant liver disease is uncommon as a result of this process, hepatic artery thrombosis caused by polyarteritis has accounted for approximately half the reported cases of infarction of the liver. Clinically apparent ischemic disease of the bowel is more frequent, and may range from massive infarction to segmental ischemia with ulceration, hemorrhage,[38] or perforation.[37, 39]

Lupus erythematosus causes gastrointestinal involvement in from 10 to 60 per cent of cases,[36, 40] usually manifest clinically as abdominal pain. Most frequently, such symptoms reflect an arteritis of smaller vessels, and massive bowel infarction is uncommon. However, segmental lesions leading to necrosis and perforation of small bowel or colon have been reported.[37] In addition, abdominal pain in lupus may be due to serositis or to acute pancreatitis, although the latter is related more to corticosteroid therapy than to lupus itself. Furthermore, there is an uncommon but well documented association of either classic ulcerative colitis or Crohn's disease with lupus erythematosus.[41] Accordingly, the appearance of gastrointestinal symptoms in patients with lupus may be particularly difficult to evaluate.

Dermatomyositis is noteworthy because of the high incidence of associated gastrointestinal malignancies in this disorder. Vasculitis does occur, however, and may be associated with ischemic bowel ulceration and hemorrhage.

In *Henoch-Schönlein purpura*, or allergic vasculitis, there is a high incidence of gastrointestinal involvement, manifest most commonly by abdominal pain and gastrointestinal bleeding, reflecting localized or segmental ischemia and ulceration. Gross infarction or perforation is rare, but has been reported.[42]

A number of less common vascular disorders have been associated with ischemic lesions of the bowel. One rare syndrome of progressive occlusive vascular disease affecting small and medium-sized arteries,[43] described initially by Köhlmeier[44] and Degos et al.,[45] involves chiefly the skin ("malignant atrophic papulosis") and intestine. It primarily affects young men, and terminates in intestinal infarction and perforation. This disease is recognized by its characteristic cutaneous lesions. Ta-

kayasu's ("pulseless") disease may also affect mesenteric arteries.[46] Vasculitis affecting the intramural arteries and arterioles also occurs in patients using enteric-coated potassium chloride tablets[47, 48] and in radiation injury to the bowel (see pp. 1406 to 1413). In either circumstance, the resulting ischemic necrosis may lead to ulceration, stricture formation, or, less commonly, perforation.

Diagnosis and Management. In general, the diagnosis of vasculitis of the bowel will be suggested more by the systemic and laboratory features of the disease than by the abdominal findings, which are nonspecific. It is of interest that, in contrast to most patients with chronic atherosclerotic mesenteric insufficiency, patients with vasculitis may have steatorrhea in the absence of symptoms;[49] the mechanism for this has not been established. A radiographic picture of mucosal ulceration or edema (thumbprinting, spiculation) may not be distinguishable from Crohn's disease in either appearance or location (Fig. 114–9). Although abdominal angiography has been employed to advantage in these disorders,[50] it has not generally been used in the acute situation.

As with other types of mesenteric vascular processes, the acute management decisions revolve to a large extent around the question of surgical exploration for possible infarction or perforation. The syndrome of Henoch-Schönlein purpura (allergic vasculitis) rarely requires surgery. However, in this as in other vascular conditions, if clinical signs of an acute abdomen are present, surgical exploration may be indicated. The problem is compounded by the fact that many patients with systemic vasculitis are already receiving corticosteroids, and these agents may mask important signs of a serious intra-abdominal process. Careful and continuing clinical, laboratory, and radiographic reassessment is mandatory in such patients, with the expectation that emergency exploration may be required at any time.

INTRAMURAL INTESTINAL HEMORRHAGE

Bleeding into the wall of the small intestine may occur in a wide variety of clinical

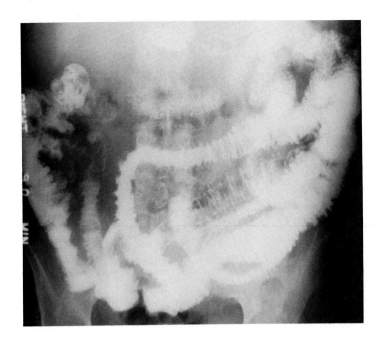

Figure 114–10. Intramural intestinal hemorrhage. This small bowel examination shows separation of loops and thickened mucosal folds, reflecting mucosal, intramural, and intramesenteric hemorrhage, occurring spontaneously in a patient on anticoagulant therapy. (Courtesy of Dr. Henry I. Goldberg.)

situations, including abdominal trauma, ischemic bowel infarction, vasculitis, and bleeding diatheses occurring spontaneously or as the result of anticoagulant therapy.[51-53] Such bleeding may be localized, with formation of a hematoma, or may be more diffuse.

In these cases associated with trauma, the intramural hemorrhage occurs almost always in the duodenum or proximal jejunum, presumably because the bowel at this location is fixed in position and may be compressed against the spine.[51, 52] Clinically, patients may present in one of two ways. A few develop severe abdominal pain, tenderness, absent bowel sounds, and leukocytosis immediately after the traumatic episode. These patients may be diagnosed erroneously as having a perforated viscus. A larger group of patients may not seek medical attention until several days after the traumatic episode, which in some circumstances may have been so slight as to have been disregarded. These patients exhibit the signs and symptoms of partial or complete high small bowel obstruction, with pain, vomiting, and, occasionally, a palpable mass caused by the presence of the hematoma.

Spontaneous intramural hemorrhage may also develop, either abruptly or over a period of several days, with cramping abdominal pain and variable tenderness, mass, or signs of intestinal obstruction. Hematemesis or melena and fever may be present.[53]

The diagnosis of intramural hemorrhage may be suggested by its characteristic, but nonspecific, radiographic features.[52, 54] On plain film, it may be possible to delineate a segment of bowel, separated from adjacent loops, with a narrowed lumen and thickened walls. Barium contrast studies show "cat's paw" or "thumbprint" defects, or a typical "coil spring" or "stacked coins" appearance (Fig. 114–10). The appearance of this lesion (also seen in bowel infarction) in a patient with heart disease who is being treated with anticoagulants may raise the dilemma as to whether one is dealing with hemorrhage or ischemia. In those traumatic cases associated with a large localized hematoma, a mass may be evident.

The treatment of patients with intramural hemorrhage varies with the clinical situation. If the patient is completely obstructed, or if there is strong evidence for peritonitis, the patient should probably be explored, particularly that group of patients seen early after trauma. In most cases, however, it is possible to manage the patient conservatively, with nasogastric suction, fluid replacement, and correction of any bleeding diathesis.[51, 53] Necrosis of the bowel wall is unusual in these patients. Usually, pain and other evidence of obstruction will subside within a few days.

ABDOMINAL AORTIC ANEURYSM

Abdominal aortic aneurysms are usually atherosclerotic in origin but may occasionally be due to syphilis, trauma, polyarteritis nodosa, or infection (mycotic aneurysm). Atherosclerotic aneurysms nearly always affect the aorta distal to the origin of the renal arteries, but may extend distally to involve the common iliac arteries as well. The aneurysm may be fusiform or saccular in shape; although the true significance of this distinction is uncertain, the latter may be more prone to rupture, an event which probably occurs in fewer than 10 per cent of cases.

CLINICAL PICTURE AND DIAGNOSIS

Clinically, "leakage" or rupture of an abdominal aneurysm is associated with pain in the abdomen, flank, or back; it may be present for several weeks preceding actual rupture. Occasionally, the pain may be worse in the recumbent position and may be relieved by sitting up or by leaning forward, thus suggesting a diagnosis of pancreatic disease.

On physical examination, a pulsatile mass is detectable, usually in the epigastrium (the bifurcation of the aorta corresponds roughly to the location of the umbilicus). The pulsations are expansile; differentiation of an aneurysm from an overlying abdominal mass with transmitted pulsations may be facilitated by demonstrating that the pulsations not only are felt directly over the mass but also displace the examining fingers laterally. A bruit may be present, but is usually of no help in diagnosis.

In the uncomplicated aneurysm, laboratory studies are not helpful. Radiographic examination, however, will often show the presence of a soft tissue mass in the region of the abdominal aorta, usually with peripheral calcification. Depending upon the size of the aneurysm, erosion of the lower dorsal and upper lumbar vertebrae or displacement of surrounding viscera, including bowel, kidneys, and ureters, may be evident.

Abdominal aortic aneurysms may rupture in one or more of several directions. Most commonly, bleeding is into the retroperitoneal tissues surrounding the aorta. The predilection for this site probably reflects erosion of the expanding vessel wall by the vertebral column. Less frequently the aneurysm may bleed into the free peritoneal cavity; in this event, shock supervenes rapidly and the outlook is extremely grave, even when appropriate therapeutic measures (transfusion and surgery) are immediately at hand. An additional site of rupture is into the small intestine, most commonly the third portion of the duodenum, presumably because in this area the intestine is fixed retroperitoneally in close proximity to the aorta itself. Such patients usually present with massive gastrointestinal bleeding, but occasionally bleeding may occur intermittently over a period of weeks.[55] Rarely abdominal aneurysms may rupture into the inferior vena cava.

TREATMENT

Treatment of an abdominal aortic aneurysm includes resection of the involved portions, including, if necessary, the common iliac arteries, and replacement with a Dacron graft.[56] There is little doubt that the patient with a ruptured aortic aneurysm requires immediate surgical intervention if he is to survive. In contrast, the patient with an asymptomatic abdominal aneurysm which has not ruptured may present a major therapeutic dilemma. Factors which must be taken into consideration include the propensity of the aneurysm to rupture and the general condition of the patient as affected by age and the presence of associated disease such as high blood pressure and coronary artery disease. In good hands (i.e., surgeons with extensive experience in aortic surgery, operating under optimal circumstances) operative mortality for an elective aneurysmectomy is 5 to 18 per cent, but it increases to 34 to 85 per cent when done as an emergency.[56-59] Thus it is desirable to avoid the latter circumstance if possible, but without subjecting patients whose aneurysm may not be a threat, or who have other potentially life-threatening cardiovascular disease, to unnecessary surgery.

It has been the general experience that aneurysms larger than 5 to 7 cm in diameter, which are increasing in size, or which have become symptomatic, have a significantly increased risk of rupturing.[57-59] Patients with such aneurysms should be considered operative candidates, regardless of age, unless there are compelling reasons which indicate that the operative risk is unacceptably high. The younger patient with an aneurysm of between 5 and 7 cm in diameter, and who is a reasonably good operative risk, could be regarded as a surgical candidate even in the absence of symptoms, but such decisions must be individualized. Asymptomatic aneurysms smaller than 4.5 cm in diameter have an extremely low risk of rupture and do not constitute an indication for surgery.[57-59] However, these aneurysms should be followed carefully, and an increase in size or the development of symptoms should be taken as indications for resection.

SUPERIOR MESENTERIC ARTERY SYNDROME

It has been suggested that, in patients of the "asthenic habitus," postprandial epigastric pain or bloating occasionally may be caused by compression of the third portion of the duodenum between the superior mesenteric artery anteriorly and the fixed retroperitoneal structures posteriorly. In such patients assumption of the knee-chest position may afford relief of symptoms, presumably because of an increase in the anatomical angle in which the duodenum lies. Although barium contrast studies indeed may be suggestive of extrinsic compression of the duodenum by the superior mesenteric artery, the validity of this syndrome remains in doubt, and surgical intervention is generally not warranted.

REFERENCES

1. Williams, L. F., Jr. Vascular insufficiency of the intestine. Gastroenterology 61:757, 1971.
2. Mikkelsen, W. P. Intestinal angina: Its surgical significance. Amer. J. Surg. 94:262, 1957.
3. Watt, J. K., Watson, W. C., and Haase, S. Chronic intestinal ischemia. Brit. Med. J. 2:199, 1967.
4. Ingelfinger, F. J. Chronic vascular insufficiency of the gastrointestinal tract: Abdominal angina. Gastroenterology 45:789, 1963.
5. Bynum, T. E., and Jacobson, E. D. Blood flow and gastrointestinal function. Gastroenterology 60:325, 1971.
6. Dardik, H., Seidenberg, B., Parker, J., and Hurwitt, E. Intestinal angina with malabsorption treated by elective re-vascularization. J.A.M.A. 194:1206, 1967.
7. Price, W. E., Rohrer, G. V., and Jacobson, E. D. Mesenteric vascular diseases. Gastroenterology 57:599, 1969.
8. Marston, A. Mesenteric arterial disease: The present position. Gut, 8:203, 1967.
9. Dunbar, J. D., Molnar, W., Beman, F. M., and Marable, S. A. Compression of the celiac trunk and abdominal aorta. Amer. J. Roent. 95:731, 1965.
10. Stoney, R. J., and Wylie, E. J. Recognition and management of visceral ischemic syndromes. Ann. Surg. 164:714, 1966.
11. Snyder, M. A., Mahoney, E. B., and Rob, C. G. Symptomatic celiac artery stenosis due to constriction by the neurofibrous tissue of the celiac ganglion. Surgery 61:372, 1967.
12. Marable, S. A., Kaplan, M. F., Beman, F. M., and Molnar, W. Celiac compression syndrome. Amer. J. Surg. 115:97, 1968.
13. Edwards, A. J., Hamilton, J. D., Nichol, W. D., Taylor, G. W., and Dawson, A. M. Experience with coeliac axis compression syndrome. Brit. Med. J. 1:342, 1970.
14. Lord, R. S., Stoney, R. J., and Wylie, E. J. Coeliac-axis compression. Lancet 2:795, 1968.
15. Derrick, J. R., Pollard, H. S., and Moore, R. M. The pattern of arteriosclerotic narrowing of the celiac and superior mesenteric arteries. Ann. Surg. 149:684, 1959.
16. Charrette, E. P., Iyengar, R. K., Lynn, R. B., Paloschi, G. B., and West, R. O. Abdominal pain associated with celiac artery compression. Surg. Gynec. Obstet. 132:1009, 1971.
17. Brennen, M. F., Clarke, A. M., and Macbeth, W. A. A. G. Infarction of the midgut associated with oral contraceptives. New Eng. J. Med. 279:1213, 1968.
18. Glotzer, D. J., and Shaw, R. S. Massive bowel infarction: An autopsy study assessing the potentialities of reconstructive vascular surgery. New Eng. J. Med. 260:162, 1959.
19. Ottinger, L. W., and Austen, W. G. A study of 136 patients with mesenteric infarction. Surg. Gynec. Obstet. 124:251, 1967.
20. Williams, L. F., Wittenberg, J., Grimes, E. T., and Byrne, J. J. Ischemic diseases of the bowel. I. Ischemia of the small bowel. Dis. Colon Rectum 13:275, 1970.
21. Bergan, J. J. Recognition and treatment of intestinal ischemia. Surg. Clin. N. Amer. 47:109, 1967.
22. Ming, S., and Levitan, R. Acute hemorrhagic necrosis of the gastrointestinal tract. New Eng. J. Med. 263:59, 1960.
23. Williams, L. F., Jr. Vascular insufficiency of the bowels. Disease-A-Month, August, 1970.

24. Arosemena, E., and Edwards, J. E. Lesions of the small mesenteric arteries underlying intestinal infarction. Geriatrics 22:122, 1967.

25. Fagin, R. R., and Kirsner, J. B. Ischemic diseases of the colon. Advan. Intern. Med. 17:343, 1971.

26. Kilpatrick, Z. M., Silverman, J. F., Betancourt, E., Farman, J., and Lawson, J. P. Vascular occlusion of the colon and oral contraceptives: Possible relation. New Eng. J. Med. 278:438, 1968.

27. Marston, A., Pheils, M. T., Thomas, M. L., and Morson, B. C. Ischemic colitis. Gut 7:1, 1966.

28. Kilpatrick, Z. M., Farman, J., Yesner, R., and Spiro, H. M. Ischemic proctitis. J.A.M.A. 205:74, 1968.

29. de Dombal, F. T., Fletcher, D. M., and Harris, R. S. Early diagnosis of ischemic colitis. Gut 10:131, 1969.

30. Byrne, J. J., Wittenberg, J., Grimes, E. T., and Williams, L. F. Ischemic diseases of the bowel. II. Ischemic colitis. Dis. Colon Rectum 13:283, 1970.

31. Miller, W. T., Scott, J., Rosato, E. F., Rosato, F. A., and Crow, H. Ischemic colitis with gangrene. Radiology 94:291, 1970.

32. Naitove, A., and Weismann, R. Primary mesenteric venous thrombosis. Ann. Surg. 161:516, 1965.

33. Civetta, J. M., and Kolodny, M. Mesenteric venous thrombosis associated with oral contraceptives. Gastroenterology 58:713, 1970.

34. Matthews, J. E., and White, R. R. Primary mesenteric venous occlusive disease. Amer. J. Surg. 122:579, 1971.

35. Schmid, F. R., Cooper, N. S., Ziff, M., and McEwen, C. Arteritis in rheumatoid arthritis. Amer. J. Med. 30:56, 1961.

36. Pollak, V., Grove, W., Kark, R., Muehrcke, R. C., Pirani, C. L., and Steck, I. E. Systemic lupus erythematosus simulating acute surgical conditions of the abdomen. New Eng. J. Med. 259:258, 1958.

37. Finkbiner, R. B., and Decker, J. P. Ulceration and perforation of the intestine due to necrotizing arteriolitis. New Eng. J. Med. 258:14, 1963.

38. Cabal, E., and Holtz, S. Polyarteritis as a cause of intestinal hemorrhage. Gastroenterology 61:99, 1971.

39. Miller, D. R., and O'Farrell, T. P. Perforation of the small intestine secondary to necrotizing vasculitis. Ann. Surg. 162:81, 1965.

40. Mendeloff, A. I., and Shulman, L. E. Gastrointestinal responses in connective tissue diseases. In Current Concepts of Clinical Gastroenterology. J. R. Gamble and D. L. Wilbur (eds.). Boston, Little, Brown and Co., 1965, pp. 107–123.

41. Kurlander, D. J., and Kirsner, J.B. The association of chronic "non-specific" inflammatory bowel disease with lupus erythematosus. Ann. Intern. Med. 60:799, 1964.

42. Rodriguez-Erdmann, F., and Levitan, R. Gastrointestinal and roentgenological manifestations of Henoch-Schönlein purpura. Gastroenterology 54:260, 1968.

43. Strole, W. E., Jr., Clark, W. H., and Isselbacher, K. J. Progressive arterial occlusive disease (Köhlmeier-Degos). New Eng. J. Med., 276:195, 1967.

44. Köhlmeier, W. Multiple Hautnekrosen bei Thromboangiitis obliterans. Arch. Dermat. Syph. 181:783, 1941.

45. Degos, R., Delort, J., and Tricot, R. Dermatite papulo-squameuse atrophiante. Bull. Soc. franç. dermat. Syph. 49:148, 281, 1942.

46. Kirshbaum, J. D. Abdominal aortitis with stenosis (Takayasu's disease) and occlusive superior mesenteric arteritis associated with renal artery stenosis and hypertension. Amer. Heart J. 80:811, 1970.

47. Allen, A. C., Boley, S. J., Schultz, L., and Schwartz, S. Potassium-induced lesions of the small bowel. II. Pathology and pathogenesis. J.A.M.A. 193:1001, 1965.

48. Schwartz, S., Boley, S., Schultz, L., and Allen, A. A survey of vascular diseases of the small intestine. Sem. Roent. 1:178, 1966.

49. Carron, D. B., and Douglas, A. P. Steatorrhoea in vascular insufficiency of the small intestine. Quart. J. Med. 34:331, 1965.

50. Phillips, J.C., and Howland, W. J. Mesenteric arteritis in systemic lupus erythematosus. J.A.M.A. 206:1569, 1968.

51. Judd, D. R., Taybi, H., and King, H. Intramural hematoma of the small bowel. Arch. Surg. 89:527, 1964.

52. Wiot, J. F. Intramural small intestinal hemorrhage—a differential diagnosis. Sem. Roent. 1:219, 1966.

53. Killian, S. T., and Heitzman, E. J. Intramural hemorrhage of small intestine due to anticoagulants. J.A.M.A. 200:591, 1967.

54. Khilnani, M. T., Marshak, R. H., Eliasoph, J., and Wolf, B. S. Intramural intestinal hemorrhage. Amer. J. Roent. 92:1061, 1964.

55. Rosato, F. E., Barker, C., and Roberts, B. Aortico-intestinal fistula. J. Thor. Cardiovasc. Surg. 53:511, 1967.

56. DeBakey, M. D., Crawford, E. S., Cooley, D. A., Morris, G. C., Royster, T. S., and Abbott, W. P. Aneurysm of abdominal aorta. Analysis of results of graft replacement therapy one to eleven years after operation. Ann. Surg. 160:622, 1964.

57. Fomon, J. J., Kurzweg, F. T., and Broadaway, R. K. Aneurysms of the aorta: A review. Ann. Surg. 165:557, 1967.

58. Bernstein, E. F., Fisher, J. C., and Varco, R. L. Is excision the optimum treatment for all abdominal aortic aneurysms? Surgery, 61:83, 1967.

59. Smith, G. Clinical aspects of aneurysms and their management. Practitioner 206:338, 1971.

Chapter 115

Diseases of the Peritoneum, Mesentery, and Diaphragm

Michael D. Bender, Robert K. Ockner

ANATOMY AND PHYSIOLOGY OF THE PERITONEUM

ANATOMY

The peritoneum is the serous membrane which lines the peritoneal cavity and its contained viscera. It forms a closed sac, except for the fimbriated ostia of the fallopian tubes, and is divided into visceral and parietal portions. The visceral peritoneum encloses the intraperitoneal organs and forms the mesenteries by which they are suspended. The parietal peritoneum lines the anterior, lateral, and posterior abdominal walls, the undersurface of the diaphragm, and the pelvic floor. Those abdominal viscera which are retroperitoneal, including the duodenum, the ascending and descending colon, and portions of the pancreas, kidneys, and adrenals, are covered anteriorly by the parietal peritoneum.

BLOOD SUPPLY

The greater part of the peritoneal surface and mesentery is supplied by the splanchnic blood vessels, and drained via the splanchnic venous system and portal vein. A smaller area is supplied by branches of the lower intercostal, subcostal, lumbar, and iliac arteries and is drained by veins which enter the inferior vena cava via the lumbar and iliac veins.

INNERVATION

The innervation of the parietal peritoneum differs from that of the visceral peritoneum. The parietal peritoneum is innervated by twigs from the same spinal nerves which supply the abdominal wall. As a result, irritation of the parietal peritoneum gives rise to afferent stimuli perceived as somatic pain, transmitted via the intercostal nerves. In contrast, there are no pain receptors in the visceral peritoneum; afferent stimuli run in the distribution of the sympathetic nervous system to the viscera. These differences account for the more precise localization of pain and definite physical signs which result from irritation of the parietal peritoneum.

The diaphragmatic peritoneum has a double innervation. The central portion is supplied by the phrenic nerve (C3 to C5), whereas the peripheral portion is innervated through intercostal nerves. Thus irritation of the diaphragmatic peritoneum may cause pain to be referred to either the

1578

shoulder (phrenic distribution) or the thoracic or abdominal wall (intercostal distribution).

PHYSIOLOGY

Movement of fluid, and of both large and small molecular weight solutes across the peritoneal membrane, appears to be accomplished by means of simple passive diffusion.[1, 2] In a number of in vitro and in vivo studies, apparent changes in membrane permeability have resulted from alterations in temperature, oxygen tension, pH, and calcium concentration,[1] as effects of various hormonal and pharmacologic agents (including vasopressin, corticosteroids, serotonin, and histamine),[1,3] and metabolic inhibitors. However, the clinical and physiological significance of these effects remains uncertain. Furthermore, changes in mesenteric blood flow and capillary permeability may have contributed to the observed changes.[4] By electron microscopy, a close continuity between the peritoneal cavity and subperitoneal capillaries is demonstrable; molecules less than 30 Å in diameter and with a molecular weight under 2000 are absorbed by capillaries and enter the portal vein, whereas heavier, larger molecules are absorbed by lymphatics.[5]

The peritoneal lymphatics play a major role in removing solid and liquid material from the peritoneal cavity, although only the diaphragmatic lymphatics have been well studied. Early experimental work showed that particles injected intraperitoneally pass between mesothelial cells and into lymphatics on the diaphragmatic surface. Electron microscopic studies of diaphragmatic peritoneum have demonstrated the presence of an anatomical arrangement which facilitates absorption from the peritoneal cavity. In areas where peritoneal mesothelial cells contact the terminal lymphatics (lacunae), gaps are present between mesothelial cells, the submesothelial basement membrane is scanty or absent, and the diaphragmatic lymphatic endothelium lacks a basement membrane. As a result of this anatomical arrangement, particles and large molecules may move through the intercellular gaps between mesothelial and endothelial cells into the terminal lymphatics, tran-

sit which may be further increased by respiratory motion.[6] The importance of these diaphragmatic lymphatics has been demonstrated in animal studies in which obliteration of the diaphragmatic peritoneum by abrasion significantly delays the absorption of serum from the peritoneal cavity and increases the propensity of portal hypertension to produce ascites.[7]

The clearance of peritoneal fluid from the abdominal cavity was first studied in animals; a rapid initial clearance followed by a constant clearance phase was documented. Studies in man, using intraperitoneal saline and labeled albumin, confirm that equilibration of saline between serum and peritoneal fluid occurs within two hours, after which fluid is absorbed at a relatively constant rate of 33 ml per hour.[8] The rate of absorption in the initial two hours varies with the osmolar gradient, and becomes constant after equilibration.[9]

DIAGNOSIS OF PERITONEAL DISEASE

HISTORY AND PHYSICAL EXAMINATION

The cardinal symptoms of peritoneal disease are abdominal pain and ascites; fever, distention, nausea, vomiting, and altered bowel habits are variably present. Direct tenderness, rebound tenderness, and involuntary spasm of the anterior abdominal musculature are the major signs of peritoneal irritation. The signs and symptoms may be less marked in the elderly or debilitated patient and will vary, depending upon the location and cause of the underlying process (vide infra). Diagnosis may be facilitated by radiology, paracentesis, biopsy, and peritoneoscopy.

RADIOLOGY

Peritoneal disease may be reflected by the presence of ascites. Large amounts of fluid, readily detectable on plain abdominal films, are manifested by abdominal haziness, increased density shifting to the pelvis on upright films, separation of bowel loops, and obliteration of the psoas shadows. Smaller amounts of fluid, from 800 to 1000 ml, may be detected by widening of the flank stripe (the line formed by the lateral colonic wall and peritoneum, and visible between the air-filled bowel lumen and the extraperitoneal fat layer) to more than 1 to 2 mm and by obliteration of the hepatic angle, i.e., the right lateral inferior margin of the liver.[10]

The peritoneum itself is difficult to evaluate radiographically. Induced pneumoperitoneum may demonstrate nodules on the parietal peritoneum; barium contrast studies may indirectly reflect involvement of visceral peritoneum by changes similar to those seen with transmural involvement of the bowel wall by other processes. Bizarre angular patterns of intestinal loops, rigidity of the bowel with diminished peristalsis, or altered mucosal patterns with filling defects or flattened folds are suggestive of primary disease of the bowel with secondary peritoneal involvement.

ABDOMINAL PARACENTESIS

Diagnostic paracentesis for obvious or suspected ascites is easily performed at the bedside with plastic catheters, and may provide valuable information with little risk. The procedure may be performed with the patient supine or sitting, after making certain that the bladder is empty. With sterile technique and under local anesthesia, the needle or catheter is introduced in the midline between the umbilicus and pubis. By entering through the avascular linea alba the risk of hemorrhage is reduced, but the catheter may be introduced laterally if necessary. Evaluation of the fluid obtained may include gross inspection and laboratory determination of protein, cell count and differential, culture, amylase, glucose, cultures for tuberculosis and fungi, cytology, Sudan stain, and lipid concentration.

PERITONEAL BIOPSY

The peritoneum can be examined histologically by means of percutaneous biopsy with a Cope or Vim-Silverman needle. In the presence of ascites, biopsy is a safe bedside technique with little morbidity. Hemorrhage is the major complication, especially in the patient with portal hypertension and enlarged intra-abdominal veins. Perforation and infection are uncommon.

Most data have been accumulated using the Vim-Silverman needle. With this needle adequate tissue is obtained in 80 to 85 per cent of attempts, and a diagnosis may be made in 30 to 45 per cent.[11] A positive diagnosis has been made in 50 to 60 per cent of cases of tuberculous peritonitis and in 25 to 40 per cent of cases of carcinoma. More recently, experience with the blunt-ended Cope needle indicates that the diagnostic yield may be increased to as high as 60 to 90 per cent.[12] The Cope needle is probably the instrument of choice because of its greater diagnostic yield and safety.

PERITONEOSCOPY

Peritoneoscopy may afford direct inspection of the peritoneum and abdominal organs, and permit biopsy of suspected pathology under direct vision. It is a relatively minor operative procedure, may be performed under local anesthesia in seriously ill patients, and involves little discomfort, morbidity, or mortality.[13] The ability to examine patients without ascites by the introduction of carbon dioxide or air is a great advantage; patients with ascites may require paracentesis in order to allow an adequate examination. A positive peritoneoscopic diagnosis may obviate the need for surgical exploration, thereby eliminating the morbidity of general anesthesia and postoperative problems, with little risk and a good diagnostic yield.

DISEASES OF THE PERITONEUM

ASCITES

PATHOPHYSIOLOGY

Ascites, the accumulation of fluid within the peritoneal cavity, may be caused by abnormalities in several physiological factors, including portal venous pressure, colloid osmotic pressure, hepatic lymph formation, splanchnic lymphatic drainage, sodium metabolism, and subperitoneal capillary permeability. Increased portal venous pressure is reflected in an increased filtration pressure at the capillary level and results in transudation of fluid at an accelerated rate. Normally, filtration pressure is balanced by a plasma colloid osmotic pressure, which primarily reflects albumin concentration. Thus a rise in portal venous pressure or a fall in plasma albumin may lead to the formation of ascites, although portal hypertension caused by extrahepatic portal venous obstruction rarely causes ascites in the absence of liver disease or hypoalbuminemia.[14]

Abnormalities of lymphatic flow have been implicated in the formation of ascites, especially in cirrhosis. Thus increased formation of hepatic lymph with extravasation into the peritoneal cavity, together with inadequate reabsorption of lymph, has been postulated as important in the genesis of ascites.[15] In support of this concept, it has been shown that albumin, newly synthesized in the liver, may enter the peritoneal cavity directly, without first having entered the peripheral circulation.[16] However, lymphatic flow may be increased to an equal degree in cirrhotic patients with and without ascites.

Renal retention of sodium and water also contributes to ascites formation. Patients with ascites tend to have increased total body water, total body exchangeable sodium, and normal or increased plasma volume. It has been suggested that renal sodium retention may be the initiating step in ascites formation, leading to expansion of plasma volume and secondarily to ascites formation as an "overflow" phenomenon.[17] Postulated mechanisms for renal sodium retention in cirrhosis include impaired hepatic inactivation of aldosterone or renin, hepatic production of a humoral stimulator of aldosterone secretion, and deficiency of an unknown natriuretic hormone. In addition to these humoral influences, alterations in renal hemodynamics, particularly intrarenal vasoconstriction which leads to a reduction in cortical perfusion, may also play a role in renal sodium retention.[18] The site of the functional defect leading to excessive renal tubular sodium reabsorption and impaired water diuresis may involve both the proximal and distal tubules.[19] The relative importance of all these mechanisms remains uncertain. Even if renal sodium retention is not the primary defect in ascites

formation, secondary hyperaldosteronism is present in the majority of patients with ascites and cirrhosis.

Finally, permeability of the subperitoneal capillaries is increased in a wide variety of inflammatory and neoplastic diseases and is probably of importance in the development of ascites caused by myxedema, ovarian disease, and allergic vasculitis. These entities are discussed in greater detail below.

CLINICAL AND LABORATORY FEATURES

Increasing abdominal distention is the major symptom of ascites, although when large amounts of fluid are present, the patient may complain of dyspnea and abdominal discomfort. On examination, the flanks bulge and a fluid wave may be demonstrable. Shifting dullness is somewhat more sensitive, but may be nonspecific. Although it is difficult to detect less than 1.5 to 2 liters of fluid, placing the patient on his hands and knees and percussing flatness over the dependent abdomen ("puddle sign") may reveal the presence of as little as 300 to 400 ml of fluid.

Laboratory analysis of the peritoneal fluid is essential for the proper evaluation of ascites. The protein concentration and specific gravity have been used to classify fluid as exudative or transudative. Fluids with protein levels above 3.0 mg per 100 ml or a specific gravity above 1.016 have been designated exudates; below those values, they are designated transudates. Diseases usually but not invariably associated with transudative ascites include congestive heart failure, inferior vena cava obstruction, Budd-Chiari syndrome, hypoalbuminemia, cirrhosis, Meigs' syndrome, and vasculitis. Exudates are common in peritoneal malignancy, tuberculous peritonitis, myxedema, pancreatic ascites, and bacterial peritonitis. However, strict reliance on this rather arbitrary division may be misleading. For example, fluid from patients with congestive heart failure may contain more than 3 g per 100 ml of protein.[20] In cirrhotic ascites, protein may exceed 2.5 g per 100 ml, depending on the location of the portal obstruction,[15] and tuberculous peritonitis is occasionally associated with a transudate.

Furthermore, specific gravity determinations are often quite inaccurate (owing to temperature changes, hygrometer variations, and other factors), and therefore should be used primarily as a means of checking the protein concentration. Thus arbitrary classification of ascites as exudative or transudative may lead to errors in diagnosis. On the other hand, the information is useful as a guide to diagnostic approach, and exceptions to the aforementioned generalizations are unusual when protein values are found to be at the high or low extremes.

Other chemistries may also help in diagnosis. Glucose values of less than 60 mg per 100 ml may suggest neoplastic effusion with a large number of free cancer cells.[21] Peritoneal fluid amylase is greatly increased in pancreatic ascites, and triglyceride levels will exceed those in plasma in chylous ascites.

A large number of red cells, especially grossly bloody ascites, raises the suspicion of neoplasm, particularly hepatoma or ovarian carcinoma. Tuberculous peritonitis, pancreatitis, hepatic vein thrombosis, and abdominal trauma may also be associated with bloody ascites. The presence of more than 250 leukocytes per mm^3 in ascitic fluid is an indication of peritoneal irritation, caused by infection, inflammation, or infiltration by tumor. Polymorphonuclear leukocytes usually reflect acute bacterial infection, whereas lymphocytes and monocytes characterize chronic inflammatory disease, especially tuberculosis. Ascites of eosinophilic enteritis and peritonitis produces a high eosinophil count in ascitic fluid.

Cytological examination is valuable and quite accurate in the evaluation of ascites caused by malignancy, especially when adequate volumes of fluid can be obtained. Overall accuracy may range from 60 to 90 per cent, and false positive Class V cytologies are rare in skilled hands.[22]

DIFFERENTIAL DIAGNOSIS OF ASCITES

The causes of ascites may be grouped into those processes in which the peritoneum is not directly involved (Table 115–1) and those in which the peritoneum itself is diseased (Table 115–2). The former group of conditions will be discussed here,

TABLE 115–1. CAUSES OF ASCITES NOT ASSOCIATED WITH PERITONEAL DISEASE

I. Portal hypertension
  A. Cirrhosis
  B. Hepatic congestion
    1. Congestive heart failure
    2. Constrictive pericarditis
    3. Inferior vena cava obstruction
    4. Hepatic vein obstruction (Budd-Chiari syndrome)
  C. Portal vein occlusion
II. Hypoalbuminemia
  A. Nephrotic syndrome
  B. Protein-losing enteropathy
  C. Malnutrition
III. Miscellaneous
  A. Myxedema
  B. Ovarian disease
    1. Meigs' syndrome
    2. Struma ovarii
    3. Ovarian overstimulation syndrome
  C. Pancreatic ascites
  D. Bile ascites
  E. Chylous ascites

TABLE 115–2. DISEASES OF THE PERITONEUM

I. Infections
  A. Tuberculous peritonitis
  B. Spontaneous bacterial peritonitis
  C. Fungal
    1. *Candida albicans*
    2. Histoplasma
  D. Parasitic
    1. Schistosomiasis
    2. Enterobius
II. Neoplasms
  A. Primary mesothelioma
  B. Secondary carcinomatosis
III. Pseudomyxoma peritonei
IV. Familial paroxysmal peritonitis
V. Miscellaneous
  A. Vasculitis
    1. SLE and other collagen-vascular diseases
    2. Allergic vasculitis (Schönlein-Henoch purpura)
    3. Köhlmeier-Degos disease
  B. Eosinophilic gastroenteritis
  C. Whipple's disease
  D. Granulomatous peritonitis
    1. Sarcoidosis
    2. Crohn's disease
    3. Starch peritonitis
  E. Gynecologic lesions
    1. Endometriosis
    2. Deciduosis
  F. Peritoneal lymphangiectasia
  G. Peritoneal loose bodies
  H. Peritoneal encapsulation

and the latter subsequently, under diseases of the peritoneum. Despite the sizable differential diagnosis of ascites, it has been the general experience that over 90 per cent of cases are due to one of four conditions, including cirrhosis, neoplasm, congestive heart failure, and tuberculosis.[20, 23] The relative frequency of these causes varies, depending upon the patient population selected for study.

Portal Hypertension. CIRRHOSIS. Cirrhosis is the most common cause of ascites in North America. Most of the pathophysiological mechanisms discussed may play a part in the etiology of cirrhotic ascites: portal hypertension, hypoalbuminemia, alteration in lymph flow, and renal retention of sodium and water. Discussion of cirrhosis is beyond the scope of this text, and the reader is referred to other sources.

CARDIAC CAUSES OF PORTAL HYPERTENSION. Diseases which cause mechanical or functional impedance to hepatic venous flow are often associated with ascites. Among these, congestive heart failure, particularly right sided, is the most frequent. Constrictive pericarditis deserves particular emphasis and should always be considered in cases of ascites of obscure origin. It usually presents with fatigue, ascites, and tender hepatomegaly, often with little peripheral edema. In the evaluation of the patient with ascites, the physical findings characteristic of this entity should be searched for: jugular venous distention with early diastolic collapse and inspiratory swelling, a diastolic knock which may be confused with a third heart sound, and pulsus paradoxus. Clear lung fields and low voltage on the electrocardiogram are often present. The diagnosis may be confirmed by cardiac fluoroscopy and cardiac catheterization.

INFERIOR VENA CAVA AND HEPATIC VEIN OBSTRUCTION (BUDD-CHIARI SYNDROME). Inferior vena cava and hepatic vein obstruction characteristically cause ascites and hepatomegaly. The Budd-Chiari syndrome may present with a varied course as an acute, subacute, or chronic illness, and may result from thrombi, intimal fibrosis, or tumor involving the hepatic veins or vena cava.[24] Thrombosis may be secondary to polycythemia vera (and other causes of hyperviscosity or thrombocytosis), hemoglo-

binopathies such as sickle cell disease, or the use of oral contraceptives.[25] Recently, a surgically remediable cause of unknown etiology, membranous obstruction of the inferior vena cava, has been reported from Japan.[26]

Presenting signs and symptoms include abdominal pain in 55 per cent, ascites in 90 to 95 per cent, and tender hepatomegaly in 70 per cent; splenomegaly and jaundice are seen in only 30 per cent. Liver function may be only mildly abnormal, with a high alkaline phosphatase or increased BSP retention. Femoral venous pressure may be elevated in the face of normal pressure in the tributaries of the superior vena cava. The diagnosis may be suggested by liver biopsy (which shows centrilobular necrosis, hepatic congestion, and eventually fibrosis and cirrhosis), but usually depends upon direct demonstration of venous occlusion. Hepatic venography may show vena caval obstruction or a narrow, occluded main hepatic vein with a "network pattern" of neighboring veins.

Hypoalbuminemia. Ascites is uncommon in patients with uncomplicated hypoalbuminemia, although it may be noted in up to 12 per cent of those with the nephrotic syndrome. Nephrotic patients with ascites have a serum albumin level of less than 2.5 per 100 ml, and often less than 1.5 per 100 ml. Protein-losing enteropathy and malnutrition are infrequent causes of hypoalbuminemic ascites in North America.

Myxedema. Myxedema is an unusual but treatable cause of clinically significant ascites, and presents with intractable exudative ascites which may respond poorly to diuretics. Patients frequently have only impaired mentation and ascites. Mild systemic changes of myxedema may be overlooked, and a number of these patients are subjected to an unnecessary laparotomy. The fluid is yellow and gelatinous, and generally has a protein of over 4 g per 100 ml. Although the pathophysiology is poorly understood, it is postulated that there is increased capillary permeability with escape of protein-rich fluid. Intravenous fluorescein causes tissue staining before, but not after, treatment with thyroxine, and protein electrophoresis of ascitic fluid is similar to the serum pattern.[27] The ascites is rapidly cleared within two to three weeks after the start of thyroxine.

Ovarian Disease. Ovarian causes of ascites, aside from carcinoma, include Meigs' syndrome and the ovarian overstimulation syndrome. Meigs' syndrome consists of ascites and hydrothorax with various benign ovarian tumors. Initially, the syndrome was described specifically with fibromas, but it now appears that cystadenomas are more common.[28] The formation of ascites in this condition has variously been ascribed to either an interrupted ovarian venous drainage with transudation or large tumors with edematous, myxoid stroma.

A rare tumor of the ovary, *struma ovarii,* is a unilateral ovarian teratoma containing thyroid tissue. Patients may present with symptoms of hyperthyroidism, ascites, or an ovarian mass. About one-third may have ascites, and about one-third demonstrate hyperthyroidism; 10 per cent have both.[29] Tumors associated with ascites are larger than 6 cm in diameter. The rich blood supply of thyroid tissue, together with edema and hemorrhage of the capsule caused by repeated twisting of the stalk, may account for the ascites. The diagnosis should be suspected if ovarian calcification is noted on abdominal X-rays and if I^{131} uptake is localized to the abdomen.

Massive ascites, pleural effusion, and hypovolemia have developed in association with enlarged ovaries after treatment with clomiphene and human menopausal gonadotropin. This "ovarian overstimulation" syndrome could be caused by transudation of fluid through an edematous ovarian stroma, but animal studies have suggested that it may actually be due to liberation of a substance from the ovary which increases capillary permeability.[30]

Pancreatic Ascites. It has become apparent that pancreatic ascites is more common than previously recognized, especially in alcoholics.[31] These patients present with intermittent abdominal pain compatible with pancreatitis, along with massive, chronic, refractory ascites. Diagnosis is not difficult, because serum amylase is elevated in 93 per cent; the ascitic fluid amylase is always elevated (with values as high as 39,000 Somogyi units). The fluid protein is over 2.5 g per 100 ml in 85 per cent, and may contain both white and

red cells. At surgery, chronic pancreatitis with a pseudocyst is usually found. Frequently, overt leakage of pancreatic secretions is evident. Excision or internal drainage procedures usually relieve the ascites, although removal of the fluid alone may help.

Bile Ascites. It is now well recognized that extravasated bile may cause chronic peritoneal fluid accumulation. After biliary tract surgery a small number of patients develop abdominal distention caused by accumulation of bile in the peritoneal cavity, but have no fever, leukocytosis, or peritoneal signs.[32] Nausea, malaise, jaundice, and acholic stools are usually present. Bile ascites may be noted as long as two months postoperatively, and is due to biliary tract leakage of any cause. Paracentesis is diagnostic, because it yields a bilious fluid and may be therapeutic if the leak is slow and small. Most often, re-exploration is necessary to repair the leak. The difference between this group and the more dramatic course of acute bile peritonitis may reflect the sterility of the extravasated bile. Experiments using germ-free animals and antibiotics show that bacteria play a major role in determining the severity of acute experimental bile peritonitis.[33]

Chylous Ascites. Chylous ascites is due to the accumulation of lipid-rich lymph in the peritoneal cavity. The diagnosis is made by recovering a turbid fluid from the abdomen which separates into layers on standing or stains positively for fat. The fluid is sterile and contains lymphocytes. Its significant lipid content (triglyceride levels exceed those of plasma) differentiates it from "pseudochyle." The latter is opalescent, does not contain large amounts of triglycerides, and is phospholipid-protein material from degenerating cells.

The cause of chylous ascites is neoplastic in 30 per cent (mainly intra-abdominal, retroperitoneal, and thoracic), inflammatory in 35 per cent (mesenteric adenitis, pancreatitis, or tuberculosis), traumatic in 11 per cent, congenital in 1 per cent and "idiopathic" in 23 per cent, among whom are patients with lymphangiectasia.[34] It may also be present in over half the patients with ascites caused by the nephrotic syndrome.[35] Chronic and acute chylous ascites differ in etiology and symptomatology. *Chronic chylous ascites* usually presents without pain, but with weight loss, hypoproteinemia, and inanition. Neoplastic disease is the cause in 80 per cent of chronic cases, and lymphomas comprise about half of these.[36]

Acute chylous peritonitis presents with the sudden onset of crampy abdominal pain in up to one-third of patients, often after a heavy meal, and localized in the right lower quadrant. Occasionally, a soft swelling may be noted in the left supraclavicular area, presumably caused by lymph extravasation in the neck. In 50 per cent of patients with the acute syndrome, laparotomy is negative except for chylous fluid, dilated lymphatics, and an edematous, inflamed mesentery and peritoneum. These are the so-called idiopathic cases.[37] Another 20 per cent demonstrate intestinal obstruction, with distention of the lacteals and weeping of chyle from the bowel surface. Trauma accounts for 15 per cent, with disruption of the cisterna chyli, and a final 15 per cent are due to rupture of chyle-containing cysts. Lymphangiography may occasionally localize the obstruction.

Congenital malformations are the cause of chylous ascites in 39 per cent of pediatric patients. These include stenosis or atresia of the lymphatics, hernia, and mesenteric cysts. In 31 per cent of pediatric patients, a cause is never found, but some of the idiopathic cases may be self-limited.[38]

The cause of chylous ascites is often discovered only at exploratory laparotomy. In patients in whom no cause is found, improvement may follow removal of chylous fluid. Internal drainage procedures or parenteral infusions of chyle are not helpful. Intravenous hyperalimentation or medium-chain triglycerides may be helpful in supporting the patient. Acute or idiopathic cases often clear spontaneously, but chronic chylous ascites may contribute to the debilitation associated with the primary disease.

TREATMENT OF ASCITES

The successful treatment of ascites often depends on the treatment of the underlying cause. In the case of cirrhotic ascites, however, the mainstays of treatment are sodium restriction and diuretics. A significant number of patients who are maintained on a sodium-restricted dietary program for days to weeks may undergo a spontaneous diuresis.[39] A well balanced diet, carefully restricted in sodium content (250 to 500 mg per day initially), is usually necessary. If the patient responds, sodium intake may be gradually liberalized. Fluid intake should be restricted if progressive weight gain or dilutional hyponatremia occurs.

Reasonable estimates of optimal diuresis have recently been provided from studies on the kinetics of endogenous ascites mobilization in cirrhotics. In cirrhotics without edema, only about 300 ml of the total daily urine volume is derived from the mobilization of ascites, and diuretics increase this only by 16 per cent, to 350 ml. With coexisting edema, a threefold increase in removal of ascites, to a maximum of about 900 ml, can be attained.[40] These findings provide a rational basis for management. Vigorous diuresis in excess of 1 liter per day cannot be expected to reduce ascites volume more rapidly than this upper limit. Rather, diuresis exceeding this amount occurs at the expense of plasma volume, and may lead to volume depletion, decreased renal perfusion, oliguria, and azotemia. There is no need to "dry out" a patient as rapidly and completely as possible, because the presence of a moderate amount of ascites is of little physiological consequence.

Diuretic agents commonly used include spironolactone (100 to 200 mg per day in divided doses), thiazide diuretics (50 to 100 mg hydrochlorothiazide per day or alternate days), furosemide (40 to 80 mg per day), or ethacrynic acid (50 to 100 mg per day). Larger doses of spironolactone may be used, monitoring the aldosterone-antagonist effect by the urinary sodium-potassium ratio. An increase in dosage of 100 mg every two to four days (up to 1000 mg daily) until the urinary sodium-potassium ratio is greater than 1, may lead to a gradual diuresis with only minimal risk of volume depletion, hypokalemia, or encephalopathy.[41] Commonly employed regimens combine spironolactone (a potassium-sparing diuretic) with a thiazide, furosemide, or ethacrynic acid.

Abdominal paracentesis of more fluid than needed for diagnostic studies (usually less than 1 liter) carries with it the risk of hypovolemia and its complications. It should rarely be used except to relieve respiratory distress or the discomfort of associated hernias or abdominal wall pain. After paracentesis of greater than 2 liters, about half the volume removed reaccumulates within 24 hours and the remainder over three to four days.[40]

Other agents such as corticosteroids, mannitol, albumin, or reinfusion of ascitic fluid have been suggested for management of refractory ascites. The clinical usefulness of these measures remains uncertain owing to side effects, expense, and lack of sustained effect. Surgical procedures such as thoracic duct cannulation, eversion of an ileal loop, bilateral adrenalectomy, or the use of a Holter valve (to drain ascites from the peritoneum into a systemic vein) have all been tried, but their value is questionable. Portasystemic shunting can reduce ascites, but the mortality and morbidity of this procedure are frequently prohibitive.

INFECTIONS OF THE PERITONEUM

TUBERCULOUS PERITONITIS

Although peritonitis is an unusual form of tuberculosis (about 0.5 per cent of patients admitted to a tuberculosis sanatorium),[42] it is one of the most important diseases involving the peritoneum. Its insidious nature and the clinical circumstances in which it occurs often cause it to be mistaken for neoplastic disease or ascites caused by cirrhosis.

Pathogenesis. Most cases of tuberculous peritonitis are not due to contiguous extension of active disease in or adjacent to the peritoneal cavity. Rather, they appear to reflect reactivation of latent tuberculous foci in the peritoneum, established at the time of earlier hematogenous spread from a primary focus, usually in the lung.[42,43] Thus many patients with tuberculous peritonitis do not have currently active pulmonary, intestinal, or genital tuberculosis. On the other hand, hematogenous spread from pulmonary or generalized miliary tuberculosis can cause concurrent tuberculous peritonitis.

Epidemiology. In the United States,

the disease is most commonly encountered in the municipal hospital setting, with its large population of cirrhotics and poorly nourished, debilitated patients.[44] There is no sex or age predilection, but from 80 to 90 per cent in reported series are black. This predilection may reflect socioeconomic rather than genetic factors.

Clinical Features. The clinical features of tuberculous peritonitis vary with the population studied. Generally, the onset is insidious, and over 70 per cent of patients have had symptoms for four months or longer. The most common complaints are constitutional, with fever, anorexia, weakness, malaise, and weight loss in 80 per cent. Abdominal pain is reported in only 50 per cent, and this is usually described as a vague, dull, diffuse discomfort. The incidence and intensity of vomiting, constipation, and diarrhea are variable. The major objective finding is ascites, which is clinically evident in 75 per cent of cases. Abdominal tenderness, usually diffuse, is present in 65 per cent; despite classic descriptions, the so-called doughy abdomen is rare. Hepatomegaly may be found in 25 per cent, and a mass caused by loculated fluid or an inflamed omentum or mesentery may be palpated in 20 per cent. Lymphadenopathy may be present. It is evident from the clinical description that the signs and symptoms of tuberculous peritonitis are nonspecific and variable. Therefore tuberculous peritonitis must be suspected in any patient with ascites, fever, unexplained constitutional symptoms, or diffuse abdominal pain or tenderness.

Laboratory Findings. Routine blood studies are rarely helpful; there is a normal white blood cell count in 70 to 90 per cent, and anemia is only variably present. The tuberculin skin test is negative in an average of 20 per cent of reported cases, although many of these are in patients with extraperitoneal and miliary disease. If tuberculosis is confined to the peritoneum, the first-strength purified protein derivative test may be positive in virtually 100 per cent.[43] A negative test may become positive during treatment, suggesting that the patient may have been anergic initially.

Other studies may prove useful, especially if disease is more generalized. Pulmonary infiltrates are seen in about 15 per cent of patients, and 40 per cent have a pleural effusion. Barium studies of the intestine, pyelograms, or salpingograms are rarely helpful, although bizarre angular or rigid small bowel loops and altered mucosal patterns may suggest mesenteric involvement. Percutaneous liver biopsy or lymph node biopsy may show granulomas, but this finding is not necessarily diagnostic of active intra-abdominal tuberculosis. It is interesting that of patients with tuberculous peritonitis, less than half will have evidence of disease elsewhere in the body.

Examination of the peritoneal fluid is the most important initial diagnostic test. Protein exceeds 2.5 g per 100 ml in 85 to 100 per cent of patients. Most patients have over 250 leukocytes per mm^3, and 90 to 100 per cent have more than 80 per cent mononuclear forms on differential count. Acid-fast stains of the peritoneal fluid will demonstrate the organisms in only about 5 per cent of patients. Results of culturing the fluid may also be disappointing, as the reported average of positive cultures is only 40 per cent. However, the yield may be improved to 80 per cent by concentrating up to 1 liter of fluid by centrifugation[43] and by inoculating guinea pigs.[44]

Peritoneal biopsy for granulomas is positive in 30 to 50 per cent of patients when using the Vim-Silverman needle, but use of the Cope needle has been reported to double this yield.[12, 43] The biopsy specimen should be cultured, but data on the yield of this procedure are limited.

The diagnosis is often suggested at peritoneoscopy by the appearance of the peritoneum, which may be studded with small granulomas. Direct biopsy through the peritoneoscope may improve the yield over that of needle biopsy by 20 to 30 per cent.[11, 43] The diagnosis is easily made at laparotomy, and this has been used as the primary diagnostic approach by some.[45, 46] Approximately 15 to 20 per cent of patients may need laparotomy to establish the diagnosis after all other efforts are negative. Laparotomy is generally well tolerated in these patients in the absence of serious contraindications.

Prognosis and Treatment. Prior to the availability of chemotherapy, the mortality rate of tuberculous peritonitis was as high as 60 per cent. However, the disease is now curable with antituberculous agents. Therapy with isoniazid and either para-aminosalicylic acid, streptomycin, or ethambutol should be continued for 18 to 24 months. Constitutional symptoms should begin to improve within one to two weeks of the onset of therapy, and fever should resolve within four weeks.

The place of corticosteroids in treatment is as yet unresolved. A three-month course of prednisone, 30 mg per day, may decrease the development of late fibrotic complications such as intestinal obstruction,[43] but the number of patients studied is small, and adequate therapy with antituberculous agents may be sufficient.[46]

SPONTANEOUS BACTERIAL PERITONITIS

Spontaneous or "primary" peritonitis is an acute or subacute bacterial infection of the peritoneum, not associated with the usual underlying etiological factors such as perforated viscus, abscess, or penetrating abdominal wound.

In the past, spontaneous peritonitis was mainly a disease of children with nephrotic syndrome, and the most common organisms were pneumococci and streptococci. In the antibiotic era primary pneumococcal or streptococcal peritonitis has become rare, although it is still occasionally reported.[47] Since the condition mimics peritonitis caused by an acute surgical emergency, laparotomy is almost always undertaken. The diagnosis is made at laparotomy and by culture of nonenteric organisms.

The diagnosis should be considered preoperatively in (1) patients with pre-existing ascites who develop fever or changing abdominal signs and symptoms; (2) patients with a focus for bacteremia, such as indwelling catheters, cellulitis, or urinary, biliary, and pulmonary infection; and (3) patients with decreased immunological competence, as in hypogammaglobulinemia. In these circumstances, preoperative paracentesis may reveal gram-positive organisms and indicate antibiotics as sole therapy.

SPONTANEOUS BACTERIAL
PERITONITIS IN CIRRHOTICS

It has become apparent that spontaneous peritonitis may occur in almost 10 per cent of cirrhotics with portal hypertension and overt ascites.[48]

In contrast to spontaneous peritonitis in noncirrhotics, about 60 per cent of causative organisms in cirrhotics are enteric, with 36 per cent being *Escherichia coli.* Pneumococci are the second most frequently cultured single organism (16 per cent), and various types of streptococci account for 24 per cent. Pseudomonas, Proteus, Aerobacter, Klebsiella, Bacteroides, Aeromonas, and Salmonella are other, less frequently cultured gram negative organisms. The prevalence of enteric organisms implicates local factors in the pathogenesis of spontaneous bacterial peritonitis. Congested lymphatics and splanchnic vessels, an edematous bowel wall, and perhaps a change in the intestinal flora may all play a part in allowing passage of bacteria through the intestinal wall. Gross intestinal lesions such as erosion or infarction are uncommon. Hematogenous spread with seeding of ascites, perhaps aided by failure of the cirrhotic liver to effectively remove bacteria from the blood stream, may also play a role. Foci of infection in the biliary tract, urine, lungs, skin, or indwelling catheters are present in 25 per cent of patients. Finally, a possible local role of systemic metabolic changes seen in cirrhosis, such as alkalosis, hypokalemia, and hypoxia, has not been documented, but these factors may contribute.

Clinical and Laboratory Features. Spontaneous peritonitis usually occurs in the setting of decompensated hepatic function; ascites is present in virtually all, jaundice and portal-systemic collaterals in 80 per cent, and azotemia in 55 per cent. As with tuberculous peritonitis, spontaneous peritonitis may be masked by the signs of cirrhosis or hepatic failure. Thirty-five per cent will have no peritoneal signs, although only 5 per cent develop completely silent peritonitis. Spontaneous peritonitis causes abdominal pain in 80 per cent, fever in 80 per cent, hypotension in 70 per cent, and encephalopathy in almost 75 per cent. For practical purposes, any deterioration of a cirrhotic patient with ascites should alert the clinician to the possibility of bacterial peritonitis.

Liver function studies are nearly always abnormal. Leukocytosis is the rule, but up to 25 per cent of patients have a normal white count. Blood cultures are positive in 75 per cent. Paracentesis remains the major diagnostic procedure, with 90 per cent having over 300 polymorphonuclear cells per mm^3. Although gram stain of the fluid is positive in only about 40 per cent, culture is positive in 90 per cent. The ascites protein usually remains under 3 g per 100 ml.

Prognosis and Treatment. A bacteriological response may be achieved with appropriate antibiotics in about 60 per cent of patients. Gram-positive cocci are most successfully treated, but there are no other clinical or laboratory features which predict successful treatment. However, delayed recognition and institution of antibiotic therapy may influence the outcome. Antibiotic concentrations in ascitic fluid in the presence of peritonitis rapidly achieve bactericidal levels after parenteral administration. Thus intraperitoneal instillation of antibiotics is unnecessary. Although drainage of the peritoneal fluid has not been well evaluated, it probably adds little to the management of spontaneous peritonitis.

Despite the successful bacteriological response in over half the patients with spontaneous peritonitis, prognosis is extremely grave. Overall survival is less than 5 per cent.

FUNGAL AND PARASITIC
INFECTION

Peritoneal inflammation caused by fungi and parasites is rare. *Candida albicans* has been reported to cause massive ascites by direct peritoneal involvement. However, this has occurred only when the organism has been able to enter the peritoneal cavity from the intestine, usually by perforation of an ulcer.[49] Recovery may follow a long course of amphotericin B.

Peritoneal involvement by *Histoplasma capsulatum* is exceedingly rare, appearing in only one of 530 patients with active histoplasmosis in a sanatorium population.[50] Peritoneal infection is noted in only 2 to 4 per cent of patients with disseminated histoplasmosis.

Parasitic infestation rarely leads to clinical peritoneal disease; its major importance lies in its ability to mimic peritoneal carcinomatosis or tuberculosis at laparotomy. Cases of granulomatous peritonitis caused by schistosomiasis have been reported, without other extraintestinal involvement. This is rarely symptomatic, and may be due to escape of eggs from intestinal veins.[51] Enterobiasis has been reported to give rise to a granulomatous peritonitis in women, apparently by migrating through the upper female genital tract.[52] Although most patients are asymptomatic, occasionally one may present with lower abdominal pain.

NEOPLASMS OF THE PERITONEUM

PRIMARY MESOTHELIOMA

Primary mesotheliomas are rare tumors arising from the epithelial and mesenchymal elements of the peritoneum.

Pathogenesis. During the last decade, asbestos exposure has been reported in 70 to 80 per cent of patients with mesotheliomas,[53, 54] approximately 30 per cent of which are peritoneal. This usually involves occupational exposure among textile workers, brakeliners, insulators, or handlers of other asbestos products. However, exposure may be indirect and limited to household or neighborhood contact. The mean time interval between exposure to asbestos and development of mesothelioma is about 35 to 40 years.[54] Although the duration of exposure is usually prolonged, it may be relatively short.

Aside from historical evidence of asbestos exposure, 60 to 80 per cent of patients with mesotheliomas tend to have pathological evidence of pulmonary asbestosis, including pulmonary fibrosis, pleural hyaline plaques, and "asbestos bodies" in the lungs. It has also been demonstrated that one-third of patients with peritoneal mesotheliomas have asbestos fibers in peritoneal tissue, if proper techniques are used to demonstrate them.[55] The significance of these findings is somewhat clouded by studies which show a large percentage (25 to 50 per cent) of the general population to have asbestos bodies and pleural plaques, but without asbestosis or mesotheliomas.[56] Furthermore, it has been recognized that the so-called asbestos bodies are nonspecific, and that identical bodies occur with at least 20 different substances.[56] Although asbestos seems to play a role in the pathogenesis of mesothelioma, the exact incidence and pathophysiological mechanism remain to be defined.

Pathology. On gross examination, primary mesotheliomas of the peritoneum may be extremely difficult to differentiate from secondary carcinomatosis of the peritoneum. They usually involve both the visceral and parietal peritoneum extensively, although they also form discrete plaques and nodules. Superficial capsular invasion of viscera and local lymph node involvement can be found, but visceral metastases are rare. A concomitant pleural mesothelioma is present in 30 to 60 per cent of patients.[55, 57]

The histological characteristics are quite variable.[55] Individual cells are rarely pleomorphic and have few mitoses. Epithelial elements predominate in 70 per cent, with tubular, papillary, sheet-like, cleft-like, or solid nest-like patterns. Sometimes mesenchymal elements predominate, with a marked fibromatous component and spindle-shaped cells. It is somewhat characteristic of mesotheliomas to have both epithelial and mesenchymal elements mixed in one tumor. A negative periodic acid–Schiff stain for mucin and a positive stain for hyaluronic acid are further suggestive, but not diagnostic, of mesothelioma. A definite diagnosis can be made only when the suggestive gross, histological and histochemical features are combined with a thorough surgical or postmortem examination to rule out an underlying primary tumor.

Clinical Aspects. Clinically, mesotheliomas present with abdominal pain and distention, ascites, nausea, vomiting, and weight loss. The diagnosis can only be suggested by cytology or peritoneal biopsy, and exploration is necessary to rule out a primary neoplasm. Prognosis is poor, with most patients surviving only one to two years after diagnosis.[57,58] Oral and intraperitoneal chemotherapy and radiation have not been helpful in the small number of patients treated.

SECONDARY CARCINOMATOSIS

Incidence and Etiology. Peritoneal involvement by spread from a primary neoplasm is one of the most common causes of peritoneal disease. Pathological study of unselected open peritoneal biopsy specimens in a large general hospital reveals that about 65 per cent are neoplastic. Over 75 per cent of these are metastatic adenocarcinoma; other tumors such as sarcomas, carcinoids, teratomas, lipomas, or nervous tissue tumors are extremely rare.[59] Malignancies of lymphoid or myeloid tissue can also infiltrate the peritoneum. Up to one-third of patients with leukemia may have peritoneal fluid, but less than 5 per cent have more than 1 liter of ascites.[60] Malignant lymphoma invades the serosa in about 20 per cent of patients, most often associated with bowel wall invasion, and may cause ascites. Peritoneal disease has been found in one-third of patients with reticulum cell sarcoma, but in only 10 per cent with Hodgkin's disease or lymphosarcoma.[61] Multiple myeloma has rarely been reported to cause peritoneal infiltration with ascites. Ascites occurs in about 10 per cent of patients with myeloid metaplasia, usually resulting from portal hypertension, cardiac disease, renal disease, or tuberculosis. Ectopic peritoneal implantation of myeloid tissue may also cause ascites, possibly because of occult splenic rupture.[62]

Pathophysiology. Although carcinomatous infiltration is among the most common causes of ascites, there has been little systematic study of its pathophysiology. Patients with ovarian cancer and peritoneal metastases demonstrate increased permeability to albumin in areas of peritoneum not involved by tumor.[63] Tumors may produce substances that increase peritoneal permeability, but this is unproved. Subserous lymphatic obstruction may play a major role in ascites formation in carcinomatosis.

Clinical Features and Diagnosis. Patients with peritoneal carcinomatosis present with ascites, diffuse abdominal pain, weight loss, and, less frequently, nausea and vomiting. Paracentesis yields fluid that may be either a transudate or exudate, and often contains red cells or gross blood.[20] The diagnosis is made most directly by cytology, peritoneal biopsy, or peritoneoscopy, as discussed above.

It is important to remember that many peritoneal diseases may present with a clinical picture mimicking peritoneal carcinomatosis. Particularly, tuberculous peritonitis and spontaneous bacterial peritonitis of cirrhosis must be ruled out, especially because they are treatable. Meigs' syndrome, myxedema, hypoalbuminemic ascites, and Budd-Chiari syndrome may be confused with peritoneal carcinomatosis in the appropriate clinical setting.

Prognosis and Therapy. Once neoplasm has spread to the peritoneum, the prognosis is poor. However, there are a number of palliative approaches which may be helpful. Instillation of cytotoxic agents may reduce the ascites in 40 to 60 per cent of patients,[65] and seems most effective when cytology is positive and the ascitic glucose level is low.[21] Cytotoxic agents kill free-floating and implanted neoplastic cells, but do not affect lymphatic obstruction. Nitrogen mustard, 5-fluorouracil and thio-TEPA have been used with about equal success.

Instillation of radioactive isotopes such as Au^{198} or P^{32} has also afforded a 40 to 60 per cent palliation rate, with Au^{198} probably somewhat superior.[64] With this modality, ascites recurs in 50 per cent in three to six months, but 10 to 20 per cent may be free of ascites for as long as one year. Isotopes are preferred by some over chemotherapeutic agents because of the lower incidence of nausea, vomiting, and bone marrow depression. The radiation effect is due to beta emission, and is limited to the peritoneal surface and to the tissues 1 to 2 mm below it. The mechanism is probably both inhibition of tumor cell growth and fibrosis of the peritoneal membrane and lymphatics.

Finally, quinacrine instillation has been used with good responses in up to 75 per cent of patients, with dosages of 400 mg for three to five days.[66] The effect of quinacrine depends on a fibrosing serositis; however, 25 to 50 per cent of patients develop fever, nausea, vomiting, pain, or ileus, thus limiting its usefulness.

PSEUDOMYXOMA PERITONEI

Etiology. Pseudomyxoma peritonei is a rare condition in which the peritoneal cavity becomes distended with a pale, translucent, semisolid material which has been shown biochemically and histochemically to be a mucin. There are two major causes of this "mucinous ascites": mucinous cystadenomas and cystadenocarcinomas of the ovary, and mucoceles of the appendix. Other less common causes include ovarian teratomas, ovarian fibromas, uterine carcinoma, mucinous adenocarcinoma of the bowel, adenocarcinoma in urachal cysts, mucoid omphalomesenteric cysts of the navel, and carcinoma of the common bile duct.[67]

Clinical and Pathologic Features. Pseudomyxoma presents primarily with increasing abdominal girth; usually there is a disparity between the amount of ascites and the clinical state of the patient. At laparotomy the peritoneal cavity is filled with mucinous material lying freely as a homogeneous mass or multiple cystic masses, whereas in other places it may be firmly attached to the peritoneum, where nests of the columnar epithelial cells characteristic of the syndrome are located. This epithelium may be quite scarce in relation to the amount of mucin present, and indeed mucin alone may be present, leading to the speculation that mucin may be produced by an altered peritoneal mesothelium.

The major point of controversy concerns the malignant nature of the epithelial cells. Mucoceles of the appendix result from obstruction of the proximal lumen of the appendix by fibrosis, with accumulation of mucus behind it; rupture can be demonstrated with the development of pseudomyxoma. Although some investigators believe that pseudomyxoma can be caused by rupture of a simple mucocele with benign epithelium,[68] others have reported that careful examination of serial sections of the appendix has shown cellular atypia, indicating that these are highly differentiated carcinomas of low biological malignancy.[69] Similarly, some have claimed that 90 to 95 per cent of mucinous cystadenomas of the ovary are benign, but others have found evidence of low-grade malignancy in a large percentage of those

tumors previously thought to be benign. Pseudomyxoma develops in large numbers of tumors with grade I malignancy, but very rarely in benign cystadenomas. Rupture of the cyst can also be demonstrated in patients who develop pseudomyxoma.

Prognosis and Therapy. Because the tumor is either benign or of low-grade malignancy, it rarely metastasizes, and the course of the disease is often long. Death is usually the result of intestinal obstruction and fistulas.[70] In recent years a more aggressive (albeit limited) combined surgical and chemotherapeutic approach has brightened the outlook. Removal of the ovary, appendix, peritoneal nodules, and omentum, evacuation of mucin, and instillation of an alkylating agent is now the treatment of choice.[71] Various other pharmacological agents have been tried without success, including trypsin, hyaluronidase, and acetylcysteine.[72]

FAMILIAL PAROXYSMAL POLYSEROSITIS (FAMILIAL MEDITERRANEAN FEVER)

Etiology and Pathogenesis. Familial paroxysmal polyserositis (FPP) is a disease characterized by recurrent episodes of acute, self-limited serositis, especially peritonitis. It is an inherited disease, transmitted as an autosomal recessive, and occurs predominantly in Mediterranean peoples (Sephardic Jews, Armenians, and Arabs). The genetic relationship is securely established, and has been thought to be associated with an inherited biochemical or metabolic defect. However, extensive studies of possible allergic, hypersensitivity, metabolic, or endocrine factors have identified neither the etiology nor the pathogenesis of FPP.[73]

Clinical Features. The onset of the disease is usually early, but 10 to 30 per cent of patients may have their first episode after the age of 20, even as late as age 47. Approximately 60 per cent of patients are males.

The disease usually appears suddenly with an attack of serositis, peritonitis in 55 per cent, arthritis in about 25 per cent, or pleuritis in 5 per cent.[74] During the course of FPP, 95 per cent eventually develop peritonitis, the sole manifestation in 30 per cent of patients.[73] The attack consists of the sudden onset of fever, usually 101 to 103° F, with localized or diffuse abdominal pain. Almost invariably there is exquisite direct abdominal tenderness, with marked rebound in two-thirds of patients. Involuntary spasm and guarding may be striking in one-quarter of patients, and may be generalized and board-like. Leukocytosis is present in almost 90 per cent, and plain film of the abdomen reveals air-fluid levels. After six to 12 hours, these signs and symptoms recede, and the patient is usually well in 24 to 48 hours. These attacks occur at irregular and unpredictable intervals, and the patient is entirely well between them. Aside from the usual rapid resolution and the recurrent nature of the disease, it presents all the characteristics of an acute surgical abdomen.

Although peritonitis is the major manifestation, during the course of FPP 40 per cent of patients develop pleuritis, 75 per cent develop arthritis (usually monarticular and rarely protracted), and 50 per cent develop an erysipelas-like erythema on the lower extremities. Pericarditis has been reported. The only fatal complication, amyloid nephropathy, has been reported to develop in about 25 per cent of patients.[74] Other investigators have found lower incidences of the joint, skin, and renal manifestations.[73]

Pathology. At peritoneoscopy or laparotomy during an acute attack the peritoneum is lusterless and hyperemic, with occasional scattered areas of fibrin-like material; the cavity contains some serous fluid. Peritoneal biopsy reveals acute inflammation with polymorphonuclear infiltration, vascular dilatation, and edema. Between attacks, the peritoneum almost always returns to normal. Rarely, organization of the exudate has led to the formation of adhesions.[74]

Prognosis and Treatment. The prognosis of FPP is excellent, with many patients followed for years with good general health despite hundreds of attacks. They may increase in frequency with age, but occasionally there are remissions or very intractable periods. The development of amyloid nephropathy heralds a poor prognosis, with subsequent renal failure and death in 90 per cent of affected patients under the age of 40.

There is no treatment of proved value in FPP.[73] It has been reported that attacks may be suppressed or intervals between attacks lengthened in 20 per cent of patients with the use of 20 mg per day of prednisone, but the side effects of this dose prohibit prolonged use in this chronic disease. Control of the acute attack has occasionally been successful with high dose steroids tapered over one week. No other medication aborts or ameliorates the course of the disease. Only pregnancy appears to be a frequent suppressant of attacks, but treatment with progestational agents has been unsuccessful.

Two types of diet therapy have been attempted. Elimination diets have rarely been of benefit. Favorable reports on the benefit of a low fat (20 gm) diet claimed a dramatic decrease in the number and severity of attacks. However, better controlled studies with larger numbers of patients have been unable to confirm these initial reports.

MISCELLANEOUS LESIONS OF THE PERITONEUM

PERITONEAL VASCULITIS

The so-called autoimmune vascular diseases (e.g., systemic lupus erythematosus [SLE], periarteritis nodosa) involve the vessels of the gut wall, but the peritoneum is usually affected after the gut wall is diseased. Although about 20 per cent of patients with SLE, periarteritis, scleroderma, and dermatomyositis develop acute abdominal problems (i.e., ulceration, hemorrhage, perforation, obstruction, or infarction), isolated peritonitis unassociated with the above is found in less than 1 per cent.[75]

Peritonitis resulting from arteritis of subserosal arteries most commonly occurs in SLE, manifesting the usual signs and symptoms of acute peritonitis and ascites. Acute lupus peritonitis is responsive to steroids, but obviously the surgeon may be forced to operate in order to rule out a surgically correctable lesion.[76] A trial of steroids may be warranted if other signs of acute SLE are present.

Allergic vasculitis caused by Schönlein-Henoch purpura rarely causes exudative ascites, and it resolves with steroid therapy.[77]

Köhlmeier-Degos disease is a rare form of systemic vasculitis affecting small and medium-sized arteries, and mainly involving the skin and gut.[78] The disease usually begins with the onset of atrophic skin lesions, but after a variable period of weeks to years is followed by abdominal pain, weight loss, and diarrhea. Obstruction of lymphatics by fibrosis of the serosa and retroperitoneum may cause malabsorption and chylous ascites. At laparotomy, atrophic patches similar to the skin lesion are found in the serosa of the bowel wall, along with a peritoneal exudate. These atrophic patches are due to thrombi of small arteries, leading to focal ischemia. Approximately 50 per cent of patients die of peritonitis (owing to infarction and perforation of the bowel) within two years after onset. Pathologically, Köhlmeier-Degos disease differs from periarteritis, in that there is deposition of fibrous tissue between the endothelium and internal elastic lamina. In periarteritis, there is usually extensive involvement of the entire wall, with aneurysm formation. (The reader is referred to pp. 1572 to 1573.)

EOSINOPHILIC PERITONITIS

Eosinophilic gastroenteritis usually presents with peripheral eosinophilia and symptoms caused by mucosal or submucosal involvement, i.e., malabsorption and obstruction. Patients may present, however, with predominantly subserosal disease and concomitant eosinophilic ascites. Paracentesis yields fluid filled with eosinophils, often well over 50 per cent. At laparotomy, a thickened, edematous serosa infiltrated with eosinophils, lymphocytes, and plasma cells is found. The response to steroids is often dramatic, with complete clearing of the ascites. (See also pp. 1066 to 1075.)

WHIPPLE'S DISEASE

The broad spectrum of Whipple's disease is discussed on pages 938 to 948. It is of note that a few patients present primarily with peritoneal manifestations. A picture very similar to tuberculous peritonitis has been described, with ascites, low-grade fever, weight loss, and multiple peritoneal nodules on peritoneoscopy.[79] Histologically, the nodules are composed of chronic inflammatory cells with periodic acid–Schiff positive material in macrophages, similar to the material found in small intestinal mucosa and other tissues. Long-term antibiotic treatment with antimicrobial agents (penicillin, tetracycline) leads to resolution of peritoneal disease and disappearance of ascites.

Whipple's disease may cause ascites by means other than direct peritoneal involvement. Indeed, 5 to 10 per cent of patients have ascites, caused by protein-losing enteropathy with hypoalbuminemia, lymphatic obstruction by involved mesenteric nodes, or rupture of dilated serosal lymphatics. Chylous ascites may also be caused by lymphatic involvement.

GRANULOMATOUS PERITONITIS

SARCOIDOSIS

Very rarely this disease affects the peritoneum, causing granulomatous peritonitis and ascites.[80] The diagnosis can only be made by exclusion, with negative mycobacterial and fungal cultures, a positive Kveim test, and perhaps lack of response to antituberculous therapy. Despite the presence of noncaseating granulomas and response to steroids, it may be reasonable to treat all patients for tuberculosis in whom the diagnosis is uncertain.

CROHN'S DISEASE

This disease rarely presents with "miliary" serosal nodules composed of noncaseating granulomas and minimal (but definite) abnormalities of the bowel wall.[81] The major importance of this rare manifestation of Crohn's disease is its confusion with tuberculous peritonitis at laparotomy.

FOREIGN BODIES

A number of foreign bodies may cause a granulomatous peritoneal reaction, the most common being starch granulomatous peritonitis.[82] This syndrome appears two to nine weeks postoperatively, but has been seen four months later. The signs and symptoms are consistent with intestinal obstruction or peritonitis, i.e., pain, tenderness, fever, nausea and vomiting, and abdominal distention. The small bowel may obstruct in about 25 per cent of patients. At laparotomy, miliary peritoneal nodules, adhesions, and ascites are found, and may be confused with carcinomatosis, especially in patients who have previously undergone an operation for cancer. Pathologically, the lesions consist of granulomas with epithelioid cells, giant cells, and an intense mononuclear infiltrate, but starch granules are easily identified by the characteristic Maltese cross. The prognosis is good, with no progression to chronic disease, although occasionally the serosal nodules may persist or adhesions may cause obstruction up to one and one-half years later. The reason that some patients develop a granulomatous reaction to starch is unclear; there is no good evidence for hypersensitivity.

GYNECOLOGIC LESIONS

Because the female genital tract opens into the peritoneal cavity, endometrial and decidual tissue occasionally implant on the peritoneum and cause symptoms. Endometriosis may involve the bowel wall and cause ascites, but symptomatic cases with only peritoneal involvement are rare.[83] Postpartum abdominal pain with peritoneal signs has been reported, caused by a diffuse peritoneal decidual reaction involving the omentum.[84]

PERITONEAL LYMPHANGIECTASIS

Peritoneal lymphangiectasis is a rare condition in which there is a communication between distended peritoneal lymphatics and the vascular system, leading to bloody ascites, hemorrhage, and death in severe cases.[85] Patients may be asymptomatic, or may present with abdominal pain or an abdominal mass caused by distended lymphatics. At laparotomy, pendunculated and nonpedunculated blood-filled cysts are found. It is not clear whether this condition is congenital or acquired.

PERITONEAL LOOSE BODIES

A small number of patients have been reported in whom loose peritoneal cysts have been found associated with nonspecific abdominal pain. These cysts are 1 to 6 cm in diameter, contain fluid, and have soft, thin walls. Their origin is considered to be peritoneal, because they are lined with mesothelial cells, and continuity of cyst pedicles to the peritoneum has been demonstrated. It has been speculated that chronic inflammation or irritation may provoke mesothelial cell proliferation and subsequent cyst formation.[86] It remains unclear whether these cysts are truly symptomatic or are just incidental findings.

PERITONEAL ENCAPSULATION

Peritoneal encapsulation is a rare developmental anomaly in which the entire small bowel is enclosed in a peritoneal sac, without other evidence of abnormality or malrotation. It has been suggested that the abnormal peritoneal sac is derived from the peritoneum of the normal umbilical hernia, the neck of which becomes adherent to the duodenum. The peritoneum of the umbilical hernia is then drawn into the abdominal cavity with the intestines when they are suddenly retracted in the twelfth gestational week. The condition is asymptomatic, although it has been associated with intermittent abdominal pain.[87]

DISEASES OF THE MESENTERY AND OMENTUM

GENERAL CLINICAL FEATURES

Patients with mesenteric disease usually present with nonspecific symptoms, such as abdominal pain, abdominal distention, or intestinal obstruction. The most frequent physical finding is a mass, which may be mobile. Associated lymphatic obstruction may cause steatorrhea, chylous ascites, or protein-losing enteropathy, with hypoalbuminemia and edema.

Although there are no specific laboratory findings, mesenteric disease may be suspected if calcifications, displacement of bowel loops, or pressure deformities are noted radiographically. However, definitive diagnosis of diseases of the mesentery and omentum usually depends upon direct inspection and biopsy, either at surgery or by means of peritoneoscopy.

MESENTERIC INFLAMMATORY DISEASE

Mesenteric inflammatory disease is composed of a spectrum ranging from inflammatory to fibrotic lesions of the mesentery, most commonly called "mesenteric panniculitis" and "retractile mesenteritis," respectively. Other terms applied to these conditions have included primary liposclerosis, lipogranuloma, isolated lipodystrophy, and mesenteric Weber-Christian disease.

Etiology and Pathogenesis. The underlying etiological agents initiating the pathological sequence may include trauma, infection, or ischemia. Malignant lymphomas have developed in several patients with mesenteric panniculitis.[88] Mesenteric panniculitis has been reported as part of generalized Weber-Christian disease involving multiple organs, but this entity is probably unrelated to isolated mesenteric inflammatory disease.

It is postulated that the underlying pathogenetic defect involves excessive growth of morphologically normal fat tissue, with subsequent degeneration, fat necrosis, and xanthogranulomatous inflammation. After the degeneration of hyperplastic mesenteric adipose tissue, lipid material, perhaps abnormal, is released from degenerating fat cells. This evokes granulomatous infiltration, with eventual progression to fibrotic scarring. Mesenteric inflammatory disease may be a nonspecific response of the mesentery to any form of injury.

Clinical Features. Mesenteric panniculitis presents with recurrent episodes of crampy abdominal pain, either localized or generalized, with weight loss, nausea, vomiting, and low-grade fever.[88] A mass is palpable in 60 per cent, with local tenderness but usually without peritoneal signs. Leukocytosis may occur. Roentgenologic evaluation may reveal displacement of intestinal segments, extrinsic pressure deformities, separation of jejunoileal loops with kinking or angulation, and rugal distortions of the mesenteric border of compressed loops.

A certain number of patients with mesenteric panniculitis apparently progress to a chronic process which is probably identical with that described as retractile mesenteritis. These patients continue to have abdominal pain, fever, and weight loss, and in addition may develop small bowel obstruction, mesenteric thrombosis, and intestinal lymphatic obstruction, with resultant ascites, steatorrhea, and protein-losing enteropathy.[89, 90]

Pathology. At laparotomy patients with mesenteric panniculitis have a thickened mesentery, most often in the mesenteric root, and almost always limited to the small bowel mesentery. Histological examination of the affected mesentery reveals infiltration of fat by macrophages with abundant foamy cytoplasm, focal lymphocytic infiltration, fat necrosis, fibrosis, and calcification.

In retractile mesenteritis, the mesentery is thickened, fibrotic, and retracted, with opalescent pale gray plaques. There is a dense collagen and fibrous tissue proliferation; less fat necrosis and inflammation are evident than in the earlier panniculitis stage. Rarely, the colonic mesentery and peritoneum may be involved with a similar fibrotic reaction.

Prognosis and Treatment. Because of the small number of patients evaluated, the prognosis and therapy of this disease are poorly defined. However, it seems that the prognosis is usually excellent, because about 75 per cent of patients in one small series became asymptomatic over a period of months to years.[88] Corticosteroids have been claimed to be useful in symptomatic treatment of mesenteric panniculitis, but it is not clear whether they change the duration of the disease or slow the progression to retractile mesenteritis.

MESENTERIC CYSTS

Etiology and Pathogenesis. Mesenteric cysts are mainly chylous lymphatic cysts; they may also be of enteric, urogenital, or celomic origin. Most authorities attribute the origin of mesenteric cysts to sequestrations of the lymphatic system, with continued growth of congenitally malformed or malpositioned lymphatics.[91] They may not be closed structures, because they can wax and wane in size and rarely rupture. Distended lymphaticovenous shunts have been demonstrated, and it is postulated that there may be congenital deficiencies in the formation or persistence of these shunts in the fine lymphaticovenous networks.[92] Trauma, lymphangitis, and obstruction probably play little role in the origin of mesenteric cysts.

Clinical Features. Mesenteric cysts usually become symptomatic relatively late, with about 75 per cent presenting after ten years of age. They are often asymptomatic, but when symptomatic the patients present with complaints related to their size and position.[91] A slowly enlarging, painless mass is found, which is round, smooth, mobile, and nontender. Occasionally, the cysts rupture, bleed, suppurate, and cause intermittent intestinal obstruction, or dysuria owing to pressure on the bladder. They may mimic appendicitis with appendiceal abscess or abdominal aneurysm with transmitted aortic pulsations; very large cysts have closely simulated free ascites. The usual treatment is enucleation or excision; the latter probably decreases the possibility of recurrence.

MESENTERIC AND OMENTAL TUMORS

Mesenteric tumors are rare tumors which may arise from any of the cellular elements of the mesentery.[93] Fibromas account for about 25 per cent; myomas, 15 per cent; lipomatous tumors, 15 per cent;' histiocytic tumors (xanthogranulomas), 15 per cent; hemangiopericytomas, 10 per cent; neurofibromas, 5 per cent; and mesenchymomas, 5 per cent. The symptoms of mesenteric tumors are nonspecific and include weight loss, abdominal pain, abdominal mass, and symptoms caused by compression of local structures. Most of the connective tissue tumors are well differentiated, low-grade fibrosarcomas which are locally invasive, and which may be cured by excision. On the other hand approximately 50 per cent of the lipomatous, histiocytic, or leiomyomatous tumors are malignant, and may metastasize.

Lymphoid tumors of the mesentery have also been described, and may be locally infiltrative. Of great interest are benign lymphoid tumors, probably hamartomatous in nature, which may present with an associated hypochromic, microcytic anemia (with no marrow iron), no evidence of blood loss, hypoferremia, resistance to iron therapy, and complete correction by removal of the tumor.[94] The etiology of the anemia and the ferrokinetics have not been extensively investigated.

Omental tumors, in contrast to mesenteric tumors, are derived from muscle in 60 per cent (leiomyomas, leiomyosarcomas, or hemangiopericytomas).[95] Abdominal pain, an abdominal mass, and weight loss are seen in patients with large symptomatic tumors (65 per cent), and ascites is more common than with mesenteric tumors. About 40 per cent of omental tumors are malignant; they also tend to produce local invasion and peritoneal implants rather than distant metastases.

MESENTERIC HERNIAS

Various forms of herniation of the mesentery result from anomalous intestinal rotation, with fusion of the mesentery and parietal peritoneum during embryonic development.[96] Mesenteric hernias present with chronic, intermittent small intestinal obstruction or acute obstruction. A palpable mass may be present in the upper abdomen. Surgical reduction is indicated in symptomatic patients.

OMENTAL TORSION AND INFARCTION

Torsion of the omentum is an acute surgical condition which usually mimics acute appendicitis or acute cholecystitis. The underlying cause of omental torsion is not clear. Predisposing factors that have been suggested are malformation of the omental pedicle, variable amounts and dispositions of omental fat, increased mobility of the right omentum, venous redundancy with omental kinking, or nonspecific inflammatory foci in the omentum.[97] Abdominal pain is the major symptom, localizing to the right lower quadrant in 80 per cent and the right upper quadrant in about 10 per cent. Nausea, vomiting, fever, abdominal mass, and leukocytosis are each present in about half the patients. At laparotomy vascular engorgement, torsion, and gangrene of the omentum are found, and are relieved by omentectomy.

Omental infarction presents a similar picture of acute right-sided abdominal pain, localized peritoneal signs, fever, and leukocytosis. A heavy omentum with infarction of the right margin is found at laparotomy, and is cured by omentectomy. Various theories have been proposed to explain the segmental nature of the infarction: anomalous venous drainage, rupture of vessels in a heavy omentum, stretching of vessels with subsequent endothelial damage and thrombosis, or disproportionate fat growth with relative ischemia.[98] Recently the finding of tenuous connections between the right omentum and the rest of the omentum has suggested that omental infarction may result from an embryological variant. The areas of infarction are in those portions of the omentum that have arisen from the ventral mesogastrium, and these have weak bands of fusion and a tenuous blood supply. When this anatomic variant is stressed by congestion or increased intra-abdominal pressure, thrombosis may result.[99]

DISEASES OF THE DIAPHRAGM

EVENTRATION

Eventration of the diaphragm is a congenital abnormality in which there is a weakness of the central portion of either the right or left leaf of the diaphragm, owing to absence of muscular tissue in that area; the peripheral musculature and phrenic innervation are intact. Eventration is often an incidental, asymptomatic radiographic finding. Most symptomatic patients present in the fourth or fifth decade of life, with nonspecific dyspepsia, epigastric discomfort or burning, and eructation.[100] Occasionally, gastric outlet obstruction may result from volvulus at the cardia or pylorus. Respiratory distress is uncommon in adults, although pulmonary function may be compromised on testing.

The diagnosis may be suggested by dullness to percussion, absent breath sounds, and the presence of bowel sounds over the affected hemidiaphragm. The trachea and heart may be pushed to the contralateral side. If the physical signs are confusing, the combination of chest films,

fluoroscopy, and pneumoperitoneum should establish the diagnosis. Symptomatic eventration responds well to surgical repair, which involves resection of the central diaphragm and closure using pericardium or synthetic mesh.

HERNIATION

Diaphragmatic hernias are due to congenital abnormalities in the formation of the diaphragm. The diaphragm is derived from four embryonic structures: the septum transversum ventrally, the pleuroperitoneal membrane and body wall laterally, and the mesoesophagus mediodorsally. Most commonly, the left pleuroperitoneal membrane fails to fuse with the septum transversum, causing a left posterolateral defect without a hernia sac. If fusion is complete but there is a failure of muscularization posterolaterally, a hernia with a sac is formed. This posterolateral wedge-shaped defect is called the foramen of Bochdalek.

Bochdalek hernias are asymptomatic in one-quarter of patients, but 50 per cent have vague, intermittent abdominal pain, and 25 per cent have chest pain, cardiovascular symptoms, and dyspnea.[101] Incarceration of intestine leads to acute, sharp substernal pain radiating to the left upper quadrant or back, along with the typical symptoms of intestinal obstruction. The hernia may also contain omentum, stomach, spleen, liver, or pancreas. The diagnosis can usually be made on lateral chest film, which reveals a blunted cardiophrenic angle, a small effusion, and a gas-filled intestinal loop. Intestinal contrast studies or pneumoperitoneum may be necessary for small hernias. Because of the danger of strangulation, surgery is always indicated in those cases with incarceration or obstruction.

Congenital defects also occur in the retrocostoxiphoid region, usually on the right, possibly because the pericardial attachment to the diaphragm is more extensive on the left. These foramen of Morgagni hernias nearly always have a hernial sac. Morgagni hernias are rarely symptomatic, but may present with epigastric discomfort, dyspepsia, or bloating. Acute symptoms are almost always due to large bowel obstruction, unlike Bochdalek hernias, although omentum and stomach may also be incarcerated.[102] Lateral chest films are usually diagnostic, and may be confirmed with barium enema. Surgical repair is necessary to prevent incarceration and strangulation.

REFERENCES

1. Berndt, W., and Gosselin, R. Differential changes in permeability of mesentery to Rb and P^{32} Amer. J. Physiol. 202:701, 1962.
2. Aune, S. Transperitoneal exchange. Scand. J. Gastroent. 5:85, 99, 161, 241, 253, 1970.
3. Shear, L., Harvey, J., and Barry, K. Peritoneal sodium transport: Enhancement by pharmacologic and physical agents. J. Lab. Clin. Med. 67:181, 1966.
4. Henderson, L., and Kintzel, J. Influence of antidiuretic hormone on peritoneal membrane area and permeability. J Clin. Invest. 50:2437, 1971.
5. Kraft, A., Tompkins, R., and Joseph, J. Peritoneal electrolyte absorption: Analysis of portal, systemic venous and lymphatic transport. Surgery 64:148, 1968.
6. French, J., Florey, H., and Maris, B. The absorption of particles by the lymphatics of the diaphragm. Quart. J. Exp. Physiol. 45: 88, 1960.
7. Raybuck, H., Allen, L., and Haims, W. Absorption of serum from the peritoneal cavity. Amer. J. Physiol. 199:1021, 1960.
8. Shear, L., Swartz, C., Shinaberger, J., and Barry, K. Kinetics of peritoneal fluid absorption in man. New Eng. J. Med. 272:123, 1965.
9. Shear, L., Castellot, J., Shinaberger, J., Poole, L., and Barry, K. Enhancement of peritoneal fluid absorption by dehydration, mercaptomerin, and vasopressin. J. Pharm. Exp. Therap. 154:289, 1966.
10. Feife, E., Gagliardi, R., and Pfister, R. The roentgenologic evaluation of ascites. Amer. J. Roent. 101:388, 1967.
11. Viranuvatti, V., Hitanant, S., Boonyapaknavig, V., Plengvanit, V., Kalayasiri, C., and Chearani, O. Peritoneal biopsy: Experience with blind and direct vision biopsy. Amer. J. Proct. 17:489, 1966.
12. Levine, H. Needle biopsy of the peritoneum in exudative ascites. Arch. Intern. Med. 120:542, 1967.
13. Steigmann, F., and Villa F. Peritoneoscopy. In Gastroenterologic Medicine, M. Paulson (ed.). Philadelphia, Lea and Febiger, 1969, pp. 294–310.
14. Atkinson, M., and Losowsky, M. The mechanism of ascites formation in chronic liver disease. Quart. J. Med. 30:153, 1961.
15. Witte, M., Witte, C., and Dumont, A. Progress in liver disease: Physiological factors involved in the causation of cirrhotic ascites. Gastroenterology 61:742, 1971.
16. Zammon, O., Oratz, M., Kessler, R., et al. Albumin to ascites: Demonstration of a direct

pathway bypassing the systemic circulation. J. Clin. Invest. 48:2074, 1969.
17. Denison, E., Lieberman, F., and Reynolds, T. 9-alpha-fluorohydrocortisone induced ascites in alcoholic liver disease. Gastroenterology 61:497, 1971.
18. Epskin, M., Berk, D., Hollenberg, N., Adams, D., Chalmers, T., Abrams, H., and Merrill, J. Renal failure in the patient with cirrhosis: The role of active vasoconstriction. Amer. J. Med. 49:175, 1970.
19. Chaimovitz, C., Szylman, P., Alroy, G., and Better, O.: Mechanism of increased renal tubular sodium reabsorption in cirrhosis. Amer. J. Med. 52:198, 1972.
20. Tavel, M. Ascites: Etiologic considerations, with emphasis on the value of several laboratory findings in diagnosis. Amer. J. Med. Sci. 237:727, 1959.
21. Clarkson, B. Relationship between cell type, glucose concentration and response to treatment in neoplastic effusions. Cancer 17:914, 1964.
22. Ceelen, G. The cytologic diagnosis of ascitic fluid. Acta Cytol. 8:175, 1964.
23. Berner, E., Fred, H., Riggs, S., and Davis, J. Diagnostic possibilities in patients with conspicuous ascites. Arch. Intern. Med. 113:687, 1964.
24. Parker, R. Occlusion of the hepatic veins in man. Medicine 38:369 1959.
25. Sterup, K., and Mosbeck, J. Budd-Chiari syndrome after taking oral contraceptives. Brit. Med. J. 4:660, 1967.
26. Takeuchi, J., Takada, A., Hasumuru, Y., Matsuda, Y., and Ikegami, F. Budd-Chiari syndrome associated with obstruction of the inferior vena cava. Amer. J. Med. 51:11, 1971.
27. Clancey, R., and MacKay I. Myxedematous ascites. Med. J. Austral. 2:415 1970.
28. Kipnis, D. Clinicopathological conference. Massive ascites due to Meigs' syndrome. Amer. J. Med. 47:125, 1969.
29. Kempers, R., Dockerty, M., Hoffman, D., and Bartholomew, L. Struma ovarii—ascitic, hyperthyroid, and asymptomatic syndromes. Ann. Intern. Med. 72:883, 1970.
30. Polishuk, W. Z., and Schenker, J. G. Ovarian overstimulation syndrome. Fertil. Steril. 20:443, 1969.
31. Scindler, S., Schafer, J., Hull, D., and Griffin, W. Chronic pancreatic ascites. Gastroenterology 59:453, 1970.
32. Rosato, E., Berkowitz, H., and Roberts, B. Bile ascites. Surg. Gynec. Obstet. 130:494, 1970.
33. Cain, J., Labat, J., and Cohn, I. Bile peritonitis in germ free dogs. Gastroenterology 53:600, 1967.
34. Vasko, J., and Tapper, R. The surgical significance of chylous ascites. Arch Surg. 95:355, 1967.
35. Lindenbaum, J., and Scheidt, S. Chylous ascites and the nephrotic syndrome. Amer. J. Med. 44:830, 1968.
36. Kelley, M., and Butt, H. Chylous ascites, an analysis of its etiology. Gastroenterology 39: 161, 1960.
37. Krizek, T., and Davis, J. Acute chylous peritonitis. Arch. Surg. 91:253, 1965.

38. Sanchez, R., Makour, G., Brennan, L., and Wooley, M.   Chylous ascites in children. Surgery 69:183, 1971.

39. Gabuzda, G.   Cirrhosis, ascites, and edema; clinical course related to management. Gastroenterology 58:546, 1970.

40. Shear, L., Ching, S., and Gabuzda, G.   Compartmentalization of ascites and edema in patients with hepatic cirrhosis. New Eng. J. Med. 282:1391, 1970.

41. Eggert, R.   Spironolactone diuresis in patients with cirrhosis and ascites. Brit. Med. J. 2:401, 1970.

42. Sohocky, S.   Tuberculous peritonitis. Amer. Rev. Resp. Dis. 95:398, 1967.

43. Singh, M., Bhargava, A., and Jain, K.   Tuberculous peritonitis. New Eng. J. Med. 281:1091, 1969.

44. Burack, W., and Hollister, R.   Tuberculous peritonitis. Amer. J. Med. 28:510, 1960.

45. Gonnella, J., and Hudson, E.   Clinical patterns of tuberculous peritonitis. Arch. Intern. Med. 117:164, 1966.

46. Borhanmanesh, F., Hekmat, K., Vaezzadeh, K., and Rezai, H.: Tuberculous peritonitis: prospective study of 32 cases in Iran. Ann. Intern. Med. 76:567, 1972.

47. Friedland, J., and Harris, M.   Primary pneumococcal peritonitis in a young adult. Amer. J. Surg. 119:737, 1970.

48. Conn, H., and Fessel, M.   Spontaneous bacterial peritonitis in cirrhosis; variations on a theme. Medicine 50:161, 1971.

49. Montemartini, C., Specchia, G., and Dander, B.   Peritonitis caused by Candida albicans. Digestion 3:368, 1970.

50. Reddy, P., Gorelick, D., Brasher, C., and Larsh, H.   Progressive disseminated histoplasmosis as seen in adults. Amer. J. Med. 48:629, 1970.

51. Blumberg, H., Srinivasan, K., and Parnes, I.   Peritoneal schistosomiasis simulating carcinoma. N. Y. State J. Med. 66:758, 1966.

52. Sjovall, A., and Aherman, M. Peritoneal granulomas in women due to the presence of Enterobius. Acta Obstet. Gynec. Scand. 47:361, 1968.

53. Lieben, J., and Pistawka, H. Mesothelioma and asbestos exposure. Arch. Environ. Health 14:559, 1967.

54. Elmes, P.   The epidemiology and clinical features of asbestosis and related diseases. Postgrad. Med. J. 42:623, 1966.

55. Hourihane, D. A biopsy series of mesotheliomata, and attempts to identify asbestos within some of the tumors. Ann. N. Y. Acad. Sci. 132:647, 1965.

56. Wright, G. Asbestos and health in 1969. Amer. Rev. Resp. Dis. 100:467, 1969.

57. Winslow, D., and Taylor, H. Malignant peritoneal mesotheliomas. Cancer 13:127, 1960.

58. Roberts, G., and Irvine, R. Peritoneal mesothelioma, a report of four cases. Brit. J. Surg. 57:645, 1970.

59. Walsch, D., and Williams, G. Surgical biopsy studies of omental and peritoneal nodules. Brit. J. Surg. 58:428, 1971.

60. Prolla, J., and Kirsner, J. The gastrointestinal lesions and complications of the leukemias. Ann. Intern. Med. 61:1084, 1964.

61. Ehrlich, A., Shilder, G., Geller, W., and Sherlock, P. Gastrointestinal manifestations of malignant lymphoma. Gastroenterology 54:1115, 1968.

62. Gorshein, D., and Brauer, M.   Ascites in myeloid metaplasia due to ectopic peritoneal implantation. Cancer 23:1403, 1969.

63. Hirabayashi, K., and Graham, J.   Genesis of ascites in ovarian cancer. Amer. J. Obstet. Gynec. 106:492, 1970.

64. O'Bryan, R., Tulley, R., Brennan, M., and San Diego, E.   Critical analysis of the control of malignant effusions with radioisotopes. Henry Ford Hosp. Med. J. 16:3, 1968.

65. Silverberg, I. Management of effusions. Oncology 24:26, 1969.

66. Dollinger, M., Krakoff, I., and Karnovsky, D.   Quinacrine in the treatment of neoplastic effusions. Ann. Intern. Med. 66:249, 1967.

67. Jones, D. Pseudomyxoma peritonei. Brit. J. Clin. Pract. 19:675, 1965.

68. Parsons, J., Gray, J., and Thorbjarnarson, B.   Pseudomyxoma peritonei. Arch. Surg. 101:545, 1970.

69. Hellsten, S.   Mucocele and carcinoma of the appendix. Acta Path. Micro. Scand. 60:473, 1964.

70. Long, R., Spratt, J., and Dowling, E. Pseudomyxoma peritonei. Amer. J. Surg. 117:162, 1969.

71. Byron, R., Yonemoto, R., King, R., et al.   The management of pseudomyxoma peritonei secondary to ruptured mucocele of the appendix. Surg. Gynec. Obstet. 122:509, 1966.

72. Rosato, F., and Seltzer, M. Pseudomyxoma peritonei, case report including in vitro mucolysis. Surgery 68:301, 1970.

73. Siegal, S.   Familial paroxysmal peritonitis: Analysis of 50 cases. Amer. J. Med. 36:893, 1964.

74. Sohar, E., Gafni, J., Pras, M., and Heller, H.   Familial Mediterranean fever: A survey of 470 cases and review of the literature. Amer. J. Med. 43:227, 1967.

75. Matolo, N., and Albo, D.   Gastrointestinal complications of collagen vascular disease. Amer. J. Surg. 122:678, 1971.

76. Pollack, V., Grove, W., Kark, R., Muehrke, R., Pirani, C., and Steck, I.   Systemic lupus erythematosus simulating acute surgical condition of the abdomen. New Eng. J. Med. 259:258, 1958.

77. Efstratapoulous, A., and Sdourgi, J.   Ascites due to allergic purpura. Lancet 2:168, 1971.

78. Lomholt, G., Hjorth, N., and Fischermann, K. Lethal peritonitis from Degos' disease. Acta Chir. Scand. 134:495, 1968.

79. Isenberg, J., Gilbert, S., and Pitcher, J.   Ascites with peritoneal involvement in Whipple's disease. Gastroenterology 60:305, 1971.

80. Wong, M., and Rosen, S.   Ascites in sarcoidosis due to peritoneal involvement. Ann. Intern. Med. 57:277, 1962.

81. Heaton, K., McCarthy, C., Huton, R., Cornes, J., and Read, A.   Miliary Crohn's disease. Gut 8:4, 1967.

82. Holmes, E., and Eggleston, J. Starch granulomatous peritonitis. Surgery 71:85, 1972.

83. Berstein, J., Perlow, V., and Brenner, J. Massive ascites due to endometriosis. Amer. J. Dig. Dis. 6:1, 1961.

84. Hulme-Moir, I., and Ross, M. A case of early postpartum abdominal pain due to a haemorrhagic deciduosis peritonei. J. Obstet. Gynaec. Brit. Cwlth. 76:746, 1969.

85. Negus, D., Whimster, I., and Wiernick, G. Peritoneal lymphangiectasis. Brit. J. Surg. 53:740, 1966.

86. Lascano, E., Villamayor, R., and Llauro, J. Loose cysts of the peritoneal cavity. Ann. Surg. 152:836, 1960.

87. Lewin K., and McCarthy L. Peritoneal encapsulation of the small intestine. Gastroenterology 59:270, 1970.

88. Ogden, W., Bradburn, D., and Rives, J. Mesenteric panniculitis: Review of 27 cases. Ann. Surg. 161:864, 1965.

89. Soergel, K., and Hensley, G. Fatal mesenteric panniculitis. Gastroenterology 51:529, 1966.

90. Aach, R., Kalin, L., and Frick, R. Obstruction of the small intestine due to retractile mesenteritis. Gastroenterology 54:594, 1968.

91. Hardin, W., and Hardy, J. Mesenteric cysts. Amer. J. Surg. 119:640, 1970.

92. Elliot, G., Kliman, M., and Elliott, K. Persistence of lymphaticovenous shunts at the level of the microcirculation; their relationship to lymphangioma of the mesentery. Ann. Surg. 172:131, 1970.

93. Yannopoulous, K., and Stout, A. P. Primary solid tumors of the mesentery. Cancer 16:914, 1963.

94. Neerhont, R., Larson, W., and Mansur, P. Mesenteric lymphoid hamartoma associated with chronic hypoferremia, anemia, growth failure and hypogammaglobulinemia. New Eng. J. Med. 280:922, 1969.

95. Stout, A. P., Hendry, J., and Purdie, F. Primary solid tumors of the great omentum. Cancer 16:231, 1963.

96. Schaefer, C., and Waugh, D. Mesentericoparietal hernia. Amer. J. Surg. 116:847, 1968.

97. Fahlund, G., and Smedley, W. Primary torsion of the greater omentum. Amer. Surg. 31:285, 1965.

98. DeLaurentis, D., Kim, D., and Hartshorn, J. Idiopathic segmental infarction of the greater omentum. Arch. Surg. 102:474, 1971.

99. Epstein, L., and Lempke, R. Primary idiopathic segmental infarction of the greater omentum. Ann. Surg. 167:437, 1968.

100. Thomas, T. Nonparalytic eventration of the diaphragm. J. Thorac. Cardiovasc. Surg. 55:586, 1968.

101. Ahrend, T., and Thompson, B. Hernia of the foramen of Bochdalek in the adult. Amer. J. Surg. 122:612, 1971.

102. Comer, T., and Clagett, O. Surgical treatment of hernia of the foramen of Morgagni. J. Thorac. Cardiovasc. Surg. 52:461, 1966.

Index

NOTE: Page numbers in *italic* type denote illustrations and tables.
Readers interested in pediatric entities, including developmental anomalies, are referred to the entries under *Children* and *Infants*.